COHEN'S

PATHWAYS *of the*
PULP

COHEN'S
PATHWAYS *of the*
PULP

ELEVENTH EDITION

EDITORS

KENNETH M. HARGREAVES, DDS, PhD, FICD, FACD

Professor and Chair
Department of Endodontics
Professor
Departments of Pharmacology, Physiology (Graduate School), and Surgery (Medical School)
President's Council Endowed Chair in Research
University of Texas Health Science Center at San Antonio
San Antonio, Texas
Diplomate, American Board of Endodontics

LOUIS H. BERMAN, DDS, FACD

Clinical Associate Professor
Department of Endodontics
School of Dentistry
University of Maryland
Baltimore, Maryland
Faculty, Albert Einstein Medical Center
Philadelphia, Pennsylvania
Private Practice, Annapolis Endodontics
Annapolis, Maryland
Diplomate, American Board of Endodontics

Web Editor

ILAN ROTSTEIN, DDS

Associate Dean of Continuing Education
Chair of the Division of Endodontics, Orthodontics, and General Practice Dentistry
Herman Ostrow School of Dentistry
University of Southern California
Los Angeles, California

ELSEVIER

ELSEVIER

3251 Riverport Lane
St. Louis, Missouri 63043

Notices

International Standard Book Number 978-0-323-09635-5

Executive Content Strategist: Kathy Falk
Professional Content Development Manager: Jolynn Gower
Senior Content Development Specialist: Courtney Sprehe
Publishing Services Manager: Julie Eddy
Senior Project Manager: Richard Barber
Design Direction: Renee Duenow

Working together
to grow libraries in
developing countries

www.elsevier.com • www.bookaid.org

Printed in Canada

Last digit is the print number: 9 8 7 6 5 4 3 2 1

About the Authors

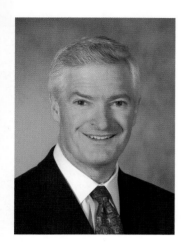

KENNETH M. HARGREAVES

Dr. Hargreaves is Professor and Chair of the Department of Endodontics at the University of Texas Health Science Center at San Antonio. He is a Diplomate of the American Board of Endodontics and maintains a private practice limited to endodontics. He is an active researcher, lecturer, and teacher and serves as the Editor-in-Chief of the Journal of Endodontics. He is principal investigator on several nationally funded grants that combine his interests in pain, pharmacology, and regenerative endodontics. He has received several awards, including a National Institutes of Health MERIT Award for pain research, the AAE Louis I. Grossman Award for cumulative publication of research studies, and two IADR Distinguished Scientist Awards.

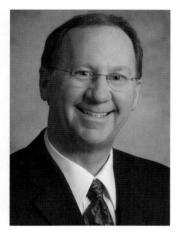

LOUIS H. BERMAN

Dr. Berman received his dental degree from the University of Maryland School of Dentistry and his Certificate in Endodontics from The Albert Einstein Medical Center. He is Clinical Associate Professor of Endodontics at the University of Maryland School of Dentistry and a Clinical Instructor and Guest Lecturer at The Albert Einstein Medical Center. He has lectured internationally in the field of endodontics and has published in several peer-reviewed international dental journals as well as co-authoring textbook chapters on numerous topics in various endodontic textbooks. He is past president of the Maryland State Association of Endodontics and is a member of the Journal of Endodontics Scientific Advisory Board. A Diplomate of the American Board of Endodontics and Fellow of the American College of Dentistry, Dr. Berman has been in full-time private practice in Annapolis, Maryland since 1983.

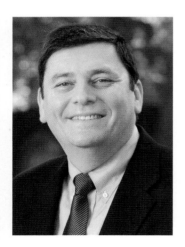

ILAN ROTSTEIN

Dr. Rotstein is Professor and Chair of Endodontics, Orthodontics, and General Practice Residency and Associate Dean at the Herman Ostrow School of Dentistry of the University of Southern California in Los Angeles. He is on the Executive Leadership Team of the School of Dentistry and ambassador member of the University of Southern California.

He has served in leadership roles for various dental organizations, including chair of the International Federation of Endodontic Associations' Research Committee, member on committees of the American Association of Endodontists, European Society of Endodontology, and as scientific reviewer for international endodontic and dental journals. He has also served as president of the Southern California Academy of Endodontists, Israel Endodontic Society, International Association for Dental Research—Israel Division, and chair of the Israel National Board of Diplomates in Endodontics.

Dr. Rotstein has published more than 150 scientific papers and research abstracts in the dental literature as well as chapters in international endodontic textbooks, including *Pathways of the Pulp, Ingle's Endodontics, Endodontics: Principles and Practice, Seltzer and Bender's Dental Pulp,* and *Harty's Endodontics in Clinical Practice.* He has lectured extensively in more than 25 countries throughout 5 continents.

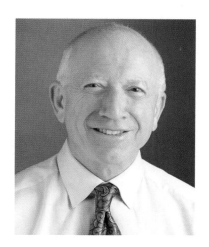

Stephen Cohen
MA, DDS, FICD, FACD

The field of endodontics would be difficult to imagine without *Pathways of the Pulp*. In speaking with colleagues across North America and around the world, it becomes clear that *Pathways* has had an immense, ubiquitous, and persistent impact on endodontics. This enduring contribution to our specialty is due to the genius of Stephen Cohen, who, together with Richard Burns, developed the most distinguished and perpetually updated evidenced-based textbook in our specialty. Their insight was to form a collaboration of the most renowned experts in our field, with expansion of the authorships for each new edition, and with an unwavering emphasis on the art and science of contemporary endodontic therapy. The result was a textbook that is both comprehensive and nuanced, which has transcended 11 editions and 14 languages since 1976. As each edition of *Pathways* evolved, it changed with the times, updating from unquestionable dogma into what was later considered the novel state of the art. Each edition progressed through the decades of endodontics and was inclusive of the next generation of technologies, philosophies, materials, devices, and instruments. As a result, with Steve as the lead editor since its inception, *Pathways of the Pulp* is considered the most comprehensive and innovative endodontic textbook available, literally defining the field of endodontics.

Stephen is an active educator, having lectured for decades around the world and serving as a Clinical Professor of Endodontics at the Arthur A. Dugoni School of Dentistry of the University of the Pacific. His passion for teaching, coupled with his distinctive authoritative voice and his vast scientific and clinical expertise, generates a highly effective combination for educating students on every facet of the endodontic specialty. His steadfast commitment in his authoring and editing of *Pathways of the Pulp* has propelled this textbook into what it is today.

In short, Dr. Stephen Cohen is a renaissance man, being both a practitioner and a teacher, whose breadth of expertise is leveraged by a passionate focus on detail and clarity. Defined by his unquestionable ethics and pursuit of perfection, Stephen's philosophy of learning, teaching, and practicing endodontics can best be summed up in his own words, as he penned in the Introduction of his last edition of *Pathways*:

"As clinicians we must meet this rich convergence of discovery and invention with an equally rich commitment to continuous learning, exposing ourselves to all the science our field has to offer. This is our duty to our founders, this is our responsibility to our patients, and this is our gift to ourselves."

Steve is a pioneer who has transformed the field of endodontics. For the tenth edition of this textbook, we recognized his legacy by renaming this textbook *Cohen's Pathways of the Pulp*. We reinforce our esteem appreciation of him by dedicating this eleventh edition to our mentor and friend, Dr. Stephen Cohen.

Kenneth M. Hargreaves and
Louis H. Berman

Contributors

Frederic Barnett, DMD
Chairman
Dental Endodontics
Albert Einstein Medical Center
Philadelphia, Pennsylvania

Bettina Basrani, DDS, PhD
Specialist in Endodontics
Associate Professor
Endodontics
University of Toronto
Toronto, Ontario, Canada

Ellen Berggreen, PhD
Speciality in Endodontics
Professor
Biomedicine
University of Bergen
Bergen, Norway

Louis H. Berman, DDS, FACD
Clinical Associate Professor
Department of Endodontics
School of Dentistry
University of Maryland
Baltimore, Maryland
Faculty, Albert Einstein Medical Center
Philadelphia, Pennsylvania
Private Practice, Annapolis Endodontics
Annapolis, Maryland
Diplomate, American Board of Endodontics

George Bogen, DDS
Lecturer
Loma Linda University, University of
California Los Angeles and NOVA
Southeastern University
Private Practice in Endodontics
Los Angeles, California

Serge Bouillaguet, DMD, PhD
Professor and Head of the Endodontic Unit
Division of Cariology and Endodontology
School of Dental Medicine
University of Geneva
Geneva, Switzerland

**Nicholas Chandler, BDS (Lond), MSc
(Manc), PhD (Lond), LDSRCS (Eng),
MRACDS (Endo), FDSRCPS (Glas),
FDSRCS (Edin), FFDRCSI FICD**
Associate Professor of Endodontics
Faculty of Dentistry
University of Otago
Dunedin, New Zealand

**Gary Shun-Pan Cheung, BDS, MDS,
MSc, FRACDS, FAMS, FHKAM,
FCDSHK, FDSRSCEd, PhD**
Professor in Endodontics
Department of Comprehensive Dental Care
Faculty of Dentistry
University of Hong Kong
Sai Ying Pun, Hong Kong

Noah Chivian, DDS, FACD, FICD
Clinical Professor
Department of Endodontics
Rutgers School of Dental Medicine
Adjunct Professor
Department of Endodontics
University of Pennsylvania
School of Dental Medicine.
Attending in Endodontics
Newark Beth Israel Medical Center
Newark, NewJersey
Diplomate, American Board of Endodontics

Jeffrey M. Coil, DMD, PhD
Director, Graduate Endodontics
Oral Biological and Medical Sciences
University of British Columbia
Vancouver, British Columbia, Canada

**Didier Dietschi, DMD, PhD,
Privat-Docent**
Senior Lecturer
School of Dental Medicine
Department of Cariology and Endodontics
University of Geneva
Geneva, Switzerland;
Adjunct Professor
School of Dentistry
Department of Comprehensive Care
Case Western Reserve University
Cleveland, Ohio

Anibal Diogenes, DDS, MS, PhD
Assistant Professor
Endodontics
University of Texas Health Science Center
at San Antonio
San Antonio, Texas

Samuel O. Dorn, DDS, FICD, FACD
Professor, Chair, and Director of Graduate
Endodontics, and the Frank B. Trice DDS
Professorship in Endodontics
Department of Endodontics
University of Texas at Houston School
of Dentistry
Houston, Texas

**Conor Durack, BDS NUI, MFD RCSI,
MClinDent (Endo), MEndo RCS (Edin)**
Endodontist and Practice Partner
Riverpoint Specialist Dental Clinic
Limerick, Ireland

Mohamed I. Fayad, DDS, MS, PhD
Diplomate, American Board of Endodontics
Clinical Associate Professor
Director of Research
Department of Endodontics
College of Dentistry
University of Illinois at Chicago
Chicago, Illinois

Bing Fan, DDS, MSc, PhD
Director
Department of Endodontics
School and Hospital of Stomatology
Wuhan University
Wuchang, Wuhan, Hubei, China

Ashraf Fouad, DDS, MS
Professor and Chair
Endodontics Prosthodontics and
Operative Dentistry
University of Maryland
Baltimore, Maryland

Inge Fristad, Cand. Odont, DDS, PhD
Department of Clinical Dentistry
University of Bergen
Bergen, Norway

Bradley H. Gettleman, DDS, MS
Private Practice of Endodontics
Glendale, Arizona
Diplomate, American Board of Endodontics

Gerald N. Glickman, DDS, MS, MBA, JD
Professor and Chair
Department of Endodontics
Texas A&M University Baylor College
of Dentistry
Dallas, Texas
Diplomate of the American Board
of Endodontics

Kishor Gulabivala, BDS, MSc, PhD
Professor
Department of Endodontology and
Restorative Dentistry
UCL Eastman Dental Institute
London, Great Britain

James L. Gutmann, DDS, Cert Endo, PhD (honoris causa), FACD, FICD, FADI
Professor Emeritus
Department of Restorative Sciences
Baylor College of Dentistry
Texas A&M University System, Health Science Center
Dallas, Texas
Diplomate of the American Board of Endodontics
Honorary Professor, School of Stomatology
Wuhan University
Wuhan, China

Kenneth M. Hargreaves, DDS, PhD, FICD, FACD
Professor and Chair
Department of Endodontics
Professor
Departments of Pharmacology, Physiology (Graduate School) and Surgery (Medical School)
President's Council Endowed Chair in Research
University of Texas Health Science Center at San Antonio
San Antonio, Texas
Diplomate, American Board of Endodontics

George T.-J. Huang, DDS, MSD, DSc
Professor
Director for Stem Cells and Regenerative Therapies
Department of Bioscience Research
College of Dentistry
University of Tennessee Health Science Center
Memphis, Tennessee

Bradford R. Johnson, DDS, MHPE
Associate Professor and Director of Postdoctoral Endodontics
Department of Endodontics
University of Illinois at Chicago
Chicago, Illinois

William Johnson, DDS, MS
Richard E. Walton Professor and Chair
Department of Endodontics
University of Iowa College of Dentistry
Iowa City, Iowa

David G. Kerns, DMD, MS
Professor and Director of Postdoctoral Periodontics
Texas A&M University—Baylor College of Dentistry
Dallas, Texas

Asma Khan, BDS, PhD
Assistant Professor
Department of Endodontics
University of North Carolina at Chapel Hill
Chapel Hill, North Carolina

James C. Kulild, DDS, MS
Professor Emeritus
Department of Endodontics
University of Missouri-Kansas City
Kansas City, Kansas

Sergio Kuttler, DDS
CEO/President
International Endodontic Institute
Fort Lauderdale, Florida
Co-Founder
International Dental Institute
Fort Lauderdale, Florida

Alan S. Law, DDS, PhD
The Dental Specialists
Lake Elmo, Minnesota

Linda G. Levin, DDS, PhD
Adjunct Associate Professor
Department of Endodontics
University of North Carolina at Chapel Hill
Chapel Hill, North Carolina

Martin D. Levin, DMD
Adjunct Associate Professor
Department of Endodontics
University of Pennsylvania
Philadelphia, Pennsylvania

Roger P. Levin, DDS
Chairman and CEO
Levin Group, Inc.
Owings Mills, Maryland

Louis M. Lin, BDS, DMD, PhD
Professor
Department of Endodontics
College of Dentistry
New York University
New York, New York

Henrietta L. Logan, PhD
Professor Emeritus
Department of Community Dentistry and Behavioral Science
University of Florida
Gainesville, Florida

Matthew Malek, DDS
Clinical Assistant Professor
Department of Endodontics
College of Dentistry
New York University
New York, New York

Donna Mattscheck, DMD
Private Practice
Portland, Oregon

Zvi Metzger, DMD
Professor Emeritus
Department of Endodontology
The Goldschleger School of Dental Medicine
Tel Aviv University
Tel Aviv, Israel

Madhu K. Nair, DMD, MS, PhD
Professor and Chairman
Department of Oral and Maxillofacial Diagnostic Sciences
University of Florida
Gainesville, Florida

Umadevi P. Nair, DMD, MDS
Clinical Assistant Professor
Department of Endodontics
University of Florida
Gainesville, Florida

Carl W. Newton, DDS, MSD
Professor
Department of Endodontics
School of Dentistry
Indiana University
Indianapolis, Indiana

Yuan-Ling Ng, BDS, MSc, PhD
Senior Clinical Lecturer in Endodontology / Programme Director in Endodontology
Restorative Dental Sciences (Endodontics)
UCL Eastman Dental Institute
University College—London
London, Great Britain

Donald R. Nixdorf, DDS, MS
Associate Professor
Diagnostic and Biological Services;
Adjunct Assistant Professor
Department of Neurology
University of Minnesota—Twin Cities
Minneapolis, Minnesota;
Research Investigator
Health Partners Institute for Education and Research
Bloomington, Minnesota

John Nusstein, DDS, MS
Professor and Chair
Division of Endodontics
College of Dentistry
The Ohio State University
Columbus, Ohio

Shanon Patel, BDS, MSc, MClinDent, FDS, MRD, PhD
Consultant Endodontist
Endodontic Postgraduate Unit
King's College London Dental Institute
London, Great Britain

Christine I. Peters, DMD
Professor
Department of Endodontics
Arthur A. Dugoni School of Dentistry
University of the Pacific
San Francisco, California

Ove A. Peters, DMD, MS, PhD
Professor and Co-chair
Department of Endodontics
Arthur A. Dugoni School of Dentistry
University of the Pacific
San Francisco, California
Diplomate, American Board of Endodontics

Al Reader, BS, DDS, MS
Professor and Program Director
Advanced Endodontics Program
College of Dentistry
The Ohio State University
Columbus, Ohio

Domenico Ricucci, MD, DDS
Private Practice
Cetraro, Italy

Isabela N. Rôças, DDS, MSc, PhD
Professor
Department of Endodontics
Head
Molecular Microbiology Laboratory
Faculty of Dentistry
Estácio de Sá University
Rio de Janeiro, Brazil

Robert S. Roda, DDS, MS
Adjunct Assistant Professor
Department of Endodontics
Baylor College of Dentistry
Dallas, Texas
Private Practice Limited to Endodontics
Scottsdale, Arizona
Diplomate, American Board of Endodontics

Paul A. Rosenberg, DDS
Professor and Director—Advanced
Education Program
Department of Endodontics
College of Dentistry
New York University
New York, New York

Ilan Rotstein, DDS
Associate Dean of Continuing Education
Chair of the Division of Endodontics,
Orthodontics and General Practice
Dentistry
Herman Ostrow School of Dentistry
University of Southern California
Los Angeles, California

Avishai Sadan, DMD, MBA
Dean
Herman Ostrow School of Dentistry
University of Southern California
Los Angeles, California

Frank Setzer, DMD, PhD, MS
Assistant Professor
Clinic Director, Endodontics
Director, Predoctoral Endodontic Program
Department of Endodontics
School of Dental Medicine
University of Pennsylvania
Philadelphia, Pennsylvania

**Asgeir Sigurdsson, DDS, MS,
Cert. Endo**
Associate Professor and Chair
Department of Endodontics
College of Dentistry
New York University
New York, New York
Diplomate of the American Board
of Endodontics

Stéphane Simon, DDS, MPhil, PhD
Senior Lecturer
Departments of Oral Biology and
Endodontics
School of Dentistry,
University of Paris Diderot (Paris7)
Paris, France

José F. Siqueira, Jr., DDS, MSc, PhD
Chairman and Professor
Department of Endodontics
Estácio de Sá University
Rio de Janeiro, Brazil

Aviad Tamse, DMD, FICD
Professor Emeritus
Department of Endodontology
Goldschlager School of Dental Medicine
Tel Aviv University
Tel Aviv, Israel

Franklin Tay, BDSc (HOns), PhD
Department of Endodontics
Georgia Regents University
Augusta, Georgia

Yoshitsugu Terauchi, DDS, Phd
CT & MicroEndodontic Center
Intellident Medical Corporation
Yamato City
Kanagawa, Japan

Martin Trope BDS, DMD
Adjunct Professor
School of Dentistry
University of North Carolina at Chapel Hill
Chapel Hill, North Carolina
Clinical Professor
School of Dentistry
University of Pennsylvania
Philadelphia, Pennsylvania

**Paula J. Waterhouse, BDS (Hons), FDS
RCS (Ed), FDS (Paed) RCS, PhD, FHEA**
School of Dental Sciences
Newcastle University
Newcastle upon Tyne, Great Britain

**John M. Whitworth, Jr., PhD, BChD,
FDSRCSEd, FDSRCS (RestDent)**
Senior Lecturer/Hon Clinical Consultant
School of Dental Sciences
Newcastle University
Newcastle upon Tyne, Great Britain

Edwin J. Zinman, DDS, JD
Private Practice of Law
Editorial Board
Journal of American Academy of
Periodontology
Former Lecturer
Department of Stomatology
School of Dentistry
University of California—San Francisco
San Francisco, California

New to This Edition

EIGHT NEW CHAPTERS

Chapter 2: Radiographic Interpretation covers imaging modalities, diagnostic tasks in endodontics, three-dimensional imaging, cone beam computed tomography, intraoperative or postoperative assessment of endodontic treatment complications, and more!

Chapter 4: Pain Control looks at two overarching topics: local anesthesia for restorative dentistry and endodontics and analgesics and therapeutic recommendations.

Chapter 11: Evaluation of Outcomes covers the reasons for evaluating treatment outcomes, outcome measurements for endodontic treatment, the outcomes of vital pulp therapy procedures, nonsurgical root canal treatment, nonsurgical retreatment, and surgical retreatment.

Chapter 16: Root Resorption looks at the histological features of root resorption, external inflammatory resorption, external cervical resorption, and internal resorption.

Chapter 19: Managing Iatrogenic Endodontic Events looks at treatment scenarios for eight different iatrogenic events: cervicofacial subcutaneous emphysema, sodium hypochlorite accidents, perforations (nonsurgical), inferior alveolar nerve injury (surgical), sinus perforation, instrument separation, apical extrusion of obturation materials, and ledge formation.

Chapter 21: Cracks and Fractures looks at three categories of cracks and fractures: cracked and fractured cusps, cracked and split teeth, and vertical root fractures, emphasizing the early diagnosis of these conditions.

Chapter 23: Vital Pulp Therapy addresses the living pulp, pulpal response to caries, procedures for generating reparative dentin, indications and materials for vital pulp therapy, MTA applications, treatment recommendations, and more!

Chapter 27: Bleaching Procedures provides a review of internal and external bleaching procedures, their impact on pulpal health/endodontic treatment, with presentations of cases and clinical protocols.

NEW CHAPTER ORGANIZATION

Chapters have been reorganized and grouped into three parts: Part I: *The Core Science of Endodontics*, Part II: *The Advanced Science of Endodontics*, and Part III: *Expanded Clinical Topics*. The seven chapters in Part 1 focus on the core clinical concepts for dental students; the chapters in Parts II and III provide the information that advanced students and endodontic residents and clinicians need to know. In addition, seven additional chapters are included in the online version.

The new organization better reflects the chronology of endodontic treatment.

EXPERT CONSULT

New features included on the Expert Consult site include:

- Seven chapters exclusively online:
  - *Chapter 24: Pediatric Endodontics: Endodontic Treatment for the Primary and Young Dentition*
  - *Chapter 25: Endodontic and Periodontic Interrelationships*
  - *Chapter 26: Effects of Age and Systemic Health on Endodontics*
  - *Chapter 27: Bleaching Procedures*
  - *Chapter 28: Understanding and Managing the Fearful Dental Patient*
  - *Chapter 29: Endodontic Records and Legal Responsibilities*
  - *Chapter 30: Key Principles of Endodontic Practice Management*

- Twelve lecture modules consisting of assigned readings, PowerPoint slides, written objectives for each lecture, and suggested examination questions. Topics covered include:
  - Diagnosis
  - Treatment planning
  - Pain control
  - Isolation
  - Cleaning and shaping
  - Obturation
  - Surgery
  - Assessment of outcomes
  - Pulp biology
  - Pathobiology
  - Emergencies
  - Restoration

- New videos and animations

Introduction

ENDODONTICS: A VIEW OF THE FUTURE

The Editors have had the privilege of "standing on the shoulders" of our generous contributors, enabling us to "look over the horizon" to gain a glimpse at our endodontic future. As we advance into the years ahead, we will incorporate even more refined and accurate improvements in pulpal diagnosis, canal cleaning and disinfection, canal obturation, and surgical enhancements.

In looking more clearly toward our impending endeavors, it becomes important to scrutinize the deficiencies of our past and present. Over the past several decades we have gone from arsenic to sodium hypochlorite, from bird droppings to gutta percha, from hand files to motor-driven files, from culturing to one-visit appointments, from two-dimensional to three-dimensional radiography, and from pulp removal to pulpal regeneration. And still, the clinical and academic controversies are pervasive. So, where will the future of our specialty take us?

With patients living longer and with the inescapable comparison of endodontics to endosseous implants, the demand for endodontic excellence has greatly increased. To that end, we suspect that future evidence-based approaches will continue to question the longevity of successful implant retention, intensifying the need for more predictable endodontic outcomes.

Surprisingly, we still base our diagnosis on a presumed and almost subjective pulpal status. Imagine a future in which endodontic diagnosis could be more objective by non-invasively scanning the pulp tissue. Imagine algorithms built into all digital radiography for interpreting and extrapolating disease processes. CBCT has made a huge impact on endodontic diagnosis, but can we enhance these digital captures with a resolution that would approach micro-computed tomography, and with less radiation? Will non-radiation imaging methods such as MRI (magnetic resonance imaging) leave the dental research clinic to provide a novel solution to address these issues? Will it be CT technology or some other form of detection for dramatically enhancing our guidance during surgical and nonsurgical treatment in order to both maximize our precision and minimize tooth structure and associated tissue removal? Considering the differences in color and consistency of the tissues within the pulp chamber, future technology may permit us to better discriminate these differences and enhance our ability for more precision when negotiating the openings to these canals. And as for clinical visualization: will there be digital or electronic enhancements of conventional loupes? Will 3-D visualization and monitor-based observation change the way we visualize and implement our procedures? During our canal cleaning and shaping, we are lucky if we can debride half of the pulpal tissues within all of the canal ramifications; however, we still use an irrigant that is so toxic by a non-selective mechanism, such that when inadvertently extruded beyond the canal system it can cause severe tissue damage. Our future technology should guide us to obtain the complete removal of organic debris within the pulpal spaces while obtaining complete canal disinfection—and without the potential morbidity from toxic non-selective chemicals. We still use files that can inadvertently separate. The resolution may be in a complete transformation in metallurgy or even the implementation of other non-metal cutting materials. Our obturation material is one of the worst filling materials in dentistry. Hopefully, the future evolution of obturation will lead us to a totally leakage-free, non-neurotoxic, and biocompatible substance that will three-dimensionally expand into *all* microscopic canal ramifications and stop when there is no more space to expand to, being limited to when it reaches the periodontal ligament. Will this obturating material be newly regenerated vital pulp?

Clearly, it is evident that our endodontic future lies in out-of-the-box thinking with the next generation of transformations coming with collaborations not just from within the biological sciences, but rather in conjunction with physicists, chemists, engineers, and a multitude of other great innovative minds. The predictability of endodontics must be incontestable, not just with better technology to guide us toward greater success, but also to better elucidate exactly when endodontics *cannot* be successful. Our future needs to focus on predictability, which will only be achieved by reinventing the wheel with disruptive technologies, rather than persisting with variations and modifications of our current convictions.

As a specialty, we have advanced by leaps and bounds since our inception, but we are still in our infancy with a brilliant future ahead of us. Since 1976 and with 11 editions, *Pathways of the Pulp* has always been about the art and science of endodontics. The dedicated contributing authors have generously given their time to meticulously describe what is considered the state of the art of our specialty. We are hopeful that future editions will guide us toward enhanced endodontic outcomes, with the never-ending pursuit of endodontic excellence.

Contents

COHEN'S
PATHWAYS *of the*
PULP

The Core Science of Endodontics

Diagnosis

LOUIS H. BERMAN | ILAN ROTSTEIN

ART AND SCIENCE OF DIAGNOSIS

Diagnosis is the art and science of detecting and distinguishing deviations from health and the cause and nature thereof.[6] The purpose of a diagnosis is to determine what problem the patient is having and why the patient is having that problem. Ultimately, this will directly relate to what treatment, if any, will be necessary. No appropriate treatment recommendation can be made until all of the *whys* are answered. Therefore, careful data gathering as well as a planned, methodical, and systematic approach to this investigatory process is crucial.

Gathering objective data and obtaining subjective findings are not enough to formulate an accurate clinical diagnosis. The data must be interpreted and processed to determine what information is significant, and what information might be questionable. The facts need to be collected with an active dialogue between the clinician and the patient, with the clinician asking the right questions and carefully interpreting the answers. In essence, the process of determining the existence of an oral pathosis is the culmination of the art and science of making an accurate diagnosis.

The process of making a diagnosis can be divided into five stages:
1. The patient tells the clinician the reasons for seeking advice.
2. The clinician questions the patient about the symptoms and history that led to the visit.
3. The clinician performs objective clinical tests.
4. The clinician correlates the objective findings with the subjective details and creates a tentative list of differential diagnoses.
5. The clinician formulates a definitive diagnosis.

This information is accumulated by means of an organized and systematic approach that requires considerable clinical judgment. The clinician must be able to approach the problem by crafting what questions to ask the patient and how to ask these pertinent questions. Careful listening is paramount to begin painting the picture that details the patient's complaint. These subjective findings combined with results of diagnostic tests provide the critical information needed to establish the diagnosis.

Neither the art nor the science is effective alone. Establishing a differential diagnosis in endodontics requires a unique blend of knowledge, skills, and ability to interpret and interact with a patient in real time. Questioning, listening, testing, interpreting, and finally answering the ultimate question of *why* will lead to an accurate diagnosis and in turn result in a more successful treatment plan.

Chief Complaint

On arrival for a dental consultation, the patient should complete a thorough registration that includes information pertaining to medical and dental history (Figs. 1-1 and 1-2). This should be signed and dated by the patient, as well as initialed by the clinician as verification that all of the submitted information has been reviewed (see Chapter 29 for more information).

The reasons patients give for consulting with a clinician are often as important as the diagnostic tests performed. Their remarks serve as initial important clues that will help the clinician to formulate a correct diagnosis. Without these direct and unbiased comments, objective findings may lead to an incorrect diagnosis. The clinician may find a dental pathosis, but it may not contribute to the pathologic condition that mediates the patient's chief complaint. Investigating these complaints may indicate that the patient's concerns are related to a medical condition or to recent dental treatment. Certain patients may

TELL US ABOUT YOUR SYMPTOMS

LAST NAME _____ FIRST NAME _____

1. Are you experiencing any pain at this time? If not, please go to question 6.   Yes _____ No _____

2. If yes, can you locate the tooth that is causing the pain?   Yes _____ No _____

3. When did you first notice the symptoms? _____

4. Did your symptoms occur suddenly or gradually? _____

5. Please check the frequency and quality of the discomfort, and the number that most closely reflects the intensity of your pain:

LEVEL OF INTENSITY (On a scale of 1 to 10) 1 = Mild 10 = Severe	FREQUENCY	QUALITY
1____2____3____4____5____6____7____8____9____10____	_____ Constant	_____ Sharp
	_____ Intermittent	_____ Dull
	_____ Momentary	_____ Throbbing
	_____ Occasional	

Is there anything you can do to relieve the pain?   Yes _____ No _____

If yes, what? _____

Is there anything you can do to cause the pain to increase?   Yes _____ No _____

If yes, what? _____

When eating or drinking, is your tooth sensitive to: Heat _____ Cold _____ Sweets _____

Does your tooth hurt when you bite down or chew?   Yes _____ No _____

Does it hurt if you press the gum tissue around this tooth?   Yes _____ No _____

Does a change in posture (lying down or bending over) cause your tooth to hurt?   Yes _____ No _____

6. Do you grind or clench your teeth?   Yes _____ No _____

7. If yes, do you wear a night guard?   Yes _____ No _____

8. Has a restoration (filling or crown) been placed on this tooth recently?   Yes _____ No _____

9. Prior to this appointment, has root canal therapy been initiated on this tooth?   Yes _____ No _____

10. Is there anything else we should know about your teeth, gums, or sinuses that would assist us in our

    diagnosis? _____

Signed: Patient or Parent _____ Date _____

FIG. 1-1 Dental history form that also allows the patient to record pain experience in an organized and descriptive manner.

TELL US ABOUT YOUR HEALTH

LAST NAME _____ **FIRST NAME** _____

How would you rate your health?   Please circle one.   Excellent   Good   Fair   Poor

When did you have your last physical exam? _____

If you are under the care of a physician, please give reason(s) for treatment.

_____

Physician's Name, Address, and Telephone Number:

Name _____ Address _____

City _____ State _____ Zip _____ Telephone _____

Have you ever had any kind of surgery?   Yes _____ No _____

If yes, what kind? _____ Date _____

_____ Date _____

Have you ever had any trouble with prolonged bleeding after surgery?   Yes _____ No _____

Do you wear a pacemaker or any other kind of prosthetic device?   Yes _____ No _____

Are you taking any kind of medication or drugs at this time?   Yes _____ No _____

If yes, please give name(s) of the medicine(s) and reason(s) for taking them:

Name _____ Reason _____

_____ _____

Have you ever had an unusual reaction to an anesthetic or drug (like penicillin)?   Yes _____ No _____

If yes, please explain: _____

Please circle any past or present illness you have had:

Alcoholism	Blood pressure	Epilepsy	Hepatitis	Kidney or liver	Rheumatic fever
Allergies	Cancer	Glaucoma	Herpes	Mental	Sinusitis
Anemia	Diabetes	Head/Neck injuries	Immunodeficiency	Migraine	Ulcers
Asthma	Drug dependency	Heart disease	Infectious diseases	Respiratory	Venereal disease

Are you allergic to Latex or any other substances or materials?   Yes _____ No _____

If so, please explain _____

If female, are you pregnant?   Yes _____ No _____

Is there any other information that should be known about your health? _____

_____

Signed: Patient or Parent _____ Date: _____

FIG. 1-2 Succinct, comprehensive medical history form designed to provide insight into systemic conditions that could produce or affect the patient's symptoms, mandate alterations in treatment modality, or change the treatment plan.

even receive initial emergency treatment for pulpal or periapical symptoms in a general hospital.[93] On occasion, the chief complaint is simply that another clinician correctly or incorrectly advised the patient that he or she had a dental problem, with the patient not necessarily having any symptoms or any objective pathosis. Therefore, the clinician must pay close attention to the actual expressed complaint, determine the chronology of events that led to this complaint, and question the patient about other pertinent issues, including medical and dental history. For future reference and in order to ascertain a correct diagnosis, the patient's chief complaint should be properly documented, using *the patient's own words*.

Medical History

The clinician is responsible for taking a proper medical history from every patient who presents for treatment. Numerous examples of medical history forms are available from a variety of sources, or clinicians may choose to customize their own forms. After the form is completed by the patient, or by the parent or guardian in the case of a minor, the clinician should review the responses with the patient, parent, or guardian and then initial the medical history form to indicate that this review has been done. The patient "of record" should be questioned at each treatment visit to determine whether there have been any changes in the patient's medical history or medications. A more thorough and complete update of the patient's medical history should be taken if the patient has not been seen for over a year.[51,52]

Baseline blood pressure and pulse should be recorded for the patient at each treatment visit. Elevation in blood pressure or a rapid pulse rate may indicate an anxious patient who may require a stress reduction protocol, or it may indicate that the patient has hypertension or other cardiovascular health problems. Referral to a physician or medical facility may be indicated. It is imperative that vital signs be gathered at each treatment visit for any patient with a history of major medical problems. The temperature of patients presenting with subjective fever or any signs or symptoms of a dental infection should be taken.[57,80,105]

The clinician should evaluate a patient's response to the health questionnaire from two perspectives: (1) those medical conditions and current medications that will necessitate altering the manner in which dental care will be provided and (2) those medical conditions that may have oral manifestations or mimic dental pathosis.

Patients with serious medical conditions may require either a modification in the manner in which the dental care will be delivered or a modification in the dental treatment plan (Box 1-1). In addition, the clinician should be aware if the patient has any drug allergies or interactions, allergies to dental products, an artificial joint prosthesis, organ transplants, or is taking medications that may negatively interact with common local anesthetics, analgesics, sedatives, and antibiotics.[80] This may seem overwhelming, but it emphasizes the importance of obtaining a thorough and accurate medical history while considering the various medical conditions and dental treatment modifications that may be necessary before dental treatment is provided.

Several medical conditions have oral manifestations, which must be carefully considered when attempting to arrive at an accurate dental diagnosis. Many of the oral soft tissue changes that occur are more related to the medications used to treat the

---

Cardiovascular: High- and moderate-risk categories of endocarditis, pathologic heart murmurs, hypertension, unstable angina pectoris, recent myocardial infarction, cardiac arrhythmias, poorly managed congestive heart failure[57,80,105]

Pulmonary: Chronic obstructive pulmonary disease, asthma, tuberculosis[80,129]

Gastrointestinal and renal: End-stage renal disease; hemodialysis; viral hepatitis (types B, C, D, and E); alcoholic liver disease; peptic ulcer disease; inflammatory bowel disease; pseudomembranous colitis[25,34,48,80]

Hematologic: Sexually transmitted diseases, HIV and AIDS, diabetes mellitus, adrenal insufficiency, hyperthyroidism and hypothyroidism, pregnancy, bleeding disorders, cancer and leukemia, osteoarthritis and rheumatoid arthritis, systemic lupus erythematosus[35,43,76,80,83,88,100,135]

Neurologic: Cerebrovascular accident, seizure disorders, anxiety, depression and bipolar disorders, presence or history of drug or alcohol abuse, Alzheimer disease, schizophrenia, eating disorders, neuralgias, multiple sclerosis, Parkinson disease[36,44,80]

---

medical condition rather than to the condition itself. More common examples of medication side effects are stomatitis, xerostomia, petechiae, ecchymoses, lichenoid mucosal lesions, and bleeding of the oral soft tissues.[80]

When developing a dental diagnosis, a clinician must also be aware that some medical conditions can have clinical presentations that mimic oral pathologic lesions.[13,28,32,74,80,102,107,133] For example, tuberculosis involvement of the cervical and submandibular lymph nodes can lead to a misdiagnosis of lymph node enlargement secondary to an odontogenic infection. Lymphomas can involve these same lymph nodes.[80] Immunocompromised patients and patients with uncontrolled diabetes mellitus respond poorly to dental treatment and may exhibit recurring abscesses in the oral cavity that must be differentiated from abscesses of dental origin.[43,76,80,83] Patients with iron deficiency anemia, pernicious anemia, and leukemia frequently exhibit paresthesia of the oral soft tissues. This finding may complicate making a diagnosis when other dental pathosis is present in the same area of the oral cavity. Sickle cell anemia has the complicating factor of bone pain, which mimics odontogenic pain, and loss of trabecular bone pattern on radiographs, which can be confused with radiographic lesions of endodontic origin. Multiple myeloma can result in unexplained mobility of teeth. Radiation therapy to the head and neck region can result in increased sensitivity of the teeth and osteoradionecrosis.[80] Trigeminal neuralgia, referred pain from cardiac angina, and multiple sclerosis can also mimic dental pain (see also Chapter 17). Acute maxillary sinusitis is a common condition that may create diagnostic confusion because it may mimic tooth pain in the maxillary posterior quadrant. In this situation the teeth in the quadrant may be extremely sensitive to cold and percussion, thus mimicking the signs and symptoms of pulpitis. This is certainly not a complete list of all the medical entities that can mimic dental disease, but it should alert the clinician that a medical problem could confuse and complicate the diagnosis of dental pathosis; this issue is discussed in more detail in subsequent chapters.

If, at the completion of a thorough dental examination, the subjective, objective, clinical testing and radiographic findings do not result in a diagnosis with an obvious dental origin, then the clinician must consider that an existing medical problem could be the true source of the pathosis. In such instances, a consultation with the patient's physician is always appropriate.

Dental History

The chronology of events that lead up to the chief complaint is recorded as the *dental history*. This information will help guide the clinician as to which diagnostic tests are to be performed. The history should include any past and present symptoms, as well as any procedures or trauma that might have evoked the chief complaint. Proper documentation is imperative. It may be helpful to use a premade form to record the pertinent information obtained during the dental history interview and diagnostic examination. Often a SOAP format is used, with the history and findings documented under the categories of *Subjective*, *Objective*, *Appraisal*, and *Plan*. There are also built-in features within some practice management software packages that allow digital entries into the patient's electronic file for the diagnostic workup (Figs. 1-3 and 1-4).

History of Present Dental Problem

The dialogue between the patient and the clinician should encompass all of the details pertinent to the events that led to the chief complaint. The clinician should direct the conversation in a manner that produces a clear and concise narrative that chronologically depicts all of the necessary information about the patient's symptoms and the development of these symptoms. To help elucidate this information, the patient is first instructed to fill out a dental history form as a part of the patient's office registration. This information will help the clinician decide which approach to use when asking the patient questions. The interview first determines *what is going on* in an effort to determine *why is it going on* for the purpose of eventually determining *what is necessary to resolve the chief complaint*.

Dental History Interview

After starting the interview and determining the nature of the chief complaint, the clinician continues the conversation by documenting the sequence of events that initiated the request for an evaluation. The dental history is divided into five basic directions of questioning: localization, commencement, intensity, provocation and attenuation, and duration.

Localization. "Can you point to the offending tooth?" Often the patient can point to or tap the offending tooth. This is the most fortunate scenario for the clinician because it helps direct the interview toward the events that might have caused any particular pathosis in this tooth. In addition, localization allows subsequent diagnostic tests to focus more on this particular tooth. When the symptoms are not well localized, the diagnosis is a greater challenge.

Commencement. "When did the symptoms first occur?" A patient who is having symptoms often remembers when these symptoms started. Sometimes the patient will even remember the initiating event: it may have been spontaneous in nature; it may have begun after a dental visit for a

restoration; trauma may be the etiology, biting on a hard object may have initially produced the symptoms, or the initiating event may have occurred concurrently with other symptoms (sinusitis, headache, chest pain, etc.). However, the clinician should resist the tendency to make a premature diagnosis based on these circumstances. The clinician should not simply assume "guilt by association" but instead should use this information to enhance the overall diagnostic process.

Intensity. "How intense is the pain?" It often helps to quantify how much pain the patient is actually having. The clinician might ask, "On a scale from 1 to 10, with 10 the most severe, how would you rate your symptoms?" Hypothetically, a patient could present with "an uncomfortable sensitivity to cold" or "an annoying pain when chewing" but might rate this "pain" only as a 2 or a 3. These symptoms certainly contrast with the type of symptoms that prevent a patient from sleeping at night. Often the intensity can be subjectively measured by what is necessary for the diminution of pain—for example, acetaminophen versus a narcotic pain reliever. This intensity level may affect the decision to treat or not to treat with endodontic therapy. Pain is now considered a standard vital sign, and documenting pain intensity (scale of 0 to 10) provides a baseline for comparison after treatment.

Provocation and attenuation. "What produces or reduces the symptoms?" Mastication and locally applied temperature changes account for the majority of initiating factors that cause dental pain. The patient may relate that drinking something cold causes the pain or possibly that chewing or biting is the only stimulus that "makes it hurt." The patient might say that the pain is only reproduced on "release from biting." On occasion, a patient may present to the dental office with a cold drink in hand and state that the symptoms can only be *reduced* by bathing the tooth in cold water. Nonprescription pain relievers may relieve some symptoms, whereas narcotic medication may be required to reduce others (see Chapter 4 for more information). Note that patients who are using narcotic as well as non-narcotic (e.g., ibuprofen) analgesics may respond differently to questions and diagnostic tests, thereby altering the validity of diagnostic results. Thus, it is important to know what drugs patients have taken in the previous 4 to 6 hours. These provoking and relieving factors may help the clinician to determine which diagnostic tests should be performed to establish a more objective diagnosis.

Duration. "Do the symptoms subside shortly, or do they linger after they are provoked?" The difference between a cold sensitivity that subsides in a few seconds and one that subsides in minutes may determine whether a clinician repairs a defective restoration or provides endodontic treatment. The duration of symptoms after a stimulating event should be recorded to establish how long the patient felt the sensation in terms of seconds or minutes. Clinicians often first test control teeth (possibly including a contralateral "normal" tooth) to define a "normal" response for the patient; thus, "lingering" pain is apparent when comparing the duration between the control teeth and the suspected tooth.

With the dental history interview complete, the clinician has a better understanding of the patient's chief complaint and can concentrate on making an objective diagnostic evaluation,

Name: (Last) _____ (First) _____ Date: _____ Tooth: _____

S. (SUBJECTIVE)
Chief Complaint:
History of Present Illness:

Nature of Pain:	None	Mild	Moderate	Severe				
Quality:	Dull	Sharp	Throbbing	Constant				
Onset:	Stim Required	Intermittent	Spontaneous					
Location:	Localized	Diffuse	Referred	Radiating to:				
Duration:	Seconds	Minutes	Hours	Constant				
Initiated by:	Cold	Heat	Sweet	Spontaneous	Palpation	Mastication	Supination	Keeps awake at night
Relieved by:	Cold	Heat	OTC-Meds	Narc-Meds				

O. (OBJECTIVE)

Extraoral:
Facial swelling: Yes No
L Nodes swollen: Yes No

Intraoral:
Soft tissues: WNL
Swelling: Yes No Mild Moderate Severe Location:
Sinus tract: Yes No Closed
Clinical crown: Restn Caries Exposure Fracture

#	Cold	Heat	EPT	Perc	Palp	Mob	Bite Stick	Dis-color	Periodontal Exam								
									MB	B	DB	DL	L	ML	Recessn	Furcation	Bleed - Probing

(Normal: N   No Response: 0   Mild: +   Moderate: ++   Severe: +++   Lingered: L   Delayed: D)

Radiographic Findings:

Alveolar Bone:	WNL	Apical lucency	Lateral lucency	Ap / Lat opacity	Crestal bone loss		
Lamina Dura:	WNL	Obscure	Broken	Widened			
Roots:	WNL	Curvature	Resorption	Perforation	Dilaceration	Fracture	Long	Sinus / IAN
Pulp Chamber:	WNL	Calcification	Pulp Stone	Exposure	Resorption	Perforation	
Pulp Canal:	WNL	Calcification	Bifurcated	Resorption	Prior RCT	Furcation Involvement	Perforation
Crown:	WNL	Caries	Restoration	Crown	Dens in dente		
Sinus Tract:	Traces to:						

A. (Assessment)

Diagnosis: Pulpal: WNL   Rev Pulpitis   Irrev Pulpitis   Necrosis   Prior RCT / Non-healing   Pulpless
              Periapical: WNL   APP   CPP   APA   CPA   Cond Osteitis
Etiology: Caries   Restoration   Prior RCT   Iatrogenic   Coronal leakage   Trauma   Perio   Elective   Resorptn   VRF
Prognosis: Good   Fair   Poor

P. (PLAN)

Endodontic: Caries control   RCT   ReTx   I&D   Apico   Apexification/genesis   Perf / Resorption Repair

Periodontal: S/RP   Crown lengthen   Root amp   Hemisection   Extraction

Restorative: Temp   Post space   B/U   P&C   Onlay / Crown   Bleach

FIG. 1-3 When taking a dental history and *performing* a diagnostic examination, often a premade form can facilitate complete and accurate documentation. (Courtesy Dr. Ravi Koka, San Francisco, CA.)

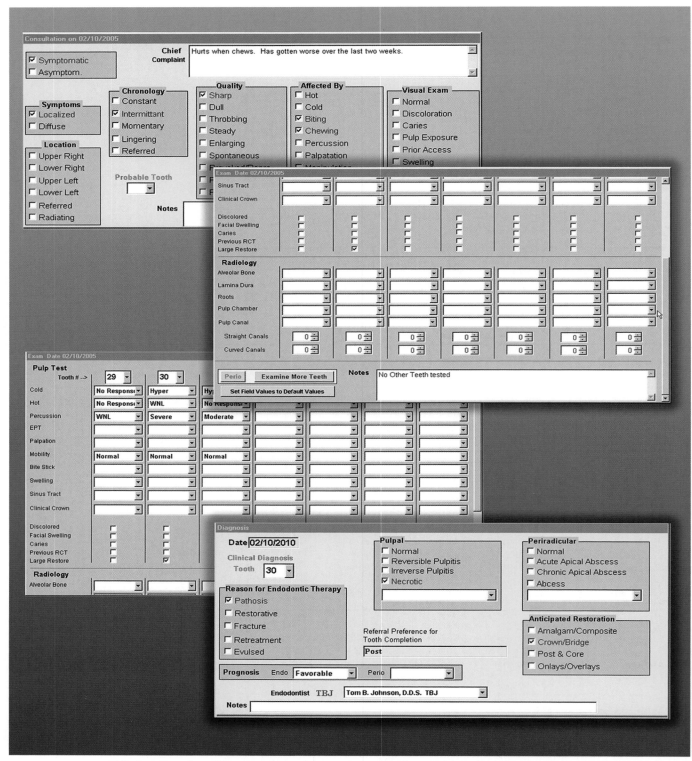

FIG. 1-4 Several practice management software packages have features for charting endodontic diagnoses using user-defined drop-down menus and areas for specific notations. Note that for legal purposes, it is desirable that all recorded documentation have the ability to be locked, or if any modifications are made after 24 hours, the transaction should be recorded with an automated time/date stamp. This is necessary so that the data cannot be fraudulently manipulated. (Courtesy PBS Endo, Cedar Park, TX.)

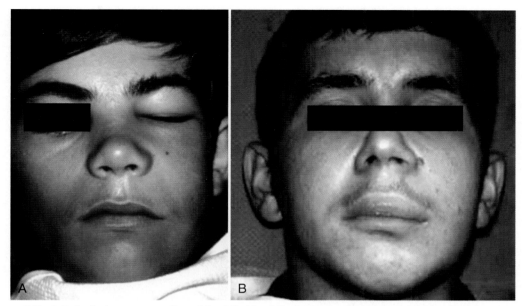

FIG. 1-5 **A,** Canine space swelling of the left side of the face extending into and involving the left eye. **B,** Swelling of the upper lip and the loss of definition of the nasolabial fold on the patient's left side, which indicates an early canine space infection.

although the subjective (and artistic) phase of making a diagnosis is not yet complete and will continue after the more objective testing and scientific phase of the investigatory process.

EXAMINATION AND TESTING

Extraoral Examination

Basic diagnostic protocol suggests that a clinician observe patients as they enter the operatory. Signs of physical limitations may be present, as well as signs of facial asymmetry that result from facial swelling. Visual and palpation examinations of the face and neck are warranted to determine whether swelling is present. Many times a facial swelling can be determined only by palpation when a unilateral "lump or bump" is present. The presence of bilateral swellings may be a normal finding for any given patient; however, it may also be a sign of a systemic disease or the consequence of a developmental event. Palpation allows the clinician to determine whether the swelling is localized or diffuse, firm or fluctuant. These latter findings will play a significant role in determining the appropriate treatment.

Palpation of the cervical and submandibular lymph nodes is an integral part of the examination protocol. If the nodes are found to be firm and tender along with facial swelling and an elevated temperature, there is a high probability that an infection is present. The disease process has moved from a localized area immediately adjacent to the offending tooth to a more widespread systemic involvement.

Extraoral facial swelling of odontogenic origin typically is the result of endodontic etiology because diffuse facial swelling resulting from a periodontal abscess is rare. Swellings of non-odontogenic origin must always be considered in the differential diagnosis, especially if an obvious dental pathosis is not found.[77] This situation is discussed in subsequent chapters.

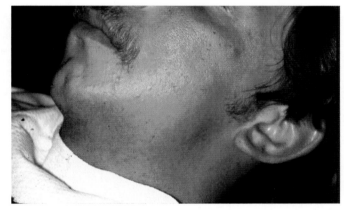

FIG. 1-6 Buccal space swelling associated with an acute periradicular abscess from the mandibular left second molar.

A subtle visual change such as loss of definition of the nasolabial fold on one side of the nose may be the earliest sign of a canine space infection (Fig. 1-5). Pulpal necrosis and periradicular disease associated with a maxillary canine should be suspected as the source of the problem. Extremely long maxillary central incisors may also be associated with a canine space infection, but most extraoral swellings associated with the maxillary centrals express themselves as a swelling of the upper lip and base of the nose.

If the buccal space becomes involved, the swelling will be extraoral in the area of the posterior cheek (Fig. 1-6). These swellings are generally associated with infections originating from the buccal root apices of the maxillary premolar and molar teeth and the mandibular premolar (Fig. 1-7) and first molar teeth. The mandibular second and third molars may also be involved, but infections associated with these two teeth are just as likely to exit to the lingual where other spaces

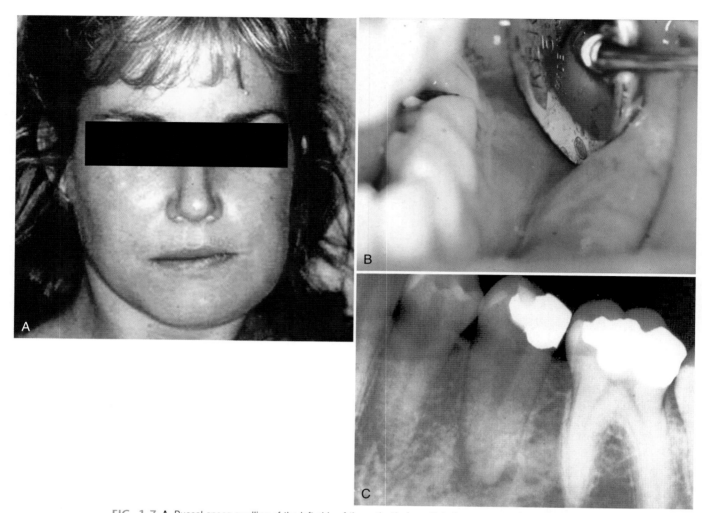

FIG. 1-7 **A,** Buccal space swelling of the left side of the patient's face. Note the asymmetry of the left side of the face. **B,** Intraoral view shows swelling present in the left posterior mucobuccal fold. **C,** This buccal space infection was associated with periradicular disease from the mandibular left second premolar. Note on the radiograph the periradicular radiolucency and large restoration associated with this tooth.

would be involved. For infections associated with these teeth, the root apices of the maxillary teeth must lie superior to the attachment of the buccinator muscle to the maxilla, and the apices of the mandibular teeth must be inferior to the buccinator muscle attachment to the mandible.[77]

Extraoral swelling associated with mandibular incisors will generally exhibit itself in the submental (Fig. 1-8) or submandibular space. Infections associated with any mandibular teeth, which exit the alveolar bone on the lingual and are inferior to the mylohyoid muscle attachment, will be noted as swelling in the submandibular space. Further discussions of fascial space infections may be found in Chapter 14.

Sinus tracts of odontogenic origin may also open through the skin of the face (Figs. 1-9 and 1-10).[2,56,64] These openings in the skin will generally close once the offending tooth is treated and healing occurs. A scar is more likely to be visible on the skin surface in the area of the sinus tract stoma than on the oral mucosal tissues (Fig. 1-10, *C* and *D*). Many patients with extraoral sinus tracts give a history of being treated by general physicians, dermatologists, or plastic surgeons with systemic or topical antibiotics or surgical procedures in

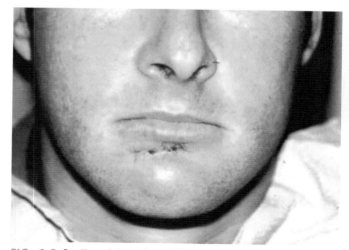

FIG. 1-8 Swelling of the submental space associated with periradicular disease from the mandibular incisors.

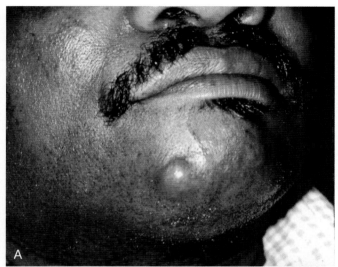

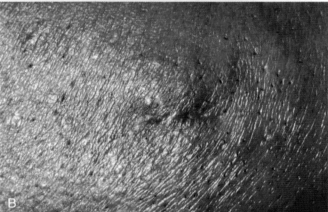

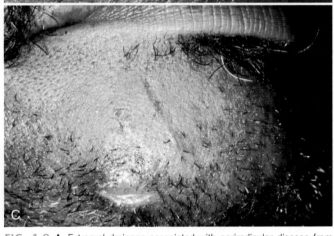

FIG. 1-9 **A,** Extraoral drainage associated with periradicular disease from the mandibular right canine. Note the parulis on the right anterior side of the face. **B,** Initial scar associated with the extraoral drainage incision after the parulis was drained and root canal therapy performed on the canine. **C,** Three-month follow-up shows healing of the incision area. Note the slight inversion of the scar tissue.

attempts to heal the extraoral stoma. In these particular cases, after multiple treatment failures, the patients may finally be referred to a dental clinician to determine whether there is a dental cause. Raising the awareness of physicians to such cases will aid in more accurate diagnosis and faster referral to the dentist or endodontist.

Intraoral Examination

The intraoral examination may give the clinician insight as to which intraoral areas may need a more focused evaluation. Any abnormality should be carefully examined for either prevention or early treatment of associated pathosis.[4,30,75,113,110,126] Swelling, localized lymphadenopathy, or a sinus tract should provoke a more detailed assessment of related and proximal intraoral structures.

Soft Tissue Examination

As with any dental examination, there should be a routine evaluation of the intraoral soft tissues. The gingiva and mucosa should be dried with either a low-pressure air syringe or a 2-by-2-inch gauze pad. By retracting the tongue and cheek, all of the soft tissue should be examined for abnormalities in color or texture. Any raised lesions or ulcerations should be documented and, when necessary, evaluated with a biopsy or referral.[82]

Intraoral Swelling

Intraoral swellings should be visualized and palpated to determine whether they are diffuse or localized and whether they are firm or fluctuant. These swellings may be present in the attached gingiva, alveolar mucosa, mucobuccal fold, palate, or sublingual tissues. Other testing methods are required to determine whether the origin is endodontic, periodontic, or a combination of these two or whether it is of nonodontogenic origin.

Swelling in the anterior part of the palate (Fig. 1-11) is most frequently associated with an infection present at the apex of the maxillary lateral incisor or the palatal root of the maxillary first premolar. More than 50% of the maxillary lateral incisor root apices deviate in the distal or palatal directions. A swelling in the posterior palate (Fig. 1-12) is most likely associated with the palatal root of one of the maxillary molars.[77]

Intraoral swelling present in the mucobuccal fold (Fig. 1-13) can result from an infection associated with the apex of the root of any maxillary tooth that exits the alveolar bone on the facial aspect and is inferior to the muscle attachment present in that area of the maxilla (see also Chapter 14). The same is true with the mandibular teeth if the root apices are superior to the level of the muscle attachments and the infection exits the bone on the facial. Intraoral swelling can also occur in the sublingual space if the infection from the root apex spreads to the lingual and exits the alveolar bone superior to the attachment for the mylohyoid muscle. The tongue will be elevated and the swelling will be bilateral because the sublingual space is contiguous with no midline separation. If the infection exits the alveolar bone to the lingual with mandibular molars and is inferior to the attachment of the mylohyoid muscle, the swelling will be noted in the submandibular space. Severe infections involving the maxillary and mandibular molars can extend into the parapharyngeal space, resulting in intraoral swelling of the tonsillar and pharyngeal areas. This can be life threatening if the patient's airway becomes obstructed.[77,80]

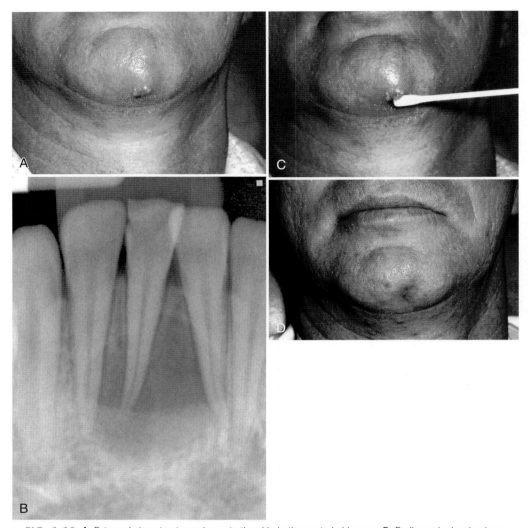

FIG. 1-10 **A,** Extraoral sinus tract opening onto the skin in the central chin area. **B,** Radiograph showing large radiolucency associated with the mandibular incisors. **C,** A culture is obtained from the drainage of the extraoral sinus tract. **D,** The healed opening of the extraoral sinus tract 1 month after root canal therapy was completed. Note the slight skin concavity in the area of the healed sinus tract.

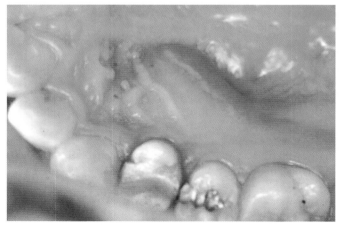

FIG. 1-11 Fluctuant swelling in the anterior palate associated with periradicular disease from the palatal root of the maxillary first premolar.

Intraoral Sinus Tracts

On occasion, a chronic endodontic infection will drain through an intraoral communication to the gingival surface and is known as a *sinus tract*.[12] This pathway, which is sometimes lined with epithelium, extends directly from the source of the infection to a surface opening, or *stoma*, on the attached gingival surface. As previously described, it can also extend extraorally. The term *fistula* is often inappropriately used to describe this type of drainage. The fistula, by definition, is actually an abnormal communication pathway between two internal organs or from one epithelium-lined surface to another epithelium-lined surface.[6]

Histologic studies have found that most sinus tracts are not lined with epithelium throughout their entire length. One study found that only 1 out of the 10 sinus tracts examined were lined with epithelium, whereas the other nine specimens were lined with granulation tissue.[55] Another study, with a larger sample size, found that two thirds of the specimens did not have epithelium extending beyond the level of the surface mucosa rete ridges.[12] The remaining specimens had some

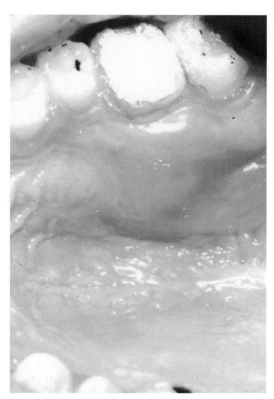

FIG. 1-12 Fluctuant swelling in the posterior palate associated with periradicular disease from the palatal root of the maxillary first molar.

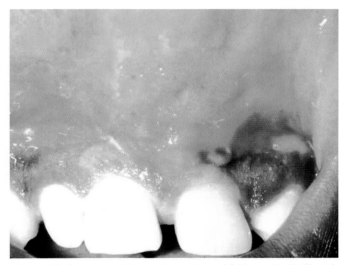

FIG. 1-13 Fluctuant swelling in the mucobuccal fold associated with periradicular disease from the maxillary central incisor.

epithelium that extended from the oral mucosa surface to the periradicular lesion.[12] The presence or absence of an epithelial lining does not seem to prevent closure of the tract as long as the source of the problem is properly diagnosed and adequately treated and the endodontic lesion has healed. Failure of a sinus tract to heal after treatment will necessitate further diagnostic procedures to determine whether other sources of infection are present or whether a misdiagnosis occurred.

In general, a periapical infection that has an associated sinus tract is not painful, although often there is a history of varying magnitudes of discomfort before sinus tract development. Besides providing a conduit for the release of infectious exudate and the subsequent relief of pain, the sinus tract can also provide a useful aid in determining the source of a given infection. Sometimes objective evidence as to the origin of an odontogenic infection is lacking. The stoma of the sinus tract may be located directly adjacent to or at a distant site from the infection. Tracing the sinus tract will provide objectivity in diagnosing the location of the problematic tooth. To trace the sinus tract, a size #25 or #30 gutta-percha cone is threaded into the opening of the sinus tract. Although this may be slightly uncomfortable to the patient, the cone should be inserted until resistance is felt. After a periapical radiograph is exposed, the origin of the sinus tract is determined by following the path taken by the gutta-percha cone (Fig. 1-14). This will direct the clinician to the tooth involved and, more specifically, to the root of the root of the tooth that is the source of the pathosis. Once the causative factors related to the formation of the sinus tract are removed, the stoma and the sinus tract will close within several days.

The stomata of intraoral sinus tracts may open in the alveolar mucosa, in the attached gingiva, or through the furcation or gingival crevice. They may exit through either the facial or the lingual tissues depending on the proximity of the root apices to the cortical bone. If the opening is in the gingival crevice, it is normally present as a narrow defect in one or two isolated areas along the root surface. When a narrow defect is present, the differential diagnosis must include the opening of a periradicular endodontic lesion, a vertical root fracture, or the presence of a developmental groove on the root surface. This type of sinus tract can be differentiated from a primary periodontal lesion because the latter generally presents as a pocket with a broad coronal opening and more generalized alveolar bone loss around the root. Other pulp testing methods may assist in verifying the source of infection.[111,112,121]

Palpation

In the course of the soft tissue examination, the alveolar hard tissues should also be palpated. Emphasis should be placed on detecting any soft tissue swelling or bony expansion, especially noting how it compares with and relates to the adjacent and contralateral tissues. In addition to objective findings, the clinician should question the patient about any areas that feel unusually sensitive during this palpation part of the examination.

A palpation test is performed by applying firm digital pressure to the mucosa covering the roots and apices. The index finger is used to press the mucosa against the underlying cortical bone. This will detect the presence of periradicular abnormalities or specific areas that produce painful response to digital pressure. A positive response to palpation may indicate an active periradicular inflammatory process. This test does not indicate, however, whether the inflammatory process is of endodontic or periodontal origin.

Percussion

Referring back to the patient's chief complaint may indicate the importance of percussion testing for this particular case. If the patient is experiencing acute sensitivity or pain on mastication, this response can typically be duplicated by individually percussing the teeth, which often isolates the symptoms to a particular tooth. Pain to percussion does not indicate that the

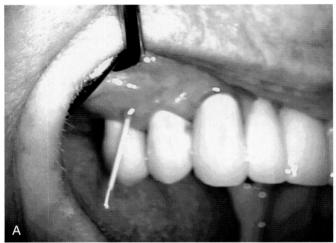

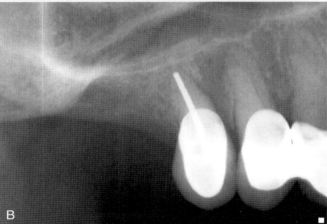

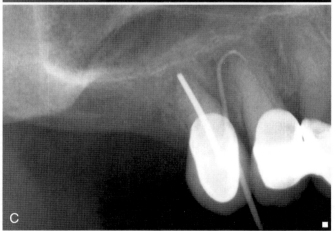

FIG. 1-14 **A,** To locate the source of an infection, the sinus tract can be traced by threading the stoma with a gutta-percha point. **B,** Radiograph of the area shows an old root canal in a maxillary second premolar and a questionable radiolucent area associated with the first premolar, with no clear indication of the etiology of the sinus tract. **C,** After tracing the sinus tract, the gutta-percha is seen to be directed to the source of pathosis, the apex of the maxillary first premolar.

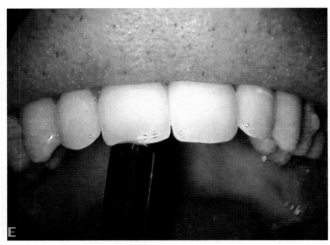

FIG. 1-15 Percussion testing of a tooth, using the back end of a mirror handle.

tooth is vital or nonvital but is rather an indication of inflammation in the periodontal ligament (i.e., symptomatic apical periodontitis). This inflammation may be secondary to physical trauma, occlusal prematurities, periodontal disease, or the extension of pulpal disease into the periodontal ligament space. The indication of where the pain originates is interpreted by the mesencephalic nucleus, receiving its information from proprioceptive nerve receptors. Although subject to debate, the general consensus is that there are relatively few proprioceptors in the dental pulp; however, they are prevalent in the periodontal ligament spaces.[24] This is why it may be difficult for the patient to discriminate the location of dental pain in the earlier stages of pathosis, when only the C fibers are stimulated. Once the disease state extends into the periodontal ligament space, the pain may become more localized for the patient; therefore, the affected tooth will be more identifiable with percussion and mastication testing.

Before percussing any teeth, the clinician should tell the patient what will transpire during this test. Because the presence of acute symptoms may create anxiety and possibly alter the patient's response, properly preparing the patient will lead to more accurate results. The contralateral tooth should first be tested as a control, as should several adjacent teeth that are certain to respond normally. The clinician should advise the patient that the sensation from this tooth is normal and ask to be advised of any tenderness or pain from subsequent teeth.

Percussion is performed by tapping on the incisal or occlusal surfaces of the teeth either with the finger or with a blunt instrument. The testing should initially be done gently, with light pressure being applied digitally with a gloved finger tapping. If the patient cannot detect significant difference between any of the teeth, the test should be repeated using the blunt end of an instrument, like the back end of a mirror handle (Fig. 1-15). The tooth crown is tapped vertically and horizontally. The tooth should first be percussed occlusally, and if the patient discerns no difference, the test should be repeated, percussing the buccal and lingual aspects of the teeth. For any heightened responses, the test should be repeated as necessary to determine that it is accurate and reproducible, and the information should be documented.

Although this test does not disclose the condition of the pulp, it indicates the presence of a periradicular inflammation.

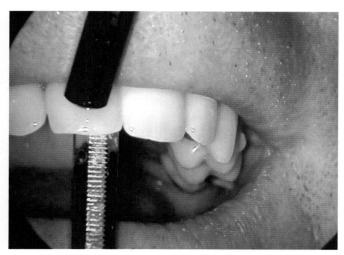

FIG. 1-16 Mobility testing of a tooth, using the back ends of two mirror handles.

An abnormal positive response indicates inflammation of the periodontal ligament that may be of either pulpal or periodontal origin. The sensitivity of the proprioceptive fibers in an inflamed periodontal ligament will help identify the location of the pain. This test should be done gently, especially in highly sensitive teeth. It should be repeated several times and compared with control teeth.

Mobility

Like percussion testing, an increase in tooth mobility is not an indication of pulp vitality. It is merely an indication of a compromised periodontal attachment apparatus. This compromise could be the result of acute or chronic physical trauma, occlusal trauma, parafunctional habits, periodontal disease, root fractures, rapid orthodontic movement, or the extension of pulpal disease, specifically an infection, into the periodontal ligament space. Tooth mobility is directly proportional to the integrity of the attachment apparatus or to the extent of inflammation in the periodontal ligament. Often the mobility reverses to normal after the initiating factors are repaired or eliminated. Because determining mobility by simple finger pressure can be visually subjective, the back ends of two mirror handles should be used, one on the buccal aspect and one on the lingual aspect of the tooth (Fig. 1-16). Pressure is applied in a facial-lingual direction as well as in a vertical direction and the tooth mobility is scored (Box 1-2). Any mobility that exceeds +1 should be considered abnormal. However, the teeth should be evaluated on the basis of how mobile they are relative to the adjacent and contralateral teeth.

Periodontal Examination

Periodontal probing is an important part of any intraoral diagnosis. The measurement of periodontal pocket depth is an indication of the depth of the gingival sulcus, which corresponds to the distance between the height of the free gingival margin and the height of the attachment apparatus below. Using a calibrated periodontal probe, the clinician should record the periodontal pocket depths on the mesial, middle, and distal aspects of both the buccal and lingual sides of the tooth, noting the depths in millimeters. The periodontal probe is "stepped" around the long axis of the tooth, progressing in 1-mm increments. Periodontal bone loss that is wide, as determined by a wide span of deep periodontal probings, is generally considered to be of periodontal origin and is typically more generalized in other areas of the mouth. However, isolated areas of vertical bone loss may be of an endodontic origin, specifically from a nonvital tooth whose infection has extended from the periapex to the gingival sulcus. Again, proper pulp testing is imperative, not just for the determination of a diagnosis but also for the development of an accurate prognosis assessment. For example, a periodontal pocket of endodontic origin may resolve after endodontic treatment, but if the tooth was originally vital with an associated deep periodontal pocket, endodontic treatment will not improve the periodontal condition. In addition, as discussed in Chapter 21, a vertical root fracture may often cause a localized narrow periodontal pocket that extends deep down the root surface. Characteristically, the adjacent periodontium is usually within normal limits.

Furcation bone loss can be secondary to periodontal or pulpal disease. The amount of furcation bone loss, as observed both clinically and radiographically, should be documented (Box 1-3). Results of pulp tests (described later) will aid in diagnosis.

Pulp Tests

Pulp testing involves attempting to make a determination of the responsiveness of pulpal sensory neurons.[62,63] The tests involve thermal or electrical stimulation of a tooth in order to obtain a subjective response from the patient (i.e., to determine whether the pulpal nerves are functional), or the tests may involve a more objective approach using devices that detect the integrity of the pulpal vasculature. Unfortunately, the quantitative evaluation of the status of pulp tissue can only be determined histologically, as it has been shown that there is not necessarily a good correlation between the objective clinical signs and symptoms and the pulpal histology.[122,123]

Thermal

Various methods and materials have been used to test the pulp's response to thermal stimuli. The baseline or normal response to either cold or hot is a patient's report that a sensation is felt but disappears immediately upon removal of the thermal stimulus. Abnormal responses include a lack of response to the stimulus, a lingering or intensification of a painful sensation after the stimulus is removed, or an immediate, excruciatingly painful sensation as soon as the stimulus is placed on the tooth.

Cold testing is the primary pulp testing method used by many clinicians today. It is especially useful for patients presenting with porcelain jacket crowns or porcelain-fused-to-metal crowns where no natural tooth surface (or much metal) is accessible. If a clinician chooses to perform this test with sticks of ice, then the use of a rubber dam is recommended, because melting ice will run onto adjacent teeth and gingiva, yielding potentially false-positive responses.

Frozen carbon dioxide (CO_2), also known as *dry ice* or *carbon dioxide snow*, or CO_2 *stick*, has been found to be reliable in eliciting a positive response if vital pulp tissue is present in the tooth.[46,98,99] One study found that vital teeth would respond to both frozen CO_2 and skin refrigerant, with skin refrigerant producing a slightly quicker response.[66] Frozen carbon dioxide has also been found to be effective in evaluating the pulpal response in teeth with full coverage crowns for which other tests such as electric pulp testing is not possible.[11] For testing purposes, a solid stick of CO_2 is prepared by delivering CO_2 gas into a specially designed plastic cylinder (Fig. 1-17). The resulting CO_2 stick is applied to the facial surface of either the natural tooth structure or crown. Several teeth can be tested with a single CO_2 stick. The teeth should be isolated and the oral soft tissues should be protected with a 2-by-2-inch gauze or cotton roll so the frozen CO_2 will not come into contact with these structures. Because of the extremely cold temperature of the frozen CO_2 ($-69°F$ to $-119°F$; $-56°C$ to $-98°C$), burns of the soft tissues can occur. It has been demonstrated on extracted teeth that frozen CO_2 application has resulted in a significantly greater intrapulpal temperature decrease than either skin refrigerant or ice.[11] Also, it appears that the application of CO_2 to teeth does not result in any irreversible damage to the pulp tissues or cause any significant enamel crazing.[61,104]

The most popular method of performing cold testing is with a refrigerant spray. It is readily available, easy to use, and provides test results that are reproducible, reliable, and equivalent to that of frozen CO_2.[46,66,96,141] One of the current products contains 1,1,1,2-tetrafluoroethane, which has zero ozone depletion potential and is environmentally safe. It has a temperature of $-26.2°C$.[66] The spray is most effective for testing purposes when it is applied to the tooth on a large #2 cotton pellet (Fig. 1-18). In one study,[65] a significantly lower intrapulpal temperature was achieved when a #2 cotton pellet was dipped or sprayed with the refrigerant compared with the result when a small #4 cotton pellet or cotton applicator was used. The sprayed cotton pellet should be applied to the mid-facial area of the tooth or crown. As with any other pulp testing method, adjacent or contralateral "normal" teeth should also be tested to establish a baseline response. It appears that frozen CO_2 and refrigerant spray are superior to other cold testing methods and equivalent or superior to the electric pulp tester for assessing pulp vitality.[11,46] However, one study found that periodontal attachment loss and gingival recession may influence the reported pain response with cold stimuli.[116]

To be most reliable, cold testing should be used in conjunction with an electric pulp tester (described later in this chapter) so that the results from one test will verify the findings of the other test. If a mature, nontraumatized tooth does not respond to both cold testing and electric pulp testing, then the pulp should be considered necrotic.[23,98,141] However, a multirooted tooth, with at least one root containing vital pulp tissue, may respond to a cold test and electric pulp test even if one or more of the roots contain necrotic pulp tissue.[98]

Another thermal testing method involves the use of heat. Heat testing is most useful when a patient's chief complaint is intense dental pain on contact with any hot liquid or food. When a patient is unable to identify which tooth is sensitive, a heat test is appropriate. Starting with the most posterior tooth in that area of the mouth, each tooth is individually isolated with a rubber dam. An irrigating syringe is filled with a liquid (most commonly plain water) that has a temperature similar to that which would cause the painful sensation. The liquid is then expressed from the syringe onto the isolated tooth to determine whether the response is normal or abnormal. The clinician moves forward in the quadrant, isolating each individual tooth until the offending tooth is located. That tooth will exhibit an immediate, intense painful response to the heat. With heat testing, a delayed response may occur, so waiting 10 seconds between each heat test will allow sufficient time for the onset of symptoms. This method can also be used to apply cold water to the entire crown for cases in which cold is the precipitating stimulus.

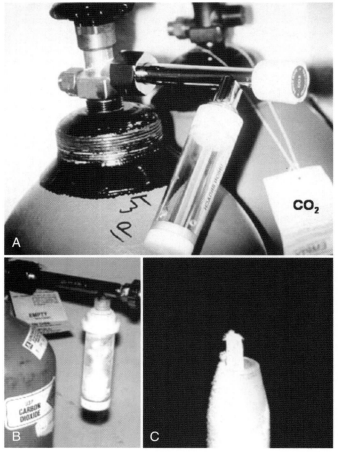

FIG. 1-17 A, Carbon dioxide tank with apparatus attached to form solid CO_2 stick/pencil. **B,** CO_2 gas being transformed into a solid stick/pencil. **C,** CO_2 stick/pencil extruded from end of a plastic carrier and ready for use.

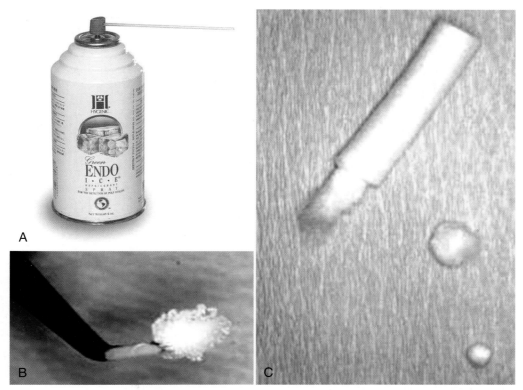

FIG. 1-18 **A,** Refrigerant spray container. **B,** A large cotton pellet made of a cotton roll or a ready-made size #2 (large) cotton pellet can be used to apply the refrigerant spray to the tooth surface. The small #4 cotton pellet does not provide as much surface area as the #2 cotton pellet, and therefore should not be used to deliver the refrigerant to the tooth surface. **C,** A large cotton pellet sprayed with the refrigerant and ready to be applied to the tooth surface. (*A,* Courtesy Coltène/Whaledent, Cuyahoga Falls, OH.)

Another method for heat testing is to apply heated gutta-percha or compound stick to the surface of the tooth. If this method is used, a light layer of lubricant should be placed onto the tooth surface before applying the heated material to prevent the hot gutta-percha or compound from adhering to the dry tooth surface. Heat can also be generated by the friction created when a dry rubber-polishing wheel is run at a high speed against the dry surface of a tooth. However, this latter method is seldom used today and is not recommended. Another approach is the use of electronic heat-testing instruments.[20]

If the heat test confirms the results of other pulp testing procedures, emergency care can then be provided. Often a tooth that is sensitive to heat may also be responsible for some spontaneous pain. The patient may present with cold liquids in hand just to minimize the pain (Fig. 1-19). In such cases, the application of cold to a specific tooth may eliminate the pain and greatly assist in the diagnosis. Typically, a tooth that responds to heat and then is relieved by cold is found to be necrotic.

Electric

Assessment of pulp neural responses (*vitality*) can also be accomplished by electric pulp testing.[79] Electric pulp testers of different designs and manufacturers have been used for this purpose. Electric pulp testers should be an integral part of any dental practice. It should be noted that the vitality of the pulp is determined by the intactness and health of the vascular supply, not by the status of the pulpal nerve fibers. Even though

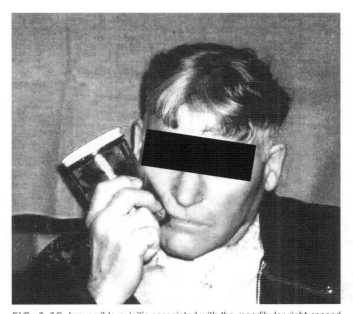

FIG. 1-19 Irreversible pulpitis associated with the mandibular right second molar. Patient has found that the only way to alleviate the pain is to place a jar filled with ice water against the right side of his face.

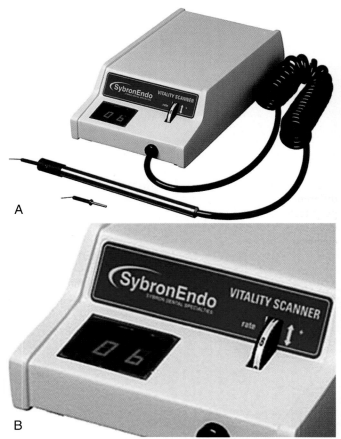

FIG. 1-20 A, Electric pulp tester with probe. The probe tip will be coated with a conducive medium such as toothpaste and placed in contact with the tooth surface. The patient will activate the unit by placing a finger on the metal shaft of the probe. **B,** View of the electric pulp tester control panel; the knob on the front right of the unit controls the rate at which the electric current is delivered to the tooth. The plastic panel on the left front displays the digital numerical reading obtained from the pulp test. The digital scale runs from 0 to 80. (Courtesy SybronEndo, Orange, CA.)

advances are being made with regard to determining the vitality of the pulp on the basis of the blood supply, this technology has not been perfected enough at this time to be used on a routine basis in a clinical setting.

The electric pulp tester has some limitations in providing predictable information about the vitality of the pulp. The response of the pulp to electric testing does not reflect the histologic health or disease status of the pulp.[122,123] A response by the pulp to the electric current only denotes that some viable nerve fibers are present in the pulp and are capable of responding. Numeric readings on the pulp tester have significance only if the number differs significantly from the readings obtained from a control tooth tested on the same patient with the electrode positioned at a similar area on both teeth. However, in most cases, the response is scored as either present or absent. Studies[122,123] have shown that electric pulp test results are most accurate when no response is obtained to any amount of electric current. This lack of response has been found most frequently when a necrotic pulp is present. In addition, false-positive and false-negative responses can occur (Box 1-4), and the clinician must take it into account when formulating the final diagnosis.

The electric pulp tester will not work unless the probe can be placed in contact with or be bridged to the natural tooth structure.[95] With the advent of universal precautions for infection control, the use of rubber gloves prevents the clinician from completing the circuit.[7] Some pulp testers may require the patient to place a finger, or fingers, on the tester probe to complete the electric circuit; however, the use of lip clips is an alternative to having patients hold the tester. Proper use of the electric pulp tester requires the evaluated teeth to be carefully isolated and dried. A control tooth of similar tooth type and location in the arch should be tested first in order to establish a baseline response and to inform the patient as to what a "normal" sensation is. The suspected tooth should be tested at least twice to confirm the results. The tip of the testing probe that will be placed in contact with the tooth structure must be coated with a water- or petroleum-based medium.[86] The most commonly used medium is toothpaste. The coated probe tip is placed in the incisal third of the facial or buccal area of the tooth to be tested.[15] Once the probe is in contact with the tooth, the patient is asked to touch or grasp the tester probe, unless a lip clip is used (Fig. 1-20, *A*). This completes the circuit and initiates the delivery of electric current to the tooth.

The patient is instructed to remove his or her finger(s) from the probe when a "tingling" or "warming" sensation is felt in the tooth. The readings from the pulp tester are recorded (Fig. 1-20, *B*) and will be evaluated once all the appropriate teeth have been tested by the electric pulp tester and the other pulp testing methods.

If a complete coverage crown or extensive restoration is present, a bridging technique can be attempted to deliver the electric current to any exposed natural tooth structure.[95] The tip of an endodontic explorer is coated with toothpaste or other appropriate medium and placed in contact with the natural tooth structure. The tip of the electric pulp tester probe is coated with a small amount of toothpaste and placed in contact with the side of the explorer. The patient completes the circuit and the testing proceeds as described previously. If no natural tooth structure is available, then an alternative pulp testing method, such as cold, should be used.

One study compared the ability of thermal and electric pulp testing methods to register the presence of vital pulp tissue.[99] The *sensitivity,* which is the ability of a test to identify teeth that are diseased, was 0.83 for the cold test, 0.86 for heat test, and 0.72 for the electric test. This means the cold test correctly identified 83% of the teeth that had a necrotic pulp, whereas heat tests were correct 86% of the time and electric pulp tests were correct only 72% of the time. This same study evaluated the *specificity* of these three tests. Specificity relates to the ability of a test to identify teeth without disease. Ninety-three percent of teeth with healthy pulps were correctly identified by both the cold and electric pulp tests, whereas only 41% of the teeth with healthy pulps were identified correctly by the heat test. From the results of the testing, it was found that the cold test had an accuracy of 86%, the electric pulp test 81%, and the heat test 71%.

Some studies have indicated there might not be a significant difference between pulp testing results obtained by electric pulp tester and those obtained by the thermal methods.[46,98,99] Cold tests, however, have been shown to be more reliable than electric pulp tests in younger patients with less developed root apices.[5,42,98] This is the reason to verify the results obtained by one testing method and compare them with results obtained by other methods. Until such time that the testing methods used to assess the vascular supply of the pulp become less time consuming and technique sensitive, thermal and electric pulp testing will continue to be the primary methods for determining pulp vitality.

Laser Doppler Flowmetry

Laser Doppler flowmetry (LDF) is a method used to assess blood flow in microvascular systems. Attempts are being made to adapt this technology to assess pulpal blood flow. A diode is used to project an infrared light beam through the crown and pulp chamber of a tooth. The infrared light beam is scattered as it passes through the pulp tissue. The Doppler principle states that the light beam's frequency will shift when hitting moving red blood cells but will remain unshifted as it passes through static tissue. The average Doppler frequency shift will measure the velocity at which the red blood cells are moving.[114]

Several studies[40,60,69,84,114,115,117] have found LDF to be an accurate, reliable, and reproducible method of assessing pulpal blood flow. One of the great advantages of pulp testing with devices such as the LDF is that the collected data are based on objective findings rather than subjective patient responses. As is discussed in Chapter 20, certain luxation injuries will cause inaccuracies in the results of electric and thermal pulp testing. LDF has been shown to be a great indicator for pulpal vitality in these cases.[130] This technology, however, is not being used routinely in the dental practice.

Pulse Oximetry

The pulse oximeter is another noninvasive device (Fig. 1-21). Widely used in medicine, it is designed to measure the oxygen concentration in the blood and the pulse rate. A pulse oximeter works by transmitting two wavelengths of light, red and infrared, through a translucent portion of a patient's body (e.g., a finger, earlobe, or tooth). Some of the light is absorbed as it passes through the tissue; the amount absorbed depends on the ratio of oxygenated to deoxygenated hemoglobin in the blood. On the opposite side of the targeted tissue, a sensor detects the absorbed light. On the basis of the difference between the light emitted and the light received, a microprocessor calculates the pulse rate and oxygen concentration in the blood.[118] The transmission of light to the sensor requires that there be no

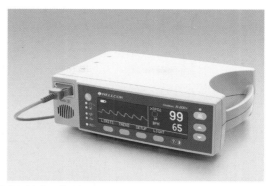

FIG. 1-21 Nellcor OxiMax N-600x pulse oximeter. (Courtesy Nellcor Puritan Bennett, Boulder, CO; now part of Covidien.)

obstruction from restorations, which can sometimes limit the usefulness of pulse oximetry to test pulp vitality.

Custom-made sensors have been developed and were found to be more accurate than electric and thermal pulp tests.[31,54] This sensor has been especially useful in evaluating teeth that have been subjected to traumatic injuries, as such teeth tend to present, especially in the short term, with questionable vitality using conventional pulp testing methods.[8,31,53]

Studies regarding the ability of pulse oximetry to diagnose pulp vitality draw various conclusions. Several studies have found pulse oximetry to be a reliable method for assessing pulp vitality.[69,70,118,125,140] Others have stated that in its present form the pulse oximeter may not be predictable in diagnosing pulp vitality.[140] Most of the problems appear to be related to the currently available technology. Some investigators have concluded that the devices used for pulp testing are too cumbersome and complicated to be used on a routine basis in a dental practice.[68,118,140]

Special Tests

Bite Test

Percussion and bite tests are indicated when a patient presents with pain while biting. On occasion, the patient may not know which tooth is sensitive to biting pressure, and percussion and bite tests may help to localize the tooth involved. The tooth may be sensitive to biting when the pulpal pathosis has extended into the periodontal ligament space, creating a *symptomatic apical periodontitis,* or the sensitivity may be present secondary to a crack in the tooth. The clinician can often differentiate between periradicular periodontitis and a cracked tooth or fractured cusp. If periradicular periodontitis is present, the tooth will respond with pain to percussion and biting tests regardless of where the pressure is applied to the coronal part of the tooth. A cracked tooth or fractured cusp will typically elicit pain only when the percussion or bite test is applied in a certain direction to one cusp or section of the tooth.[22,108]

For the bite test to be meaningful, a device should be used that will allow the clinician to apply pressure to individual cusps or areas of the tooth. A variety of devices have been used for bite tests, including cotton tip applicators, toothpicks, orangewood sticks, and rubber polishing wheels. There are several devices specifically designed to perform this test. The Tooth Slooth (Professional Results, Laguna Niguel, CA) (Fig. 1-22) and FracFinder (Hu-Friedy, Oakbrook, IL) are just two of the commercially available devices used for the bite test. As with all pulp tests, adjacent and contralateral teeth should

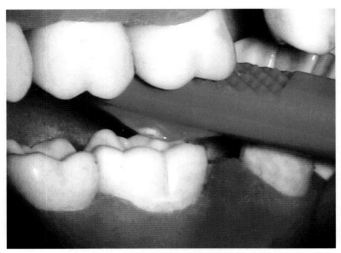

FIG. 1-22 To determine which tooth, or tooth part, is sensitive to mastication, having the patient bite on a specially designed bite stick is often helpful.

be used as controls so that the patient is aware of the "normal" response to these tests. The small cupped-out area on these instruments is placed in contact with the cusp to be tested. The patient is then asked to apply biting pressure with the opposing teeth to the flat surface on the opposite side of the device. The biting pressure should be applied slowly until full closure is achieved. The firm pressure should be applied for a few seconds; the patient is then asked to release the pressure quickly. Each individual cusp on a tooth can be tested in a like manner. The clinician should note whether the pain is elicited during the pressure phase or on quick release of the pressure. A common finding with a fractured cusp or cracked tooth is the frequent presence of pain upon release of biting pressure.

Test Cavity

The test cavity method for assessing pulp vitality is not routinely used since, by definition, it is an invasive irreversible test. This method is used only when all other test methods are deemed impossible or the results of the other tests are inconclusive. An example of a situation in which this method can be used is when the tooth suspected of having pulpal disease has a full coverage crown. If no sound tooth structure is available to use a bridging technique with the electric pulp tester and cold test results are inconclusive, a small class I cavity preparation is made through the occlusal surface of the crown. This is accomplished with a high-speed #1 or #2 round bur with proper air and water coolant. The patient is not anesthetized while this procedure is performed, and the patient is asked to respond if any painful sensation is felt during the drilling procedure. If the patient feels pain once the bur contacts sound dentin, the procedure is terminated and the class I cavity preparation is restored. This sensation signifies only that there is some viable nerve tissue remaining in the pulp, not that the pulp is totally healthy. If the patient fails to feel any sensation when the bur reaches the dentin, this is a good indication that the pulp is necrotic and root canal therapy is indicated.

Staining and Transillumination

To determine the presence of a crack in the surface of a tooth, the application of a stain to the area is often of great assistance.

It may be necessary to remove the restoration in the tooth to better visualize a crack or fracture. Methylene blue dye, when painted on the tooth surface with a cotton tip applicator, will penetrate into cracked areas. The excess dye may be removed with a moist application of 70% isopropyl alcohol. The dye will indicate the possible location of the crack.

Transillumination using a bright fiberoptic light probe to the surface of the tooth may be very helpful (Fig. 1-23). Directing a high-intensity light directly on the exterior surface of the tooth at the cementum-enamel junction (CEJ) may reveal the extent of the fracture. Teeth with fractures block transilluminated light. The part of the tooth that is proximal to the light source will absorb this light and glow, whereas the area beyond this fracture will not have light transmitted to it and will show as gray by comparison.[101] Although the presence of a fracture may be evident using dyes and transillumination, the depth of the fracture cannot always be determined.

Selective Anesthesia

When symptoms are not localized or referred, the diagnosis may be challenging. Sometimes the patient may not even be able to specify whether the symptoms are emanating from the maxillary or mandibular arch. In these instances, when pulp testing is inconclusive, *selective anesthesia* may be helpful.

If the patient cannot determine which arch the pain is coming from, then the clinician should first selectively anesthetize the maxillary arch. This should be accomplished by using a periodontal ligament (intraligamentary) injection. The injection is administered to the most posterior tooth in the quadrant of the arch that may be suspected, starting from the distal sulcus. The anesthesia is subsequently administered in an anterior direction, one tooth at a time, until the pain is eliminated. If the pain is not eliminated after an appropriate period of time, then the clinician should similarly repeat this technique on the mandibular teeth below. It should be understood that periodontal ligament injections may anesthetize an adjacent tooth and thus are more useful for identifying the arch rather than the specific tooth.

Radiographic Examination and Interpretation

Intraoral Radiographs

The radiographic interpretation of a potential endodontic pathosis is an integral part of endodontic diagnosis and prognosis assessment. Few diagnostic tests provide as much useful information as dental radiography. For this reason, the clinician is sometimes tempted to prematurely make a definitive diagnosis based solely on radiographic interpretation. However, the image should be used only as one sign, providing important clues in the diagnostic investigation. When not coupled with a proper history and clinical examination and testing, the radiograph alone can lead to a misinterpretation of normality and pathosis (Fig. 1-24). Because treatment planning will ultimately be based on the diagnosis, the potential for inappropriate treatment may frequently exist if the radiograph alone is used for making final diagnosis. The clinician should not subject the patient to unnecessary multiple radiation exposures; two pretreatment images from different angulations are often sufficient. Under extenuating circumstances, however, especially when the diagnosis is difficult, additional exposures may be necessary to determine the presence of multiple roots,

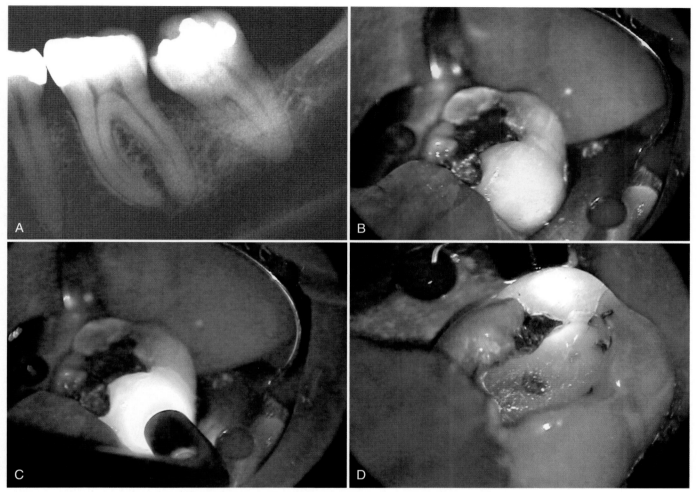

FIG. 1-23 Sometimes there is no clear indication of why a tooth is symptomatic. This radiograph shows a mandibular second molar with a moderately deep restoration (A); the pulp tests nonvital. Without any transillumination, a fracture cannot be detected (B). However, by placing a high-intensity light source on the tooth surface, a root fracture can be observed on the buccal surface (C) and the distal-lingual surface (D).

multiple canals, resorptive defects, caries, restoration defects, root fractures, and the extent of root maturation and apical development.

The radiographic appearance of endodontic pathosis can sometimes be highly subjective. In a study by Goldman and colleagues, there was only 50% agreement among interpreters for the radiographic presence of pathosis.[49] When the cases were reevaluated several months later, the same evaluators agreed with their own original diagnosis less than 85% of the time.[50] This further emphasizes the necessity for additional objective diagnostic tests, as well as the importance of obtaining and comparing older radiographs.

For standard two-dimensional radiography, clinicians basically project x-radiation through an object and capture the image on a recording medium, either x-ray film or a digital sensor. Much like casting a shadow from a light source, the image appearance may vary greatly depending on how the radiographic source is directed. Thus, the three-dimensional interpretation of the resulting two-dimensional image requires not only knowledge of normality and pathosis but also advanced knowledge of how the radiograph was exposed. By virtue of "casting a shadow," the anatomic features that are closest to the film (or sensor) will move the least when there is a change in the horizontal or vertical angulation of the radiation source (Fig. 1-25). This may be helpful in determining the existence of additional roots, the location of pathosis, and the unmasking of anatomic structures. Changes in the horizontal or vertical angulation may help elucidate valuable anatomic and pathologic information; it also has the potential to hide important information. An incorrect vertical angulation may cause the buccal roots of a maxillary molar to be masked by the zygomatic arch. An incorrect horizontal angulation may cause roots to overlap with the roots of adjacent teeth, or it may incorrectly create the appearance of a one-rooted tooth, when two roots are actually present.

In general, when endodontic pathosis appears radiographically, it appears as bone loss in the area of the periapex. The pathosis may present merely as a widening or break in the lamina dura—the most consistent radiographic finding when a tooth is nonvital[67]—or it may present as a radiolucent area at the apex of the root or in the alveolar bone adjacent to the exit of a lateral or furcation accessory canal. On occasion there may be no radiographic change at all, even in the presence of a disease process in the alveolar bone.

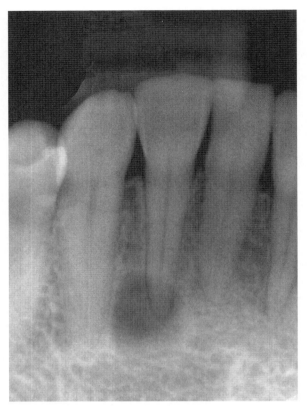

FIG. 1-24 Radiograph showing what appears to be a mandibular lateral incisor associated with periapical lesion of a nonvital tooth. Although pulp necrosis can be suspected, the tooth tested vital. In this case, the appearance of apical bone loss is secondary to a cementoma.

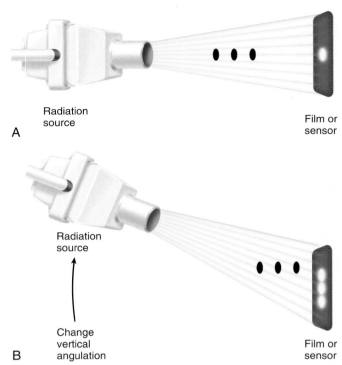

FIG. 1-25 Radiographic images are only two-dimensional, and often it is difficult to discriminate the relative location of overlapping objects. **A,** When the source of radiation is directly perpendicular to overlapping objects, the image is captured without much separation of the objects. However, when the radiation source is at an angle to offset the overlapping objects, the image is captured with the objects being viewed as separated. **B,** The object that is closest to the film (or sensor) will move the least, with the object closest to the radiation source appearing farthest away.

Two-dimensional dental radiography has two basic short-comings: the lack of early detection of pathosis in the cancellous bone, because of the density of the cortical plates, and the influence of the superimposition of anatomic structures. Variability in the radiographic expression of an osseous pathosis has much to do with the relative location of the root of the tooth and how it is oriented with respect to the cortical and cancellous bone. Radiographic changes from bone loss will not be detected if the loss is only in cancellous bone.[16] However, the radiographic evidence of pathosis will be observed once this bone loss extends to the junction of the cortical and cancellous bone. In addition, certain teeth are more prone to exhibit radiographic changes than others, depending on their anatomic location.[17] The radiographic appearance of endodontic pathosis is correlated with the relationship of the periapex of the tooth and its juxtaposition to the cortical-cancellous bone junction. The apices of most anterior and premolar teeth are located close to the cortical-cancellous bone junction. Therefore, periapical pathosis from these teeth is exhibited sooner on the radiograph. By comparison, the distal roots of mandibular first molars and both roots of mandibular second molars are generally positioned more centrally within the cancellous bone, as are maxillary molars, especially the palatal roots. Periapical lesions from these roots must expand more before they reach the cortical-cancellous bone junction and are recognized as radiographic pathosis. For these reasons, it is important not to exclude the possibility of pulpal pathosis in situations in which there are no radiographic changes.

Many factors can influence the quality of the radiographic interpretation, including the ability of the person exposing the radiograph, the quality of the radiographic film, the quality of the exposure source, the quality of the film processing, and the skill with which the film is viewed. Controlling all of these variables can be a difficult challenge but is paramount for obtaining an accurate radiographic interpretation.

Digital Radiography
Digital radiography has been available since the late 1980s and has recently been refined with better hardware and more user-friendly software. It has the ability to capture, view, magnify, enhance, and store radiographic images in an easily reproducible format that does not degrade over time. Significant advantages of digital radiographs over conventional radiographs include lower radiation doses, instant viewing, convenient manipulation, efficient transmission of an image via the Internet, simple duplication; and easy archiving.

Digital radiography uses no x-ray film and requires no chemical processing. Instead, a *sensor* is used to capture the image created by the radiation source. This sensor is either directly or wirelessly attached to a local computer, which interprets this signal and, using specialized software, translates the signal into a two-dimensional digital image that can be displayed, enhanced, and analyzed. The image is stored in the patient's file, typically in a dedicated network server, and can be recalled as needed. Further information about digital radiography may be found in Chapter 2.

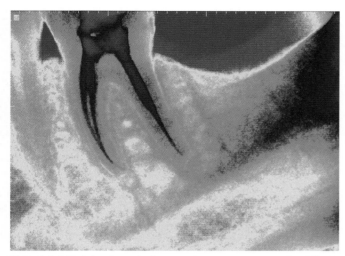

FIG. 1-26 Digital radiography has an advantage over conventional film in that the image can be enhanced and colorized, a useful tool for patient education.

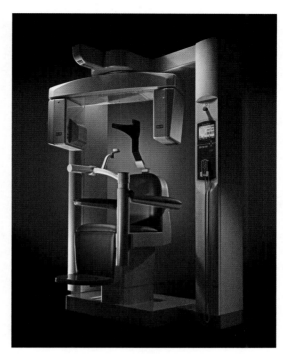

FIG. 1-27 Cone-beam volumetric tomography, using the 3D Accuitomo 80. (Courtesy J. Morita USA, Irvine, CA.)

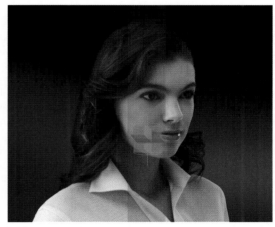

FIG. 1-28 Cone-beam volumetric tomography has the ability to capture, store, and present radiographic images in various horizontal and vertical planes. (Courtesy J. Morita USA, Irvine, CA.)

The viewing of a digital radiographic image on a high-resolution monitor allows for rapid and easy interpretation for both the clinician and the patient. The image appears almost instantly, with no potential for image distortion from improper chemical processing. The clinician can magnify different areas on the radiograph and then digitally enhance the image in order to better visualize certain anatomic structures; in some cases the image can even be colorized, a useful tool for patient education (Fig. 1-26).

In the past, x-ray film has had a slightly better resolution than most digital radiography images, at about 16 line pairs per millimeter (lp/mm).[87] Some sensor manufacturers, however, now claim to offer resolutions beyond that of conventional film. Under the best of circumstances, the human eye can see only about 10 lp/mm, which is the lowest resolution for most dental digital radiography systems. Digital sensors are much more sensitive to radiation than conventional x-ray film and thus require 50% to 90% less radiation in order to acquire an image, an important feature for generating greater patient acceptance of dental radiographs.

The diagnostic quality of this expensive technology has been shown to be comparable to, but not necessarily superior to, perfectly exposed and perfectly processed conventional film-based radiography.[39,73,97] Furthermore, it was found that the interpretation of a digital radiograph can be subjective, similar to that of the conventional film.[134] Factors that appear to have the most impact on the interpretation of the image are the years of experience of the examiner and familiarity of the operator with the given digital system.[134]

Cone-Beam Computerized Tomography

Limitations in conventional two-dimensional radiography promulgated a need for three-dimensional imaging, known as *cone-beam computerized tomography* (CBCT) (also known as *cone-beam volumetric tomography* [CBVT]) or as *cone-beam volumetric imaging* [CBVI]. Although a form of this technology has existed since the early 1980s,[106] specific devices for dental use first appeared almost two decades later.[90] Most of these machines are similar to a dental panoramic radiographic device, whereby the patient stands or sits as a cone-shaped

radiographic beam is directed to the target area with a reciprocating capturing sensor on the opposite side (Fig. 1-27). The resulting information is digitally reconstructed and interpreted to create an interface whereby the clinician can three-dimensionally interpret "slices" of the patient's tissues in a multitude of planes (Figs. 1-28 and 1-29).[37,33] The survey of the scans can be interpreted immediately after the scan. Various software applications have been used to enable the images to be sent to other clinicians. This is accomplished either in printed format or with portable and transferable software that can be used interactively by another clinician.

In general, many dental applications only require a limited field of vision, confining the study to the maxilla and mandible.

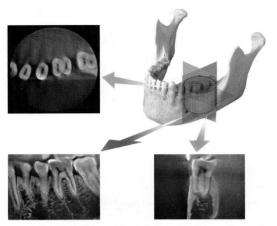

FIG. 1-29 Cone-beam volumetric tomography has the advantage of being able to detect pathosis in the bone or associated with the teeth without the obstruction of anatomic structures. The planes of vision may be axial, sagittal, or coronal. (Courtesy J. Morita USA, Irvine, CA.)

However, many devices have the ability to provide a full field of vision for viewing more regional structures. Clinicians should thoroughly understand the ethical and medical-legal ramifications of doing scans with full fields of view. Incidental nondental findings have been seen from these scans, such as intracranial aneurysms, that when undetected could be life threatening.[91]

The radiation source of CBCT is different from that of conventional two-dimensional dental imaging in that the radiation beam created is conical in shape. Also, conventional digital dental radiography is captured and interpreted as *pixels,* a series of dots that collectively produces an image of the scanned structure. For CBCT, the image is instead captured as a series of three-dimensional pixels, known as *voxels.* Combining these voxels gives a three-dimensional image that can be "sliced" into various planes, allowing for specific evaluations never before possible without a necropsy (Fig. 1-30). One of the advantages of using a device that has a limited field of vision is that the voxel size can be less than half that of a device using a full field of vision, thereby increasing the resolution of the resulting image and providing for a more accurate interpretation of anatomic structures and pathologic conditions. The development of limited field of vision devices has also contributed to decreasing the costs of these relatively expensive machines, making them more practical for dental office use.[41]

Compared with two-dimensional radiographs, CBCT can clearly visualize the interior of the cancellous bone without the superimposition of the cortical bone. Studies show that CBCT is much more predictable and efficient in demonstrating anatomic landmarks, bone density, bone loss, periapical lesions, root fractures, root perforations and root resorptions.[1,21,26,27,38,47,71,78,81,85,92,94,128,131,142]

The superimposition of anatomic structures can also mask the interpretation of alveolar defects. Specifically, the maxillary sinus, zygoma, incisive canal and foramen, nasal bone, orbit, mandibular oblique ridge, mental foramen, mandibular mentalis, sublingual salivary glands, tori, and the overlap of adjacent roots may either obscure bone loss or mimic bone loss, making an accurate interpretation of conventional radiography sometimes difficult or impossible. Several studies have

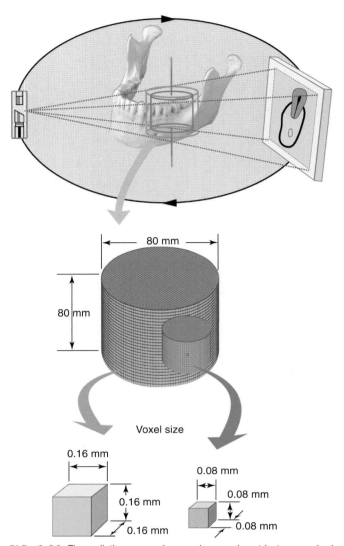

FIG. 1-30 The radiation source in cone-beam volumetric tomography is conical. The receiving sensor captures the image as "voxels," or three-dimensional pixels of information, allowing digital interpretation.

demonstrated the advantages of CBCT in the differential diagnosis of such structures from pathologic conditions.[21,29,71,137]

Cone-beam computerized tomography should not be seen as a replacement for conventional dental radiography, but rather as a diagnostic adjunct. The advantage of conventional dental radiography is that it can visualize most of the structures in one image. CBCT can show great detail in many planes of vision but can also leave out important details if the "slice" is not in the area of existing pathosis (Fig. 1-31). There is a promising future for the use of CBCT for endodontic diagnosis and treatment. It has already proven invaluable in the detection of dental and nondental pathoses (Fig. 1-32). For a further review of CBCT and radiography, see Chapter 2.

Magnetic Resonance Imaging (MRI)

MRI has also been suggested for dental diagnosis. It may offer simultaneous three-dimensional hard- and soft-tissue imaging of teeth without ionizing radiation.[58] The use of MRI in endodontics is still limited.

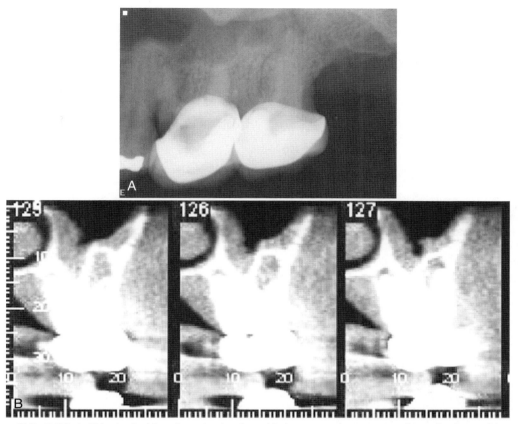

FIG. 1-31 **A,** This standard two-dimensional radiographic image reveals recurrent caries under the mesial margin of the maxillary first molar. However, the patient localized pain to mastication on the maxillary second molar. **B,** Cone-beam volumetric tomography revealed an apical radiolucency associated with the maxillary second molar. The bone loss was obscured on the two-dimensional radiograph by the maxillary sinus, zygoma, and cortical bone.

Cracks and Fractures

The wide variety of types of cracks and fractures in teeth and their associated signs and symptoms often make their diagnosis difficult. The extensiveness of the crack or fracture line may directly alter the prognosis assessment for a given tooth and should be examined before treatment decision making. Certain types of cracks may be as innocent as a superficial enamel craze line, or they may be as prominent as a fractured cusp. The crack may progress into the root system to involve the pulp, or it may split the entire tooth into two separate segments. The crack may be oblique, extending cervically, such that once the coronal segment is removed the tooth may or may not be restorable. Any of these situations may present with mild, moderate, or severe symptoms or possibly no symptoms at all.

Crack Types

There have been many suggestions in the literature of was to classify cracks in teeth. By defining the type of crack present, an assessment of the prognosis may be determined and treatment alternatives can be planned (see Chapter 21). Unfortunately, it is often extremely difficult to determine how extensive a crack is until the tooth is extracted.

Cracks in teeth can be divided into three basic categories:

♦ Craze lines
♦ Fractures (also referred to as *cracks*)
♦ Split tooth/roots

Craze lines are merely cracks in the enamel that do not extend into the dentin and either occur naturally or develop after trauma. They are more prevalent in adult teeth and usually occur more in the posterior teeth. If light is transilluminated through the crown of such a tooth, these craze lines may show up as fine lines in the enamel with light being able to transmit through them, indicating that the crack is only superficial. The use of optical coherence tomography (OCT) has also been suggested for detection of enamel cracks.[59] Craze lines typically will not manifest with symptoms. No treatment is necessary for craze lines unless they create a cosmetic issue.

Fractures extend deeper into the dentin than superficial craze lines and primarily extend mesially to distally, involving the marginal ridges. Dyes and transillumination are helpful for visualizing potential root fractures.

Symptoms from a fractured tooth range from none to severe pain. A fracture in the tooth does not necessarily dictate that the tooth has split into two pieces; however, left alone or especially with provocations such as occlusal prematurities, the fracture may progress into a split root. A fractured tooth may be treated by a simple restoration, endodontics (nonsurgical or surgical), or even extraction, depending on the extent and orientation of the fracture, the degree of symptoms, and whether the symptoms can be eliminated. This makes the clinical management of fractured teeth difficult and sometimes unpredictable.

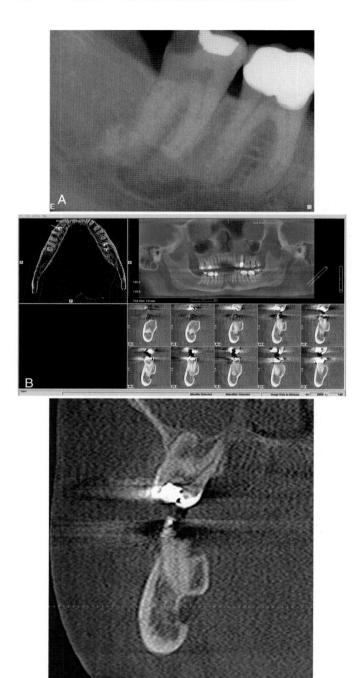

FIG. 1-32 **A,** Periapical radiograph showing a large apical radiolucency associated with the mandibular second molar. Apical pathosis should be ruled out. **B,** Cone-beam volumetric tomography revealed salivary indentation of the mandible in the area apical and lingual to the mandibular second molar, consistent with a Stafne defect. **C,** Enlargement of coronal section in the area of the mandibular second molar and the Stafne defect located on the lingual aspect of the mandible.

A definitive combination of factors, signs, and symptoms that, when collectively observed, allows the clinician to conclude the existence of a specific disease state is termed a *syndrome*. However, given the multitude of signs and symptoms that fractured roots can present with, it is often difficult to achieve an objective definitive diagnosis. For this reason, the

terminology of *cracked tooth syndrome*[22,108] should be avoided.[6] The subjective and objective factors seen in cases of fractured teeth will generally be diverse; therefore, a tentative diagnosis of a fractured tooth will most likely be more of a prediction. Once this prediction is made, the patient must be properly informed as to any potential decrease in prognosis of the pending dental treatment. Because treatment options for repairing fractured teeth have only a limited degree of success, early detection and prevention, and proper informed consent, are crucial.[9,10,72,119,120,124,132]

Split tooth/roots occur when a fracture extends from one surface of the tooth to another surface of the tooth, with the tooth separating into two segments. If the split is more oblique, it is possible that once the smaller separated segment is removed, the tooth might still be restorable—for example, a fractured cusp. However, if the split extends below the osseous level, the tooth may not be restorable and endodontic treatment may not result in a favorable prognosis.

Proper prognosis assessment is imperative before any dental treatment but is often difficult in cases of cracked teeth. Because of the questionable long-term success from treating cases of suspected or known fractures, the clinician should be cautious in making the decision to continue with treatment and should avoid endodontic treatment in cases of a definitive diagnosis of split roots.

Vertical Root Fractures

One of the more common reasons for recurrent endodontic pathosis is the *vertical root fracture,* a severe crack in the tooth that extends longitudinally down the long axis of the root (Figs. 1-33 and 1-34). Often it extends through the pulp and to the periodontium. It tends to be more centrally located within the tooth, as opposed to being more oblique, and typically traverses through the marginal ridges. These fractures may be present before endodontic treatment, secondary to endodontic treatment, or may develop after endodontic treatment has been completed. Because diagnosing these vertical root fractures may be difficult, they often go unrecognized. Therefore, diagnosing the existence and extent of a vertical root fracture is imperative before any restorative or endodontic treatment is done, as it can dramatically affect the overall success of treatment.

A patient who consents to endodontic treatment must be informed if the tooth has a questionable prognosis. The clinician must be able to interpret the subjective and objective findings that suggest a vertical root fracture or split tooth, be able to make a prediction as to the eventual potential of healing, and convey this information to the patient. A more detailed discussion on vertical root fractures is described in Chapter 21.

Perforations

Root perforations are clinical complications that may lead to treatment failure. When root perforation occurs, communications between the root canal system and either periradicular tissues or the oral cavity may reduce the prognosis of treatment. Root perforations may result from extensive carious lesions, resorption, or operator error occurring during root canal instrumentation or post preparation.

The treatment prognosis of root perforations depends on the size, location, time of diagnosis and treatment, degree of periodontal damage, as well as the sealing ability and biocompatibility of the repair material.[45] It has been recognized that

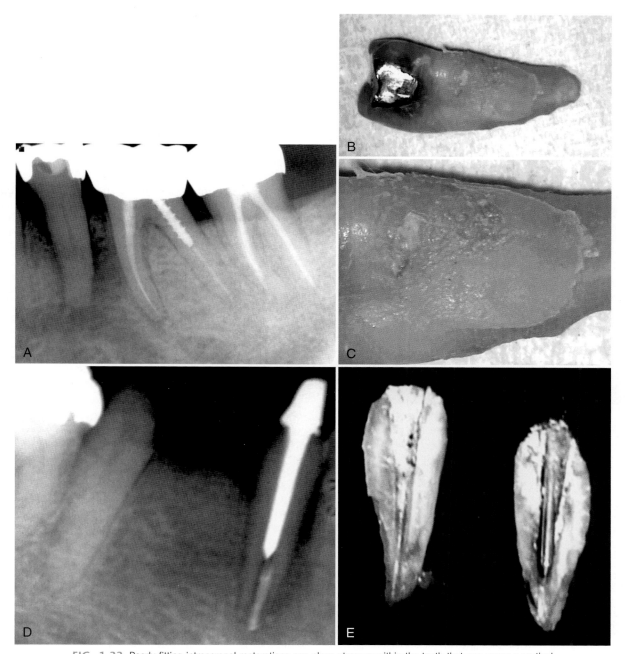

FIG. 1-33 Poorly fitting intracoronal restorations can place stresses within the tooth that can cause a vertical root fracture. **A,** This radiograph of a mandibular second premolar (with a gold inlay) reveals extensive periapical and periradicular bone loss, especially on the distal aspect. **B,** The tooth pulp tested nonvital, and there was an associated 12-mm-deep, narrow, isolated periodontal pocket on the buccal aspect of the tooth. After the tooth was extracted, the distal aspect was examined. **C,** On magnification (×16) the distal aspect of the root revealed an oblique vertical root fracture. Similarly, the placement of an ill-fitting post may exert intraradicular stresses on a root that can cause a fracture to occur vertically. **D,** This radiograph depicts a symmetrical space between the obturation and the canal wall, suggesting a vertical root fracture. **E,** After the tooth is extracted, the root fracture can be easily observed.

treatment success depends mainly on immediate sealing of the perforation and appropriate infection control. Among the materials that are commonly used to seal root perforations are mineral trioxide aggregate (MTA), Super EBA, intermediate restorative material (IRM), glass ionomer cements, and composites. The topic of perforations is further discussed in Chapter 19.

CLINICAL CLASSIFICATION OF PULPAL AND PERIAPICAL DISEASES

Many attempts have been made over the years to develop classifications of pulpal and periapical disease. However, studies have shown that making a correlation between clinical signs and symptoms and the histopathology of a given clinical

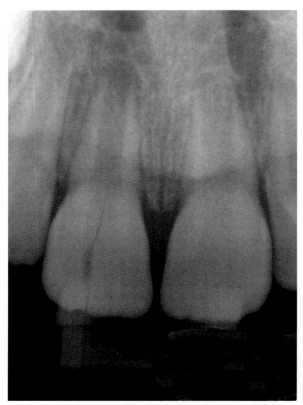

FIG. 1-34 Physical trauma from sports-related injuries or seizure-induced trauma, if directed accordingly, may cause a vertical root fracture in a tooth. This fracture occurred in a 7-year-old child secondary to trauma from a grand mal seizure.

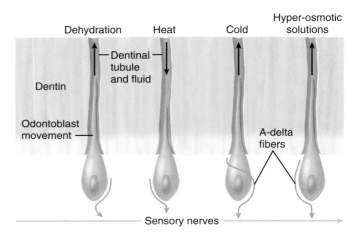

Dentin tubule fluid movement

FIG. 1-35 Dentinal tubules are filled with fluid that, when stimulated, will cause sensation. Temperature changes, air, and osmotic changes can provoke the odontoblastic process to induce the stimulation of underlying A-delta fibers.

condition is challenging.[122,123] Therefore, *clinical* classifications have been developed in order to formulate treatment plan options. In the most general terms, the objective and subjective findings are used to classify the suspected pathosis, with the assigned designations merely representing the presence of healthy or diseased tissue.

The terminology and classifications that follow are based on those suggested by the American Association of Endodontists in 2012.[6]

Pulpal Disease

Normal Pulp

This is a clinical diagnostic category in which the pulp is symptom-free and normally responsive to pulp testing.[6] Teeth with normal pulp do not usually exhibit any spontaneous symptoms. The symptoms produced from pulp tests are mild, do not cause the patient distress, and result in a transient sensation that resolves in seconds. Radiographically, there may be varying degrees of pulpal calcification but no evidence of resorption, caries, or mechanical pulp exposure. No endodontic treatment is indicated for these teeth.

Pulpitis

This is a clinical and histologic term denoting inflammation of the dental pulp, clinically described as reversible or irreversible and histologically described as acute, chronic, or hyperplastic.[6]

Reversible Pulpitis

This is a clinical diagnosis based on subjective and objective findings indicating that the inflammation should resolve and the pulp return to normal.[6] When the pulp within the tooth is irritated so that the stimulation is uncomfortable to the patient but reverses quickly after irritation, it is classified as *reversible pulpitis*. Causative factors include caries, exposed dentin, recent dental treatment, and defective restorations. Conservative removal of the irritant will resolve the symptoms. Confusion can occur when there is exposed dentin, without evidence of pulp pathosis, which can sometimes respond with sharp, quickly reversible pain when subjected to thermal, evaporative, tactile, mechanical, osmotic, or chemical stimuli. This is known as *dentin* (or *dentinal*) *sensitivity* (or *hypersensitivity*). Exposed dentin in the cervical area of the tooth accounts for most of the cases diagnosed as dentin sensitivity.[103]

As described in Chapter 12, fluid movement within dentinal tubules can stimulate the odontoblasts and associated fast-conducting A-delta nerve fibers in the pulp, which in turn produce sharp, quickly reversible dental pain (Fig. 1-35). The more open these tubules are (e.g., from a newly exposed preparation, dentin decalcification, periodontal scaling, tooth-bleaching materials, or coronal tooth fractures), the more the tubule fluid will move and, subsequently, the more the tooth will display dentin sensitivity when stimulated. When making a diagnosis, it is important to discriminate this dentin sensitivity sensation from that of reversible pulpitis, which would be secondary to caries, trauma, or new or defective restorations. Detailed questioning about recent dental treatment and a thorough clinical and radiographic examination will help to separate dentin sensitivity from other pulpal pathosis, as the treatment modalities for each are completely different.[18]

Irreversible Pulpitis

As the disease state of the pulp progresses, the inflammatory condition of the pulp can change to *irreversible pulpitis*. At this stage, treatment to remove the diseased pulp will be necessary. This condition can be divided into the subcategories of *symptomatic* and *asymptomatic* irreversible pulpitis.

Symptomatic Irreversible Pulpitis

This is a clinical diagnosis based on subjective and objective findings indicating that the vital inflamed pulp is incapable of healing.[6] Teeth that are classified as having *symptomatic irreversible pulpitis* exhibit intermittent or spontaneous pain. Rapid exposure to dramatic temperature changes (especially to cold stimuli) will elicit heightened and prolonged episodes of pain even after the thermal stimulus has been removed. The pain in these cases may be sharp or dull, localized, diffuse, or referred. Typically, there are minimal or no changes in the radiographic appearance of the periradicular bone. With advanced irreversible pulpitis, a thickening of the periodontal ligament may become apparent on the radiograph, and there may be some evidence of pulpal irritation by virtue of extensive pulp chamber or root canal space calcification. Deep restorations, caries, pulp exposure, or any other direct or indirect insult to the pulp, recently or historically, may be present. It may be seen radiographically or clinically or may be suggested from a complete dental history. Patients who present with symptomatic anterior teeth for which there are no obvious etiologic factors should be also questioned regarding past general anesthesia or endotracheal intubation procedures.[3,127,138] In addition, patients should be questioned about a history of orthodontic treatment. Typically, when symptomatic irreversible pulpitis remains untreated, the pulp will eventually become necrotic.[109,139]

Asymptomatic Irreversible Pulpitis

This is a clinical diagnosis based on subjective and objective findings indicating that the vital inflamed pulp is incapable of healing.[6] The patient, however, does not complain of any symptoms. On occasion, deep caries will not produce any symptoms, even though clinically or radiographically the caries may extend well into the pulp. Left untreated, the tooth may become symptomatic or the pulp will become necrotic. In cases of *asymptomatic irreversible pulpitis,* endodontic treatment should be performed as soon as possible so that symptomatic irreversible pulpitis or necrosis does not develop and cause the patient severe pain and distress.

Pulp Necrosis

This is a clinical diagnostic category indicating death of the dental pulp. The pulp is usually nonresponsive to pulp testing.[6] When pulpal *necrosis* (or *nonvital pulp*) occurs, the pulpal blood supply is nonexistent and the pulpal nerves are nonfunctional. It is the only clinical classification that directly attempts to describe the histologic status of the pulp (or lack thereof). This condition is subsequent to symptomatic or asymptomatic irreversible pulpitis. After the pulp becomes completely necrotic, the tooth will typically become asymptomatic until such time when there is an extension of the disease process into the periradicular tissues. With pulp necrosis, the tooth will usually not respond to electric pulp tests or to cold stimulation. However, if heat is applied for an extended period of time, the tooth may respond to this stimulus. This response could possibly be related to remnants of fluid or gases in the pulp canal space expanding and extending into the periapical tissues.

Pulpal necrosis may be partial or complete and it may not involve all of the canals in a multirooted tooth. For this reason, the tooth may present with confusing symptoms. Pulp testing over one root may give no response, whereas over another root it may give a positive response. The tooth may also exhibit symptoms of symptomatic irreversible pulpitis. Pulp necrosis, in the absence of restorations, caries, or luxation injuries, is likely caused by a longitudinal fracture extending from the occlusal surface and into the pulp.[19]

After the pulp becomes necrotic, bacterial growth can be sustained within the canal. When this infection (or its bacterial byproducts) extends into the periodontal ligament space, the tooth may become symptomatic to percussion or exhibit spontaneous pain. Radiographic changes may occur, ranging from a thickening of the periodontal ligament space to the appearance of a periapical radiolucent lesion. The tooth may become hypersensitive to heat, even to the warmth of the oral cavity, and is often relieved by applications of cold. As previously discussed, this may be helpful in attempting to localize a necrotic tooth (i.e., by the application of cold one tooth at a time) when the pain is referred or not well localized.

Previously Treated

This is a clinical diagnostic category indicating that the tooth has been endodontically treated and the canals are obturated with various filling materials other than intracanal medicaments.[6] In this situation, the tooth may or may not present with signs or symptoms but will require additional nonsurgical or surgical endodontic procedures to retain the tooth. In most such situations, there will no longer be any vital or necrotic pulp tissue present to respond to pulp testing procedures.

Previously Initiated Therapy

This is a clinical diagnostic category indicating that the tooth has been previously treated by partial endodontic therapy (e.g., pulpotomy, pulpectomy).[6] In most instances, the partial endodontic therapy was performed as an emergency procedure for symptomatic or asymptomatic irreversible pulpitis cases. In other situations, these procedures may have been performed as part of vital pulp therapy procedures, traumatic tooth injuries, apexification, or apexogenesis therapy. At the time these cases present for root canal therapy it would not be possible to make an accurate pulpal diagnosis because all, or part, of the pulp tissue has already been removed.

Apical (Periapical) Disease

Normal Apical Tissues

This classification is the standard against which all of the other apical disease processes are compared. In this category the patient is asymptomatic and the tooth responds normally to percussion and palpation testing. The radiograph reveals an intact lamina dura and periodontal ligament space around all the root apices.

Periodontitis

This classification refers to an inflammation of the periodontium.[6] When located in the periapical tissues it is referred to as apical periodontitis. Apical periodontitis can be subclassified to symptomatic apical periodontitis and asymptomatic apical periodontitis.

Symptomatic Apical Periodontitis

This condition is defined as an inflammation, usually of the apical periodontium, producing clinical symptoms including a painful response to biting or percussion or palpation. It might or might not be associated with an apical radiolucent area.[6]

This tooth may or may not respond to pulp vitality tests, and the radiograph or image of the tooth will typically exhibit at least a widened periodontal ligament space and may or may not show an apical radiolucency associated with one or all of the roots.

Asymptomatic Apical Periodontitis

This condition is defined as inflammation and destruction of apical periodontium that is of pulpal origin, appears as an apical radiolucent area, and does not produce clinical symptoms.[6] This tooth does not usually respond to pulp vitality tests, and the radiograph or image of the tooth will exhibit an apical radiolucency. The tooth is generally not sensitive to biting pressure but may "feel different" to the patient on percussion. Manifestation of persistent apical periodontitis may vary among patients.[89]

Acute Apical Abscess

This condition is defined as an inflammatory reaction to pulpal infection and necrosis characterized by *rapid onset*, spontaneous pain, tenderness of the tooth to pressure, pus formation, and swelling of associated tissues.[6] A tooth with an *acute apical abscess* will be acutely painful to biting pressure, percussion, and palpation. This tooth will not respond to any pulp vitality tests and will exhibit varying degrees of mobility. The radiograph or image can exhibit anything from a widened periodontal ligament space to an apical radiolucency. Swelling will be present intraorally and the facial tissues adjacent to the tooth will almost always present with some degree of swelling. The patient will frequently be febrile, and the cervical and submandibular lymph nodes may exhibit tenderness to palpation.

Chronic Apical Abscess

This condition is defined as an inflammatory reaction to pulpal infection and necrosis characterized by *gradual onset*, little or no discomfort, and the intermittent discharge of pus through an associated sinus tract.[6] In general, a tooth with a *chronic apical abscess* will not present with clinical symptoms. The tooth will not respond to pulp vitality tests, and the radiograph or image will exhibit an apical radiolucency. Usually the tooth is not sensitive to biting pressure but can "feel different" to the patient on percussion. This entity is distinguished from asymptomatic apical periodontitis because it will exhibit intermittent drainage through an associated sinus tract.

REFERRED PAIN

The perception of pain in one part of the body that is distant from the actual source of the pain is known as *referred pain*. Whereas pain of nonodontogenic origin can refer pain to the teeth, teeth may also refer pain to other teeth as well as to other anatomic areas of the head and neck (see Chapters 4 and 17). This may create a diagnostic challenge, in that the patient may insist that the pain is from a certain tooth or even from an ear when, in fact, it is originating from a distant tooth with pulpal pathosis. Using electronic pulp testers, investigators found that patients could localize *which* tooth was being stimulated only 37.2% of the time and could narrow the location to three teeth

only 79.5% of the time, illustrating that patients may have a difficult time discriminating the exact location of pulpal pain.[44]

Referred pain from a tooth is usually provoked by an intense stimulation of pulpal C fibers, the slow conducting nerves that when stimulated cause an intense, slow, dull pain. Anterior teeth seldom refer pain to other teeth or to opposite arches, whereas posterior teeth may refer pain to the opposite arch or to the periauricular area but seldom to the anterior teeth.[14] Mandibular posterior teeth tend to transmit referred pain to the periauricular area more often than maxillary posterior teeth. One study showed that when second molars were stimulated with an electric pulp tester, patients could discriminate accurately which arch the sensation was coming from only 85% of the time, compared with an accuracy level of 95% with first molars and 100% with anterior teeth.[136] The investigators also pointed out that when patients first feel the sensation of pain, they are more likely to accurately discriminate the origin of the pain. With higher levels of discomfort, patients have less ability to accurately determine the source of the pain. Therefore, in cases of diffuse or referred pain, the history of where the patient first felt the pain may be significant.

Because referred pain can complicate a dental diagnosis, the clinician must be sure to make an accurate diagnosis to protect the patient from unnecessary dental or medical treatment. If after all the testing procedures are complete and it is determined that the pain is not of odontogenic origin, then the patient should be referred to an orofacial pain clinic for further testing. For further information on pain of nonodontogenic origin, see Chapter 17.

SUMMARY

Endodontics is a multifaceted specialty, with much emphasis on how cases are clinically treated. Clinicians have increased their ability to more accurately perform endodontic procedures by way of increased visualization using the operating microscope, precise apical foramen detection using electronic apex locators, enhanced imaging techniques using digital radiography, and more. Practices have incorporated more refined canal cleaning and shaping techniques by using ultrasonics and rotary-driven nickel titanium files facilitated with computer-assisted electronic handpieces. Many other advancements have also been introduced with the objective of achieving an optimal result during endodontic treatment. However, these advancements are useless if an incorrect diagnosis is made. Before the clinician ever considers performing any endodontic treatment, the following questions must be answered:

- Is the existing problem of dental origin?
- Are the pulpal tissues within the tooth pathologically involved?
- Why is the pulpal pathosis present?
- What is the prognosis?
- What is the appropriate form of treatment?

Testing, questioning, and reasoning are combined to achieve an accurate diagnosis and to ultimately form an appropriate treatment plan. The art and science of making this diagnosis are the first steps that must be taken before initiating any endodontic treatment.

REFERENCES

1. Abella F, Patel S, Duran-Sindreu F, et al: Evaluating the periapical status of teeth with irreversible pulpitis by using cone-beam computed tomography scanning and periapical radiographs, *J Endod* 38:1588, 2012.

2. Abuabara A, Zielak JC, Schramm CA, Baratto-Filho F: Dental infection simulating skin lesion, *An Bras Dermatol* 87:619, 2012.

3. Adolphs N, Kessler B, von Heymann C, et al: Dentoalveolar injury related to general anaesthesia: a 14 years review and a statement from the surgical point of view based on a retrospective analysis of the documentation of a university hospital, *Dent Traumatol* 27:10, 2011.

4. Al-Hezaimi K, Naghshbandi J, Simon JH, Rotstein I: Successful treatment of a radicular groove by intentional replantation and Emdogain therapy: four years follow-up, *Oral Surg Oral Med Oral Pathol Oral Radiol Endodon* 107:e82, 2009.

5. Alomari FA, Al-Habahbeh R, Alsakarna BK: Responses of pulp sensibility tests during orthodontic treatment and retention, *Int Endod J* 44:635, 2011.

6. American Association of Endodontists: *Glossary of endodontic terms*, ed 8, Chicago, 2012, American Association of Endodontists.

7. Anderson RW, Pantera EA: Influence of a barrier technique on electric pulp testing, *J Endod* 14:179, 1988.

8. Andreasen J, Andreasen F, Andreasen L, editors: *Textbook and color atlas of traumatic injuries to the teeth*, ed 4, Philadelphia, 2008, Wiley Blackwell.

9. Andreasen JO, Ahrensburg SS, Tsillingaridis G: Root fractures: the influence of type of healing and location of fracture on tooth survival rates: an analysis of 492 cases, *Dent Traumatol* 28:404, 2012.

10. Arakawa S, Cobb CM, Rapley JW, Killoy WJ, et al: Treatment of root fracture by CO_2 and Nd:YAG lasers: an in vitro study, *J Endod* 22:662, 1996.

11. Augsburger RA, Peters DD: In vitro effects of ice, skin refrigerant, and CO_2 snow on intrapulpal temperature, *J Endod* 7:110, 1981.

12. Baumgartner JC, Picket AB, Muller JT: Microscopic examination of oral sinus tracts and their associated periapical lesions, *J Endod* 10:146, 1984.

13. Beltes C, Zachou E: Endodontic management in a patient with vitamin D-resistant Rickets, *J Endod* 38:255, 2012.

14. Bender IB: Pulpal pain diagnosis: a review, *J Endod* 26:175, 2000.

15. Bender IB, Landau MA, Fonsecca S, Trowbridge HO: The optimum placement-site of the electrode in electric pulp testing of the 12 anterior teeth, *J Am Dent Assoc* 118:305, 1989.

16. Bender IB, Seltzer S: Roentgenographic and direct observation of experimental lesions in bone. Part I, *J Am Dent Assoc* 62:152, 1961.

17. Bender IB, Seltzer S: Roentgenographic and direct observation of experimental lesions in bone. Part II, *J Am Dent Assoc* 62:708, 1961.

18. Berman LH: Dentinal sensation and hypersensitivity: a review of mechanisms and treatment alternatives, *J Periodontol* 56:216, 1984.

19. Berman LH, Kuttler S: Fracture necrosis: diagnosis, prognosis assessment, and treatment recommendations, *J Endod* 36:442, 2010.

20. Bierma MK, McClanahan S, Baisden MK, Bowles WR: Comparison of heat-testing methodology, *J Endod* 38:1106, 2012.

21. Bornstein MM, Lauber R, Sendi P, von Arx T: Comparison of periapical radiography and limited cone-beam computed tomography in mandibular molars for analysis of anatomical landmarks before apical surgery, *J Endod* 37:151, 2011.

22. Cameron CE: The cracked tooth syndrome: additional findings, *J Am Dent Assoc* 93:971, 1981.

23. Chen E, Abbottt PV: Evaluation of accuracy, reliability, and repeatability of five dental pulp tests, *J Endod* 37:1619, 2011.

24. Chiego DJ, Cox CF, Avery JK: H-3 HRP analysis of the nerve supply to primate teeth, *Dent Res* 59:736, 1980.

25. Cleveland JL, Gooch BF, Shearer BG, Lyerla RL: Risk and prevention of hepatitis C virus infection, *J Am Dent Assoc* 130:641, 1999.

26. Costa FF, Gaia BF, Umetsubo OS, Cavalcanti MGP: Detection of horizontal root fracture with small-volume cone-beam computed tomography in the presence and absence of intracanal metallic post, *J Endod* 37:1456, 2011.

27. Costa FF, Gaia BF, Umetsubo OS, et al: Use of large-volume cone-beam computed tomography in identification and localization of horizontal root fracture in the presence and absence of intracanal metallic post, *J Endod* 38:856, 2012.

28. Costa FWG, Rodrigues RR, Batista ACB: Multiple radiopaque mandibular lesions in a patient with Apert syndrome, *J Endod* 38:1639, 2012.

29. Cotton TP, Geisler TM, Holden DT, Schwartz SA, et al: Endodontic applications of cone-beam volumetric tomography, *J Endod* 33:1121, 2007.

30. Dankner E, Harari D, Rotstein I: Dens evaginatus of anterior teeth: literature review and radiographic survey of 15,000 teeth, *Oral Surg Oral Med Oral Pathol* 81:472, 1996.

31. Dastmalchi N, Jafarzadeh H, Moradi S: Comparison of the efficacy of a custom-made pulse oximeter probe with digital electric pulp tester, cold spray, and rubber cup for assessing pulp vitality, *J Endod* 38:1182, 2012.

32. Davido N, Rigolet A, Kerner S, et al: Case of Ewing's sarcoma misdiagnosed as a periapical lesion of maxillary incisor, *J Endod* 37:259, 2011.

33. Deepak BS, Subash TS, Narmatha VJ, et al: Imaging techniques in endodontics: an overview, *J Clin Imaging Sci* 2:13, 2012.

34. DeRossi SS, Glick M: Dental considerations for the patient with renal disease receiving hemodialysis, *J Am Dent Assoc* 127:211, 1996.

35. DeRossi SS, Glick M: Lupus erythematosus: considerations for dentistry, *J Am Dent Assoc* 129:330, 1998.

36. Dirks SJ, Paunovich ED, Terezhalmy GT, Chiodo LK: The patient with Parkinson's disease, *Quint Int* 34:379, 2003.

37. Durack C, Patel S: Cone beam computed tomography in endodontics, *Braz Dent J* 23:179, 2012.

38. Edlund M, Nair MK, Nair UP: Detection of vertical root fractures by using cone-beam computed tomography: a clinical study, *J Endod* 37:768, 2011.

39. Eikenerg S, Vandre R: Comparison of digital dental x-ray systems with self-developing film and manual processing for endodontic file length determination, *J Endod* 26:65, 2000.

40. Evans D, Reid J, Strang R, Stirrups D: A comparison of laser Doppler flowmetry with other methods of assessing the vitality of traumatized anterior teeth, *Endod Dent Traumatol* 15:284, 1999.

41. Farman AG, Levato CM, Scarfe WC: A primer on cone beam CT. *Inside Dentistry* 1:90, 2007.

42. Filippatos CG, Tsatsoulis IN, Floratos S, Kontakiotis EG: A variability of electric pulp response threshold in premolars: a clinical study, *J Endod* 38:144, 2012.

43. Fouad AF: Diabetes mellitus as a modulating factor of endodontic infections, *J Dent Educ* 67:459, 2003.

44. Friend LA, Glenwright HD: An experimental investigation into the localization of pain from the dental pulp, *Oral Surg Oral Med Oral Pathol* 25:765, 1968.

45. Fuss Z, Trope M: Root perforations: classification and treatment choices based on prognostic factors, *Endod Dent Traumatol* 12:255, 1996.

46. Fuss Z, Trowbridge H, Bender IB, Rickoff B, Sorin S: Assessment of reliability of electrical and thermal pulp testing agents, *J Endod* 12:301, 1986.

47. Ganz SD: Cone beam computed tomography-assisted treatment planning concepts, *Dent Clin North Am* 55:515, 2011.

48. Gillcrist JA: Hepatitis viruses A, B, C, D, E and G: implications for dental personnel, *J Am Dent Assoc* 130:509, 1999.

49. Goldman M, Pearson A, Darzenta N: Endodontic success: who is reading the radiograph? *Oral Surg Oral Med Oral Pathol* 33:432, 1972.

50. Goldman M, Pearson A, Darzenta N: Reliability of radiographic interpretations, *Oral Surg Oral Med Oral Pathol* 38:287, 1974.

51. Goodchild JH, Glick M: A different approach to medical risk assessment, *Endod Topics* 4:1, 2003.

52. Goon WW, Jacobsen PL: Prodromal odontalgia and multiple devitalized teeth caused by a herpes zoster infection of the trigeminal nerve: report of case, *J Am Dent Assoc* 116:500, 1988.

53. Gopikrishna V, Tinagupta K, Kandaswamy D: Comparison of electrical, thermal and pulse oximetry methods for assessing pulp vitality in recently traumatized teeth, *J Endod* 33:531, 2007.

54. Gopikrishna V, Tinagupta K, Kandaswamy D: Evaluation of efficacy of a new custom-made pulse oximeter dental probe in comparison with electrical and thermal tests for assessing pulp vitality, *J Endod* 33:411, 2007.

55. Harrison JW, Larson WJ: The epithelized oral sinus tract, *Oral Surg Oral Med Oral Pathol* 42:511, 1976.

56. Heling I, Rotstein I: A persistent oronasal sinus tract of endodontic origin, *J Endod* 15:132, 1989.

57. Herman WW, Konzelman JL, Prisant LM: New national guidelines on hypertension, *J Am Dent Assoc* 135:576, 2004.

58. Idiyatullin D, Corum C, Moeller S, et al: Dental magnetic resonance imaging: making the invisible visible, *J Endod* 37:745, 2011.

59. Imai K, Shimada Y, Sadr A, et al: Noninvasive cross-sectional visualization of enamel cracks by optical coherence tomography *in vitro*, *J Endod* 38:1269, 2012.

60. Ingolfsson AER, Tronstad L, Riva CE: Reliability of laser Doppler flowmetry in testing vitality of human teeth, *Endod Dent Traumatol* 10:185, 1994.

61. Ingram TA, Peters DD: Evaluation of the effects of carbon dioxide used as a pulp test. Part 2: in vivo effect on canine enamel and pulpal tissues, *J Endod* 9:296, 1983.

62. Jafarzadeh H, Abbott PV: Review of pulp sensibility tests. Part I: general information and thermal tests, *Int Endod J* 43:738, 2010.

63. Jafarzadeh H, Abbott PV: Review of pulp sensibility tests. Part II: electric pulp tests and test cavities, *Int Endod J* 43:945, 2010.

64. Johnson BR, Remeikis NA, Van Cura JE: Diagnosis and treatment of cutaneous facial sinus tracts of dental origin, *J Am Dent Assoc* 130:832, 1999.

65. Jones DM: Effect of the type carrier used on the results of dichlorodifluoromethane application to teeth, *J Endod* 25:692, 1999.

66. Jones VR, Rivera EM, Walton RE: Comparison of carbon dioxide versus refrigerant spray to determine pulpal responsiveness, *J Endod* 28:531, 2002.

67. Kaffe I, Gratt BM: Variations in the radiographic interpretation of the periapical dental region, *J Endod* 14:330, 1988.

68. Kahan RS, Gulabivala K, Snook M, Setchell DJ: Evaluation of a pulse oximeter and customized probe for pulp vitality testing, *J Endod* 22:105, 1996.

69. Karayilmaz H, Kirzioglu Z: Comparison of the reliability of laser Doppler flowmetry, pulse oximetry and electric pulp tester in assessing the pulp vitality of human teeth, *J Oral Rehabil* 38:340, 2011.

70. Kataoka SH, Setzer FC, Gondim-Junior E, et al: Pulp vitality in patients with intraoral and oropharyngeal malignant tumors undergoing radiation therapy assessed by pulse oximetry, *J Endod* 37:1197, 2011.

71. Katz J, Chaushu G, Rotstein I: Stafne's bone cavity in the anterior mandible: a possible diagnosis challenge, *J Endod* 27:304, 2001.

72. Kawai K, Masaka N: Vertical root fracture treated by bonding fragments and rotational replantation, *Dent Traumatol* 18:42, 2002.

73. Khocht A, Janal M, Harasty L, Chang K: Comparison of direct digital and conventional intraoral radiographs in detecting alveolar bone loss, *J Am Dent Assoc* 134:1468, 2003.

74. Koivisto T, Bowles WR, Rohrer M: Frequency and distribution of radiolucent jaw lesions: a retrospective analysis of 9,723 cases, *J Endod* 38:729, 2012.

75. Kusgoz A, Yildirim T, Kayipmaz S, Saricaoglu S: Nonsurgical endodontic treatment of type III dens invaginatus in maxillary canine: an 18-month follow up, *Oral Surg Oral Med Oral Pathol Oral Radiol Endodon* 107:e103, 2009.

76. Lalla RV, D'Ambrosio JA: Dental management considerations for the patient with diabetes mellitus, *J Am Dent Assoc* 132:1425, 2001.

77. Laskin DM: Anatomic considerations in diagnosis and treatment of odontogenic infections, *J Am Dent Assoc* 69:308, 1964.

78. Liang YH, Li G, Wesselink PR, Wu MK: Endodontic outcome predictors identified with periapical radiographs and cone-beam computed tomography scans, *J Endod* 37:326, 2011.

79. Lin J, Chandler NP: Electric pulp testing: a review, *Int Endod J* 41:365, 2008.

80. Little JW, Falace DA, Miller CS, Rhodus NL: *Dental management of the medically compromised patient*, ed 8, St. Louis, 2013, Elsevier Mosby.

81. Lofthag-Hansen S, Huumonen S, Gröndahl K, Gröndahl HG: Limited cone-beam CT and intraoral radiography for the diagnosis of periapical pathology, *Oral Surg Oral Med Oral Pathol Oral Radiol Endod* 103:114, 2007.

82. Marder MZ: The standard of care for oral diagnosis as it relates to oral cancer, *Compend Contin Educ Dent* 19:569, 1998.

83. Mattson JS, Cerutis DR: Diabetes mellitus: a review of the literature and dental implications, *Comp Cont Educ Dent* 22:757, 2001.

84. Mesaros S, Trope M, Maixner W, Burkes EJ: Comparison of two laser Doppler systems on the measurement of blood flow of premolar teeth under different pulpal conditions, *Int Endod J* 30:167, 1997.

85. Metska ME, Aartman IHA, Wesselink PR, Özor AR: Detection of vertical root fractures *in vivo* in endodontically treated teeth by cone-beam computed tomography scans, *J Endod* 38:1344, 2012.

86. Michaelson RE, Seidberg BH, Guttuso J: An in vivo evaluation of interface media used with the electric pulp tester, *J Am Dent Assoc* 91:118, 1975.

87. Miles DA, VanDis ML: Advances in dental imaging, *Dent Clin North Am* 37:531, 1993.

88. Miller CS, Little JW, Falace DA: Supplemental corticosteroids for dental patients with adrenal insufficiency: reconsideration of the problem, *J Am Dent Assoc* 132:1570, 2001.

89. Morsani JM, Aminoshariae A, Han YW: Genetic predisposition to persistent apical periodontitis, *J Endod* 37:455, 2011.

90. Mozzo P, Proccacci A, et al: A new volumetric CT machine for dental imaging based on the cone-beam technique: preliminary results, *Eur Radiol* 8:1558, 1998.

91. Nair M, Pettigrew J, Mancuso A: Intracranial aneurysm as an incidental finding, *Dentomaxillofac Radiol* 36:107, 2007.

92. Nakata K, Naitob M, Izumi M, et al: Effectiveness of dental computed tomography in diagnostic imaging of periradicular lesion of each root of a multirooted tooth: a case report, *J Endod* 32:583, 2007.

93. Nalliab RP, Allareddy V, Elangovan S, et al: Hospital emergency department visits attributed to pulpal and periapical disease in the United States in 2006, *J Endod* 37:6, 2011.

94. Özer SY: Detection of vertical root fractures by using cone beam computed tomography with variable voxel sizes in an *in vitro* model, *J Endod* 37:75: 2011.

95. Pantera EA, Anderson RW, Pantera CT: Use of dental instruments for bridging during electric pulp testing, *J Endod* 18:37, 1992.

96. Pantera EA, Anderson RW, Pantera CT: Reliability of electric pulp testing after pulpal testing with dichlorodifluoromethane, *J Endod* 19:312, 1993.

97. Paurazas SM, Geist JR, Pink FE: Comparison of diagnostic accuracy of digital imaging using CCD and CMOS-APS sensors with E-speed film in the detection of periapical bony lesions, *Oral Surg Oral Med Oral Pathol Oral Radiology Endodon* 44:249, 2000.

98. Peters DD, Baumgartner JC, Lorton L: Adult pulpal diagnosis. 1. Evaluation of the positive and negative responses to cold and electric pulp tests, *J Endod* 20:506, 1994.

99. Petersson K, Soderstrom C, Kiani-Anaraki M, Levy G: Evaluation of the ability of thermal and electric tests to register pulp vitality, *Endod Dent Traumatol* 15:127, 1999.

100. Pinto A, Glick M: Management of patients with thyroid disease: oral health considerations, *J Am Dent Assoc* 133:849, 2002.

101. Pitts DL, Natkin E: Diagnosis and treatment of vertical root fractures, *J Endod* 9:338, 1983.

102. Poeschl PW, Crepaz V, Russmueller G, et al: Endodontic pathogens causing deep neck space infections: clinical impact of different sampling techniques and antibiotic susceptibility, *J Endod* 37:1201, 2011.

103. Rees JS, Addy M: A cross-sectional study of dentine hypersensitivity, *J Clin Periodontol* 29:997, 2002.

104. Rickoff B, Trowbridge H, Baker J, Fuss Z, et al: Effects of thermal vitality tests on human dental pulp, *J Endod* 14:482, 1988.

105. Riley CK, Terezhalmy GT: The patient with hypertension, *Quint Int* 32:671, 2001.

106. Robb RA, Sinak LJ, Hoffman EA, et al: Dynamic volume imaging of moving organs, *J Med Syst* 6:539, 1982.

107. Rodrigues CD, Villar-Neto MJC, Sobral APV, et al: Lymphangioma mimicking apical periodontitis, *J Endod* 37:91, 2011.

108. Rosen H: Cracked tooth syndrome, *J Prosthet Dent* 47:36, 1982.

109. Rotstein I, Engel G: Conservative management of a combined endodontic-orthodontic lesion, *Endod Dent Traumatol* 7:266, 1991.

110. Rotstein I, Moshonov J, Cohenca N: Endodontic therapy for a fused mandibular molar, *Endod Dent Traumatol* 13:149, 1997.

111. Rotstein I, Simon HS: Diagnosis, prognosis and decision-making in the treatment of combined periodontal-endodontic lesions, *Periodontol 2000* 34:165, 2004.

112. Rotstein I, Simon HS: The endo-perio lesion: a critical appraisal of the disease condition, *Endodon Topics* 13:34, 2006.

113. Rotstein I, Stabholz A, Heling I, Friedman S: Clinical considerations in the treatment of dens invaginatus, *Endod Dent Traumatol* 3:249, 1987.

114. Roykens H, Van Maele G, DeMoor R, Martens L: Reliability of laser Doppler flowmetry in a 2-probe assessment of pulpal blood flow, *Oral Surg Oral Med Oral Pathol Oral Radiol Endodon* 87:742, 1999.

115. Rud J, Omnell KA: Root fractures due to corrosion: diagnostic aspects, *Scand J Dent Res* 78:397, 1970.

116. Rutsatz C, Baumhardt SG, Feldens CA, et al: Response of pulp sensibility test is strongly influenced by periodontal attachment loss and gingival recession, *J Endod* 38:580, 2012.

117. Sasano T, Nakajima I, Shohi N, et al: Possible application of transmitted laser light for the assessment of human pulpal vitality, *Endod Dent Traumatol* 13:88, 1997.

118. Schnettler JM, Wallace JA: Pulse oximetry as a diagnostic tool of pulp vitality, *J Endod* 17:488, 1991.

119. Schwartz RS: Mineral trioxide aggregate: a new material for endodontics, *J Am Dent Assoc* 130:967, 1999.

120. Selden HS: Repair of incomplete vertical root fractures in endodontically treated teeth: in vivo trials, *J Endod* 22:426, 1996.

121. Seltzer S, Bender IB, Nazimov H: Differential diagnosis of pulp conditions, *Oral Surg Oral Med Oral Pathol* 19:383, 1965.

122. Seltzer S, Bender IB, Ziontz M: The dynamics of pulp inflammation: correlations between diagnostic data and actual histologic findings in the pulp. Part I, *Oral Surg Oral Med Oral Pathol* 16:846, 1963.

123. Seltzer S, Bender IB, Ziontz M: The dynamics of pulp inflammation: correlations between diagnostic data and actual histologic findings in the pulp. Part II, *Oral Surg Oral Med Oral Pathol* 16:969, 1963.

124. Seo DG, Yi YA, Shin AJ, Park JW: Analysis of factors associated with cracked teeth, *J Endod* 38:288, 2012.

125. Setzer FC, Kataoka SH, Natrielli F, et al: Clinical diagnosis of pulp inflammation based on pulp oxygenation rates measured by pulse oximetry, *J Endod* 38:880, 2012.

126. Simon JHS, Dogan H, Ceresa LM, Silver GK: The radicular groove: it's potential clinical significance, *J Endod* 26:295, 2000.

127. Simon JHS, Lies J: Silent trauma, *Endod Dent Traumatol* 15:145, 1999.

128. Shemesh H, Cristescu RC, Wesselink PR, Wu MK: The use of cone-beam computed tomography and digital periapical radiographs to diagnose root perforations, *J Endod* 37:513, 2011.

129. Steinbacher DM, Glick M: The dental patient with asthma: an update and oral health considerations, *J Am Dent Assoc* 132:1229, 2001.

130. Stroblitt H, Gojer G, Norer B, Emshoff R: Assessing revascularization of avulsed permanent maxillary incisors by laser Doppler flowmetry, *J Am Dent Assoc* 134:1597, 2003.

131. Suebnukarn S, Rhienmora P, Haddawy P: The use of cone-beam computed tomography and virtual reality simulation for pre-surgical practice in endodontic microsurgery, *Int Endod J* 45:627, 2012.

132. Sugaya T, Kawanami M, Noguchi H, et al: Periodontal healing after bonding treatment of vertical root fracture, *Dent Traumatol* 17:174, 2001.

133. Tatlidil R, Gözübüyük MM: Mucinous adenocarcinoma of lung presenting as oral metastases: a case report and literature review, *J Endod* 37:110, 2011.

134. Tewary S, Luzzo J, Hartwell G: Endodontic radiography: who is reading the digital radiograph, *J Endod* 37:919, 2011.

135. Treister N, Glick M: Rheumatoid arthritis: a review and suggested dental care considerations, *J Am Dent Assoc* 130:689, 1999.

136. Van Hassel HJ, Harrington GW: Localization of pulpal sensation, *Oral Surg Oral Med Oral Pathol* 28:753, 1969.

137. Velvart P, Hecker H, Tillinger G: Detection of the apical lesion and the mandibular canal in conventional radiography and computed tomography, *Oral Surg Oral Med Oral Pathol Oral Radiol Endodon* 92:682, 2001.

138. Vogel J, Stubinger S, Kaufmann M: Dental injuries resulting from tracheal intubation: a retrospective study, *Dent Traumatol* 25:73, 2009.

139. Von Böhl M, Ren Y, Fudalej PS, Kuijpers-Jagtman AM: Pulpal reactions to orthodontic force application in humans: a systematic review, *J Endod* 38:1463, 2012.

140. Wallace JA, Schnettler JM: Pulse oximetry as a diagnostic tool of pulpal vitality, *J Endod* 17:488, 1993.

141. Weisleder R, Yamauchi S, Caplan DJ, et al: The validity of pulp testing: a clinical study, *J Am Dent Assoc* 140:1013, 2009.

142. Zou X, Liu D, Yue L, Wu M: The ability of cone-beam computerized tomography to detect vertical root fractures in endodontically treated and nonendodontically treated teeth: a report of 3 cases, *Oral Surg Oral Med Oral Pathol Oral Radiol Endodon* 111:797, 2011.

CHAPTER 2

Radiographic Interpretation

MADHU K. NAIR | MARTIN D. LEVIN | UMADEVI P. NAIR

CHAPTER OUTLINE

RADIOGRAPHIC INTERPRETATION

Interpretation of information captured by radiographic imaging modalities is central to the diagnostic process. It is very important to capture a diagnostically useful image using appropriate exposure parameters and view it with interactive manipulation of brightness and contrast or window/level (for cone beam computed tomography [CBCT] studies) in an optimal environment to adequately evaluate anatomy and diagnose pathoses. Accurate interpretation of root and canal morphology, determination of radiographic canal length, diagnosis of radicular and periradicular disease (Fig. 2-1), and postsurgical and long-term evaluation of the outcome of endodontic treatment are some of the routine diagnostic imaging tasks in endodontics.[181] Systematic and methodical interpretation processes must be followed for all images. Recognition of anatomy, anatomic variants, and pathologic conditions or deviations from normal is important. Various imaging modalities exist in radiology. Some use ionizing radiation, whereas others use ultrasonic waves (ultrasonography, or US) or powerful external magnetic fields (magnetic resonance imaging, or MRI). Interventional and noninterventional imaging modalities are also available. Imaging modalities using ionizing radiation are most frequently used in endodontic diagnoses. The different image capture modalities include conventional intraoral film and the more modern digital receptors.

Imaging Modalities

Digital radiography using electronic sensors or photostimulable phosphor (PSP) plates is widely used in endodontics. The advantages of using digital sensors over film are many. Significant advantages include noteworthy dose reduction (especially in comparison with D-speed film used with round collimation); almost instantaneous generation of high-resolution digital images with resolution approaching or equaling that of film for specific diagnostic tasks; the ability to postprocess images for enhanced diagnostic outcomes; elimination of variables associated with wet processing of conventional film; ease of transmission and of archiving and retrieving images from databases or picture archiving and communication systems (PACS); facilitation of use of an all-electronic patient record[123,188]; reduced exposure of personnel to hazardous chemicals; and reduced environmental impact.

Digital imaging modalities in endodontics use different image capture technologies, which include a charge-coupled device (CCD), a complementary metal oxide semiconductor (CMOS), or a PSP (also sometimes referred to as an indirect acquisition modality). Film images also can be digitized using a flatbed scanner or CCD/CMOS-based cameras mounted on a camera stand, with images captured using a frame grabber from a mounted, lighted platform.

CCD-based solid-state sensors were used extensively in endodontics initially. However, the earlier generation sensors had

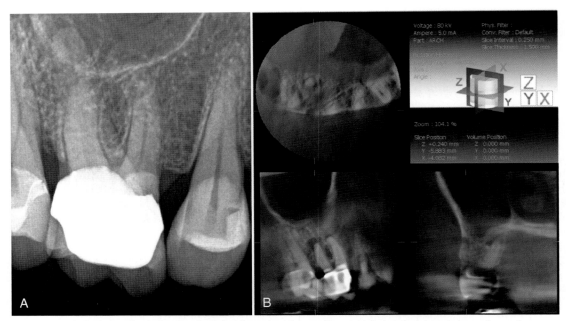

FIG. 2-1 A, A well-angulated periapical radiograph of the maxillary right first molar taken during a diagnostic appointment for endodontic evaluation of the maxillary right quadrant. At first glance, there is little radiographic evidence of significant or periradicular change. **B,** Contemporaneous CBCT image of same tooth gives an entirely different perspective; periapical changes are visible on all three roots in all three anatomic planes of section. (*B taken* with J. Morita Veraviewepocs 3D [J. Morita, Osaka, Japan]).

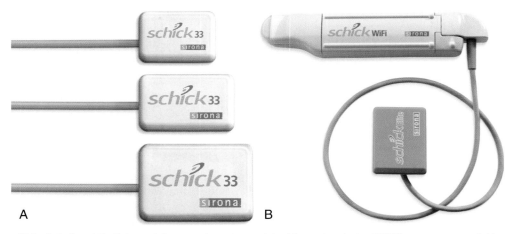

FIG. 2-2 A and B, High-resolution complementary metal oxide semiconductor (CMOS) sensors are available from many manufacturers. Note that Figure B shows wireless CMOS sensors transmit images to the chairside workstation by 2.4 GHz radio frequency. (Courtesy SIRONA DENTAL SYSTEMS, Long Island City, NY.)

a smaller active area and limited x-ray absorption and conversion efficiency, in addition to being bulky. Sensors use an array of radiation-sensitive elements that generate electric charges proportionate to the amount of incident radiation. To reduce the amount of radiation needed to capture an image, a light-sensitive array was developed that uses a scintillation layer laid on top of the CCD chip or added with a fiberoptic coupling. The generated charge is read out in a "bucket brigade" fashion and transferred to an analog-to-digital converter in the frame grabber assembly of the workstation. The digital information is processed, and an image is formed. CMOS-based sensors, on the other hand, have an active transistor at each element location. The area available for signal generation is relatively less,

and there is a fixed pattern noise. These sensors are less expensive to manufacture and have been shown to be equally useful for specific diagnostic tasks.[4] Unlike the CCD, the CMOS chip requires very little electrical energy; therefore, no external power supply is needed to support USB utilization, and wireless applications are feasible. Wireless sensors are available (Fig. 2-2). However, radiofrequency interference may be a problem with these sensors. The current WiFi sensor is less bulky and has a wire attached to it that enables transmission via 802.11 b/g standard. It uses a lithium-ion polymer battery that can last for approximately 100 exposures.

Yet another type of sensor uses PSPs for image capture. PSP technology is also referred to as *computed radiography* (CR).[94,169]

Unlike the CCD and CMOS sensors, PSP sensors are wireless. The phosphor is activated by a process called *doping*, which enables charges to be generated and stored when exposed to radiation. A latent image is stored in the sensor, and a PSP reader with a laser beam of specific wavelength is used to read out the image. Previously captured images can be erased by exposing the PSP sensor to white light. PSP plates can be damaged easily by scratching, but they are not as expensive as CCD or CMOS sensors. Incomplete erasure of the image can lead to ghost images when the plate is reused, and delayed processing can result in a decrease in image clarity.[2] PSP-based sensors are used in high-volume scenarios. Spatial resolution is lower with this type of sensor, but it has a wider dynamic range. These sensors can tolerate a wider range of exposures to produce a diagnostically useful image.

Radiation dose continues to be a concern with all imaging studies. The lowest possible dose must be delivered for each study. Most dental offices would not be in compliance with the latest recommendations of the National Council for Radiation Protection (NCRP) on reducing the radiation dose from intraoral radiographs (Box 2-1). Two terms have been specifically defined in the NCRP's report. The terms *shall* and *shall not* indicate that adherence to the recommendation would be in compliance with the standards of radiation safety. The terms *should* and *should not* indicate prudent practice and acknowledge that exceptions may be made in certain circumstances. In addition, the report establishes nine new recommendations for image processing of conventional film.

A strong argument can be made for clinicians to switch to a direct digital radiography (DDR) system to avoid all the drastic changes necessary to ensure compliance with the new recommendations. Even though restriction of an intraoral dental x-ray beam is mandated by federal law to a circle no greater than 7 cm, rectangular collimation has been proven to significantly reduce the radiation dose to the patient.

The American Dental Association (ADA) Council on Scientific Affairs has made the following statement:

> Tissue area exposed to the primary x-ray beam should not exceed the minimum coverage consistent with meeting diagnostic requirements and clinical feasibility. For periapical and bitewing radiography, rectangular collimation should be used whenever possible because a round field beam used with a rectangular image receptor produces ... unnecessary radiation exposure to the patient.[1]

Image Characteristics and Processing

Spatial resolution achieved with current generation digital sensors is equally good or better than that of conventional intraoral radiographic film. Intraoral film has a resolution of 16 line pairs per millimeter (lp/mm) as measured using a resolution tool, and it increases to 20 to 24 lp/mm with magnification. *Spatial resolution* is defined as the ability to display two objects that are close to each other as two separate entities. *Contrast resolution* is defined as the ability to differentiate between areas on the image based on density. Most diagnostic tasks in endodontics require a high-contrast resolution.[121] However, image quality is not just a function of spatial resolution. The choice of appropriate exposure parameters, sensor properties, the image processing used, and viewing conditions and modalities directly affect diagnostic accuracy.

Postprocessing of images may be carried out to alter image characteristics. Radiographs need not be reexposed if image quality is not adequate. Diagnostic information can be teased out of the image if appropriate image processing is used. However, the original image must be acquired with optimal exposure parameters to accomplish meaningful image processing.[178] Suboptimally exposed images cannot be processed to yield diagnostic information, which may lead to a reduction in the diagnostic accuracy of the image. Image enhancement must be task specific. Signal-to-noise ratio (SNR) must be optimized to extract necessary information from the image. The bit-depth of images also has a direct relationship to image quality. It indicates the number of shades of gray that the sensor can capture for display. For example, an 8-bit image can depict 256 shades of gray. Most sensors are 12 or 14 bits in depth, capturing 4,096 or 65,536 shades of gray, respectively. If the sensor captures several thousand shades of gray, the image can be manipulated through enhancement techniques to display those shades of gray that best depict the anatomy of interest. The human visual system is limited in the number of shades of gray that can be read at any point in time. Therefore, image

---

BOX 2-1

Recommendations of the National Council on Radiation Protection

1. Dentists must examine their patients before ordering or prescribing x-ray images (this is not a new guideline).
2. The use of leaded aprons on patients shall not be required if all other recommendations in this report are rigorously followed (read full Report #145).
3. Thyroid shielding shall be used for children and should be provided for adults when it will not interfere with the examination (e.g., panoramic imaging).
4. Rectangular collimation of the beam, which has been recommended for years, shall be routinely used for periapical radiographs. Each dimension of the beam, measured in the plane of the image receptor, should not exceed the dimension of the image receptor by more than 2% of the source-to-image receptor distance. Similar collimation should be used, when feasible, for bitewing radiographs.
5. Image receptors of speeds slower than ANSI speed Group E films shall not be used for intraoral radiography. Faster receptors should be evaluated and adopted if found acceptable. For extraoral radiography, high-speed (400 or greater) rare earth screen-film systems or digital-imaging systems of equivalent or greater speed shall be used.
6. Dental radiographic films shall be developed according to the film manufacturer's instructions using the time-temperature method. In practical application, this means that sight development (reading wet x-ray films at the time of the procedure) shall not be used.
7. Radiographic techniques for digital imaging shall be adjusted for the minimum patient dose required to produce a signal-to-noise ratio sufficient to provide image quality to meet the purpose of the examination.
8. Clinicians designing new offices or remodeling existing locations will need shield protection to be provided by a qualified expert.

Modified from the National Council on Radiation Protection and Measurements: *Radiation protection in dentistry,* Report #145, Bethesda, Md, 2003. Available at: www.ncrppublications.org/Reports/145.

enhancement is a must for all images, so as to delineate signals of interest through manipulation of the grayscale. Most endodontic tasks require a high contrast and thus a shorter grayscale.

Digital radiographs can be saved in different file formats. Several file formats are available: DICOM (*Digital Imaging and Communications in Medicine*); tiff (*tagged image file format*); jpeg (*joint photographic experts group*); gif (*graphics interchange format*); BMP (*Windows' bitmap image file*); PNG (*portable network graphics*); and so on. There also are several proprietary formats. "Lossy" and "lossless" compression schemes can be used for saving images, although lossless compression is preferred.[58]

Digital Imaging and Communications in Medicine (DICOM)

DICOM is a set of international standards established in 1985 by the American College of Radiology (ACR) and the National Electrical Manufacturers Association (NEMA)[46,175] to address the issue of vendor-independent data formats and data transfers for digital medical images.[77] The ADA has promoted the interoperability of dental images through the efforts of its Working Group 12.1.26. DICOM serves as a standard for the transferal of radiologic images and other medical information between computers, allowing digital communication between systems from various manufacturers and across different platforms (e.g., Apple iOS or Microsoft Windows).[78] The DICOM standard provides for several hundred attribute fields in the record header, which contains information about the image (e.g., pixel density, dimensions, and number of bits per pixel), in addition to relevant patient data and medical information. Although earlier versions did not specify the exact order and definition of the header fields, each vendor is required to publish a DICOM conformance statement, which gives the location of pertinent data. The big hurdle is to support medical and dental consultations between two or more locations with different imaging software. With DICOM in place, dental clinicians can change vendors and maintain database interoperability. Most software vendors are striving to achieve full DICOM compliance, and some have achieved at least partial compliance. However, proprietary DICOM images are still produced in different systems, with the capability to export in universal DICOM format as needed. Diagnostic images are best saved as DICOM files to preserve image fidelity or as tiff files with no compression. Diagnosis suffers when images undergo lossy compression.[50,103,180]

Based on the DICOM model, the ADA Standards Committee on Dental Informatics has identified four basic goals for electronic standards in dentistry: (1) interoperability, (2) electronic health record design, (3) clinical workstation architecture, and (4) electronic dissemination of dental information.[7] The dental profession must continue to promote DICOM compatibility so that proprietary software and file types do not hinder communication and risk making data obsolete.

DIAGNOSTIC TASKS IN ENDODONTICS

Working Length Determination

Digital imaging systems perform as well as intraoral film or better for working length determination.[121] No significant difference was noted between measurements made on digital

images.[99] Older studies compared the early generation digital sensors with limited bit-depth to D-speed films, and the films showed better performance. It is important to analyze the type of sensor used, software, processing, video card and monitor, and viewing conditions to determine whether the sensor is good for a specific diagnostic task. Calibration improves the diagnostic accuracy.[108] Likewise, the use of optimal processing parameters improves image quality to the extent of making a significant difference in the diagnostic outcome. For instance, density plot analysis was shown to help with endodontic file measurements.[146] The major advantage of direct digital radiography (CCD, CMOS) is that the dose is significantly less compared with that required for film. The use of DDR, therefore, is justified when its performance is comparable to that of film with no statistically significant differences.[101]

The three types of measurement generally available with digital imaging software are (1) linear measurement, the distance between two points in millimeters (Fig. 2-3); (2) angle measurement, the angle between two lines; and (3) area measurement, the area of the image or a segment of the image. Because magnification and distortion errors play a significant role in the accuracy of two-dimensional (2D) radiographic measurement, both film and digital systems are subject to parallax error. However, a study that compared endodontic file length images of human teeth taken with a custom jig suggested that "measurement error was significantly less for the digital images than the film-based images."[49] This was true even though, as the authors pointed out, the measurement differences may not have been clinically significant. Sophisticated calibration algorithms are under development, and accurate measurement of parallel images should be more feasible in the future.[30]

Diagnosis and Healing

Image enhancement of direct and indirect digital radiographs based on the diagnostic task at hand has been shown to increase diagnostic accuracy compared to film-based images, which cannot be enhanced.[2,190] Posttreatment endodontic evaluation of healing of apical radiolucent areas is a challenge. Early changes indicating healing and bone fill are difficult to detect on conventional or digital radiographs. However, bone fill can be detected using more sensitive techniques, such as digital subtraction radiography, in which two images, separated in time but acquired with the exact same projection geometry and technique factors, can be subtracted from one another to tease out subtle changes in the periodontium and surrounding bone. Subtraction techniques are difficult to carry out in routine clinical practice because they are technique sensitive and can yield incorrect information if not performed accurately. Several studies have shown the usefulness of subtraction radiography using digital sensors.[117,129,194]

Three-Dimensional Imaging

Computed tomography (CT) was introduced by Sir Godfrey Hounsfield in the 1970s. *Tomography* refers to "slice imaging," in which thin slices of the anatomy of interest are captured and synthesized manually or using an algorithm. CT makes use of automated reconstruction. Medical-grade CT used a translate-rotate image acquisition scheme as the technology developed, but the modality always resulted in higher radiation dose delivery because of redundancy of data capture, in addition to longer scan times with the potential for motion artifact.

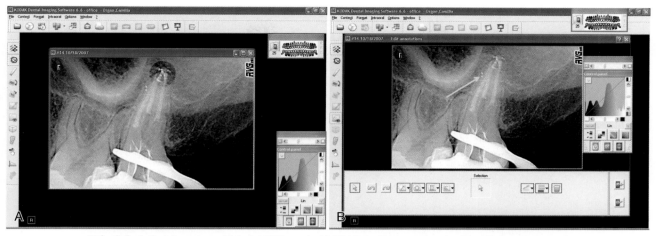

FIG. 2-3 **A,** Certain regions of interest (ROI) can be highlighted with a preset contrast tool that can be moved around the image. **B,** Preprogramed filters that enhance sharpness and contrast can be selected to optimize the image acquired. (Courtesy Carestream Dental LLC, Atlanta, GA.)

Multiple detectors and x-ray sources were used in later generations of CT units to reduce scanning times. The increased radiation dose, artifacts from metallic restorations, cost of scanning, long acquisition times, and lack of adequate dental-specific software have been drawbacks limiting the use of the technology in dentistry until recently. The advent of cone beam volumetric computed tomography (CBVCT) introduced a faster, low-dose, low-cost, high-contrast imaging modality that could capture information in three dimensions using a limited field of view.

CBVCT, or cone beam CT (CBCT), is a relatively new diagnostic imaging modality that has been recently added to the endodontic imaging armamentarium. This modality uses a cone beam instead of a fan-shaped beam in multidetector computed tomography (MDCT), acquiring images of the entire volume as it rotates around the anatomy of interest. Compared with MDCT images, CBCT offers relatively high-resolution, isotropic images, allowing effective evaluation of root canal morphology and other subtle changes within the root canal system. Even though the resolution is not as high as that of conventional radiographs (18 microns), the availability of three-dimensional (3D) information, the relatively higher resolution, and a significantly lower dose compared to MDCT make CBCT the imaging modality of choice in challenging situations demanding localization and characterization of root canals.

The adoption of advanced imaging modalities such as CBCT for select diagnostic tasks is becoming popular with clinicians performing endodontic procedures. Two-dimensional grayscale images, whether conventional film based or digital, cannot accurately depict the full 3D representation of the teeth and supporting structures. In fact, traditional images are poor representations of even the pulpal anatomy. They grossly underestimate canal structure and often cannot accurately visualize periapical changes, especially where there is thick cortical bone, as in the presence of anatomic obstructions (Fig. 2-4, *A*). CBCT, however, allows the clinician to view the tooth and pulpal structures in thin slices in all three anatomic planes: axial, sagittal, and coronal. This capability alone allows visualization of periapical pathoses and root morphology previously impossible to assess (Fig. 2-4, *B* and *C*). Several tools available in CBCT, such as the ability to change the vertical or horizontal angulation of the image in real time, in addition to thin-slice, grayscale data of varying thicknesses, will never be available for conventional or even digital radiography. Furthermore, the use of CBCT data to view the region of interest in three anatomic planes of section at very low x-ray doses has never been as easy or accessible as it is today.

Microcomputed tomography (micro-CT) has also been evaluated in endodontic imaging.[87,144,145] Comparison of the effects of biomechanical preparation on the canal volume of reconstructed root canals in extracted teeth using micro-CT data was shown to assist with characterization of morphologic changes associated with these techniques.[145] Peters et al.[144] used micro-CT to evaluate the relative performance of nickel-titanium (Ni-Ti) instruments after the shaping of root canals of varying preoperative canal geometry (for examples, see Chapter 6). A study to examine the potential and accuracy of micro-CT for imaging of filled root canals showed it to be a highly accurate and nondestructive method for the evaluation of root canal fillings and its constituents. The qualitative and quantitative correlations between histologic and micro-CT examination of root canal fillings were high.[87] However, it is important to note that micro-CT remains a research tool and cannot be used for human imaging in vivo.

This chapter discusses the principles, applications, imaging attributes, image artifacts, and potential liability of adopting CBCT technology for endodontic procedures. Given this information, the student of endodontics will begin to realize the significant advantages, limitations, and diagnostic and treatment planning capabilities of this radiographic imaging modality.

PRINCIPLES OF CONE BEAM COMPUTED TOMOGRAPHY

Three important parameters of cone beam imaging are described in the following sections:
- Voxel size
- Field of view (FOV)
- Slice thickness/measurement accuracy

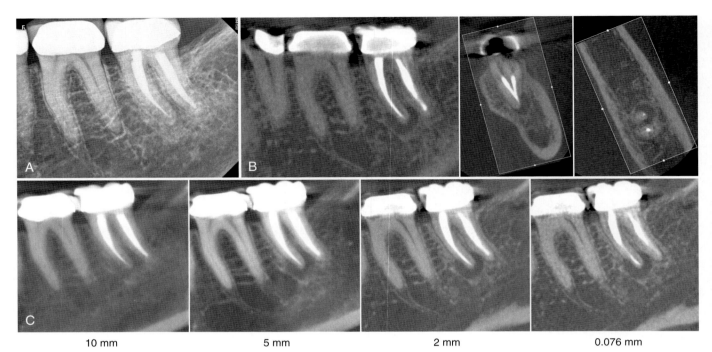

10 mm   5 mm   2 mm   0.076 mm

FIG. 2-4 This case demonstrates the difficulty in assessing lesions in the mandibular posterior region when there is a dense cortex. This well-angulated periapical radiograph (A) does not clearly show any radiolucencies associated with the mandibular left second molar, for which the patient has presented for evaluation and possible retreatment. The CBCT corrected sagittal, coronal, and axial reconstructed multiplanar views (B, *left to right,* sagittal, coronal, and axial views) show previous endodontic treatment, with a 6-mm diameter radiolucency with a well-defined, mildly corticated border, centered over a point on the buccal aspect of the root, 2 mm coronal to the apex; these are features consistent with an apical rarefying osteitis. The ray sum images of the sagittal view, where the image is "thinned" by decreasing the number of adjacent voxels using postprocessing software, simulates a curvilinear projection, showing diminishing superimposition (C, *left to right,* image layer of 10 mm, 5 mm, 2 mm, and 0.076 mm). (Data acquired and reformatted at 0.076 mm voxel size using a CS 9000 3D unit [Carestream Dental, Atlanta, Ga].)

Voxels and Voxel Sizes

Voxels are cuboidal elements that constitute a 3D volume, unlike pixels, which are 2D. Data are acquired and represented in three dimensions using voxels. Unlike with medical computed tomography (MDCT), cone beam units acquire x-ray information using low kV and low mA exposure parameters in a single pass from 180 to 360 degrees of rotation around the anatomy of interest. Medical scanners use higher voltages of 120 kV or more and current of about 400 mA. Several units used in maxillofacial imaging use significantly lower exposure parameters (Figs. 2-5 to 2-7). The x-ray dose for all cone beam units is significantly lower than the dose received from a MDCT unit. Image attributes are also different in that volumes are reconstructed from isotropic voxels; that is, the images are constructed from volumetric detector elements that are cubical in nature and have the same dimensions of length, width, and depth. These voxel sizes can be as small as 0.076 to 0.6 mm.[118] By comparison, MDCT slice data are 0.5 mm to 1 cm thick. Fig. 2-8 illustrates the difference between a pixel and a voxel, the difference between an anisotropic pixel of MDCT and an isotropic pixel (voxel) of CBCT, and how the pixel data are acquired from both modalities.

The patient is positioned on a gantry in an MDCT unit, and images are acquired multiple slices at a time, which

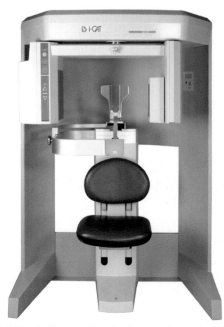

FIG. 2-5 i-CAT unit. (Courtesy Imaging Sciences International, Hatfield, Pa.)

the patient. A typical CBCT examination would expose the patient to only about 20 to 500 μSv in a single study, whereas a typical medical examination of the head would approach 2100 μSv[2] because the image data are gathered one section at a time. Therefore, soft tissue imaging is better with MDCT because the signal intensity is higher. However, this is not a requirement for dental diagnostic tasks because hard tissue visualization is more important. Consequently, CBCT data have a much higher resolution than MDCT data for hard tissue visualization because of the smaller voxel sizes that medical-grade scanners are incapable of achieving at a significantly lower dose. Increased noise is observed as a result of volumetric acquisition, but the SNR is maintained at a desirable level that facilitates adequate diagnosis based on hard tissue signals.

Field of View

The field of view (FOV) (Figs. 2-9 and 2-10) ranges from as small as a portion of a dental arch to an area as large as the entire head. The selection of the FOV depends on several factors. Among the most important are the following:
- Diagnostic task
- Type of patient
- Spatial resolution requirements

Diagnostic Task

The diagnostic task is the single most important determinant of the FOV in any imaging study. Based on the outcome of the clinical assessment, history, and evaluation of previous and other available imaging studies, a segment of the jaw or a larger area may need to be imaged using an appropriate FOV. If systemic conditions or generalized disorders are suspected, a larger FOV is sometimes required. For most endodontic purposes, a limited FOV can be used, if no signs or symptoms of systemic conditions are reported or noted. Under no circumstances should a screening study be done using a large FOV in the absence of signs and symptoms justifying the procedure. Several multifunctional cone beam units are available that allow the clinician to acquire several image types. Image quality has a direct impact on the diagnostic outcome; therefore, the choice of an FOV should be made carefully. Figure 2-11 illustrates the advantages of using multiple image types for an endodontic case.

Additional benefits of CBCT imaging software include allowing the clinician to format the volume to generate an image that looks like a panoramic radiograph. Conventional panoramic machines, although not commonly used by endodontists, use the focal trough, or zone of sharpness, to position patients so as to minimize distortion along multiple axes. All inherent problems associated with panoramic imaging, including distortion, magnification, blurring, ghost shadows, and other artifacts, can be expected on the resulting image if patient positioning is not accurate. With CBCT, such artifacts are not generated, resulting in a distortion-free panoramic reconstruction (Fig. 2-12). However, it must be noted that CBCTs should not be generated in patients requiring a panoramic radiograph alone, because of dose concerns.

Newer hybrid units, such as the CS 9300 3D Extraoral Imaging System (Carestream Dental, Atlanta, Georgia), have a wide range of FOV choices for a variety of diagnostic tasks, in addition to a conventional panoramic imaging option

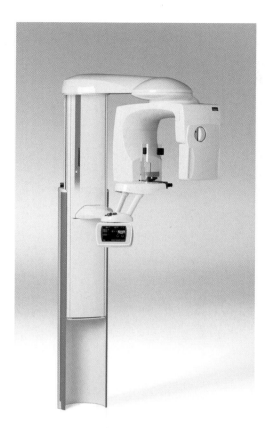

A

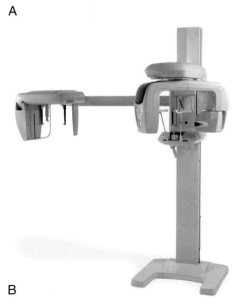

B

FIG. 2-6 **A**, Planmeca ProMax 3D. **B**, J. Morita Veraviewepocs 3D. (**A** courtesy Planmeca Oy, Helsinki, Finland; **B** courtesy J. Morita Corp, Osaka, Japan.)

prolongs the acquisition time. The number of slices acquired is a direct function of the sensor array configuration. Spiral CT uses continuous translator motion of the gantry as images are acquired, thus shortening the acquisition time. This results in significantly higher absorbed x-ray doses for

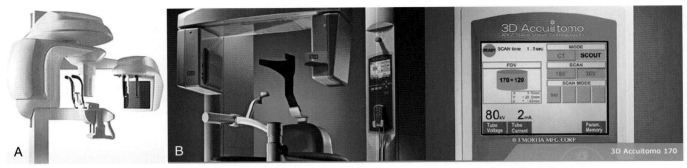

FIG. 2-7 **A**, CS 9000 3D and CS 8100 Extraoral imaging systems. **B**, Morita Accu-i-tomo 170. (**A** Courtesy Carestream Dental LLC, Atlanta, GA; **B** Courtesy J Morita, Irvine, CA.)

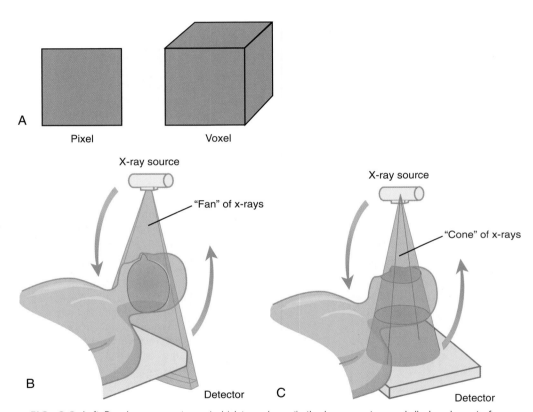

FIG. 2-8 *Left,* Drawing represents a *pixel* (picture element), the image capture and display element of any traditional digital image displayed on the computer. Shades of gray or color are displayed in these pixels to represent a 2D image. *Right,* Drawing represents a *voxel* (volume element). Voxels in CBCT are isometric and have the same dimension or length on all sides. They are very small (from 0.076 to 0.60 microns) and are the capture elements for cone beam imaging devices. Principles of conventional fan beam and cone beam computed tomography are presented in (**B**) and (**C**), respectively. (**B** and **C** from Babbush CA: *Dental implants: the art and science,* ed 2, St Louis, 2011, Elsevier/Saunders.)

(Fig. 2-13). The CS 9000 unit offers the lowest voxel size of 76 microns, whereas the CS 9300 can resolve down to 90 microns, with a range extending to 500 microns for larger FOV studies. Likewise, the Morita 3D Accuitomo 80 (J. Morita USA, Irvine, California) generates isotropic voxels of 80 microns. Although not necessary for use in every case, this technology, when appropriate, improves visualization and ultimately leads to better care in select situations. A record of exposure and doses must be maintained for each patient.

Type of Patient

Patient size and thus the amount of regional anatomy captured in the study also help determine the FOV. The smallest possible FOV must be chosen for the task at hand. Just because a

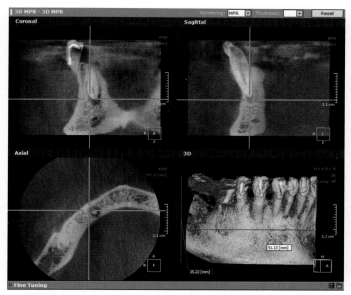

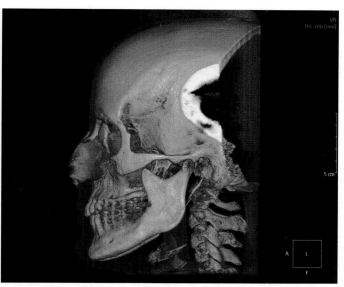

FIG. 2-9 Multiplanar and 3D color reconstructed views of the mandibular quadrant taken on a CBCT machine with a volume size of 37 × 50 mm. (Data acquired and reformatted at 0.076 mm voxel size using a CS 9000 3D unit [Carestream Dental, Atlanta, Ga].)

FIG. 2-10 Image of entire head (17 × 23 cm) from a large FoV machine. (Image acquired with i-CAT unit [Imaging Sciences International, Hatfield, Pa].)

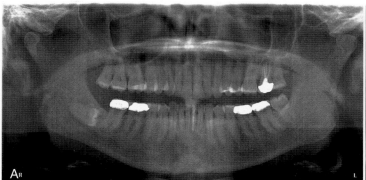

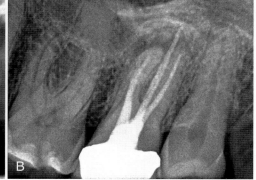

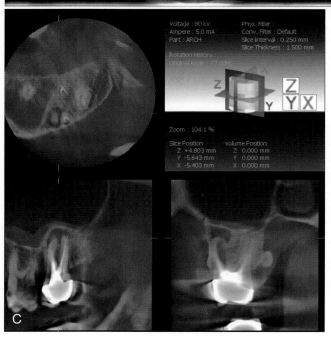

FIG. 2-11 **A,** Panoramic 2D image exposed with the J. Morita Veraviewepocs 3D for evaluation of the mandibular left central incisor. Other radiographic findings also were revealed, including the horizontal bony impaction of the mandibular right third molar and a possible lesion of endodontic origin associated with the endodontically treated maxillary left second molar. Data available from the scan allowed a 3D reconstruction to be made for areas of concern. **B,** Periapical radiograph of the maxillary left second molar on the same patient revealed a periapical area of low attenuation in the region of the periapex of the mesiobuccal root. In this case, also, changes could be evaluated in greater detail with CBCT imaging. **C,** CBCT of the maxillary left second molar revealed detailed periapical and periradicular changes in all three orthogonal planes of the section, specifically illustrating the lesion of endodontic origin associated with the mesiobuccal root. Examination of the width of the mesiobuccal root in both the axial and coronal views (buccolingually) showed that the mesiobuccal root possibly had two canals and that only a single canal was treated during the initial endodontic therapy. (Data acquired and reformatted at 0.076 mm voxel size using a CS 9000 3D unit [Carestream Dental, Atlanta, Ga].)

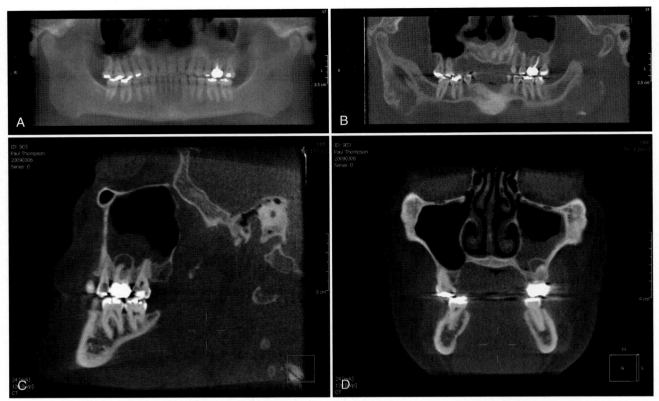

FIG. 2-12 **A,** This reconstructed panoramic image from CBCT data approximates the view one would see with a conventional panoramic radiograph. It is somewhat difficult to see the lesion on the maxillary left first molar. **B,** This thin-slice pseudopanoramic image shows the lesion more precisely because the thin slice (0.10 mm) removes most of the anatomic superimposition. These slices of the maxillary left first molar show the lesion in sagittal (**C**) and coronal (**D**) views, confirming the features seen in the pseudopanoramic view.

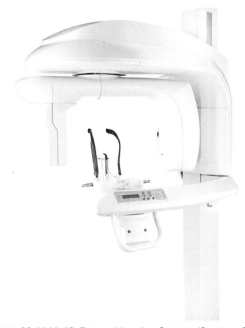

FIG. 2-13 CS 9300 3D Extraoral Imaging System. (Courtesy Carestream Dental LLC, Atlanta, GA.)

clinician owns a cone beam machine does *not* mean that every patient should be exposed to a cone beam study.[119] If previous studies are available, they need to be evaluated first in a recall patient. Use of imaging in children must be minimized. Cone beam machines with smaller FOVs can somewhat limit the radiation dose to critical organs and tissues of the head and neck in these cases.

Spatial Resolution Requirements

All endodontic imaging procedures require high spatial resolution. Assessment of canal structure, canal length, and lesions of endodontic origin (LEOs)[160] showing apical change, in addition to an understanding of possible revision cases, are important tasks requiring minute detail. If CBCT is used, the data acquisition should be performed at the smallest voxel size: the smaller the voxel size, the higher the spatial resolution. Many of the larger stand-alone cone beam machines, such as the i-CAT (Imaging Sciences International, Irvine, California), default to a 0.4 mm voxel size. This voxel size is inadequate for high spatial detail. However, these units often have a voxel size selection option that allows smaller voxel sizes to be used during the image acquisition. The absolute maximum voxel size for endodontic imaging should be 0.2 mm.[35] Units typically use voxel sizes of 0.076 to 0.16 mm for their native image capture (Fig. 2-14).

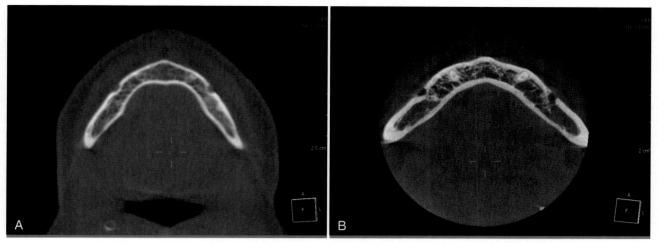

FIG. 2-14 **A**, Axial slice from data obtained with a 0.4 mm voxel size. Compare the trabecular pattern and outline of the mental foramina to the same location in an axial slice from data obtained with a 0.16 mm voxel size (**B**).

IMAGING TASKS IMPROVED OR SIMPLIFIED BY CONE BEAM VOLUMETRIC COMPUTED TOMOGRAPHY

The Executive Opinion of the American Academy of Oral and Maxillofacial Radiology and, later, the position paper on the use of CBCT in endodontics jointly developed by the American Association of Endodontists (AAE) and the American Academy of Oral and Maxillofacial Radiology (AAOMR), list indications for potential use in selected cases, including evaluation of the anatomy and complex morphology, differential diagnosis of complex pathoses with certain qualifiers, intraoperative or postoperative assessment of endodontic treatment, dentoalveolar trauma, resorption, presurgical case planning, and dental implant case planning.[34] Use of CBCT must be determined on a case-by-case basis only. These indications do not in any way mandate the use of CBCT for every case that falls into one of the preceding categories. For endodontic treatment and assessments, there are at least five primary imaging tasks in which CBCT scans have a distinct advantage over traditional 2D radiographs. These tasks include evaluation of the following factors:

1. Differential diagnosis
   a. Lesions of endodontic origin
   b. Lesions of nonendodontic origin
   c. Diagnosis of endodontic treatment failures
   d. Vertical root fractures
2. Evaluation of anatomy and complex morphology
   a. Anomalies
   b. Root canal system morphology
3. Intraoperative or postoperative assessment of endodontic treatment complications
   a. Overextended root canal obturation material
   b. Separated endodontic instruments
   c. Calcified canal identification
   d. Localization of perforation
4. Dentoalveolar trauma
5. Internal and external root resorption
6. Presurgical case planning
7. Dental implant case planning
8. Assessment of endodontic treatment outcomes

Differential Diagnosis

Lesions of Endodontic Origin

Clinical endodontic diagnosis relies on subjective and objective information collected during patient examinations. Diagnosis of the pulpal status of the teeth can sometimes be challenging if adequate radiographic information is unavailable. It is fundamental to understand that lesions of endodontic origin arise secondary to pulpal breakdown products and form adjacent to canal portals of exit.[155,161] These radiolucent lesions, formed as a result of loss of bone mineralization, can and do form three dimensionally anywhere along the root surface anatomy.[154] A 30% to 40% mineral content loss is needed for these lesions to be visualized on conventional radiographs.[116] Furthermore, the thickness of the cortical plate covering the lesion may significantly affect the radiographic appearance of the lesion on a conventional image.[192] In a comparative investigation of the use of CBCT and periapical (PA) radiography in the evaluation of the periodontal ligament (PDL), Pope et al.[148a] showed that necrotic teeth examined with CBCT had widened PDLs, but healthy, vital teeth showed significant variation. They called for further investigation to determine whether health and disease can be appropriately judged by the use of CBCT in epidemiologic investigations.

Digital subtraction radiography (DSR) has been observed to increase diagnostic capability; observers identified incipient periapical lesions in more than 70% of the cases.[116] Before the advent of CBCT, clinicians were unable to routinely visualize the presence, specific location, and extensiveness of periapical bone loss using conventional radiography.[107] This was especially true in areas with superimposition of anatomic structures. Visual obstruction from anatomic features, such as buccal bone and the malar process over the apices of maxillary roots, simply "disappears" when the examiner can scroll through the slices of the bone from facial to palatal in 0.1 mm sections while also changing axial orientations. CBCT showed significantly higher rates of detection of

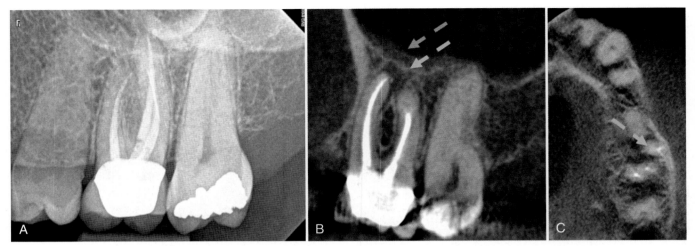

FIG. 2-15 A 62-year-old female was referred for evaluation and possible treatment for chronic continuous dentoalveoar pain (CCDAP) in the maxillary left region. The patient could alleviate this condition by placing a moist cotton roll in the adjacent vestibule to prevent the buccal mucosa from contacting the alveolus supporting the maxillary teeth in this area. This condition began after a history of local anesthetic administration, persisted for 1 year, and led to three successive new crowns and endodontic treatment on the "offending tooth," in an effort to remedy the condition without improvement. The response to endodontic tests, TMJ, and myofascial evaluations were normal. Application of topical xylocaine resulted in cessation of pain for 15 minutes. A PA radiograph (A) showed a root-treated, maxillary left first molar with no apparent radiographic lesion. A limited FOV CBCT of the maxillary left posterior was exposed. The corrected sagittal view (B) showed an approximately 4 mm, well-defined oval, mildly corticated area of low attenuation (radiolucent) centered over the apex of the mesiobuccal root and extending to the junction of the middle and apical third of the mesiobuccal root (yellow arrow). There was a mild mucositis (green arrow). There was a previously untreated mesioaccessory canal (C) and a mild mucositis. A diagnosis of neuropathic pain and a chronic apical periodontitis was made. Daily application of topical ketamine, gabapentin, and clonidine was prescribed. Endodontic revision of the maxillary left first molar was performed 3 months after the patient was stabilized with the topical medications. (Data acquired and reformatted at 0.076 mm voxel size using a CS 9000 3D [Carestream Dental, LLC, Atlanta, GA].)

periapical lesions in maxillary molars and premolars compared to PA radiography.[109]

Lesions of Nonendodontic Origin

Differential diagnosis of periapical pathology is crucial to endodontic treatment planning. Substantial evidence in the literature points to a significant chance that lesions of the tooth-supporting structures are nonendodontic in origin, such as periapical cemento-osseous dysplasia; central giant cell granulomas; simple bone cysts; odontogenic cysts, tumors, or malignancies; and neuropathic pain (Fig. 2-15).*

Neuropathic orofacial pain or atypical odontalgia (AO), also known as *chronic continuous dentoalveolar pain* (CCDAP)[131a] and *persistent idiopathic facial pain* (PDAP),[80a] is related to a tooth, teeth, or pain at an extraction site where no clinical or radiographic pathosis is evident. Two systematic reviews of AO showed the incidence of persistent pain of more than 6 months' duration after nonsurgical and surgical endodontic treatment, excluding local inflammatory causes, was 3.4%.[130a] The pathophysiology of this pain is uncertain, but it is hypothesized to involve deafferentation of peripheral sensory neurons in predisposed patients. The diagnosis of AO is challenging and depends on the patient history and clinical examination findings, in addition to the absence of radiographic findings. In some cases the symptoms from AP and AO are closely related.

Pigg et al.[146a] conducted a study of 20 patients with AO. All of the patients had at least one tooth in the region of discomfort that had undergone invasive treatment; 21 of 30 teeth had undergone endodontic treatment. These researchers found that 60% had no periapical lesions, and among those who did, CBCT showed 17% more periapical lesions than conventional radiography. This study demonstrated that CBCT may be a useful supplement to 2D radiography (see Fig. 2-15).

The 3D radiographic appearance of a periapical lesion provides additional information about the lesion's relationship to the tooth and other anatomic structures (e.g., the vascular bundle) and about the aggressiveness of the lesion. This information, along with pulp sensitivity testing, is useful for adequate treatment planning and management of these conditions.

Diagnosis of Endodontic Treatment Failures

Failure of previous endodontic therapy can be attributed to various factors, such as procedural errors, missed canals, or persistent periapical pathosis. Knowledge of the cause of failure is pertinent to the treatment of these cases because it allows the cause to be adequately rectified. With the advent of CBCT, in select cases of retreatment in which the cause of failure is otherwise undetectable, adequate information may be collected to apply to the treatment plan (Fig. 2-16). The technology is most useful in detecting uninstrumented and unfilled

---

*References 28, 54, 56, 81, 130, 143, 151, and 152.

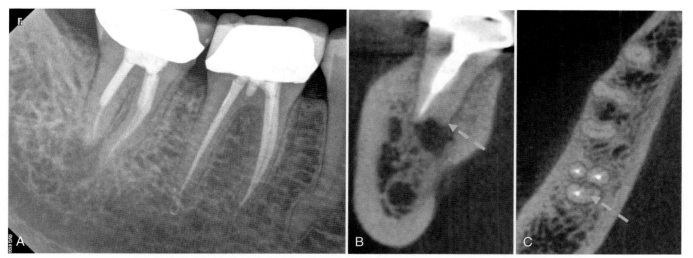

FIG. 2-16 This 38-year-old female patient presented for evaluation and treatment of a symptomatic mandibular right second molar, which had been endodontically treated more than 10 years previously. This tooth was sensitive to percussion and biting forces; periodontal findings were normal. Microscopic examination of the exposed dentin was negative for a vertical fracture. The PA radiograph **(A)** showed the previous endodontic treatment; a post present in the distal canal; and an approximately 5 mm diameter, unilocular, diffuse area of low density centered at the periapex of the distal root. Contemporaneous CBCT sagittal **(B)** and axial **(C)** images revealed a previously untreated distobuccal canal. (Data acquired and reformatted at 0.076 mm voxel size using a CS 9000 3D unit [Carestream Dental, Atlanta, Ga].)

canals, extension of the root canal filling, and the presence and extent of periradicular bone loss. The sensitivity of CBCT and PA radiographs for diagnosing strip perforations in root-filled teeth has been shown to be low.[51] Radiopaque filling materials in the root canals of endodontically treated teeth can produce streak artifacts, which can mimic fracture lines or perforations.[166,198]

Vertical Root Fractures

Vertical root fractures (VRFs) that run along the long axis of a tooth are often difficult to diagnose clinically. The prevalence of VRF in endodontically treated teeth has been reported to range from 8.8% to 13.4%.[61,174,196] These fractures typically run in the buccolingual direction and are confined to the roots, making it difficult to visualize the fracture. Visualizing the fracture on a conventional radiograph is possible when the x-ray beam is parallel to the plane of the fracture.[153] Challenges in diagnosis with regard to the extent and exact location of the fracture often lead to unwarranted extraction of teeth. Since the introduction of CBCT to dentistry, various reports of the application of the technology to detect vertical root fractures have been published. The reported sensitivity for detection of VRFs has ranged from 18.8% to 100%[115]; by comparison, conventional radiographs have a reported sensitivity of approximately 37%[48,75] (Fig. 2-17). CBCT has been used to visualize VRFs in controlled clinical studies in which clinical diagnosis was difficult.[48] Vertical root fractures were successfully detected at a spatial resolution ranging from 76 to 140 microns. However, only a limited number of units provide such high resolution. A comparison of various CBCT units for the detection of VRFs demonstrated that the units with flat panel detectors (FPDs) were superior to the image intensifier tube/charge-coupled device (IIT/CCD)–based detectors; the smaller FOV and the ability to view axial

slices also improved detection of VRFs.[76] Continued improvement of sensor technology, including the use of FPDs, has resulted in enhanced resolution. Voxel dimensions are smaller in these units. Detection of vertical root fractures with thickness ranging from 0.2 to 0.4 mm was found to be more accurate with CBCT than with digital radiography.[133,138] The presence of root canal filling in the teeth lowers the specificity of CBCT in detecting vertical root fractures[75,76,95]; this has been attributed to the radiopaque material causing streak artifacts that mimic fracture lines.[198]

Evaluation of Anatomy and Complex Morphology

The precise location and visualization of dental anomalies, root morphology, and canal anatomy are vastly improved with CBCT data. Root curvature, additional roots, and anomalies within the canals themselves (e.g., obstructions, narrowing, bifurcation) are made more apparent when all three anatomic planes of section are available for review, especially with the capability of narrowing the slice thickness to as little as 0.076 mm. Visual obstruction from anatomic features such as buccal bone and the malar process over the apices of maxillary roots simply will "disappear" when you can scroll through the slices of the bone from facial to palatal in 0.076 mm sections while also changing axial orientations (Fig. 2-18).

Dental Anomalies

The use of CBCT technology has been reported in the diagnosis and treatment planning of various dental anomalies (e.g., dens invaginatus) that often have complex morphologic presentations.[131] The prevalence of dens invaginatus was as high as 6.8% in the adolescent Swedish population studied.[14] The complex nature of the anomaly presents a diagnostic challenge

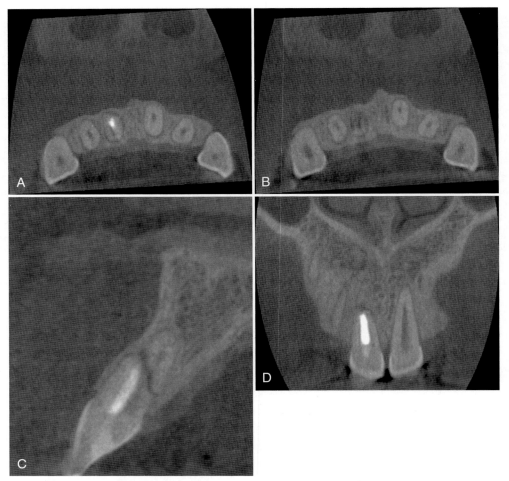

FIG. 2-17 Root fracture in an endodontically obturated maxillary right central incisor. **A,** Axial view with artifacts from a highly attenuating (opaque) obturant. **B,** View without artifacts from obturant. **C,** Oblique parasagittal view. **D,** Paracoronal view. (Data acquired and reformatted at 0.076 mm voxel size using a CS 9000 3D unit [Carestream Dental, Atlanta, Ga].)

when conventional radiographs are used.[137] In case reports in which CBCT was used for diagnosis and treatment planning, treatment options included conservative endodontic treatment of the invagination, surgical treatment of the periapical pathology, and complete revascularization of the dens after removal of the invagination (Fig. 2-19).[124,185]

Root Canal System Morphology

As the adage goes, nature seldom makes a straight line and never makes two of the same. This statement is dramatically illustrated in the evaluation of root canal system morphology. With ever-present unusual and atypical root shapes and numbers, there is sometimes a need to look further than what a clinician can see or imagine with 2D radiography (Fig. 2-20). Variations in root canal morphology have been studied using various in vitro techniques.[57,147,182,183] The results of these studies point to the fact that there is significant variation in the root canal morphology among various ethnic population groups.[3,72,73,128,187] CBCT has been reported to be comparable to canal staining and clearing techniques for identification of the root canal morphology,[125] and CBCT studies report variation in the root canal morphology among various ethnic groups.[126,173,197,199]

INTRAOPERATIVE OR POSTOPERATIVE ASSESSMENT OF ENDODONTIC TREATMENT COMPLICATIONS

Materials Extending Beyond the Root Canal

CBCT scans provide the opportunity to map endodontic treatment complications through the examination of 3D representations of the teeth and supporting structures in different planes. Few high-level studies related to the effects of endodontic treatment complications have been published in the endodontic literature.[176] However, it is generally recognized that overfilling of the root canal, causing damage to vital structures such as the inferior alveolar neurovascular bundle (IAN) (Fig. 2-21) or the maxillary sinus, can cause significant morbidity.[24,25,60,64]

Endodontic therapy undertaken in close proximity to the IAN should receive special attention because direct trauma, mechanical compression, chemical neurotoxicity, and an increase in temperature greater than 10° C may cause irreversible damage.[51,68,71,179] Scolozzi et al.[162] reported that sensory disturbances can include pain, anesthesia, paresthesia,

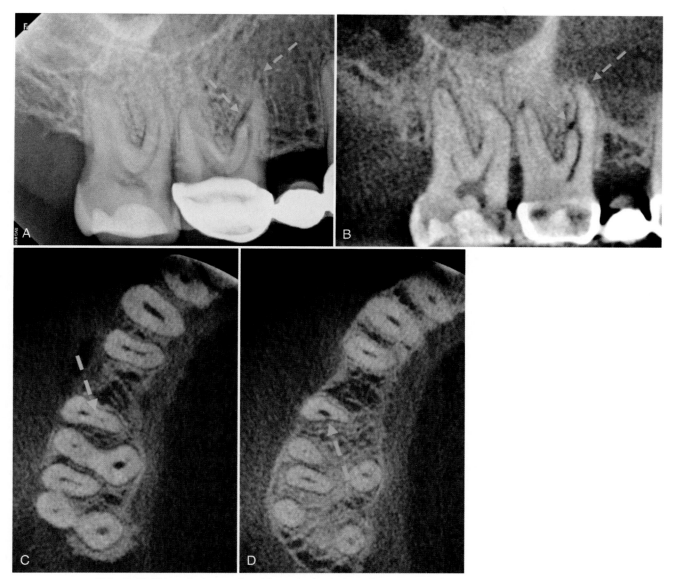

FIG. 2-18 This patient was referred for evaluation and possible treatment after emergency pulp extirpation performed by others. The location of the physiologic terminus and radiographic apex did not appear to coincide even remotely in the PA radiograph (**A**), so a CBCT-aided assessment was required. A CBCT scan was able to clearly show the exact location of the canal terminus and radiographic apex (**B**), the presence of a mesioaccessory canal with an isthmus (**C**), and the oval canal (**D**), facilitating treatment of this case. (Courtesy Dr. Anastasia Mischenko, Chevy Chase, Md. Data acquired and reformatted at 0.076 mm voxel size using a CS 9000 3D unit [Carestream Dental, Atlanta, Ga].)

hypoesthesia, and dysesthesia.[162] The IAN is located in the cribriform bone-lined mandibular canal and courses obliquely through the ramus of the mandible and horizontally through the mandible body to the mental foramen and the incisive foramen.[8] There are many anatomic variations of the IAN, including the anterior loop and bifid mandibular canals.[35] Kovisto et al.[97] used CBCT measurements from 139 patients to show that the apices of the mandibular second molar were closest to the IAN. In females, the mesial root of the second molar was closer than in males, and the distances in all roots measured increased with the age of the patient. There was a high correlation between the measurements from left to right

side in the same patient; an average distance of 1.51 to 3.43 mm in adults.[97] Procedures involving the mandibular second molar were most likely to cause nerve damage.[106] Further research is required to clarify the risks and benefits of CBCT when endodontic treatment is contemplated on teeth with a proximal relationship between the IAN and root apices. Porgrel[148] treated 61 patients with involvement of the IAN after root canal therapy during a 7-year period. Eight patients were asymptomatic; 42 patients were seen for mild symptoms or were examined more than 3 months postoperatively, with only 10% experiencing improvement. Five patients underwent surgical treatment before 48 hours elapsed and recovered completely.

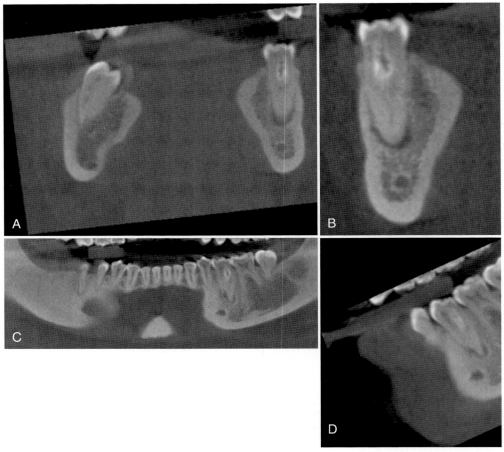

FIG. 2-19 **A,** Dens in dente of the mandibular left second bicuspid; coronal slice. **B,** Coronal view. **C,** Panoramic reconstruction from CBCT. **D,** Sagittal view. (Data acquired and reformatted at 0.076 mm voxel size using a CS 9000 3D unit [Carestream Dental, Atlanta, Ga].)

Six patients underwent surgery between 10 days and 3 months, with four experiencing partial recovery; the remaining two had no improvement.[148]

New imaging technologies, such as high-resolution magnetic resonance imaging (MRI-HR) and magnetic resonance neurography (MRN), promise to improve isolation of the IAN from the neighboring artery and vein contained within the inferior alveolar bony canal. MRN studies have documented the ability to demonstrate nerve continuity and localize extraneural nerve compression before surgical nerve exploration. Postoperative periapical radiographs should be exposed on the day of endodontic treatment completion or a suspected iatrogenic event, and any suspected compromise of the IAN or other vital structures should be evaluated immediately. In all cases in which trauma to the IAN is suspected from periapical or panoramic radiography or by the report of symptoms consistent with nerve injury, exposure of a CBCT image volume should be considered. It is generally accepted that immediate surgical debridement should be attempted to maximize recovery.[51,149] With the introduction of MRI algorithms for dental diagnostic purposes, it is expected that this imaging modality will be increasingly used in diagnostic and treatment planning. MRI has the capability to demonstrate vascularity to the tooth of interest, in addition to the presence of inflammatory exudates in the apical regions, without exposing the patient to ionizing radiation. Receiver coils are being developed to enhance the image quality of maxillofacial and dental magnetic resonance studies.

The accidental introduction of root canal instruments, irrigating solutions, obturation material, and root tips into the maxillary sinus has been reported. Serious consequences associated with the intrusion of foreign bodies into the maxillary sinus include pain, paresthesia, and aspergillosis, a rare but well-documented complication of endodontic treatment.[16a] Guivarc'h et al.[71a] reported that the overextension of heavy metal–containing root canal sealers, such as zinc oxide eugenol cement, may promote fungal infection in immunocompromised patients, leading to bone destruction and damage to adjacent structures. This case report described the use of computed tomography to assess the patient before surgery and at 6 months.[71a] The use of CBCT as an aid in the localization and retrieval of an extreme overextension of thermoplasticized injectable gutta-percha into the sinus and contiguous soft tissues has been described by Brooks and Kleinman.[26]

Fractured Instruments

Instrument fracture can occur at any stage of endodontic treatment, and in any canal location. The incidence of this complication, reported in clinical studies on a per canal or per tooth basis, ranges from 0.39% to 5.0%.[44,135] Molars are

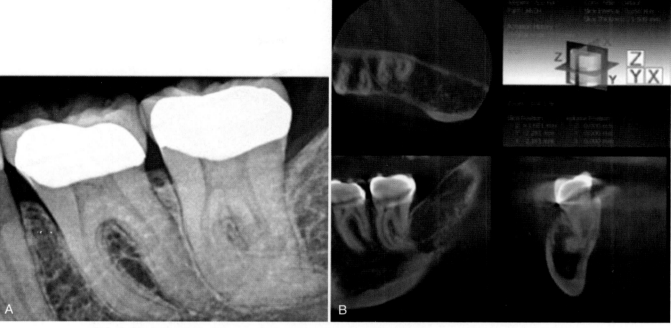

FIG. 2-20 **A,** Mandibular left second molar referred for endodontic evaluation and possible treatment. This 2D radiograph reveals significant pulp stones and canal calcification developing not only in the coronal aspect of the root canal system, but also extending down the visible distal canal. The apical third of the canal system appears unusual and dilacerated. Cone beam volumetric tomography (CBVT) would be beneficial in visualizing the root canal anatomy, so as to create the ideal endodontic access. **B,** Single slice of the CBVT image for tooth #18. Information about the direction of the root canal anatomy is provided in all three planes of the section: axial, coronal, and sagittal. Interestingly, the axial slice shows that the mesial lingual root actually traverses buccally as it approaches its terminal extent. This is valuable information for the clinician before the entire root canal system is cleaned and shaped; it also establishes a higher degree of treatment predictability.

predominantly affected by instrument fracture, with the highest incidence found in the apical third of mandibular molars.[4,40,103,127]

A systematic review and meta-analysis showed that when endodontic treatment was performed at a high technical standard, instrument fracture did not significantly reduce the prognosis. More specifically, when no initial radiographic periapical lesion was present initially, 92.4% of cases remained healthy; when a periapical lesion was present initially, 80.7% of periapical lesions showed radiographic healing. However, the presence or absence of periradicular lesions on preoperative and postoperative examinations was based on planar radiographic assessments, which calls these findings into question.[134] Other studies showed that the chances of endodontic failure increased if the canal system could not be thoroughly disinfected, if a periradicular periodontitis was present, or if technical standards were compromised.[39,91,168,170] Use of CBCT to triangulate the retained instrument and assess the canal shape, especially in cases in which the operating microscope does not allow direct visualization, can be helpful in formulating a removal strategy. If the fractured instrument is lodged in the lingual aspect of a ribbon-shaped canal, for example, an instrument may be inserted toward the buccal to bypass and remove the imbedded instrument without forcing the fragment further apically. Without the use of CBCT, intracanal instruments can be reliably removed or bypassed in 85.3% of cases if straight-line access is possible; however, reliable removal or bypass is possible in only 47.7% of cases if the instrument is not visible (Fig. 2-22).[127] When a separated instrument is lodged in the apical third of a root canal, the chances of retrieval are the lowest, but the apical terminus may be adequately sealed by treatment of an anastomosing canal, if present.[63] The possibility of instrument removal based on CBCT triangulation has not been published to date.

Calcified Canals

According to the Pew Research Center, 10,000 U.S. individuals will reach the age of 65 every day until 2030, and the nation's 65-year-old and over cohort will grow to 81 million in 2050, up from 37 million in 2005 (also see Chapter 26).[82] This aging population will present increasing challenges for dental clinicians because calcification of the root canal system increases as part of the natural aging process,[69] possibly leading to more untreated canals that may serve as a niche for microorganisms.[19,88] Pulp chambers in the crown of the tooth decrease in size, forming more rapidly on the roof and floor of posterior teeth.[184] Typically, root canals calcify at the coronal aspect first, with decreasing calcification as the canal travels apically. Magnification and illumination are essential tools for the identification and treatment of calcified canals, but CBCT can assist in the perioperative treatment of such conditions.[16] Preoperative assessment of calcified teeth using CBCT can suggest the best tactic for locating calcified canals in the chamber floor and

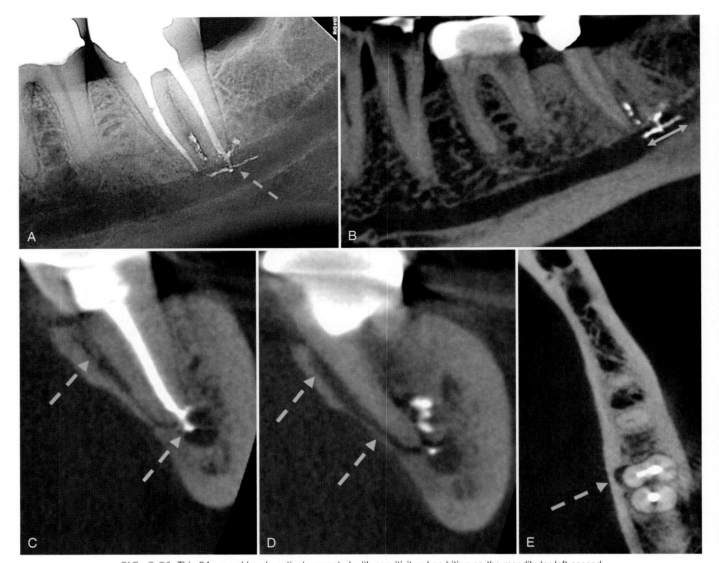

FIG. 2-21 This 64-year-old male patient presented with sensitivity when biting on the mandibular left second molar. The history included endodontic revision more than 6 months earlier and subsequent transient paresthesia and dysesthesia along the distribution of the inferior alveolar nerve, which persisted for 1 week after the retreatment. The results of periodontal probing and microscopic examination of the exposed root surface at the sulcus were normal. The PA radiograph showed the approximate location of the excess radiopaque material, a feature consistent with extruded sealer (**A**, *yellow arrow*). The length of approximately 3.4 mm and the true location of the offending material in the mandibular canal were assessed in the corrected sagittal view (**B**, *yellow arrow*) and corrected cross-sectional view (**C**, *yellow arrow*). The corrected cross-sectional view also showed a lesion of low attenuation extending from the apex to an area near the crest of the alveolus with erosion of the lingual cortical plate (**C**, *blue arrow*; **D**, *yellow arrows*). The same lesion was shown in the corrected axial view (**E**, *yellow arrow*). Examination of the extracted tooth revealed a vertical fracture at the lingual aspect of the distal root. (Data acquired and reformatted at 0.076 mm voxel size using a CS 9000 3D unit [Carestream Dental, Atlanta, Ga].)

roots using software-based measurement tools. The insertion of radiopaque markers, such as instruments or obturation material, can facilitate reliable canal localization using available multiplanar reformations. The increased sensitivity and specificity provided by CBCT can also assist in the determination of the periapical status of calcified root canals that may not require measures that can lead to procedural errors, such as off-course access, instrument fracture, or root perforation.[83] The difficulty in locating calcified canals can be further compounded by morphologic anomalies associated with gender

and ethnic origin.[163] CBCT can be an important adjunct to magnification and illumination in these cases.

Perforations

A *perforation* is defined as a "mechanical or pathologic communication between the root canal system and external tooth surface"[6]; it is usually associated with an iatrogenic event,[159] accounting for about 10% of all nonhealed cases.[85] Root perforations can be caused by a post preparation, the search for a calcified canal, a strip perforation, or an attempt to retrieve a

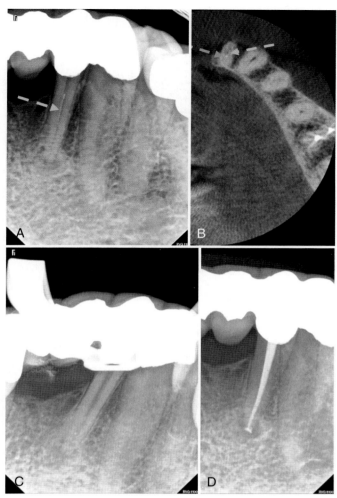

FIG. 2-22 Unexpected torsional and flexural failure of endodontic instruments can occur during instrumentation. This PA radiograph (**A**) shows a separated stainless steel hand file located at the midroot of the mandibular left lateral incisor in a patient referred for revision therapy. To aid development of a retreatment strategy, CBCT was used to localize the instrument (**B**, *yellow arrow*) in the lingual canal. The patient's buccal canal was identified (**B**, *green arrow*), and subsequent instrumentation allowed removal of the offending instrument segment (**C**), leading to successful completion of treatment (**D**). (Data acquired and reformatted at 0.076 mm voxel size using a CS 9000 3D unit [Carestream Dental, Atlanta, Ga].)

fractured instrument. They are often difficult to localize with conventional imaging because no information about the buccolingual dimension can be obtained.[195] Shemesh et al.[166] compared the sensitivity and specificity of CBCT scans with two-angulation periapical imaging using phosphor plates to assess the likelihood of detecting root or strip perforations after root canal treatment with laterally compacted gutta-percha and sealer. They found that the two methods showed similar specificity, but the CBCT image volumes showed higher sensitivity. Single-angulated periapical radiographs (PAs) showed 40% of the perforations, and two-angled PAs showed 63%, suggesting that if PAs alone are used, two-angled images were superior. There was no significant difference in the detection of root perforations between PA and CBCT radiography. The researchers noted that the results may have been affected by the small

size of the perforations and that the method of obturation did not favor extravasation of obturation material.[166] CBCT images suffer from beam hardening artifact resulting from root canal obturation and restorative materials (e.g., gutta-percha, posts, and perforation repair materials), which creates challenges to the interpretation of root integrity. An approach advocated by Bueno et al.[29] suggested that a map-reading strategy of viewing sequential axial slices reduces the beam hardening effect. Newer root canal obturation materials with lower radiopacity profiles and improved CBCT software algorithms are expected to reduce artifact formation in the future.

Dentoalveolar Trauma

Systematic epidemiologic data suggest that facial trauma is a common occurrence, resulting in injuries to the dentition in 57.8% of household and play accidents, 50.5% of sports accidents, 38.6% of work-related accidents, 35.8% of acts of violence, and 34.2% of traffic accidents, with 31% unspecified.[62] The prevalence of traumatic dental injuries varies according to the population studied, but these injuries occur most commonly in children 7 to 10 years of age (also see Chapter 20).[13] Dental traumatic injuries affect one fourth of all schoolchildren and almost one third of adults, and most injuries occur before the age of 19.[65] Maxillary central incisors sustain approximately 80% of all dental traumatic injuries, followed by maxillary lateral incisors and mandibular incisors.[9] The most common type of traumatic dental injuries in the primary dentition are luxation injuries, whereas crown fractures are the predominant dental injury to the permanent dentition.[98] Determination of the extent of injury to the dentinopulpal complex requires a methodical approach that evaluates the teeth, periodontium, and associated structures (Fig. 2-23) and may result in significant long-term complications.[5,42]

Injuries to the orofacial complex can cause dental trauma that results in the following injuries to the primary and permanent dentition: (1) infraction; (2) crown fracture, uncomplicated and complicated; (3) crown/root fracture; (4) root fracture; (5) concussion; (6) subluxation; (7) lateral luxation; (8) intrusion; (9) extrusion; and (10) avulsion.[12] The International Association of Dental Traumatology's guidelines for the management of traumatic dental injures suggest that CBCT may be beneficial when used to assess and monitor healing in patients after dental traumatic injuries, especially in cases of lateral luxation and root fracture.[45] (These guidelines can be reviewed at *www.dentaltraumaguide.org*.) Intra-alveolar root fractures generally affect the permanent dentition of males and are relatively uncommon, accounting for 0.5% to 7% of dental impact injuries.[12,41,67,132] Root-fractured teeth are a challenging condition to diagnose, and the limitations of planar radiography have been well documented in the dental literature.[38,45,96,136] A systematic retrospective study showed that maxillary central (68%) and lateral (27%) incisors were primarily affected, with only limited occurrence in mandibular incisors (5%). This retrospective study concluded that CBCT allowed improved treatment planning compared with PA imaging alone.[191] At least seven systematic laboratory studies and one systematic in vivo animal study reported significantly improved accuracy for the detection of root fractures when CBCT was compared with periapical radiography.* In a systematic clinical study,

---

*References 75, 76, 84, 114, 133, and 189.

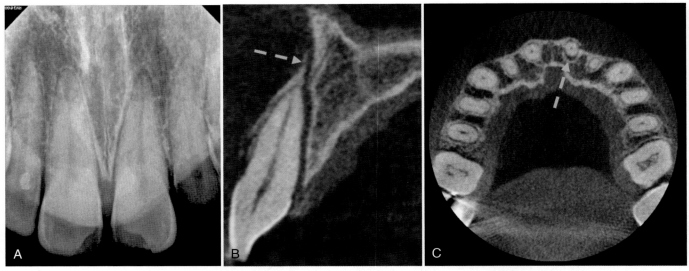

FIG. 2-23 After a traumatic injury to the maxillary right and left central incisors, crown fractures were noted. The PA radiograph showed an extrusive luxation injury in the maxillary left central incisor (**A**). The alveolar fracture (**B**, *yellow arrow*) and true extent of the displacement (**C**, *yellow arrow*) became evident with CBCT. (Data acquired and reformatted at 0.076 mm voxel size using a CS 9000 3D unit [Carestream Dental, Atlanta, Ga].)

Bornstein et al.[23] examined 38 patients with 44 permanent teeth that sustained intra-alveolar fractures. In the study sample reported, 68.2% of teeth had oblique fractures that extended to the cervical third of the root, contradicting the findings of previous studies conducted with periapical imaging alone. CBCT imaging offered improved visualization of the location and angulation of root fractures compared to periapical and occlusal intraoral radiographs.[23]

Several of these studies suggest that lower resolution scans using voxel sizes in excess of 0.3 mm may not improve radiographic assessments.[76,189] A study by Wang et al.[186] showed that the sensitivity and specificity of PA radiography for root fractures were 26.3% and 100%, respectively; the findings for CBCT were 89.5% and 97.5%, respectively. CBCT images of root-filled teeth showed lower sensitivity and unchanged specificity, whereas 2D images showed the same sensitivity and specificity.[186] CBCT allows for the management of traumatic injuries in which a root fracture or alveolar fracture is suspected by providing undistorted multiplanar views of the dentition and supporting bone without the superimposition of anatomic structures.[37,107,157] CBCT image volumes provide superior sensitivity in detecting intra-alveolar root fractures compared with multiple PA radiographs; this allows for the detection of dental and alveolar displacements, including damage to other perioral structures, such as the maxillary sinus and nasal floor.[89] The presence of root canal fillings and posts affected the specificity of the findings as a result of artifact generation.[76,114] Outcome measurements of a region of interest can be compared over time with greater geometric accuracy using CBCT.[74]

The healing of root fractures is influenced by many factors, most prominently the stage of root development, with immature roots showing better healing than mature roots.[59] Other factors that influence healing are the extent of dislocation and repositioning, type of splinting, use of antibiotics, and location of the fracture on the root. The long-term survival of teeth with intra-alveolar root fractures was evaluated in a systematic study by Andreasen et al.[11] This study showed that the type of healing (e.g., hard tissue fusion, PDL interposition with and without bone) and the location of the fracture on the root had the most influence on tooth loss. CBCT should be considered when placement of individual PA radiographs will adversely affect patient management; PA radiographs will produce a higher radiation dose for assessment of the region of interest; or intra-alveolar fracture of the root or supporting structures is suspected and sufficient information cannot be obtained with conventional radiography.[89]

The decision to use CBCT imaging for assessment of traumatic injuries should be based on the diagnostic yield expected and in accordance with the "as low as reasonably achievable" (ALARA) principle. CBCT scan volumes that use the most appropriate detector size and shape, beam projection geometry, and beam collimation should be selected to produce high-resolution images and reduce x-radiation exposure whenever possible.[158] In all cases, it should be recognized that children and young adults are more susceptible to the effects of radiation than adults, and CBCT studies should answer specific clinical questions that cannot be answered by lower dose PA and panoramic imaging technologies.[79] New technologies that allow for comparison of matched CBCT images in a serial fashion at a reduced dose have been tested. This technology promises a dose reduction of 10 to 40 times by using the initial scan as prior knowledge and adaptive prior image constrained compressed sensing (APICCS) algorithms to greatly reduce the number of projections and x-ray tube current levels required (Fig. 2-24).[100]

Internal and External Root Resorption

Most clinicians are aware, and ideally communicate to their patients, that the long-term prognosis for teeth with extensive root resorption may be unpredictable. Endodontic treatment can often resolve these defects, and early diagnosis and treatment typically mean an improved prognosis. CBCT imaging of these resorptive lesions provides the clinician with enhanced

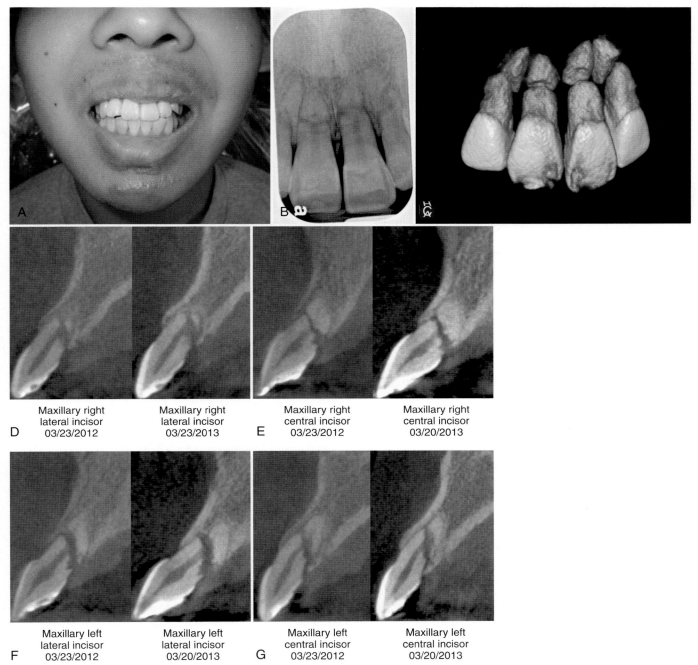

Maxillary right lateral incisor 03/23/2012	Maxillary right lateral incisor 03/23/2013
Maxillary right central incisor 03/23/2012	Maxillary right central incisor 03/20/2013
Maxillary left lateral incisor 03/23/2012	Maxillary left lateral incisor 03/20/2013
Maxillary left central incisor 03/23/2012	Maxillary left central incisor 03/20/2013

FIG. 2-24 Horizontal root fractures resulting from trauma (**A**) were evident in this 22-year-old male patient, who was referred with a contemporaneous film–based PA radiograph (**B**) for evaluation and possible treatment 9 months after trauma to his maxillary lateral and central incisors. Since the trauma, the teeth had been stabilized with a ribbon-type splint on the palatal surface; they were of normal color and responded to all pulp tests within normal limits. There was slight mobility in all of the traumatized teeth. The true nature of the root fractures (**C**, 3D reconstructed view) was evident in the corrected sagittal views of the maxillary right lateral (**D**) and central (**E**) incisors, and in the maxillary left central (**F**) and lateral (**G**) incisors. Temporal examination revealed no changes at the initial presentation, 12-month, and 30-month reevaluations (left to right in each group). Task-specific exposure parameters allowed each successive CBCT image volume to be exposed with lower kVp and mA, resulting in a 20% radiation dose reduction. (Data acquired and reformatted at 0.076 mm voxel size using a CS 9000 3D unit [Carestream Dental, Atlanta, Ga].)

information so that more appropriate treatment planning options are available.

As described in Chapter 16, root resorption (RR) results in the loss of dentin, cementum, or bone by the action of clastic cells.[15] In the primary dentition, RR is caused by normal physiologic processes, except when resorption is premature; in the permanent dentition, it is caused by inflammatory processes.[36,52,141] The successful management of RR in the adult dentition depends on clinical and radiographic examination leading to early detection and accurate diagnosis.[142] Unfortunately, teeth affected by RR have a poor prognosis if the causative lesion is not treated.[140] Although parallax intraoral imaging techniques can be helpful in localizing RR,[86] only CBCT assessments can provide the true size and position of all resorptive defects in the region of interest.[36,140] Intraoral imaging produced false-negative results in 51.9% of cases studied and false-positive results in 15.3%.[122] The interpretation of RR should rely on the least invasive test that can reliably detect the occurrence of the condition.[140] The use of CBCT in the evaluation of RR eliminates structure superimposition and compression of 3D features. Patel et al.[140] compared the sensitivity and specificity of PA imaging with CBCT scans using the receiver operating characteristic (ROC) curve, a standard measure of diagnostic performance. PA imaging showed satisfactory (Az 0.78) accuracy, whereas CBCT showed perfect results (Az 1.00).[140]

Although the literature describes many classification systems, this section divides inflammatory root resorption into two groups, according to location: internal root resorption (IRR) and external root resorption (ERR).[177] IRR is a relatively rare occurrence that is usually detected on routine diagnostic PA or panoramic radiographs.[102,139] It is characterized by structural changes in the tooth that appear as oval or round radiolucent enlargements of the pulp canal, usually with smooth, well-defined margins.[32] IRR is usually asymptomatic, associated with pulpal necrosis coronal to the resorptive lesion and vital or partially vital pulps where active.[140] These lesions can easily be confused with extracanal invasive cervical resorption because the radiographic appearance of the two lesions can be identical. CBCT is helpful for diagnosing the location and exact size of IRR. In a study by Estrela et al.,[52] 48 PA radiographs and CBCT scans were exposed on 40 individuals.[52] IRR was detected in 68.8% of PA radiographs, whereas CBCT scans showed 100% of the lesions. Conventional radiographs were able to detect only lesions between 1 and 4 mm in 52.1% of the images, whereas CBCT was able to show 95.8% of the lesions. This finding was in agreement with other studies that demonstrated the value of tomographic analysis.[36,105] In a study by Kim et al.,[92] the extent and location of the IRR was accurately reproduced with the fabrication of a rapid prototyping tooth model. Although relatively few systematic studies on artificially induced IRR have been reported because of the difficulty in creating such defects, Kamburoglu and Kursun[90] concluded that high-resolution CBCT imaging performed better than low-resolution CBCT imaging in detecting simulated small internal resorptive lesions.

ERR is typically idiopathic, but severe luxation and avulsion injuries can result in lesions that may progress rapidly, and early treatment is recommended.[47] The recommended timing of radiographic examinations using CBCT has not been established with a strong evidence grade. Many ERR cases involve young patients, in whom the radiation dose is critical, and

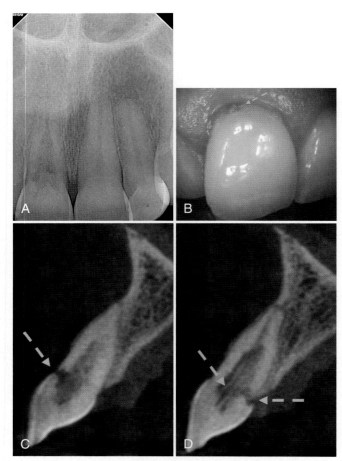

FIG. 2-25 Invasive cervical resorption, a form of external resorption, was evaluated in this patient after a PA radiographic image (**A**) and visual examination (**B**) showed pathognomonic signs of this lesion. A CBCT image was exposed to determine the true extent of resorption and also restorability. The lesion showed a perforative defect at the CEJ on the facial (**C**, *yellow arrow*) and palatal (**D**, *yellow arrow*) aspects. An intact layer of predentin (**D**, *blue arrow*) is a hallmark of this condition. (Data acquired and reformatted at 0.076 mm voxel size using a CS 9000 3D unit [Carestream Dental, Atlanta, Ga].)

multiple scans would be difficult to justify. ERR can be classified as surface resorption, external inflammatory resorption, external replacement resorption, external cervical resorption, and transient apical breakdown (Fig. 2-25).[141] These lesions are always associated with bony resorption, making comparability of laboratory studies problematic because the lesions lack the changes in the periodontal membrane and associated bony changes that would improve visualization. Differentiation between IRR and ERR is challenging, even with multiple changes in x-ray angulation. The early stages of ERR were difficult to view with conventional radiography, and lesions less than 0.6 mm in diameter and 0.3 mm in depth could not be detected. Medium-sized lesions were visible in 6 of 13 cases, with improved visualization for proximal lesions without regard to the root third being examined.[10]

ERR is difficult to detect if the lesion is confined to the buccal, palatal, or lingual surfaces of the root.[20,66] Liedke et al.[105] conducted systematic diagnostic performance tests and showed similar sensitivity and specificity among the different voxel sizes studied (0.4, 0.3, and 0.2 mm); however, the likelihood ratio showed better probability of correct identification of ERR with either 0.3 or 0.2 mm scans. These researchers suggested the use of a 0.3 mm voxel size protocol, rather than a 0.2 mm one, to reduce scanning time and the resulting dose.[105] Although voxel size is an important consideration, the SNR of different detectors, the radiation dose, viewing conditions, and the processing algorithms also affect detection probability.

Even though many in vitro studies have been performed on the ability of CBCT to detect RR, additional evaluations that use in vivo methodology will add to the cumulative knowledge.

PRESURGICAL VISUALIZATION

Surgical endodontic treatment is often performed in cases of endodontic nonhealing when nonsurgical retreatment is not possible. In the past, conventional and digital 2D PA radiographs were the only means of assessing the apical region. Unfortunately, the information available from these images may not adequately prepare the clinician to resolve the pathosis surgically. For example, the clinician may be unable to observe whether the lesion has perforated the buccal or palatal cortical plates, as in the example that follows, or even observe which root or roots are involved. Presurgical confusion is

resolved with cone beam imaging. Multiplanar views allow the clinician to see the defect and suspected causes from the axial, sagittal, and coronal aspects; 3D grayscale or color imaging helps the clinician visualize the entire defect before the incision is made. This is an immense improvement over conventional imaging (Fig. 2-26).

The relationship of the teeth and the associated pathology to important anatomic landmarks must be taken into consideration in the treatment planning for endodontic surgical procedures. These anatomic landmarks include, but are not limited to, the maxillary sinus, the mandibular canal, the mental foramen, the incisive canal, and the buccal and lingual/palatine cortical plate. The close proximity of the maxillary posterior teeth to the sinus has been linked to maxillary sinusitis of odontogenic origin; changes in the maxillary sinus have ranged from thickening of the schneiderian membrane to actual accumulation of fluid in the sinuses.[110,111,113] The relationship of the roots of the posterior teeth to the sinus during presurgical treatment planning and the changes within the sinus can be best appreciated with the use of CBCT images.[22,111,165]

The relationship of the roots of the mandibular posterior teeth and associated periapical pathology to the mandibular canal, the presence of an anterior loop, and the distance of the mandibular canal from the buccal and lingual cortical plates are pertinent pieces of information when surgical procedures in mandibular posterior teeth are planned.[21] The 3D nature of

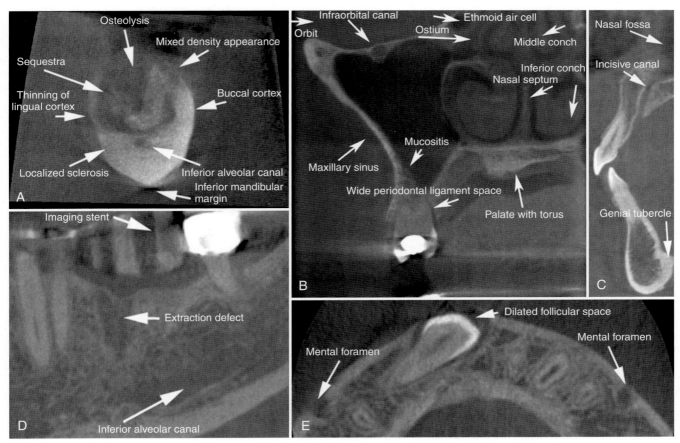

FIG. 2-26 **A** to **W,** Anatomic landmarks on CBCT images acquired using CS 9000, CS 9300, and i-CAT units. (Carestream Dental, Atlanta, Ga [CS 9000 and CS 9300 units]; and Imaging Sciences International, Hatfield, Pa [i-CAT unit].)

Continued

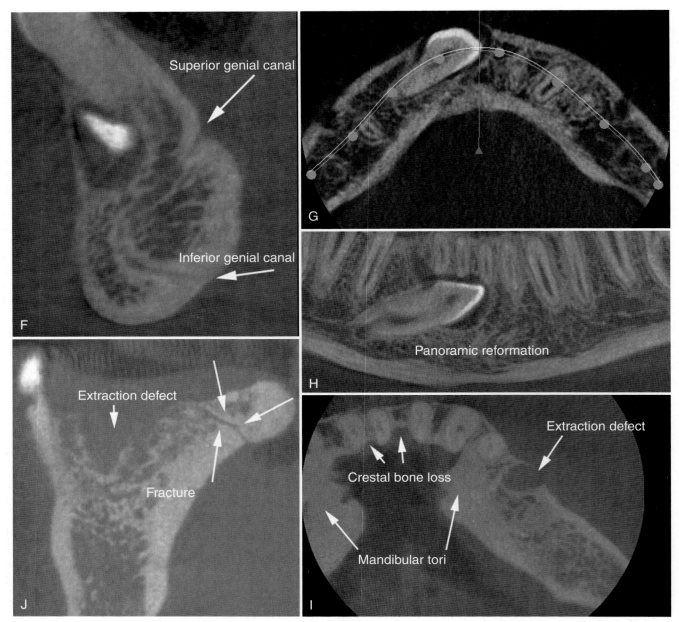

FIG. 2-26, cont'd

this relationship can best be assessed using CBCT.[93] A potential difference in the location of the mandibular canal with respect to age and gender has been reported.[97,167]

Outcomes Assessment

Endodontic treatment outcome predictors using PA radiographs and CBCT imaging have been shown to vary and also are influenced by patient inclusion and exclusion criteria.[104] Historically, PA radiographs and physical examinations were used to determine the success of endodontic treatment, and the absence of posttreatment periradicular radiolucencies and symptoms was considered the criterion for success. However, these planar imaging–based studies have resulted in an overestimation of successful outcomes, compared to CBCT assessments,[192a] because apical periodontitis confined within the cancellous bone or lesions covered by a thick

cortex may be undetectable with conventional radiographic assessments.[18] Additional discrepancies between PA radiography and CBCT have resulted from geometric distortion, limiting comparisons of time-based evaluations, even with careful attention to paralleling technique factors.[112] A clinical study comparing the sensitivity, specificity, predictive values, and accuracy of PA and panoramic radiography and CBCT imaging in 888 consecutive patients showed that the prevalence of apical periodontitis in root-treated teeth was 17.6%, 35.3% and 63.3%, respectively. Conventional radiography showed increased accuracy when the evaluation of larger lesions was assessed.[53]

Outcome predictors identified with PA radiographs and CBCT scans may be different depending on the research performed. Liang et al.[104] retrospectively evaluated 115 endodontically treated teeth with vital pulps 2 years after treatment.

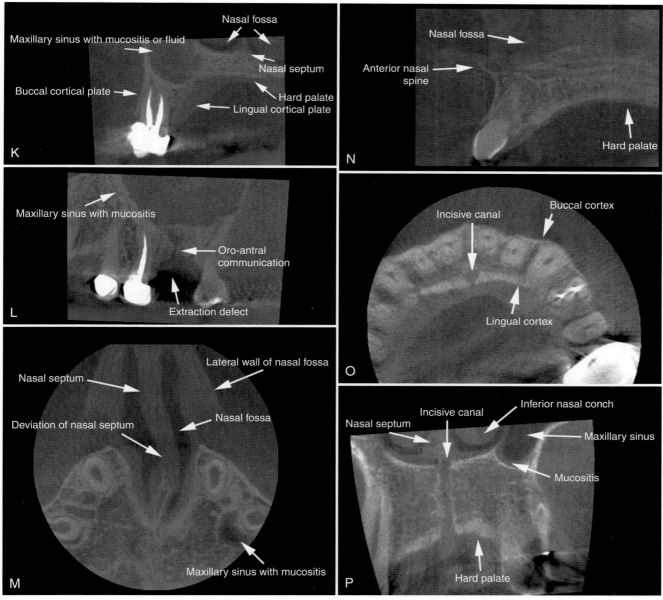

FIG. 2-26, cont'd *Continued*

The authors noted that the recall rate of 36% was comparable to that in other studies, but the result may have been affected because patients with symptomatic or already extracted teeth may not have responded. This lost-to-follow-up cohort significantly reduced the level of evidence.[59a] PA radiography identified periapical lesions in only 12.6% of teeth compared to CBCT images, which identified 25.9% of teeth with periapical lesions. In multivariate logistic regression analysis, the extent of root fillings and density were outcome predictors when using PA imaging, whereas density of root fillings and quality of the coronal restoration were outcome predictors when using CBCT scans. The use of cross-sectional tomography in endodontic treatment is not yet supported by high-level studies that show improved outcomes for patients.

The predictive value and diagnostic accuracy of radiologic assessments are critical to the practice of dentistry, and the diagnostic value of radiographs depends on the radiograph's ability to show the histology of apical periodontitis (AP). De Paula-Silva et al.[43] evaluated the periapex of 83 root-treated and untreated dogs' teeth using PA radiography, CBCT scans, and histopathologic analysis. PA radiography detected AP in 71% of roots; CBCT scans detected AP in 84%; and histologic analysis detected AP in 93%. These findings, corroborated by other studies,[27,70,150] emphasized the low negative predictive value (NPV) of PA radiography at 0.25, showing that when the periapical tissues had a normal appearance, 75% actually had AP. CBCT scans resulted in an NPV almost two times higher than that for PA radiography; however, CBCT scans were not able to detect some AP that was confined to the apical foramen or had little volumetric bone loss. The positive predictive value was the same for PA radiography and CBCT scans compared with histologic examination, but true positive and true

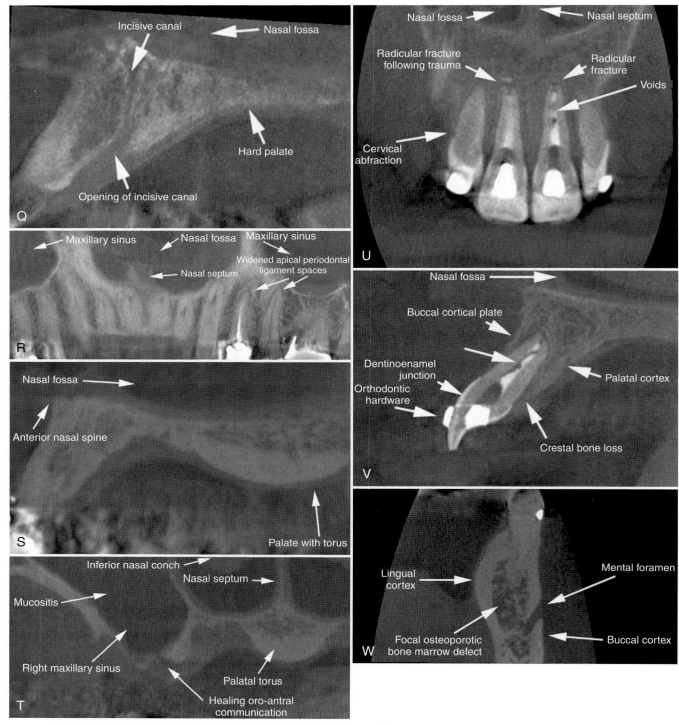

FIG. 2-26, cont'd

negative diagnosis of AP using CBCT scans occurred in 92% of cases.

Determination of healing or nonhealing in individual cases should depend on the clinical and radiographic findings, adjusted for risk factors for the patient, radiation dose, and cost (Fig. 2-27). For patients who are medically complex and subject to possible increased detriment from apical periodontitis (i.e., patients with altered immune systems, such as those

undergoing chemotherapy or anti-HIV protocols or who have risk factors associated with prosthetic joints and/or infective endocarditis), these factors should be considered in the decision on whether to use CBCT. The American Academy of Periodontology has published a position paper stating that periodontal disease might contribute to adverse systemic health conditions.[156] The scientific basis for the relationship of AP and adverse systemic health conditions has not been

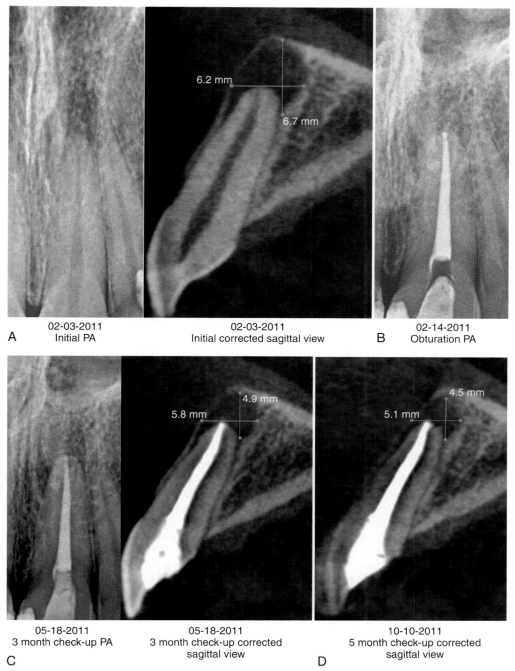

A 02-03-2011 Initial PA	02-03-2011 Initial corrected sagittal view	**B** 02-14-2011 Obturation PA
05-18-2011 3 month check-up PA	05-18-2011 3 month check-up corrected sagittal view	10-10-2011 5 month check-up corrected sagittal view
C		**D**

FIG. 2-27 This series of radiographs shows a maxillary left central incisor several months after a bicycle accident. The patient complained of significant discomfort and mobility with slight swelling in the periapical region. The preoperative PA radiograph (**A**, *left*) and contemporaneous CBCT image (**A**, *right,* corrected sagittal view) showed an approximately 6 mm, well-defined periapical radiolucency with a noncorticated diffuse border, centered over the apex, consistent with a periradicular periodontitis. No root or alveolar fractures were observed. A postoperative PA radiograph (**B**) showed satisfactory canal obturation. At a 3-month checkup visit, the patient complained of continued sensitivity to touch and mobility. There was excessive contact with the opposing incisor, which was adjusted. Because the 3-month checkup PA radiograph (**C**, *left*) showed no change in the periradicular radiolucency, a CBCT image (**C**, *right,* corrected sagittal view) was required to assess healing. The periradicular radiolucency was smaller, consistent with progress in healing. A subsequent 5-month CBCT image (**D**, corrected sagittal view) showed continued healing. Consistent with the as low as reasonably achievable (ALARA) principle, no PA radiograph was exposed. (Data acquired and reformatted at 0.076 mm voxel size using a CS 9000 3D unit [Carestream Dental, Atlanta, Ga].)

established[33]; however, new associations between AP and systemic health should be predicated on research that uses CBCT in the detection of endodontic disease.[193]

IMPLANT SITE ASSESSMENTS

Successful endosseous implant site assessment requires the development of a prosthetically driven approach,[130b] with special emphasis on the evaluation of bone volume, the osseous topography, and the location of anatomic structures in relation to positioning of the implant. The AAOMR has published advisory recommendations suggesting all radiographic studies should interface with the dental and medical histories, clinical examinations, and treatment planning. Panoramic radiography, which may be supplemented by PA radiography, should be used for initial imaging assessments. Cross-sectional imaging, including CBCT, should not be used as an initial imaging examination. The AAOMR affirms the need for cross-sectional imaging in the preoperative diagnostic phase, recommending CBCT because it provides the highest diagnostic yield at an acceptable radiation dose risk. CBCT should be used at the smallest FOV necessary, with optimized technique factors, to minimize radiation dose in accordance with the ALARA principle.[177a]

CBCT allows for precise planning and delivery of implants that can reproduce the anatomy with submillimetric accuracy, leading to improved outcomes.[171] The use of CBCT to assess linear measurements, proximity to vital anatomic structures, mapping of the alveolar ridge topography, and fabrication of surgical guides is supported by the dental literature. The use of CBCT to gauge bone density, provide intraoperative surgical navigation, and assess implant integration is generally considered an area that requires further research.[17]

Virtual implant planning using CBCT data allows clinicians to visualize the result before the commencement of treatment, facilitating the virtual investigation of multiple treatment scenarios until the best plan is attained. The evaluation of bone dimensions, bone quality, the long axis of the alveolar bone, internal anatomy, and jaw boundaries; the detection of pathologic features; and the transfer of radiographic information are the main imaging goals. Pathoses of the jaws, such as retained root tips, inflammatory lesions, cysts, and tumors, in addition to extraoral structures, such as the sinuses and temporomandibular joints (TMJs), must also be assessed.[80] CBCT imaging should be considered to evaluate implant sites in the region of teeth with a high likelihood of periradicular pathosis.[200]

IMAGE PERCEPTION AND VIEWING ENVIRONMENT

Medical image perception is an important area of knowledge, and ongoing research relies on an understanding of perceptual issues, such as psychological factors, dwell time, visual search physiology, search tactics, appreciation for the reading environment, and fatigue factors, to increase search satisfaction. Understanding these issues may improve the ability to interpret and report on dental radiographic findings.[155a]

The increasing use of digital radiography in the dental environment has led to a sea change in workflow and the necessity for new ways to view and document radiographic images. Simple to accomplish, but important to improve, are the viewing conditions for softcopy interpretation, including moderately reduced ambient lighting, ranging from 25 to 40 lux.[110a]

FUTURE OF CBCT

The first decade of the twenty-first century saw the development of a wide range of CBCT applications, especially in dentistry. Lower radiation dose, higher spatial resolution, smaller FOV, and relatively lower cost may contribute to CBCT becoming the standard of care in 3D dentomaxillofacial imaging in selected cases. CBCT systems are increasingly being used in medical applications, such as operating rooms, emergency departments, intensive care units, and private otolaryngology offices. Operating room–based C-arm systems have been in use for a number of years, with applications in interventional angiography, cancer surgery, vascular surgery, orthopedic surgery, neurosurgery, and radiotherapy.[55] Applications in otolaryngology and mammography are common, and imaging of extremities in weight-bearing scenarios is under development. Many of these applications rely on systems that use task-specific protocols that benefit from CBCT's 2D flat panel detectors, which allow for a single rotation of the source to generate a study of the region of interest, as opposed to complex MDCTs that use redundant imaging via multiple slice acquisitions to generate a 3D volume.[164]

The introduction of new, high-performance, flat-panel detectors and software algorithms centering on improving the noise-power spectrum and noise-equivalent quanta will continue to increase the utility of CBCT systems in the future. Areas of research include (1) image perception and image quality assessment, to better understand how physicians and dentists analyze radiographic images and thereby improve diagnostic decision making[172]; (2) iterative reconstruction that uses sophisticated algorithms to reduce artifacts; (3) known-component reconstructions that use a model-based 3D image reconstruction and iterative software to reduce image artifacts in the presence of metallic devices such as screws and implants; (4) image registration to align tissues for image-guided surgery and outcomes assessment,[120] (5) image-guided procedures that provide up-to-the-minute surgical navigation; and (6) segmentation to allow discrimination between normal and diseased tissues and permit volumetric measurements (Fig. 2-28).

CONCLUSIONS

Digital radiography has several advantages and has become an indispensable diagnostic tool for many dentists in daily practice. Once the digital image appears on the monitor, the dental x-ray software allows image enhancement, which should be used with caution and based on the diagnostic task. Inappropriate use of enhancement has been shown to adversely affect diagnosis.[121] If digital radiographs are exported using various software packages created for graphic design and image manipulation, digital information can be altered, added, or removed. The DICOM standard has been accepted as the universal standard for image transmission and archiving, so that each image can be transmitted and stored without the use of proprietary software that would seriously limit its distribution. DICOM ensures that all images are readable in any viewing software without loss of fidelity or diagnostic information. Image enhancement features of digital radiography allow

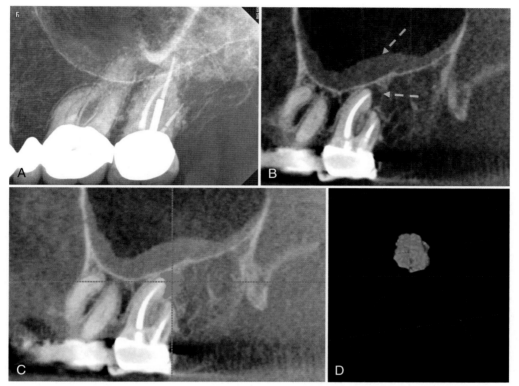

FIG. 2-28 The problem of superimposition of unrelated structures onto the features of interest is reduced when tomographic slices are used instead of images in which an entire volume of data is compressed into a planar image. This PA radiographic image **(A)** of the maxillary left second molar shows no radiographic indicators of pathosis. A contemporaneously exposed CBCT image **(B,** corrected sagittal view) shows a 4.3 × 1.9 mm, well-defined unilocular, noncorticated area of low attenuation centered over the apex of the mesiobuccal root, consistent with a periradicular periodontitis *(yellow arrow)*. There is a moderate mucositis in the region of the maxillary sinus adjacent to this tooth *(blue arrow)*. Experimental semiautomated segmentation of this image using active contour methods (ITK-SNAP) allowed for measurement of the true volume of the lesion **(C)** and for future temporal comparisons based on volumetric measurements **(D)**. This lesion measured 85,112 voxels and 38.1044 cubic mm. (Data acquired and reformatted at 0.076 mm voxel size using a CS 9000 3D unit [Carestream Dental, Atlanta, Ga]; volumetric segmentation and measurement using ITK-SNAP [Radiology Department, School of Medicine, University of Pennsylvania].)

mishandling of images, leading to potential abuse. Published studies illustrate the potential for fraudulent use of digital radiography.[31]

There is a dearth of studies related to the diagnostic performance of the different sensor types currently available on the market. Slight to moderate differences in spatial resolution capabilities exist. With rapid advancement in sensor technology and frequent software upgrades, selection of one system over another for a specific diagnostic task may appear challenging. A review of the most commonly used solid-state sensors notes that most systems perform comparably with intraoral film and also allow for postprocessing of images, which is not possible with film-based images. Other factors that assume significance in this context are the availability of technical and customer support, frequency of both hardware and software upgrades, dimensions of the sensor and its active area, number of sensors needed in a practice (and thus cost issues), the detector quantum efficiency (DQE), and conformance to the DICOM standard for seamless integration with other systems. CCD/CMOS sensors appear to offer the best contrast and spatial resolution, in addition to facilitating

instantaneous image capture, and therefore are recommended for endodontic applications. Careful and appropriate image processing further helps tease out the signal of interest. In an enterprise-wide setting or in larger private practices that have multiple specialty areas, PSP-based sensors may be more cost effective for large volume imaging (e.g., full mouth series of radiographs). However, at least one or two CCD/CMOS-based systems should be available for faster image acquisition, such as for endodontic purposes and intraoperative procedures.

It is recommended that the literature be constantly reviewed for updates on digital radiography and advanced imaging modalities for specific endodontic applications because hardware and software upgrades continue to make rapid progress. Previous studies have shown that most digital images performed comparably to conventional intraoral film for a variety of diagnostic tasks. Most of these studies were done with earlier generation sensors. The advances in sensor technology have resulted in greatly enhanced image quality, and this trend is expected to continue. Also of interest in the future will be the use of task-based, appropriate image processing parameters that result in a reduced radiation dose and significant enhancement of the diagnostic information. Automation of this process will result in faster and more consistent image processing based on the diagnostic task. Such procedures are routinely carried out in medical radiology.

Three-dimensional imaging will continue to be used extensively as sensor characteristics improve and more user-friendly software is introduced. As bit-depth and spatial resolution of images increase, CBCT will continue to be explored for more applications in endodontics. Image interpretation also is important. Occult pathology and incidental findings in adjacent regions can be easily missed or go unrecognized by those who have not received specific training in the interpretation of regional anatomy. Image processing can greatly alter signal characteristics, thus rendering the task fairly challenging. Besides, if other pathoses are discovered, additional imaging may be necessary, including MRI, nuclear medicine studies, or even MDCT for evaluation of soft tissues, with and without the use of contrast.

The advent of 3D imaging has provided the endodontist with tools that were not available until now, facilitating interactive image manipulation and enhancement and thus significantly increasing the amount of information that can be gleaned from a volume. Lack of distortion, magnification, artifacts associated with conventional radiography, and the relative low radiation dose compared to medical-grade CT will result in more clinicians adopting such technology to enable accurate diagnoses and treatment planning, in addition to long-term follow-up and the evaluation of healing. Judicious use of CBCT and all other imaging modalities using ionizing radiation is advocated. The AAE/AAOMR position paper provides recommendations for the use of CBCT in endodontics.[34] That position paper is presented at the end of this chapter.

When the clinician works with different vendor products, it is important to have a quality assurance program in place. This is not being done currently. Additionally, accreditation of stand-alone imaging laboratories is now a requirement for reimbursement of medical and dental diagnostic procedures from government agencies and some major third-party insurance providers. Several states are considering enforcing this requirement to prevent abuse of CBCT.

Likewise, definitive referral criteria are lacking. Indications, contraindications, and choice of alternate imaging modalities need to be considered before CBCT is used. There is a learning curve to this technology, and appropriate positioning, choice of exposure parameters (and thus the effective dose), reconstruction schemes, choice of postprocessing algorithms based on diagnostic task, voxel sizes, and cost must be considered. The literature contains few studies to help us formulate definitive guidelines for the use of CBCT in dentistry.

It is equally important to record the doses associated with each study. Accreditation criteria have been developed by the Intersocietal Accreditation Commission for cone beam CT in dentistry that are useful for ensuring the safe use of these units. The lowest possible dose must be imparted to the patient as part of a radiologic examination to minimize stochastic effects that have no known threshold for expression. No dose can be considered a "safe dose." The benefits of any radiographic study must outweigh the risks. All studies must be interpreted fully because signals from adjacent areas may appear in the volume of interest, including small FOV studies. Retakes can be avoided by adhering to protocol selection based on the task at hand. The ALARA principle must be followed, regardless of the dose values reported by the vendor, to optimize the dose for the specific examination. Use of thyroid collars and lead aprons is recommended in the NCRP guidelines, as long as they do not interfere with image acquisition.

Joint Position Statement of the American Association of Endodontists and the American Academy of Oral and Maxillofacial Radiology on the Use of Cone Beam Computed Tomography in Endodontics: 2015 Update

This statement was prepared by the Special Committee to Revise the Joint AAE/AAOMR Position Statement on Use of CBCT in Endodontics, and approved by the AAE Board of Directors and AAOMR Executive Council in May 2015.

INTRODUCTION

This updated joint position statement of the American Association of Endodontists (AAE) and the American Academy of Oral and Maxillofacial Radiology (AAOMR) is intended to provide scientifically-based guidance to clinicians regarding the use of cone beam computed tomography (CBCT) in endodontic treatment and reflects new developments since the 2010 statement.[1] The guidance in this statement is not intended to substitute for a clinician's independent judgment in light of the conditions and needs of a specific patient.

Endodontic disease adversely affects quality of life and can produce significant morbidity in afflicted patients. Radiography is essential for the successful diagnosis of odontogenic and non-odontogenic pathoses, treatment of the root canal systems of a compromised tooth, biomechanical instrumentation, evaluation of final canal obturation, and assessment of healing.

Until recently, radiographic assessments in endodontic treatment were limited to intraoral and panoramic radiography. These radiographic technologies provide two-dimensional representations of three-dimensional anatomic structures. If any element of the geometric configuration is compromised, the image may demonstrate errors.[2] In more complex cases, radiographic projections with different beam angulations can allow parallax localization. However, complex anatomy and surrounding structures can render interpretation of planar images difficult.

The advent of CBCT has made it possible to visualize the dentition, the maxillofacial skeleton, and the relationship of anatomic structures in three dimensions.[3] CBCT, as with any technology, has known limitations, including a possible higher radiation dose to the patient. Other limitations include

potential for artifact generation, high levels of scatter and noise, and variations in dose distribution within a volume of interest.[4]

CBCT should be used only when the patient's history and a clinical examination demonstrate that the benefits to the patient outweigh the potential risks. CBCT should not be used routinely for endodontic diagnosis or for screening purposes in the absence of clinical signs and symptoms. Clinicians should use CBCT only when the need for imaging cannot be met by lower dose two-dimensional (2D) radiography.

VOLUME SIZE(S)/FIELD OF VIEW

There are numerous CBCT equipment manufacturers, and several models are available. In general, CBCT is categorized into large, medium and limited-volume units based on the size of their "field of view" (FOV). The size of the FOV describes the scan volume of CBCT machines. That volume determines the extent of anatomy included. It is dependent on the detector size and shape, beam projection geometry, and the ability to collimate the beam. To the extent practical, FOV should only slightly exceed the dimensions of the anatomy of interest.

Generally, the smaller the FOV, the lower the dose associated with the study. Beam collimation limits the radiation exposure to the region of interest and helps ensure that an optimal FOV can be selected based on disease presentation. Smaller scan volumes generally produce higher resolution images. Because endodontics relies on detecting small alterations such as disruptions in the periodontal ligament space, optimal resolution should be sought.[5]

The principal limitations of large FOV CBCT imaging are the size of the field irradiated and the reduced resolution compared to intraoral radiographs and limited volume CBCT units with inherent small voxel sizes.[5] The smaller the voxel size, the higher is the spatial resolution. Moreover, the overall scatter generated is reduced due to the limited size of the FOV. Optimization of the exposure protocols keeps doses to a minimum without compromising image quality. If a low-dose protocol can be used for a diagnostic task that requires lower resolution, it should be employed, absent strong indications to the contrary.

In endodontics, the area of interest is limited and determined prior to imaging. For most endodontic applications, limited FOV CBCT is preferred to medium or large FOV CBCT because there is less radiation dose to the patient, higher spatial resolution, and shorter volumes to be interpreted.

DOSE CONSIDERATIONS

Selection of the most appropriate imaging protocol for the diagnostic task must be consistent with the ALARA principles that every effort should be made to reduce the effective radiation dose to the patient "as low as reasonably achievable." Because radiation dose for a CBCT study is higher than that for an intraoral radiograph, clinicians must consider overall radiation dose over time. For example, will acquiring a CBCT study now eliminate the need for additional imaging procedures in the future? It is recommended to use the smallest possible FOV, the smallest voxel size, the lowest mA setting (depending on the patient's size), and the shortest exposure time in conjunction with a pulsed exposure-mode of acquisition.

If extension of pathoses beyond the area surrounding the tooth apices or a multifocal lesion with possible systemic etiology is suspected, and/or a non-endodontic cause for devitalization of the tooth is established clinically, appropriate larger field of view protocols may be employed on a case-by-case basis.

There is a special concern with overexposure of children (up to and including 18 year-olds) to radiation, especially with the increased use of CT scans in medicine. The AAE and the AAOMR support the Image Gently Campaign led by the Alliance for Radiation Safety in Pediatric Imaging. The goal of the campaign is, "to change practice; to raise awareness of the opportunities to lower radiation dose in the imaging of children." Information on use of CT is available at http://www.imagegently.org/Procedures/ComputedTomography.aspx

INTERPRETATION

If a clinician has a question regarding image interpretation, it should be referred to an oral and maxillofacial radiologist.[6]

RECOMMENDATIONS

The following recommendations are for limited FOV CBCT scans.

Diagnosis

Endodontic diagnosis is dependent upon thorough evaluation of the patient's chief complaint, history, and clinical and radiographic examination. Preoperative radiographs are an essential part of the diagnostic phase of endodontic therapy. Accurate diagnostic imaging supports the clinical diagnosis.

Recommendation 1: Intraoral radiographs should be considered the imaging modality of choice in the evaluation of the endodontic patient.

Recommendation 2: Limited FOV CBCT should be considered the imaging modality of choice for diagnosis in patients who present with contradictory or non-specific clinical signs and symptoms associated with untreated or previously endodontically-treated teeth.

Rationale:

◆ In some cases, the clinical and planar radiographic examinations are inconclusive. Inability to confidently determine the etiology of endodontic pathosis may be attributed to limitations in both clinical vitality testing and intraoral radiographs to detect odontogenic pathoses. CBCT imaging has the ability to detect periapical pathosis before it is apparent on 2D radiographs.[7]

◆ Preoperative factors such as the presence and true size of a periapical lesion play an important role in endodontic treatment outcome. Success, when measured by radiographic criteria, is higher when teeth are endodontically treated before radiographic signs of periapical disease are detected.[8]

◆ Previous findings have been validated in clinical studies in which primary endodontic disease detected with intraoral radiographs and CBCT was 20% and 48%, respectively. Several clinical studies had similar findings, although with slightly different percentages.[9,10] Ex vivo experiments in which simulated periapical lesions were created yielded similar results.[11,12] Results of in vivo animal studies, using histologic assessments as the gold standard also showed similar results observed in human clinical and ex-vivo studies.[13]

◆ Persistent intraoral pain following root canal therapy often presents a diagnostic challenge. An example is persistent dentoalveolar pain also known as atypical odontalgia.[14] The diagnostic yield of conventional intraoral radiographs and CBCT scans was evaluated in the differentiation between patients presenting with suspected atypical odontalgia vs. symptomatic apical periodontitis, without radiographic evidence of periapical bone destruction.[15] CBCT imaging detected 17% more teeth with periapical bone loss than conventional radiography.

Initial Treatment

Preoperative:

Recommendation 3: Limited FOV CBCT should be considered the imaging modality of choice for initial treatment of teeth with the potential for extra canals and suspected complex morphology, such as mandibular anterior teeth, and maxillary and mandibular premolars and molars, and dental anomalies.

Intraoperative:

Recommendation 4: If a preoperative CBCT has not been taken, limited FOV CBCT should be considered as the imaging modality of choice for intra-appointment identification and localization of calcified canals.

Postoperative:

Recommendation 5: Intraoral radiographs should be considered the imaging modality of choice for immediate postoperative imaging.

Rationale:

◆ Anatomical variations exist among different types of teeth. The success of non-surgical root canal therapy depends on identification of canals, cleaning, shaping and obturation of root canal systems as well as quality of the final restoration.

- 2D imaging does not consistently reveal the actual number of roots and canals. In studies, data acquired by CBCT showed a very strong correlation between sectioning and histologic examination.[16,17]
- In a 2013 study, CBCT showed higher mean values of specificity and sensitivity when compared to intraoral radiographic assessments in the detection of the MB2 canal.[18]

Non-Surgical Retreatment

Recommendation 6: Limited FOV CBCT should be considered the imaging modality of choice if clinical examination and 2D intraoral radiography are inconclusive in the detection of vertical root fracture (VRF).

Rationale:

- In non-surgical retreatment, the presence of a vertical root fracture significantly decreases prognosis. In the majority of cases, the indication of a vertical root fracture is more often due to the specific pattern of bone loss and periodontal ligament space enlargement than direct visualization of the fracture. CBCT may be recommended for the diagnosis of vertical root fracture in unrestored teeth when clinical signs and symptoms exist.
- Higher sensitivity and specificity were observed in a clinical study where the definitive diagnosis of vertical root fracture was confirmed at the time of surgery to validate CBCT findings, with sensitivity being 88% and specificity 75%.[19] Several case series studies have concluded that CBCT is a useful tool for the diagnosis of vertical root fractures. In vivo and laboratory studies[20,21] evaluating CBCT in the detection of vertical root fractures agreed that sensitivity, specificity, and accuracy of CBCT were generally higher and reproducible. The detection of fractures was significantly higher for all CBCT systems when compared to intraoral radiographs. However, these results should be interpreted with caution because detection of vertical root fracture is dependent on the size of the fracture, presence of artifacts caused by obturation materials and posts, and the spatial resolution of the CBCT.

Recommendation 7: Limited FOV CBCT should be the imaging modality of choice when evaluating the non-healing of previous endodontic treatment to help determine the need for further treatment, such as non-surgical, surgical or extraction.

Recommendation 8: Limited FOV CBCT should be the imaging modality of choice for non-surgical re-treatment to assess endodontic treatment complications, such as overextended root canal obturation material, separated endodontic instruments, and localization of perforations.

Rationale:

- It is important to evaluate the factors that impact the outcome of root canal treatment. The outcome predictors

identified with periapical radiographs and CBCT were evaluated by Liang et al.[22] The results showed that periapical radiographs detected periapical lesions in 18 roots (12%) as compared to 37 on CBCT scans (25%). 80% of apparently short root fillings based on intraoral radiographs images appeared flush on CBCT. Treatment outcome, length and density of root fillings and outcome predictors determined by CBCT showed different values when compared with intraoral radiographs.

- Accurate treatment planning is an essential part of endodontic retreatment. Incorrect, delayed or inadequate endodontic diagnosis and treatment planning places the patient at risk and may result in unnecessary treatment. Treatment planning decisions using CBCT versus intraoral radiographs were compared to the gold standard diagnosis.[23] An accurate diagnosis was reached in 36%-40% of the cases with intraoral radiographs compared to 76%-83% with CBCT. A high level of misdiagnosis was noted in invasive cervical resorption and vertical root fracture. In this study, the examiners altered their treatment plan after reviewing the CBCT in 56%-62.2% of the cases, thus indicating the significant influence of CBCT.

Surgical Retreatment

Recommendation 9: Limited FOV CBCT should be considered as the imaging modality of choice for pre-surgical treatment planning to localize root apex/apices and to evaluate the proximity to adjacent anatomical structures.

Rationale:

The use of CBCT has been recommended for treatment planning of endodontic surgery.[24,25] CBCT visualization of the true extent of periapical lesions and their proximity to important vital structures and anatomical landmarks is superior to that of periapical radiographs.

Special Conditions

a. Implant Placement:

Recommendation 10: Limited FOV CBCT should be considered as the imaging modality of choice for surgical placement of implants.[26]

b. Traumatic Injuries:

Recommendation 11: Limited FOV CBCT should be considered the imaging modality of choice for diagnosis and management of limited dento-alveolar trauma, root fractures, luxation, and/or displacement of teeth and localized alveolar fractures, in the absence of other maxillofacial or soft tissue injury that may require other advanced imaging modalities.[27]

c. Resorptive Defects:

Recommendation 12: Limited FOV CBCT is the imaging modality of choice in the localization and differentiation of external and internal resorptive defects and the determination of appropriate treatment and prognosis.[28,29]

REFERENCES

1. American Association of Endodontists; American Academy of Oral and Maxillofacial Radiology. Use of cone-beam computed tomography in endodontics Joint Position Statement of the American Association of Endodontists and the American Academy of Oral and Maxillofacial Radiology. Oral Surg Oral Med Oral Pathol Oral Radiol Endod 2011;111(2):234-7.
2. Grondahl HG, Huumonen S. Radiographic manifestations of periapical inflammatory lesions. Endodontic Topics 2004;8:55-67.
3. Patel S, Durack C, Abella F, Shemesh H, Roig M, Lemberg K. Cone beam computed tomography in Endodontics—a review. Int Endod J 2015;48:3-15.
4. Suomalainen A, Pakbaznejad Esmaeili E, Robinson S. Dentomaxillofacial imaging with panoramic views and cone beam CT. Insights imaging 2015;6:1-16.
5. Venskutonis T, Plotino G, Juodzbalys G, Mickevičienė L. The importance of cone-beam computed tomography in the management of endodontic problems: a review of the literature. J Endod 2014;40(12):1895-901.
6. Carter L, Farman AG, Geist J, Scarfe WC, Angelopoulos C, Nair MK, Hildebolt CF, Tyndall D, Shrout M. American Academy of Oral and Maxillofacial Radiology executive opinion statement on performing and interpreting diagnostic cone beam computed tomography. Oral Surg Oral Med Oral Pathol Oral Radiol Endod 2008;106(4):561-2.
7. De Paula-Silva FW, Wu MK, Leonardo MR, da Silva LA, Wesselink PR. Accuracy of periapical radiography and cone-beam computed tomography scans in diagnosing apical periodontitis using histopathological findings as a gold standard. J Endod 2009;35(7):1009-12.
8. Friedman S. Prognosis of initial endodontic therapy. Endodontic Topics 2002;2:59-98.
9. Patel S, Wilson R, Dawood A, Mannocci F. The detection of periapical pathosis using periapical radiography and cone beam computed tomography—part 1: preoperative status. Int Endod J 2012;8:702-10.
10. Abella F, Patel S, Duran-Sindreu F, Mercad M, Bueno R, Roig M. Evaluating the periapical status of teeth with irreversible pulpitis by using cone-beam computed tomography scanning and periapical radiographs. J Endod 2012;38(12):1588-91.

11. Cheung G, Wei L, McGrath C. Agreement between periapical radiographs and cone-beam computed tomography for assessment of periapical status of root filled molar teeth. Int Endod J 2013;46(10):889-95.
12. Sogur E, Grondahl H, Bakst G, Mert A. Does a combination of two radiographs increase accuracy in detecting acid-induced periapical lesions and does it approach the accuracy of cone-beam computed tomography scanning? J Endod 2012;38(2):131-6.
13. Patel S, Dawood A, Mannocci F, Wilson R, Pitt Ford T. Detection of periapical bone defects in human jaws using cone beam computed tomography and intraoral radiography. Int Endod J 2009;42(6):507-15.
14. Nixdorf D, Moana-Filho E. Persistent dento-alveolar pain disorder (PDAP): Working towards a better understanding. Rev Pain 2011;5(4):18-27.
15. Pigg M, List T, Petersson K, Lindh C, Petersson A. Diagnostic yield of conventional radiographic and cone-beam computed tomographic images in patients with atypical odontalgia. Int Endod J 2011;44(12):1365-2591.
16. Blattner TC, Goerge N, Lee CC, Kumar V, Yelton CGJ. Efficacy of CBCT as a modality to accurately identify the presence of second mesiobuccal canals in maxillary first and second molars: a pilot study. J Endod 2010;36(5):867-70.
17. Michetti J, Maret D, Mallet J-P, Diemer F. Validation of cone beam computed tomography as a tool to explore root canal anatomy. J Endod 2010;36(7):1187-90.
18. Vizzotto MB, Silveira PF, Arús NA, Montagner F, Gomes BP, Da Silveira HE. CBCT for the assessment of second mesiobuccal (MB2) canals in maxillary molar teeth: effect of voxel size and presence of root filling. Int Endod J 2013;46(9):870-6.
19. Edlund M, Nair MK, Nair UP. Detection of vertical root fractures by using cone-beam computed tomography: a clinical study. J Endod 2011;37(6):768-72.
20. Metska ME, Aartman IH, Wesselink PR, Özok AR. Detection of vertical root fracture in vivo in endodontically treated teeth by cone-beam computed tomography scans. J Endod 2012;38(10):1344-7.
21. Brady E, Mannocci F, Wilson R, Brown J, Patel S. A comparison of CBCT and periapical radiography for

the detection of vertical root fractures in non-endodontically treated teeth. Int Endod J 2014;47(8):735-46.
22. Liang H, Li Gang, Wesselink P, Wu M. Endodontic outcome predictors identified with periapical radiographs and cone-beam computed tomography scans. J Endod 2011;37(3):326-31.
23. Ee J, Fayad IM, Johnson B. Comparison of endodontic diagnosis and treatment planning decisions using cone-beam volumetric tomography versus periapical radiography. J Endod 2014;40(7):910-6.
24. Venskutonis T, Plotino G, Tocci L, Gambarini G, Maminskas J, Juodzbalys G. Periapical and endodontic status scale based on periapical bone lesions and endodontic treatment quality evaluation using cone-beam computed tomography. J Endod 2015;41(2):190-6.
25. Low KM, Dula K, Bürgin W, Arx T. Comparison of periapical radiography and limited cone-beam tomography in posterior maxillary teeth referred for apical surgery. J Endod 2008;34(5):557-62.
26. Tyndall D, Price J, Tetradis S, Ganz S, Hildebolt C, Scarf W. Position statement of the American Academy of Oral and Maxillofacial Radiology on selection criteria for the use of radiology in dental implantology with emphasis on cone beam computed tomography. Oral Surg Oral Med Oral Pathol Oral Radiol 2012June;113(6):817-26.
27. May JJ, Cohenca N, Peters OA. Contemporary management of horizontal root fractures to the permanent dentition: diagnosis, radiologic assessment to include cone-beam computed tomography. Pediatric Dentistry 2013;35:120-4.
28. Estrela C, Bueno MR, De Alencar AH, Mattar R, Valladares Neto J, Azevedo BC, De Araújo Estrela CR. Method to evaluate Inflammatory Root Resorption by using Cone Beam computed tomography. J Endod 2009;35(11):1491-7.
29. Durack C, Patel S, Davies J, Wilson R, Mannocci F. Diagnostic accuracy of small volume cone beam computed tomography and intraoral periapical radiography for the detection of simulated external inflammatory root resorption. Int Endod J 2011Feb;44(2):136-47.

Special Committee to Revise the Joint AAE/AAOMR Position Statement on Use of Limited FOV CBCT in Endodontics

Mohamed I. Fayad, Co-Chair, AAE
Martin D. Levin, AAE
Richard A. Rubinstein, AAE
Craig S. Hirschberg, AAE Board Liaison

Madhu Nair, Co-Chair, AAOMR
Erika Benavides, AAOMR
Axel Ruprecht, AAOMR
Sevin Barghan, AAOMR

REFERENCES

1. Affairs ADACoS: An update on radiographic practices: information and recommendations, ADA Council on Scientific Affairs, *J Am Dent Assoc* 132:235, 2001.
2. Akdeniz BG, Sogur E: An ex vivo comparison of conventional and digital radiography for perceived image quality of root fillings, *Int Endod J* 38:397, 2005.
3. Alavi AM, Opasanon A, Ng YL, Gulabivala K: Root and canal morphology of Thai maxillary molars, *Int Endod J* 35:478, 2002.
4. Al-Fouzan KS: Incidence of rotary ProFile instrument fracture and the potential for bypassing in vivo, *Int Endod J* 36:864, 2003.
5. Al-Hadlaq SM, Al-Turaiki SA, Al-Sulami U, Saad AY: Efficacy of a new brush-covered irrigation needle in removing root canal debris: a scanning electron microscopic study, *J Endod* 32:1181, 2006.

6. American Association of Endodontists: *Glossary of endodontic terms*, ed 7, Chicago, 2003, The Association.
7. American Dental Association moves forward on electronic standards, *ADA News* 30, August 1999.
8. Anderson LC, Kosinski TF, Mentag PJ: A review of the intraosseous course of the nerves of the mandible, *J Oral Implantol* 17:394, 1991.
9. Andreasen FM, Andreasen JO: Crown fractures. *Textbook and color atlas of traumatic injuries to the teeth*, ed 3, Copenhagen, 1994, Munksgaard, pp 257-277.
10. Andreasen FM, Sewerin I, Mandel U, Andreasen JO: Radiographic assessment of simulated root resorption cavities, *Endod Dent Traumatol* 3:21, 1987.
11. Andreasen JO, Ahrensburg SS, Tsilingaridis G: Root fractures: the influence of type of healing and location of

fracture on tooth survival rates: an analysis of 492 cases, *Dent Traumatol* 28:404, 2012.
12. Andreasen JO, Andreasen FM, Andersson L: *Textbook and color atlas of traumatic injuries to the teeth*, Copenhagen, 2007, Munksgaard/John Wiley & Sons.
13. Andreasen JO, Ravn JJ: Epidemiology of traumatic dental injuries to primary and permanent teeth in a Danish population sample, *Int J Oral Surg* 1:235, 1972.
14. Backman B, Wahlin YB: Variations in number and morphology of permanent teeth in 7-year-old Swedish children, *Int J Paediatr Dent* 11:11, 2001.
15. Bakland LK: Root resorption, *Dent Clin North Am* 36:491, 1992.
16. Ball RL, Barbizam JV, Cohenca N: Intraoperative endodontic applications of cone beam computed tomography, *J Endod* 39:548, 2013.

16a. Beck-Mannagetta J, Necek D, Grasserbauer M: Solitary aspergillosis of maxillary sinus: a complication of dental treatment, *Lancet* 2:1260, 1983.

17. Benavides E, Rios HF, Ganz SD, et al: Use of cone beam computed tomography in implant dentistry: the International Congress of Oral Implantologists consensus report, *Implant Dent* 21:78, 2012.

18. Bender IB: Factors influencing the radiographic appearance of bony lesions, *J Endod* 8:161, 1982.

19. Bergenholtz G: Micro-organisms from necrotic pulp of traumatized teeth, *Odontol Revy* 25:347, 1974.

20. Borg E, Kallqvist A, Grondahl K, Grondahl HG: Film and digital radiography for detection of simulated root resorption cavities, *Oral Surg Oral Med Oral Pathol Oral Radiol Endod* 86:110, 1998.

21. Bornstein MM, Lauber R, Sendi P, von Arx T: Comparison of periapical radiography and limited cone beam computed tomography in mandibular molars for analysis of anatomical landmarks before apical surgery, *J Endod* 37:151, 2011.

22. Bornstein MM, Wasmer J, Sendi P, et al: Characteristics and dimensions of the schneiderian membrane and apical bone in maxillary molars referred for apical surgery: a comparative radiographic analysis using limited cone beam computed tomography, *J Endod* 38:51, 2012.

23. Bornstein MM, Wolner-Hanssen AB, Sendi P, von Arx T: Comparison of intraoral radiography and limited cone beam computed tomography for the assessment of root-fractured permanent teeth, *Dent Traumatol* 25:571, 2009.

24. Bouillaguet S, Wataha JC, Tay FR, et al: Initial in vitro biological response to contemporary endodontic sealers, *J Endod* 32:989, 2006.

25. Bratel J, Jontell M, Dahlgren U, Bergenholtz G: Effects of root canal sealers on immunocompetent cells in vitro and in vivo, *Int Endod J* 31:178, 1998.

26. Brooks JK, Kleinman JW: Retrieval of extensive gutta-percha extruded into the maxillary sinus: use of 3-dimensional cone beam computed tomography, *J Endod* 39:1189, 2013.

27. Brynolf I: A histological and roentgenological study of periapical region of human upper incisors, *Odontol Revy* 18(Suppl 11):1, 1967.

28. Bueno MR, De Carvalhosa AA, Castro PH, et al: Mesenchymal chondrosarcoma mimicking apical periodontitis, *J Endod* 34:1415, 2008.

29. Bueno MR, Estrela C, De Figueiredo JA, Azevedo BC: Map-reading strategy to diagnose root perforations near metallic intracanal posts by using cone beam computed tomography, *J Endod* 37:85, 2011.

30. Burger CL, Mork TO, Hutter JW, Nicoll B: Direct digital radiography versus conventional radiography for estimation of canal length in curved canals, *J Endod* 25:260, 1999.

31. Calberson FL, Hommez GM, De Moor RJ: Fraudulent use of digital radiography: methods to detect and protect digital radiographs, *J Endod* 34:530, 2008.

32. Caliskan MK, Turkun M: Prognosis of permanent teeth with internal resorption: a clinical review, *Endod Dent Traumatol* 13:75, 1997.

33. Caplan DJ: Epidemiologic issues in studies of association between apical periodontitis and systemic health, *Endod Topic* 8:15, 2008.

34. Special Committee to Revise the Joint AAE/AAOMR Position Statement on Use of CBCT in Endodontics: Joint position statement of the American Association of Endodontists and the American Academy of Oral and Maxillofacial Radiology on the use of cone beam computed tomography in endodontics: 2015 Update. Approved by the AAE Board of Directors and AAOMR Executive Council, May, 2015.

35. Claeys V, Wackens G: Bifid mandibular canal: literature review and case report, *Dentomaxillofac Radiol* 34:55, 2005.

36. Cohenca N, Simon JH, Mathur A, Malfaz JM: Clinical indications for digital imaging in dento-alveolar trauma. Part 2. Root resorption, *Dent Traumatol* 23:105, 2007.

37. Cohenca N, Simon JH, Roges R, et al: Clinical indications for digital imaging in dentoalveolar trauma. Part 1. Traumatic injuries, *Dent Traumatol* 23:95, 2007.

38. Cotton TP, Geisler TM, Holden DT, et al: Endodontic applications of cone beam volumetric tomography, *J Endod* 33:1121, 2007.

39. Crump MC, Natkin E: Relationship of broken root canal instruments to endodontic case prognosis: a clinical investigation, *J Am Dent Assoc* 80:1341, 1970.

40. Cuje J, Bargholz C, Hulsmann M: The outcome of retained instrument removal in a specialist practice, *Int Endod J* 43:545, 2010.

41. Davidovich E, Heling I, Fuks ABL: The fate of a mid-root fracture: a case report, *Dent Traumatol* 21:170, 2005.

42. Day PF, Duggal MSL: A multicentre investigation into the role of structured histories for patients with tooth avulsion at their initial visit to a dental hospital, *Dent Traumatol* 19:243, 2003.

43. de Paula-Silva FW, Wu MK, Leonardo MR, et al: Accuracy of periapical radiography and cone beam computed tomography scans in diagnosing apical periodontitis using histopathological findings as a gold standard, *J Endod* 35:1009, 2009.

44. Di Fiore PM, Genov KA, Komaroff E, et al: Nickel-titanium rotary instrument fracture: a clinical practice assessment, *Int Endod J* 39:700, 2006.

45. Diangelis AJ, Andreasen JO, Ebeleseder KA, et al: International Association of Dental Traumatology guidelines for the management of traumatic dental injuries. Part 1. Fractures and luxations of permanent teeth, *Dent Traumatol* 28:2, 2012.

46. DICOM: Digital imaging and communications in medicine (DICOM). Part 1. Introduction and overview. Accessed July 26, 2009. Available at: ftp://medical.nema.org/medical/dicom/2008/08_01pu.pdf.

47. Durack C, Patel S, Davies J, et al: Diagnostic accuracy of small volume cone beam computed tomography and intraoral periapical radiography for the detection of simulated external inflammatory root resorption, *Int Endod J* 44:136, 2011.

48. Edlund M, Nair MK, Nair UP: Detection of vertical root fractures by using cone beam computed tomography: a clinical study, *J Endod* 37:768, 2011.

49. Eikenberg S, Vandre R: Comparison of digital dental x-ray systems with self-developing film and manual processing for endodontic file length determination, *J Endod* 26:65, 2000.

50. Eraso FE, Analoui M, Watson AB, Rebeschini R: Impact of lossy compression on diagnostic accuracy of radiographs for periapical lesions, *Oral Surg Oral Med Oral Pathol Oral Radiol Endod* 93:621, 2002.

51. Escoda-Francoli J, Canalda-Sahli C, Soler A, et al: Inferior alveolar nerve damage because of overextended endodontic material: a problem of sealer cement biocompatibility? *J Endod* 33:1484, 2007.

52. Estrela C, Bueno MR, De Alencar AH, et al: Method to evaluate inflammatory root resorption by using cone beam computed tomography, *J Endod* 35:1491, 2009.

53. Estrela C, Bueno MR, Leles CR, et al: Accuracy of cone beam computed tomography and panoramic and periapical radiography for detection of apical periodontitis, *J Endod* 34:273, 2008.

54. Eversole LR, Leider AS, Hansen LS: Ameloblastomas with pronounced desmoplasia, *J Oral Maxillofac Surg* 42:735, 1984.

55. Fahrig R, Fox AJ, Lownie S, Holdsworth DW: Use of a C-arm system to generate true three-dimensional computed rotational angiograms: preliminary in vitro and in vivo results, *Am J Neuroradiol* 18:1507, 1997.

56. Faitaroni LA, Bueno MR, De Carvalhosa AA, et al: Ameloblastoma suggesting large apical periodontitis, *J Endod* 34:216, 2008.

57. Fan B, Gao Y, Fan W, Gutmann JL: Identification of a C-shaped canal system in mandibular second molars. II. The effect of bone image superimposition and intraradicular contrast medium on radiograph interpretation, *J Endod* 34:160, 2008.

58. Farman AG, Avant SL, Scarfe WC, et al: In vivo comparison of Visualix-2 and Ektaspeed Plus in the assessment of periradicular lesion dimensions, *Oral Surg Oral Med Oral Pathol Oral Radiol Endod* 85:203, 1998.

59. Feely L, Mackie IC, Macfarlane T: An investigation of root-fractured permanent incisor teeth in children, *Dent Traumatol* 19:52, 2003.

59a. Fletcher RH, Fletcher SW, editors: *Clinical epidemiology: the essentials*, Baltimore, 2005, Lippincott Williams & Wilkins.

60. Forman GH, Rood JP: Successful retrieval of endodontic material from the inferior alveolar nerve, *J Dent* 5:47, 1997.

61. Fuss Z, Lustig J, Tamse A: Prevalence of vertical root fractures in extracted endodontically treated teeth, *Int Endod J* 32:283, 1999.

62. Gassner R, Bosch R, Tuli T, Emshoff R: Prevalence of dental trauma in 6000 patients with facial injuries: implications for prevention, *Oral Surg Oral Med Oral Pathol Oral Radiol Endod* 87:27, 1999.

63. Gencoglu N, Helvacioglu D: Comparison of the different techniques to remove fractured endodontic instruments from root canal systems, *Eur J Dent* 3:90, 2009.

64. Geurtsen W, Leyhausen G: Biological aspects of root canal filling materials: histocompatibility, cytotoxicity, and mutagenicity, *Clin Oral Investig* 1:5, 1997.

65. Glendor U: Epidemiology of traumatic dental injuries: a 12 year review of the literature, *Dent Traumatol* 24:603, 2008.

66. Goldberg F, De Silvio A, Dreyer C: Radiographic assessment of simulated external root resorption cavities in maxillary incisors, *Endod Dent Traumatol* 14:133, 1998.

67. Gomes AP, de Araujo EA, Goncalves SE, Kraft R: Treatment of traumatized permanent incisors with crown and root fractures: a case report, *Dent Traumatol* 17:236, 2001.

68. Gonzalez-Martin M, Torres-Lagares D, Gutierrez-Perez JL, Segura-Egea JJ: Inferior alveolar nerve paresthesia after overfilling of endodontic sealer into the mandibular canal, *J Endod* 36:1419, 2010.

69. Goodis HE, Rossall JC, Kahn AJ: Endodontic status in older US adults: report of a survey, *J Am Dent Assoc* 132:1525; quiz, 95; 2001.

70. Green TL, Walton RE, Taylor JK, Merrell P: Radiographic and histologic periapical findings of root canal treated teeth in cadaver, *Oral Surg Oral Med Oral Pathol Oral Radiol Endod* 83:707, 1997.

71. Grotz KA, Al-Nawas B, de Aguiar EG, et al: Treatment of injuries to the inferior alveolar nerve after endodontic procedures, *Clin Oral Investig* 2:73, 1998.

71a. Guivarc'h M, Ordioni U, Catherine J-H, et al: Implications of endodontic-related sinus aspergillosis in a patient treated by infliximab: a case report, *J Endod* 41:125, 2015.

72. Gulabivala K, Aung TH, Alavi A, Ng YL: Root and canal morphology of Burmese mandibular molars, *Int Endod J* 34:359, 2001.

73. Gulabivala K, Opasanon A, Ng YL, Alavi A: Root and canal morphology of Thai mandibular molars, *Int Endod J* 35:56, 2002.

74. Gutteridge DL: The use of radiographic techniques in the diagnosis and management of periodontal diseases, *Dentomaxillofac Radiol* 24:107, 1995.

75. Hassan B, Metska ME, Ozok AR, et al: Detection of vertical root fractures in endodontically treated teeth by a cone beam computed tomography scan, *J Endod* 35:719, 2009.

76. Hassan B, Metska ME, Ozok AR, et al: Comparison of five cone beam computed tomography systems for the detection of vertical root fractures, *J Endod* 36:126, 2010.

77. Hargreaves KM, Geisler T, Henry M, Wang Y: Regeneration potential of the young permanent tooth: what does the future hold? *Pediatr Dent* 30:253, 2008.

78. Hargreaves KM, Giesler T, Henry M, Wang Y: Regeneration potential of the young permanent tooth: what does the future hold? *J Endod* 34(Suppl 7):S51, 2008.

79. Hatcher DC: Operational principles for cone beam computed tomography, *J Am Dent Assoc* 141(Suppl 3):3S, 2010.

80. Hatcher DC: Cone beam CT for pre-surgical assessment of implant sites, *AADMRT Newsletter*, Summer, 2005. Accessed August 2, 2013. Available at: http://aadmrt.com/static.aspx?content=currents/hatcher_summer_05.

80a. Headache Classification Subcommittee, International Headache Society: The international classification of headache disorders: second edition, *Cephalgia* 24:9, 2004.

81. Hopp RN, Marchi MT, Kellermann MG, et al: Lymphoma mimicking a dental periapical lesion, *Leuk Lymphoma* 53:1008, 2012.

82. Pew Research Center: US population projections: 2005-2050. Available at: www.pewhispanic.org/2008/02/11/us-population-projections-2005-2050.

83. Hulsmann M, Rummelin C, Schafers F: Root canal cleanliness after preparation with different endodontic handpieces and hand instruments: a comparative SEM investigation, *J Endod* 23:301, 1997.

84. Iikubo M, Kobayashi K, Mishima A, et al: Accuracy of intraoral radiography, multidetector helical CT, and limited cone beam CT for the detection of horizontal tooth root fracture, *Oral Surg Oral Med Oral Pathol Oral Radiol Endod* 108:e70, 2009.

85. Ingle JI: A standardized endodontic technique utilizing newly designed instruments and filling materials, *Oral Surg Oral Med Oral Pathol* 14:83, 1961.

86. Jacobs R, Mraiwa N, Van Steenberghe D, et al: Appearance of the mandibular incisive canal on panoramic radiographs, *Surg Radiol Anat* 26:329, 2004.

87. Jung M, Lommel D, Klimek J: The imaging of root canal obturation using micro-CT, *Int Endod J* 38:617, 2005.

88. Kakehashi S, Stanley HR, Fitzgerald RJ: The effects of surgical exposures of dental pulps in germ-free and conventional laboratory rats, *Oral Surg Oral Med Oral Pathol* 20:340, 1965.

89. Kamburoglu K, Ilker Cebeci AR, Grondahl HG: Effectiveness of limited cone beam computed tomography in the detection of horizontal root fracture, *Dent Traumatol* 25:256, 2009.

90. Kamburoglu K, Kursun S: A comparison of the diagnostic accuracy of CBCT images of different voxel resolutions used to detect simulated small internal resorption cavities, *Int Endod J* 43:798, 2010.

91. Kerekes K, Tronstad L: Long-term results of endodontic treatment performed with a standardized technique, *J Endod* 5:83, 1979.

92. Kim E, Kim KD, Roh BD, et al: Computed tomography as a diagnostic aid for extracanal invasive resorption, *J Endod* 29:463, 2003.

93. Kim TS, Caruso JM, Christensen H, Torabinejad M: A comparison of cone beam computed tomography and direct measurement in the examination of the mandibular canal and adjacent structures, *J Endod* 36:1191, 2010.

94. Kitagawa H, Scheetz JP, Farman AG: Comparison of complementary metal oxide semi-conductor and charge-coupled device intraoral x-ray detectors using subjective image quality, *Dentomaxillofac Radiol* 32:408, 2003.

95. Khedmat S, Rouhi N, Drage N, et al: Evaluation of three imaging techniques for the detection of vertical root fractures in the absence and presence of gutta-percha root fillings, *Int Endod J* 45:1004, 2012.

96. Kositbowornchai S, Nuansakul R, Sikram S, et al: Root fracture detection: a comparison of direct digital radiography with conventional radiography, *Dentomaxillofac Radiol* 30:106, 2001.

97. Kovisto T, Ahmad M, Bowles WR: Proximity of the mandibular canal to the tooth apex, *J Endod* 37:311, 2011.

98. Kramer PF, Zembruski C, Ferreira SH, Feldens CA: Traumatic dental injuries in Brazilian preschool children, *Dent Traumatol* 19:299, 2003.

99. Lamus F, Katz JO, Glaros AG: Evaluation of a digital measurement tool to estimate working length in endodontics, *J Contemp Dent Pract* 2:24, 2001.

100. Lee H, Xing L, Davidi R, et al: Improved compressed sensing-based cone beam CT reconstruction using adaptive prior image constraints, *Phys Med Biol* 57:2287, 2012.

101. Leddy BJ, Miles DA, Newton CW, Brown CE Jr: Interpretation of endodontic file lengths using RadioVisiography, *J Endod* 20:542, 1994.

102. Levin L, Trope M: Root resorption. In Hargreaves KM, Goodis HE, editors: *Seltzer and Bender's dental pulp*, Chicago, 2002, Quintessence Publishing, pp 425-448.

103. Li G, Sanderink GC, Welander U, et al: Evaluation of endodontic files in digital radiographs before and after employing three image processing algorithms, *Dentomaxillofac Radiol* 33:6, 2004.

104. Liang YH, Li G, Wesselink PR, Wu MK: Endodontic outcome predictors identified with periapical radiographs and cone beam computed tomography scans, *J Endod* 37:326, 2011.

105. Liedke GS, da Silveira HE, da Silveira HL, et al: Influence of voxel size in the diagnostic ability of cone beam tomography to evaluate simulated external root resorption, *J Endod* 35:233, 2009.

106. Littner MM, Kaffe I, Tamse A, Dicapua P: Relationship between the apices of the lower molars and mandibular canal: a radiographic study, *Oral Surg Oral Med Oral Pathol* 62:595, 1986.

107. Lofthag-Hansen S, Huumonen S, Grondahl K, Grondahl HG: Limited cone beam CT and intraoral radiography for the diagnosis of periapical pathology, *Oral Surg Oral Med Oral Pathol Oral Radiol Endod* 103:114, 2007.

108. Loushine RJ, Weller RN, Kimbrough WF, Potter BJ: Measurement of endodontic file lengths: calibrated versus uncalibrated digital images, *J Endod* 27:779, 2001.

109. Low KM, Dula K, Burgin W, von Arx T: Comparison of periapical radiography and limited cone beam tomography in posterior maxillary teeth referred for apical surgery, *J Endod* 34:557, 2008.

110. Lu Y, Liu Z, Zhang L, et al: Associations between maxillary sinus mucosal thickening and apical periodontitis using cone beam computed tomography scanning: a retrospective study, *J Endod* 38:1069, 2012.

110a. McEntee M, Brennan P, Evanoff M, et al: Optimum ambient lighting conditions for the viewing of softcopy radiological images, *roc. SPIE* 6146, Medical Imaging 2006: Image Perception, Observer Performance, and Technology Assessment, 61460W (March 17, 2006); doi:10.1117/12.660137.

111. Maillet M, Bowles WR, McClanahan SL, et al: Cone beam computed tomography evaluation of maxillary sinusitis, *J Endod* 37:753, 2011.

112. Marmulla R, Wortche R, Muhling J, Hassfeld S: Geometric accuracy of the NewTom 9000 Cone Beam CT, *Dentomaxillofac Radiol* 34:28, 2005.

113. Mehra P, Murad H: Maxillary sinus disease of odontogenic origin, *Otolaryngol Clin North Am* 37:347, 2004.

114. Melo SL, Bortoluzzi EA, Abreu M Jr, et al: Diagnostic ability of a cone beam computed tomography scan to assess longitudinal root fractures in prosthetically treated teeth, *J Endod* 36:1879, 2010.

115. Metska ME, Aartman IH, Wesselink PR, Ozok AR: Detection of vertical root fractures in vivo in endodontically treated teeth by cone beam computed tomography scans, *J Endod* 38:1344, 2012.

116. Miguens SA Jr, Veeck EB, Fontanella VR, da Costa NP: A comparison between panoramic digital and digitized images to detect simulated periapical lesions using radiographic subtraction, *J Endod* 34:1500, 2008.

117. Mikrogeorgis G, Lyroudia K, Molyvdas I, et al: Digital radiograph registration and subtraction: a useful tool for the evaluation of the progress of chronic apical periodontitis, *J Endod* 30:513, 2004.

118. Miles D: *Color atlas of cone beam volumetric imaging for dental applications*, Hanover Park, Ill, 2008, Quintessence.

119. Miles DA, Danforth RA: A clinician's guide to understanding cone beam volumetric imaging. *Academy of Dental Therapeutics and Stomatology*, Special Issue, pp 1-13, 2007. Available at: www.ineedce.com.

120. Mirota DJ, Uneri A, Schafer S, et al: Evaluation of a system for high-accuracy 3D image-based registration of endoscopic video to C-arm cone beam CT for image-guided skull base surgery, *IEEE Trans Med Imaging* 32:1215, 2013.

121. Nair MK, Nair UP: Digital and advanced imaging in endodontics: a review, *J Endod* 33:1, 2007.

122. Nance RS, Tyndall D, Levin LG, Trope M: Diagnosis of external root resorption using TACT (tuned-aperture computed tomography), *Endod Dent Traumatol* 16:24, 2000.

123. Naoum HJ, Chandler NP, Love RM: Conventional versus storage phosphor-plate digital images to visualize the root canal system contrasted with a radiopaque medium, *J Endod* 29:349, 2003.

124. Narayana P, Hartwell GR, Wallace R, Nair UP: Endodontic clinical management of a dens invaginatus case by using a unique treatment approach: a case report, *J Endod* 38:1145, 2012.

125. Neelakantan P, Subbarao C, Subbarao CV: Comparative evaluation of modified canal staining and clearing technique, cone beam computed tomography, peripheral quantitative computed tomography, spiral computed tomography, and plain and contrast medium-enhanced digital radiography in studying root canal morphology, *J Endod* 36:1547, 2010.

126. Neelakantan P, Subbarao C, Subbarao CV, Ravindranath M: Root and canal morphology of mandibular second molars in an Indian population, *J Endod* 36:1319, 2010.

127. Nevares G, Cunha RS, Zuolo ML, Bueno CE: Success rates for removing or bypassing fractured instruments: a prospective clinical study, *J Endod* 38:442, 2012.

128. Ng YL, Aung TH, Alavi A, Gulabivala K: Root and canal morphology of Burmese maxillary molars, *Int Endod J* 34:620, 2001.

129. Nicopoulou-Karayianni K, Bragger U, Patrikiou A, et al: Image processing for enhanced observer agreement in the evaluation of periapical bone changes, *Int Endod J* 35:615, 2002.

130. Nixdorf DR, Moana-Filho EJ, Law AS, et al: Frequency of nonodontogenic pain after endodontic therapy: a systematic review and meta-analysis, *J Endod* 36:1494, 2010.

130a. Nixdorf DR, Moana-Filho EJ, Law AS, et al: Frequency of persistent tooth pain after root canal therapy: a systematic review and meta-analysis, *J Endod* 36:224, 2010.

130b. Norton MR, et al: Guidelines of the Academy of Osseointegration for the provision of dental implants and associated patient care, *Int J Oral Maxillofac Implants* 25:620, 2010.

131. Oehlers FA: Dens invaginatus (dilated composite odontome). II. Associated posterior crown forms and pathogenesis, *Oral Surg Oral Med Oral Pathol* 10:1302, 1957.

131a. Ohrback R, List T, Goulet JP, Svensson P: Recommendations from the International Consensus Workshop: convergence on an orofacial pain taxonomy, *J Oral Rehab* 37:807, 2010.

132. Orhan K, Aksoy U, Kalender A: Cone beam computed tomographic evaluation of spontaneously healed root fracture, *J Endod* 36:1584, 2010.

133. Ozer SY: Detection of vertical root fractures of different thicknesses in endodontically enlarged teeth by cone beam computed tomography versus digital radiography, *J Endod* 36:1245, 2010.

134. Panitvisai P, Parunnit P, Sathorn C, Messer HH: Impact of a retained instrument on treatment outcome: a systematic review and meta-analysis, *J Endod* 36:775, 2010.

135. Parashos P, Gordon I, Messer HH: Factors influencing defects of rotary nickel-titanium endodontic instruments after clinical use, *J Endod* 30:722, 2004.

136. Patel S: New dimensions in endodontic imaging. Part 2. Cone beam computed tomography, *Int Endod J* 42:463, 2009.

137. Patel S: The use of cone beam computed tomography in the conservative management of dens invaginatus: a case report, *Int Endod J* 43:707, 2010.

138. Patel S, Brady E, Wilson R, et al: The detection of vertical root fractures in root filled teeth with periapical radiographs and CBCT scans, *Int Endod J* 46:1140, 2013.

139. Patel S, Dawood A: The use of cone beam computed tomography in the management of external cervical resorption lesions, *Int Endod J* 40:730, 2007.

140. Patel S, Dawood A, Wilson R, et al: The detection and management of root resorption lesions using intraoral radiography and cone beam computed tomography: an in vivo investigation, *Int Endod J* 42:831, 2009.

141. Patel S, Ford TP: Is the resorption external or internal? *Dent Update* 34:218, 2007.

142. Patel S, Kanagasingam S, Pitt Ford T: External cervical resorption: a review, *J Endod* 35:616, 2009.

143. Peters E, Lau M: Histopathologic examination to confirm diagnosis of periapical lesions: a review, *J Can Dent Assoc* 69:598, 2003.

144. Peters OA, Peters CI, Schonenberger K, Barbakow F: ProTaper rotary root canal preparation: effects of canal anatomy on final shape analysed by micro CT, *Int Endod J* 36:86, 2003.

145. Peters OA, Schonenberger K, Laib A: Effects of four Ni-Ti preparation techniques on root canal geometry assessed by microcomputed tomography, *Int Endod J* 34:221, 2001.

146. Piepenbring ME, Potter BJ, Weller RN, Loushine RJ: Measurement of endodontic file lengths: a density profile plot analysis, *J Endod* 26:615, 2000.

146a. Pigg M, List T, Petersson K, Lindh C, et al: Diagnostic yield of conventional radiographic and cone beam computed tomographic images in patients with atypical odontalgia, *Int Endod J* 44:1092, 2011.

147. Pineda F, Kuttler Y: Mesiodistal and buccolingual roentgenographic investigation of 7,275 root canals, *Oral Surg Oral Med Oral Pathol* 33:101, 1972.

148. Pogrel MA: Damage to the inferior alveolar nerve as the result of root canal therapy, *J Am Dent Assoc* 138:65, 2007.

148a. Pope O, Sathorn C, Parashos P: A comparative investigation of cone beam computed tomography and periapical radiography in the diagnosis of a healthy periapex, *J Endod* 40:360, 2014.

149. Renton T: Prevention of iatrogenic inferior alveolar nerve injuries in relation to dental procedures, *Dent Update* 37:350, 2010.

150. Ricucci D, Langeland K: Apical limit of root canal instrumentation and obturation. Part 2. A histological study, *Int Endod J* 31:394, 1998.

151. Rodrigues CD, Estrela C: Traumatic bone cyst suggestive of large apical periodontitis, *J Endod* 34:484, 2008.

152. Rodrigues CD, Villar-Neto MJ, Sobral AP, et al: Lymphangioma mimicking apical periodontitis, *J Endod* 37:91, 2011.

153. Rud J, Omnell KA: Root fractures due to corrosion: diagnostic aspects, *Scand J Dent Res* 78:397, 1970.

154. Ruddle CJ: Endodontic diagnosis, *Dent Today* 21:90-92, 94, 96-101; quiz 01, 78; 2002.

155. Ruddle CJ: Endodontic disinfection-tsunami irrigation, *Endod Prac*, Feb 7, 2008.

155a. Samei E, Krupinski E, editors: *Medical imaging: perception and techniques*, Cambridge, UK, 2010, Cambridge University Press.

156. Scannapieco FA: Position paper of the American Academy of Periodontology: periodontal disease as a potential risk factor for systemic diseases, *J Periodontol* 69:841, 1998.

157. Scarfe WC: Imaging of maxillofacial trauma: evolutions and emerging revolutions, *Oral Surg Oral Med Oral Pathol Oral Radiol Endod* 100(Suppl 2):S75, 2005.

158. Scarfe WC, Levin MD, Gane D, Farman AG: Use of cone beam computed tomography in endodontics, *Int J Dent* 63:45, 2009.

159. Schafer E, Al Behaissi A: pH changes in root dentin after root canal dressing with gutta-percha points containing calcium hydroxide, *J Endod* 26:665, 2000.

160. Schilder H: Cleaning and shaping the root canal, *Dent Clin North Am* 18:269, 1974.

161. Schilder H: Canal debridement and disinfection. In Cohen S, Burns C, editors: *Pathways of the pulp*, St Louis, 1976, Mosby, pp 111-133.

162. Scolozzi P, Lombardi T, Jaques B: Successful inferior alveolar nerve decompression for dysesthesia following endodontic treatment: report of 4 cases treated by mandibular sagittal osteotomy, *Oral Surg Oral Med Oral Pathol Oral Radiol Endod* 97:625, 2004.

163. Sert S, Bayirli GS: Evaluation of the root canal configurations of the mandibular and maxillary permanent teeth by gender in the Turkish population, *J Endod* 30:391, 2004.

164. Siewerdsen JH, Jaffray DA: Cone beam computed tomography with a flat-panel imager: effects of image lag, *Med Phys* 26:2635, 1999.

165. Sharan A, Madjar D: Correlation between maxillary sinus floor topography and related root position of posterior teeth using panoramic and cross-sectional computed tomography imaging, *Oral Surg Oral Med Oral Pathol Oral Radiol Endod* 102:375, 2006.

166. Shemesh H, Cristescu RC, Wesselink PR, Wu MK: The use of cone beam computed tomography and digital periapical radiographs to diagnose root perforations, *J Endod* 37:513, 2011.

167. Simonton JD, Azevedo B, Schindler WG, Hargreaves KM: Age- and gender-related differences in the position of the inferior alveolar nerve by using cone beam computed tomography, *J Endod* 35:944, 2009.

168. Sjogren U, Hagglund B, Sundqvist G, Wing K: Factors affecting the long-term results of endodontic treatment, *J Endod* 16:498, 1990.

169. Sonoda M, Takano M, Miyahara J, Kato H: Computed radiography utilizing scanning laser stimulated luminescence, *Radiology* 148:833, 1983.

170. Spili P, Parashos P, Messer HH: The impact of instrument fracture on outcome of endodontic treatment, *J Endod* 31:845, 2005.

171. Stratemann SA, Huang JC, Maki K, et al: Comparison of cone beam computed tomography imaging with physical measures, *Dentomaxillofac Radiol* 37:80, 2008.

172. Swets JA: *Signal detection theory and ROC analysis in psychology and diagnostics: collected papers*, Mahwah, NJ, 1996, Lawrence Erlbaum Associates.

173. Tian YY, Guo B, Zhang R, et al: Root and canal morphology of maxillary first premolars in a Chinese subpopulation evaluated using cone beam computed tomography, *Int Endod J* 45:996, 2012.

174. Toure B, Faye B, Kane AW, et al: Analysis of reasons for extraction of endodontically treated teeth: a prospective study, *J Endod* 37:1512, 2011.

175. Torabinejad M: *Endodontics: principles and practice*, St Louis, 2009, Saunders.

176. Torabinejad M, Bahjri K: Essential elements of evidence-based endodontics: steps involved in conducting clinical research, *J Endod* 31:563, 2005.

177. Tronstad L: Root resorption: etiology, terminology and clinical manifestations, *Endod Dent Traumatol* 4:241, 1988.

177a. Tyndall DA: Position statement of the American Academy of Oral and Maxillofacial Radiology on selection criteria for the use of radiology in dental implantology with emphasis on cone beam computed tomography, *Oral Surg Oral Med Oral Pathol Oral Radiol* 113:817, 2012.

178. Tyndall DA, Ludlow JB, Platin E, Nair M: A comparison of Kodak Ektaspeed Plus film and the Siemens Sidexis digital imaging system for caries detection using receiver operating characteristic analysis, *Oral Surg Oral Med Oral Pathol Oral Radiol Endod* 85:113, 1998.

179. Valmaseda-Castellon E, Berini-Aytes L, Gay-Escoda C: Inferior alveolar nerve damage after lower third molar surgical extraction: a prospective study of 1117 surgical extractions, *Oral Surg Oral Med Oral Pathol Oral Radiol Endod* 92:377, 2001.

180. Versteeg CH, Sanderink GC, Lobach SR, van der Stelt PF: Reduction in size of digital images: does it lead to less detectability or loss of diagnostic information? *Dentomaxillofac Radiol* 27:93, 1998.

181. Versteeg KH, Sanderink GC, van Ginkel FC, van der Stelt PF: Estimating distances on direct digital images and conventional radiographs, *J Am Dent Assoc* 128:439, 1997.

182. Vertucci FJ: Root canal morphology of mandibular premolars, *J Am Dent Assoc* 97:47, 1978.

183. Vertucci FJ: Root canal anatomy of the human permanent teeth, *Oral Surg Oral Med Oral Pathol* 58:589, 1984.

184. Vertucci FJ: Root canal morphology and its relationship to endodontic procedures, *Endod Topics* 10:3, 2005.

185. Vier-Pelisser FV, Pelisser A, Recuero LC, et al: Use of cone beam computed tomography in the diagnosis, planning and follow up of a type III dens invaginatus case, *Int Endod J* 45:198, 2012.

186. Wang P, Yan XB, Lui DG, et al: Detection of dental root fractures by using cone beam computed tomography, *Dentomaxillofac Radiol* 40:290, 2011.

187. Weng XL, Yu SB, Zhao SL, et al: Root canal morphology of permanent maxillary teeth in the Han nationality in Chinese Guanzhong area: a new modified root canal staining technique, *J Endod* 35:651, 2009.

188. Wenzel A, Grondahl HG: Direct digital radiography in the dental office, *Int Dent J* 45:27, 1995.

189. Wenzel A, Haiter-Neto F, Frydenberg M, Kirkevang LL: Variable-resolution cone beam computerized tomography with enhancement filtration compared with intraoral photostimulable phosphor radiography in detection of transverse root fractures in an in vitro model, *Oral Surg Oral Med Oral Pathol Oral Radiol Endod* 108:939, 2009.

190. Westphalen VP, Gomes de Moraes I, Westphalen FH, et al: Conventional and digital radiographic methods in the detection of simulated external root resorptions: a comparative study, *Dentomaxillofac Radiol* 33:233, 2004.

191. Wolner-Hanssen AB, von Arx T: Permanent teeth with horizontal root fractures after dental trauma: a retrospective study, *Schweiz Monatsschr Zahnmed* 120:200, 2010.

192. Wu MK, Dummer PM, Wesselink PR: Consequences of and strategies to deal with residual post-treatment root canal infection, *Int Endod J* 39:343, 2006.

192a. Wu M-K, Shemesh H, Wesselink PR: Limitations of previously-published systematic reviews evaluating the outcome of endodontic treatment, *Int Endod J* 42:656, 2009.

193. Cotti E, Dessi C, Piras A, Mercuro G: Can a chronic dental infection be considered a cause of cardiovascular disease? A review of the literature, *Int J Cardiol* (2010). doi:10.1016/j.ijcard.2010.08.011.

194. Yoshioka T, Kobayashi C, Suda H, Sasaki T: An observation of the healing process of periapical lesions by digital subtraction radiography, *J Endod* 28:589, 2002.

195. Young GR: Contemporary management of lateral root perforation diagnosed with the aid of dental computed tomography, *Aust Endod J* 33:112, 2007.

196. Zadik Y, Sandler V, Bechor R, Salehrabi R: Analysis of factors related to extraction of endodontically treated teeth, *Oral Surg Oral Med Oral Pathol Oral Radiol Endod* 106:e31, 2008.

197. Zhang R, Wang H, Tian YY, et al: Use of cone beam computed tomography to evaluate root and canal morphology of mandibular molars in Chinese individuals, *Int Endod J* 44:990, 2011.

198. Zhang Y, Zhang L, Zhu XR, et al: Reducing metal artifacts in cone beam CT images by preprocessing projection data, *Int J Radiat Oncol Biol Phys* 67:924, 2007.

199. Zheng Q, Zhang L, Zhou X, et al: C-shaped root canal system in mandibular second molars in a Chinese population evaluated by cone beam computed tomography, *Int Endod J* 44:857, 2011.

200. Zhou W, Han C, Li D, et al: Endodontic treatment of teeth induces retrograde periimplantitis, *Clin Oral Implants Res* 20:1326, 2009.

CHAPTER 3

Case Selection and Treatment Planning

PAUL A. ROSENBERG | MATTHEW MALEK

CHAPTER OUTLINE

Common Medical Findings That May Influence Endodontic Treatment Planning
Cardiovascular Disease
Diabetes
Pregnancy
Malignancy
Medication-Related Osteonecrosis of the Jaws (MRONJ)
Human Immunodeficiency Virus (HIV) and Acquired Immunodeficiency Syndrome (AIDS)
End-Stage Renal Disease and Dialysis
Prosthetic Implants
Behavioral and Psychiatric Disorders
Psychosocial Evaluation

Development of the Endodontic Treatment Plan
Endodontic Prognosis
Single-Visit versus Multiple-Visit Treatment
Interdisciplinary Treatment Planning
Periodontal Considerations
Surgical Considerations
Restorative and Prosthodontic Considerations
Endodontic Therapy or Dental Implant
Other Factors That May Influence Endodontic Case Selection
Anxiety
Scheduling Considerations

The process of case selection and treatment planning begins after a clinician has diagnosed an endodontic problem. The clinician must determine whether the patient's oral health needs are best met by providing endodontic treatment and maintaining the tooth or by advising extraction. The use of rotary instruments, ultrasonics, and microscopy as well as new materials has made it possible to predictably retain teeth that previously would have been extracted. In addition, even teeth that have failed initial endodontic treatment can often be successfully retreated using nonsurgical or surgical procedures.

Increased knowledge concerning the importance of anxiety control, premedication with a nonsteroidal anti-inflammatory drug (NSAID) or acetaminophen, profound local anesthesia, appropriate occlusal adjustment, and biology-based clinical procedures enables clinicians to complete endodontic procedures without intraoperative or posttreatment pain.

Questions concerning tooth retention and possible referral can be answered only after a complete patient evaluation. The evaluation must include assessment of medical, psychosocial, and dental factors as well as consideration of the relative complexity of the endodontic procedure. Although most medical conditions do not contraindicate endodontic treatment, some can influence the course of treatment and require specific modifications. A number of valuable texts are available that review the subject of dental care for the medically compromised patient.[14,48,110] The American Academy of Oral Medicine

(Edmonds, WA) has an excellent website (www.aaom.com) that can be used to elicit information about medically compromised patients.

Perhaps the most important advice for a clinician who plans to treat a medically compromised patient is to be prepared to communicate with the patient's physician. The proposed treatment can be reviewed, and medical recommendations should be documented. Fig. 3-1 depicts a sample medical consultation letter that can be modified as necessary.

The American Society of Anesthesiologists (ASA; Park Ridge, IL) Physical Status Classification system is commonly used to express medical risk (Box 3-1). The ASA classification system remains the most widely used assessment method for preanesthetic patients despite some inherent limitations to its use as a peritreatment risk predictor. This classification system is a generally accepted and useful guide for pretreatment assessment of relative risk but does not advise appropriate treatment modifications. The clinician should go beyond the classification system and gather more information from the patient and physician, including the patient's compliance with suggested medication, frequency of physician visits, and most recent visit.

Typical questions include the following: *Do you take medication as prescribed by your physician?* Or, *when was the last time you were examined by your physician?* Other systems have been proposed that would better reflect the increasing number of

Michael White, MD
1 Walker Street
Brown City, OK

Dear Dr. White,

Your patient, Ms. Mary Smith, presented for consultation on August 10, 2009, concerning tooth #19. The tooth is asymptomatic at this time, but a small (4 mm x 3 mm), well-circumscribed periradicular radiolucency associated with the palatal root was noted on radiographic examination. The tooth was tested for vitality using thermal and electrical modalities and found to be nonvital, indicating an odontogenic cause for the lesion. The tooth will require endodontic treatment in order to be maintained. The prognosis for nonsurgical endodontic treatment in this case is good. I anticipate that her dental medication plan would include lidocaine with epinephrine for anesthesia and ibuprofen for postoperative pain control.

In a review of the patient's medical history she noted that she is being treated for a malignancy of the thyroid gland and is undergoing radiation therapy. She was unable to provide more specific information about her treatment.

I would appreciate information regarding her ability to undergo endodontic treatment at this time. Please call me if there is further information that you would require concerning the dental treatment to be provided. Thank you.

Yours truly,

Peter Jones, DDS

FIG. 3-1 Sample medical consultation letter.

BOX 3-1

American Society of Anesthesiologists Physical Status Classification System

P1: Normal, healthy patient; no dental management alterations required

P2: Patient with mild systemic disease that does not interfere with daily activity or who has a significant health risk factor (e.g., smoking, alcohol abuse, gross obesity)

P3: Patient with moderate to severe systemic disease that is not incapacitating but may alter daily activity

P4: Patient with severe systemic disease that is incapacitating and a constant threat to life

From: www.asahq.org/clinical/physicalstatus.htm.

---

medically complex patients treated by clinicians as Americans live longer.[35] Regardless of the classification system used, these generalized guidelines need to be individualized for the patient under care.

An alternative means of considering risk assessment is to review the following issues:

- History of allergies
- History of drug interactions, adverse effects
- Presence of prosthetic valves, joints, stents, pacemakers, and so on
- Antibiotics required (prophylactic or therapeutic)
- Hemostasis (normal expected, modification to treatment)
- Patient position in chair
- Infiltration or block anesthesia with or without vasoconstrictor
- Significant equipment concerns (radiographs, ultrasonics, electrosurgery)

- Emergencies (potential for occurrence, preparedness)
- Anxiety (past experiences and management strategy)

A review of these areas provides the clinician with essential background data before initiating treatment.

COMMON MEDICAL FINDINGS THAT MAY INFLUENCE ENDODONTIC TREATMENT PLANNING

Cardiovascular Disease

Patients with some forms of cardiovascular disease are vulnerable to physical or emotional stress that may be encountered during dental treatment, including endodontics. Patients may be confused or ill informed concerning the specifics of their particular cardiovascular problem. In these situations, consultation with the patient's physician is mandatory before the initiation of endodontic treatment. "For patients with symptoms of unstable angina or those who have had an MI [myocardial infarction] within the past 30 days (major risk category), elective care should be postponed."[48] One study found "no significant increase in the risk of experiencing a second vascular event after dental visits, including those that involved invasive procedures, in periods up to 180 days after a first recorded ischemic stroke, transient ischemic attack (TIA) or acute MI."[94]

The use of vasoconstrictors in local anesthetics poses potential problems for patients with ischemic heart disease. In these patients, local anesthetics without vasoconstrictors may be used as needed. If a vasoconstrictor is necessary, patients with intermediate clinical risk factors (i.e., a past history of MI without ischemic symptoms) and those taking nonselective beta-blockers can safely be given up to 0.036 mg epinephrine (two cartridges containing 1:100,000 epinephrine) at one appointment. For patients at higher risk (i.e., those who have had an MI within the past 7 to 30 days and unstable angina), the use of vasoconstrictors should be discussed with the physician.[48]

Vasoconstrictors may interact with some antihypertensive medications and should be used only after consultation with the at-risk patient's physician. Local anesthetic agents with minimal or no vasoconstrictors are usually adequate for non-surgical endodontic procedures[48] (see also Chapter 4). A systematic review of the cardiovascular effects of epinephrine concluded that the increased risk for adverse events among uncontrolled hypertensive patients was low, and the reported adverse events associated with epinephrine use in local anesthetics was minimal.[4] Another review highlighted the advantages of including a vasoconstrictor in the local anesthesia and stated that "pain control was significantly impaired in those patients receiving the local anesthetic without the vasoconstrictor as compared to those patients receiving the local anesthetic with vasoconstrictor."[13]

A patient who has specific heart conditions may be susceptible to an infection of the heart valves, induced by a bacteremia. This infection is called *infective* or *bacterial endocarditis* and is potentially fatal. In 2008, the American College of Cardiology and American Heart Association (AHA) Task Force on Practice Guidelines published an update on their previous guidelines, which focused on infectious endocarditis. This guideline stated that "prophylaxis against infective endocarditis is reasonable for the following patients at highest risk for adverse outcomes from infective endocarditis who undergo dental procedures that involve manipulation of either gingival tissue or the periapical region of teeth or perforation of the oral mucosa: patients with prosthetic cardiac valves or prosthetic material used for cardiac valve repair . . . , patients with previous infective endocarditis . . . [and] patients with congenital heart disease."[71]

The specific recommendations are summarized in a reference guide by the American Association of Endodontists (AAE; Chicago, IL), found online at www.aae.org/uploadedfiles/publications_and_research/guidelines_and_position_statements/antibioticprophylaxisquickrefguide.pdf). Because the AHA periodically revises its recommended antibiotic prophylactic regimen for dental procedures, it is essential that the clinician stay current concerning this important issue. There is a low compliance rate among at-risk patients regarding their use of the suggested antibiotic coverage before dental procedures. Therefore, the clinician must question patients concerning their compliance with the prescribed prophylactic antibiotic coverage before endodontic therapy. If a patient has not taken the antibiotic as recommended, it may be administered up to 2 hours after the procedure.[71]

Patients with artificial heart valves are considered susceptible to bacterial endocarditis. Consulting the patient's physician in such cases regarding antibiotic premedication is essential. Some physicians elect to administer parenteral antibiotics in addition to or in place of the oral regimen.

A dentist may be the first to detect elevated blood pressure if he or she routinely evaluates blood pressure before treatment. Furthermore, patients receiving treatment for hypertension may not be controlled adequately because of poor compliance or inappropriate drug therapy. Abnormal blood pressure readings may be the basis for physician referral.

Some patients may be disposed to serious life-threatening complications due to stress. Acute heart failure during a stressful dental procedure in a patient with significant valvular disease and heart failure or the development of infectious endocarditis represent two such life-threatening disorders.[91] Careful evaluation of patients' medical histories including the cardiac status of patients, the use of appropriate prophylactic antibiotics, and stress reduction strategies will minimize the risk of serious cardiac sequelae.

There is a widespread belief among dentists and physicians that oral anticoagulation therapy in which patients receive drugs such as warfarin (Coumadin) must be discontinued before dental treatment to prevent serious hemorrhagic complications, especially during and after surgical procedures. Aspirin is a drug commonly used as an anticoagulant on a daily basis without the supervision of a physician. Clinical studies do not support the routine withdrawal of anticoagulant therapy before dental treatment for patients who are taking such medications.[10,39,48]

When patients report they are receiving an anticoagulant medication, they can benefit from the clinician using the following guidelines:

- Identify the reason why the patient is receiving anticoagulant therapy.
- Assess the potential risk versus benefit of altering the drug regimen.
- Know the laboratory tests used to assess anticoagulation levels (i.e., the international normalized ratio [INR] value should be 3.5 or less for patients who are taking warfarin to safely undergo dental or surgical endodontic procedures).[48] Be familiar with methods used to obtain hemostasis both intraoperatively and postoperatively.
- Be familiar with the potential complications associated with prolonged or uncontrolled bleeding.
- Consult the patient's physician to discuss the proposed dental treatment and to determine the need to alter the anticoagulant regimen.

Another cardiac complication may occur in patients with Hodgkin disease or breast cancer, who often receive irradiation to the chest as an element of treatment. Although the therapy often cures the malignancy, it has been implicated in causing late-onset heart disease that may influence the development of a treatment plan and subsequent treatment. Dentists must identify patients who have received irradiation to the chest and consult with patients' physicians to determine whether that therapy has damaged the heart valves or coronary arteries. Patients with radiation-induced valvular disease may require prophylactic antibiotics when undergoing specific dental procedures that are known to cause a bacteremia and a heightened risk of developing endocarditis. Patients with radiation-induced coronary artery disease should be administered only limited amounts of local anesthetic agents containing a vasoconstrictor. They may require the administration of sedative agents and cardiac medications to preclude ischemic episodes. Consultation with the patient's physician is an appropriate response when a patient presents with a history that includes prior radiation to the chest.[29]

Diabetes

The Centers for Disease Control and Prevention (CDC, Atlanta, GA) in 2011 reported that 25.8 million people, or 8.3% of the U.S. population, have diabetes. There were also about 1.9 million people aged 20 years or older newly diagnosed with diabetes in 2010. (See Centers for Disease Control and

Prevention *Diabetes Fact Sheet*, available at http://cdc.gov/diabetes/pubs/estimates11.htm#2, 2011.) Diabetes is the seventh leading cause of death in the United States,[61] and, according to the *Diabetes Fact Sheet*, the risk for death among people with diabetes is about twice that of people of similar age but without diabetes. It is likely that patients with diabetes who require endodontic treatment will be increasingly common.

Diabetes mellitus appears to have multiple causes and several mechanisms of pathophysiology.[48] It can be thought of as a combination of diseases that share the key clinical feature of glucose intolerance. Patients with diabetes, even those who are well controlled, require special consideration during endodontic treatment. The patient with well-controlled diabetes, who is free of serious complications such as renal disease, hypertension, or coronary atherosclerotic disease, is a candidate for endodontic treatment. However, special considerations exist in the presence of acute infections. The non–insulin-controlled patient may require insulin, or the insulin dose of some insulin-dependent patients may have to be increased.[79] When surgery is required, consultation with the patient's physician is advisable in order to consider adjustment of the patient's insulin dosage, antibiotic prophylaxis, and dietary needs during the posttreatment period.

The clinician should ask patients with diabetes who self-monitor their glucose levels to bring a glucometer to each visit. If pretreatment glucose levels are below normal fasting range (80 to 120 mg/dl), it may be appropriate to take in a carbohydrate source.[100] A source of glucose (e.g., glucose tablets, orange juice, or soda) should be available if signs of insulin shock (hypoglycemic reaction caused by overcontrol of glucose levels) occur.[48] Signs and symptoms of hypoglycemia include confusion, tremors, agitation, diaphoresis, and tachycardia.[100] The clinician can avoid a hypoglycemic emergency by taking a complete, accurate history of the time and amount of the patient's insulin and meals. When questions arise concerning the appropriate course to follow, the patient's physician should be contacted or treatment deferred.

Appointments should be scheduled with consideration given to the patient's normal meal and insulin schedule.[79] Usually, a patient with diabetes who is well managed medically and is under good glycemic control without serious complications such as renal disease, hypertension, or coronary atherosclerotic heart disease can receive any indicated dental treatment.[57] However, patients with diabetes who have serious medical complications may need a modified dental treatment plan. For instance, although prophylactic antibiotics generally are not required, it "may be prescribed a patient with brittle (very difficult to control) diabetes for whom an invasive procedure is planned but whose oral health is poor and the fasting plasma glucose exceeds 200 mg/dL."[48] Local anesthesia would not be an issue in the presence of well-controlled diabetes, "but for patients with concurrent hypertension or history of recent myocardial infarction, or with a cardiac arrhythmia, the dose of epinephrine should be limited to no more than two cartridges containing 1:100,000 epinephrine."[48]

Inadequate diabetic control may predispose such patients to several oral infections, including dental pulp infection.[45] One study determined that although apical periodontitis may be significantly more prevalent in untreated teeth in patients with type 2 diabetes, the disease does not seem to influence the response to root canal treatment.[52] However, other studies suggest that diabetes is associated with a decrease in the success

of endodontic treatment in cases with pretreatment periradicular lesions.[12,28] In a prospective study on the impact of systemic diseases on the risk of tooth extraction, it has been also shown that an increased risk of tooth extraction after nonsurgical root canal treatment was significantly associated with diabetes mellitus, hypertension, and coronary heart disease.[103] Patients with diabetes and other systemic diseases may be best served by referral to an endodontist for treatment planning.

Pregnancy

Although pregnancy is not a contraindication to endodontics, it does modify treatment planning. Protection of the fetus is a primary concern when administration of ionizing radiation or drugs is considered. Of all the safety aids associated with dental radiography, such as high-speed film, digital imaging, filtration, and collimation, the most important is the protective lead apron with thyroid collar.[5,107] Although drug administration during pregnancy is a controversial subject, Box 3-2 presents commonly used dental drugs usually compatible with both pregnancy and breast-feeding. Based on U.S. Food and Drug Administration pregnancy risk factor definitions,[35] local anesthetics administered with epinephrine generally are considered safe for use during pregnancy and are assigned to the pregnancy risk classification categories B and C. (See www.fda.gov/Drugs/DevelopmentApprovalProcess/DevelopmentResources/Labeling/ucm093310.htm.) Few anxiolytics are considered safe to use during pregnancy. However, a single, short-term exposure to nitrous oxide–oxygen (N_2O-O_2) for less than 35 minutes is not thought to be associated with any human fetal anomalies, including low birth weight.[48] If a need exists for antibiotic therapy, penicillins, cephalosporins, and macrolides are considered first-line agents.

The analgesic of choice during pregnancy had been acetaminophen (category B).[78] However, a link between acetaminophen and childhood asthma has been suggested. Research has found that "the use of acetaminophen in middle to late but not early pregnancy may be related to respiratory symptoms in the first year of life."[74] This finding, although not completely validated, should be discussed with pregnant patients when an analgesic is being considered. Aspirin and nonsteroidal anti-inflammatory drugs also convey risks for constriction of the ductus arteriosus, as well as for postpartum hemorrhage and delayed labor.[78]

A major concern is that a drug may cross the placenta and be toxic or teratogenic to the fetus. In addition, any drug that is a respiratory depressant can cause maternal hypoxia, resulting in fetal hypoxia, injury, or death. Ideally, no drug should be administered during pregnancy, especially during the first trimester. If a specific situation makes adherence to this rule

---

BOX 3-2

Partial List of Drugs Usually Compatible with Both Pregnancy and Breast-Feeding

- Local anesthetics including lidocaine, etidocaine, and prilocaine
- Many antibiotics including penicillins, clindamycin, and azithromycin
- Acetaminophen
- Acyclovir
- Prednisone
- Antifungals including fluconazole and nystatin

difficult, then the clinician should review the appropriate current literature and discuss the case with the physician and patient.[11,55,60]

Further considerations exist during the postpartum period if the mother breast-feeds her infant. A clinician should consult the responsible physician before using any medications for the nursing mother. Alternative considerations include using minimal dosages of drugs, having the mother bank her milk before treatment, having her feed the child before treatment, or suggesting the use of a formula for the infant until the drug regimen is completed. Limited data are available on drug dosages and the effects on breast milk.[48]

In terms of treatment planning, elective dental care is best avoided during the first trimester because of the potential vulnerability of the fetus. The second trimester is the safest period in which to provide routine dental care. Complex surgical procedures are best postponed until after delivery.

Malignancy

Some malignancies may metastasize to the jaws and mimic endodontic pathosis, whereas others can be primary lesions (Fig. 3-2). The most common malignancies metastasize to the jaws are breast, lung, thyroid, and prostate.[53] A panoramic radiograph and a cone-beam computer tomography image are useful in providing an overall view of all dental structures. When a clinician begins an endodontic procedure on a tooth with a well-defined apical radiolucency, it might be assumed to result from a nonvital pulp. Pulp testing is essential to confirm a lack of pulp vitality in such cases. A vital response in such cases indicates a nonodontogenic lesion.

Careful examination of pretreatment radiographs from different angulations is important because lesions of endodontic origin would not be expected to be shifted away from the radiographic apex in the various images. Alternative methods, such a cone-beam computed tomography (CBC), may provide important diagnostic information (see Chapter 2).

A useful website for the differential diagnosis of radiographic lesions (Oral Radiographic Differential Diagnosis [ORAD] II) is available online at www.orad.org/index.html. A definitive diagnosis of periradicular lesions can be made only after biopsy. When a discrepancy exists between the initial diagnosis and clinical findings, consultation with an endodontist is advisable.

Patients undergoing chemotherapy or radiation to the head and neck may have impaired healing responses.[48] Treatment should be initiated only after the patient's physician has been

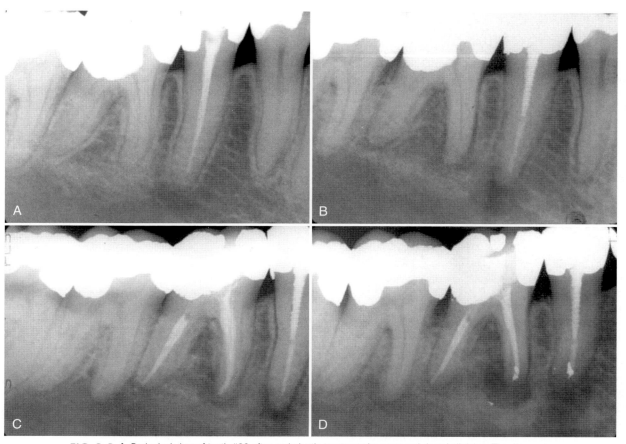

FIG. 3-2 A, Periapical view of tooth #29 after endodontic treatment by a general dental clinician. The diagnosis was irreversible pulpitis. **B,** Patient was referred to an endodontist 4 months later to evaluate radiolucencies of teeth #29 and #30. Symptoms indicated irreversible pulpitis of tooth #30, with concurrent lower right lip and chin paresthesia. Past medical history revealed breast cancer in remission. **C,** Nonsurgical endodontics was performed on tooth #30. Immediate referral was made to an oncologist/oral surgeon for biopsy to rule out nonodontogenic origin of symptoms. **D,** Surgical posttreatment radiograph of teeth #29 and #30. The biopsy report confirmed metastatic breast cancer. (Courtesy Dr. R. Sadowsky, Dr. L. Adamo, and Dr. J. Burkes.)

consulted. A dialogue among the dentist, physician, and patient is required prior to determining whether a tooth or teeth should be extracted or endodontically treated prior to radiation.

The effect of the external beam of radiation therapy on normal bone is to decrease the number of osteocytes, osteoblasts, and endothelial cells, thus decreasing blood flow. Pulps may become necrotic from this impaired condition.[48] Toxic reactions during and after radiation and chemotherapy are directly proportional to the amount of radiation or dosage of cytotoxic drug to which the tissues are exposed. Delayed toxicities can occur several months to years after radiation therapy.

Oral infections and any potential problems should be addressed before initiating radiation. It is advised that symptomatic nonvital teeth be endodontically treated at least 1 week before initiating radiation or chemotherapy, whereas treatment of asymptomatic nonvital teeth may be delayed.[48] The outcome of endodontic treatment should be evaluated within the framework of the toxic results of radiation and drug therapy. The white blood cell (WBC) count and platelet status of a patient undergoing chemotherapy should also be reviewed before endodontic treatment. In general, routine dental procedures can be performed if the granulocyte count is greater than 2000/mm[3] and the platelet count is greater than 50,000/mm[3]. If urgent care is needed and the platelet count is below 50,000/mm[3], consultation with the patient's physician is required.[48]

Medication-Related Osteonecrosis of the Jaws (MRONJ)

Bisphosphonates offer great benefits to patients at risk of bone metastases and in the prevention and treatment of osteoporosis, although this and other drugs (e.g., denosumab) are associated with a rare occurrence of osteonecrosis.

To distinguish medication-related osteonecrosis of the jaws (MRONJ) from other delayed healing conditions, the following working definition of MRONJ has been adopted by the American Association of Oral and Maxillofacial Surgeons (AAOMS): Patients may be considered to have MRONJ if all of the following three characteristics are present (see American Association of Oral and Maxillofacial Surgeons: Position paper on Bisphosphonate-Related Osteonecrosis of the Jaw—2014 update, available at www.aaoms.org/docs/position_papers/mronj_position_paper.pdf?pdf=MRONJ-Position-Paper):

1. Current or previous treatment with an antiresorptive drug such as a bisphosphonate or an antiangiogenic drug (e.g., sunitinib [Sutent], sorafenib [Nexavar], bevacizumab [Avastin], or sirolimus [Rapamune]
2. Exposed, necrotic bone in the maxillofacial region that has persisted for more than 8 weeks
3. No history of radiation therapy to the jaws

A patient's risk of developing osteonecrosis of the jaw while receiving oral bisphosphonates appears to be low, but there are factors known to increase the risk for MRONJ (Box 3-3). According to the American Association of Endodontists (available at www.aae.org/uploadedFiles/Publications_and_Research/Guidelines_and_Position_Statements/bisphosonatesstatement.pdf, 2012), such risks include a history of taking bisphosphonates, especially intravenous (IV) formulations, previous history of cancer, and a history of a traumatic dental procedure. In addition to the usual risk factors, patients receiving high-dose IV bisphosphonates for more than 2 years are at most risk for developing osteonecrosis of the jaw.

BOX 3-3

Risk Factors for Development of Bisphosphonate-Associated Osteonecrosis

- History of taking bisphosphonates for more than 2 to 3 years, especially with intravenous therapy
- History of cancer, osteoporosis, or Paget disease
- History of traumatic dental procedure
- Patient more than 65 years of age
- History of periodontitis
- History of chronic corticosteroid use
- History of smoking
- History of diabetes

It has been reported that patients with multiple myeloma and metastatic carcinoma to the skeleton who are receiving intravenous, nitrogen-containing bisphosphonates are at greatest risk for osteonecrosis of the jaws. These patients represent 94% of published cases. The mandible is more commonly affected than the maxilla (2:1 ratio), and 60% of cases are preceded by a dental surgical procedure.[108] Treatment outcomes of MRONJ are unpredictable, and prevention strategies are extremely important.

Management of high-risk patients might include nonsurgical endodontic treatment of teeth that otherwise would be extracted. The combination of orthodontic extrusion and bloodless extraction—exfoliation of the extruded roots after their movement—has also been suggested with the aim of minimizing trauma and enhancing the health of the surrounding tissues in patients at risk of developing MRONJ or when a patient refuses to undergo conventional tooth extraction.[95]

For patients at higher risk of MRONJ, surgical procedures such as extractions, endodontic surgery, or placement of dental implants should be avoided. (See www.aae.org/uploadedFiles/Publications_and_Research/Guidelines_and_Position_Statements/bisphosonatesstatement.pdf, 2012.) Sound oral hygiene and regular dental care may be the best approach to lowering the risk of MRONJ. Patients taking bisphosphonates and undergoing endodontic therapy should sign an informed consent form, inclusive of the risks, benefits, and alternative treatment plans. The following recommendations have been suggested to reduce the risk of MRONJ associated with endodontic treatment[58]:

- Apply a 1-minute mouth rinse with chlorhexidine prior to the start of the treatment with the aim of lowering the bacterial load of the oral cavity.
- Avoid the use of anesthetic agents with vasoconstrictors in order to prevent impairment of tissue vascularization.
- Work under aseptic conditions, including removing of all caries and placement of rubber dam prior to intracanal procedures.
- Avoid damage to the gingival tissues during the placement of rubber dam.
- Avoid maintaining patency of the apical foramen to prevent bacteremia.
- Use techniques that reduce the risk of overfilling and overextension.

Aggressive use of systemic antibiotics is indicated in the presence of an infection in a patient taking bisphosphonates.[48] Discontinuing bisphosphonate therapy may not eliminate any risk of developing MRONJ.[51,54,56] Some clinicians have proposed use of the CTX (C-terminal telopeptide of type I collagen α_1 chain) test (Quest Diagnostics, Madison, NJ) for assessing the risk of developing bone osteonecrosis (BON). For patients who have developed MRONJ, close coordination with an oral maxillofacial surgeon or oncologist is highly recommended.

An astute awareness of the potential risk of MRONJ in patients receiving bisphosphonate therapy is critical. Increased attentiveness to the prevention, recognition, and management of MRONJ will allow the clinician to make the best treatment decisions. Our knowledge of MRONJ is developing rapidly and it is essential that the clinician monitor the literature for changes in treatment protocols.[51,54,56]

Human Immunodeficiency Virus (HIV) and Acquired Immunodeficiency Syndrome (AIDS)

From 1987 through 1994, HIV disease mortality increased and reached a plateau in 1995. Subsequently, the mortality rate for this disease decreased an average of 33% per year from 1995 through 1998, and 5.5% per year from 1999 through 2009.[61] This dramatic improvement seems to be due to the use of a combination of highly active antiretroviral therapy (HAART) and improved preventive strategies.[48]

It is important, when treating patients with AIDS, that the clinician understand the patient's level of immunosuppression, drug therapies, and the potential for opportunistic infections. Although the effect of HIV infection on long-term prognosis of endodontic therapy is unknown, it has been demonstrated that clinicians may not have to alter their short-term expectations for periapical healing in patients infected with HIV.[77] The clinical team must also minimize the possibility of transmission of HIV from an infected patient, and this is accomplished by adherence to universal precautions. (See Universal Precautions for Prevention of Transmission of HIV and Other Bloodborne Infections, available at www.cdc.gov/niosh/topics/bbp/universal.html.)

Although saliva is not the main route for transmission of HIV, the virus has been found in saliva and its transmission through saliva has been reported.[33] Infected blood can transmit HIV, and during some procedures it may become mixed with saliva. Latex gloves and eye protection are essential for the clinician and staff. HIV can be transmitted by needlestick or via an instrument wound, but the frequency of such transmission is low, especially with small-gauge needles. Nevertheless, "Patients at high risk for AIDS and those in whom AIDS or HIV has been diagnosed should be treated in a manner identical to that for any other patient—that is, with standard precautions."[48]

A vital aspect of treatment planning for the patient with HIV/AIDS is to determine the current CD4[+] lymphocyte count and level of immunosuppression. In general, patients having a CD4[+] cell count exceeding 350 cells/mm^3 may receive all indicated dental treatments. Patients with a CD4[+] cell count of less than 200 cells/mm^3 or severe neutropenia (neutrophil count lower than 500/μL) will have increased susceptibility to opportunistic infections and may be effectively medicated with prophylactic drugs. White blood cell and differential counts, as well as a platelet count, should be ordered before any surgical procedure is undertaken. Patients with severe thrombocytopenia may require special measures (platelet replacement) before

surgical procedures. Care in prescribing medications must also be exercised with any medications after which the patient may experience adverse drug effects, including allergic reactions, toxic drug reactions, hepatotoxicity, immunosuppression, anemia, serious drug interactions, and other potential problems. The practitioner should also be aware of oral manifestations of the disease as far as it concerns diagnosis and treatment planning. For instance, candidiasis of the oral mucosa, Kaposi sarcoma, hairy leukoplakia of the lateral borders of the tongue, herpes simplex virus (HSV), herpes zoster, recurrent aphthous ulcerations, linear gingival erythema, necrotizing ulcerative periodontitis, necrotizing stomatitis, oral warts, facial palsy, trigeminal neuropathy, salivary gland enlargement, xerostomia, and melanotic pigmentation are all reported to be associated with HIV infection. It is essential that consultation with the patient's physician occurs before performing surgical procedures or initiating complex treatment plans.[48,86]

End-Stage Renal Disease and Dialysis

Consultation with the patient's physician is important before dental care is initiated for patients being treated for end-stage renal disease. Depending on the patient's status and the presence of other diseases common to renal failure (e.g., diabetes mellitus, hypertension, and systemic lupus erythematosus), dental treatment may be best provided in a hospital setting. The goal of dental care for patients being treated for end-stage renal disease is to slow the progression of dental disease and preserve the patient's quality of life.[48,76]

The most recent American Heart Association guidelines do not include a recommendation for prophylactic antibiotics before invasive dental procedures for patients receiving dialysis with intravascular access devices, unless an abscess is being incised and drained.[3,48] Because controversy exists about the need for prophylactic antibiotics, consultation with the physician is important for patients receiving hemodialysis and those who have known cardiac risk factors. When prophylaxis is used, the standard regimen of the American Heart Association is recommended.[3]

Some drugs frequently used during endodontic treatment are affected by dialysis. Drugs metabolized by the kidneys and nephrotoxic drugs should be avoided. Both aspirin and acetaminophen are removed by dialysis and require a dosage adjustment in patients with renal failure. Amoxicillin and penicillin also require dosage adjustment as well as a supplemental dosage subsequent to hemodialysis.[76] It is advisable to consult the patient's physician concerning specific drug requirements during endodontic treatment. Endodontic treatment is best scheduled on the day after dialysis. On the day of dialysis, patients are generally fatigued and could have a bleeding tendency.[48]

Chronic renal failure is a disorder that may stimulate secondary hyperparathyroidism that can cause a variety of bone lesions. In some instances, these lesions appear in the periapical region of teeth and can lead to a misdiagnosis of a lesion of endodontic origin.[50]

Prosthetic Implants

Patients with prosthetic implants are frequently treated in dental practices. The question concerning the need for antibiotic prophylaxis to prevent infection of the prosthesis has been debated for many years. A statement was issued jointly in 2003 by the American Dental Association (ADA; Chicago, IL) and the American Academy of Orthopaedic Surgeons (AAOS; Rosemont, IL) in an attempt to clarify the issue.[1] The statement concluded that scientific evidence does not support the need for antibiotic prophylaxis for dental procedures to prevent prosthetic joint infections. It went on to state that antibiotic prophylaxis is not indicated for dental patients with pins, plates, and screws, nor is it routinely indicated for most patients with total joint replacements. However, the statement indicated that some "high-risk patients" who are at increased risk for infection and undergoing dental procedures likely to cause significant bleeding should receive antibiotic prophylactic treatment. Such patients would include those who are immunocompromised or immunosuppressed, who have insulin-dependent (type 1) diabetes, who are in the first 2 years following joint replacement, or who have previous joint infections, malnourishment, or hemophilia.[1] The advisory statement concludes that the final decision on whether to provide antibiotic prophylaxis is the responsibility of the clinician, who must consider potential benefits and risks.[1] It should be noted that although endodontics has been shown to be a possible cause of bacteremia,[19,90] the risk is minimal in comparison with extractions, periodontal surgery, scaling, and prophylaxis.[72] In February 2009, the AAOS published a statement entitled "Antibiotic Prophylaxis for Bacteremia in Patients with Joint Replacements." In this updated publication it was stated: "Given the potential adverse outcomes and cost of treating an infected joint replacement, the AAOS recommends that clinicians consider antibiotic prophylaxis for all total joint replacement patients prior to any invasive procedure that may cause bacteremia." (See American Academy of Orthopaedic Surgeons: AAOS releases new statement on antibiotics after arthroplasty, www.aaos.org/news/aaosnow/may09/cover2.asp, 2012.)

However, the American Academy of Oral Medicine's (AAOM) position on this statement is that the "2009 information statement is more an opinion than an official guideline, AAOM believes that it should not replace the 2003 joint consensus statement prepared by the relevant organizations: the ADA, the AAOS and the Infectious Disease Society of America (IDSA)."[49] In 2012, an evidenced-based guideline was published that included recommendations of the AAOS-ADA clinical practice guideline for Prevention of Orthopaedic Implant Infection in Patients Undergoing Dental Procedures. This guideline stated that there is limited evidence for discontinuing the practice of routinely prescribing prophylactic antibiotics for patients with hip and knee prosthetic joint implants undergoing dental procedures. (See American Academy of Orthopaedic Surgeons: Prevention of orthopaedic implant infection in patients undergoing dental procedures, available at www.aaos.org/research/guidelines/PUDP/PUDP_guideline.pdf, 2012.)

Consultation with the patient's physician on a case-by-case basis is advisable to assess the need for prophylaxis.

Behavioral and Psychiatric Disorders

Stress reduction is an important factor in the treatment of patients with behavioral and psychiatric disorders. Sensitivity to the patient's needs must be part of the dental team's approach. Significant drug interactions and side effects are associated with tricyclic antidepressants, monoamine oxidase inhibitors, and antianxiety medications.[48] Consultation with physicians in such cases is essential before using sedatives, hypnotics, antihistamines, or opioids.

Psychosocial Evaluation

The initial visit, during which medical and dental histories are gathered, provides an opportunity to consider the patient's psychosocial status. Although some patients may want to maintain a tooth with a questionable prognosis, others may lack the ability to comprehend the potential risks and benefits. It would be a mistake to lead patients beyond what they can appreciate, and patients should not be allowed to dictate treatment that has a poor prognosis.

The clinician should also assess the patient's level of anxiety as an important part of preparation for the procedure to follow. It is reasonable to assume that most patients are anxious to some degree, especially when they are about to undergo endodontic treatment. A conversation describing the procedure and what the patient can expect is an important part of an anxiety-reduction protocol. It is well documented that a high level of anxiety is a predictor of poor anesthesia and posttreatment pain.[15,62] More than 200 studies indicate that behavioral intervention for the highly anxious patient before treatment decreases anxiety before and after surgery, reduces posttreatment pain, and accelerates recovery.[15]

DEVELOPMENT OF THE ENDODONTIC TREATMENT PLAN

The strategic value of a tooth in question should be considered before presenting alternative treatment plans to the patient. Although some decisions may be straightforward, considering alternative treatment options can be challenging as the clinician weighs multiple factors that will play a role in determining the ultimate success or failure of the case. Referral of the patient to a specialist should be considered when the complexity of a procedure is beyond the ability of a clinician. Factors that affect endodontic prognosis, including periodontal and restorative considerations, must be considered. The alternative of a dental implant is another choice when the endodontic prognosis is poor.

ENDODONTIC PROGNOSIS

Prognostic studies have identified a number of preoperative factors affecting the outcome of primary endodontic treatment. In a systematic review, it was determined that the absence of periapical radiolucency improves the outcome of root canal treatment significantly. The same study also showed that tooth vitality does not have an impact on the endodontic prognosis, as long as the periapex is healthy.[70] Studies have shown that the size of the radiolucency may also affect the outcome of endodontic treatment.[31,70] Another study found that the existence of sinus tract, narrow but deep periodontal probing depth, pain, and discharging sinus have a significant effect on the outcome of nonsurgical root canal treatment.[67] Preoperative pain is not only one of the most important predictors for postoperative pain,[64] it also has an impact on tooth survival after endodontic treatment.[68]

These findings suggest that all preexisting signs and symptoms that could affect the prognosis of treatment, along with the prognostic factors associated with other disciplines—which will be discussed in the next segment—should be taken into consideration when developing a treatment plan. It is of utmost importance that the prognosis and risks and benefits of the treatment be relayed to the patient before the initiation of the treatment as well.

There is a general belief that the prognoses for retreatment cases are less than those for primary treatment, but this is not universally supported. In a systematic review it was suggested that the outcome of retreatment cases should be similar to treatment cases as long as access to the apical infection can be reestablished.[65] However, there is some evidence indicating that the incidence of postoperative pain and flare-up is higher in retreatment cases in comparison to treatments.[36] The presence of preoperative periapical lesion, apical extent of root filling, and quality of coronal restoration has been proved to significantly affect the outcome of retreatment cases.[65]

Retreatment cases offer a particular set of challenges to the clinician (Figs. 3-3 and 3-4), and this topic is covered extensively in Chapter 8. Important questions to be considered before retreatment include the following:

◆ Why did the treatment fail?
◆ Can the point of bacterial entry to the canal space be identified?
◆ Are prior radiographs available for review?
◆ Is there an obvious procedural problem that can be corrected?
◆ Is the canal system readily accessible for reentry?
◆ Are there additional factors (other than endodontic) that may have contributed to the failure?
◆ Is the tooth critical to the treatment plan?
◆ Does the patient understand the prognosis for the tooth and want to attempt retreatment?

A retreatment plan should be developed after the clinician has determined the cause of failure and weighed other factors that may affect the prognosis (e.g., root fracture, defective restoration) (Figs. 3-5 to 3-8). Retreatment cases may require surgical endodontics in combination with nonsurgical retreatment. Referral to a specialist is often helpful when planning treatment for complex cases. If retreatment (with or without surgery) on a tooth with a new restoration is being considered, it must be weighed against the possibility of an implant. Many variables must be considered before a reasonable conclusion can be reached.

Single-Visit versus Multiple-Visit Treatment

Some vital cases are suitable for single-visit treatment. The number of roots, time available, and the clinician's skills are factors to be considered. Severity of the patient's symptoms is

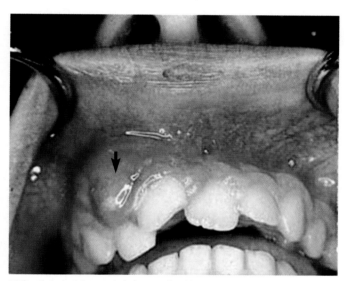

FIG. 3-3 Incision and drainage should be performed on this fluctuant swelling (*arrow*) in conjunction with canal instrumentation.

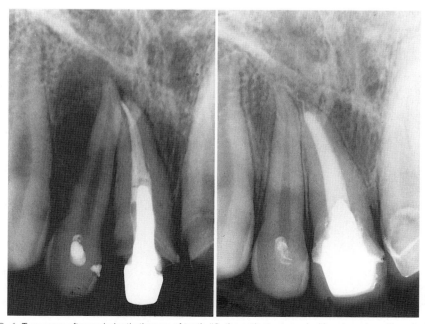

FIG. 3-4 Two years after endodontic therapy of tooth #8, the patient returned with pain and swelling. A clinician mistakenly began endodontic access on tooth #7, without confirming the apparent radiographic diagnosis by sensibility testing. Tooth #7 was vital, and tooth #8 was successfully retreated after removal of the post. (Courtesy Dr. Leon Schertzer.)

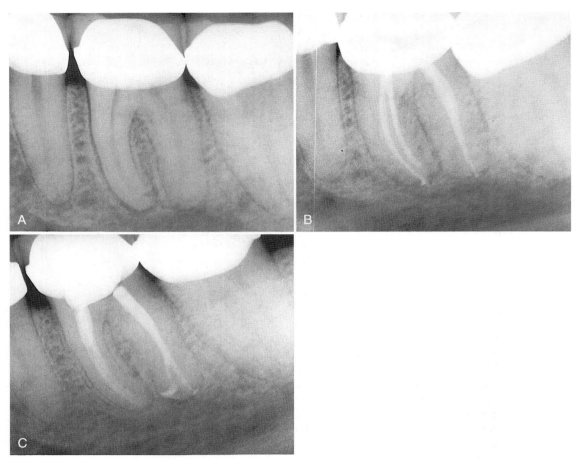

FIG. 3-5 Many years after endodontic treatment of tooth #19, the patient returned with a chief complaint of pain and an inability to chew with the tooth. Despite the radiographic appearance of excellent endodontic treatment, the tooth was retreated and the patient's pain disappeared. Note the unusual distal root anatomy, which was not apparent during the initial procedure. **A,** Initial radiograph. **B,** Completion of initial endodontic therapy. **C,** Retreatment.

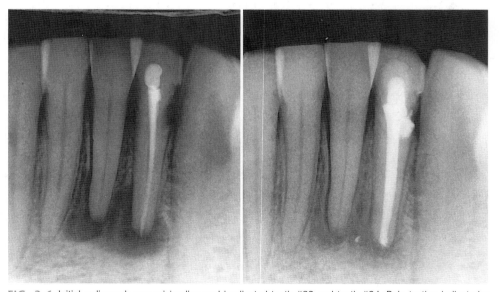

FIG. 3-6 Initial radiograph was misleading and implicated tooth #23 and tooth #24. Pulp testing indicated a vital pulp in tooth #24, and it was not treated. Retreatment of #23 resulted in healing of the periradicular lesion. (Courtesy Dr. Leon Schertzer.)

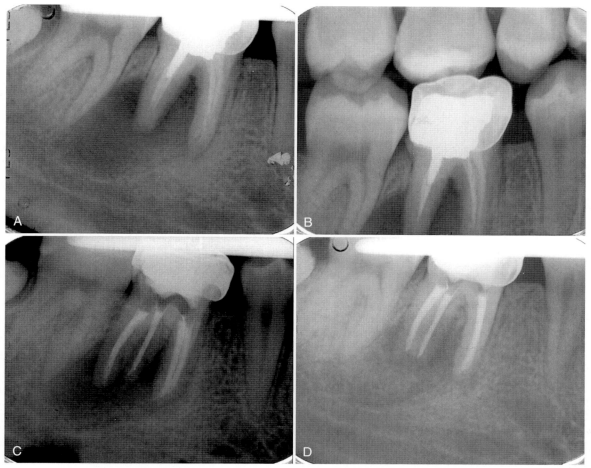

FIG. 3-7 Nonsurgical retreatment of tooth #30. An additional root was located and treated. **A,** Note inadequate endodontic treatment and large periapical lesion. **B,** Bitewing radiograph. **C,** Retreatment after post removal. **D,** Eighteen-month recall radiograph indicates periapical healing.

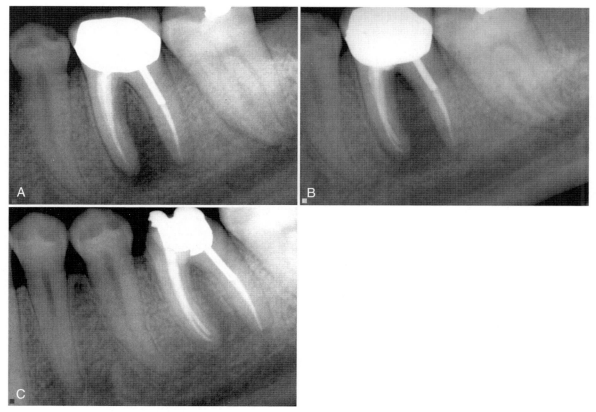

FIG. 3-8 Despite several exacerbations during endodontic retreatment, this case responded rapidly after the completion of therapy. Radiographic evaluation indicates a good periapical response after only 4 months.

another important consideration. For example, a patient in severe pain, with or without swelling, should not experience a long visit including access, instrumentation, and obturation. Treatment in such cases should be directed at alleviating pain, with filling of the canal postponed until a later visit. The clinician's judgment of what the patient can comfortably tolerate (regarding duration of the visit) is made on a case-by-case basis.

There are advantages in having a patient return for a second visit, after initially presenting with an endodontic emergency due to pain or swelling with or without a stoma. The second visit allows the clinician to determine the effect of the treatment on inflamed and infected tissues. Deferring the filling of the canal(s) leads to a shorter initial visit for the emergency patient.

Although some studies have reported less posttreatment pain in single-visit cases,[26,80,96] a systematic review found that the incidence of postobturation discomfort was similar in the single- and multiple-visit approaches.[27] In another systematic review it was concluded that there was a lack of compelling evidence indicating a significantly different prevalence of post-treatment pain/flare-up with either single- or multiple-visit root canal treatment.[85] Differences in research methodology explain the conflict in these findings.

Regarding the healing rate of single- and multiple-visit cases, a systematic review found that there was no detectable difference in the effectiveness of root canal treatment in terms of radiologic success between single and multiple visits.[27] A more recent systematic review also found that the healing rate of single- and multiple-visit root canal treatment is similar for infected teeth.[96]

Teeth with nonvital pulps and apical periodontitis pose a microbiologic problem. It is important to avoid pushing bacterial debris into the periapical tissues. Agreement is lacking concerning the appropriateness of single-visit endodontics for treating these patients. Some have postulated that the intervisit use of an antimicrobial dressing is essential to thoroughly disinfect the root canal system.[92,93,99] In contrast, other researchers have found no statistically significant difference in success when using the single-visit or multiple-visit approach to the nonvital tooth with apical periodontitis.[27,31,59,73,75,106] A systematic review found that, single-visit root canal treatment appeared to be slightly more effective than multiple-visit treatment (6.3% higher healing rate). However, the difference between these two treatment regimens was not statistically significant.[84] This is a complicated issue because the inability to detect differences between groups might also be due to variations in research methodology, including sample size, duration of follow-up, and treatment methods.

It is possible that total elimination of bacteria may not be absolutely necessary for healing. Perhaps maximal reduction of bacteria, effective root canal filling, and a timely satisfactory coronal restoration can result in a high level of clinical success. However, regardless of the number of appointments, effective bacteriologic disinfection of the root canal system is critical.[46]

Treatment planning for an endodontic case should be based on biologic considerations. Patients who present with acute symptoms present a different set of biologic issues than those with an asymptomatic tooth. Swelling associated with an abscess, cellulitis, or presence of a stoma represent signs of pathologic processes. The biologic significance of these conditions should be considered before determining specific goals for each visit.

Developing specific goals at each visit helps to organize the treatment. For example, for an uncomplicated molar or premolar, some clinicians will set a specific goal for the first visit that includes access and thorough instrumentation while deferring the obturation to a second visit. Uncomplicated single-rooted, vital teeth may be planned for a single-visit approach. It is important that ample time be allowed so that the procedure can be adequately completed without undue stress.

These recommendations have a biologic basis. Biologically, it is not reasonable to partially instrument root canal systems, thereby leaving residual inflamed pulpal remnants or necrotic debris in the canal, because such remnants may cause pain and be susceptible to infection. The clinician would be well advised to begin canal instrumentation only if time permits the extirpation of all pulp tissue and debridement of the root canal system.

Although in most cases the clinical procedures required to complete endodontic treatment can be accomplished in a single visit, that does not mean it is the better course of treatment. What can be done and what should be done represent two very different approaches to endodontic treatment planning. The patient's systemic health, level of anxiety, and symptoms, as well as the complexity of the root canal system, are factors that must be considered.

A study concerning the outcome of initial treatment noted the complexity of treating apical periodontitis.[31] The author commented:

Treatment of this disease cannot be improved merely by changing treatment techniques. Because apical periodontitis results from interactions between microorganisms, their environment and the host immune system, only use of effective modifiers of any of these three factors might significantly improve the outcome of treatment.

INTERDISCIPLINARY TREATMENT PLANNING

Periodontal Considerations

Extensive periodontal lesions may complicate endodontic prognosis. Lesions with endodontic and periodontal components may necessitate consultation with an endodontist or periodontist in order to gather more information about the tooth's prognosis.

A 4-year retrospective study found that attachment loss and periodontal status affected endodontic prognosis of endodontically treated molars.[87] It is crucial that the dental practitioner be aware of the periodontal factors that may influence the prognosis of endodontic treatment, such as root perforations, bone loss, and clinical attachment loss.

When establishing the prognosis of a tooth with an endodontic/periodontal lesion, there are essential factors to be considered. Determination of pulp vitality and the extent of the periodontal defect are central to establishing the prognosis and developing a treatment plan for a tooth with an endodontic/periodontal lesion (see also Chapter 25).

In primary endodontic disease, the pulp is nonvital (Figs. 3-9 and 3-10), whereas in primary periodontal disease, the pulp retains vitality. True combined endodontic-periodontal disease occurs less frequently. The combined lesion is found

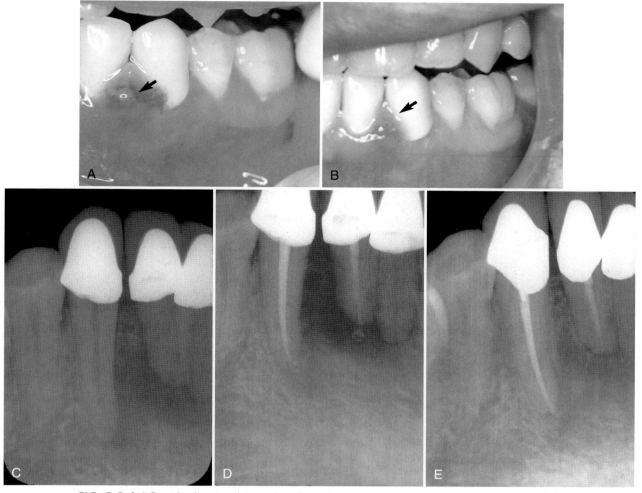

FIG. 3-9 **A,** Inflamed, edematous interproximal tissue *(arrow)* caused by acute endodontic pathosis. **B,** Soft tissue healing *(arrow)* 3 days after initiation of endodontic treatment. **C,** Periradicular pathosis. **D,** Completed endodontic therapy. **E,** Periradicular healing at 1-year recall.

when the endodontic disease process advances coronally and joins with a periodontal pocket progressing apically. There is significant attachment loss with this type of lesion, and the prognosis is guarded.[81] The radiographic appearance of combined endodontic-periodontal lesions may be similar to that of a vertically fractured tooth. Therapy for true combined lesions requires both endodontic and periodontal therapy. Sequencing of treatment is based on addressing the initial chief complaint.

The prognosis and treatment of each type of endodontic-periodontal disease vary. Primary endodontic disease should be treated solely by endodontic therapy, and the prognosis is usually good. Primary periodontal disease should be treated only by periodontal therapy, and the prognosis varies depending on the severty of the disease and patient's response to treatment.[81]

Pathogenesis of the lesion can be better understood after sensibility testing, periodontal probing, radiographic assessment, and evaluation of dental history. When extensive prostheses are planned, the potential risk of including a tooth with a questionable prognosis must be considered. It is not prudent to incorporate a chronic problem into a new complex prosthesis (Fig. 3-11).

Surgical Considerations

Surgical evaluation is particularly valuable in the diagnosis of lesions that may be nonodontogenic. Biopsy is the definitive means of diagnosing osseous pathosis, which may mimic a lesion of endodontic origin. When retreatment is being considered, the clinician must determine whether nonsurgical, surgical, or combined treatment is appropriate. This decision is influenced by the presence of complex restorations, posts, and the radiographic assessment of prior endodontic therapy.

Endodontic surgery is most often performed in an attempt to improve the apical seal and correct failure of nonsurgical therapy. Bacteria are the essential cause of failure. It is important that the clinician determine the bacterial path of ingress. For example, a deficient restoration or recurrent decay will result in microleakage into the root canal space. Unless that issue is addressed, apical surgery may not be predictable (Fig. 3-12).

When a deficient restoration is identified, it must be replaced to prevent continued bacterial penetration. Endodontic surgery (see Chapter 9) may also be performed as a primary procedure when there are complications such as calcific metamorphosis. In those cases, by using surgery as primary therapy, an apical seal can be established while preserving the crown of the tooth.

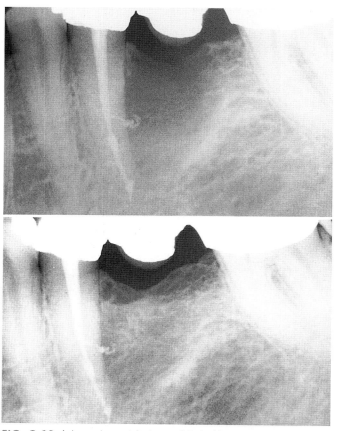

FIG. 3-10 A large, bony defect associated with tooth #20 healed after endodontic therapy. The tooth was nonvital, and no significant periodontal probing depth indicated pulpal disease.

The treatment plan for these cases is determined after reviewing multiple radiographs and considering the possibility of completing nonsurgical therapy without destroying an otherwise functional crown or natural tooth. Endodontic surgery without prior nonsurgical therapy should be a treatment of last resort and only when nonsurgical treatment is not possible.

Reviewing the best available evidence for alternative treatments is an important aspect of treatment planning for a tooth with failed endodontics. Evidence concerning healing potential after endodontic surgery is an important consideration in the management of posttreatment disease.[30] Numerous studies

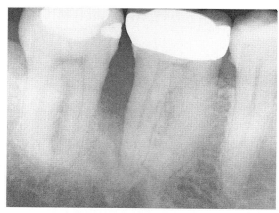

FIG. 3-11 Tooth #30 has a poor prognosis. Periodontal probing reached the apex of the distal root. Extraction is indicated and should be done as soon as possible to prevent further damage to the mesial bone associated with tooth #31. Implant site preservation is another consideration in treatment planning for this case.

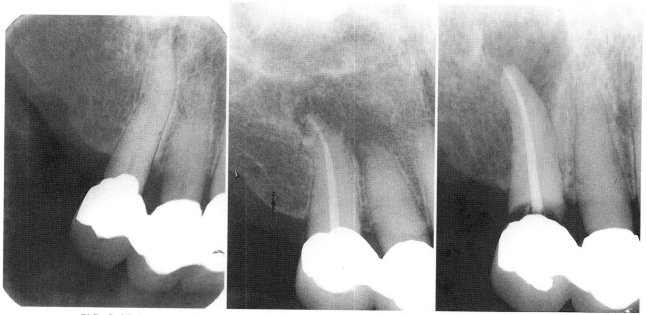

FIG. 3-12 Four years after endodontic therapy, the patient complained of pain and swelling associated with tooth #6. The initial impression was that apical surgery was indicated. However, further radiographs revealed the true cause of the endodontic failure. The initial endodontic access through the crown or caries damaged the coronal seal and recurrent decay followed.

have examined the outcome of apical surgery and the results vary considerably.[101,104,112] This variability may reflect actual outcome differences or reflect variations in case selection techniques, recall periods, and methodology.

One prospective study indicated that there is an increased odds ratio for disease persistence for teeth with larger pretreatment lesions and pretreatment root canal filling of adequate length.[104] Another study found that patients presenting with pain at the initial examination before surgery had a significantly lower rate of healing at the 1-year follow-up compared with patients who did not have pain at the initial examination.[101]

It should also be noted that the periodontal condition of the tooth, including the interproximal bone levels and the amount of marginal bone loss, has been shown to significantly affect the long-term prognosis of periapical surgery.[102,105] Moreover, it has been shown that isolated endodontic lesions have much higher success rates at the 1- to 5-year follow-up (95.2%) in comparison with endodontic-periodontal combined lesions (77.5%).[40]

Dramatic changes in surgical technique and materials have occurred: The advent of microscopy, endoscopy, and ultrasonics, as well as improved retrograde filling materials, represents important modifications of surgical technique. An outcome study comparing traditional root-end surgery (TRS) and endodontic microsurgery (EMS) found that the probability of success for EMS was 1.58 times greater than the probability of success for TRS.[89] Another study comparing the EMS techniques with and without the use of higher magnification found that the difference of probability of success between the groups was statistically significant for molars, but no significant difference was found for the premolar or anterior teeth.[88] Cone-beam computed tomography has proved to be of value in some surgical cases. It produces three-dimensional images of a tooth, pathosis, and adjacent anatomic structures. It is beneficial for localizing the mandibular canal,[42] mental foramen, maxillary sinus, and nasal cavity.[16]

Restorative and Prosthodontic Considerations

A satisfactory restoration may be jeopardized by a number of factors. Subosseous root caries (perhaps requiring crown lengthening), poor crown-to-root ratio, and extensive periodontal defects or misalignment of teeth may have serious effects on the final restoration. These problems must be recognized before endodontic treatment is initiated. For complex cases, a restorative treatment plan should be in place before initiating endodontic treatment (see Chapter 22). Some teeth may be endodontically treatable but nonrestorable, or they may represent a potential restorative complication because of a large prosthesis. Reduced coronal tooth structure under a full-coverage restoration makes endodontic access more difficult because of reduced visibility and lack of radiographic information about the anatomy of the chamber. It is not unusual for restorations to be compromised during endodontic access (see Fig. 3-12). Whenever possible, restorations should be removed before endodontic treatment.

Full coverage restorations are usually suggested after endodontic treatment. In a systematic review on tooth survival following nonsurgical root canal treatment, four factors were found to be of significance in tooth survival[66]:

- A crown restoration after root canal treatment
- Tooth having both mesial and distal proximal contacts
- Tooth not functioning as an abutment for removable or fixed prosthesis
- Tooth type or specifically nonmolar teeth

Another systematic review found that the odds for healing of apical periodontitis increase with both adequate root canal treatment and adequate restorative treatment. However, poorer clinical outcomes may be expected with adequate root filling/inadequate coronal restoration and inadequate root filling/adequate coronal restoration, with no significant difference in the odds of healing between these two combinations.[34] These findings suggest that the quality of the coronal restoration is as important as the quality of the root canal treatment. Therefore, to increase the success of the treatment, it is strongly suggested that the clinician discuss the restorative plan of the tooth with both the patient and—if it is a referred patient—with the referring dentists before initiation of treatment.

Endodontic Therapy or Dental Implant

The successful evolution of dental implants as a predictable replacement for missing teeth has had a positive impact on patient care. A clinician now has an additional possibility to consider when developing a treatment plan for a patient with a missing tooth or teeth. More challenging is the decision concerning whether or not to provide endodontic therapy for a tooth with a questionable prognosis or extract and use a single-tooth implant as a replacement. Numerous studies have evaluated both nonsurgical endodontic therapy[18,69,70,82,97,98] and endosseous dental implants.[2,17,37,47]

It is not possible to compare outcome studies because of variations in research methodologies, follow-up periods, and criteria associated with determining success or failure. A review of outcome studies points to the need for randomized controlled trials with standardized or similar methodologies that could provide a higher level of evidence to use in answering important clinical prognostic questions.

A synthesis of available evidence indicates that both primary root canal treatment and single-tooth implants are highly predictable procedures when treatment is appropriately planned and implemented. A study assessed clinical and radiographic success of initial endodontic therapy of 510 teeth over a 4- to 6-year period. It was found that 86% of teeth healed and 95% remained asymptomatic and functional.[18] Another study considered the outcomes of endodontic treatment on 1,462,936 teeth. More than 97% of teeth were retained after 8 years.[82] In a similar study it was found that overall, 89% of the 4744 teeth were retained in the oral cavity 5 years after the endodontic retreatment.[83] A study concerning the outcome of endodontic therapy on 1312 patients in general practice with a mean follow-up time of 3.9 years found a combined failure rate of 19.1%, concluding that "failure rates for endodontic therapy are higher than previously reported in general practices, according to results of studies based on dental insurance claims data."[7]

The American Dental Association's Council on Scientific Affairs has reported high survival rates for endosseous implants. An evaluation of 10 studies with more than 1400 implants demonstrated survival rates ranging from 94.4% to 99% with a mean survival rate of 96.7%.[2] With such high survival rates reported for endodontics and single-tooth implants, a clinician must consider a multiplicity of factors within the context of the best available evidence. Most current studies indicate no significant difference in the long-term prognosis between restored endodontically treated teeth and single-tooth implants.[37]

In a retrospective cross-sectional comparison of initial non-surgical endodontic treatment and single-tooth implants, it was suggested that restored endodontically treated teeth and single-tooth implant restorations have similar survival rates, although the implant group showed a longer average and median time to obtain function and a higher incidence of posttreatment complications requiring subsequent treatment intervention.[20] A review summarized the best available evidence concerning factors influencing treatment planning involving preservation of a tooth with endodontic therapy or replacement by a single-tooth implant. Factors considered included prosthetic restorability of the natural tooth, quality of bone, aesthetic concerns, cost-to-benefit ratio, systemic factors, potential for adverse effects, and patient preferences.[37] The authors concluded that "endodontic treatment of teeth represents a feasible, practical and economical way to preserve function in a vast array of cases and that dental implants serve as a good alternative in selected indications in which prognosis is poor."[37]

Aside from treatment outcome, there are other factors involved in any treatment that the practitioner has to consider when making a treatment planning decision. In a study evaluating the quality of life of endodontically treated versus implant treated patients, the results showed a high rate of satisfaction with both treatment modalities.[32] One study found that comparing to endodontic molar retreatment and fixed partial dentures, implant-supported restoration, despite its high survival rate, has been shown to be the least cost-effective treatment option.[41] Another study found that "endodontically treated natural teeth may provide more effective occlusal contact during masticatory function compared with implant-supported restorations, leading to more efficient mastication."[109]

Another important factor is the patient's health status. Implants require a surgical procedure that may not be possible due to the patient's medical status. One area of concern is diabetes mellitus. However, it has been shown that dental implant osseointegration can be accomplished in these subjects as long as they have good glycemic control.[38]

It seems clear that patients are best served by retaining their natural dentition as long as the prognosis for long-term retention is positive. It is not reasonable to extract a tooth if endodontics with a good prognosis can be completed. It is also not reasonable for a patient to invest in root canal therapy, a post, and a crown if the prognosis is highly questionable and an implant with a good prognosis can be placed. An important advantage of providing endodontic therapy is to allow rapid return of the patient's compromised dentition to full function and aesthetics. This rapid return is in marked contrast to the use of provisional restorations associated with dental implants while waiting for osseous integration. The challenge is to weigh all pretreatment variables and reach a reasonable conclusion concerning the prognosis for tooth retention or implant placement.

Interestingly, some endodontic advanced education programs are now including implant training in their curricula. This training will enable the endodontist to provide more value to the patient and referring the dental clinician as treatment plans are determined. Such dually trained endodontists will be well positioned to provide endodontic therapy or place an implant as best serves the patient.

OTHER FACTORS THAT MAY INFLUENCE ENDODONTIC CASE SELECTION

A variety of factors may complicate proposed endodontic therapy. Calcifications, dilacerations, or resorptive defects may compromise endodontic treatment of a tooth with potentially strategic value (Fig. 3-13). The inability to isolate a tooth is also a problem and may result in bacterial contamination of the root canal system. Extra roots and canals pose a particular

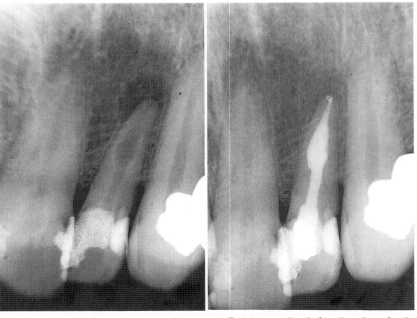

FIG. 3-13 Resorptive defects can be successfully treated. Early intervention, before there is perforation of the root, increases the chance of success. (Courtesy Dr. Leon Schertzer.)

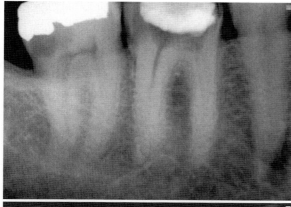

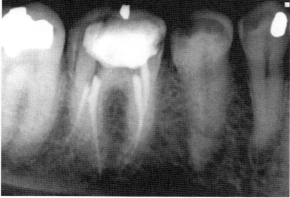

FIG. 3-14 The presence of curved roots and multiple canals is a complicating factor.

anatomic challenge that radiographs do not always reveal (Fig. 3-14). A bitewing radiograph is useful in providing an accurate image of the pulp chambers of posterior teeth. The clinician should recognize these potential problems and be able to manage and factor them into the decision concerning the tooth's prognosis, including the possibility that the patient should be referred to a specialist.

Another consideration is the stage of maturity of the tooth. Primary and immature permanent teeth may have a pulpal pathosis caused by caries or trauma; preserving these young teeth is essential. Premature loss of an anterior tooth can lead to malocclusion, predispose the patient to tongue habits, impair aesthetics, and damage the patient's self-esteem. (See Chapters 20 and 24 for further information.)

Some clinicians use a simple formula for determining which endodontic cases they treat and which they refer to a specialist. The number of roots may be the determining factor in a decision concerning referral, or the key factor may be the chronic or acute status of the case. Others consider the complexity of the ultimate prosthesis as a factor in considering an endodontic referral. The most important variables in determining whether to refer a patient to a specialist are the skills of the clinician and the complexity of the case.

The American Association of Endodontists (AAE) developed guidelines for assessing endodontic case difficulty (available at www.aae.org/uploadedFiles/Publications_and _Research/Guidelines_and_Position_Statements/ 2006CaseDifficultyAssessmentFormB_Edited2010.pdf) (see Fig. 2-1). The AAE Endodontic Case Difficulty Assessment

Form enables a clinician to assign a level of difficulty to a particular case. The form describes cases with minimal, moderate, and high degrees of difficulty. This form lists criteria that can be used to identify cases that should be referred to a specialist. The use of surgical operating microscopes, endoscopes, and ultrasonics enables the specialist to predictably treat teeth that would not previously have been treatable.

Anxiety

Anxiety presents a problem at many levels of dental care (see also Chapter 28). Avoidance of dental treatment due to anxiety appears to be associated with significant deterioration of oral and dental health.[111] Even at the diagnostic stage, severe anxiety may confuse the process.[23] Several studies support the hypothesis that pain or fear of pain is a primary source of anxiety as well as an obstacle to seeking dental care.[44,111] Also, highly anxious patients appear to be more sensitive to pain.[24,43] High levels of anxiety have been found to negatively affect clinical procedures including local anesthesia.[62] In 2009, Binkley tested the hypothesis that having natural red hair color, which is caused by variants of the melanocortin-1 receptor (*MC1R*) gene, could predict a patient's experiencing dental care–related anxiety and dental care avoidance.[8] She found that participants with *MC1R* gene variants reported significantly more dental care–related anxiety and fear of dental pain than did participants with no *MC1R* gene variants. A more recent study confirmed the relationship between the red hair phenotype and anxiety. However, this study found no association between the red hair phenotype and the success of local anesthesia.[21]

It has been demonstrated that dental anxiety and expectation of pain had a profound effect on a patient's ability to understand information provided.[25] A person's cognitive ability to process information is significantly affected by stress.[25] A study found that 40% of patients who had minor oral surgery did not remember receiving both written and verbal instructions, contributing to 67% noncompliance with antibiotic prescriptions.[9] Patients' anxiety can compromise their understanding of complex treatment plans. Decisions made by a patient concerning options involving tooth retention or loss may be markedly affected by anxiety.

Unfortunately, the impact that a high level of anxiety can have on patient's cognition, local anesthesia, and intraoperative and postoperative experiences is not always recognized. A landmark medical study found that pretreatment discussion of surgical treatments and associated discomfort reduced by 50% the need for posttreatment morphine and reduced the time to discharge.[22] Existing research has focused primarily on the effect of pretreatment information on reducing anxiety and stress during surgery.[25]

More than 200 studies indicate that preemptive behavioral intervention decreases anxiety before and after surgery, reduces posttreatment pain intensity and intake of analgesics, and accelerates recovery.[15] A calm setting, reassurance by the clinician and explanation of the treatment plan, as well as a discussion about pain prevention strategies are all important steps even before treatment starts.[63] A written description as well as a verbal description of the proposed treatment are helpful. It may also be of value to have a family member or friend accompany the patient for a discussion of the treatment plan.

Scheduling Considerations

If a vital case is to be treated by a multivisit approach, it is suggested that the clinician allow 5 to 7 days between canal instrumentation and obturation to allow periradicular tissues to recover. When a vital case is to be treated in a single visit, adequate time must be scheduled so that the clinician can comfortably complete the procedure. Because profound inferior alveolar nerve block anesthesia can require approximately 15 to 20 minutes, it is wise to include that time when scheduling a patient's appointment (see also Chapter 4).

Appointments to fill nonvital cases should be scheduled approximately 1 week after instrumentation to maximize the antimicrobial effect of the intracanal dressing when calcium hydroxide is used.[6,92,93] Acute (pain or swelling) nonvital cases should be seen every 24 to 48 hours to monitor the patient's progress and bring the acute symptoms under control. Further cleaning and shaping are important components of the treatment as the clinician seeks to eliminate persistent microbes in the canal system. Long delays between visits contribute to the development of resistant microbial strains and should be avoided.

REFERENCES

1. American Dental Association and American Academy of Orthopaedic Surgeons: Antibiotic prophylaxis for dental patients with total joint replacements. *J Am Dent Assoc* 134:895, 2003.
2. American Dental Association Council of Scientific Affairs: Dental endosseous implants: an update, *J Am Dent Assoc* 135:92, 2004.
3. Baddour LM, Bettmann MA, Bolger AF, et al: Nonvalvular cardiovascular device-related infections, *Circulation* 108:2015, 2003.
4. Bader JD, Bonito AJ, Shugars DA, et al: A systematic review of cardiovascular effects of epinephrine on hypertensive dental patients, *Oral Surg Oral Med Oral Pathol Oral Radiol Endod* 93:648, 2002.
5. Bean LR, Devore WD: The effect of protective aprons in dental roentgenography, *Oral Surg Oral Med Oral Pathol* 28:505, 1969.
6. Bergenholtz GH-BP, Reit C: *Textbook of Endodontology*, Oxford, 2003, Blackwell.
7. Bernstein SD, Horowitz AJ, Man M, et al: Outcomes of endodontic therapy in general practice: a study by the practitioners engaged in applied research and learning network, *J Am Dent Assoc* 43:478, 2012.
8. Binkley CJ, Beacham A, Neace W, et al: Genetic variations associated with red hair color and fear of dental pain, anxiety regarding dental care and avoidance of dental care, *J Am Dent Assoc* 140:896, 2009.
9. Blinder D, Rotenberg L, Peleg M, et al: Patient compliance to instructions before oral surgical procedures, *Int J Oral Maxillofac Surg* 30:216, 2001.
10. Brennan MT, Valerin MA, Noll JL, et al: Aspirin use and post-operative bleeding from dental extractions. *J Dent Res* 87:740, 2008.
11. Briggs GG, Freeman RK, Yaffe SJ: *Drugs in pregnancy and lactation: a reference guide in fetal and neonatal risk*, ed 8, Philadelphia, 2009, Lippincott Williams & Wilkins.
12. Britto LR, Katz J, Guelmann M, et al: Periradicular radiographic assessment in diabetic and control individuals, *Oral Surg Oral Med Oral Pathol Oral Radiol Endod* 96:449, 2003.
13. Brown RS, Rhodus NL: Epinephrine and local anesthesia revisited, *Oral Surg Oral Med Oral Pathol Oral Radiol Endod* 100:401, 2005.
14. Burket LW, Greenberg MS, Glick M, et al: *Burket's oral medicine*, ed 11, Hamilton, BC, 2008, Decker.
15. Carr DB, Goudas LC: Acute pain, *Lancet* 353:2051, 1999.
16. Cotton TP, Geisler TM, Holden DT, et al: Endodontic applications of cone-beam volumetric tomography, *J Endod* 33:1121, 2007.
17. Creugers NH, Kreulen CM, Snoek PA, et al: A systematic review of single-tooth restorations supported by implants, *J Dent* 28:209, 2000.
18. de Chevigny C, Dao TT, Basrani BR, et al: Treatment outcome in endodontics: the Toronto study—phase 4: initial treatment, *J Endod* 34:258, 2008.

19. Debelian GJ, Olsen I, Tronstad L: Bacteremia in conjunction with endodontic therapy, *Endod Dent Traumatol* 11:142, 1995.
20. Doyle SL, Hodges JS, Pesun IJ, et al: Retrospective cross sectional comparison of initial nonsurgical endodontic treatment and single-tooth implants, *J Endod* 32:822, 2006.
21. Droll BM, Drum M, Nusstein J, et al: Anesthetic efficacy of the inferior alveolar nerve block in red-haired women, *J Endod* 38:1564, 2012.
22. Egbert LD, Battit GE, Welch CS, et al: Reduction of postoperative pain by encouragement and instruction of patients. a study of doctor-patient rapport, *N Engl J Med* 270:825,1964.
23. Eli I: Dental anxiety: a cause for possible misdiagnosis of tooth vitality, *Int Endod J* 26:251, 1993.
24. Eli I, Schwartz-Arad D, Baht R, et al: Effect of anxiety on the experience of pain in implant insertion, *Clin Oral Implants Res* 14:115, 2003.
25. Eli I, Schwartz-Arad D, Bartal Y: Anxiety and ability to recognize clinical information in dentistry, *J Dent Res* 87:65, 2008.
26. Fava LR: One-appointment root canal treatment: incidence of postoperative pain using a modified double-flared technique, *Int Endod J* 24:258, 1991.
27. Figini L, Lodi G, Gorni F, et al: Single versus multiple visits for endodontic treatment of permanent teeth: a Cochrane systematic review, *J Endod* 34:1041, 2008.
28. Fouad AF, Burleson J: The effect of diabetes mellitus on endodontic treatment outcome: data from an electronic patient record, *J Am Dent Assoc* 134:43, 2003.
29. Friedlander AH, Sung EC, Child JS: Radiation-induced heart disease after Hodgkin's disease and breast cancer treatment: dental implications, *J Am Dent Assoc* 134:1615, 2003.
30. Friedman S: Considerations and concepts of case selection in the management of post-treatment endodontic disease (treatment failure). *Endod Top* 1:54, 2002.
31. Friedman S: Prognosis of initial endodontic therapy, *Endod Top* 1:54, 2002.
32. Gatten DL, Riedy CA, Hong SK, et al: Quality of life of endodontically treated versus implant treated patients: a University-based qualitative research study, *J Endod* 37:903, 2011.
33. Gaur AH, Dominguez KL, Kalish ML, et al: Practice of feeding premasticated food to infants: a potential risk factor for HIV transmission, *Pediatrics* 124:658, 2009.
34. Gillen BM, Looney SW, Gu LS, et al: Impact of the quality of coronal restoration versus the quality of root canal fillings on success of root canal treatment: a systematic review and meta-analysis, *J Endod* 37:865, 2011.
35. Goodchild JH, Glick M: A different approach to medical risk assessment, *Endod Top* 4:1, 2003.
36. Imura N, Zuolo ML: Factors associated with endodontic flare-ups: a prospective study, *Int Endod J* 28:261, 1995.

37. Iqbal MK, Kim S: A review of factors influencing treatment planning decisions of single-tooth implants versus preserving natural teeth with nonsurgical endodontic therapy, *J Endod* 34:519, 2008.
38. Javed F, Romanos GE: Impact of diabetes mellitus and glycemic control on the osseointegration of dental implants: a systematic literature review, *J Periodontol* 80:1719, 2009.
39. Jeske AH, Suchko GD: Lack of a scientific basis for routine discontinuation of oral anticoagulation therapy before dental treatment, *J Am Dent Assoc* 134:1492, 2003.
40. Kim E, Song JS, Jung IY, et al: Prospective clinical study evaluating endodontic microsurgery outcomes for cases with lesions of endodontic origin compared with cases with lesions of combined periodontal-endodontic origin, *J Endod* 34:546, 2008.
41. Kim SG, Solomon C: Cost-effectiveness of endodontic molar retreatment compared with fixed partial dentures and single-tooth implant alternatives, *J Endod* 37:321, 2011.
42. Kim TS, Caruso JM, Christensen H, et al: A comparison of cone-beam computed tomography and direct measurement in the examination of the mandibular canal and adjacent structures, *J Endod* 36:1191, 2010.
43. Klages US, Kianifard S, Ulusoy O, et al: Anxiety sensitivity as predictor of pain in patients undergoing restorative dental procedures, *Community Dent Oral Epidemiol* 34:139, 2006.
44. Lahmann C, Schoen R, Henningsen P, et al: Brief relaxation versus music distraction in the treatment of dental anxiety: a randomized controlled clinical trial, *J Am Dent Assoc* 139:317, 2008.
45. Lima SMF, Grisi DC, Kogawa EM: Diabetes mellitus and inflammatory pulpal and periapical disease: a review, *Int Endod J* 46:1, 2013.
46. Lin LM, Lin J, Rosenberg PA, et al: One-appointment endodontic therapy: biological considerations, *J Am Dent Assoc* 138:1456, 2007.
47. Lindh T, Gunne J, Tillberg A, et al: A meta-analysis of implants in partial edentulism, *Clin Oral Implants Res* 9:80, 1998.
48. Little JW, Falace DA, Miller CS, et al: *Dental management of the medically compromised patient*, ed 8, St. Louis, 2012, Mosby.
49. Little JW, Jacobson JJ, Lockhart PB, et al: The dental treatment of patients with joint replacements: a position paper from the American Academy of Oral Medicine, *J Am Dent Assoc* 141:667, 2010.
50. Loushine, RJ, Weller RN, Kimbrough WF, et al: Secondary hyperparathyroidism: a case report, *J Endod* 29:272, 2003.
51. Markiewicz MR, Margarone JE, Campbell JH, et al: Bisphosphonate-associated osteonecrosis of the jaws: a review of current knowledge, *J Am Dent Assoc* 136:1669, 2005.

52. Marotta PS, Fontes TV, Armada L, et al: Type 2 diabetes mellitus and the prevalence of apical periodontitis and endodontic treatment in an adult Brazilian population, *J Endod* 38:297, 2012.

53. McDaniel RK, Luna MA, Stimson PG: Metastatic tumors in the jaws, *Oral Surg Oral Med Oral Pathol* 31:380, 1971.

54. Melo MD, Obeid G: Osteonecrosis of the jaws in patients with a history of receiving bisphosphonate therapy: strategies for prevention and early recognition, *J Am Dent Assoc* 136:1675, 2005.

55. Michalowicz BS, DiAngelis AJ, Novak MJ, et al: Examining the safety of dental treatment in pregnant women, *J Am Dent Assoc* 139:685, 2008.

56. Migliorati CA, Casiglia J, Epstein J, et al: Managing the care of patients with bisphosphonate-associated osteonecrosis: an American Academy of Oral Medicine position paper, *J Am Dent Assoc* 136:1658, 2005.

57. Miley DD, Terezhalmy GT: The patient with diabetes mellitus: etiology, epidemiology, principles of medical management, oral disease burden, and principles of dental management, *Quintessence Int* 36:779, 2005.

58. Moinzadeh AT, Shemesh H, Neircynk NA, et al: Bisphosphonates and their clinical implications in endodontic therapy, *Int Endod J* 46:391, 2012.

59. Molander A, Warfvinge J, Reit C, et al: Clinical and radiographic evaluation of one- and two-visit endodontic treatment of asymptomatic necrotic teeth with apical periodontitis: a randomized clinical trial, *J Endod* 33:1145, 2007.

60. Moore PA: Selecting drugs for the pregnant dental patient, *J Am Dent Assoc* 129:1281, 1998.

61. Murphy SL, Xu J, Kochanek KD: Deaths: Preliminary data for 2010, *National Vital Statistics Reports* 60:1, 2012.

62. Nakai Y, Milgrom P, Mancl L, et al: Effectiveness of local anesthesia in pediatric dental practice, *J Am Dent Assoc* 131:1699, 2000.

63. Ng SK, Chau AW, Leung WK: The effect of pre-operative information in relieving anxiety in oral surgery patients, *Community Dent Oral Epidemiol* 32:227, 2004.

64. Ng YL, Glennon JP, Setchell DJ, et al: Prevalence of and factors affecting post-obturation pain in patients undergoing root canal treatment, *Int Endod J* 37:381, 2004.

65. Ng YL, Mann V, Gulabivala K: Outcome of secondary root canal treatment: a systematic review of the literature, *Int Endod J* 41:1026, 2008.

66. Ng YL, Mann V, Gulabivala K: Tooth survival following non-surgical root canal treatment: a systematic review of the literature, *Int Endod J* 43:171, 2010.

67. Ng YL, Mann V, Gulabivala K: A prospective study of the factors affecting outcomes of nonsurgical root canal treatment—part 1: periapical health, *Int Endod J* 44:583, 2011.

68. Ng YL, Mann V, Gulabivala K: A prospective study of the factors affecting outcomes of non-surgical root canal treatment: part 2: tooth survival, *Int Endod J* 44:610, 2011.

69. Ng YL, Mann V, Rahbaran S, et al: Outcome of primary root canal treatment: systematic review of the literature—part 1. Effects of study characteristics on probability of success, *Int Endod J* 40:921, 2007.

70. Ng YL, Mann V, Rahbaran S, et al: Outcome of primary root canal treatment: systematic review of the literature—Part 2. Influence of clinical factors, *Int Endod J* 41:6, 2008.

71. Nishimura RA, Carabello BA, Faxon DP, et al: ACC/AHA 2008 guideline update on valvular heart disease: focused update on infective endocarditis: a report of the American College of Cardiology/American Heart Association Task Force on Practice Guidelines: endorsed by the Society of Cardiovascular Anesthesiologists, Society for Cardiovascular Angiography and Interventions, and Society of Thoracic Surgeons, *Circulation* 118:887, 2008.

72. Pallasch TJ, Slots J: Antibiotic prophylaxis and the medically compromised patient, *Periodontol* 10:107, 1996.

73. Penesis VA, Fitzgerald PI, Fayad MI, et al: Outcome of one-visit and two-visit endodontic treatment of necrotic teeth with apical periodontitis: a randomized controlled trial with one-year evaluation, *J Endod* 34:251, 2008.

74. Persky V, Piorkowski J, Hernandez E, et al: Prenatal exposure to acetaminophen and respiratory symptoms in the first year of life, *Ann Allergy Asthma Immunol* 101:271, 2008.

75. Peters LB, Wesselink PR: Periapical healing of endodontically treated teeth in one and two visits obturated in the presence or absence of detectable microorganisms, *Int Endod J* 35:660, 2002.

76. Proctor R, Kumar N, Stein A, et al: Oral and dental aspects of chronic renal failure, *J Dent Res* 84:199, 2005.

77. Quesnell BT, Alves M, Hawkinson RW Jr, et al: The effect of human immunodeficiency virus on endodontic treatment outcome, *J Endod* 31:633, 2005.

78. Rayburn WF, Amanze AC: Prescribing medications safely during pregnancy, *Med Clin North Am* 92:1227, 2008.

79. Rhodus NL, Vibeto BM, Hamamoto DT: Glycemic control in patients with diabetes mellitus upon admission to a dental clinic: considerations for dental management, *Quintessence Int* 36:474, 2005.

80. Roane JB, Dryden JA, Grimes EW: Incidence of postoperative pain after single- and multiple-visit endodontic procedures, *Oral Surg Oral Med Oral Pathol* 55:68, 1983.

81. Rotstein I, Simon JH: The endo-perio lesion: a crisitcal appraisal of the disease condition, *Endod Top* 13:34, 2006.

82. Salehrabi R, Rotstein I: Endodontic treatment outcomes in a large patient population in the USA: an epidemiological study, *J Endod* 30:846, 2004.

83. Salehrabi R, Rotstein I: Epidemiologic evaluation of the outcomes of orthograde endodontic retreatment, *J Endod* 36:790, 2010.

84. Sathorn C, Parashos P, Messer HH: Effectiveness of single- versus multiple-visit endodontic treatment of teeth with apical periodontitis: a systematic review and meta-analysis, *Int Endod J* 38:347, 2005.

85. Sathorn C, Parashos P, Messer HH: The prevalence of postoperative pain and flare-up in single- and multiple-visit endodontic treatment: a systematic review, *Int Endod J* 41:91, 2008.

86. Scully C, Cawson RA: *Medical problems in dentistry*, ed 5, Edinburgh, 2005, Churchill Livingstone.

87. Setzer FC, Boyer KR, Jeppson JR, et al: Long-term prognosis of endodontically treated teeth: a retrospective analysis of preoperative factors in molars, *J Endod* 37:21, 2011.

88. Setzer FC, Kohli MR, Shah SB, et al: Outcome of endodontic surgery: a meta-analysis of the literature—part 2: comparison of endodontic microsurgical techniques with and without the use of higher magnification, *J Endod* 38:1, 2012.

89. Setzer FC, Shah SB, Kohli MR, et al: Outcome of endodontic surgery: a meta-analysis of the literature—part 1: comparison of traditional root-end surgery and endodontic microsurgery, *J Endod* 36:1757, 2010.

90. Siqueira JF: Endodontic infections: concepts, paradigms, and perspectives, *Oral Surg Oral Med Oral Pathol Oral Radiol Endod* 94:281, 2002.

91. Sirois DA, Fatahzadeh M: Valvular heart disease, *Oral Surg Oral Med Oral Pathol Oral Radiol Endod* 91:15, 2001.

92. Sjögren U, Figdor D, Perrson S, et al: Influence of infection at the time of root filling on the outcome of endodontic treatment of teeth with apical periodontitis, *Int Endod J* 30:297, 1997.

93. Sjogren U, Hagglund B, Sundqvist G, et al: Factors affecting the long-term results of endodontic treatment, *J Endod* 16:498, 1990.

94. Skaar D, O'Connor H, Lunos S, et al: Dental procedures and risk of experiencing a second vascular event in a Medicare population, *J Am Dent Assoc* 143:1190, 2012.

95. Smidt A, Lipovetsky-Adler M, Sharon E: Forced eruption as an alternative to tooth extraction in long-term use of oral bisphosphonates: review, risks and technique, *J Am Dent Assoc* 143:1303, 2012.

96. Su Y, Wang C, Ye L: Healing rate and post-obturation pain of single- versus multiple-visit endodontic treatment for infected root canals: a systematic review, *J Endod* 37:125, 2011.

97. Torabinejad M, Goodacre CJ: Endodontic or dental implant therapy: the factors affecting treatment planning, *J Am Dent Assoc* 137:973, 2006.

98. Torabinejad M, Kutsenko D, Machnick TK, et al: Levels of evidence for the outcome of nonsurgical endodontic treatment, *J Endod* 31:637, 2005.

99. Vera J, Siqueira JF, Ricucci D, et al: One- versus two-visit endodontic treatment of teeth with apical periodontitis: a histobacteriologic study, *J Endod* 38:1040, 2012.

100. Vernillo AT: Diabetes mellitus: relevance to dental treatment, *Oral Surg Oral Med Oral Pathol Oral Radiol Endod* 91:263, 2001.

101. von Arx T, Jensen SS, Hanni S: Clinical and radiographic assessment of various predictors for healing outcome 1 year after periapical surgery, *J Endod* 33:123, 2007.

102. von Arx T, Jensen SS, Hanni S: Five-year longitudinal assessment of the prognosis of apical microsurgery, *J Endod* 38:570, 2012.

103. Wang CH, Chueh LH, Chen SC, et al: Impact of diabetes mellitus, hypertension, and coronary artery disease on tooth extraction after nonsurgical root canal treatment, *J Endod* 37:1, 2011.

104. Wang N, Knight K, Dao T, et al: Treatment outcome in endodontics—The Toronto Study. Phases I and II: apical surgery, *J Endod* 30:751, 2004.

105. Wang Q, Cheung GSP, Ng RPY: Survival of surgical endodontic treatment performed in a dental teaching hospital: a cohort study, *Int Endod J* 37:764, 2004.

106. Weiger R, Rosendahl R, Lost C: Influence of calcium hydroxide intracanal dressings on the prognosis of teeth with endodontically induced periapical lesions, *Int Endod J* 33:219, 2000.

107. White SC: 1992 assessment of radiation risk from dental radiography, *Dentomaxillofac Radiol* 21:118, 1992.

108. Woo SB, Hellstein JW, Kalmar JR, et al: Narrative systematic review: bisphosphonates and osteonecrosis of the jaws, *Ann Intern Med* 144:753, 2006.

109. Woodmansey KF, Ayik M, Buschang PH, et al: Differences in masticatory function in patients with endodontically treated teeth and single-implant-supported prostheses: a pilot study, *J Endod* 35:10, 2009.

110. Wynn RL, Meiller TF, Crossley HL: *Drug information handbook for dentistry: including oral medicine for medically-compromised patients & specific oral conditions*, ed 18, Hudson, OH, 2012, Lexi-Comp.

111. Yu SM, Bellamy HA, Kogan MD, et al: Factors that influence receipt of recommended preventive pediatric health and dental care, *Pediatrics* 110:73, 2002.

112. Zuolo ML, Ferreira MO, Gutmann JL: Prognosis in periradicular surgery: a clinical prospective study, *Int Endod J* 33:91, 2000.

CHAPTER 4

Pain Control

AL READER | JOHN NUSSTEIN | ASMA KHAN

CHAPTER OUTLINE

I. LOCAL ANESTHESIA FOR RESTORATIVE DENTISTRY AND ENDODONTICS

Effective local anesthesia is the bedrock of pain control in endodontics and restorative dentistry. Regardless of the clinician's skills, both treatment and patient management are difficult or impossible to deliver without effective pain control. This chapter reviews the pharmacology of local anesthetics and the relative advantages and limitations of various anesthetics and routes of administration. Other chapters in this book provide complementary information on the use of local anesthetics in diagnosis (see Chapter 1) and the treatment of emergency patients (see Chapter 18). The authors assume that the reader is familiar with various anesthetic injection techniques; several excellent texts are available for review regarding this point.[195,262,353]

MECHANISMS OF ACTION FOR ANESTHETICS

Most dental pharmacology courses teach that local anesthetics block sodium channels by partitioning into two types, the uncharged basic form of the molecule (RN), which crosses cell membranes, and the charged acid form of the molecule (RNH$^+$), which binds to the inner pore of the sodium channel. As a first approximation, this model is reasonably accurate. However, molecular research has demonstrated the existence of at least nine subtypes of voltage-gated sodium channels (VGSCs) that differ in their expression pattern, biophysical properties, and roles in mediating peripheral pain (Table 4-1). These channels have a clear clinical relevance.[39,170,241] Indeed, several groups of patients have been described with genetic mutations to a VGSC, with significant reported effects on pain sensitivity.

The broad class of VGSCs can be divided into channels that are blocked by a toxin (tetrodotoxin [TTX]) and those that are resistant to the toxin (TTX-R). Most TTX-R channels are found primarily on nociceptors (e.g., Na$_v$ 1.8 and Na$_v$ 1.9).[433] These channels also are relatively resistant to local anesthetics and are sensitized by prostaglandins.[148] As is explained later in the chapter, the presence of TTX-R sodium channels may explain why local anesthetics are less effective when administered to patients with odontalgia. Many of the adverse effects of local anesthetics are attributed to their ability to block other VGSCs expressed in the central nervous system (CNS) or heart (see Table 4-1).

VGSCs consist of an alpha and a beta subunit. The alpha subunit serves as a voltage sensor, leading to channel activation and sodium ion passage when the channel detects an electrical field. The biologic basis for an electrical pulp tester, therefore, is the generation of a small electrical field across the dental pulp that can activate VGSCs.[170] Interestingly, sensitization of TTX-R channels by prostaglandins lowers the activation threshold and increases the number of sodium ions that flow through the channel.[148] Put another way, an inflammation-induced elevation in prostaglandin levels sensitizes TTX-R channels, leading to greater activation with weaker stimuli. This may explain the increased responsiveness to electrical pulp testing seen in patients with irreversible pulpitis.

Local anesthetics have other mechanisms that may contribute to their pharmacology for treating odontogenic pain. For example, local anesthetics modulate certain G protein–coupled receptors (GPCRs). The GPCRs are a major class of cell membrane receptors, and many classes of dental drugs (e.g., opioids, catecholamines) and endogenous mediators produce their effects by activating specific GPCRs and their related second messenger pathways. Studies suggest that local anesthetics inhibit the G-alpha-q ($G_{\alpha q}$) class of GPCRs, which includes receptors activated by inflammatory mediators such as bradykinin.[183] Local anesthetics may therefore block the actions of a major hyperalgesic agent.

Other studies have indicated that local anesthetics potentiate the actions of the G-alpha-i ($G_{\alpha i}$) class of GPCRs.[32] This could have a major effect in potentiating the actions of vasoconstrictors, including the newly recognized analgesic role that vasoconstrictors play in inhibiting pulpal nociceptors.[43,169] Prolonged alteration of GPCR function might explain why analgesia obtained with long-acting local anesthetics persists well beyond the period of anesthesia.[78,104,300] More research is needed on this exciting aspect of local anesthetic pharmacology.

CLINICALLY AVAILABLE LOCAL ANESTHETICS

The most common forms of injectable local anesthetics are in the amide class. In 2003, the American Dental Association specified a uniform color code for dental cartridges to prevent confusion among brands (Table 4-2). Local anesthetics can be divided roughly into three types: short duration (30 minutes of pulpal anesthesia), intermediate duration (60 minutes of pulpal anesthesia), and long duration (over 90 minutes of pulpal anesthesia). However, clinical anesthesia does not always follow these guidelines, depending on whether the local anesthetic is used as a block or for infiltration. For example, bupivacaine is classified as a long-acting agent, and when it is used in an inferior alveolar nerve (IAN) block, this is true.[112] However, when it is used for infiltration for anterior teeth, it

TABLE 4-1

Voltage-Gated Sodium Channels and Pain

Channel Subtype	Tissue Expression	Tetrodotoxin Sensitive	Peripheral Role in Pain
Na$_v$ 1.1	Central nervous system (CNS), sensory neurons	Yes	?
Na$_v$ 1.2	CNS	Yes	No
Na$_v$ 1.3	CNS	Yes	No
Na$_v$ 1.4	Muscle	Yes	No
Na$_v$ 1.5	Heart	Somewhat	No
Na$_v$ 1.6	CNS, sensory neurons	Yes	?
Na$_v$ 1.7	CNS, sensory neurons	Yes	?
Na$_v$ 1.8	Sensory neurons	No	Yes
Na$_v$ 1.9	Sensory neurons	No	Yes

TABLE 4-2

Local Anesthetics Available in the United States*

Anesthetic	Vasoconstrictor	Dental Cartridge Color Codes†	Maximum Allowable Dose	Typical Maximum Dose
2% Lidocaine	1:100,000 epinephrine	Red	13	8
2% Lidocaine	1:50,000 epinephrine	Green	13	8
2% Lidocaine	Plain (no vasoconstrictor)	Light blue	8	8
2% Mepivacaine	1:20,000 levonordefrin	Brown	11	8
3% Mepivacaine	Plain (no vasoconstrictor)	Tan	7	5½
4% Prilocaine	1:200,000 epinephrine	Yellow	5½	5½
4% Prilocaine	Plain (no vasoconstrictor)	Black	5½	5½
0.5% Bupivacaine	1:200,00 epinephrine	Blue	10	10
4% Articaine	1:100,000 epinephrine	Gold	7	7
4% Articaine	1:200,000 epinephrine	Silver	7	7

*This table provides the maximum dosage in two formats. The maximum allowable dose generally is approached only with complex oral and maxillofacial surgical procedures. The typical maximum dose is the usual outer envelope of drug dosage for most endodontic, surgical, and restorative dental procedures. Both columns show the number of cartridges that would be required for an adult weighing 67.5 kg (150 pounds).
†Uniform dental cartridge color codes were mandated by the American Dental Association in June, 2003.

has a shorter duration of anesthetic action than 2% lidocaine with 1:100,000 epinephrine[81,156] (this is discussed in more detail later in the chapter).

SELECTION OF A LOCAL ANESTHETIC: POSSIBLE ADVERSE EFFECTS, MEDICAL HISTORY, AND PREOPERATIVE ANXIETY

Possible Adverse Effects

Possible adverse reactions to local anesthetics can be divided into six major categories: cardiovascular reactions, systemic effects, methemoglobinemia, peripheral nerve paresthesia, allergic reactions to the anesthetic and/or latex, and reactions to anesthetics containing a sulfite antioxidant. These reactions range from fairly common (e.g., tachycardia after intraosseous injection of 2% lidocaine with 1:100,000 epinephrine) to extremely rare (e.g., allergic reactions to lidocaine).

Cardiovascular Reactions

Although classic research studies have reported that large dosages or intravenous (IV) injections of local anesthetics were required to produce cardiovascular effects,[192,419] it now is well recognized that even comparatively small amounts of epinephrine can induce measurable tachycardia after nerve block or intraosseous injection.[113,150,358] Several authors have reported increases in heart rate with infiltration injections and nerve blocks using 2% lidocaine with 1:100,000 epinephrine[2,172,236,375,418]; others have reported that no significant changes in heart rate occurred or that the changes were clinically insignificant.[282,413,422] When specific information was given on dosing and heart rate increases, several studies found mean heart rate increases.[2,172,235,418] Two studies found increases on average of about 4 beats/min with approximately 20 μg of epinephrine[172,235]; three studies recorded increases of 10 to 15 beats/min with 45 to 80 μg of epinephrine[2,235,375]; and one study found increases of approximately 21 beats/min using 144 μg.[418] Increasing the amount of epinephrine in an infiltration or block injection, therefore, increases the likelihood of an elevated heart rate.

Tachycardia after injection is primarily a pharmacologic effect. The cardiovascular effects are the result of alpha-adrenoceptor stimulation by systemic distribution of the vasoconstrictor throughout the vascular compartment. The patient may also report heart palpitations associated with anxiety or fear and may experience transient tachycardia and changes in blood pressure. Large doses or inadvertent IV injection may lead to lidocaine toxicity and CNS depression.[115,308] To reduce this risk, the clinician should always aspirate before making the injection, inject slowly, and use dosages within accepted guidelines. The maximal dosages for local anesthetics are listed in Table 4-2.

Systemic Effects

Acute toxicity from an overdose of a local anesthetic often is the result of inadvertent IV administration or of a cumulative large dose (e.g., repeated injections). As shown in Table 4-1, VGSCs are found in the CNS and the myocardium, the two major sites of anesthetic-induced toxicity. Although systemic effects from a local anesthetic are rare, they can include an initial excitatory phase (e.g., muscle twitching, tremors, grand mal convulsions) and a subsequent depressive phase (e.g., sedation, hypotension, and respiratory arrest).[86,115] It should be noted that symptomatic management (possibly including cardiopulmonary resuscitation [CPR], airway support, and supplemental oxygen) is the primary response to this adverse event.[229,233] An acute hypotensive crisis with respiratory failure also has been interpreted as the result of hypersensitivity to local anesthetics[62]; these patients should be evaluated with allergy testing. To reduce the risk of systemic effects from anesthetics, the clinician must always aspirate before giving the injection and must use dosages within accepted guidelines (see Table 4-2). Finder and Moore[115] proposed a "rule of 25" as a simple means of remembering maximal local anesthetic dosages: with currently formulated local anesthetic cartridges, it generally is safe to use one cartridge of local anesthetic for every 25 pounds of patient weight (e.g., six cartridges for a patient weighing 150 pounds [67.5 kg]).

Methemoglobinemia

Metabolism of certain local anesthetics (e.g., prilocaine, benzocaine, articaine, and to a lesser extent lidocaine) can produce a metabolite that causes methemoglobinemia; this effect often occurs several hours after injection of the local anesthetic.[265,439] Typical signs and symptoms include cyanosis, dyspnea, emesis, and headache. In a study on benzocaine-induced methemoglobinemia, 67% of reported adverse effects of benzocaine were associated with methemoglobinemia; of these events, 93% occurred with spray formulations of benzocaine, and only one case involved the gel formulation.[301] To reduce the risk of methemoglobinemia, clinicians should take care to refrain from giving excessive dosages of local anesthetics.

Peripheral Nerve Paresthesia

Postinjection paresthesia is a rare adverse effect of local anesthetics.[161,265,453] The incidence of paresthesia (which involved the lip and/or tongue) associated with articaine and prilocaine was higher than that found with either lidocaine or mepivacaine.[132,140,161] Another study evaluated patients referred with a diagnosis of damage to the inferior alveolar and/or lingual nerve that could only have resulted from an IAN block.[345] In 35% of these cases, the paresthesia was caused by a lidocaine formulation, and in 30%, it was caused by an articaine formulation. The conclusion was that there was not a disproportionate nerve involvement from articaine, although this interpretation does not account for large differences in clinical usage of the two local anesthetics. However, with any paresthesia, documentation of the patient's reported area of altered sensation, the type of altered sensation (e.g., anesthesia, paresthesia, dysesthesia), and regular follow-up are important.[463]

Allergic Reactions to Local Anesthetics and Latex

The amide local anesthetics appear to have little immunogenicity and therefore have an extremely low rate of allergic reactions.[382] One study included more than 140 patients specifically referred for allergy testing because of adverse effects after injection of a local anesthetic; none of these patients had hypersensitivity reactions to intradermal local anesthetics,[368] but case reports of hypersensitivity reactions after administration of local anesthetics have been published.[41,62,302,382] Some concern has been raised that the rubber latex stopper in dental anesthetic cartridges might be a source of allergen to patients allergic to latex. In a review of this literature (1966 to 2001), Shojaei and Haas[385] concluded that some evidence for exposure to the latex allergen exists, although no causal study has been published.

Local anesthetic formulations that contain vasoconstrictors also contain sulfite to prevent oxidation of this agent. Sulfite-induced reactions came to prominence with the report of six deaths after exposure to salad bars or homemade wine.[20] Common reported signs and symptoms include allergic-like reactions, such as urticaria, bronchospasm, and anaphylaxis. Risk factors include an active history of asthma (perhaps 5% of asthmatics are at risk) and atopic allergy. The use of local anesthetics without vasoconstrictors is a possible alternative with these patients. No sulfite reaction in dental practice has ever been documented, possibly because the amount of sulfite in local anesthetic cartridges is relatively small.

EFFECTS OF SYSTEMIC DISEASES OR CONDITIONS ON LOCAL ANESTHETICS

It has been stated that vasoconstrictors should be avoided in patients with high blood pressure (higher than 200 mmHg systolic or 115 mmHg diastolic), cardiac dysrhythmias, unstable angina, less than 6 months since myocardial infarction or cerebrovascular accident, or severe cardiovascular disease.[262] However, these conditions are contraindications to routine dental treatment. Patients taking antidepressants, nonselective beta-blocking agents, medicine for Parkinson disease, and

cocaine have a potential for problems.[262,353] In patients taking these medications, plain mepivacaine (3% Carbocaine) can be used for the inferior alveolar nerve block.

Alcoholics have been found to be more sensitive to painful stimulation.[406] Alcoholics with a history of depression/unhappiness may also have reduced pulpal anesthesia.[116] In contrast, alcoholics in recovery may not be at increased risk for inadequate pain control with local anesthesia.[116]

Any of the commonly available local anesthetics are safe for use in pregnant or lactating women.[162] The most important aspect of care with pregnant patients is to eliminate the source of pain by performing the indicated endodontic treatment; this reduces the need for systemic medications.[162]

Local anesthetics may interact with a patient's medications, so a thorough review of the medical history is an absolute requirement. Potential drug-drug interactions occur primarily with the vasoconstrictors in local anesthetic formulations (Table 4-3). Judicious use of local anesthetic solutions without vasoconstrictors (e.g., 3% mepivacaine) is a reasonable alternative for adult patients.

Studies have found that women try to avoid pain more than men, accept it less, and fear it more.[99,114,249,303] One study found that women find postsurgical pain more intense than males, but men are more disturbed than women by low levels of pain that lasts several days.[303] Another study found gender differences in analgesia for postoperative endodontic pain.[374] Anxiety

TABLE 4-3

Possible Drug Interactions with Vasoconstrictors

Drugs	Possible Adverse Effects	Recommendations
Tricyclic Antidepressants		
Amitriptyline, doxepin	Increased cardiovascular responses	Reduce or eliminate vasoconstrictors
Nonselective Beta-Blockers		
Nadolol, propranolol	Hypertension, bradycardia	Reduce or eliminate vasoconstrictors
Recreational Drugs		
Cocaine	Hypertension, myocardial infarction, dysrhythmias	Instruct patient to abstain from drug use for 48 hours before procedure; do not use vasoconstrictors
COMT Inhibitors		
Entacapone, tolcapone	Increased cardiovascular responses	Reduce or eliminate vasoconstrictors
Antiadrenergic Drugs		
Guanadrel, guanethidine	Increased cardiovascular responses	Reduce or eliminate vasoconstrictors
Nonselective Alpha-Adrenergic Blockers		
Chlorpromazine, clozapine, haloperidol	Increased cardiovascular responses	Reduce or eliminate vasoconstrictors
Digitalis		
Digoxin	Dysrhythmias (especially with large dosage of vasoconstrictor)	Reduce or eliminate vasoconstrictor
Hormone		
Levothyroxine	Dysrhythmias (especially with large dosage of vasoconstrictor)	*Euthyroid:* No precaution *Hyperthyroid:* Reduce or eliminate vasoconstrictors
Monoamine Oxidase Inhibitors		
Furazolidone, linezolid, selegiline, tranylcypromine	No interaction	None

Modified from Naftalin L, Yagiela JA: Vasoconstrictors: indications and precautions, *Dent Clin North Am* 46:733, 2002.
COMT, Catecholamine *O*-methyl transferase.

may also modulate differences in pain responses between males and females. In addition, pain threshold response varies greatly at different stages of the menstrual cycle.[42] Other studies have shown that women report greater pain relief from kappa opioid agonists (e.g., pentazocine) after endodontic treatment.[420] We should be aware that women might react differently to pain than men.[114]

CLINICAL ANESTHESIA AND ROUTES OF ANESTHETIC ADMINISTRATION

Recognition is growing that evidence-based therapeutics offers an excellent source of information that should become an aspect of treatment in conjunction with the practitioner's clinical skills and the patient's particular needs. In many areas of dentistry, this is a limited concept because few randomized, placebo-controlled, double-blind clinical trials have been conducted. However, this is not the case with dental pharmacology. The astute clinician can make informed decisions on various local anesthetics and routes of injection based on a large collection of well-designed clinical trials. The following discussion focuses on the clinical aspects of local anesthesia, with special emphasis on restorative dentistry and endodontics.

IMPORTANT CLINICAL FACTORS IN LOCAL ANESTHESIA

Traditional Methods of Confirming Anesthesia

Traditional methods of confirming anesthesia usually involve questioning the patient ("Is your lip numb?"), soft tissue testing (e.g., lack of mucosal responsiveness to a sharp explorer), or simply beginning treatment. However, these approaches may not be effective for determining pulpal anesthesia.[60,179,277,424]

Determining Pulpal Anesthesia in Asymptomatic Vital Teeth

Anesthesia in asymptomatic vital teeth can be measured more objectively by applying a cold refrigerant (Fig. 4-1) or by using an electrical pulp tester (EPT), as described in Chapter 1 (Fig. 4-2). Application of cold or the electrical pulp tester can be used to test the tooth under treatment for pulpal anesthesia before a clinical procedure is started.[56,100,201,257]

Determining Pulpal Anesthesia in Symptomatic Vital Teeth

In symptomatic (painful) vital teeth and after administration of a local anesthetic, testing with a cold refrigerant or an electrical pulp tester can be used to evaluate pulpal anesthesia before an endodontic procedure is started.[68,100,323,355] If the patient responds to the stimulus, pulpal anesthesia has not been obtained, and supplemental anesthetic should be administered. However, in patients presenting for an emergency appointment with a painful vital tooth (e.g., symptomatic irreversible pulpitis), the lack of a response to pulp testing may not guarantee pulpal anesthesia.[100,323,355] Therefore, if a patient experiences pain when the endodontic procedure is started,

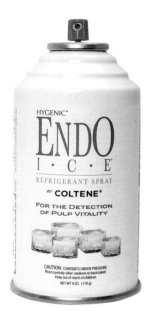

FIG. 4-1 A cold refrigerant may be used to test for pulpal anesthesia before the start of a clinical procedure. (Coltène/Whaledent Inc., Cuyahoga Falls, OH.)

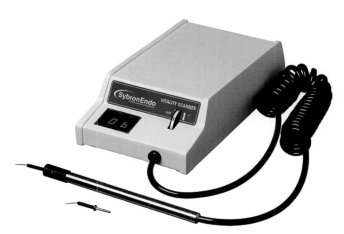

FIG. 4-2 An electrical pulp tester also may be used to test for pulpal anesthesia before a clinical procedure is started. (Courtesy SybronEndo, Corporation Orange, CA.)

supplemental anesthetic is indicated, regardless of the responsiveness to pulpal testing. If the chamber is necrotic and the canals are vital, no objective test can predict the level of clinical anesthesia.

Patient Who Has Had Previous Difficulty with Anesthesia

Anesthesia is more likely to be unsuccessful in patients who report a history of previous difficulty with anesthesia.[214] These patients generally make comments such as, "Novocaine doesn't work on me" or "It takes a lot of shots to get my teeth numb." A good clinical practice is to ask the patient if dentists previously have had difficulty obtaining anesthesia. If the answer is yes, supplemental injections should be considered.

Failure to Achieve Anesthesia in Patients with Pain

Obtaining anesthesia is often difficult in patients with endodontic pain of pulpal origin. A number of explanations have been proposed for this.[170] One is that conventional anesthetic techniques do not always provide profound pulpal anesthesia, and patients with preexisting hyperalgesia may be unable to tolerate any noxious input. Another explanation relates to the theory that inflamed tissue has a lower pH, which reduces the amount of the base form of anesthetic that penetrates the nerve membrane. Consequently, less of the ionized form is available in the nerve to achieve anesthesia. However, this explanation does not account for the mandibular molar with pulpitis that is not readily blocked by an inferior alveolar injection administered at some distance from the area of inflammation. Correlating localized inflammatory changes with failure of the IAN block is difficult.

Another explanation for failure is that nerves arising from inflamed tissue have altered resting potentials and decreased excitability thresholds.[51,427] Two studies demonstrated that local anesthetics were unable to prevent impulse transmission because of these lowered excitability thresholds.[292,427] Another factor might be the TTX-R sodium channels, which are resistant to the action of local anesthetics,[373] are increased in inflamed dental pulp,[399,431,433] and are sensitized by prostaglandins.[148] A related factor is the increased expression of sodium channels.[399,431,433]

Finally, patients in pain are often apprehensive, which lowers the pain threshold. Therefore, practitioners should consider supplemental techniques (e.g., intraosseous injections[320,323,332,355] or periodontal ligament injections[68]) if an IAN block fails to provide pulpal anesthesia for patients with irreversible pulpitis.

Use of Topical Anesthetics

Fear of needle insertion is a major cause of apprehension in dental patients.[234,289,290] Although some studies have demonstrated the effectiveness of topical anesthetics,[146,175,186,312,372] others have shown no significant pain reduction.[146,222,270] Interestingly, one study showed that patients who thought they were receiving a topical anesthetic anticipated less pain regardless of whether they actually received the anesthetic.[270] The most important aspect of a topical anesthetic may not be its clinical effectiveness, but rather its psychological effect on the patient, who believes the practitioner is doing everything possible to prevent pain.

Reversing the Action of Local Anesthetics

Phentolamine mesylate (0.4 mg in a 1.7-ml cartridge [Ora-Verse, Novalar Pharmaceuticals, San Diego, California]) is a recently developed agent that shortens the duration of soft tissue anesthesia. The duration of soft tissue anesthesia is longer than pulpal anesthesia and is often associated with difficulty eating, drinking, and speaking.[176,245] The best use of OraVerse is after dental procedures when postoperative pain is not a concern. Asymptomatic endodontic patients may benefit from the use of a reversal agent when they have speaking engagements or important meetings or must perform in musical or theatrical events.[121] Therefore, OraVerse may be used to shorten the duration of soft tissue anesthesia if the patient presents with an asymptomatic tooth and little postoperative pain is anticipated.[121]

INFERIOR ALVEOLAR NERVE BLOCK FOR RESTORATIVE DENTISTRY

2% Lidocaine and 1 : 100,000 Epinephrine

Because failure occurs most often with the IAN block,[214] factors that modify mandibular anesthesia must be carefully reviewed. The technique for administering an IAN block can be reviewed in available textbooks.[195,262] The following discussion reviews the expected outcomes after administration of a conventional IAN block to asymptomatic patients using 1.8 ml of 2% lidocaine with 1 : 100,000 epinephrine (Xylocaine, Lignospan, Octocaine). Although anesthesia requirements vary among dental procedures, the following discussion concentrates on *pulpal* anesthesia in asymptomatic patients and thus is directly relevant to endodontic therapy.

Anesthetic Success

One way to define anesthetic success for nerve blocks is the percentage of subjects who achieve two consecutive nonresponsive readings on electrical pulp testing within 15 minutes and continuously sustain this lack of responsiveness for 60 minutes. In other words, the objective is to achieve anesthesia within 15 minutes and to have it last 1 hour. This endpoint is as important for restorative dentistry as it is for endodontic treatment, so it is used as a benchmark for clinically significant information from research on local anesthetics. Using this criterion, the percentage of cases in which anesthesia was obtained after IAN block injections ranged from 10% (central incisor) to 65% (second molar).* It is important to note that all patients from these studies reported a positive lip sign (e.g., profound lip numbness); therefore, profound lip numbness *does not* predict pulpal anesthesia. However, lack of soft tissue anesthesia is a useful indicator that the block injection was not administered accurately for that patient. Missed blocks occur in about 5% of cases, and the clinician should readminister the nerve block before continuing with treatment.

Anesthetic Failure

Anesthetic failure can be defined as the percentage of subjects who never achieved two consecutive nonresponsive EPT readings at any time during a 60-minute period. Using this criterion, anesthetic failure rates ranged from 17% (second molar) to 58% (central incisor).†

Noncontinuous Anesthesia

Another measure of mandibular anesthesia is noncontinuous anesthesia, which may be related to the action of the anesthetic solution on the nerve membrane (blocking and unblocking the sodium channels). This occurs in about 12% to 20% of patients.‡

Slow Onset

After a conventional IAN block injection, the onset of pulpal anesthesia occurs within 10 to 15 minutes in most cases (Fig. 4-3).§ Slow onset can be defined as the percentage of

---

*References 60, 165, 179, 277, 322, 353, and 424.
†References 60, 112, 165, 179, 277, 322, 353, 388, 424, and 425.
‡References 60, 158, 165, 179, 277, 322, 353, and 424.
§References 60, 112, 165, 179, 277, 322, 353, 388, 424, and 425.

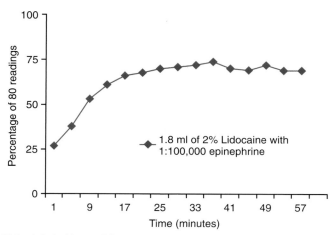

FIG. 4-3 Incidence of first mandibular molar anesthesia as determined by lack of response to electrical pulp testing at the maximum setting (percentage of 80 readings) across time for 60 minutes.

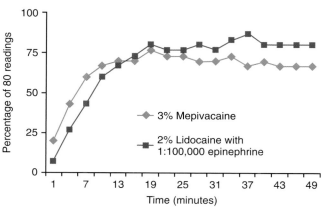

FIG. 4-4 Incidence of first mandibular molar anesthesia: comparison of 3% mepivacaine to 2% lidocaine with 1:100,000 epinephrine. Results were determined by lack of response to electrical pulp testing at the maximum setting (percentage of 80 readings) across time for 50 minutes. No significant difference between the two solutions was noted.

subjects who achieved a nonresponsive EPT reading after 15 minutes. In mandibular teeth, slow onset occurs in 12% to 20% of patients.

Duration

The duration of action for pulpal anesthesia in the mandible is very good.* If patients are anesthetized initially, anesthesia usually persists for approximately 2½ hours.[112] Figure 4-3 depicts the time course for complete pulpal anesthesia for an asymptomatic first molar, as defined by the percentage of patients who did not respond to a stimulus (EPT) across time for 60 minutes. Most patients achieved pulpal anesthesia within 15 minutes and had a duration of anesthesia of at least 1 hour, but the success rate was not 100% for the population.

ALTERNATIVE ANESTHETIC SOLUTIONS FOR THE INFERIOR ALVEOLAR NERVE BLOCK

Plain Solutions: 3% Mepivacaine (Carbocaine, Polocaine, Scandonest) and 4% Prilocaine (Citanest Plain)

In a study of volunteers without dental pathosis, anesthesia from IAN injection of 3% mepivacaine plain and 4% prilocaine plain was as effective as that from 2% lidocaine with 1:100,000 (Fig. 4-4).[277] A clinical study of patients with irreversible pulpitis also found that 3% mepivacaine and 2% lidocaine with 1:100,000 epinephrine were equivalent for IAN blocks.[68] These findings support the selection of 3% mepivacaine as a local anesthetic when medical conditions or drug therapies suggest caution in the administration of solutions containing epinephrine.

4% Prilocaine with 1:200,000 Epinephrine (Citanest Forte) and 2% Mepivacaine with 1:20,000 Levonordefrin (Carbocaine with Neo-Cobefrin)

In a study of volunteers without dental pathosis, IAN injection of 4% prilocaine with 1:200,000 epinephrine or 2% mepivacaine with 1:20,000 levonordefrin worked as well as 2% lidocaine with 1:100,000 epinephrine in achieving pulpal anesthesia.[179]

Levonordefrin has 75% alpha activity and only 25% beta activity, making it seemingly more attractive than epinephrine (50% alpha activity and 50% beta activity).[262] However, levonordefrin is marketed as a 1:20,000 concentration in dental cartridges.[262] Clinically, the higher concentration of levonordefrin makes it equipotent to epinephrine in clinical and systemic effects,[158,179] so 1:20,000 levonordefrin offers no clinical advantage over 1:100,000 epinephrine.

Articaine with 1:100,000 Epinephrine (Septocaine, Articadent, Zorcaine)

Articaine has been reported to be a safe and effective local anesthetic.[378] It was approved for use in the United States in April, 2000, and is marketed as a 4% solution with either 1:100,000 or 1:200,000 epinephrine.[265,299] Articaine is classified as an amide. It has a thiophene ring (instead of a benzene ring, as do the other amide local anesthetics) and an extra ester linkage, which results in hydrolysis of articaine by plasma esterases.[271] A number of studies have evaluated articaine and concluded that it is safe when used in appropriate doses.* Lidocaine and articaine have the same maximal dose of 500 mg for adult patients (recommended dose, 6.6 to 7 mg/kg), but the maximum number of cartridges is different because of the differences in drug concentration (see Table 4-2).[262]

---

*References 60, 112, 165, 179, 277, 322, 353, 388, 424, and 425.

*References 82, 178, 193, 263, 265, 293, 328, 389, and 449.

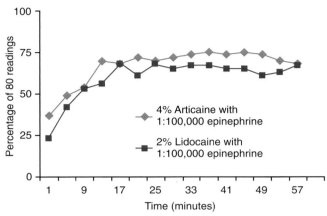

FIG. 4-5 Incidence of first mandibular molar anesthesia: comparison of 4% articaine with 1:100,000 epinephrine to 2% lidocaine with 1:100,000 epinephrine. Results were determined by lack of response to electrical pulp testing at the maximum setting (percentage of 80 readings) across time for 60 minutes. No significant difference between the two solutions was noted.

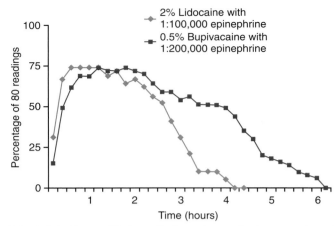

FIG. 4-6 Incidence of first mandibular molar anesthesia: comparison of 0.5% bupivacaine with 1:200,000 epinephrine to 2% lidocaine with 1:100,000 epinephrine. Results were determined by lack of response to electrical pulp testing at the maximum setting (percentage of 80 readings) across time for 6 hours. The bupivacaine solution showed a longer duration of anesthesia than the lidocaine solution.

Clinical Effectiveness of Articaine for Inferior Alveolar Nerve Blocks

The available literature indicates that articaine is equally effective for IAN blocks when statistically compared to other local anesthetics.* In comparing the anesthetic efficacy of 4% articaine with 1:100,000 epinephrine to 2% lidocaine with 1:100,000 epinephrine for IAN blocks, one study found that the two solutions were not significantly different (Fig. 4-5).[288] Two studies found no difference in efficacy between 4% articaine with 1:100,000 and 1:200,000 epinephrine.[299,412] In summary, repeated clinical trials have failed to demonstrate any statistical superiority of articaine over lidocaine for IAN blocks.

Articaine and Uncorroborated Insurance Carrier Warning

A letter was sent to thousands of U.S. dentists in 2006 by insurer Emery and Webb/Ace USA stating, "... we have noticed an increase in reversible and, in some cases, nonreversible paresthesias (with Septocaine) ... We are writing you to alert you to these events in hopes that you will not fall victim to one of these incidents."[261] Knowledgeable dentists and educators communicated their concerns, and a Notice of Retraction was issued:

> Unfortunately, we at Emery & Webb discovered upon further review, and subsequent to the mailings, that both documents contained inaccuracies and an alarmist tone, which was not warranted ... Emery and Webb has not noted an increase in malpractice claims or lawsuits in connection with articaine ... It should be made clear that Emery and Webb has not conducted any scientific investigation, sampling, testing, or other investigation of the articaine anesthetic, and has no independent knowledge or data which would restrict the use of the product.[261]

Astute clinicians should be very careful of Web chat sites and colleagues' clinical endorsements, because they may not accurately reflect the correct information regarding articaine.

Long-Acting Anesthetics

Clinical trials with bupivacaine (Marcaine) and etidocaine (Duranest) have been conducted in patients undergoing oral surgery,[84,371] endodontic treatment,[104,300] and periodontic treatment.[78,254] Etidocaine was withdrawn from the market by Dentsply Pharmaceuticals (York, Pennsylvania). Bupivacaine was found to have a slower onset of pulpal anesthesia than lidocaine for IAN blocks.[112] Generally, bupivacaine provides prolonged analgesia and is indicated when postoperative pain is anticipated, but not all patients want lip numbness for an extended period.[371] Patients should be questioned about their preference. Although bupivacaine has a somewhat slower onset than lidocaine, its duration of pulpal anesthesia in the mandible is almost twice as long (approximately 4 hours; Fig. 4-6).[112]

Ropivacaine (Naropin), a relatively new long-acting local anesthetic, is a structural homolog of bupivacaine.[223] A number of studies have shown that ropivacaine has a lower potential for toxic CNS and cardiovascular effects than bupivacaine but produces equivalent pharmacologic effects.[223] Ropivacaine and levobupivacaine are being developed as potentially new local anesthetics based on their stereochemistry. Both are S-isomers and are thought to cause less toxicity than the racemic mixture of bupivacaine currently marketed.[392] A clinical trial has indicated that levobupivacaine showed significantly better postoperative pain control at 4 and 24 hours after infiltration injection than ropivacaine.[331] Because of their decreased potential for cardiac and CNS toxicity, ropivacaine and levobupivacaine may replace bupivacaine with epinephrine in clinical dental practice.

Buffered Lidocaine

Buffering lidocaine using sodium bicarbonate raises the pH of the anesthetic solution. In medicine there is evidence that buffering lidocaine results in less pain during the injection.[55,164]

---

*References 64, 95, 159, 160, 263, 264, 288, 421, and 450.

In dentistry, some studies[15,16,44,210] found that buffered lidocaine produced less pain on injection and a faster onset of anesthesia. However, other dental studies[350,435] did not find less pain on injection or a faster onset with buffered lidocaine for IAN block. Using a commercial buffering system (Onpharma, Los Gatos, California) in asymptomatic subjects, one study[266] found a reduction in onset time and injection pain, whereas another study[180] found no difference in these measurements. In symptomatic patients with a diagnosis of pulpal necrosis and associated acute swelling, no significant decrease in pain of infiltrations or significant decrease in pain of an incision and drainage procedure was found when the buffered anesthetic formulation was used.[29] Most patients who had the incision and drainage procedure experienced moderate to severe pain.

Use of Mannitol

An Ohio State University research group studied the use of mannitol to increase the efficacy of nerve blocks. Mannitol, a hyperosmotic sugar solution, is thought to temporarily disrupt the protective covering (perineurium) of sensory nerves, allowing the local anesthetic to gain entry to the innermost part of the nerve.[22] These researchers found that the use of mannitol in combination with lidocaine increased anesthetic success in IAN blocks about 15% to 20% but did not provide complete pulpal anesthesia for restorative or endodontic treatment.[239,398,443] The drug combination may be introduced sometime in the future.

ALTERNATIVE INJECTION SITES

Gow-Gates and Vazirani-Akinosi Techniques

Some clinicians have reported that the Gow-Gates technique[154] has a higher success rate than the conventional IAN block injection,[259,262] but controlled experimental studies have failed to show superiority of the Gow-Gates technique.[11,149,294,411] Neither has the Vazirani-Akinosi technique[12,149,262] been found superior to the standard inferior alveolar injection.[149,271,394,411,460] In a small study of 21 patients, no difference was found between lidocaine (11 patients) and articaine (10 patients) formulations for the Gow-Gates injection in patients with irreversible pulpitis.[384] Another study found the Gow-Gates technique had a higher success rate (52%) than the Vazirani-Akinosi technique (41%) in patients with irreversible pulpitis.[4] Further research is indicated with both techniques in patients presenting with symptomatic irreversible pulpitis. The Vazirani-Akinosi technique is indicated for cases involving a limited mandibular opening (trismus).

Incisive Nerve Block/Infiltration at the Mental Foramen

The incisive nerve block is successful 80% to 83% of the time in anesthetizing the premolar teeth for about 20-30 minutes.[30,202,313,437] It is not effective for the central and lateral incisors.[313]

Lidocaine Infiltrations

Labial or lingual infiltration injections of a lidocaine solution alone are not effective for pulpal anesthesia in the mandible.[118,281,459]

Articaine Infiltrations

Articaine is significantly better than lidocaine for buccal infiltration of the mandibular first molar.[75,203,205,362] However, articaine alone does not predictably provide pulpal anesthesia of the first molar. There is no difference between 4% articaine with 1:100,000 and 1:200,000 epinephrine for buccal infiltration.[275]

In anterior teeth, buccal and lingual infiltrations of articaine provide initial pulpal anesthesia, but the anesthesia declines over 60 minutes.[190,326]

ATTEMPTS TO INCREASE SUCCESS OF THE INFERIOR ALVEOLAR NERVE BLOCK

Increasing the Volume of Anesthetic

One possible method for increasing anesthetic success could be to double the injection volume of local anesthetic solution. However, increasing the volume of 2% lidocaine with epinephrine to 3.6 ml (two cartridges) does not increase the incidence of pulpal anesthesia with the IAN block (Fig. 4-7).[322,455]

Increasing the Epinephrine Concentration

A second approach for increasing the success of the IAN block could be to increase the concentration of epinephrine. However, when this technique was evaluated in clinically normal teeth, no advantage was seen in using a higher concentration (1:50,000 versus 1:100,000) of epinephrine.[80,425]

Addition of Hyaluronidase

Hyaluronidase reduces the viscosity of the injected tissue, permitting a wider spread of injected fluids.[21] Early studies in dentistry found that an IAN block was more easily attained and was more complete when hyaluronidase was added to an anesthetic solution.[230,258] A recent study found that hyaluronidase may increase the duration of the effects of lidocaine.[377] However, a controlled clinical trial found that adding hyaluronidase to a lidocaine solution with epinephrine did not statistically increase the incidence of pulpal anesthesia in IAN blocks.[360] In addition, hyaluronidase increased the occurrence of adverse effects (i.e., increased pain and trismus).[360]

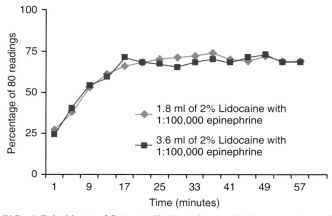

FIG. 4-7 Incidence of first mandibular molar anesthesia: comparison of 1.8 ml and 3.6 ml of 2% lidocaine with 1:100,000 epinephrine. Results were determined by lack of response to electrical pulp testing at the maximum setting (percentage of 80 readings) across time for 60 minutes. No significant difference between the two volumes was noted.

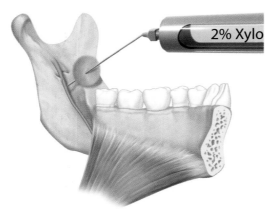

FIG. 4-8 Injection site for the mylohyoid nerve block.

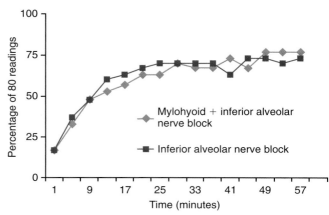

FIG. 4-9 Incidence of first mandibular molar anesthesia: comparison of the combination mylohyoid infiltration plus the inferior alveolar nerve block to the inferior alveolar nerve block alone. Results were determined by lack of response to electrical pulp testing at the maximum setting (percentage of 80 readings) across time for 60 minutes. No significant difference between the two techniques was noted.

CARBONATED ANESTHETIC SOLUTIONS

Experimentally, carbonated anesthetic solutions are more effective because the anesthetic is trapped in the nerve.[60] In addition, carbon dioxide (CO_2) has a synergistic relationship with local anesthetics and a direct depressant action on nerves.[60] However, a controlled clinical study was unable to demonstrate a superior effect of lidocaine hydrocarbonate in IAN blocks.[60]

Diphenhydramine as a Local Anesthetic Agent

Diphenhydramine (Benadryl) has been advocated for patients who are allergic to commonly used local anesthetics. Two studies found that diphenhydramine was less effective than lidocaine for extractions.[286,432] Another study found that the combinations of lidocaine/diphenhydramine with epinephrine, and diphenhydramine with epinephrine, were significantly less effective for pulpal anesthesia than lidocaine with epinephrine for IAN blocks.[440] These researchers also found that the diphenhydramine solutions were more painful on injection and had a high incidence of moderate postoperative pain.

Addition of Meperidine to Lidocaine

Two studies found that the addition of meperidine (Demerol) to a lidocaine formulation did not increase the success of the IAN block.[37,151]

FACTORS IN FAILURE OF THE INFERIOR ALVEOLAR NERVE BLOCK

Accessory Innervation: Mylohyoid Nerve

The mylohyoid nerve is the accessory nerve most often cited as a cause of failure of mandibular anesthesia.[127,441] A controlled clinical trial compared the IAN block alone to a combination of the IAN block and a mylohyoid nerve block using 2% lidocaine with 1:100,000 epinephrine (Fig. 4-8), which was aided by the use of a peripheral nerve stimulator.[66] The investigators found that the mylohyoid injection did not significantly enhance pulpal anesthesia of the IAN block (Fig. 4-9), so the study does not support the hypothesis that the mylohyoid nerve is a major factor in failure of the IAN block.

Accuracy of Injection

It has been theorized that an inaccurate injection contributes to inadequate mandibular anesthesia, but a number of studies determined that the use of ultrasound, a peripheral nerve stimulator, or radiographs to guide needle placement for IAN blocks did not result in more successful pulpal anesthesia.[35,134,165,387] The authors of these studies speculated that the anesthetic solution migrated along the path of least resistance, which was determined by fascial planes and structures encountered in the pterygomandibular space. These studies highlight an important clinical point: Lack of pulpal anesthesia is not necessarily the result of an inaccurate injection.

Needle Deflection

Needle deflection has been proposed as a cause of failure with the IAN block.[70,83,182] Several in vitro studies have shown that beveled needles tend to deflect toward the nonbeveled side (i.e., away from the bevel).* To compensate for this, a bidirectional needle rotation technique using the computer-controlled local anesthetic delivery system (CCLAD) (Milestone Scientific, Livingston, New Jersey) has been proposed in which the CCLAD handpiece assembly and needle are rotated in a fashion similar to the rotation of an endodontic hand file.[182] The technique was found to reduce deflection during insertion of the needle. A controlled clinical trial compared the anesthetic success of the conventional IAN block using two needle insertion methods.[224] However, no significant difference in anesthetic success was seen when the needle bevel was oriented away from the mandibular ramus (so that the needle would deflect toward the mandibular foramen [50% success]) compared with the bidirectional CCLAD needle rotation technique (56% success).[224] Neither technique resulted in an acceptable rate of anesthetic success in patients with symptomatic irreversible pulpitis.

Needle Bevel and Success

In asymptomatic subjects, the orientation of the needle bevel away or toward the mandibular ramus for an IAN block did

*References 13, 70, 83, 182, 199, and 363.

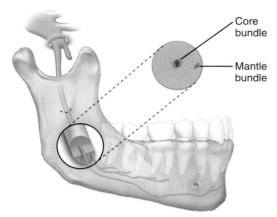

FIG. 4-10 **Central core theory.** The axons in the mantle bundle supply the molar teeth, and those in the core bundle supply the anterior teeth. The extraneural local anesthetic solution diffuses from the mantle to the core. (Modified and redrawn from De Jong RH: *Local anesthetics,* St Louis, 1994, Mosby.)

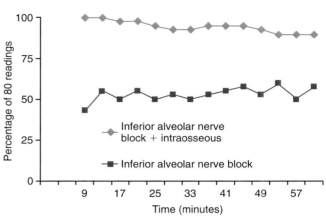

FIG. 4-11 Incidence of first mandibular molar anesthesia: comparison of the combination intraosseous injection of 2% lidocaine with 1:100,000 epinephrine plus the inferior alveolar nerve block to the inferior alveolar nerve block alone. Results were determined by lack of response to electrical pulp testing at the maximum setting (percentage of 80 readings) across time for 60 minutes. The combination technique was significantly better at all postinjection times.

not affect anesthetic success or failure.[405] Therefore, the use of commercial needles with markers to indicate the needle bevel is not necessary.

Speed of Injection and Success

A slow inferior alveolar nerve block increases success over a fast injection[204] but not for patients diagnosed with irreversible pulpitis.[9]

Cross-Innervation

Cross-innervation from the contralateral inferior alveolar nerve has been implicated in failure to achieve anesthesia in anterior teeth after an IAN injection. Experimentally, cross-innervation occurs in incisors[367,458] but plays a very small role in failure of an IAN block.

Red Hair

In medicine, red-haired females have shown reduced subcutaneous efficacy of lidocaine and increased requirements for desflurane.[102] However, in dentistry, having red hair was unrelated to success rates of the inferior alveolar nerve block,[102] although it has been shown to be associated with higher levels of dental anxiety.[102]

A Theory on Why Failure Occurs with the Inferior Alveolar Nerve Block in Restorative Dentistry

The central core theory may be the best explanation of why failure occurs with the IAN block.[85,407] According to this theory, nerves on the outside of the nerve bundle supply molar teeth, and nerves on the inside of the nerve bundle supply anterior teeth (Fig. 4-10). Even if deposited at the correct site, the anesthetic solution may not diffuse into the nerve trunk and reach all nerves to produce an adequate block. Although this theory may explain the higher experimental failure rates with the IAN block in anterior teeth compared with posterior teeth,* it does not explain the increased failure rate observed in painful teeth.

ENHANCEMENT OF MANDIBULAR ANESTHESIA FOR RESTORATIVE DENTISTRY

Supplemental Articaine Infiltrations

An important clinical finding is that an articaine infiltration of the first molar, premolars, and anterior teeth after an IAN block should provide pulpal anesthesia for approximately 1 hour.[163,206,326] The second molar may require a supplemental intraosseous (IO) or intraligamentary (IL) injection to achieve success.

Supplemental Intraosseous Anesthesia

Supplemental IO injections of lidocaine and mepivacaine with vasoconstrictors allow quick onset and increase the success of the inferior alveolar nerve block for approximately 60 minutes (Fig. 4-11).[103,158] The addition of a supplemental IO injection reduced the incidence of slow onset of pulpal anesthesia to zero compared with the IAN block alone (18% incidence).[103] Using 3% mepivacaine plain for IO injection results in pulpal anesthesia for approximately 30 minutes (Fig. 4-12).[137]

Supplemental Intraligamentary Anesthesia

Supplemental IL injections of 2% lidocaine with 1:100,000 epinephrine increase the success of the inferior alveolar nerve block, but the duration is approximately 23 minutes.[61]

MAXILLARY ANESTHESIA FOR RESTORATIVE DENTISTRY

Descriptions of conventional techniques for maxillary anesthesia are available for review in numerous articles and textbooks.[195,262]

2% Lidocaine with 1:100,000 Epinephrine

As a frame of reference, the most commonly used injection for anesthetization of maxillary teeth is infiltration with a cartridge of 2% lidocaine with 1:100,000 epinephrine.

---

*References 60, 112, 165, 179, 277, 322, 353, 388, 424, and 425.

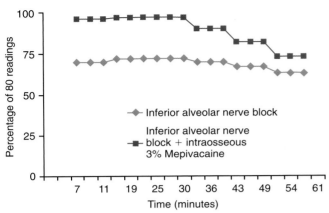

FIG. 4-12 Incidence of first mandibular molar anesthesia: comparison of the combination intraosseous injection with 3% mepivacaine plus the inferior alveolar nerve block to the inferior alveolar nerve block alone. Results were determined by lack of response to electrical pulp testing at the maximum setting (percentage of 80 readings) across time for 60 minutes. The combination technique proved significantly better for approximately 30 minutes.

Anesthetic Success

Infiltration results in a fairly high incidence of successful pulpal anesthesia (around 87% to 92%).* However, some patients may not be anesthetized because of individual variations in response to the drug administered, operator differences, and variations of anatomy and tooth position.

Onset of Pulpal Anesthesia

Pulpal anesthesia usually occurs in 3 to 5 minutes.[†]

Duration of Pulpal Anesthesia

The duration of pulpal anesthesia is a problem with maxillary infiltrations.[‡] Pulpal anesthesia of the anterior teeth declines after about 30 minutes, with most losing anesthesia by 60 minutes.[§] In premolars and first molars, pulpal anesthesia is good until about 40-45 minutes and then it starts to decline.[||] Additional local anesthetic should be administered depending on the duration of the procedure and the tooth group affected.

Time Course of Pulpal Anesthesia for the Maxillary First Molar

Figure 4-13 shows the time course for complete pulpal anesthesia for an asymptomatic first molar, as defined by the percentage of patients who do not respond at all to an EPT stimulus over time. Some patients had a slow onset of anesthesia until around 11 minutes. The overall success rate (no response at the device's highest setting) is 95% to 100%, with peak effects observed at around 30 minutes after injection.

---

*References 48, 108, 156, 211, 246, 272, 287, 324, 334, 353, and 381.
[†]References 48, 108, 156, 211, 246, 272, 287, 324, 334, 353, and 381.
[‡]References 48, 108, 156, 211, 246, 272, 287, 324, 334, 353, and 381.
[§]References 48, 108, 156, 211, 246, 272, 287, 324, 334, 353, and 381.
[||]References 48, 108, 156, 211, 246, 272, 287, 324, 334, 353, and 381.

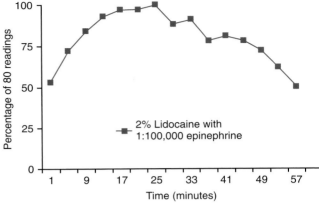

FIG. 4-13 Incidence of first maxillary molar anesthesia, as determined by lack of response to electrical pulp testing at the maximum setting (percentage of 80 readings) across time for 60 minutes.

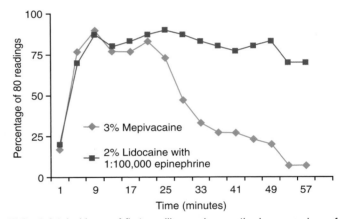

FIG. 4-14 Incidence of first maxillary molar anesthesia: comparison of 3% mepivacaine to 2% lidocaine with 1:100,000 epinephrine. Results were determined by lack of response to electrical pulp testing at the maximum setting (percentage of 80 readings) across time for 60 minutes. The 3% mepivacaine showed a shorter duration of anesthesia than the lidocaine solution.

Significance of Lip Numbness

Soft tissue anesthesia (lip or cheek numbness) is not necessarily related to the duration of pulpal anesthesia. Pulpal anesthesia does not last as long as soft tissue anesthesia.[156,272,287]

ALTERNATIVE ANESTHETIC SOLUTIONS FOR INFILTRATIONS

Plain Solutions: 3% Mepivacaine (Carbocaine, Polocaine, Scandonest) and 4% Prilocaine (Citanest Plain)

Anesthesia duration is shorter with these solutions.[211,272] Therefore, use these for procedures of short duration (10 to 15 minutes) (Fig. 4-14). These agents are generally not as safe as solutions with vasoconstrictors if *large* volumes are administered because they are rapidly absorbed systemically, resulting in excessive plasma concentrations and possible toxic reactions.[262]

4% Prilocaine with 1 : 200,000 Epinephrine (Citanest Forte), 2% Mepivacaine with 1 : 20,000 Levonordefrin (Carbocaine with Neo-Cobefrin), and 4% Articaine with 1 : 100,000 Epinephrine (Septocaine, Articadent, Zorcaine)

These formulations are similar to 2% lidocaine with 1 : 100,000 epinephrine.[108,211,246]

0.5% Bupivacaine with Epinephrine (Marcaine)

Success rates (no response to EPT) with bupivacaine range from 80% to 95% in the maxillary lateral incisor, compared with 50% in the maxillary second premolars.[81,156,223,410] Although bupivacaine provides long-term anesthesia with the IAN block, it *does not* provide prolonged pulpal anesthesia with maxillary infiltration injection.[81,156,223] In the lateral incisor, bupivacaine has a shorter duration of pulpal anesthesia than lidocaine.[81,156] In the first molar, bupivacaine's duration of pulpal anesthesia is equivalent to that of lidocaine.[156] Neither agent provides pulpal anesthesia for an hour.[81,156]

EXTENDING THE DURATION OF PULPAL ANESTHESIA FOR MAXILLARY TEETH

Increasing the Solution Volume

A two-cartridge volume of 2% lidocaine with epinephrine extends the duration of pulpal anesthesia but not for 60 minutes.[287]

Increasing the Epinephrine Concentration

Increasing the epinephrine concentration to 1 : 50,000 epinephrine increases duration for the lateral incisor but not the first molar.[272] Duration was not 60 minutes in either teeth.[272]

Repeating the Infiltration

Adding another cartridge of 2% lidocaine with epinephrine at 30 minutes in anterior teeth and 45 minutes in posterior teeth significantly improves the duration of pulpal anesthesia and may be the best way to extend the duration of pulpal anesthesia (Fig. 4-15).[381]

ALTERNATIVE MAXILLARY INJECTION TECHNIQUES FOR RESTORATIVE DENTISTRY

Posterior Superior Alveolar (PSA) Nerve Block

The PSA nerve block anesthetizes the second molars and about 80% of first molars.[257,343] An additional mesial infiltration injection may be necessary to anesthetize the first molar. Generally, the PSA block injection is not advocated for routine restorative procedures. An infiltration of the molars is preferred.

Infraorbital Nerve Block

The infraorbital nerve block results in lip numbness but does not predictably anesthetize incisor pulps.[33,209] It usually anesthetizes the canines and premolars, but the duration is less than 1 hour.[33,209] Essentially, this injection technique is the

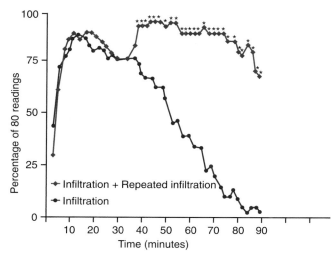

FIG. 4-15 Incidence of maxillary lateral incisor pulpal anesthesia using an initial infiltration and a repeated infiltration 30 minutes later (both infiltrations used 1.8 ml of 2% lidocaine with 1 : 100,000 epinephrine). Results were determined by lack of response to electrical pulp testing at the maximum setting (percentage of 80 readings). The repeated infiltration injection significantly prolonged the duration of pulpal anesthesia.

same as an infiltration injection over the premolar teeth for pulpal anesthesia. Generally, the infraorbital injection is not advocated for routine restorative procedures. An infiltration of the individual maxillary teeth is preferred.

Second Division Nerve Block

The second division nerve block usually anesthetizes pulps of molars and some second premolars but does not predictably anesthetize first premolars, canines, or lateral and central incisors.[47,117] The high tuberosity technique is preferred to the greater palatine approach because it is easier and less painful.[47] Generally, the second division nerve block is not advocated for routine restorative procedures. An infiltration of the individual teeth is preferred.

Palatal–Anterior Superior Alveolar (P-ASA) Nerve Block

Traditionally, maxillary anterior teeth have been anesthetized with an infiltration injection near the apex of the target tooth. In the late 1990s, the P-ASA injection, a site-specific injection for maxillary anterior teeth, was introduced.[125,126] The P-ASA injection involves a palatal injection into the incisive canal; it derives its name from the injection's supposed ability to anesthetize both the right and left anterior superior alveolar nerves (Fig. 4-16). Unfortunately, the injection technique does not provide predictable pulpal anesthesia for the incisors and canines[50] and is often painful.[318]

Anterior Middle Superior Alveolar (AMSA) Nerve Block

The AMSA injection is another new technique for anesthetizing maxillary teeth.[123,124,126,130] The AMSA injection site is located palatally at a point that bisects the premolars and is approximately halfway between the midpalatine raphe and the crest of the free gingival margin (Fig. 4-17). The AMSA injection

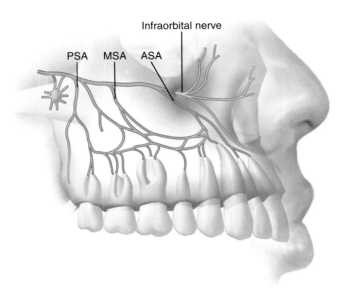

FIG. 4-16 Distribution of the maxillary division of the trigeminal nerve, showing the anterior superior alveolar (ASA) nerve, the middle superior alveolar (MSA) nerve, and the posterior superior alveolar (PSA) nerve.

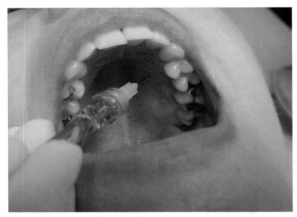

FIG. 4-17 Palatal injection site for the anterior middle superior alveolar (AMSA) injection.

supposedly can anesthetize both the anterior and middle superior alveolar nerves[123,124,126] (see Fig. 4-16), resulting in unilateral anesthesia of the maxillary central and lateral incisors, canines, and first and second premolars. Unfortunately, the injection technique does not provide predictable pulpal anesthesia for these maxillary teeth[247] and is often painful.[321]

Pain, Inflammation, and Anxiety
Results differ from the normal when anesthesia is given to patients with any of these conditions.

SUPPLEMENTAL ANESTHESIA FOR RESTORATIVE DENTISTRY IN THE MANDIBLE AND MAXILLA

Indications
A supplemental injection is used if the standard injection is not effective. It is useful to repeat an initial injection only if the patient is not exhibiting the "classic" signs of soft tissue

anesthesia (e.g., numbness of the lip). Generally, if the classic signs are present, reinjection is not very effective.[208] For example, after the inferior alveolar nerve block, the patient develops lip, chin, and tongue numbness and quadrant "deadness" of the teeth. A useful procedure is to pulp test the tooth with a cold refrigerant or an electrical pulp tester before the cavity preparation is begun.[56,100] If the patient feels pain to cold, a supplemental injection is indicated. To think that reinjection using the inferior alveolar nerve block approach will be successful is wishful thinking; failure the first time is usually followed by failure on the second attempt. Clinicians may think another injection is helpful because the patient sometimes achieves pulpal anesthesia after the second injection, but the patient may simply be experiencing slow onset of pulpal anesthesia from the first injection.

The clinician should go directly to a supplemental technique. Three such injections are *the infiltration injection; the IO injection; and the IL injection (formerly called the periodontal ligament [PDL] injection).*

Infiltrations

Additional Infiltration of Lidocaine in the Maxilla
Because the duration of pulpal anesthesia for infiltration in the maxilla is not 60 minutes, adding an additional cartridge of 2% lidocaine with 1:100,000 epinephrine at 30 minutes in the anterior teeth and at about 45 minutes in premolar and molar teeth significantly improves the duration of pulpal anesthesia. This is an important clinical finding and may be the best way to extend the duration of pulpal anesthesia in maxillary teeth.[381]

Additional Infiltration of Articaine in the Mandible
Another important clinical finding is that an articaine infiltration of the first molar, premolars, and anterior teeth after an inferior alveolar nerve block should provide pulpal anesthesia for approximately 1 hour.[163,206,326] The second molar may require a supplemental IO or IL injection to achieve success.

Intraosseous Anesthesia
The IO injection is a supplemental technique that has been shown to be effective through substantial research and clinical usage. It is particularly useful in conjunction with a conventional injection when it is likely that supplemental anesthesia will be necessary (e.g., in mandibular second molar teeth).[103,137,158] The IO injection allows placement of a local anesthetic directly into the cancellous bone adjacent to the tooth. When a primary IO injection was compared with an infiltration injection, the IO technique showed a quicker onset and a shorter duration of anesthesia (Fig. 4-18).[324]

The Stabident IO system (Fairfax Dental Inc., Miami, Florida) is composed of a slow-speed, handpiece-driven perforator and a solid 27-gauge wire with a beveled end that drills a small hole through the cortical plate (Fig. 4-19). The anesthetic solution is delivered to cancellous bone through the 27-gauge, ultrashort injector needle placed into the hole made by the perforator (Fig. 4-20).

The X-Tip IO anesthetic delivery system (Dentpsly International, York, Pennsylvania) consists of an X-tip that separates into two parts, the drill and the guide sleeve (Fig. 4-21). The drill, a special hollow needle, leads the guide sleeve through the cortical plate; it then is separated from the guide sleeve and withdrawn. The remaining guide sleeve is designed to accept a 27-gauge needle for injection of the anesthetic

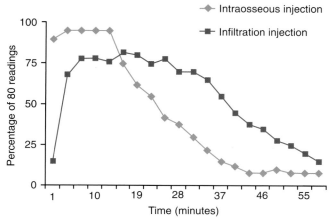

FIG. 4-18 **Incidence of anesthesia for intraosseous and infiltration injections.** Results were determined by lack of response to electrical pulp testing at the maximum setting (percentage of 80 readings) across time for 60 minutes. The intraosseous injection showed a quicker onset and a shorter duration of anesthesia.

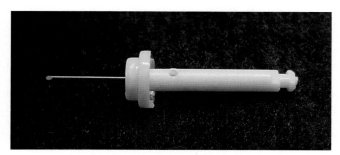

FIG. 4-19 The Stabident perforator, a solid, 27-gauge wire with a beveled end that is placed in a slow-speed handpiece.

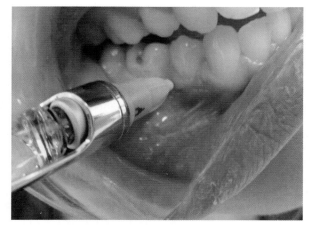

FIG. 4-20 The anesthetic solution is delivered to the cancellous bone through the needle placed into the hole made by the perforator.

solution (Fig. 4-22). The guide sleeve is removed after the IO injection is complete.

The technique for IO injection of anesthetic using the Stabident or X-Tip system can be reviewed in the systems' instruction manuals or in published papers.[67,138,356-358]

Success

Supplemental IO injections of lidocaine and mepivacaine with vasoconstrictors allow quick onset and increase the success of

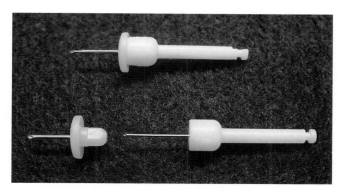

FIG. 4-21 The X-Tip anesthetic delivery system consists of an X-tip *(top)* that separates into two parts: the drill (a special hollow needle) and the guide sleeve component *(bottom)*.

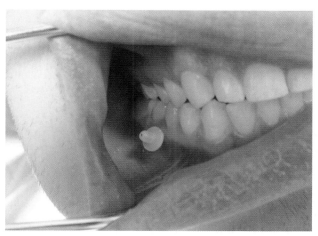

FIG. 4-22 Anesthetic solution is injected through the X-tip guide sleeve.

the inferior alveolar nerve block for approximately 60 minutes (see Fig. 4-11).[103,158] The addition of a supplemental IO injection reduced the incidence of slow onset of pulpal anesthesia to zero compared with the IAN block alone (18% incidence).[103] Using 3% mepivacaine plain results in pulpal anesthesia for approximately 30 minutes (see Fig. 4-12).[137]

Failure

If the anesthetic solution flows out of the perforation site (backflow), anesthetization will not occur.[139] Reperforation or use of another perforation site is a practical way to gain access to the cancellous bone in such cases. In fewer than 10% of cases, constricted cancellous spaces may limit the distribution of the anesthetic solution around the apices of the teeth.* In such cases, failure may result even if the anesthetic solution is delivered intraosseously.

Perforator Breakage

In about 1% of cases, the metal perforator separates from the plastic shank during use.[67,103,139,320,356-358] The metal wire is easily removed with a hemostat. This separation usually occurs during a difficult perforation (e.g., dense cortical bone); the wire probably is heated excessively, causing the plastic hub to melt. No perforator breakage (metal perforator breaking into parts) has been reported in numerous controlled clinical studies.[67,103,139,320,356-358] However, excessive torquing of the

*References 67, 103, 139, 158, 320, 323, 355-358, and 402.

perforator laterally by an inexperienced operator may result in breakage.

Optimal Location for Injection Site

Injection at a site distal to the tooth to be anesthetized produces the best anesthesia.* Maxillary and mandibular second molars are an exception to this rule. A mesial site should be selected for these teeth because of the increased thickness of the cortical plate in the mandible and the difficulty with perforation and needle placement at a distal site.

Onset of Anesthesia

The onset of anesthesia is immediate, which eliminates the waiting period.†

Site Selection: Attached Gingiva or Alveolar Mucosa

Both the Stabident and X-Tip IO systems instruct the user to locate the perforation site in attached gingiva. This gingival site allows the perforation to be made through a minimal thickness of cortical bone and generally is equidistant between adjacent root structures. However, because the guide sleeve remains in place with the X-Tip system, two studies have successfully used it in alveolar mucosa at a more apical location.[139,320] The X-Tip system has a definite clinical advantage over the Stabident system because the X-Tip perforation may be made at an apical location in unattached gingiva. If the Stabident system is used apically in alveolar mucosa, the hole created for delivering the anesthetic solution is almost impossible to find. The clinician may want to consider using the X-Tip system in an apical location in specific clinical situations. For example, when periodontal pocketing does not allow perforation into cancellous bone through the more coronal attached gingiva or when interproximal space is lacking (i.e., roots are too close together), the X-Tip system can be used to achieve pulpal anesthesia. If the Stabident system fails, the clinician may want to consider using the X-Tip apically to achieve pulpal anesthesia.

Care must be taken during IO injection to avoid insertion in areas of the roots and other critical structures, such as the mental foramen.

Injection Discomfort

When the IO injection is used as a primary injection, pain is experienced about a fourth of the time.[67,138,356-358] When the IO injection is used as a supplemental injection, fewer patients experience pain.[103,137,158,356,402]

Duration

With a primary IO injection, the duration of pulpal anesthesia declines steadily over an hour.[67,358] There is an even shorter duration with 3% mepivacaine compared with 2% lidocaine with 1:100,000 epinephrine.[358] With a supplemental IO injection of lidocaine after the inferior alveolar nerve block in patients without pain, the duration of pulpal anesthesia is very good for an hour.[103,158] A solution of 3% mepivacaine used as a supplemental IO injection results in a shorter anesthetic duration.[137]

Repeating the Intraosseous Injection

Repeating the IO injection, using 1.4 ml of 2% lidocaine with 1:100,000 epinephrine 30 minutes after the initial IO injection, provides an additional 15 to 20 minutes of pulpal anesthesia, similar to the duration of the initial IO injection.[198]

Use of Bupivacaine for Intraosseous Anesthesia

In an attempt to increase the duration of pulpal anesthesia with IO injections, some clinicians may consider using long-acting anesthetics. Bupivacaine (Marcaine) is a long-acting anesthetic, but only for IAN blocks. Long-acting anesthetics do not show an extended duration of anesthesia when injected by the IO or maxillary infiltration routes.[81,156,185,402] Bupivacaine has cardiotoxic effects[28] and for IO anesthesia basically is equivalent to 2% lidocaine with epinephrine in terms of efficacy, duration, and heart rate effects. Therefore, bupivacaine offers no advantage clinically and should not be used for IO anesthesia.

Systemic Effects of Intraosseous Injection

A transient increase in heart rate has been reported in 46% to 93% of cases involving Stabident and X-Tip IO injection of solutions containing epinephrine or levonordefrin.* Four clinical trials using techniques such as objective electrocardiographic recordings and pulse oximetry have shown that subjects experienced a transient tachycardia (mean increase of 12 to 32 beats/min) after Stabident IO injection of 1.8 ml of 2% lidocaine with 1:100,000 epinephrine, 1.8 ml of 2% mepivacaine with 1:20,000 levonordefrin, or 1.8 ml of 1.5% etidocaine with 1:200,000 epinephrine.[57,158,359,402] Another clinical trial reported transient tachycardia after IO injection, but not with infiltration injection, of 1.8 ml of 2% lidocaine with 1:100,000 epinephrine in the maxillary anterior region.[444] Generally, all these studies showed that the heart rate returned to baseline readings within 4 minutes in most patients. Therefore, injection of anesthetic solutions containing vasoconstrictors, using either the Stabident or X-Tip system, results in a transient tachycardia. No significant change in diastolic, systolic, or mean arterial blood pressure has been observed with IO injection of 2% lidocaine with 1:100,000 epinephrine.[57,359]

An IO injection of 1.4 ml of 2% lidocaine with 1:100,000 epinephrine with the CCLAD (CompuDent, Milestone Scientific, Livingston, New Jersey) at a fast rate resulted in a significantly higher heart rate compared to a slow solution deposition using either the CCLAD or a traditional syringe.[408]

Clinical Significance of Increased Heart Rate

Although the patient is likely to notice the transient tachycardia that occurs after Stabident or X-Tip IO injection of 2% lidocaine with 1:100,000 epinephrine, it generally is not clinically significant in healthy patients.[359] The clinical significance, cardiovascular effects, and contraindications to the use of vasoconstrictors in IO injections have been reviewed.[359]

Lack of Heart Rate Effect of 3% Mepivacaine in Intraosseous Anesthesia

No significant tachycardia occurs when 3% mepivacaine is used for IO anesthesia.[137,359] Clinicians should keep in mind that this anesthetic is an alternative for IO injection in

---

*References 67, 103, 139, 158, 356-358, and 402.
†References 67, 103, 139, 158, 356-358, and 402.

*References 67, 103, 139, 158, 320, 323, 356-358, and 402.

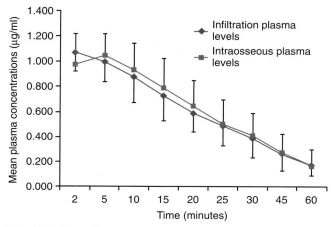

FIG. 4-23 Mean plasma concentrations of lidocaine for the intraosseous and infiltration injection techniques. No statistical differences were seen between the two techniques at any time period.

patients whose medical condition or drug therapy suggests caution in the use of solutions containing epinephrine or levonordefrin.[137,359]

Plasma Levels of Lidocaine After Intraosseous Injection

Some authors have cautioned that administration of an overly large volume of local anesthetic with an IO injection could lead to overdose reactions.[189] One experimental study using volunteers found that injection of 1.8 ml of 2% lidocaine with 1:100,000 epinephrine produced venous plasma levels of lidocaine that were the same for maxillary anterior IO and infiltration injections (Fig. 4-23).[444] Although systemic concentrations of vasoconstrictors have a short-lived effect on the heart rate, the plasma concentration of lidocaine delivered with IO injection is no more than that delivered with infiltration, so the IO technique should not be considered an intravascular injection with regard to lidocaine. Also, if it were an intravascular injection, little or no anesthetic effect would be demonstrated; that is, all the local anesthetic solution would be carried into the vascular system, with none left for pulpal anesthesia. Obviously, clinical and experimental studies have demonstrated clinical anesthesia with IO techniques.* Therefore, the precautions for the maximum amount of lidocaine for an infiltration injection would seem to apply to an IO injection.

Postoperative Discomfort

When IO injections are given with the Stabident system, either as a primary or a supplemental technique, most patients report no or only mild pain; approximately 2% to 15% report moderate pain.[67,158,356-358] Less postoperative discomfort is reported for the Stabident IO injection than for IL injection.[379]

One study found that significantly more men experienced postoperative pain with the X-Tip system than with the Stabident system.[138] The authors interpreted these results as being due to the denser, more mineralized bone in the posterior mandible in men and to the fact that the diameter of the X-Tip perforating system is larger than that of the Stabident perforator, meaning the X-Tip system generates more frictional heat during perforation.

---

*References 67, 103, 139, 320, 323, and 355-358.

Postoperative Problems

With the Stabident system, fewer than 5% of patients develop swelling or exudate at the site of perforation.[67,158,356-358] The X-Tip system may show a higher incidence of postoperative swelling clinically.[138] With both systems, swelling or exudate (or both) may persist for weeks after the injection, but this resolves with time.[67,138,158,356-358] Slow healing of perforation sites may be the result of overheating of the bone caused by pressure during perforation.

With both the Stabident and X-Tip systems, approximately 4% to 15% of patients report that for a few days, the tooth "feels high" during chewing.[67,138,158,356-358] This feeling most likely is an increased awareness to biting that results from soreness in the area caused by damage from perforation or inflammation of the bone. The incidence of this feeling for the IO injection is lower than that reported for the IL injection (36% to 49%).[79,379]

Medical Contraindications

Patients taking antidepressants, nonselective beta-blocking agents, medicine for Parkinson disease, and cocaine should not receive IO injections of solutions containing epinephrine or levonordefrin.[353] Three percent mepivacaine plain is preferred.

Intraligamentary Anesthesia

The IL injection is another technique that is used if a conventional injection is unsuccessful.[397,428] The technique for IL injection of anesthesia is reviewed in a number of published papers and textbooks.

Success

For use as a primary injection, IL injections have a reported success rate of about 75% in mandibular and maxillary posterior teeth, with a duration of pulpal anesthesia of 10 to 15 minutes.[379,436] Success rates are low in anterior teeth.[280,379,436]

For use as a supplemental injection (standard techniques have failed to provide adequate anesthesia), good success rates are achieved, but the duration of pulpal anesthesia is approximately 23 minutes.[61]

Mechanism of Action

An IL injection forces anesthetic solutions through the cribriform plate into the marrow spaces around the tooth.[101,129,352,396,430] The primary route is *not* via the periodontal ligament, and unlike the intrapulpal (IP) injection,[38,423] the mechanism of action is not a pressure anesthesia.[105,296] The IL injection should be considered an intraosseous injection.

Back-Pressure

Studies have shown that the most important factor for anesthetic success with an IL injection is injection under *strong back-pressure*.[396,428] Pressure is necessary to force the solution into the marrow spaces.

Anesthetic Solutions

A vasoconstrictor significantly increases the efficacy of an IL injection.[155,213,228,278,379] Injection of a vasoconstrictor alone (1:100,000 epinephrine) does not produce pulpal anesthesia.[379] Anesthetic solutions with reduced vasoconstrictor concentrations (bupivacaine with 1:200,000 epinephrine) are not very effective with this technique.[155,200,213] Articaine is equivalent to lidocaine.[34]

Amount of Solution Delivered

Usually about 0.2 ml of solution is deposited with each mesial and distal injection, using a traditional or pressure syringe. The exact amount is not always known because some of the anesthetic solution may escape from the sulcus during the injection.

Injection Discomfort

When the IL injection is used as a primary injection, needle insertion and injection have the potential to be painful about a third of the time.[296,379,436] The IL injection may be quite painful in maxillary anterior teeth[436] and should not be used in these teeth; infiltration is preferred. The potential for pain with the IL technique is greatly reduced when the injection is used as a supplemental injection after an inferior alveolar nerve block.[61]

Onset of Anesthesia

The onset of anesthesia is immediate with an IL injection,* which means no waiting period is required for the anesthesia to take effect. If anesthesia is still not adequate, reinjection is necessary.

Duration

Experimental studies with the EPT have shown that when the IL injection is given as a primary injection, the duration of profound pulpal anesthesia is approximately 10 to 20 minutes.[296,379,436] When the injection is used as a supplemental technique in asymptomatic teeth after an IAN block, the duration of pulpal anesthesia is approximately 23 minutes.[61]

New Technology for Intraligamentary Injections: CCLAD

A computer-assisted local anesthetic delivery system, introduced by Milestone Scientific, can be used to administer an IL injection. The CCLAD (also called *CompuDent* or *The Wand*) accommodates a standard local anesthetic cartridge that is linked by sterile microtubing to a disposable, penlike handpiece with a Luer-Lok needle (Fig. 4-24). The device is activated by a foot control, which automates the infusion of local anesthetic solution at a controlled rate. The fast rate delivers 1.4 ml of solution in 1 minute. The slow rate delivers 1.4 ml of solution in approximately 4 minutes, 45 seconds. The slow rate is used for the IL injection.

Anesthetic Success of the IL Injection Using the CCLAD

An experimental study compared the anesthetic efficacy of primary IL injection of 1.4 ml of 4% articaine with 1:100,000 epinephrine and 1.4 ml of 2% lidocaine with 1:100,000 epinephrine administered with a CCLAD in the mandibular first molar.[34] Successful pulpal anesthesia (two consecutive maximum EPT readings) was obtained 86% of the time with the articaine solution and 74% of the time with the lidocaine solution. No significant difference was seen between the articaine and lidocaine solutions. The duration of pulpal anesthesia ranged from 31 to 34 minutes, longer than the 10 minutes recorded in a similar study using a pressure syringe and 0.4 ml of a lidocaine solution.[436] Therefore, the CCLAD system offers the advantage of increasing the duration of pulpal anesthesia; however, the anesthesia slowly decreases over 60 minutes.

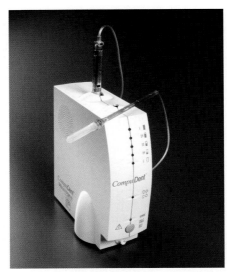

FIG. 4-24 Wand computer-assisted local anesthetic delivery unit (The Wand/CompuDent). The handpiece assembly and microtubing are also shown. (Courtesy Milestone Scientific, Livingston, NJ.)

Postoperative Discomfort

When the IL injection is used as a primary technique, postoperative pain occurs in a third to three quarters of patients, with a duration of 14 hours to 3 days.[79,296,379,397,428,436] There is no difference between articaine and lidocaine.[34] The discomfort is related to damage from needle insertion rather than to the pressure of depositing the solution.[79] About a fourth of patients report that their tooth feels "high" in occlusion.[379,436]

Systemic Effects

When a high-pressure syringe was used in dogs, IL injection of solutions containing epinephrine caused cardiovascular responses similar to those seen with IV injections.[395] Clinical studies using a high-pressure syringe in human beings found that IL injections of such solutions did not significantly change the heart rate, rhythm, or amplitude or the blood pressure.[53,317] These studies support the conclusion that IL injections do not cause significant changes in heart rate in human beings.

Other Factors

Different needle gauges (25, 27, or 30 gauge) are equally effective.[428] Special pressure syringes have been marketed but have not been proven more effective than a standard syringe.[379,428,436]

Safety of the Periodontium

Clinical and animal studies have demonstrated the relative safety of the IL injection technique.* Minor transient damage occurs only at the site of needle penetration, and the tissue subsequently undergoes repair. In rare cases, periodontal abscesses and deep pocket formation have occurred after IL injections.[61,436] A small clinical risk of periodontal abscess formation and bone loss exists with this technique, and although these effects are rare, the clinician should be aware of them. Localized areas of root resorption after IL injections have also been reported.[339,361]

---

*References 79, 296, 379, 397, 428, and 436.

*References 45, 128, 129, 135, 255, 296, 340, 379, 428, and 436.

Safety of the Pulp

Clinical and animal studies have shown that IL injections have no permanent effect on the pulp.* However, IL injection of a solution with epinephrine produces a rapid, prolonged decrease in blood flow.[228] Some have suggested that using this injection technique during restorative procedures could result in accumulation of inflammatory mediators that would not be effectively removed because of the reduced blood flow.[228] This hypothesis was directly tested, and the IL injection of an anesthetic solution containing a vasoconstrictor in conjunction with a deep cavity preparation did *not* produce a more severe reaction than in controls (cavity preparation only).[344] Rather, the depth of the cavity preparation was the most important factor dictating pulpal responses. IL injections are therefore unlikely to cause pulpal necrosis.

Safety in Primary Teeth

One study has shown that IL injection of primary teeth may cause enamel hypoplasia of the developing permanent teeth.[45] The effect noted was not caused by the injection technique, but by the anesthetics used; that is, the cytotoxic anesthetic agents bound to the enamel matrix in the developing tooth germ. The same effect seemingly would be produced by an infiltration injection next to the developing tooth, so the recommendation that IL injections be used with great care on primary teeth close to developing permanent teeth[45] may not be correct.

Safety in Periodontally Involved Sites

IL injections have been shown to be safe in cases of mild to moderate gingival inflammation or incipient periodontitis.[76]

Avulsion

In a letter to the editor of the *Journal of the American Dental Association*, Nelson[311] reported on the avulsion of a tooth after IL injections. However, *no* clinical or experimental study has reported avulsion or loosening of teeth with this technique.[296,379,436] Avulsion should not be a concern with IL injections.

LOCAL ANESTHESIA FOR ENDODONTICS

For an emergency patient presenting with a tooth diagnosed with symptomatic irreversible pulpitis, anesthesia is administered with a standard IAN block. The patient reports classic signs of anesthesia (lip numbness and a dull feeling of the tooth or quadrant). After isolation, access preparation is begun. When the bur is in enamel, the patient feels nothing. Once the bur enters dentin (or possibly not until the pulp is exposed), the patient feels sharp pain. Obviously, pulpal anesthesia is not profound, and additional anesthetic is required. The following discussion outlines useful information for anesthetizing these endodontic patients.

Success of the Inferior Alveolar Nerve Block in Patients Presenting with Symptomatic Irreversible Pulpitis

Endodontic clinical studies of mandibular posterior teeth in patients with irreversible pulpitis have shown success occurs

14% to 57% of the time.* Articaine is not superior to lidocaine in this group of patients.[64,364,415] Nor is bupivacaine statistically superior to lidocaine.[376]

Some authors have suggested that a two-cartridge volume is better than a one-cartridge volume.[7] However, others did not find a statistically significant difference between one- and two-cartridge volumes.[336] In addition, a number of studies have used a two-cartridge volume, and success rates are similar to those for a one-cartridge volume.[122,253,330,390]

The epinephrine concentration in 2% lidocaine does not seem to make a difference in success in patients with symptomatic irreversible pulpitis.[8]

Success of Maxillary Molar Infiltration in Patients Presenting with Irreversible Pulpitis

Endodontic clinical studies of maxillary posterior buccal infiltrations in patients presenting with irreversible pulpitis have shown success occurs 54% to 88% of the time.[6,207,323] Although some authors have found a difference between articaine and lidocaine,[401] others have not.[27,207,370,384]

Asymptomatic Irreversible Pulpitis Versus Symptomatic Irreversible Pulpitis

Patients who have spontaneous pain and have moderate to severe pain at an emergency visit (symptomatic irreversible pulpitis) have less successful anesthesia after an inferior alveolar nerve block than patients who do not have spontaneous pain or only have pain when the tooth is stimulated (asymptomatic irreversible).[23] It is important to distinguish between these patients, because the success rates differ.

Supplemental Techniques

Infiltrations
Supplemental Buccal, Lingual, or Buccal Plus Lingual Infiltrations of Articaine

Although the infiltration of articaine is effective in restorative dentistry as a supplemental technique (after the inferior alveolar nerve block),[163] its use in endodontically involved teeth does not result in predictable pulpal anesthesia.[273,330,390] Success rates in studies have ranged from 38% to 84%, with most studies reporting success rates less than 60%.† A buccal infiltration of lidocaine is also not effective (65% success).[336]

Buccal infiltration alone, buccal plus lingual infiltrations alone (or after an inferior alveolar nerve block) do not result in complete pulpal anesthesia.‡ Therefore, IO and IL injections are the preferred techniques for supplemental anesthesia, and the IP injection is indicated when the IO or IL injection is not successful.

Intraosseous Anesthesia
Success in Symptomatic Irreversible Pulpitis

High success rates (around 90%) have been reported when the IO injection was used as a supplemental injection with

---

*References 251, 296, 342, 361, 379, and 436.

---

*References 3, 8, 26, 64, 68, 98, 131, 188, 197, 224, 226, 273, 295, 323, 330, 335, 355, 364, 391, 404, and 415.
†References 3, 4, 98, 273, 330, and 390.
‡References 3, 4, 10, 98, 109, and 346.

irreversible pulpitis.[36,273,320,323,330] There is no difference between lidocaine and articaine.[36] Three percent mepivacaine has an 80% success rate, which increases to 98% with a second IO injection of 3% mepivacaine.[355]

An initial supplemental IO injection of 0.45 to 0.9 ml of 2% lidocaine with 1 : 100,000 epinephrine was successful in 79% of posterior mandibular teeth.[332] A second IO injection of the remaining cartridge increased the success rate to 91%. Therefore, initially giving a quarter to a half cartridge of 2% lidocaine with 1 : 100,000 epinephrine was less successful than initially giving a full cartridge.

Although some authors[338,354] have suggested an IO injection alone successfully anesthetizes patients presenting with irreversible pulpitis, it is very doubtful that this would be successful.[36,273,320,323,330]

Anesthetic Success in Symptomatic Teeth with Totally Necrotic Pulps and Radiolucent Areas

No study has investigated the use of IO anesthesia in patients with symptomatic teeth, totally necrotic pulps, and radiolucent areas. In a preliminary study performed at Ohio State, anesthetic solution deposition was very painful in these teeth, and the study had to be terminated.

Anesthetic Success in Partially Vital Teeth

The IO injection should work in teeth in which the chamber is necrotic, the canals are vital or partially vital, and widening of the periodontal ligament can be seen radiographically. A recent history of hot and cold sensitivity should differentiate this condition from that of a necrotic tooth experiencing an acute exacerbation (Phoenix abscess).

Injection Pain with Intraosseous Injection in Patients with Irreversible Pulpitis

Generally the Stabident system produces a very low incidence of moderate pain from perforation and solution deposition in asymptomatic patients.[67,138,356-358] A higher incidence was reported when the system was used to make IO injections in mandibular posterior teeth with symptomatic irreversible pulpitis. Up to 9% of patients reported moderate to severe pain after perforation, and 5% to 31% reported moderate to severe pain during deposition of the anesthetic solution.[323,355]

With the X-Tip system, 48% of patients with symptomatic irreversible pulpitis had moderate to severe pain with perforation, and 27% had moderate pain with solution deposition.[320] Patients with irreversible pulpitis may experience a transient but moderate to severe pain on perforation and solution deposition when either the Stabident or X-Tip system is used. The higher pain ratings, compared with those for asymptomatic teeth, are probably related to preexisting peripheral or central sensitization, which leads to increased pain responsiveness and preoperative anxiety.

Duration in Mandibular Teeth

In patients with irreversible pulpitis, supplemental IO injection using either the Stabident or X-Tip system provided anesthesia for the entire débridement appointment.[320,323,355]

Intraligamentary Anesthesia
Success

The overall success of supplemental IL injections in achieving pulpal anesthesia for endodontic procedures has been reported to be 50% to 96%.[68,260,397,428] As a primary anesthetic technique, IL injection produced a 50% to 79% success rate.[212,260] If a first IL injection fails, reinjection results in a success rate of 92%.[428] Similar results have been reported by other investigators.[397] IL injection is not successful in mandibular anterior teeth.[280,436] In addition, supplemental IL injections are not as successful as supplemental IO injections.[208,461]

Anesthetic Success of the IL Injection Using the CCLAD in Symptomatic Patients Presenting with Irreversible Pulpitis

A supplemental IL injection, administered with a CCLAD system in mandibular posterior teeth diagnosed with irreversible pulpitis after failure of an IAN injection, produced a 56% anesthesia success rate.[319] These results were somewhat disappointing because the CCLAD should have been capable of delivering approximately 1.4 ml of anesthetic solution with the IL injection by consistent maintenance of a precise flow rate.

Injection Discomfort

When the IL injection is given as a supplemental injection to anesthetize symptomatic vital teeth (i.e., in symptomatic irreversible pulpitis), the patient may have moderate pain.[100] Patients should be informed of this possibility.

Selective Anesthesia

Although some have reported that the IL injection can be used in the differential diagnosis of pulpally involved teeth,[256,386] experimental studies have shown that adjacent teeth may also become anesthetized with IL injection for a single tooth.[296,379,436] Therefore, the IL injection should *not* be used for differential diagnosis.

Duration

When the IL injection is used as a supplemental technique in endodontic therapy, the clinician must work fairly quickly and be prepared to reinject if profound anesthesia dissipates.

Intrapulpal Injection

In about 5% to 10% of mandibular posterior teeth with irreversible pulpitis, supplemental IO or IL injections, even when repeated, do not produce profound anesthesia; pain persists when the pulp is entered. This is an indication for an IP injection.

The major drawback of the IP injection technique is that the needle and injection are made directly into a vital and very sensitive pulp; this injection is often moderately to severely painful.[323] Because endodontic research offers more successful methods of supplemental anesthesia, the IP injection should be given only after all other supplemental techniques have failed. Another disadvantage of the technique is the possible duration of pulpal anesthesia (15 to 20 minutes). The bulk of the pulpal tissue must be removed quickly, at the correct working length, to prevent recurrence of pain during instrumentation. Yet another disadvantage is that the pulp obviously must be exposed to allow direct injection. Anesthetic problems frequently occur before exposure while the clinician is still working in dentin.*

---

*References 273, 319, 320, 323, 330, 355, and 390.

The advantage of the IP injection is that it produces profound anesthesia if given under back-pressure.[38,423] The onset of anesthesia is immediate, and no special syringes or needles are required. The methods for this technique can be found in many excellent endodontic textbooks. As mentioned previously, strong back-pressure is a major factor in achieving successful IP anesthesia.[38,423] Depositing the anesthetic solution passively into the chamber is insufficient because the solution does not diffuse throughout the pulp.

MANAGEMENT OF ANESTHESIA IN ENDODONTIC CASES

Symptomatic Irreversible Pulpitis

When symptomatic irreversible pulpitis is a factor, the teeth that are most difficult to anesthetize are the mandibular molars, followed by the mandibular premolars, the maxillary molars and premolars, and the mandibular anterior teeth. The fewest problems arise in the maxillary anterior teeth.

In some teeth, irreversible pulpitis is the condition in the apical portion of the canals; the tissue in the chamber is necrotic and does not respond to pulp testing. The pulp chamber can be entered easily, but when attempts are made to place a file to length, severe pain results. IO or IL injections are helpful in these cases, and an IP injection may be used. However, irreversible pulpitis must be differentiated from a symptomatic necrotic tooth with a distinct apical abscess. In the latter condition, it is doubtful if IO or IL injections would be effective, and these injections may be quite painful, and bacteria may be forced into the periapical tissues by an IP injection.

Anesthetizing Mandibular Posterior Teeth

Until the 1980s, before supplemental IO and IL injections became popular, clinicians would administer the conventional IAN block and long buccal injection (molars). After signs of soft tissue anesthesia became evident, the pain abated and the patient relaxed. Local anesthesia produced the classic soft tissue signs and relieved the painful symptoms, but pain frequently resulted when the access opening was begun or the pulp was entered. Currently, this pain has been significantly reduced with supplemental techniques.

Timing of Supplemental IO Injection

Integration of the results of many clinical trials has changed the paradigm for anesthesia in patients with symptomatic irreversible pulpitis. Considering the high failure rate of the IAN block in patients with these teeth, now, after administering an anesthetic conventionally and observing signs of soft tissue anesthesia (which is required for a successful supplemental injection), the tooth is tested with cold refrigerant. If the result is negative, the clinician may proceed with access; if the result is positive, an IO injection is administered before the rubber dam is placed. The patient should be informed that the tooth is not as anesthetized as desired and that a little extra anesthetic will ensure his or her comfort. The clinician then explains that this extra anesthetic is placed next to the tooth and that the patient may feel some discomfort during the injection. Before the supplemental IO injection, a buccal infiltration of a cartridge of 4% articaine with 1:100,000 epinephrine is given over the tooth to reduce the pain of the IO injection. Because the supplemental IO injection is more successful than the

supplemental IL injection for mandibular teeth with irreversible pulpitis,[208,461] the supplemental IO injection has replaced the IL injection. In addition, because negative testing with a cold refrigerant may not always indicate profound pulpal anesthesia, clinicians may proceed directly to an IO injection once soft tissue anesthesia is obtained. This technique significantly reduces pain and allows treatment to start sooner.

Many practitioners do not use this regimen because clinicians essentially do what they were taught in their initial clinical training, and sometimes change can be difficult. For example, a 1998 study in the *Journal of the American Medical Association* urged the use of anesthesia during circumcision[19]; nevertheless, up to 96% of baby boys don't receive anesthesia. Because many physicians were taught during their residencies not to administer anesthesia, changing their practice philosophy probably will be a slow process. This is a common problem in many health care disciplines, and it emphasizes the need for practitioners to stay current with recent advances.

Supplemental IO Injection: Use 3% Mepivacaine or 2% Lidocaine with 1:100,000 Epinephrine?

As a starting point, the authors recommend using 1.8 ml of 3% mepivacaine plain (e.g., 3% Carbocaine) for the IO injection. The basis for this recommendation is not the cardiovascular risks associated with anesthetic solutions containing a vasoconstrictor, but rather the results of clinical research, which indicate that 3% mepivacaine is reasonably effective and has no clinical side effect of increased heart rate.[137,359] A few patients may overreact to the heart rate increase produced by solutions containing epinephrine, making treatment difficult or time-consuming, because the patient must be calmed before treatment can begin. However, many clinicians also use 2% lidocaine with 1:100,000 epinephrine for IO anesthesia. Clinicians may want to experiment to determine which anesthetic solution (3% mepivacaine or 2% lidocaine with epinephrine) works best for them.

After anesthesia has been obtained, the rubber dam is placed, and the access preparation is slowly begun. The patient should be assured that the procedure will be stopped if he or she feels pain.

If the initial pain occurs in dentin, the rubber dam is removed and another cartridge of 3% mepivacaine is administered, which should be successful.[355] Again, the clinician should make sure that lip anesthesia has developed from the IAN block and that the anesthetic solution is deposited into medullary bone.

If the initial pain occurs when the pulp is entered, the rubber dam is removed and another cartridge of 3% mepivacaine is administered. If the patient still has pain, an IP injection is given. Some practitioners modify the access preparation under these conditions by creating a straight-line channel that directly opens the pulp tissue with little lateral access preparation (i.e., creating an entry hole the size of a #2 round bur). This provides quick access to the pulp, and the small size of the access facilitates IP injection with back-pressure if this technique is indicated. Usually, once the pulp is removed, further pain is minimal, owing to the longer duration of mandibular anesthesia.*

---

*References 60, 112, 277, 313, 332, and 424.

Anesthetizing Mandibular Anterior Teeth

An inferior alveolar injection is given and the tooth is tested with cold refrigerant. If the result is negative, the clinician may proceed with access; if the result is positive, an IO injection is administered before access is begun (the IL injection does not work well in mandibular anterior teeth).[280,436] Before the supplemental IO injection, a labial infiltration of a cartridge of 4% articaine with 1:100,000 epinephrine is given over the tooth to reduce the pain of the IO injection. If pain is felt upon access, the IO injection is repeated. If this is unsuccessful, an IP injection is added.

Anesthetizing Maxillary Posterior Teeth

The initial anesthetic dose of 2% lidocaine with 1:100,000 epinephrine is doubled (to 3.6 ml) for the buccal infiltration.[287] A small amount of anesthetic solution is usually administered palatally for the rubber dam retainer. Although fewer anesthetic problems develop with the maxillary molars and premolars than with the mandibular posterior teeth, the clinician should be aware that they can occur.[6,323] The tooth is tested with cold refrigerant. If the result is negative, the clinician may proceed with access; if the result is positive, an IO or IL injection is administered before access is begun. If pain is felt during the access, the IO or IL injection is repeated. In some cases, an IP injection may be needed. Occasionally, pain is experienced in the palatal canal of molars. Infiltration over the palatal apex with 0.5 ml of anesthetic solution enhances pulpal anesthesia and may prove helpful.[157]

The duration of anesthesia in the maxilla is less than that in the mandible.[156,287,381] Therefore, if pain is experienced during instrumentation or obturation, additional primary and/or supplemental injections are necessary.

Anesthetizing Maxillary Anterior Teeth

Anesthetic is administered initially as a labial infiltration and occasionally as a palatal infiltration for the rubber dam retainer. The tooth is tested with cold refrigerant. If the result is negative, the clinician may proceed with access; if the result is positive, an IO injection is administered before access is begun. Rarely is an IO injection needed. The duration of anesthesia may be less than 1 hour. An additional infiltration injection may be necessary if the patient experiences pain during the later stages of instrumentation or obturation.[156,287,381]

Anesthetizing Symptomatic Teeth with Total Pulpal Necrosis and Periapical Abscess

Symptomatic teeth with total pulp necrosis and periapical radiolucencies are an indicator of pain in the periapical tissue. These teeth may be painful to manipulation and movement during treatment and require extra care. For mandibular teeth, the IAN block (and long buccal injection for molar teeth) is given in all situations. For maxillary teeth with no swelling, anesthetic is administered with conventional infiltration. If soft-tissue swelling is present (i.e., cellulitis or abscess), infiltration should be done on either side of the swelling, or a block could be administered (second division nerve block, PSA nerve block, or infraorbital nerve block). These provide some degree of bone and soft tissue anesthesia. After signs of anesthesia are observed, the rubber dam is placed, and the access is begun *slowly*. The pulp chamber usually can be entered without causing the patient discomfort if the tooth is not torqued excessively. Hand and rotary file shaping can be performed without causing much pain if instruments are used with gentleness and care.

Occasionally, the conventional injections do not provide profound anesthesia, particularly in the maxillary teeth. Although results from clinical trials are lacking for treatment of this region, anecdotal experience suggests that careful consideration of a supplemental injection, consisting of an additional palatal infiltration injection, may be helpful.[348]

In patients with severe preoperative pain, a long-acting anesthetic (e.g., bupivacaine) may help control postoperative pain in mandibular teeth but is not very successful in maxillary teeth.[81,156] However, the duration of analgesia in the mandible is usually not so long to preclude prescribing oral analgesics.[112]

Anesthetizing Asymptomatic Teeth with Total Pulp Necrosis and Periapical Radiolucencies

Asymptomatic teeth are the easiest to anesthetize. Although it may be tempting to proceed without anesthesia, vital sensitive tissue (ingrowth of periapical tissue into canal) may be encountered in the apical portion of canals or placement of files may cause pressure and extrusion of fluid periapically. The conventional injections are administered: IAN block and long buccal injection (for molars), infiltration injections for maxillary teeth. The clinician then proceeds with access and file placement. The patient usually is comfortable in such cases. Rarely, some discomfort may be felt during canal preparation, requiring an IO or IL injection. An IP injection should not be given, because bacteria and debris may be forced from the canal into the periapical tissue. Additional infiltration may be necessary in the maxilla if anesthesia begins to wear off.

Interim Treatment for Irreversible Pulpitis Using Pulpotomy

Patients often have to decide between extraction and endodontic treatment for irreversible pulpitis. Because of financial circumstances, patients may choose extraction if they are only presented with two choices. One study performed pulpotomies in patients with irreversible pulpitis and restored the teeth with intermediate restorative material (IRM) or IRM base/glass ionomer core.[274] They found pain was present in 10% of patients at 6 months and in 22% at 12 months. Although not ideal, the third option of pulpotomy and temporary restoration may allow the patient time to find the means to finance complete endodontic treatment.[87,218,274]

Pain Reduction in Irreversible Pulpitis When Endodontic Treatment Is Impossible

Endodontic débridement (pulpectomy or pulpotomy) most predictably relieves the pain of irreversible pulpitis.[240,329] When débridement is not possible, clinicians may prescribe strong analgesics and antibiotics in an attempt to relieve the pain. Unfortunately, the pain persists, and antibiotics have no effect on the pain of untreated irreversible pulpitis.[309] One clinical trial evaluated pain reduction in untreated irreversible pulpitis by giving an IO injection of Depo-Medrol (a long-acting methylprednisolone).[136] Clinically, the authors found that Depo-Medrol reduced the pain to manageable levels for up to 7 days before the patient received endodontic treatment, supporting this as a method for controlling a patient's pain until definitive endodontic treatment can be performed.

Oral Conscious Sedation with Triazolam (Halcion) and Alprazolam (Xanax)

Patients who are anxious have reduced pain tolerance[253] and may be harder to anesthetize. Oral conscious sedation is beneficial in reducing patient's anxiety. However, as shown by two studies, triazolam and alprazolam are *not* a way to reduce pain during endodontic or dental treatment.[226,253] Profound local anesthesia is still required to control the patient's pain.

Conscious Sedation with Nitrous Oxide

Nitrous oxide provides conscious sedation for apprehensive dental patients. Moreover, nitrous oxide provides a mild analgesic effect. A recent study showed administration of 30% to 50% nitrous oxide resulted in a statistically significant increase in the success of the IAN block in patients presenting with symptomatic irreversible pulpitis.[404]

Preemptive Nonsteroidal Antiinflammatory Drugs (NSAIDs)

Rationale for Preemptive NSAID Use in Patients Presenting with Irreversible Pulpitis

Administering NSAIDs 1 hour before anesthetic administration has been proposed to increase the success of the IAN block in patients presenting with irreversible pulpitis. The rationale is that prostaglandin induces sensitization of peripheral nociceptors.[174,327] Interventions with NSAIDs reduce the overall concentration of prostaglandins and lead to reduced activation of these receptors.[327] It has been shown that prostaglandin E_2 (PGE_2) is reduced in the pulps of patients presenting with irreversible pulpitis when NSAIDs were taken.[341]

Preemptive NSAID Use in Mandibular Posterior Teeth with Symptomatic Irreversible Pulpitis

An early study[291] of preemptive ibuprofen use found higher success rates of the IAN block using tooth sensitivity levels (TSLs). However, the assumption of pulpal anesthesia was not tested by accessing the endodontically involved teeth. Preemptive lornoxicam (8 mg) significantly improved the efficacy of the IAN block, but diclofenac (50 mg) did not.[347] The use of preemptive ketorolac had no significant effect on the success rate of the IAN block.[5,197,284] One study used preemptive oral ketamine and found that the requirements for the number of anesthetic cartridges were reduced when compared to a placebo.[216] However, the assumption of pulpal anesthesia was not tested by accessing the involved teeth.

A number of other studies[5,131,187,330,390] have demonstrated that preemptive administration of 600 mg or 800 mg ibuprofen, a combination of 800 mg ibuprofen and 1000 mg acetaminophen, or a combination of acetaminophen/hydrocodone did not statistically improve the success of the IAN block in patients presenting with symptomatic irreversible pulpitis.

However, preemptive NSAIDs have been shown to improve anesthesia in other studies.[316,333] In addition, a meta-analysis

seemed to indicate an effect from preemptive NSAIDs in the treatment of irreversible pulpitis.[248] A simple explanation for these disparate findings is lacking, and more studies are needed on this topic.

Preemptive NSAID Use in Mandibular Posterior Teeth with Asymptomatic Irreversible Pulpitis

In one study[333] of patients presenting with no spontaneous pain at the endodontic appointment (asymptomatic irreversible pulpitis), preoperative administration of 600 mg ibuprofen or 75 mg indomethacin increased the success of the IAN block (78% and 62%, respectively) over a placebo (32%). However, as shown by Argueta-Figueroa et al.,[23] success rates are higher in patients with asymptomatic irreversible pulpitis. Another study of patients who presented with asymptomatic irreversible pulpitis[383] found that 400 mg of ibuprofen, 0.5 mg dexamethasone, and a placebo resulted in success rates of 25%, 38%, and 13%, respectively. However, the success rates with either ibuprofen or dexamethasone would not ensure profound pulpal anesthesia without supplemental injection of a local anesthetic.

Preemptive NSAID Use in Maxillary First Molars with Symptomatic Irreversible Pulpitis

One study[351] compared preemptive NSAIDs in maxillary teeth and found success rates of 93% for an 800-mg dose of ibuprofen, 90% for a 100-mg dose of aceclofenac, and 73% for 1000 mg of paracetamol. All these were significantly better than a placebo (26% success).

Patient Satisfaction with Painful Dental Procedures

Studies[131,253,404] have shown that patients were moderately or completely satisfied with endodontic treatment even though moderate to severe pain was experienced. Patient satisfaction may be related to the "bedside manner" of the dentist or to satisfaction with the emergency procedure, which they hoped would abate their discomfort. This is an important finding clinically because it helps explain why patients accept painful dental and medical procedures.

ANESTHESIA FOR SURGICAL PROCEDURES

Incision for Drainage

Clinicians should always attempt to achieve some degree of anesthesia before performing an incision and drainage procedure because patients tolerate such procedures better. In the mandible, a conventional IAN injection and long buccal injection are given. In the maxilla, 1.8 ml of 2% lidocaine with 1:100,000 epinephrine is infiltrated on both sides of the facial swelling. As an alternative, because we are mostly concerned with soft tissue anesthesia, a PSA or second division nerve block can be used for premolar and molar teeth and an infraorbital injection given for anterior teeth. For palatal swelling, 0.5 ml of 2% lidocaine with 1:100,000 epinephrine is infiltrated over the greater palatine foramen (molar and premolar teeth) or nasopalatine foramen (anterior teeth). These injections should not be given if swelling is present over the foramen; infiltration should be done on either side of the swelling. The Wand system reduces the pain of palatal injections. Generally, the computer-assisted injection system causes less pain than the conventional syringe technique for AMSA, palatal, and IAN block injections.*

Profound anesthesia is usually difficult to achieve in these cases,[29] and this must be explained to the patient. The swelling is not injected because traditionally it has been believed that injection directly into a swelling is contraindicated. Reasons for this included the possible spread of infection and the contention that the inflamed tissue's lower pH would make the anesthetic solution less effective. These ideas may have some merit, but swellings are not injected basically because it is *very* painful and relatively ineffective. An area of cellulitis has an increased blood supply, and an anesthetic injected into this area is largely carried away into the systemic circulation, which diminishes the anesthetic's local effectiveness. Also, edema and purulence may dilute the solution. (See Chapter 18 for additional information on incision and drainage procedures.)

Periapical Surgery

Most periapical surgery should be performed by an endodontist because he or she has received advanced training in the surgical procedures, periapical bone anatomy of the mandible and maxilla, use of magnification technologies, complex canal anatomy, and advanced microsurgical techniques for retrograde preparation and filling.

In the mandible, the inferior alveolar and long buccal injections are reasonably effective. Additional buccal infiltration injections in the vestibule may be useful to achieve vasoconstriction, particularly in the mandibular anterior region. In the maxilla, infiltration injections are generally effective; usually larger volumes are necessary to provide anesthesia over the surgical field. If the area of operation is inflamed, anesthesia may not be totally successful.

After the flap has been reflected, if anesthesia is inadequate, attempts to enhance or regain anesthesia (through additional infiltrations or injecting the sensitive area) are not particularly effective. The effectiveness of surgical anesthesia is decreased by half compared to anesthesia for nonsurgical procedures because when the clinician reflects a flap and opens into bone, the anesthetic solution is diluted by bleeding and removed by irrigation.[454]

Use of a long-acting anesthetic has been advocated for surgery.[84,371] In the mandible, this is reasonably effective. In the maxilla, long-acting agents have a shorter duration of anesthesia and decreased epinephrine concentrations, which result in more bleeding during surgery.[78,454]

Administration of a long-acting anesthetic after periapical surgery has been suggested.[262] However, postsurgical pain is usually not severe and can be managed by analgesics.[279]

SUMMARY AND FUTURE DIRECTIONS FOR EFFECTIVE ANESTHESIA

The emergence of evidence-based dentistry has rapidly drawn interest across all fields of dentistry. Fortunately, the large number of high-quality, randomized, controlled studies in anesthesia and analgesia provide a wealth of information supporting evidence-based recommendations. The practitioner must focus on high-quality research when making clinical decisions. This section of the chapter adopted the evidence-based approach in providing a comprehensive summary of

local anesthetic clinical trials for the treatment of patients with endodontic pain.

The prudent practitioner knows that there is no "magic bullet" in pain control. Rather, the clinician must be knowledgeable about the advantages and disadvantages of several anesthetic-vasoconstrictor combinations and the various routes of injection. Clearly, judicious selection of local anesthetics, delivered through multiple sites of injection, is likely to provide predictable anesthesia with minimal exposure to side effects.

Research continues in the development of new or improved anesthetics. Investigations on extended-duration anesthetic formulations suggest that local anesthetics may prove useful for treating postprocedural pain.[141,462] In the future, clinicians may be able to provide anesthesia of a specific area for a day or maybe a number of days using liposomal-encapsulated anesthetic agents. The timing of anesthesia would be tailored by how the liposome is formulated to dissolve and the amount of drug in the liposome.

In addition, capsaicin and transient receptor potential vanilloid-1 (TRPV-1) agonists and antagonists may in the future be used in the clinical management of pain associated with inflammation.[144,232,237]

New modes of delivery of drugs are also being studied. Microneedles may be used in the future to deliver topical or local anesthetics across mucosal surfaces painlessly.[14,331,451]

II. ANALGESICS AND THERAPEUTIC RECOMMENDATIONS

NON-NARCOTIC ANALGESICS

Management of endodontic pain is multifactorial and directed at reducing the peripheral and central components of hyperalgesia through combined endodontic procedures and pharmacotherapy. A major class of drugs for managing endodontic pain is non-narcotic analgesics, which include both NSAIDs and acetaminophen. NSAIDs have been shown to be very effective in managing pain of inflammatory origin and, by virtue of their binding to plasma proteins, actually exhibit increased delivery to inflamed tissue via the extravasation of plasma proteins.[49,92,168,171] Although these drugs classically are thought to produce analgesia through peripheral mechanisms, the CNS is believed to be an additional site of action.[267,409] NSAIDs inhibit the synthesis of prostaglandins by blocking the enzyme cyclooxygenase (COX) which has two known isoforms, COX-1 and COX-2. Some researchers have proposed that a splice variant of COX-1 (i.e., COX-3) is expressed predominantly in the CNS and is the major site of action of acetaminophen.[59,231,325,380] However, recent studies[177] indicate that the antipyretic and analgesic effects of acetaminophen do not involve inhibition of COX-3; they are more likely exerted through effects of an active metabolite on CNS cannabinoid receptors,[18] and this metabolite appears to act by blocking a calcium channel ($Ca_V3.2$).[225]

Numerous NSAIDs are available for management of pain and inflammation (Table 4-4). Unfortunately, comparatively few studies (particularly for endodontic pain) directly compare one NSAID to another for analgesia and side-effect liability. The lack of comprehensive comparative studies in endodontic models means that only general recommendations can be made, and clinicians are encouraged to

---

*References 145, 181, 349, and 456.

TABLE 4-4

Summary of Selected Non-Narcotic Analgesics

Analgesic	Trade Name	Dose Range (mg)	Daily Dose (mg)
Acetaminophen	Tylenol and others	325-650	4000
Aspirin	Many	325-1000	4000
Diclofenac potassium	Cataflam	50-100	150-200
Diflunisal	Dolobid	250-1000	1500
Etodolac	Lodine	200-400	1200
Fenoprofen	Nalfon	200	1200
Flurbiprofen	Ansaid	50-100	200-300
Ibuprofen	Motrin et al.	200-800	2400 (Rx)
Ketoprofen	Orudis	25-75	300 (Rx)
Ketorolac*	Toradol Sprix	30-60 (oral) 31.5	60 126 mg
Naproxen	Naprosyn	250-500	1500
Naproxen Na	Anaprox and others	220-550	1650 (Rx)

Modified from Cooper SA: Treating acute dental pain, *Postgrad Dent* 2:7, 1995.
Note: Cyclooxygenase-2 (COX-2) inhibitors are not included (see text).
Rx, Prescription strength.
*A new package insert for ketorolac tablets includes the instructions that the drug should be used only as a transition from injectable ketorolac and for no longer than 5 days. The package insert for intranasal ketorolac states that for patients 65 years of age or older, renally impaired patients, and patients weighing less than 50 kg, the dose should be limited to 15.75 mg, and the maximum daily dose should be limited to 63 mg.

familiarize themselves with several of these drugs. Ibuprofen generally is considered the prototype of contemporary NSAIDs and has a well-documented efficacy and safety profile.[89] Other NSAIDs may offer certain advantages over ibuprofen. For example, etodolac (i.e., Lodine) has reduced gastrointestinal (GI) irritation,[25] and ketoprofen (i.e., Orudis) has been shown in some studies to be somewhat more analgesic than ibuprofen.[73] An intranasal formulation of ketorolac tromethamine (Sprix, Regency Therapeutics, Shirley, New York) is now available and provides significant pain relief within 30 minutes of administration in patients with endodontic pain.[420] Recent studies suggest that in addition to inhibiting cyclooxygenase, ketorolac and diclofenac inhibit peripheral N-methyl-D-aspartate (NMDA) receptors, which may contribute to their analgesic effects.[54,96] The advantages of NSAIDs include their well-established analgesic efficacy for inflammatory pain. Many of the NSAIDs listed in Table 4-4 have been shown to be more effective than traditional acetaminophen and opioid combinations such as acetaminophen with codeine.[72,89,417]

A 2002 paper represents the first systematic review comparing all endodontic pain studies evaluating oral NSAIDs.[184] This study also provides a framework for other investigators interested in conducting systematic reviews for endodontic research. The authors concluded that NSAIDs combined with other drugs (e.g., flurbiprofen with tramadol[97]) or pretreatment and posttreatment application of NSAIDs provides effective pain control. Although relatively new to endodontic research,

systematic reviews of analgesic drugs in inflammatory pain models have been conducted for several years. Table 4-5 lists the results of a large ongoing systematic review of the relative efficacy of analgesics in inflammatory pain conditions. Importantly, the data are generated based on postoperative patients having moderate to severe pain, and the number needed to treat (NNT) is based on the relative superiority of the analgesic over placebo for producing a 50% relief in pain. These data, therefore, constitute important, clinically relevant information for clinicians who want to compare the relative efficacy of posttreatment analgesics. Of course, other issues, such as the potential adverse effects of drugs and the patient's medical history, must be considered when a treatment plan for postendodontic pain is developed.

The introduction of selective inhibitors of COX-2 offered the potential for both analgesic and antiinflammatory benefits and reduced GI irritation.[91,227] Oral surgery pain studies evaluating COX-2 inhibitors have indicated that rofecoxib (i.e., Vioxx) has significant analgesic efficacy in this model.[106] In one study, a 50-mg dose of rofecoxib produced analgesia equivalent to 400 mg of ibuprofen, with the two drugs displaying similar times for onset of analgesia.[106] Expression of COX-2 is increased in inflamed human dental pulp,[310] and a COX-2 inhibitor (rofecoxib) is analgesic in patients with endodontic pain. However, most selective COX-2 inhibitors have been withdrawn from the market due to prothrombic adverse effects, and the only coxib still available, celecoxib, has not received approval by the U.S. Food and Drug Administration (FDA) for treatment of acute inflammatory pain. Concern has been raised that the COX-2 inhibitors may also display at least some GI irritation in patients with preexisting GI disease.[426]

Another major concern centers on the recognized prothrombic adverse effects of the COX-2 inhibitors. This debate originally started when patients randomized to 50 mg/day of rofecoxib in the VIGOR study had a fivefold increase in thromboembolic cardiovascular (CV) events compared to 1000 mg/day of naproxen.[40] The debate continued until the demonstration of an increased risk for prothrombic events after long-term administration of rofecoxib, which led to the withdrawal of this drug from the market in 2004.[110] Two meta-analyses have examined the CV safety of traditional NSAIDs and COX-2 inhibitors. Kearney et al.[217] conducted a meta-analysis of 138 randomized trials, and McGettigan and Henry[276] conducted a meta-analysis of 23 controlled observational studies.[217,276] Kearney et al.[217] estimated a relative risk for CV events associated with COX-2 to be 1.42 (95% CI, 1.64 to 2.91). Naproxen was found to have no significant adverse effects on the CV system in both meta-analyses. Diclofenac (Voltaren) is a relatively COX-2–selective drug and seems to have a degree of COX-2 selectivity similar to that of celecoxib. Diclofenac was associated with increased CV events. In the randomized trial analysis, there was an increase in CV risk with high-dose ibuprofen. Based on the available data, the FDA has requested that manufacturers of all prescription products containing nonselective NSAIDs revise their product labeling to include (1) a boxed warning regarding the potential serious adverse CV events and the serious, potentially life-threatening GI adverse events associated with the use of this class of drugs; (2) a contraindication to use in patients who have recently undergone coronary artery bypass surgery; and (3) a medication guide for patients regarding the potential for CV and GI adverse events associated with the use of this class of drugs.

TABLE 4-5

Oxford League Table of Analgesic Efficacy*

Analgesic[†]	Number of Patients in Comparison	Percentage with at Least 50% Pain Relief	NNT	Lower Confidence Interval	Higher Confidence Interval
Ibuprofen (800 mg)	76	100	1.6	1.3	2.2
Ketorolac (60 mg) (IM)	116	56	1.8	1.5	2.3
Diclofenac (100 mg)	548	69	1.8	1.6	2.1
Oxycodone IR (5 mg) + acetaminophen (500 mg)	150	60	2.2	1.7	3.2
Diclofenac (50 mg)	738	63	2.3	2	2.7
Naproxen (440 mg)	257	50	2.3	2	2.9
Oxycodone IR (15 mg)	60	73	2.3	1.5	4.9
Ibuprofen (600 mg)	203	79	2.4	2	4.2
Ibuprofen (400 mg)	5456	55	2.5	2.4	2.7
Aspirin (1200 mg)	279	61	2.4	1.9	3.2
Oxycodone IR (10 mg)	315	66	2.6	2	3.5
Ketorolac (10 mg) + acetaminophen (650 mg)	790	50	2.6	2.3	3.1
Ibuprofen (200 mg)	3248	48	2.7	2.5	2.9
Naproxen (500/550)	784	52	2.7	2.3	3.3
Diclofenac (50 mg)	1296	57	2.7	2.4	3.1
Diclofenac (25 mg)	204	54	2.8	2.1	4.3
Demerol (100 mg) (IM)	364	54	2.9	2.3	3.9
Tramadol (150 mg)	561	48	2.9	2.4	3.6
Morphine (10 mg) (IM)	946	50	2.9	2.6	3.6
Naproxen (500/550 mg)	169	46	3	2.2	4.8
Naproxen (220/250 mg)	202	45	3.4	2.4	5.8
Ketorolac (30 mg) (IM)	359	53	3.4	2.5	4.9
Acetaminophen (500 mg)	561	61	3.5	2.2	13.3
Acetaminophen (600/650 mg) + codeine (60 mg)	1123	42	4.2	3.4	5.3
Acetaminophen (650 mg) + dextropropoxyphene (65 mg hydrochloride or 100 mg napsylate)	963	38	4.4	3.5	5.6
Aspirin (600/650 mg)	5061	38	4.4	4	4.9
Acetaminophen (600/650 mg)	1886	38	4.6	3.9	5.5
Tramadol (100 mg)	882	30	4.8	3.8	6.1
Tramadol (75 mg)	563	32	5.3	3.9	8.2
Aspirin (650 mg) + codeine (60 mg)	598	25	5.3	4.1	7.4
Oxycodone IR (5 mg) + acetaminophen (325 mg)	149	24	5.5	3.4	
Ketorolac (10 mg) (IM)	142	48	5.7	3	53
Acetaminophen (300 mg) + codeine (30 mg)	379	26	5.7	4	9.8
Tramadol (50 mg)	770	19	8.3	6	13
Codeine (60 mg)	1305	15	16.7	11	48
Placebo	>10,000	18	N/A	N/A	N/A

Modified from http://www.medicine.ox.ac.uk/bandolier/booth/painpag/acutrev/analgesics/lftab.html (Accessed August 10, 2015.)
IM, Intramuscular; NA, not applicable; NNT, number needed to treat.
*Analgesics are listed in descending order from most to least effective based on the number needed to treat (NNT). The NNT reflects the superiority of an analgesic over a placebo treatment; therefore an analgesic with a lower NNT has greater efficacy than an analgesic with a higher NNT. The NNT is calculated for the proportion of patients with at least 50% pain relief over 4 to 6 hours compared with placebo in randomized, double-blind, and single-dose studies in patients with moderate to severe pain. The 95% confidence interval contains the upper and lower estimates of the NNT with a 95% chance of accuracy.
[†]Drugs were given orally except where noted.

The available data do not suggest an increased risk of serious CV events for the short-term, low-dose use of NSAIDs available over the counter, but the FDA has requested changes to the label to better inform consumers about the safe use of these products. Given this situation and reasonable alternative NSAIDs, we recommend against the use of COX-2 inhibitors for the treatment of patients with routine endodontic pain.

Limitations and Drug Interactions

Clinicians should educate themselves not only on the efficacy of the non-narcotic analgesics, but also on their limitations and interactions with other drugs.[52] For example, NSAIDs exhibit an analgesic ceiling that limits the maximal level of analgesia and induces side effects, including those affecting the GI system (3% to 11% incidence) and the CNS (1% to 9% incidence of dizziness and headache). NSAIDs are contraindicated in patients with ulcers and aspirin hypersensitivity.[63,65,125,396] They also are associated with severe GI complications, and the risk of adverse effects increases with an increasing lifetime-accumulated dose of these drugs and concurrent intake of aspirin, steroids, or coumadin.[24,93,242,442] A strategy for avoiding GI bleeding associated with NSAIDs is to use a proton pump inhibitor (PPI). A combination of a PPI (esomeprazole magnesium) with naproxen (Vimovo, Patheon/Astrozenica, Wilmington, Delaware) is now available. Although this is a cost-effective approach, it does not protect the lower GI tract.[400] Another approach is to use a histamine receptor H$_2$ antagonist in combination with an NSAID. The combination of famotidine (an H$_2$-receptor antagonist) and ibuprofen (Duexis, Horizon Pharma, Northbrook, Illinois) was recently approved by the FDA. The NSAIDs have been reported to interact with a number of other drugs (Table 4-6).

Acetaminophen and opioid combination drugs are alternatives for patients unable to take NSAIDs.[71] Further information is available on the pharmacology and adverse effects of this important class of drugs.[52,69,93,133,452] Other resources are also available for evaluation of drug interactions, including Internet drug search engines, such as *rxlist.com*, *Epocrates.com*, and *Endodontics.UTHSCSA.edu*.

Acetaminophen

Acetaminophen (*N*-acetyl *p*-aminophenol) is one of the most commonly used analgesic and antipyretic drugs. Acetaminophen alone is not comparable to ibuprofen in relieving moderate to severe pain; however, a combination of ibuprofen and acetaminophen may provide greater pain relief than either drug alone. In a randomized, double-blind, placebo-controlled study, patients who had undergone pulpectomy were administered a single dose of either a combination of acetaminophen (1000 mg) and ibuprofen (600 mg) or ibuprofen (600 mg) alone. The combination of the two analgesics provided greater pain relief in the immediate postoperative period (8 hours) than ibuprofen (600 mg) alone.[285]

Acetaminophen is one of the most common drugs found in combination products for the relief of pain and symptoms of cold or flu. It is considered safe when taken at normal doses, but in higher doses, acetaminophen causes liver toxicity and is associated with nearly half of the cases of acute liver failure in the United States.[244] Most acetaminophen is conjugated in the liver to form inactive metabolites. A small portion is metabolized by the cytochrome P450 system to form *N*-acetyl-*p*-benzoquinone imine (NAPQI), which is very toxic but is

TABLE 4-6

Summary of Selected Drug Interactions with Nonsteroidal Antiinflammatory Drugs (NSAIDs)

Drug	Possible Effect
Angiotensin-converting enzyme (ACE) inhibitors	Reduced antihypertensive effectiveness of captopril (and especially indomethacin)
Anticoagulants	Increase in prothrombin time or bleeding with anticoagulants (e.g., coumarins)
Beta-blockers	Reduced antihypertensive effects (e.g., propranolol, atenolol, pindolol)
Cyclosporine	Increased risk of nephrotoxicity
Digoxin	Increase in serum digoxin levels (especially ibuprofen, indomethacin)
Dipyridamole	Increased water retention (especially indomethacin)
Hydantoins	Increased serum levels of phenytoin
Lithium	Increased serum levels of lithium
Loop diuretics	Reduced effectiveness of loop diuretics (e.g., furosemide, bumetanide)
Methotrexate	Increased risk of toxicity (e.g., stomatitis, bone marrow suppression)
Penicillamine	Increased bioavailability (especially indomethacin)
Sympathomimetics	Increased blood pressure (especially indomethacin with phenylpropanolamine)
Thiazide diuretics	Reduced antihypertensive effectiveness

Data from Facts and Comparisons: *Drug facts and comparisons,* ed 54, St Louis, 2000, Facts and Comparisons; Gage T, Pickett F: *Mosby's dental drug reference,* ed 5, St Louis, 2000, Mosby; and Wynn R, Meiller T, Crossley H: *Drug information handbook for dentistry,* Hudson, Ohio, 2000, Lexi-Comp.

generally detoxified by glutathione and converted into nontoxic compounds. Large doses of acetaminophen saturate the main route of metabolism, causing more acetaminophen to be converted to NAPQI. Liver injury occurs once glutathione becomes depleted and NAPQI is allowed to accumulate. To minimize this risk, it has been recommended that healthy adults not take more than 3 g (3000 mg) of acetaminophen in a 24-hour period (*www.tylenolprofessional.com/extra-strength-tylenol-dosage-faq.html*). The FDA mandated that by 2014, manufacturers of oral prescription acetaminophen combination medicines limit the maximum amount of acetaminophen to 325 mg per tablet. The FDA also requires a boxed warning to be added to the label of all oral prescription drug products that contain acetaminophen. (A boxed warning, the strongest warning that the FDA requires, indicates that the drug carries a significant risk of serious adverse effects).

OPIOID ANALGESICS

Opioids are potent analgesics and are often used in dentistry in combination with acetaminophen, aspirin, or ibuprofen. Most clinically available opioids activate mu opioid receptors at several important sites in the brain and on afferent neurons. Studies indicate that they activate peripheral opioid receptors in dental pulp and that IL injection of morphine significantly

TABLE 4-7

Selected Opioid Combination Analgesic Drugs

Formulation	Trade Name*	Possible Rx
APAP 300 mg and codeine 30 mg	Tylenol with codeine no. 3	2 tabs q4h
APAP 500 mg and hydrocodone 5 mg	Vicodin, Lortab 5/500	1-2 tabs q6h
APAP 325 mg and oxycodone 5 mg	Percocet	1 tab q6h
APAP 500 mg and oxycodone 5 mg	Tylox	1 tab q6h
ASA 325 mg and codeine 30 mg	Empirin with codeine no. 3	2 tabs q4h
ASA 325 mg and oxycodone 5 mg	Percodan	1 tab q6h

APAP, Acetaminophen; *ASA*, aspirin; *Rx*, prescription.
*Several generics are available for most formulations.

TABLE 4-8

Analgesic Doses of Representative Opioids

Opioid	Dose Equivalent to Codeine 60 mg
Codeine	60 mg
Oxycodone	5-6 mg
Hydrocodone	10 mg
Dihydrocodeine	60 mg
Propoxyphene HCl	102 mg
Propoxyphene-N	146 mg
Meperidine	90 mg
Tramadol	50 mg

Modified from Troullos E, Freeman R, Dionne RA: The scientific basis for analgesic use in dentistry, *Anesth Prog* 33:123, 1986.
HCl, Hydrochloride; *N*, napsylate.

reduces pain in endodontic patients and in other inflammatory pain states.[94,111,167] Gender-dependent differences appear to exist in responsiveness to at least the kappa opioid agonists.[142] In a randomized, controlled clinical trial, women taking a combination of pentazocine and naloxone had significantly less postoperative endodontic pain than men taking the same medications.[374]

Although opioids are effective as analgesics for moderate to severe pain, their use is generally limited by their adverse side effects, which can include nausea, emesis, dizziness, drowsiness, and the potential for respiratory depression and constipation. Chronic use is associated with tolerance and dependence. Because the dosage is limited by side effects, these medications are almost always used in combination drugs to manage dental pain. A combination formulation is preferred because it permits a lower dose of the opioid, thereby reducing side effects (Table 4-7).

Codeine is often considered the prototype opioid for orally available combination drugs. Most studies have found that the 60-mg dose of codeine (the amount in two tablets of Tylenol with codeine no. 3) produces significantly more analgesia than placebo, although it often produces less analgesia than either aspirin 650 mg or acetaminophen 600 mg.[71,72,168] In general, patients taking only 30 mg of codeine report about as much analgesia as those taking a placebo.[31,417] Table 4-8 provides comparable doses of other opioids equivalent to 60 mg of codeine.

CORTICOSTEROIDS

Posttreatment pain or flare-up after endodontic treatment can be attributed to inflammation, infection, or both in the periradicular tissues. Establishing patency and subsequently débriding and shaping the root canal system may irritate the periradicular tissues and inadvertently introduce bacteria, bacterial products, necrotic pulp tissue, or caustic irrigating solution through apical foramina.

In response to this irritation, inflammatory mediators (e.g., prostaglandins [PGs], leukotrienes, bradykinin, platelet-activating factor, substance P) are released into the tissues surrounding the apical area of the tooth. As a result, pain fibers are directly stimulated or sensitized, and an increase in vascular dilation and permeability results in edema and increased interstitial tissue pressure.

Glucocorticosteroids are known to reduce the acute inflammatory response by suppressing vasodilation, migration of polymorphonuclear (PMN) leukocytes, and phagocytosis and by inhibiting formation of arachidonic acid from neutrophil and macrophage cell membrane phospholipids, thus blocking the COX and lipoxygenase pathways and respective synthesis of PGs and leukotrienes. It is not surprising that a number of investigations have evaluated the efficacy of corticosteroids (administered via either intracanal or systemic routes) in the prevention or control of postoperative endodontic pain or flare-ups.[268]

Intracanal Administration

Several studies have evaluated intracanal administration of steroids. In 50 consecutive patients requiring nonsurgical root canal treatment of vital teeth, one investigator alternately placed a dexamethasone solution or saline placebo as intracanal medicaments after the root canals had been cleaned and shaped.[307] Pretreatment pain ratings were collected, as were ratings at 24, 48, and 72 hours after treatment. Results indicated a significant reduction in pain at 24 hours but no significant difference at 48 and 72 hours. In a similar double-blind clinical trial, intracanal placement of a 2.5% steroid solution or saline placebo on completion of instrumentation resulted in a significant reduction of the incidence of postoperative pain in teeth in which the pulp was vital.[58] When the pulp was necrotic, however, there was no significant difference between the steroid and placebo in reducing postoperative discomfort.

Another study found no significant difference in the flare-up rate when either formocresol, Ledermix (a corticosteroid antibiotic paste), or calcium hydroxide was placed as an intracanal medicament in strict sequence, irrespective of the presence or absence of symptoms or radiographic signs of apical periodontitis.[416] However, a large-scale clinical trial of 223 patients reported significantly less posttreatment pain in patients after intracanal administration of Ledermix compared with either calcium hydroxide or no intracanal dressing.[107] Intracanal steroids appear to have significant effects for reducing postoperative pain.[365]

Systemic Administration

Some studies have evaluated the systemic route of administration of corticosteroids on posttreatment pain or flare-ups. In one double-blind, randomized, placebo-controlled study, dexamethasone (4 mg/ml) or saline was injected intramuscularly at the conclusion of a single-visit endodontic appointment or at the first visit of a multivisit procedure.[269] The results indicated that the steroid significantly reduced the incidence and severity of pain at 4 hours when compared with the placebo. No difference in pain was seen at the 24- and 48-hour time points.

In a similar study, 106 patients with irreversible pulpitis and acute periradicular periodontitis were given an intraoral intramuscular injection of dexamethasone at different doses, either on completion of a single-visit endodontic treatment or after the first visit of a multivisit procedure.[250] Systemic administration of dexamethasone was shown to significantly reduce the severity of pain at 4 and 8 hours, with an optimum dose between 0.07 and 0.09 mg/kg. However, no significant reduction in the severity of pain was noted at 24, 48, and 72 hours, and no overall effect was seen on the incidence of pain. Another study compared the effect an IL injection of methylprednisolone, mepivacaine, or placebo in preventing posttreatment endodontic pain.[215] The results showed that methylprednisolone significantly reduced postoperative pain within a 24-hour follow-up period.

In a double-blind placebo-controlled study, patients with irreversible pulpitis were given 4 mg of dexamethasone or placebo by means of a supraperiosteal injection at the apex of the treated tooth after pulpectomy.[283] This is an injection technique that most clinicians would be familiar with (as opposed to intramuscular injection). Posttreatment pain was significantly reduced in the steroid group during the first 24 hours. There was no difference at 48 hours.

Yet another study evaluated the effect of IO injection of methylprednisolone or placebo in patients with irreversible pulpitis. Highly significant pain reduction in the steroid group was maintained for 7 days after a single injection.[143]

Animal studies have histologically evaluated the antiinflammatory effects of corticosteroids on inflamed periradicular tissues. In one study, after an acute inflammatory reaction was induced in the molar teeth of rats by overextending endodontic instruments, sterile saline or dexamethasone was infiltrated supraperiosteally into the buccal vestibule adjacent to the treated teeth. Dexamethasone significantly reduced the number of neutrophils present and thus had an antiinflammatory effect on the periradicular tissues of the treated teeth.[315]

Other studies of systemic administration have evaluated the effect of oral administration of corticosteroids on the incidence and severity of posttreatment endodontic pain. In a double-blind, controlled clinical trial, 50 patients randomly received either 0.75 mg of dexamethasone or a placebo tablet orally after initial endodontic treatment.[238] Oral dexamethasone significantly reduced posttreatment pain after 8 and 24 hours compared with placebo. A follow-up study evaluated the effect a larger oral dose of dexamethasone (i.e., 12 mg given every 4 hours) on the severity of posttreatment endodontic pain.[147] Results showed that dexamethasone was effective in reducing posttreatment endodontic pain up to 8 hours after the treatment was completed; no effect on the severity of pain was seen at 24 and 48 hours after treatment. In a double-blind study comparing etodolac and dexamethasone, the perioperative administration of oral dexamethasone was comparable to that of etodolac in reducing pain after endodontic surgery. In a randomized clinical trial,[252] 40 patients received a single dose of prednisolone (30 mg) or placebo 30 minutes before initiation of endodontic treatment. Prednisolone significantly reduced posttreatment pain at 6, 12, and 24 hours compared to placebo.[194]

Collectively, these studies on systemic steroid administration indicate that corticosteroids reduce the severity of posttreatment endodontic pain compared with placebo treatment. However, given the relative safety/efficacy relationship between steroids and NSAIDs, most investigators choose an NSAID as the drug of first choice for postoperative pain control.

ANTIBIOTICS

Because bacteria are involved in endodontic cases with apical periodontitis, the incidence of a posttreatment infection or flare-up is a concern to clinicians providing endodontic treatment. Prescribing an antibiotic to prevent such an occurrence might make sense, but use of antibiotics is controversial for several reasons.[119] First, overprescribing of antibiotics, especially when these drugs are not indicated, has led to increased bacterial resistance and patient sensitization. Second, antibiotics have been mistakenly prescribed for patients with severe pain who have a vital tooth (i.e., when bacteria are unlikely to be a causative factor in periradicular pain).[457] Third, even when bacteria are likely to be present, data from controlled clinical trials provide little or no support for the hypothesis that antibiotics reduce pain.[218]

A series of clinical studies evaluated the efficacy of prophylactically administered systemic antibiotics for preventing posttreatment endodontic flare-ups. Working on the premise that the incidence of infectious flare-ups after endodontic treatment is 15%, Morse et al.[305] randomly prescribed a prophylactic dose of either penicillin or erythromycin to patients after endodontic treatment of teeth with a diagnosis of necrotic pulp and chronic periradicular periodontitis (no placebo was used). The results showed that the overall incidence of flare-ups was 2.2%, with no difference between penicillin and erythromycin. Similar results were obtained in a study in which dental students (instead of private practitioners) provided the endodontic treatment.[1] Outcomes found a 2.6% incidence of flare-up, with no statistically significant differences between penicillin and erythromycin. However, neither the original nor the follow-up study was a randomized, placebo-controlled clinical trial. This observation appears to be highly significant for clinical recommendations because in general, randomized controlled studies fail to detect any analgesic benefit to antibiotics, whereas open-label or historical control studies often report profound effects.[119]

To determine whether the timing of administration of an antibiotic altered the occurrence of flare-ups and pain unassociated with flare-ups, researchers analyzed components of two separate prospective studies of patients undergoing endodontic treatment for teeth with necrotic pulps and chronic periradicular periodontitis. In the first study, prophylactic penicillin was provided; in the second study, patients were instructed to take penicillin (or erythromycin if they were allergic to penicillin) at the first sign of swelling.[304,305] The authors concluded that prophylactic administration of antibiotics is preferable to having the patient take antibiotics at the first sign of an infection.

Another study of similar design compared the incidence of flare-up when a cephalosporin or erythromycin was given prophylactically.[306] When the data from previous studies were pooled and retrospectively compared, the authors concluded that prophylactically administered antibiotics, including cephalosporins, significantly reduced the incidence of flare-ups in endodontic cases involving necrotic pulp and chronic periradicular periodontitis. However, these studies have been questioned because of the lack of concurrent placebo-treated groups and the use of historical controls.

In a multicenter, two-part clinical study, 588 consecutive patients received one of nine medications or placebos and were monitored for 72 hours after treatment.[414] The results showed that ibuprofen, ketoprofen, erythromycin, penicillin, and penicillin plus methylprednisolone significantly reduced the severity of pain within the first 48 hours after treatment. The second part of the study then evaluated the incidence of posttreatment pain after obturation of the same teeth in the first phase of the study.[414] Although only 411 of the original 588 patients participated in this phase, they were randomly given the same medications or placebo after completion of the obturation appointment. The incidence of posttreatment pain was lower after obturation (5.83%) than after cleaning and shaping (21.76%) of the root canal system, and no significant difference was found in the effectiveness of the various medications and placebo in controlling posttreatment pain after obturation.

Walton and Chiappinelli[429] were concerned that previous studies were uncontrolled, retrospective, or carried out on different patient groups at different times and with different treatment modalities. They conducted a randomized, prospective, double-blind clinical trial to test the hypothesis that an antibiotic (e.g., penicillin) can prevent a posttreatment endodontic flare-up.[429] Eighty patients with teeth that had necrotic pulp and chronic periradicular periodontitis were randomly divided into three groups. In the first two groups, either penicillin or a placebo was administered 1 hour before and 6 hours after the individual appointments on a double-blind basis. Upon completion of the individual appointments, which included débridement, shaping, and possibly obturation of the root canal system, the patients completed questionnaires at 4, 8, 12, 24, and 48 hours. No significant difference was found among the three groups in the incidence of flare-ups, pain, or swelling. The authors concluded that the use of prophylactic penicillin offers no benefit for postoperative pain or flare-up, and prophylactic administration of penicillin should not be used routinely in patients undergoing endodontic treatment of necrotic teeth and chronic periradicular periodontitis.

In another randomized, prospective, placebo-controlled clinical study, a group of investigators examined whether supplemental penicillin reduced symptoms or shortened the course of recovery of emergency patients diagnosed with necrotic pulp and acute apical abscess.[120] Patients were randomly given penicillin, a placebo, or no medication. Using a visual analog scale, the subjects then evaluated their postoperative pain and swelling for up to 72 hours. No significant difference was found among the three groups. Recovery occurred as a result of endodontic treatment alone.

It is well recognized that antibiotics may be indicated for the management of infections of endodontic origin. However, a review of the available literature indicates that prophylactic use is contraindicated in immunocompetent patients with no systemic signs of infection and with swelling localized to the vestibule. Controlled clinical studies indicate that antibiotics offer little or no benefit for pain reduction under these circumstances, but they may be indicated for immunocompromised patients and for patients with systemic signs and symptoms of an infection or an infection that has spread into the fascial spaces of the head and neck.

PAIN MANAGEMENT STRATEGIES

When managing pain in an individual patient, the skilled clinician must customize the treatment plan, balancing the general principles of endodontics, mechanisms of hyperalgesia, and pain management strategies with the particular factors of the individual patient (e.g., medical history, concurrent medications).[171,219,220,369,393]

Effective management of endodontic pain starts with the "three Ds": *diagnosis*, *definitive* dental treatment, and *drugs* (Box 4-1). Comprehensive reviews on *diagnosis* and *definitive* dental treatment (e.g., incision and drainage, pulpectomy) are provided elsewhere in this text (Chapters 1, 6, 9, and 18). As described earlier in this chapter, the management of endodontic pain should focus on the removal of peripheral mechanisms of hyperalgesia and allodynia (see Box 4-1). This generally requires treatment that removes and reduces causative factors (e.g., bacterial and immunologic factors). For example, both pulpotomy and pulpectomy have been associated with substantial reduction in patient reports of pain compared to pretreatment pain levels.[97,173,274,337] However, pharmacotherapy often is required to reduce continued nociceptor input (e.g., NSAIDs, local anesthetics) and suppress central hyperalgesia (e.g., NSAIDs, opioids).

Pretreatment

Treatment with an NSAID before a procedure has been shown to have a significant benefit in many studies[89,191] but not all.[314] The rationale for pretreatment is to block the development of hyperalgesia by reducing the input from peripheral nociceptors. For patients who cannot take NSAIDs, pretreatment with acetaminophen also has been shown to reduce postoperative pain.[298] Patients can be pretreated 30 minutes before the procedure with either an NSAID (e.g., ibuprofen 400 mg or flurbiprofen 100 mg) or with acetaminophen 1000 mg.[97,191,298]

Long-Acting Local Anesthetics

A second pharmacologic approach for pain management is the use of long-acting local anesthetics, such as bupivacaine and ropivacaine. Clinical trials indicate that long-acting local anesthetics not only provide anesthesia during the procedure, but

---

BOX 4-1

Considerations for Effective "Three D" Pain Control

1. Diagnosis
2. Definitive dental treatment
3. Drugs
   - Pretreat with nonsteroidal antiinflammatory drugs (NSAIDs) or acetaminophen when appropriate.
   - Use long-acting local anesthetics when indicated.
   - Use a flexible prescription plan.
   - Prescribe "by the clock" rather than as needed.

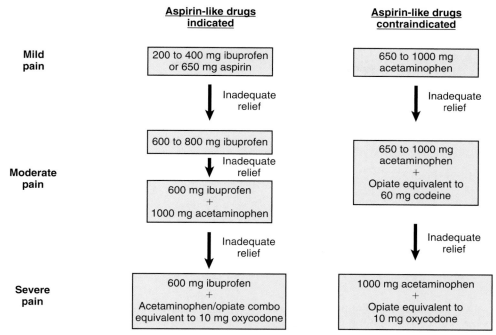

	Aspirin-like drugs indicated	**Aspirin-like drugs contraindicated**

Mild pain

200 to 400 mg ibuprofen or 650 mg aspirin

650 to 1000 mg acetaminophen

↓ Inadequate relief

↓ Inadequate relief

Moderate pain

600 to 800 mg ibuprofen

↓ Inadequate relief

600 mg ibuprofen + 1000 mg acetaminophen

650 to 1000 mg acetaminophen + Opiate equivalent to 60 mg codeine

↓ Inadequate relief

↓ Inadequate relief

Severe pain

600 mg ibuprofen + Acetaminophen/opiate combo equivalent to 10 mg oxycodone

1000 mg acetaminophen + Opiate equivalent to 10 mg oxycodone

FIG 4-25 A flexible analgesic strategy.

also significantly delay the onset of posttreatment pain compared with local anesthetics that contain lidocaine.[77,89,152,153,196] Administration of long-acting local anesthetics by block injection has been shown to reduce posttreatment pain for 2 to 7 days after the oral procedure[152,153,196] because an afferent barrage of nociceptors can induce central hyperalgesia.[445-447] The analgesic benefit of long-acting local anesthetics is more prominent with block injections than infiltration injections, but the clinician should also be aware of adverse effects attributed to these agents.[28,297]

Flexible Plan

A third pharmacologic approach is the use of a flexible plan for prescribing analgesics (Fig. 4-25).* A flexible prescription plan serves to minimize both postoperative pain and side effects. Given these goals, the clinician's strategy is twofold: (1) to achieve a maximally effective dose of the non-narcotic analgesic (either an NSAID or acetaminophen for patients who cannot take NSAIDs); and (2) in the rare cases in which the patient still has moderate to severe pain, to consider adding drugs that increase the NSAID's analgesia. Because of its predictive value, the presence of preoperative pain or mechanical allodynia may be an indicator that such NSAID combinations should be considered.

Most, but not all, studies report that combining an NSAID with acetaminophen 1000 mg alone (i.e., no opioid) produces nearly twice the analgesic response as just the NSAID.[46,74,285,434] Administration of ibuprofen 600 mg with acetaminophen 1000 mg produced significant relief of posttreatment endodontic pain compared to ibuprofen alone or placebo (Fig. 4-26). However, in a recent study, the analgesic effect of a combination of ibuprofen 600 mg with acetaminophen 1000 mg did not differ from that of acetaminophen alone.[434] Studies have also shown that concurrent administration of an NSAID and

an acetaminophen-opioid combination drug provided significantly greater analgesia than an NSAID alone.[46,403] The concurrent administration of acetaminophen and NSAIDs appears to be well tolerated, with no detectable increase in side effects or alterations in pharmacokinetics.[46,243,403,448]

In cases of moderate to severe pain, an NSAID may need to be administered with an opioid. Two general methods are used to combine NSAIDs and opioids to achieve the analgesic benefits of both. The first involves an alternating regimen of an NSAID followed by an acetaminophen-opioid combination.[17,72] Aspirin and opioid combinations are not used in this alternating schedule because of the potential for NSAID/aspirin interactions. The second method involves administration of a single drug consisting of an NSAID-opioid combination. For example, a tablet of Vicoprofen contains both ibuprofen (200 mg) and hydrocodone (7.5 mg). Postoperative pain studies have shown that this combination was about 80% more effective for analgesia than ibuprofen (200 mg) alone, with about the same incidence of side effects.[438] Other opioids can be added to an NSAID for increased analgesia. Ibuprofen 400 mg with a 10-mg oxycodone tablet produces significantly greater analgesia than ibuprofen alone.[90] A study on posttreatment endodontic pain demonstrated short-term benefits of the combination of flurbiprofen and tramadol.[97] Other NSAID and opioid combinations have also been evaluated.[93] However, the results of clinical trials on the use of NSAIDs alone and combined with acetaminophen (see Fig. 4-26) suggest that opioid combinations may be required only rarely.

Not all patients require concurrent use of NSAIDs with acetaminophen-opioid combinations or combinations of an NSAID and opioid. The basic premise of a flexible prescription plan is that the analgesic prescribed is matched to the patient's need. The major advantage of a flexible plan is that the clinician is prepared for those rare cases when additional pharmacotherapy is indicated to increase the efficacy of pain control. As mentioned, preoperative hyperalgesia may be an indicator

---

*References 17, 72, 166, 168, 171, 219, 221, and 417.

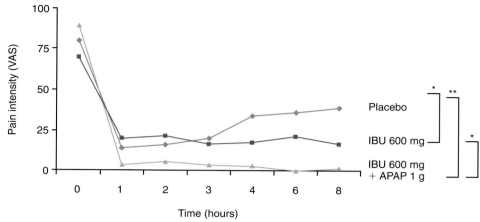

FIG. 4-26 Comparison of ibuprofen 600 mg with acetaminophen 1000 mg to ibuprofen alone or to placebo treatment in postendodontic pain patients. (From Menhinick KA, Gutmann JL, Regan JD, et al: The efficacy of pain control following nonsurgical root canal treatment using ibuprofen or a combination of ibuprofen and acetaminophen in a randomized, double-blind, placebo-controlled study, *Int Endod J* 37:531, 2004.)

for more comprehensive pharmacotherapy. When considering the combination of various analgesics, the clinician must make sure to use dosing regimens that do not exceed any of the drugs' maximum daily dosage.

FUTURE DIRECTIONS

COX-inhibiting nitric oxide (NO) donors (CINODs), a new class of NSAIDs, have an NO-donating moiety. These drugs, also known as NO-NSAIDs, were developed with the idea that the released NO would lead to improved vascular tone and mucosal blood flow, thus attenuating the adverse effects of NSAIDs on GI mucosa and blood pressure. Although none of the CINODS have been approved by the FDA yet, they may be available in the near future.

Current use of analgesics has been driven by clinical trials to arrive at doses that obtain the desired level of pain relief with acceptable side-effect profiles. After administration, drugs are absorbed and distributed to their site of action, where they interact with functional targets. They then undergo metabolism and eventual excretion. All of the steps along the way are influenced by a variety of environmental and genetic factors. The ability to predict how a patient's genome may affect the efficacy of a given analgesic drug is being discovered in the field of pain pharmacogenomics (for a review, see Rollason et al.[366]).

One example relevant to pain control in dentistry is the variable efficacy of codeine in a specific population. Many analgesic drugs are metabolized by the cytochrome P450 (CYP) family of hepatic enzymes, and the genes that encode for their biosynthesis have been identified. Codeine is a prodrug that is demethylated to produce morphine, which is responsible for its analgesic action. This demethylation is catalyzed by the enzyme cytochrome P402D6. It has been estimated that 6% to 7% of the Caucasian population has a nonfunctional CYP2D6 mutant allele, making them poor metabolizers of codeine to morphine.[88] These patients may be aware that codeine is ineffective in their systems from past experience and may request a different (usually more potent) form of narcotic. The clinician may suspect drug-seeking behavior, when in fact there is a biochemical reason for their request. Given the current state of clinical DNA analysis, it is not incomprehensible to envision a time when rapid (chairside) genomic evaluation will lead to specific recommendations for analgesic prescription.

SUMMARY

The information and recommendations provided in this chapter were selected to aid the clinician in the management of acute endodontic pain. Clinical judgment must also take into account other sources of information—the patient history, concurrent medications, the nature of the pain, and the overall treatment plan—when determining the best means of alleviating patient pain. An effective approach to managing endodontic pain demands integration of general principles of pain mechanisms and management with thorough, individualized clinical assessment.

REFERENCES

1. Abbott A, et al: A prospective randomized trial on efficacy of antibiotic prophylaxis in asymptomatic teeth with pulpal necrosis and associated periapical pathosis, *Oral Surg* 66:722, 1988.
2. Aelig W, Laurence D, O'Neil R, Verrill P: Cardiac effects of adrenaline and felypressin as vasoconstrictors in local anaesthesia for oral surgery under diazepam sedation, *Br J Anaesth* 42:174, 1970.
3. Aggarwal V, Jain A, Kabi D: Anesthetic efficacy of supplemental buccal and lingual infiltrations of articaine and lidocaine after an inferior alveolar nerve block in patients with irreversible pulpitis, *J Endod* 35:925, 2009.
4. Aggarwal V, Singla M, Kabi D: Comparative evaluation of anesthetic efficacy of Gow-Gates mandibular conduction anesthesia, Vazirani-Akinosi technique, buccal-plus-lingual infiltrations, and conventional inferior alveolar nerve anesthesia in patients with irreversible pulpitis, *Oral Surg Oral Med Oral Pathol Oral Radiol Endod* 109:303, 2010.
5. Aggarwal V, Singla M, Kabi D: Comparative evaluation of effect of preoperative oral medication of ibuprofen and ketorolac on anesthetic efficacy of inferior alveolar nerve block with lidocaine in patients with irreversible pulpitis: a prospective, double-blind, randomized trial, *J Endod* 36:375, 2010.
6. Aggarwal V, Singla M, Miglani S, et al: A prospective, randomized, single-blind comparative evaluation of anesthetic efficacy of posterior alveolar nerve blocks, buccal infiltrations, and buccal plus palatal infiltrations in patients with irreversible pulpitis, *J Endod* 37:1491, 2011.

7. Aggarwal V, Singla M, Miglani S, Kohli S: Comparative evaluation of 1.8 mL and 3.6 mL of 2% lidocaine with 1:200,000 epinephrine for inferior alveolar nerve block in patients with irreversible pulpitis: a prospective, randomized single-blind study, *J Endod* 38:753, 2012.

8. Aggarwal V, Singla M, Miglani S, Kohli S: Comparison of the anesthetic efficacy of epinephrine concentrations (1:80,000 and 1:200,000) on 2% lidocaine for inferior alveolar nerve block in patients with symptomatic irreversible pulpitis: a randomized, double-blind clinical trial, *Int Endod J* 47:373, 2014.

9. Aggarwal V, Singla M, Miglani S, et al: A prospective, randomized single-blind evaluation of effect of injection speed on anesthetic efficacy of inferior alveolar nerve block in patients with symptomatic irreversible pulpitis, *J Endod* 38:1578, 2012.

10. Aggarwal V, Singla M, Rizvi A, Miglani S: Comparative evaluation of local infiltration of articaine, articaine plus ketorolac, and dexamethasone on anesthetic efficacy of inferior alveolar nerve block with lidocaine in patients with irreversible pulpitis, *J Endod* 37:445, 2011.

11. Agren E, Danielsson K: Conduction block analgesia in the mandible: a comparative investigation of the techniques of Fischer and Gow-Gates, *Swed Dent J* 5:91, 1981.

12. Akinosi J: A new approach to the mandibular nerve block, *Br J Oral Surg* 15:83, 1977.

13. Aldous J: Needle deflection: a factor in the administration of local anesthetics, *J Am Dent Assoc* 77:602, 1968.

14. Al-Qallaf B, Das DB: Optimizing microneedle arrays to increase skin permeability for transdermal drug delivery, *Ann N Y Acad Sci* 1161:83, 2009.

15. Al-Sultan AF: Effectiveness of pH adjusted lidocaine versus commercial lidocaine for maxillary infiltration anesthesia, *Al-Rafidain Dent J* 4:34, 2004.

16. Al-Sultan AF, Fathie WK, Hamid RS: A clinical evaluation on the alkalization of local anesthetic solution in periapical surgery, *Al-Rafidain Dent J* 6:71, 2006.

17. American Association of Endodontists: *Post-endodontic pain control*, Chicago, 1995, The Association.

18. Anderson B: Paracetamol (acetaminophen): mechanisms of action, *Paediatr Anaesth* 18:915, 2008.

19. Andersson C: Local anesthesia for infants undergoing circumcision, *JAMA* 279:1170, 1998.

20. US Food and Drug Administration: New sulfite regulations, *FDA Drug Bull* 16:17, 1986.

21. Wyeth Laboratories: *Wydase lyophilized hyaluronidase 150 units [package insert]*, Philadelphia, 2004, Wyeth Laboratories.

22. Antonijevic I, Mousa S, Schafer M, Stein C: Perineurial defect and peripheral opioid analgesia in inflammation, *J Neurosci* 15:165, 1995.

23. Argueta-Figueroa L, Arzate-Sosa G, Mendieta-Zeron H: Anesthetic efficacy of articaine for inferior alveolar nerve blocks in patients with symptomatic versus asymptomatic irreversible pulpitis, *Gen Dent* 60:e39, 2012.

24. Arnold J, Salom I, Berger A: Comparison of gastrointestinal microbleeding associated with use of etodolac, ibuprofen, indomethacin, and naproxen in normal subjects, *Curr Ther Res* 37:730, 1985.

25. Asarch T, Allen K, Petersen B, Beiraghi S: Efficacy of a computerized local anesthesia device in pediatric dentistry, *Pediatr Dent* 21:421, 1999.

26. Ashraf H, Kazem M, Dianat O, Noghrehkar F: Efficacy of articaine versus lidocaine in block and infiltration anesthesia administered in teeth with irreversible pulpitis: a prospective, randomized, double-blind study, *J Endod* 39:6, 2013.

27. Atasoy UO, Alacam T: Efficacy of single buccal infiltrations for maxillary first molars in patients with irreversible pulpits: a randomized controlled trial, *Int Endod J* 47:222, 2014.

28. Bacsik C, Swift J, Hargreaves K: Toxic systemic reactions of bupivacaine and etidocaine, *Oral Surg Oral Med Oral Pathol Oral Radiol Endod* 79:18, 1995.

29. Balasco M, Drum M, Reader A, et al: Buffered lidocaine for incision and drainage: a prospective,

30. Batista da Silva C, Berto LA, Volpato MC, et al: Anesthetic efficacy of articaine and lidocaine for incisive/mental nerve block, *J Endod* 36:438, 2010.

31. Beaver W: Mild analgesics: a review of their clinical pharmacology, *Am J Med Sci* 251:576, 1966.

32. Benkwitz C, Garrison JC, Linden J, et al: Lidocaine enhances G alpha I protein function, *Anesthesiology* 99:1093, 2003.

33. Berberich G, Reader A, Drum M, et al: A prospective, randomized, double-blind comparison of the anesthetic efficacy of 2% lidocaine with 1:100,000 and 1:50,000 epinephrine and 3% mepivacaine in the intraoral, infraorbital nerve block, *J Endod* 35:1498, 2009.

34. Berlin J, Nusstein J, Reader A, et al: Efficacy of articaine and lidocaine in a primary intraligamentary injection administered with a computer-controlled local anesthetic delivery system, *Oral Surg Oral Med Oral Pathol Oral Radiol Endod* 99:361, 2005.

35. Berns J, Sadove M: Mandibular block injection: a method of study using an injected radiopaque material, *J Am Dent Assoc* 65:736, 1962.

36. Bigby J, Reader A, Nusstein J, et al: Articaine for supplemental intraosseous anesthesia in patients with irreversible pulpitis, *J Endod* 32:1044, 2006.

37. Bigby J, Reader A, Nusstein J, Beck M: Anesthetic efficacy of lidocaine/meperidine for inferior alveolar nerve blocks in patients with irreversible pulpitis, *J Endod* 33:7, 2007.

38. Birchfield J, Rosenberg PA: Role of the anesthetic solution in intrapulpal anesthesia, *J Endod* 1:26, 1975.

39. Black JA, Liu S, Tanaka M, et al: Changes in the expression of tetrodotoxin-sensitive sodium channels within dorsal root ganglia neurons in inflammatory pain, *Pain* 108:237, 2004.

40. Bombardier C, Laine L, Reicin A, et al: Comparison of upper gastrointestinal toxicity of rofecoxib and naproxen in patients with rheumatoid arthritis; VIGOR Study Group, *N Engl J Med* 343:1520, 2000.

41. Bosco DA, Haas DA, Young ER, Harrop KL: An anaphylactoid reaction following local anesthesia: a case report, *Anesth Pain Control Dent* 2:87, 1993.

42. Bowles WR, Burke R, Sabino M, et al: Sex differences in neuropeptide content and release from rat dental pulp, *J Endod* 37:1098, 2011.

43. Bowles WR, Flores CM, Jackson DL, Hargreaves KM: Beta 2-adrenoceptor regulation of CGRP release from capsaicin-sensitive neurons, *J Dent Res* 82:308, 2003.

44. Bowles WH, Frysh H, Emmons R: Clinical evaluation of buffered local anesthetic, *Gen Dent* 43:182, 1995.

45. Brannstrom M, Lindskog S, Nordenvall K: Enamel hypoplasia in permanent teeth induced by periodontal ligament anesthesia of primary teeth, *J Am Dent Assoc* 109:735, 1984.

46. Breivik E, Barkvoll P, Skovlund E: Combining diclofenac with acetaminophen or acetaminophen-codeine after oral surgery: a randomized, double-blind, single oral dose study, *Clin Pharmacol Ther* 66:625, 1999.

47. Broering R, Reader A, Drum M, et al: A prospective, randomized comparison of the anesthetic efficacy of the greater palatine and high tuberosity second division nerve blocks, *J Endod* 35:1337, 2009.

48. Brunetto PC, Ranali J, Ambrosano GMB, et al: Anesthetic efficacy of 3 volumes of lidocaine with epinephrine in maxillary infiltration anesthesia, *Anesth Prog* 55:29, 2008.

49. Bunczak-Reeh M, Hargreaves K: Effect of inflammation on delivery of drugs to dental pulp, *J Endod* 24:822, 1998.

50. Burns Y, Reader A, Nusstein J, et al: Anesthetic efficacy of the palatal-anterior superior alveolar injection, *J Am Dent Assoc* 135:1269, 2004.

51. Byers MR, Taylor PE, Khayat BG, Kimberly CL: Effects of injury and inflammation on pulpal and periapical nerves, *J Endod* 16:78, 1990.

52. Byrne B: Drug interactions: a review and update, *Endod Topics* 4:9, 2004.

53. Cannell H, Kerwala C, Webster K, Whelpton R: Are intraligamentary injections intravascular? *Br Dent J* 175:281, 1993.

54. Cairns BE, Dong XD, Wong H, Svensson P: Intramuscular ketorolac inhibits activation of rat peripheral NMDA receptors, *J Neurophysiol* 107:3308, 2012.

55. Cepeda MS, Tzortzopoulou A, Thackrey M, et al: Adjusting the pH of lidocaine for reducing pain on injection (review), *Cochrane Database Syst Rev* 8:12, 2010.

56. Certosimo A, Archer R: A clinical evaluation of the electric pulp tester as an indicator of local anesthesia, *Oper Dent* 21:25, 1996.

57. Chamberlain T, Davis R, Murchison D, et al: Systemic effects of an intraosseous injection of 2% lidocaine with 1:100,000 epinephrine, *Gen Dent* 48:299, 2000.

58. Chance K, Lin L, Shovlin F, Skribner J: Clinical trial of intracanal corticosteroid in root canal therapy, *J Endod* 13:466, 1987.

59. Chandrasekharan NV, Dai H, Roos KL, et al: COX-3, a cyclooxygenase-1 variant inhibited by acetaminophen and other analgesic/antipyretic drugs: cloning, structure, and expression [see comment], *Proc Natl Acad Sci U S A* 99:13926, 2002.

60. Chaney MA, Kerby R, Reader A, et al: An evaluation of lidocaine hydrocarbonate compared with lidocaine hydrochloride for inferior alveolar nerve block, *Anesth Prog* 38:212, 1991.

61. Childers M, Reader A, Nist R, et al: Anesthetic efficacy of the periodontal ligament injection after an inferior alveolar nerve block, *J Endod* 22:317, 1996.

62. Chiu CY, Lin TY, Hsia SH, et al: Systemic anaphylaxis following local lidocaine administration during a dental procedure, *Pediatr Emerg Care* 20:178, 2004.

63. Chng H, Pitt Ford T, McDonald F: Effects of prilocaine local anesthetic solutions on pulpal blood flow in maxillary canines, *Endod Dent Traumatol* 12:89, 1996.

64. Claffey E, Reader A, Nusstein J, et al: Anesthetic efficacy of articaine for inferior alveolar nerve blocks in patients with irreversible pulpitis, *J Endod* 30:568, 2004.

65. Clark K, Reader A, Beck M, Meyers W: Anesthetic efficacy of an infiltration injection in mandibular anterior teeth following an inferior alveolar nerve block, *Anesth Prog* 49:49, 2002.

66. Clark S, Reader A, Beck M, Meyers WJ: Anesthetic efficacy of the mylohyoid nerve block and combination inferior alveolar nerve block/mylohyoid nerve block, *Oral Surg Oral Med Oral Pathol Oral Radiol Endod* 87:557, 1999.

67. Coggins R, Reader A, Nist R, et al: Anesthetic efficacy of the intraosseous injection in maxillary and mandibular teeth, *Oral Surg Oral Med Oral Pathol Oral Radiol Endod* 81:634, 1996.

68. Cohen H, Cha B, Spangberg L: Endodontic anesthesia in mandibular molars: a clinical study, *J Endod* 19:370, 1993.

69. *Drug facts and comparisons*, St Louis, 2000, Facts and Comparisons, Inc.

70. Cooley R, Robison S: Comparative evaluation of the 30-gauge dental needle, *Oral Surg Oral Med Oral Pathol* 48:400, 1979.

71. Cooper S: New peripherally acting oral analgesics, *Ann Rev Pharmacol Toxicol* 23:617, 1983.

72. Cooper S: Treating acute dental pain, *Postgrad Dent* 2:7, 1995.

73. Cooper S, Berrie R, Cohn P: The analgesic efficacy of ketoprofen compared to ibuprofen and placebo, *Adv Ther* 5:43, 1988.

74. Cooper SA: The relative efficacy of ibuprofen in dental pain, *Compend Contin Educ Dent* 7:580, 1986.

75. Corbett IP, Kanaa MD, Whitworth JM, Meechan JG: Articaine infiltration for anesthesia of mandibular first molars, *J Endod* 34:514, 2008.

76. Cromley N, Adams D: The effect of intraligamentary injections on diseased periodontiums in dogs, *Gen Dent* 39:33, 1991.

77. Crout R, Koraido G, Moore P: A clinical trial of long-acting local anesthetics for periodontal surgery, *Anesth Prog* 37:194, 1990.

78. Crout RJ, Koraido G, Moore PA: A clinical trial of long-acting local anesthetics for periodontal surgery, *Anesth Prog* 37:194, 1990.

79. D'Souza J, Walton R, Peterson L: Periodontal ligament injection: an evaluation of extent of anesthesia and postinjection discomfort, *J Am Dent Assoc* 114:341, 1987.

80. Dagher FB, Yared GM, Machtou P: An evaluation of 2% lidocaine with different concentrations of epinephrine for inferior alveolar nerve block, *J Endod* 23:178, 1997.

81. Danielsson K, Evers H, Nordenram A: Long-acting local anesthetics in oral surgery: an experimental evaluation of bupivacaine and etidocaine for oral infiltration anesthesia, *Anesth Prog* 32:65, 1985.

82. Daublander M, Muller R, Lipp M: The incidence of complications associated with local anesthesia in dentistry, *Anesth Prog* 44:132, 1997.

83. Davidson M: Bevel-oriented mandibular injections: needle deflection can be beneficial, *Gen Dent* 37:410, 1989.

84. Davis W, Oakley J, Smith E: Comparison of the effectiveness of etidocaine and lidocaine as local anesthetic agents during oral surgery, *Anesth Prog* 31:159, 1984.

85. DeJong R: Neural blockade by local anesthetics, *J Am Dent Assoc* 238:1383, 1997.

86. Dernedde M, Furlan D, Verbesselt R, et al: Grand mal convulsion after an accidental intravenous injection of ropivacaine, *Anesth Analg* 98:521, 2004.

87. DeRosa T: A retrospective evaluation of pulpotomy as an alternative to extraction, *Gen Den* 54:37, 2006.

88. Diogenes A, Akopian AN, Hargreaves KM: NGF upregulates TRPA1: implications for orofacial pain, *J Dent Res* 86:550, 2007.

89. Dionne R: Suppression of dental pain by the preoperative administration of flurbiprofen, *Am J Med Sci* 80:41, 1986.

90. Dionne R: Additive analgesic effects of oxycodone and ibuprofen in the oral surgery model, *J Oral Maxillofac Surg* 57:673, 1999.

91. Dionne R: COX-2 inhibitors: better than ibuprofen for dental pain? *Compendium* 20:518, 1999.

92. Dionne RA: Additive analgesic effects of oxycodone and ibuprofen in the oral surgery model, *J Oral Maxillofac Surg* 57:673, 1999.

93. Dionne RA, Berthold C: Therapeutic uses of non-steroidal anti-inflammatory drugs in dentistry, *Crit Rev Oral Biol Med* 12:315, 2000.

94. Dionne RA, Lepinski AM, Gordon SM, et al: Analgesic effects of peripherally administered opioids in clinical models of acute and chronic inflammation, *Clin Pharmacol Ther* 70:66, 2001.

95. Donaldson D, James-Perdok L, Craig B, et al: A comparison of Ultracaine DS (articaine HCl) and Citanest forte (prilocaine HCl) in maxillary infiltration and mandibular nerve block, *J Can Dent Assoc* 53:38, 1987.

96. Dong XD, Svensson P, Cairns BE: The analgesic action of topical diclofenac may be mediated through peripheral NMDA receptor antagonism, *Pain* 15:36, 2009.

97. Doroshak A, Bowles W, Hargreaves K: Evaluation of the combination of flurbiprofen and tramadol for management of endodontic pain, *J Endod* 25:660, 1999.

98. Dou L, Luo J, Yang D: Anaesthetic efficacy of supplemental lingual infiltration of mandibular molars after inferior alveolar nerve block plus buccal infiltration in patients with irreversible pulpitis, *Int Endod J* 120:42, 2012.

99. Dougher MJ, Goldstein D: Induced anxiety and pain, *J Anxiety Disord* 1:259, 1987.

100. Dreven LJ, Reader A, Beck M, et al: An evaluation of an electric pulp tester as a measure of analgesia in human vital teeth, *J Endod* 13:233, 1987.

101. Dreyer WP, van Heerden JD, de V Joubert JJ: The route of periodontal ligament injection of local anesthetic solution, *J Endod* 9:471, 1983.

102. Droll B, Drum M, Nusstein J, et al: Anesthetic efficacy of the inferior alveolar nerve block in red-haired women, *J Endod* 38:1564, 2012.

103. Dunbar D, Reader A, Nist R, et al: Anesthetic efficacy of the intraosseous injection after an inferior alveolar nerve block, *J Endod* 22:481, 1996.

104. Dunsky JL, Moore PA: Long-acting local anesthetics: a comparison of bupivacaine and etidocaine in endodontics, *J Endod* 10:457, 1984.

105. Edwards R, Head T: A clinical trial of intraligamentary anesthesia, *J Dent Res* 68:1210, 1989.

106. Ehrich E, et al: Characterization of rofecoxib as a cyclooxygenase inhibitor and demonstration of analgesia in the dental pain model, *Clin Pharmacol Ther* 65:336, 1999.

107. Ehrmann EH, Messer HH, Adams GG: The relationship of intracanal medicaments to postoperative pain in endodontics, *Int Endod J* 36:868, 2003.

108. Evans G, Nusstein J, Drum M, et al: A prospective, randomized, double-blind comparison of articaine and lidocaine for maxillary infiltrations, *J Endod* 34:389, 2008.

109. Fan S, Chen WL, Pan CB, et al: Anesthetic efficacy of inferior alveolar nerve block plus buccal infiltration or periodontal ligament injections with articaine in patients with irreversible pulpitis, *Oral Surg Oral Med Oral Pathol Oral Radiol Endod* 108:89, 2009.

110. US Food and Drug Administration: MedWatch: Rofecoxib

111. Fehrenbacher J, Sun XX, Locke E, et al: Capsaicin-evoked iCGRP release from human dental pulp: a model system for the study of peripheral neuropeptide secretion in normal healthy tissue, *Pain* 144:253, 2009.

112. Fernandez C, Reader A, Beck M, Nusstein J: A prospective, randomized, double-blind comparison of bupivacaine and lidocaine for inferior alveolar nerve blocks, *J Endod* 31:499, 2005.

113. Fernieini EM, Bennett JD, Silverman DG, Halaszynski TM: Hemodynamic assessment of local anesthetic administration by laser Doppler flowmetry, *Oral Surg Oral Med Oral Pathol Oral Radiol Endod* 91:526, 2001.

114. Fillingim R, Edwards R: The relationship of sex and clinical pain to experimental pain responses, *Pain* 83:419, 1999.

115. Finder R, Moore PA: Adverse drug reactions to local anesthesia, *Dent Clin North Am* 46:747, 2002.

116. Fiset L, Leroux B, Rothen M, et al: Pain control in recovering alcoholics: effects of local anesthesia, *J Stud Alcohol* 58:291, 1997.

117. Forloine A, Drum M, Reader A, et al: A prospective, randomized, double-blind comparison of the anesthetic efficacy of two percent lidocaine with 1:100,000 epinephrine and three percent mepivacaine in the maxillary high tuberosity second division nerve block, *J Endod* 36:1770, 2010.

118. Foster W, McCartney M, Reader A, Beck M: Anesthetic efficacy of buccal and lingual infiltrations of lidocaine following an inferior alveolar nerve block in mandibular posterior teeth, *Anesth Prog* 54:163, 2007.

119. Fouad A: Are antibiotics effective for endodontic pain? An evidence-based review, *Endod Topics* 3:52, 2002.

120. Fouad A, Rivera E, Walton R: Penicillin as a supplement in resolving the localized acute apical abscess, *Oral Surg Oral Med Oral Pathol* 81:590, 1996.

121. Fowler S, Nusstein J, Drum M, et al: Reversal of soft-tissue anesthesia in asymptomatic endodontic patients: a preliminary, prospective, randomized, single-blind study, *J Endod* 37:1353, 2011.

122. Fowler S, Reader A: Is the volume of 3.6 mL better than 1.8 mL for inferior alveolar nerve blocks in patients with symptomatic irreversible pulpitis? *J Endod* 39:970, 2013.

123. Friedman M, Hochman M: A 21st century computerized injection system for local pain control, *Compendium* 18:995, 1997.

124. Friedman M, Hochman M: The AMSA injection: a new concept for local anesthesia of maxillary teeth using a computer-controlled injection system, *Quintessence Int* 29:297, 1998.

125. Friedman M, Hochman M: P-ASA block injection: a new palatal technique to anesthetize maxillary anterior teeth, *J Esthetic Dent* 11:63, 1999.

126. Friedman M, Hochman M: Using AMSA and P-ASA nerve blocks for esthetic restorative dentistry, *Gen Dent* 5:506, 2001.

127. Frommer J, Mele F, Monroe C: The possible role of the mylohyoid nerve in mandibular posterior tooth sensation, *J Am Dent Assoc* 85:113, 1972.

128. Froum SJ, Tarnow D, Caiazzo A, Hochman MN: Histologic response to intraligament injections using a computerized local anesthetic delivery system: a pilot study in mini-swine, *J Periodontol* 71:1453, 2000.

129. Fuhs QM, Walker WA III, Gough RW, et al: The periodontal ligament injection: histological effects on the periodontium in dogs, *J Endod* 9:411, 1983.

130. Fukayama H, Yoshikawa F, Kohase H, et al: Efficacy of anterior and middle superior alveolar (AMSA) anesthesia using a new injection system: the Wand, *Quintessence Int* 34:537, 2003.

131. Fullmer S, Drum M, Reader A, et al: Effect of preoperative acetaminophen/hydrocodone on the efficacy of the inferior alveolar nerve block in patients with symptomatic irreversible pulpitis: a prospective, randomized, double-blind, placebo-controlled study, *J Endod* 40:1, 2014.

132. Gaffen AS, Haas DA: Retrospective review of voluntary reports of nonsurgical paresthesia in dentistry, *J Can Dent Assoc* 75:579, 2009.

133. Gage T, Pickett F: *Mosby's dental drug reference*, ed 4, St Louis, 2000, Mosby.

134. Galbreath J: Tracing the course of the mandibular block injection, *Oral Surg Oral Med Oral Pathol* 30:571, 1970.

135. Galili D, Kaufman E, Garfunkel AA, Michaeli Y: Intraligamental anesthesia: a histological study, *Int J Oral Surg* 13:511, 1984.

136. Gallatin E, Reader A, Nist R, Beck M: Pain reduction in untreated irreversible pulpitis using an intraosseous injection of Depo-Medrol, *J Endod* 26:633, 2000.

137. Gallatin E, Stabile P, Reader A, et al: Anesthetic efficacy and heart rate effects of the intraosseous injection of 3% mepivacaine after an inferior alveolar nerve block, *Oral Surg Oral Med Oral Pathol Oral Radiol Endod* 89:83, 2000.

138. Gallatin J, Nusstein J, Reader A, et al: A comparison of injection pain and postoperative pain of two intraosseous anesthetic techniques, *Anesth Prog* 50:111, 2003.

139. Gallatin J, Reader A, Nusstein J, et al: A comparison of two intraosseous anesthetic techniques in mandibular posterior teeth, *J Am Dent Assoc* 134:1476, 2003.

140. Garisto GA, Gaffen AS, Lawrence HP, et al: Occurrence of paresthesia after dental local anesthetic administration in the United States, *J Am Dent Assoc* 141:836, 2010.

141. Garry MG, Jackson DL, Geier HE, et al: Evaluation of the efficacy of a bioerodible bupivacaine polymer system on antinociception and inflammatory mediator release, *Pain* 82:49, 1999.

142. Gear R, et al: Kappa-opioids produce significantly greater analgesia in women than in men, *Nat Med* 2:1248, 1996.

143. Geborek P, Mansson B, Wollheim FA, Moritz U: Intraarticular corticosteroid injection into rheumatoid arthritis knees improves extensor muscles strength, *Rheum Int* 9:265, 1990.

144. Gerner P, Binshtok AM, Wang CF, et al: Capsaicin combined with local anesthetics preferentially prolongs sensory/nociceptive block in rat sciatic nerve, *Anesthesiology* 109:872, 2008.

145. Gibson RS, Allen K, Hutfless S, Beiraghi S: The Wand vs traditional injection: a comparison of pain related behaviors, *Pediatr Dent* 22:458, 2000.

146. Gill C, Orr D: A double-blind crossover comparison of topical anesthetics, *J Am Dent Assoc* 98:213, 1979.

147. Glassman G, Krasner P, Morse DR, et al: A prospective randomized double-blind trial on efficacy of dexamethasone for endodontic interappointment pain in teeth with asymptomatic inflamed pulps, *Oral Surg Oral Med Oral Pathol* 67:96, 1989.

148. Gold M, Reichling D, Shuster M, Levine J: Hyperalgesic agents increase a tetrodotoxin-resistant Na+-current in nociceptors, *Proc Natl Acad Sci U S A* 93:1108, 1996.

149. Goldberg S, Reader A, Drum M, et al: A comparison of the anesthetic efficacy of the conventional inferior alveolar, Gow-Gates and Vazirani-Akinosi techniques, *J Endod* 34:1306, 2008.

150. Goldstein DS, Dionne R, Sweet J, et al: Circulatory, plasma catecholamine, cortisol, lipid, and psychological responses to a real-life stress (third molar extractions): effects of diazepam sedation and of inclusion of epinephrine with the local anesthetic, *Psychosom Med* 44:259, 1982.

151. Goodman A, Reader A, Nusstein J, et al: Anesthetic efficacy of lidocaine/meperidine for inferior alveolar nerve blocks, *Anesth Prog* 53:131, 2006.

152. Gordon SM: Blockade of peripheral neuronal barrage reduces postoperative pain, *Pain* 306:264, 1997.

153. Gordon SM, Brahim JS, Dubner R, et al: Attenuation of pain in a randomized trial by suppression of peripheral nociceptive activity in the immediate postoperative period, *Anesth Analg* 95:1351, 2002.

154. Gow-Gates G: Mandibular conduction anesthesia: a new technique using extra-oral landmarks, *Oral Surg Oral Med Oral Pathol* 36:321, 1973.

155. Gray R, Lomax A, Rood J: Periodontal ligament injection: with or without a vasoconstrictor? *Br Dent J* 162:263, 1987.

156. Gross R, McCartney M, Reader A, Beck M: A prospective, randomized, double-blind comparison of bupivacaine and lidocaine for maxillary infiltrations, *J Endod* 33:1021, 2007.

157. Guglielmo A, Drum M, Reader A, Nusstein J: Anesthetic efficacy of a combination palatal and buccal infiltration of the maxillary first molar, *J Endod* 37:460, 2011.

158. Guglielmo A, Reader A, Nist R, et al: Anesthetic efficacy and heart rate effects of the supplemental intraosseous injection of 2% mepivacaine with 1:20,000 levonordefrin, *Oral Surg Oral Med Oral Pathol Oral Radiol Endod* 87:284, 1999.

159. Haas D, Harper D, Saso M, Young E: Comparison of articaine and prilocaine anesthesia by infiltration in maxillary and mandibular arches, *Anesth Prog* 37:230, 1990.

160. Haas D, Harper D, Saso M, Young E: Lack of differential effect by Ultracaine (articaine) and Citanest (prilocaine) in infiltration anaesthesia, *J Can Dent Assoc* 57:217, 1991.

161. Haas DA, Lennon D: A 21 year retrospective study of reports of paresthesia following local anesthetic administration, *J Can Dent Assoc* 61:319, 1995.

162. Haas DA, Pynn BR, Sands TD: Drug use for the pregnant or lactating patient, *Gen Dent* 48:54, 2000.

163. Haase A, Reader A, Nusstein J, et al: Comparing anesthetic efficacy of articaine versus lidocaine as a supplemental buccal infiltration of the mandibular first molar after an inferior alveolar nerve block, *J Am Dent Assoc* 139:1228, 2008.

164. Hanna MN, Elhassan A, Veloso PM, et al: Efficacy of bicarbonate in decreasing pain on intradermal injection of local anesthetics: a meta analysis, *Reg Anesth Pain Med* 34:122, 2009.

165. Hannan L, Reader A, Nist R, et al: The use of ultrasound for guiding needle placement for inferior alveolar nerve blocks, *Oral Surg Oral Med Oral Pathol Oral Radiol Endod* 87:658, 1999.

166. Hargreaves K: Neurochemical factors in injury and inflammation in orofacial tissues. In Lund JP, Lavigne GJ, Dubner R, Sessle BJ, editors: *Orofacial pain: basic sciences to clinical management*, Chicago, 2000, Quintessence.

167. Hargreaves K, Joris J: The peripheral analgesic effects of opioids, *J Am Pain Soc* 2:51, 1993.

168. Hargreaves K, Troullos E, Dionne R: Pharmacologic rationale for the treatment of acute pain, *Dent Clin North Am* 31:675, 1987.

169. Hargreaves KM, Jackson DL, Bowles WR: Adrenergic regulation of capsaicin-sensitive neurons in dental pulp, *J Endod* 29:397, 2003.

170. Hargreaves KM, Keiser K: Local anesthetic failure in endodontics: mechanisms and management, *Endod Topics* 1:26, 2003.

171. Hargreaves KM, Keiser K: New advances in the management of endodontic pain emergencies, *J Calif Dental Assoc* 32:469, 2004.

172. Hasse AL, Heng MK, Garrett NR: Blood pressure and electrocardiographic response to dental treatment with use of local anesthesia, *J Am Dent Assoc* 113:639, 1986.

173. Hasselgren G, Reit C: Emergency pulpotomy: pain relieving effect with and without the use of sedative dressings, *J Endod* 15:254, 1989.

174. Henry MA, Hargreaves KM: Peripheral mechanisms of odontogenic pain, *Dent Clin North Am* 51:19, 2007.

175. Hersh E, Houpt M, Cooper S, et al: Analgesic efficacy and safety of an intraoral lidocaine patch, *J Am Dent Assoc* 127:1626, 1996.

176. Hersh E, Moore P, Papas A, et al: Reversal of soft-tissue local anesthesia with phentolamine mesylate in adolescents and adults, *J Am Dent Assoc* 139:1080, 2008.

177. Hersh EV, Lally ET, Moore PA: Update on cyclooxygenase inhibitors: Has a third COX isoform entered the fray? *Curr Med Res Opin* 21:1217, 2005.

178. Hidding J, Khoury F: General complications in dental local anesthesia, *Dtsch Zahnarztl Z* 46:831, 1991.

179. Hinkley SA, Reader A, Beck M, Meyers WJ: An evaluation of 4% prilocaine with 1:200,000 epinephrine and 2% mepivacaine with 1:20,000 levonordefrin compared with 2% lidocaine with 1:100,000 epinephrine for inferior alveolar nerve block, *Anesth Prog* 38:84, 1991.

180. Hobeich P, Simon S, Schneiderman E, He J: A prospective, randomized, double-blind comparison of the injection pain and anesthetic onset of 2% lidocaine with 1:100,000 epinephrine buffered with 5% and 10% sodium bicarbonate in maxillary infiltrations, *J Endod* 39:597, 2013.

181. Hochman M, Chiarello D, Hochman CB, et al: Computerized local anesthetic delivery vs traditional syringe technique: subjective pain response, *NY State Dent J* 63:24, 1997.

182. Hochman M, Friedman M: In vitro study of needle deflection: a linear insertion technique versus a bidirectional rotation insertion technique, *Quintessence Int* 31:33, 2000.

183. Hollmann MW, Herroeder S, Kurz KS, et al: Time-dependent inhibition of G protein-coupled receptor signaling by local anesthetics, *Anesthesiology* 100:852, 2004.

184. Holstein A, Hargreaves KM, Niederman R: Evaluation of NSAIDs for treating post-endodontic pain, *Endod Topics* 3:3, 2002.

185. Hull T, Rothwell B: Intraosseous anesthesia comparing lidocaine and etidocaine (abstract), *J Dent Res* 77:197, 1998.

186. Hutchins H, Young F, Lackland D, Fishburne C: The effectiveness of topical anesthesia and vibration in alleviating the pain of oral injections, *Anesth Prog* 44:87, 1997.

187. Ianiro SR, Jeansonne JB, McNeal SF, Eleazer PD: The effect of preoperative acetaminophen or a combination of acetaminophen and ibuprofen on the success of the inferior alveolar nerve block for teeth with irreversible pulpitis, *J Endod* 33:11, 2007.

188. Idris M, Sakkir N, Naik KG, Jayaram NK: Intraosseous injection as an adjunct to conventional local anesthetic techniques: a clinical study, *J Conserv Dent* 17:432, 2014.

189. Ingle J, Bakland L: *Endodontics*, vol 5, Hamilton, Ontario, 2002, Decker.

190. Jaber A, Whitworth JM, Corbett IP, et al: The efficacy of infiltration anaesthesia for adult mandibular incisors: a randomized double-blind cross-over trial comparing articaine and lidocaine buccal and buccal plus lingual infiltrations, *Br Dent J* 209:E16, 2010.

191. Jackson D, Moore P, Hargreaves K: Preoperative nonsteroidal anti-inflammatory medication for the prevention of postoperative dental pain, *J Am Dent Assoc* 119:641, 1989.

192. Jage J: Circulatory effects of vasoconstrictors combined with local anesthetics, *Anesth Pain Control Dent* 2:81, 1993.

193. Jakobs W, Ladwig B, Cichon P, et al: Serum levels of articaine 2% and 4% in children, *Anesth Prog* 42:113, 1995.

194. Jalalzadeh SM, Mamavi A, Shahriari S, et al: Effect of pretreatment prednisolone on postendodontic pain: a double-blind parallel-randomized clinical trial, *J Endod* 36:978, 2010.

195. Jastak J, Yagiela J: *Local anesthesia of the oral cavity*, New York, 1995, Elsevier Health Science.

196. Jebeles JA, Reilly JS, Gutierrez JF, et al: Tonsillectomy and adenoidectomy pain reduction by local bupivacaine infiltration in children, *Int J Pediatr Otorhinolaryngol* 25:149, 1993.

197. Jena A, Shashirekha G: Effect of preoperative medications on the efficacy of inferior alveolar nerve block in patients with irreversible pulpitis: a placebo-controlled study, *J Conserv Dent* 16:171, 2013.

198. Jensen J, Nusstein J, Drum M, et al: Anesthetic efficacy of a repeated intraosseous injection following a primary intraosseous injection, *J Endod* 34:126, 2008.

199. Jeske A, Boschart B: Deflection of conventional versus nondeflecting dental needles in vitro, *Anesth Prog* 32:62, 1985.

200. Johnson G, Hlava G, Kalkwarf K: A comparison of periodontal intraligamental anesthesia using etidocaine HCL and lidocaine HCL, *Anesth Prog* 32:202, 1985.

201. Jones VR, Rivera EM, Walton RE: Comparison of carbon dioxide versus refrigerant spray to determine pulpal responsiveness, *J Endod* 28:531, 2002.

202. Joyce AP, Donnelly JC: Evaluation of the effectiveness and comfort of incisive nerve anesthesia given inside or outside the mental foramen, *J Endod* 19:409, 1993.

203. Jung IY, Kim JH, Kim ES, et al: An evaluation of buccal infiltrations and inferior alveolar nerve blocks in pulpal anesthesia for mandibular first molars, *J Endod* 34:11, 2008.

204. Kanaa MD, Meechan JG, Corbett IP, Whitworth JM: Speed of injection influences efficacy of inferior alveolar nerve blocks: a double-blind randomized controlled trial in volunteers, *J Endod* 32:919, 2006.

205. Kanaa MD, Whitworth JM, Corbett IP, Meechan JG: Articaine and lidocaine mandibular buccal infiltration anesthesia; a prospective randomized double-blind cross-over study, *J Endod* 32:296, 2006.

206. Kanaa MD, Whitworth JM, Corbett IP, Meechan JG: Articaine buccal infiltration enhances the effectiveness of lidocaine inferior alveolar nerve block, *Int Endod J* 42:238, 2009.

207. Kanaa MD, Whitworth JM, Meechan JG: A comparison of the efficacy of 4% articaine with 1:100,000 epinephrine and 2% lidocaine with 1:80,000 epinephrine in achieving pulpal anesthesia in maxillary teeth with irreversible pulpitis, *J Endod* 38:279, 2012.

208. Kanaa MD, Whitworth JM, Meechan JG: A prospective trial of different supplementary local anesthetic techniques after failure of inferior alveolar nerve block in patients with irreversible pulpitis in mandibular teeth, *J Endod* 38:421, 2012.

209. Karkut B, Reader A, Drum M, et al: A comparison of the local anesthetic efficacy of the extraoral versus the intraoral infraorbital nerve block, *J Am Dent Assoc* 141:185, 2010.

210. Kashyap VM, Desai R, Reddy PB, Menon S: Effect of alkalinisation of lignocaine for intraoral nerve block on

pain during injection, and speed of onset of anaesthesia, *Br J Oral Maxillofac Surg* 49:e72, 2011.

211. Katz S, Drum M, Reader A, et al: A prospective, randomized, double-blind comparison of 2% lidocaine with 1:100,000 epinephrine, 4% prilocaine with 1:200,000 epinephrine and 4% prilocaine for maxillary infiltrations, *Anesth Prog* 57:45, 2010.

212. Kaufman E, Galili D, Garfunkel A: Intraligamentary anesthesia: a clinical study, *J Pros Dent* 49:337, 1983.

213. Kaufman E, Solomon V, Rozen L, Peltz R: Pulpal efficacy of four lidocaine solutions injected with an intraligamentary syringe, *Oral Surg Oral Med Oral Pathol Oral Radiol Endod* 78:17, 1994.

214. Kaufman E, Weinstein P, Milgrom P: Difficulties in achieving local anesthesia, *J Am Dent Assoc* 108:205, 1984.

215. Kaufman E, et al: Intraligamentary injection of slow-release methylprednisolone for the prevention of pain after endodontic treatment, *Oral Surg Oral Med Oral Pathol* 77:651, 1994.

216. Kaviani N, Khademi A, Ebtehaj I, Mohammadi Z: The effect of orally administered ketamine on requirement for anesthetics and postoperative pain in mandibular molar teeth with irreversible pulpitis, *J Oral Sci* 53:461, 2011.

217. Kearney PM, Baigent C, Godwin J, et al: Do selective cyclo-oxygenase-2 inhibitors and traditional non-steroidal anti-inflammatory drugs increase the risk of atherothrombosis? Meta-analysis of randomised trials [see comment], *Br Med J* 332:1302, 2006.

218. Keenan JV, Farman A, Fedorowicz Z, Newton JT: A Cochrane systematic review finds no evidence to support the use of antibiotics for pain relief in irreversible pulpitis, *J Endod* 32:87, 2006.

219. Keiser K: Strategies for managing the endodontic pain patient, *Texas Dent J* 120:250, 2003.

220. Keiser K, Hargreaves K: Building effective strategies for the management of endodontic pain, *Endod Topics* 3:93, 2002.

221. Keiser K, Hargreaves KM: Strategies for managing the endodontic pain patient, *J Tenn Dent Assoc* 83:24, 2003.

222. Keller B: Comparison of the effectiveness of two topical anesthetics and a placebo in reducing injection pain, *Hawaii Dent J* 16:10, 1985.

223. Kennedy M, Reader A, Beck M, Weaver J: Anesthetic efficacy of ropivacaine in maxillary anterior infiltration, *Oral Surg Oral Med Oral Pathol Oral Radiol Endod* 91:406, 2001.

224. Kennedy S, Reader A, Nusstein J, et al: The significance of needle deflection in success of the inferior alveolar nerve block in patients with irreversible pulpitis, *J Endod* 29:630, 2003.

225. Kerckhove N, Mallet C, François A, et al: Cav3.2 calcium channels: the key protagonist in the supraspinal effect of paracetamol, *Pain* 155:764, 2014.

226. Khademi AA, Saatchi M, Minaiyan M, et al: Effect of preoperative alprazolam on the success of inferior alveolar nerve block for teeth with irreversible pulpitis, *J Endod* 38:1337, 2012.

227. Khan AA, Dionne RA: The COX-2 inhibitors: new analgesic and anti-inflammatory drugs, *Dent Clin North Am* 46:679, 2002.

228. Kim S: Ligamental injection: a physiological explanation of its efficacy, *J Endod* 12:486, 1986.

229. Kindler CH, Paul M, Zou H, et al: Amide local anesthetics potently inhibit the human tandem pore domain background K+ channel TASK-2 (KCNK5), *J Pharmacol Exp Ther* 306:84, 2003.

230. Kirby C, Eckenhoff J, Looby J: The use of hyaluronidase with local anesthetic agents in nerve block and infiltration anesthesia, *Surgery* 25:101, 1949.

231. Kis B, Snipes A, Bari F, Busija DW: Regional distribution of cyclooxygenase-3 mRNA in the rat central nervous system, *Brain Res Mol Brain Res* 126:78, 2004.

232. Kissin I: Vanilloid-induced conduction analgesia: selective, dose-dependent, long-lasting, with a low level of potential neurotoxicity, *Anesth Analg* 107:271, 2008.

233. Klein SM, Pierce T, Rubin Y, et al: Successful resuscitation after ropivacaine-induced ventricular fibrillation, *Anesth Analg* 97:901, 2003 [erratum appears in *Anesth Analg* 98:200, 2004].

234. Kleinknecht R, Klepac R, Alexander L: Origins and characteristics of fear of dentistry, *J Am Dent Assoc* 86:842, 1993.

235. Knoll-Kohler E, Frie A, Becker J, Ohlendorf D: Changes in plasma epinephrine concentration after dental infiltration anesthesia with different doses of epinephrine, *J Dent Res* 68:1098, 1989.

236. Knoll-Kohler E, Knoller M, Brandt K, Becker J: Cardiohemodynamic and serum catecholamine response to surgical removal of impacted mandibular third molars under local anesthesia: a randomized double-blind parallel group and crossover study, *J Oral Maxillofac Surg* 49:957, 1991.

237. Knotkova H, Pappagallo M, Szallasi A: Capsaicin (TRPV1 agonist) therapy for pain relief: farewell or revival? *Clin J Pain* 24:142, 2008.

238. Krasner P, Jackson E: Management of posttreatment endodontic pain with oral dexamethasone: a double-blind study, *Oral Surg Oral Med Oral Pathol* 62:187, 1986.

239. Kreimer T, Kiser R II, Reader A, et al: Anesthetic efficacy of combinations of 0.5 mol/L mannitol and lidocaine with epinephrine for inferior alveolar nerve blocks in patients with symptomatic irreversible pulpitis, *J Endod* 38:598, 2012.

240. Krupinski J, Krupinska A: Dental pulp analgesia before its amputation or removal, *Czas Stomatol* 29:383, 1976.

241. Lai J, Porreca J, Hunter J, Gold M: Voltage-gated sodium channels and hyperalgesia, *Ann Rev Pharmacol* 44:371, 2004.

242. Laine L, Bombardier C, Hawkey CJ, et al: Stratifying the risk of NSAID-related upper gastrointestinal clinical events: results of a double-blind outcomes study in patients with rheumatoid arthritis, *Gastroenterology* 123:1006, 2002.

243. Lanza F, et al: Effect of acetaminophen on human gastric mucosal injury caused by ibuprofen, *Gut* 27:440, 1986.

244. Larson AM, Polson J, Fontana RJ, et al: Acute liver failure study G: Acetaminophen-induced acute liver failure: results of a United States multicenter, prospective study [see comment], *Hepatology* 42:1364, 2005.

245. Laviola M, McGavin S, Freer G, et al: Randomized study of phentolamine mesylate for reversal of local anesthesia, *J Dent Res* 87:635, 2008.

246. Lawaty I, Drum M, Reader A, Nusstein J: A prospective, randomized, double-blind comparison of 2% mepivacaine with 1:20,000 levonordefrin versus 2% lidocaine with 1:100,000 epinephrine for maxillary infiltrations, *Anesth Prog* 57:139, 2010.

247. Lee S, Reader A, Nusstein J, et al: Anesthetic efficacy of the anterior middle superior alveolar (AMSA) injection, *Anesth Prog* 51:80, 2004.

248. Li C, Yang X, Ma X, et al: Preoperative oral nonsteroidal anti-inflammatory drugs for the success of the inferior alveolar nerve block in irreversible pulpitis treatment: a systematic review and meta-analysis based on randomized controlled trials, *Quintessence Int* 43:209, 2012.

249. Liddell A, Locker D: Gender and age differences in attitudes to dental pain and dental control, *Community Dent Oral Epidemiol* 25:314, 1997.

250. Liesinger A, Marshall F, Marshall J: Effect of variable doses of dexamethasone on posttreatment endodontic pain, *J Endod* 19:35, 1993.

251. Lin L, et al: Periodontal ligament injection: effects on pulp tissue, *J Endod* 11:529, 1985.

252. Lin S, Levin L, Emodi O, et al: Etodolac versus dexamethasone effect in reduction of postoperative symptoms following surgical endodontic treatment: a double-blind study, *Oral Surg Oral Med Oral Pathol Oral Radiol Endod* 101:814, 2006.

253. Lindemann MRA, Nusstein J, Drum M, Beck M: Effect of sublingual triazolam on the efficacy of the inferior alveolar nerve block in patients with irreversible pulpitis, *J Endod* 34:1167, 2008.

254. Linden E, Abrams H, Matheny J, et al: A comparison of postoperative pain experience following periodontal surgery using two local anesthetic agents, *J Periodontol* 57:637, 1986.

255. List G, et al: Gingival crevicular fluid response to various solutions using the intraligamentary injection, *Quint Int* 19:559, 1988.

256. Littner MM, Tamse A, Kaffe I: A new technique of selective anesthesia for diagnosing acute pulpitis in the mandible, *J Endod* 9:116, 1983.

257. Loetscher C, Melton D, Walton R: Injection regimen for anesthesia of the maxillary first molar, *J Am Dent Assoc* 117:337, 1988.

258. Looby J, Kirby C: Use of hyaluronidase with local anesthetic agents in dentistry, *J Am Dent Assoc* 38:1, 1949.

259. Malamed S: The Gow-Gates mandibular block: evaluation after 4,275 cases, *Oral Surg Oral Med Oral Pathol* 51:463, 1981.

260. Malamed S: The periodontal ligament (PDL) injection: an alternative to inferior alveolar nerve block, *Oral Surg Oral Med Oral Pathol* 53:117, 1982.

261. Malamed S: Articaine versus lidocaine: the author responds, *Calif Dent J* 35:383, 2007.

262. Malamed S: *Handbook of local anesthesia*, ed 6, St Louis, 2012, Mosby/Elsevier.

263. Malamed S, Gagnon S, Leblanc D: A comparison between articaine HCl and lidocaine HCl in pediatric dental patients. *Pediatr Dent* 22:307, 2000.

264. Malamed S, Gagnon S, Leblanc D: Efficacy of articaine: a new amide local anesthetic, *J Am Dent Assoc* 131:635, 2000.

265. Malamed SF, Gagnon S, Leblanc D: Articaine hydrochloride: a study of the safety of a new amide local anesthetic, *J Am Dent Assoc* 132:177, 2001.

266. Malamed SF, Tavana S, Falkel M: Faster onset and more comfortable injection with alkalinized 2% lidocaine with epinephrine 1:100,000, *Compend Suppl* 34:10, 2013.

267. Malmberg A, Yaksh T: Antinociceptive actions of spinal nonsteroidal anti-inflammatory agents on the formalin test in rats, *J Pharmacol Exp Ther* 263:136, 1992.

268. Marshall G: Consideration of steroids for endodontic pain, *Endod Topics* 3:41, 2002.

269. Marshall J, Walton R: The effect of intramuscular injection of steroid on posttreatment endodontic pain, *J Endod* 10:584, 1984.

270. Martin M, Ramsay D, Whitney C, et al: Topical anesthesia: differentiating the pharmacological and psychological contributions to efficacy, *Anesth Prog* 41:40, 1994.

271. Martinez G, Benito P, Fernandez C, et al: A comparative study of direct mandibular nerve block and the Akinosi technique, *Med Oral* 8:143, 2003.

272. Mason R, Drum M, Reader A, et al: A prospective, randomized, double-blind comparison of 2% lidocaine with 1:100,000 and 1:50,000 epinephrine and 3% mepivacaine for maxillary infiltrations. *J Endod* 35:1173, 2009.

273. Matthews R, Drum M, Reader A, et al: Articaine for supplemental buccal mandibular infiltration anesthesia in patients with irreversible pulpitis when the inferior alveolar nerve block fails, *J Endod* 35:343, 2009.

274. McDougal RA, Delano EO, Caplan D, Sigurdsson A: Success of an alternative for interim management of irreversible pulpitis, *J Am Dent Assoc* 135:1707, 2004.

275. McEntire M, Nusstein J, Drum M, et al: Anesthetic efficacy of 4% articaine with 1:100,000 epinephrine versus 4% articaine with 1:200,000 epinephrine as a primary buccal infiltration in the mandibular first molar, *J Endod* 37:450, 2011.

276. McGettigan P, Henry D: Cardiovascular risk and inhibition of cyclooxygenase: a systematic review of the observational studies of selective and nonselective inhibitors of cyclooxygenase 2 [see comment], *JAMA* 296:1633, 2006.

277. McLean C, Reader A, Beck M, Meyers WJ: An evaluation of 4% prilocaine and 3% mepivacaine compared with 2% lidocaine (1:100,000 epinephrine) for inferior alveolar nerve block, *J Endod* 19:146, 1993.

278. Meechan J: A comparison of ropivacaine and lidocaine with epinephrine for intraligamentary anesthesia, *Oral Surg Oral Med Oral Pathol Oral Radiol Endod* 93:469, 2002.

279. Meechan J, Blair G: The effect of two different local anaesthetic solutions on pain experience following apicoectomy, *Br Dent J* 175:410, 1993.

280. Meechan J, Ledvinka J: Pulpal anesthesia for mandibular central incisor teeth: a comparison of infiltration and intraligamentary injections, *Int Endod J* 35:629, 2002.

281. Meechan JG, Kanaa MD, Corbett IP, et al: Pulpal anesthesia for permanent first molar teeth: a double-blind randomized cross-over trial comparing buccal and buccal plus lingual infiltration injections in volunteers, *Int Endod J* 39:764, 2006.

282. Meechan JG, Rawlins MD: The effects of two different dental local anesthetic solutions on plasma potassium levels during third molar surgery, *Oral Surg Oral Med Oral Pathol* 66:650, 1988.

283. Mehrvarzfar P, Shababi B, Sayyad R, et al: Effect of supraperiosteal injection of dexamethasone on postoperative pain, *Aust Endod J* 34:25, 2008.

284. Mellor AC, Dorman ML, Girdler NM: The use of an intra-oral injection of ketorolac in the treatment of irreversible pulpitis, *Int Endod J* 38:789, 2005.

285. Menhinick K, Gutmann J, Regan J, et al: The efficacy of pain control following nonsurgical root canal treatment using ibuprofen or a combination of ibuprofen and acetaminophen in a randomized, double-blind, placebo-controlled study, *Int Endod J* 37:531, 2003.

286. Meyer R, Jakubowski W: Use of tripelennamine and diphenhydramine as local anesthetics, *J Am Dent Assoc* 69:112, 1964.

287. Mikesell A, Drum M, Reader A, Beck M: Anesthetic efficacy of 1.8 mL and 3.6 mL of 2% lidocaine with 1:100,000 epinephrine for maxillary infiltrations, *J Endod* 34:121, 2008.

288. Mikesell P, Nusstein J, Reader A, et al: A comparison of articaine and lidocaine for inferior alveolar nerve blocks, *J Endod* 31:265, 2005.

289. Milgrom P, Coldwell S, Getz T, et al: Four dimensions of fear of dental injections, *J Am Dent Assoc* 128:756, 1997.

290. Milgrom P, Fiset L, Melnick S, Weinstein P: The prevalence and practice management consequences of dental fear in a major US city, *J Am Dent Assoc* 116:61, 1988.

291. Modaresi J, Dianat O, Mozayeni MA: The efficacy comparison of ibuprofen, acetaminophen-codeine, and placebo premedication therapy on the depth of anesthesia during treatment of inflamed teeth, *Oral Surg Oral Med Oral Pathol* 102:399, 2006.

292. Modaresi J, Dianat O, Soluti A: Effect of pulp inflammation on nerve impulse quality with or without anesthesia, *J Endod* 34:438, 2008.

293. Moller R, Covine B: Cardiac electrophysiologic effects of articaine compared with bupivacaine and lidocaine, *Anesth Analg* 76:1266, 1993.

294. Montagnese TA, Reader A, Melfi R: A comparative study of the Gow-Gates technique and a standard technique for mandibular anesthesia, *J Endod* 10:158, 1984.

295. Monterio MR, Groppo FC, Haiter-Neto F, et al: Four percent articaine buccal infiltration versus 2% lidocaine inferior alveolar nerve block for emergency root canal treatment in mandibular molars with irreversible pulpitis: a randomized clinical study, *Int Endod J* 48:145, 2014.

296. Moore KD, Reader A, Meyers WJ: A comparison of the periodontal ligament injection using 2% lidocaine with 1:100,000 epinephrine and saline in human mandibular premolars, *Anesth Prog* 34:181, 1987.

297. Moore P: Long-acting local anesthetics: a review of clinical efficacy in dentistry, *Compendium* 11:24, 1990.

298. Moore P, et al: Analgesic regimens for third molar surgery: pharmacologic and behavioral considerations, *J Am Dent Assoc* 113:739, 1986.

299. Moore PA, Boynes SG, Hersh EV, et al: Dental anesthesia using 4% articaine 1:200,000 epinephrine: two clinical trials, *J Am Dent Assoc* 137:1572, 2006.

300. Moore PA, Dunsky JL: Bupivacaine anesthesia: a clinical trial for endodontic therapy, *Oral Surg Oral Med Oral Pathol* 55:176, 1983.

301. Moore TJ, Walsh CS, Cohen MR: Reported adverse event cases of methemoglobinemia associated with benzocaine products, *Arch Intern Med* 164:1192, 2004.

302. Morais-Almeida M, Gaspar A, Marinho S, Rosado-Pinto J: Allergy to local anesthetics of the amide group with tolerance to procaine, *Allergy* 58:827, 2003.

303. Morin C, Lund JP, Villarroel T, et al: Differences between the sexes in post-surgical pain, *Pain* 85:79, 2000.

304. Morse D, et al: Infectious flare-ups and serious sequelae following endodontic treatment: a prospective randomized trial on efficacy of antibiotic prophylaxis in cases of asymptomatic pulpal-periapical lesions, *Oral Surg Oral Med Oral Pathol* 64:96, 1987.

305. Morse D, et al: Prophylactic penicillin versus erythromycin taken at the first sign of swelling in cases of asymptomatic pulpal-periapical lesions: a comparative analysis, *Oral Surg Oral Med Oral Pathol* 65:228, 1988.

306. Morse D, et al: A comparison of erythromycin and cefadroxil in the prevention of flare-ups from asymptomatic teeth with pulpal necrosis and associated periapical pathosis, *Oral Surg Oral Med Oral Pathol* 69:619, 1990.

307. Moskow A, et al: Intracanal use of a corticosteroid solution as an endodontic anodyne, *Oral Surg Oral Med Oral Pathol* 58:600, 1984.

308. Naftalin L, Yagiela J: Vasoconstrictors: indications and precautions, *Dent Clin North Am* 46:733, 2002.

309. Nagle D, Reader A, Beck M, Weaver J: Effect of systemic penicillin on pain in untreated irreversible pulpitis, *Oral Surg Oral Med Oral Pathol Oral Radiol Endod* 90:636, 2000.

310. Nakanishi T, Shimuzu H, Matsuo T: Immunohistochemical analysis of cyclooxygenase-2 in human dental pulp (abstract), *J Dent Res* 78:142, 1999.

311. Nelson P: Letter to the editor, *J Am Dent Assoc* 103:692, 1981.

312. Nicholson JW, Berry TG, Summitt JB, et al: Pain perception and utility: a comparison of the syringe and computerized local injection techniques, *Gen Dent* 49:167, 2001.

313. Nist RA, Reader A, Beck M, Meyers WJ: An evaluation of the incisive nerve block and combination inferior alveolar and incisive nerve blocks in mandibular anesthesia, *J Endod* 18:455, 1992.

314. Niv D: Intraoperative treatment of postoperative pain. In Campbell JN, editor: *Pain 1996: an updated review*, Seattle, 1996, IASP Press.

315. Nobuhara WK, Carnes DL, Gilles JA: Anti-inflammatory effects of dexamethasone on periapical tissues following endodontic overinstrumentation, *J Endod* 19:501, 1993.

316. Noguera-Gonzalez D, Cerda-Cristerna B, Chavarria-Bolanos D, et al: Efficacy of preoperative ibuprofen on the success of inferior alveolar nerve block in patients with symptomatic irreversible pulpitis: a randomized controlled clinical trial, *Int Endo J* 46:56, 2013.

317. Nusstein J, Berlin J, Reader A, et al: Comparison of injection pain, heart rate increase and post-injection pain of articaine and lidocaine in a primary intraligamentary injection administered with a computer-controlled local anesthetic delivery system, *Anesth Prog* 51:126, 2004.

318. Nusstein J, Burns Y, Reader A, et al: Injection pain and postinjection pain of the palatal-anterior superior alveolar injection, administered with the Wand Plus system, comparing 2% lidocaine with 1:100,000 epinephrine to 3% mepivacaine, *Oral Surg Oral Med Oral Pathol Oral Radiol Endod* 97:164, 2004.

319. Nusstein J, Claffey E, Reader A, et al: Anesthetic effectiveness of the supplemental intraligamentary injection, administered with a computer-controlled local anesthetic delivery system, in patients with irreversible pulpitis, *J Endod* 31:354, 2005.

320. Nusstein J, Kennedy S, Reader A, et al: Anesthetic efficacy of the supplemental X-tip intraosseous injection in patients with irreversible pulpitis, *J Endod* 29:724, 2003.

321. Nusstein J, Lee S, Reader A, Weaver J: Injection pain and postinjection pain of the anterior middle superior alveolar injection administered with the Wand or conventional syringe, *Oral Surg Oral Med Oral Pathol Oral Radiol Endod* 98:124, 2004.

322. Nusstein J, Reader A, Beck FM: Anesthetic efficacy of different volumes of lidocaine with epinephrine for inferior alveolar nerve blocks, *Gen Dent* 50:372; quiz, 376; 2002.

323. Nusstein J, Reader A, Nist R, et al: Anesthetic efficacy of the supplemental intraosseous injection of 2% lidocaine with 1:100,000 epinephrine in irreversible pulpitis, *J Endod* 24:487, 1998.

324. Nusstein J, Wood M, Reader A, et al: Comparison of the degree of pulpal anesthesia achieved with the intraosseous injection and infiltration injection using 2% lidocaine with 1:100,000 epinephrine, *Gen Dent* 53:50, 2005.

325. Nusstein JM, Beck M: Effectiveness of 20% benzocaine as a topical anesthetic for intraoral injections, *Anesth Prog* 50:159, 2003.

326. Nuzum FM, Drum M, Nusstein J, et al: Anesthetic efficacy of articaine for combination labial plus lingual infiltrations versus labial infiltration in the mandibular lateral incisor, *J Endod* 36:952, 2010.

327. Obrien TP, Roszkowski MT, Wolff LF, et al: Effect of a non-steroidal anti-inflammatory drug on tissue levels of immunoreactive prostaglandin E_2, immunoreactive leukotriene, and pain after periodontal surgery, *J Periodontol* 67:1307,1996.

328. Oertel R, Ebert U, Rahn R, Kirch W: The effect of age on pharmacokinetics of the local anesthetic drug articaine, *Reg Anesth Pain Med* 24:524, 1999.

329. Oguntebi B, DeSchepper E, Taylor T, et al: Postoperative pain incidence related to the type of emergency treatment of symptomatic pulpitis, *Oral Surg Oral Med Oral Pathol Oral Radiol Endod* 73:479, 1992.

330. Oleson M, Drum M, Reader A, et al: Effect of preoperative ibuprofen on the success of the inferior alveolar nerve block in patients with irreversible pulpitis, *J Endod* 36:379, 2010.

331. Papagiannopoulou P, Argiriadou H, Georgiou M, et al: Preincisional local infiltration of levobupivacaine vs ropivacaine for pain control after laparoscopic cholecystectomy, *Surg Endosc* 17:1961, 2003.

332. Parente SA, Anderson RW, Herman WW, et al: Anesthetic efficacy of the supplemental intraosseous injection for teeth with irreversible pulpitis, *J Endod* 24:826, 1998.

333. Parirokh M, Ashouri R, Rekabi AR, et al: The effect of premedication with ibuprofen and indomethacin on the success of inferior alveolar nerve block for teeth with irreversible pulpitis, *J Endod* 36:1450, 2010.

334. Parirokh M, Sadeghi A, Nakhaee N, et al: Effect of topical anesthesia on pain during infiltration injection and success of anesthesia for maxillary central incisors, *J Endod* 38:1553, 2012.

335. Parirokh M, Sadr S, Nakhaee N, et al: Efficacy of supplemental buccal infiltrations and intraligamentary injections to inferior alveolar nerve blocks in mandibular first molars with asymptomatic irreversible pulpitis: a randomized controlled trial, *Int Endod J* 47:926, 2014.

336. Parirokh M, Satvati SA, Sharifi R, et al: Efficacy of combining a buccal infiltration with an inferior alveolar nerve block for mandibular molars with irreversible pulpitis, *Oral Surg Oral Med Oral Pathol Oral Radiol Endod* 109:468, 2010.

337. Penniston S, Hargreaves K: Evaluation of periapical injection of ketorolac for management of endodontic pain, *J Endod* 22:55, 1996.

338. Pereira LA, Groppo FC, Bergamaschi CD, et al: Articaine (4%) with epinephrine (1:100,000 or 1:200,000) in intraosseous injections in symptomatic irreversible pulpitis of mandibular molars: anesthetic efficacy and cardiovascular effects, *Oral Surg Oral Med Oral Pathol Oral Radiol Endod* 116:e85, 2013.

339. Pertot W, Dejou J: Bone and root resorption: effects of the force developed during periodontal ligament injections in dogs, *Oral Surg Oral Med Oral Pathol* 74:357, 1992.

340. Peterson J, Matsson L, Nation W: Cementum and epithelial attachment response to the sulcular and periodontal ligament injection techniques, *Pediatr Dent* 5:257, 1983.

341. Petrini M, Ferrante M, Ciavarelli L, et al: Prostaglandin E₂ to diagnose reversible from irreversible pulpitis, *Int J Immunopathol Pharmacol* 25:157, 2012.

342. Peurach J: Pulpal response to intraligamentary injection in cynomolgus monkey, *Anesth Prog* 32:73, 1985.

343. Pfeil L, Drum M, Reader A, et al: Anesthetic efficacy of 1.8 milliliters and 3.6 milliliters of 2% lidocaine with 1:100,000 epinephrine for posterior superior alveolar nerve blocks, *J Endod* 36:598, 2010.

344. Plamondon T, Walton R, Graham G, et al: Pulp response to the combined effects of cavity preparation and periodontal ligament injection, *Oper Dent* 15:86, 1990.

345. Pogrel M: Permanent nerve damage from inferior alveolar nerve blocks: an update to include articaine, *Calif Dent J* 35:217, 2007.

346. Poorni S, Veniashok B, Senthilkumar AD, et al: Anesthetic efficacy of four percent articaine for pulpal anesthesia by using inferior alveolar nerve block and buccal infiltration techniques in patients with irreversible pulpitis: a prospective randomized double-blind clinical trial, *J Endod* 37:1603, 2011.

347. Prasanna N, Subbarao CV, Gutmann JL: The efficacy of pre-operative oral medication of lornoxicam and diclofenac potassium on the success of inferior alveolar nerve block in patients with irreversible pulpitis: a double-blind, randomized controlled trial, *Int Endod J* 44:330, 2011.

348. Premdas C, Pitt Ford T: Effect of palatal injections on pulpal blood flow in premolars, *Endod Dent Traumatol* 11:274, 1995.

349. Primosch R, Brooks R: Influence of anesthetic flow rate delivered by the Wand local anesthetic system on pain response to palatal injections, *Am J Dent* 15:15, 2002.

350. Primosch RE, Robinson L: Pain elicited during intraoral infiltration with buffered lidocaine, *Am J Dent* 9:5, 1996.

351. Ramachandran A, Khan SI, Mohanavelu D, Kumar KS: The efficacy of pre-operative oral medication of paracetamol, ibuprofen, and aceclofenac on the success of maxillary infiltration anesthesia in patients with irreversible pulpitis: a double-blind, randomized controlled clinical trial, *J Conserv Dent* 15:310, 2012.

352. Rawson R, Orr D: Vascular penetration following intraligamental injection, *J Oral Maxillofac Surg* 43:600, 1985.

353. Reader A, Nusstein J, Drum M: *Successful local anesthesia for restorative dentistry and endodontics*, Hanover Park, Ill, 2011, Quintessence.

354. Reemers T, Glickman G, Spears R, He J: The efficacy of the IntraFlow intraosseous injection as a primary anesthesia technique, *J Endod* 34:280, 2008.

355. Reisman D, Reader A, Nist R, et al: Anesthetic efficacy of the supplemental intraosseous injection of 3% mepivacaine in irreversible pulpitis, *Oral Surg Oral Med Oral Pathol Oral Radiol Endod* 84:676, 1997.

356. Reitz J, Reader A, Nist R, et al: Anesthetic efficacy of a repeated intraosseous injection given 30 minutes following an inferior alveolar nerve block/intraosseous injection, *Anesth Prog* 45:143, 1998.

357. Reitz J, Reader A, Nist R, et al: Anesthetic efficacy of the intraosseous injection of 0.9 mL of 2% lidocaine (1:100,000 epinephrine) to augment an inferior alveolar nerve block, *Oral Surg Oral Med Oral Pathol Oral Radiol Endod* 86:516, 1998.

358. Replogle K, Reader A, Nist R, et al: Anesthetic efficacy of the intraosseous injection of 2% lidocaine (1:100,000 epinephrine) and 3% mepivacaine in mandibular first molars, *Oral Surg Oral Med Oral Pathol Oral Radiol Endod* 83:30, 1997.

359. Replogle K, Reader A, Nist R, et al: Cardiovascular effects of intraosseous injections of 2% lidocaine with 1:100,000 epinephrine and 3% mepivacaine, *J Am Dent Assoc* 130:649, 1999.

360. Ridenour S, Reader A, Beck M, Weaver J: Anesthetic efficacy of a combination of hyaluronidase and lidocaine with epinephrine in inferior alveolar nerve blocks, *Anesth Prog* 48:9, 2001.

361. Roahen JO, Marshall FJ: The effects of periodontal ligament injection on pulpal and periodontal tissues, *J Endod* 16:28, 1990.

362. Robertson D, Nusstein J, Reader A, Beck M: Anesthetic efficacy of articaine and lidocaine in buccal infiltration injections of the mandibular first molar, *J Am Dent Assoc* 138:1104, 2007.

363. Robison SF, Mayhew RB, Cowan RD, Hawley RJ: Comparative study of deflection characteristics and fragility of 25-, 27-, and 30-gauge short dental needles, *J Am Dent Assoc* 109:920, 1984.

364. Rogers BS, Botero TM, McDonald NJ, et al: Efficacy of articaine versus lidocaine as a supplemental buccal infiltration in mandibular molars with irreversible pulpitis: a prospective, randomized, double-blind study, *J Endod* 40:753, 2014.

365. Rogers MJ, Johnson BR, Remeikis NA, BeGole EA: Comparison of effect of intracanal use of ketorolac tromethamine and dexamethasone with oral ibuprofen on post treatment endodontic pain, *J Endod* 25:381, 1999.

366. Rollason V, Samer C, Piguet V, et al: Pharmacogenetics of analgesics: toward the individualization of prescription, *Pharmacogenomics* 9:905, 2008.

367. Rood J: The nerve supply of the mandibular incisor region, *Br Dent J* 143:227, 1977.

368. Rood JP: Adverse reaction to dental local anesthetic injection: "allergy" is not the cause, *Br Dent J* 189:380, 2000.

369. Rosenberg P: Clinical strategies for managing endodontic pain, *Endod Topics* 3:78, 2002.

370. Rosenberg PA, Amin KG, Zibari Y, Lin LM: Comparison of 4% articaine with 1:100,000 epinephrine and 2% lidocaine with 1:100,000 epinephrine when used as a supplemental anesthetic, *J Endod* 33:403, 2007.

371. Rosenquist J, Rosenquist K, Lee P: Comparison between lidocaine and bupivacaine as local anesthetics with diflunisal for postoperative pain control after lower third molar surgery, *Anesth Prog* 35:1, 1988.

372. Rosivack R, Koenigsberg S, Maxwell K: An analysis of the effectiveness of two topical anesthetics, *Anesth Prog* 37:290, 1990.

373. Roy M, Nakanishi T: Differential properties of tetrodotoxin-sensitive and tetrodotoxin-resistant sodium channels in rat dorsal root ganglion neurons, *J Neurosci* 12:2104, 1992.

374. Ryan JF, Jureidini B, Hodges JS, et al: Gender differences in analgesia for endodontic pain, *J Endod* 34:552, 2008.

375. Salomen M, Forsell H, Sceinin M: Local dental anesthesia with lidocaine and adrenalin: effects on plasma catecholamines, heart rate, and blood pressure, *Int J Oral Maxillofac Surg* 17:392, 1988.

376. Sampaoi RM, Carnaval TG, Lanfredi CB, et al: Comparison of the anesthetic efficacy between bupivacaine and lidocaine in patients with irreversible pulpitis of mandibular molar, *J Endod* 38:594, 2012.

377. Satish SV, Shetty KP, Kilaru K, et al: Comparative evaluation of the efficacy of 2% lidocaine containing 1:200,000 epinephrine with and without hyaluronidase (75 IU) in patients with irreversible pulpitis, *J Endod* 39:1116, 2013.

378. Schertzer E, Malamed S: Articaine vs lidocaine, *J Am Dent Assoc* 131:1248, 2000.

379. Schleder JR, Reader A, Beck M, Meyers WJ: The periodontal ligament injection: a comparison of 2% lidocaine, 3% mepivacaine, and 1:100,000 epinephrine to 2% lidocaine with 1:100,000 epinephrine in human mandibular premolars, *J Endod* 14:397, 1988.

380. Schwab JM, Schluesener HJ, Meyermann R, Serhan CN: COX-3 the enzyme and the concept: steps towards highly specialized pathways and precision therapeutics? *Prostaglandins Leukot Essent Fatty Acids* 69:339, 2003.

381. Scott J, Drum M, Reader A, et al: Efficacy of a repeated infiltration to prolong duration of pulpal anesthesia in maxillary lateral incisors, *J Am Dent Assoc* 140:318, 2009.

382. Seng G, Kraus K, Cartridge G: Confirmed allergic reactions to amide local anesthetics, *Gen Den* 44:52, 1996.

383. Shahi S, Mokhtari H, Rahimi S, et al: Effect of premedication with ibuprofen and dexamethasone on success rate of inferior alveolar nerve block for teeth with asymptomatic irreversible pulpitis: a randomized clinical trial, *J Endod* 39:160, 2013.

384. Sherman MG, Flax M, Namerow K, Murray PE: Anesthetic efficacy of the Gow-Gates injection and maxillary infiltration with articaine and lidocaine for irreversible pulpitis, *J Endod* 34:656, 2008.

385. Shojaei A, Haas D: Local anesthetic cartridges and latex allergy: a literature review, *J Can Dent Assoc* 68:622, 2002.

386. Simon D, Jacobs L, Senia E, Walker W: Intraligamentary anesthesia as an aid in endodontic diagnosis, *Oral Surg Oral Med Oral Pathol* 54:77, 1982.

387. Simon F, Reader A, Drum M, et al: A prospective, randomized single-blind study of the anesthetic efficacy of the inferior alveolar nerve block administered with a peripheral nerve stimulator, *J Endod* 36:429, 2010.

388. Simon F, Reader A, Meyers W, et al: Evaluation of a peripheral nerve stimulator in human mandibular anesthesia (abstract), *J Dent Res* 69:278, 1990.

389. Simon M, Gielen M, Alberink N, et al: Intravenous regional anesthesia with 0.5% articaine, 0.5% lidocaine, or 0.5% prilocaine: a double-blind randomized clinical study, *Reg Anesth* 22:20, 1997.

390. Simpson M, Drum M, Reader A, et al: Effect of preoperative ibuprofen/acetaminophen on the success of the inferior alveolar nerve block in patients with symptomatic irreversible pulpitis, *J Endod* 37:593, 2011.

391. Singla M, Subbiya A, Aggarwal V, et al: Comparison of the anesthetic efficacy of different volumes of 4% articaine (1.8 and 3.6 mL) as supplemental buccal infiltration after failed inferior alveolar nerve block, *Int Endod J* 48:103, 2015.

392. Sinnott CJ, Strichartz GR: Levobupivacaine versus ropivacaine for sciatic nerve block in the rat, *Reg Anesth Pain Med* 28:294, 2003.

393. Siqueira J, Barnett F: Interappointment pain: mechanisms, diagnosis, and treatment, *Endod Topics* 3:93, 2004.

394. Sisk A: Evaluation of the Akinosi mandibular block technique in oral surgery, *Oral Maxillofac Surg* 44:113, 1986.

395. Smith G, Pashley D: Periodontal ligament injection: evaluation of systemic effects, *Oral Surg Oral Med Oral Pathol* 56:571, 1983.

396. Smith G, Walton R: Periodontal ligament injections: distribution of injected solutions, *Oral Surg Oral Med Oral Pathol* 55:232, 1983.

397. Smith G, Walton R, Abbott B: Clinical evaluation of periodontal ligament anesthesia using a pressure syringe, *J Am Dent Assoc* 107:953, 1983.

398. Smith S, Reader A, Drum M, et al: Anesthetic efficacy of a combination of 0.5 M mannitol plus 127.2 mg of lidocaine with 50 μg epinephrine in inferior alveolar nerve blocks: a prospective randomized, single-blind study, *Anesth Prog* 60(1):3, 2013.

399. Sorensen H, Skidmore L, Rzasa R, et al: Comparison of pulpal sodium channel density in normal teeth to diseased teeth with severe spontaneous pain (abstract), *J Endod* 30:287, 2004.

400. Spiegel BM, Chiou CF, Ofman JJ: Minimizing complications from nonsteroidal antiinflammatory drugs: cost-effectiveness of competing strategies in varying risk groups, *Arthritis Rheum* 53:185, 2005.

401. Srinivasan N, Kavitha M, Loganathan CS, Padmini G: Comparison of anesthetic efficacy of 4% articaine and 2% lidocaine for maxillary buccal infiltration in patients with irreversible pulpitis, *Oral Surg Oral Med Oral Pathol Oral Radiol Endod* 107:133, 2009.

402. Stabile P, Reader A, Gallatin E, et al: Anesthetic efficacy and heart rate effects of the intraosseous injection of 1.5% etidocaine (1 : 200,000 epinephrine) after an inferior alveolar nerve block, *Oral Surg Oral Med Oral Pathol Oral Radiol Endod* 89:407, 2000.

403. Stambaugh J, Drew J: The combination of ibuprofen and oxycodone/acetaminophen in the management of chronic cancer pain, *Clin Pharmacol Ther* 44:665, 1988.

404. Stanley W, Drum M, Nusstein J, et al: Effect of nitrous oxide on the efficacy of the inferior alveolar nerve block in patients with symptomatic irreversible pulpitis, *J Endod* 38:565, 2012.

405. Steinkruger G, Nusstein J, Reader A, et al: The significance of needle bevel orientation in success of the inferior alveolar nerve block, *J Am Dent Assoc* 137:1685, 2006.

406. Stewart SH, Finn PR, Pihi RO: A dose-response study of the effects of alcohol on the perceptions of pain and discomfort due to electric shock in men at high familial-genetic risk for alcoholism, *Psychopharmacology* 119:261, 1995.

407. Strichartz G: Molecular mechanisms of nerve block by local anesthetics, *Anesthesiology* 45:421, 1967.

408. Susi L, Reader A, Nusstein J, et al: Heart rate effects of intraosseous injections using slow and fast rates of anesthetic solution deposition, *Anesth Prog* 55:9, 2008.

409. Svensson CI, Yaksh TL: The spinal phospholipase-cyclooxygenase-prostanoid cascade in nociceptive processing, *Ann Rev Pharmacol Toxicol* 42:553, 2002.

410. Teplitsky P, Hablichek C, Kushneriuk J: A comparison of bupivacaine to lidocaine with respect to duration in the maxilla and mandible, *J Can Dent Assoc* 53:475, 1987.

411. Todorovic L, Stajcic Z, Petrovic V: Mandibular versus inferior alveolar dental anaesthesia: clinical assessment of 3 different techniques, *Int J Oral Maxillofac Surg* 15:733, 1986.

412. Tofoli GR, Ramacciato JC, de Oliveira PC, et al: Comparison of effectiveness of 4% articaine associated with 1 : 100,000 or 1 : 200,000 epinephrine in inferior alveolar nerve block, *Anesth Prog* 50:164, 2003.

413. Tolas AG, Pflug AE, Halter JB: Arterial plasma epinephrine concentrations and hemodynamic responses after dental injection of local anesthetic with epinephrine, *J Am Dent Assoc* 104:41, 1982.

414. Torabinejad M, et al: Effectiveness of various medications on postoperative pain following root canal obturation, *J Endod* 20:427, 1994.

415. Tortamano IP, Siviero M, Costa CG, et al: A comparison of the anesthetic efficacy of articaine and lidocaine in patients with irreversible pulpitis, *J Endod* 35:165, 2009.

416. Trope M: Relationship of intracanal medicaments to endodontic flare-ups, *Endod Dent Traumatol* 6:226, 1990.

417. Troullos E, Freeman R, Dionne R: The scientific basis for analgesic use in dentistry, *Anesth Prog* 33:123, 1986.

418. Troullos ES, Goldstein DS, Hargreaves KM, Dionne RA: Plasma epinephrine levels and cardiovascular response to high administered doses of epinephrine contained in local anesthesia, *Anesth Prog* 34:10, 1987.

419. Troullos ES, Hargreaves KM, Goldstein DS, et al: Epinephrine suppresses stress-induced increases in plasma immunoreactive beta-endorphin in humans, *J Clin Endocrinol Metab* 69:546, 1989.

420. Turner CL, Eggleston GW, Lunos S, et al: Sniffing out endodontic pain: use of an intranasal analgesic in a randomized clinical trial, *J Endod* 37:439, 2011.

421. Vahatalo K, Antila H, Lehtinen R: Articaine and lidocaine for maxillary infiltration anesthesia, *Anesth Prog* 40:114, 1993.

422. Vanderheyden PJ, Williams RA, Sims TN: Assessment of ST segment depression in patients with cardiac disease after local anesthesia, *J Am Dent Assoc* 119:407, 1989.

423. VanGheluwe J, Walton R: Intrapulpal injection: factors related to effectiveness, *Oral Surg Oral Med Oral Pathol* 19:38, 1997.

424. Vreeland DL, Reader A, Beck M, et al: An evaluation of volumes and concentrations of lidocaine in human inferior alveolar nerve block, *J Endod* 15:6, 1989.

425. Wali M, Drum M, Reader A, Nusstein J: Prospective, randomized, single-blind study of the anesthetic efficacy of 1.8 and 3.6 milliliters of 2% lidocaine with 1 : 50,000 epinephrine for the inferior alveolar nerve block, *J Endod* 36:1459, 2010.

426. Wallace J: Selective COX-2 inhibitors: Is the water becoming muddy? *Trends Pharmacol Sci* 20:4, 1999.

427. Wallace JA, Michanowicz AE, Mundell RD, Wilson EG: A pilot study of the clinical problem of regionally anesthetizing the pulp of an acutely inflamed mandibular molar, *Oral Surg Oral Med Oral Pathol* 59:517, 1985.

428. Walton R, Abbott B: Periodontal ligament injection: a clinical evaluation, *J Am Dent Assoc* 103:571, 1981.

429. Walton R, Chiappinelli J: Prophylactic penicillin: effect on posttreatment symptoms following root canal treatment of asymptomatic periapical pathosis, *J Endod* 19:466, 1993.

430. Walton RE: Distribution of solutions with the periodontal ligament injection: clinical, anatomical, and histological evidence, *J Endod* 12:492, 1986.

431. Warren CA, Mok L, Gordon S, et al: Quantification of neural protein in extirpated tooth pulp, *J Endod* 34:7, 2008.

432. Welborn J, Kane J: Conduction anesthesia using diphenhydramine HCl, *J Am Dent Assoc* 69:706, 1964.

433. Wells JE, Bingham V, Rowland KC, Hatton J: Expression of Nav1.9 channels in human dental pulp and trigeminal ganglion, *J Endod* 33:1172, 2007.

434. Wells LK, Drum M, Nusstein J, et al: Efficacy of Ibuprofen and ibuprofen/acetaminophen on postoperative pain in symptomatic patients with a pulpal diagnosis of necrosis, *J Endod* 37:1608, 2011.

435. Whitcomb M, Drum M, Reader A, et al: A prospective, randomized double-blind study of the anesthetic efficacy of sodium bicarbonate buffered 2% lidocaine with 1 : 100,000 epinephrine in inferior alveolar nerve blocks, *Anesth Prog* 57:59, 2010.

436. White JJ, Reader A, Beck M, Meyers WJ: The periodontal ligament injection: a comparison of the efficacy in human maxillary and mandibular teeth, *J Endod* 14:508, 1988.

437. Whitworth J, Kanna MD, Corbett IP, Meechan JG: Influence of injection speed on the effectiveness of incisive/mental nerve block: a randomized, controlled, double-blind study in adult volunteers, *J Endod* 33:1149, 2007.

438. Wideman G, et al: Analgesic efficacy of a combination of hydrocodone with ibuprofen in postoperative pain, *Clin Pharmacol Ther* 65:66, 1999.

439. Wilburn-Goo D, Lloyd L: When patients become cyanotic: acquired methemoglobinemia, *J Am Dent Assoc* 130:826, 1999.

440. Willett J, Reader A, Drum M, et al: The anesthetic efficacy of diphenhydramine and the combination of diphenhydramine/lidocaine for the inferior alveolar nerve block, *J Endod* 34:1446, 2009.

441. Wilson S, Johns P, Fuller P: The inferior alveolar and mylohyoid nerves: an anatomic study and relationship to local anesthesia of the anterior mandibular teeth, *J Am Dent Assoc* 108:350, 1984.

442. Wolf M, Lichtenstein D, Singh G: Gastrointestinal toxicity of nonsteroidal antiinflammatory drugs, *New Engl J Med* 340:1888, 1999.

443. Wolf R, Reader A, Drum M, et al: Anesthetic efficacy of combinations of 0.5 m mannitol and lidocaine with epinephrine in inferior alveolar nerve blocks: a prospective randomized, single-blind study, *Anesth Prog* 58:157, 2011.

444. Wood M, Reader A, Nusstein J, et al: Comparison of intraosseous and infiltration injections for venous lidocaine blood concentrations and heart rate changes after injection of 2% lidocaine with 1 : 100,000 epinephrine, *J Endod* 31:435, 2005.

445. Woolf C: Evidence for a central component of post-injury pain hypersensitivity, *Nature* 306:686, 1983.

446. Woolf C: Windup and central sensitization are not equivalent, *Pain* 66:105, 1996.

447. Woolf C: Transcriptional and posttranslational plasticity and the generation of inflammatory pain, *Proc Natl Acad Sci U S A* 96:7723, 1999.

448. Wright C, et al: Ibuprofen and acetaminophen kinetics when taken concurrently, *Clin Pharmacol Ther* 34:707, 1983.

449. Wright G, Weinberger S, Friedman C, et al: The use of articaine local anesthesia in children under 4 years of age: a retrospective report, *Anesth Prog* 36:268, 1989.

450. Wright G, Weinberger S, Marti R, Plotzke O: The effectiveness of infiltration anesthesia in the mandibular primary molar region, *Pediatr Dent* 13:278, 1991.

451. Wu Y, Qiu Y, Zhang S, et al: Microneedle-based drug delivery: studies on delivery parameters and bio-compatibility, *Biomed Microdevices* 10:601, 2008.

452. Wynn R, Meiller T, Crossley H: *Drug information handbook for dentistry*, Hudson, Ohio, 2000, Lexi-Comp.

453. Wynn RL, Bergman SA, Meiller TF: Paresthesia associated with local anesthetics: a perspective on articaine, *Gen Dent* 51:498, 2003.

454. Yamazaki S, Seino H, Ozawa S, et al: Elevation of a periosteal flap with irrigation of the bone for minor oral surgery reduces the duration of action of infiltration anesthesia, *Anesth Prog* 53:8, 2006.

455. Yared GM, Dagher FB: Evaluation of lidocaine in human inferior alveolar nerve block, *J Endod* 23:575, 1997.

456. Yesilyurt CBG, Tasdemir T: Summary of: pain perception during inferior alveolar injection administered with the Wand or conventional syringe, *Br Dent J* 205:258, 2008.

457. Yingling NM, Byrne BE, Hartwell GR: Antibiotic use by members of the American Association of Endodontists in the year 2000: report of a national survey, *J Endod* 28:396, 2002.

458. Yonchak T, Reader A, Beck M, et al: Anesthetic efficacy of infiltrations in mandibular anterior teeth, *Anesth Prog* 48:55, 2001.

459. Yonchak T, Reader A, Beck M, et al: Anesthetic efficacy of unilateral and bilateral inferior alveolar nerve blocks to determine cross innervation in anterior teeth, *Oral Sur Oral Med Oral Pathol Oral Radiol Endod* 92: 132, 2001.

460. Yucel E, Hutchison I: A comparative evaluation of the conventional and closed mouth technique for inferior alveolar nerve block, *Aust Dent J* 40:15, 1995.

461. Zarei M, Ghoddusi J, Sharifi E, et al: Comparison of the anesthetic efficacy of and heart rate changes after periodontal ligament or intraosseous X-tip injection in mandibular molars: a randomized controlled clinical trail, *Int Endod J* 45:921, 2012.

462. Zhang JM, Li H, Munir MA: Decreasing sympathetic sprouting in pathologic sensory ganglia: a new mechanism for treating neuropathic pain using lidocaine, *Pain* 109:143, 2004.

463. Zorian EV, Sharagin NV: Comparative evaluation of the topical action of anesthetics on the dental tissues in experimental conditions, *Stomatologiia* 53:1, 1974.

CHAPTER 5

Tooth Morphology, Isolation, and Access

JAMES L. GUTMANN | BING FAN

CHAPTER OUTLINE

The dental pulp presents with a variety of configurations and shapes throughout the dentition. Therefore, a thorough knowledge of tooth morphology, careful interpretation of radiographic documentation, and adequate access to and exploration of the pulpal space are prerequisites for all root canal procedures, whether nonsurgical or surgical.[182] To enhance this exploration and interpretation, magnification and illumination are indispensable. This chapter describes and illustrates tooth morphology and explains the techniques necessary to achieve unobstructed, direct access to the root canal system. The clinician is challenged to perform adequate enlarging, shaping,

cleaning, disinfection, and obturation of the pulpal space to achieve predictable outcomes with root canal procedures. However, the optimal result is difficult to achieve if the access is not prepared properly. Therefore, knowledge of the complexity of the root canal system is essential to understand the principles and problems encountered in access preparation.

The complexity of the root canal system is best understood by the integration of formative knowledge of tooth anatomy and the interpretation of radiographic documentation. Careful evaluation of two or more periapical radiographs, exposed at different horizontal angulations of the x-ray cone, is essential.

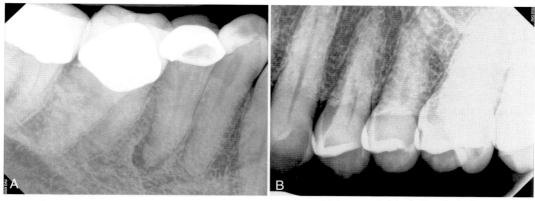

FIG. 5-1 **A,** Abrupt disappearance of the large canal in the mandibular first premolar indicates a canal bifurcation. **B,** The same is true for the maxillary first premolar.

These divergently exposed radiographs along with cone-beam computed tomography (CBCT) scans in some clinical situations (see Chapter 2) provide important information about root canal morphology. However, the inclination of the x-ray tube significantly influences the ability to detect variable root canal systems present in many teeth. For example, in premolars, if the horizontal angle is varied by either 20 or 40 degrees, the number of root canals seen in the maxillary first and second premolars and the mandibular first premolars coincides with the number of canals actually present.[134] However, in the mandibular second premolar, only the 40-degree horizontal angle correctly identifies the root canal morphology. The careful reading and interpretation of each radiograph before and during root canal procedures is necessary because many teeth present with unusual canal morphology. Unfortunately, the interpretation of traditional radiographs may not always result in the correct morphologic assessment, particularly when only a buccolingual view is taken. In one study, 790 extracted mandibular incisors and premolars were radiographed to assess the incidence of canal bifurcation in a root.[147] When the *fast break* guideline was used (i.e., interpreting a sudden disappearance or narrowing of a canal as a sign of canal division, such as bifurcation [Fig. 5-1]), the result was failure to identify one third of these divisions from a single radiographic view. Thus, evaluation of the root canal system is most accurate when the information from several radiographic views is integrated with a thorough clinical exploration of the interior and exterior of the tooth. Alternatively, the recent development of micro-computed tomography (μCT) scanning of teeth has greatly increased clinical assessment of these complexities and three-dimensional (3D) relationships found in root canal systems.

The main objectives of root canal procedures are adequate enlargement, shaping, cleaning, and disinfection of all pulpal spaces, along with obturation of these spaces with an acceptable filling material. At times a root canal or its elaborate, complex system may go undetected, which results in failure to achieve the stated objectives. Therefore, the use of a vast array of tools, in particular magnification and illumination, is essential to accomplish these objectives on a more predictable basis.

Initially important aids for determining pulp space morphology, in particular the pulp chamber and location of root canal orifices, include multiple pretreatment radiographs, CBCTs, examination of the pulp chamber floor with a sharp explorer, visual assessment of color changes in the dentin,

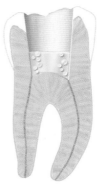

FIG. 5-2 Allowing sodium hypochlorite (NaOCl) to remain in the pulp chamber may help locate a calcified root canal orifice. Tiny bubbles may appear in the solution, indicating the position of the orifice. This is best observed through magnification.

troughing of anatomic grooves with ultrasonic tips, staining the chamber floor with 1% methylene blue dye, performing a sodium hypochlorite "champagne bubble" test (Fig. 5-2), visualizing the pulp chamber anatomy from established documents,[107] and root canal bleeding points. Sequential application of 17% aqueous ethylene diaminetetraacetic acid (EDTA) and 95% ethanol has been recommended for effective cleaning and drying of the pulp chamber floor before visual inspection.[207]

Specifically, the use of the dental operating microscope (DOM), which is intended to provide superior magnification, increased lighting, and enhanced visibility,[182] is recommended to determine the location of root canal orifices in the properly prepared coronal access (Fig. 5-3). Removal of dentin that may obscure the location of these orifices is also enhanced with better visualization with the DOM. The DOM also improves the identification of extra canals (e.g., the mesiopalatal canal found in many first and second maxillary molars) and has been shown to be superior to the use of the naked eye and magnifying loupes for this assessment.[14,187] Additional studies have noted that use of the DOM improves the detection of mesiopalatal canals to more than 90% in maxillary first molars and 60% in maxillary second molars.[108,207] These evaluative studies demonstrate that magnification and illumination greatly enhance the identification of the pulp chamber morphology and ultimately enable the clinician to achieve better outcomes within each of the stated objectives for root canal procedures.

As with all advances in technology, however, there are varying points of concurrence and disagreement. For example, one group of investigators determined that dental loupes and the DOM were equally effective for locating mesiopalatal canals in maxillary molars,[29] whereas other studies determined that the DOM did not significantly enhance the ability to locate canals.[80] However, there appears to be consensus that the DOM enhances the locating of canals by magnifying and illuminating the grooves in the pulpal floor and by distinguishing the color differences in the dentin of the floor and walls.[41,107]

COMPONENTS OF THE ROOT CANAL SYSTEM

The dental pulp is often referred to as the root canal system, as opposed to a simple tube or circular space, due to its complexity (Fig. 5-4). The outline of this system generally corresponds to the external contour of the tooth. However, factors such as physiologic aging, pathosis, trauma, and occlusion all can modify its dimensions through the production of dentin

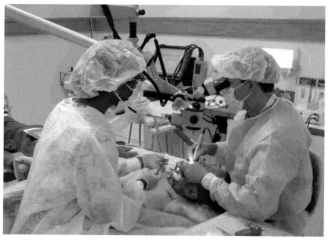

FIG. 5-3 The dental operating microscope (DOM) has vastly improved locating the position of the coronal canal anatomy.

or reparative (irregular secondary, irritation, and tertiary) dentin (Fig. 5-5).[199] The root canal system is divided into two portions: the pulp chamber, located in the anatomic crown of the tooth, and the pulp or root canal (or canals), found in the anatomic root. Other notable features are the pulp horns; accessory, lateral, and furcation canals; canal orifices; apical deltas; and apical foramina. The pulp horns are important because the pulp in them is often exposed by caries, trauma, or mechanical invasion, which usually necessitates vital pulp or root canal procedures. Also, the pulp horns undergo rapid mineralization, along with reduction of the size and shape of the pulp chamber because of the formation of reparative dentin over time.

The root canal begins as a funnel-shaped canal orifice, generally at or just apical to the cervical line, and ends at the apical foramen, which opens onto the root surface at or within 3 mm of the center of the root apex.* Nearly all root canals are curved, particularly in a faciolingual direction. These curves may pose problems during enlargement and shaping procedures because they are not evident on a standard two-dimensional (2D) radiograph. Angled views are often necessary to determine their presence, direction, and severity. A curvature may be a gradual curve of the entire canal or a sharp curvature near the apex. Double S-shaped canal curvatures also can occur. In most cases, the number of root canals corresponds to the number of roots; however, an oval root may have more than one canal.

Accessory canals are minute canals that extend in a horizontal, vertical, or lateral direction from the pulp space to the periodontium. In 74% of cases they are found in the apical third of the root, in 11% in the middle third, and in 15% in the cervical third.[223] Accessory canals contain connective tissue and vessels but do not supply the pulp with sufficient circulation to form a collateral source of blood flow. They are formed by the entrapment of periodontal vessels in Hertwig's epithelial root sheath during calcification.[46] They may play a significant role in the communication of disease processes, serving as avenues for the passage of irritants, primarily from the pulp to

---

*References 30, 81, 83, 170, 223, and 227.

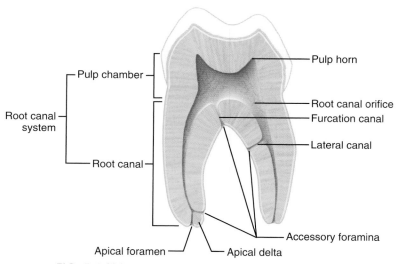

FIG. 5-4 Major anatomic components of the root canal system.

Labels: Pulp chamber · Root canal system · Root canal · Apical foramen · Apical delta · Pulp horn · Root canal orifice · Furcation canal · Lateral canal · Accessory foramina

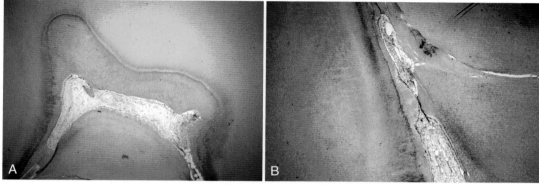

FIG. 5-5 **A**, Formation of reparative dentin and reduction of the pulp chamber space. **B**, Calcific narrowing and closing of a root canal as it leaves the pulp chamber. (From Gutmann JL, Lovdahl PE: *Problem solving in endodontics,* ed 5, St Louis, 2011, Elsevier.)

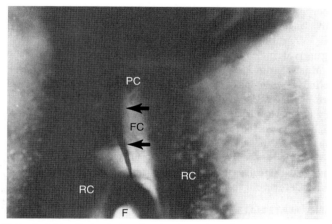

FIG. 5-6 Mandibular first molar showing a furcation canal *(FC, arrows). F,* Furcation; *PC,* pulp chamber floor; *RC,* root canal.

FIG. 5-7 Accessory canals occur in three distinct patterns in the mandibular first molars. **A**, In 13% a single furcation canal extends from the pulp chamber to the intraradicular region. **B**, In 23% a lateral canal extends from the coronal third of a major root canal to the furcation region (80% extend from the distal root canal). **C**, About 10% have both lateral and furcation canals.

the periodontium, although communication of inflammatory processes may occur from either tissue.

Accessory canals that are present in the bifurcation or trifurcation of multirooted teeth are referred to as *furcation canals* (Fig. 5-6).[223,226] These channels form as a result of the entrapment of periodontal vessels during the fusion of the diaphragm, which becomes the pulp chamber floor.[46] In mandibular molars these canals occur in three distinct patterns (Fig. 5-7). Tables 5-1 and 5-2 present the incidence of furcation canals for each tooth.

Based on scanning electron microscopy (SEM) studies, the diameter of furcation openings in mandibular molars varies from 4 to 720 m.[224] The number of furcation canals ranges from none to more than 20 per specimen. Foramina on both the pulp chamber floor and the furcation surface were found in 36% of maxillary first molars, 12% of maxillary second molars, 32% of mandibular first molars, and 24% of mandibular second molars (Fig. 5-8). Mandibular teeth have a higher incidence of foramina involving both the pulp chamber floor and the furcation surface (56%) than do maxillary teeth (48%). No relationship was found between the incidence of accessory foramina and the occurrence of pulp chamber calcification or the distance from the chamber floor to the furcation. Radiographs usually fail to show the presence of furcation and lateral canals in the coronal portion of these roots. In one study involving 200 permanent molars, the pulp chamber floor was stained with 0.5% basic fuscin dye. Patent furcation canals were detected in 24% of maxillary and mandibular first molars, 20% of mandibular second molars, and 16% of maxillary second molars.[87] Pulpal inflammation can communicate to the periodontium via these canals, and the result is furcation lesions in the absence of demonstrable periodontal disease. Likewise, the long-term presence of periodontal furcation lesions may influence the viability of the coronal or radicular pulp tissue when these aberrant channels are present.[84]

ROOT CANAL ANATOMY

The knowledge of common root canal morphology and its frequent variations is a basic requirement for success during root canal procedures. The significance of canal anatomy has been underscored by studies that demonstrated that the natural variations in canal geometry had a greater effect on the changes that occurred during enlargement and shaping than did the instrumentation techniques used to achieve these objectives.[167-169]

From the early works of Preiswerk[175] in 1912, Fasoli and Arlotta[67] in 1913, and Hess and Zurcher[90] in 1917, to more recent studies[33,82,100,190] demonstrating the anatomic complexities of the root canal system, data indicate that a root with a

TABLE 5-1

Morphology of the Maxillary Permanent Teeth*

Tooth	Root	Number of Teeth	Canals with Lateral Canals	Position of Lateral Canals				Transverse Anastomosis Between Canals	Position of Transverse Anastomosis			Position of Apical Foramen		Apical Deltas
				Cervical	Middle	Apical	Furcation		Cervical	Middle	Apical	Central	Lateral	
Central	—	100	24	1	6	93	—	—	—	—	—	12	88	1
Lateral	—	100	26	1	8	91	—	—	—	—	—	22	78	3
Canine	—	100	30	0	10	90	—	—	—	—	—	14	86	3
First premolar	—	400	49.5	4.7	10.3	74	11	34.2	16.4	58	25.6	12	88	3.2
Second premolar	—	200	59.5	4	16.2	78.2	1.6	30.8	18.8	50	31.2	22.2	77.8	15.1
First molar	MB	100	51	10.7	13.1	58.2	↑	52	10	75	15	24	76	8
	DB	100	36	10.1	12.3	59.6	18	0	0	0	0	19	81	2
	P	100	48	9.4	11.3	61.3	→	0	0	0	0	18	82	4
Second molar	MB	100	50	10.1	14.1	65.8	↑	21	8	72	20	12	88	3
	DB	100	29	9.1	13.3	67.6	10	0	0	0	0	17	83	2
	P	100	42	8.7	11.2	70.1	→	0	0	0	0	19	81	4

From Vertucci FJ: Root canal anatomy of the human permanent teeth, *Oral Surg Oral Med Oral Pathol* 58:589, 1984.
DP, Distobuccal; *MB*, mesiobuccal; *P*, palatal.
*Figures represent percentage of the total.

TABLE 5-2

Morphology of the Mandibular Permanent Teeth*

Tooth	Root	Number of Teeth	Canals with Lateral Canals	Position of Lateral Canals				Transverse Anastomosis Between Canals	Position of Transverse Anastomosis			Position of Apical Foramen		Apical Deltas
				Cervical	Middle	Apical	Furcation		Cervical	Middle	Apical	Central	Lateral	
Central	—	100	20	3	12	85	—	—	—	—	—	25	75	5
Lateral	—	100	18	2	15	83	—	—	—	—	—	20	80	6
Canine	—	100	30	4	16	80	—	—	—	—	—	30	70	8
First premolar	—	400	44.3	4.3	16.1	78.9	0.7	32.1	20.6	52.9	26.5	15	85	5.7
Second premolar	—	400	48.3	3.2	16.4	80.1	0.3	30	0	66.7	33.3	16.1	83.9	3.4
First molar	Mesial	100	45	10.4	12.2	54.4	← 23 →	63	12	75	13	22	78	10
	Distal	100	30	8.7	10.4	57.9		55	10	72	18	20	80	14
Second molar	Mesial	100	49	10.1	13.1	65.8	← 11 →	31	10	77	13	19	81	6
	Distal	100	34	9.1	11.6	68.3		16	11	74	15	21	79	7

From Vertucci FJ: Root canal anatomy of the human permanent teeth, *Oral Surg Oral Med Oral Pathol* 58:589, 1984.
*Figures represent percentage of the total.

FIG. 5-8 **A,** Electron photomicrograph of the pulp chamber floor of a mandibular first molar. Multiple accessory foramina can be seen *(arrows)*, ranging from 20 to 140 μm. (×20.) **B,** Electron photomicrograph of the furcation surface of a mandibular first molar. Multiple accessory foramina can be seen on the furcation surface. (×30.). *D,* Distal canal; *M,* mesial canals.

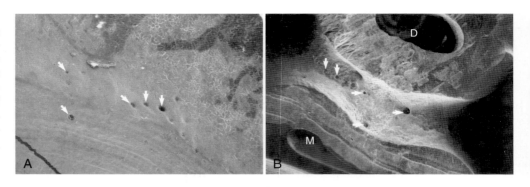

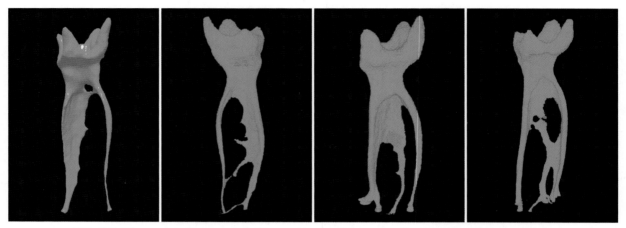

FIG. 5-9 Microcomputed tomography (μCT) scans show multiple canal configurations, depicting the complexity of the root canal system.

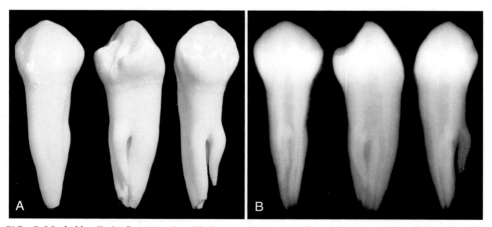

FIG. 5-10 **A,** Mandibular first premolar with three separate roots trifurcating in the midroot. **B,** Radiograph of the three views. Small canals diverging from the main canal create a configuration that is difficult to prepare and obturate biomechanically.

tapering canal and a single foramen is the exception rather than the rule. Investigators have shown multiple foramina, additional canals, fins, deltas, intercanal connections, loops, C-shaped canals, and furcation and lateral canals in most teeth (Fig. 5-9).* Consequently, complex anatomy must be considered the norm. The first premolar in Fig. 5-10, *A,* is a good example of complex anatomy. The extra root is not obvious in a pretreatment radiograph (Fig. 5-10, *B*). Figure 5-11 shows a cross-section of a similar tooth. This tooth has a fine, ribbon-shaped canal system instead of two distinct canals. Both these teeth present challenges for locating the canal and for achieving the previously stated objectives for root canal procedures.

Typically, root canals take variable pathways throughout, coursing from the orifice to the apex. The pulp canal system is complex, and canals may branch, divide, and rejoin. Weine[238]

---

*References 48, 53, 154, 170, 196, and 223.

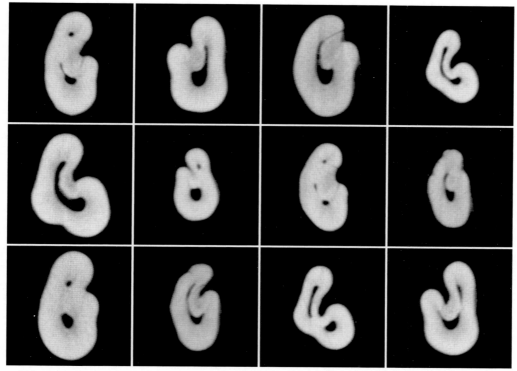

FIG. 5-11 Cross sections of teeth similar to those seen in Fig. 5-10 amplify the unique nature of the root canal system, particularly its ribbon and C-shaped configurations.

categorized the root canal systems in any root into four basic types. Other studies,[225] using cleared teeth in which the root canal systems had been stained with hematoxylin dye, found a much more complex canal system. In doing so the authors identified eight pulp space configurations, which can be briefly described as follows (Fig. 5-12):

Type I: A single canal extends from the pulp chamber to the apex (1).

Type II: Two separate canals leave the pulp chamber and join short of the apex to form one canal (2-1).

Type III: One canal leaves the pulp chamber and divides into two in the root; the two then merge to exit as one canal (1-2-1).

Type IV: Two separate, distinct canals extend from the pulp chamber to the apex (2).

Type V: One canal leaves the pulp chamber and divides short of the apex into two separate, distinct canals with separate apical foramina (1-2).

Type VI: Two separate canals leave the pulp chamber, merge in the body of the root, and separate short of the apex to exit as two distinct canals (2-1-2).

Type VII: One canal leaves the pulp chamber, divides and then rejoins in the body of the root, and finally separates into two distinct canals short of the apex (1-2-1-2).

Type VIII: Three separate, distinct canals extend from the pulp chamber to the apex (3).

The anatomic variations present in these teeth are listed in Tables 5-1 and 5-2. The only tooth that showed all eight possible configurations was the maxillary second premolar.

The percentages of human permanent teeth with these variable canal configurations are presented in Tables 5-3 and 5-4.

Similar observations have been described in large population studies with the exceptions that one canal was found in 23% of maxillary laterals, 55% of mesiobuccal roots of maxillary second molars, and 30% of distal roots of mandibular second molars.[33,242] Differences in these studies, from the types described by Weine, may be due to variations in the ethnic and racial populations studied. Other studies that were ethnic, racial, or gender-specific based have indicated wide variations in canal morphology, which sometimes appeared more often in specific teeth.* These authors concluded that gender, racial, and ethnic aspects should be considered in the pretreatment evaluation for root canal procedures (Fig. 5-13).

In addition to in vitro morphologic studies, a large number of case reports has described a variety of complex canal configurations (see Tables 5-8 to 5-27 online at the Expert Consult site). Reports of complex anatomy from both in vitro and in vivo investigations contribute to the adage that it is easier to recognize an anatomic feature if one is already prepared to see it. With the availability of CBCT, many more irregular and challenging root canal anatomies have been identified.[168,217]

One well-recognized ethnic variant is the higher incidence of single-rooted and C-shaped mandibular second molars in Native American and Asians populations (Fig. 5-14).[62,63,130,131] However, this is not always the case, as the occurrence of two canals in the mesiobuccal root of maxillary first molars in Japanese patients is similar to that described for other ethnic groups.[239] All this information makes it clear that the clinician is confronted daily with highly complex and variable root canal systems.

---

*References 82, 100, 190, 219, 229-231, and 236.

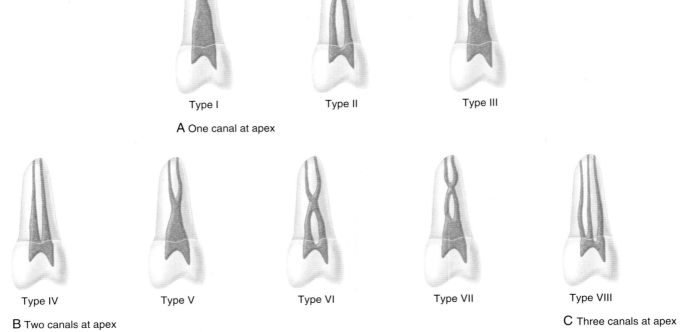

Type I

Type II

Type III

A One canal at apex

Type IV

Type V

Type VI

Type VII

Type VIII

B Two canals at apex

C Three canals at apex

FIG. 5-12 Diagrammatic representation of canal configurations based on the work of Vertucci.

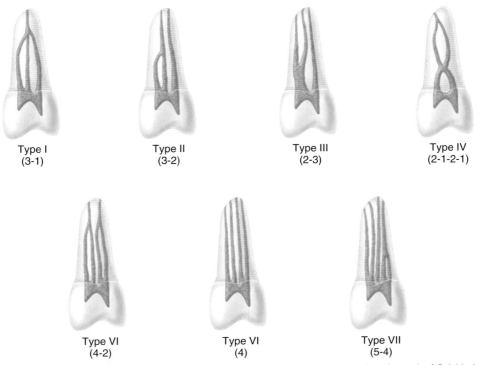

Type I
(3-1)

Type II
(3-2)

Type III
(2-3)

Type IV
(2-1-2-1)

Type VI
(4-2)

Type VI
(4)

Type VII
(5-4)

FIG. 5-13 Diagrammatic representation of supplemental canal configurations based on the work of Gulabivala and colleagues on a Burmese population.

TABLE 5-3

Classification and Percentage of Root Canals in the Maxillary Teeth

Tooth	Number of Teeth	Type I (1) Canals	Type II (2-1) Canals	Type III (1-2-1) Canals	Total with One Canal at Apex	Type IV (2) Canals	Type V (1-2) Canals	Type VI (2-1-2) Canals	Type VII (1-2-1-2) Canals	Total with Two Canals at Apex	Type VIII (3) Canals	Total with Three Canals at Apex
Maxillary central	100	100	0	0	100	0	0	0	0	0	0	0
Maxillary lateral	100	100	0	0	100	0	0	0	0	0	0	0
Maxillary canine	100	100	0	0	100	0	0	0	0	0	0	0
Maxillary first premolar	400	8	18	0	26	62	7	0	0	69	5	5
Maxillary second premolar	200	48	22	5	75	11	6	5	2	24	1	1
Maxillary First Molar												
Mesiobuccal	100	45	37	0	82	18	0	0	0	18	0	0
Distobuccal	100	100	0	0	100	0	0	0	0	0	0	0
Palatal	100	100	0	0	100	0	0	0	0	0	0	0
Maxillary Second Molar												
Mesiobuccal	100	71	17	0	88	12	0	0	0	12	0	0
Distobuccal	100	100	0	0	100	0	0	0	0	0	0	0
Palatal	100	100	0	0	100	0	0	0	0	0	0	0

From Vertucci FJ: Root canal anatomy of the human permanent teeth, *Oral Surg Oral Med Oral Pathol* 58:589, 1984.

TABLE 5-4

Classification and Percentage of Root Canals in the Mandibular Teeth

Tooth	Number of Teeth	Type I (1) Canals	Type II (2-1) Canals	Type III (1-2-1) Canals	Total with One Canal at Apex	Type IV (2) Canals	Type V (1-2) Canals	Type VI (2-1-2) Canals	Type VII (1-2-1-2) Canals	Total with Two Canals at Apex	Type VIII (3) Canals	Total with Three Canals at Apex
Mandibular central incisor	100	70	5	22	97	3	0	0	0	3	0	0
Mandibular lateral incisor	100	75	5	18	98	2	0	0	0	2	0	0
Mandibular canine	100	78	14	2	94	6	0	0	0	6	0	0
Mandibular first premolar	400	70	0	4	74	1.5	24	0	0	25.5	0.5	0.5
Mandibular second premolar	400	97.5	0	0	97.5	0	2.5	0	0	2.5	0	0
Mandibular first molar												
Mesial	100	12	28	0	40	43	8	10	0	59	1	1
Distal	100	70	15	0	85	5	8	2	0	15	0	0
Mandibular second molar												
Mesial	100	27	38	0	65	26	9	0	0	35	0	0
Distal	100	92	3	0	95	4	1	0	0	5	0	0

From Vertucci FJ: Root canal anatomy of the human permanent teeth, *Oral Surg Oral Med Oral Pathol* 58:589, 1984.

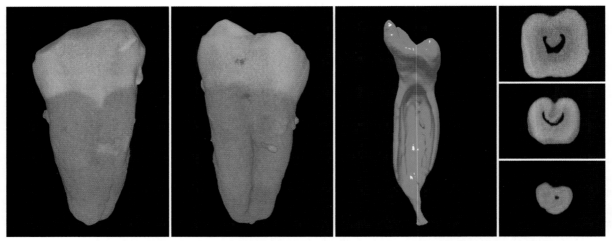

FIG. 5-14 Common variant of a C-shaped canal anatomy found in Native Americans and Asian populations.

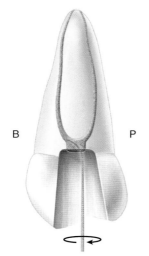

FIG. 5-15 An oval orifice must be explored with apically curved small instruments. When trying to locate the buccal canal, the clinician should place the file tip in the orifice with the tip curved to the buccal side. To explore for the palatal canal, a curved file tip is placed toward the palate. *B,* Buccal; *P,* palatal.

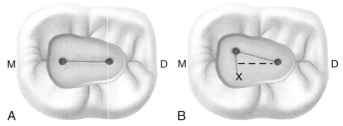

FIG. 5-16 **A,** In a mandibular second molar with two canals, both orifices are in the mesiodistal midline. **B,** If two orifices are not directly in the mesiodistal midline, a search should be made for another canal on the opposite side in the area of "X." *D,* Distal; *M,* mesial.

Clinical Determination of the Root Canal Configuration

Coronal Considerations

Examination of the pulp chamber floor can reveal clues to the location of orifices and to the type of canal system present. It is important to note that if only one canal is present, it usually is located in the center of the access preparation. All such orifices, particularly if oval shaped, should be explored thoroughly with small, stiff K-files that have a smooth to sharp bend in the apical 1 to 2 mm (C files and C+ files, Dentsply Tulsa Dental Specialties, Tulsa, Oklahoma, and Dentsply Maillefer, Ballaigues, Switzerland, respectively). If only one orifice is found and it is not in the center of the root, another orifice probably exists, and the clinician should search for it on the opposite side (Fig. 5-15). The relationship of the two orifices to each other is also significant (Fig. 5-16). The closer they are, the greater the chance the two canals join at some point in the body of the

root. As the distance between orifices in a root increases, the greater is the chance the canals will remain separate. The more separation between orifices, the less the degree of canal curvature.[40] The direction a file takes when introduced into an orifice is also important. If the first file inserted into the distal canal of a mandibular molar points either in a buccal or lingual direction, a second canal is present. If two canals are present, they will be smaller than a single canal. (See μCTs and cross sections of all tooth groups later in this chapter. In addition, rotational videos of these groups can be found online as Videos 5-1 through 5-16 at the Expert Consult site.)

Midroot Considerations

As the canal leaves the coronal portion of the root and blends into the midroot portion, many changes can occur, including fins, webs, culs-de-sac, and isthmuses (also called *anastomoses*). These structures are narrow, ribbon-shaped communications between two root canals that contain pulp or pulpally derived tissue, or they may represent a communication between two canals that split in the midroot portion of the canal. These structures contain variable amounts of tissue, and when the pulp is infected, they often contain bacteria and their byproducts. In one study, isthmuses in the mesiobuccal root of maxillary first molars were found most often 3 to 5 mm from the root apex.[244] A complete or partial isthmus was found at the 4-mm level 100% of the time. In another study, partial isthmuses were found more often than complete ones.[213]

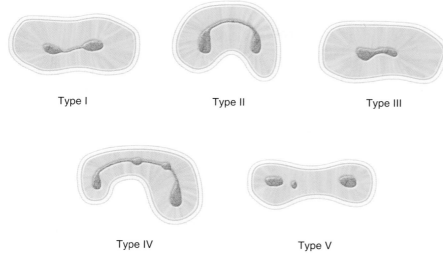

Type I   Type II   Type III

Type IV   Type V

FIG. 5-17 Schematic representation of isthmus classifications described by Kim and colleagues. Type I is an incomplete isthmus; it is a faint communication between two canals. Type II is characterized by two canals with a definite connection between them (complete isthmus). Type III is a very short, complete isthmus between two canals. Type IV is a complete or incomplete isthmus between three or more canals. Type V is marked by two or three canal openings without visible connections. (From Kim S, Pecora G, Rubinstein R, Dorscher-Kim J: *Color atlas of microsurgery in endodontics,* Philadelphia, 2001, Saunders.)

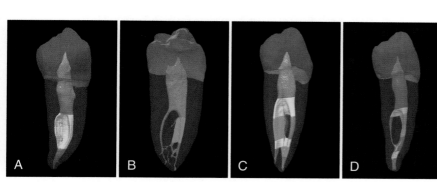

A   B   C   D

FIG. 5-18 μCT scans of mandibular premolars reflect a wide variation in canal morphology, moving from coronal to apical sections The red color indicates a non–C-shaped canal space; yellow indicates a semilunar canal shape; and green indicated a continuous C-shaped configuration.

Isthmuses are found in 15% of anterior teeth; in maxillary premolar teeth, they are found in 16% at the 1-mm level from the apex and in 52% at the 6-mm level, which puts them primarily in the middle third of the canal (Fig. 5-17). The prevalence of an isthmus increases in the mesiobuccal root of the maxillary first molar, from 30% to 50% near the junction of middle and apical thirds of the root. Eighty percent of the mesial roots of mandibular first molars have these communications at the apical to middle third junction, with the distal root display more in the apical third.

Another change that often occurs in the midroot portion is the splitting of a single canal into two or more canals, along with a wide variation in canal morphology. Likewise, canals often join in this area, starting as coronally two separate canals (Fig. 5-18).

Whenever a root contains two canals that join to form one, the lingual/palatal canal generally is the one with direct access to the apex, although this may require radiographic verification. When one canal separates into two, the division is buccal and palatal/lingual, and the lingual canal generally splits from the main canal at a sharp angle, sometimes nearly a right angle (Fig. 5-19). One study[197] recommended visualizing this configuration as a lower case letter "h". The buccal canal is the straight-line portion of the h; the lingual canal exists about midroot at a sharp angle from the buccal canal. In these situations modification of the access to develop an unobstructed passage of instruments into the lingual canal is indicated.

Although the splitting of one canal into two presents challenges for the clinician, of greater concern is the very small

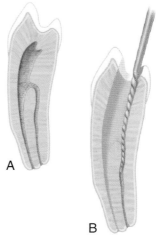

A

B

FIG. 5-19 A, Mesial view of a mandibular premolar with a type V canal configuration. The lingual canal separates from the main canal at nearly a right angle. B, This anatomy requires widening of access in a lingual direction to achieve straight-line access to the lingual canal. This should be done with a DOM.

canal that may split off, at times at almost a 90 degree angle, and cannot be located tactilely or even under magnification with the DOM. Although these canals may join the main canal at some point apically, some of them exit separately. This is not uncommon in teeth with C-shaped canals.

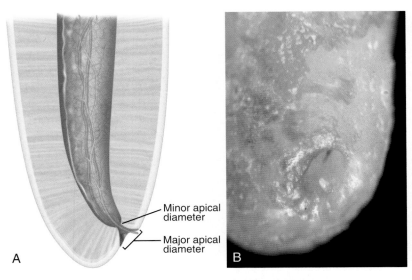

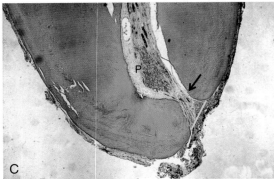

FIG. 5-20 **A,** Morphology of the root apex. From its orifice the canal tapers to the apical constriction, or minor apical diameter, which generally is considered the narrowest part of the canal. From this point the canal widens as it exits the root at the apical foramen, or major apical diameter. The space between the minor and major apical diameters is funnel shaped. **B,** Clinical view of major apical foramen. **C,** Histologic view of the canal constriction and canal foramen. (**B** and **C** from Gutmann JL, Lovdahl PE: *Problem solving in endodontics,* ed 5, St Louis, 2011, Elsevier.)

Apical Considerations

The classic concept of apical root anatomy is based on three anatomic and histologic landmarks in the apical region of a root: the apical constriction (AC), the cementodentinal junction (CDJ), and the apical foramen (AF). Kuttler's description of the anatomy of the root apex has the root canal tapering from the canal orifice to the AC, which generally is 0.5 to 1.5 mm coronal to the AF (Fig. 5-20).[109] The AC generally is considered the part of the root canal with the smallest diameter; it also is the reference point clinicians use most often as the apical termination for enlarging, shaping, cleaning, disinfecting, and filling. Violation of this area with instruments or filling materials is not recommended for long-term, successful outcomes.

The CDJ is the point in the canal where cementum meets dentin; it is also the point where pulp tissue ends and periodontal tissues begin. The location of the CDJ in the root canal varies considerably. It generally is not in the same area as the AC, and estimates place it approximately 1 mm from the AF.[184,200]

From the AC, or minor apical diameter, the canal widens as it approaches the AF, or major apical diameter. The space between the major and minor diameters has been described as funnel shaped or hyperbolic, or as having the shape of a morning glory. The mean distance between the major and minor apical diameters is 0.5 mm in a young person and 0.67 mm in an older individual.[109] The distance is greater in older individuals because of the buildup of cementum.

The AF is the "circumference or rounded edge, like a funnel or crater, that differentiates the termination of the cemental canal from the exterior surface of the root."[109] The diameter of the foramen is 502 μm in individuals 18 to 25 years of age and 681 μm in those over age 55, which demonstrates the growth of the AF with age.[109] By comparison, these sizes are larger than the cross-sectional diameter of #50 and #60 root canals files, respectively. The AF does not normally exit at the anatomic apex, but rather is offset 0.5 to 3 mm. This variation is more marked in older teeth through cementum apposition. Studies have shown that the AF coincides with the apical root vertex in 17% to 46% of cases.*

The location and diameter of the CDJ differ from those of the AF in maxillary anterior teeth.[174] Extension of cementum from the AF into the root canal differs considerably, even when opposite canal walls are compared. Cementum reaches the same level on all canal walls in only 5% of cases. The greatest extension generally occurs on the concave side of the canal curvature. This variability confirms that the CDJ and the AC generally are not in the same area and that the CDJ should be considered just a variable junction at which two histologic tissues meet in the root canal (Fig. 5-21). The diameter of the canal at the CDJ varies considerably; it was determined to be 353 μm for the central incisors, 292 μm for the lateral incisors, and 298 μm for the canines.[167] These measures approximate the size of #30 to #35 root canal files.

In maxillary anterior teeth, the root apex and main AF coincided in 17% of examined central incisors and canines and

---

*References 30, 81, 83, 170, 182, 208, 223, and 227.

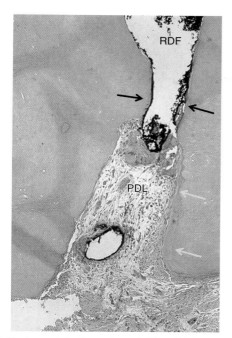

FIG. 5-21 Root apex following root canal filling *(RCF)* short of the actual root length. Histologic evidence shows that hard tissue *(black arrows)* has formed from the cells of the periodontal ligament *(PDL)* adjacent to the root filling material. Cementum formation on the internal aspect of the apical foramen is indicated by the yellow arrows. These findings accentuate the variable nature of the apical tissues. (From Gutmann JL, Lovdahl PE: *Problem solving in endodontics,* ed 5, St Louis, 2011, Elsevier.)

TABLE 5-6

Size of Main Apical Foramina	
Teeth	**Mean Value (μm)**
Maxillary incisors	289.4
Mandibular incisors	262.5
Maxillary premolars	210
Mandibular premolars	268.25
Maxillary molars	
Palatal	298
Mesiobuccal	235.05
Distobuccal	232.2
Mandibular molars	
Mesial	257.5
Distal	392

From Morfis A, Sylaras SN, Georgopoulou M, et al: Study of the apices of human permanent teeth with the use of a scanning electron microscope, *Oral Surg Oral Med Oral Pathol* 77:172, 1994.

TABLE 5-5

Mean Perpendicular Distance from Root Apex to Apical Constriction with Mesiodistal and Labiolingual Diameters at Constriction			
Tooth	**Mesiodistal (mm)**	**Labiolingual (mm)**	**Vertical (mm)**
Central incisor	0.37	0.428	0.863
Lateral incisor	0.307	0.369	0.825
Canine	0.313	0.375	1.01

From Mizutani T, Ohno N, Nakamura H: Anatomical study of the root apex in the maxillary anterior teeth, *J Endod* 18:344, 1992.

in 7% of lateral incisors.[139] Both the root apex and the AF of the central incisors and canines were displaced distolabially, whereas those of the lateral incisors were displaced distolingually. The perpendicular distance from the root apex to the AC and both mesiodistal and labiolingual root canal diameters at the AC are shown in Table 5-5. The labiolingual diameter in all maxillary anterior teeth is approximately 50 μm more than the mesiodistal diameter. This has definite implications for intracanal root canal procedures because only the mesiodistal diameter is evident on radiographs.

Scanning electron microscopy has been used to determine the number and size of main apical foramina, their distance from the anatomic apex, and the size of accessory foramina. Morfis et al.[145] observed that more than one main foramen was found in all teeth except the palatal root of maxillary molars

and the distal root of mandibular molars. No main foramen was seen in 24% of maxillary premolars and 26% of maxillary incisors. The mesial roots of mandibular molars (50%) and maxillary premolars (48%) and the mesial roots of maxillary molars (42%) had the highest percentage of multiple main foramina. This finding is consistent with observations that blunted roots usually have more than one root canal. The mean values for the size of the main foramen are listed in Table 5-6. Sizes ranged from 210 μm for the maxillary premolars to 392 μm for the distal roots of the mandibular molars. All groups of teeth had at least one accessory foramen. The maxillary premolars had the most and the largest accessory foramina (mean value, 53 μm) and the most complicated apical morphologic makeup. The mandibular premolars had strikingly similar characteristics, a possible reason root canal procedures may fail in premolar teeth.

The morphology of the apical third of the root reflects multiple anatomic variations, including numerous accessory canals; areas of resorption and repaired resorption; attached, embedded, and free pulp stones; varying amounts of reparative dentin; and varying root canal diameters (Table 5-7).[140,141] Primary dentinal tubules are found less often than in the coronal dentin and are more or less irregular in direction and density. Some areas are completely devoid of tubules. Fine tubular branches (300 to 700 μm in diameter) that run at a 45-degree angle to the main tubules and microbranches (25 to 200 μm in diameter) that run at a 90-degree angle to the main tubules are often present (Fig. 5-22). This variable nature of the apical structure and significant absence of dentinal tubules may lead to reduced chances of bacterial invasion into the dentinal walls; however, it also presents challenges for all root canal procedures, from cleaning and disinfection to obturation.

Clinically, considerable controversy exists over the exact termination point for root canal procedures in the apical third of the root; clinical determination of apical canal morphology is difficult at best.[84,193] The existence of an AC may be more conceptual than real. Several studies have reported that a traditional single AC was present less than half the time, particularly when apical root resorption and periradicular pathosis were factors.[44,55,192,238] The apical portion of the root canal often

TABLE 5-7

Median Canal Diameter 1, 2, and 5 mm from Apex

Tooth (Canal) Position	Buccal/Lingual			Mesial/Distal		
	1 mm	2 mm	5 mm	1 mm	2 mm	5 mm
Maxillary						
Central incisor	0.34	0.47	0.76	0.3	0.36	0.54
Lateral incisor	0.45	0.6	0.77	0.33	0.33	0.47
Canine	0.31	0.58	0.63	0.29	0.44	0.5
Premolar						
Single canal	0.37	0.63	1.13	0.26	0.41	0.38
Buccal	0.3	0.4	0.35	0.23	0.31	0.31
Palatal	0.23	0.37	0.42	0.17	0.26	0.33
Molar						
Single mesiobuccal	0.43	0.46	0.96	0.22	0.32	0.29
First mesiobuccal	0.19	0.37	0.46	0.13	0.27	0.32
Second mesiobuccal	0.19	0.31	0.38	0.16	0.16	0.16
Distobuccal	0.22	0.33	0.49	0.17	0.25	0.31
Palatal	0.29	0.4	0.55	0.33	0.4	0.74
Mandibular						
Incisor	0.37	0.52	0.81	0.25	0.25	0.29
Canine	0.47	0.45	0.74	0.36	0.36	0.57
Premolar						
Single	0.35	0.4	0.76	0.28	0.32	0.49
Buccal	0.2	0.34	0.36	0.23	0.29	0.41
Palatal	0.13	0.32	0.37	0.18	0.21	0.17
Molar						
Single M	0.45	0.8	2.11	0.22	0.3	0.29
Mesiobuccal	0.4	0.42	0.64	0.21	0.26	0.32
Mesiolingual	0.38	0.44	0.61	0.28	0.24	0.35
Distal	0.46	0.5	1.07	0.35	0.34	0.59

From Wu M-K, R'oris A, Barkis D, Wesselink P: Prevalence and extent of long oval canals in the apical third, *Oral Surg Oral Med Oral Pathol Oral Radiol Endod* 89:739, 2000.

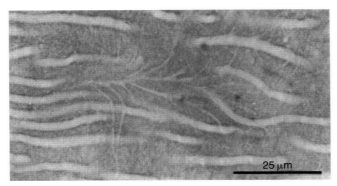

FIG. 5-22 Fine tubules and microbranches can be seen in the apical part of the root. (From Mjör IA, Nordahl I: The density and branching of dentinal tubules in human teeth, *Arch Oral Biol* 41:401, 1996.)

is tapered, or the walls are parallel to each other, or the canal has multiple constrictions.[55] Weine[238] recommended the following termination points: 1 mm from the apex when no bone or root resorption has occurred; 1.5 mm from the apex when only bone resorption has occurred; and 2 mm from the apex when both bone and root resorption are present.

Locating the AC and AF is difficult clinically; for this reason, some researchers contend that the radiographic apex is a more reliable reference point.[250] These authors recommend that root canal procedures terminate at or within 3 mm of the radiographic apex, depending on the pulpal diagnosis. For vital cases, clinical and biologic evidence indicates that a favorable point at which to terminate therapy is 2 to 3 mm short of the radiographic apex.[103,195] This leaves an apical pulp stump, which prevents extrusion of irritating filling materials into the periradicular tissues. However, what is not recognized commonly among clinicians is that this so-called pulp stump is actually not pulp tissue, but rather periodontal tissue that can ensure apical healing with cementum over the root end (see Fig. 5-21). On the other hand, pulp necrosis, bacteria and their byproducts, and biofilms may be present in the apical root canal, which may negate healing if they are not removed thoroughly during root canal procedures. Studies have shown that in these cases, a better success rate is achieved when therapy ends at or within 2 mm of the radiographic apex.[102,103,195] When the intracanal procedures ended short of the 2-mm point or extended past the radiographic apex, the success rate declined by 20%. For revision of procedural failures, apical procedures should extend to or preferably 1 to 2 mm short of the radiographic apex to prevent overextension of instruments and filling materials into the periradicular tissues (see Chapters 6 and 8).

Many investigators who have evaluated apical and periradicular tissues after root canal procedures concluded that the most favorable prognosis was obtained when procedures were terminated at the AC, and the worst prognosis was produced by treatment that extended beyond the AC.[113-116,180] Procedures terminated more than 2 mm from the AC had the second worst prognosis. These findings occurred with root canal procedures in teeth with both vital and necrotic pulps and when bacteria were present beyond the AF. Sealer or gutta-percha (or both) in the periradicular tissues, lateral canals, and apical ramifications may cause a severe inflammatory reaction. However, it is difficult to locate the AC clinically, which is why some studies direct clinicians to terminate all procedures at or beyond the radiographic apex, thereby filling all apical ramifications and lateral canals.[186] This dictate is empirically based, and CBCT evaluation of procedures previously thought to be successful has allowed identification of more posttreatment disease.[158]

Although the apical limit of instrumentation and obturation during root canal procedures continues to be the subject of major controversy, modern electronic apex locators can help the clinician determine the approximate working length of the root canal with greater assuredness. The ultimate challenges are that the two hallmarks of the apical region are its variability and unpredictability. The tremendous variation in canal shapes and diameters complicates enlargement and shaping procedures in all dimensions. Success in these goals depends on the anatomy of the root canal system, the dimensions of the canal walls, use of the appropriate instruments within these confines, and the operator's skill and experience.

OBJECTIVES AND GUIDELINES FOR ACCESS CAVITY PREPARATION

Objectives

Access to the complex root canal system is the first and arguably the most important phase of any nonsurgical root canal procedure.[84,212] The objectives of access cavity preparation are to (1) remove all caries when present, (2) conserve sound tooth structure, (3) unroof the pulp chamber completely, (4) remove all coronal pulp tissue (vital or necrotic), (5) locate all root canal orifices, and (6) achieve straight- or direct-line access to the apical foramen or to the initial curvature of the canal. If done properly, a thorough assessment of the restorative needs of every tooth can be made (e.g., the need for crown lengthening, a post, or simply a bonded core or composite to ensure the structural integrity of the tooth after root canal procedures).

A properly prepared access cavity creates a smooth, straight-line path to the canal system and ultimately to the apex or position of the first curvature (Fig. 5-23, *A*). Straight-line access provides the best chance of débridement of the entire canal space; it reduces the risk of instrument breakage[143]; and it results in straight entry into the canal orifice, with the line angles forming a funnel that drops smoothly into the canal (or canals). Projection of the canal center line to the occlusal surface of the tooth indicates the location of the line angles (Fig. 5-23, *B*). Connection of the line angles creates the outline form. Modifications of the access outline form may be needed to facilitate location of canals and to create a convenient form for the planned procedures.

KEY STEPS TO CONSIDER IN ACCESS PREPARATION

Visualization of the Likely Internal Anatomy

Internal tooth anatomy dictates access shape; therefore, the first step in preparing an access cavity is visualization of the position of the pulp space in the tooth. This visualization requires evaluation of angled periapical radiographs and examination of the tooth anatomy at the coronal, cervical, and root levels. Although only two-dimensional, diagnostic radiographs help the clinician estimate the position of the pulp chamber, the degree of chamber calcification, the number of roots and canals, and the approximate canal length. Palpation along the attached gingiva may aid in the determination of root location and direction. This information, when considered together, guides the clinician in the direction of the bur that is chosen to begin cutting the access cavity.

Evaluation of the Cementoenamel Junction and Occlusal Tooth Anatomy

Traditionally, access cavities have been prepared in relation to the occlusal anatomy. However, complete reliance on the occlusal/lingual anatomy is dangerous because this morphology can change as the crown is destroyed by caries and reconstructed with various restorative materials. Likewise, the root may not be perpendicular to the occlusal surface of the tooth; thus complete dependence on the occlusal or lingual anatomy may explain the occurrence of some procedural errors, such as coronal perforations along the cervical line or into the furcation. Krasner and Rankow[107] found that the cementoenamel junction (CEJ) was the most important anatomic landmark for determining the location of pulp chambers and root canal orifices. Their study demonstrated the existence of a specific and consistent anatomy of the pulp chamber floor. These authors proposed guidelines, or spatial concepts, that apply to the 3D assessment of the pulp chamber anatomy and that can help the clinician determine the number and location of orifices on the chamber floor (see Fig. 5-23, *B*).

Centrality: The floor of the pulp chamber is always located in the center of the tooth at the level of the CEJ.

Concentricity: The walls of the pulp chamber are always concentric to the external surface of the tooth at the level of the CEJ; that is, the external root surface anatomy reflects the internal pulp chamber anatomy.

Location of the CEJ: The distance from the external surface of the clinical crown to the wall of the pulp chamber is the same throughout the circumference of the tooth at the level of the CEJ, making the CEJ the most consistent repeatable landmark for locating the position of the pulp chamber.

Symmetry: Except for the maxillary molars, canal orifices are equidistant from a line drawn in a mesiodistal direction through the center of the pulp chamber floor. Except for the maxillary molars, canal orifices lie on a line perpendicular to a line drawn in a mesiodistal direction across the center of the pulp chamber floor.

Color change: The pulp chamber floor is always darker in color than the walls.

Orifice location: The orifices of the root canals are always located at the junction of the walls and the floor; the

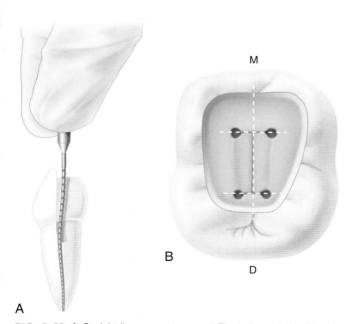

FIG. 5-23 A, Straight-line access to a canal. The instrument should not be deflected until it reaches the initial canal curvature. In some cases coronal tooth structure must be sacrificed to obtain direct access to the pulp chamber. **B,** Diagrammatic representation of centrality and concentricity of symmetry and location of canal orifices. *D,* Distal; *M,* mesial.

orifices of the root canals are always located at the angles in the floor-wall junction; and the orifices of the root canals are always located at the terminus of the roots' developmental fusion lines.

More than 95% of the teeth these investigators examined conformed to these spatial relationships.[107] Slightly less than 5% of mandibular second and third molars did not conform because of the occurrence of C-shaped anatomy.

Preparation of the Access Cavity Through the Lingual and Occlusal Surfaces

Access cavities on anterior teeth usually are prepared through the lingual tooth surface, and those on posterior teeth are prepared through the occlusal surface. These approaches are the best for achieving straight-line access while reducing esthetic and restorative concerns. Some authors have recommended that the traditional anterior access for mandibular incisors be moved from the lingual surface to the incisal surface in selected cases[135]; this allows better access to the lingual canal and improves canal débridement (Fig. 5-24). In

teeth that are lingually inclined or rotated, this is often the preferred choice for access and is performed before the dental dam is placed, or careful alignment of the root is determined before a bur is used.[84] Likewise, initial access through crowns may be better achieved without a dental dam in place so that the inclination of the root can be visualized; this information can be used as an indicator of the direction of the long axis of the treated tooth. Furthermore, canal identification and partial enlargement before dental dam placement may be beneficial in some cases. The Micro-Opener (Dentsply Maillefer) (Fig. 5-25, A) and EndoHandle with Find and File instruments (Venta Innovative Dental Products, Logan, Utah) (Fig. 5-25, B) are excellent instruments for locating canal orifices and developing the canal pathway when a dental dam has not been placed. These flexible, stainless steel hand instruments have variably tapered tips and permit not only canal identification, but also initial pathway formation when indicated. The former has offset handles that provide enhanced visualization of the pulp chamber, whereas the latter permits the use of a wide variety of instruments of different sizes.

Removal of All Defective Restorations and Caries before Entry Into the Pulp Chamber

Removal of all defective restorations and caries before entering the root canal system is essential for many reasons.[84] Hidden caries or fractures are often identified, and the ability to determine the restorability of the tooth is enhanced. In this respect it is not uncommon, before entering the pulp chamber, to stop with the access opening preparation in favor of a crown lengthening procedure or adding a bonded buildup. Subsequently, the tooth will be much easier to isolate before entry into the pulp chamber, and sound restorative margins will have been identified. In some cases, an extraction may be indicated because of tooth fracture or unrestorability (Fig. 5-26). Ultimately, with an open preparation, canals are much easier to locate, especially under enhanced illumination and magnification, and intracanal procedures are facilitated. Studies have indicated that clinicians were about 40% more likely to miss fractures, caries, and marginal breakdown if restorations were not completely removed.[1] Working through a clean access also

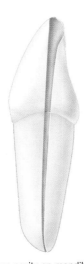

FIG. 5-24 An incisal access cavity on mandibular anterior teeth may allow for improved straight-line access and canal débridement.

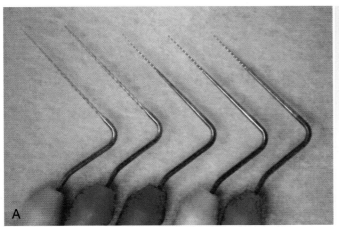

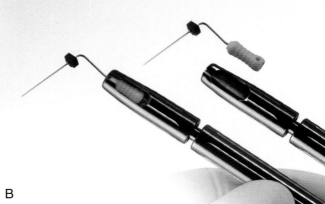

FIG. 5-25 **A,** Set of Micro-Openers (Dentsply Maillefer) for canal identification and enlargement. **B,** Similar tool but with changeable instruments that are placed in the EndoHandle (Courtesy Venta Endo) and can be positioned straight or at different angles.

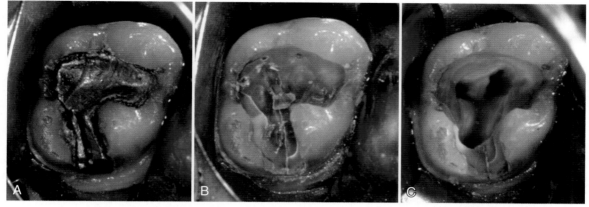

FIG. 5-26 **A,** Maxillary molar requiring root canal procedure. **B,** Removal of the amalgam reveals a vertical fracture on the palatal margin. **C,** Complete cleaning and shaping of the canals. Fracture lines are still visible, but no probings are present. (From Gutmann JL, Lovdahl PE: *Problem solving in endodontics,* ed 5, St Louis, 2011, Elsevier.)

prevents restorative debris from becoming dislodged and inadvertently pushed into the canal system.

Removal of Unsupported Tooth Structure

Along with the removal of caries and restorations, unsupported tooth structure should be removed to prevent tooth fracture during or between procedures. Although unnecessary removal of sound tooth structure should be avoided, oftentimes the access shape may have to be modified to facilitate canal location and intracanal procedures.

Preparation of Access Cavity Walls that Do Not Restrict Straight- or Direct-Line Passage of Instruments to the Apical Foramen or Initial Canal Curvature

Sufficient tooth structure must be removed to allow instruments to be placed easily into each canal orifice without interference from canal walls, particularly when a canal curves severely or leaves the chamber floor at an obtuse angle. Hence, access design depends not only on the orifice location, but also on the position and curvature of the entire canal. The walls of the root canal, rather than the walls of the access preparation, must guide the passage of instruments into the canal. Failure to follow this guideline results in treatment errors, including root perforation, misdirection of an instrument from the main canal (ledge formation), instrument separation, or creation of an incorrect canal shape (apical transportation).

Inspection of the Pulp Chamber Walls and Floor

Magnification is particularly important during initial root canal procedures, especially for determining the location of canals and removing tissue and calcifications from the pulp chamber. Illumination provided by the use of many magnification tools, in particular the DOM, aids in the initial negotiation of constricted, curved, and partially calcified canals. Enhanced vision allows the clinician to see internal dentin color changes and subtle landmarks that may not be visible to the unaided eye, including previously hidden cracks and decay. Surgical loupes

and endodontic endoscopes[12] are also available to help in locating intricate root canal systems. In most cases, after dental dam placement, in addition to magnification, a sharp endodontic explorer (DG-16) is used to locate canal orifices and to determine their angle of departure from the pulp chamber.

Tapering of Cavity Walls and Evaluation of Space Adequacy for a Coronal Seal

A proper access cavity generally has tapering walls, with its widest dimension at the occlusal surface. In such a preparation, occlusal forces do not push the temporary restoration into the cavity and disrupt the seal. A minimum 3.5 mm of temporary filling material (e.g., Cavit; 3M ESPE, St. Paul, Minnesota) is needed to provide an adequate coronal seal for a short time.[237] Recently, canal orifice plugs of composite, glass ionomer, and mineral trioxide aggregate (ProRoot MTA, Dentsply Tulsa Dental Specialties) have shown promise in reducing the risk of bacterial contamination of the canal system when microleakage occurs at the coronal-restorative margins.[96]

MECHANICAL PHASES OF ACCESS CAVITY PREPARATION

The preparation of an access cavity requires the following equipment:
- Magnification and illumination
- Handpieces
- Burs
- Endodontic explorers
- Endodontic spoon
- Ultrasonic unit and tips

Magnification and Illumination

The access cavity is best prepared with the use of magnification and an appropriate light source. In lieu of a DOM, surgical loupes with an auxiliary light source are highly recommended.

Handpieces

Good tactile awareness is essential to perform most phases of access preparation with a high-speed handpiece. In many cases,

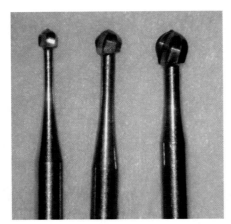

FIG. 5-27 Access burs: #2, #4, and #6 round carbide burs.

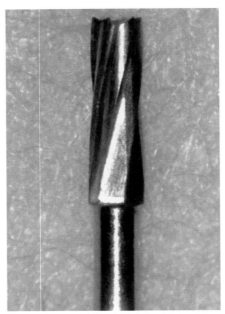

FIG. 5-28 Access bur: #57 fissure carbide bur.

the use of a slow-speed handpiece is indicated, which is especially helpful in the careful excavation of caries located in the area of the anticipated access opening. For challenging access cavity preparations, especially those involving calcified and receded pulp chambers, even experienced clinicians may sacrifice cutting speed and efficiency in favor of the increased cutting control of the slow-speed handpiece or an ultrasonic tip.

Burs

Numerous burs have been developed exclusively for access cavity preparation. Providing a detailed, unabridged list of these burs would be difficult, and most clinicians have their own set of preferred access burs. To meet the overall needs in this regard, various companies have developed access kits with a large variety of burs (Dentsply Tulsa Dental Specialities; SS White, Lakewood, New Jersey; SybronEndo, Orange, California; Ultradent Products, Inc., South Jordan, Utah). In reality, creating an access cavity that meets the previously stated guidelines is more important than worrying about which burs are used in the process. This discussion, therefore, covers some of the more common access burs.

Round carbide burs (sizes #2, #4, and #6) (Fig. 5-27) are used extensively in the preparation of access cavities. They are used to excavate caries and to create the initial external outline shape. They also are useful for penetrating through the roof of the pulp chamber and for removing the roof. Some clinicians prefer to use a fissure carbide bur (Fig. 5-28) or a diamond bur with a rounded cutting end (Fig. 5-29) to perform these procedures. The advantage of the fissure carbide and diamond round-end burs is that they also can be used for some of the axial wall extensions of the access cavity preparation. However, when these burs are used for this purpose by inexperienced clinicians, their cutting ends can gouge the pulp floor and axial walls.

Fissure carbide and diamond burs with safety tips (i.e., noncutting ends) (Fig. 5-30) are safer choices for axial wall extensions. They can be used to extend and favorably orient the axial walls of the pulp chamber. Because they have no cutting end, the burs can be allowed to extend to the pulp floor, and the entire axial wall can be moved and oriented all in one plane from the enamel surface to the pulp floor. Such a technique produces axial walls free of gouges as the final access extensions are created. Fissure carbide and diamond burs also can be used to level off cusp tips and incisal edges,

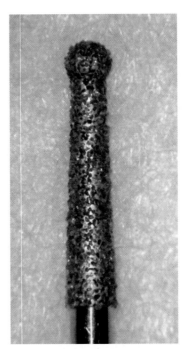

FIG. 5-29 Access bur: Round-end cutting tapered diamond bur.

which are used as reference points for the working length determination.

Round diamond burs (sizes #2 and #4) (Fig. 5-31) are needed when the access must be made through porcelain or metalloceramic restorations.[84] Diamond burs are less traumatic to porcelain than carbide burs and are more likely to penetrate the porcelain without cracking or fracturing it. They should always be used with water spray to control heat buildup in porcelain restorations. After penetrating the porcelain with a diamond bur, a carbide bur, such as a transmetal bur (Dentsply Maillefer) (Fig. 5-32), is used for metal or dentin penetration because of this bur's greater cutting efficiency.[84]

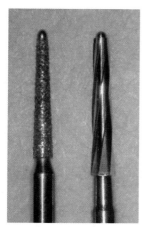

FIG. 5-30 Access burs: Safety-tip tapered diamond bur *(left);* safety-tip tapered carbide bur *(right)*.

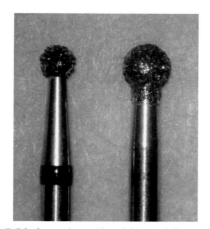

FIG. 5-31 Access burs: #2 and #4 round diamond burs.

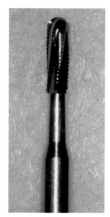

FIG. 5-32 Access bur: Transmetal bur.

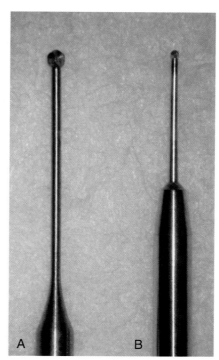

FIG. 5-33 Access burs. **A,** Mueller bur. **B,** LN bur or Extendo Bur.

A significant trend in restorative dentistry is the increased use of zirconia-based crowns and onlays. Zirconia has different mechanical and thermal characteristics than metal. Carbide burs do not cut zirconia efficiently or safely. Zirconia is a brittle material and when cut can develop cracks that propagate through the framework and lead to eventual failure of the crown or onlay. Diamond bur manufacturers are aware of these issues, and they are currently introducing medium- and fine-grit diamond burs that efficiently cut zirconia (Komet USA, Savannah, Georgia; Prima Dental Gloucester, England; SS White). These diamond burs should be used with copious water spray to minimize heat buildup in the zirconia crowns during access preparations.[84] Also, some diamond burs may degrade rapidly when cutting through zirconia and should be thrown away after one use.

Many teeth requiring access cavity preparations have metal restorations that must be penetrated. These restorations may be amalgams, all-metal cast restorations, or metal copings of porcelain fused to metal crowns. As previously mentioned, a transmetal bur is excellent for cutting through metal because of its exceptional cutting efficiency. To penetrate a metallic restoration, a new transmetal bur is recommended for each restoration, together with copious water spray for maximal cutting effect.

When a receded pulp chamber and calcified orifice are identified, or to locate and identify the canal orifice, countersinking or cutting into the root is often indicated. Extended-shank round burs, such as the Mueller bur (Brasseler USA, Savannah, Georgia) (Fig. 5-33, *A*) or Extendo Bur (Dentsply Tulsa Dental Specialties), also known as the LN bur (Dentsply Maillefer) (Fig. 5-33, *B*), can be used. The Munce Discovery bur (CJM Engineering, Santa Barbara, California) is similar to the Mueller bur but has a stiffer shaft and is available in smaller head sizes. The extra-long shank of these burs moves the head of the handpiece away from the tooth, improving the clinician's visibility during this delicate procedure. As an alternative, ultrasonic units offer good visibility with precision cutting.

Once the orifices have been located, they should be flared or enlarged and blended into the axial walls of the access cavity. This process permits the intracanal instruments used during the enlargement and shaping procedures to penetrate the canal effortlessly. Some clinicians might consider this task part of the

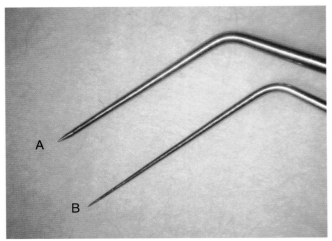

FIG. 5-34 **A,** Access instruments: DG-16 endodontic explorer. **B,** JW-17 endodontic explorer.

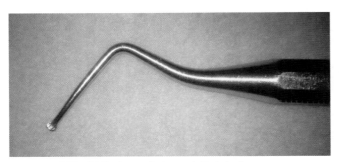

FIG. 5-35 Access instrument: Endodontic spoon.

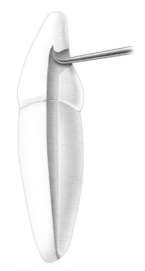

FIG. 5-36 Removal of the pulp horn is evaluated with a #17 operative explorer.

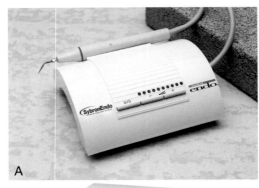

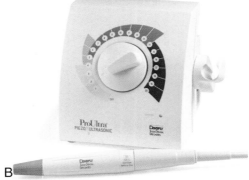

FIG. 5-37 **A,** Endo ultrasonic unit (MiniEndo II). **B,** ProUltra Piezo Ultrasonic. (**A** courtesy SybronEndo, Orange, Calif; **B** courtesy DENTSPLY Tulsa Dental Specialties, Tulsa, Okla.)

canal enlargement and shaping phase; however, when done before deep canal penetration, it establishes a well-prepared access opening and may prevent subsequent error.

Endodontic Explorer and Spoon

Various hand instruments are useful for preparing access cavities. The DG-16 endodontic explorer (Fig. 5-34, *A*) is used to identify canal orifices and to determine canal angulation. An alternative, the JW-17 endodontic explorer (Fig. 5-34, *B*) (CK Dental Industries, Orange, California) serves the same purpose, but its thinner, stiffer tip can be useful for identifying the possible location of a calcified canal. A sharp endodontic spoon, which comes in different sizes (Fig. 5-35) can be used to remove coronal pulp and carious dentin. A #17 operative explorer, which can also be found as a doubled-ended instrument with the DG-16, is useful for detecting any remaining overhang from the pulp chamber roof, particularly in the area of a pulp horn of anterior teeth (Fig. 5-36). Failure to remove this overhang, along with the propensity for it to harbor tissue debris, often leads to tooth discoloration, especially in teeth restored only with bonded palatal composite.

Ultrasonic Unit and Tips

Ultrasonic units (Fig. 5-37) and tips specifically designed for activities during access opening preparation are extremely valuable. Ultrasonic tips from various manufacturers can be used to trough and deepen developmental grooves, remove tissue, and explore for canals. Ultrasonic systems provide

outstanding visibility compared with traditional handpiece heads, which typically obstruct vision. Fine ultrasonic tips, such as Sine Tips, ProUltra Tips, and Smart X BUC Tips (Dentsply Tulsa Dental Specialties; Dentsply Maillefer; and SybronEndo, respectively), are smaller than round burs, and their abrasive coatings or variable surfaces permit careful shaving away of dentin and calcifications during exploration for canal orifices.

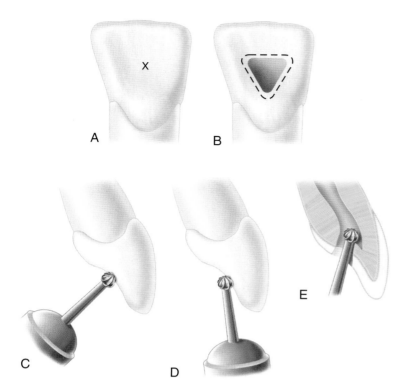

FIG. 5-38 **A,** In anterior teeth the starting location for the access cavity is the center of the anatomic crown on the lingual surface *(X)*. **B,** Preliminary outline form for anterior teeth. The shape should mimic the expected final outline form, and the size should be half to three fourths the size of the final outline form. **C,** The angle of penetration for the preliminary outline form is perpendicular to the lingual surface. **D,** The angle of penetration for initial entry into the pulp chamber is nearly parallel to the long axis of the root. **E,** Completion of removal of the pulp chamber roof; a round carbide bur is used to engage the pulp horn, cutting on a lingual withdrawal stroke.

ACCESS CAVITY PREPARATIONS

Anterior Teeth

The following discussion outlines the steps for maxillary and mandibular anterior teeth. Tooth-specific access concerns are illustrated and discussed in the section Morphology of and Access Cavity Preparations for Individual Teeth, later in the chapter.

External Outline Form

Once caries and restorations have been removed as necessary to establish sound tooth margins, an initial external outline opening is cut on the lingual surface of the anterior tooth. This step may also be performed during the removal of caries and restorations. For an intact tooth, cutting commences at the center of the lingual or palatal surface of the anatomic crown (Fig. 5-38, *A*). A #2 or #4 round bur or a tapered fissure bur may be used to penetrate the enamel and slightly into the dentin (approximately 1 mm). An outline form is developed that is similar in geometry to an ideal access shape for the particular anterior tooth (Fig. 5-38, *B*); it is half to three quarters the projected final size of the access cavity. Because most of this step involves removal of enamel, the high-speed handpiece is used for cutting efficiency. The bur is directed perpendicular to the lingual surface as the external outline opening is created (Fig. 5-38, *C*).

Penetration of the Pulp Chamber Roof

Experienced clinicians usually penetrate the pulp chamber roof using a high-speed handpiece; however, less experienced clinicians may find the increased tactile sensation of a slow-speed handpiece a safer option. Continuing with the same round or tapered fissure bur, the angle of the bur is rotated from perpendicular to the lingual/palatal surface to parallel to the long axis of the root (see Fig. 5-38, *D*). Penetration into the tooth continues along the root's long axis until the roof of the pulp chamber is penetrated; frequently, a drop into the chamber effect is felt when this occurs. Measuring the distance from the incisal edge to the roof of the pulp chamber on a dimensionally accurate pretreatment radiograph may serve as guide in limiting penetration and possibly preventing a perforation. If the drop-in effect is not felt at this depth, an endodontic explorer can be used to probe the depth of the access, using magnification or the DOM. Often a small opening into the chamber is present, or the dentin is very thin and the explorer penetrates into the chamber. The depth and angle of penetration should be assessed for any deviation away from the long axis of the root in both the mesiodistal and buccolingual dimensions, and the penetration angle should be realigned if necessary. Angled radiographs can be used to assess progress at any time if any confusion or doubt exists. A little caution and concern at this stage can prevent a mishap.

Removal of the Chamber Roof

Once the pulp chamber has been penetrated, the remaining roof is removed by catching the end of a round bur under the lip of the dentin roof and cutting on the bur's withdrawal stroke (see Fig. 5-38, *E*). Because each tooth has a unique pulp chamber anatomy, working in this manner enables the internal pulp anatomy to dictate the external outline form of the access opening. In teeth with irreversible pulpitis, pulp tissue hemorrhage can impair vision during this process. In such cases, as soon as sufficient roof structure has been removed to allow instrument access, the coronal pulp should be amputated at the orifice level with a spoon or round bur and the chamber irrigated copiously with sodium hypochlorite. If the hemorrhage continues, a tentative canal length can be established by measuring the pretreatment radiograph. A small broach coated

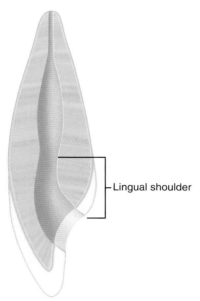

FIG. 5-39 Lingual shoulder of the anterior tooth, extending from the cingulum to 2 mm apical to the orifice.

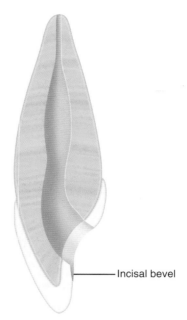

FIG. 5-40 Placing an incisal bevel on the lingual surface of a maxillary anterior tooth can lead to fracture of the permanent restoration during occlusal function.

with a chelating agent then can be used loosely in the canal to grasp and sever the pulp at a more apical level. Copious irrigation with sodium hypochlorite helps control hemorrhage. Subsequently, the chamber roof, including the pulp horns, is removed and all internal walls are flared to the lingual surface of the tooth. Complete roof removal is confirmed with a #17 operative explorer if no "catches" are identified as the explorer tip is withdrawn from the pulp chamber along the mesial, distal, and facial walls.

Removal of the Lingual Shoulder and Coronal Flaring of the Orifice

Once the orifice or orifices have been identified and confirmed, the lingual shoulder or ledge is removed. This is a shelf of dentin that extends from the cingulum to a point approximately 2 mm apical to the orifice (Fig. 5-39). Its removal improves straight-line access and allows for more intimate contact of files with the canal's walls for effective shaping and cleaning. In addition, its removal from mandibular anterior teeth may often expose an extra orifice and canal.

The contemporary approach to flaring the orifice involves the use of rotary nickel-titanium (NiTi) orifice openers that allow rapid, safe removal of the lingual ledge, following the manufacturer's directions for use (DFUs). When used properly, these openers allow refinement of the orifice shape or help to enhance straight-line access to the canal with minimal removal of dentin. Although there may be subtle differences in these instruments from manufacturer to manufacturer, proper application achieves the same objective. A time-tested and traditional way to achieve the same goal involves the use of a tapered, safety-tip diamond or carbide bur or a Gates-Glidden bur. However, use of these instruments may result in excessive removal of cervical dentin. When a fine, safety-tip diamond bur is used, the tip is placed approximately 2 mm apical to the canal orifice and inclined to the lingual during rotation to slope the lingual shoulder. The bur should be placed so as to avoid putting a bevel on the incisal edge of the access preparation (Fig. 5-40). When Gates-Glidden burs are used, the largest that

can be placed passively 2 mm apical to the orifice is used first. During rotation, gentle pressure is applied on the bur as it cuts against the lingual shoulder and then is withdrawn. The size of these burs can be increased sequentially, depending on the size of the canal, with repeated shaping of the lingual wall until the lingual shoulder of dentin has been eliminated in anterior teeth. During this process, the orifice is often concomitantly flared so that it is contiguous with all walls of the access preparation. If this is not achieved, use of the orifice openers is recommended.

Straight-Line Access Determination

After removal of the lingual shoulder and flaring of the orifice, straight-line access must be determined. Ideally, a small intracanal file can reach the apical foramen or the first point of canal curvature with no deflections. Unnecessary deflection of the file can result in numerous consequences related to loss of instrument control. Deflected instruments function under more stress than those with minimal or no deflection pressure and are more susceptible to separation during enlargement and shaping (Fig. 5-41). Deflected instruments also lack access to critical areas of the canal and therefore do not function effectively. Without straight-line access, procedural errors (e.g., ledging, transportation, and zipping) may occur, but this is primarily seen with the use of hand files or larger NiTi instruments (Fig. 5-42).

If the lingual shoulder has been removed properly and a file still binds on the incisal edge, the access cavity should be extended further incisally until the file is not deflected (Fig. 5-43). The final position of the incisal wall of the access cavity is determined by two factors: (1) complete removal of the pulp horns and (2) straight-line access.

Visual Inspection of the Access Cavity

Appropriate magnification and illumination should be used to inspect and evaluate the completed access cavity. Although this

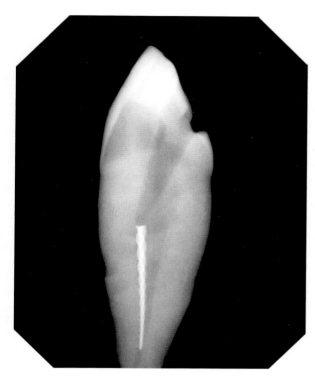

FIG. 5-41 Separation of a rotary endodontic instrument as a result of underextended access preparation rather than canal binding.

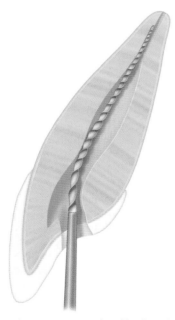

FIG. 5-42 Inadequate access preparation. The lingual shoulder was not removed, and incisal extension is incomplete. The file has begun to deviate from the canal in the apical region, creating a ledge.

can be done during any stage of the preparation, it should always be done at this point. The axial walls at their junction with the orifice must be inspected for grooves that might indicate an additional canal. The orifice and coronal portion of the canal must be evaluated for a bifurcation.

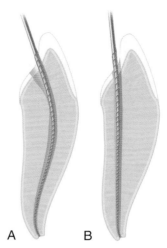

FIG. 5-43 **A**, The lingual ledge of dentin remains, deflecting the file toward the labial wall. As a result, portions of the lingual canal wall will not be shaped and cleaned. **B**, Removal of the lingual ledge results in straight-line access.

Refinement and Smoothing of Restorative Margins

The final step in the preparation of an access cavity is to refine and smooth the cavosurface margins. Rough or irregular margins can contribute to coronal leakage through a permanent or temporary restoration. Proper restorative margins are important because anterior teeth may not require a crown as the final restoration. Smooth cavosurface margins allow the placement of a composite resin restoration with the precision necessary to minimize coronal leakage. Such leakage could jeopardize the success of the root canal procedure.

Another factor to consider regarding the access margin of a maxillary anterior tooth is that the final composite resin restoration will be placed on a functional tooth surface. The incisal edges of the mandibular anterior teeth slide over these maxillary lingual surfaces during excursive jaw movements. Therefore, the restorative margins of an access cavity in maxillary anterior teeth should be created to allow a bulk of restorative material at the margin. Butt joint margins are indicated, rather than beveled margins, which produce thin composite edges that can fracture under functional loads and ultimately result in coronal leakage. If the anterior tooth requires a crown as the final restoration, the cavosurface margin becomes a less critical factor, although if it is not restored in a timely fashion, breakdown and leakage may occur.

Individual Anterior Teeth

See the figures in the section Morphology of and Access Cavity Preparations for Individual Teeth, later in this chapter.

Posterior Teeth

Preparing access cavities on posterior teeth is similar to the process for anterior teeth, but significant differences warrant a separate discussion.[84] Posterior teeth requiring root canal procedures typically have been heavily restored or the carious process was extensive. Such conditions, along with the complex pulp anatomy and position of posterior teeth in the oral cavity, can make the access process challenging.

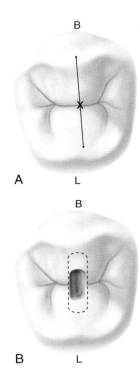

FIG. 5-44 **A,** Starting location for access to the maxillary premolar *(X).* **B,** Initial outline form *(dark area)* and projected final outline form *(dashed line).* *B,* Buccal; *L,* lingual.

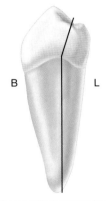

FIG. 5-45 The crown of a mandibular premolar is tilted lingually relative to the root. *B,* Buccal; *L,* lingual.

External Outline Form

Removal of caries and existing restorations from a posterior tooth requiring a root canal procedure often results in the development of an acceptable access outline form. However, if the tooth is intact, the access starting location must be determined for an intact tooth. The pulp chamber of posterior teeth is positioned in the center of the tooth at the level of the CEJ. Therefore, in maxillary premolars, the point of entry that determines the external outline form is on the central groove between the cusp tips (Fig. 5-44). Crowns of mandibular premolars are tilted lingually relative to their roots (Fig. 5-45); therefore, the starting location must be adjusted to compensate

for this tilt (Fig. 5-46). In mandibular first premolars, the starting location is halfway up the lingual incline of the buccal cusp on a line connecting the cusp tips. Mandibular second premolars require less of an adjustment because they have less lingual inclination. The starting location for this tooth is one third the way up the lingual incline of the buccal cusp on a line connecting the buccal cusp tip and the lingual groove between the lingual cusps.

To determine the starting location for molar access cavity preparations, the mesial-distal and apical-coronal boundary limitations for this outline must be determined (Fig. 5-47). Evaluation of bite-wing radiographs is an accurate method of assessing the mesiodistal extensions of the pulp chamber (Fig. 5-48). The mesial boundary for both the maxillary and mandibular molars is a line connecting the mesial cusp tips. Pulp chambers are rarely found mesial to this imaginary line. A good initial distal boundary for maxillary molars is the oblique ridge. For mandibular molars, the initial distal boundary is a line connecting the buccal and lingual grooves. For molars the correct starting location is on the central groove halfway between the mesial and distal boundaries.

Penetration through the enamel into the dentin (approximately 1 mm) is achieved with a #2 or #4 round bur for premolars and a #4 or #6 round bur for molars. A tapered fissure bur may be used instead of round burs. The bur is directed perpendicular to the occlusal table, and an initial outline shape is created at about half to three fourths its projected final size. The premolar shape is oval and widest in the buccolingual dimension. The molar shape is also oval initially; it is widest in a buccolingual dimension for maxillary molars and in a mesiodistal direction for mandibular molars. The final outline shape for molars is approximately triangular (for three canals) or rhomboid (for four canals); however, the canal orifices dictate the position of the corners of these geometric shapes. Therefore, until the orifices have been located, the initial outline form should be left as roughly oval.

Penetration of the Pulp Chamber Roof

Once initial penetration into the pulp chamber has been achieved, the angle of penetration changes from perpendicular to the occlusal table to an angle appropriate for penetration through the roof of the pulp chamber. In premolars the angle is parallel to the long axis of the root or roots, both in the mesiodistal and buccolingual directions. Failure to analyze this penetration angle carefully can result in gouging or perforation because premolar roots often are tilted relative to the occlusal plane. In molars the penetration angle should be toward the largest canal because the pulp chamber space usually is largest just occlusal to the orifice of this canal. Therefore, in maxillary molars, the penetration angle is toward the palatal orifice, and in mandibular molars, it is toward the distal orifice (Fig. 5-49).

As with anterior teeth, penetration is limited to the distance measured on a pretreatment radiograph to just penetrate the roof of the pulp chamber. If the drop-in effect is not felt at this depth, a careful evaluation of the angle of penetration is necessary before going deeper into the chamber. In multirooted posterior teeth, lateral and furcation perforations may occur rapidly without attention to 3D detail during this penetration. As with anterior teeth, aggressive probing with an endodontic explorer at any time during the penetration often can help locate the pulp chamber.

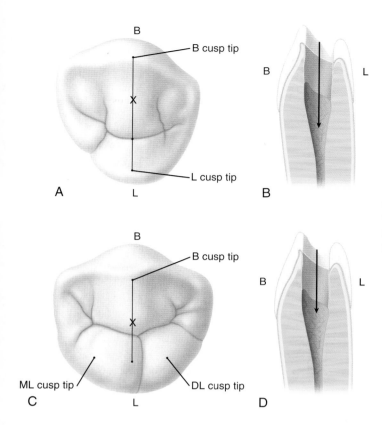

FIG. 5-46 **A,** Mandibular first premolar and access starting location *(X)* (occlusal view). **B,** Mandibular first premolar and starting location (proximal view). **C,** Mandibular second premolar and access starting location *(X)* (occlusal view). **D,** Mandibular second premolar and starting location (proximal view). *B,* Buccal; *DL,* distolingual; *L,* lingual; *ML,* mesiolingual.

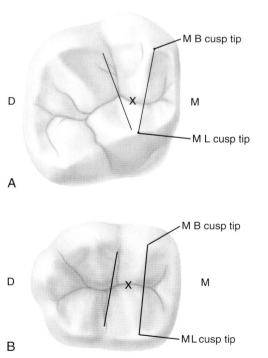

FIG. 5-47 **A,** Mesial and distal boundary of a maxillary molar with the access starting location *(X).* **B,** Mesial and distal boundary of a mandibular molar showing the access starting location *(X). D,* Distal; *M,* mesial; *MB,* mesiobuccal; *ML,* mesiolingual.

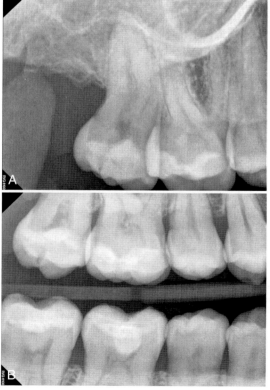

FIG. 5-48 **A,** Periapical radiograph of the teeth in the maxillary right quadrant. **B,** Bite-wing radiograph of the same teeth provides a clearer delineation of the pulpal morphology.

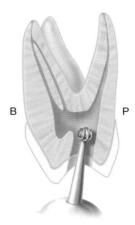

FIG. 5-49 Angle of penetration toward the largest canal (palatal) in a maxillary molar. *B,* Buccal; *P,* palatal.

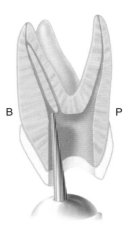

FIG. 5-51 Safety-tip carbide bur is used to shape the axial wall in one plane from the orifice to the cavosurface margin. *B,* Buccal; *P,* palatal.

FIG. 5-50 **A,** Pulp roof/pulp horn removal. The round bur hooks under the lip of the pulp horn. **B,** The bur is rotated and withdrawn in an occlusal direction to remove the lip. **C,** Removal of a cervical dentin bulge. A Gates-Glidden bur is placed just apical to the orifice and withdrawn in a distoocclusal direction. **D,** A safety-tip tapered diamond bur is used to blend and funnel the axial wall from the cavosurface margin to the orifice.

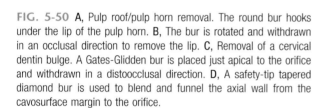

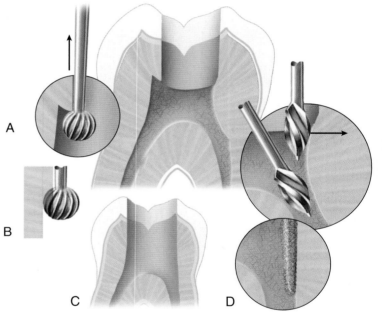

Removal of the Chamber Roof

The bur of choice is used to remove the roof of the pulp chamber completely, including all pulp horns (Fig. 5-50, *A* and *B*). Visibility problems caused by pulpal hemorrhage should be handled as described in the previous section for anterior teeth. The goal is to funnel the corners of the access cavity directly into the orifices, and a safety-tip diamond or carbide bur (Multi Bur, Dentsply Tulsa Dental Specialties) performs this task nicely (Fig. 5-50, *C* and *D*); it can be set on the pulp floor and the entire axial wall shaped at one time, with little or no apical pressure (Fig. 5-51). These burs are passed between the orifices along the axial walls to remove the roof, taper the internal walls, and create the desired external outline shape simultaneously.

Identification of All Canal Orifices

In posterior teeth with multiple canals, the canal orifices play an important role in determining the final extensions of the

external outline form of the access cavity. Ideally, the orifices are located at the corners of the final preparation to facilitate all of the root canal procedures (Fig. 5-52). Internally, the access cavity should have all orifices positioned entirely on the pulp floor and should not extend into an axial wall. Extension of an orifice into the axial wall creates a "mouse hole" effect (Fig. 5-53), which indicates internal underextension and impedes straight-line access. In such cases the orifice must be repositioned onto the pulp floor without interference from axial walls.

Removal of the Cervical Dentin Bulges and Orifice and Coronal Flaring

In posterior teeth the internal impediments to an ideal access opening are the cervical dentin ledges or bulges and the natural coronal canal constriction.[84] The cervical bulges are shelves of dentin that frequently overhang orifices in posterior teeth, restricting access into root canals and accentuating existing canal curvatures.[117] They can develop from mesial, distal, buccal, and lingual walls inward. These bulges can be removed safely with burs or ultrasonic instruments. The removal instruments should be placed at the orifice level, and light pressure should be used to cut laterally toward the dentin bulge to remove the overhanging ledge (Fig. 5-54). After removal of the ledge, the orifice and constricted coronal portion of the canal can be flared with NiTi orifice openers, Gates-Glidden burs, or large, tapered rotary instruments (.10/.12), which are used in a sweeping upward motion with minimal lateral pressure away from the furcation. As the orifice is enlarged, it should be tapered and blended into the axial wall so that an explorer can slide down the corner of the external outline form, down the axial wall, and into the orifice without encountering any obstructions (see Fig. 5-54).

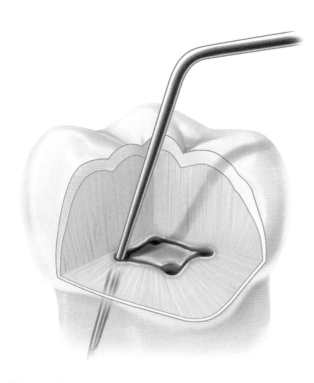

FIG. 5-52 An endodontic explorer is used to search for canal orifices.

Straight-Line Access Determination

Straight-line access is paramount to successful shaping, especially given the complexity of the root canal systems in posterior teeth. Files must have unimpeded access to the apical foramen or the first point of canal curvature to perform properly. Therefore, each canal must have straight-line access, and adjustments must be made accordingly (see Fig. 5-54, O).

Visual Inspection of the Pulp Chamber Floor

The floor and walls must be inspected, using appropriate magnification and illumination, to ensure that all canal orifices are visible and no roof overhangs are present (Fig. 5-55).

Refinement and Smoothing of the Restorative Margins

In both temporary and interim permanent restorations, the restorative margins should be refined and smoothed to minimize the potential for coronal leakage. The final permanent restoration of choice for posterior teeth that have undergone a root canal procedure is generally a crown or onlay, although this may vary, depending on the opposing dentition and patient function.

Individual Posterior Teeth

See the figures in the section Morphology of and Access Cavity Preparations for Individual Teeth, later in the chapter.

CHALLENGING ACCESS PREPARATIONS

Teeth with Minimal or No Clinical Crown

Forming an access cavity on a tooth with little or no clinical crown might seem to be a simple procedure. For example, in young teeth, traumatic fractures often expose the pulp chamber, making access preparation easy. However, in older teeth with previous caries or large restorations, the pulp chambers typically have receded or calcified (Fig. 5-56). Loss of significant coronal anatomy to guide penetration angles can make access quite difficult. A thorough evaluation of these teeth clinically and their root angulation on pretreatment radiographs is essential. Pulp chambers are located at the center of the crown at the level of the CEJ. Access often is started without a dental dam in place so that root eminences can be visualized and palpated as access preparation progresses (Fig. 5-57). Every effort is made to stay centered within the root for the best

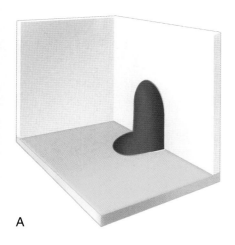

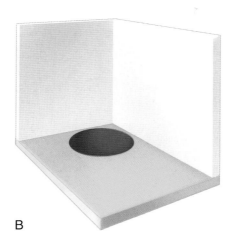

FIG. 5-53 **A**, Mouse hole effect caused by extension of the orifice into the axial wall. **B**, Orifice that lies completely on the pulp floor.

A   B

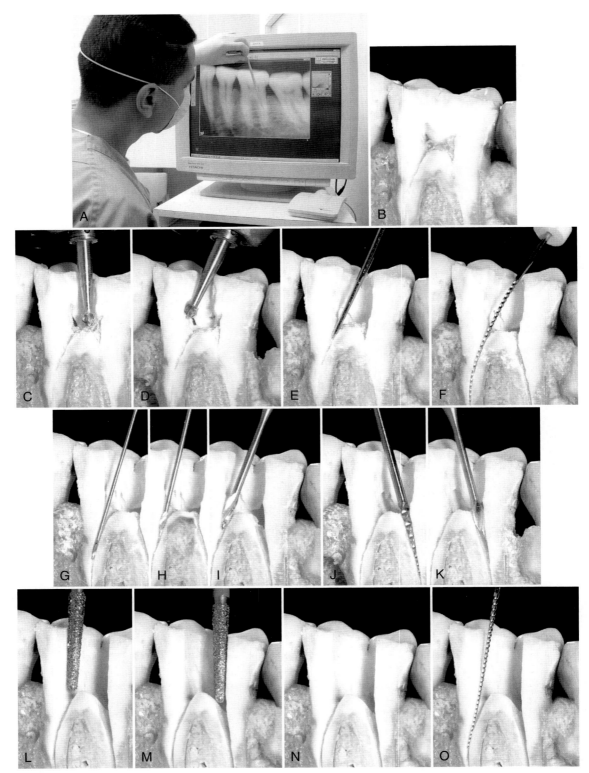

FIG. 5-54 **A,** Evaluation of the pretreatment radiograph. **B,** Clinical evaluation of the tooth. **C,** Penetration of the pulp roof. **D,** Removal of the pulp roof/pulp horns with a round carbide bur. **E,** Location of the orifice with a Mueller or LN bur. **F,** Exploration of the canal with a small K-file. **G to I,** Flaring of the orifice/coronal third of the mesial canal with Gates-Glidden burs. **J,** Flaring of the orifice/coronal third of the distal canal with a #.12 taper nickel-titanium rotary file. **K,** Flaring of the orifice/coronal third of the distal canal with a Gates-Glidden bur. **L,** Funneling of the mesial axial wall from the cavosurface margin to the mesial orifice. **M,** Funneling of the distal axial wall from the cavosurface margin to the distal orifice. **N,** Completed access preparation. **O,** Verification of straight-line access.

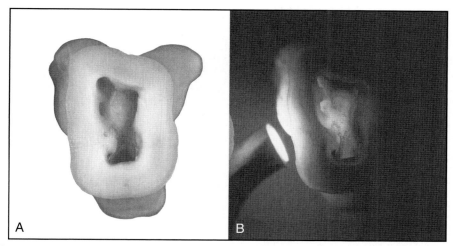

FIG. 5-55 A fiberoptic light can be applied to the cervical aspect of the crown to help obtain maximal visibility with magnification. Transillumination often reveals landmarks otherwise invisible to the unaided eye.

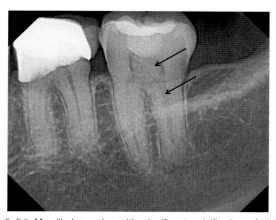

FIG. 5-56 Mandibular molar with significant calcification of the pulp chamber and canal spaces *(arrows)*.

chance of locating the pulp canal.[25] The depth of penetration needed to reach the pulp canal is measured on a pretreatment radiograph. If this depth is reached without locating the canal, two radiographs should be taken before the process proceeds. A straight-on radiograph shows whether the preparation is deviating in a mesial or distal direction. Applying the buccal object rule, an angled radiograph shows a buccal or lingual deviation in penetration. After checking these radiographs, the operator can alter the penetration angle, if necessary, while penetrating apically. As soon as the pulp canal is identified, the dental dam must be placed and the access preparation finalized, using the guidelines discussed previously.

Heavily Restored Teeth (Including Those with Full Coronal Coverage)

Restorative materials often alter the external anatomic landmarks on the crown of a tooth, making access preparation difficult. Restorative materials and full crowns rarely reproduce the original tooth anatomy in the exact same position. The crown-to-root angulation often is altered when large restorations or crowns correct occlusal discrepancies (Fig. 5-58). Most restorative materials block the passage of light into the

internal aspects of the tooth, resulting in poor visibility during preparation of the access cavity. All these factors, singly or together, complicate the preparation of access cavities on heavily restored teeth (Fig. 5-59).[1] The DOM and transillumination of the cervical area of a heavily restored tooth can greatly improve visibility and reveal landmarks that otherwise would be missed (see Fig. 5-55).

In most cases, complete removal of large restorations is the wisest course, and treatment should be planned accordingly (Fig. 5-60). These restorations often have leaking, defective margins or recurrent caries, or both. Removing the restoration enhances visibility of the internal anatomic structures through direct visualization and increased light penetration. With increased visibility, recurrent caries and fracture lines on the pulp chamber walls or floor can be seen, especially with the DOM. Clinicians are 40% more likely to miss these anomalies when restorations are not removed completely.[1] Better visibility also makes locating receded or calcified canals easier.

Coronal leakage often occurs when parts of large restorations are left in the tooth because the restorations are loosened by the vibration of the access drilling. Furthermore, removal of these restoration remnants prevents pieces of the restorative material from falling into the root canal. Instruments can rub against restoration fragments during the root canal procedures, creating filings that can be carried into the canal system. Thorough removal prevents these problems.

Complete removal of an extensive restoration from the cervical region of the tooth permits more direct access to the root canal or canals. For example, class V restorations often cause calcifications in the coronal portion of the canal, making location of the canal through the occlusal approach quite difficult. Removal of the class V restoration allows more direct access to the canal, which makes location and penetration much easier. Any remaining canals can be managed through the traditional occlusal access cavity (Fig. 5-61).

When an extensive restoration is a full metalloceramic or partial veneer crown, the restoration must be evaluated thoroughly. If any concerns arise about recurrent decay or leaking margins, the crown should be removed before an access cavity is formed. Removal of the crown allows elimination of all recurrent caries and improves the visibility of the pulp spaces.

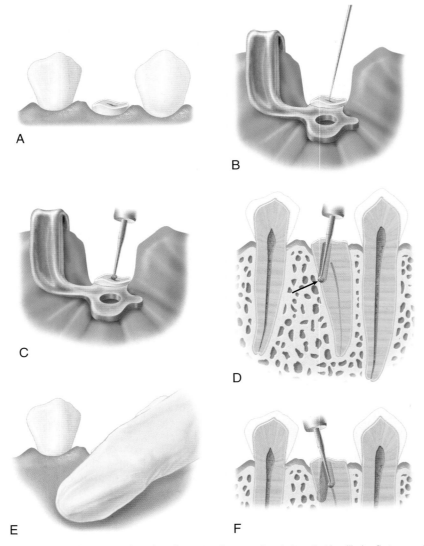

A

B

C

D

E

F

FIG. 5-57 Access cavity preparation when the anatomic crown is missing. **A,** Mandibular first premolar with the crown missing. **B,** An endodontic explorer fails to penetrate the calcified pulp chamber. **C,** A long-shank round bur is directed in the assumed long axis of the root. **D,** Perforation of the root wall *(arrow)*, resulting from failure to consider root angulation. **E,** Palpation of the buccal root anatomy without a dental dam in place to determine root angulation. **F,** Correct bur angulation after repair of the perforation with mineral trioxide aggregate (MTA). The dental dam is placed as soon as the canal has been identified.

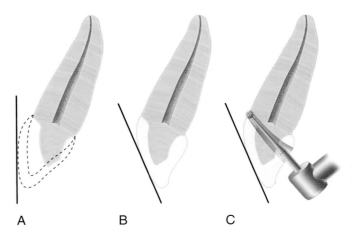

FIG. 5-58 Access cavity error resulting from alteration of the original tooth contours by a full veneer crown. **A,** Original crown contour of the tooth. **B,** A full veneer crown is used to change the original crown contour for esthetic purposes. **C,** Access perforation resulting from reliance on the full veneer crown contour rather than the long axis of the root.

A   B   C

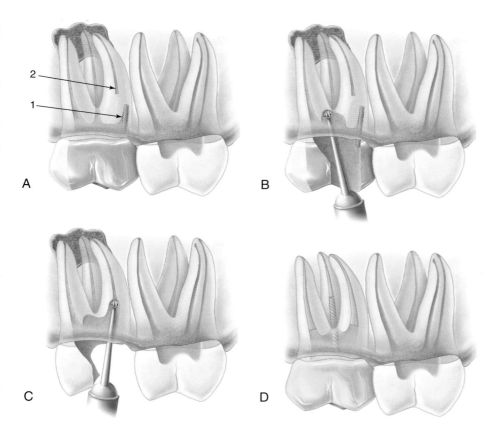

A

B

C

D

FIG. 5-59 **A,** In a heavily restored maxillary second molar that requires root canal therapy, the clinician may attempt access to the canals. Pre-treatment radiographs demonstrate three important factors: (1) a reinforcing pin is in place *(arrow);* (2) at least two thirds of the coronal portion is restorative material; and (3) the mesio-buccal canal appears calcified *(arrow).* These factors suggest complete excavation. **B,** A patient may ask the clinician to attempt an unexcavated search for the canals; this may result in a furcal perforation, compromising the prognosis. In such cases the patient should be engaged in the decision to continue treatment, which unquestionably involves removal of the existing restoration. **C,** A safer, more conservative approach is to remove the amalgam, the pin, and any old cements. Careful excavation, using enhanced vision, results in access to the pulp chamber. **D,** The clinician now can perform sound root canal therapy, followed by internal reinforcement and full coverage.

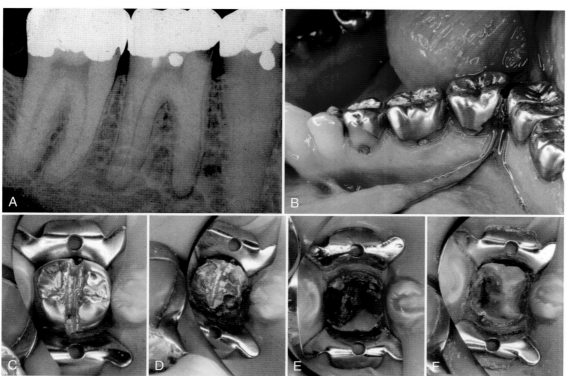

FIG. 5-60 **A,** Radiograph showing apical lesions on both roots and recurrent caries under the mesial margin of the crown. **B,** Clinical photograph of the crown and tissues that appear normal. **C,** Cutting of the crown from the tooth. **D,** Crown has been removed, and decay is evident around the core restoration. **E,** Removal of the old restoration shows significant decay. **F,** Final excavation, which allows for evaluation of the tooth structure and facilitates direct access to the pulp chamber. (From Gutmann JL, Lovdahl PE: *Problem solving in endodontics,* ed 5, St Louis, 2011, Elsevier.)

Development of an access through an intact metalloceramic crown should be done with caution. When such restorations are placed, they often change the crown-to-root angulation to correct preexisting occlusal discrepancies. Metalloceramic crowns often alter previous tooth rotation. Both these situations make the preparation of access cavities challenging. Pretreatment radiographs can be helpful, but the metal in the full veneer crown usually masks the underlying pulp chamber. In these situations the best approach is to stay as centered in the tooth as possible, using all available clinical and radiographic information. The DOM and transillumination of the CEJ are valuable aids in this process.

Metalloceramic crowns are best penetrated with new, sharp carbide burs. Round burs work well, but tungsten carbide transmetal burs are more efficient. These crosscut fissure burs are specifically designed to cut through metal restorative materials. Porcelain or metalloceramic restorations must be handled delicately to minimize the potential for fracture (Fig. 5-62). Whatever the nature of the crown, efforts should be made to avoid being too conservative. Attempting to save the crown often leads to an underextended preparation. All the guidelines for access cavity preparations discussed earlier must be followed. When the preparation is complete, the margins and internal spaces must be evaluated for caries, leakage, and fractures.

Access in Teeth with Calcified Canals

Often a 2D pretreatment radiograph may be interpreted as showing total or nearly total calcification of the pulp chamber and radicular canal spaces (see Fig. 5-56). Unfortunately, these spaces have adequate room to allow passage of millions of microorganisms. Chronic inflammatory processes (e.g., caries, medications, occlusal trauma, and aging) often cause pulpal degeneration and concomitant narrowing of the root canal system.[84] Although the coronal portion of the canal may appear diminished significantly, canals often become less calcified as they approach the root apex. Despite these perceived 2D anatomic alterations, many canals do exist, and attempts must be made to manage them to the canal terminus.

Chambers and roots that demonstrate significant calcifications may present problems with locating, penetrating, and

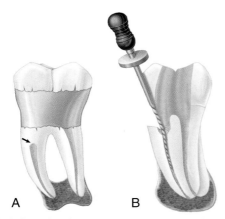

FIG. 5-61 A, Extensive class V restoration necessitated by root caries and periodontal disease that led to canal calcification *(arrow).* **B,** Access to the canal is occluded by calcification. Removal of the facial restoration may be required to obtain access from the buccal surface.

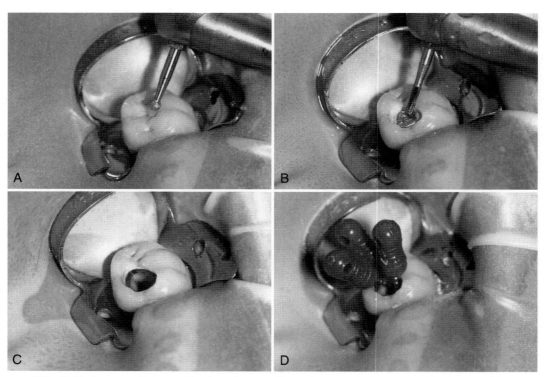

FIG. 5-62 Access cavity preparation through a metalloceramic crown. **A,** A round diamond bur is used to penetrate the porcelain. **B,** Following the access outline with the round diamond bur, a transmetal bur is used to cut through the metal. **C,** Prepared access cavity allowing direct approach to the canals. **D,** Files are placed on the access cavity walls without impingement.

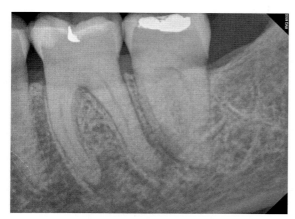

FIG. 5-63 Mandibular molar with what appears to be almost complete calcification of the pulp chamber and root canals. However, pathosis is present, which indicates the presence of bacteria and some necrotic tissue in the apical portion of the roots.

negotiating the pulpal spaces.[84] The use of magnification and transillumination, as well as careful examination of color changes and pulp chamber shapes, assists in locating the canals (Fig. 5-63). However, the search for the root canal orifices should be made only after the pulp chamber has been completely prepared and its floor has been cleaned and dried (95% denatured ethanol may be useful for drying the floor and enhancing visibility). A fiberoptic light directed through the CEJ can reveal subtle landmarks and color changes that may not otherwise be visible. The chamber floor is darker in color than its walls, and developmental grooves connecting orifices are lighter in color than the chamber floor. Awareness of these color differences when searching for calcified orifices is essential, especially when searching for canal orifices that are located at the angles formed by the floor and walls and at the end points of developmental grooves. Additional methods to help locate calcified root canals include staining the pulp chamber floor with 1% methylene blue dye, performing the sodium hypochlorite "champagne bubble" test (see Fig. 5-2) and searching for canal bleeding points. These approaches are enhanced when the area is viewed through magnification.

In teeth with significant calcifications that obscure and block the root canal, the calcified material must be removed slowly down the root. Long, thin ultrasonic tips should be used under the high magnification of a DOM to avoid removing too much tooth structure. As the clinician proceeds apically, exposure of two radiographs should be considered, one from the straight-on direction and the other from an angled direction. A very small piece of lead foil placed at the apical extent of the penetration can provide a radiographic reference.

Uncovering canals that contain calcified material is a challenge. When the canal is located, a small K-file (#6, #8, or #10 or, preferably, a C or C+ file [Dentsply Tulsa and Maillefer, respectively]) coated with a chelating agent should be introduced into the canal to determine patency. These instruments provide added stiffness to the shaft for better penetration. The file should not be removed until some canal enlargement has occurred. The file should be used in short up-and-down movements and in a selective circumferential filing motion, with most of the lateral pressure directed away from the furcation. This enlarges the coronal aspect of the canal safely and moves it laterally, to avoid thinning of the dentin wall adjacent to the

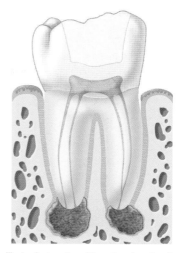

FIG. 5-64 Mandibular first molar with a class I restoration, calcified canals, and periradicular radiolucencies. Presumably a pulp exposure has occurred, resulting in calcification and ultimate necrosis of the pulp tissue.

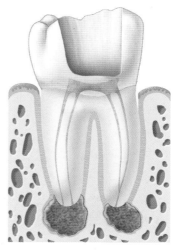

FIG. 5-65 Excavation of a restoration and base material. The cavity preparation is extended toward the assumed location of the pulp chamber, keeping in mind that pulp chambers are located in the center of the tooth at the level of the cementoenamel junction *(CEJ).*

furcation. It also creates a path of insertion for larger files and for preflaring burs. Figs. 5-64 through 5-69 illustrate several methods that can be used to locate calcified spaces. For the most successful results, the sequence should be followed as shown.

If the canal orifice cannot be found, it is wise to stop excavating the dentin to avoid weakening the tooth structure or perforating into the periodontal ligament. Management of these problems can be found in Chapter 19. There is no rapid technique or solution for dealing with calcified root canals.[84] Painstaking removal of small amounts of dentin with the aid of the DOM and radiographic confirmation has proved to be the safest approach.

Crowded or Rotated Teeth

Traditional access preparations may not be possible in patients with crowded teeth. The decision about an alternative approach

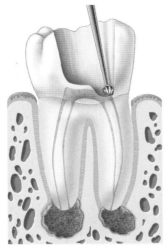

FIG. 5-66 Use a long-shank #2 or #4 round bur to remove dentin and attempt to locate calcified canals.

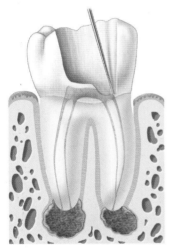

FIG. 5-67 An endodontic explorer is used to probe the pulp floor. A straight ultrasonic tip may be used to remove dentin. Angled radiographs must be taken to monitor progress.

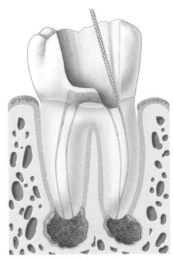

FIG. 5-68 At the first indication of a canal space, the smallest instrument (i.e., a #.06 or #.08 C or C+ file or micro openers) should be introduced into the canal. Gentle passive movement, both apical and rotational, often produces some penetration. A slight pull, signaling resistance, usually is an indication that the canal has been located. This should be confirmed by radiographs.

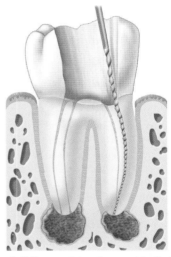

FIG. 5-69 A small K-file negotiates the canal to its terminus. An apex locator or radiograph is used to confirm the file's position.

must be based on straight-line access principles and conservation of tooth structure. In certain circumstances a buccal access preparation may be the treatment of choice (Fig. 5-70).[84] Modern restorative materials have made repair of this access esthetically acceptable.

Rotated teeth can present problems during access cavity preparation because of the altered crown-to-root relationships. According to a study by Moreinis,[144] diagnostic periapical radiographs, although only 2D, are indispensable for "determining the anatomic relationship of the crown to the root and the angle of the root in the arch." When these factors are identified, reasonable variations in the access opening must be visualized before the tooth is entered. Perforations in rotated teeth during access preparation usually occur because of faulty angulation of the bur with respect to the long axis of the root.

Other problems can occur when tooth angulations are not considered during preparation of an access cavity. Such problems include the following:

- Mistaken identification of an already located canal, resulting in a search in the wrong direction for additional canals. Whenever a difficult canal is located, a file should be placed in the canal and an angled radiograph taken. This determines which canal has been located. A search for another canal orifice can then begin in the correct direction.
- Failure to locate a canal or extra canals.
- Excessive gouging of coronal or radicular tooth structure.
- Instrument separation during attempts to locate an orifice.
- Failure to débride all pulp tissue from the chamber.

The best way to handle any these problems is to prevent them from occurring. A thorough radiographic examination is

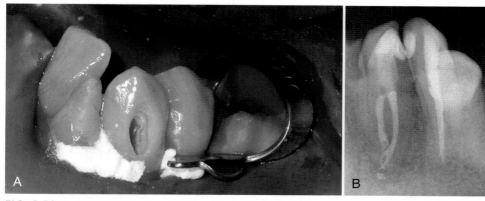

FIG. 5-70 **A,** Access cavity on crowded mandibular anterior teeth. The access preparation is cut through the buccal surface on the canine. The lateral incisor has also been accessed through the buccal surface; root canal procedures were performed, and the access cavity was permanently restored with composite. **B,** Obturation.

crucial. The initial outline form occasionally can be created without the dental dam, which facilitates positioning of the bur with the long axis of the tooth. Bur penetration for both depth and angulation should be confirmed frequently with radiographs.

ERRORS IN ACCESS CAVITY PREPARATION

Unfortunately, errors can occur in the preparation of an access cavity. Most are the result of failure to follow the access guidelines; others reflect a lack of understanding of the internal and external tooth morphology. Common errors are discussed and illustrated in Figs. 5-71 through 5-73 and detailed extensively elsewhere in this text and other publications.[84]

MORPHOLOGY OF AND ACCESS CAVITY PREPARATIONS FOR INDIVIDUAL TEETH

The anatomy shown in the following figures was obtained from human teeth through the use of recently developed 3D imaging techniques. The teeth were scanned in a high-resolution, microcomputer-assisted tomographic scanner. The data were then manipulated with proprietary computer programs to produce the 3D reconstructions and visualization. The following individuals and sources are recognized to have contributed greatly to this endeavor.

The 3D reconstructed images in this chapter were obtained from the tooth and canal morphology database at the School of Stomatology, Wuhan University, China. The database was established by Dr. Bing Fan's group and supported by the National Natural Science Foundation of China (grant no. 30572042, 30872881, 81070821) and the Key Technologies R&D Programme of Hubei Province of China (grant no. 2007AA302B06). The microcomputed tomography machine used for scanning was the μCT-50, Scanco Medical, Bassersdorf, Switzerland. The multiple softwares used for 3D reconstruction included 3D-Doctor (Able Software Corp., Lexington, Massachusetts) and VGStudio MAX (Volume Graphics GmbH, Heidelberg, Germany).

Radiographs: Courtesy Dr. L. Stephen Buchanan, Santa Barbara, California; Dr. John Khademi, Durango, Colorado; Dr. Raed S. Kasem, Clearwater, Florida; Dr. Gary Manasse, Jacksonville, Florida; Dr. Michael DeGrood, DeBary, Florida; and Dr. Kevin Melker, Clearwater, Florida.

Access cavity illustrations: Designed and formatted by Dr. Richard Burns, San Mateo, California; and Dr. Eric Herbranson, San Leandro, California.

All tables in this section that provide literature documentation for the studies on root canal anatomy are available online at the Expert Consult site and can be accessed accordingly.

Maxillary Central Incisor

The root canal system outline of the maxillary central incisor reflects the external surface outline (Fig. 5-74). A newly erupted central incisor has three pulp horns, and the pulp chamber is wider mesiodistally than buccolingually. A lingual shoulder usually is present, and it must be removed to gain access to the lingual wall of the root canal. The lingual shoulder prevents direct access to the root canal and deflects files labially, often resulting in a ledge or perforation. In cross section, the root canal at the CEJ is triangular in young teeth and oval in older teeth. It gradually becomes round as it approaches the apical foramen (see Table 5-8 online at the Expert Consult site). The μCT scans of this tooth are seen in Fig. 5-75. (See Video 5-1 online at the Expert Consult site for rotational views of these teeth.)

The external access outline form for the maxillary central incisor is a rounded triangle with its base toward the incisal aspect (Figs. 5-76 through 5-79). The width of the triangular base is determined by the distance between the mesial and distal pulp horns. The mesial and distal external walls should converge toward the cingulum. All internal walls should funnel to the root canal orifice. If the lingual shoulder has been removed properly, the entire orifice should be seen through the access opening. The incisal internal wall should approach the lingual surface of the tooth in a near butt joint to allow for a bulk of restorative material on this functional surface.

Variation

The outline form of the access cavity changes to a more oval shape as the tooth matures and the pulp horns recede because the mesial and distal pulp horns are less prominent.

Maxillary Lateral Incisor

The pulp chamber outline of the maxillary lateral incisor is similar to that of the maxillary central incisor; however, it is

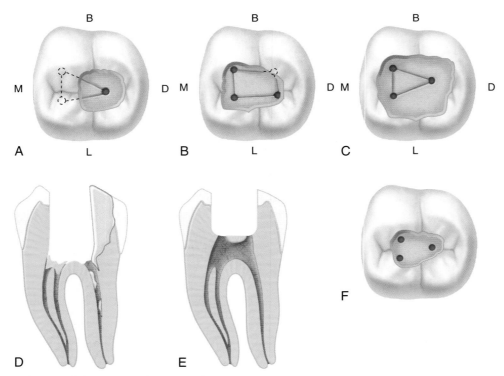

FIG. 5-71 A, Poor access placement and inadequate mesial extension leave both mesial orifices uncovered. Information about the position and location of pulp chambers can be obtained through evaluation of pretreatment radiographs, especially bite-wing radiographs, and assessment of the tooth anatomy at the cementoenamel junction (CEJ). **B,** Inadequate extension of the distal access cavity leaves the distobuccal canal orifice unexposed. All developmental grooves must be traced to their termination and must not be allowed to disappear into an axial wall. **C,** Gross overextension of the access cavity weakens the coronal tooth structure and compromises the final restoration. This mistake results from failure to determine correctly the position of the pulp chamber and the angulation of the bur. **D,** Allowing debris to fall into canal orifices results in an iatrogenic mishap. Amalgam fillings and dentin debris block canal orifices, preventing proper shaping and cleaning. Complete removal of the restoration and copious irrigation help prevent this problem. **E,** Failure to remove the roof of the pulp chamber is a serious underextension error; the pulp horns have been exposed. Bite-wing radiographs are excellent aids in determining vertical depth. **F,** Access preparation in which the roof of the pulp chamber remains and the pulp horns have been mistaken for canal orifices. The whitish color of the roof, the depth of the access cavity, and the lack of developmental grooves are clues to this underextension. Root canal orifices generally are positioned at or slightly apical to the CEJ. *B,* Buccal; *D,* distal; *L,* lingual; *M,* mesial.

smaller, and two or no pulp horns may be present (Fig. 5-80). This tooth is wider mesiodistally than buccolingually. A cross section at the CEJ shows a pulp chamber centered in the root, and its shape may be triangular, oval, or round. From the CEJ the pulp canal becomes round in cross section in the midroot and apical areas. The lingual shoulder of dentin must be removed before instruments can be used to explore the canal (see Table 5-9 online at the Expert Consult site). The µCT scans of this tooth are shown in Fig. 5-81. (See Video 5-2 online at the Expert Consult site for rotational views of these teeth.) Normally only one root canal is present, but other variations have been reported.

The external access outline form for the maxillary lateral incisor may be a rounded triangle or an oval, depending on the prominence of the mesial and distal pulp horns (Figs. 5-82 through 5-84). When the horns are prominent, the rounded triangular shape is compressed mesiodistally relative to a central incisor, producing a more slender triangle. The outline form usually is oval if the mesial and distal pulp horns are not

prominent. All other aspects of the access preparation are the same as those for the central incisor.

The maxillary lateral incisor often has anomalies. One such variation in form is the presence of a palatal radicular or developmental groove (Fig. 5-85).[121,153-155,161-164] Although this groove may be present on the roots of all anterior teeth, it is more common in the maxillary lateral incisor. There is generally direct communication between the groove and the pulp cavity, and this occurs primarily through dentinal tubules.

Dens invaginatus, another anomaly, has been classified into three types based on severity, ranging from simple to more complex.[194] Type 1 is an invagination that is confined to the crown. Type 2 is an invagination that extends past the CEJ but does not involve the periradicular tissues. Type 3 is an invagination that extends beyond the CEJ and can have a second apical foramen. Often both surgical and nonsurgical root canal procedures are necessary to properly manage this condition.*

---

*References 155, 167, 170, 178, 179, 181, 182, 188, 195, and 208.

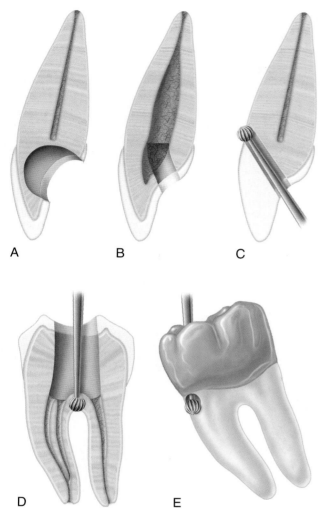

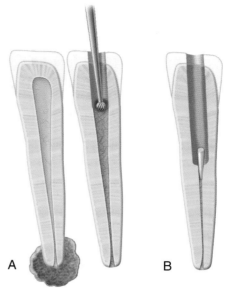

FIG. 5-73 **A,** The most embarrassing error, with the greatest potential for medical and legal damage, is entering the wrong tooth because of incorrect dental dam placement. When the crowns of teeth appear identical, the clinician should mark the tooth with a felt-tip marker before placing the dental dam. **B,** Burs and files can be broken if used with an improper motion, excessive pressure, or before the access cavity has been properly prepared. A broken instrument may lock into the canal walls, requiring excessive removal of tooth structure to retrieve it. On occasion, fragments may not be retrievable.

FIG. 5-72 **A,** Overzealous tooth removal caused by improper bur angulation and failure to recognize the lingual inclination of the tooth. This results in weakening and mutilation of the coronal tooth structure, which often leads to coronal fractures. **B,** Inadequate opening; the access cavity is positioned too far to the gingival, with no incisal extension. This can lead to bur and file breakage, coronal discoloration because the pulp horns remain, inadequate instrumentation and obturation, root perforation, canal ledging, and apical transportation. **C,** Labial perforation caused by failure to extend the preparation to the incisal before the bur shaft entered the access cavity. **D,** Furcation perforation caused by failure to measure the distance between the occlusal surface and the furcation. The bur bypasses the pulp chamber and creates an opening into the periodontal tissues. Perforations weaken the tooth and cause periodontal destruction. To ensure a satisfactory result, they must be repaired as soon as they are made. **E,** Perforation of the mesial tooth surface caused by failure to recognize that the tooth was tipped and failure to align the bur with the long axis of the tooth. This is a common error in teeth with full crowns. Even when these perforations are repaired correctly, they usually cause a permanent periodontal problem because they occur in a difficult maintenance area.

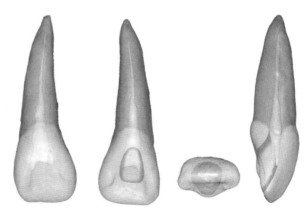

FIG. 5-74 Maxillary central incisor. Average time of eruption—7 to 8 years; average age of calcification—10 years; average length—22.5 mm. Root curvature (most common to least common): straight, labial, distal.

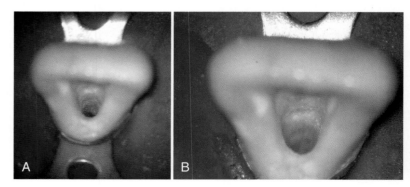

FIG. 5-75 μCT scans of maxillary central incisors. **A,** Common anatomic presentation. **B,** Central incisor with a lateral canal, which is common. **C,** Rare multiple-canal variation. All teeth are shown from both a buccal (vestibular) and a proximal perspective, along with the cross-sectional anatomy at the coronal, middle, and apical levels. (See Video 5-1 online at the Expert Consult site for rotational views of these teeth.)

FIG. 5-76 Access cavity for a maxillary central incisor as viewed through the dental operating microscope. **A,** ×3.4 magnification. **B,** ×8.4 magnification.

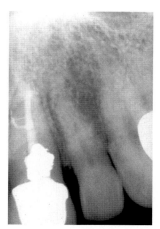

FIG. 5-77 Curved accessory canal with intersecting straight lateral canal.

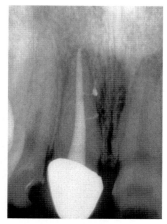

FIG. 5-79 Double lateral canals.

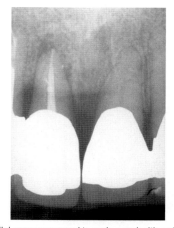

FIG. 5-78 Parallel accessory canal to main canal with a simple lateral canal.

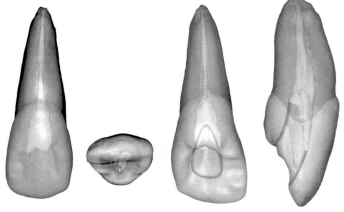

FIG. 5-80 Maxillary lateral incisor. Average time of eruption—8 to 9 years; average age of calcification—11 years; average length—22 mm. Root curvature (most common to least common): distal, straight.

Maxillary Canine

The root canal system of the maxillary canine is similar in many ways to that of the maxillary incisors (Fig. 5-86). A major difference is that it is wider labiolingually than mesiodistally. Another difference is that it has no pulp horns. Its smallest pointed incisal edge corresponds to the single cusp. The pulp chamber outline at the CEJ is oval. A lingual shoulder is present, which may prevent shaping and cleaning of the root canal in its lingual dimension. From this point, the root canal remains oval until it approaches the apical third of the root, where it becomes constricted. Because of this oval shape, the clinician must take care to circumferentially file labially and palatally to shape and clean the canal properly.[124] Usually one root canal is present, although two canals have been reported (see Table 5-10 online at the Expert Consult site). The μCT scans for the maxillary canine can be seen in Fig. 5-87. (See Video 5-3 online at the Expert Consult site) for rotational views of these teeth. The thin buccal bone over the canine eminence often disintegrates, and fenestration is an occasional anatomic finding.

The external access outline form is oval or slot shaped because no mesial or distal pulp horns are present (Figs. 5-88 through 5-90). The mesiodistal width of the slot is determined by the mesiodistal width of the pulp chamber. The incisogingival dimension is determined by straight-line access factors and removal of the lingual shoulder. The incisal extension often approaches to within 2 to 3 mm of the incisal edge to allow for straight-line access. The incisal wall meets the lingual surface of the canine in a butt joint to provide adequate thickness for restorative material because this tooth is heavily involved in excursive occlusal guidance and function. All internal walls funnel to the orifice.

Maxillary First Premolar

Most maxillary first premolars have two root canals, regardless of the number of roots (Fig. 5-91). Ethnicity plays a factor in that Asian people have a higher incidence of one canal than do other ethnic groups.[120,156]

A furcation groove or developmental depression on the palatal aspect of the buccal root is another anatomic feature. Its prevalence has been reported as 62% to 100%.[97,112,211] This groove may pose a risk to root canal and restorative procedures in this tooth.[118] At the deepest part of the invagination, the average dentin thickness was found to be 0.81 mm.

The pulp chamber of the maxillary first premolar is considerably wider buccolingually than mesiodistally. In the buccolingual dimension, the chamber outline shows a buccal and a

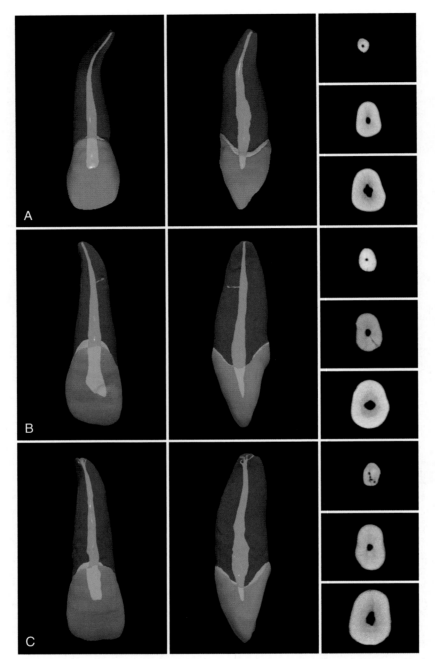

FIG. 5-81 μCT scans of maxillary lateral incisors. **A,** Common anatomic presentation. **B,** Lateral incisor with a large lateral canal, which is common. **C,** Lateral incisor with an apical delta. All teeth are shown from both a buccal (vestibular) and a proximal perspective, along with the cross-sectional anatomy at the coronal, middle, and apical levels. (See Video 5-2 online at the Expert Consult site for rotational views of these teeth.)

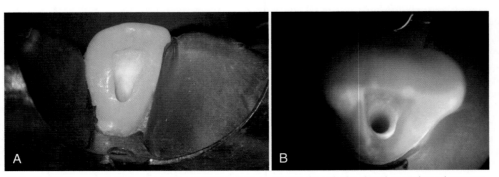

FIG. 5-82 Access cavity for a maxillary lateral incisor as viewed through the dental operating microscope. **A,** ×3.4 magnification. **B,** ×5.1 magnification with cervical fiberoptic transillumination.

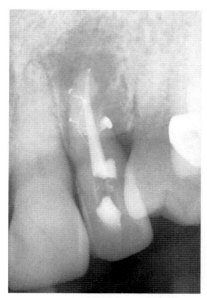

FIG. 5-83 Lateral incisor with a canal loop and multiple lateral canals with associated lesions.

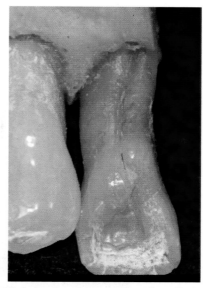

FIG. 5-85 Cadaver specimen showing a lingual/palatal groove.

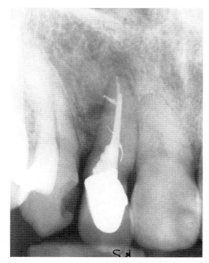

FIG. 5-84 Multiple accessory foramina.

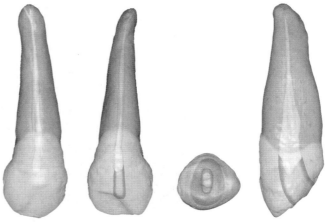

FIG. 5-86 Maxillary canine. Average time of eruption—10 to 12 years; average age of calcification—13 to 15 years; average length—26.5 mm. Root curvature (most common to least common): distal, straight, labial.

palatal pulp horn. The buccal pulp horn usually is larger. From the occlusal level, the chamber maintains a width similar that of the floor, which is located just apical to the cervical line. The palatal orifice is slightly larger than the buccal orifice. In cross section at the CEJ, the palatal orifice is wider buccolingually and kidney shaped because of its mesial concavity. From the floor, two root canals take on a round shape at midroot and rapidly taper to their apices, usually ending in extremely narrow, curved root canals. The palatal canal usually is slightly larger than the buccal canal. The maxillary first premolar may have one, two, or three roots and canals; it most often has two (see Table 5-11 online at the Expert Consult site). The μCT scans for the maxillary first premolar can be seen in Fig. 5-92. (See Video 5-4 available online at the Expert Consult site for rotational views of these teeth.)

If two canals are present, they are labeled buccal and palatal; three root canals are designated mesiobuccal, distobuccal, and palatal. Directional positioning of small files can help identify the anatomy. The roots are considerably shorter and thinner than in the canines. In double-rooted teeth, the roots most often are the same length. The buccal root is often found to be fenestrated through the cortical plate of bone; this can pose both nonsurgical and surgical treatment challenges.

The access preparation for the maxillary first premolar is oval or slot shaped (Figs. 5-93 through 5-96). It also is wide buccolingually, narrow mesiodistally, and centered mesiodistally between the cusp tips. In fact, the mesiodistal width should correspond to the mesiodistal width of the pulp chamber. The buccal extension typically is two thirds to three fourths up the buccal cusp incline. The palatal extension is approximately halfway up the palatal cusp incline. The buccal and palatal walls funnel directly into the orifices. Because of the mesial concavity of the root, the clinician must take care

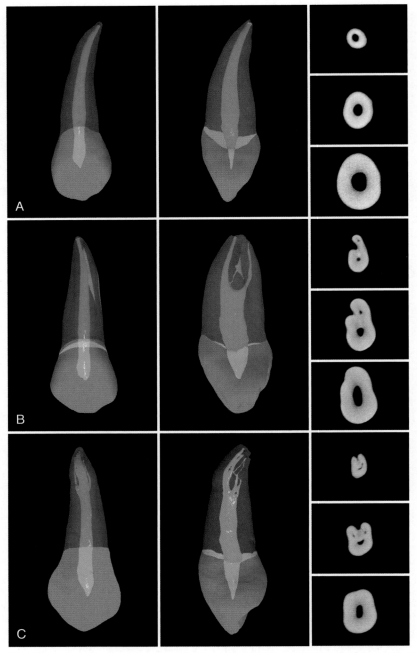

FIG. 5-87 μCT scans for the maxillary canine. **A,** Common anatomic presentation. **B,** Canine with two roots. **C,** Canine with significant deviations of the canal system in the apical thirdAll teeth are shown from both a buccal (vestibular) and a proximal perspective, along with the cross-sectional anatomy at the coronal, middle, and apical levels. (See Video 5-3 online at the Expert Consult site for rotational views of these teeth.)

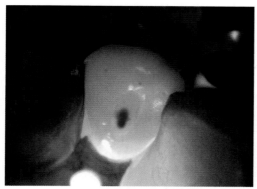

FIG. 5-88 Access cavity for a maxillary canine as viewed through the dental operating microscope. (×5.1 magnification with cervical fiberoptic transillumination.)

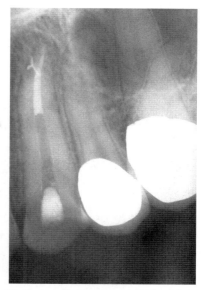

FIG. 5-90 Canine with lateral canal dividing into two canals.

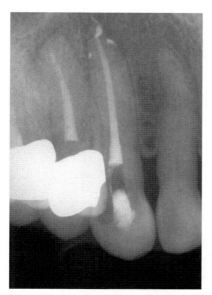

FIG. 5-89 Canine with multiple accessory foramina.

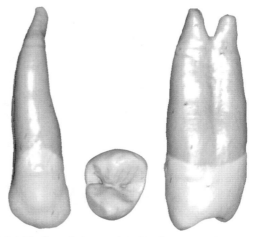

FIG. 5-91 Maxillary first premolar. Development and anatomic data: average time of eruption—10 to 11 years; average age of calcification—12 to 13 years; average length—20.6 mm. Root curvature (most common to least common): buccal root—lingual, straight, buccal; palatal root—straight, buccal, distal; single root—straight, distal, buccal.

not to overextend the preparation in that direction because this could result in perforation.

Variation

When three canals are present, the external outline form becomes triangular, with the base on the buccal aspect. The mesiobuccal and distobuccal corners of the triangle should be positioned directly over the corresponding canal orifices.

Maxillary Second Premolar

The root canal system of the maxillary second premolar is wider buccolingually than mesiodistally (Fig. 5-97). This tooth may have one, two, or three roots and canals (see Table 5-12 online at the Expert Consult site). Two or three canals can occur in a single root.[68] The scans for the maxillary second premolar can be seen in Fig. 5-98. (See Video 5-5 online at the Expert Consult site for rotational views of these teeth.) Directional positioning of small files can help identify the anatomy. The mesiodistal and buccolingual aspects of the pulp chamber are similar to those of the first premolar. A buccal and a palatal

pulp horn are present; the buccal pulp horn is larger. A single root is oval and wider buccolingually than mesiodistally. The canal or canals remain oval from the pulp chamber floor and taper rapidly to the apex. The roots of the maxillary second premolar are approximately as long as those of the first premolar, and apical curvature is common, particularly with large maxillary sinus cavities.

When two canals are present in this tooth, the maxillary second premolar access preparation is nearly identical to that of the first premolar. Because this tooth usually has one root, if two canals are present, they are nearly parallel to each other, and the external outline form must have a greater buccolingual extension, to permit straight-line access to these canals, than with the first premolar with two roots and diverging canals. If only one canal is present, the buccolingual extension is less

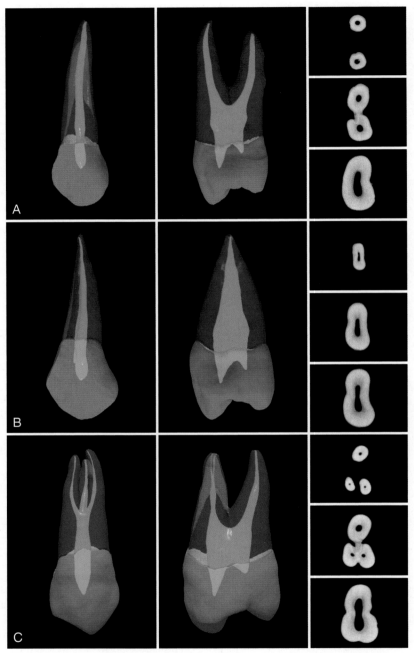

FIG. 5-92 μCT scans of maxillary first premolars. **A,** Common anatomic presentation of this tooth showing two roots. **B,** Premolar with only one canal. **C,** Premolar with three roots. All teeth are shown from both a buccal (vestibular) and a proximal perspective, along with the cross-sectional anatomy at the coronal, middle, and apical levels. (See Video 5-4 online at the Expert Consult site for rotational views of these teeth.)

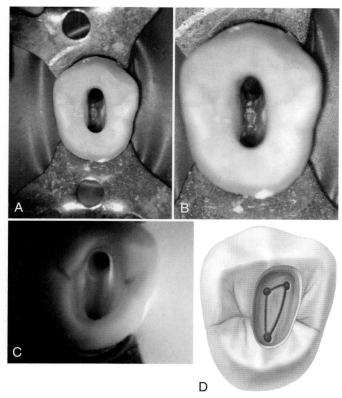

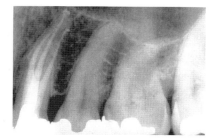

FIG. 5-96 Three canals.

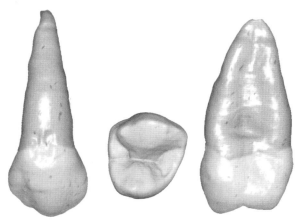

FIG. 5-93 Access cavity for a maxillary first premolar as viewed through the dental operating microscope. **A,** ×3.4 magnification. **B,** ×5.1 magnification. **C,** ×8.4 magnification with cervical fiberoptic transillumination. **D,** Schematic representation of a three-canal access preparation.

FIG. 5-97 Maxillary second premolar. Average time of eruption—10 to 12 years; average age of calcification—12 to 14 years; average length—21.5 mm. Root curvature (most common to least common): distal, bayonet, buccal, straight.

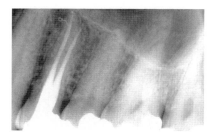

FIG. 5-94 Lateral bony lesion associated with a filled lateral canal.

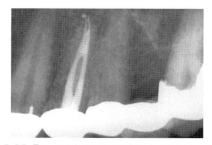

FIG. 5-95 Two canals that have fused and then redivided.

and corresponds to the width between the buccal and palatal pulp horns (Figs. 5-99 through 5-102). If three canals are present, the external access outline form is the same triangular shape illustrated for the maxillary first premolar.

Maxillary First Molar

The maxillary first molar is the largest tooth in volume and one of the most complex in root and canal anatomy (Fig. 5-103).[50] The pulp chamber is widest in the buccolingual dimension, and four pulp horns are present (mesiobuccal, mesiopalatal, distobuccal, and distopalatal). The pulp chamber's cervical outline form has a rhomboid shape, sometimes with rounded corners. The mesiobuccal angle is an acute angle; the distobuccal angle is an obtuse angle; and the palatal angles are basically right angles. The palatal canal orifice is centered palatally; the distobuccal orifice is near the obtuse angle of the pulp chamber floor; and the main mesiobuccal canal orifice is buccal and mesial to the distobuccal orifice and is positioned within the acute angle of the pulp chamber. The mesiopalatal canal orifice (also referred to as the *MB-2*) is located palatal and mesial to the mesiobuccal orifice. A line drawn to connect the three main canal orifices—the mesiobuccal orifice, distobuccal orifice, and palatal orifice—forms a triangle, known as the *molar triangle*.

The three individual roots of the maxillary first molar (i.e., mesiobuccal root, distobuccal root, and palatal root) form a tripod. The palatal root is the longest, has the largest diameter, and generally offers the easiest access. It can contain one, two,

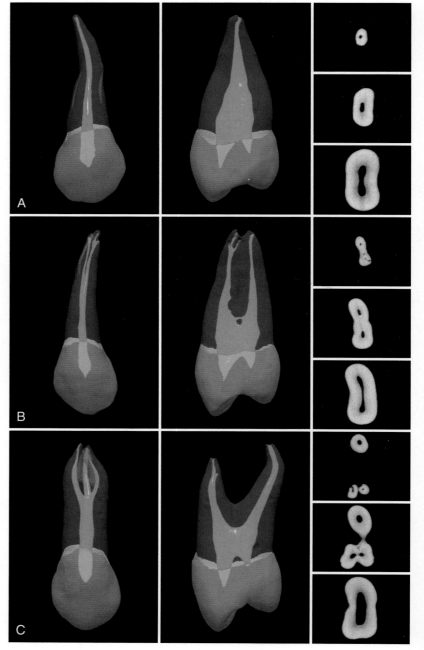

FIG. 5-98 μCT scans of maxillary second premolars. A, Common anatomic presentation showing one canal. B, Second premolar with two canals and an apical delta. C, Second premolar with three roots/canals that divide at the junction of the middle and apical third of the main root. All teeth are shown from both a buccal (vestibular) and a proximal perspective, along with the cross-sectional anatomy at the coronal, middle, and apical levels. (See Video 5-5 online at the Expert Consult site for rotational views of these teeth.)

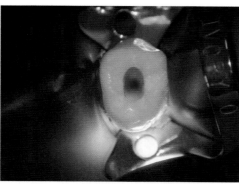

FIG. 5-99 Access cavity for a maxillary second premolar as viewed through the dental operating microscope. (×5.1 magnification with cervical fiberoptic transillumination.)

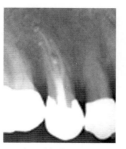

FIG. 5-100 Second premolar with three canals and a large lateral canal.

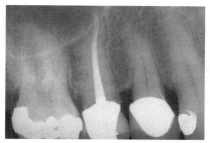

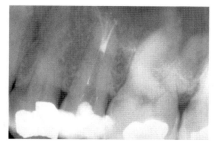

FIG. 5-101 Single canal that has divided into two canals.

FIG. 5-102 Single canal that has split into three canals.

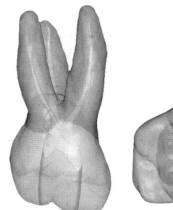
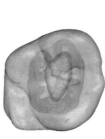
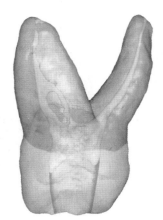
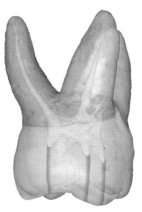

FIG. 5-103 Maxillary first molar. Average time of eruption—6 to 7 years; average age of calcification—9 to 10 years; average length—20.8 mm. Root curvature (most common to least common): mesiobuccal root—distal, straight; distobuccal root—straight, mesial, distal; palatal root—buccal, straight.

or three root canals (see Table 5-13 online at the Expert Consult site). The palatal root often curves buccally at the apical one third, which may not be obvious on a standard periapical radiograph. From its orifice the palatal canal is flat, ribbonlike, and wider in a mesiodistal direction. The distobuccal root is conical and may have one or two canals (see Table 5-14 online at the Expert Consult site). From its orifice, the canal (or canals) first is oval and then becomes round as it approaches the apical third of the root. The mesiobuccal root has generated more research and clinical investigation than any other root in the mouth.[202] It may have one, two, or three root canals (see Table 5-15 online at the Expert Consult site). A single mesiobuccal canal is oval and wider buccolingually; two or three canals are more circular. In general, a concavity exists on the distal aspect of the mesiobuccal root, which makes this wall thin. The μCT scans for the maxillary first molar can be seen in Fig. 5-104. (See Video 5-6 online at the Expert Consult site for rotational views of these teeth.) The DOM has been used to study the location and pathway of the mesiopalatal canal in maxillary first and second molars.[80] The clinician must always keep in mind that the location of this canal varies greatly; it generally is located mesial to or directly on a line between the mesiobuccal and palatal orifices, within 3.5 mm palatally and 2 mm mesially of the mesiobuccal orifice (Figs. 5-105 and 5-106). These authors[80] found that not all mesioopalatal orifices lead to a true canal. A true orifice for this canal was present in only 84% of molars in which a second orifice was identified (Fig. 5-107).[205]

Negotiation of the mesiopalatal canal often is difficult; a ledge of dentin covers its orifice, the orifice has a mesiobuccal inclination on the pulp floor, and the canal's pathway often takes one or two abrupt curves in the coronal part of the root. Most of these obstructions can be eliminated by troughing or countersinking with ultrasonic tips mesially and apically along the mesiobuccal pulpal groove (Figs. 5-108 through 5-111). This procedure may shift the canal mesially, meaning that the access wall also must be moved farther mesially. Troughing can easily be 0.5 to 3 mm deep, and care must be taken to avoid furcal wall perforation in this root. Apical to the troughing level. the canal may be straight or may curve sharply to the distobuccal, buccal, or palatal.

Because the maxillary first molar almost always has four canals, the access cavity has a rhomboid shape, with the corners corresponding to the four orifices (see Fig. 5-108). One study demonstrated that the access cavity should not extend into the mesial marginal ridge.[246] Distally, the preparation can invade the mesial portion of the oblique ridge, but it should not penetrate through the ridge. The buccal wall should be parallel to a line connecting the mesiobuccal and distobuccal orifices and not to the buccal surface of the tooth.

Maxillary Second Molar

Coronally, the maxillary second molar closely resembles the maxillary first molar (Fig. 5-112). The root and canal anatomy are similar to those of the first molar, although there are differences. The distinguishing morphologic feature of the

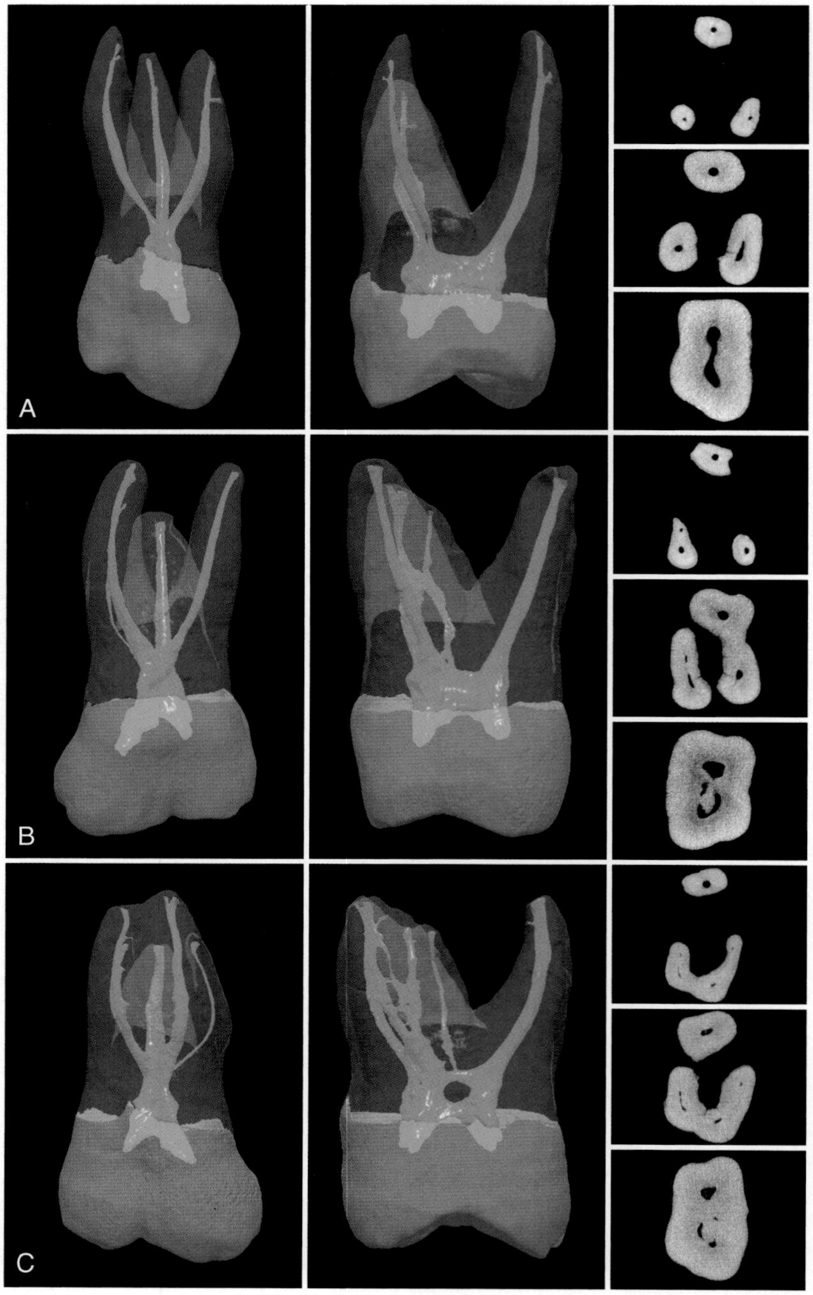

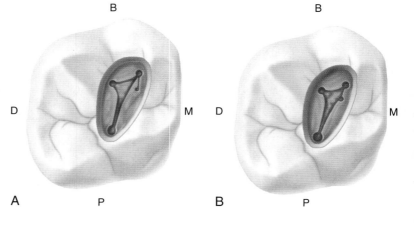

FIG. 5-104 μCT scans of maxillary first molars. **A**, Common anatomic presentation showing accessory/lateral canals. **B**, First molar with four canals, with mesiobuccal and mesio-palatal sharing an anastomosis in the midroot. **C**, Maxillary molar with four pulp horns, five canals, and significant anastomoses between the canals. All teeth are shown from both a buccal (vestibular) and a proximal perspective, along with the cross-sectional anatomy at the coronal, middle, and apical levels. (See Video 5-6 online at the Expert Consult site for rotational views of these teeth.)

FIG. 5-105 The two locations of the second mesiobuccal (MB-2) canal orifices in a maxillary first molar. *B,* Buccal; *D,* distal; *M,* mesial; *P,* palatal.

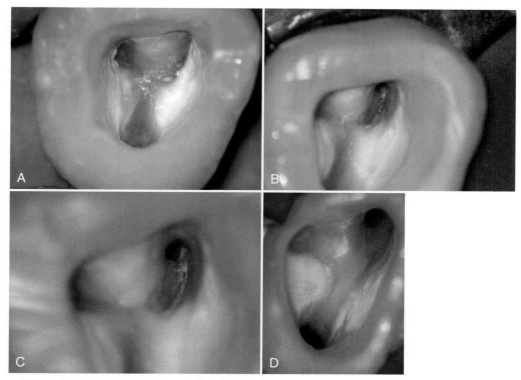

FIG. 5-106 Access cavity for a maxillary first molar as viewed through the dental operating microscope. A, Four apparent orifices, with a projection of dentin covering the mesial groove. (×3.4.) B, Removal of the mesial projection and troughing of the mesial groove to locate the second mesiobuccal *(MB-2)* canal. (×5.1.) C, Despite deepening of the mesial groove, the MB-2 canal cannot be located. (×8.5.) D, The MB-2 canal cannot be found even after removal of the mesial groove. (×13.6.)

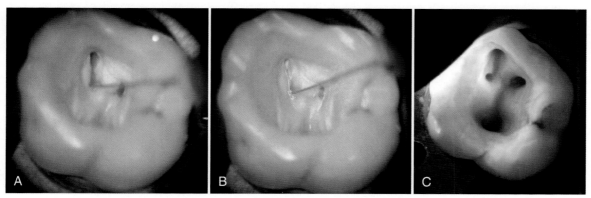

FIG. 5-107 Access preparation for a maxillary first molar as viewed through the dental operating microscope. A, Four apparent orifices located under ×3.4 magnification. B, Second mesiobuccal canal is located by deepening the mesial groove. (×5.1.) C, Four distinct canal orifices can be seen. (×5.1 magnification with cervical fiberoptic transillumination.)

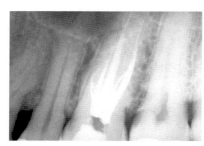

FIG. 5-108 Four canals with loops and accessory canals.

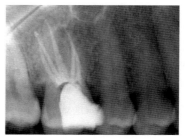

FIG. 5-109 Two canals in both buccal roots with a common foramen in each root.

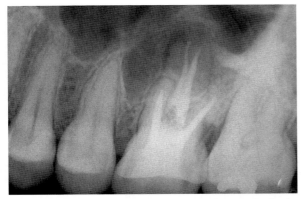

FIG. 5-110 Two separate canals in palatal root. (Courtesy Dr. Paulo Nogueira, São Paulo, Brazil.)

maxillary second molar is that its three roots are grouped closer together and are sometimes fused. Also, they generally are shorter than the roots of the first molar and not as curved. The second molar usually has one canal in each root; however, it may have two or three mesiobuccal canals, one or two disto-buccal canals, or two palatal canals (see Tables 5-16 to 5-18 online at the Expert Consult site). Four canals are less likely to be present in the second molar than in the first molar. The μCT scans for the maxillary second molar can be seen in Fig. 5-113. (See Video 5-7 online at the Expert Consult site for rotational views of these teeth.) The three main orifices usually form a flat triangle and sometimes almost a straight line (Figs. 5-114 through 5-118). The mesiobuccal canal orifice is located more to the buccal and mesial than in the first molar; the disto-buccal orifice approaches the midpoint between the mesio-buccal and palatal orifices[250]; and the palatal orifice usually is

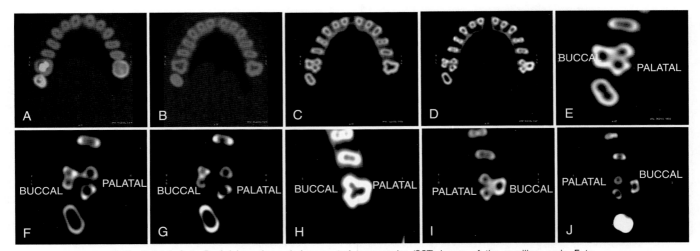

FIG. 5-111 A to D, Axial section spiral computed tomography (SCT) image of the maxillary arch. E to G, Enlarged axial section SCT image of tooth #3 showing two palatal roots and two canals in the fused buccal root. H to J, Enlarged axial section SCT image of tooth #14 showing the two palatal roots and a single canal in the fused buccal root. (From Gopikrishna V, Reuben J, Kandaswamy D: Endodontic management of a maxillary first molar with two palatal roots and a fused buccal root diagnosed with spiral computed tomography: a case report, *Oral Surg Oral Med Oral Pathol Oral Radiol Endod* 105:e74, 2008.)

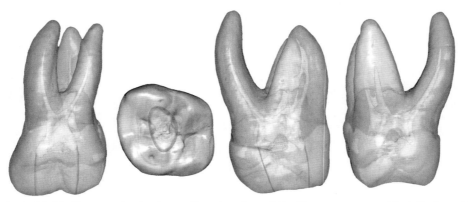

FIG. 5-112 Maxillary second molar. Average time of eruption—11 to 13 years; average age of calcification—14 to 16 years; average length—20 mm. Root curvature (most common to least common): mesiobuccal root—distal, straight; distobuccal root—straight, mesial, distal; palatal root—straight, buccal.

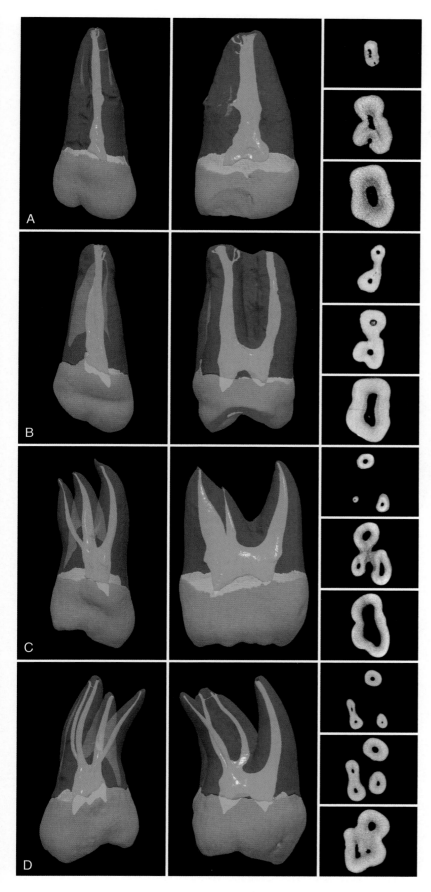

FIG. 5-113 μCT scans of maxillary second molars; four possible variations. **A,** Uncommon anatomic presentation of this tooth with one canal. **B,** Second molar with two canals. **C,** Second molar with three canals. **D,** Second molar with four distinct canals. All teeth are shown from both a buccal (vestibular) and a proximal perspective, along with the cross-sectional anatomy at the coronal, middle, and apical levels. (See Video 5-7 online at the Expert Consult site for rotational views of these teeth.)

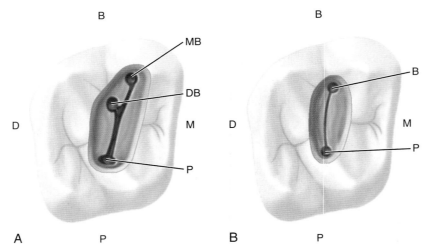

FIG. 5-114 **A,** Three canal orifices in a maxillary second molar. **B,** Two canal orifices in a maxillary second molar. *B,* Buccal; *P,* palatal; *D,* distal, *DB,* distobuccal; *M,* medial; *MB,* mesiobuccal.

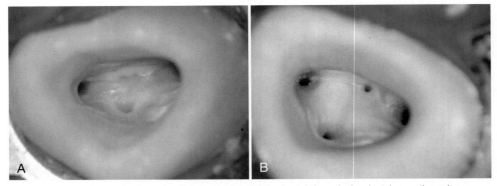

FIG. 5-115 Access cavity for a maxillary second molar as viewed through the dental operating microscope. **A,** Dentin projection covering the mesial aspect of the floor of the pulp chamber. (×8.4.) **B,** Fourth canal orifice (second mesiobuccal, *MB-2*), which was identified after removal of the dentin projection and troughing of the groove connecting the MB-1 orifice and the palatal *(P)* canal orifice. (×8.4.)

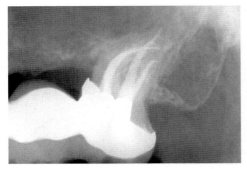

FIG. 5-116 Severely curved mesiobuccal root with a right-angle curve in the distobuccal *(DB)* root.

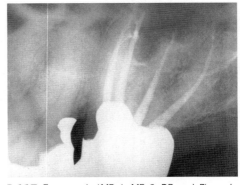

FIG. 5-117 Four canals (*MB-1, MB-2, DB,* and *P*) can be seen.

located at the most palatal aspect of the root. In general, the canal orifices in the maxillary second molar are closer mesially to each other than they are in the maxillary first molar.

The floor of the pulp chamber is markedly convex, which gives the canal orifices a slight funnel shape. On occasion the canals curve into the chamber at a more horizontal angle, requiring removal of a lip of dentin so that a canal can be

entered more in a direct line with the axis. Teeth with two canals usually have a buccal and a palatal canal of equal length and diameter (see Fig. 5-114, *B*). These parallel root canals are frequently superimposed radiographically, but they can be imaged by exposing the radiograph from a distal angle. To enhance radiographic visibility, especially when interference arises from the malar process, a more perpendicular and distoangular radiograph may be exposed. When two roots are present, each root may have one canal, or the buccal root may have two canals that join before reaching a single foramen. One study found that two palatal roots and two palatal canals occur in 1.47% of these teeth.[166]

When four canals are present, the access cavity preparation of the maxillary second molar has a rhomboid shape and is a smaller version of the access cavity for the maxillary first molar (see Fig. 5-115). If only three canals are present, the access cavity is a rounded triangle with the base to the buccal. As with the maxillary first molar, the mesial marginal ridge need not be invaded. Because the tendency in maxillary second molars is for the distobuccal orifice to move closer to a line connecting the mesiobuccal and palatal orifices, the triangle becomes more obtuse and the oblique ridge usually is not invaded.

If only two canals are present, the access outline form is oval and widest in the buccolingual dimension. Its width corresponds to the mesiodistal width of the pulp chamber, and the oval usually is centered between the mesial pit and the mesial edge of the oblique ridge.

Maxillary Third Molar

Loss of the maxillary first and second molars often is the reason the third molar must be considered a strategic abutment (Fig. 5-119). Careful examination of the root morphology is important before treatment is determined. The radicular anatomy of the third molar is completely unpredictable, and it may be

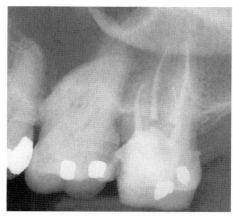

FIG. 5-118 Four canals with two distinct palatal roots and canals.

advisable to explore the root canal morphology to evaluate the likelihood and degree of success. Even so, many third molars have adequate root formation; given reasonable accessibility, they can serve well as functioning dentition after root canal therapy.

The root anatomy of the maxillary third molar varies greatly. This tooth can have one to four roots and one to six canals, and C-shaped canals also can occur. The third molar usually has three roots and three root canals (see Table 5-19 online at the Expert Consult site). The tooth may be tipped significantly to the distal, the buccal, or both, which creates an even greater access problem than with the second molar. The μCT scans for the maxillary molar can be seen in Fig. 5-120. (See Video 5-8 online at the Expert Consult site for rotational views of these teeth.)

The access cavity form for the third molar can vary greatly. Because the tooth typically has one to three canals, the access preparation can be anything from an oval that is widest in the buccolingual dimension to a rounded triangle similar to that used for the maxillary second molar. All the canal orifices often lie nearly in a straight line as the distobuccal orifice moves even closer to the line connecting the mesiobuccal and palatal orifices. The resultant access cavity is an oval or highly obtuse triangle (Figs. 5-121 and 5-122).

Mandibular Central and Lateral Incisors

The root canal systems and access cavities for the two mandibular incisors are so similar they are discussed together (Fig. 5-123). As with the maxillary incisors, a lingual shoulder must be eliminated to allow direct-line access. The shoulder conceals the orifice to a second canal that, if present, is found immediately beneath it. Unlike the maxillary incisors, the pulp outline of the mandibular incisors is wider labiolingually. At the CEJ the pulp outline is oval and wider labiolingually than mesiodistally. At midroot the canal outline is still oval, but the canal is more constricted and narrower labiolingually. Most mandibular incisors have a single root with what radiographically appears to be a long, narrow canal. However, it is a broad canal labiolingually. Often a dentinal bridge is present in the pulp chamber that divides the root into two canals. The two canals usually join and exit through a single apical foramen, but they may persist as two separate canals. On occasion one canal branches into two canals, which subsequently rejoin into a single canal before reaching the apex (see Table 5-20 online

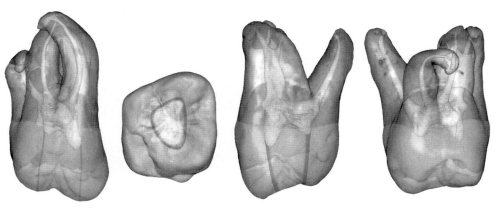

FIG. 5-119 Maxillary third molar. Average time of eruption—17 to 22 years; average age of calcification—18 to 25 years; average length—17 mm.

FIG. 5-120 μCT scans of maxillary third molars show a range of anatomic variations; A, Single-canal tooth. B, Two-rooted third molar. C, Two-rooted, three-canal third molar with significant root curvatures. D, Three-rooted, four-canal third molar. All teeth are shown from both a buccal (vestibular) and a proximal perspective, along with the cross-sectional anatomy at the coronal, middle, and apical levels. (See Video 5-8 online at the Expert Consult site for rotational views of these teeth.)

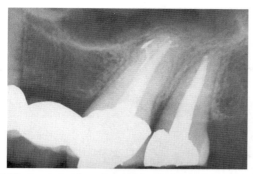

FIG. 5-121 Canals that have fused into a single canal. Multiple accessory canals can be seen in the second molar.

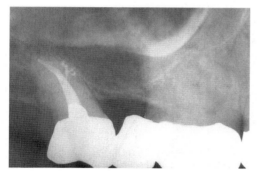

FIG. 5-122 Distal bridge abutment with major accessory canal.

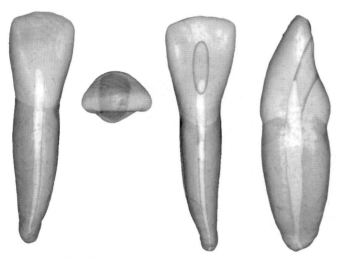

FIG. 5-123 Mandibular central/lateral incisors. Average time of eruption—6 to 8 years; average age of calcification—9 to 10 years; average length—20.7 mm. Root curvature (most common to least common): straight, distal, labial.

at the Expert Consult site). The scans of the mandibular central incisor can be seen in Fig. 5-124. The scans for the mandibular lateral incisors can be seen in Fig. 5-125. (See Videos 5-9 and 5-10 online at the Expert Consult site for rotational views of these teeth.)

One study determined that a relationship existed between crown size and the incidence of bifid root canals in these teeth.[234,235] Double root canals occur more often in teeth with a smaller index.

The mandibular incisors, because of their small size and internal anatomy, may be the most difficult access cavities to prepare. The external outline form may be triangular or oval, depending on the prominence of the mesial and distal pulp horns (Figs. 5-126 through 5-128). When the form is triangular, the incisal base is short and the mesial and distal legs are long incisogingivally, creating a long, compressed triangle. Without prominent mesial and distal pulp horns, the oval external outline form also is narrow mesiodistally and long incisogingivally. One study[152] determined that by age 40 years, the mandibular incisor pulp chamber has decreased in size sufficiently to justify an oval access cavity routinely. Complete removal of the lingual shoulder is critical because this tooth often has two canals that are buccolingually oriented, and the lingual canal most often is missed. To avoid missing this canal, the access preparation is extended well into the cingulum gingivally. Because the lingual surface of this tooth is not involved with occlusal function, restoration of the access opening with butt joint junctions between the internal walls and the lingual surface is not required.

Mandibular Canine

The root canal system of the mandibular canine is very similar to that of the maxillary canine, except that the dimensions are smaller, the root and root canal outlines are narrower in the mesiodistal dimension, and the mandibular canine occasionally has two roots and two root canals located labially and lingually (Fig. 5-129) (see Table 5-21 online at the Expert Consult site). The μCT scans of the mandibular canine can be seen in Fig. 5-130. (See Video 5-11 online at the Expert Consult site for rotational views of these teeth.) A fourth type is seen in subsequent Figs. 5-131 to 5-135.[222]

The root canal of the mandibular cuspid is narrow mesiodistally but usually very broad buccolingually. A lingual shoulder must be removed to gain access to the lingual wall of the root canal or to the entrance of a second canal. The lingual wall is almost slitlike compared with the larger buccal wall, which makes the canal a challenge to shape and clean.

The access cavity for the mandibular canine is oval or slot shaped (see Fig. 5-131). The mesiodistal width corresponds to the mesiodistal width of the pulp chamber. The incisal extension can approach the incisal edge of the tooth for straight-line access, and the gingival extension must penetrate the cingulum to allow a search for a possible lingual canal.

Mandibular First Premolar

As a group, the mandibular premolars present anatomic challenges because of the extreme variations in their root canal morphology (Fig. 5-136).[123,157,252] The root canal system of the mandibular first premolar is wider buccolingually than mesiodistally.[253] Two pulp horns are present: a large, pointed buccal horn and a small, rounded lingual horn. At the cervical line the root and canal are oval; this shape tends to become round as the canal approaches the middle of the root. If two canals are present, they tend to be round from the pulp chamber to their foramen. In another anatomic variation, a single, broad root canal may bifurcate into two separate root canals. Direct access to the buccal canal usually is possible, whereas the lingual canal may be quite difficult to find. The lingual canal tends to diverge from the main canal at a sharp angle. In addition, the lingual inclination of the crown tends to direct files

Text continued on p. 190

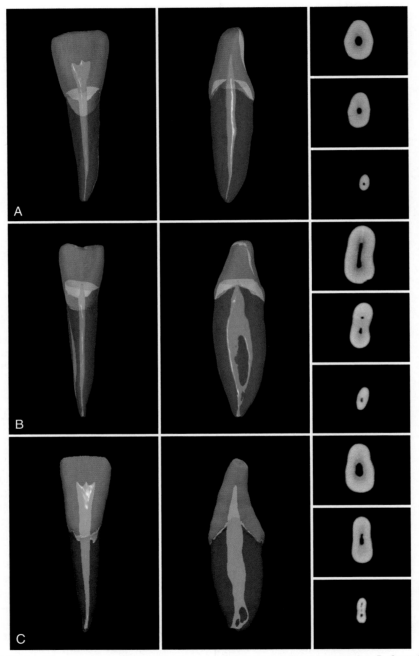

FIG. 5-124 μCT scans of mandibular central incisors. **A,** Common anatomic presentation. **B,** Central incisor with two canals. **C,** Central incisor with an apical delta. All teeth are shown from both a buccal (vestibular) and a proximal perspective, along with the cross-sectional anatomy at the coronal, middle, and apical levels. (See Video 5-9 online at the Expert Consult site for rotational views of these teeth.)

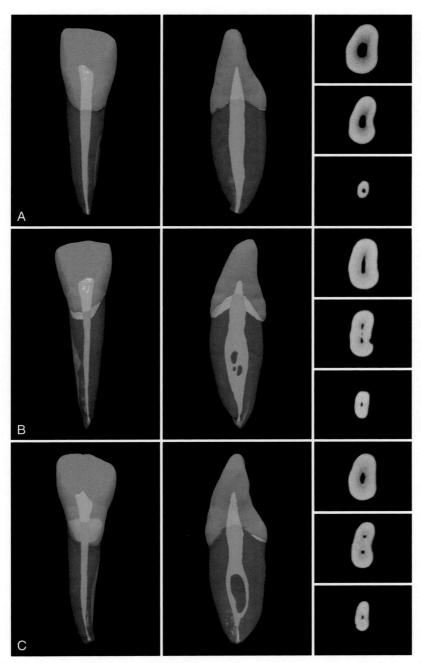

FIG. 5-125 μCT scans of mandibular lateral incisors. **A,** Common anatomic presentation. **B,** Lateral incisor with broad, thin buccolingual anatomy. **C,** Lateral incisor in which the canal splits into two but returns to form one canal apically. All teeth are shown from both a buccal (vestibular) and a proximal perspective, along with the cross-sectional anatomy at the coronal, middle, and apical levels. (See Video 5-10 online at the Expert Consult site for rotational views of these teeth.)

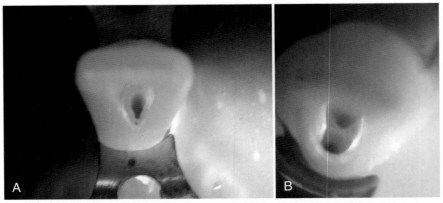

FIG. 5-126 Access cavity for mandibular incisors as viewed through the dental operating microscope. **A,** One canal orifice. (×8.5 magnification with cervical fiberoptic transillumination.) **B,** Two canal orifices. (×8.5 magnification with cervical fiberoptic transillumination.)

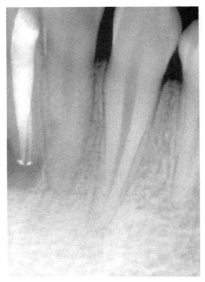

FIG. 5-127 Double-rooted mandibular lateral incisor.

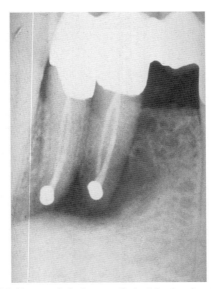

FIG. 5-128 Two canals in the mandibular lateral and central incisors.

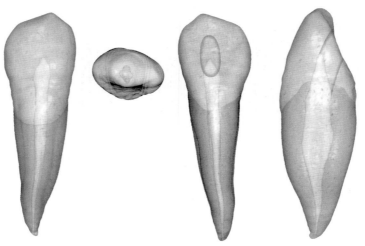

FIG. 5-129 Mandibular canine. Average time of eruption—9 to 10 years; average age of calcification—13 years; average length—25.6 mm. Root curvature (most common to least common): straight, distal, labial.

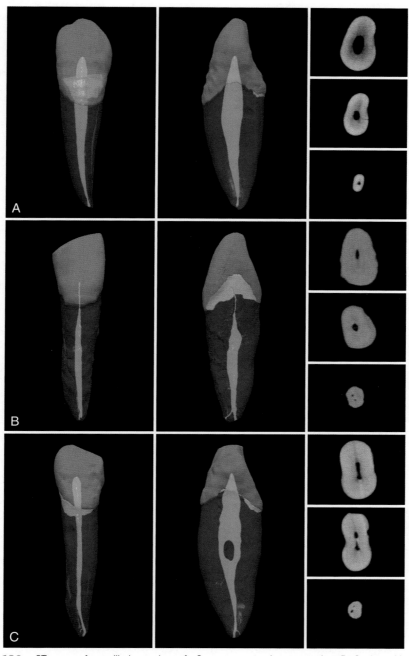

FIG. 5-130 μCT scans of mandibular canines. **A,** Common anatomic presentation. **B,** Canine with an extra apical canal. **C,** Canine that splits into two but returns to one canal apically. All teeth are shown from both a buccal (vestibular) and a proximal perspective, along with the cross-sectional anatomy at the coronal, middle, and apical levels. A fourth type is seen in Figs. 5-133 through 5-135. (See Video 5-11 online at the Expert Consult site for rotational views of these teeth.)

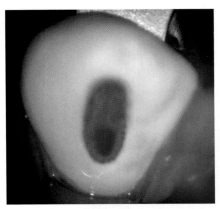

FIG. 5-131 Access preparation for a mandibular canine as viewed through the dental operating microscope. (×5.1.)

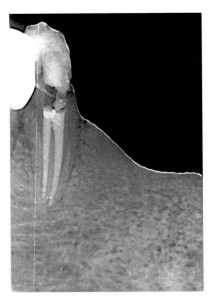

FIG. 5-134 Two separate root canals.

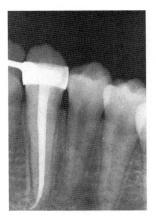

FIG. 5-132 One canal with a sharp mesial curvature at the apex.

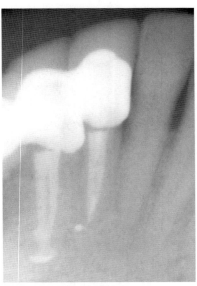

FIG. 5-135 Mandibular canine and lateral incisor with two canals.

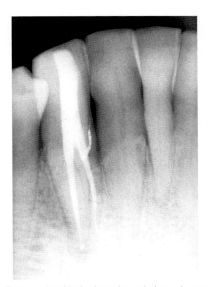

FIG. 5-133 Two canals with the lateral canal above the crest of bone; the lateral canal is probably responsible for the pocket depth.

buccally, making location of a lingual canal orifice more difficult. To counter this situation, the clinician may need to extend the lingual wall of the access cavity farther lingually; this makes the lingual canal easier to locate. The mandibular first premolar sometimes may have three roots and three canals (see Table 5-22 online at the Expert Consult site). Multiple studies have reported C-shaped canal anatomy in this tooth.[13,65,67] The μCT scans for the mandibular first premolar can be seen in Fig. 5-137. (See Video 5-12 online at the Expert Consult site for rotational views of these teeth.)

The oval external outline form of the mandibular first premolar typically is wider mesiodistally than its maxillary counterpart, making it more oval and less narrow (Figs. 5-138 through 5-141). Because of the lingual inclination of the crown, buccal extension can nearly approach the tip of the buccal cusp to achieve straight-line access. Lingual extension

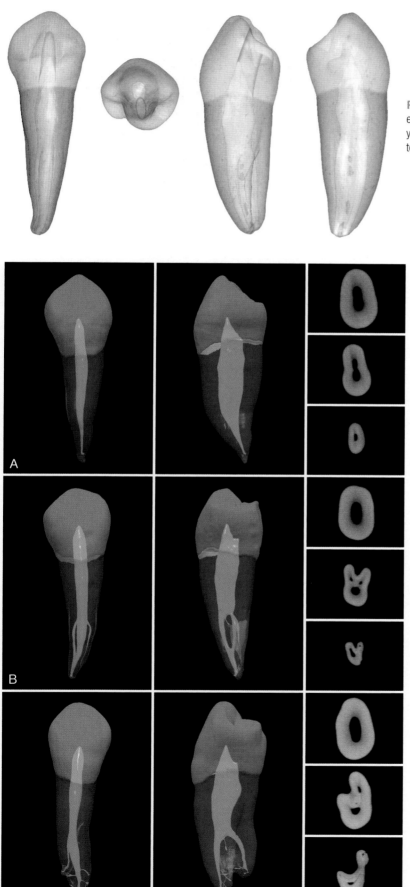

FIG. 5-136 Mandibular first premolar. Average time of eruption—10 to 12 years; average age of calcification—12 to 13 years; average length—21.6 mm. Root curvature (most common to least common): straight, distal, buccal.

FIG. 5-137 μCT scans of mandibular first preomlars. **A,** Common anatomic presentation. **B,** First premolar with significant canal deviations in the middle to apical third before returning to a single large canal apically and a small deviating canal to the proximal. **C,** First premolar with a branching main canal lingually and multiple accessory canals. All teeth are shown from both a buccal (vestibular) and a proximal perspective, along with the cross-sectional anatomy at the coronal, middle, and apical levels. (See Video 5-12 online at the Expert Consult site for rotational views of these teeth.)

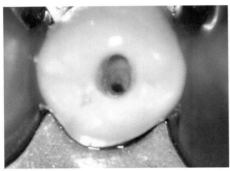

FIG. 5-138 Access cavity for a mandibular first premolar as viewed through the dental operating microscope: one orifice. (×5.1.)

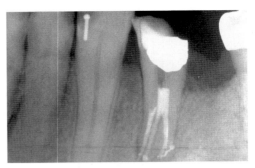

FIG. 5-141 Three canals.

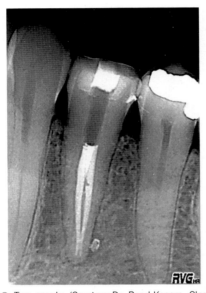

FIG. 5-139 Two canals. (Courtesy Dr. Raed Kasem, Clearwater, Fla.)

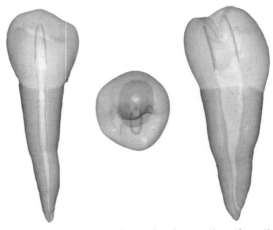

FIG. 5-142 Mandibular second premolar. Average time of eruption—11 to 12 years; average age of calcification—13 to 14 years; average length—22.3 mm. Root curvature (most common to least common): straight, distal, buccal.

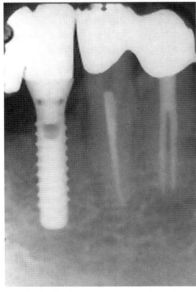

FIG. 5-140 Single canal that has divided into two.

barely invades the poorly developed lingual cusp incline. Mesiodistally the access preparation is centered between the cusp tips. Often the preparation must be modified to allow access to the complex root canal anatomy frequently seen in the apical half of the tooth root.

Mandibular Second Premolar

The mandibular second premolar is similar to the first premolar, with the following differences: the lingual pulp horn usually is larger; the root and root canal are more often oval than round; the pulp chamber is wider buccolingually; and the separation of the pulp chamber and root canal normally is distinguishable compared with the more regular taper in the first premolar (Fig. 5-142). The canal morphology of the mandibular second premolar is similar to that of the first premolar with its many variations: two, three, and four canals and a lingually tipped crown. Fortunately, these variations are found less often in the second premolar (see Table 5-23 online at the Expert Consult site). The μCT scans for the mandibular second premolar can be seen in Fig. 5-143. (See Video 5-13 online at the Expert Consult site for rotational views of these teeth.) The access cavity form for the mandibular second premolar varies

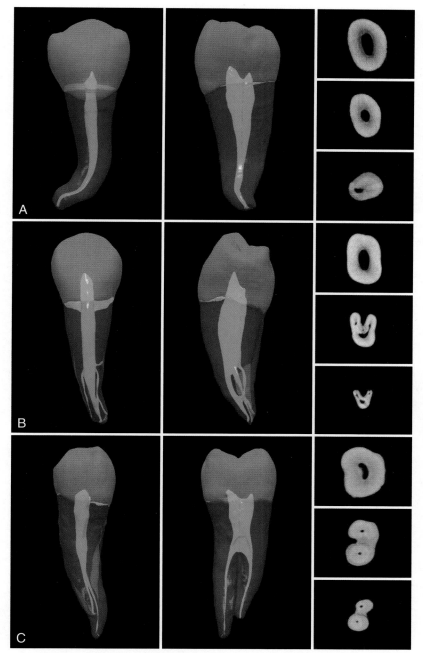

FIG. 5-143 μCT scans of mandibular second premolars. **A,** Common anatomic presentation. **B,** Second premolar with significant canal deviations in the middle to apical third. **C,** Second premolar with fused root that exhibits two distinct canals. All teeth are shown from both a buccal (vestibular) and a proximal perspective, along with the cross-sectional anatomy at the coronal, middle, and apical levels. (See Video 5-13 online at the Expert Consult site for rotational views of these teeth.)

in at least two ways in its external anatomy. First, because the crown typically has a smaller lingual inclination, less extension up the buccal cusp incline is required to achieve straight-line access. Second, the lingual half of the tooth is more fully developed; therefore, the lingual access extension typically is halfway up the lingual cusp incline.[54] The mandibular second premolar can have two lingual cusps, sometimes of equal size. When this occurs, the access preparation is centered mesiodistally on a line connecting the buccal cusp and the lingual groove between

the lingual cusp tips. When the mesiolingual cusp is larger than the distolingual cusp, the lingual extension of the oval outline form is just distal to the tip of the mesiolingual cusp (Figs. 5-144 through 5-149).

Mandibular First Molar

The earliest permanent posterior tooth to erupt, the mandibular first molar seems to be the tooth that most often requires an endodontic procedure (vital pulp capping, pulpotomy, root

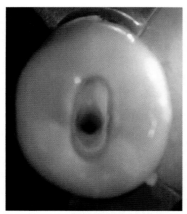

FIG. 5-144 Access cavity for a mandibular second premolar as viewed through the dental operating microscope: one canal orifice. (×5.1 magnification with cervical fiberoptic transillumination.)

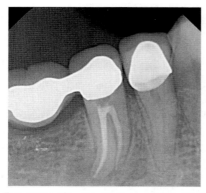

FIG. 5-145 Two canals. (Courtesy Dr. Haider Al Zubaidi, Ocala, Fla.)

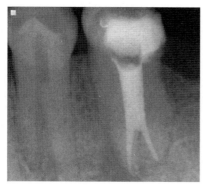

FIG. 5-146 Single canal that has divided at the apex. (Courtesy Dr. Haider Al Zubaidi, Ocala, Fla.)

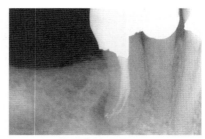

FIG. 5-147 Single canal that has divided and crossed over at the apex.

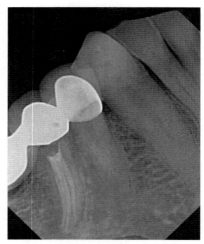

FIG. 5-148 Three separate canals. (Courtesy Dr. Haider Al Zubaidi, Ocala, Fla.)

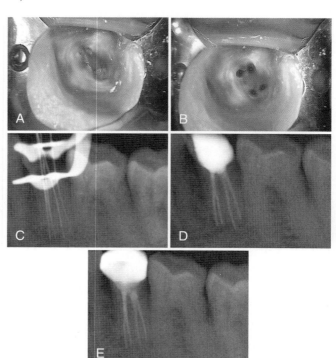

FIG. 5-149 A, Initial access opening. B, Access opening showing orifices of the four root canals. C, Working length determination. D, Immediate posttreatment radiograph. E, Recall radiograph 1 year posttreatment. (From Sachdeva GS, Ballal S, Gopikrishna V, Kandaswamy D: Endodontic management of a mandibular second premolar with four roots and four root canals with the aid of spiral computed tomography: a case report, *J Endod* 34:104, 2008.)

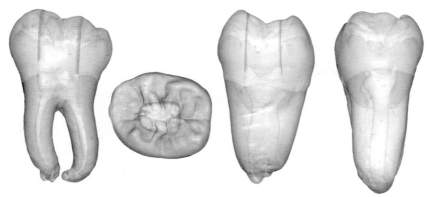

FIG. 5-150 Mandibular first molar. Average time of eruption—6 years; average age of calcification—9 to 10 years; average length—21 mm. Root curvature (most common to least common): mesial root—distal, straight; distal root—straight, distal.

canal); therefore, its morphology has received a great deal of attention (Fig. 5-150).[261] It often is extensively restored, and it is subjected to heavy occlusal stress. Consequently, the pulp chamber frequently has receded or is calcified. The tooth usually has two roots, but occasionally it has three, with two or three canals in the mesial root and one, two, or three canals in the distal root (see Tables 5-24 and 5-25 online at the Expert Consult site). The μCT scans of the mandibular first molar can be seen in Fig. 5-151. (See Video 5-14 online at the Expert Consult site for rotational views of these teeth.)

The canals in the mesial root are the mesiobuccal and mesiolingual canals. A middle mesial (MM) canal sometimes is present in the developmental groove between the other mesial canals,[148] but it may only represent a wide anastomosis between the two mesial canals.[54] The incidence of an MM canal ranges from 1%[223] to 15%.[77,209] The canals in the distal root include the distal canal (if only one canal is present) and the distobuccal and distolingual and middle distal canals (if more than one is present).[75] The orifices to these canals are connected by a developmental groove. Orifices to all canals usually are located in the mesial two thirds of the crown, and the pulp chamber floor is roughly trapezoid or rhomboid. Usually four pulp horns are present.

The presence of two separate distal roots is rare, but this does occur. In such cases the distolingual root is smaller than the distobuccal root and usually more curved. Also, the distolingual root often has a sharp apical hook toward the buccal side that is not obvious on radiographs (Fig. 5-152). The mesial root, the wider of the two roots, curves mesially from the cervical line to the middle third of the root and then angles distally to the apex. The buccal and lingual surfaces are convex throughout their length, whereas the distal surface of the mesial root and the mesial surface of the distal root have a root concavity, which makes the dentin wall very thin.

The mesial canal orifices usually are well separated in the main pulp chamber and connected by a developmental groove.[40] The mesiobuccal orifice is commonly under the mesiobuccal cusp, whereas the mesiolingual orifice generally is found just lingual to the central groove. On occasion an middle mesial canal orifice is present in the groove between the two mesial orifices (Figs. 5-152 through 5-159). The clinician must always check for such an orifice after shaping and cleaning the main root canals. A bur is used to remove any protuberance from the mesial axial wall that would prevent direct access to the

developmental groove between the two mesial orifices. Magnification is a tremendous aid during the exploration of this developmental groove with the sharp tip of an endodontic explorer. If a depression or orifice is located, the groove can be troughed with ultrasonic tips, at the expense of the mesial aspect, until a small file can negotiate the space.

When only one distal canal is present, the orifice is oval buccolingually and the opening generally is located distal to the buccal groove. This orifice usually can be explored from the mesial with either an endodontic explorer or a small K-file. If the file tip takes a sharp turn in a distobuccal or distolingual direction, the clinician should search for yet another orifice; in rare cases a mesiodistal canal orifice is present.

If three main root canals are present in this tooth, each is oval in the cervical and middle thirds of the root and round in the apical third. If two canals (distobuccal and distolingual) are present in the distal root, they usually are more round than oval for their entire length. The mesial root canals usually are curved, with the greatest curvature in the mesiobuccal canal. This canal can have a significant curvature in the buccolingual plane that may not be apparent on radiographs. Such a curvature usually can be detected with precurved pathfinder instruments.

Multiple accessory foramina may be located in the furcation of the mandibular molars. These foramina usually are impossible to clean and shape directly; they are rarely seen, except occasionally on a posttreatment radiograph if they have been filled with root canal sealer or thermoplastic filling material. Because sodium hypochlorite solutions can dissolve organic debris, the pulp chamber should be thoroughly exposed to allow the solution to reach the tiny openings. Fractures occasionally occur, which are quite visible with magnification, on proximal marginal ridges and extend down the root or under the lingual cusps.

The access cavity for the mandibular first molar typically is trapezoid or rhomboid, regardless of the number of canals present.[247] When four or more canals are present, the corners of the trapezoid or rhombus should correspond to the positions of the main orifices. Mesially the access need not invade the marginal ridge, except if access to the tooth itself is compromised. Distal extension must allow straight-line access to the distal canal or canals. The buccal wall forms a straight connection between the mesiobuccal and distobuccal orifices, and the lingual wall connects the mesiolingual and distolingual orifices without bowing.

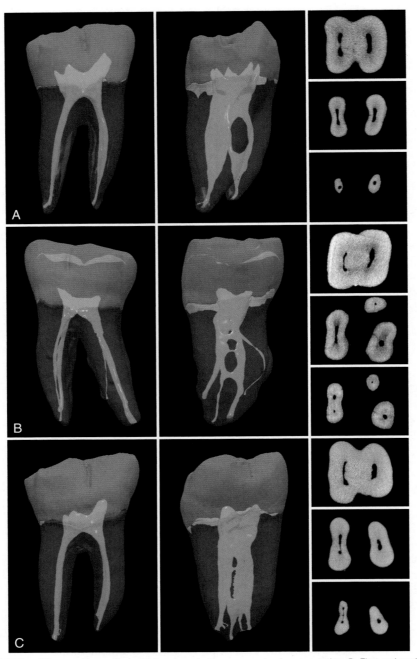

FIG. 5-151 μCT scans of mandibular first molars. **A,** Common anatomic presentation. **B,** First molar with three main canals and a deviant fourth canal/fourth root. **C,** First molar with wide connections or anastomoses between the mesial canals, demonstrating multiple canal exits. All teeth are shown from both a buccal (vestibular) and a proximal perspective, along with the cross-sectional anatomy at the coronal, middle, and apical levels. (See Video 5-14 online at the Expert Consult site for rotational views of these teeth.)

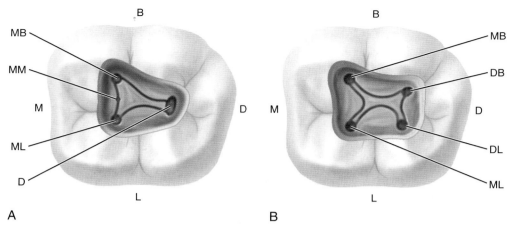

A

B

FIG. 5-152 Access cavities for the mandibular first molar. **A,** Three mesial canal orifices and one distal canal orifice. **B,** Two mesial and two distal canal orifices. *B,* Buccal; *D,* distal, distal orifice; *DB,* distobuccal orifice; *DL,* distolingual orifice; *L,* labial; *M,* mesial; *MB,* mesiobuccal orifice; *ML,* mesiolingual orifice; *MM,* middle mesial orifice.

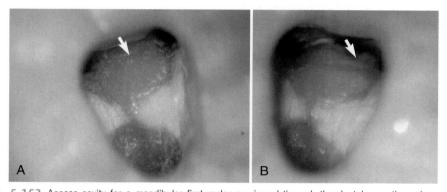

FIG. 5-153 Access cavity for a mandibular first molar as viewed through the dental operating microscope. **A,** Three canal orifices (*MB, ML,* and *D*) and a dentinal projection *(arrow)* can be seen. (×5.1.) A possible middle mesial *(MM)* orifice may be present along the mesial groove. **B,** Troughing of the mesial groove allows identification of the MM canal orifice *(arrow).* (×5.1.)

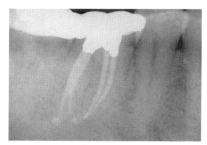

FIG. 5-154 Two mesial and two distal canals.

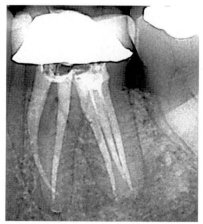

FIG. 5-155 Three canals in the distal root. (Courtesy Dr. Raed Kasem, Clearwater, Fla.)

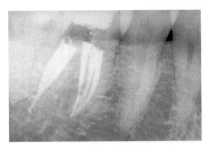

FIG. 5-156 Three mesial canals.

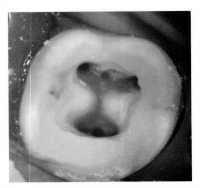

FIG. 5-157 Three orifices in the mesial root and three orifices in the distal root. (Courtesy Dr. Haider Al Zubaidi, Ocala, Fla.)

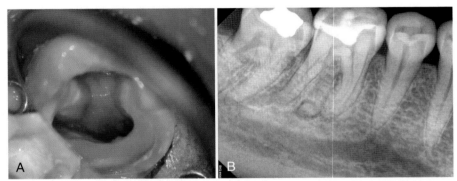

FIG. 5-158 **A,** Radix entomolaris. Notice lingual position of its orifice in relation to the two canals in the distal root. **B,** Radiograph with obvious radix entomolaris on mandibular first molar that curves to the buccal. The reader is referred to a recent publication that details extensively this type of anatomy (see following credit for part **B**). (**A** courtesy Dr. William J. Aippersbach, Venice, Fla; **B** from Abella F, Patel S, Durán-Sindreu F et al: Mandibular first molars with disto-lingual roots: review and clinical management, *Int Endod J* 45:963, 2012.)

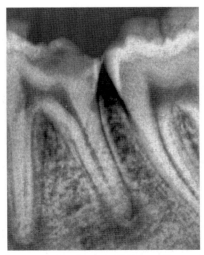

FIG. 5-159 Pretreatment radiograph. Notice position and appearance of the distolingual root. (Courtesy Dr. William J. Aippersbach, Venice, Fla.)

A variation in root morphology is the presence of an extra distolingual root.[203] Usually this root has a type 1 canal configuration. Two thirds of the first mandibular molars found in a Chinese population had this variation.[251] Similarly, this distolingual root occurred in 4% of mandibular first molars of a Kuwaiti population.[159] These results confirm the observation that East Asian populations have more three-rooted mandibular first molars than do other racial groups.[8]

Mandibular molars, mainly first molars, may also have an additional root located lingually or buccally. Although this is a rare occurrence in Caucasian populations, it is more common in Asian populations.[220] The radix entomolaris (RE) is a supernumerary root located distolingually in mandibular molars (see Fig. 5-158),[10,32] whereas the radix paramolaris (RP) is an extra root located mesiobuccally. Each root usually contains a single root canal. The orifice of the RE is located distolingually to mesiolingually from the main canal or canals of the distal root; the orifice of the RP is located mesiobuccally to distobuccally from the main mesial root canals. A dark line or groove from the main root canal on the pulp chamber floor leads to

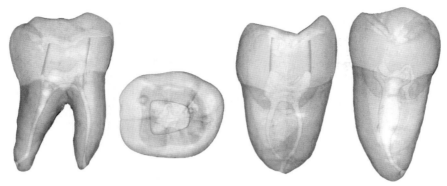

FIG. 5-160 Mandibular second molar. Average time of eruption—11 to 13 years; average age of calcification—14 to 15 years; average length—19.8 mm. Root curvature (most common to least common): mesial root—distal, straight; distal root—straight, distal, mesial, buccal; single root—straight, distal, bayonet, lingual.

these orifices.[32] These anatomic variations present definite challenges to therapy because of their orifice inclination and root canal curvature. The canal can be straight, may have a coronal curvature, or can have separate coronal and apical curvatures.[52]

Mandibular Second Molar

The mandibular second molar is somewhat smaller coronally than the first molar and tends to be more symmetric (Fig. 5-160). This tooth is identified by the proximity of its roots. The two roots often sweep distally in a gradual curve, with the apices close together. In some cases only one root is present. The degree of canal curvature and the configuration were studied in the mesial roots of 100 randomly selected mandibular first and second molars; 100% of the specimens showed curvature in both buccolingual and mesiodistal views.[45]

The pulp chamber and canal orifices of the mandibular second molar generally are not as large as those of the first molar. This tooth may have one, two, three, or four root canals (see Table 5-26 online at the Expert Consult site). The μCT scans for the mandibular second molar can be seen in Fig. 5-161. (See Video 5-15 online at the Expert Consult site for rotational views of these teeth.) Figs. 5-162 through 5-166 provide additional variations and views of this tooth.

The two mesial orifices are located closer together. In some mandibular second molars with single or fused roots, a file placed in the mesiobuccal canal may appear to be in the distal canal. This happens because the two canals sometimes are connected by a semicircular slit, a variation of the C-shaped canal[137,234,262] that often occurs in this tooth. The distal aspect of the mesial root and the mesial aspect of the distal root have concavities.

Mandibular second molars may have one to six canals, although the most prevalent configurations are two, three, and four canals (see Fig. 5-162). When three canals are present, the access cavity is similar to that for the mandibular first molar, although perhaps a bit more triangular and less rhomboid. The distal orifice is less often ribbon shaped buccolingually; therefore, the buccal and lingual walls converge more aggressively distally to form a triangle. The second molar may have only two canals, one mesial and one distal, in which case the orifices are nearly equal in size and line up in the buccolingual center of the tooth. The access cavity for a two-canal second molar is rectangular, wide mesiodistally and narrow buccolingually. The access cavity for a single-canal mandibular second molar is oval and is lined up in the center of the occlusal surface.

Mandibular Third Molar

The mandibular third molar is anatomically unpredictable and must be evaluated on the basis of its root formation (Fig. 5-167).[110] Fused short, severely curved, or malformed roots often support well-formed crowns. This tooth may have one to four roots and one to six canals (see Table 5-27 online at the Expert Consult site). The μCT scans for the mandibular third molar can be seen in Fig. 5-168. (See Video 5-16 online at the Expert Consult site for rotational views of these teeth.) Additional variations are seen in Figs. 5-169 through 5-171.

C-shaped canals also can occur (Fig. 5-172). Most of these teeth can be successfully root treated, regardless of anatomic irregularities; however, the long-term prognosis is determined by the root surface volume in contact with bone. The clinician must weigh the benefit of treatment against the prognosis.

The anatomy of the mandibular third molar is unpredictable; therefore, the access cavity can take any of several shapes. When three or more canals are present, a traditional rounded triangle or rhomboid shape is typical. When two canals are present, a rectangular shape is used. For single-canal molars, an oval shape is customary.

Teeth with C-Shaped Root Canal Systems

The main cause for C-shaped roots and canals is the failure of Hertwig's epithelial root sheath to fuse on either the buccal or lingual root surface (Fig. 5-173). The C-shaped canal system can assume many variations in its morphology (Fig. 5-174, A). Further cross section of types I, II, and III are seen in Fig. 5-174, B to D. The original classification[133] has been modified and has produced a more detailed description of C-shaped root and canal morphology. The C-shaped canal configuration can vary along the root depth so that the appearance of the orifices may not be good predictors of the actual canal anatomy.[62,64,137,234,262]

Category I (C1): The shape is an uninterrupted "C" with no separation or division (see Fig. 5-163, A).

Category II (C2): The canal shape resembles a semicolon resulting from a discontinuation of the "C" outline (see

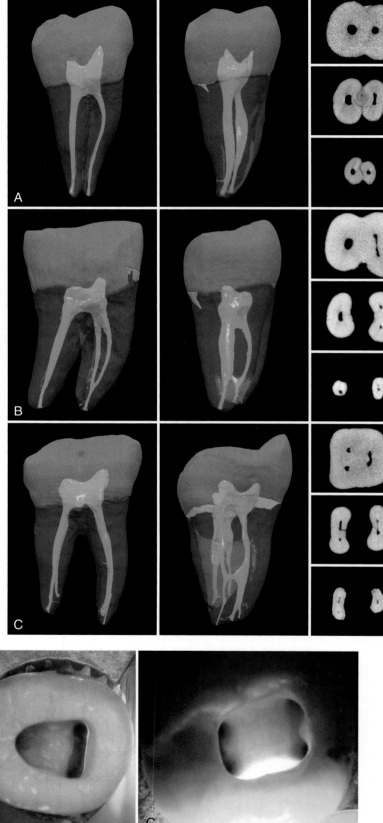

FIG. 5-161 μCT scans of mandibular second molars. **A,** Two-canal second molar with fused roots. **B,** Second molar with three initial canals ending in one canal apically in both roots. **C,** Second molar with four distinct canals. All teeth are shown from both a buccal (vestibular) and a proximal perspective, along with the cross-sectional anatomy at the coronal, middle, and apical levels. (See Video 5-15 online at the Expert Consult site for rotational views of these teeth.)

FIG. 5-162 Access cavity for a mandibular second molar as viewed through the dental operating microscope. **A,** Two canal orifices (*M* and *D*). (×5.1.) **B,** Three canal orifices (*MB, ML,* and *D*). (×3.4 magnification with cervical fiberoptic transillumination.) **C,** Four canal orifices identified (*MB, ML, DB,* and *DL*). (×5.1 magnification with cervical fiberoptic transillumination.)

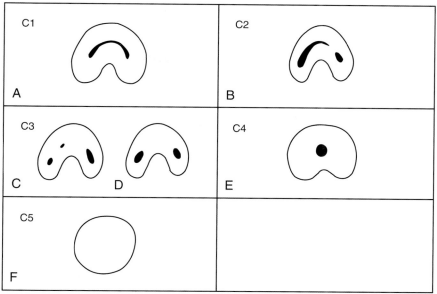

FIG. 5-163 Classification of C-shaped canal configuration. (From Fan B, Cheung G, Fan M, Gutmann J: C-shaped canal system in mandibular second molars. I. Anatomical fractures, *J Endod* 30:899, 2004.)

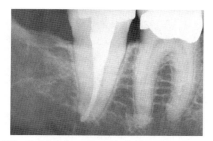

FIG. 5-164 Anastomosis of all canals into one.

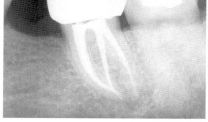

FIG. 5-166 Fusion of mesial canals at the apex.

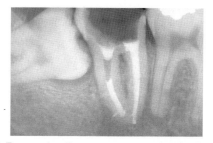

FIG. 5-165 Two canals with an accessory canal at the distal root apex.

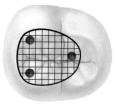

FIG. 5-167 Mandibular third molar. Average time of eruption—17 to 21 years; average age of calcification—18 to 25 years; average length—18.5 mm.

Fig. 5-163, *B*), but either angle α or β should be no less than 60 degrees.

Category III (C3): Two or three separate canals (see Fig. 5-163, *C* and *D*) and both angles, α and β, are less than 60 degrees.

Category IV (C4): Only one round or oval canal is in the cross-section (see Fig. 5-163, *E*).

Category V (C5): No canal lumen can be observed (is usually seen near the apex only) (see Fig. 5-163, *F*).

The **C**-shaped root canal system was first reported in 1979 in a maxillary molar.[43] Most **C**-shaped canals occur in the mandibular second molar (Figs. 5-175 through 5-180),[234] but

they also have been reported in the mandibular first molar,[146] the maxillary first and second molars, and the mandibular first premolar.* One study reported the incidence of **C**-shaped canal anatomy in maxillary first molars as 2 in 2175 (0.092%); this study also determined that the DB and palatal orifices were connected by a common groove (see Fig. 5-176, *B*).[53] Investigators who examined 309 Chinese maxillary second molars found **C**-shaped root canals in 4.9%.[254]

C-shaped mandibular molars are so named because of the cross-sectional morphology of their fused roots and their root

---

*References 62, 63, 65, 66, 146, 150, 252, 253, 261, and 262.

FIG. 5-168 μCT scans of mandibular third molars represent multiple variations for this tooth. A, Single C-shaped type canal. B, Complex anatomy with significant canal curvatures apically. C, Three canals that curve in multiple directions. D, Flattened, ribbon-shaped canals with significant apical curvatures. All teeth are shown from both a buccal (vestibular) and a proximal perspective, along with the cross-sectional anatomy at the coronal, middle, and apical levels. (See Video 5-16 online at the Expert Consult site for rotational views of these teeth.)

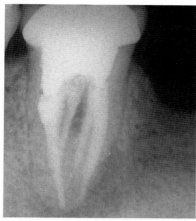

FIG. 5-169 Five canals. (Courtesy Dr. Paulo Nogueira, São Paulo, Brazil.)

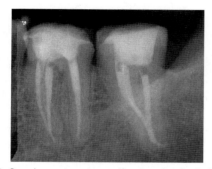

FIG. 5-170 Complex root anatomy. (Courtesy Dr. Paulo Nogueira, São Paulo, Brazil.)

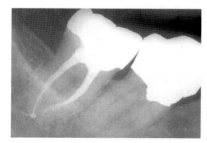

FIG. 5-171 Complex apical anatomy.

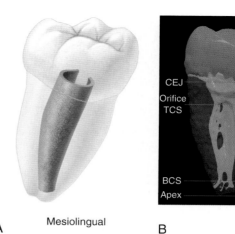

A   Mesiolingual   B

FIG. 5-172 A, Diagram of a C-shaped canal anatomy: one continuous canal from pulp chamber floor to apex. B, One large canal moving from the top of the C-shaped canal *(TCS)* to the apical-most or bottom of C-shaped canal *(BCS)*, encompassing most of the canal space.

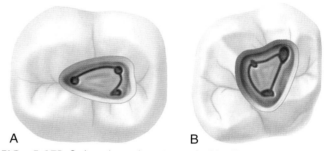

A   B

FIG. 5-173 C-shaped canal anatomy. A, Mandibular second molar. B, Maxillary first molar.

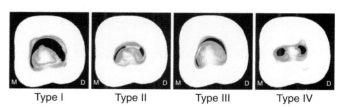

Type I   Type II   Type III   Type IV

FIG. 5-174 Types of pulpal floor. *M,* Mesial side; *D,* distal side. (From Min Y, Fan B, Cheung G, Gutmann J, Fan M: C-shaped canal system in mandibular second molars. III. The morphology of the pulp chamber floor, *J Endod* 32:1155, 2006.)

canals. Instead of having several discrete orifices, the pulp chamber of a molar with a C-shaped root canal system is a single, ribbon-shaped orifice with an arc of 180 degrees or more. It starts at the mesiolingual line angle and sweeps around either to the buccal or the lingual to end at the distal aspect of the pulp chamber (see Fig. 5-176, *A*). Below the orifice, the root structure can show a wide range of anatomic variations. These can be classified into two basic types: those with a single, ribbon-like, C-shaped canal from orifice to apex, and those with three or more distinct canals below the usual C-shaped orifice. Fortunately, molars with a single swath of canal are the exception rather than the rule. More common is the second type, with discrete canals that take unusual forms.[43] Other investigators determined that C-shaped canals in mandibular second molars can vary in shape and number along the root length.[136]

One study reported a case of a mandibular first molar with a normal mesiolingual orifice and a C-shaped groove that ran continuously from the mesiobuccal orifice along the buccal wall to the distal canal orifice.[18] The groove ran continuously down the root to the apical third, where it divided into two canals. Other researchers reported a C-shaped groove in a mandibular first molar that extended from the DL to the DB orifice and across the buccal surface to the MB orifice.[26] The ML orifice remained separate. Four separate apical foramina were noted. One investigator evaluated 811 endodontically treated mandibular second molars and found that 7.6% had C-shaped canals.[239] Several variants of the C-shaped canal

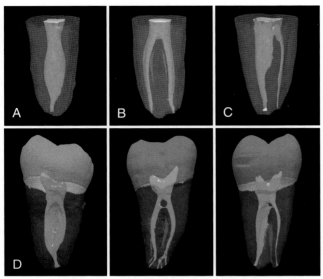

FIG. 5-175 Three-dimensional classification of C-shaped canal configuration. **A**, Merging type. **B**, Symmetrical type. **C**, Asymmetrical type. **D**, Additional C-shaped canal variations. (From Gao Y, Fan B, Cheung G, Gutmann J, Fan M: C-shaped canal system in mandibular second molars. IV. Morphological analysis and transverse measurement, *J Endod* 32:1062, 2006.)

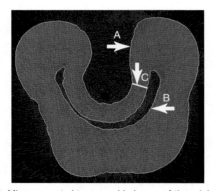

FIG. 5-176 Microcomputed tomographic image of the minimal wall thickness measurement. *A,* Outer root surface. *B,* Inner canal wall. *C,* Thinnest wall thickness. (From Gao Y, Fan B, Cheung G, Gutmann J, Fan M: C-shaped canal system in mandibular second molars. IV. Morphological analysis and transverse measurement, *J Endod* 32:1062, 2006.)

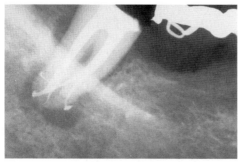

FIG. 5-177 Mandibular second molar with multiple foramina (see also Fig. 5-172, *D*).

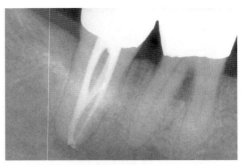

FIG. 5-178 Mandibular second molar with interconnecting canal anatomy.

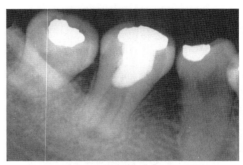

FIG. 5-179 Pretreatment appearance of a mandibular first molar with a C-shaped canal (see also Fig. 5-175, *D*).

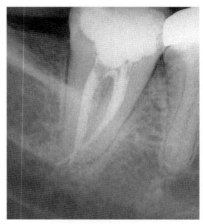

FIG. 5-180 Root canal obturation showing the ribbonlike canal space. (Courtesy Dr. Paulo Nogueira, São Paulo, Brazil.)

morphology were noted, the most common being two or three canals that merged and exited as one canal.[239]

Significant ethnic variation can be seen in the incidence of C-shaped root canal systems. This anatomy is much more common in Asians than in the Caucasian population. Investigators in Japan[106] and China[254] found a 32% incidence of C-shaped canals. Others found the occurrence of C-shaped canals in a Chinese population to be 23% in mandibular first molars and 32% in mandibular second molars.[254,255,257] Another study found a 19% rate in mandibular second molars in Lebanese subjects[85] and an 11% rate in a Saudi Arabian population.[6] Mandibular molars in a Burmese population were found to have C-shaped canals in 22% of teeth.[82] Another investigation found that 33% of Koreans had a C-shaped canal morphology in mandibular second molars.[105,189]

Four types of pulpal floors were found in mandibular second molars[137]:

Type I: A peninsula-like floor with continuous C-shaped orifice (see Fig. 5-174).

Type II: A buccal, striplike dentin connection between the peninsula-like floor and the buccal wall of the pulp chamber that separates the C-shaped groove into mesial (M) and distal (D) orifices. Sometimes the mesial orifice is separated into a mesiobuccal (MB) orifice and a mesiolingual (ML) orifice by another striplike dentin connection between the peninsula-like floor and the mesial wall of the pulp chamber (most common) (see Fig. 5-174).

Type III: Only one mesial, striplike dentin connection between the peninsula-like floor and the M wall, which separates the C-shaped groove into a small ML orifice and a large MB-D orifice. The MB-D orifice was formed by the merging of the MB orifice and the D orifice (second most common) (see Fig. 5-174).

Type IV: Non–C-shaped floors. One distal canal orifice and one oval or two round mesial canal orifices are present (least common) (see Fig. 5-174).

Not all C-shaped mandibular second molars with C-shaped canal systems have a C-shaped pulpal floor. This makes diagnosis difficult. However, radiographically a tooth with a C-shaped canal system always has a fused root with a longitudinal groove in the middle of the root.[63] Furthermore, there are three types of C-shaped canal systems in mandibular second molars (see Fig. 5-175).[73]

Type I (merging type): Canals merge to one main canal before exiting at the apical foramen

Type II (symmetric type): Separated mesial and distal canals in each root exit as separate canals

Type III (asymmetric type): Separated mesial and distal canals, with the distal canal having a long isthmus across the furcation area

The minimal wall thickness in the middle and apical parts of type III and in the apical part of type II makes these regions danger zones for canal enlargement procedures (see Fig. 5-176).[73]

Another study on mandibular molars found that there is a higher risk of root perforation at the thinner lingual walls of C-shaped canals during shaping and after canal preparation procedures. Both buccal and lingual canal walls were frequently narrower at the mesial locations.[36]

The access cavity for teeth with a C-shaped root canal system varies considerably and depends on the pulp morphology of the specific tooth. Teeth with C-shaped anatomy pose a considerable technical challenge; therefore, use of the DOM during all treatment phases is recommended.

REFERENCES

1. Abbott PV: Assessing restored teeth with pulp and periapical diseases for the presence of cracks, caries, and marginal breakdown, *Aust Dent J* 49:33, 2004.
2. Acosta Vigouraux SA, Trugeda Bosaans SA: Anatomy of the pulp chamber floor of the permanent maxillary first molar, *J Endod* 4:214, 1978.
3. al Shalabi RM, Omer OE, Glennon J, et al: Root canal anatomy of maxillary first and second permanent molars, *Int Endod J* 33:405, 2000.
4. Alapati S, Zaatar El, Shyama M, Al-Zuhair N: Maxillary canine with two root canals, *Med Princ Pract* 15:74, 2006.
5. Alavi AM, Opasanon A, Ng Y-L, Gulabivala K: Root and canal morphology of Thai maxillary molars, *Int Endod J* 35:478, 2002.
6. Al-Fougan KS: C-shaped root canals in mandibular second molars in a Saudi Arabian population, *Int Endod J* 34:499, 2002.
7. Al-Nazhan S: Two root canals in a maxillary central incisor with enamel hypoplasia, *J Endod* 17:469, 1991.
8. Al-Nazhan S: Incidence of fourth canal in root canal treated mandibular first molars in a Saudi Arabian sub-population, *Int Endod J* 32:49, 1999.
9. Al-Qudah AA, Awawdeh LA: Root canal morphology of mandibular incisors in a Jordanian population, *Int Endod J* 39:873, 2006.
10. Attam K, Nawal RR, Utneja S, Talwar S: Radix entomolaris in mandibular first molars in Indian population: a review and case reports, *Case Rep Dent* 1-7, article ID 595494, 2012.
11. Awawdeh LA, Al-Qudah AA: Root form and canal morphology of mandibular premolars in a Jordanian population, *Int Endod J* 41:240, 2008.
12. Bahcall JK, Barss JT: Fiberoptic endoscope usage for intracanal visualization, *J Endod* 27:128, 2001.
13. Baisden MK, Kulilid JC, Weller RN: Root canal configuration of the mandibular first premolar, *J Endod* 18:505, 1992.
14. Baldassari-Cruz LA, Lilly JP, Rivera EM: The influence of dental operating microscopes in locating the mesiolingual canal orifice, *Oral Surg Oral Med Oral Pathol Oral Radiol Endod* 93:190, 2002.
15. Baratto-Filho F, Fariniuk LF, Ferreira EF, et al: Clinical and macroscopic study of maxillary molars with two palatal roots, *Int Endod J* 35:796, 2002.
16. Barbizam JVB, Ribeiro RG, Filho MT: Unusual anatomy of permanent maxillary molars, *J Endod* 30:668, 2004.
17. Barkhordar RA, Sapone J: Surgical treatment of a three-rooted maxillary second premolar: report of a case, *Oral Surg Oral Med Oral Pathol* 63:614, 1987.
18. Barnett F: Mandibular molar with C-shaped canal, *Dent Traumatol* 2:79, 1986.
19. Baugh D, Wallace J: Middle mesial canal of the mandibular first molar: a case report and literature review, *J Endod* 30:185, 2004.
20. Beatty RG: A five-canal maxillary first molar, *J Endod* 10:156, 1984.
21. Beatty RG, Interian CM: A mandibular first molar with five canals: report of case, *J Am Dent Assoc* 111:769, 1985.
22. Beatty RG, Krell K: Mandibular molars with five canals: report of two cases, *J Am Dent Assoc* 114:802, 1987.
23. Benenati FW: Maxillary second molars with two palatal canals and a palatogingival groove, *J Endod* 11:308, 1985.
24. Benjamin KA, Dowson J: Incidence of two root canals in human mandibular incisor teeth, *Oral Surg Oral Med Oral Pathol* 38:122, 1974.
25. Bjørndal L, Carlsen O, Thuesen G, et al: External and internal macromorphology in 3D reconstructed maxillary molars using computerized x-ray microtomography, *Int Endod J* 32:3, 1999.
26. Bolger WL, Schindler WG: A mandibular first molar with a C-shaped root configuration, *J Endod* 14:515, 1998.
27. Bond JL, Hartwell G, Portell FR: Maxillary first molar with six canals, *J Endod* 14:258, 1988.
28. Bram SM, Fleisher R: Endodontic therapy in a mandibular second bicuspid with four canals, *J Endod* 17:513, 1991.
29. Buhrley LJ, Barrows MJ, BeGole EA, Wenckus CS: Effect of magnification on locating the MB-2 canal in maxillary molars, *J Endod* 28:324, 2002.
30. Burch JG, Hulen S: The relationship of the apical foramen to the anatomic apex of the tooth root, *Oral Surg Oral Med Oral Pathol* 34:262, 1972.
31. Cabo-Valle M, Gonzalez-Gonzalez JM: Maxillary central incisor with two root canals: an unusual presentation, *J Oral Rehabil* 28:797, 2001.
32. Calberson FL, DeMoor RJ, Deroose CA: The radix entomolaris and paramolaris: a clinical approach in endodontics, *J Endod* 33:58, 2007.
33. Calişkan MK, Pehlivan Y, Sepetçioğlu F, et al: Root canal morphology of human permanent teeth in a Turkish population, *J Endod* 21:200, 1995.
34. Carnes EJ, Skidmore AE: Configurations and deviation of root canals of maxillary first premolars, *Oral Surg Oral Med Oral Pathol* 36:880, 1973.
35. Cecic P, Hartwell G, Bellizzi R: The multiple root canal system in the maxillary first molar: a case report, *J Endod* 8:113, 1982.
36. Chai WL, Thong YL: Cross-sectional morphology and minimum canal wall widths in C-shaped roots of mandibular molars, *J Endod* 30:509, 2004.
37. Chan K, Yew SC, Chao SY: Mandibular premolars with three root canals: two case reports, *Int Endod J* 25:261, 1992.
38. Christie WH, Peikoff MD, Acheson DW: Endodontic treatment of two maxillary lateral incisors with anomalous root formation, *J Endod* 7:528, 1981.
39. Christie WH, Peikoff MD, Fogel HM: Maxillary molars with two palatal roots: a retrospective clinical study, *J Endod* 17:80, 1991.
40. Cimilli H, Mumcu G, Cimilli T, et al: Correlation between root canal patterns, *Oral Surg Oral Med Oral Pathol Oral Radiol Endod* 102:e16, 2006.
41. Coelho de Carvalho MC, Zuolo ML: Orifice locating with a microscope, *J Endod* 26:532, 2000.
42. Collins IJ: Maxillary lateral incisor with two roots, *Aust Endod J* 27:37, 2001.
43. Cooke HG, Cox FL: C-shaped canal configurations in mandibular molars, *J Am Dent Assoc* 99:836, 1979.

44. Coolidge ED: Anatomy of the root apex in relation to treatment problems, *J Am Dent Assoc* 16:1456, 1929.

45. Cunningham CJ, Senia ES: A three-dimensional study of canal curvature in the mesial roots of mandibular molars, *J Endod* 18:294, 1992.

46. Cutright DE, Bhaskar SN: Pulpal vasculature as demonstrated by a new method, *Oral Surg Oral Med Oral Pathol* 27:678, 1969.

47. da Costa LF, Sousa Neto MD, Fidel SR: External and internal anatomy of mandibular molars, *Braz Dent J* 7:33, 1996.

48. Dankner E, Friedman S, Stabholz A: Bilateral C-shape configuration in maxillary first molars, *J Endod* 16:601, 1990.

49. D'Arcangelo C, Varvara G, De Fazio P: Root canal treatment in mandibular canines with two roots: a report of two cases, *Int Endod J* 34:331, 2001.

50. Degerness RA, Bowles WR. Dimension, anatomy and morphology of the mesiobuccal root canal system in maxillary molars, *J Endod* 36:985, 2010.

51. DeGrood ME, Cunningham CJ: Mandibular molar with five canals: report of a case, *J Endod* 23:60, 1997.

52. DeMoor RJ, Calberson FL: The radix entomolaris in mandibular first molars: an endodontic challenge, *Int Endod J* 37:789, 2004.

53. DeMoor RJG: C-shaped root canal configuration in maxillary first molars, *Int Endod J* 35:200, 2002.

54. DeMoor RJG, Calberson FLG: Root canal treatment in a mandibular second premolar with three root canals, *J Endod* 31:310, 2005.

55. Dummer PMH, McGinn JH, Rees DG: The position and topography of the apical canal constriction and apical foramen, *Int Endod J* 17:192, 1984.

56. El Deeb ME: Three root canals in mandibular second premolars: literature review and a case report, *J Endod* 8:376, 1982.

57. England MC Jr, Hartwell GR, Lance JR: Detection and treatment of multiple canals in mandibular premolars, *J Endod* 17:174, 1991.

58. Eskoz N, Weine FS: Canal configuration of the mesiobuccal root of the maxillary second molar, *J Endod* 21:38, 1995.

59. Fabra-Campos H: Unusual root anatomy of mandibular first molars, *J Endod* 11:568, 1985.

60. Fabra-Campos H: [Upper lateral incisor with two canals], *Endodoncia* 9:104, 1991.

61. Fahid A, Taintor JF: Maxillary second molar with three buccal roots, *J Endod* 14:181, 1988.

62. Fan B, Cheung GSP, Fan M, et al: C-shaped canal system in mandibular second molars. I. Anatomical fractures, *J Endod* 30:899, 2004.

63. Fan B, Cheung GSP, Fan M, et al: C-shaped canal system in mandibular second molars. II. Radiographic features, *J Endod* 30:904, 2004.

64. Fan B, Pan Y, Gao Y, et al: Three-dimensional morphologic analysis of isthmuses in the mesial roots of mandibular molars, *J Endod* 36:1866, 2010.

65. Fan B, Yang J, Gutmann JL, Fan M: Root canal systems in mandibular first premolars with C-shaped root configurations. I. Microcomputed tomography mapping of the radicular groove and associated root canal cross sections, *J Endod* 34:1337, 2008.

66. Fan B, Ye WH, Xie EZ, et al: Three-dimensional morphological analysis of C-shaped canals in mandibular first premolars in a Chinese population, *Int Endod J* 45:1035,2012.

67. Fasoli G, Arlotta A: Su ll' anatomia del canali radicolari del denti umani, *L Stomatol* 11, 1913.

68. Ferreira CM, de Moraes IG, Bernardineli N: Three-rooted maxillary second premolar, *J Endod* 26:105, 2000.

69. Fischer GM, Evans CE: A three rooted mandibular second premolar, *Gen Dent* 40:139, 1992.

70. Fogel HM, Peikoff MD, Christie WH: Canal configuration in the mesiobuccal root of the maxillary first molar: a clinical study, *J Endod* 20:135, 1994.

71. Friedman S, Moshonov J, Stabholz A: Five root canals in a mandibular first molar, *Dent Traumatol* 2:226, 1986.

72. Funato A, Funato H, Matsumoto K: Mandibular central incisor with two root canals, *Dent Traumatol* 14:285, 1998.

73. Gao Y, Fan B, Cheung GSP, et al: C-shaped canal system in mandibular second molars. IV. Morphological analysis and transverse measurement, *J Endod* 32:1062, 2006.

74. Genovese FR, Marsico EM: Maxillary central incisor with two roots: a case report, *J Endod* 29:220, 2003.

75. Ghoddusi J, Naghavi N, Zarei M, Rohani E: Mandibular first molar with four distal canals, *J Endod* 33:1481, 2007.

76. Gilles J, Reader A: An SEM investigation of the mesiolingual canal in human maxillary first and second molars, *Oral Surg Oral Med Oral Pathol* 70:638, 1990.

77. Goel NK, Gill KS, Taneja JR: Study of root canal configuration in mandibular first permanent molars, *J Indian Soc Pedod Prev Dent* 8:12, 1991.

78. Gonzalez-Plata RR, Gonzalez-Plata EW: Conventional and surgical treatment of a two-rooted maxillary central incisor, *J Endod* 29:422, 2003.

79. Gopikrishna V, Reuben J, Kandaswamy D: Endodontic management of a maxillary first molar with two palatal roots and a fused buccal root diagnosed with spiral computed tomography: a case report, *Oral Surg Oral Med Oral Pathol Oral Radiol Endod* 105:e74, 2008.

80. Görduysus MO, Görduysus M, Friedman S: Operating microscope improves negotiation of second mesiobuccal canals in maxillary molars, *J Endod* 27:683, 2001.

81. Green D: Double canals in single roots, *Oral Surg Oral Med Oral Pathol* 35:689, 1973.

82. Gulabivala K, Aung TH, Alavi A, Mg Y-L: Root and canal morphology of Burmese mandibular molars, *Int Endod J* 34:359, 2001.

83. Gutierrez JH, Aguayo P: Apical foraminal openings in human teeth: number and location, *Oral Surg Oral Med Oral Pathol Oral Radiol Endod* 79:769, 1995.

84. Gutmann JL, Lovdahl PE: *Problem solving in endodontics*, ed 5, St Louis, 2011, Elsevier.

85. Haddad GY, Nehma WB, Ounsi HF: Diagnosis, classification and frequency of C-shaped canals in mandibular second molars in the Lebanese population, *J Endod* 25:268, 1999.

86. Hartwell G, Bellizzi R: Clinical investigation of in vivo endodontically treated mandibular and maxillary molars, *J Endod* 8:555, 1982.

87. Haznedaroglu F, Ersev H, Odaba H, et al: Incidence of patent furcal accessory canals in permanent molars of a Turkish population, *Int Endod J* 36:515, 2003.

88. Heling B: A two-rooted maxillary central incisor, *Oral Surg Oral Med Oral Pathol* 43:649, 1977.

89. Heling I, Gottlieb-Dadon I, Chandler NP: Mandibular canine with two roots and three root canals, *Dent Traumatol* 11:301, 1995.

90. Hess W, Zurcher E: *The anatomy of root canals of the teeth of the permanent and deciduous dentitions*, New York, 1925, William Wood.

91. Holtzman L: Root canal treatment of mandibular second premolar with four root canals: a case report, *Int Endod J* 31:364, 1998.

92. Hülsman M: Mandibular first premolars with three root canals, *Endod Dent Traumatol* 6:189, 1990.

93. Hülsmann M: A maxillary first molar with two distobuccal root canals, *J Endod* 23:707, 1997.

94. Imura N, Hata GI, Toda T: Two canals in mesiobuccal roots of maxillary molars, *Int Endod J* 31:410, 1998.

95. Jacobsen EL, Dick K, Bodell R: Mandibular first molars with multiple mesial canals, *J Endod* 20:610, 1994.

96. Jenkins S, Kulild J, Williams K, et al: Sealing ability of three materials in the orifice of root canal systems obturated with gutta-percha, *J Endod* 32:225, 2006.

97. Joseph I, Varma BR, Bhat KM: Clinical significance of furcation anatomy of the maxillary first premolar: a biometric study on extracted teeth, *J Periodontol* 67:386, 1996.

98. Karagöz-Kucukay I: Root canal ramifications in mandibular incisors and efficacy of low-temperature injection thermoplasticized gutta-percha filling, *J Endod* 20:236, 1994.

99. Kartal N, Ozcelik B, Cimilli H: Root canal morphology of maxillary premolars, *J Endod* 24:417, 1998.

100. Kartal N, Yanikoglu FC: Root canal morphology of mandibular incisors, *J Endod* 18:562, 1992.

101. Kasahara E, Yasuda E, Yamamoto A, Anzai M: Root canal systems of the maxillary central incisor, *J Endod* 16:158, 1990.

102. Kerekes K, Tronstad L: Long-term results of endodontic treatment performed with a standardized technique, *J Endod* 5:83, 1979.

103. Kerekes K, Tronstad L: Morphometric observations in root canals of human premolars, *J Endod* 3:74, 1997.

104. Kerekes K, Tronstad L: Morphometric observations on root canals of human premolars, *J Endod* 3:417, 1998.

105. Kim Y, Lee SJ, Woo J: Morphology of maxillary first and second molars analyzed by cone-beam computed tomography in a Korean population: variations in the number of roots and canals and the incidence of fusion, *J Endod* 38:1063, 2012.

106. Kotoku K: Morphological studies on the roots of the Japanese mandibular second molars, *Shika Gakuho* 85:43, 1985.

107. Krasner P, Rankow HJ: Anatomy of the pulp chamber floor, *J Endod* 30:5, 2004.

108. Kulild JC, Peters DD: Incidence and configuration of canal systems in the mesiobuccal root of maxillary first and second molars, *J Endod* 16:311, 1990.

109. Kuttler Y: Microscopic investigation of root apexes, *J Am Dent Assoc* 50:544, 1955.

110. Kuzekanani M, Haghani J, Nosrati H: Root and canal morphology of mandibular third molars in an Iranian population, *J Dent Res Dent Clin Dent Prospects* 6:85, 2012.

111. Lambruschini GM, Camps J: A two-rooted maxillary central incisor with a normal clinical crown, *J Endod* 19:95, 1995.

112. Lammertyn PA, Rodfigo SB, Brunotto M, Crosa M: Furcation groove of maxillary first premolar, thickness, and dentin structures, *J Endod* 35:814, 2009.

113. Langeland K: *Tissue changes in the dental pulp: an experimental histologic study*, Oslo, 1957, Oslo University Press.

114. Langeland K: The histopathologic basis in endodontic treatment, *Dent Clin North Am* 11:49, 1967.

115. Langeland K: Tissue response to dental caries, *Dent Traumatol* 3:149, 1987.

116. Langeland K: Reacción tisular a los materiales de obturación del conducto. In Guldener PHA, Langeland K, editors: *Endodoncia*, Barcelona, 1995, Springer-Verlag Ibérica.

117. Leeb J: Canal orifice enlargement as related to biomechanical preparation, *J Endod* 9:463, 1983.

118. Li J, Li L, Pan Y: Anatomic study of the buccal root with furcation groove and associated root canal shape in maxillary first premolars by using microcomputed tomography, *J Endod* 9:265, 2013.

119. Lin W-C, Yang S-F, Pai S-F: Nonsurgical endodontic treatment of a two-rooted maxillary central incisor, *J Endod* 32:478, 2006.

120. Loh HS: Root morphology of the maxillary first premolar in Singaporeans, *Aust Endod J* 43:399, 1998.

121. Low D: Unusual maxillary second premolar morphology: a case report, *Quintessence Int* 32:626, 2001.

122. Lu T-Y, Yang S-F, Pai S-F: Complicated root canal morphology of mandibular first premolars in a Chinese population using cross section method, *J Endod* 32:932, 2006.

123. Lui N, Li X, Liu N, et al: A micro-computed tomography study of the root canal morphology of the mandibular first premolar in a population from southwestern China, *Clin Oral Investig* 7:999, 2012 (Epub ahead of print)

124. Lumley PJ, Walmsley AD, Walton RE, Rippin JW: Cleaning of oval canals using ultrasonics and sonic instrumentation, *J Endod* 19:453, 1993.

125. Macri E, Zmener O: Five canals in a mandibular second premolar, *J Endod* 26:304, 2000.

126. Madeira MC, Hetem S: Incidence of bifurcations in mandibular incisors, *Oral Surg Oral Med Oral Pathol* 36:589, 1973.

127. Mader CL, Konzelman JL: Double-rooted maxillary central incisors, *Oral Surg Oral Med Oral Pathol* 50:99, 1980.

128. Maggiore F, Jou YT, Kim S: A six canal maxillary first molar: case report, *Int Endod J* 35:486, 2002.

129. Mangani F, Ruddle CJ: Endodontic treatment of a "very particular" maxillary central incisor, *J Endod* 20:560, 1994.

130. Manning SA: Root canal anatomy of mandibular second molars. I, *Int Endod J* 23:34, 1990.

131. Manning SA: Root canal anatomy of mandibular second molars. II. C-shaped canals, *Int Endod J* 23:40, 1990.

132. Martinez-Berná A, Ruiz-Badanelli P: Maxillary first molars with six canals, *J Endod* 9:375, 1983.

133. Martinez-Berná A, Badanelli P: Mandibular first molars with six root canals, *J Endod* 11:348, 1985.

134. Martinez-Lozano MA, Forner-Navarro L, Sanchez-Cortes JL: Analysis of radiologic factors in determining premolar root canal systems, *Oral Surg Oral Med Oral Pathol Oral Radiol Endod* 88:719, 1999.

135. Mauger MJ, Waite RM, Alexander JB, Schindler WG: Ideal endodontic access in mandibular incisors, *J Endod* 25:206, 1999.

136. Melton DC, Krell KV, Fuller MW: Anatomical and histological features of C-shaped canals in mandibular second molars, *J Endod* 17:384, 1991.

137. Min Y, Fan B, Cheung GSP, et al: C-shaped canal system in mandibular second molars. III. The morphology of the pulp chamber floor, *J Endod* 32:1155, 2006.

138. Miyashita M, Kasahara E, Yasuda E, et al: Root canal system of the mandibular incisor, *J Endod* 23:479, 1997.

139. Mizutani T, Ohno N, Nakamura H: Anatomical study of the root apex in the maxillary anterior teeth, *J Endod* 18:344, 1992.

140. Mjör IA, Nordahl I: The density and branching of dentinal tubules in human teeth, *Arch Oral Biol* 41:401, 1996.

141. Mjör IA, Smith MR, Ferrari M, Mannocei F: The structure of dentin in the apical region of human teeth, *Int Endod J* 34:346, 2001.

142. Moayedi S, Lata D: Mandibular first premolar with three canals, *Endodontology* 16:26, 2004.

143. Monnan G, Smallwood ER, Gulabivala K: Effects of access cavity location and design on degree and distribution of instrumented root canal surface in maxillary anterior teeth, *Int Endod J* 34:176, 2001.

144. Moreinis SA: Avoiding perforation during endodontic access, *J Am Dent Assoc* 98:707, 1979.

145. Morfis A, Sylaras SN, Georgopoulou M, et al: Study of the apices of human permanent teeth with the use of a scanning electron microscope, *Oral Surg Oral Med Oral Pathol* 77:172, 1994.

146. Nallapati S: Three canal mandibular first and second premolars: a treatment approach—a case report, *J Endod* 31:474, 2005.

147. Nattress BR, Martin DM: Predictability of radiographic diagnosis of variations in root canal anatomy in mandibular incisor and premolar teeth, *Int Endod J* 24:58, 1991.

148. Navarro LF, Luzi A, Garcia AA, Garcia AH: Third canal in the mesial root of permanent mandibular first molars: review of the literature and presentation of 3 clinical reports and 2 in vitro studies, *Med Oral Patol Oral Cir Bucal* 12:E605, 2007.

149. Neaverth EJ, Kotler LM, Kaltenbach RF: Clinical investigation (in vivo) of endodontically treated maxillary first molars, *J Endod* 13:506, 1987.

150. Newton CW, McDonald S: A C-shaped canal configuration in a maxillary first molar, *J Endod* 10:397, 1984.

151. Ng YL, Aung TH, Alavi A, Gulabivala K: Root and canal morphology of Burmese maxillary molars, *Int Endod J* 34:620, 2001.

152. Nielsen CJ, Shahmohammadi K: The effect of mesio-distal chamber dimension on access preparation in mandibular incisors, *J Endod* 31:88, 2005.

153. Nosonowitz DM, Brenner MR: The major canals of the mesiobuccal root of the maxillary first and second molars, *NY J Dent* 43:12, 1973.

154. Okumura T: Anatomy of the root canals, *Trans Seventh Int Dent Cong* 1:170, 1926.

155. Orguneser A, Kartal N: Three canals and two foramina in a mandibular canine, *J Endod* 24:444, 1998.

156. Özcan E, Çolak H, Hamid M: Root and canal morphology of maxillary first premolars in a Turkish population, *J Dent Sci* 7:390, 2012.

157. Park J-B, Kim N, Park S, et al: Evaluation of root anatomy of permanent mandibular premolars and molars in a Korean population with cone-beam computed tomography, *Eur J Dent* 7:94, 2013.

158. Patel S, Wilson R, Dawood A, et al: The detection of periapical pathosis using digital periapical radiography and cone beam computed tomography. Part 2. A 1-year post-treatment follow-up, *Int Endod J* 45:711, 2012.

159. Pattanshetti N, Gaidhane M, Al Kandari AM: Root and canal morphology of the mesiobuccal and distal roots of permanent first molars in a Kuwait population: a clinical study, *Int Endod J* 41:755, 2008.

160. Patterson JM: Bifurcated root of upper central incisor, *Oral Surg Oral Med Oral Pathol* 29:222, 1970.

161. Pecora JD, Santana SVS: Maxillary lateral incisor with two roots: case report, *Braz Dent J* 2:151, 1991.

162. Pecora JD, Saquy PC, Sousa Neto MD, Woelfel JB: Root form and canal anatomy of maxillary first premolars, *Braz Dent J* 2:87, 1991.

163. Pecora JD, Sousa Neto MD, Saquy PC, Woelfel JB: In vitro study of root canal anatomy of maxillary second premolars, *Braz Dent J* 3:81, 1992.

164. Pecora JD, Sousa Neto MD, Saquy PC: Internal anatomy, direction and number of roots and size of mandibular canines, *Braz Dent J* 4:53, 1993.

165. Pecora JD, Woelfel JB, Sousa Neto MD, Issa EP: Morphologic study of the maxillary molars. II. Internal anatomy, *Braz Dent J* 3:53, 1992.

166. Peikoff MD, Christie WH, Fogel HM: The maxillary second molar: variations in the number of roots and canals, *Int Endod J* 29:365, 1996.

167. Peters OA, Laib A, Gohring TN, Barbakow F: Changes in root canal geometry after preparation assessed by high-resolution computed tomography, *J Endod* 27:1, 2001.

168. Peters OA, Laib A, Rüegsegger P, Barbakow F: Three-dimensional analysis of root canal geometry by high resolution computed tomography, *J Dent Res* 79:1405, 2000.

169. Peters OA, Peters CI, Schonenberger K, Barbakow F: ProTaper rotary root canal preparation: assessment of torque force in relation to canal anatomy, *Int Endod J* 36:93, 2003.

170. Pineda F, Kuttler Y: Mesiodistal and buccolingual roentgenographic investigation of 7275 root canals, *Oral Surg Oral Med Oral Pathol* 33:101, 1972.

171. Plotino G: A mandibular third molar with three mesial roots: a case report, *J Endod* 34:224, 2008.

172. Pomeranz H, Eidelman DL, Goldberg MG: Treatment considerations of the middle mesial canal of mandibular first and second molars, *J Endod* 7:565, 1981.

173. Pomeranz H, Fishelberg G: The secondary mesiobuccal canal of maxillary molars, *J Am Dent Assoc* 88:119, 1974.

174. Ponce EH, Vilar Fernandez JA: The cemento-dentino-canal junction, the apical foramen, and the apical constriction: evaluation by optical microscopy, *J Endod* 29:214, 2003.

175. Preiswerk G. *Lehrbuch und Atlas der Konservierenden Zahnheilkunde*, München, 1912, JF Lehmann's Verlag.

176. Rankine-Wilson RW, Henry P: The bifurcated root canal in lower anterior teeth, *J Am Dent Assoc* 70:1162, 1965.

177. Reeh ES: Seven canals in a lower first molar, *J Endod* 24:497, 1998.

178. Rhodes JS: A case of an unusual anatomy of a mandibular second premolar with four canals, *Int Endod J* 34:645, 2001.

179. Ricucci D: Three independent canals in the mesial root of a mandibular first molar, *Dent Traumatol* 13:47, 1997.

180. Ricucci D, Langeland K: Apical limit of root canal instrumentation and obturation. Part 2. A histologic study, *Int Endod J* 31:394, 1998.

181. Rödig T, Hülsmann M: Diagnosis and root canal treatment of a mandibular second premolar with three root canals, *Int Endod J* 36:912, 2003.

182. Rubinstein R, Kim S: Long-term follow-up of cases considered healing 1 year after apical microsurgery, *J Endod* 28:378, 2002.

183. Rwenyonyi CM, Kutesa AM, Muwazi LM, Buwembo W: Root and canal morphology of maxillary first and second permanent molar teeth in a Ugandan population, *Int Endod J* 40:679, 2007.

184. Saad AY, Al-Yahya AS: The location of the cementodentinal junction in single-rooted mandibular first premolars from Egyptian and Saudi patients: a histologic study, *Int Endod J* 36:541, 2003.

185. Sachdeva GS, Ballal S, GopiKrishna V, Kandas Wamy D: Endodontic management of a mandibular second premolar with four roots and four root canals with the aid of spiral computed tomography: a case report, *J Endod* 34:104, 2008.

186. Schilder H: Filling root canals in three dimensions, *Dent Clin North Am* 11:723, 1967.

187. Schwarze T, Baethge C, Stecher T, Geurtsen W: Identification of second canals in the mesiobuccal root of maxillary first and second molars using magnifying loupes or an operating microscope, *Aust Endod J* 28:57, 2002.

188. Seidberg BH, Altman M, Guttuso J, Suson M: Frequency of two mesiobuccal root canals in maxillary first molars, *J Am Dent Assoc* 87:852, 1973.

189. Seo MS, Park DS: C-shaped root canals of mandibular second molars in a Korean population: clinical observation and in vitro analysis, *Int Endod J* 37:139, 2004.

190. Sert S, Bayirli GS: Evaluation of the root canal configurations of the mandibular and maxillary permanent teeth by gender in the Turkish population, *J Endod* 30:391, 2004.

191. Shin SJ, Park JW, Lee JK, Hwang SW: Unusual root canal anatomy in maxillary second molars: two case reports, *Oral Surg Oral Med Oral Pathol Oral Radiol Endod* 104:e61, 2007.

192. Sidow SJ, West LA, Liewehr FR, Loushine RJ: Root canal morphology of human maxillary and mandibular third molars, *J Endod* 26:675, 2000.

193. Simon JHS: The apex: how critical is it? *Gen Dent* 42:330, 1994.

194. Sinai IH, Lustbader S: A dual-rooted maxillary central incisor, *J Endod* 10:105, 1984.

195. Sjögren U, Hägglund B, Sundqvist G, Wing K: Factors affecting the long-term results of endodontic treatment, *J Endod* 16:498, 1990.

196. Skidmore AE, Bjørndal AM: Root canal morphology of the human mandibular first molar, *Oral Surg Oral Med Oral Pathol* 32:778, 1971.

197. Slowey RE: Root canal anatomy: road map to successful endodontics, *Dent Clin North Am* 23:555, 1979.

198. Smadi L, Khraisat A: Detection of a second mesiobuccal canal in the mesiobuccal roots of maxillary first molar teeth, *Oral Surg Oral Med Oral Pathol Oral Radiol Endod* 103:e77, 2007.

199. Smith AJ: Dentin formation and repair. In Hargreaves KM, Goodis HE, editors: *Seltzer and Bender's dental pulp*, Chicago, 2002, Quintessence.

200. Smulson MH, Hagen JC, Ellenz SJ: Pulpoperiapical pathology and immunologic considerations. In Weine FS, editor: *Endodontic therapy*, ed 5, St Louis, 1996, Mosby.

201. Soares JA, Leonardo RT: Root canal treatment of three-rooted maxillary first and second premolars: a case report, *Int Endod J* 36:705, 2003.

202. Spagnuolo G, Ametrano G, D'Antò V, et al: Microcomputed tomography analysis of mesiobuccal orifices and major apical foramen in first maxillary molars, *Open Dent J* 6:118, 2012.

203. Sperber GH, Moreau JL: Study of the number of roots and canals in Senegalese first permanent mandibular molars, *Int Endod J* 31:117, 1998.

204. Sponchiado EC, Ismail HAA, Braga MRL, et al: Maxillary central incisor with two-root canals: a case report, *J Endod* 32:1002, 2006.

205. Stabholz A, Goultschin J, Friedman S, Korenhouser S: Crown-to-root ratio as a possible indicator of the presence of a fourth root canal in maxillary first molars, *Israel J Dent Sci* 1:85, 1984.

206. Stroner WF, Remeikis NA, Carr GB: Mandibular first molar with three distal canals, *Oral Surg Oral Med Oral Pathol* 57:554, 1984.

207. Stropko JJ: Canal morphology of maxillary molars: clinical observations of canal configurations, *J Endod* 25:446, 1990.

208. Subay RK, Kayatas M: Dens invaginatus in an immature lateral incisor: a case report of complex endodontic treatment, *Oral Surg Oral Med Oral Pathol Oral Radiol Endod* 102:e37, 2006.

209. Sundaresh KJ, Srinivasan R, Mallikarjuna R, Rajalbandi S. Endodontic management of middle mesial canal of the mandibular molar, *BMJ Case Rep* 2013. pii: bcr2012008261, doi: 10.1136/br-2012-008261

210. Sykaras S, Economou P: [Root canal morphology of the mesio-buccal root of the maxillary first molar], *Odontostomatol Proodos* 24:99, 1970.

211. Tamse A, Katz A, Pilo R: Furcation groove of buccal root of maxillary first premolars: a morphometric study, *J Endod* 26:359, 2000.

212. Taylor GN: Techniiche per la preparazione e l'otturazione intracanalare, *La Clinica Odontoiatrica del Nord America* 20:566, 1988.

213. Teixeira FB, Sano CL, Gomes BP, et al: A preliminary in vitro study of the incidence and position of the root canal isthmus in maxillary and mandibular first molars, *Int Endod J* 36:276, 2003.

214. Thews ME, Kemp WB, Jones CR: Aberrations in palatal root and root canal morphology of two maxillary first molars, *J Endod* 5:94, 1979.

215. Thomas RP, Moule AJ, Bryant R: Root canal morphology of maxillary permanent first molar teeth at various ages, *Int Endod J* 26:257, 1993.

216. Thompson BH, Portell FR, Hartwell GR: Two root canals in a maxillary lateral incisor, *J Endod* 11:353, 1985.

217. Tian Y-Y, Guo B, Zhang R, et al: Root and canal morphology of maxillary first premolars in a Chinese subpopulation evaluated using cone-beam computed tomography, *Int Endod J* 45:996, 2012.

218. Todd HW: Maxillary right central incisor with two root canals, *J Endod* 2:227, 1976.

219. Trope M, Elfenbein L, Tronstad L: Mandibular premolars with more than one root canal in different race groups, *J Endod* 12:343, 1986.

220. Tu M-G, Tsai C-C, Jou M-J, et al: Prevalence of three rooted mandibular first molars among Taiwanese individuals, *J Endod* 33:1163, 2007.

221. Ulusoy OI, Görgül G: Endodontic treatment of a maxillary second molar with two palatal roots: a case report, *Oral Surg Oral Med Oral Pathol Oral Radiol Endod* 104:e95, 2007.

222. Versiani MA, Pécora JD, Sousa-Neto MD: The anatomy of two-rooted mandibular canines determined using micro-computed tomography, *Int Endod J* 44:682, 2011.

223. Vertucci FJ: Root canal anatomy of the human permanent teeth, *Oral Surg Oral Med Oral Pathol* 58:589, 1984.

224. Vertucci FJ, Anthony RL: A scanning electron microscopic investigation of accessory foramina in the furcation and pulp chamber floor of molar teeth, *Oral Surg Oral Med Oral Pathol* 62:319, 1986.

225. Vertucci FJ, Seelig A, Gillis R: Root canal morphology of the human maxillary second premolar, *Oral Surg Oral Med Oral Pathol* 38:456, 1974.

226. Vertucci FJ, Williams RG: Furcation canals in the human mandibular first molar, *Oral Surg Oral Med Oral Pathol* 38:308, 1974.

227. Von der Lehr WN, Marsh RA: A radiographic study of the point of endodontic egress, *Oral Surg Oral Med Oral Pathol Oral Radiol Endod* 35:705, 1973.

228. Von der Vyver PJ, Traub AJ: Maxillary central incisor with two root canals: a case report, *J Dent Assoc South Afr* 50:132, 1995.

229. Walker RT: Root form and canal anatomy of maxillary first premolars in a southern Chinese population, *Dent Traumatol* 3:130, 1987.

230. Walker RT: Root form and canal anatomy of mandibular first molars in a southern Chinese population, *Dent Traumatol* 4:19, 1988.

231. Walker RT: Root form and canal anatomy of mandibular first premolars in a southern Chinese population, *Dent Traumatol* 4:226, 1988.

232. Walker RT: The root canal anatomy of mandibular incisors in a southern Chinese population, *Int Endod J* 21:218, 1988.

233. Walvekar SV, Behbehani JM: Three root canals and dens formation in a maxillary lateral incisor: a case report, *J Endod* 23:185, 1997.

234. Wang Y, Guo J, Yang HB, et al: Incidence of C-shaped root canal systems in mandibular second molars in the native Chinese population by analysis of clinical methods, *Int J Oral Sci* 4:161, 2012.

235. Warren EM, Laws AJ: The relationship between crown size and the incidence of bifid root canals in mandibular incisor teeth, *Oral Surg Oral Med Oral Pathol* 52:425, 1981.

236. Wasti F, Shearer AC, Wilson NH: Root canal systems of the mandibular and maxillary first permanent molar teeth of South Asian Pakistanis, *Int Endod J* 34:263, 2001.

237. Webber RT, del Rio CE, Brady JM, Segall RO: Sealing quality of a temporary filling material, *Oral Surg Oral Med Oral Pathol* 46:123, 1978.

238. Weine FS, editor: *Endodontic therapy*, p 243, ed 5, St Louis, 1996, Mosby.

239. Weine FS; Members of the Arizona Endodontic Association: The C-shaped mandibular second molar: incidence and other considerations, *J Endod* 24:372, 1998.

240. Weine FS, Hayami S, Hata G, Toda T: Canal configuration of the mesiobuccal root of the maxillary first molar of a Japanese subpopulation, *Int Endod J* 32:79, 1999.

241. Weine FS, Healy HJ, Gerstein H, Evanson L: Canal configuration in the mesiobuccal root of the maxillary first molar and its endodontic significance, *Oral Surg Oral Med Oral Pathol* 28:419, 1969.

242. Weine FS, Pasiewicz RA, Rice RT: Canal configuration of the mandibular second molar using a clinically oriented in vitro method, *J Endod* 14:207, 1988.

243. Weisman MI: A rare occurrence: a bi-rooted upper canine, *Aust Endod J* 26:119, 2000.

244. Weller NR, Niemczyk SP, Kim S: Incidence and position of the canal isthmus. Part 1. Mesiobuccal root of the maxillary first molar, *J Endod* 21:380, 1995.

245. Weller RN, Hartwell G: The impact of improved access and searching techniques on detection of the mesiolingual canal in maxillary molars, *J Endod* 15:82, 1989.

246. Wells DW, Bernier WE: A single mesial canal and two distal canals in a mandibular second molar, *J Endod* 10:400, 1984.

247. Wilcox LR, Walton RE, Case WB: Molar access: shape and outline according to orifice location, *J Endod* 15:315, 1989.

248. Wong M: Maxillary first molar with three palatal canals, *J Endod* 17:298, 1991.

249. Wu M-K, Barkis D, R'oris A, Wesselink PR: Does the first file to bind correspond to the diameter of the canal in the apical region? *Int Endod J* 35:264, 2002.

250. Wu M-K, Wesselink P, Walton R: Apical terminus location of root canal treatment procedures, *Oral Surg Oral Med Oral Pathol Oral Radiol Endod* 89:99, 2000.

251. Xuan H, Haibing Y, Guoju LI, et al: A study of the distobuccal root canal orifice of the maxillary second molars in Chinese individuals evaluated by cone-beam computed tomography, *J Appl Oral Sci* 20:563, 2012.

252. Xuan Y, Bin G, Ke-Zeng L, et al: Cone-beam computed tomography study of root and canal morphology of mandibular premolars in a western Chinese population, *BMC Med Imag* 12:18, 2012.

253. Yang H, Cheng Tian C, Li G, et al: A cone-beam computed tomography study of the root canal morphology of mandibular first premolars and the location of root canal orifices and apical foramina in a Chinese subpopulation, *J Endod* 39:435, 2013.

254. Yang Z-P, Yang S-F, Lee G: The root and root canal anatomy of maxillary molars in a Chinese population, *Dent Traumatol* 4:215, 1998.

255. Yang Z-P, Yang S-F, Lin YL: C-shaped root canals in mandibular second molars in a Chinese population, *Dent Traumatol* 4:160, 1988.

256. Yang ZP: Multiple canals in a mandibular first premolar: case report, *Aust Dent J* 39:18, 1994.

257. Yew SC, Chan K: A retrospective study of endodontically treated mandibular first molars in a Chinese population, *J Endod* 19:471, 1993.

258. Yoshioka T, Villegas JC, Kobayashi C, Suda H: Radiographic evaluation of root canal multiplicity in mandibular first premolars, *J Endod* 30:73, 2004.

259. Zaatar EI, al Anizi SA, al Duwairi Y: A study of the dental pulp cavity of mandibular first permanent molars in the Kuwait population, *J Endod* 24:125, 1998.

260. Zaatar EI, Al-Kandari AM, Alhomaidah S, Al Yasin IM: Frequency of endodontic treatment in Kuwait: radiographic evaluation of 846 endodontically treated teeth, *J Endod* 23:453, 1997.

261. Zhang R, Wang H, Tian YY, et al: Use of cone-beam computed tomography to evaluate root and canal morphology of mandibular molars in Chinese individuals, *Int Endod J* 44:990, 2011.

262. Zheng Q, Zhang L, Zhou X, et al: C-shaped root canal system in mandibular second molars in a Chinese population evaluated by cone-beam computed tomography, *Int Endod J* 44:857, 2011.

263. Zillich R, Dowson J: Root canal morphology of mandibular first and second premolars, *Oral Surg Oral Med Oral Pathol* 36:738, 1973.

CHAPTER 6

Cleaning and Shaping the Root Canal System

OVE A. PETERS | CHRISTINE I. PETERS | BETTINA BASRANI

CHAPTER OUTLINE

Clinical endodontics encompasses a number of treatments, but they have in common the goal of preventing and treating microbial contamination of pulps and root canal systems. Treatment of traumatic dental injuries and prophylactic treatment of vital pulps are fundamentally different from pulpectomies and root canal instrumentation of teeth with infected pulps (see Chapter 1 for more details on diagnosis).

Endodontic therapy is directed toward one specific set of aims: to cure or prevent periradicular periodontitis.[355,526] The ultimate aim is for patients to retain their natural teeth in function and aesthetics.

To date, many treatment modalities, including the use of nickel-titanium rotary instruments, have not consistently provided a statistically relevant impact on treatment outcomes.[375] This poses a problem in the age of evidence-based therapy, because new therapeutic techniques should deliver improved clinical results over standard procedures. However, the few pertinent clinical trials[99,375,387] and numerous in vitro studies do suggest that certain practices in canal preparation and disinfection are more appropriate than others. This chapter will summarize relevant information.

Orthograde root canal treatment is a predictable and usually highly successful procedure, both in relatively straightforward (Fig. 6-1) and more complex cases (Fig. 6-2). Studies and reviews report favorable outcome rates of up to 95% for the treatment of teeth diagnosed with irreversible pulpitis[39,103,157] and positive outcome rates of up to 85% for infected, necrotic teeth.[102,158,345,375,408]

Microorganisms can breach dental hard-tissue barriers through several avenues, the most common being dental caries (Fig. 6-3). Shaping and cleaning procedures (Box 6-1) as part of root canal treatment are directed against microbial challenges to the root canal system. However, disinfection per se does not guarantee long-term retention of root canal-treated teeth; there is good evidence that this outcome is closely related to placement of an adequate coronal restoration.[21,346,400,425] Moreover, the impact of preservation of radicular structural strength should not be underestimated.[172]

PRINCIPLES OF CLEANING AND SHAPING

Endodontists agree that a major biologic aim of root canal therapy is to address apical periodontitis by disinfection and subsequent sealing of root canal systems. However, considerable disagreement exists over how this goal should be achieved. Although the terms *cleaning* and *shaping* are often used to describe root canal treatment procedures,[417] reversing the order to *shaping* and *cleaning* more correctly reflects the fact that enlarged canals direct and facilitate the cleaning action of irrigants and the removal of infected dentin.

Planktonic microorganisms in the pulp cavity and coronal root canal may be readily killed by irrigants early in a

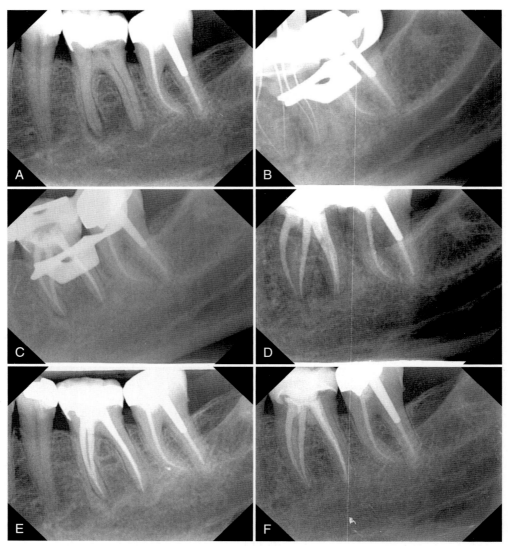

FIG. 6-1 Effect of routine root canal treatment of a mandibular molar. **A,** Pretreatment radiograph of tooth #19 shows radiolucent lesions adjacent to both mesial and distal root apices. **B,** Working length radiograph shows two separate root canals in the mesial root and two merging canals in the distal root. **C,** Posttreatment radiograph after shaping of root canal systems with nickel-titanium rotary files and obturation with thermoplasticized gutta-percha. **D,** Six-month recall radiograph after restoration of tooth #19 with an adhesively inserted full ceramic crown; some periradicular bone fill can be seen. **E,** One-year recall radiograph displays evidence of additional periradicular healing. **F,** Five-year recall radiograph; tooth not only is periapically sound but also clinically asymptomatic and fully functional.

BOX 6-1

Basic Objectives in Cleaning and Shaping

The primary objectives in cleaning and shaping the root canal system are to do the following:
- Remove infected soft and hard tissue
- Give disinfecting irrigants access to the apical canal space
- Create space for the delivery of medicaments and subsequent obturation
- Retain the integrity of radicular structures

procedure, but bacteria in less accessible canal areas or in biofilms still can elicit or maintain apical periodontitis. In everyday practice, these bacteria can be targeted only after mechanical root canal preparation.

Mechanical Objective

An ideal mechanical objective of root canal instrumentation is complete and centered incorporation of the original canals into the prepared shape, meaning that all root canal surfaces are mechanically prepared (*green areas* in Fig. 6-4, *A* and *B*). This goal is unlikely to be met with current techniques.[359,386]

Preparation errors such as deviations, zipping, and perforations should be absent. Although these negative effects of canal

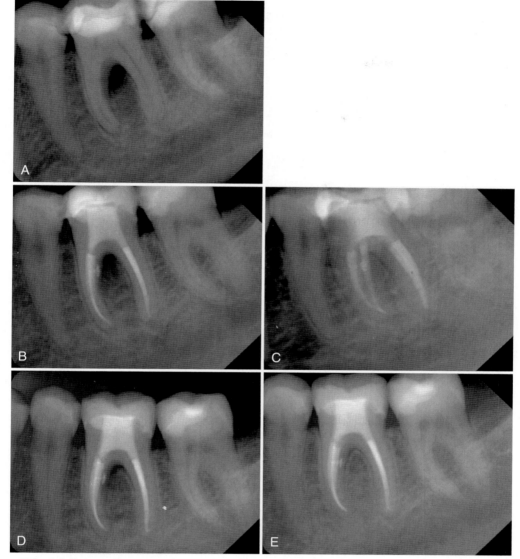

FIG. 6-2 Root canal treatment in a case of apical and interradicular pathosis. **A,** Pretreatment radiograph of tooth #19 shows an interradicular lesion. **B-C,** Posttreatment radiographs after root canal preparation and obturation. Note the lateral canal in the coronal third of the root canal. **D-E,** Two-month recall radiograph suggests rapid healing. (Courtesy Dr. H. Walsch.)

shaping and other procedural mishaps (discussed later) per se may not affect the probability of a favorable outcome,[290] they leave parts of the root canal system inaccessible for disinfection and are undesirable for that reason alone.

Another important mechanical objective is to retain as much cervical and radicular dentin as possible so as not to weaken the root structure, thereby preventing root fractures. Before root canal shaping, dentin wall thickness dimensions of 1 mm and below have been demonstrated in anatomic studies.[127,164] Straightening of canal paths can lead to thinning of curved root walls (Fig. 6-5). Although no definitive minimal radicular wall thickness has been established, 0.3 mm is considered critical by some authors.[287] To avoid overpreparation and outright perforations, adequate access cavity preparation and optimal enlargement of the coronal third of the root canal has to be ascertained (discussed later).

Biologic Objective

Schilder suggested that canals should be prepared to a uniform and continuous taper[445]; however, this guideline was aimed at facilitating obturation rather than targeting antimicrobial efficacy. For optimal disinfection, the preparation shape and antimicrobial efficacy are intimately related through the removal of infected pulp and dentin (Fig. 6-6) and creation of space for delivery of irrigants.

Traditionally, fluids have been dispensed passively into root canals by syringe and needle (Fig. 6-7). When delivered with passive needle irrigation, solutions have been shown to progress only 1 mm farther than the tip of the needle.[189,396,426] Enlarged apical canals and finer needles are likely to allow increasingly deeper needle placement, and this improves debridement and disinfection of canals.[5,12,147,532] However,

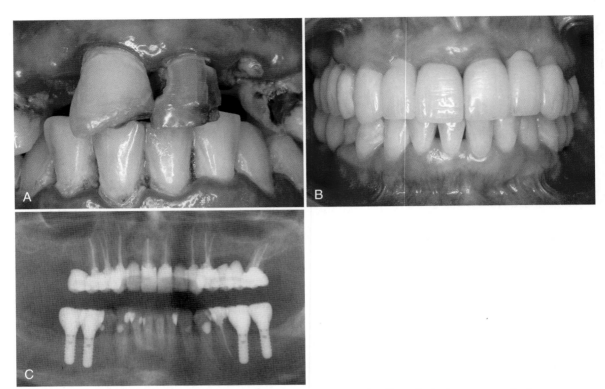

FIG. 6-3 Root canal therapy as part of a comprehensive treatment plan. The patient, who was recovering from intravenous drug addiction, requested restorative dental treatment. Because of extensive decay, several teeth had to be extracted, and nine teeth were treated endodontically. Root canal treatment was aided by nickel-titanium rotary instruments, and obturation was done with lateral compaction of gutta-percha and AH26 as the sealer. Microsurgical retrograde therapy was performed on tooth #8, and the distobuccal root of #14 had to be resected. Metal-free adhesively luted restorations were placed, and missing mandibular teeth were replaced by implants. **A,** Pretreatment intraoral status, showing oral neglect. **B,** Posttreatment intraoral status at 4-year follow-up, showing fully functional, metal-free, tooth-colored reconstructions. **C,** Panoramic radiograph at 4-year recall shows sound periradicular tissues in relation to endodontically treated teeth. (Restorations done by Dr. Till N. Göhring.)

thorough cleaning of the most apical part of any preparation remains difficult,[561] especially in narrow and curved canals.[16,211,404]

Technical Objective

Although a continuous taper that encompasses the original shape and curvature of a given root canal is an accepted goal, final apical preparation size remains a much-disputed entity in root canal therapy, as does final taper of the preparation.[47] Arguments were made for better disinfection with larger sizes (i.e., #50 or greater)[89,415] in combination with smaller tapers of .02 to .05. Others found no difference whether the selected final size was small or large.[105,570] A self-adjusting file was introduced,[327] which does not prepare canals to a specific normed size; its debridement effect is thought to result from a greater radicular wall contact, notably in buccolingually wide canals.[361]

Clinical Issues

A wide spectrum of possible strategies exists for attaining the goal of removing the canal contents and eliminating infection. Lussi and colleagues introduced an approach to removing canal contents and accomplishing disinfection that did not

involve the use of a file: the noninstrumentation technique.[303,304] This system consisted of a pump, a hose, and a special valve that was cemented into the access cavity (Fig. 6-8, *A*) to provide oscillation of irrigation solutions (1% to 3% sodium hypochlorite) at a reduced pressure. Although several in vitro studies suggested that canals can be cleaned and subsequently filled using this noninvasive system (see Fig. 6-8, *B* and *C*),[304,305] preliminary clinical results have not been as convincing (see Fig. 6-8, *D*).[25]

At the opposite end of the spectrum is a treatment technique that essentially removes all intraradicular infection through extraction of the tooth in question (see Fig. 6-8, *E* and *F*). Almost invariably, periradicular lesions heal after extraction of the involved tooth.

Clinical endodontic therapy takes place somewhere along this spectrum of treatment strategies. This is reflected in some of the controversies that surround the cleaning and shaping process, such as how large the apical preparation should be and what are the correct diameter, length, and taper.[250] Once the decision has been made to initiate endodontic treatment, the clinician must integrate his or her knowledge of dental anatomy, immunology, and bioengineering science with clinical information.

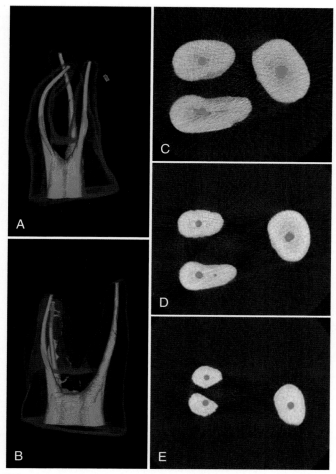

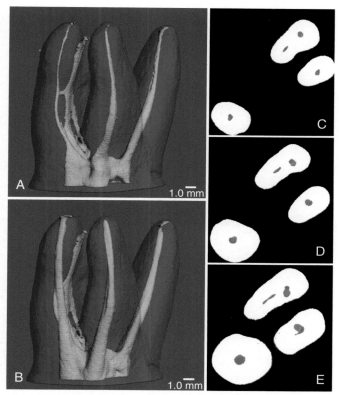

FIG. 6-5 Example of excessive thinning of dental structure during root canal treatment. **A-B,** Microcomputed tomography reconstructions show pretreatment and posttreatment root canal geometry of a maxillary molar. **C-E,** Cross sections of the coronal, middle, and apical thirds with pretreatment canal cross sections. Note the transportation and thinning, in particular, in the main mesiobuccal canal.

FIG. 6-4 Example of a desired shape, with the original root canal fully incorporated into the prepared outline. **A-B,** Microcomputed tomography reconstructions in clinical and mesiodistal views of a maxillary molar prepared with a NiTi rotary system. The *green area* indicates the pretreatment shape, and the *red area* indicates the posttreatment shape. Areas of *mixed red and green* indicate no change (i.e., no removal of radicular dentin). **C-E,** Cross sections of the coronal, middle, and apical thirds; the pretreatment cross sections *(green)* are encircled by the posttreatment outlines *(red)* in most areas. (*A-B,* From Hübscher W, Barbakow F, Peters OA: Root-canal preparation with FlexMaster: canal shapes analysed by micro-computed tomography, *Int Endod J* 36:740, 2003.)

Endodontic therapy has been compared to a chain of events, wherein the chain is only as strong as each individual link. For the purposes of this chapter, shaping and cleaning of the root canal system is considered a decisive link, because shaping determines the efficacy of subsequent procedures. It includes mechanical debridement, the creation of space for the delivery of medicaments, and optimized canal geometries for adequate obturation.[373] These tasks are attempted within a complex anatomic framework, as recognized in the early 20th century by Walter Hess[218] (Fig. 6-9; see also Chapter 5 for a complete description of root canal anatomy).

A clinician must choose appropriate strategies, instruments, and devices to overcome challenges and accomplish precise preparation in shape, length, and width. This allows endodontic therapy to address various forms of the disease processes described previously (Fig. 6-10). Recall radiographs taken at appropriate intervals predictably demonstrate longevity and favorable outcomes (see Figs. 6-1, 6-2, and 6-11) if a systematic approach to root canal shaping is adhered to (see Box 6-1).

Endodontic files traditionally have been manufactured according to empiric designs, and most instruments still are conceived based on individual clinicians' philosophies rather than developed through an evidence-based approach. Similar to the development of composite resins in restorative dentistry, the development of new files is a fast and market-driven process. With new instruments becoming available, the clinician may find it difficult to pick the file and technique most suitable for an individual case. Clinicians must always bear in mind that all file systems have benefits and weaknesses. Ultimately, clinical experience, handling properties, usage safety, and case outcomes, rather than marketing or the inventor's name, should decide the fate of a particular design. The following section describes typical instruments used in root canal shaping.

ENDODONTIC INSTRUMENTS

General Characteristics

Design Elements

Root canal preparation instruments such as K-files and nickel-titanium rotary instruments follow certain design principles

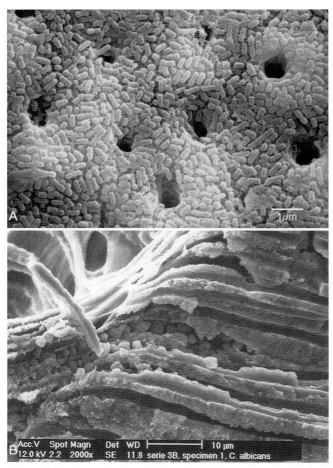

FIG. 6-6 Presence of microorganisms inside the main root canal and dentinal tubules. **A**, Scanning electron micrograph of a root canal surface shows a confluent layer of rod-shaped microbes (×3000). **B**, Scanning electron micrograph of a fractured root with a thick smear layer and fungi in the main root canal and dentinal tubules. (*A*, Courtesy Professor C. Koçkapan. *B*, Courtesy Professor T. Waltimo.)

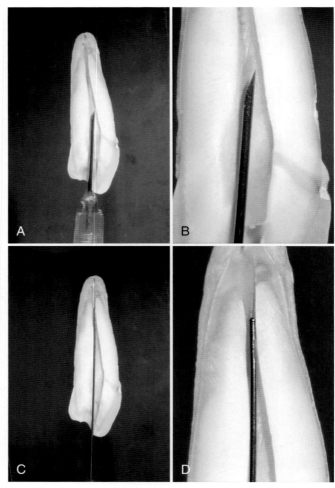

FIG. 6-7 Irrigation needles inserted into prepared root canals. **A-B**, A 27-gauge needle barely reaches the middle third. **C-D**, A 30-gauge, side-venting needle reaches the apical third in adequately enlarged canals.

that relate to drills and reamers used for work in wood and metal, respectively, whereas other instruments such as broaches and Hedström files do not find a direct technologic correlate. Design elements such as the tip, flutes, and cross sections are considered relevant for files and reamers used in rotary motion. These pertinent aspects are briefly described next; for a more detailed review, the reader is referred to the literature.[181,420,427,483]

Tip Design

In root canal preparation, an instrument tip has two main functions: to guide the file through the canal and to aid the file in penetrating deeper into the canal. A clinician unfamiliar with the tip design, in particular of a rotary instrument, may do either of the following: (1) transport the canal (if the tip is capable of enlarging and is used too long in one position in a curved canal) or (2) encounter excessive torsion and break the file (if a noncutting tip is forced into a canal with a smaller diameter than the tip).

The angle and radius of its leading edge and the proximity of the flute to its actual tip end determines the cutting ability

of a file tip. Cutting ability and file rigidity determine the propensity to transport the canal. The clinician must keep in mind that as long as a flexible file with a noncutting tip is engaged, 360-degree canal transportation is unlikely to occur.[410]

Studies have indeed shown that tip design affects file control, efficiency, and outcome in the shaping of root canal systems.[330,331] The tip of the original K-file resembled a pyramid; instrument tips have been described as *cutting, noncutting,* and *partially cutting,* although no clear distinction exists among the three types (Fig. 6-12).

Noncutting tips, also called *Batt tips,* are created by grinding and smoothing the apical end of the instrument (see Fig. 6-12, *A*). A tip modification was introduced with the Flex-R file, which was manufactured fully by grinding so that the transitional angles were smoothed laterally between the tip and the instrument's working parts.[411] Similar techniques are required to manufacture NiTi K-files.[512]

For NiTi rotary files, typically rounded noncuttings tips are used (see Fig. 6-12, *B*), which effectively prevent preparation errors that were found with earlier so-called safe cutting tips.[236] One exception to this rule is the type of rotary

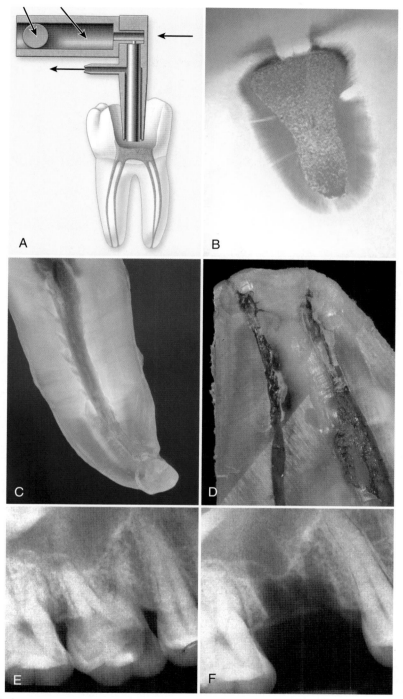

FIG. 6-8 Spectrum of strategies for accomplishing the primary aim of root canal treatment: elimination of infection. **A,** Schematic diagram of minimally invasive therapy using the noninstrumentation technique (NIT). **B,** Example of teeth cleaned in vitro using NIT. Note the clean intracanal surface, which is free of adhering tissue remnants. **C-D,** Examples of teeth cleaned in vivo and later extracted to investigate the clinical effects of NIT. Note the relatively clean, tissue-free canal space in **C** and the significant tissue revealed by rhodamine B staining in **D. E-F,** Course of maximally invasive therapy; apically involved tooth #30 was extracted, effectively removing the source of periradicular inflammation. (*A-B,* Courtesy Professor A. Lussi. *C-D,* Courtesy Professor T. Attin. *E-F,* Courtesy Dr. T. Kaya.)

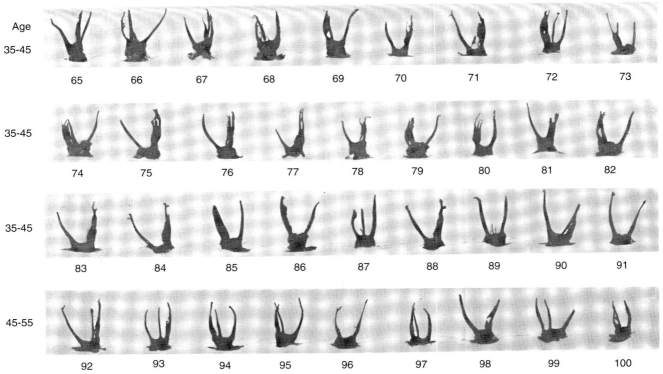

Age
35-45

65 66 67 68 69 70 71 72 73

35-45

74 75 76 77 78 79 80 81 82

35-45

83 84 85 86 87 88 89 90 91

45-55

92 93 94 95 96 97 98 99 100

FIG. 6-9 Panel of 36 anatomic preparations of maxillary molars from the classic work by Professor Walter Hess of Zurich. Note the overall variability of root canal systems and the decrease of canal dimensions with age. (From Hess W: *The anatomy of the root canals of teeth of the permanent dentition,* London, 1925, John Bale, Sons & Danielsson.)

specifically designed as a retreatment instrument; cutting tips in that case facilitate removal of the existing root canal filling material and are sufficiently safe.

Longitudinal and Cross-Sectional Design

The *flute* of the file is the groove in the working surface used to collect soft tissue and dentin chips from the wall of the canal. The effectiveness of a flute depends on its depth, width, configuration, and surface finish. The surface with the greatest diameter that follows the groove (where the flute and land intersect) as it rotates forms the *leading (cutting) edge,* or the *blade* of the file. The cutting edge forms and deflects chips along the wall of the canal and severs or snags soft tissue. Its effectiveness depends on its angle of incidence and sharpness.

Some instruments have a feature between trailing and cutting edge that forms a larger contact area with the radicular wall; this surface is called a radial land (Fig. 6-13). Such a land is thought to reduce the tendency of the file to thread into the canal. It also supports the cutting edge and limits the depth of cut; its position relative to the opposing cutting edge and its width determine its effectiveness. On the other hand, landed files are typically less cutting efficient compared to triangular cross sections.[380]

To reduce frictional resistance, some of the surface area of the land that rotates against the canal wall may be reduced to form the *relief.* The angle the cutting edge forms with the long axis of the file is called the *helical angle* (see Fig. 6-13).

If a file is sectioned perpendicular to its long axis, the *rake angle* is the angle formed by the leading edge and the radius of the file through the point of contact with the radicular wall. If the angle formed by the leading edge and the surface to be cut is 90 degrees, the rake angle is said to be neutral. The rake angle may be *negative* or *scraping* (Fig. 6-14, *A*) or *positive* or *cutting* (Fig. 6-14, *C*).

The *cutting angle* is considered a better indication of a file's cutting ability and is determined by measuring the angle formed by the leading edge of the file and a tangent to the radicular wall in the point of contact. The clearance angle corresponds to the cutting angle at the trailing edge of the file and, in case of reciprocating action, becomes the cutting angle. The sum of cutting angle and rake angle is 90 degrees.

The *pitch* of the file is the distance between a point on the leading edge and the corresponding point on the adjacent leading edge (the distance from one "spiral twist" to the next) (see Fig. 6-13). The smaller the pitch or the shorter the distance between corresponding points, the more spirals the file has and the greater the helix angle. Although K-files have a constant pitch typically in the range of 1 mm, many NiTi rotaries have a variable pitch, one that changes along the working surface. When variable pitch is used, usually tighter spirals are located close to the tip of the file and more space between the flutes is located toward the coronal part of the file. A longitudinal section through an instrument reveals the *core* (see Fig. 6-13). The outer diameter of a tapered instrument increases from the file tip toward the handle; depending

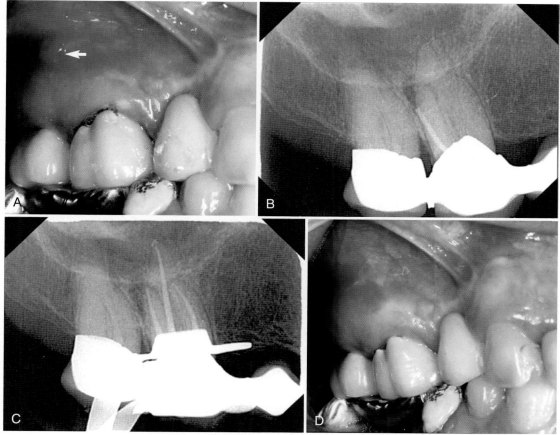

FIG. 6-10 Sinus tract as a sign of a chronic apical abscess and effect of routine root canal treatment. **A,** Intraoral photograph of left maxillary region with draining sinus tract *(arrow)* periapical to tooth #14. **B,** Pretreatment radiograph with gutta-percha point positioned in the sinus tract, pointing toward the distobuccal root of #14. **C,** Finished root canal fillings after 2 weeks of calcium hydroxide dressing. **D,** Intraoral photograph of the same region as in **A,** showing that the sinus tract had closed by the time obturation was performed.

on core dimensions, the flute may become proportionately deeper, resulting in a *core taper* that may be different from the *external taper*.

The cutting angles, helix angles, and external and core tapers may vary along the working surface of the file, and the ratios of these quantities can vary among instruments of the same series. A change in any of these features may influence the file's effectiveness or its propensity for breakage as it progresses into the canal space.

Taper

The taper usually is expressed as the amount the file diameter increases each millimeter along its working surface from the tip toward the file handle. For example, a size #25 file with a .02 taper would have a 0.27-mm diameter 1 mm from the tip, a 0.29-mm diameter 2 mm from the tip, a 0.31 mm diameter 3 mm from the tip, and so forth. Instruments can have constant or variable taper: Some manufacturers express the taper in terms of percentage (e.g., a .02 instrument has been said to have a 2% taper; Fig. 6-15). Current instrument developments include variations in helical angle, pitch, and taper along the cutting portion, which along with variations in alloy and rotational speed (rpm) all affect cutting behavior.[380] The ability

to determine cross-sectional diameter at a given point on a file can help the clinician determine the file size in the point of curvature and the relative stress being placed on the instrument. Instruments with greater tapers are designed so that the tip of the instrument functions as a guide and the middle and coronal part of the instrument's working part is the one engaging the canals walls.

ISO Norms

Standardized specifications have been established to improve endodontic instrument quality.[238] For example, the International Standards Organization (ISO) has worked with the Fédération Dentaire Internationale (FDI) to define specifications. These standards are designated with an ISO number. The American Dental Association (ADA) also has been involved in this effort, as has the American National Standards Institute (ANSI); these standards are designated with an ANSI number. However, new instrument designs have resulted in a need for reconsideration of the standards.

Two ISO standards pertain to endodontic instruments. ISO No. 3630-1 deals with K-type files as does ANSI No. 28), Hedström files (ANSI No. 58), and barbed broaches and rasps (ANSI No. 63). ISO No. 3630-3 deals with condensers,

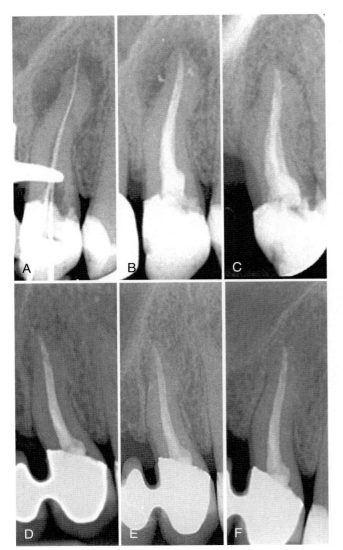

FIG. 6-11 Relationship of radicular anatomy and endodontic disease as shown by filled accessory canals. **A,** Working length radiograph of tooth #13 shows lesions mesially and distally but not apically. **B,** Posttreatment radiograph shows the accessory anatomy. **C,** Six-month recall radiograph before placement of the restoration. **D,** Two-year recall radiograph after resection of the mesiobuccal root of tooth #14 and placement of a fixed partial denture. Excess sealer appears to have been resorbed, forming a distal residual lesion. **E,** Four-year recall radiograph shows almost complete bone fill. **F,** Seven-year recall radiograph; tooth #14 is radiologically sound and clinically within normal limits.

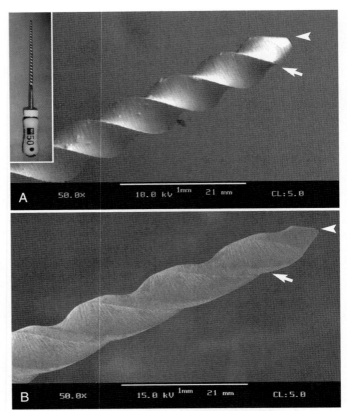

FIG. 6-12 Comparison of the flute geometry and tip configuration of a hand file *(inset)* and a NiTi rotary instrument. **A,** K-file with sharp cutting edges *(arrow)* and Batt tip *(arrowhead)*. **B,** GT rotary file with rounded, noncutting tip *(arrowhead),* smooth transition, and guiding radial lands *(arrow).*

pluggers, and spreaders (ANSI No. 71); however, the term *ISO-normed instruments* is often used as a synonym for K-files (see Fig. 6-15).

One important feature of ISO-normed hand instruments is a defined increase in tip diameter of 0.05 or 0.1 mm, depending on the instrument size (Fig. 6-16). ISO-normed K- and Hedström files (Fig. 6-17) are available in different lengths (21, 25, and 31 mm), but all have a 16-mm-long section of cutting flutes (see Figs. 6-12 and 6-15). The cross-sectional diameter at the first rake angle of any file is labeled D0. The point 1 mm coronal to D0 is D1, the point 2 mm coronal to D0 is D2, and so on up to D16. The D16 point is the largest diameter of an

ISO-normed instrument. Each file derives its numeric name from the diameter at D0 and is assigned a specific color code (see Fig. 6-15).

Another aspect of ISO files is the standard taper of 0.32 mm over 16 mm of cutting blades, or 0.02 mm increase in diameter per millimeter of flute length (.02 taper). Thus, a size #10 instrument has a diameter of 0.1 mm at D0 and a corresponding diameter of 0.42 mm at D16 [0.1 mm + (16 * 0.02 mm)]. For a size #50 instrument, the diameters are 0.5 mm at D0 and 0.82 mm at D16.

The ISO-normed design is a simplification that has specific disadvantages, and it may explain the clinical observation that enlarging a root canal from size #10 to #15 is more difficult than the step from size #55 to #60. The introduction of K-type files with tip sizes between the ISO-stipulated diameters seemed to solve the problem. However, the use of such files is not universally recommended, perhaps because the approved machining tolerance of ±0.02 mm could negate any intended advantages. Moreover, although ±0.02 mm tolerance is stipulated by the ISO norm, most manufacturers do not adhere to it.[253,449,499,581]

Another suggested modification relates to tips with a constant 29% percentage of diameter increments. This sizing pattern creates smaller instruments that carry less of a workload. However, the intended advantage is offset by larger diameters, because the 29% increase between successive files is

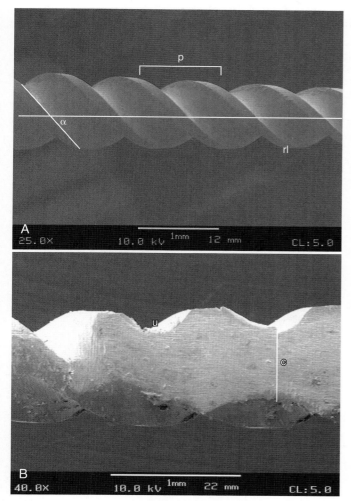

FIG. 6-13 Design characteristics of nickel-titanium rotary instruments. **A,** Lateral view showing the details of the helical angle, pitch *(p),* and the presence of guiding areas, or radial lands *(rl)* (scanning electron micrograph [SEM], ×25). **B,** Ground working part of the instrument in **A,** showing U-shaped excavations and the dimension of the instrument core *(c).*

actually greater than the percentage change found in the ISO file series.

Further changes to the numbering system for files with different sizes have been implemented by several manufacturers. One system has introduced "half" sizes in the range of #15 through #60, resulting in instruments in sizes #15, #17.5, #20, #22.5, and so on.

Alloys

There are currently two principally different types of alloys used for endodontic instruments, stainless steel and nickel-titanium. Most manually operated endodontic instruments are fabricated from stainless steel and have considerable resistance to fracture. A clinician who is careful in applying force and adheres to a strict program of discarding instruments after use should have few instrument fractures. Stainless steel files are comparably inexpensive so that adequate cleaning and sterilization for reuse of files in sizes up to #60 may not be cost effective. If this is the case, files in the range up to #60 may be considered disposable instruments.[490]

Several burs and instruments designed for slow-speed handpiece operation such as Gates Glidden drills, Peeso burs, and pilot drills for intraradicular posts are also manufactured from stainless steel. Instruments designed for rotary root canal instrumentation, however, are typically made of nickel-titanium.[454] This alloy offers unique properties, specifically flexibility and corrosion resistance.

Physical and Chemical Properties of Steel and Nickel Titanium Alloys

Basic engineering terms relate to metals and their behavior when used to manufacture endodontic instruments. Stress-strain diagrams describe the response of metal wires under loading depending on their crystal configuration (Fig. 6-18).

During the development of the equiatomic *nitinol* [this acronym is derived from *ni*ckel-*ti*tanium investigated at the *N*aval *O*rdinance *L*aboratory] alloy (55% [by weight] nickel and 45% [by weight] titanium), several effects were noted that relate to its specific crystal arrangement with two stable main phases, *austenite* and *martensite* (Fig. 6-19): a shape memory effect as temperature- and strain-dependent pseudoelasticity, all attributable to specific thermodynamic properties of the new alloy.[77,133,356,517]

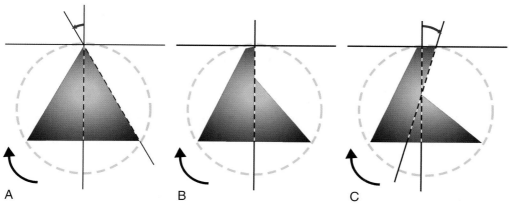

FIG. 6-14 The rake angle of an endodontic file can be negative (**A**), neutral (**B**) or positive (**C**).

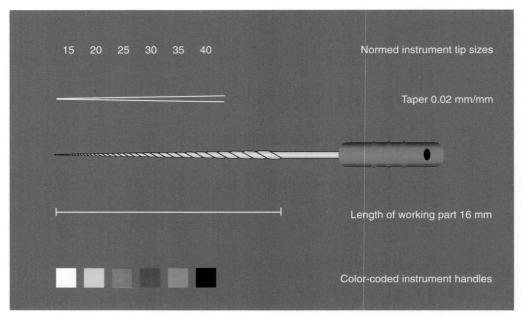

FIG. 6-15 Schematic drawing of an ISO-normed hand instrument size #35. Instrument tip sizing, taper, and handle colors are regulated by the ISO/ANSI/ADA norm.

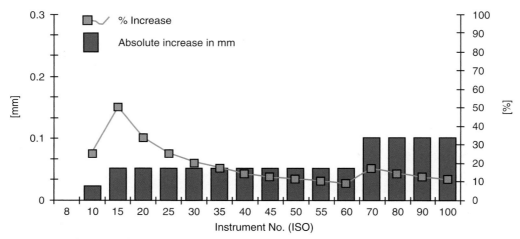

FIG. 6-16 Increase in tip diameter in absolute figures and in relation to the smaller file size. Note the particularly large increase from size #10 to size #15.

Walia and colleagues thought that the pseudoelastic properties of 55-nitinol might prove advantageous in endodontics and initially tested hand instruments.[542] They found that size #15 NiTi instruments were two to three times more flexible than stainless steel instruments; moreover, the instruments showed superior resistance to angular deflection.[542]

Furthermore, hardly any plastic deformation of cutting flutes was recorded when an instrument was bent up to 90 degrees, and forces required to bend endodontic files to 45 degrees were reduced by 50% with NiTi.[454,542] Serene and colleagues speculated that heat, probably during sterilization cycles, could even restore the molecular structure of used NiTi files, resulting in an increased resistance to fracture.[454] Such a behavior is claimed to occur for current martensitic instruments.[377]

These unusual properties are the result of a molecular crystalline phase transformation in specific crystal structures of the austenitic and martensitic phases of the alloy.[517] External stresses transform the austenitic crystalline form of NiTi into a martensitic crystalline structure that can accommodate greater stress without increasing the strain. As a result, a NiTi file has transformational elasticity, also known as *pseudoelasticity,* or the ability to return to its original shape after being deformed (see Fig. 6-19, *B*). This property dictates that typically NiTi instruments are manufactured by milling rather than twisted; twisting incorporates plastic deformation and is used, for example, to produce stainless steel K-files.

Similar to the application of deforming forces, heat can also result in phase transformation (see Fig. 6-19, *A*) from austenite to martensite and vice versa.[209,329] Moreover, thermal conditions during the production of the raw wire can be used to modify its properties, most important of which is its flexibility.[192,461] For austenitic endodontic instruments, a recoverable

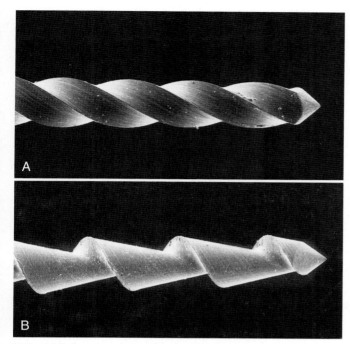

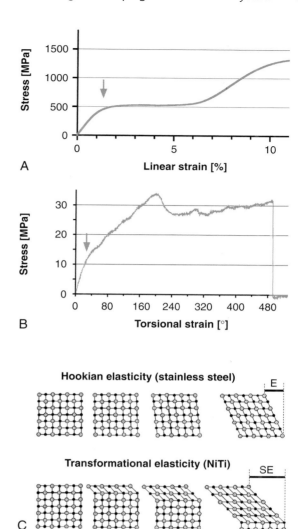

FIG. 6-17 Scanning electron micrographs of endodontic hand files fabricated by twisting (K-file size #40, **A**) and grinding (Hedström file #50, **B**). (Both images courtesy Dentsply Maillefer, Ballaigues, Switzerland).

FIG. 6-18 Stress-strain behavior of nickel-titanium alloy. **A**, Schematic diagram of linear extension of a NiTi wire. **B**, Torque to failure test of a size #60, #.04 taper ProFile NiTi instrument. Note the biphasic deformation, indicated by arrows in **A-B**. **C**, Comparison of stainless steel and nickel-titanium crystal lattices under load. Hookian elasticity accounts for the elastic behavior *(E)* of steel, whereas transformation from martensite to austenite and back occurs during the pseudoelastic *(PE)* behavior of NiTi alloy. (*C*, Modified from Thompson SA: An overview of nickel-titanium alloys used in dentistry, *Int Endod J* 33:297, 2000.)

elastic response of up to 7% is expected (Fig. 6-20). However, more martensitic instruments will have less of an elastic range and are more likely to plastically deform during use.[377,461]

Experiments designed to test fracture resistance demonstrate physical properties of endodontic instruments; following the pertinent ISO norm, 3630-1 graphs such as those shown in Fig. 6-20 are generated and compared among different designs.

Attempts to improve the NiTi alloy continue, and reports indicate that new NiTi alloys may be five times more flexible than currently used alloys.[225,461] NiTi instruments may have imperfections such as milling marks, metal flash, or rollover.[135,454,524,542] Some researchers have speculated that fractures in NiTi instruments originate at such surface imperfections.[11]

Surface irregularities may provide reservoirs of corrosive substances, most notably sodium hypochlorite (NaOCl). Chloride corrosion may lead to micropitting[428] and possibly subsequent fracture in NiTi instruments.[202] Immersion in various disinfecting solutions for extended periods (e.g., overnight soaking) produced corrosion of NiTi instruments and subsequent decreased torsional resistance.[350,486] For ProTaper,[52] RaCe, and ProFile385 instruments, 2-hour immersion damaged the integrity of the alloy. Other authors did not find a corrosion-related effect on K3-files[36] or ProFile instruments.[120]

Regular reprocessing procedures do not seem to significantly affect NiTi rotary instruments.[293,330,503] In one study, only limited material loss occurred when NiTi LightSpeed instruments were immersed in 1% and 5% NaOCl for 30 to 60 minutes.[84] Corrosion of NiTi instruments used in the clinical setting, therefore, might not significantly contribute to fracture except when the instruments are immersed in warmed NaOCl for longer than 60 minutes. In the majority of studies,

sterilization procedures do not appear to negatively impact torsional strength[221,464] or fatigue resistance[79,220] of most NiTi instruments: austenitic[538] and martensitic[92] alloy behaved grossly similarly in this aspect.

There is an ongoing discussion over the impact of other aspects of clinical usage on the mechanical properties of NiTi rotaries. Most likely, clinical usage leads to some changes in the alloy, potentially through work hardening.[10,254]

Another strategy to improve surface characteristics is electropolishing; also surface coatings and ion implantation have been tried. Electropolishing is a process that removes surface irregularities such as flash and bur marks. It is thought to improve material properties, specifically fatigue and corrosion resistance; however, the evidence for both these claims is

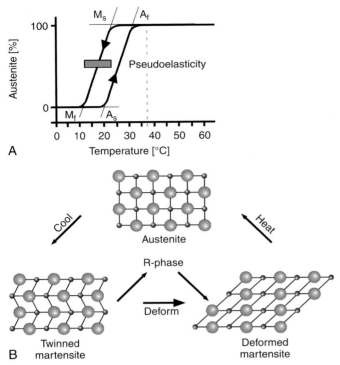

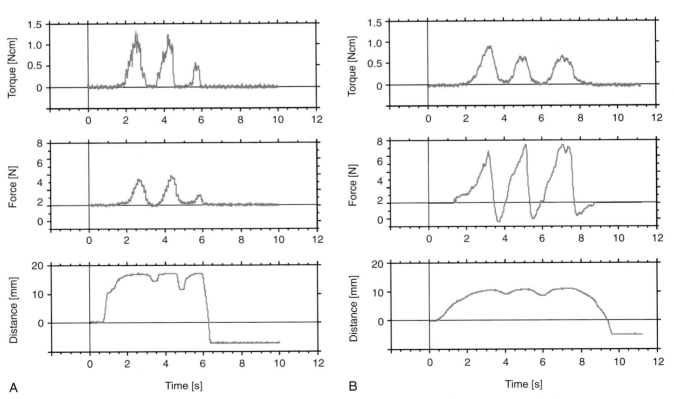

FIG. 6-19 Pseudoelastic behavior of Nickel titanium is based on the two main crystal configurations, martensite and austenite, which depend on temperature (**A**) and applied strain (**B**). Formation of the respective configuration initiates at the start temperatures, M_s and A_s.

mixed. One study found an extension of fatigue life for electropolished instruments,[20] whereas others found no improvement of fatigue resistance of electropolished instruments.[78,100,217] Boessler and colleagues suggested a change in cutting behavior with an increase of torsional load after electropolishing.[59]

Corrosion resistance of electropolished NiTi rotaries is also controversial. One study found superior corrosion resistance for electropolished RaCe instruments,[63] whereas another study demonstrated similar corrosion susceptibility for RaCe and nonelectropolished ProFile instruments.[385] Attempts have been made to improve surface quality by coating it with titanium nitride.[398,438] The latter process also seems to have a beneficial effect on cutting efficiency.[438]

Perhaps more relevant than surface treatment are modification of the base alloy that significantly alter material properties within the atomic ratio.[369] The first commercialized alloy was M-Wire (SportsWire, Langley, OK), which was shown to have higher fatigue resistance with similar torsional strength.[249] More recently, instrument are produced through production process that include annealing and cooling steps to create instruments that, after cold working during the production process, are more martensitic during dental treatment, as defined by their M_s temperature (see Fig. 6-19, *A*). Under clinical conditions these alloys are more flexible[510] and present higher fatigue resistance.[377] Examples are the newly introduced gold and blue alloys types (Dentsply Tulsa Dental Specialties, Tulsa, OK) or so-called controlled memory alloy used in Hyflex instruments (Coltene Endo, Cuyahoga Falls, OH).

FIG. 6-20 Physical factors (torque, axial force, and insertion depth) that affect root canal instrumentation documented with a torque-testing platform. **A**, ProFile size #45, #.04 taper used in a mildly curved canal of a single-rooted tooth, step-back after apical preparation to size #40. **B**, FlexMaster size #35, #.06 taper used in a curved distobuccal canal of a maxillary first molar, crown-down during the initial phase of canal preparation.

Manually Operated Instruments

Endodontic trays contain many items familiar from general dentistry but certain hand instruments are designed specifically for endodontic procedures. This includes instruments employed for procedures inside the pulp space, for example hand and engine-driven instruments for root canal preparation, and energized instruments for root canal shaping. Special instruments and devices for root canal obturation are selected for filling prepared canal spaces.

K-Type Instruments

Manually operated instruments are generically called *files*. Defined by function, files are instruments that enlarge canals with apico-coronal insertion and withdrawal motions.

Historically, root canal instruments were manufactured from carbon steel. Subsequently, the use of stainless steel greatly improved the quality of instruments. More recently, K-type files manufactured from NiTi were introduced (NiTi-Flex, Dentsply Maillefer, Ballaigues, Switzerland).

Files were first mass produced by the Kerr Manufacturing Co. of Romulus, Michigan, in the early 1900s, hence the name "K-type" file (or K-file) and K-type reamer (K-reamer). K-files and K-reamers were manufactured by the same process—that is, by twisting square or triangular metal blanks along their long axis, producing partly horizontal cutting blades (see Fig. 6-17, *A*). Three or four equilateral, flat surfaces were ground at increasing depths on the sides of a piece of wire, producing a tapered pyramidal shape. The wire then was stabilized on one end, and the distal end was rotated to form the spiral instrument. The number of sides and the number of spirals determine whether the instrument is best suited for filing or reaming. Generally, a three-sided configuration with fewer spirals (e.g., 16 per 16-mm working portion) is used for reaming (i.e., cutting and enlarging canals with rotational motions). A file has more flutes per length unit (e.g., 20) than a reamer, whereas a three- sided or triangular configuration is generally more flexible than a four-sided one.[437]

K-type instruments are useful for penetrating and enlarging root canals. Generally, a reaming motion (i.e., constant file rotation) causes less transportation than a filing motion (translational or "in and out" motion).[171,482] (*Transportation* is defined here as the excessive loss of dentin from the outer wall of a curved canal in the apical segment, as described in more detail later.)

Stainless steel K-files may be precurved by overbending. This procedure subjects the file to substantial strain and should therefore be done carefully. Permanent deformation occurs when the flutes become wound more tightly or opened more widely (Fig. 6-21). When such deformation occurs, the instrument should no longer be used; file fracture is likely to occur during clockwise motion after plastic deformation.[456]

Interestingly, although the force required for failure is the same in both directions of rotation,[271,278] failure occurs in the counterclockwise direction at half the number of rotations required for failure in the clockwise direction. Therefore, K-type instruments should be operated more carefully when pressure is applied in a counterclockwise direction.

Cross-sectional analysis of a K-file reveals why this design allows careful application of clockwise and counterclockwise rotational and translational working strokes: the cross section is symmetrical with negative rake angles, allowing dentin to be adequately cut in both clockwise and counter-clockwise direction.

Reamers are instruments that are similar to K-files in overall design, but they have fewer cutting flutes per mm of the working surface. They are more appropriate for twisting motion and are less frequently used today.[437]

H-Type Instruments

H-type instruments, also known as Hedström files (see Fig. 6-17, *B*), are milled from round, stainless steel blanks. These files are very efficient for translational strokes,[437] because of a positive rake angle and a blade with a cutting rather than a scraping angle. Rotational working movements are strongly discouraged because of the possibility of fracture. Hedström

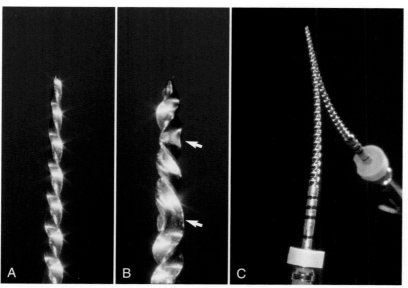

FIG. 6-21 Deformation of endodontic instruments manufactured from nickel-titanium alloy. **A** and **B**, Intact and plastically deformed ProFile instruments (*arrow* indicates areas of permanent deformation). **C**, ProFile instrument placed on a mirror to illustrate elastic behavior.

files up to size #25 can be efficiently used to relocate canal orifices and, with adequate filing strokes, to remove overhangs. Similarly, wide oval canals can be instrumented with Hedström files as well as with rotary instruments. On the other hand, overzealous filing can lead to considerable thinning of the radicular wall and strip perforations (Fig. 6-22). As with stainless steel K-files, Hedström files have been described as disposable instruments.[490]

Bending Hedström files results in points of greater stress concentration than in K-type instruments. These prestressed areas may lead to the propagation of cracks and ultimately fatigue failure.[200] Note that clinically, fatigue fractures may occur without visible signs of deformation.

Hedström files are produced by grinding a single continuous flute into a tapered blank. Computer-assisted machining technology has allowed the development of H-type instruments with complex forms. This process, called *multiaxis grinding*, allows adjustment of the rake angle, helix angle, multiple flutes, and tapers and is also used to fabricate the majority of NiTi instruments. Because the H-file generally has sharper edges than the K-file, it has a tendency to thread into the canal during rotation, particularly if the instrument's blades are nearly parallel. Awareness of threading-in forces is important to avoid instrument failure.

Effectiveness and Wear of Instruments

The ability of an endodontic hand instrument to cut and machine dentin is essential; however, no standards exist for either the cutting or the machining effectiveness of endodontic files, nor have clear requirements been established for resistance to wear. In any study of the effectiveness of an instrument, two factors must be investigated: (1) effectiveness in cutting or breaking loose dentin and (2) effectiveness in machining dentin.

Attempts have been made to evaluate the effectiveness of an instrument when used with a linear movement.[437,442] Collectively, these studies showed that instruments might differ significantly, not only when comparing brands and types but also within one brand and type. For K-files, effectiveness varies 2 to 12 times between files of the same brand. This variation for Hedström files is greater, ranging from 2.5 to more than 50 times.[498] The greater variation among Hedström files is easy to understand because the H-file is the result of more individual grinding during manufacture than the conventional K-file, which is difficult to alter much during the manufacturing process. For example, during the grinding of a Hedström file, the rake angle can be modified to neutral or even slightly positive; this is impossible to achieve with a K-file.

During canal preparation, a file's rake edge shaves off dentin that accumulates in the grooves between the rake edges. The deeper and larger this space, the longer the stroke can be before the instrument is riding on its own debris, making it ineffective.

These design variations and the rake angle of the edges determine the effectiveness of a Hedström file. Of the hybrid files, the K-Flex (SybronEndo, Orange, CA) file has properties similar to those of K-files. The Flex-R file (Integra Miltex, York, PA), which is a ground instrument with a triangular cross section similar to a K-file, more closely resembles a Hedström file in its variations in cutting behavior. It also is more effective at substrate removal than the K-files but cannot measure up to the H-files' ability to machine radicular dentin.[498]

Barbed Broaches

Barbed broaches (Fig. 6-23) are produced in a variety of sizes and color codes. They are manufactured by cutting sharp, coronally angulated barbs into metal wire blanks. Broaches are intended to remove vital pulp from root canals, and in cases of mild inflammation, they work well for severing pulp at the constriction level *in toto*. The use of broaches has declined since the advent of NiTi rotary instruments, but broaching occasionally may be useful for expediting emergency procedures (see Chapter 18) and removing materials (e.g., cotton pellets or absorbent points) from root canals.

Low-Speed Engine-Driven Instruments

Burs

Specialized burs are available for endodontic access cavities. These burs are used in both high-speed and slow-speed handpieces and are manufactured from stainless steel. Access cavity preparation and used materials are described in detail in Chapter 5.

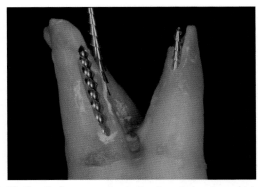

FIG. 6-22 Result of an overenthusiastic attempt at root canal treatment of a maxillary second molar with large stainless steel files. Multiple strip perforations occurred; consequently, the tooth had to be extracted.

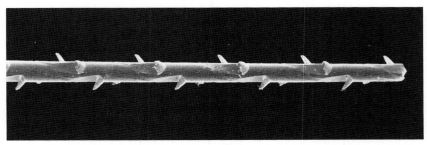

FIG. 6-23 Scanning electron micrograph of a barbed broach. (Moyco Union Broach, York, PA.)

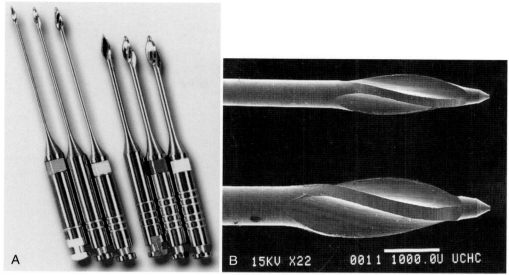

FIG. 6-24 **A,** Various Gates-Glidden (GG) burs made of stainless steel and scanning electron micrograph (**B,** working tip). (**A,** From Johnson WT: *Color atlas of endodontics,* St Louis, 2002, Saunders.)

Gates-Glidden Drills

Gates-Glidden (GG) drills (Fig. 6-24) have been used for more than 100 years without noteworthy design changes. Gates Glidden drills are typically used to enlarge coronal canal areas.[119] When misused, GG drills can dramatically reduce radicular wall thickness.[173,242]

GG drills are sized from 1 to 6 (with corresponding diameters of 0.5 to 1.5 mm); the number of rings or color-coding on the shank identifies the specific drill size. GG instruments are available in various lengths and by several manufacturers. Each instrument has a long, thin shaft with parallel walls and a short, oval cutting head with safety tips (Fig. 6-24, *B*); these drills are produced in stainless steel and NiTi varieties. Because of their design and physical properties,[68] GG drills are side-cutting instruments; they can be used to cut dentin as they are withdrawn from the canal (i.e., on the outstroke).[417] Used this way, their cutting action can deliberately be directed away from external root concavities in single-rooted and furcated teeth. GG drills should be used only in the straight portions of a canal.[522]

Two procedural sequences have been proposed: with the step-down technique, the clinician starts with a large drill and progresses to smaller ones; conversely, with the step-back technique, the clinician starts with a small drill and progresses to larger ones. With the step-down approach, the clinician must select a GG instrument with a diameter that allows introduction into the respective orifice and progression for about 1 mm. The subsequent smaller instruments progress deeper into the canal until the coronal third has been preenlarged. This technique efficiently opens root canal orifices and works best when canals exit the access cavity without severe angulations. Opened orifices simplify subsequent cleaning and shaping procedures and help establish a smooth glide path from the access cavity into the root canal system.

With the step-back approach, a small GG instrument is introduced into the canal, and dentin is removed on the outstroke. This process is repeated with the next larger GG instrument, which is again worked shorter than the preceding smaller one. In this way, the coronal third of the root canal is enlarged and dentin overhangs are removed.

When used adequately, GG instruments are inexpensive, safe, and clinically beneficial tools. Gates-Glidden drills may be used safely and to their fullest potential at 750 to 1500 rpm. High revolutions per minute (rpm), excessive pressure, an incorrect angle of insertion, and the use of GG instruments to aggressively drill into canals have resulted in mishaps such as strip perforation. The preferred mode of action for GG drills is against the outer canal wall, away from the canal curvature. Also, cyclic fatigue may cause GG instruments to fracture when used in curved canal areas, and the short cutting heads may fracture with high torsional loads. As with nickel-titanium rotary instruments, GG drills work best when used in electric gear reduction handpieces rather than with air motors.

Peeso Drills (Reamers)

Peeso drills are typically used in root canal preparation either for coronal flaring or during post preparation. These drill are at this point manufactured mostly from stainless steel by milling similar to the Gates Gliddens. Peeso drills are also used in the electric slow-speed handpiece; the rotational speed is the range of 800 to 1200 rpm; the cutting flutes are more parallel and longer compared to GG drills but shorter than the 16 mm prescribed for ISO-normed hand files. Peeso drills are classified as type P and type B-l, as defined by ISO norm 3630-2.[299] The sizing for these drills is also numbers 1 to 6, similar to GGs. Peeso drills are available with cutting and noncutting tips and should be used with caution to avoid excessive preparation and thinning of radicular dentin walls.[4]

Engine-Driven Instruments for Canal Preparation

Instrument Types

Engine-driven instruments for root canal preparation made of stainless steel have been in use for more than half a century—for the first decades, mainly in handpieces that permitted reciprocation (alternating clockwise-counterclockwise motion). The major two problems with this type of instrument were canal transportation (discussed later) and file fracture. This

TABLE 6-1

Grouping of Instruments According to Their Mode of Cutting and Details

Group	Enlargement Potential	Preparation Errors	Fracture Resistance	Clinical Performance
I ProFile[1], ProSystem GT, GTX[1], Quantec[2], Pow-R[3], Guidance[4], K3[2] LightSpeed var.[2]	+, Depending in sizes, often time consuming	++ Low incidence, usually <150 μm canal transportation	+/– Fatigue + Torsional load, depending on system	++ Good, depending on treatment conditions; no difference between instruments shown so far, except for inexperienced clinicians, who perform better with landed instruments
II ProTaper var.[1], RaCe[5], Hero 642[6], FlexMaster[7], Mtwo[7], Sequence[8], Alpha[9]... ProFile Vortex[1] Twisted File[1]	+/–, Good with use of hybrid techniques	+/–, Overall more demanding in clinicians' ability	+ Fatigue +/– Torsional load, depending on taper, handling	
III, EndoEZE AET[12], Liberator[11]... WaveOne[1], Reciproc[7] OneShape[6] SAF	Limited	Varies, Liberator— EndoEZE AET— WaveOne, Reciproc+	Varies + with WaveOne, Reciproc	Varies

Manufacturers:
Grouping of instruments according to their mode of cutting and details about manufacturers. Group I consists of radial-landed instruments with reaming action. Group II instruments have a triangular cross section and cutting action. Group III is made up of instruments with unusual geometry, movement, or sequence.

changed with the advent of NiTi rotaries from about the early 1990s; the much more flexible alloy allowed continuous rotation and reduced both canal preparation errors and instrument fracture compared to earlier engine driven techniques.

Currently, more than 50 types of rotary instrument systems have been described and more continue to be developed. The instruments vary greatly in terms of design, alloy used, and recommended cutting movement (Table 6-1). Various built-in features may help prevent procedural errors, increase efficiency, and improve the quality of canal shaping.

For example, a longer pilot tip may guide the instrument and help to stay centered in the canal long axis. Alternatively, a file can be given an asymmetric cross section to help maintain the central axis of the canal.

Another direction of instrument development is the prevention of instrument fractures (Fig. 6-25). There are several ways to modify an instrument to make it less likely to fracture; for example, increasing the core diameter will increase torsional resistance. Another approach is to use a torque-limiting motor (discussed later). Alternatively, a zero taper or nearly parallel and fluted working portion of the file can be provided for curved canals so that the apical portion of the canal can be enlarged without undue file stress and compression of debris. More recently a reciprocation motion was reapplied to NiTi rotary instruments to prevent threading-in and instrument fractures in general.

Yet another, more recent, direction of instrument development is to improve shaping as it relates to circumferential root canal wall contact. One example for this strategy is a file manufactured from an expandable and flexible hollow NiTi tube, the so-called Self-adjusting File (ReDent-Nova, Ra'anana, Israel, Israel) (Fig. 6-26). More recently, a substantial S-shape was superimposed onto a flexible NiTi rotary that provides a larger envelope of motion while maintaining a limited maximum flute diameter (TRUShape, Dentsply Tulsa Dental Specialties).

Marketed files vary greatly in terms of their specific design characteristics, such as tip sizing, taper, cross section, helix angle, and pitch (see Fig. 6-13). Some of the early systems have

been removed from the market or relegated to minor roles; others, such as ProFile (Dentsply Tulsa Dental Specialties), are still successfully used. More recently added instruments vary in cross-sectional and longitudinal design (Fig. 6-27). However, the extent to which clinical outcome changes (if any) will depend on design characteristics is difficult to forecast.[375,381]

Most instruments described in the following section are manufactured by a grinding process, although some are produced by laser etching and yet others by plastic deformation under specific heating and cooling processes. Surface quality has been considered an important detail because cracks that arise from superficial defects may play a role in instrument fracture.[11] Moreover, surface defects such as metal flash and rollover are common in unused NiTi instruments.[135,314]

Many variables and physical properties influence the clinical performance of NiTi rotaries.[272,374,454,512] Clinical practice has generated much of what is known about NiTi instruments, including reasons for instrument fracture[33] and instrument sequences. These instruments have substantially reduced the incidence of relevant canal shaping errors,[387] but they are also thought to fracture somewhat more easily than hand instruments.

Table 6-1 and the following sections describe the instrument groups most widely used for root canal preparation at this point in time. Most basic strategies apply to all NiTi rotary instruments, regardless of the specific design or brand. However, three design groups need to be analyzed separately: group I, instruments designed for passive preparation; group II, rotary instruments designed for active cutting; and group III, unique designs that do not fit in either group I or group II.

Group I: Passive Preparation; Presence of Radial Lands
The first commercially successful rotary instruments were ProFile (Dentsply Tulsa Dental Specialties), LightSpeed (marketed in its current form by SybronEndo), and GT rotaries (Dentsply Tulsa Dental Specialties) and have in common a cross section with so-called radial lands. These are created by three round excavations, also known as the U-shape. The

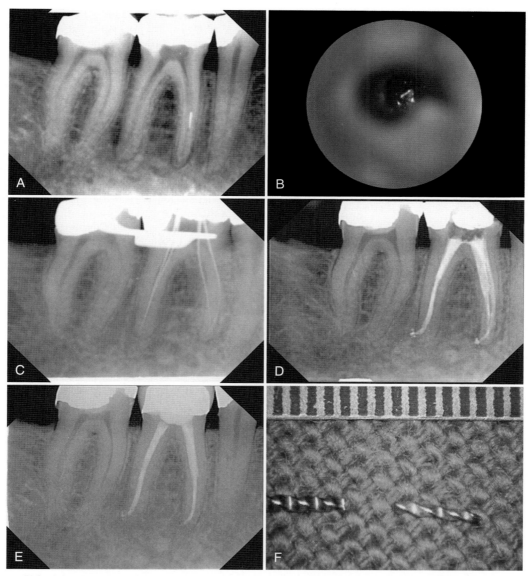

FIG. 6-25 Removal of a fractured NiTi instrument from a mesiolingual canal of a mandibular molar. **A,** Fragment located in the middle third of the root. **B,** Clinical aspect of the fragment after enlargement of the coronal third of the root canal with modified Gates-Glidden drills, visualized with an operating microscope (×25). **C,** Radiograph taken after removal of the fragment; four hand files have been inserted into the canals. **D,** Final radiograph shows slight widening of the coronal third of the mesiolingual canal and fully sealed canal systems. A full crown was placed immediately after obturation. **E,** Recall radiograph 5 years after obturation shows sound periradicular tissues. **F,** Removed fragment and separated file (gradation of ruler is 0.5 mm).

design of the instrument tip and also the lateral file surface (radial land) guide the file as it progresses apically. This makes rotaries listed in group I fairly safe regarding preparation errors. On the other hand, it results in a reaming action rather than cutting of dentin and this makes them inefficient. Moreover, the smear layer produced with radial-landed rotaries is different in consistency and amount compared to the debris and smear created by cutting files.[366,573]

LightSpeed

The LightSpeed file, developed by Drs. Steve Senia and William Wildey in the early 1990s and now also known as LS1, was introduced as an instrument different from all others because of its long, thin, noncutting shaft and short anterior cutting head. The same design principles apply to the currently available LSX instrument (SybronEndo) that is manufactured not by milling but by a stamping process. A full set consists of 25 LightSpeed LS1 instruments in sizes #20 to #100, including half sizes (e.g., 22.5, 27.5); LSX does not have half sizes, and a set includes sizes #20 to #80.

The original LightSpeed is a widely researched NiTi rotary instrument,[50,392,394,459,513,514] and most reports have found that the system has a low incidence of overall and specific preparation errors. One report found similar shaping abilities for LSX and LightSpeed LS1 assessed with a double-exposure technique.[240]

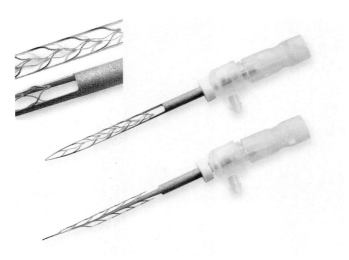

FIG. 6-26 The SAF instrument. The instrument is made as a hollow, thin NiTi lattice cylinder that is compressed when inserted into the root canal and adapts to the canal's cross section. It is attached to a vibrating handpiece. Continuous irrigation is applied through a special hub on the side of its shank. Inset shows the abrasive surface of the instrument. (Courtesy ReDent-Nova, Ra'anana, Israel.)

ProFile

The ProFile system (Dentsply Tulsa Dental Specialties) was introduced by Dr. Ben Johnson in 1994. ProFile instruments have increased tapers compared with conventional hand instruments. The ProFile system was first sold as the "Series 29" hand instruments in .02 taper, but it soon became available in .04 and .06 tapers. The tips of the ProFile Series 29 rotary instruments had a constant proportion of diameter increments (29%). Later, a ProFile series with ISO-sized tips (Dentsply Maillefer) was developed and marketed in Europe.

Cross sections of a ProFile instrument show a U-shape design with radial lands (Fig. 6-28) and a parallel central core. Lateral views show a 20-degree helix angle, a constant pitch, and bullet-shaped noncutting tips (see Fig. 6-12). Together with a slightly negative rake angle, this configuration facilitates a reaming action on dentin rather than cutting. Also, debris is transported coronally and is effectively removed from the root canals.

ProFile instruments shaped canals without major preparation errors in a number of in vitro investigations.[74,75,515,516] A slight improvement in canal shape was noted when .04 and .06 tapered instruments were used in an alternating fashion.[73] Loss

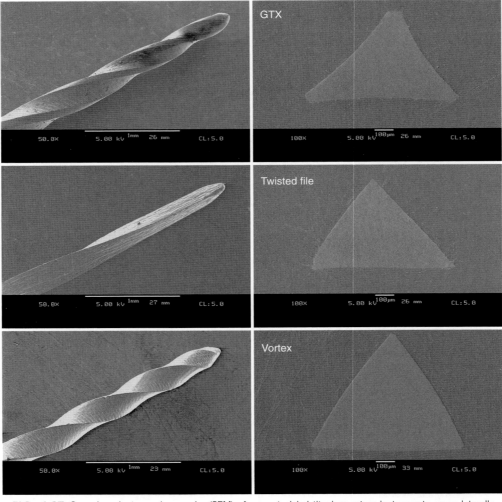

FIG. 6-27 Scanning electron micrographs (SEM) of current nickel titanium rotary instruments, seen laterally (left panel, ×50) and in cross sections (right panel, ×100). Note the radial landed cross section of the GTX instrument

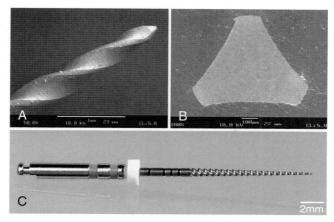

No. of instruments/ set	Tip sizes	Size increments	r.p.m. (recommended)	Lengths
Orifice Shapers: 6	20-80	10; from 60: 20	150 to 350, low apical force, torque to fracture and working torque dependent on instrument size	19 mm
ProFile .06: 6	15-40	5		21 mm, 25 mm, some 31 mm
ProFile .04: 9	15-90	5; from #45: 15; from #60: 30		
ProFile .02: 6	15-45	5		
Profile Series 29	13-100	Varies, 29%		21 mm, 25 mm

FIG. 6-28 Design features of a ProFile instrument. **A,** Lateral view (scanning electron micrograph [SEM], ×50). **B,** Cross section (SEM, ×200). **C,** Lateral view. **D,** Design specifications.

of working length did not exceed 0.5 mm[73-75,515,516] and was not affected by the use of .06 tapered instruments.[73] Comparative assessments in vitro suggested that ProFile prepared mesial canals in mandibular molars with less transportation than K3 and RaCe.[9]

A more recent addition to the ProFile family of instruments was Vortex (Dentsply Tulsa Dental Specialties). The major change lies in the nonlanded cross section, whereas tip sizes and tapers are similar to existing ProFiles, hence these files are placed in group 2 (discussed later).

GT and GTX Files

The Greater Taper, or GT file, was introduced by Dr. Steve Buchanan in 1994. This instrument incorporates a radial landed cross-sectional design and was marketed as ProFile GT (Dentsply Tulsa Dental Specialties). The system was first produced as a set of four hand-operated files and later as engine-driven files. The instruments came in four tapers (.06, .08, .10, and .12), and the maximum diameter of the working part was 1 mm. The design limited the maximum shank diameter and decreased the length of the cutting flutes with increasing taper. The instruments had a variable pitch and a growing number of flutes in progression to the tip; the apical instrument diameter was 0.2 mm. Instrument tips were noncutting and rounded; these design principles are mostly still present in the current incarnation, the GTX instrument. The main differences are the M-Wire alloy type used and minor design and handling changes.

Studies on GT files found that the prepared shape stayed centered and was achieved with few procedural errors.[173,208] A shaping assessment using micro-computed tomography [μCT; see Fig. 6-4 as an example)] showed that GT files machined statistically similar canal wall areas compared with ProFile and LightSpeed preparations.[386] These walls were homogeneously planed and smooth.[366,573] The more recently introduced GTX variant is manufactured from M-Wire and does not appear to have significantly improved physical properties[254] or shaping capacity.[241] GT instruments were available for small (tip size #20), medium (tip size #30), and large canal diameters (tip size #40).

K3

In a sequence of design developments by their inventor, Dr. McSpadden, the Quantec 2000 files were followed by the Quantec SC, the Quantec LX, and the current K3 system (all by SybronEndo). The overall design of the K3 is similar to that of the ProFile in that it includes instruments with .02, .04, and .06 tapers. The most obvious difference between the Quantec and K3 models is the K3's unique cross-sectional design: a slightly positive rake angle for greater cutting efficiency, wide radial lands, and a peripheral blade relief for reduced friction. Unlike the Quantec, a two-flute file, the K3 features a third radial land to help prevent threading-in.

In the lateral aspect, the K3 has a variable pitch and variable core diameter, which provide apical strength. This intricate design is relatively difficult to manufacture, resulting in some metal flash.

Like most other current instruments, the K3 features a round safety tip, but the file is about 4 mm shorter than other files (although it has the same length of cutting flutes) because of the so-called Axxess handle. The instruments are coded by ring color and number.

Tested in vitro, K3's shaping ability seems to be similar to that of the ProTaper[51] and superior to that achieved with hand instruments.[440] More recently, when curved canals in lower molars were shaped to a size #30 .06,[14] K3 files had less canal transportation in a modified Bramante model than RaCe but more than ProFile.

Summary

Radial landed rotary instruments are considered very safe, even when accidentally taken beyond the confines of the root canal. Fracture resistance to torsional loading and cyclic varies depending on specific instrument design. The limited cutting efficacy of these files was perceived as a downside and is a reason that the market share has diminished.[55] However, their excellent track record in clinical applications and research continues to support the use of rotaries listed in group I.

Group II: Active Cutting; Triangular Cross Section

Rotaries in group II all have a more active cutting flute design in common. Radial lands are absent (see Fig. 6-13), and this fact results in a higher cutting efficacy. This translates to a higher potential for preparation errors, in particular when the instrument is taken through the apical foramen, thus eliminating the guide derived from the noncutting tip.

ProTaper Universal

The ProTaper system originally comprised six instruments: three shaping files and three finishing files. This set is now complemented by two larger finishing files and a separate set of three rotaries tailored to retreatment procedures. The instruments were designed by Drs. Cliff Ruddle, John West, and Pierre Machtou. In cross sections, ProTaper shows a convex triangle with sharp cutting edges and no radial lands. The cross section of finishing files F3, F4, and F5 is slightly relieved for increased flexibility. The three shaping files have tapers that increase coronally, and the reverse pattern is seen in the five finishing files.

Shaping files nos. 1 and 2 have tip diameters of 0.185 mm and 0.2 mm, respectively, 14-mm-long cutting blades, and partially active tips. The finishing files (F1-F5) have tip diameters of 0.2, 0.25, 0.3, 0.4, and 0.5 mm, respectively, between D0 and D3, and the apical tapers are .07, .08, .09, .05, and .04, respectively. The finishing files have rounded noncutting tips.

Two aspects of handling have been emphasized for ProTaper. The first is the preparation of a glide path, either manually[368] or with special rotary instruments.[53] An enlargement to a size approaching the subsequent rotaries' tips, at least larger than the file's core diameter, prevents breakage and allows assessment of the canal size.[368] This means that the glide path should correspond to a size #15 or #20. The second specific recommendation is the use of a more laterally directed "brushing" working stroke. Such a stroke allows the clinician to coronally direct larger files away from danger zones and counteract any "threading-in" effect.[58] Both usage elements should be

considered good practice for other instruments, particularly for more actively cutting ones.[391]

In a study using plastic blocks, ProTaper created acceptable shapes more quickly than GT rotary, ProFile, and Quantec instruments,[573] but it also created somewhat more aberrations. This was recently corroborated comparing preparations of mesial root canals in mandibular molars ex vivo with ProTaper Universal to Alpha (Gebr. Brasseler GmbH & Co. KG-Komet, Lemgo, Germany).[536] In a comparison of ProTaper and K3 instruments (SybronEndo), Bergmans and colleagues found few differences, with the exception of some transportation by the ProTaper into the furcation region.[51] A study using µCT showed that the ProTaper created consistent shapes in constricted canals, without obvious preparation errors, although wide canals may be insufficiently prepared with this system.[384] It has been recommended that ProTaper be combined with less tapered, more flexible rotaries to reduce apical transportation.[244]

A newer version of this system, called ProTaper Next was introduced in 2013. Current research suggests that mechanical properties of these instruments, manufactured from M-Wire, are better than ProTaper Universal.[23,138,370]

No data are currently available on shaping outcomes or clinical results.

HERO 642, HERO Shaper

Several systems in group II (see Table 6-1) were designed with positive rake angles, which provide greater cutting efficiency. HERO instruments (MicroMega, Besançon, France) are an example. The original version was known as HERO 642 (the acronym HERO stands for high elasticity in rotation), and the name has now changed into HERO Shaper, with little apparent differences in the instrument design.

Cross sections of HERO instruments show geometries similar to those of an H-file without radial lands. Tapers of .02, .04, and .06 are available in sizes ranging from #20 to #45. The instruments are relatively flexible but maintain an even distribution of force into the cutting areas.[528,529] HERO instruments have a progressive flute pitch and a noncutting passive tip, similar to other NiTi rotary systems. The instruments are coded by handle color.

Research with HERO files indicates a shaping potential similar to that of the FlexMaster[230] (VDW, Munich, Germany) and ProFile,[164] although in one study HERO files induced more changes in cross-sectional anatomy.[179] HERO instruments also caused some aberrations when used in simulated canals with acute curves,[517] but they were safer than Quantec SC instruments (SybronEndo).[236] More recently, HERO Shapers had a better centering ability compared to RaCe instruments in resin blocks.[28] Using a modified Bramante technique in vitro, earlier HERO 642 and current HERO Shaper rotaries showed no differences in canal cross sections before and after shaping.[28]

FlexMaster

The FlexMaster file system is currently unavailable in the United States but popular in Europe. It features .02, .04, and .06 tapers. The cross sections have a triangular shape, with sharp cutting edges and no radial lands. This makes for a relatively solid instrument core and active cutting ability. The overall manufacturing quality seems high, with minimal metal flash and rollover.

FlexMaster files have rounded, passive tips; the tip diameters range from 0.15 to 0.7 mm for .02 instruments and 0.15

to 0.4 mm for .04 and .06-tapered files. In addition to the standard set, the Intro file is available, which has a .11 taper and a 9-mm cutting part. The instruments are marked with milled rings on the instrument shaft, and the manufacturer provides a system box that indicates sequences for narrow, medium-size, and wide canals.

Several studies indicate that the FlexMaster allows centered preparations in both constricted and wider canals[227] and that it performed on par with other systems.[230,550] Clinical studies confirmed that the FlexMaster showed superior shaping characteristics compared with K-files.[441] Also, novice dental students were able to shape plastic blocks successfully with the FlexMaster after a short training period.[484,485] Tested in a well-described model of simulated canals, FlexMaster instruments led to few aberrations but took longer than preparations with RaCe files.[325] Moreover, FlexMaster appeared to be less effective than RaCe in removing dye from the walls of simulated canals prepared to size #30 but were more effective than ProFile.[446]

RaCe, BioRaCe, BT Race

The RaCe file has been manufactured since 1999 by FKG and was later distributed in the United States by Brasseler (Savannah, GA). The name, which stands for *reamer* with *alternating cutting edges*, describes just one design feature of this instrument. Light microscopic imaging of the file shows flutes and reverse flutes alternating with straight areas; this design is aimed at reducing the tendency of files to thread into a root canal. Cross sections are triangular or square for .02 instruments with size #15 and #20 tips. The lengths of cutting parts vary from 9 to 16 mm.

The surface quality of RaCe instruments has been modified by electropolishing, and the two largest files (size #35, .08 taper and size #40, .10 taper) are also available in stainless steel. The tips are round and noncutting, and the instruments handles are color-coded and marked by and milled rings. RaCe instruments have been marketed in various packages to address small and large canals; recently they are sold as BioRaCe, purportedly to allow larger preparation sizes, with an emphasis on the use of .02 tapered instruments.

Few results of in vitro experiments comparing RaCe to other contemporary rotary systems are available.[443,444] Canals in plastic blocks and in extracted teeth were prepared by the RaCe system with less transportation than with ProTaper files.[443] In another study, ProTaper and RaCe performed similarly when canals were prepared to an apical size #30.[360] When preparing to a size #40, RaCe files prepared canals rapidly and with few aberrations or instrument deformities.[397] The newer BioRaCe instrument sequence utilizes .02 tapered instruments to promote larger apical sizes. As with any rotary system, this is also possible in a hybrid hand-rotary technique. BioRace instruments prepared S-shaped canals in plastic blocks (to size #40) similarly to ProTaper and MTwo but were superior when combined with S-Apex.[62] In a clinical study, Rocas and colleagues found no significant differences between NiTi hand file preparation and BioRace regarding the reduction of bacterial load.[413] A new variant, BT RaCe, has been introduced and incorporates different tip designs, as well as different sequences.

EndoSequence

The EndoSequence rotary instrument is produced by FKG in Switzerland and marketed in the United States by Brasseler. This instrument adheres to the conventional length of the cutting flutes, 16 mm, and to larger tapers, .04 and .06,

to be used in a crown-down approach. The overall design, including the available tapers and cross sections, is thus similar to many other files; however, the manufacturer claims that a unique longitudinal design (called alternating wall contact points [ACP]) reduces torque requirements and keeps the file centered in the canal. It also has varying, comparatively small helical angles. Another feature of the EndoSequence design is an electrochemical treatment after manufacturing, similar to that of RaCe files, resulting in a smooth, polished surface. This is thought to promote better fatigue resistance, hence a rotational speed of 600 rpm is recommended for EndoSequence.[264] Most in vitro results, however, suggest that EndoSequence is not superior to other files in cyclic fatigue resistance.[217,277,401]

Twisted File

In 2008, SybronEndo presented the first fluted NiTi file manufactured by plastic deformation, a process similar to the twisting process that is used to produce stainless steel K-files: the Twisted File (TF). According to the manufacturer, a thermal process allows twisting during a phase transformation into the so-called R-phase of nickel-titanium. The instrument is currently available with a size tip from #25 to #50 and in tapers from .04 to .12.

The unique production process is thought to result in superior physical properties; indeed, early studies suggested significantly better fatigue resistance when size #25 .06 taper Twisted Files were compared to K3 instruments of the same size GTX instrument.[163] Moreover, as determined by bending tests according to the ISO norm for hand instruments, 3630-1, Twisted Files size #25 .06 taper were more flexible than ProFiles of the same size.[162] Others found similar levels for fatigue resistance for TF and Profile of similar size.[277]

A more recent development for TF is the use of an electric motor that allows different file movement, both continuous rotation and reciprocation, depending on the clinical situation (TF Adaptive, SybronEndo).

ProFile Vortex

Profile Vortex files are manufactured from NiTi. Two versions are on the market, one made from M-Wire and another from so-called blue wire (Vortex Blue, which showed greater resistance to cyclic fatigue and increased torque resistance), and they have varying helical angles to counteract the tendency of nonlanded files to thread into the root canal. Vortex instruments are recommended to be used at 500 rpm; higher rotational speed results in less torque generated.[37] Canal preparation with ProFile Vortex in vitro was similar to other rotary instruments.[83,563] Vortex instruments are available in sizes #15 to #50 and in .04 and .06 tapers.

MTwo

This instrument, originally sold in Italy by Sweden e Martina, was put onto the European market in 2004. The instrument has a two-fluted S-shaped cross section. The original strategy allowed for three distinct shaping approaches after the use of a basic sequence with tip sizes from #10 to #25 and tapers ranging from .04 to .06. Subsequent enlargement was meant to create apical sizes up to #40 .04 or, alternatively, to #25 .07 or to larger apical sizes with so-called apical files. MTwo is a well-researched and cutting-efficient instrument; clinically it is an example for the so-called single length technique. Canal shapes with MTwo were similar to other contemporary root canal instruments, either in rotation or reciprocation.[80]

Summary

The market share for rotary files without radial lands continues to expand because of perceived higher efficacy. The overall incidence of clinically relevant preparation errors (details are discussed later) appears to be low, in spite of more aggressive cutting by files without radial lands. Instrument fractures remain a concern, as does the tendency of continuously rotating instruments to thread or pull into the canal, specifically as working length is approached.

Group III, Special Cases

WaveOne, Reciproc

A way to mitigate problems with continuous rotation (e.g., taper lock, fatigue fracture, threading-in) is to return to reciprocation, which had been used decades ago (e.g., in the Giromatic handpiece).[233] A case report[566] described this approach using ProTaper F2 in reciprocation. Based on experiments evaluating the maximal rotational angle before plastic deformation for the selected instrument, a forward angle of 144 degrees followed by a reverse rotation of 72 degrees was recommended.[566] This cycle continues at 400 rpm until working length is reached.

Subsequently two instruments specifically designed for reciprocation were brought to the market: WaveOne (Tulsa Dentsply Dental Specialties) and Reciproc (VDW, currently not available in the United States). WaveOne instruments are available in three tip sizes, #21, #25, and #40, with tapers of .06 and .08, respectively. Corresponding sizes for Reciproc are tips of #25, #40, and #50 with tapers of .08, .06, and .05, respectively. Both instruments feature variable tapers that are largest toward the tips. The main WaveOne cross section is triangular, similar to ProTaper, whereas Reciproc is a two-fluted file with a design similar to MTwo.

Special motors are used for both systems to provide reciprocation action with alternating counterclockwise and clockwise rotations of about 150 to 170 and 30 to 50 degrees, respectively.[151]

Both files are machined with left-leaning flutes; therefore, the cutting direction for both is clockwise. One problem that may occur with this design is the transportation of dentin debris into the apical area, rather than moving debris coronally. There is mixed evidence for this phenomenon[81,124] in vitro. Clinically, frequent careful cleaning of the cutting blades with a moist gauze is recommended.

The shaping ability of these systems, according to current in vitro data, seems similar to that of established systems with continuous rotation.[80,324,537]

Self-Adjusting File

The self-adjusting file (SAF; ReDent-Nova) represents a different approach, both in file design and mode of operation.[327] The file is really a cylindrical, hollow device, designed as a thin-walled NiTi lattice with a lightly abrasive surface (see Fig. 6-26). An initial glide path is established up to a #20 K-file to allow the insertion of the SAF file. The file is proposed to be compressed from its 1.5 mm diameter into dimensions equivalent to those of a #25 K-file. It is operated with a handpiece that generates in-and-out vibrations (4000 per minute) and 0.4 mm amplitudes. As noted, the file is hollow, which allows

for continuous irrigation through the file while operated in the root canal.

In vitro data for this system suggest that indeed more wall contact is made compared to rotary files,[361,382] resulting in better debridement and antimicrobial efficacy.[289,472] Shaping quality is also on par with rotary instruments.[382,537]

Endo-Eze

The Giromatic handpiece (MicroMega), a rotary instrument system in use since 1969, delivers 3000 quarter-turn reciprocating movements per minute. Special rasps and barbed broaches made from stainless steel were most often used in Giromatic handpieces, but K-type and H-type instruments may also be used. The preparation quality with this system was insufficient in curved canals, and the technique fell into disregard.[233]

The Endo-Eze file system (Ultradent, South Jordan, UT) is a more recently introduced addition using a similar motion, provided by special equipment or an original Giromatic handpiece. The set has four engine-driven instruments that are designed to clean the middle third of the canal. The sizes and tapers are #10 and #13, with tapers ranging from 0.02 to 0.04. In this system, the use of stainless steel hand instruments is suggested for the apical third of the canal.

Preparation quality in curved canals appeared to be inferior to NiTi rotaries.[349,358] In straight canals, Endo-EZE performed similar to FlexMaster.[419]

Sonic and Ultrasonic Instruments

An alternative way of instrumenting root canals was introduced when clinicians became able to activate files by electromagnetic ultrasonic energy. Piezoelectric ultrasonic units are also available for this purpose. These units activate an oscillating sinusoidal wave in the file with a frequency of about 30 kHz.

Two types of units, ultrasonic and sonic, are marketed. Ultrasonic devices, which operate at 25 to 30 kHz, include the magnetostrictive Cavi-Endo (Dentsply Caulk, Milford, DE), the piezoelectric ENAC (Osada, Tokyo), the EMS Piezon Master 400 (Electro Medical Systems, Vallée de Joux, Switzerland), and the P5 Neutron (Acteon Satelec, Merignac Cedex, France) (Fig. 6-29). Sonic devices, which operate at 2 to 3 kHz, include the Sonic Air MM 1500 (MicroMega), the Megasonic 1400 (Megasonic Corp, House Springs, MO), and the Endostar (Syntex Dental Products, Valley Forge, PA).

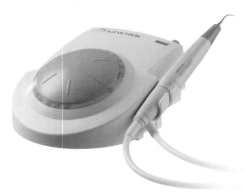

FIG. 6-29 Example of an ultrasonic unit. (Neutron P5 piezoelectric, courtesy Acteon Satelec, Merignac Cedex, France).

Ultrasonic device holders can fit regular types of instrument blanks (e.g., K-files), whereas sonic devices use special inserts known as Rispi-Sonic, Shaper-Sonic, Trio-Sonic, or Heli-Sonic files.

Although similar in function, piezoelectric units have some advantages over the magnetostrictive systems. For example, piezoelectric devices generate little heat, so no cooling is needed for the handpiece. Magnetostrictive systems, however, generate considerable heat, and a special cooling system is needed in addition to the cooling effect provided by root canal irrigation. Working without water-cooling becomes essential when using an operating microscope, because the water spray may obstruct visualization.

The piezoelectric transducer transfers more energy to the file than does the magnetostrictive system, making it more cutting efficient. The file in an ultrasonic device vibrates in a sinus wave–like fashion. A standing wave has areas with maximal displacement (i.e., antinodes) and areas with no displacement (i.e., nodes). The tip of the instrument exhibits an antinode. If powered too high, especially with no contact with the canal wall, the instrument may break because of the intense vibration. Therefore, files must be used only for a short time, must remain passive within the canal, and the power must be controlled carefully. The frequency of breakage in files used for longer than 10 minutes may be as high as 10%, and the breakage normally occurs at the nodes of vibrations.[7] Ultrasonic devices have been linked to a higher incidence of preparation errors and to reduced radicular wall thickness.[298,321,582]

Summary

An abundance of NiTi systems is currently on the market. Table 6-1 lists these instruments systematically and illustrates some of the most relevant properties. Most systems included in Table 6-1 have files with tapers greater than the .02 stipulated by the ISO norm. Differences exist in tip designs, cross sections, and manufacturing processes. In vitro tests have continued to identify the effect of specific designs on shaping capabilities and fracture resistance. A desirable goal is the instrumentation of more canal surface, in an effort to make biofilm more susceptible to subsequent chemical disinfection. At the same time, instrumentation paradigms that conserve more dentin appear desirable to promote long-term function.[172] Meaningful differences in clinical outcomes in regard to various specific design variations have yet to be ascertained.[187,375,443]

Motors

Motors for rotary instruments have become more sophisticated since the simple electric motors of the first generation in the early 1990s (Fig. 6-30, *A*). Electric motors with gear reduction are most suitable for rotary NiTi systems, because they ensure a constant rpm level and constant torque. They can also be programmed to provide alternative rotation patterns, for example, reciprocation with freely selectable angles of rotation.[151] Electric motors often have presets for rpm and torque and are capable of delivering torques much higher than those required to break tips. Some authors think that torque-controlled motors (see Fig. 6-30, *B* to *D*) increase operational safety.[160] Others have suggested that such motors may mainly benefit inexperienced clinicians.[569] These motors probably do not reduce the risk of fracture caused by cyclic fatigue, and even if the torque is below the fracture load at D3, a fracture at a smaller diameter (D2) is still possible.

To complicate matters further, a differential exists between torque at failure at D3 and the working torque needed to operate an instrument effectively (Fig. 6-31 and Box 6-2).[57,374,383,432] In many cases the working torque is greater than the torque required to fracture the instrument's tip.

This differential between working torque and tip fracture load is especially large, with files having a taper equal to or greater than .06; therefore, these files are rather ineffective in

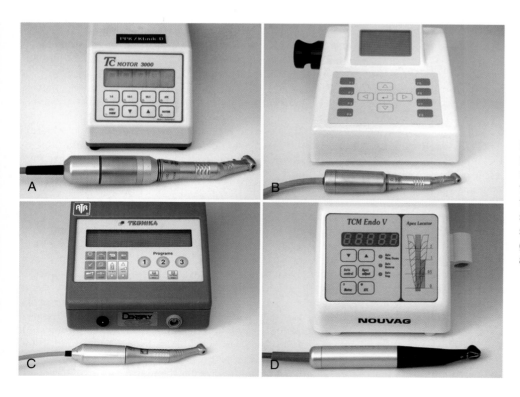

FIG. 6-30 Examples of motors used with rotary nickel-titanium endodontic instruments. **A,** First-generation motor without torque control. **B,** Fully electronically controlled second-generation motor with sensitive torque limiter. **C,** Frequently used simple torque-controlled motor. **D,** Newer-generation motor with built-in apex locator and torque control.

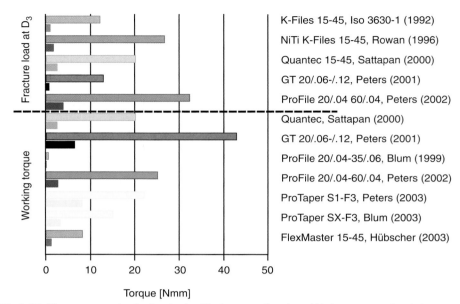

FIG. 6-31 Diagram comparing fracture loads at D_3 *(upper section of graph)* to torques occurring during preparation of root canals *(lower section of graph)*. Filled columns represent the largest file in each set, and open columns show the scores of the most fragile file (see text and Box 6-3 for details).

BOX 6-2

Instrument Breakage with Torsional Load (MacSpadden Factor)

For rotary instrument tips, susceptibility to breakage is governed by the quotient of torque needed to fracture divided by working torque. Simply put, the larger the value, the safer the file.

---

most torque-controlled motors. Future motors will likely offer more microprocessor controlled features—for example, information about the specific instrument being used, such as the presets and the usage history.

Certain motors have built-in apex locators (see Fig. 6-30, *D*). This type of motor may be programmed to stop a rotary instrument when working length is reached or go into reverse gear. Similar changes in movement can occur in an adaptive fashion, depending on the torsional load that the instrument experiences in the root canal. The TF Adaptive motor (SybronEndo) is an example for this technology.

Some of the factors, besides the motor itself, that may influence the incidence of fracture in engine-driven NiTi rotary instruments are lubrication, specific instrument motion, and speed of rotation. It cannot be overemphasized that NiTi rotary instruments should be used only in canals that have been flooded with irrigant. Although lubricants such as RC-Prep (Premier Dental Products Co., Plymouth Meeting, PA) and Glyde (Dentsply Maillefer) have been recommended in the past, their benefit may be restricted to plastic blocks[19] and less relevant when rotary instruments engage dentin surfaces. Moreover, experimental data for dentin suggest that the use of lubricants fails to reduce torque values during simulated canal preparation.[61,376] Finally, because of chemical interactions between NaOCl and ethylenediamine tetra-acetic acid (EDTA),[183] alternating irrigants and using lubricants that

contain EDTA may even be counterproductive. Details in irrigation solution interactions are described later in this chapter.

For instrument motion, some manufacturers recommend a pecking, up-and-down motion. This not only prevents threading in of the file, it is also thought to distribute stresses away from the instrument's point of maximum flexure, where fatigue failure would likely occur.[285,394] However, such in-and-out movements did not significantly enhance the life span of ProFile .04 taper or GT rotary instruments rotated around a 5-mm radius cylinder with a 90-degree curve.[374,379] Furthermore, large variations were noted in the lengths of the fractured segments.[226,530] This suggests that ductile fractures may originate at points of surface imperfections. Files made of more martensitic alloy tend to work better with longer sweeping or brushing strokes. The notion of "brushing" is not directly related to a paintbrush motion, as this would predispose a file to bending and subsequent fatigue.[391] It rather refers to stroking against the wall away from the danger zone, the inner curvature of a curved root.

Rotational speed may influence instrument deformation and fracture. Some studies indicated that ProFile instruments with ISO-norm tip diameters failed more often at higher rotational speed,[131,159] whereas other studies did not find speed to be a factor.[116,252] For Vortex, 300 rpm reduced the generated torque and force; this higher rpm preset did not result in an increase of instrument fractures in vitro.[37]

Clinicians must fully understand the factors that control the forces exerted on continuously rotating NiTi instruments (Box 6-3). To minimize the risk of fracture and prevent taper lock, motor-driven rotary instruments should not be forced in an apical direction. Similarly, acute apical curves limit the use of instruments with higher tapers because of the risk of cyclic fatigue. The incidence of instrument fracture can be reduced to an absolute minimum if clinicians use data from well-designed torque and stress studies. Adequate procedural strategies, such as an adequate glide path, a detailed knowledge of anatomic structures, with avoidance of extreme canal

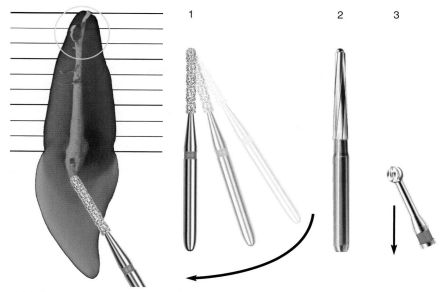

FIG. 6-32 Sequence of instruments used for optimal preparation of an access cavity (e.g., in an incisor). A parallel-sided diamond or steel bur is used to remove overlying enamel in a 90-degree angle toward the enamel surface *(1)*. The bur is then tilted vertically to allow straight-line access to the root canal *(arrow)*. A bur with a noncutting tip (e.g., Endo-Z bur or ball-tipped diamond bur) is then used to refine access *(2)*. Overhangs or pulp horns filled with soft tissue are finally cleared with a round bur used in a brushing or pulling motion *(3)*.

BOX 6-3

Factors Governing the Potential for Nickel-Titanium Rotary Instrument Fractures

- Clinician's handling (most important)
- Combination of torsional load, bending, and axial fatigue
- Root canal anatomy
- Manufacturing process and quality

---

configurations, and specific instrumentation sequences may also improve shaping results.

Certain procedures have evolved for removing fractured instruments from root canals (see Fig. 6-25); these are discussed in detail elsewhere in this book (see Chapters 8 and 19). Most of those methods require the use of additional equipment, such as a dental operating microscope and ultrasonic units. However, the best way to deal with instrument fracture is prevention. An understanding of the anatomy of the root canal system, together with a clear plan for selecting, sequencing, and using shaping instruments, can certainly help prevent procedural mishaps.

STEPS OF CLEANING AND SHAPING

Access: Principles

Access cavity preparation is essential for root canal treatment and is described in detail elsewhere in this book (Chapter 5). It should be emphasized at this point that mishaps during access (e.g., perforation) significantly affect the long-term outcome of a root canal treated tooth. Overenlargement or gouging during access significantly reduces structural strength[402] and may lead to root fracture and nonrestorable conditions.

Rationally, the use of a cylindrical diamond bur, followed by a tapered fluted bur with noncutting tip and perhaps a small round bur, is recommended (Fig. 6-32). One experiment suggested that more conservative access cavities, in particular in premolars, may increase fracture resistance and permit similar shaping outcomes.[270] The use of ultrasonically powered tips under magnification is aimed at achieving ideal access cavities (Fig. 6-33), including discovery and perhaps relocation of the canal orifices.

Coronal Preflaring

The extension of an access cavity into the coronal-most portion of the root canal is called *coronal flaring*. If a canal is constricted, mineralized, or difficult to access, flaring the coronal portion prior to any deep entry into the root canal is beneficial. This canal modification should be preceded by a scouting step, in which a small (e.g., size #10) K-file is passively placed several millimeters into the root canal. Tools for preflaring include Gates Gliddens (Fig. 6-34) and dedicated NiTi instruments (Fig. 6-35). Both step-back and step-down sequences have been recommended for Gates Gliddens, whereas NiTi rotaries are typically used in a crown-down sequence. More recently, specific orifice shaping rotaries have been developed that are used as a single instrument, rather than a sequence.

The use of laterally cutting NiTi rotaries allows the clinician to modify the root canal orifice to form a receptacle for subsequent instrumentation. This is related to removal of coronal mineralization and to relocation of the canal pathway by removal of dentin overhangs. For example, a second mesiobuccal canal typically exits the pulp chamber toward the mesial under a dentin shelf and then curves toward the distal. It is this curve in a small canal that often leads to formation of a ledge, which in turn prevents shaping to length.

Preenlargement of the coronal half to two thirds of a root canal allows files unimpeded access to the apical one third and

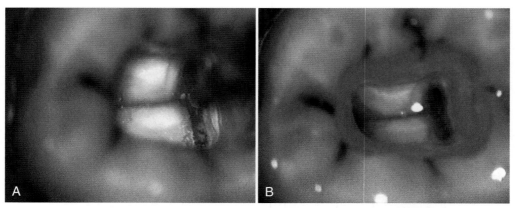

FIG. 6-33 Clinical views of an access cavity in a mandibular molar. **A,** As seen through an operating microscope (×20). **B,** Modification with an ultrasonically activated tip.

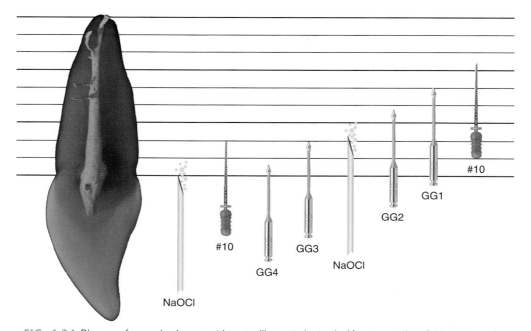

FIG. 6-34 Diagram of coronal enlargement in a maxillary anterior tooth. After preparation of the access cavity (see Fig. 6-32) and copious irrigation, Gates-Glidden burs are used in a step-down manner to enlarge the orifice and provide straight-line access into the middle third of the canal. Precurved size #10 K-files are used to explore the canal path and dimension.

gives the clinician better tactile control in directing small, adequately precurved negotiating files (Fig. 6-36).

One of the purported benefits of early coronal flaring is access of disinfecting irrigation solutions, but this has not been confirmed in experiments. On the other hand, a documented benefit of coronal flaring is mitigation of working length changes during canal preparation.[496]

Comparatively little is known about the efficacy of individual flaring instruments. One study compared the cutting efficacy of radial-landed and triangular cross sections.[338,380] The latter were shown to be more cutting efficient compared to radial-landed design; somewhat surprisingly, flexible martensitic alloy was cutting more rapidly compared to conventional NiTi alloys.

Patency File

A *patency file* is a small K-file (usually a size #10 or #15) that is passively extended slightly beyond the apical foramen. The use of a patency file has been suggested for most rotary techniques. This step is thought to remove accumulated debris, to help maintain working length, and to translate into greater clinical success.[345] One concern with the patency file was that instead of having a cleaning effect, the file would push contaminated debris through the foramen. However, an in vitro study suggested that the risk of inoculation was minimal when canals were filled with NaOCl.[243] Maintaining patency throughout an endodontic procedure does not lead to an increase in posttreatment symptoms.[22] Only initial clinical evidence exists favoring the use of a patency file; however, experience suggests

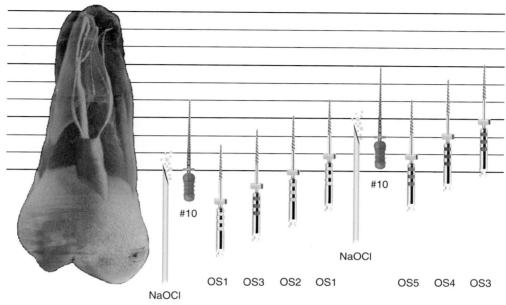

FIG. 6-35 Diagram of coronal enlargement in a more complicated maxillary posterior tooth. This maxillary molar presents several difficulties, including a narrow mesiobuccal canal that exits the pulp cavity at an angle. A possible approach in a case involving difficult entry into the root canal system is to use a small orifice shaper (OS1) after ensuring a coronal glide path with a K-file. Use of a sequence of orifice shapers (OS3 to OS1) then allows penetration into the middle third of the root canal. Wider canals can accept a second sequence of orifice shapers. Copious irrigation and securing a glide path with a size #10 K-file are prerequisites for use of NiTi rotary instruments.

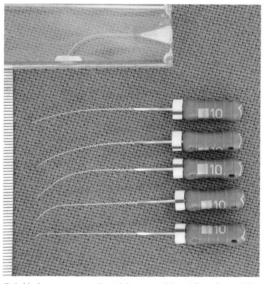

FIG. 6-36 Various precurved, stainless steel hand files for pathfinding and gauging. Compare the curves in the instruments to the ones in a plastic training block (gradation of ruler is 0.5 mm).

that this technique involves relatively little risk and provides some benefit as long as small files are used carefully.

Working Length Determination

Devices

Radiographs, tactile sensation, the presence of moisture on paper points, and knowledge of root morphology have been used to determine the length of root canal systems. Following earlier experiments by Custer,[110] Sunada developed the first commercialized electronic apex locator,[501] suggesting that the apical foramen could be localized using a direct electric current. Currently, the electronic apex locator is considered an accurate tool for determining working length.[153] One study reported that the use of electronic apex locators in a dental student clinic resulted in a higher quality of obturation length control and an overall reduction in the number of radiographs taken.[152] However, these devices must not be considered flawless, because several variables are known to affect their accuracy. For example, immature roots can present problems.[234] Once roots mature (i.e., form a narrow apical foramen) and instruments are able to contact the canal walls, an electronic apex locator's accuracy greatly improves. Some investigators have found no statistical difference between roots with vital and necrotic tissue.[175,319] Because apical root resorption is prevalent in necrotic cases with longstanding apical lesions,[541] it may be concluded that apical resorption does not have a significant effect on the accuracy of electronic apex locators.

Some clinicians have advocated the use of the electronically determined working length in lieu of working length estimations using the placement of a file in the canal and a radiograph. However, combined use of both of these techniques has been shown to result in greater accuracy.[136] Furthermore, radiographs may add essential anatomic information that could be missed if electronic apex locators are used exclusively.

The first two generations of electronic apex locators were sensitive to the contents of the canal and irrigants used during treatment. The development of an algorithm called the *ratio measurement method* distinguished the third generation of apex locators.[263] To arrive at this method, the impedance of the canal was measured with two current sources of different frequencies, and a quotient was determined using the electrical potentials proportional to each impedance.[263] This study found that

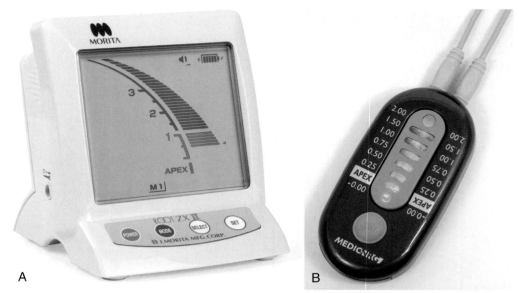

FIG. 6-37 A, Root ZX apex locator with lip clip and file holder. **B,** NRG miniature electronic apex locator. (*A,* Courtesy J Morita, Irvine, CA. *B,* Courtesy MedicNRG, Kibutz Afikim, Israel.)

electrolytes did not have a significant effect on the accuracy of the unit. This means that clinically canal contents need not be dried, but fluids in contact with crowns or coronal metallic restoration materials could conduct currents and lead to false results.

Some third-generation apex locators are the Endex Plus, or Apit (Osada, Los Angeles, CA), the Root ZX (J. Morita, Kyoto, Japan),[153,276] and the Neosono Ultima EZ (Acteon Satelec). The Endex Plus device uses 1 and 5 kHz and provides apex location based on subtraction. The Root ZX emits currents at frequencies of 8 and 0.4 kHz and provides apex location based on the resulting quotient. In addition to latest model apex locators, manufacturers have developed smaller models (Fig. 6-37, *B*).

Apex locators are generally safe to use; however, manufacturers' instructions state that they should not be used on patients with pacemakers without consulting the patient's cardiologist. However, when connected directly to cardiac pacemakers in vitro, electronic apex locators did not interfere with the function of the pacemaker,[165] and they did not interfere with the functioning of any of the cardiac devices tested in a clinical study under electrocardiogram monitoring.[556]

Strategies

Anatomic studies and clinical experience suggest that typically teeth are 19 to 25 mm long. Most clinical crowns are approximately 10 mm long, and most roots range from 9 to 15 mm in length. Roots, therefore, can be divided into thirds that are 3 to 5 mm long. An important issue in root canal treatment is the apical end point of the prepared shape in relation to the apical anatomy. Traditional treatment has held that canal preparation and subsequent obturation should terminate at the *apical constriction,* the narrowest diameter of the canal (Fig. 6-38). This point is thought to coincide with the cementodentinal junction (CDJ) (see Chapter 12) and is based on histologic sections and ground specimens. However, the position and anatomy of the CDJ vary considerably from tooth to tooth, from root to root, and from wall to wall in each canal.

Moreover, the CDJ cannot be located precisely on radiographs. For this reason, some have advocated terminating the preparation in necrotic cases at 0.5 to 1 mm short of the radiographic apex and 1 to 2 mm short[206,407,562] in cases involving irreversible pulpitis. Although there is no definitive validation for this strategy at present,[435] well-controlled follow-up studies seem to support it.[476,478]

Working to shorter lengths may lead to the accumulation and retention of debris, which in turn may result in apical blockage (Fig. 6-39). If the path to the apex is blocked, working to short lengths may contribute to procedural errors such as apical perforations and fractured instruments. Such obstacles (which consist of collagen fibers, dentin mud, and, most important, residual microbes) in apical canal areas are a major cause of persistent or recurrent apical periodontitis,[196,342,466] or *post-treatment disease*[156,559] (also see Chapters 14 and 15).

Using an electronic apex locator has helped clinicians identify the position of apical foramina more accurately and allow safe canal shaping as close as 0.5 mm to the canal terminus.

Canal Enlargement/Preparation

Rationale

Like the position of the apical constriction, apical diameters are difficult to assess clinically.[274] Some have recommended gauging canal diameters by passing a series of fine files apically until one fits snugly. However, such an approach is likely to result in underestimation of the diameter.[555] This is a crucial point because the initial canal size is a major determinant for the desired final apical diameter.

An ongoing debate exists between those who prefer smaller apical preparations combined with tapered shapes and those who favor larger apical preparations for better removal of infected dentin and to allow irrigation fluids access to the apical areas (Table 6-2). Both sides stress the importance of maintaining the original path of the canal during preparation; otherwise, bacteria in the apical one-third of the root canal may not be reached by sufficient amounts of an antimicrobial agent.[335] Investigators demonstrated a higher percentage of

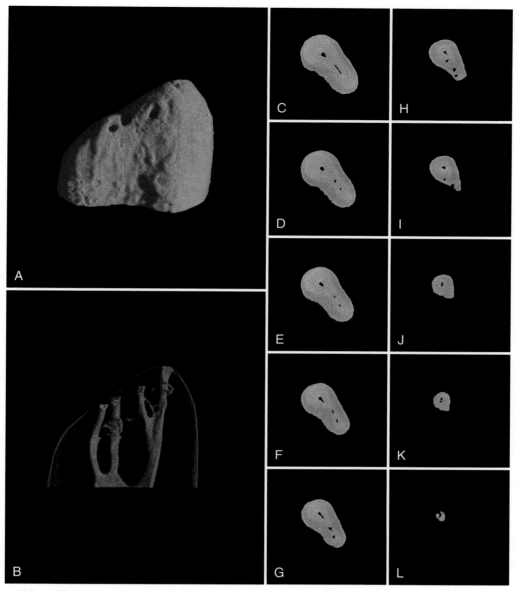

FIG. 6-38 Microcomputed tomographic scan of anatomy of the apical 5 mm of a mesiobuccal root (8 μm resolution). A-B, Three-dimensional reconstruction of outer contour and root canal systems. C-L, Cross sections of root at 0.5 mm apart.

TABLE 6-2

Characteristics of Wide and Narrow Apical Preparations

Root Canal Preparation	Benefits	Drawbacks
Narrow apical size	Minimal risk of canal transportation and extrusion of irrigants or filling material Can be combined with tapered preparation to counteract some drawbacks Less compaction of hard tissue debris in canal spaces	Little removal of infected dentin Questionable rinsing effect in apical areas during irrigation Possibly compromised disinfection during interappointment medication Not ideal for lateral compaction
Wide apical size	Removal of infected dentin Access of irrigants and medications to apical third of root canal	Risk of preparation errors and extrusion of irrigants and filling material Not ideal for thermoplastic obturation

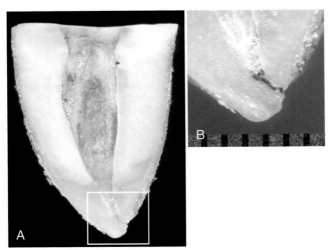

FIG. 6-39 Presence of dentin dust as a possible source of microbial irritation. Tooth #18 underwent root canal therapy. The clinician noted an apical blockage but was unable to bypass it. Unfortunately, intense pain persisted and at the patient's request, the tooth was extracted a week later. **A,** Mesial root of tooth #18; mesial dentin has been removed. **B,** Magnified view (×125) of rectangle in **A** shows an apical block (gradation of ruler is 0.5 mm).

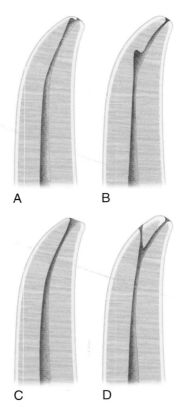

FIG. 6-40 Schematic diagrams showing the most common preparation errors. **A,** Apical zip. **B,** Ledge. **C,** Apical zip with perforation. **D,** Ledge with perforation.

bacterial elimination in single-root canal systems by using a combination of significant enlargement of the apical third and NaOCl irrigation.[89] Preparation errors (e.g., zips, canal transportation) may occur in larger preparations, with both stainless steel and NiTi instruments (Fig. 6-40).

Thorough disinfection of the apical part of a root canal is essential, because this area is most likely to harbor residual intraradicular bacteria.[343] Wider apical preparations remove potentially infected dentin, allowing the delivering needle and subsequently the antimicrobial irrigant to penetrate the root canal more deeply.[101,147]

A study investigating rotary NiTi files of three tapers (.06, .08, and .10) with file tips in sizes #20, #30, and #40 showed that size #20 instruments left significantly more debris in the apical third compared with size #40 instruments.[532] On the other hand, a study in which half the samples were prepared to a size #25 file and the other half to a size #40 file found no statistically significant difference in bacterial growth after instrumentation, with no growth observed after 1 week of treatment with a Ca(OH)$_2$ dressing.[570] Step-down sequences with additional apical enlargement to ISO size #35 and a serial step-back technique with no apical enlargement were compared, using NaOCl and EDTA as irrigants. Here, no significant difference was detected in colony-forming units with or without apical enlargement.[105] These researchers concluded that dentin removal in the apical third might be unnecessary if a suitable coronal taper is achieved.

Despite the disagreement over the appropriate width of a preparation (see Table 6-2), these studies suggest that root canal preparations should be confined to the canal space, should be sufficiently wide, and should incorporate the original root canal cross sections (see Fig. 6-4).

Traditional cleaning and shaping strategies (e.g., the step-back technique) focused immediate preparation of the apical third of the root canal system, followed by various flaring techniques to facilitate obturation.[180,436,518] In an attempt to reach the canal terminus, the clinician first selected a small file,

placed an appropriate curve on the instrument, and then tried to work the file to full length. If the terminus could not be reached, the file was removed and, after irrigation, either the same file or a smaller one was inserted. However, not infrequently, full length was not obtained, either because of blockage or because of coronal binding.

Coronal binding is caused by overhangs at the orifice level and when the canal is less tapered than an instrument, making it bind coronally. Moreover, a straight root often contains a curved canal, such as buccal and lingual curvatures that cannot be seen on radiographs.[109,389] In addition, passing a precurved negotiating file through a coronally tight canal will straighten the instrument.[487]

Various instrumentation sequences have been developed for hand and rotary instruments; these are discussed later in this chapter. However, the shape of the access cavity is *the* prerequisite that must be optimized before any canal preparation can take place (see Chapter 5).

As stated previously, preparation of an adequate access cavity (see Fig. 6-32) may involve the use of a cylindrical diamond or fissure bur, a safety-ended drill for additional enlargement, and round burs to remove overhangs on outward strokes. The access cavity shape must allow instruments unimpeded access to the middle third of the root canal system. Ultrasonically powered instruments used under an operating microscope greatly facilitate removal of mesial dentin shelves in mandibular molars (see Fig. 6-33, *A* and *B*) and other teeth. Preexisting restorations allow for ideal access cavities that serve as reservoirs of irrigants (see Fig. 6-33, *C*).

Basic cleaning and shaping strategies for root canal preparation can be categorized as crown-down, step-back, apical widening, and hybrid techniques. In a crown-down approach, the clinician passively inserts a large instrument into the canal up to a depth that allows easy progress. The next smaller instrument is then used to progress deeper into the canal; the third instrument follows deeper again, and this process continues until the terminus is reached. Both hand and rotary instruments may be used in a crown-down manner. However, instrument sets with various tip diameters and tapers allow the use of either decreasing tapers or decreasing diameters for apical progress. Debate continues as to which of those strategies is superior for avoiding taper lock; currently, no compelling evidence favors either of them.

In the step-back approach, working lengths decrease in a stepwise manner with increasing instrument size. This prevents less flexible instruments from creating ledges in apical curves while producing a taper for ease of obturation.

As discussed previously, the aim of apical widening is to fully prepare apical canal areas for optimal irrigation efficacy and overall antimicrobial activity. Apical enlargement has been broken down into three phases: preenlargement, apical enlargement, and apical finishing.[545]

Most rotary techniques require a crown-down approach to minimize torsional loads,[57] and they reduce the risk of instrument fracture. Used sequentially, the crown-down technique can help enlarge canals further. All basic techniques described so far may be combined into a hybrid technique to eliminate or reduce the shortcomings of individual instruments.

Root canal preparation can be broken down into a series of steps that parallel the insertion depths of individual instruments. Anatomic studies and clinical experience suggest that most teeth are 19 to 25 mm long. Most clinical crowns are approximately 10 mm long, and most roots range from 9 to 15 mm in length. Roots, therefore, can be divided into thirds that are 3 to 5 mm long.

Provided adequate tools are used and the access cavity design is appropriate, excessive thinning of radicular structures can be avoided (see Fig. 6-5). Vertical root fractures and perforations are possible outcomes of excessive removal of radicular dentin in zones that have been termed *danger zones*.[15] Overenthusiastic filing, for example, may lead to more procedural errors (see Figs. 6-22 and 6-40). On the other hand, ideal preparation forms without any preparation errors and with circular incorporation of the original canal cross sections may be achieved with suitable techniques (see Fig. 6-4).

Dedicated NiTi instruments have been introduced or suggested for coronal preenlargement, such as the ProFile orifice shapers, GT accessory files, the ProTaper SX, the FlexMaster Intro file, and the size #40, .10 taper or size #35, .08 taper RaCe files. These instruments are better suited than GGs and safer for more difficult cases (see Figs. 6-34 and 6-35).

Techniques
Standardized Technique
The standardized technique adopts the same working length definition for all instruments introduced into a root canal. It therefore relies on the inherent shape of the instruments to impart the final shape to the canal. Negotiation of fine canals is initiated with lubricated fine files in a so-called watch-winding movement. These files are advanced to working length and worked either in the same hand movement or with

"quarter-turn-and-pull" until a next larger instrument may be used. Conceptually, the final shape should be predicted by the last instrument used (Fig. 6-41). A single matching gutta-percha point may then be used for root canal filling. In reality, this concept is often violated: curved canals shaped with the standardized technique will be wider than the last used instrument,[14] exacerbated by the pulling portion of the hand movement. Moreover, adequate compaction of gutta-percha in such small a taper (~.02) is difficult or impossible[13] (see Chapter 7).

The standardized technique was hampered by the very standardization of the instruments used to perform the technique. Specifically, the similar size increment by 0.05 mm up to size 55 was clinically more difficult to achieve moving from size #10 to size #15, compared to the step from size #40 to #45. In very small files (sizes #6 to #10), the problem is partly resolved by several key points: (1) apical dimensions are such that a size #6 file does not significantly remove dentin other than in severely calcified cases; (2) a size #8 file taken 0.5 to 1 mm long to establish patency (discussed later in the chapter) contacts the desired end point of the preparation with a diameter approaching the tip size of a #10 file; (3) similarly, placing a size #10 file just minutely through the foramen eases the way for passive insertion of the subsequent #15 file to full length.[417]

Step-Back Technique
Realizing the importance of a shape larger than that produced with the standardized approach, one investigator suggested the step-back technique,[552] incorporating a stepwise reduction of the working length for larger files, typically in 1-mm or 0.5-mm steps, resulting in flared shapes with 0.05 and 0.10 taper, respectively (Fig. 6-42). Incrementally reducing the working length when using larger and stiffer instruments also reduced the incidence of preparation errors, in particular in curved canals. This concept appeared to be clinically very effective.[339]

Although the step-back technique was primarily designed to avoid preparation errors in curved canals, it applies to the preparation of apparently[109,439] straight canals as well. Several modifications of the step-back technique have been described over the years. Another investigator advocated the insertion of progressively larger hand instruments as deep as they would passively go in order to explore and provide some enlargement prior to reaching the working length.[518]

Step-Down Technique
Other investigators described a different approach.[174] They advocated shaping the coronal aspect of a root canal first, before apical instrumentation commenced. This technique is intended to minimize or eliminate the amount of necrotic debris that could be extruded through the apical foramen during instrumentation.[146] Moreover, by first flaring the coronal two thirds of the canal, apical instruments are unimpeded through most of their length. This in turn may facilitate greater control and less chance of zipping near the apical constriction.[280]

Crown-Down Technique
Numerous modifications of the original step-down technique have been introduced, including the description of the crown-down technique.[150,317,433] The more typical step-down technique includes the use of a stainless steel K-file exploring the apical constriction and establishing working length. In

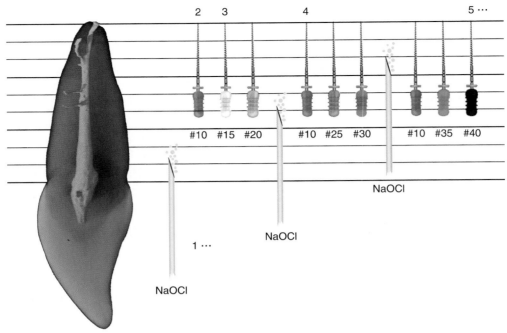

FIG. 6-41 Root canal instrumentation with hand files: Part I. After the orifice has been accessed and copious irrigation performed *(1)*, the working length (WL) is determined. A size #10 or #15 K-file is advanced to the desired apical preparation end point, aided by an electronic apex locator *(2)*. The apical canal areas are then enlarged with K-files *(3)* used in the balanced force technique (see Fig. 9-43). Frequent, copious irrigation with sodium hypochlorite is mandatory to support antimicrobial therapy. Frequent recapitulation with fine K-files is recommended to prevent blockage *(4)*. Apical enlargement is complete to the desired master apical file (MAF) size *(5)*, which depends on pretreatment canal sizes and individual strategy. Typically, size #40 or larger may be reached in anterior teeth, as in this example. File sizes larger than #20 may be used with NiTi instruments (e.g., NiTiFlex).

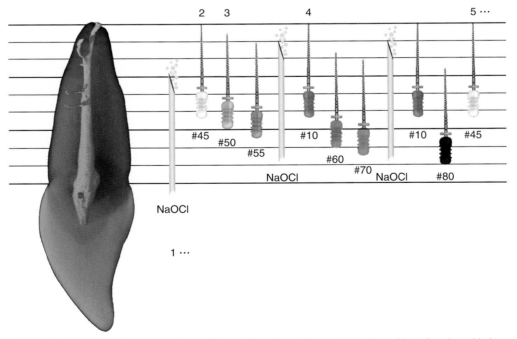

FIG. 6-42 Root canal instrumentation with hand files: Part II. Frequent irrigation with sodium hypochlorite *(1)* is more efficient after the working length (WL) is reached, because irrigation needles may penetrate deeper into the canal. Canal taper is increased to further improve antimicrobial efficiency and to simplify subsequent obturation. Hand instruments are set to decreasing working length in 0.5 mm increments (step-back) from the master apical file (MAF) *(2 and 3)*. A fine K-file is used to recapitulate to WL during the procedure *(4),* and the MAF is used as a final recapitulation *(5)* to ensure that remaining dentin chips have been removed.

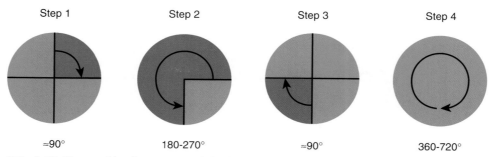

Step 1   Step 2   Step 3   Step 4

≈90°   180-270°   ≈90°   360-720°

FIG. 6-43 Diagram of handle movements during balanced force hand preparation. **Step 1:** After pressureless insertion of a Flex-R or NiTiFlex K-file, the instrument is rotated clockwise 90 degrees, using only light apical pressure. **Step 2:** The instrument is rotated counterclockwise 180 to 270 degrees; sufficient apical pressure is used to keep the file at the same insertion depth during this step. Dentin shavings are removed with a characteristic clicking sound. **Step 3:** This step is similar to step 1 and advances the instrument more apically. **Step 4:** After two or three cycles, the file is loaded with dentin shavings and is removed from the canal with a prolonged clockwise rotation.

contrast, a crown-down technique relies more on coronal flaring and then determination of the working length later in the procedure.

To ensure penetration during step-down, one may have to enlarge the coronal third of the canal with progressively smaller GG drills or with other rotary instruments. Irrigation should follow the use of each instrument and recapitulation after every other instrument. To properly enlarge the apical third and to round out ovoid shape and lateral canal orifices, a reverse order of instruments may be used starting with a size #20 (for example) and enlarging this region to a size #40 or #50 (for example). The tapered shape can be improved by stepping back up the canal with larger instruments, bearing in mind all the time the importance of irrigation and recapitulation.

The more typical crown-down, or double-flare, technique[150] consisted of an exploratory action with a small file, a crown-down portion with K-files of descending sizes, and an apical enlargement to size #40 or similar. The original technique included stepping back in 1-mm increments with ascending file sizes and frequent recapitulations with a small K-file and copious irrigation. It is further emphasized that significant wall contact should be avoided in the crown-down phase to reduce hydrostatic pressure and the possibility of blockage. Several studies demonstrated more centered preparations in teeth with curved root canals shaped with a modified double-flare technique and Flex-R files compared to shapes prepared with K-files and step-back technique.[434,433] A double-flare technique was also suggested for ProFile rotary instruments.[447]

Balanced Force Technique

Regarding hand movements, a general agreement exists that the so-called balanced force technique creates the least canal aberrations with K-files. This technique has been described as a series of rotational movements for Flex-R files,[412] but it can also be used for K-files and other hand instruments such as GT hand files. Many explanations have been offered for the obvious and undisputed efficacy of the balanced force approach,[94,275,439] but general agreement exists that it provides excellent canal-centering ability, superior to other techniques with hand instruments.[30,71,283]

The balanced force technique involves three principle steps.[412] The first step (after passive insertion of an instrument into the canal) is a clockwise rotation of about 90 degrees to

engage dentin (Fig. 6-43). In the second step, the instrument is held in the canal with adequate axial force and rotated counterclockwise to break loose the engaged dentin chips from the canal wall; this produces a characteristic clicking sound. Classically, in the third step, the file is removed with a clockwise rotation to be cleaned; however, because files used with the balanced force technique are not precurved, every linear outward stroke essentially is a filing stroke and may lead to some straightening of the canal path. Therefore, in many cases, the clinician may advance farther apically rather than withdrawing the file, depending on the grade of difficulty.

Rotary Instrumentation

NiTi rotary instruments are an invaluable adjunct in the preparation of root canals, although hand instruments may be able to enlarge some canals just as efficiently when used in appropriate sequences. Hand instruments should be used only after coronal preenlargement (e.g., with GG drills). After preenlargement, the access cavity and canals are flooded with irrigant, and a precurved scouting file is advanced into the canal. A lubricant when using hand instruments can help prevent apical blockage in this early stage. Once the working length has been established (aided by an electronic apex locator and radiographically verified), apical preparation to begins to facilitate a glide path for subsequent rotary instrumentation (Fig. 6-44).

The term *glide path* has been used in endodontics since the early 2000s[384] and relates to securing an open pathway to the canal terminus that subsequent engine-driven instruments can follow. The typical minimum glide path is a size #15 to #20 K-file and should be confirmed with a straight, not precurved file. Various small engine-driven instruments were introduced to simplify this process, such as Pathfiles (Dentsply Maillefer),[53] Scout RaCe (FKG Dentaire SA, La Chaux-de-Fonds Switzerland),[344] and G-file (MicroMega).[112] Copious irrigation and frequent recapitulations with a smaller file to working length may be required, and in some instances, clinicians must devise creative strategies using small crown-down or step-back sequences.

Fig. 6-45 illustrates the development of two different shapes in the mesial root canals of a mandibular molar, clearly showing that substantial areas of the root canal surface in either case are not instrumented, even when apical size #50 or 0.09 taper are reached (see the red areas in Fig. 6-45, *G* and *I*).

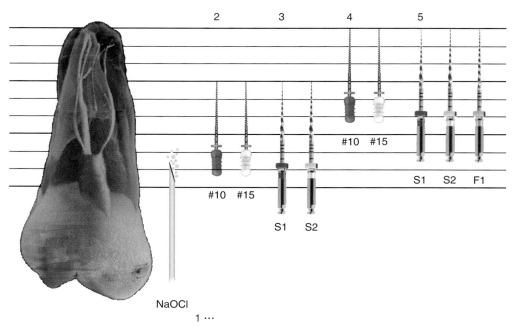

FIG. 6-44 Instrumentation of root canals with ProTaper instruments. After irrigation and scouting (*1* and *2*), the coronal thirds are enlarged with shaping files S1 and S2. Hand files then are used to determine the WL and to secure a glide path. Apical preparation is completed with S1 and S2. Finishing files are used to the desired apical width.

Specific NiTi Instrumentation Techniques
Crown Down
This was the dominant approach for many years and is still being used, for example, for ProFile and several others (ProFile Vortex, HERO 642, K3, and FlexMaster). It must be noted that the manufacturers' instructions for these systems vary somewhat, and the instructions for GT rotary, RaCe, and the Twisted File vary even more. Clinicians should always read the manufacturers' instructions for details on working with those instruments.

Working length is determined after any coronal preenlargement , and an open glide path is secured with K-files up to size #15 or #20, depending on the canal anatomy. If canal size permits, canal preparation begins with .06 taper instruments in descending tip diameters.[57] In more difficult small canals, .06 tapers are followed by .04-tapered instruments, also with descending tip diameters. Apical preparation is performed either with multiple shaping waves, as suggested for GT rotary files,[76] or in a step-back manner.[445] Recapitulation with a small hand file is recommended throughout the preparation.

Single Length
The approach for ProTaper Universal and ProTaper Next instruments differs from that for many other NiTi rotary files (except MTwo, WaveOne and Reciproc) in that no traditional crown-down procedure is performed (see Fig. 6-44).

Size #10 and #15 hand files are passively inserted into the coronal two thirds of a root canal as path-finding files, which confirm the presence of a smooth, reproducible glide path. This step is essential for ProTaper shaping instruments, because they are mostly side cutters and have fine, fragile tips.

Shaping files S1 and S2 are then passively inserted into the scouted canal spaces, which have been filled with irrigant (preferably NaOCl). If necessary, the SX file can be used at this stage to relocate orifices or remove obstructing dentin. After each shaping file is used, the canals are reirrigated, and a size #10 file is used to recapitulate to break up debris and move it into solution. This process is repeated until the depth of the path-finding #10 or #15 file is reached.

After irrigation, the apical third is fully negotiated and enlarged to at least a size #15 K-file, and the working length is confirmed (see Fig. 6-44). Depending on the canal anatomy, the rest of the apical preparation can be done with engine-driven ProTaper shaping and finishing hand files. As an alternative, handles can be placed on these instruments so that they can be used for the balanced force technique.

ProTapers S1 and S2 are then carried to the full working length, still in a floating, brushing motion. The working length should be confirmed after irrigation and recapitulation with a K-file, aided by an electronic apex locator or radiographs. Because of the progressive taper and more actively cutting flutes higher up in the ProTaper design, interferences in the middle and coronal thirds are removed at this stage.

The preparation is finished with one or more of the ProTaper finishing files, used in a nonbrushing manner; because of their decreasing taper, these files will reach the working length passively. Recapitulation and irrigation conclude the procedures (see Fig. 6-44).

LightSpeed Technique
Since the introduction of LightSpeed instruments, the manufacturer's guidelines have changed. This section presents a version used for the original LightSpeed rather than the LS variant (Fig. 6-46).

After access and coronal preenlargement with the instrument of choice, working lengths are obtained, and apical enlargement is done with at least a loose-fitting size #15 K-file. LSX instruments are then slowly advanced to working length

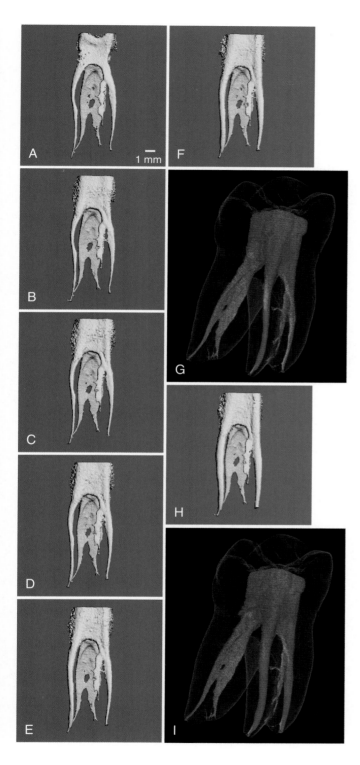

1 mm

FIG. 6-45 Stepwise enlargement of mesial root canal systems in an extracted mandibular molar demonstrated with microcomputed tomography (μCT) reconstructions. The buccal canal *(left)* was prepared with a Light-Speed (LS) instrument, and the lingual canal *(right)* was shaped with a ProTaper (PT) instrument. **A,** Pretreatment view from the mesial aspect. Note the additional middle canal branching from the lingual canal into the coronal third. **B,** Initial preparation and opening of the orifices, aided by ultrasonically powered instruments. **C,** First step of root canal preparation, up to LightSpeed size #20 and ProTaper shaping file S1. **D,** Further enlargement to LS size #30 and PT shaping file S2. **E,** Apical preparation to LS size #40 and PT finishing file F1. **F,** Additional enlargement to LS size #50 and PT finishing file F2. **G,** Superimposed μCT reconstructions comparing the initial canal geometry *(in green)* with the shape reached after use of the instruments shown in **F. H,** Final shape after step-back with LS instruments and PT finishing file F3. **I,** Superimposed μCT reconstructions comparing initial geometry and final shape. Note the slight ledge in the buccal canal after LS preparation and some straightening in the lingual canal after PT preparation.

All LightSpeed instruments are used in the following way: a slow, continuous apical movement is used until the blade binds; after a momentary pause, the blade is advanced further with intermittent ("pecking") motions.

Technique with the Self-Adjusting File

For this unusual file, a coronal flaring step—for example, with a G—precedes exploration with small K-files, including verification of patency and determining of working length. A glide path to a size #20 is considered appropriate; then the selected self-adjusting file is introduced into the canal with continuous irrigation through the center of the hollow file at a rate of approximately 5 ml/min. This maintains a continuous flow of active irrigant that carries with its outflow tissue debris and the dentin mud generated by the file. One file is used throughout the procedure. It is initially compressed into the root canal and gradually enlarges while cleaning and shaping the canal.

The file can rotate passively around its long axis and is guided by the operator to working length. The file is initially compressed into the root canal and gradually enlarges while cleaning and shaping the canal. The suggested time frame of instrumentation per canal dictates the final size and is approximately 3 to 4 minutes.[60] Obturation may commence with various techniques that allow plastifying gutta-percha (see Chapter 7).

Hybrid Techniques

For some time, combining various NiTi preparation systems have been suggested[89,545] to address certain shortcomings of current instruments (Box 6-4). Although many combinations are possible, the most popular and useful ones involve coronal preenlargement followed by different additional apical preparation sequences. However, clinicians must keep in mind that anatomic variations in each canal must be addressed individually with specific instrument sequences. Most important, oval canals extend deep into the apical area,[505,551,560] and apical foramina may in fact be oval in most cases.[70] Naturally, a rotating file can produce a round canal at best (Fig. 6-47); therefore, a strategy must be devised for adequately shaping oval canals without overly weakening radicular structure (compare Figs. 6-4 and 6-5). One hybrid approach completely prepared 95%

while registering tactile feedback. The first instrument that experiences resistance 4 mm short of working length is the final apical size; it is then advanced to working length like the smaller instruments before. The next larger instrument is placed to 4 mm short of working length. This prepares the apical 5 mm for a matching SimpliFill obturator (SybronEndo). Midroot shaping is then accomplished with sequentially larger LSX instruments. Finally, the so-called master apical rotary, or MAR, is used to recapitulate to the working length.

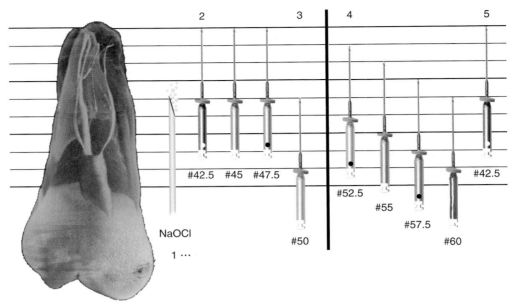

FIG. 6-46 Finishing of LightSpeed preparations to allow obturation. With the canal system flooded *(1)*, apical preparation *(2)* is continued until an LS instrument requires 12 pecks to reach the working length (WL). The next LS instrument *(3)* then is used to a point 4 mm short of the WL to prepare for LightSpeed's SimpliFill obturation system. Alternatively, canals may be flared for other root canal filling techniques by preparing with each subsequent instrument 1 mm shorter *(5)*.

BOX 6-4

Benefits of Using a Combination of Instruments for Endodontic Therapy

- Instruments can be used in a manner that promotes their individual strengths and avoids their weaknesses (most important).
- Hand instruments secure a patent glide path.
- Tapered rotary instruments efficiently enlarge coronal canal areas.
- Less tapered instruments allow additional apical enlargement.

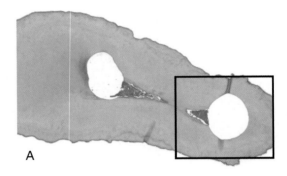

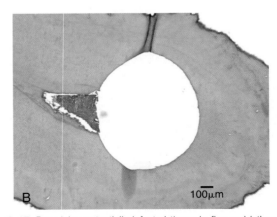

or more of all such canals and resulted in extremely wide apical sizes that may be difficult to achieve with most instrument systems.[255,257,256]

Histologic slides (see Fig. 6-47) and µCT reconstructions show critical areas that were not mechanically prepared despite the use of various individual rotary techniques. The aim of hybridizing NiTi rotary techniques, therefore, is to increase apical size using a fast and safe clinical procedure.

Various clinicians have used this type of hybrid procedure in their practices (see Figs. 6-2 and 6-10). The principle involves the use of a variety of instruments: for example, GG drills and K-files for establishing straight-line access; ProTaper instruments for body shaping and apical preenlargement; NiTi K-files or LightSpeed instruments for apical widening; and various instruments for final smoothing.[545]

After a stainless steel file has confirmed a smooth glide path into the coronal two thirds, irrigation and mechanical preparation with a sequence of ProTaper shaping files opens and preenlarges the apical third (Fig. 6-48). Once the working length has been established, the apical third is flooded with

FIG. 6-47 Remaining potentially infected tissue in fins and isthmus configuration after preparation with rotary instruments. **A,** Cross section through a mesial root of a mandibular molar, middle to coronal third of the root. Both canals have been shaped; the left one is transported mesially (×10). **B,** Magnified view of rectangle in **A**. Note the presence of soft tissue in the isthmus area (×63). (Courtesy Professor H. Messer.)

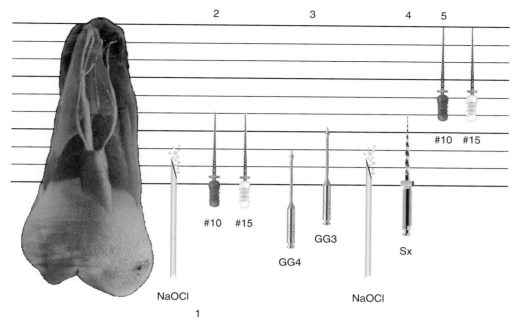

FIG. 6-48 Hybrid technique: Part I. After irrigation *(1)* and scouting *(2)*, GG drills *(3)* or ProTaper SX files *(4)* are used for coronal preenlargement and to secure straight-line access to the middle third. Precurved K-files are then used to explore and determine the working length *(5)*.

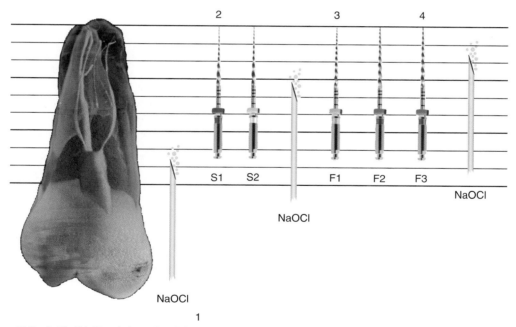

FIG. 6-49 Hybrid technique: Part II. In canal systems flooded with irrigant *(1)*, ProTaper shaping instruments S1 and S2 *(2)* and then finishing instruments F1 and F2 *(3)* are used to preenlarge the apical third, allowing irrigants access to the canals. Finishing instrument F3 may be used if feasible *(4)*.

NaOCl and further enlarged with ProTaper finishing files F1 and F2. The F3 ProTaper finishing file is relatively inflexible, and because of its side-cutting action, it should be used with caution in curved canals (Fig. 6-49). Further enlargement is possible with the F4 and F5 instruments, but these files may not be used in more acutely curved canals. The effectiveness of techniques combining different rotary instruments in enlarging canals recently was documented using superimposed root canal cross sections (Fig. 6-50). This method can help identify insufficiently prepared areas and weakening of the radicular structure.

A different approach, using, for example, NiTi K-files, .02 tapered rotaries (e.g., RaCe), or LightSpeed LSX (Fig. 6-51), may be also advantageous if larger sizes are desired. Finally, the overall shape may be smoothed with either engine-driven or handheld instruments. Handheld ProTaper or GT instruments may aid removal of acute apical curvatures or ledges and provide access to apical canal areas for irrigants.

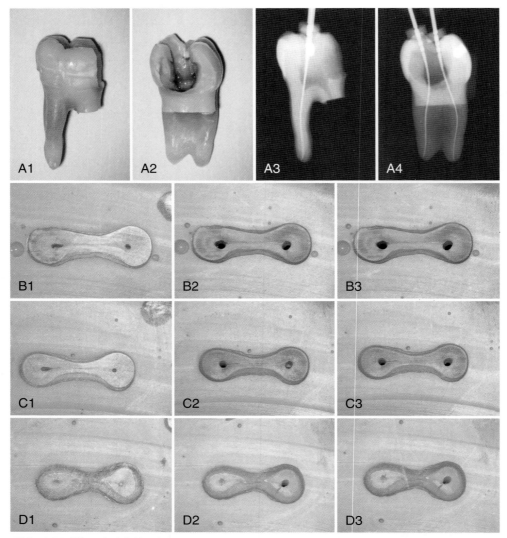

FIG. 6-50 Effect of a hybrid technique on root canal anatomy studied in a Bramante model. **A1-A4**, Both mesial canals of an extracted mandibular molar have been instrumented. Canal cross sections are shown before instrumentation (**B1-D1**). **B2-D2**, Cross sections after preenlargement with a ProTaper F3 file (*left canal*) and a size #45, #.02 taper instrument *(right canal)*. The final apical sizes were LightSpeed (LS) #50 and size #50, #.02 taper in the left and the right canal, respectively. (Courtesy Drs. S. Kuttler, M. Gerala, and R. Perez.)

Some hybrid systems seem to work better than others, but the deciding factors are likely the root canal anatomy and an adequate preparation goal.

Most cases requiring root canal therapy lend themselves to canal preparation with many different systems. Depending on the individual anatomy and the clinician's strategy, various sequences may be used. Mesiobuccal roots of the maxillary molar can show substantial curvature; rotary instrumentation or hybrid techniques allow preservation of the curvature and optimal enlargement. Occasionally hand instruments other than ISO-normed files are used in these cases to ensure a smooth, tapered shape or to eliminate ledges.

Final Apical Enlargement

Conceptually, file sizes during canal preparation were termed *initial apical file, master apical file,* and *final file* (or IAF, MAF, and FF, respectively). The first file to bind, the IAF, is supposed to give clinicians a guide in determining the final size of their canal preparation. On the other hand, many current instrumentation techniques have, due to their design, predefined final sizes—for example, WaveOne shaping aims at final sizes #25 .08 taper and #40, .08 taper.

Whichever apical size was conceptually aimed for, after shaping the overall canal to a tapered form, the apical size at that point should be assessed during apical gauging. K-files or K-Flexofiles are often recommended for this step; the files should be gently moved toward the working length (WL), and the binding point should be noted. The presence of an apical narrowing would translate into the fact that the WL may be reached without shaping effort with the desired size during gauging; however, the next larger size will stay back by a small distance. Finally, it should be verified that patency is maintained.

If apical gauging suggests that the canal is undershaped, additional enlargement is done with any technique appropriate to the specific anatomy of the root canal, often necessitating a hybrid technique.

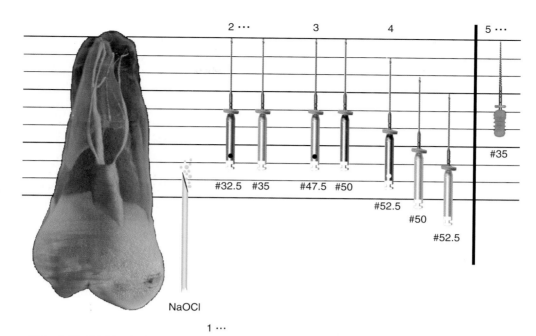

FIG. 6-51 Hybrid technique: Part III. Under irrigation *(1)*, LightSpeed instruments may be used to enlarge substantially *(2* and *3)* and to flare the apical section *(4)*. NiTi hand instruments *(5)* may be used similarly (see text for a more detailed explanation).

DISINFECTION OF THE ROOT CANAL SYSTEM

Hydrodynamics of Irrigation

Irrigation dynamics refers to how irrigants flow, penetrate, and readily exchange within the root canal system as well as the forces they produce. A better understanding of the fluid dynamics of different modes of irrigation will contribute to achieving predictable disinfection of the root canal system. Hence, in endodontic disinfection, the process of delivery is as important as the antibacterial characteristics of the irrigants.[65]

Irrigation is defined as "to wash out a body cavity or wound with water or a medicated fluid" and aspiration as "the process of removing fluids or gases from the body with a suction device." Disinfectant, meanwhile, is defined as "an agent that destroys or inhibits the activity of microorganisms that cause disease."[106]

The objectives of irrigation in endodontics are mechanical, chemical, and biologic. The mechanical and chemical objectives are as follows: (1) flush out debris, (2) lubricate the canal, (3) dissolve organic and inorganic tissue, and (4) prevent the formation of a smear layer during instrumentation or dissolve it once it has formed.[42] The mechanical effectiveness will depend on the ability of irrigation to generate optimum streaming forces within the entire root-canal system. The chemical effectiveness will depend on the concentration of the antimicrobial irrigant, the area of contact, and the duration of interaction between irrigant and infected material.[65] The final efficiency of endodontic disinfection will depend on its chemical and mechanical effectiveness.[190]

The biologic function of irrigants is related to their antimicrobial effects. In principle, irrigants should (1) have a high efficacy against anaerobic and facultative microorganisms in their planktonic state and in biofilms, (2) inactivate endotoxin, and (3) be nontoxic when they come in contact with vital tissues, and (4)b not cause an anaphylactic reaction.[42]

Efficiency of root canal irrigation in terms of debris removal and eradication of bacteria depends on several factors: penetration depth of the needle, diameter of the root canal, inner and outer diameter of the needle, irrigation pressure, viscosity of the irrigant, velocity of the irrigant at the needle tip, and type and orientation of the needle bevel (Fig. 6-52).

Penetration Depth of the Needle

The size and length of the irrigation needle—in relation to root canal dimensions—is of utmost importance for the effectiveness of irrigation.

Diameter of the Root Canal

The apical diameter of the canal has an impact on needle penetration depth (see earlier in this chapter for details regarding apical preparation size (see Fig. 6-7, Table 6-2).[72,578]

Inner and Outer Diameter of the Needle (Fig. 6-53, *A* and *B*)

The external needle diameter is of relevance for the depth of introduction into the root canal and for rigidity of the tip, an important consideration for irrigation of curved canals. Common 27 gauge injection needles have an external diameter of 0.42 mm, but smaller irrigation tips with external diameters of 0.32 mm (30 gauge) are available.[235] The Stropko Flexi-Tip (30 gauge) needle is fabricated from nickel-titanium to improve penetration into curved root canals.[205]

Irrigation Pressure

The internal diameter determines the pressure necessary for moving the syringe plunger. The speed of the plunger

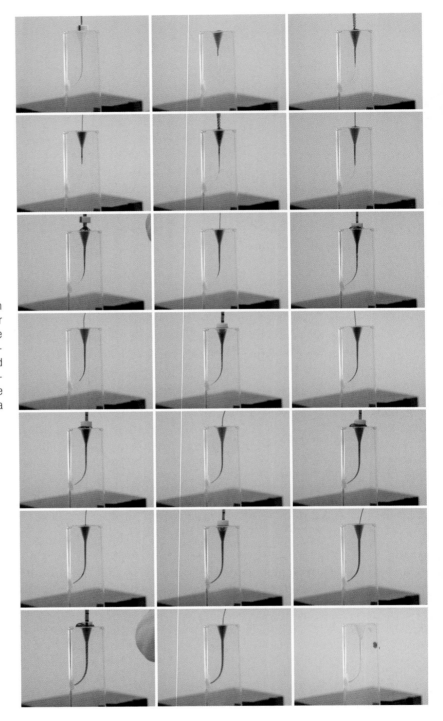

FIG. 6-52 Irrigation and movement of irrigants depends on canal shape. Sequential enlargement of a canal in clear plastic block was performed with a sequence of ProFile instruments in accordance with the manufacturer's recommendations. Alternating irrigation with blue and red fluid was done after each preparation step. Note the apical presence of irrigant after sufficient shape has been provided. Note the distribution of fluid immediately after irrigation with a 30-gauge needle.

determines the velocity with which the irrigant is extruded. Narrow needles require more pressure onto the plunger and extrude the irrigant with higher velocity than large needle sizes, which extrude greater amounts of irrigants but cannot be introduced as deep.

Type and Orientation of the Bevel of the Needle
To improve safety of irrigation and prevent extrusion of the irrigant through the apical foramen, some needles release the solution via lateral openings and have a closed, safe-ended tip.

The orientation of the bevel is crucial to produce a turbulence effect on the dentinal wall of the canal. Side-vented and double side-vented needles lead to maximum shear stress concentrated on the wall facing the outlet (the proximal outlet for the double side-vented).[67]

Irrigants

An optimal irrigant would have all of the characteristics considered beneficial in endodontics but none of the negative or harmful properties. Presently, no solution can be regarded

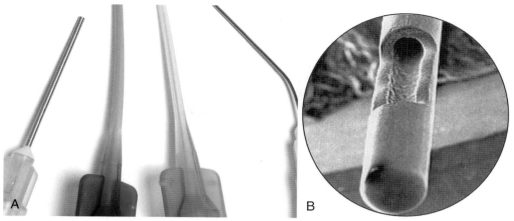

FIG. 6-53. **A**, Various types of needles for root canal irrigation. Shown are examples with open end and closed end, side vented. These are manufactured from plastic and stainless steel. **B**, SEM image of 30 gauge safety needle. (Courtesy Dr. F. Tay.)

BOX 6-5

Benefits of Using Irrigants in Root Canal Treatment

- Removal of particulate debris and wetting of the canal walls
- Destruction of microorganisms
- Dissolution of organic debris
- Opening of dentinal tubules by removal of the smear layer
- Disinfection and cleaning of areas inaccessible to endodontic instruments

BOX 6-6

Properties of an Ideal Irrigant for Root Canal Treatment

An ideal irrigant should do the following:
- Be an effective germicide and fungicide
- Be nonirritating to the periapical tissues
- Remain stable in solution
- Have a prolonged antimicrobial effect
- Be active in the presence of blood, serum, and protein derivatives of tissue
- Have low surface tension
- Not interfere with repair of periapical tissues
- Not stain tooth structure
- Be capable of inactivation in a culture medium
- Not induce a cell-mediated immune response
- Be able to completely remove the smear layer, and be able to disinfect the underlying dentin and its tubules
- Be nonantigenic, nontoxic, and noncarcinogenic to tissue cells surrounding the tooth
- Have no adverse effects on the physical properties of exposed dentin
- Have no adverse effects on the sealing ability of filling materials
- Have a convenient application
- Be relatively inexpensive

---

as optimal. However, combined use of selected irrigation products greatly contribute to successful outcome of treatment (Box 6-5 and Box 6-6).

Sodium Hypochlorite

NaOCl is the most commonly used irrigating solution[332] because of its an antibacterial capacity and the ability to dissolve necrotic tissue, vital pulp tissue, and the organic components of dentin and biofilms in a fast manner.[453]

NaOCl solution is frequently used as a disinfectant or a bleaching agent. It is the irrigant of choice in endodontics, owing to its efficacy against pathogenic organisms and pulp digestion, and satisfies most of the preferred characteristics stated earlier.[332]

History

Hypochlorite was first produced in 1789 in France. Hypochlorite solution was used as a hospital antiseptic that was sold under the trade names Eusol and Dakin's solution. Dakin recommended NaOCl as a buffered 0.5% solution for the irrigation of wounds during World War I.[114] Coolidge[108] later introduced NaOCl to endodontics an intracanal irrigation solution.[575]

Mode of Action

When sodium hypochlorite contacts tissue proteins, nitrogen, formaldehyde, and acetaldehyde are formed. Peptide links are fragmented and proteins disintegrate, permitting hydrogen in the amino groups (-NH-) to be replaced by chlorine (-NCl-) forming chloramines; this plays an important role for the antimicrobial effectiveness. Necrotic tissue and pus are dissolved and the antimicrobial agent can better reach and clean the infected areas.

In 2002 Estrela reported that sodium hypochlorite exhibits a dynamic balance (Fig. 6-54)[142]:

1. Saponification reaction: Sodium hypochlorite acts as an organic and fat solvent that degrades fatty acids and transforms them into fatty acid salts (soap) and glycerol (alcohol), reducing the surface tension of the remaining solution.
2. Neutralization reaction: Sodium hypochlorite neutralizes amino acids by forming water and salt. With the exit of hydroxyl ions, the pH is reduced.
3. Hypochlorous acid formation: When chlorine dissolves in water and it is in contact with organic matter, it forms

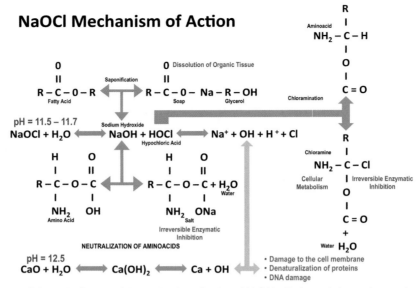

NaOCl Mechanism of Action

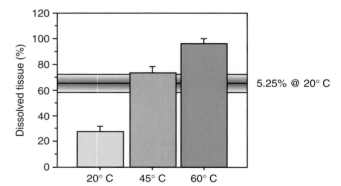

FIG. 6-54 Schematic diagram of the mechanism of action of NaOCl with the main interactions and properties highlighted. (Courtesy Dr. A. Manzur.)

hypochlorous acid. It is a weak acid with the chemical formula HClO that acts as an oxidizer. Hypochlorous acid (HOCl⁻) and hypochlorite ions (OCl⁻) lead to amino acid degradation and hydrolysis.

4. Solvent action: Sodium hypochlorite also acts as a solvent, releasing chlorine that combines with protein amino groups (NH) to form chloramines (chloramination reaction). Chloramines impede cell metabolism; chlorine is a strong oxidant and inhibits essential bacterial enzymes by irreversible oxidation of SH groups (sulfydryl group).[142]

5. High pH: Sodium hypochlorite is a strong base (pH > 11). The antimicrobial effectiveness of sodium hypochlorite, based on its high pH (hydroxyl ions action), is similar to the mechanism of action of calcium hydroxide. The high pH interferes in cytoplasmic membrane integrity due to irreversible enzymatic inhibition, biosynthetic alterations in cellular metabolism, and phospholipid degradation observed in lipidic peroxidation.[142]

Allergic Reactions to Sodium Hypochlorite

Although few reports have been published on allergic reactions to NaOCl,[144,198] real allergies to NaOCl are unlikely to occur, as both Na and Cl are essential elements in the physiology of the human body. It must be remembered that the hypochlorous acid (active component of the sodium hypochlorite) is a chemical substance that is elaborated by neutrophils in the process of phagocytosis; it may create local tissue damage when it is produced in excess (liquefaction necrosis: purulent exudate) but does not cause allergic responses. Nevertheless, hypersensitivity and contact dermatitis may occur in rare situations. A case report describes a serious chemical burn in an endodontist's eye caused by accidental contact with 3.5% NaOCl used as an irrigant during root canal.[403]

When hypersensitivity to NaOCl is suspected or confirmed, chlorhexidine should not be used either because of its chlorine content. For individuals who genetically have more possibilities than the normal population to generate allergies to multiple elements (allergies to food or to latex), a skin test

FIG. 6-55 Effect of heating on the ability of 0.5% sodium hypochlorite (NaOCl) to dissolve pulp tissue: NaOCl heated to 113° F (45° C) dissolved pulp tissue as well as the positive control (5.25% NaOCl) did. When the NaOCl was heated to 140° F (60° C), almost complete dissolution of tissue resulted. (Modified from Sirtes G, Waltimo T, Schaetzle M, Zehnder M: The effects of temperature on sodium hypochlorite short-term stability, pulp dissolution capacity, and antimicrobial efficacy, *J Endod* 31:669, 2005.)

for both NaOCl and CHX may be indicated. The use of an alternative irrigant with high antimicrobial efficacy, such as iodine potassium iodide, should be considered, assuming there is no known allergy to that irrigant. Solutions such as alcohol or tap water are less effective against microorganisms and do not dissolve vital or necrotic tissue; however, Ca(OH)₂ could be used as a temporary medicament because it dissolves both vital and necrotic tissue.[18,207]

Temperature

Increasing the temperature of low-concentration NaOCl solutions improves their immediate tissue-dissolution capacity (Fig. 6-55).[575] Furthermore, heated hypochlorite solutions remove organic debris from dentin shavings more efficiently. Bactericidal rates for NaOCl solutions, the capacity of human pulp dissolution, and increased efficacy were detailed in several

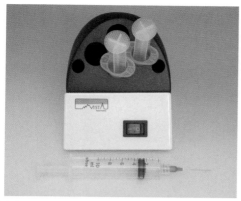

FIG. 6-56 Device for heating syringes filled with irrigation solution (e.g., sodium hypochlorite) before use. (Courtesy Vista Dental Products, Racine, WI.)

studies.[475] There are various devices to preheat NaOCl syringes (Fig. 6-56); however, it was demonstrated that as soon as the irrigant touches the root canal system, the temperature reaches the body temperature.[579] Therefore, some authors recommend in situ heating of NaOCl. This can be done by activating ultrasonic or sonic tips to the NaOCl inside the root canal for a couple of minutes (see irrigation timings, discussed later). Macedo and colleagues stated that the efficacy of NaOCl on dentin is improved by refreshment, ultrasonic activation, and exposure time.[307] In this investigation, a 10° C temperature rise during ultrasonic activation was insufficient to increase the reaction rate. However, no clinical studies are available at this point to support the use of heated NaOCl.[42,104]

Concentrations

NaOCl is used in concentrations between 0.5% and 6% for root canal irrigation. Controversy exists over recommended concentrations of sodium hypochlorite during root canal treatment. Some in vitro studies have shown that NaOCl in higher concentrations is more effective against *Enterococcus faecalis* and *Candida albicans*.[177,395,547] In contrast, clinical studies have indicated both low and high concentrations to be equally effective in reducing bacteria from the root canal system.[87,111] NaOCl in higher concentrations has a better tissue-dissolving ability.[204] However, in lower concentrations when used in high volumes it can be equally effective.[336,470] Higher concentrations of NaOCl are more toxic than lower concentrations.[491] However, due to the confined anatomy of the root canal system, higher concentrations have successfully been used during root canal treatment, with a low incidence of mishaps.

In summary, if lower concentrations are to be used for intracanal irrigation, it is recommended that the solution be used in higher volume and in more frequent intervals to compensate for the limitations in effectiveness.[470]

Instrumentation coupled with an antimicrobial irrigant, such as NaOCl, has been shown to yield more negative cultures than instrumentation alone.[86,323,364,372,463] However, even with the use of NaOCl, removal of bacteria from the root canal systems following instrumentation remains an elusive goal.

Grossman observed pulp tissue dissolution capacity and reported that 5% sodium hypochlorite dissolved this tissue in between 20 minutes and 2 hours.[185] The dissolution of bovine pulp tissue by sodium hypochlorite (0.5, 1.0, 2.5, and 5.0%)

was studied in vitro under different conditions.[142] The study yielded the following conclusions:

1. The velocity of dissolution of the bovine pulp fragments was directly proportional to the concentration of the sodium hypochlorite solution and was greater without the surfactant;
2. variations in surface tension, from beginning to end of pulp dissolution, were directly proportional to the concentration of the sodium hypochlorite solution and greater in the solutions without surfactant. Solutions without surfactant presented a decrease in surface tension and those with surfactant an increase;
3. in heated sodium hypochlorite solutions, dissolution of the bovine pulp tissue was more rapid;
4. the greater the initial concentration of the sodium hypochlorite solutions, the smaller was the reduction of its pH.[142]

Time

There is conflicting evidence regarding the time course of the antibacterial effect of NaOCl.[42,195] In some articles hypochlorite is reported to kill the target microorganism in seconds, even at low concentrations, whereas other reports have published considerably longer times for the killing of the same species.[185] Such differences are likely a result of several factors: the presence of organic matter during experiments has a detrimental effect on the antibacterial activity of NaOCl. Haapasalo and colleagues showed that the presence of dentin caused marked delays in the killing of *Enterococcus faecalis* by 1% NaOCl.[193] Morgental and colleagues reported similar findings.[337]

Many of the earlier studies were performed in the presence of an unknown amount of organic matter. When such confounding factors are eliminated, it has been shown that NaOCl kills the target microorganisms rapidly even at low concentrations of less than 0.1%.[195,539] However, in vivo the presence of organic matter (inflammatory exudate, tissue remnants, and microbial biomass) consumes NaOCl and weakens its effect. Therefore, continuous replenishing of irrigation solution and allowing sufficient contact time are important factors for the effectiveness of NaOCl.[195]

The chlorine ion, which is responsible for the dissolving and antibacterial capacity of NaOCl, is unstable and consumed rapidly during the first phase of tissue dissolution, probably within 2 minutes,[336] which provides another reason for continuous replenishment. This should especially be considered in view of the fact that rotary root canal preparation techniques have expedited the shaping process. The optimal time that a hypochlorite irrigant at a given concentration needs to remain in the canal system is an issue yet to be resolved.[575]

Toxicity

If inadvertently NaOCl is extruded through the apex, severe accidents may occur (Fig. 6-57, A-C). It is important to recognize the symptoms and act accordingly. After an accident with NaOCl, the following can be expected: severe pain, edema of neighboring soft tissues, possible extension of edema over the injured half of face and upper lip, profuse bleeding from root canal, profuse interstitial bleeding with hemorrhage of skin and mucosa (ecchymosis), chlorine taste and irritation of throat after injection into maxillary sinus, secondary infection possible, and reversible anesthesia or paresthesia is possible. To manage these lesions, the clinician should inform the patient and control pain with local anesthesia and analgesics.

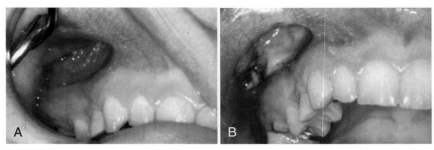

FIG. 6-57 Toxic effect of sodium hypochlorite on periradicular tissues. After root canal treatment of tooth #3, the patient reported pain. **A,** On a return visit, an abscess was diagnosed and incised. **B,** Osteonecrosis was evident after 3 weeks.

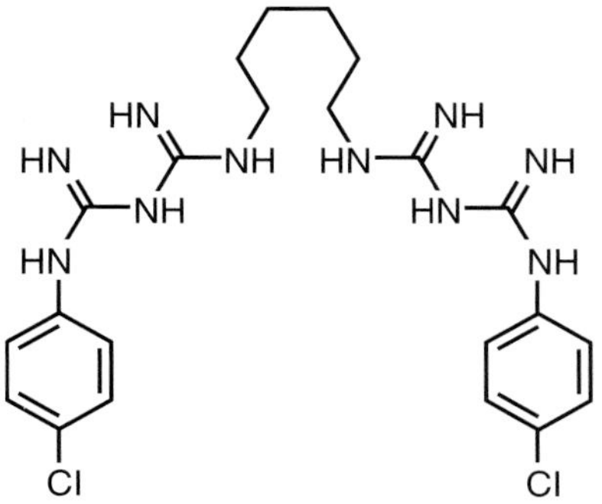

FIG. 6-58 Schematic drawing of the chlorhexidine molecule.

The application of extraoral cold compresses to reduce swelling is also effective. After 1 day, warm compresses and frequent warm mouth rinses for stimulation of local systemic circulation should be used. Patients should be recalled daily to monitor recovery. The use of antibiotics is not obligatory and is recommended only in cases of high risk or evidence of secondary infection. The administration of antihistamine is also not obligatory, and the use of corticosteroids is controversial. Further endodontic therapy with sterile saline or chlorhexidine as root canal irrigants and referral to a hospital in case of worsening symptoms were suggested.[260]

Chlorhexidine
History
Chlorhexidine (CHX) was developed in the UK and first marketed as an antiseptic cream.[148] It has been used for general disinfection purposes and the treatment of skin, eye, and throat infections in both humans and animals.[148,294] It has been used as an irrigant and medicament in endodontics for more than a decade.[309,333,363]

Molecular Structure
CHX is a strongly basic molecule with a pH between 5.5 and 7 that belongs to the polybiguanide group and consists of two symmetric four-chlorophenyl rings and two bisbiguanide groups connected by a central hexamethylene chain. CHX digluconate salt is easily soluble in water and very stable[184] (Fig. 6-58).

Mode of Action
Chlorhexidine, because of its cationic charges, is capable of electrostatically binding to the negatively charged surfaces of bacteria,[117] damaging the outer layers of the cell wall and

rendering it permeable.[214,229,228] CHX is a wide-spectrum antimicrobial agent, active against gram-positive, gram-negative bacteria and yeasts.[129]

Depending on its concentration, CHX can have both bacteriostatic and bactericidal effects. At high concentrations, CHX acts as a detergent; and exerts its bactericidal effect by damaging the cell membrane and causes precipitation of the cytoplasm. At low concentrations, CHX is bacteriostatic, causing low molecular-weight substances (i.e., potassium and phosphorus) to leak out without the cell being permanently damaged.[43]

Substantivity
Because of the cationic nature of the CHX molecule, it can be absorbed by anionic substrates such as the oral mucosa and tooth structure.[308,312,414,527] CHX is readily adsorbed onto hydroxyapatite and teeth. Studies have shown that the uptake of CHX onto teeth is reversible.[222] This reversible reaction of uptake and release of CHX leads to substantive antimicrobial activity and is referred to as *substantivity*. This effect depends on the concentration of CHX. At low concentrations of 0.005% to 0.01%, only a constant monolayer of CHX is adsorbed on the tooth surface, but at higher concentrations (>0.02%), a multilayer of CHX is formed on the surface, providing a reservoir of CHX that can rapidly release the excess into the environment as the concentration of CHX in the surrounding environment decreases.[139] Time and concentration of CHX can influence the antibacterial substantivity, and the conclusions are inconsistent. Some studies demonstrated that 4% CHX has greater antibacterial substantivity than 0.2% after a 5-minute application.[333] Other studies stated that CHX should be left for more than 1 hour in the canal to be adsorbed by the dentin.[291] Komorowski and colleagues suggested that a 5-minute application of CHX did not induce substantivity, so dentin should be treated with CHX for 7 days.[265] However, when Paquette and Malkhassian,[364] in their in vivo study, medicated the canals with either liquid or gel forms of CHX for 1 week, neither of them could achieve total disinfection. Therefore, residual antimicrobial efficacy of CHX in vivo still remains to be demonstrated.

Cytotoxicity
CHX is normally used at concentrations between 0.12% and 2%. Löe and colleagues[294] demonstrated that at these concentrations, CHX has a low level of tissue toxicity, both locally and systemically. When 2% CHX was used as a subgingival irrigant, no apparent toxicity was noted on gingival tissues.[295,488] Additionally, CHX rinses have been suggested to promote healing

of periodontal wounds after surgery.[24] These reports were the basis of many studies that assumed that CHX will be tolerated on periapical tissues with a similar response than in the gingival tissues.[245] When compared CHX and NaOCl into subcutaneous tissues of guinea pigs and rats, an inflammatory reaction developed; however, the toxic reaction from CHX was less than that of NaOCl.[352,571] Moreover, a reduced incidence of alveolar osteitis was found when CHX was applied as a rinse in the extraction sites of the third molars on the day of surgery and several days after.[91] Allergic and anaphylactic reactions to CHX were reported in only a few articles.[166,351] It is important to mention that patients that are allergic to NaOCl may be also allergic to CHX.

On the other hand, some controversial results were found. Some studies demonstrated that CHX is cytotoxic to some lines of cultured human skin fibroblasts.[219] It has been reported that CHX has a higher cytotoxicity profile than povidone iodine when studied in osteoblastic human alveolar bone.[88] Also, when CHX was injected in the hind paw of mice, it could induce severe toxic reactions.[149]

Finally, when CHX is mixed with NaOCl, parachloroaniline (PCA) is formed.[46] The toxicity level of CHX on periapical tissues when applied in the root canals, especially with other irrigants, merits further investigation.

Chlorhexidine as an Endodontic Irrigant

CHX has been extensively studied as an endodontic irrigant and intracanal medication, both in vivo[35,292,311,364,564] and in vitro.[41,44,45,141,245,265,273,281,282,469,471,506,540,574]

The antibacterial efficacy of CHX as an irrigant is concentration dependent. It has been demonstrated that 2% CHX has a better antibacterial efficacy than 0.12% CHX in vitro.[45] When comparing with the effectiveness with NaOCl, controversial results can be found. NaOCl has an obvious advantage over CHX with the dissolution capacity of organic matter that CHX lacks; therefore, even though in vitro studies suggest some advantages with the use of CHX, as soon as organic and dental tissue is added, NaOCl is clearly preferable.

The antibacterial effectiveness of CHX in infected root canals has been investigated in several in vivo studies. Investigators reported that 2.5% NaOCl was significantly more effective than 0.2% CHX when the infected root canals were irrigated for 30 minutes with either of the solutions.[409]

In a controlled and randomized clinical trial, the efficacy of 2% CHX liquid was tested against saline using culture technique. All the teeth were initially instrumented and irrigated using 1% NaOCl. Then either 2% CHX liquid or saline was applied as a final rinse. The authors reported a further reduction in the proportion of positive cultures in the CHX group. Their results showed a better disinfection of the root canals using CHX compared to saline as a final rinse.[574]

The antibacterial efficacy of 2% CHX gel was tested against 2.5% NaOCl in teeth with apical periodontitis, with the bacterial load assessed using a real-time quantitative polymerase chain reaction (RTQ-PCR) and colony forming units (CFUs). The bacterial reduction in the NaOCl group was significantly greater than that for the CHX group when measured by RTQ-PCR. Based on culture technique, bacterial growth was detected in 50% of the CHX group cases compared to 25% in the NaOCl group.[540] On the other hand, another study based on this culture technique revealed no significant difference between the antibacterial efficacy of 2.5% NaOCl and 0.12% CHX

liquid when used as irrigants during the treatment of infected canals.[469,471]

In a systematic review, Ng and colleagues demonstrated that abstaining from using 2% CHX as an adjunct irrigant to NaOCl was associated with superior periapical healing.[345] Unlike NaOCl, CHX lacks a tissue-dissolving property. Therefore, NaOCl is still considered the primary irrigating solution in endodontics.

Chlorhexidine as an Intracanal Medication

CHX as intracanal medication has been the focus of many in vitro[38,128,265,281,468] CHX used as intracanal medicament has at least as good or even better antimicrobial efficacy than $Ca(OH)_2$.[468] and it was shown to be very effective in eliminating a biofilm of E. faecalis.[288]

When in vivo studies are analyzed,[35,115,123,140,292,311,364,580] some controversial results were found. On one hand, CHX, inhibits experimentally induced inflammatory external root resorption when applied for 4 weeks.[292] In infected root canals, it was shown to reduce bacteria as effectively as $Ca(OH)_2$ when applied for 1 week.[34] Because of its substantivity, CHX has the potential to prevent bacterial colonization of root canal walls for prolonged periods of time.[245,265] It was demonstrated that its effect depended on the concentration of CHX but not on its mode of application, which may be as a liquid or gel.[44]

In vivo, results can be different; one of the reasons for this is that researchers[193] developed an experimental model using dentin powder particles to investigate the possible inactivation of some antibacterial medicaments when they come in contact with dentin. They showed that dentin powder had inhibitory effects on all medicaments tested. The effect was dependent on the concentration of the medicament and the duration of contact. The effect of $Ca(OH)_2$ was totally abolished by the presence of dentin powder. The effect of 0.05% CHX and 1% NaOCl was reduced but not totally eliminated by the presence of dentin. No inhibition could be measured when full-strength solutions of CHX and IKI were used.

An in vivo investigation assessed the antibacterial efficacy of three different intracanal medications: camphorated paramonochlorophenol, $Ca(OH)_2$, and 0.12% CHX liquid by applying them for 1 week in single-rooted teeth of patients with apical periodontitis. The proportions of positive cultures were not significantly different among the tested medications, but they were slightly lower in teeth medicated with CHX (0.12%) liquid than those medicated with camphorated paramonochlorophenol or $Ca(OH)_2$.[35] Another in vivo study evaluated antibacterial effectiveness of 2% CHX liquid as an intracanal medication in teeth with apical periodontitis. The authors concluded that a moderate increase in bacterial counts during a medication period of 7 to 14 days that was similar to outcomes seen and reported for $Ca(OH)_2$ by Peters and colleagues.[364, 372] On the other hand, an alternative investigation[311] demonstrated no significant differences among the medication groups. Intracanal medication with $Ca(OH)_2$, 2% CHX gel, or a mixture of $Ca(OH)_2$/CHX applied for 7 days did not reduce the bacterial concentration beyond what was achieved after chemomechanical preparation using 1% NaOCl. Other research showed that a final rinse with MTAD and medication with 2%CHX gel, did not reduce bacterial counts beyond levels achieved by a chemomechanical preparation using NaOCl.[310]

Chlorhexidine Mixed with Calcium Hydroxide

To enhance the properties of both CHX and Ca(OH)₂, their combination was analyzed in several in vitro and in vivo studies. The high pH of Ca(OH)₂ was unaffected when combined with CHX.[46] However, the results have not been conclusive. Some in vitro studies have reported an improved antibacterial action when both agents were combined,[45,145,575] whereas other studies reported contradictory results.[199]

The combination of CHX and Ca(OH)₂ showed good antimicrobial properties when tested in animal studies.[480] When studied in vivo in patients with apical periodontitis, the results showed similar antibacterial efficacy of each medicament alone or in combination.[311] In another clinical study, when 0.12% CHX was used during cleaning and shaping and an intracanal medication with Ca(OH)₂/0.12% CHX was left in the canals for 7 days, it was found that using 0.12% CHX solution as an irrigant significantly reduced the number of intracanal bacteria, but it failed to render the canals bacteria free.[465] Therefore, it seems that the usefulness of mixing Ca(OH)₂ with CHX remains controversial.

Chlorhexidine and Coronal Penetration of Bacteria

Several studies analyzed the property of antibacterial substantivity and bacterial penetration.[178] It was demonstrated that placement of intracanal medication delays bacterial penetration because of the physical barrier alongside the antibacterial action of the medicament. Gomes and colleagues,[178] in a laboratory study, investigated the time required for recontamination of the root canal system of teeth with coronal restorations medicated with Ca(OH)₂, 2% CHX gel, or a combination of both and concluded that if medication is present, retardation of microorganism invasion was seen. Overall, because of its substantivity, CHX as an intracanal medicament/irrigant may delay the coronal recontamination of the root canal system, but more in vivo studies are needed to corroborate these results.

Interaction between CHX, NaOCl, and EDTA

NaOCl and CHX when in contact produce a change of color and a precipitate (Fig. 6-59, A and B). The reaction is dependent of the concentration of NaOCl. The higher the concentration of NaOCl, the more precipitate is generated in the presence of 2% CHX.[46] Furthermore, concerns have been raised that the color change may have some clinical relevance because of staining, and the resulting precipitate might interfere with the seal of the root obturation. Basrani and colleagues evaluated

the chemical nature of this precipitate and reported the formation of 4-chloroaniline (PCA).[46] Furthermore, a study using time-of-flight secondary ion mass spectrometry (TOF-SIMS) analysis shows the penetration of PCA inside dentinal tubules. PCA has been shown to be toxic in humans with short-term exposure, resulting in cyanosis, which is a manifestation of methemoglobin formation. The combination of NaOCl and CHX causes color changes and formation of a possibly toxic insoluble precipitate that may interfere with the seal of the root obturation. Alternatively, the canal can be dried using paper points before the final CHX rinse.[575]

The combination of CHX and EDTA produces a white precipitate, so a group of investigators[399] did a study to determine whether the precipitate involves the chemical degradation of CHX. The precipitate was produced and redissolved in a known amount of dilute trifluoroacetic acid. Based on the results, CHX was found to form a salt with EDTA rather than undergoing a chemical reaction.

Chlorhexidine and Dentin Bonding

Researchers evaluated the effect of CHX on resin-dentin bond stability ex vivo.[90] They concluded that autodegradation of collagen matrices can occur in resin-infiltrated dentin, but this may be prevented by the application of a synthetic protease inhibitor such as CHX.[90] Because of its broad-spectrum matrix metalloproteinase (MMP)-inhibitory effect, CHX may significantly improve resin-dentin bond stability.[90]

Allergic Reactions to Chlorhexidine

Allergic responses to CHX are rare, and there are no reports of reactions following root canal irrigation with CHX.[27,235] Several studies have reported the sensitization rate to be approximately 2%.[268] However, some allergic reactions such as anaphylaxis, contact dermatitis, and urticaria have been reported following direct contact to mucosal tissue or open wounds.[134,388,451,479]

Decalcifying Agents

Debris is defined as dentin chips or residual vital or necrotic pulp tissue attached to the root canal wall. Smear layer was defined by the American Association of Endodontists in 2003 as a surface film of debris retained on dentin or another surface after instrumentation with either rotary instruments or endodontic files; it consists of dentin particles, remnants of vital or necrotic pulp tissue, bacterial components, and retained irrigants. Although it has been viewed as an impediment to irrigant penetration into dentinal tubules (Fig. 6-60), there is

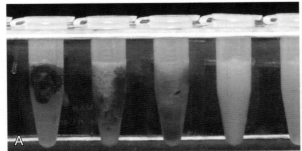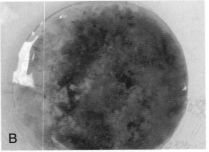

FIG. 6-59 Red precipitate forming after contact between NaOCl and chlorhexidine. **A,** When 2% CHX is mixed with different concentration of NaOCl, a change of color and precipitate occurs. The higher the concentration of NaOCl, the larger is the precipitate formation. **B,** Detail of the interaction between 2% CHX and 5%NaOCl.

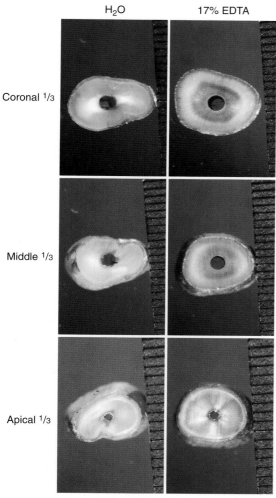

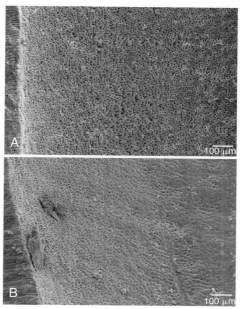

FIG. 6-61 Example of canals with minimal smear layer. **A**, Middle third after irrigation with 17% ethylenediaminetetraacetic acid (EDTA) and 2.5% sodium hypochlorite (NaOCl). **B**, Apical third with some particulate debris.

FIG. 6-60 Penetration of irrigants into dentinal tubules after root canal preparation with different dentin pretreatments. *Left column,* Irrigation with tap water and then with blue dye. *Right column,* Smear layer is removed with 17% EDTA, applied in high volume and with a 30-gauge needle, followed by irrigation with blue dye. Note the comparable diffusion of dye in the apical sections, whereas dye penetrated deeper into the dentin in the two coronal sections.

still a controversy about the influence of smear layer on the outcome of endodontic treatment. Some researchers emphasize the importance on removing the smear layer to allow irrigants, medications, and sealers to penetrate dentinal tubules and improve disinfection. On the other hand, other researchers focused on keeping the smear layer as a protection for bacterial invasion, apical and coronal micro leakage, bacterial penetration of the tubules, and the adaptation of root canal materials. The majority of the conclusions on smear layer are based on in vitro studies. A clinical study by Ng and colleagues[345] found that the use of EDTA significantly increased the odds of success of retreatment cases twofold.

Ethylenediamine Tetra-Acetic Acid

Ethylenediamine tetra-acetic acid, widely abbreviated as EDTA, is an aminopolycarboxylic acid and a colorless, water-soluble solid EDTA is often suggested as an irrigation solution because it can chelate and remove the mineralized portion of the smear layer (Fig. 6-61). It is a polyaminocarboxylic acid with the formula $[CH_2N(CH_2CO_2H)_2]_2$. Its prominence as a chelating agent arises from its ability to sequester di- and tricationic metal ions such as Ca^{2+} and Fe^{3+}. After being bound by EDTA, metal ions remain in solution but exhibit diminished reactivity.[494]

History

The compound was first described in 1935 by Ferdinand Munz, who prepared the compound from ethylenediamine and chloroacetic acid. Chelating agents were introduced into endodontics as an aid for the preparation of narrow and calcified root canals in 1957 by Nygaard-Østby.[232] Today, EDTA is mainly synthesized from ethylenediamine (1,2-diaminoethane), formaldehyde (methanal), and sodium cyanide.[232,494]

Mode of Action

On direct exposure for extended time, EDTA extracts bacterial surface proteins by combining with metal ions from the cell envelope, which can eventually lead to bacterial death.[232] Chelators such as EDTA form a stable complex with calcium. When all available ions have been bound, equilibrium is formed and no further dissolution takes place; therefore, EDTA is self-limiting.[232]

Applications in Endodontics

EDTA alone normally cannot remove the smear layer effectively; a proteolytic component, such as NaOCl, must be added to remove the organic components of the smear layer.[176] For root canal preparation, EDTA has limited value alone as an irrigation fluid.[176] EDTA is normally used in a concentration of 17% and can remove the smear layers when in direct contact with the root canal wall for less than 1 minute. Even though EDTA has self-limited action, if it is left in the canal for longer or NaOCl is used after EDTA, erosion of dentin has been demonstrated (Fig. 6-62).

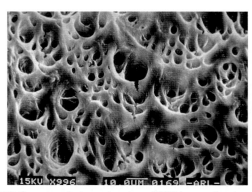

FIG. 6-62 Scanning electron microscope (SEM) image of root canal dentin exposed to 2 minutes of EDTA.

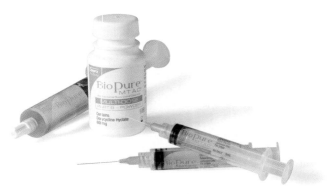

FIG 6-63 Container with BioPure MTAD. (Courtesy Dentsply Tulsa Dental Specialties, Tulsa, OK.)

Although citric acid appears to be slightly more potent at similar concentration than EDTA, both agents show high efficiency in removing the smear layer. In addition to their cleaning ability, chelators may detach biofilms adhering to root canal walls.[188] This may explain why an EDTA irrigant proved to be highly superior to saline in reducing intracanal microbiota despite the fact that its antiseptic capacity is relatively limited.[188] Antiseptics such as quaternary ammonium compounds (EDTAC) or tetracycline antibiotics (MTAD) (see the discussion on the combination of irrigants, presented later) have been added to EDTA and citric acid irrigants, respectively, to increase their antimicrobial capacity. The clinical value of this, however, is questionable. EDTAC shows similar smear-removing efficacy as EDTA, but it is more caustic.

The effect of chelators in negotiating narrow, tortuous, calcified canals to establish patency depends on both canal width and the amount of active substance available, since the demineralization process continues until all chelators have formed complexes with calcium.[232,452,577] Therefore, studies should be read with cautious because one study can show demineralization up to a depth of 50 μ m into dentin,236 but other reports demonstrated significant erosion after irrigation with EDTA.[519]

A comparison of bacterial growth inhibition showed that the antibacterial effects of EDTA were stronger than citric acid and 0.5% NaOCl but weaker than 2.5% NaOCl and 0.2% CHX.[467] EDTA had a significantly better antimicrobial effect than saline solution. It exerts it strongest effect when used synergistically with NaOCl, although no disinfecting effect on colonized dentin could be demonstrated.[212]

Interaction of EDTA and NaOCl

Investigators studied the interactions of EDTA with NaOCl.[183] They concluded that EDTA retained its calcium-complex ability when mixed with NaOCl, but EDTA caused NaOCl to lose its tissue-dissolving capacity, with virtually no free chlorine detected in the combinations. Clinically, this suggests that EDTA and NaOCl should be used separately. In an alternating irrigating regimen, copious amounts of NaOCl should be administered to wash out remnants of the EDTA. In modern endodontics, EDTA is used once the cleaning and shaping is completed for around 1 minute. It can be activated with ultrasonic activation for better penetration in dentinal tubules. It should be taken into consideration that an increase in the temperature of EDTA is not desirable. Chelators have a temperature range within which they work best. When EDTA is heated from 20° to 90°, the calcium binding capacity decreases.[576]

HBPT

HEBP (1-hydroxyethylidene-1, 1-bisphosphonate; also called etidronic acid) is a weak chelator.[575] It is a potential alternative to EDTA because it has no short-term reactivity with NaOCl. It can be used in combination with NaOCl without affecting its proteolytic or antimicrobial properties.[575] It is nontoxic,[26,125] and it is used in medicine to treat bone diseases.[362]

Combination of Irrigants and Added Detergent
Surface Tension
Irrigants with low surface tension have better wettabilty, and it is assumed that they may penetrate better in dentinal tubules and anatomic irregularities. Detergents (e.g., Tween 80) are added to irrigants to lower their surface tension. However, Boutsioukis and Kishen did not find support for this rationale,[65] perhaps because the effect of surface tension is important only at the interface between two immiscible fluids (e.g., between irrigant and an air bubble, but not between irrigant and dentinal fluid). Studies have also confirmed that surfactants do not enhance the ability of NaOCl to dissolve pulp tissue[251] or the efficacy of common chelators to remove calcium or smear layer.[65,125,300,577]

BioPure MTAD and Tetraclean
Two new irrigants based on a mixture of antibiotics, citric acid, and a detergent have been developed. These irrigants are capable of removing both the smear layer and organic tissue from the infected the root canal system.[520] MTAD (Fig. 6-63), introduced by Torabinejad and Johnson at Loma Linda University in 2003,[520] is an aqueous solution of 3% doxycycline, a broad-spectrum antibiotic; 4.25% citric acid, a demineralizing agent; and 0.5% polysorbate 80 detergent (Tween 80).[520] It is mixed as a liquid and powder prior to use. MTAD has been recommended in clinical practice as a final rinse after completion of conventional chemomechanical preparation.[48,248,457,458,520,521]

Tetraclean (Ogna Laboratori Farmaceutici, Muggio, Italy) is a combination product similar to MTAD. The two irrigants differ in the concentration of antibiotics (doxycycline 150 mg/5 ml for MTAD and 50 mg/5 ml for Tetraclean) and the kind of detergent (Tween 80 for MTAD, polypropylene glycol for Tetraclean).

Mode of Action
All tetracyclines are derivatives of four ringed nuclei that differ structurally in regard to the chemical groups at the 2, 5, 6, and

7 positions. These derivatives exhibit different characteristics such as absorption, protein binding, metabolism, excretion, and degree of activity against susceptible organism.[210] Tetracyclines inhibit protein synthesis by reversibly binding to the 30S subunit of bacterial ribosome in susceptible bacteria. It is effective against *Aa. capnocytophaga*, *P. gingivalis*, and *P. intermedia* and affects both gram-positive and gram-negative (more gram-negative effect) types. Tetracycline is a bacteriostatic antibiotic, but in high concentrations, tetracycline may also have a bactericidal effect. Doxycycline, citric acid, and Tween 80 together may have a synergistic effect on the disruption of the bacterial cell wall and on the cytoplasmic membrane.

Smear Layer Removal

In two studies, the efficacy of MTAD or EDTA in the removal of the smear layer was confirmed, but no significant difference between these two solutions was reported.[507,508]

Antibacterial Efficacy

Earlier in vitro research on MTAD showed its antimicrobial efficacy over conventional irrigants.[118,267,507,508,521] Torabinejad and colleagues found that MTAD was effective in killing *E. faecalis* up to 200× dilution.[117] Shabahang and Torabinejad showed that the combination of 1.3% NaOCl as a root canal irrigant and MTAD as a final rinse was significantly more effective against *E. faecalis* than the other regimens.[458] A study using extracted human teeth contaminated with saliva showed that MTAD was more effective than 5.25% NaOCl in disinfection of the teeth. In contrast to the previously mentioned studies, later research suggested less than optimal antimicrobial activity of MTAD.[170,248,258] Krause and colleagues,[267] using bovine tooth sections, showed that 5.25% NaOCl was more effective than MTAD in disinfection of dentin disks inoculated with *E. faecalis*.[458,468]

Clinical Trials

Malkhassain and colleagues, in a clinical controlled trial of 30 patients, reported that the final rinse with MTAD did not reduce the bacterial counts in infected canals beyond levels achieved by a chemomechanical preparation using NaOCl alone.[310]

Protocol for Use

MTAD was developed as a final rinse to disinfect the root canal system and remove the smear layer. The effectiveness of MTAD to completely remove the smear layer is enhanced when a low concentration of NaOCl (1.3%) is used as an intracanal irrigant before placing 1 ml of MTAD in a canal for 5 minutes and rinsing it with an additional 4 ml of MTAD as the final rinse.[457]

QMiX

QMiX was introduced in 2011; it is one of the new combination products introduced for root canal irrigation (Fig. 6-64). It is recommended to be used at the end of instrumentation, after NaOCl irrigation. According to the patent[194] QMix contains a CHX-analog, Triclosan (N-cetyl-N,N,N-trimethylammonium bromide), and EDTA as a decalcifying agent; it is intended as antimicrobial irrigant as well as an agent to remove canal wall smear layers and debris.

Protocol

QMiX is suggested as a final rinse. If sodium hypochlorite was used throughout the cleaning and shaping, saline can rinse out NaOCl to prevent the formation of PCA.

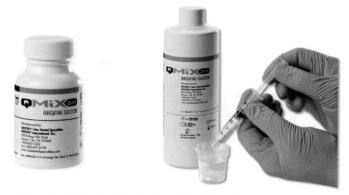

FIG 6-64 QMiX 2in1. Combination of C, EDTA and detergent. QMiX irrigating solution is a single solution used as a final rinse after bleach for one-step smear layer removal and disinfection. (Courtesy Dentsply Tulsa Dental Specialties, Tulsa, OK.)

Smear Layer Removal

Stojic and colleagues investigated the effectiveness of smear layer removal by QMiX using scanning electron microscopy.[500] QMiX removed smear layer equally well as EDTA. Dai and colleagues examined the ability of two pH versions of QMiX to remove canal wall smear layers and debris using an open canal design.[113] Within the limitations of an open-canal design, the two experimental QMiX versions are as effective as 17% EDTA in removing canal wall smear layers after the use of 5.25% NaOCl as the initial rinse.

Antibacterial Efficacy and Effect on Biofilms

Stojic and colleagues assessed,[500] in a laboratory experimental model, the efficacy of QMiX against *Enterococcus faecalis* and mixed plaque bacteria in planktonic phase and biofilms. QMiX and 1% NaOCl killed all planktonic *E. faecalis* and plaque bacteria in 5 seconds. QMiX and 2% NaOCl killed up to 12 times more biofilm bacteria than 1% NaOCl ($P < .01$) or 2% CHX ($P < .05$; $P < .001$). Wang and colleagues compared the antibacterial effects of different disinfecting solutions on young and old *E. faecalis* biofilms in dentin canals using a novel dentin infection model and confocal laser scanning microscopy.[548] Six percent NaOCl and QMiX were the most effective disinfecting solutions against the young biofilm, whereas against the 3-week-old biofilm, 6% NaOCl was the most effective followed by QMiX. Both were more effective than 2% NaOCl and 2% CHX. Morgental and colleagues showed that QMiX was less effective than 6% NaOCl and similar to 1%NaOCl in bactericidal action.[337] According to their in vitro study, it appears that the presence of dentin slurry has the potential to inhibit most current antimicrobials in the root canals system,

Moreover, Ordinola and colleagues found that several endodontic irrigants containing antimicrobial compounds such as chlorhexidine (QMiX), cetrimide, maleic acid, iodine compounds, or antibiotics (MTAD) lacked an effective antibiofilm activity when the dentin was infected intraorally.[353] The irrigant solutions 4% peracetic acid and 2.5% to 5.25% sodium hypochlorite decreased significantly the number of live bacteria in biofilms, providing also cleaner dentin surfaces ($P < .05$). They concluded that several chelating agents containing antimicrobials could not remove or kill significantly biofilms developed on intraorally infected dentin, with the exception of sodium hypochlorite and 4% peracetic acid. Dissolution ability is mandatory for an appropriate eradication of biofilms attached to dentin.

Clinical Trials

The efficacy and biocompatibility of QMiX was demonstrated via nonclinical in vitro and ex vivo studies. Further clinical research from independent investigators is needed to corroborate the findings.

Iodine Potassium Iodide

Iodine potassium iodide (IKI) is a root canal disinfectant that is used in concentrations ranging from 2% to 5%. IKI kills a wide spectrum of microorganisms found in root canals but shows relatively low toxicity in experiments using tissue cultures.[491] Iodine acts as an oxidizing agent by reacting with free sulfhydryl groups of bacterial enzymes, cleaving disulfide bonds. E. faecalis often is associated with therapy-resistant periapical infections (see Chapter 15), and combinations of IKI and CHX may be able to kill $Ca(OH)_2$-resistant bacteria more efficiently. One study evaluated the antibacterial activity of a combination of $Ca(OH)_2$ with IKI or CHX in infected bovine dentin blocks.[473] Although $Ca(OH)_2$ alone was unable to destroy E. faecalis inside dentinal tubules, $Ca(OH)_2$ mixed with either IKI or CHX effectively disinfected dentin. Others demonstrated that IKI was able to eliminate E. faecalis from bovine root dentin when used with a 15-minute contact time.[32] An obvious disadvantage of iodine is a possible allergic reaction in some patients. Although iodine is not generally considered an allergen, some patients are hypersensitive to this compound and may be considered to have an iodine "allergy."

Intracanal Medication

When treatment cannot be completed in one appointment (see Chapters 3 and 14), the surviving intracanal bacteria proliferate between appointments.[85,546] Therefore, an intracanal medication that will restrict bacterial regrowth, supply continued disinfection, and create a physical barrier can be advantageous.

Calcium Hydroxide

Calcium hydroxide is the most popular intracanal medication in use. Hermann introduced it in 1920.[215,216] Although its use was well documented for its time, evidence of its efficacy in clinical endodontics is controversial. A series of articles promoted the antibacterial efficacy of $Ca(OH)_2$ in human root canals.[85,87] Subsequent studies substantiated these reports,[354,477] and the routine use of $Ca(OH)_2$ as an interappointment intracanal medicament became widespread.[429]

However, newer clinical studies and systematic reviews failed to show a clear benefit of $Ca(OH)_2$ to further eliminate bacterial from the root canal.[372,429] $Ca(OH)_2$ mostly is used as slurry of $Ca(OH)_2$ in a water base; at body temperature, less than 0.2% of the $Ca(OH)_2$ is dissolved into Ca^{++} and OH^- ions. Because $Ca(OH)_2$ needs water to dissolve, water should be used as the vehicle for the $Ca(OH)_2$ paste. In contact with air, $Ca(OH)_2$ forms calcium carbonate ($CaCO_3$). However, this is an extremely slow process and of little clinical significance. $Ca(OH)_2$ paste, with a significant amount of calcium carbonate, feels granular because the carbonate has a very low solubility.[422,477]

$Ca(OH)_2$ is a slow-acting antiseptic; direct-contact experiments in vitro show that a 24-hour contact period is required for complete killing of enterococci.[422,477] Another study of 42 patients found that NaOCl canal irrigation reduced the bacteria level by only 61.9%, but use of $Ca(OH)_2$ in the canals for 1 week resulted in a 92.5% reduction.[463] These researchers concluded that $Ca(OH)_2$ should be used in infected cases to more predictably obtain disinfection.

In addition to killing bacteria, $Ca(OH)_2$ has the beneficial ability to hydrolyze the lipid moiety of bacterial lipopolysaccharides (LPS), thereby inactivating the biologic activity of the lipopolysaccharide and reducing its effect.[424,423] This is a desirable effect because dead cell wall material remains after the bacteria have been killed and can continue to stimulate inflammatory responses in the periradicular tissue.

The main characteristics of $Ca(OH)_2$ include limited solubility, high pH, use as a broad-spectrum antimicrobial agent, and the ability to sustain antimicrobial action for long periods.

Other Uses of $Ca(OH)_2$

Long-term calcium hydroxide treatment can be used to induce apexification of the immature tooth with pulpal necrosis before placing an obturation material such as gutta-percha in the root canal system.[155] Also, in cases where revascularization is desired, $Ca(OH)_2$ can be used instead of antibiotic pastes (for more details, see the discussion presented later in the chapter and Chapter 10).

Clinical Protocol

Calcium hydroxide should be in contact with the tissue to act. $Ca(OH)_2$ powder may be mixed with sterile water or saline and placed into the canal with using a lentulo paste filler.[371] Alternatively, the mix may be applied from sterile, single-dose packages (e.g., Calasept [J.S. Dental, Ridgefield, CT], Calcijet [Centrix, Shelton, CT], and DT Temporary Dressing [Global Dental Products, North Bellmore, NY]) (Fig. 6-65). The mixture should be thick to carry as many $Ca(OH)_2$ particles as possible; however, it should not be overdried to retain enough moisture and to promote continued dissociation with a resulting high pH. For maximum effectiveness, the root canal should be filled homogeneously to the working length.

Limitations of Calcium Hydroxide

There are some concerns regarding the use of $Ca(OH)_2$. The handling and proper placement of $Ca(OH)_2$ present a challenge to the average clinician.[296,474] Moreover, the removal of $Ca(OH)_2$ is frequently incomplete,[306] resulting in a residue covering 20% to 45% of the canal wall surfaces, even after copious irrigation with saline, NaOCl, or EDTA.[276] Residual $Ca(OH)_2$ can shorten the setting time of zinc oxide eugenol–based endodontic sealers.[315] Most notably, it may interfere with the seal of the root filling and compromise the quality of treatment. An additional concern is that $Ca(OH)_2$ is not totally effective against several endodontic pathogens, including E. faecalis and Candida albicans.[547] The ability of $Ca(OH)_2$ to completely eradicate bacteria from the root canal has been questioned. For example, in vitro studies have shown that dentin can inactivate the antibacterial activity of $Ca(OH)_2$,[193,393] and one clinical study has shown that the number of bacteria-positive canals actually increased after $Ca(OH)_2$ medication.[372] Other studies have also indicated that $Ca(OH)_2$ could not predictably eliminate bacteria or that cultures changed from negative to positive after $Ca(OH)_2$ placement.[372,546]

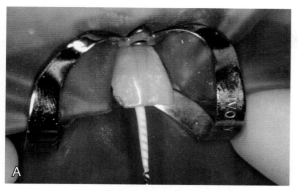
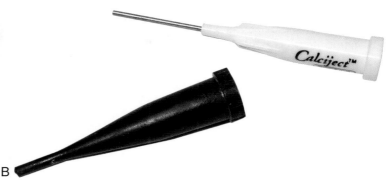

FIG. 6-65 A, Application of calcium hydroxide paste in the canal with a lentulo spiral. B, Calciject is a calcium hydroxide prefilled, easy-to-use, single-dose syringe system. Centrix NeedleTube cartridges can be used for direct syringe injection into the root canal. (A, Courtesy Dr. S. Friedman. B, Courtesy Centrix, Shelton, CT.)

When different studies report inconsistent results, a systematic review and meta-analysis technique can clarify conflicting research data and the current state of knowledge regarding specific issues. Therefore, based on the current best available evidence, $Ca(OH)_2$ has limited effectiveness in eliminating bacteria from human root canals when assessed by culture techniques. The quest for better antibacterial protocols and sampling techniques must continue to ensure that bacteria can be been reliably eradicated prior to obturation.

Phenolic Preparations

Phenol (C_6H_5OH) and phenolic preparation used to be commonly used intracanal medicament in endodontics. It was thought that because of their volatile properties, they could penetrate dentinal tubules and anatomic irregularities. However, later it was demonstrated that these compounds have a short life span, and their volatility can diffuse through the temporary fillings and also through the periapical tissue causing toxicity. Despite the severe toxicity of phenolic preparations, derivatives of phenol, such as paramonochlorophenol (C_6H_4OHCl), thymol ($C_6H_3OHCH_3C_3H_7$), and cresol ($C_6H_4OHCH_3$), remain available. Currently, $Ca(OH)_2$ or no medication is preferred.[167] Phenol is a nonspecific protoplasm poison that has an optimal antibacterial effect at 1% to 2%. Many dental preparations use much too high a concentration of phenol (e.g., in the range of 30%).[167] At such a concentration, the antimicrobial effect in vivo is lower than optimal and of very short duration.[326] Derivatives of phenol are stronger antiseptics and more toxic than phenol. Phenolic compounds are available as camphorated solutions.[491,492] Camphorated solutions result in a less toxic phenolic compound because they slow the release of toxins to the surrounding tissues. Studies in vitro have shown that phenol and phenol derivatives are highly toxic to mammalian cells, and their antimicrobial effectiveness does not sufficiently balance their toxicity.[491,492] Phenols are ineffective antiseptics under clinical conditions.[85,137]

Formaldehyde

Formaldehyde, used as formocresol, is highly toxic, mutagenic, and carcinogenic; however, it has been used extensively in endodontic therapy.[284] These formulations are still being recommended for use in pediatric dentistry when treating deciduous teeth. The formaldehyde component of formocresol may vary substantially between 19% and 37%. Tricresol formalin,

another formaldehyde preparation, contains 10% tricresol and 90% formaldehyde.[284] All of these preparations have a formaldehyde content well above the 10% normally used for fixation of pathologic specimens. Formaldehyde is volatile and releases antimicrobial vapors when applied to a cotton pellet for pulp chamber disinfection. All formaldehyde preparations are potent toxins with an antimicrobial effectiveness much lower than their toxicity.[492,493] There is no clinical reason to use formocresol as an antimicrobial agent for endodontic treatment, based on what is known at this time. The alternatives are better antiseptics with significantly lower toxicity.[492,493]

Halogens

Chlorinated solutions have been used for many years to irrigate root canals. They are also used as intracanal dressings in the form of chloramine-T, an N-chloro-tosylamide sodium salt. Iodine, in the form of IKI, is a very effective antiseptic solution with low tissue toxicity. IKI is an effective disinfectant for infected dentin and can kill bacteria in infected dentin in 5 minutes in vitro.[422] IKI releases vapors with a strong antimicrobial effect. The solution can be prepared by mixing 2 g of iodine in 4 g of potassium iodide; this mixture then is dissolved in 94 ml of distilled water. Tincture of iodine (5%) has proved to be one of the few reliable agents for disinfecting rubber dam and tooth surfaces during the preparation of an aseptic endodontic workfield.[334]

Chlorhexidine

CHX is also used as an intracanal medication and was discussed extensively earlier in this chapter.

Steroids

Steroids have been used locally, within the root canal system, to reduce pain and inflammation. Ledermix (Riemser Arzneimittel AG, Insel Riems, Germany) is a commercially available product that was developed about 1960 by Prof. André Schroeder.[450] The active ingredients are the potent anti-inflammatory corticoid triamcinolone acetonide in combination with the broad-spectrum antibiotic demeclocycline. It is an intracanal medicament paste popularly used in some countries. Ledermix paste has been advocated as an initial dressing, particularly if the patient presents with endodontic symptoms.[450] Ledermix paste contains triamcinolone acetonide as an anti-inflammatory agent, at a concentration of 1%.[261] The clinical effect is a rapid relief of pain associated with acute inflammatory conditions of the pulp and periodontium.

Ledermix paste is a nonsetting, water-soluble paste material for use as root canal medicament or as a direct or indirect pulp-capping agent. The mechanism of action of this substance is based on inhibition of the ribosomal protein synthesis in the bacteria. The release and dentin diffusion characteristics of triamcinolone from Ledermix paste when used as a root canal medicament have been investigated under different conditions.[1-3] Collectively, these studies show that triamcinolone is released from Ledermix paste in the root canal and can reach the systemic circulation via diffusion through dentinal tubules, lateral canals, and the apical foramen. Also, because of its root resorption inhibition property, it was tested for replanted teeth in dogs. The results showed that the groups treated with Ledermix, triamcinolone, and demeclocycline had significantly more favorable healing and more remaining root structure than the group filled with gutta-percha and sealer (positive control).[95]

Triple-Antibiotic Paste

The triple-antibiotics regimen, composed of metronidazole, ciprofloxacin, and minocycline, was first tested[430] for its effectiveness against *Escherichia coli*–infected dentin in vitro. The same research group also tested its bactericidal efficacy against microbes from carious dentin and infected pulp. They found that the mixture of antibiotics is sufficiently potent to eradicate the bacteria.[511] The clinical effectiveness of the triple-antibiotic paste in the disinfection of immature teeth with apical periodontitis has been reported.[557] One potential concern of using an intracanal antibiotic paste is that it may cause bacterial resistance. Additionally, intracanal use of minocycline can cause tooth discoloration, creating potential cosmetic complications. For this reason, a dual paste (metronidazole, ciprofloxacin) and, alternatively, abandonment of this protocol in favor of $Ca(OH)_2$ have been considered.[279] Another reason for such a change could be the reported high toxicity to stem cells of paste prepared from antibiotic powder.[418]

Bioactive Glass

Research is under way in the use of bioactive glass as an intracanal medicament. In one study,[578] the glass used was composed of 53% SiO_2 (w/w), 23% Na_2O, 20% CaO, and 4% P_2O_5 and was prepared from reagent-grade Na_2CO_3, $CaHPO_4$, $2H_2O$, $CaCO_3$, and Belgian sand. When used in root canals, bioactive glass was found to kill bacteria, but the mechanism of action was not pH related, and dentin did not seem to alter its effect.[578] Some newer obturating materials (e.g., Resilon; Pentron Clinical Technologies, Wallingford, CT) contain bioactive glass.

Lubricants

In root canal treatment, lubricants are mostly used to emulsify and keep in suspension debris produced by mechanical instrumentation. Although irrigation solutions serve as lubricants for hand instrumentation, special gel-type substances are also marketed. Two of these are wax-based RC-Prep, which contains EDTA and urea peroxide, and glycol-based Glyde. Another purported function of lubricants is to facilitate the mechanical action of endodontic hand or rotary files. A study evaluating the effects of lubrication on cutting efficiency found that tap water and 2.5% NaOCl solutions increased cutting efficiency compared with dry conditions.[572] The authors of this study

cited the ability of an irrigant to remove debris as the factor for the increased efficiency. Similarly, a reduction of torque scores was found when canals in normed dentin disks were prepared with ProFile and ProTaper instruments under irrigation, but the use of a gel-type lubricant resulted in similar torques as in dry, nonlubricated canals.[61,376]

In summary, irrigation is an indispensable step in root canal treatment to ensure disinfection. NaOCl is the irrigant of choice because of its tissue-dissolving and disinfecting properties. EDTA or other chelators should be used at the end of a procedure to remove the smear layer, followed by a final flush with NaOCl for 1 minute for maximum cleaning efficiency and to minimize dentin erosion. This strategy also minimizes inactivation of NaOCl by chemical interactions.

Disinfection Devices and Techniques

Syringe Delivery

Application of an irrigant into a canal by means of a syringe and needle allows exact placement, replenishing of existing fluid, rinsing out of larger debris particles, as well as allowing direct contact to microorganisms in areas close to the needle tip. In passive syringe irrigation, the actual exchange of irrigant is restricted to 1 to 1.5 mm apical to the needle tip, with fluid dynamics taking place near the needle outlet.[66,575] Volume and speed of fluid flow are proportional to the cleansing efficiency inside a root canal.[66] Therefore, both the diameter and position of the needle outlet determine successful chemomechanical debridement; placement close to working length is required to guarantee fluid exchange at the apical portion of the canal, but close control is required to avoid extrusion.[66,224,322] Therefore, the choice of an appropriate irrigating needle is important. Although larger-gauge needles allows a quicker and larger amount of fluid exchange, the wider diameter does not allow cleaning of the apical and narrower areas of the root canal system (see irrigation dynamics earlier in this chapter) (see Fig. 6-7). Excess pressure or binding of needles into canals during irrigation with no possibility of backflow of the irrigant should be avoided under all circumstances[231] to prevent extrusion into periapical spaces. In immature teeth with wide apical foramina or when the apical constriction no longer exists, special care must be taken to prevent irrigation extrusion and potential accidents.[111]

There are different sizes and types of irrigation needles. The size of the irrigation needle[101] should be chosen depending on the canal size and taper.[89,328,347] Most root canals that have not been instrumented are too narrow to be reached effectively by disinfectants, even when fine irrigation needles are used (see Figs. 6-7 and 6-52). Therefore, effective cleaning of the root canal must include intermittent agitation of the canal content with a small instrument[320,535] to prevent debris from accumulating at the apical portion of the root canal (see Fig 6-47).

Preparation size[328] and taper[105] ultimately determine how close a needle can be placed to the final apical millimeters of a root canal. Open-ended needles are recommended over the end open needles to prevent extrusion of the irrigant. Some needles and suction tips may be attached to the air/water syringe to increase both the speed of irrigant flow and the volume of irrigant. Examples include the Stropko Irrigator (Vista Dental Products), which is an adapter that connects to the air/water syringe and accepts standard Luer-lock needle tips for irrigant removal and application as well as air-drying.

Manually Activated Irrigation

Liquid placed inside the root canal more effectively reaches crevices and mechanically untouched areas if it is agitated inside the root canal. Corono-apical movements of the irrigation needle,[231] stirring movements with small endodontic instruments,[320,535] and manual push-pull movements using a fitted master gutta-percha cone have been recommended.[225]

Other than conventional irrigation, additional techniques for endodontic disinfection have been proposed and tested, including laser systems and gaseous ozone. Several new devices for endodontic irrigation or disinfection have been introduced, among which are the EndoActivator System (Dentsply Tulsa Dental Specialties), passive ultrasonic irrigation, EndoVac (Discus Dental Inc., Culver City, CA), the Safety-Irrigator (Vista Dental Products, Racine, WI), the Self-adjusting File (discussed earlier), photoactivation disinfection, and ozone. These new devices use pressure, vacuum, oscillation, or a combination with suction.

Sonically Activated Irrigation

The EndoActivator System uses safe, noncutting polymer tips in an easy-to-use subsonic hand piece to quickly and vigorously agitate irrigant solutions during endodontic therapy (Fig. 6-66).

In one study,[130] the safety of various intracanal irrigation systems was analyzed by measuring the apical extrusion of irrigant. The authors concluded that EndoActivator had a minimal statistically insignificant amount of irrigant extruded out of the apex in comparison with manual, ultrasonic, and Rinsendo (Dürr Dental, Bietigheim-Bissingen, Germany) groups.[130]

When cleanliness of the root canal walls was analyzed, [421] investigators suggested that both passive sonic or ultrasonic irrigation rendered root canals significantly cleaner than manual preparation in comparison with manual syringe irrigation.[82,533] When comparing sonic with ultrasonic irrigation, the results can be controversial. The majority of the studies benefit ultrasonic irrigation.[246,421] The difference lies in the oscillating movements: sonic devices range between 1500 Hz and 6000 Hz, and ultrasonic equipment requires vibrations greater than 20,000 Hz.[246,302,497] If sonic devices are left in the canal for longer periods of time, better cleaning effects can be found. Sonic or ultrasonic irrigation may be carried out with activated smooth wires or plastic inserts, endodontic instruments, or activated irrigation needles. Examples include EndoSonor (Dentsply Maillefer) and EndoSoft ESI (EMS Electro Medical Systems, Nyon, Switzerland) inserts, IrriSafe (Acteon Satelec), the EndoActivator System (Dentsply Tulsa Dental Specialties), and the Vibringe sonic syringe (Vibringe B.V., Amsterdam, Netherlands). Inadvertent cavitation of root canal walls has not been observed with sonic activation of instruments.[320]

Passive Ultrasonic Irrigation

Richman was the first to introduce ultrasonic devices in endodontics.[405] The files are driven to oscillate at ultrasonic frequencies of 25 to 30 kHz to mechanically prepare the root canal walls.[543,544] (See the discussion presented earlier in this chapter for more details.) It has been shown that ultrasonically driven files are effective to activate the irrigation liquids inside the root canal system by inducing acoustic streaming and cavitation.

Two types of ultrasonic irrigation have been described in the literature: one where irrigation is combined with simultaneous ultrasonic instrumentation (UI) and another without simultaneous instrumentation, called *passive ultrasonic irrigation* (PUI).[8,554] During UI, the file is intentionally brought into contact with the root canal wall. But because of the complex canal anatomy, the UI will never contact the entire wall and it may result in uncontrolled cutting of the root canal walls without effective disinfection.[8,373,560] In a study by Macedo,[307] instrument oscillation frequency, ultrasonic power, and file taper determined the occurrence and extent of cavitation. Some degree of cavitation occurred between the file and canal surface and reached lateral canals and isthmuses.

Passive ultrasonic irrigation (PUI) was first described by Weller and colleagues[554] The term *passive* is related to the noncutting action of the ultrasonically activated file.[8] PUI relies on the transmission of acoustic energy from an oscillating file or smooth wire to an irrigant in the root canal.

PUI should be introduced in the canal once that the root canal system has a final apical size and taper. A fresh solution of irrigant should be introduced and a small file or smooth wire (for example, size #15) is ultrasonically activated. Because the root canal has already been shaped, the file or wire can move more freely,[416,534,535] and the irrigant can penetrate into the apical part of the root canal system,[269] with the cleaning effect being more significant.[301] Using this noncutting methodology, the potential to create aberrant shapes within the root canal are reduced to a minimum. Obviously, a file larger than a #15 or #20 will require a wide root canal to reduce oscillation dampening by wall contact.

Ultrasonic activation of the irrigant seems to improve debridement of the root canal system in vitro, and the results in vivo present some controversy. Therefore, objective guidelines regarding their risks and benefits have not been ascertained.[286,575] Ultrasonic activation of the irrigant can be intermittent or continue. The ProUltra PiezoFlow (Dentsply Tulsa Dental Specialties) has been introduced to irrigate and activate the liquids at the same time. The device consists mainly of an ultrasonically energized needle connected to a reservoir of sodium hypochlorite (NaOCl). This continuous ultrasonic irrigation (CUI) system allows simultaneous continuous irrigant delivery and ultrasonic activation; unlike PUI,

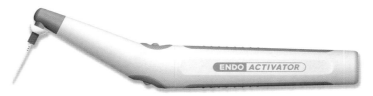

FIG. 6-66 The EndoActivator, a sonic frequency system. (Courtesy Dentsply Tulsa Dental Specialties, Tulsa, OK.)

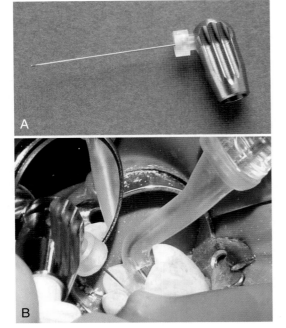

FIG. 6-67 The EndoVac system: magnification of the closed-ended micro-cannula (**A**), and clinical view of the EndoVac system combined with the Safety-Irrigator (**B**). (*A,* Courtesy Discus Dental Inc., Culver City, CA. *B,* Courtesy Dr. A. Azarpazhooh.)

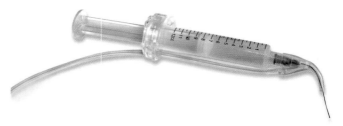

FIG. 6-68 The Safety-Irrigator. (Courtesy Vista Dental Products, Racine, WI.)

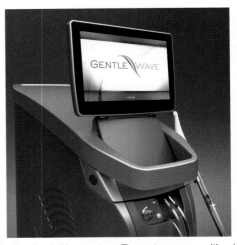

FIG. 6-69 The GentleWave system. The system uses multisonic energy to develop a broad section of waves within the irrigation solution to clean inside the roots canal system. It has two main components: a handpiece and a console (shown in figure). (Courtesy Sonendo, Inc, Laguna Hills, CA.)

it does not require the intermittent replenishment of irrigant between ultrasonic file activations. Research shows better elimination of debris and better penetration of irrigant into dentinal tubules.[6,93,247]

Negative Apical Pressure

Another approach to afford better access of irrigation solution to the apical portion of the canal is so-called negative-pressure irrigation (Fig. 6-67). Here, irrigant is delivered into the access chamber, and a very fine needle connected to the dental unit's suction device is placed into the root canal. Excess irrigant from the access cavity is then transported apically and ultimately removed via suction. First, a macrocannula, equivalent to an ISO size #55, .02 taper instrument, removes coronal debris. Subsequently, a microcannula, equivalent to a size #32, .02 taper, removes particles lodged close to working length. Such a system is commercially available (EndoVac, Discus Dental) and may prove a valuable adjunct in canal disinfection.[348] One of the main characteristics of the system is the safety. Many studies proved that EndoVac will not extrude irrigation solution through the apex. On the other hand, because the irrigation is deposited in the coronal area, the irrigant flow in the apical last millimeters of the canal is very passive, and some concerns were expressed that flow is laminar and passive in the apical region. In one study, the apical negative pressure mode of irrigation generated the lowest wall shear stress.[96]

Another device that makes use of pressure-suction technology is the RinsEndo system (Dürr Dental, Bietigheim-Bissingen, Germany). It aspirates the delivered rinsing solution into an irrigation needle that is placed close to working length and at the same time activates the needle with oscillations of 1.6 Hz amplitude.[69,322]

Safety-Irrigator

The Safety-Irrigator (Vista Dental Products) is an irrigation/evacuation system that apically delivers the irrigant under positive pressure through a thin needle containing a lateral opening and evacuates the solution through a large needle at the root canal orifice (Fig. 6-68). The Safety-Irrigator features a large coronal evacuation tube, enabling the user to safely irrigate and evacuate simultaneously. It fits any standard Luer-lock syringe. Designed to limit risk of NaOCl accidents, this "negative-pressure" irrigation device comes fully assembled and fitted with a side-vented irrigating needle for added safety. This system was tested in vitro to evaluate the removal of dentin debris from artificially made grooves in standardized root canals and showed that there was no significant difference among the manual dynamic activation (MDA) with a nontapered gutta-percha cone, the Safety Irrigator, and the apical negative pressure irrigation. These techniques produced better cleaning efficacy than syringe irrigation (P < .005) but significantly worse than MDA with a tapered cone (P < .05). Continuous ultrasonic irrigation was significantly better than all the other techniques tested in this study (P < .001).[247]

Gentle Wave System

Sonendo Inc. develops a so-called multisonic cleaning technology (Gentle Wave, Fig. 6-69) that only requires pulp chamber access. This system is noninstrumentational and being tested clinically with, according to the company, promising results. It appears to have the potential to reach inaccessible canal areas with significantly more cleaned surface than other systems. A first in vitro study shows the potential of the system to debride better than conventional needle irrigation or ultrasonically activated irrigation.[197]

Laser-Activated Irrigation

Lasers are widely used in dentistry and include diode, Nd:YAG, erbium, and CO_2, which produces radiation in both the near- and far-infrared electromagnetic spectrum.[186] Laser devices have been proposed to improve the efficacy of irrigants.[186] Lasers have been studied for their ability to clean and effectively disinfect root canals. The Er:YAG laser wavelength (2940 nm) has the highest absorption in water and a high affinity to hydroxyapatite, which makes it suitable for use in root canal treatment.[107]

Laser energy may be used to activate irrigant solutions in different ways—for example, at a molecular level, as in photo-activated disinfection (PAD), or at a bulk flow level, as in laser-activated irrigation (LAI). Several studies in vivo and ex vivo have indicated that laser activated irrigation is promising for removing smear layer[168] and dentin debris[121,122] in less time than PUI. The mechanism of action[56] is based on the generation of a secondary cavitation effect with expansion and successive implosion of fluids.[56]

These results are in agreement with data related to a new erbium laser technique that used a photon-induced photo-acoustic streaming (PIPS) of irrigants. In that technique, the laser tip is placed into the coronal access opening of the pulp chamber only and is kept stationary without advancing into the orifice of the canal.[132] The use of a newly designed tapered and stripped tip with specific minimally ablative laser settings is required, resulting in low energy (20 mJ), a pulse repetition rate of 15 Hz, and a very short pulse duration (50 μs). The difference in laser penetration and bacterial killing is attributed to the difference in the degree of absorption of different wavelengths of light within the dentin. Bergmans and colleagues concluded in their in vivo study that the Nd:YAG laser irradiation is not an alternative but a possible supplement to existing protocols for canal disinfection, as the properties of laser light may allow a bactericidal effect beyond 1 mm of dentine.[49] Endodontic pathogens that grow as biofilms, however, are difficult to eradicate even upon direct laser exposure.[65]

Photoactivation Disinfection

Photodynamic therapy (PDT) or light-activated therapy (LAT) may have endodontic applications because of its antimicrobial effectiveness.[203] In principle, antimicrobial photodynamic therapy (APDT) is a two-step procedure that involves the introduction of a photosensitizer (step 1: photosensitization of the infected tissue) followed by light illumination (step 2: irradiation of the photosensitized tissue) of the sensitized tissue, which would generate a toxic photochemistry on the target cell, leading to cell lysis. Each of these elements used independently will not have any action, but together they have a synergism effect to produce antibacterial action. Indeed, in vitro experiments showed promising results when used as an adjunct disinfected device. Shresta and Kishen concluded that the tissue inhibitors existing within the root canal affected the antibacterial activity of PDT at varying degrees,[462] and further

research is required to enhance their antimicrobial efficacy in an endodontic environment.

Antibacterial Nanoparticles

Nanoparticles are microscopic particles with one or more dimensions in the range of 1 to 100 nm. Nanoparticles are recognized to have properties that are unique from their bulk or powder counterparts. Antibacterial nanoparticles have been found to have a broad spectrum of antimicrobial activity and a far lower propensity to induce microbial resistance than antibiotics. Such nanoparticles in endodontics are being studied in different ways, such as mixed with irrigants, photo-sensitizer, and sealers.[259] Currently, the consensus is that the successful application of nanoparticles in endodontics will depend on both the effectiveness of antimicrobial nanoparticles and the delivery method used to disperse these particles into the anatomic complexities of the root canal system.

Superoxidized Water

Superoxidized water,[191] also called electrochemically activated water[313,481] or oxidative potential water,[208,455] is effectively saline that has been electrolyzed to form superoxidized water, hypochlorous acid, and free chlorine radicals. It is commercially available as Sterilox (Sterilox Technologies, Radnor, PA). This solution is nontoxic to biologic tissues yet able to kill microorganisms. The solution is generated by electrolyzing saline solution, a process no different than that used in the commercial production of NaOCl.[154] The difference, however, is that the solution accumulating at the anode is harvested as the anolyte and that at the cathode as the catholyte. These solutions display properties that are dependent on the strength of the initial saline solution, the applied potential difference, and the rate of generation. The technology that allows harvesting of the respective solutions resides in the design of the anode and the cathode and originates either in Russia (electrochemically activated water) or in Japan (oxidative potential water).[312,313] Although the solutions bear different names, the principles in the manufacturing process appear to be similar.

The use of superoxidized water is sparsely described in the endodontic literature but shows early promise. The solutions from both technologies have been tested for their ability to debride root canals,[208,313] remove smear layer,[455,481] and kill bacteria[223] and bacterial spores.[297] Results are favorable and show biocompatibility with vital systems.[237]

Anolyte and catholyte solutions generated from one such technology (Radical Waters Halfway House 1685, South Africa) have shown promise as antibacterial agents against laboratory-grown, single-species biofilm models.[169] Such solutions have been recommended as suitable for removing biofilms in dental unit water lines[312] and have even been marketed for this purpose. Cautious clinicians may prefer to wait for more studies to demonstrate safety and efficacy under ordinary clinical setting conditions before adopting newer, less tested irrigating solutions.

CRITERIA TO EVALUATE CLEANING AND SHAPING

Well-Shaped Canals

The main aims of canal shaping are to directly remove tissues and microbial irritants and to provide sufficient geometrical space for subsequent obturation (see Table 6-2). To achieve these goals, the prepared canal should include the original canal (see the red areas in Fig. 6-4); there should be an apical narrowing and the canal should be tapered. These concepts were popularized by Schilder[445] and are still maintained today.[17,258]

Therefore, a well-shaped canal is defined more specifically by the absence of procedural errors (discussed later) and the achievement of disinfection; more recently another element was added to this equation, the retention of as much tooth structure as feasible.[172]

A clinician can often determine whether a canal is adequately shaped by examining radiographs and relying on clinical experience—for example, when fitting a cone. At this time the feel would be of tug-back, a slight resistance to pull; a radiograph should show a symmetrical canal-shape lateral of the cone, the presence of an intact apical narrowing, and no thinned-out radicular wall sections.

Using magnification, clinicians should inspect the canal orifice and the coronal third of each shaped canal for clean canal walls.[367] Immediately after irrigation with sodium hypochlorite, an absence of visible turbidity and effervescence should be noted. If present, these phenomena, along with visible deposits on the canal walls, are indicative of organic matter still in suspension or adherent to the radicular walls.

Signs of Mishaps

Instrument Fracture

Most reports suggest that manual endodontic file fracture or rotary instrument fracture occur at a rate of approximately 1% to 6% and 0.4% to 5%, respectively.[365,495,531] Such fractures are untoward events and perceived as such by clinicians.[55] Evidently, retained instrument fragments limit access of disinfecting irrigants to the root canal system, possibly impeding sufficient elimination of microorganisms.[196] However, the current clinical evidence does not suggest that the presence of a retained instrument must result in a significantly higher rate of failing root canal treatments when done by specialists.[495]

In general, instruments used in rotary motion break into two distinct modes: torsional and flexural.[374,431,530] Torsional fracture occurs when an instrument tip is locked in a canal while the shank continues to rotate, thereby exerting enough torque to fracture the tip. This also may occur when instrument rotation is sufficiently slowed in relation to the cross-sectional diameter. In contrast, flexural fracture occurs when the cyclic loading leads to metal fatigue. This problem precludes the manufacture of continuously rotating stainless steel endodontic instruments, because steel develops fatal fatigue after only a few cycles.[454] NiTi instruments can withstand several hundred flexural cycles before they fracture,[201,285,394,530,567] but they still can fracture in the endodontic setting after a low (i.e., below 10,000) number of cycles.[97]

Repeated loading and cyclic fatigue tests for endodontic instruments are not described in pertinent norms. Initially, rotary instruments such as Gates-Glidden burs and Peeso reamers were tested with a superimposed bending deflection.[68] In GG burs, a 2-mm deflection of the instrument tip resulted in fatigue life spans ranging from 21,000 revolutions (size #1 burs) to 400 revolutions (size #6 burs).[68] In another study, stainless steel and NiTi hand files were rotated to failure in steel tubes with an acute 90-degree bend and an unspecified radius.[454]

Under these conditions, size #40 stainless steel instruments fractured after fewer than 20 rotations, whereas various NiTi files of the same size withstood up to 450 rotations.

Cyclic fatigue was also evaluated for ProFile .06 taper instruments using a similar device.[567,568] The number of rotations to failure for unused control instruments ranged from 1260 (size #15 files) to 900 (size #40 files). These scores did not change when the instruments were tested under simulated clinical conditions such as repeated sterilization and contact with 2.5% NaOCl. Subsequently, control instruments were compared with a group of instruments used in the clinical setting in five molar cases[568]; again, no significant differences were found in resistance to cyclic fatigue.

One study used a different testing method involving tempered metal cylinders with radii of 5 mm and 10 mm that produced a 90-degree curve.[201] The researchers reported fatigue fractures for size #15, .04 taper ProFile instruments after about 2800 cycles with the 10 mm cylinders. In size #40, .04 taper ProFile instruments, fractures occurred after about 500 cycles with the 5-mm cylinders. In comparison, size #15, .06 taper ProFile instruments also failed after about 2800 revolutions with the 10-mm cylinders, but failure occurred in size #40, .06 taper ProFile specimens after only 223 cycles with the 5-mm cylinders.

Rotary NiTi instruments with larger tapers and sizes consistently fractured after fewer rotations,[390] and although the radius of the curves was halved, fatigue life was reduced by 400%. Another investigation reported similar results for selected HERO instruments,[201] and the findings were confirmed by other tests on GT rotary instruments. Size #20, .06 taper GT files failed after 530 rotations in a 90-degree curve with a 5-mm radius; size #20, .12 taper GT files failed after 56 rotations under the same conditions.[378]

Reuse of rotary instruments depends on safety, specifically on assessment of fatigue and also the potential to properly clean NiTi surfaces.[36,63,350,357,460,486,489,525] Specific instruments perform differently in this regard, as fatigue depends more on the amount of metal in cross section at the point of stress concentration[182,523] than on the specifics of instrument design.[98]

On the other hand, manufacturers constantly claim that their instrument has been equipped with design elements that render it more fatigue resistant. For example, LightSpeed LSX is manufactured without a milling process. However, no data have been published regarding its fatigue resistance. GTX is manufactured from a novel NiTi alloy, M-Wire, to increase its fatigue resistance.[249] However, investigators could not confirm these findings.[266] Similarly, another study did not find the Twisted File,[277] which is not milled and hence thought to be fatigue resistant,[163] to perform better than conventionally manufactured ProFile rotaries. Another feature, electropolishing (discussed earlier), does not appear to confer a significantly increased fatigue resistance to EndoSequence[277,401] and RaCe.[523,525,565] One possible reason for these variable outcomes is the different testing environments used in vitro[100]; clinically, even greater variability is to be expected.

Attempts have been made to use tests according to norms and specifications described for stainless steel hand instruments such as K-files and Hedström files,[239] as no comparable norms exist for instruments used in continuous rotary motion. Consequently, a number of models have been devised to assess specific properties of NiTi rotary instruments, including torque at failure, resistance against cyclic fatigue, and others

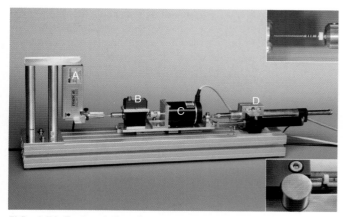

FIG. 6-70 Testing platform for analysis of various factors during simulated canal preparation with rotary endodontic instruments. Labeled components are a force transducer (**A**), a torque sensor (**B**), a direct-drive motor (**C**), and an automated feed device (**D**). For specific tests, a cyclic fatigue phantom or a brass mount compliant with ISO No. 3630-1 *(insets)* may be attached.

(Fig. 6-70). These systems may simultaneously assess torque at failure, working torque axial force, and cyclic fatigue.

According to the norms mentioned previously, torque at failure is recorded with the apical 3 mm of the instrument firmly held in the testing device while the instrument's handle is rotated. A wide variety of rotary NiTi endodontic instruments have been tested in this way—for example, ProFile NiTi rotary files in ISO sizes #25, #30, and #35 (.04 taper) fractured at 0.78, 1.06, and 1.47 Ncm, respectively.[503]

Investigators reported similar scores when instruments were forced to fracture in plastic blocks with simulated curved canals.[504] In a different setup, GT rotary instruments (size #20, .06 taper to size #20, .12 taper) fractured at 0.51 and 1.2 Ncm, respectively.[378] These values are somewhat lower than data obtained from the same but slightly modified torque bench,[254] pointing to the importance of experimental conditions for torque and fatigue measurements.

Compared with NiTi instruments with tapered flutes, LightSpeed instruments had lower torque to fracture (0.23 to 2 Ncm).[318] No such data are currently available for Light-Speed LSX.

When analyzing clinical factors involved in instrument fracture, one must consider both torsional load and cyclic fatigue.[431] However, these are not separate entities, especially in curved canals.[64] Working an instrument with high torque may lower resistance to cyclic fatigue.[161] Conversely, cyclic prestressing has been shown to reduce the torsional resistance of ProTaper finishing files,[530] as well as K3[31] and MTwo.[390] Also, cyclic fatigue occurs not only in the lateral aspect when an instrument rotates in a curved canal but also axially when an instrument is bound and released by canal irregularities.[54]

The torque generated during canal preparation depends on a variety of factors, and an important one is the contact area.[57] The size of the surface area contacted by an endodontic instrument is influenced by the instrumentation sequence or by the use of instruments with different tapers.[448] A crown-down approach is recommended to reduce torsional loads (and thus the risk of fracture) by preventing a large portion of the tapered rotating instrument from engaging root dentin (known as *taper lock*).[57,569]

The clinician can further modify torque by varying axial pressure, because these two factors are related448 (see Fig. 6-20). In fact, a light touch is recommended for all current NiTi instruments to avoid forcing the instrument into taper lock. The same effect might occur in certain anatomic situations, such as when canals merge, dilacerate, and divide.

The torsional behavior of NiTi rotary endodontic instruments cannot be described properly without advanced measurement systems and a new set of norms. However, the clinician must be able to interpret correctly the stress-strain curves for all rotary NiTi instruments used in the clinical setting to be able to choose an appropriate working torque and axial force.

Therefore, a careful evaluation should be performed before the attempt is made to remove any retained fragment (see Fig. 6-25). In fact, Ward and colleagues suggested that any attempt of fragment removal be made only when the fragment is located coronal of a significant root canal curve and thus visible with the aid of magnification.[549]

There are sophisticated means and strategies to remove retained fragments, which are described in detail in Chapter 19.

Of note, assessment of physical parameters governing rotary root canal preparation was considered crucial because NiTi rotary in vitro had increased risk of fracture compared with K-files. Some clinicians also describe instrument fracture as a main issue for concern.[55]

In a study using plastic blocks, as many as 52 ProFile Series 29 instruments became permanently deformed.[515] Three fractures were reported in a subsequent study on ISO-norm ProFile taper .04 instruments, and three other instruments were distorted.[75] An even higher fracture incidence was shown in a study on rotary instruments used in plastic blocks in a specially designed testing machine.[509] These findings were supported by two studies in which high fracture incidences were reported for LightSpeed and Quantec rotary instruments used in a clinical setting.[33,431]

On the other hand, as stated previously, a retrospective clinical study suggested similar outcomes with and without retained instrument fragments[495]; moreover, others' experience suggests that the number of rotary instrument fractures is lower than previously estimated.[126,262,558] Removal of such fragments is possible in many situations, but there is also the potential for further damage (e.g., perforation) rather than successful removal.[502,558] Consequently, a benefit-versus-risk analysis should be carried out prior to attempts to remove NiTi instrument fragments to address the reasons and the clinical consequences of instrument fracture.

Canal Transportation

Perhaps the most frequent adverse outcomes during canal shaping are aberrations from the original canal path. Much has been written on the appearance of such aberrations using labels as zip and elbow formation, ledging, perforation, stripping, and others.[553]

Canal transportation is at the root of all these clinical problems and may be defined as "the removal of canal wall structure on the outside curve in the apical half of the canal due to the tendency of files to restore themselves to their original linear shape during canal preparation."[17]

As files tend to straighten in the canal, transportation typically occurs toward the inner (or convex) radicular wall at midroot. Such a shift of the canal axis during shaping results in excessive loss of dentin and may ultimately result in perforation, whereas apical transportation may lead to zipping or apical perforation (see Fig. 6-40).

Conceptually, any canal preparation will shift the canal axis, which is often determined as the center of gravity in cross sections. It has been held that a transportation of about 100 to 150 μm may be clinically acceptable.[233]

If canal transportation has led to ledge formation, subsequent instruments will bypass the area of the ledge only when adequately precurved. In case of rotary instrumentation, hand-operated instruments of comparable size are then recommended (Fig. 6-71).

Perforation

As indicated earlier, perforation may be the ultimate result of canal transportation when it occurs within the root canal system. Other perforations are those in the access cavity; a discussion of access cavity preparation may be found in Chapter 5. Obviously, the preparation of mineralized canals requires advanced operator skills and is facilitated by magnification (Fig. 6-72).

Three types of perforations can be defined: strip perforations that occur toward the furcation in multirooted teeth (also known as "danger zones"[15]), perforations associated with canal curvatures, and perforations though the apical foramen.

Blockage

A canal may become impassable during the process of cleaning and shaping due to two distinct, but often connected, occurrences. A ledge is a dentinal shelf that is created by shaping instruments that straighten and dig into the convex side of the canal wall. In less severe cases, ledges can be corrected and smoothed out with precurved instruments. This condition may lead to false paths and impede optimal obturation when working length cannot be reached with master cones.

A blockage refers mainly to a root canal area that is filled with densely compacted debris or collagenous pulp remnants (see Fig. 6-39). It may also be caused by other obstacles such as a fractured files or remnants of a preexisting coronal or radicular filling materials. Clinically the presence of ledge or

block is signaled by the inability of a straight flexible instrument to penetrate deeper into the root canal; however, this needs to be differentiated from a small or mineralized canal, which causes longer portions of the instrument's cutting flutes to bind.

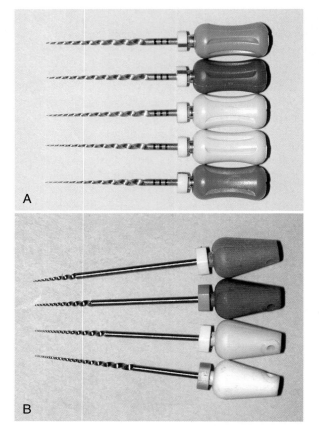

FIG. 6-71 Instruments with increased taper that can be used by hand. **A,** ProTaper instruments with special handles attached to rotary instrument shanks. **B,** GT hand instruments.

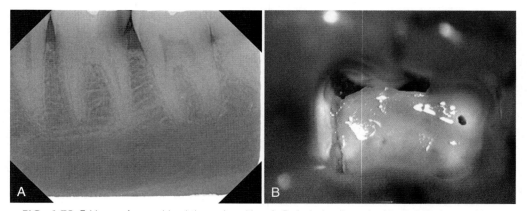

FIG. 6-72 Evidence of coronal hard-tissue deposition. **A,** Periapical radiograph of tooth #19 shows evidence of reduced coronal and radicular pulp space. **B,** Intraoral photograph, taken through an operating microscope (×25), of access cavity of the tooth shown in **A**; note the calcific metamorphosis.

Obviously, such a blockage prevents the apical canal portion from being disinfected. For details of strategies to deal with ledge and blockage, please refer to Chapter 19.

Another reason for a perceived blockage may be an abrupt canal curvature.

SAMPLE PROTOCOL FOR CONTEMPORARY CLEANING AND SHAPING PROCEDURES

- Using well-angulated preoperative radiographs, analyze case difficulty under well-established parameters.
- Place rubber dam and estimate working length.
- Prepare a conservative access cavity sufficient to reveal all root canal orifices.
- Scout canals with a #10 K-file in the presence of a lubricant.
- If the selected series of rotary instruments advances easily to the estimated working length (WL), confirm patency and determine WL using an electronic apex locator.
- If the instruments meet resistance and the file does not progress gently to WL, use a dedicated NiTi instrument; it is prudent to modify the orifice to create a coronal receptacle for the subsequent rotaries. Negotiate, confirm patency, and determine WL.
- Create a reproducible glide path to WL with appropriate instruments.
- Irrigate with sodium hypochlorite throughout the shaping procedure.
- Advance the selected series of rotary instruments (based on canal anatomy) passively in the presence of sodium hypochlorite to shape the middle third. When shaping canals that have a larger buccal-lingual dimension, consider shaping as two canals.

- Clean cutting flutes routinely upon removal, and remove debris with an alcohol-moistened gauze. If the selected rotary does not progress easily, remove irrigant, recapitulate with a #10 K-file, and choose a different, often smaller, instrument.
- Use copious irrigation, and reverify canal patency and working length throughout and upon completion of shaping. Gauge the size of the foramen with an appropriate hand file.
- Protocol for irrigation:
  - Irrigate using copious amounts of sodium hypochlorite.
  - Activate the irrigant.
  - Select irrigation solution for smear layer management.
  - Perform the final irrigation.
- Dry the canal thoroughly and obturate with a technique that promotes a three-dimensional fill.
- Restore the endodontically treated tooth in a timely manner.

SUMMARY

Cleaning and shaping are important, interdependent steps in root canal treatment. Cleaning, as demonstrated by an intracanal surface free of smear layer, can be done only after root canals have been sufficiently enlarged to accommodate adequate irrigation needles. Canal preparation is optimized when mechanical aims are fulfilled and enlargement is acceptable; such aims include avoiding both significant preparation errors and weakening of the radicular structure, which can result in fractures.

Taken together and performed to a high standard, the procedures described in this chapter lay the foundation for biologic success in both straightforward (Fig. 6-73) and more

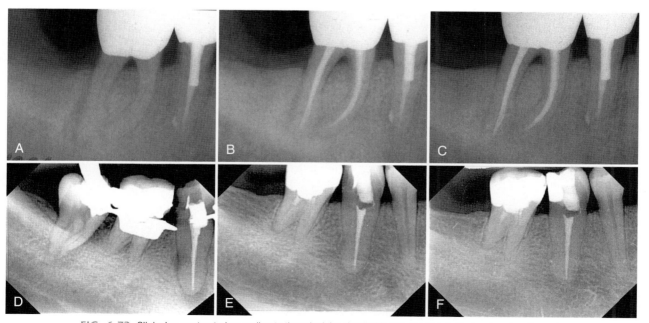

FIG. 6-73 Clinical cases treated according to the principles detailed in this chapter. **A,** Pretreatment radiograph of tooth #30 with a periradicular lesion. **B,** Postobturation radiograph. **C,** Two-year follow-up radiograph shows osseous healing. **D,** Immediate postobturation radiograph of tooth #29 shows both a periapical and a lateral osseous lesion. **E-F,** One-year and three-year follow-up radiographs show progressing osseous healing. Note the imperfect obturation of tooth #30.

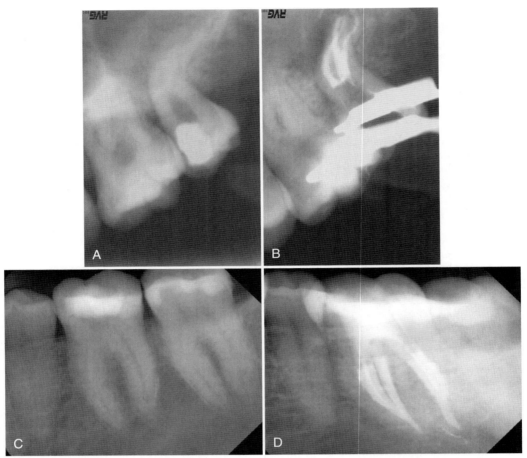

FIG. 6-74 Complicated clinical cases treated with hybrid techniques. **A,** Pretreatment radiograph of tooth #16 indicates laceration and significant curvature of all roots. **B,** Posttreatment radiograph shows multiple planes of curvature. **C,** Pretreatment radiograph of tooth #19, which was diagnosed with irreversible pulpitis. **D,** Angulated posttreatment radiograph shows three canals in the mesiobuccal root canal system, all of which were prepared to apical size #50. (*A-B,* Courtesy T. Clauder. *C-D,* Courtesy Dr. H. Walsch.)

complicated (Fig. 6-74) clinical cases. Recall radiographs confirm favorable outcomes or biologic success (i.e., prevention or healing of periradicular periodontitis) over the years. Similarly, adherence to the principles discussed leads to predictable outcomes for root canal treatments.

ACKNOWLEDGMENTS

The authors are grateful to Paul Singh, DDS; Ana Arias, DDS, PhD; Dr. Gevik Malkhassian, DDS, MSc FRCD(C); and Mr. Nicholas Epelbaum, BSc, for their invaluable help in preparing this text.

REFERENCES

1. Abbott PV, Heithersay GS, Hume WR: Release and diffusion through human tooth roots in vitro of corticosteroid and tetracycline trace molecules from Ledermix paste, *Endod Dent Traumatol* 4:55, 1988.
2. Abbott PV, Hume WR, Heithersay GS: Barriers to diffusion of Ledermix paste in radicular dentine, *Endod Dent Traumatol* 5:98, 1989.
3. Abbott PV, Hume WR, Heithersay GS: Effects of combining Ledermix and calcium hydroxide pastes on the diffusion of corticosteroid and tetracycline through human tooth roots in vitro, *Endod Dent Traumatol* 5:188, 1989.
4. Abou-Rass M, Jann JM, Jobe D, Tsutsui F: Preparation of space for posting: effect on thickness of canal walls and incidence of perforation in molars, *J Am Dent Assoc* 104:634, 1982.
5. Abou-Rass M, Piccinino MV: The effectiveness of four clinical irrigation methods on the removal of root canal debris, *Oral Surg Oral Med Oral Pathol* 54:323, 1982.
6. Adcock J, Sidow S, Looney S, et al: Histologic evaluation of canal and isthmus debridement efficacies of two different irrigant delivery techniques in a closed system, *J Endod* 37:544, 2011.
7. Ahmad M: An analysis of breakage of ultrasonic files during root canal instrumentation, *Endod Dent Traumatol* 5:78, 1989.
8. Ahmad M, Pitt Ford TJ, Crum LA: Ultrasonic debridement of root canals: acoustic streaming and its possible role, *J Endod* 13:490, 1987.
9. Al-Sudani D, Al-Shahrani S: A comparison of the canal centering ability of ProFile, K3, and RaCe nickel-titanium rotary systems, *J Endod* 32:1198, 2006.
10. Alapati SB, Brantley WA, Nusstein JM, et al: Vickers hardness investigation of work-hardening in used NiTi rotary instruments, *J Endod* 32:1191, 2006.
11. Alapati SB, Brantley WA, Svec TA, et al: Scanning electron microscope observations of new and used nickel-titanium rotary files, *J Endod* 29:667, 2003.
12. Albrecht LJ, Baumgartner JC, Marshall JG: Evaluation of apical debris removal using various sizes and tapers of ProFile GT files, *J Endod* 30:425, 2004.
13. Allison DA, Weber CR, Walton RE: The influence of the method of canal preparation on the quality of apical and coronal obturation, *J Endod* 5:298, 1979.

14. Alodeh MH, Doller R, Dummer PM: Shaping of simulated root canals in resin blocks using the step-back technique with K-files manipulated in a simple in/out filling motion, *Int Endod J* 22:107, 1989.

15. Alodeh MH, Dummer PM: A comparison of the ability of K-files and Hedstrom files to shape simulated root canals in resin blocks, *Int Endod J* 22:226, 1989.

16. Amato M, Vanoni-Heineken I, Hecker H, Weiger R: Curved versus straight root canals: the benefit of activated irrigation techniques on dentin debris removal, *Oral Surg Oral Med Oral Pathol Oral Radiol Endod* 111:529, 2011.

17. Amercian Association of Endodontists: Glossary of endodontic terms, 2012. Available at: www.aae.org/glossary.

18. Andersen M, Lund A, Andreasen JO, Andreasen FM: In vitro solubility of human pulp tissue in calcium hydroxide and sodium hypochlorite, *Endod Dent Traumatol* 8:104, 1992.

19. Anderson DN, Joyce AP, Roberts S, Runner R: A comparative photoelastic stress analysis of internal root stresses between RC Prep and saline when applied to the Profile/GT rotary instrumentation system, *J Endod* 32:222, 2006.

20. Anderson MA, Price JW, Parashos P: Fracture resistance of electropolished rotary nickel-titanium endodontic instruments, *J Endod* 33:1212, 2007.

21. Aquilino SA, Caplan DJ: Relationship between crown placement and the survival of endodontically treated teeth, *J Prosthet Dent* 87:256, 2002.

22. Arias A, Azabal M, Hidalgo JJ, de la Macorra JC: Relationship between postendodontic pain, tooth diagnostic factors, and apical patency, *J Endod* 35:189, 2009.

23. Arias A, Singh R, Peters OA: Torque and force induced by ProTaper Universal and ProTaper Next during shaping of large and small root canals in extracted teeth, *J Endod* 40:973, 2014.

24. Asboe-Jorgensen V, Attstrom R, Lang NP, Loe H: Effect of a chlorhexidine dressing on the healing after periodontal surgery, *J Periodontol* 45:13, 1974.

25. Attin T, Buchalla W, Zirkel C, Lussi A: Clinical evaluation of the cleansing properties of the noninstrumental technique for cleaning root canals, *Int Endod J*, 35:929, 2002.

26. Aubut V, Pommel L, Verhille B, et al: Biological properties of a neutralized 2.5% sodium hypochlorite solution, *Oral Surg Oral Med Oral Pathol Oral Radiol Endod* 109:e120, 2010.

27. Autegarden JE, Pecquet C, Huet S, et al: Anaphylactic shock after application of chlorhexidine to unbroken skin, *Contact Derm* 40:215, 1999.

28. Aydin C, Inan U, Yasar S, et al: Comparison of shaping ability of RaCe and Hero Shaper instruments in simulated curved canals, *Oral Surg Oral Med Oral Pathol Oral Radiol Endod* 105:e92, 2008.

29. Azarpazhooh A, Limeback H: The application of ozone in dentistry: a systematic review of literature, *J Dent* 36:104, 2008.

30. Backman CA, Oswald RJ, Pitts DL: A radiographic comparison of two root canal instrumentation techniques, *J Endod* 18:19, 1992.

31. Bahia MG, Melo MC, Buono VT: Influence of cyclic torsional loading on the fatigue resistance of K3 instruments, *Int Endod J* 41:883, 2008.

32. Baker NE, Liewehr FR, Buxton TB, Joyce AP: Antibacterial efficacy of calcium hydroxide, iodine potassium iodide, Betadine, and Betadine scrub with and without surfactant against *E faecalis* in vitro, *Oral Surg Oral Med Oral Pathol Oral Radiol Endod* 98:359, 2004.

33. Barbakow F, Lutz F: The "Lightspeed" preparation technique evaluated by Swiss clinicians after attending continuing education courses, *Int Endod J* 30:46, 1997.

34. Barbosa CA, Goncalves RB, Siqueira JF Jr, De Uzeda M: Evaluation of the antibacterial activities of calcium hydroxide, chlorhexidine, and camphorated paramonochlorophenol as intracanal medicament. A clinical and laboratory study, *J Endod* 23:297, 1997.

35. Barbosa CAM, Goncalves RB, Siqueira JF, DeUzeda M: Evaluation of the antibacterial activities of calcium hydroxide, chlorhexidine, and camphorated paramonochlorophenol as intracanal medicament. A clinical and laboratory study, *J Endod* 23:297, 1997.

36. Barbosa FO, Gomes JA, de Araujo MC: Influence of sodium hypochlorite on mechanical properties of K3 nickel-titanium rotary instruments, *J Endod* 33:982, 2007.

37. Bardsley S, Peters CI, Peters OA: The effect of three rotational speed settings on torque and apical force with vortex rotary instruments in vitro, *J Endod* 37:860, 2011.

38. Barthel CR, Zimmer S, West G, Roulet JF: Bacterial leakage in obturated root canals following the use of different intracanal medicaments, *Endod Dent Traumatol* 16:282, 2000.

39. Basmadjian-Charles CL, Farge P, Bourgeois DM, Lebrun T: Factors influencing the long-term results of endodontic treatment: a review of the literature, *Int Dent J* 52:81, 2002.

40. Reference deleted in proofs.

41. Basrani B, Ghanem A, Tjaderhane L: Physical and chemical properties of chlorhexidine and calcium hydroxide-containing medications, *J Endod* 30:413, 2004.

42. Basrani B, Haapasalo M: Update on endodontic irrigating solutions, *Endod Topics* 27:74, 2012.

43. Basrani B, Lemonie C: Chlorhexidine gluconate, *Aust Endod J* 31:48, 2005.

44. Basrani B, Santos JM, Tjäderhane L, et al: Substantive antimicrobial activity in chlorhexidine-treated human root dentin, *Oral Surg Oral Med Oral Pathol Oral Radiol Endod* 94:240, 2002.

45. Basrani B, Tjaderhane L, Santos JM, et al: Efficacy of chlorhexidine- and calcium hydroxide-containing medicaments against *Enterococcus faecalis* in vitro, *Oral Surg Oral Med Oral Pathol Oral Radiol Endod* 96:618, 2003.

46. Basrani BR, Manek S, Sodhi RN, et al: Interaction between sodium hypochlorite and chlorhexidine gluconate, *J Endod* 33:966, 2007.

47. Baugh D, Wallace J: The role of apical instrumentation in root canal treatment: a review of the literature, *J Endod* 31:330, 2005.

48. Beltz RE, Torabinejad M, Pouresmail M: Quantitative analysis of the solubilizing action of MTAD, sodium hypochlorite, and EDTA on bovine pulp and dentin, *J Endod* 29:334, 2003.

49. Bergmans L, Moisaidis P, Teughels W, et al: Bactericidal effect of Nd:YAG laser irradiation on some endodontic pathogens ex vivo, *Int Endod J* 39:547, 2006.

50. Bergmans L, Van Cleynenbreugel J, Beullens M, et al: Smooth flexible versus active tapered shaft design using NiTi rotary instruments, *Int Endod J* 35:820, 2002.

51. Bergmans L, Van Cleynenbreugel J, Beullens M, et al: Progressive versus constant tapered shaft design using NiTi rotary instruments, *Int Endod J* 36:288, 2003.

52. Berutti E, Angelini E, Rigolone M, et al: Influence of sodium hypochlorite on fracture properties and corrosion of ProTaper rotary instruments, *Int Endod J* 39:693, 2006.

53. Berutti E, Cantatore G, Castellucci A, et al: Use of nickel-titanium rotary PathFile to create the glide path: comparison with manual preflaring in simulated root canals, *J Endod* 35:408, 2009.

54. Best S, Watson P, Pilliar R, et al: Torsional fatigue and endurance limit of a size 30.06 ProFile rotary instrument, *Int Endod J* 37:370, 2004.

55. Bird DC, Chambers D, Peters OA: Usage parameters of nickel-titanium rotary instruments: a survey of endodontists in the United States, *J Endod* 35:1193, 2009.

56. Blanken J, De Moor RJ, Meire M, Verdaasdonk R: Laser induced explosive vapor and cavitation resulting in effective irrigation of the root canal. Part 1: a visualization study, *Lasers Surg Med* 41:514, 2009.

57. Blum JY, Cohen A, Machtou P, Micallef JP: Analysis of forces developed during mechanical preparation of extracted teeth using Profile NiTi rotary instruments, *Int Endod J* 32:24, 1999.

58. Blum JY, Machtou P, Ruddle C, Micallef JP: Analysis of mechanical preparations in extracted teeth using ProTaper rotary instruments: value of the safety quotient, *J Endod* 29:567, 2003.

59. Boessler C, Paqué F, Peters OA: The effect of electropolishing on torque and force during simulated root canal preparation with ProTaper shaping files, *J Endod* 35:102, 2009.

60. Boessler C, Paqué F, Peters OA: Root canal preparation with a novel nickel-titanium instrument evaluated with micro-computed tomography: canal surface preparation over time, *J Endod* 36:1068, 2010.

61. Boessler C, Peters OA, Zehnder M: Impact of lubricant parameters on rotary instrument torque and force, *J Endod* 33:280, 2007.

62. Bonaccorso A, Canatatore G, Condorelli GG, et al: Shaping ability of four nickel-titanium rotary instruments in simulated S-shaped canals, *J Endod* 35:883, 2009.

63. Bonaccorso A, Tripi TR, Rondelli G, et al: Pitting corrosion resistance of nickel-titanium rotary instruments with different surface treatments in seventeen percent ethylenediaminetetraacetic acid and sodium chloride solutions, *J Endod* 34:208, 2008.

64. Booth JR, Scheetz JP, Lemons JE, Eleazer PD: A comparison of torque required to fracture three different nickel-titanium rotary instruments around curves of the same angle but of different radius when bound at the tip, *J Endod* 29:55, 2003.

65. Boutsioukis C, Kishen A: Fluid dynamics of syringe-based irrigation to optimise anti-biofilm efficacy in root-canal disinfection, *Roots: Int Mag Endod* 2012:22, 2012.

66. Boutsioukis C, Lambrianidis T, Kastrinakis E: Irrigant flow within a prepared root canal using various flow rates: a computational fluid dynamics study, *Int Endod J* 42:144, 2009.

67. Boutsioukis C, Lambrianidis T, Verhaagen B, et al: The effect of needle-insertion depth on the irrigant flow in the root canal: evaluation using an unsteady computational fluid dynamics model, *J Endod* 36:1664, 2010.

68. Brantley WA, Luebke NH, Luebke FL, Mitchell JC: Performance of engine-driven rotary endodontic instruments with a superimposed bending deflection: V. Gates Glidden and Peeso drills, *J Endod* 20:241, 1994.

69. Braun A, Kappes D, Kruse F, Jepsen S: Efficiency of a novel rinsing device for the removal of pulp tissue in vitro, *Int Endod J* 38, 2005.

70. Briseno Marroquin B, El-Sayed MA, Willershausen-Zönnchen B: Morphology of the physiological foramen: I. Maxillary and mandibular molars, *J Endod* 30:321, 2004.

71. Briseno Marroquin B, Pistorius A, Willershausen-Zönnchen B: Canal transportation caused by a new instrumentation technique and three standard techniques, *J Endod* 22:406, 1996.

72. Brunson M, Heilborn C, Johnson DJ, Cohenca N: Effect of apical preparation size and preparation taper on irrigant volume delivered by using negative pressure irrigation system, *J Endod* 36:721, 2010.

73. Bryant ST, Dummer PMH, Pitoni C, et al: Shaping ability of .04 and .06 taper ProFile rotary nickel-titanium instruments in simulated root canals, *Int Endod J* 32:155, 1999.

74. Bryant ST, Thompson SA, Al-Omari MA, Dummer PM: Shaping ability of ProFile rotary nickel-titanium instruments with ISO sized tips in simulated root canals: Part 1, *Int Endod J* 31:275, 1998.

75. Bryant ST, Thompson SA, Al-Omari MA, Dummer PM: Shaping ability of ProFile rotary nickel-titanium instruments with ISO sized tips in simulated root canals: Part 2, *Int Endod J* 31:282, 1998.

76. Buchanan LS: The standardized-taper root canal preparation: Part 2, GT file selection and safe handpiece-driven file use, *Int Endod J* 34:63, 2001.

77. Buehler WH, Gilfrich JV, Wiley RC: Effect of low temperature phase changes on the mechanical properties of alloys near composition NiTi, *J Appl Phys* 34:1475, 1963.

78. Bui T, Mitchell JC, Baumgartner JC: Effect of electropolishing ProFile nickel-titanium rotary instruments on cyclic fatigue resistance, torsional resistance, and cutting efficiency, *J Endod* 34:190, 2008.

79. Bulem ÜK, Kecici AD, Guldass HE: Experimental evaluation of cyclic fatigue resistance of four different nickel-titanium instruments after immersion in sodium hypochlorite and/or sterilization, *J Appl Oral Sci* 21:505, 2013.

80. Bürklein S, Hinschitza K, Dammaschke T, Schäfer E: Shaping ability and cleaning effectiveness of two single-file systems in severely curved root canals of extracted teeth: Reciproc and WaveOne versus Mtwo and ProTaper, *Int Endod J* 45:449, 2012.

81. Bürklein S, Schäfer E: Apically extruded debris with reciprocating single-file and full-sequence rotary instrumentation systems, *J Endod* 38:850, 2012.

82. Burleson A, Nusstein J, Reader A, Beck M: The in vivo evaluation of hand/rotary/ultrasound instrumentation in necrotic, human mandibular molars, *J Endod* 33:782, 2007.

83. Burroughs JR, Bergeron BE, Roberts MD, et al: Shaping ability of three nickel-titanium endodontic file systems in simulated S-shaped root canals, *J Endod* 38:1618, 2012.

84. Busslinger A, Sener B, Barbakow F: Effects of sodium hypochlorite on nickel-titanium Lightspeed instruments, *Int Endod J* 31:290, 1998.

85. Byström A, Claesson R, Sundqvist G: The antibacterial effect of camphorated paramonochlorophenol, camphorated phenol and calcium hydroxide in the treatment of infected root canals, *Endod Dental Traumatol* 1:170, 1985.

86. Byström A, Sundqvist G: Bacteriologic evaluation of the effect of 0.5 percent sodium hypochlorite in endodontic therapy, *Oral Surg Oral Med Oral Pathol* 55:307, 1983.

87. Byström A, Sundqvist G: The antibacterial action of sodium hypochlorite and EDTA in 60 cases of endodontic therapy, *Int Endod J* 18:35, 1985.

88. Cabral CT, Fernandes MH: In vitro comparison of chlorhexidine and povidone-iodine on the long-term proliferation and functional activity of human alveolar bone cells, *Clin Oral Invest* 11:155, 2007.

89. Card SJ, Sigurdsson A, Ørstavik D, Trope M: The effectiveness of increased apical enlargement in reducing intracanal bacteria, *J Endod* 28:779, 2002.

90. Carrilho MR, Carvalho RM, de Goes MF, et al: Chlorhexidine preserves dentin bond in vitro, *J Dent Res* 86:90, 2007.

91. Caso A, Hung LK, Beirne OR: Prevention of alveolar osteitis with chlorhexidine: a meta-analytic review, *Oral Surg Oral Med Oral Pathol Oral Radiol Endod* 99:155, 2005.

92. Casper RB, Roberts HW, Roberts MD, et al: Comparison of autoclaving effects on torsional deformation and fracture resistance of three innovative endodontic file systems, *J Endod* 37:1572, 2011.

93. Castelo-Baz P, Martín-Biedma B, Cantatore G, et al: In vitro comparison of passive and continuous ultrasonic irrigation in simulated lateral canals of extracted teeth, *J Endod* 38:688, 2012.

94. Charles TJ, Charles JE: The "balanced force" concept for instrumentation of curved canals revisited, *Int Endod J* 31:166, 1998.

95. Chen H, Teixeira FB, Ritter AL, et al: The effect of intracanal anti-inflammatory medicaments on external root resorption of replanted dog teeth after extended extra-oral dry time, *Dent Traumatol* 28:74, 2008.

96. Chen JE, Nurbaksh B, Layton G, et al: Irrigation dynamics associated with positive pressure, apical negative pressure and passive ultrasonic irrigations: a computational fluid dynamics analysis, *Aust Endod J* 40:54, 2014.

97. Cheung GS: Instrument fractures: mechanisms, removal of fragments, and clinical outcomes, *Endod Topics* 16:1, 2009.

98. Cheung GS, Darvell BW: Low-cycle fatigue of NiTi rotary instruments of various cross-sectional shapes, *Int Endod J* 40:626, 2007.

99. Cheung GS, Liu CS: A retrospective study of endodontic treatment outcome between nickel-titanium rotary and stainless steel hand filing techniques, *J Endod* 35, 2009.

100. Cheung GS, Shen Y, Darvell BW: Does electropolishing improve the low-cycle fatigue behavior of a nickel-titanium rotary instrument in hypochlorite? *J Endod* 33:1217, 2007.

101. Chow TW: Mechanical effectiveness of root canal irrigation, *J Endod* 9:475, 1983.

102. Chugal N, Clive JM, Spångberg LSW: Endodontic infection: some biologic and treatment factors associated with outcome, *Oral Surg Oral Med Oral Pathol Oral Radiol Endod* 96:81, 2003.

103. Chugal NM, Clive JM, Spångberg LS: A prognostic model for assessment of the outcome of endodontic treatment: effect of biologic and diagnostic variables, *Oral Surg Oral Med Oral Pathol Oral Radiol Endod* 91:342, 2001.

104. Cohenca N: *Disinfection of root canal systems: the treatment of apical periodontitis*, Hoboken, NJ, 2014, Wiley Blackwell.

105. Coldero LG, McHugh S, MacKenzie D, Saunders WP: Reduction in intracanal bacteria during root canal preparation with and without apical enlargement, *Int Endod J* 35:437, 2002.

106. *Collins English Dictionary*, ed 11, England, 2003, HarperCollins.

107. Coluzzi DJ: Fundamentals of dental lasers: science and instruments, *Dent Clin North Am* 48:751, 2004.

108. Coolidge ED: The diagnosis and treatment of conditions resulting from diseased dental pulps, *J Natl Dent Assoc* 6:337, 1919.

109. Cunningham CJ, Senia ES: A three-dimensional study of canal curvatures in the mesial roots of mandibular molars, *J Endod* 18:294, 1992.

110. Custer C: Exact methods for locating the apical foramen, *J Natl Dent Assoc* 5:815, 1918.

111. Cvek M, Nord CE, Hollender L: Antimicrobial effect of root canal debridement in teeth with immature root: a clinical and microbiologic study, *Odontol Revy* 27:1, 1976.

112. D'Amario M, Baldi M, Petricca R, et al: Evaluation of a new nickel-titanium system to create the glide path in root canal preparation of curved canals, *J Endod* 39:1581, 2013.

113. Dai L, Khechen K, Khan S, et al: The effect of QMix, an experimental antibacterial root canal irrigant, on removal of canal wall smear layer and debris, *J Endod* 37:80, 2011.

114. Dakin HD: On the use of certain antiseptic substances in the treatment of infected wounds, *Br Med J* 28:318, 1915.

115. Dammaschke T, Schneider U, Stratmann U, et al: Effect of root canal dressings on the regeneration of inflamed periapical tissue, *Acta Odontol Scand* 63:143, 2005.

116. Daugherty DW, Gound TG, Comer TL: Comparison of fracture rate, deformation rate, and efficiency between rotary endodontic instruments driven at 150 rpm and 350 rpm, *J Endod* 27:93, 2001.

117. Davies A: The mode of action of chlorhexidine, *J Periodont Res Suppl* 12:68, 1973.

118. Davis JM, Maki J, Bahcall JK: An in vitro comparison of the antimicrobial effects of various endodontic medicaments on *Enterococcus faecalis*, *J Endod* 33:567, 2007.

119. Davis RD, Marshall JG, Baumgartner JC: Effect of early coronal flaring on working length change in curved canals using rotary nickel-titanium versus stainless steel instruments, *J Endod* 28:438, 2002.

120. de Castro Martins R, Bahia MG, Buono VT, Horizonte B: The effect of sodium hypochlorite on the surface characteristics and fatigue resistance of ProFile nickel-titanium instruments, *Oral Surg Oral Med Oral Pathol Oral Radiol Endod* 102:99, 2006.

121. de Groot SD, Verhaagen B, Versluis M, et al: Laser-activated irrigation within root canals: cleaning efficacy and flow visualization, *Int Endod J* 42:1077, 2009.

122. De Moor RJ, Blanken J, Meire M, Verdaasdonk R: Laser induced explosive vapor and cavitation resulting in effective irrigation of the root canal. Part 2: evaluation of the efficacy, *Lasers Surg Med* 41:520, 2009.

123. De Rossi A, Silva LA, Leonardo MR, et al: Effect of rotary or manual instrumentation, with or without a calcium hydroxide/1% chlorhexidine intracanal dressing, on the healing of experimentally induced chronic periapical lesions, *Oral Surg Oral Med Oral Pathol Oral Radiol Endod* 99:628, 2005.

124. De-Deus G, Brandão MC, Barino B, et al: Assessment of apically extruded debris produced by the single-file ProTaper F2 technique under reciprocating movement, *Oral Surg Oral Med Oral Pathol Oral Radiol Endod* 110:390, 2010.

125. De-Deus G, Namen F, Galan J, Zehnder M: Soft chelating irrigation protocol optimizes bonding quality of Resilon/Epiphany root fillings, *J Endod* 34:703, 2008.

126. DeFiore PM, Genov KA, Komaroff E, et al: Nickel-titanium rotary instrument fracture: a clinical practice assessment, *Int Endod J* 39:700, 2006.

127. Degerness RA, Bowles WR: Dimension, anatomy and morphology of the mesiobuccal root canal system in maxillary molars, *J Endod* 36:985, 2010.

128. Delany GM, Patterson SS, Miller CH, Newton CW: The effect of chlorhexidine gluconate on the root canal flora of freshly extracted necrotic teeth, *Oral Surg Oral Med Oral Pathol* 53:518, 1982.

129. Denton GW: Chlorhexidine. In Block SS, editor: *Disinfection, sterilization and preservation*, ed 4, Philadelphia, 1991, Lea & Febiger, p 274.

130. Desai P, Himel V: Comparative safety of various intracanal irrigation systems, *J Endod* 35:545, 2009.

131. Dietz DB, Di Fiore PM, Bahcall JK, Lautenschlager EP: Effect of rotational speed on the breakage of nickel-titanium rotary files, *J Endod* 26:68, 2000.

132. DiVito E, Peters OA, Olivi G: Effectiveness of the erbium: YAG laser and new design radial and stripped tips in removing the smear layer after root canal instrumentation, *Lasers Med Sci* 27:273, 2012.

133. Duerig TW: Some unresolved aspects of nitinol, *Med Sci Eng A* 438-440:69, 2006.

134. Ebo DG, Stevens WJ, Bridts CH, Matthieu L: Contact allergic dermatitis and life-threatening anaphylaxis to chlorhexidine, *J Allergy Clin Immunol* 101:128, 1998.

135. Eggert C, Peters O, Barbakow F: Wear of nickel-titanium Lightspeed instruments evaluated by scanning electron microscopy, *J Endod* 25:494, 1999.

136. ElAyouti A, Weiger R, Lost C: The ability of root ZX apex locator to reduce the frequency of overestimated radiographic working length, *J Endod* 28:116, 2002.

137. Ellerbruch ES, Murphy RA: Antimicrobial activity of root canal medicament vapors, *J Endod* 3:189, 1977.

138. Elnaghy AM: Cyclic fatigue resistance of ProTaper Next nickel-titanium rotary files, *Int Endod J* 47:1034, 2014.

139. Emilson CG, Ericson T, Heyden G, Magnusson BC: Uptake of chlorhexidine to hydroxyapatite, *J Periodont Res Suppl* 12:17, 1973.

140. Ercan E, Dalli M, Duulgergil CT, Yaman F: Effect of intracanal medication with calcium hydroxide and 1% chlorhexidine in endodontic retreatment cases with periapical lesions: an in vivo study, *J Formos Med Assoc* 106:217, 2007.

141. Ercan E, Ozekinci T, Atakul F, Gül K: Antibacterial activity of 2% chlorhexidine gluconate and 5.25% sodium hypochlorite in infected root canal: in vivo study, *J Endod* 30:84, 2004.

142. Estrela C, Estrela CR, Barbin EL, et al: Mechanism of action of sodium hypochlorite, *Braz Dent J* 13:113, 2002.

143. Estrela C, Estrela CR, Decurcio DA, et al: Antimicrobial efficacy of ozonated water, gaseous ozone, sodium hypochlorite and chlorhexidine in infected human root canals, *Int Endod J* 40:85, 2007.

144. Eun HC, Lee AY, Lee YS: Sodium hypochlorite dermatitis, *Contact Dermatitis* 11:45, 1984.

145. Evans MD, Baumgartner JC, Khemaleelakul SU, Xia T: Efficacy of calcium hydroxide: chlorhexidine paste as an intracanal medication in bovine dentin, *J Endod* 29:338, 2003.

146. Fairbourn DR, McWalter GM, Montgomery S: The effect of four preparation techniques on the amount of apically extruded debris, *J Endod* 13:102, 1987.

147. Falk KW, Sedgley CM: The influence of preparation size on the mechanical efficacy of root canal irrigation in vitro, *J Endod* 31:742, 2005.

148. Fardal O, Turnbull RS: A review of the literature on use of chlorhexidine in dentistry, *J Am Dent Assoc* 112:863, 1986.

149. Faria G, Celes MR, De Rossi A, et al: Evaluation of chlorhexidine toxicity injected in the paw of mice and added to cultured l929 fibroblasts, *J Endod* 33:715, 2007.

150. Fava LR: The double-flared technique: an alternative for biomechanical preparation, *J Endod* 9:76, 1983.

151. Fidler A: Kinematics of 2 reciprocating endodontic motors: the difference between actual and set values, *J Endod* 40:990, 2014.

152. Fouad AF, Hopson JR, Martins JB, et al: Effects of electronic dental instruments on patients with cardiac pacemakers, *J Endod* 16:188, 1990.

153. Fouad AF, Krell KV, McKendry DJ, et al: Clinical evaluation of five electronic root canal length measuring instruments, *J Endod* 16:446, 1990.

154. Frais S, Ng YL, Gulabivala K: Some factors affecting the concentration of available chlorine in commercial sources of sodium hypochlorite, *Int Endod J* 34:206, 2001.

155. Frank AL: Therapy for the divergent pulpless tooth by continued apical formation, *J Am Dent Assoc* 72:87, 1966.

156. Friedman S: Management of post-treatment endodontic disease: a current concept of case selection, *Aust Endod J* 26:104, 2000.

157. Friedman S: Prognosis of initial endodontic therapy, *Endod Topics* 2:59, 2002.

158. Friedman S, Abitbol T, Lawrence HP: Treatment outcome in endodontics: the Toronto study. Phase 1: Initial treatment, *J Endod* 29:787, 2003.

159. Gabel WP, Hoen M, Steiman HR, et al: Effect of rotational speed on nickel-titanium file distortion, *J Endod* 25:752, 1999.

160. Gambarini G: Rationale for the use of low-torque endodontic motors in root canal instrumentation, *Endod Dental Traumatol* 16:95, 2000.

161. Gambarini G: Cyclic fatigue of nickel-titanium rotary instruments after clinical use with low- and high-torque endodontic motors, *J Endod* 27:772, 2001.

162. Gambarini G, Gerosa R, De Luca M, et al: Mechanical properties of a new and improved nickel-titanium alloy for endodontic use: an evaluation of file flexibility, *Oral Surg Oral Med Oral Pathol Oral Radiol Endod* 105:798, 2008.

163. Gambarini G, Grande NM, Plotino G, et al: Fatigue resistance of engine-driven rotary nickel-titanium instruments produced by new manufacturing methods, *J Endod* 34:1003, 2008.

164. Garala M, Kuttler S, Hardigan P, et al: A comparison of the minimum canal wall thickness remaining following preparation using two nickel-titanium rotary systems, *Int Endod J* 36:636, 2003.

165. Garofalo RR, Ede EN, Dorn SO, Kuttler S: Effect of electronic apex locators on cardiac pacemaker function, *J Endod* 28:831, 2002.

166. Garvey LH, Roed-Petersen J, Husum B: Anaphylactic reactions in anaesthetised patients: four cases of chlorhexidine allergy, *Acta Anaesthesiol Scand* 45:1290, 2001.

167. Gatewood RS, Himel VT, Dorn SO: Treatment of the endodontic emergency: a decade later, *J Endod* 16:284, 1990.

168. George R, Meyers IA, Walsh LJ: Laser activation of endodontic irrigants with improved conical laser fiber tips for removing smear layer in the apical third of the root canal, *J Endod* 34:1524, 2008.

169. Ghori S, Gulabivala K, Premdas C, Spratt DA: Evaluation of the antimicrobial efficacy of electrochemically activated water on selected isolates from the root canal, *Int Endod J* 85, 2002.

170. Giardino L, Ambu E, Savoldi E, et al: Comparative evaluation of antimicrobial efficacy of sodium hypochlorite, MTAD, and Tetraclean against Enterococcus faecalis biofilm, *J Endod* 33:852, 2007.

171. Glosson CR, Haller RH, Dove B, del Rio CE: A comparison of root canal preparations using Ni-Ti hand, Ni-Ti engine-driven, and K-Flex endodontic instruments, *J Endod* 21:146, 1995.

172. Gluskin A, Peters CI, Peters OA: Minimally invasive endodontics: challenging prevailing paradigms, *Br Dent J* 216:347, 2014.

173. Gluskin AH, Brown DC, Buchanan LS: A reconstructed computerized tomographic comparison of Ni-Ti rotary GT files versus traditional instruments in canals shaped by novice operators, *Int Endod J* 34:476, 2001.

174. Goerig AC, Michelich RJ, Schultz HH: Instrumentation of root canals in molar using the step-down technique, *J Endod* 8:550, 1982.

175. Goldberg F, De Silvio AC, Manfre S, Nastri N: In vitro measurement accuracy of an electronic apex locator in teeth with simulated apical root resorption, *J Endod* 28:461, 2002.

176. Goldman M, Kronman JH, Goldman LB, et al: New method of irrigation during endodontic treatment, *J Endod* 2:257, 1976.

177. Gomes BP, Ferraz CC, Vianna ME, et al: In vitro antimicrobial activity of several concentrations of sodium hypochlorite and chlorhexidine gluconate in the elimination of Enterococcus faecalis, *Int Endod J* 34:424, 2001.

178. Gomes BP, Sato E, Ferraz CC, et al: Evaluation of time required for recontamination of coronally sealed canals medicated with calcium hydroxide and chlorhexidine, *Int Endod J* 36:604, 2003.

179. Gonzalez-Rodriguez MP, Ferrer-Luque CM: A comparison of Profile, Hero 642, and K3 instrumentation systems in teeth using digital imaging analysis, *Oral Surg Oral Med Oral Pathol Oral Radiol Endod* 97:112, 2004.

180. Goodman A, Reader A, Beck M, et al: An in vitro comparison of the efficacy of the step-back technique versus a step-back/ultrasonic technique in human mandibular molars, *J Endod* 11:249, 1985.

181. Grande NM, Plotino G, Butti A, et al: Modern endodontic NiTi systems: morphological and technical characteristics. Part I: "new generation" Ni-Ti systems, *Endod Ther* 5:11, 2005.

182. Grande NM, Plotino G, Pecci R, et al: Cyclic fatigue resistance and three-dimensional analysis of instruments from two nickel-titanium systems, *Int Endod J* 39:755, 2006.

183. Grawehr M, Sener B, Waltimo T, Zehnder M: Interactions of ethylenediamine tetraacetic acid with sodium hypochlorite in aqueous solutions, *Int Endod J* 36:411, 2003.

184. Greenstein G, Berman C, Jaffin R: Chlorhexidine: an adjunct to periodontal therapy, *J Periodontol* 57:370, 1986.

185. Grossman L, Meiman B: Solution of pulp tissue by chemical agent, *J Am Dent Assoc* 28:223, 1941.

186. Gu LS, Kim JR, Ling J, et al: Review of contemporary irrigant agitation techniques and devices, *J Endod* 35:791, 2009.

187. Guelzow A, Stamm O, Martus P, Kielbassa AM: Comparative study of six rotary nickel-titanium systems and hand instrumentation for root canal preparation, *Int Endod J* 38:743, 2005.

188. Gulabivala K: *personal communication*, 2009.

189. Gulabivala K, Ng Y-L, Gilbertson M, Eames I: The fluid mechanics of root canal irrigation, *Physiol Meas* 31:R49, 2010.

190. Gulabivala K, Patel B, Evans G, Ng Y-L: Effects of mechanical and chemical procedures on root canal surfaces, *Endod Topics* 10:103, 2005.

191. Gulabivala K, Stock CJ, Lewsey JD, et al: Effectiveness of electrochemically activated water as an irrigant in an infected tooth model, *Int Endod J* 37:624, 2004.

192. Gutmann JL, Gao Y: Alteration in the inherent metallic and surface properties of nickel-titanium root canal instruments to enhance performance, durability and safety: a focused review, *Int Endod J* 45:113, 2011.

193. Haapasalo HK, Sirén EK, Waltimo TMT, et al: Inactivation of local root canal medicaments by dentine: an in vitro study, *Int Endod J* 22:126, 2000.

194. Haapasalo M, inventor: The University Of British Columbia, assignee. Composition and method for irrigation of a prepared dental root canal. USA, 2008.

195. Haapasalo M, Shen Y, Qian W, Gao Y: Irrigation in endodontics, *Dent Clin North Am* 54:291, 2010.

196. Haapasalo M, Udnaes T, Endal U: Persistent, recurrent, and acquired infection of the root canal system post-treatment, *Endod Topics* 6:29, 2003.

197. Haapasalo M, Wang Z, Shen Y, et al: Tissue dissolution by a novel multisonic ultracleaning system and sodium hypochlorite, *J Endod* 40:1178, 2014.

198. Habets JM, Geursen-Reitsma AM, Stolz E, van Joost T: Sensitization to sodium hypochlorite causing hand dermatitis, *Contact Dermatitis* 15:140, 1986.

199. Haenni S, Schmidlin PR, Müller B, et al: Chemical and antimicrobial properties of calcium hydroxide mixed with irrigating solutions, *Int Endod J* 36:100, 2003.

200. Haikel Y, Gasser P, Allemann C: Dynamic fracture of hybrid endodontic hand instruments compared with traditional files, *J Endod* 17:217, 1991.

201. Haikel Y, Serfaty R, Bateman G, et al: Dynamic and cyclic fatigue of engine-driven rotary nickel-titanium endodontic instruments, *J Endod* 25:434, 1999.

202. Haikel Y, Serfaty R, Wilson P, et al: Mechanical properties of nickel-titanium endodontic instruments and the effect of sodium hypochlorite treatment, *J Endod* 24:731, 1998.

203. Hamblin MR, Hasan T: Photodynamic therapy: a new antimicrobial approach to infectious disease? *Photochem Photobiol Sci* 3:436, 2004.

204. Hand RE, Smith ML, Harrison JW: Analysis of the effect of dilution on the necrotic tissue dissolution property of sodium hypochlorite, *J Endod* 4:60, 1978.

205. Hargreaves KM: *Cohen's pathways of the pulp expert consult*, St. Louis, 2010, Mosby.

206. Hasselgren G: Where shall the root filling end? *NY St Dent J* 60:34, 1994.

207. Hasselgren G, Olsson B, Cvek M: Effects of calcium hydroxide and sodium hypochlorite on the dissolution of necrotic porcine muscle tissue, *J Endod* 14:125, 1988.

208. Hata G, Hayami S, Weine FS, Toda T: Effectiveness of oxidative potential water as a root canal irrigant, *Int Endod J* 34:308, 2001.

209. Hayashi Y, Yoneyama T, Yahata Y, et al: Phase transformation behaviour and bending properties of hybrid nickel-titanium rotary endodontic instruments, *Int Endod J* 40:247, 2007.

210. Haznedaroglu F, Ersev H: Tetracycline HCl solution as a root canal irrigant, *J Endod* 27:738, 2001.

211. Heard F, Walton RE: Scanning electron microscope study comparing four root canal preparation techniques in small curved canals, *Int Endod J* 30:323, 1997.

212. Heling I, Chandler NP: Antimicrobial effect of irrigant combinations within dentinal tubules, *Int Endod J* 31:8, 1998.

213. Hems RS, Gulabivala K, Ng YL, et al: An in vitro evaluation of the ability of ozone to kill a strain of *Enterococcus faecalis*, *Int Endod J* 38:22, 2005.

214. Hennessey TS: Some antibacterial properties of chlorhexidine, *J Periodont Res Suppl* 12:61, 1973.

215. Hermann B: *Calciumhydroxyd als Mittel zum Behandeln und Füllen von Zahnwurzelkanälen,* Germany, 1920, University of Würzburg.

216. Hermann BW: Dentin obliteration der wurzelkanäle nach behandlung mit calcium, *Zahnärtzl Rundschau* 888, 1930.

217. Herold KS, Johnson BR, Wenckus CS: A scanning electron microscopy evaluation of microfractures, deformation and separation in EndoSequence and Profile nickel-titanium rotary files using an extracted molar tooth model, *J Endod* 33:712, 2007.

218. Hess W: Formation of root canals in human teeth, *J Natl Dent Assoc* 3:704, 1921.

219. Hidalgo E, Dominguez C: Mechanisms underlying chlorhexidine-induced cytotoxicity, *Toxicol In Vitro* 15:271, 2001.

220. Hilfer PB, Bergeron BE, Mayerchak MJ, et al: Multiple autoclave cycle effects on cyclic fatigue of nickel-titanium rotary files produced by new manufacturing methods, *J Endod* 37:72, 2011.

221. Hilt BR, Cunningham CJ, Shen C, Richards N: Torsional properties of stainless-steel and nickel-titanium files after multiple autoclave sterilizations, *J Endod* 26:76, 2000.

222. Hjeljord LG, Rolla G, Bonesvoll P: Chlorhexidine-protein interactions, *J Periodont Res Suppl* 12:11, 1973.

223. Horiba N, Hiratsuka K, Onoe T, et al: Bactericidal effect of electrolyzed neutral water on bacteria isolated from infected root canals, *Oral Surg Oral Med Oral Pathol Oral Radiol Endod* 87:83, 1999.

224. Hsieh YD, Gau CH, Kung Wu SF, et al: Dynamic recording of irrigating fluid distribution in root canals using thermal image analysis, *Int Endod J* 40:11, 2007.

225. Huang TY, Gulabivala K, Ng YL: A bio-molecular film ex-vivo model to evaluate the influence of canal dimensions and irrigation variables on the efficacy of irrigation, *Int Endod J* 41:60, 2008.

226. Hübscher W, Barbakow F, Peters OA: Root canal preparation with FlexMaster: asessment of torque and force in relation to canal anatomy, *Int Endod J* 36:883, 2003.

227. Hübscher W, Barbakow F, Peters OA: Root canal preparation with FlexMaster: canal shapes analysed by micro-computed tomography, *Int Endod J* 36:740, 2003.

228. Hugo WB, Longworth AR: Some aspects of the mode of action of chlorhexidine, *J Pharmacol* 16:655, 1964.

229. Hugo WB, Longworth AR: The effect of chlorhexidine on the electrophoretic mobility, cytoplasmic constituents, dehydrogenase activity and cell walls of *Escherichia coli* and *Staphylococcus aureus, J Pharm Pharmacol* 18:569, 1966.

230. Hülsmann M, Gressmann G, Schäfers F: A comparative study of root canal preparation using FlexMaster and HERO 642 rotary Ni-Ti instruments, *Int Endod J* 36:358, 2003.

231. Hülsmann M, Hahn W: Complications during root canal irrigation–literature review and case reports, *Int Endod J* 33:186, 2000.

232. Hülsmann M, Heckendorff M, Lennon A: Chelating agents in root canal treatment: mode of action and indications for their use, *Int Endod J* 36:810, 2003.

233. Hülsmann M, Peters OA, Dummer PMH: Mechanical preparation of root canals: shaping goals, techniques and means, *Endod Topics* 10:30, 2005.

234. Hülsmann M, Pieper K: Use of an electronic apex locator in the treatment of teeth with incomplete root formation, *Endod Dent Traumatol* 5:238, 1989.

235. Hülsmann M, Rödig T, Nordmeyer S: Complications during root canal irrigation, *Endod Topics* 16:27, 2007.

236. Hülsmann M, Schade M, Schäfers F: A comparative study of root canal preparation with HERO 642 and Quantec SC rotary Ni-Ti instruments, *Int Endod J* 34:538, 2001.

237. Ichikawa K, Nakamura HK, Ogawa N, et al: R&D of long-term life support system by using electrochemically activated biofilm reactor of aquatic animals for space examinations, *Biol Sci Space* 13:348, 1999.

238. Ingle JI: A standardized endodontic technique using newly development instruments and filling materials, *Oral Surg Oral Med Oral Pathol* 14:83, 1961.

239. International Organization for Standardization: Dental root-canal instruments. Part 1: Files, reamers, barbed broaches, rasps, paste carriers, explorers and cotton broaches, Geneva, 1992.

240. Iqbal MK, Banfield B, Lavorini A, Bachstein B: A comparison of LightSpeed LS1 and LightSpeed LSX root canal instruments in apical transportation and length control in simulated root canals, *J Endod* 33:268, 2007.

241. Iqbal MK, Floratos S, Hsu YK, Karabucak B: An in vitro comparison of Profile GT and GTX nickel-titanium rotary instruments in apical transportation and length control in mandibular molar, *J Endod* 36:302, 2010.

242. Isom TL, Marshall JG, Baumgartner JC: Evaluation of root thickness in curved canals after flaring, *J Endod* 21:368, 1995.

243. Izu KH, Thomas SJ, Zhang P, et al: Effectiveness of sodium hypochlorite in preventing inoculation of periapical tissue with contaminated patency files, *J Endod* 30:92, 2004.

244. Javaheri HH, Javaheri GH: A comparison of three Ni-Ti rotary instruments in apical transportation, *J Endod* 33:284, 2007.

245. Jeansonne MJ, White RR: A comparison of 2.0% chlorhexidine gluconate and 5.25% sodium hypochlorite as antimicrobial endodontic irrigants, *J Endod* 20:276, 1994.

246. Jensen SA, Walker TL, Hutter JW, Nicoll BK: Comparison of the cleaning efficacy of passive sonic activation and passive ultrasonic activation after hand instrumentation in molar root canals, *J Endod* 25:735, 1999.

247. Jiang LM, Lak B, Eijsvogels LM, et al: Comparison of the cleaning efficacy of different final irrigation techniques, *J Endod* 38:838, 2012.

248. Johal S, Baumgartner JC, Marshall FJ: Comparison of the antimicrobial efficacy of 1.3% NaOCl/BioPure MTAD to 5.25% NaOCl/15% EDTA for root canal irrigation, *J Endod* 33:48, 2007.

249. Johnson E, Lloyd A, Kuttler S, Namerow K: Comparison between a novel nickel-titanium alloy and 508 nitinol on the cyclic fatigue life of ProFile 25/.04 rotary instruments, *J Endod* 34:1406, 2008.

250. Jou YT, Karabucak B, Levin J, Liu D: Endodontic working width: current concepts and techniques, *Dent Clin North Am* 48:323, 2004.

251. Jungbluth H, Peters C, Peters O, et al: Physicochemical and pulp tissue dissolution properties of some household bleach brands compared with a dental sodium hypochlorite solution, *J Endod* 38:372, 2012.

252. Karagöz-Küçükay I, Ersev H, Engin-Akkoca E, et al: Effect of rotational speed on root canal preparation with Hero 642 rotary Ni-Ti instruments, *J Endod* 29:447, 2003.

253. Keate KC, Wong M: Comparison of endodontic file tip quality, *J Endod* 16:486, 1990.

254. Kell T, Arzarpazhooh A, Peters OA, et al: Torsional profiles of new and used 20/.06 GT series X and GT rotary endodontic instruments, *J Endod* 35:1278, 2009.

255. Kerekes K, Tronstad L: Morphometric observations on root canals of human anterior teeth, *J Endod* 3:24, 1977.

256. Kerekes K, Tronstad L: Morphometric observations on the root canals of human molars, *J Endod* 3:114, 1977.

257. Kerekes K, Tronstad L: Morphometric observations on root canals of human premolars, *J Endod* 3:74, 1977.

258. Kho P, Baumgardner JC: A comparison of the antimicrobial efficacy of NaOCl/Biopure MTAD versus NaOCl/EDTA against Enterococcus faecalis, *J Endod* 32:652, 2006.

259. Kishen A: Advanced therapeutic options for endodontic biofilms, *Endod Topics* 22:99, 2012.

260. Kishor N: Oral tissue complications during endodontic irrigation-a literature review, *NY St Dent J* 79, 2013.

261. Klotz MD, Gerstein H, Bahn AN: Bacteremia after topical use of prednisolone in infected pulps, *J Am Dent Assoc* 71:871, 1965.

262. Knowles KI, Hammond NB, Biggs SG, Ibarrola JL: Incidence of instrument separation using LightSpeed rotary instruments, *J Endod* 32:14, 2006.

263. Kobayashi C, Suda H: New electronic canal measuring device based on the ratio method, *J Endod* 20:111, 1994.

264. Koch KA, Brave DG: Real World Endo Sequence file, *Dent Clin North Am* 48:159, 2004.

265. Komorowski R, Grad H, Wu XY, Friedman S: Antimicrobial substantivity of chlorhexidine-treated bovine root dentin, *J Endod* 26:315, 2000.

266. Kramkowski TR, Bahcall J: An in vitro comparison of torsional stress and cyclic fatigue resistance of ProFile GT and ProFile GT Series X rotary nickel-titanium files, *J Endod* 35:404, 2009.

267. Krause TA, Liewehr FR, Hahn CL: The antimicrobial effect of MTAD, sodium hypochlorite, doxycycline, and citric acid on *Enterococcus faecalis, J Endod* 33:28, 2007.

268. Krautheim AB, Jermann TH, Bircher AJ: Chlorhexidine anaphylaxis: case report and review of the literature, *Contact Dermatitis* 50:113, 2004.

269. Krell KV, Johnson RJ: Irrigation patterns of ultrasonic endodontic files. Part II. Diamond coated files, *J Endod* 14:535, 1988.

270. Krishan NR, Paque F, Ossareh A, et al: Impacts of conservative endodontic cavity on root canal instrumentation efficacy and resistance to fracture assessed in incisors, premolars, and molars, *J Endod* 40:8, 1160-1166, 2014.

271. Krupp JD, Brantley WA, Gerstein H: An investigation of the torsional and bending properties of seven brands of endodontic files, *J Endod* 10:372, 1984.

272. Kuhn G, Jordan L: Fatigue and mechanical properties of nickel-titanium endodontic instruments, *J Endod* 28:716, 2002.

273. Kuruvilla JR, Kamath MP: Antimicrobial activity of 2.5% sodium hypochlorite and 0.2% chlorhexidine gluconate separately and combined, as endodontic irrigants, *J Endod* 24:472, 1998.

274. Kuyk JK, Walton RE: Comparison of the radiographic appearance of root canal size to its actual diameter, *J Endod* 16:528, 1990.

275. Kyomen SM, Caputo AA, White SN: Critical analysis of the balanced force technique in endodontics, *J Endod* 20:332, 1994.

276. Lambrianidis T, Margelos J, Beltes P: Removal efficiency of calcium hydroxide dressing from the root canal, *J Endod* 25:85, 1999.

277. Larsen CM, Watanabe I, Glickman GN, He J: Cyclic fatigue analysis of a new generation of nickel titanium rotary instruments, *J Endod* 35:401, 2009.

278. Lautenschlager EP, Jacobs JJ, Marshall GW Jr, Heuer MA: Brittle and ductile torsional failures of endodontic instruments, *J Endod* 3:175, 1977.

279. Law A: Considerations for regeneration procedures, *J Endod* 39:S44, 2013.

280. Leeb J: Canal orifice enlargement as related to biomechanical preparation, *J Endod* 9:463, 1983.

281. Lenet BJ, Komorowski R, Wu XY, et al: Antimicrobial substantivity of bovine root dentin exposed to different chlorhexidine delivery vehicles, *J Endod* 26:652, 2000.

282. Leonardo MR, Tanomaru Filho M, Silva LA, et al: In vivo antimicrobial activity of 2% chlorhexidine used as a root canal irrigating solution, *J Endod* 25:167, 1999.

283. Leseberg DA, Montgomery S: The effects of Canal Master, Flex-R, and K-Flex instrumentation on root canal configuration, *J Endod* 17:59, 1991.

284. Lewis BB, Chestner SB: Formaldehyde in dentistry: a review of mutagenic and carcinogenic potential, *J Am Dent Assoc* 103:429, 1981.

285. Li UM, Lee BS, Shih CT, et al: Cyclic fatigue of endodontic nickel titanium rotary instruments: static and dynamic tests, *J Endod* 28:448, 2002.

286. Liang YH, Jiang LM, Jiang L, et al: Radiographic healing after a root canal treatment performed in single-rooted teeth with and without ultrasonic activation of the irrigant: a randomized controlled trial, *J Endod* 39:1218, 2013.

287. Lim SS, Stock CJ: The risk of perforation in the curved canal: anticurvature filing compared with the stepback technique, *Int Endod J* 20:33, 1987.

288. Lima KC, Fava LR, Siqueira JF Jr: Susceptibilities of Enterococcus faecalis biofilms to some antimicrobial medications, *J Endod* 27:616, 2001.

289. Lin J, Shen Y, Haapasalo M: A comparative study of biofilm removal with hand, rotary nickel-titanium, and self-adjusting file instrumentation using a novel in vitro biofilm model, *J Endod* 39:658, 2013.

290. Lin LM, Rosenberg PA, Lin J: Do procedural errors cause endodontic treatment failure? *J Am Dent Assoc* 136:187, 2005.

291. Lin S, Zuckerman O, Weiss EI, et al: Antibacterial efficacy of a new chlorhexidine slow release device to disinfect dentinal tubules, *J Endod* 29:416, 2003.

292. Lindskog S, Pierce AM, Blomlof L: Chlorhexidine as a root canal medicament for treating inflammatory lesions in the periodontal space, *Endod Dent Traumatol* 14:186, 1998.

293. Linsuwanont P, Parashos P, Messer HH: Cleaning of rotary nickel-titanium endodontic instruments, *Int Endod J* 37:19, 2004.

294. Loe H: Does chlorhexidine have a place in the prophylaxis of dental diseases? *J Periodont Res Suppl* 12:93, 1973.

295. Loe H, Schiott CR: The effect of mouthrinses and topical application of chlorhexidine on the development of dental plaque and gingivitis in man, *J Periodont Res* 5:79, 1970.

296. Lohbaur U, Dahl U, Dasch W, Petschelt A: Calcium release and pH of gutta-percha points containing calcium hydroxide, *J Dent Res* 272, 2001.

297. Loshon CA, Melly E, Setlow B, Setlow P: Analysis of the killing of spores of Bacillus subtilis by a new disinfectant, Sterilox, *J Appl Microbiol* 91:1051, 2001.

298. Loushine RJ, Weller RN, Hartwell GR: Stereomicroscopic evaluation of canal shape following hand, sonic, and ultrasonic instrumentation, *J Endod* 15:417, 1989.

299. Luebke NH, Brantley WA, Sabri ZI, Luebke JH: Physical dimensons, torsional performance and metallurgical properties of rotary endodontic instruments. III. Peeso drills, *J Endod* 18:13, 1992.

300. Lui JN, Kuah HG, Chen NN: Effect of EDTA with and without surfactants or ultrasonics on removal of smear layer, *J Endod* 33:472, 2007.

301. Lumley PJ, Walmsley AD: Effect of precurving on the performance of endosonic K files, *J Endod* 18:232, 1992.

302. Lumley PJ, Walmsley AD, Walton RE, Rippin JW: Cleaning of oval canals using ultrasonic or sonic instrumentation, *J Endod* 19:453, 1993.

303. Lussi A, Messerli L, Hotz P, Grosrey J: A new non-instrumental technique for cleaning and filling root canals, *Int Endod J* 28:1, 1995.

304. Lussi A, Nussbacher U, Grosrey J: A novel noninstrumented technique for cleansing the root canal system, *J Endod* 19:549, 1993.

305. Lussi A, Portmann P, Nussbacher U, et al: Comparison of two devices for root canal cleansing by the noninstrumentation technology, *J Endod* 25:9, 1999.

306. Ma JZ, Shen Y, Al-Ashaw AJ, et al: Micro-computed tomography evaluation of the removal of calcium hydroxide medicament from C-shaped root canals of mandibular second molars, *Int Endod J* in press, 2014.

307. Macedo R, Verhaagen B, Rivas DF, et al: Cavitation measurement during sonic and ultrasonic activated irrigation, *J Endod* 40:580, 2014.

308. Magnusson B, Heyden G: Autoradiographic studies of 14C-chlorhexidine given orally in mice, *J Periodont Res Suppl* 12:49, 1973.

309. Malkhassian G: Antibacterial effectiveness of a final rinse with MTAD and intracanal medication with 2% chlorhexidine gel in teeth with apical periodontitis: University of Toronto, Canada, 2007.

310. Malkhassian G, Manzur AJ, Legner M, et al: Antibacterial efficacy of MTAD final rinse and two percent chlorhexidine gel medication in teeth with apical periodontitis: a randomized double-blinded clinical trial, *J Endod* 35:1483, 2009.

311. Manzur A, González AM, Pozos A, et al: Bacterial quantification in teeth with apical periodontitis related to instrumentation and different intracanal medications: a randomized clinical trial, *J Endod* 33:114, 2007.

312. Marais JT, Brozel VS: Electro-chemically activated water in dental unit water lines, *Br Dent J* 187:154, 1999.

313. Marais JT, Williams WP: Antimicrobial effectiveness of electro-chemically activated water as an endodontic irrigation solution, *Int Endod J* 34:237, 2001.

314. Marending M, Lutz F, Barbakow F: Scanning electron microscope appearances of Lightspeed instruments used clinically: a pilot study. *Int Endod J* 31:57, 1998.

315. Margelos J, Eliades G, Verdelis C, Palaghias G: Interaction of calcium hydroxide with zinc oxide-eugenol type sealers: a potential clinical problem, *J Endod* 23:43, 1997.

316. Margolis HC, Moreno EC, Murphy BJ: Importance of high pKA acids in cariogenic potential of plaque, *J Dent Res* 64:786, 1985.

317. Marshall FJ, Pappin JB: *A crown-down pressureless preparation root canal enlargement technique*, Technique Manual, Portland, OR, 1980, Oregon Health Sciences University.

318. Marsicovetere ES, Burgess JO, Clement DJ, del Rio CE: Torsional testing of the Lightspeed nickel-titanium instrument system, *J Endod* 22:681, 1996.

319. Mayeda DL, Simon JH, Aimar DF, Finley K: In vivo measurement accuracy in vital and necrotic canals with the Endex apex locator, *J Endod* 19:545, 1993.

320. Mayer BE, Peters OA, Barbakow F: Effects of rotary instruments and ultrasonic irrigation on debris and smear layer scores: a scanning electron microscopic study, *Int Endod J* 35:582, 2002.

321. McCann JT, Keller DL, LaBounty GL: Remaining dentin/cementum thickness after hand or ultrasonic instrumentation, *J Endod* 16:109, 1990.

322. McGill S, Gulabivala K, Mordan N, Ng YL: The efficacy of dynamic irrigation using a commercially available system (RinsEndo) determined by removal of a collagen "bio-molecular film" from an ex vivo model, *Int Endod J* 41:602, 2008.

323. McGurkin-Smith R, Trope M, Caplan D, Sigurdsson A: Reduction of intracanal bacteria using GT rotary instrumentation, 5.25% NaOCl, EDTA, and Ca(OH)2, *J Endod* 31:359, 2005.

324. McRay B, Cox TC, Cohenca N, et al: A micro-computed tomography-based comparison of the canal transportation and centering ability of ProTaper Universal rotary and WaveOne reciprocating files, *Quintessence Int* 45:101, 2014.

325. Merrett SJ, Bryant ST, Dummer PM: Comparison of the shaping ability of RaCe and FlexMaster rotary nickel-titanium systems in simulated canals, *J Endod* 32:960, 2006.

326. Messer HH, Feigal RJ: A comparison of the antibacterial and cytotoxic effects of parachlorophenol, *J Dent Res* 64:818, 1985.

327. Metzger Z, Teperovich E, Zary R, et al: The Self-adjusting File (SAF). Part 1: respecting the root canal anatomy—a new concept of endodontic files and its implementation, *J Endod* 36:679, 2010.

328. Mickel AK, Chogle S, Liddle J, et al: The role of apical size determination and enlargement in the reduction of intracanal bacteria, *J Endod* 33:21, 2007.

329. Miyai K, Ebihara A, Hayashi Y, et al: Influence of phase transformation on the torsional and bending properties of nickel-titanium rotary endodontic instruments, *Int Endod J* 39:119, 2006.

330. Mize SB, Clement DJ, Pruett JP, Carnes DL Jr: Effect of sterilization on cyclic fatigue of rotary nickel-titanium endodontic instruments, *J Endod* 24:843, 1998.

331. Mizutani T, Ohno N, Nakamura H: Anatomical study of the root apex in the maxillary anterior teeth, *J Endod* 18:344, 1992.

332. Mohammadi Z: Sodium hypochlorite in endodontics: an update review, *Int Dent J* 58:329, 2008.

333. Mohammadi Z, Abbott PV: The properties and applications of chlorhexidine in endodontics, *Int Endod J* 42:288, 2009.

334. Möller AJ: Microbiological examination of root canals and periapical tissues of human teeth. Methodological studies, *Odont Tids* 74(suppl):1, 1966.

335. Möller AJ, Fabricius L, Dahlén G, et al: Influence on periapical tissues of indigenous oral bacteria and necrotic pulp tissue in monkeys, *Scan J Dent Res* 89:475, 1981.

336. Moorer WR, Wesselink PR: Factors promoting the tissue dissolving capability of sodium hypochlorite, *Int Endod J* 15:187, 1982.

337. Morgental RD, Singh A, Sappal H, et al: Dentin inhibits the antibacterial effect of new and conventional endodontic irrigants, *J Endod* 39, 2013.

338. Morgental RD, Vier-Pelisser FV, Kopper PMP, et al: Cutting efficiency of conventional and martensitic nickel-titanium instruments for coronal flaring, *J Endod* 39:1634, 2013.

339. Mullaney TP: Instrumentation of finely curved canals, *Dent Clin North Am* 23:575, 1979.

340. Müller P, Guggenheim B, Schmidlin PR: Efficacy of gasiform ozone and photodynamic therapy on a multispecies oral biofilm in vitro, *Eur J Oral Sci* 115:77, 2007.

341. Nagayoshi M, Kitamura C, Fukuizumi T, et al: Antimicrobial effect of ozonated water on bacteria invading dentinal tubules, *J Endod* 30:778, 2004.

342. Nair PN: On the causes of persistent apical periodontitis: a review. *Int Endod J* 39:249, 2006.

343. Nair PN, Sjögren U, Krey G, et al: Intraradicular bacteria and fungi in root-filled, asymptomatic human teeth with therapy-resistant periapical lesions: a long-term light and electron microscopic follow-up study, *J Endod* 16:580, 1990.

344. Nakagawa RK, Alves JL, Buono VT, Bahia MGA: Flexibility and torsional behaviour of rotary nickel-titanium PathFile, RaCe ISO 10, Scout RaCe and stainless steel K-File hand instruments, *Int Endod J* 47:290, 2014.

345. Ng YL, Mann V, Gulabivala K: A prospective study of the factors affecting outcomes of nonsurgical root canal treatment: part 1: periapical health, *Int Endod J* 44:583, 2011.

346. Ng YL, Mann V, Gulabivala K: A prospective study of the factors affecting outcomes of non-surgical root canal treatment: part 2: tooth survival, *Int Endod J* 44:610, 2011.

347. Nguy D, Sedgley C: The influence of canal curvature on the mechanical efficacy of root canal irrigation in vitro using real-time imaging of bioluminescent bacteria, *J Endod* 32:1077, 2006.

348. Nielsen BA, Baumgartner JC: Comparison of the EndoVac system to needle irrigation of root canals, *J Endod* 33:611, 2007.

349. Nordmeyer S, Schnell V, Hülsmann M: Comparison of root canal preparation using Flex Master Ni-Ti and Endo-Eze AET stainless steel instruments, *Oral Surg Oral Med Oral Pathol Oral Radiol Endod* 2010.

350. O'Hoy PY, Messer HH, Palamara JE: The effect of cleaning procedures on fracture properties and corrosion of NiTi files, *Int Endod J* 36:724, 2003.

351. Okano M, Nomura M, Hata S, et al: Anaphylactic symptoms due to chlorhexidine gluconate, *Arch Dermatol* 125:50, 1989.

352. Oncag O, Hosgor M, Hilmioglu S, et al: Comparison of antibacterial and toxic effects of various root canal irrigants, *Int Endod J* 36:423, 2003.

353. Ordinola-Zapata R, Bramante CM, Brandao Garcia R, et al: The antimicrobial effect of new and conventional endodontic irrigants on intra-orally infected dentin, *Acta Odontol Scand* epub ahead of print, 2012.

354. Ørstavik D, Haapasalo M: Disinfection by endodontic irrigants and dressings of experimentally infected dentinal tubules, *Endod Dental Traumatol* 6:142, 1990.

355. Ørstavik D, Pitt Ford TR: *Essential endodontology: prevention and treatment of apical periodontitis*, Oxford, UK, 1998, Blackwell Science.

356. Otsuka K, Ren X: Physical metallurgy of Ti–Ni-based shape memory alloys, *Progr Mat Sci* 50:511, 2005.

357. Ounsi HF, Salameh Z, Al-Shalan T, et al: Effect of clinical use of the cyclic fatigue resiatance of ProTaper nickel-titanium rotary instruments, *J Endod* 33:737, 2007.

358. Paqué F, Barbakow F, Peters OA: Root canal preparation with Endo-Eze AET: changes in root canal shape assessed by micro-computed tomography, *Int Endod J* 38:456, 2005.

359. Paqué F, Ganahl D, Peters OA: Effects of root canal preparation on apical geometry assessed by micro-computed tomography, *J Endod* 35:1056, 2009.

360. Paqué F, Musch U, Hülsmann M: Comparison of root canal preparation using RaCe and ProTaper rotary Ni-Ti instruments, *Int Endod J* 38:8, 2005.

361. Paqué F, Peters OA: Micro-computed tomography evaluation of the preparation of long oval root canals in mandibular molars with the Self-Adjusting File, *J Endod* 37:517, 2011.

362. Paqué F, Rechenberg DK, Zehnder M: Reduction of hard-tissue debris accumulation during rotary root canal instrumentation by etidronic acid in a sodium hypochlorite irrigant, *J Endod* 38:692, 2012.

363. Paquette L. The effectiveness of chlorhexidine gluconate as an intracanal medication in endodontics: an in vivo microbiological study, University of Toronto, Canada; 2004.

364. Paquette L, Legner M, Fillery ED, Friedman S: Antibacterial efficacy of chlorhexidine gluconate intracanal medication in vivo, *J Endod* 33:788, 2007.

365. Parashos P, Messer H: Rotary NiTi instrument fracture and its consequences, *J Endod* 32:1031, 2006.

366. Park H: A comparison of Greater Taper files, ProFiles, and stainless steel files to shape curved root canals, *Oral Surg Oral Med Oral Pathol Oral Radiol Endod* 91:715, 2001.

367. Parris J, Wilcox L, Walton R: Effectiveness of apical clearing: histological and radiographical evaluation, *J Endod* 20:219, 1994.

368. Patino PV, Biedma BM, Liebana CR, et al: The influence of a manual glide path on the separation of NiTi rotary instruments, *J Endod* 31:114, 2005.

369. Pereira EJ, Gomes RO, Leroy AM, et al: Mechanical behavior of M-Wire and conventional NiTi wire used to manufacture rotary endodontic instruments, *Dent Mater* 29:e318, 2013.

370. Pereira ESJ, Singh R, Arias A, Peters OA: In vitro assessment of torque and force generated by novel ProTaper Next Instruments during simulated canal preparation, *J Endod* 39:1615, 2013.

371. Peters CI, Koka RS, Highsmith S, Peters OA: Calcium hydroxide dressings using different preparation and application modes: density and dissolution by simulated tissue pressure, *Int Endod J* 38:889, 2005.

372. Peters LB, van Winkelhoff AJ, Buijs JF, Wesselink PR: Effects of instrumentation, irrigation and dressing with calcium hydroxide on infection in pulpless teeth with periapical bone lesions, *Int Endod J* 35:13, 2002.

373. Peters OA: Current challenges and concepts in the preparation of root canal systems: a review, *J Endod* 30:559, 2004.

374. Peters OA, Barbakow F: Dynamic torque and apical forces of ProFile .04 rotary instruments during preparation of curved canals, *Int Endod J* 35:379, 2002.

375. Peters OA, Barbakow F, Peters CI: An analysis of endodontic treatment with three nickel-titanium rotary root canal preparation techniques, *Int Endod J* 37:849, 2004.

376. Peters OA, Boessler C, Zehnder M: Effect of liquid and paste-type lubricants on torque values during simulated rotary root canal instrumentation, *Int Endod J* 38:223, 2005.

377. Peters OA, Gluskin AK, Weiss RA, Han JT: An in vitro assessment of the physical properties of novel Hyflex nickel-titanium rotary instruments, *Int Endod J* 45:1027, 2012.

378. Peters OA, Kappeler S, Bucher W, Barbakow F: Maschinelle Aufbereitung gekrümmter Wurzelkanäle: Messaufbau zur Darstellung physikalischer Parameter, *Schw Monatsschr Zahnmed* 111:834, 2001.

379. Peters OA, Kappeler S, Bucher W, Barbakow F: Engine-driven preparation of curved root canals: measuring cyclic fatigue and other physical parameters, *Aust Endod J* 28:11, 2002.

380. Peters OA, Morgental RD, Schulze KA, et al: Determining cutting efficiency of nickel-titanium coronal flaring instruments used in lateral action, *Int Endod J* 47:505, 2014.

381. Peters OA, Paqué F: Current developments in rotary root canal instrument technology and clinical use: a review, *Quintessence Int* 41:479, 2010.

382. Peters OA, Paqué F: Root canal preparation of maxillary molars with the self-adjusting file: a micro-computed tomography study, *J Endod* 37:53, 2011.

383. Peters OA, Peters CI, Schönenberger K, Barbakow F: ProTaper rotary root canal preparation: assessment of torque and force in relation to canal anatomy, *Int Endod J* 36:93, 2003.

384. Peters OA, Peters CI, Schönenberger K, Barbakow F: ProTaper rotary root canal preparation: effects of canal anatomy on final shape analysed by micro CT, *Int Endod J* 36:86, 2003.

385. Peters OA, Roelicke JO, Baumann MA: Effect of immersion in sodium hypochlorite on torque and fatigue resistance of nickel-titanium instruments, *J Endod* 33:589, 2007.

386. Peters OA, Schönenberger K, Laib A: Effects of four NiTi preparation techniques on root canal geometry assessed by micro computed tomography, *Int Endod J* 34:221, 2001.

387. Pettiette MT, Delano EO, Trope M: Evaluation of success rate of endodontic treatment performed by students with stainless-steel K-files and nickel-titanium hand files, *J Endod* 27:124, 2001.

388. Pham NH, Weiner JM, Reisner GS, Baldo BA: Anaphylaxis to chlorhexidine. Case report. Implication of immunoglobulin E antibodies and identification of an allergenic determinant, *Clin Exp Allergy* 30:1001, 2000.

389. Pineda F, Kuttler Y: Mesiodistal and buccolingual roentgenographic investigation of 7,275 root canals, *Oral Surg Oral Med Oral Pathol* 33:101, 1972.

390. Plotino G, Grande NM, Sorci E, et al: A comparison of cyclic fatigue between used and new Mtwo Ni–Ti rotary instruments, *Int Endod J* 39:716, 2006.

391. Plotino G, Grande NM, Sorci E, et al: Influence of a brushing working stroke on the fatigue life of NiTi rotary instruments, *Int Endod J* 40:45, 2007.

392. Portenier I, Lutz F, Barbakow F: Preparation of the apical part of the root canal by the Lightspeed and step-back techniques, *Int Endod J* 31:103, 1998.

393. Portenier I, Waltimo T, Ørstavik D, Haapasalo H: Killing of Enterococcus faecalis by MTAD and chlorhexidine digluconate with or without cetrimide in the presence or absence of dentine powder or BSA, *J Endod* 32:138, 2006.

394. Pruett JP, Clement DJ, Carnes DL Jr: Cyclic fatigue testing of nickel-titanium endodontic instruments, *J Endod* 23:77, 1997.

395. Radcliffe CE, Potouridou L, Qureshi R, et al: Antimicrobial activity of varying concentrations of sodium hypochlorite on the endodontic microorganisms Actinomyces israelii, A. naeslundii, Candida albicans and Enterococcus faecalis, *Int Endod J* 37:438, 2004.

396. Ram Z: Effectiveness of root canal irrigation, *Oral Surg Oral Med Oral Pathol* 44:306, 1977.

397. Rangel S, Cremonese R, Bryant S, Dummer PM: Shaping ability of RaCe rotary nickel-titanium instruments in simulated root canals, *J Endod* 31:460, 2005.

398. Rapisarda E, Bonaccorso A, Tripi TR, et al: The effect of surface treatments of nickel-titanium files on wear and cutting efficiency, *Oral Surg Oral Med Oral Pathol Oral Radiol Endod* 89:363, 2000.

399. Rasimick BJ, Nekich M, Hladek MM, et al: Interaction between chlorhexidine digluconate and EDTA, *J Endod* 34:1521, 2008.

400. Ray HA, Trope M: Periapical status of endodontically treated teeth in relation to the technical quality of the root filling and the coronal restoration, *Int Endod J* 28:12, 1995.

401. Ray JJ, Kirkpatrick TC, Rutledge RE: Cyclic fatigue of EndoSequence and K3 rotary files in a dynamic model, *J Endod* 33:1469, 2007.

402. Reeh ES, Messer HH: Long-term paresthesia following inadvertent forcing of sodium hypochlorite through perforation in maxillary incisor, *Endod Dental Traumatol* 5:200, 1989.

403. Regalado Farreras DC, Garcia Puente C, Estrela C: Chemical burn in an endodontist's eye during canal treatment, *J Endod* 40:1275, 2014.

404. Reynolds MA, Madison S, Walton RE, et al: An in vitro histological comparison of the step-back, sonic, and ultrasonic instrumentation techniques in small, curved root canals, *J Endod* 13:307, 1987.

405. Richman MJ: The use of ultrasonics in root canal therapy and root resection, *J Dent Med* 12:12, 1957.

406. Rickard GD, Richardson R, Johnson T, et al: Ozone therapy for the treatment of dental caries, *Cochrane Database Syst Rev* Cd004153, 2004.

407. Ricucci D, Langeland K: Apical limit of root canal instrumentation and obturation, part 2. A histological study, *Int Endod J* 31:394, 1998.

408. Ricucci D, Russo J, Rutberg M, et al: A prospective cohort study of endodontic treatments of 1,369 root canals: results after 5 years, *Oral Surg Oral Med Oral Pathol Oral Radiol Endod* 112:825, 2011.

409. Ringel AM, Patterson SS, Newton CW, et al: In vivo evaluation of chlorhexidine gluconate solution and sodium hypochlorite solution as root canal irrigants, *J Endod* 8:200, 1982.

410. Roane JB: Principles of preparation using the balanced force technique. In Hardin J, editor: *Clark's clinical dentistry*, Philadelphia, 1991, JB Lippincott, p 1.

411. Roane JB, Powell SE: The optimal instrument design for canal preparation, *J Am Dent Assoc* 113:596, 1986.

412. Roane JB, Sabala CL, Duncanson MG Jr: The "balanced force" concept for instrumentation of curved canals, *J Endod* 11:203, 1985.

413. Rocas IN, Lima KC, Siqueira JF Jr: Reduction in bacterial counts in infected root canals after rotary or hand nickel-titanium instrumentation—a clinical study, *Int Endod J* 46:681, 2013.

414. Rolla G, Loe H, Schiott CR: The affinity of chlorhexidine for hydroxyapatite and salivary mucins, *J Periodont Res* 5:90, 1970.

415. Rollison S, Barnett F, Stevens RH: Efficacy of bacterial removal from instrumented root canals in vitro related to instrumentation technique and size, *Oral Surg Oral Med Oral Pathol Oral Radiol Endod* 94:366, 2002.

416. Roy RA, Ahmad M, Crum LA: Physical mechanisms governing the hydrodynamic response of an oscillating ultrasonic file, *Int Endod J* 27:197, 1994.

417. Ruddle C: Cleaning and shaping the root canal system. In Cohen S, Burns RC, editors: *Pathways of the pulp*, ed 8, St. Louis MO, 2002, Mosby, p 231.

418. Ruparel NB, Teixeira FB, Ferraz CC, Diogenes A: Direct effect of intracanal medicaments on survival of stem cells of the apical papilla, *J Endod* 38:1372, 2012.

419. Rüttermann S, Virtej A, Janda R, Raab WH: Preparation of the coronal and middle third of oval root canals with a rotary or an oscillating system, *Oral Surg Oral Med Oral Pathol Oral Radiol Endod* 104:852, 2007.

420. Rzhanov EA, Belyeva TS: Design features of rotary root canal instruments, *ENDO (Lond)* 6:29, 2012.

421. Sabins RA, Johnson JD, Hellstein JW: A comparison of the cleaning ability of short-term sonic and ultrasonic passive irrigation after hand instrumentation in molar root canals, *J Endod* 29:674, 2003.

422. Safavi E, Spångberg LS, Langeland K: Root canal dentinal tubule disinfection, *J Endod* 16:207, 1990.

423. Safavi KE, Nichols FC: Effect of calcium hydroxide on bacterial lipopolysaccharide, *J Endod* 19:76, 1993.

424. Safavi KE, Nichols FC: Alteration of biological properties of bacterial lipopolysaccharide by calcium hydroxide treatment, *J Endod* 20:127, 1994.

425. Salehrabi R, Rotstein I: Endodontic treatment outcomes in a large patient population in the USA: an epidemiological study, *J Endod* 30:846, 2004.

426. Salzgeber RM, Brilliant JD: An in vivo evaluation of the penetration of an irrigating solution in root canals, *J Endod* 3:394, 1977.

427. Sanghvi Z, Mistry K: Design features of rotary instruments in endodontics, *J Ahmedabad Dent Coll* 2:6, 2011.

428. Sarkar NK, Redmond W, Schwaninger B, Goldberg AJ: The chloride corrosion behaviour of four orthodontic wires, *J Oral Rehab* 10:121, 1983.

429. Sathorn C, Parashos P, Messer HH: Effectiveness of single- versus multiple-visit endodontic treatment of teeth with apical periodontitis: a systematic review and meta-analysis, *Int Endod J* 38:347, 2005.

430. Sato I, Ando-Kurihara N, Kota K, Iwaku M, et al: Sterilization of infected root-canal dentine by topical application of a mixture of ciprofloxacin, metronidazole and minocycline in situ, *Int Endod J* 29:118, 1996.

431. Sattapan B, Nervo GJ, Palamara JE, Messer HH: Defects in rotary nickel-titanium files after clinical use, *J Endod* 26:161, 2000.

432. Sattapan B, Palamara JE, Messer HH: Torque during canal instrumentation using rotary nickel-titanium files, *J Endod* 26:156, 2000.

433. Saunders WP, Saunders EM: Effect of noncutting tipped instruments on the quality of root canal preparation using a modified double-flared technique, *J Endod* 18:32, 1992.

434. Saunders WP, Saunders EM: Comparison of three instruments in the preparation of the curved root canal using the modified double-flared technique, *J Endod* 20:440, 1994.

435. Schaeffer MA, White RR, Walton RE: Determining the optimal obturation length: a meta-analysis of literature, *J Endod* 31:271, 2005.

436. Schäfer E: Effects of four instrumentation techniques on curved canals: a comparison study, *J Endod* 22:685, 1996.

437. Schäfer E: Root canal instruments for manual use: a review, *Endod Dental Traumatol* 13:51, 1997.

438. Schäfer E: Effect of physical vapor deposition on cutting efficiency of nickel-titanium files, *J Endod* 28:800, 2002.

439. Schäfer E, Diey C, Hoppe W, Tepel J: Roentgenographic investigation of frequency and degree of canal curvatures in human permanent teeth, *J Endod* 28:211, 2002.

440. Schäfer E, Florek H: Efficiency of rotary nickel-titanium K3 instruments compared with stainless steel hand K-flexofile. Part 1. Shaping ability in simulated curved canals, *Int Endod J* 36:199, 2003.

441. Schäfer E, Schulz-Bongert U, Tulus G: Comparison of hand stainless steel and nickel titanium rotary instrumentation: a clinical study, *J Endod* 30:432, 2004.

442. Schäfer E, Tepel J: Cutting efficiency of Hedstrom, S and U files made of various alloys in filing motion, *Int Endod J* 29:302, 1996.

443. Schäfer E, Vlassis M: Comparative investigation of two rotary nickel-titanium instruments: ProTaper versus RaCe. Part 1: Shaping ability in simulated curved canals, *Int Endod J* 37:229, 2004.

444. Schäfer E, Vlassis M: Comparative investigation of two rotary nickel-titanium instruments: ProTaper versus RaCe. Part 2. Cleaning effectiveness and shaping ability in severely curved root canals of extracted teeth, *Int Endod J* 37:239, 2004.

445. Schilder H: Cleaning and shaping the root canal, *Dent Clin North Am* 18:269, 1974.

446. Schirrmeister JF, Strohl C, Altenburger MJ, et al: Shaping ability and safety of five different rotary nickel-titanium instruments compared with stainless steel hand instrumentation in simulated curved root canals, *Oral Surg Oral Med Oral Pathol Oral Radiol Endod* 101:807, 2006.

447. Schrader C, Ackermann M, Barbakow F: Step-by-step description of a rotary root canal preparation technique, *Int Endod J* 32:312, 1999.

448. Schrader C, Peters OA: Analysis of torque and force during step-back with differently tapered rotary endodontic instruments in vitro, *J Endod* 31:120, 2005.

449. Schrader C, Sener B, Barbakow F: Evaluating the sizes of Lightspeed instruments, *Int Endod J* 31:295, 1998.

450. Schroeder A: [Ledermix 1962—Ledermix today. Evaluation after 13 years of experience], *Zahnarztl Prax* 26:195, 1975.

451. Scully C, Ng YL, Gulabivala K: Systemic complications due to endodontic manipulations, *Endod Topics* 4:60, 2003.

452. Seidberg BH, Schilder H: An evaluation of EDTA in endodontics, *Oral Surg Oral Med Oral Pathol* 37:609, 1974.

453. Senia ES, Marshall FJ, Rosen S: The solvent action of sodium hypochlorite on pulp tissue of extracted teeth, *Oral Surg Oral Med Oral Pathol* 31:96, 1971.

454. Serene TP, Adams JD, Saxena A: *Nickel-titanium instruments: applications in endodontics*, St. Louis, 1995, Ishiaku EuroAmerica.

455. Serper A, Calt S, Dogan AL, et al: Comparison of the cytotoxic effects and smear layer removing capacity of oxidative potential water, NaOCl and EDTA, *J Oral Sci* 43:233, 2001.

456. Seto BG, Nicholls JI, Harrington GW: Torsional properties of twisted and machined endodontic files, *J Endod* 16:355, 1990.

457. Shabahang S, Pouresmail M, Torabinejad M: In vitro antimicrobial efficacy of MTAD and sodium hypochlorite, *J Endod* 29:450, 2003.

458. Shabahang S, Torabinejad M: Effect of MTAD on Enterococcus faecalis-contaminated root canals of extracted human teeth, *J Endod* 29:576, 2003.

459. Shadid DB, Nicholls JI, Steiner JC: A comparison of curved canal transportation with balanced force versus lightspeed, *J Endod* 24:651, 1998.

460. Shen Y, Cheung GS, Bian Z, Peng B: Comparison of defects in ProFile and ProTaper systems after clinical use, *J Endod* 32:61, 2006.

461. Shen Y, Zhou HM, Zheng Y-F, et al: Current challenges and concepts of the thermomechanical treatment of nickel-titanium instruments, *J Endod* 39:163, 2013.

462. Shresta A, Kishen A: The effect of tissue inhibitors on the antibacterial activity of chitosan nanoparticles and photodynamic therapy, *J Endod* 38:1275, 2012.

463. Shuping GB, Ørstavik D, Sigurdsson A, Trope M: Reduction of intracanal bacteria using nickel-titanium rotary instrumentation and various medications, *J Endod* 26:751, 2000.

464. Silvaggio J, Hicks ML: Effect of heat sterilization on the torsional properties of rotary nickel-titanium endodontic files, *J Endod* 23:731, 1997.

465. Sipert CR, Hussne RP, Nishiyama CK, Torres SA: In vitro antimicrobial activity of Fill Canal, Sealapex, Mineral Trioxide Aggregate, Portland cement and EndoRez, *Int Endod J* 38:539, 2005.

466. Siqueira JF Jr: Aetiology of root canal treatment failure: why well-treated teeth can fail, *Int Endod J* 34:1, 2001.

467. Siqueira JF Jr, Batista MM, Fraga RC, de Uzeda M: Antibacterial effects of endodontic irrigants on black-pigmented gram-negative anaerobes and facultative bacteria, *J Endod* 24:414, 1998.

468. Siqueira JF Jr, de Uzeda M: Intracanal medicaments: evaluation of the antibacterial effects of chlorhexidine, metronidazole, and calcium hydroxide associated with three vehicles, *J Endod* 23:167, 1997.

469. Siqueira JF Jr, Paiva SS, Rocas IN: Reduction in the cultivable bacterial populations in infected root canals by a chlorhexidine-based antimicrobial protocol, *J Endod* 33:541, 2007.

470. Siqueira JF Jr, Rocas IN, Favieri A, Lima KC: Chemomechanical reduction of the bacterial population in the root canal after instrumentation and irrigation with 1%, 2.5%, and 5.25% sodium hypochlorite, *J Endod* 26:331, 2000.

471. Siqueira JF Jr, Rocas IN, Paiva SS, et al: Bacteriologic investigation of the effects of sodium hypochlorite and chlorhexidine during the endodontic treatment of teeth with apical periodontitis, *Oral Surg Oral Med Oral Pathol Oral Radiol Endod* 104:122, 2007.

472. Siqueira JFJ, Alves FR, Almeida BM, et al: Ability of chemomechanical preparation with either rotary instruments or self-adjusting file to disinfect oval-shaped root canals, *J Endod* 36:1860, 2010.

473. Siren EK, Haapasalo MPP, Waltimo TMT, Ørstavik D: In vitro antibacterial effect of calcium hydroxide combined with chlorhexidine or iodine potassium iodide on Enterococcus faecalis, *Eur J Oral Sci* 112:326, 2004.

474. Siren EK, Lavonious E, Kontakiotis E: Effects of Ca(OH)2 gutta-percha points on bacteria in root canals, *J Dent Res* 543, 2000.

475. Sirtes G, Waltimo T, Schaetzle M, Zehnder M: The effects of temperature on sodium hypochlorite short-term stability, pulp dissolution capacity, and antimicrobial efficacy, *J Endod* 31:669, 2005.

476. Sjögren U, Figdor D, Persson S, Sundqvist G: Influence of infection at the time of root filling on the outcome of endodontic treatment of teeth with apical periodontitis, *Int Endod J* 30:297, 1997.

477. Sjögren U, Figdor D, Spångberg L, Sundqvist G: The antimicrobial effect of calcium hydroxide as a short-term intracanal dressing, *Int Endod J* 24:119, 1991.

478. Sjögren U, Hagglund B, Sundqvist G, Wing K: Factors affecting the long-term results of endodontic treatment, *J Endod* 16:498, 1990.

479. Snellman E, Rantanen T: Severe anaphylaxis after a chlorhexidine bath, *J Am Acad Dermatol* 40:771, 1999.

480. Soares JA, Leonardo MR, da Silva LA, et al: Effect of rotary instrumentation and of the association of calcium hydroxide and chlorhexidine on the antisepsis of the root canal system in dogs, *Braz Oral Res* 20:120, 2006.

481. Solovyeva AM, Dummer PM: Cleaning effectiveness of root canal irrigation with electrochemically activated anolyte and catholyte solutions: a pilot study, *Int Endod J* 33:494, 2000.

482. Song YL, Bian Z, Fan B, et al: A comparison of instrument-centering ability within the root canal for three contemporary instrumentation techniques, *Int Endod J* 37:265, 2004.

483. Sonntag D: Schneidengeometrie und Efficienz vollrotierender Nickel-Titan-Feilen (in German), *Endodontie* 12:229, 2003.

484. Sonntag D, Delschen S, Stachniss V: Root-canal shaping with manual and rotary Ni-Ti files performed by students, *Int Endod J* 36:715, 2003.

485. Sonntag D, Guntermann A, Kim SK, Stachniss V: Root canal shaping with manual stainless steel files and rotary Ni-Ti files performed by students, *Int Endod J* 36:246, 2003.

486. Sonntag D, Peters OA: Effect of prion decontamination protocols on nickel-titanium rotary surfaces, *J Endod* 33:442, 2007.

487. Southard DW, Oswald RJ, Natkin E: Instrumentation of curved molar root canals with the Roane technique, *J Endod* 13:479, 1987.

488. Southard SR, Drisko CL, Killoy WJ, et al: The effect of 2% chlorhexidine digluconate irrigation on clinical parameters and the level of Bacteroides gingivalis in periodontal pockets, *J Periodontol* 60:302, 1989.

489. Spanaki-Voreadi AP, Kerezoudis NP, Zinelis S: Failure mechanism of ProTaper Ni-Ti rotary instruments during

clinical use: fractographic analysis, *Int Endod J* 39:171, 2006.

490. Spångberg L: Instruments, materials, and devices. In Cohen S, Burns RC, editors: *Pathways of the pulp*, ed 7, St. Louis, MO, 1998, Mosby, p 476.

491. Spångberg L, Engström B, Langeland K: Biologic effects of dental materials. 3. Toxicity and antimicrobial effect of endodontic antiseptics in vitro, *Oral Surg Oral Med Oral Pathol* 36:856, 1973.

492. Spångberg L, Rutberg M, Rydinge E: Biologic effects of endodontic antimicrobial agents, *J Endod* 5:166, 1979.

493. Spångberg LS, Barbosa SV, Lavigne GD: AH 26 releases formaldehyde, *J Endod* 19:596, 1993.

494. Spencer NCO, Sunday JJ, Georgina OKEO, et al: Comparative stabilizing effects of some anticoagulants on fasting blood glucose of diabetics and non-diabetics, determined by spectrophotometry (glucose oxidase), *Asian J Med Sc* 3:234, 2011.

495. Spili P, Parashos P, Messer HH: The impact of instrument fracture on outcome of endodontic treatment, *J Endod* 31:845, 2005.

496. Stabholz A, Rotstein I, Torabinejad M: Effect of preflaring on tactile detection of the apical constriction, *J Endod* 21:92, 1995.

497. Stamos DE, Squitieri ML, Costas JF, Gerstein H: Use of ultrasonics in single-visit endodontic therapy, *J Endod* 13:246, 1987.

498. Stenman E, Spångberg LS: Machining efficiency of Flex-R, K-Flex, Trio-Cut, and S Files, *J Endod* 16:575, 1990.

499. Stenman E, Spångberg LS: Root canal instruments are poorly standardized, *J Endod* 19:327, 1993.

500. Stojic S, Shen Y, Qian W, et al: Antibacterial and smear layer removal ability of a novel irrigant, QMiX, *J Endod* 45:363, 2012.

501. Sunada I: New method for measuring the length of the root canal, *J Dent Res* 41:375, 1962.

502. Suter B, Lussi A, Sequiera P: Probability of removing fractured instruments from root canals, *Int Endod J* 38:112, 2005.

503. Svec TA, Powers JM: Effects of simulated clinical conditions on nickel-titanium rotary files, *J Endod* 25:759, 1999.

504. Svec TA, Powers JM: A method to assess rotary nickel-titanium files, *J Endod* 26:517, 2000.

505. Tan BT, Messer HH: The quality of apical canal preparation using hand and rotary instruments with specific criteria for enlargement based on initial apical file size, *J Endod* 28:658, 2002.

506. Tanomaru Filho M, Leonardo MR, da Silva LA: Effect of irrigating solution and calcium hydroxide root canal dressing on the repair of apical and periapical tissues of teeth with periapical lesion, *J Endod* 28:295, 2002.

507. Tay FR, Hosoya Y, Loushine RJ, et al: Ultrastructure of intraradicular dentin after irrigation with BioPure MTAD. II. The consequence of obturation with an epoxy resin-based sealer, *J Endod* 32:473, 2006.

508. Tay FR, Pashley DH, Loushine RJ, et al: Ultrastructure of smear layer-covered intraradicular dentin after irrigation with BioPure MTAD, *J Endod* 32:218, 2006.

509. Tepel J: *Experimentelle Untersuchungen über die maschinelle Wurzelkanalaufbereitung*, Berlin, Germany, 2000, Quintessenz Verlags-GmbH.

510. Testarelli L, Plotino G, Al-Sudani D, et al: Bending properties of a new nickel-titanium alloy with a lower percent by weight of nickel, *J Endod* 37:1293, 2011.

511. Thibodeau B, Teixeira F, Yamauchi M, et al: Pulp revascularization of immature dog teeth with apical periodontitis, *J Endod* 33:680, 2007.

512. Thompson SA: An overview of nickel-titanium alloys used in dentistry, *Int Endod J* 33:297, 2000.

513. Thompson SA, Dummer PM: Shaping ability of Lightspeed rotary nickel-titanium instruments in simulated root canals. Part 1, *J Endod* 23:698, 1997.

514. Thompson SA, Dummer PM: Shaping ability of Lightspeed rotary nickel-titanium instruments in simulated root canals. Part 2, *J Endod* 23:742, 1997.

515. Thompson SA, Dummer PM: Shaping ability of ProFile.04 Taper Series 29 rotary nickel-titanium instruments in simulated root canals. Part 1, *Int Endod J* 30:1, 1997.

516. Thompson SA, Dummer PM: Shaping ability of ProFile.04 Taper Series 29 rotary nickel-titanium instruments in simulated root canals. Part 2, *Int Endod J* 30:8, 1997.

517. Thompson SA, Dummer PM: Shaping ability of Hero 642 rotary nickel-titanium instruments in simulated root canals: Part 2, *Int Endod J* 33:255, 2000.

518. Torabinejad M: Passive step-back technique: a sequential use of ultrasonic and hand instruments, *Oral Surg Oral Med Oral Pathol Oral Radiol Endod* 77:402, 1994.

519. Torabinejad M, Cho Y, Khademi AA, et al: The effect of various concentrations of sodium hypochlorite on the ability of MTAD to remove the smear layer, *J Endod* 29:233, 2003.

520. Torabinejad M, Johnson WB, inventors; Torabinejad, M, Johnson WB, assignee: Irrigation solution and methods for use, December 25, 2003.

521. Torabinejad M, Shabahang S, Aprecio RM, Kettering JD: The antimicrobial effect of MTAD: an in vitro investigation, *J Endod* 29:400, 2003.

522. Torabinejad M, Walton R: *Principles and practice of endodontics*, ed 4, St. Louis, 2008, Saunders.

523. Tripi TR, Bonaccorso A, Condorelli GG: Cyclic fatigue of different nickel-titanium endodontic rotary instruments, *Oral Surg Oral Med Oral Pathol Oral Radiol Endod* 102:e106, 2006.

524. Tripi TR, Bonaccorso A, Tripi V, et al: Defects in GT rotary instruments after use: an SEM study, *J Endod* 27:782, 2001.

525. Troian CH, So MV, Figueiredo JA, Oliveira EP: Deformation and fracture of RaCe and K3 endodontic instruments according to the number of uses, *Int Endod J* 39:616, 2006.

526. Trope M: The vital tooth: its importance in the study and practice of endodontics, *Endod Topics* 5:1, 2003.

527. Turesky S, Warner V, Lin PS, Soloway B: Prolongation of antibacterial activity of chlorhexidine adsorbed to teeth: effect of sulfates, *J Periodontol* 48:646, 1977.

528. Turpin YL, Chagneau F, Bartier, et al: Impact of torsional and bending inertia on root canal instruments, *J Endod* 27:333, 2001.

529. Turpin YL, Chagneau F, Vulcain JM: Impact of two theoretical cross-sections on torsional and bending stresses of nickel-titanium root canal instrument models, *J Endod* 26:414, 2000.

530. Ullmann CJ, Peters OA: Effect of cyclic fatigue on static fracture loads in ProTaper nickel-titanium rotary instruments, *J Endod* 31:183, 2005.

531. Ungerechts C, Bårdsen A, Fristad I: Instrument fracture in root canals: where, why, when and what? A study from a student clinic, *Int Endod J* 47:183, 2014.

532. Usman N, Baumgartner JC, Marshall JG: Influence of instrument size on root canal debridement, *J Endod* 30:110, 2004.

533. van der Sluis LW, Versluis M, Wesselink PR: Passive ultrasonic irrigation of the root canal: a review of the literature, *Int Endod J* 40:415, 2007.

534. van der Sluis LW, Wu MK, Wesselink PR: A comparison between a smooth wire and a K-file in removing artificially placed dentine debris from root canals in resin blocks during ultrasonic irrigation, *Int Endod J* 38:593, 2005.

535. van der Sluis LW, Wu MK, Wesselink PR: The efficacy of ultrasonic irrigation to remove artificially placed dentine debris from human root canals prepared using instruments of varying taper, *Int Endod J* 38:764, 2005.

536. Vaudt J, Bitter K, Neumann K, Kielbassa AM: Ex vivo study on root canal instrumentation of two rotary nickel-titanium systems in comparison to stainless steel hand instruments, *Int Endod J* 42:22, 2009.

537. Versiani MA, Leoni GB, Steier L, et al: Micro-computed tomography study of oval-shaped canals prepared with the self-adjusting file, Reciproc, WaveOne, and ProTaper universal systems, *J Endod* 39:1060, 2013.

538. Viana AC, Gonzales BM, Buono VT, Bahia MG: Influence of sterilization on mechanical properties and fatigue resistance of nickel-titanium rotary endodontic instruments, *Int Endod J* 39:709, 2006.

539. Vianna ME, Gomes BP, Berber VB, et al: In vitro evaluation of the antimicrobial activity of chlorhexidine and sodium hypochlorite, *Oral Surg Oral Med Oral Pathol Oral Radiol Endod* 97:79, 2004.

540. Vianna ME, Horz HP, Gomes BP, Conrads G: In vivo evaluation of microbial reduction after chemo-mechanical preparation of human root canals containing necrotic pulp tissue, *Int Endod J* 39:484, 2006.

541. Vier FV, Figueiredo JA: Prevalence of different periapical lesions associated with human teeth and their correlation with the presence and extension of apical external root resorption, *Int Endod J* 35:710, 2002.

542. Walia HM, Brantley WA, Gerstein H: An initial investigation of the bending and torsional properties of nitinol root canal files, *J Endod* 14:346, 1988.

543. Walmsley AD: Ultrasound and root canal treatment: the need for scientific evaluation, *Int Endod J* 20:105, 1987.

544. Walmsley AD, Williams AR: Effects of constraint on the oscillatory pattern of endosonic files, *J Endod* 15:189, 1989.

545. Walsch H: The hybrid concept of NiTi rotary instrumentation, *Dent Clin North Am* 48:183, 2004.

546. Waltimo T, Trope M, Haapasalo M, Ørstavik D: Clinical efficacy of treatment procedures in endodontic infection control and one year follow-up of periapical healing, *J Endod* 31:863, 2005.

547. Waltimo TM, Ørstavik D, Siren EK, Haapasalo MP: In vitro susceptibility of Candida albicans to four disinfectants and their combinations, *Int Endod J* 32:421, 1999.

548. Wang Z, Shen Y, Haapasalo M: Effectiveness of endodontic disinfecting solutions against young and old Enterococcus faecalis biofilms in dentin canals, *J Endod* 38:1376, 2012.

549. Ward JR, Parashos P, Messer HH: Evaluation of an ultrasonic technique to remove fractured rotary nickel-titanium endodontic instruments from root canals: clinical cases, *J Endod* 29:764, 2003.

550. Weiger R, Bruckner M, ElAyouti A, Löst C: Preparation of curved root canals with rotary FlexMaster instruments compared to Lightspeed instruments and NiTi hand files, *Int Endod J* 36:483, 2003.

551. Weiger R, El Ayouti A, Löst C: Efficiency of hand and rotary instruments in shaping oval root canals, *J Endod* 28:580, 2002.

552. Weine FS, Healey HJ, Gerstein H, Evanson L: Pre-curved files and incremental instrumentation for root canal enlargement, *J Can Dent Assoc* 36:155, 1970.

553. Weine FS, Kelly RF, Lio PJ: The effect of preparation procedures on original canal shape and on apical foramen shape, *J Endod* 1:255, 1975.

554. Weller RN, Brady JM, Bernier WE: Efficacy of ultrasonic cleaning, *J Endod* 6:740, 1980.

555. West JD, Roane JB: Cleaning and shaping the root canal system. In Cohen S, Burns RC, editors: *Pathways of the pulp*, ed 7, St. Louis, MO, 1998, Mosby, p 203.

556. Wilson BL, Broberg C, Baumgardner JC, et al: Safety of electronic apex locators and pulp testers in patients with implanted cardiac pacemakers or cardioverter/defibrillators, *J Endod* 32:847, 2006.

557. Windley W 3rd, Teixeira F, Levin L, et al: Disinfection of immature teeth with a triple antibiotic paste, *J Endod* 31:439, 2005.

558. Wolcott S, Wolcott J, Ishley D, et al: Separation incidence of ProTaper rotary instruments: a large cohort clinical evaluation, *J Endod* 32:1139, 2006.

559. Wu MK, Dummer PM, Wesselink PR: Consequences of and strategies to deal with residual post-treatment root canal infection, *Int Endod J* 39:343, 2006.

560. Wu MK, van der Sluis LW, Wesselink PR: The capability of two hand instrumentation techniques to remove the inner layer of dentine in oval canals, *Int Endod J* 36:218, 2003.

561. Wu MK, Wesselink PR: Efficacy of three techniques in cleaning the apical portion of curved canals, *Oral Surg Oral Med Oral Pathol Oral Radiol Endod* 79:492, 1995.

562. Wu MK, Wesselink PR, Walton RE: Apical terminus location of root canal treatment procedures, *Oral Surg Oral Med Oral Pathol Oral Radiol Endod* 89:99, 2000.

563. Yamamura B, Cox TC, Heddaya B, et al: Comparing canal transportation and centering ability of endosequence and vortex rotary files by using micro-computed tomography, *J Endod* 38:1121, 2012.

564. Yamashita JC, Tanomaru Filho M, Leonardo MR, et al: Scanning electron microscopic study of the cleaning ability of chlorhexidine as a root-canal irrigant, *Int Endod J* 36:391, 2003.

565. Yao JH, Schwartz SA, Beeson TJ: Cyclic fatigue of three types of rotary nickel-titanium files in a dynamic model, *J Endod* 32:55, 2006.

566. Yared G: Canal preparation using only one Ni-Ti rotary instrument: preliminary observations, *Int Endod J* 41:339, 2008.

567. Yared GM, Bou Dagher FE, Machtou P: Cyclic fatigue of Profile rotary instruments after simulated clinical use, *Int Endod J* 32:115, 1999.

568. Yared GM, Bou Dagher FE, Machtou P: Cyclic fatigue of Profile rotary instruments after clinical use, *Int Endod J* 33:204, 2000.

569. Yared GM, Bou Dagher FE, Machtou P: Failure of ProFile instruments used with high and low torque motors, *Int Endod J* 34:471, 2001.

570. Yared GM, Dagher FE: Influence of apical enlargement on bacterial infection during treatment of apical periodontitis, *J Endod* 20:535, 1994.

571. Yesilsoy C, Whitaker E, Cleveland D, et al: Antimicrobial and toxic effects of established and potential root canal irrigants, *J Endod* 21:513, 1995.

572. Yguel-Henry S, Vannesson H, von Stebut J: High precision, simulated cutting efficiency measurement of endodontic root canal instruments: influence of file configuration and lubrication, *J Endod* 16:418, 1990.

573. Yun HH, Kim SK: A comparison of the shaping abilities of 4 nickel-titanium rotary instruments in simulated root canals, *Oral Surg Oral Med Oral Pathol Oral Radiol Endod* 95:228, 2003.

574. Zamany A, Safavi K, Spångberg LS: The effect of chlorhexidine as an endodontic disinfectant, *Oral Surg Oral Med Oral Pathol Oral Radiol Endod* 96:578, 2003.

575. Zehnder M: Root canal irrigants, *J Endod* 32:389, 2006.

576. Zehnder M, Paqué F: Disinfection of the root canal system during root canal re-treatment, *Endod Topics*, 19, 2008.

577. Zehnder M, Schmidlin PR, Sener B, Waltimo TM: Chelation in root canal therapy reconsidered, *J Endod* 31:817, 2005.

578. Zehnder M, Soderling E, Salonen J, Waltimo T: Preliminary evaluation of bioactive glass S53P4 as an endodontic medication in vitro, *J Endod* 30:220, 2004.

579. Zeltner M, Peters OA, Paqué F: Temperature changes during ultrasonic irrigation with different inserts and modes of activation, *J Endod* 35:573, 2009.

580. Zerella JA, Fouad AF, Spångberg LS: Effectiveness of a calcium hydroxide and chlorhexidine digluconate mixture as disinfectant during retreatment of failed endodontic cases, *Oral Surg Oral Med Oral Pathol Oral Radiol Endod* 100:756, 2005.

581. Zinelis S, Magnissalis EA, Margelos J, Lambrianidis T: Clinical relevance of standardization of endodontic files dimensions according to the ISO 3630-1 specification, *J Endod* 28:367, 2002.

582. Zmener O, Banegas G: Comparison of three instrumentation techniques in the preparation of simulated curved root canals, *Int Endod J* 29:315, 1996.

CHAPTER 7

Obturation of the Cleaned and Shaped Root Canal System

WILLIAM JOHNSON | JAMES C. KULILD | FRANKLIN TAY

CHAPTER OUTLINE

IMPORTANCE OF EFFECTIVELY SEALING THE ROOT CANAL SYSTEM

Success in endodontic treatment was originally based on the triad of debridement, thorough disinfection, and obturation, with all aspects equally important. At present, successful root canal treatment is based on broader principles. These include diagnosis and treatment planning; knowledge of anatomy and morphology; the traditional concepts of debridement, thorough disinfection, and obturation; the coronal restoration, and three-dimensional imaging of the healing of teeth with preexisting periapical pathosis. A meta-analysis of factors influencing the efficacy of primary root canal treatment found that the following four factors influenced success: the absence of a pretreatment periapical lesion, root canal fillings with no voids, obturation to within 2.0 mm of the apex, and an adequate coronal restoration.[265]

In an early radiographic study of success and failure, Ingle and colleagues[179] indicated that 58% of treatment failures were due to incomplete obturation. Unfortunately, teeth that are poorly obturated are often poorly prepared. Procedural errors such as loss of length, canal transportation, perforations, loss of coronal seal, and vertical root fracture may have occurred. These procedural errors have been shown to adversely affect the apical seal.[420]

Since the classic study by Ingle and colleagues, great emphasis has been placed on developing materials and techniques for obturating the radicular space. Various experimental methods have been used to assess microleakage after obturation, including radioisotopes,[102] dyes,[188] bacteria,[68] proteins,[248] endotoxins,[68] glucose penetration,[276] and computerized fluid filtration.[385] These methodologies have employed a variety of in vitro conditions, experimental periods that often produce conflicting results with unclear clinical implications.[113,426] There is general consensus that treatment outcomes cannot be predicted from the results of in vitro dye leakage models.[268,296,373] Even the results of microbial leakage studies have recently been challenged, due to flaws in experimental designs.[306,307] Fortunately, tooth retention rates after root canal treatment are high despite the varied conditions, materials, and techniques employed.[74,218,322] Circumstantial evidence indicates that the cleaning and shaping procedures provide an aseptic environment. With this elimination of the etiology for pathosis, the method of obturation becomes less critical.

A primate study of infected teeth with apical periodontitis demonstrated non-healing in 28% of the teeth with no bacteria after cleaning and shaping, whereas the presence of bacteria after cleaning and shaping resulted in 79% being classified as not healed.[119] When no bacteria were present, healing occurred regardless of the quality of the obturation. When bacteria were present at the time of obturation, there was a correlation between the quality of obturation and nonhealing. These results emphasized the role of bacteria in apical pathosis and the importance of cleaning and shaping procedures.

In a controlled animal study,[318] periapical lesions were created by removing the pulp and leaving the teeth open to the oral cavity. In the control group, the canals were cleaned and shaped before obturation with gutta-percha and a resin sealer. The teeth of the experimental group were cleaned and shaped as in the control group but left unobturated. At 190 days, the animals were killed and histological evaluations were performed. There was no difference in the healing between the instrumented and obturated teeth and the instrumented and unobturated teeth. The results emphasized the importance of cleaning and shaping in eliminating bacteria. Although obturation may not influence the short-term success rates, results may be different in long-term studies if coronal leakage were to occur.[314]

To date, there is no effective method for determining whether cleaning and shaping procedures have been effective. The criteria of clean dentinal filings and/or enlargement beyond the first file to bind at working length proved to be unreliable.[402] Although the length of preparation has been emphasized, the irregular canal diameter (the forgotten dimension) may be a more significant factor in success and failure.[181] Evidence indicates canals are often underprepared in the apical one-third.[67] Historically, culturing has been employed and obturation delayed until a "negative" culture was obtained. In contemporary endodontic treatment, culturing has been abandoned during routine care.[329] With vital pulp tissues, bacteria are not a major concern. In necrotic cases, the organisms involved in the disease process are primarily facultative or obligate anaerobes that may not grow in culture. Molecular microbiologic techniques (polymerase chain reaction) have demonstrated that a variety of organisms are present that do not grow in culture.[10,315,362] The role these organisms play in the disease process is not well understood.[257] The reader is referred to Chapters 14 and 15 for a fuller discussion.

The process of cleaning and shaping determines both the degree of disinfection and the ability to obturate the radicular space. Obturation is therefore a reflection of the cleaning and shaping and is evaluated on the basis of length, taper, density, level of gutta-percha removal, and the coronal seal (i.e., an adequate provisional restoration) (Fig. 7-1). It is not possible to assess the quality of the seal established during obturation with a radiograph, and it is important to remember that no material or technique prevents leakage.[2,153] Indeed, obtaining an impervious seal may not be feasible because of the porous tubular structure of dentin[2] and canal irregularities.

The primary etiology of pulpal and periradicular pathosis is, as discussed in Chapter 15, bacterial.[191,253] Pulpal remnants, necrotic tissue, bacteria, and bacterial by-products remaining in the inaccessible areas of a cleaned and shaped canal system could initiate and/or perpetuate a lesion because the host defense mechanisms are unable to remove them. Studies indicate that root canal systems cannot be completely cleaned and disinfected.[165,359,425] Obturation of the radicular space is necessary to eliminate leakage. Obturation reduces coronal leakage and bacterial contamination, seals the apex from the periapical tissue fluids, and entombs the remaining irritants in the canal.[412]

Coronal leakage has also been proposed to contribute to treatment failure based on in vitro leakage studies.[389,392] The clinical implication is that retreatment has to be performed in those teeth that are not restored permanently after 3 months of root canal treatment. This controversial issue has been recently challenged.[33,310,311] Although a coronal seal may be produced by a well-filled root filling, a coronal restoration with margins that prevent bacteria penetration, or both, data derived from a retrospective clinical study[305] suggest that a favorable treatment outcome may be achieved even in poorly filled root canals when the quality of the coronal restoration is adequate. Data produced by this retrospective study overtly challenged the rationale of endodontics. The data stimulated intense research and discussions for almost two decades on whether the quality of the coronal restoration is more significant than the quality of root canal treatment in eliminating apical periodontitis. A recent systematic review and meta-analysis of the results derived from nine similar studies indicate that poor quality root canal treatment and poor quality coronal restorations have similar odds (i.e., likelihood in non-statistical terms) in adversely affecting the healing of apical periodontitis.[137] Based on the best available evidence currently available, the odds for healing of apical periodontitis increase with both adequate root canal treatment and adequate restorative treatment.[137] It must be emphasized that these two factors were examined in isolation in those studies. While these postoperative prognostic factors are certainly important, as exemplified by the data derived from a prospective clinical study,[262,263] other preoperative and intraoperative prognostic factors also contributed significantly to periapical healing in primary and secondary root canal treatment. Nevertheless, maintaining an effective coronal seal through optimal filling of the instrumented radicular space and placing an appropriate restoration, as discussed in Chapter 22, should be considered essential components of successful root canal treatment.[168,180]

Clinicians are concerned with whether it is more appropriate to place a permanent restorative material instead of a temporary material to prevent leakage.[234,393] This is a controversial issue, as previous studies failed to provide definitive evidence to demonstrate that the presence of a permanent restoration will contribute to the long-term success of root canal treatment when those canals are optimally filled.[76,321] These results were supported by a more recent prospective clinical study that examined the factors affecting the outcomes of nonsurgical root canal treatment.[262] In this study, the authors found that the type of coronal restoration had no significant influence on periapical healing, as long as those restorations are of good quality. Paradoxically, the same group of authors reported in a separate study that cast restorations, when compared with temporary restorations, significantly improved the survival of teeth that had undergone primary or secondary root canal treatment.[263] This may be due to protection of remaining, weakened tooth structure by full-coverage cast restorations that enabled those teeth to function longer. Regarding the necessity for retreatment of root-filled teeth without permanent restorations, there is no clear evidence to justify that retreatment has to be performed in teeth in which a temporary

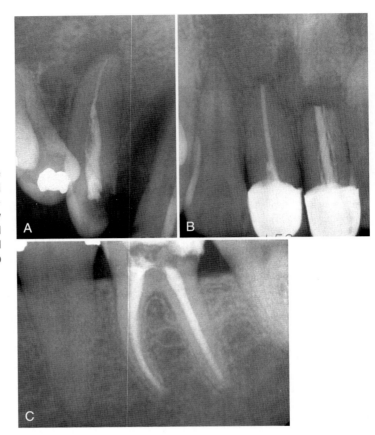

FIG. 7-1 Examples of inadequate obturation. **A,** Maxillary right canine with adequate length but lacking density and no coronal seal. Central incisor is filled to adequate length, but obturation exhibits voids. **B,** Maxillary central incisors. Maxillary right central incisor exhibits a lack of density and taper. Maxillary left central incisor has voids and unfilled canal space. **C,** Mandibular left first molar with adequate obturation; provisional restoration shows poor adaptation on the distal because of the failure to remove caries.

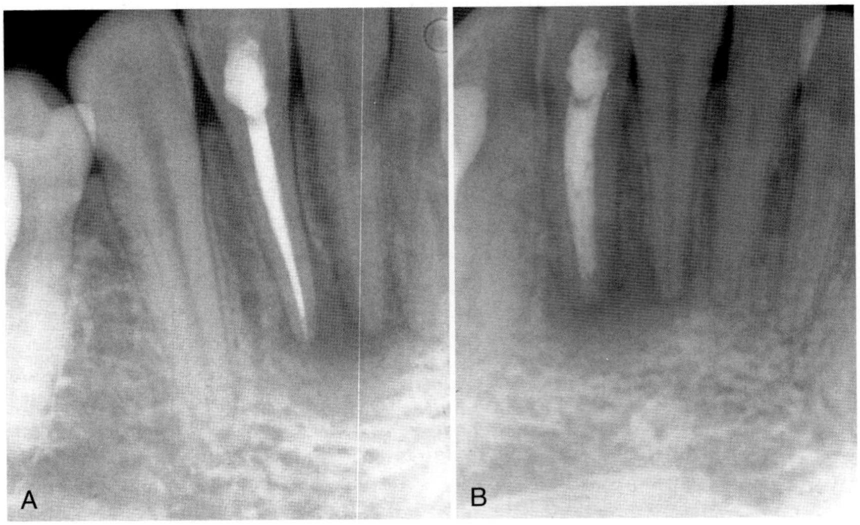

FIG. 7-2 **A,** Posttreatment radiograph of a mandibular left lateral incisor with ostensibly adequate obturation. **B,** Angled view reveals voids.

restoration has been inserted for more than three months, solely because of the suspicion of microleakage.[195] One may consider replacing the temporary restoration with a new coronal restoration immediately and to observe the tooth for at least three months before placing a permanent crown.[195]

Three-dimensional obturation of the radicular space is essential to long-term success. The canal system should be sealed apically, coronally, and laterally. Various methods have been advocated for obturation. Unfortunately, all materials and techniques result in some degree of leakage.[426] Although

a poorly obturated canal and leakage are correlated, radiographic evaluation of obturation does not correlate well with leakage.[154,199] An adequate two-dimensional radiographic appearance of the obturation may not correlate with an adequate seal (Fig. 7-2).[110] Variation in radiographic interpretation by the clinician, the overlying osseous structures, and the lack of uniformity in the obturation materials are significant variables.[36,106,107,199,388]

The diagnostic outcome of root canal treatment is based on clinical and radiographic findings. In a series of prospective studies, the Toronto group evaluated success and failure of root canal treatment at 4 to 6 years after completion of treatment. For primary root canal treatment,[91,121,127,241] teeth with pre-existing apical periodontitis were found to have a lower healing rate (82%) compared with teeth without periapical radiolucency (93%). Better outcomes were associated with teeth without periapical radiolucency, with single roots, and without mid-treatment complications such as root perforation. Teeth were treated by using flared preparation and vertical compaction of warm gutta-percha or step-back preparation and lateral compaction. Differences were noted with the adequacy of the fill and the treatment technique. Adequate length had a higher success rate (87%) when compared with inadequate length (77%). The flared preparation and vertical compaction had a higher success rate (90%) when compared with step-back preparation and lateral compaction (80%). For secondary nonsurgical root canal treatment,[92,120] teeth with pre-existing apical periodontitis were also found to have a lower healing rate (80%) compared with teeth without periapical radiolucency (93%). Better outcomes were achieved in teeth with inadequate previous root filling, without perforation and radiolucency. Similar results were reported in a more recent prospective clinical study that examined the effects of primary or secondary root canal treatment on periapical healing.[262] The percentage of roots with complete periapical healing after primary (83%) or secondary (80%) root canal treatment was similar. Absence of preoperative apical periodontitis was identified as one of the prognostic factors affecting primary or secondary root canal treatment. In the presence of apical periodontitis, treatment prognosis was significantly improved by the presence of a smaller lesion. These studies are in agreement with earlier work[364,374] indicating preexisting apical pathosis as a major factor reducing a favorable prognosis and highlighted obturation technique as a factor influencing success and failure.[364]

Although periapical radiographs have been used to examine healing of post-treatment apical periodontitis since 1922,[264] their suitability for evaluating the outcomes of root canal treatment has recently been challenged, in that previously reported outcomes based on this assessment modality may have overestimated the healing rates of apical periodontitis.[97,118,423] Imaging with periapical radiographs produces a two-dimensional superimposition of a three-dimensional structure; partially healed periapical lesions that are confined within the cancellous bone alone are not usually detected using periapical radiographs.[32] With the advent of cone-beam computed tomography (CBCT), a better diagnosis of periapical lesions within the cancellous bone can be made. This is because CBCT softwares create reconstructed images from slices of data in any plane and location of the volume of interest, thus eliminating the lack of three-dimensional assessment and anatomical noise which hampers the accuracy of periapical radiography. This results in a higher signal-to-noise ratio and image contrast, and improves the detection of periapical radiolucencies.[283,335] Although the use of CBCT may not be practical for every clinical case, the significance in adopting this novel imaging technology for assessing the healing of apical periodontitis after primary root canal treatment can be demonstrated in a recent one-year follow-up study.[284] Diagnosis using CBCT revealed a lower healed and healing rate for primary root canal treatment compared with the use of digital radiography. Complete resolution of periapical radiolucency was found to be 93% using periapical radiography and 74% for CBCT. For those teeth with preexisting periapical radiolucency, reconstructed CBCT images also showed more failures (14%) when compared with the use of periapical radiographs (10%). In another follow-up study, the technical quality of root canal fillings and the associated treatment outcome were evaluated two years post-treatment, using both periapical radiography and CBCT.[226] Complete absence of post-treatment periapical radiolucency was observed in CBCT scans in 81% and 49% of adequate and inadequate root fillings, respectively, as compared to 87% and 61% revealed by periapical radiographs. Preoperative apical periodontitis and the quality of root filling were identified by both periapical radiographs and CBCT as significant prognosis predictors. The combined use of periapical radiography and CBCT imaging confirmed that satisfactory root fillings were associated with a favorable outcome. The results of this work emphasized that developing good technical skills for obturating root canals should not be underscored, and that suitable canal obturation methods should be developed to achieve more compacted, void-free filling materials and at the correct length.

HISTORICAL PERSPECTIVES

The achievement of a "hermetic seal" is often cited as a major goal of root canal treatment. According to accepted dictionary definitions, the word *hermetic* means sealed against the escape or entry of *air*—or made airtight by fusion or sealing. However, root canal seals are commonly evaluated for *fluid* leakage—a parameter used to praise or condemn obturation materials and techniques. This occurs both apically and coronally. Somehow, the term *hermetic* has crept into endodontic nomenclature in a manner probably quite similar to the invention of an airtight seal. A god of wisdom, learning, and magic in ancient Egypt, Thoth, better known as Hermes Trismegistus (Hermes thrice greatest), is credited with this invention.[343] His significant contribution to civilization allowed the preservation of oils, spices, aromatics, grains, and other necessities in previously porous, earthenware vessels. A simple wax seal of the vessel walls helped to create the "hermetic seal." Endodontically speaking, the term *hermetic* is inappropriate; instead, terms such as *fluid-tight, fluid-impervious,* or *bacteria-tight* seals are more contemporary.

In 1924, Hatton indicated: "Perhaps there is no technical operation in dentistry or surgery where so much depends on the conscientious adherence to high ideals as that of pulp canal filling."[162] The essence of this statement had been significantly influenced by years of trial and error in both the techniques and materials used to obturate the prepared root canal system. Much of the frustration and challenge that emanated from this concern, however, was due to the lack of development in root canal preparation techniques coupled with indictments of the "focal infection" craze of that era.[178]

Before 1800, root canal filling, when done, was limited to gold. Subsequent obturations with various metals, oxychloride of zinc, paraffin, and amalgam resulted in various degrees of success and satisfaction.[203] In 1847, Hill developed the first gutta-percha root canal filling material known as "Hill's stopping."[203] The preparation, which consisted principally of bleached gutta-percha and carbonate of lime and quartz, was patented in 1848 and introduced to the dental profession. In 1867, Bowman made claim (before the St. Louis Dental Society) of the first use of gutta-percha for canal filling in an extracted first molar.[12]

References to the use of gutta-percha for root canal obturation before the turn of the twentieth century were few and vague. In 1883, Perry claimed that he had been using a pointed gold wire wrapped with some soft gutta-percha (the origin of the present-day core carrier technique?).[289] He also began using gutta-percha rolled into points and packed into the canal. The points were prepared by cutting base plate gutta-percha into slender strips, warming them with a lamp, laying them on his operating case, and rolling them with another flat surface (a contemporary technique still used by a few to custom roll a large cone?). Perry then used shellac warmed over a lamp and rolled the cones into a point of desired size, based on canal shape and length. Before placing the final gutta-percha point, he saturated the tooth cavity with alcohol; capillary attraction let the alcohol run into the canal, softening the shellac so that the gutta-percha could be packed (the forerunner of a chemical-softening technique?).

In 1887, the S.S. White Company began to manufacture gutta-percha points.[193] In 1893, Rollins introduced a new type of gutta-percha to which he added vermilion.[405] Because vermilion is pure oxide of mercury and therefore dangerous in quantity, many people justifiably criticized this technique.

With the introduction of radiographs for the assessment of root canal obturations, it became painfully obvious that the canal was not cylindrical, as earlier imagined, and that additional filling material was necessary to fill the observed voids. At first, hard-setting dental cements were used, but these proved unsatisfactory. It was also thought that the cement used should possess strong antiseptic action, hence the development of many phenolic or formalin-type paste cements. The softening and dissolution of the gutta-percha to serve as the cementing agent, through the use of resins was introduced by Callahan in 1914.[60] Subsequently a multitude of various pastes, sealers, and cements were created in an attempt to discover the best possible sealing agent for use with gutta-percha.

Over the past 70 to 80 years, the dental community has seen attempts to improve on the nature of root canal obturation with these cements and with variations in the delivery of gutta-percha to the prepared canal system. During this era, the impetus for these developments was based heavily on the continued belief in the concept of focal infection, elective localization, the hollow-tube theory, and the concept that the primary cause for failure of root canal treatment was the apical percolation of fluids, and microorganisms, into a poorly obturated root canal system.[102,317] From this chronological perspective of technical and scientific thought, this chapter clarifies and codifies contemporary concepts in the obturation of the cleaned and shaped root canal system.

TIMING OF OBTURATION

Factors influencing the appropriate time to obturate a tooth include the patient's signs and symptoms, status of the pulp and periradicular tissue, the degree of difficulty, and patient management.

Vital Pulp Tissue

At present, the consensus is that one-step treatment procedures are acceptable when the patient exhibits a completely or partially vital pulp.[123,328,372] Removal of the normal or inflamed pulp tissue and performance of the procedure under aseptic conditions should result in a successful outcome because of the relative absence of bacterial contamination. Obturation at the initial visit also precludes contamination as a result of leakage during the period between patient visits.

Elective root canal treatment for restorative reasons can be completed in one visit provided the pulp is vital, to some degree, and time permits. Obturation of root canals in patients whose condition is urgent depends on the pretreatment diagnosis. When pain occurs as the result of irreversible pulpitis, obturation can occur at the initial visit because removal of the vital tissue will generally resolve the patient's pain.

Necrotic Pulp Tissue

Patients who present with pulp necrosis with or without asymptomatic periradicular pathosis (asymptomatic apical periodontitis, chronic apical abscess, condensing osteitis) may be treated in one visit, based on the best available information. When patients present with acute symptoms caused by pulp necrosis and acute periradicular abscess, obturation is generally delayed until the patient is asymptomatic. However, more than 20 years ago, investigators demonstrated that cases with soft-tissue swelling could be completed in one visit with appropriate endodontic treatment, incision for drainage, and a regimen of antibiotics.[366] Management of these patients, however, may be more difficult should problems persist or become worse after the completion of treatment.

During the 1970s, there was concern about the timing of obturation. Performing endodontic treatment in one visit was controversial. Conventional wisdom suggested that patients would have a higher incidence of posttreatment pain. However, recent clinical studies[252,285,292] and systematic reviews[123,328,372] indicate that there is no significant difference in the healing rates of apical periodontitis between single-visit and multiple-visit root canal treatment. Patients experience less frequency of short-term post-obturation pain after single-visit than those having multiple-visit root canal treatment.[372]

In contrast to teeth with vital pulp tissue, teeth exhibiting pulp necrosis frequently exhibit bacterial contamination and may require a different approach to treatment. Sjögren and colleagues raised questions regarding the long-term prognosis of teeth exhibiting necrotic pulp tissue and apical periodontitis treated in a single-visit.[363] In their clinical study, the authors thoroughly instrumented 55 infected teeth with apical pathosis, using only 0.5% sodium hypochlorite (NaOCl) [*Editor's note*: Today, stronger concentrations of NaOCl are more commonly used. The reader is referred to Chapter 14 for a fuller discussion of this issue]. Before obturation, cultures were obtained, using anaerobic bacteriologic techniques. After cleaning and shaping, bacteria could be detected in 22 teeth. Complete healing occurred in 94% of cases that yielded a negative culture, whereas the rate of successful treatment of teeth with positive cultures before obturation was 68%, a statistically significant difference.

With the introduction of the concept of biofilms, other investigators examined the intracanal microbial status of sixteen mesial roots of human mandibular first molars with primary apical periodontitis immediately after one-visit root canal treatment.[258] In that study, the instrumented canals were irrigated with 5.25% NaOCl and 17% ethylenediaminetetraacetic acid (EDTA), and obturated with gutta-percha and zinc oxide–eugenol cement. The apical portion of the root of each tooth was removed by flap-surgery and prepared for correlative light and transmission electron microscopy examination. Fourteen of the 16 root-treated teeth revealed residual intracanal infection after instrumentation, antimicrobial irrigation, and obturation. The microbes existed mostly as biofilms in inaccessible recesses of instrumented main canals, the intercanal isthmus, and accessory canals.

In a more recent histobacteriological study, the in vivo microbiological status of the mesial roots of mandibular molars with primary apical periodontitis was examined after single-visit or two-visit root canal treatment.[397] Those roots were instrumented and irrigated with 5% NaOCl, 17% EDTA, and 2% chlorhexidine. In the single-visit group, the canals were immediately obturated, whereas in the two-visit group, calcium hydroxide dressing was placed in the canals for one week prior to obturation. In the single-visit group, no canal, out of the six canals examined, was completely free of bacteria. Residual biofilms were identified in the main canal, isthmus, apical ramifications, and dentinal tubules. In the two-visit group, two out of seven roots were rendered bacteria-free. Residual biofilms were found predominantly in the isthmus and ramifications, intermixed with necrotic tissues and debris. Taken together, these 3 studies illustrate that microbes are extremely difficult to eliminate within the complex root canal system, and that the use of an inter-appointment antimicrobial dressing resulted in improved microbiological status of the root canal system when compared with the single-visit protocol.

Calcium hydroxide has been advocated as an antimicrobial and temporary dressing in necrotic cases that cannot be treated in one visit[363] because investigators noted that bacteria in instrumented, unfilled canals can multiply and reach their pretreatment numbers in 2 to 4 days.[57] Nevertheless, the ability of calcium hydroxide to completely eradicate microbial species from the root canal system has recently been questioned. In vitro studies demonstrated that the antibacterial activity of calcium hydroxide can be inactivated by dentin.[156,297] Other clinical studies showed that the number of bacteria-positive canals did not decrease after the use of calcium hydroxide as an inter-appointment dressing.[291,401] A systematic review and meta-analysis of 8 clinical studies concluded that calcium hydroxide is useful but has limited effectiveness in completely eliminating bacteria from human root canals when assessed by culture techniques.[330] Although calcium hydroxide has a wide range of antimicrobial activity against common endodontic pathogens and is an effective anti-endotoxin agent, it is less effective against *Entercoccus faecalis* and *Candida albicans*.[251] Alternative inter-appointment dressings such as the use of chlorhexidine gel, calcium hydroxide in chlorhexidine gel, or triantibiotic paste (metronidazole, minocycline, and ciprofloxacin) has been proposed, with dichotomous results.[95,271,361,403] While there are clinical trials to support the use of calcium hydroxide or alternative inter-appointment dressings, they do not reduce bacteria load beyond levels already achieved by canal preparation with NaOCl.[238,240,360] It is fair to say inter-appointment antimicrobial dressings are fairly well accepted by clinicians in cases that cannot be treated in a single visit.

In general, obturation can be performed after cleaning and shaping procedures when the canal can be dried and the patient is not experiencing swelling. An exception is the presence or persistence of exudation from the canal. Obturation of a canal that cannot be dried is contraindicated. Procedural concerns also dictate the time of obturation. Difficult cases may require more time for preparation and can be managed more uneventfully in multiple appointments. Patients may require multiple short appointments because of medical conditions, their psychological state of mind, and fatigue.

LENGTH OF OBTURATION

One of the controversies in endodontics that remains unresolved is the apical limit of root canal treatment and obturation.[33,309] Early studies identified the dentinocemental junction as the apical limit for obturation. However, this histologic landmark cannot be determined clinically, and it has been found to be irregular within the canal. The dentinocemental junction may be several millimeters higher on the mesial canal wall when compared with the distal wall. In addition, the dentinocemental junction does not coincide with the narrowest portion of the canal or apical constriction. The reader is referred to Chapter 5 for more information about this anatomy.

Traditionally, the apical point of termination has been approximately 1 mm from the radiographic apices as determined by radiographs. Kuttler noted that the apical anatomy consists of the major diameter of the foramen and the minor diameter of the constriction (Fig. 7-3),[212] with the apical constriction identified as the narrowest portion of the canal. The average distance from the foramen to the constriction was found to be 0.5 mm, with the foramen varying in distance from the apex up to 2.5 mm. Kuttler also noted that the foramen-to-constriction distance increases with age because of cementum deposition. Supporting this finding, other investigators found that the location of the foramen was not at the apex. Deviations occurred in 92% of the roots and averaged 0.6 mm.[56] Another study noted the average apex-to-constriction distance was 0.9 mm and that 95% of the constrictions were between 0.5 and 1 mm in diameter[108]; this study also noted that the classic apical anatomy described by Kuttler was present in only 46% of the teeth. Other variations identified were the tapering constriction, the multiconstriction, and the parallel constriction. Other investigators examined 230 roots of permanent teeth stereomicroscopically and with radiographs.[37] Results of this study indicated a deviation of the foramen from the apex in 76% of the roots with microscopy and 57% with radiography; the mean distance was 1 mm.

A later study found that no foramina coincided with the longitudinal axis of the root, with the distance ranging from 0.2 to 3.8 mm (Fig. 7-4).[152] Root resorption is an additional factor in length determination. Resorption is more common

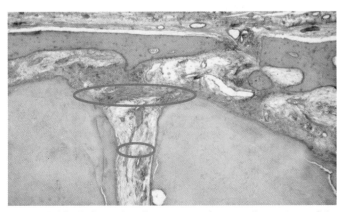

FIG. 7-3 Histologic section of a root apex, demonstrating anatomy of the classic foramen and constriction.

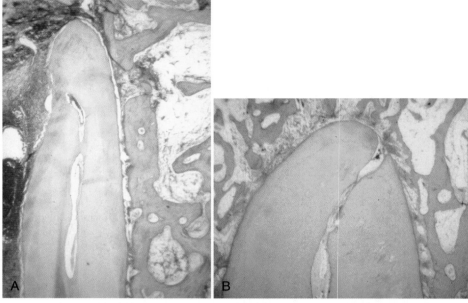

FIG. 7-4 Histologic sections demonstrating the foramen exiting short of the root apex.

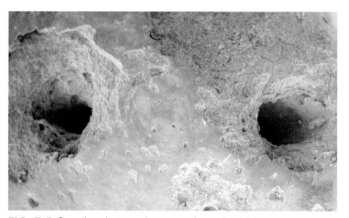

FIG. 7-5 Scanning electron microscopy of a tooth exhibiting a necrotic pulp and apical pathosis and resorption.

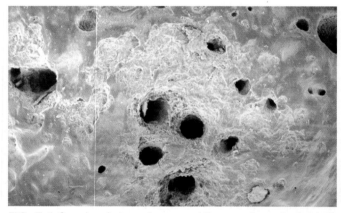

FIG. 7-6 Scanning electron microscopy of the apex of an extracted tooth that was removed because of pulp necrosis. Note the multiple accessory foramina and resorption.

with necrosis and apical bone resorption, and this can result in loss of the constriction (Fig. 7-5).[122,239] On the basis of these findings it appears that canals filled to the radiographic apex reflect an overextension of the obturating material. If overextension occurs that cannot be retrieved, and there appears to be resultant nerve damage, the practitioner is obligated to refer the patient to a qualified practitioner skilled in cases of this type.[139]

A study by the Toronto group on the prognosis of retreatment identified perforation,[92] pretreatment periradicular disease, and adequate length of the root canal filling as factors significantly influencing success and failure. The authors speculated that canals filled more than 2 mm short harbored necrotic tissue, bacteria, and irritants that when re-treated could be cleaned and sealed. The success rate for negotiating the apical unfilled canal was 74%.

Controversy also exists regarding the role accessory canals play in success and failure (Fig. 7-6). A scanning electron microscopy (SEM) study of the apical anatomy of each tooth group except the third molars noted no pattern for foraminal

openings[151]; the number of accessory canals ranged from 1 to 16. Although lateral canals can be associated with pathosis, one study that examined root-treated teeth from human cadavers reported no relationship between unfilled lateral canals and periradicular pathosis.[20] Accessory/lateral canals are often obturated by chance and only serendipitously identified on the posttreatment radiograph (Fig. 7-7).

A later histobacteriological study also found no evidence to support that lateral canals must be filled to achieve a successful long-term treatment outcome (Fig. 7-8).[313] In cases with vital pulps, forcing obturation materials into lateral canals resulted in unnecessary damage to the periradicular tissues with consequential inflammation. In cases with nonvital, infected pulps in which lateral canals appeared radiographically filled, they were actually not sealed or disinfected, and the remaining tissue in the ramification was inflamed and enmeshed with the filling material. This, however, does not mean that lateral canals should not be optimally debrided and disinfected by

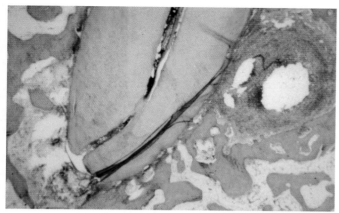

FIG. 7-7 Histologic section of a mesial root of a mandibular molar with a lateral canal present and associated lesion. Will the lesion resolve after the removal of the main canal contents, or will the lesion persist because of necrotic pulpal remnants in the lateral canal? The question remains unanswered.

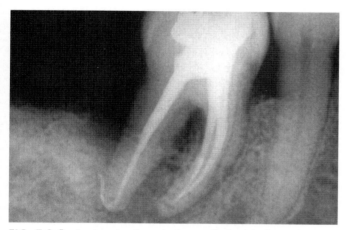

FIG. 7-8 Posttreatment radiograph of a mandibular right first molar with a lateral canal associated with the distal root.

contemporary irrigant delivery and agitation techniques to reduce microbes and/or biofilms that reside within those spaces, prior to obturation of the canal space with root-filling materials and sealers.

The importance of length control in obturation relates to extrusion of root-filling materials. In a quantitative systematic review of the literature,[338] the authors critically analyzed 12 outcome studies that fulfilled the following criteria: i) a minimum follow-up period of two years; ii) data available on termination of obturation/instrumentation; iii) adequate definition of treatment failure; iv) data available on success/failure of root canal therapy in relation to the obturation/instrumentation length; and v) presence or absence of periapical radiolucency. The 12 studies were classified into three categories based on the obturation length from the radiographic apex: A) 0-1 mm; B) >1 mm but <3 mm; and C) obturated past the radiographic apex, including sealer. From the 12 studies, only four studies that included data that could be placed into the three length categories were further subjected to meta-analysis. Results of the meta-analysis indicated that the success rate in group A (obturated 0-1 mm from apex) was marginally

better than group C (obturated past apex) by 29%. Although group A had better success than group B (obturated >1 mm short), the difference was not statistically significant. The authors concluded that a better success rate was achieved when treatment involved obturation short of the apex.

The aforementioned results derived from the sophisticated meta-analysis of multiple publications highlighted the data presented in the classic work performed by Sjögren and coworkers on healing of root-treated teeth with necrotic pulps and periapical lesions 8 to 10 years after treatment.[364] When those teeth were filled within 2 mm of the apex, 94% revealed normal periapical conditions with the use of periapical radiography at the follow-up examination. Conversely, roots with excess root fillings and those with fillings more than 2 mm short of the apex had significantly lower success rates of 76% and 68%, respectively.

Similar results were also reported in a prospective clinical study on the healing[262] and survival[263] of teeth that had undergone primary or secondary root canal treatment for 2 to 4 years. Absence of root-filling extrusion was found to be a highly significant postoperative prognostic factor affecting the success of both primary and secondary root canal treatment.[262] With respective to tooth survival, extrusion of gutta-percha root filling did not have any effect on tooth survival within the first 22 months, but significantly increased the risk of tooth loss beyond 22 months.[263] This prognostic factor was common to both primary and secondary root canal treatment. The authors attributed the delayed effect of extrusion of gutta-percha root filling on tooth survival to the possibility of sub-critical cracks created by excessive forces during compaction of gutta-percha, which eventually propagated during function and ultimately resulted in catastrophic failure.

On the basis of biologic and clinical principles, the conclusions derived from studies performed for more than two decades apart are all agreeable, in that instrumentation and obturation should not extend beyond the apical foramen.[259] This was also demonstrated in a histologic study which evaluated 41 human root-filled teeth from 36 patients.[312] In six cases exhibiting overfills, histologic examination revealed severe inflammation.

Whereas the guideline of 1 mm from the radiographic apex remains rational when using radiographs, the point of apical termination of the preparation and obturation remains empirical. The use of an apex locator in conjunction with radiographs and sound clinical judgment makes this decision more logical. The need to compact the gutta-percha and sealer against the apical dentin matrix (constriction of the canal) is necessary to prevent extrusion of materials into the periapical tissues. Deciding where the apical constriction of the canal lies is based on the clinician's basic knowledge of apical anatomy, tactile sensation, radiographic interpretation, apex locators, apical bleeding, and (if not anesthetized) the patient's response.

PREPARATION FOR OBTURATION

During the cleaning and shaping process, organic pulpal materials and inorganic dentinal debris accumulate on the canal wall, producing an amorphous irregular smear layer (Fig. 7-9).[25,244,281] As shown in one of these studies, the smear layer is superficial with a thickness of 1 to 5 μm.[244] This superficial debris can be packed into the dentinal tubules to various distances.[1]

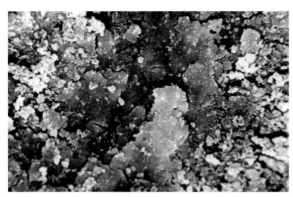

FIG. 7-9 Scanning electron microscopy of a prepared canal wall. The tubules are covered with a smear layer of organic and inorganic material.

In cases of necrosis this layer may also be contaminated with bacteria and their by-products. For example, one study found that bacteria can extend 10 to 150 μm into the dentinal tubules of necrotic teeth.[346] Another study noted that capillary action and fluid dynamics play a role in packing debris into the tubules.[3] Another investigation noted a mean penetration of 479 μm after a 28-day incubation period.[287]

The smear layer is not a complete barrier to bacteria but may act as a physical barrier, decreasing bacterial penetration into tubules. This was illustrated by a study demonstrating that removal of the smear layer permitted colonization of the dentinal tubules at a significantly higher rate when compared with leaving the smear layer in place.[104]

The smear layer may also interfere with adhesion and penetration of sealers into dentinal tubules.[410] Evidence indicates that sealer penetration into dentinal tubules does not occur when the smear layer is present.[132,277] For example, one study found that removal of the smear layer permitted Roth 811 (Roth International, Ltd., Chicago, IL), Calciobiotic root canal sealer (CRCS; Coltène/Whaledent, Cuyahoga Falls, Ohio), and Sealapex (SybronEndo, Orange, California) to penetrate to between 35 and 80 μm, whereas the presence of the smear layer obstructed tubular penetration of all sealers.[208] Other studies found that smear layer removal increased bond strength and reduced microleakage in teeth obturated with AH-26 (DENTSPLY Maillefer, Ballaigues, Switzerland).[111,133] Another investigation found that a combination of smear layer removal, AH-26 as the sealer, and vertical compaction of gutta-percha had a cumulative effect in reducing leakage.[386]

There does not appear to be a consensus on removing the smear layer before obturation.[70,347,353] The advantages and disadvantages of the smear layer remain controversial; however, growing evidence supports removal of the smear layer before obturation.[177,353] The organic debris present in the smear layer might constitute a substrate for bacterial growth.[281] It has been suggested that the smear layer prohibits sealer contact with the canal wall and permits leakage.[29] Bacterial penetration in the presence of a smear layer in canals obturated with thermoplasticized gutta-percha and sealer has been shown to be significantly higher than with smear layer removal before obturation.[281] An additional consideration is the presence of viable bacteria that remain in the dentinal tubules and use the smear layer for sustained growth and activity.[49] Removal of the smear layer introduces the possibility of reinfecting the dentinal tubules if leakage occurs.[347] However, one study demonstrated

that bacteria present before obturation are not viable after obturation.[99]

The smear layer may also interfere with the action of irrigants used as disinfectants.[272] When the smear layer is not removed, it may slowly disintegrate and dissolve around leaking obturation materials, or it may be removed by bacterial by-products such as acids and enzymes.[347]

The smear layer may interfere with the adhesion and penetration of root canal sealers. It also may prevent gutta-percha penetration during thermoplastic techniques.[155] Significant tubular penetrations of gutta-percha and sealers have been reported with thermoplasticized obturations[155] and with dentin-bonded composite resins.[221] Removal of the smear layer also enhances the adhesion of sealers to dentin and tubular penetration.[221,267,347,409] Root canal filling materials adapt better to the canal walls after smear layer removal.[101,267,409,410,411]

One investigation examined the penetration depth of three different root canal sealers into the dentinal tubules with and without the smear layer. Scanning electron microscopy of extracted single-rooted human teeth obturated by lateral compaction of gutta-percha, using AH Plus (DENTSPLY Maillefer), Apexit (Ivoclar Vivadent, Schaan, Liechtenstein), and Roth 811, demonstrated that the smear layer prohibited the sealers from penetrating dentinal tubules. Smear layer removal allowed the penetration of all sealers to occur to various depths.[205] Another study found that removal of the smear layer reduced both coronal and apical leakage regardless of the sealer tested.[79]

Another study examined the smear layer and the passage of bacteria through and around obturating materials,[77] using human maxillary incisors obturated with gutta-percha and AH-26. The teeth were exposed to standardized bacterial suspensions containing *Fusobacterium nucleatum, Campylobacter rectus,* and *Peptostreptococcus micros* for a period of 60 days, using a leakage model employing upper and lower chambers. Results indicated that 60% of the samples in which the smear layer was not removed demonstrated bacterial leakage. There was no leakage in specimens from which the smear layer was removed.

An additional method for removing the smear layer involves sonic and ultrasonic instruments. In early studies of ultrasonic instrumentation, investigators noted the technique was effective in removing the smear layer.[84] Another investigator also demonstrated smear layer removal with ultrasonication and NaOCl.[63] One study compared the cleaning efficacy of short-term sonic and ultrasonic passive irrigation with 5.25% NaOCl after hand instrumentation in the apical 3 to 6 mm of maxillary molar root canals.[319] Passive sonic or ultrasonic irrigation for 30 seconds resulted in significantly cleaner canals than hand filing alone, and ultrasonic irrigation produced significantly cleaner canals than irrigation. However, other studies found ultrasonication and NaOCl to be ineffective in removing the smear layer.[24,400] In a more recent study, a group of investigators reported that the use of the Vibringe, EndoActivator, or needle irrigation did not significantly improve sealer penetration when compared with conventional irrigation.[43]

After the completion of cleaning and shaping procedures, removal of the smear layer is generally accomplished by irrigating the canal with 17% disodium ethylenediaminetetraacetic acid (EDTA) and 5.25% NaOCl (Fig. 7-10).[25] Chelators remove the inorganic components, leaving the organic tissue elements intact. Sodium hypochlorite is necessary for removal of the

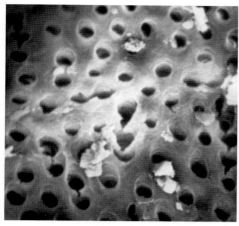

FIG. 7-10 Scanning electron microscopy of the canal wall after removal of the smear layer with 17% EDTA and 5.25% sodium hypochlorite.

remaining organic components. Citric acid has also been shown to be an effective method for removing the smear layer,[16,23,170,337] as has tetracycline.[19,164]

Chelating agents were introduced to endodontic treatment by Nygaard-Østby in 1957 for treatment of calcified narrow root canals.[266] Ethylenediaminetetraacetic acid is the chelating solution customarily used in endodontic treatment. It is available in both liquid and paste forms with common concentrations between 15% and 17%.[177] A detergent is frequently added to the liquid to decrease surface tension, to increase the cleaning ability, and to enhance the bactericidal action of the solution.[399] The effectiveness of EDTA is related to time of application, the pH, and the concentration.[254,266]

Demineralization results in increased dentin permeability[150] because of the removal of the smear layer and plugs and enlargement of the tubules. It appears that the tubular enlargement is due to selective removal of the peritubular dentin.[175] The action of chelators and acids appears to be more effective in the coronal and middle thirds of the root and is reduced apically.[177,228] This reduced activity may be a reflection of canal size.[210] This is a clinical concern because of the more irregular structure of dentin in the apical third. Another investigation demonstrated marked variations in the apical portion of the root,[250] including accessory root canals, areas of resorption and repaired resorptions, pulp stones, irregular or absent primary tubules, irregular secondary dentin, and cementum-like tissue lining the apical root canal wall. The variable structure of the apical region of human teeth presents challenges to the use of endodontic obturation techniques requiring adhesives, because this may influence the dentin bonding ability in the apical region.[250]

Ethylenediaminetetraacetic acid appears to be biocompatible when used clinically[266]; however, irreversible decalcification of periapical bone and neuroimmunologic disturbances have been noted.[342] Extrusion of both NaOCl and EDTA in clinical treatment should be avoided.[163,282,380]

The recommended time for removal of the smear layer is 1 to 5 minutes.[62,177,337] The small particles of the smear layer are primarily inorganic with a high surface-to-mass ratio that facilitates removal by acids and chelators. Investigators have found that a 1-minute exposure to 10 mL of EDTA was adequate to remove the smear layer and that a 10-minute

exposure caused excessive removal of both peritubular and intratubular dentin.[62]

The use of EDTA in combination with NaOCl is recommended[371,381] and may enhance the cleaning[228] and antimicrobial effects of these solutions when compared with using them alone.[58] Although the use of EDTA alone does not cause erosion of the canal wall dentin, it should be noted the adjunctive use of NaOCl with EDTA may result in erosion of the intraradicular dentin, depending on the timing and the concentrations of irrigants employed.[236,300,345,433]

New smear layer–removing irrigants are commercially available that combine calcium chelation of the inorganic component of the smear layer with antimicrobial activities. Examples of these irrigants include BioPure MTAD (DENSPLY Tulsa Dental Specialties)[349] and QMix 2in1 Irrigating Solution (DENSPLY Tulsa Dental Specialties).[86]

THE IDEAL ROOT CANAL FILLING

Various endodontic materials have been advocated for obturation of the radicular space. Most techniques employ a core material and sealer. Regardless of the core material a sealer is essential to every technique and helps achieve a fluid-tight seal.

The American Association of Endodontists' *Guide to Clinical Endodontics* outlines contemporary endodontic treatment.[8] Nonsurgical root canal treatment of permanent teeth "involves the use of biologically acceptable chemical and mechanical treatment of the root canal system to promote healing and repair of the periradicular tissues." The process is accomplished under aseptic conditions with rubber dam isolation. Regarding obturation, the guide states, "Root canal sealers are used in conjunction with a biologically acceptable semi-solid or solid obturating material to establish an adequate seal of the root canal system." In this area the guidelines indicate that "Paraformaldehyde-containing paste or obturating materials have been shown to be unsafe. Root canal obturation with paraformaldehyde-containing materials is below the standard of care for endodontic treatment" (Fig. 7-11). Chapter 29 gives further information about this issue.

Assessment of nonsurgical treatment is based primarily on the posttreatment radiographic examination. The radiographic criteria for evaluating obturation include the following categories: length, taper, density, gutta-percha and sealer removal to the facial cementoenamel junction in anterior teeth and to the canal orifice in posterior teeth, and an adequate provisional or definitive restoration (Fig. 7-12).

Quality assurance is accomplished through a careful evaluation of treatment procedures. Only by this approach can deficiencies be identified and corrected. Although the anatomy and morphology of the radicular space vary tremendously, the obturated root canal should reflect the original canal shape. Procedural errors in preparation, such as loss of length, ledging, apical transportation, apical perforation, stripping perforation, and separated instruments, may not be correctable. Errors in obturation, such as length, voids, inadequate removal of obturation materials, and temporization, may be correctable.

Radiographic interpretation may vary among clinicians because of differences in radiopacity in root canal sealer/cements, constituents in specific brands of gutta-percha, interpretation of voids in vivo versus in vitro,[431] the overlying bony anatomy, radiographic angulation, and the limited two-dimensional view of the obturated root canal or canals.

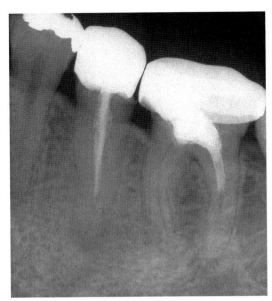

FIG. 7-11 A periapical radiograph of a mandibular left second premolar and first molar, demonstrating Sargenti paste root canal treatment. In addition to the toxic material, the technique often accompanies inadequate cleaning and shaping procedures.

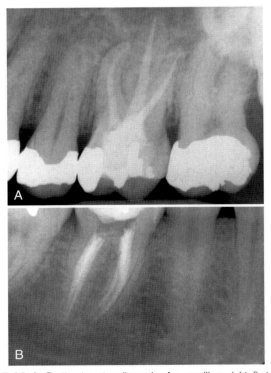

FIG. 7-12 A, Posttreatment radiograph of a maxillary right first molar, demonstrating adequate length, density, and taper. B, Posttreatment radiograph of a mandibular right first molar with an adequate obturation.

An often overlooked aspect in the assessment of root canal obturation is the density of the apical portion of the fill.[153] The apical third of the canal may be filled with a sea of root canal cement and a single master cone or poorly compacted mass of previously softened gutta-percha. Radiographically, the apical

third of the canal appears less radiodense. An ill-defined outline to the canal wall is evident, along with obvious gaps or voids in the filling material or its adaptation to the confines of the canal. Because of the use of highly radiopaque root canal sealers/cements, the apical portion may be filled only with sealer, giving the clinician the false impression of a dense, three-dimensional obturation with gutta-percha.

Root canal sealers vary in radiopacity.[304,379] Some contain silver particles or significant amounts of barium sulfate to enhance their radiopacity. Although these components may enhance visualization of anatomic structures such as lateral canals, it is important to realize they do not increase the sealing ability of the sealer and the quality of the obturation. They may also give the impression that a canal is well obturated when voids are masked by the density of the sealer. It is erroneous to claim that obturations with highly radiopaque sealers are better than those made with less radiopaque materials. This type of comparison and claim to superiority are both unfounded and unwarranted. The radiographic appearance or aesthetic appearance of the obturated canal system should be secondary to meticulous cleaning and shaping. Although assessment of the root canal obturation is based on radiographic findings, root canal sealers do not have to be highly radiopaque to be effective.

TYPES OF SEALERS

Root canal sealers are necessary to seal the space between the dentinal wall and the obturating core interface. Sealers also fill voids and irregularities in the root canal, lateral and accessory canals, and spaces between gutta-percha points used in lateral condensation. Sealers also serve as lubricants during the obturation process. Grossman outlined the properties of an ideal sealer (Box 7-1).[149] At present no sealer satisfies all the criteria.

Sealers should be biocompatible and well tolerated by the periradicular tissues.[367] All sealers exhibit toxicity when freshly mixed; however, their toxicity is greatly reduced on setting.[214] Sealers are resorbable when exposed to tissues and tissue fluids.[14] Tissue healing and repair generally appear unaffected by most sealers, provided there are no adverse breakdown products of the sealer over time.[42,50-52,54] Breakdown products from the

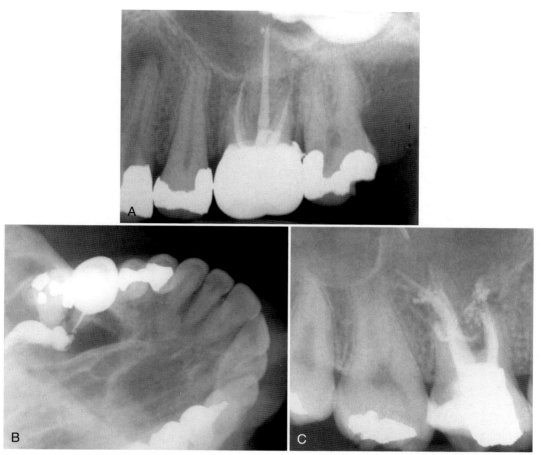

FIG. 7-13 **A,** Extrusion of sealer evident on this posttreatment radiograph of a maxillary first molar. The separated lentulo spiral in the mesiobuccal root indicates a possible method of sealer placement. **B,** Maxillary occlusal film demonstrates that the sealer is located in the maxillary sinus. Correction by nonsurgical techniques is not possible. **C,** Maxillary right first molar with extrusion of the sealer and gutta-percha.

sealers may have an adverse effect on the proliferative capability of periradicular cell populations.[146] As a result, sealers should not be placed routinely in the periradicular tissues as part of an obturation technique.[214] Although an osteogenic response has been observed with calcium hydroxide–based root canal sealers,[172,365,376,390] the ability of these sealers to sustain a high pH over time has been questioned.[207]

The most popular sealers are zinc oxide–eugenol formulations, calcium hydroxide sealers, glass ionomer sealers, resin-based (epoxy resin or methacrylate resin) sealers, and the recently introduced calcium silicate–based sealers. Despite claims by the manufacturers on the advantages of each class of sealers, there are no evidence-based data, based on randomized clinical trials, demonstrating the superiority of one class of sealer over another. Regardless of the sealer selected, all exhibit toxicity until they have set. For this reason, extrusion of sealers into the periradicular tissues should be avoided (Fig. 7-13).

Zinc Oxide and Eugenol

Zinc oxide–eugenol sealers have a history of successful use over an extended period of time. Zinc oxide–eugenol sealers will resorb if extruded into the periradicular tissues.[14] They exhibit a slow setting time,[6] shrinkage on setting,[192] solubility,[290] and they can stain tooth structure.[90,209,394] An advantage to this sealer group is antimicrobial activity.[4,18,167,249]

An early zinc oxide–eugenol sealer was introduced by Rickert and Dixon.[308] This powder/liquid sealer contained silver particles for radiopacity. Although it was possible to demonstrate the presence of lateral and accessory canals the sealer had the distinct disadvantage of staining tooth structure if not completely removed. Marketed as Pulp Canal Sealer (SybronEndo) and Pulp Canal Sealer EWT (extended working time), this sealer is popular with clinicians using thermoplastic techniques. Procosol (Procosol, Inc., Philadelphia, Pennsylvania) is a modification of Rickert's formula in which the silver particles have been removed (zinc oxide, hydrogenated resin, bismuth subcarbonate and barium sulfate; liquid eugenol).

Grossman modified the formulation and introduced a non-staining formula in 1958 (Table 7-1).[148] This is the formulation in Roth's Sealer (Roth International) Tubli-Seal (SybronEndo) is a catalyst/base zinc oxide–eugenol sealer that is convenient to mix but has a faster setting time when compared with the liquid/powder sealers. Tubli-Seal EWT provides an extended working time. Wach's Sealer (Balas Dental, Chicago, Illinois) contains Canada balsam, which gives the material a sticky or tacky property that softens the gutta-percha into a more homogeneous mass when used with lateral compaction.

Although zinc oxide–eugenol sealers possess marked cytotoxic and tissue-irrigating potencies in ex vivo cell culture

TABLE 7-1

Formula for Zinc Oxide–Eugenol Root Canal Sealer	
Powder	**Liquid**
Zinc oxide	42 parts
Staybelite resin	27 parts
Bismuth subcarbonate	15 parts
Barium sulfate	15 parts
Sodium borate, anhydrous	1 part

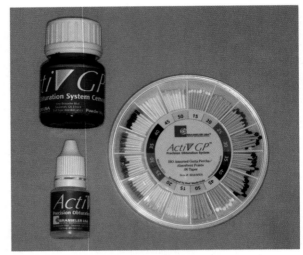

FIG. 7-14 Activ GP (Brasseler USA) glass ionomer–coated gutta-percha points and sealer.

studies,[134] their clinical usefulness has been well demonstrated in an in vivo animal model,[129] as well as in retrospective human clinical studies.[83] This discrepancy between the results of in vitro and in vivo cytotoxicity testing may be explained by the fact that most cell culture systems are represented by only one cell type (i.e. no cell-cell interactions) which is often monoclonal in origin. Another important issue to consider is the fact that culture conditions are not homeostatic and there is no elimination of toxic substances as there would be in vivo. By contrast, the human body possesses a lymphatic system and periapical defenses such as polymorphonuclear leukocytes, plasma cells, and macrophages to help eliminate toxic substances.[61] These mechanisms do not exist in a culture plate and must be taken into account for interpretations of the results of cell culture–based cytotoxicity studies reported in the endodontic literature.

Calcium Hydroxide Sealers

Calcium hydroxide sealers were developed for therapeutic activity. It was thought that these sealers would exhibit antimicrobial activity and have osteogenic–cementogenic potential. Unfortunately, these actions have not been demonstrated.[100,251] Solubility is required for release of calcium hydroxide and sustained activity. This is inconsistent with the purpose of a sealer. Calciobiotic root canal sealer (CRCS) is a zinc oxide–eugenol sealer with calcium hydroxide as one ingredient. Sealapex (SybronEndo) is a catalyst/base system. The base contains zinc oxide, calcium hydroxide, butyl benzene, sulfonamide, and zinc stearate. The catalyst contains barium sulfate and titanium dioxide as radiopacifiers in addition to resin, isobutyl salicylate, and aerosol R972. Apexit and Apexit Plus (Ivoclar Vivadent) consist of an activator (disalicylate, bismuth hydroxide/bismuth carbonate, and fillers) and a base (calcium hydroxide, hydrated colophonium [i.e., pine resin], and fillers).

Noneugenol Sealers

Developed from a periodontal dressing, Nogenol (GC America, Alsip, Illinois) is a root canal sealer without the irritating effects of eugenol. The base contains zinc oxide, barium sulfate, and bismuth oxychloride.

Glass Ionomer Sealers

Glass ionomers have been advocated for use in obturation because of their dentin-bonding properties. Ketac-Endo (3M ESPE, St. Paul, Minnesota) enables adhesion between the material and the canal wall.[128] It is also difficult to properly treat the dentinal walls in the apical and middle thirds with

conditioning agents to receive the glass ionomer sealer. A disadvantage of glass ionomers is that they must be removed if retreatment is required.[229] This sealer has minimal antimicrobial activity.[167]

Activ GP (Brasseler USA, Savannah Georgia) consists of a glass ionomer–impregnated gutta-percha cone with a glass ionomer external coating and a glass ionomer sealer (Fig. 7-14). Available in 0.04 and 0.06 tapered cones, the sizes are laser verified to ensure a more precise fit. This single cone technique is designed to provide a bond between the dentinal canal wall and the master cone (monoblock). A bacterial leakage study comparing Activ GP/glass ionomer sealer, Resilon/Epiphany, and gutta-percha (GP)/AH Plus demonstrated no statistically significant differences at 65 days.[125]

Resin Sealers

Resin sealers have a long history of use, provide adhesion, and do not contain eugenol. There are two major categories: epoxy resin–based and methacrylate resin–based sealers.

Epoxy Resin Sealers

AH-26 (DENTSPLY DeTrey, Konstanz, Germany) is a slow-setting epoxy resin that was found to release formaldehyde when setting.[204,368] AH Plus (DENTSPLY DeTrey) is a modified formulation of AH-26 in which formaldehyde is not released (Fig. 7-15).[222] The sealing abilities of AH-26 and AH Plus appear comparable.[96] AH Plus is an epoxy resin–amine based system that comes in two tubes. The epoxide paste tube contains a diepoxide (bisphenol A diglycidyl ether) and fillers as the major ingredients, while the amine paste tube contains a primary monoamine, a secondary diamine, a disecondary diamine, silicone oil, and fillers as the major ingredients. It exhibits a working time of approximately 4 hours.

Methacrylate Resin Sealers

Four generations of methacrylate resin–based root canal sealers have been marketed for commercial use.[200,278] The first generation of hydrophilic methacrylate resin–based material (Hydron; Hydron Technologies, Inc., Boca Raton, Florida) was designed for en masse root filling and appeared in the mid 1970s when

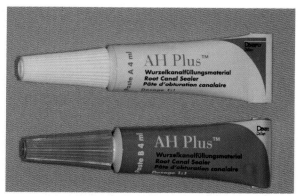

FIG. 7-15 AH Plus sealer is a resin formulation. (Courtesy DENTSPLY DeTrey, Konstanz, Germany.)

scientific foundations behind dentin bonding were at their infancy stage of development. The major component of Hydron was poly[2-hydroxyethyl methacrylate] (poly[HEMA]), which was injected into a root canal and polymerized in situ within the canal space without the adjunctive use of a root-filling material. Hydron became obsolete in the 1980s as subsequent clinical findings were unacceptable.[215]

Prior to the advent of contemporary methacrylate resin–based sealers that are specifically designed for endodontic application, there had been sporadic attempts on the use of low viscosity resin composites (i.e., resin cements) and dentin bonding agents as sealers for root-filling materials. Leonard and coworkers were the first to demonstrate, with the use of an etch-and-rinse technique (citric acid–ferric chloride etchant known as 10:3 solution), the formation of a hybrid layer in radicular dentin with C&B-Metabond (Parkell Inc., Edgewood, New York), an adhesive resin cement for cementation of indirect restorations and prostheses.[221] Following the marketing of self-priming, self-etching and self-adhesive resin cement technologies in restorative dentistry, functionally analogous, low viscosity methacrylate resin–based root canal sealers have since been available for use in endodontics. This type of bondable root canal sealers has been aggressively promoted with the highly desirable property of creating monoblocks within the root canal space.[383] The term monoblock refers to the idealized scenario in which the canal space becomes perfectly filled with a gap-free, solid mass that consists of different materials and interfaces, with the purported advantages of simultaneously improving the seal and fracture resistance of the filled canals.

The second generation of bondable sealer is nonetching and hydrophilic in nature and does not require the adjunctive use of a dentin adhesive. It is designed to flow into accessory canals and dentinal tubules to facilitate resin tag formation for retention and seal after smear layer removal with NaOCl and EDTA. EndoREZ (Ultradent Products Inc., South Jordan, Utah) is a dual-cured radiopaque hydrophilic methacrylate sealer that contains non-acidic diurethane dimethacrylate. The addition of triethyleneglycol dimethacrylate to the sealer composition renders it hydrophilic, so that it may be used in the wet environment of the root canal system and be very effective in penetrating dentinal tubules and forming long resin tags.[34,382] The sealer was found to seal best when applied to slightly moist intraradicular dentin.[440] EndoREZ is recommended for use with either a conventional gutta-percha cone or with specific EndoREZ points (resin-coated gutta-percha). A retrospective clinical and radiographic study evaluating the 10-year treatment outcome of one-visit root canal treatment using gutta-percha and the EndoREZ sealer reported accumulative probability of success of 92.1% after 10 years.[439] The authors concluded that EndoREZ may be recommended as an alternative to other commonly used root canal sealers. Unfortunately, no additional root canal sealer was used in that study for comparison.

New generations of self-etching (third generation) and self-adhesive (fourth generation) resin cements have been introduced to restorative dentists to simplify bonding procedures. They became commercially available shortly after the introduction of those resin cement systems. The third generation self-etching sealers contain a self-etching primer and a dual-cured resin composite root canal sealer. The use of self-etching primers reintroduced the concept of incorporating smear layers created by hand/rotary instruments along the sealer-dentin interface. An acidic primer is applied to the dentin surface that penetrates through the smear layer and demineralizes the superficial dentin. The acidic primer is air-dried to remove the volatile carrier and then a dual-cured moderately filled flowable resin composite sealer is applied and polymerized. Provided that these materials are sufficiently aggressive to etch through thick smear layers, the technique sensitivity of bonding to root canals may be reduced when smear layers are inadvertently retained in the apical third of instrumented canal walls.

Third-generation methacrylate resin–based sealers that incorporate the use of self-etching primers became popularized following the introduction of Resilon (Resilon Research LLC, Madison, Connecticut), a dimethacrylate-containing polycaprolactone-based thermoplastic root-filling material.[355] In RealSeal (SybronEndo), the self-etching primers are supplied as a single-bottle system and contain 2-acrylamido-2-methyl-propanesulfonic acid (AMPS) as the functional acidic monomer. The functional acidic monomer, solvent, water that is necessary for ionization of the acidic monomers, and self-cured catalysts are incorporated into "one-component" (i.e., incorporated inside a single bottle). This is similar to the so-called "one-component" type all-in-one adhesives that are currently available in restorative dentistry. The sealer that is used after application of the self-etching primer consists of bisphenol-A-glycidyldimethacrylate (BisGMA), ethoxylated BisGMA, urethane dimethacrylate (UDMA), and hydrophilic methacrylate with calcium hydroxide, barium sulfate, barium glass, bismuth oxychloride, and silica.[186] An ethoxylated bisphenol-A-dimethacrylate (EBPADMA)–based resinous solvent (e.g., RealSeal Thinning Resin, SybronEndo) is also available for adjusting the sealer viscosity.[301]

The fourth-generation methacrylate resin–based sealers (e.g., MetaSEAL, Parkell Inc.; RealSeal SE, SybronEndo) is functionally analogous to a similar class of recently introduced self-adhesive resin luting cements in that they have further eliminated the separate etching/bonding step.[302] Acidic resin monomers that are originally present in dentin adhesive primers are now incorporated into the resin-based sealer/cement to render them self-adhesive to dentin substrates. The combination of an etchant, a primer, and a sealer into an all-in-one self-etching, self-adhesive sealer is advantageous in that it reduces the application time as well as errors that may occur during each bonding step. MetaSEAL is the first commercially available fourth-generation self-adhesive dual-curable sealer.[217]

The liquid component of MetaSEAL comprises 4-META, HEMA and difunctional methacrylate monomers. The powder contains zirconium oxide as spherical radiopaque fillers, silica nanofillers, and a hydrophilic initiator. The inclusion of an acidic resin monomer, 4-methacryloyloxyethyl trimellitate anhydride (4-META), makes the sealer self-etching and hydrophilic in nature and promotes monomer diffusion into the underlying intact dentin to produce a hybrid layer after polymerization. According to the manufacturer, MetaSEAL is recommended exclusively for cold compaction and single-cone techniques and supports the use of either Resilon or gutta-percha as a root-filling material. The sealer purportedly bonds to thermoplastic root-filling materials as well as radicular dentin via the creation of hybrid layers in both substrates. MetaSEAL is also marketed as Hybrid Bond SEAL (Sun Medical Co. Ltd., Shiga, Japan) in Japan and had been reported to produce equivalent or slightly inferior sealing properties as conventional non-bonding epoxy resin-based sealers.[30,269]

RealSeal SE is the simplified dual-cured version of RealSeal and uses a polymerizable methacrylate carboxylic acid anhydride (i.e., 4-META) as the acidic resin monomer.[15,201,237] It contains EBPADMA, HEMA, BisGMA, benzoyl peroxide, tertiary amine, photoinitiators, silane-treated barium borosilicate glass, silica, bismuth oxychloride, Ca-Al-F silicate, tricalcium phosphate as additional components. It may be used with Resilon cones or pellets using cold lateral or warm vertical techniques, or with RealSeal 1, a carrier-based Resilon obturator system.[166]

Silicone Sealers

RoekoSeal (Coltène/Whaledent) is a polydimethylsiloxane that has been reported to expand slightly on setting.[273]

GuttaFlow and GuttaFlow2 (Coltène/Whaledent) are cold flowable matrices that are triturated. They consist of gutta-percha in particulate form (less than 30 μm) added to RoekoSeal (Fig. 7-16). The material is provided in capsules for trituration. The technique involves injection of the material into the canal, followed by placement of a single master cone. The material provides a working time of 15 minutes and it cures in 25 to 30 minutes. Evidence suggests that the material fills canal irregularities with consistency[435] and is biocompatible,[45,116] but the setting time is inconsistent and may be delayed by final irrigation with sodium hypochlorite.[45] The sealing

ability appears comparable to other techniques in some studies and inferior in others.[45,47,206,276,396]

Calcium Silicate Sealers

A new category of root canal sealers based on mineral trioxide aggregate (MTA) has recently been commercially available. These sealers are an outgrowth of the popularity of MTA materials, which are based on tricalcium silicate, a hydraulic (water-setting) powder used for various surgical and vital pulp therapy treatments.[279,280] This type of root canal sealer is attractive because of the bioactivity that has been reported for MTA-type materials,[131,384] which are also known for being hydrophilic.[65]

Calcium silicate sealers include some of the same hydraulic compounds found in Portland cement, primarily tricalcium silicate and dicalcium silicate powder.[65] The first use of hydraulic calcium silicate materials in dentistry dates to 1878, when a German, Dr. Witte, published a case report on using Portland cement to fill root canals.[103] Tricalcium silicate–based materials did not come into common practice until the 1990s, when Mineral Trioxide Aggregate (MTA) was introduced. MTA is a hydraulically active powder that contains primarily tricalcium silicate, dicalcium silicate, and a radiopaque powder, often bismuth oxide. Because of staining of crown dentin by the bismuth oxide component, which may be rendered brown (in NaOCl), gray (in chlorhexidine) or even black (in glutaraldehyde), the radiopacifier has now been replaced with other materials such as zirconia dioxide (zirconia) or tantalum oxide in some commercial formulations. The radiopaque agent, bismuth oxide, zirconia, or tantalum oxide, is important, without which MTA would not be distinguishable on a radiograph. Minor phases of tricalcium aluminate and calcium sulfate are often present. Some MTA-type products contain calcium carbonate, or tetracalcium aluminoferrite. The term MTA is used here to denote all the tri- and dicalcium silicate products.

Tricalcium silicate cements/sealers set by reaction with water and form a highly alkaline (pH of about 12) mixture consisting of a rigid matrix of calcium silicate hydrates and calcium hydroxide.[89] These hydrates form on the surface of the original calcium silicate particles and hydration gradually penetrates inward. When tricalcium silicate cement sets, the dimensional change is less than 0.1% expansion, which helps with creating a barrier, and is especially important for endodontics. Setting time for tricalcium silicate cements is lengthy, about 165 minutes for the initial set and less than 6 hours for the final set, which has been a major drawback for using them in some indications, but not for its use as a sealer. The consistency of the MTA products with water has not been suitable for use as a sealer. Also, the coarseness of the first MTA products, intended for surgical use, has meant they were not suitable for use as a sealer, as their film thickness was too high (>50 μm).

Four tricalcium silicate sealers are currently commercially available: MTA Fillapex (Ângelus Indústria de Produtos Odontlógicos Ltda; Londrina, Paraná, Brazil),[44,143,255,438] iRoot SP (Innovative BioCeramix Inc., Vancouver, Canada; aka Endosequence BC sealer; Brasseler USA),[44,66,231,432,434] Endo CPM Sealer (EGEO SRL, Buenos Aires, Argentina),[141,142,255,336,378] and MTA Plus (Avalon Biomed, Bradenton, Florida). The MTA Plus may be used as a cement[220,334] or a sealer by adjusting the powder:liquid ratio. Table 7-2 lists what is known about the components of these sealers. Other experimental tricalcium

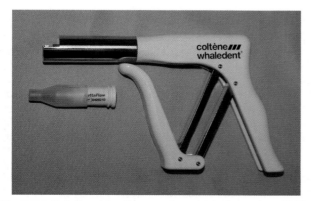

FIG. 7-16 GuttaFlow trituration capsule and injection syringe (Coltène/Whaledent).

TABLE 7-2

Composition of Tricalcium Silicate Root Canal Sealers

Generex B ProRoot Endo Sealer	MTA Fillapex	Endosequence BC Sealer (iRoot SP)	Endo CPM Sealer	MTA Plus
Powder/gel	Dual paste	Single paste	Powder/gel	Powder/gel
Mineral trioxide aggregate (MTA) powder with enhanced radiopacity Water-based gel	Salicylate resin Diluent resin Natural resin Bismuth oxide Silica MTA Pigments	Zirconium oxide Calcium silicates Calcium phosphate monobasic $(CaH_4P_2O_8)$ Calcium hydroxide Filler Thickening agents	MTA powder Silicon dioxide Calcium carbonate Bismuth oxide Barium sulfate Propylene glycol alginate Propylene glycol Sodium citrate Calcium chloride Active ingredients	MTA powder Water-based gel

silicate sealers include Generex B (aka ProRoot Endo Sealer),[404] MTAS[64] and MTA Flow.[130] The iRoot SP is premixed and MTA Fillapex has two pastes that are combined in a mixing tip. The Endo CPM Sealer and MTA Plus sealer are powder/gel systems that the user can mix to the consistency desired. The available materials' descriptions are vague; for instance, MTA Fillapex has "natural or diluent resins," with "filler and thickening agents." However, what is believed to be in common is that tricalcium silicate powder is a component of all four sealers.

The MTA Fillapex and iRoot SP sealers have non-aqueous vehicles in which the powders are dispersed. For the tricalcium silicate particles to contribute to sealing, they must become hydrated in the tooth by exchange of the non-aqueous vehicle for water in the root canal. EndoCPM Sealer and MTA Plus sealer rely on mixing with water-based gels just before use, without a non-aqueous resin. The proportions of the tricalcium silicate powders are not known in any of these materials, but are most likely to be highest in MTA Plus because no inert liquid vehicle is included. The inert vehicle is the liquid medium in the pastes of MTA Fillapex and iRoot SP that does not react with the powder. The bioactivity of MTA-type materials has made the use of tricalcium silicate powders in sealers of interest. The possibility of extrusion past the apex with a bioactive material leads to the supposition that healing in the periapical area would occur more readily with a tricalcium silicate product. However, two of the sealers have the tricalcium silicate powders dispersed in a non-reactive organic medium, which may detract from the potential benefit of the bioactive powder. To date, no peer-reviewed papers have been published to establish the benefits of tricalcium silicate powders in sealers in human clinical studies; all studies and reports are based on in vitro testing and in vivo animal models. Calcium carbonate is added to Endo CPM Sealer to reduce the pH from 12.5 to 10.0 after setting. By doing so, the manufacturer claimed that surface necrosis in contact with the material is reduced, thereby optimizing the conditions for the enzymatic action of alkaline phosphatase.[142]

The physical properties of some of these sealers have been published. Table 7-3 contains values that are known for comparison to the ISO 6876/ADA 57 methods and requirements and the AH Plus sealer. The flow, film thicknesses, solubility, dimensional stability, and radiopacity of the new sealers meet the ISO 6876 requirements. The flow of these sealers varies, but so do the values for AH Plus. The dimensional stability is excellent. The solubility of the sealers is higher than AH Plus, which may be attributed to the formation of partially soluble calcium hydroxide within the set tricalcium silicate. The radiopacities are less than AH Plus, which is known for its radiopacity.

The working and setting times of the iRoot SP and MTA Plus materials are longer than the MTA Fillapex sealer. iRoot SP has the longest setting time, and requires diffusion of water from the dentinal tubules into the sealer to set.[256] In a test where water was added to the EndoSequence BC sealer (i.e., iRoot SP), the setting time was reduced to about 150 hours, but the hardness was significantly diminished.[231] The Endosequence BC sealer has been tested for strengthening teeth when used with glass ionomer–coated cones and found to be stronger in vitro.[135]

Biocompatibility tests have been performed with some of these sealers. Endosequence BC sealer was more cytotoxic than AH Plus root canal sealer; the time to become noncytotoxic as judged from mitochondrial enzymatic (succinic dehydrogenase) activity was 5 weeks for Endosequence BC sealer and 3 weeks for AH Plus sealer.[231] Another study found that after setting, the cytotoxicity of MTA Fillapex decreased and the sealer presents suitable bioactivity to stimulate hydroxyapatite nucleation.[323]

Medicated Sealers

Sealers containing paraformaldehyde are strongly contraindicated in endodontic treatment (Fig. 7-17). Although the lead and mercury components may have been removed from these zinc oxide–eugenol formulations over time, the severely toxic paraformaldehyde content has remained a constant. These sealers are not approved by the U.S. Food and Drug Administration[12] and are unacceptable under any circumstances in clinical treatment because of the severe and permanent toxic effects on periradicular tissues.[348] A paste containing 6.5% paraformaldehyde as well as lead and mercury was advocated for use by Sargenti[325-327] and originally marketed as N-2. Lead has been reported in distant organ systems when N-2 is placed within the radicular space.[274] In another study the investigators reported the same results regarding systemic distribution of the paraformaldehyde component of N-2.[38] Removal of the heavy metals resulted in a new formulation: RC2B. Other

TABLE 7-3

Physical Properties of Tricalcium Silicate Root Canal Sealers

Quality	ISO 6876-2001 ADA 57 Requirement	AH Plus*†	MTA Fillapex†	Endosequence BC Sealer	MTA Plus White, Gray‡
Flow (mm)	>20	21, 40	25, 29	23	31
Film thickness (μm)	<50	16	24	22	47
Solubility	<3%	0.1	1.1	2.9	1.9
Dimensional stability	−1% to +0.1%	−0.04	−0.7	+0.09	+0.05
Radiopacity	>3 mm Al				4.9, 5.5
Working time (hours)	No requirement	4:00, 5:30	0:45, 0:30	2:40	0:20
Setting time (hours)	No requirement	11:30, 5:10	2:30, 2:15	>24	10:00

*An epoxy resin–based sealer included for comparative purposes.
†Measured by two authors.
‡If one value is given, white and gray versions of MTA Plus are equal.

paraformaldehyde sealers include Endomethasone, SPAD, and Reibler's paste. The toxic in vivo effects of these materials on the pulp and periapical tissues have been demonstrated over time.[80,261]

In addition to the toxic nature of the material, clinicians employing the material place it with a lentulo spiral. Overextension has resulted in osteomyelitis and paresthesia.[117,202] One of these studies reported irreversible neurotoxicity, manifested as dysesthesia, in cases where paraformaldehyde pastes were forced through the apical foramen into the periapical tissues.[202] The reader is referred to Chapter 29 for further discussion about this harmful material and technique.

SEALER PLACEMENT

Various methods of sealer placement have been advocated, including the master cone, lentulo spirals, files and reamers, and ultrasonics. Investigators compared sealer placement using a file rotated counterclockwise, the lentulo spiral (Fig. 7-18), an ultrasonic file, and coating the master gutta-percha cone.[413] Placement did not differ with the various techniques; however, the investigators noted the most variation in sealer coating was in the apical area.[413] Another study compared sealer placement with a K-type file, the lentulo spiral, and using the master cone in curved canals. Results demonstrated no significant differences in the techniques after obturation; no technique covered more than 62.5% of the canal wall surface.[158] Other investigators reported that ultrasonics produced the best sealer distribution when used circumferentially.[369] These findings were supported by another study that reported ultrasonic placement to be superior to manual placement techniques.[1]

In the past, it has been assumed that instrumented canals need to be thoroughly dried prior to obturation with root-filling materials and sealers. Indeed, there were leakage studies reporting that a better apical seal might be achieved by drying the canals with 95% ethanol prior to obturation.[370] A recent study reported that for some root canal sealers (iRoot SP, AH Plus, Epiphany and MTA Fillapex), better adhesion to the dentinal walls might be achieved by leaving the canals slightly moist (i.e., drying the canals with low vacuum via a Luer-Lok adapter for 5 seconds, followed by one paper point for one second).[256] Similar results were also reported with the use of the EndoREZ sealer.[440] This, however, does not mean that

canals should remain totally flooded with water prior to obturation, because such a level of residual moisture would adversely affect the adhesiveness of those root canal sealers to intraradicular dentin.[256]

The method of obturation does not seem to affect the sealer distribution on the canal wall in the apical portion of the canal; however, lateral compaction results in better distribution in the mid-coronal areas when compared with warm vertical compaction.[422] Another well-controlled study reported that none of five evaluated obturation techniques resulted in uniform sealer distribution along the entire length of the core obturation material.[176] Evidence indicates that the method of obturation affects the sealer penetration into tubules. This was exemplified by a study reporting that thermoplastic techniques produced deeper sealer penetration into tubules.[94] Removal of the smear layer enhances sealer penetration into the dentinal tubules.[93]

CORE MATERIALS

Although a variety of core materials have been used in conjunction with a sealer/cement, the most common method of obturation involves gutta-percha as a core material. Regardless of the obturating technique, emphasis should be placed on the process of cleaning and shaping the canal. The materials and techniques described do not routinely create an impervious seal of the canal system; all materials leak to some extent.[2] The choice of the obturation technique(s) depends on the unique circumstances with which each case presents.

The properties of an ideal obturation material have been outlined by Grossman (Box 7-2).[149] Historically, a variety of materials have been employed to obturate the root canal space. Solids, semisolid materials, and pastes have been employed. A common solid material used in the past was the silver cone.

Silver Cones

Jasper introduced cones made of silver, which he claimed produced the same success rate as gutta-percha and were easier to use.[183] The rigidity provided by the silver cones made them easier to place and permitted more predictable length control; however, their inability to fill the irregularly shaped root canal system permitted leakage (Fig. 7-19). Silver cones were believed to possess an oligodynamic property which, if true,

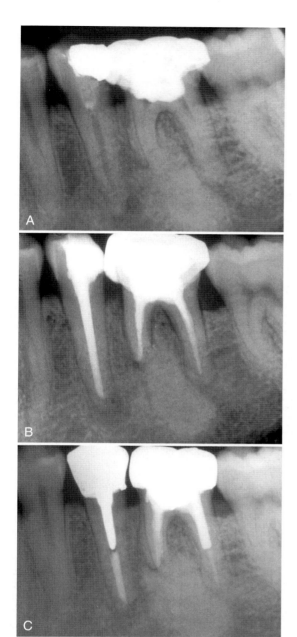

FIG. 7-17 Patient treated with Sargenti paste in her mandibular left second premolar and first molar. **A,** Pretreatment radiograph exhibits an osteolytic response associated with the premolar and a proliferative response associated with the molar. **B,** Posttreatment radiograph of the teeth. **C,** One-year follow-up radiograph exhibiting osseous regeneration apical to the second premolar.

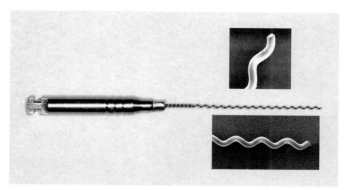

FIG. 7-18 Lentulo spiral used for sealer placement during obturation.

BOX 7-2

Properties of an Ideal Obturation Material

- ◆ Easily manipulated and provides ample working time
- ◆ Dimensionally stable with no shrinkage once inserted
- ◆ Seals the canal laterally and apically, conforming to its complex internal anatomy
- ◆ Nonirritating to the periapical tissues
- ◆ Impervious to moisture and nonporous
- ◆ Unaffected by tissue fluids—no corrosion or oxidization
- ◆ Inhibits bacterial growth
- ◆ Radiopaque and easily discernible on radiographs
- ◆ Does not discolor tooth structure
- ◆ Sterile
- ◆ Easily removed from the canal if necessary

would have resulted in the destruction of microbes within the root canal system. Unfortunately, it was not true. Moreover, when silver points contact tissue fluids or saliva, they corrode.[48] The corrosion products have been found to be cytotoxic and produce pathosis or impede periapical healing.[344]

With the introduction of rigid silver cones it became possible to easily place them to length. This resulted in clinicians often failing to properly clean and shape the canal before obturation. Treatment failures were the result of leakage and failure to remove the irritants from the root canal system. The use of silver cones today is considered to be below the standard of care in contemporary endodontic practice. For further information about this material and technique, the reader is referred to Chapter 29.

Gutta-Percha

Gutta-percha is the most popular core material used for obturation. Major advantages of gutta-percha are its plasticity, ease of manipulation, minimal toxicity, radiopacity, and ease of removal with heat or solvents. Disadvantages include its lack of adhesion to dentin and, when heated, shrinkage upon cooling. Gutta-percha is the *trans*-isomer of polyisoprene (rubber) and exists in two crystalline forms (α and β).[144] In the unheated β phase, the material is a solid mass that is compactable. When heated, the material changes to the α phase and becomes pliable and tacky and can be made to flow when pressure is applied. A disadvantage to the α phase is that the material shrinks on setting.[340]

Gutta-percha cones consist of approximately 20% gutta-percha, 65% zinc oxide, 10% radiopacifiers, and 5% plasticizers.[126] Attempts have been made to make gutta-percha more antimicrobial by the addition of materials such as iodoform,[75] calcium hydroxide,[230] chlorhexidene,[233] and tetracycline.[247] The clinical effectiveness of adding these materials has not been demonstrated. Moreover, to exert an antimicrobial pharmacological effect, the active ingredient must leach out of the gutta-percha, which could have a detrimental effect on long-term sealability.

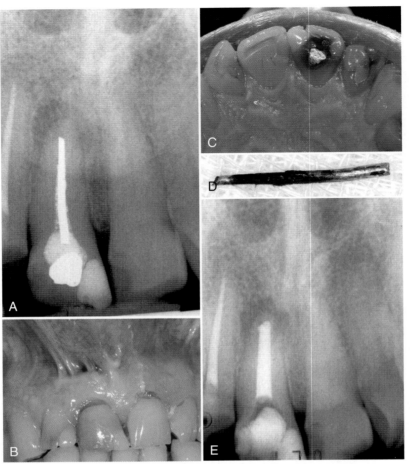

FIG. 7-19 Silver cones are advocated for ease of placement and length control. **A,** Radiograph of a facial maxillary right central incisor obturated with a silver cone. **B,** Tissue discoloration indicating corrosion and leakage. **C,** Lingual view indicates coronal leakage. **D,** Corroded silver cone removed from the tooth. **E,** Posttreatment radiograph of the tooth.

Unlike rubber, room temperature gutta-percha cannot be condensed or made to flow. Compaction results in transmission of forces to the material and the canal wall equally and may result in root fracture. Gutta-percha can be made to flow if it is modified by either heat or solvents such as chloroform. This permits adaptation to the irregularities of the canal walls.

The α form of gutta-percha melts when heated above 65°C. When cooled extremely slowly, the α form will recrystallize. Routine cooling results in the recrystallization of the β form. Although the mechanical properties for the two forms are the same, when α-phase gutta-percha is heated and cooled, it undergoes less shrinkage, making it more dimensionally stable for thermoplasticized techniques. The use of α-phase gutta-percha for obturation has increased as thermoplastic techniques have become more common.

Gutta-percha cones are available in standardized and non-standardized sizes. Standardized sizes conform to requirements contained in specifications published by the International Organization of Standardization (ISO) or ADA American National Standards Institute (ADA ANSI). The nonstandard nomenclature refers to the dimensions of the tip and body (Fig. 7-20). A fine-medium cone has a fine tip with a medium body. Standardized cones are designed to match the taper of stainless steel and nickel-titanium instruments (Figs. 7-21 and 7-22). A size

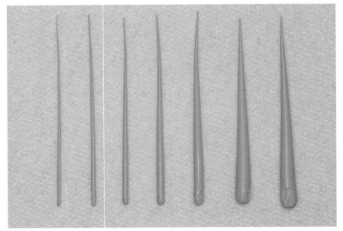

FIG. 7-20 Nonstandard gutta-percha cones: extra fine, fine fine, fine, medium fine, fine medium, medium, large, and extra large.

40, 0.04 taper cone has a tip of 0.4 mm and a taper of 0.04 mm per millimeter. Unfortunately ISO and ADA ANSI standards allow tolerances and, coupled with a less than completely accurate manufacturing process, the actual cone size varies as does the tip and taper of the master apical file.[140,243]

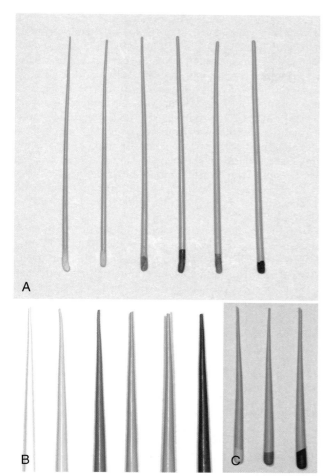

FIG. 7-21 **A**, Standard gutta-percha cone sizes #15 to #40. **B**, Standard cones #.06, taper sizes #15 to #40. **C**, Standard cones Protaper F1, F2, F3.

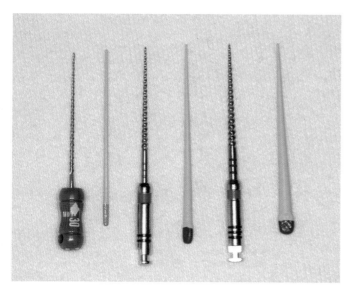

FIG. 7-22 Size #30 standard gutta-percha points exhibiting #.02, #.04, and #.06 tapers.

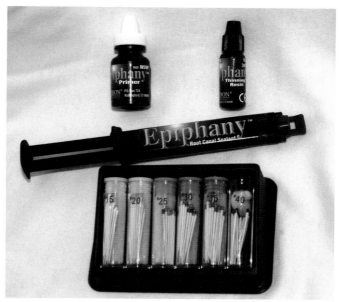

FIG. 7-23 Epiphany system with the primer, thinning resin, sealant, and standard Resilon points. (Courtesy Pentron Clinical Technologies, Wallingford, Conn.)

Although gutta-percha points cannot be heat sterilized, a study reported that gutta-percha points can be sterilized by placing in 5.25% NaOCl for one minute. This study also reported that 2% glutaraldehyde, 2% chlorhexidine, and 70% ethyl alcohol were not effective in killing *Bacillus subtilis* spores, one of the hallmark organisms used for testing effective antimicrobial effectiveness.[359]

Activ GP

Activ GP (Brasseler USA) consists of gutta-percha cones impregnated on the external surface with glass ionomer (see Fig. 7-14). Single cones are used with a glass ionomer sealer. Available in 0.04 and 0.06 taper cones, the sizes are laser-verified to help ensure a more precise fit. The single cone technique is designed to provide a bond between the dentinal canal wall and the master cone. A bacterial leakage study comparing Activ GP/glass ionomer sealer, Resilon/Epiphany, and gutta-percha/AH Plus demonstrated no statistically significant differences in leakage at 65 days.[125]

Resilon

The resin-based obturation systems RealSeal (SybronEndo), and Resinate (Obtura Spartan, Algonquin, Illinois) have been introduced as alternatives to gutta-percha (Figs. 7-23 and 7-24). Resilon is a high-performance industrial polyester that has been adapted for dental use.

The resin sealer bonds to a Resilon core, and attaches to the etched root surface. The manufacturer claims that this forms a "monoblock" (Fig. 7-25). With traditional obturation techniques, there is a gutta-percha–sealer interface and a tooth-sealer interface. With Resilon the resin sealer bonds to both the canal wall and the Resilon cone. Whether a monoblock is achievable remains controversial.[303] An in-depth review article on the subject of monoblocks indicates that with current materials and techniques, the monoblock has yet to be achieved.[383]

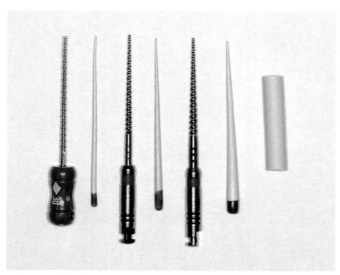

FIG. 7-24 Resilon #.02, #.04, and #.06 tapered points and a thermoplastic plug for use in the Obtura system.

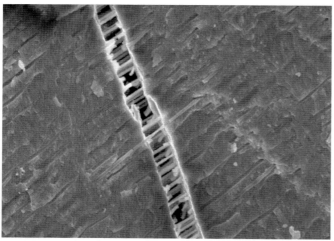

FIG. 7-25 Scanning electron microscopy view of Resilon tags extending into the dentinal tubules.

The system resembles gutta-percha and can be placed by lateral compaction, warm lateral or vertical compaction, thermoplastic injection, or with a core-carrier technique. It consists of a resin core material (Resilon) composed of polyester, difunctional methacrylate resin, bioactive glass, radiopaque fillers, and a resin sealer. Resilon is nontoxic, nonmutagenic, and biocompatible. The core material is available in nonstandard and standard cones and pellets for use in thermoplastic techniques (see Fig. 7-24).

After cleaning and shaping procedures an appropriate master cone is placed into the prepared canal and a radiograph image is exposed to verify the apical position. Because NaOCl may affect the bond strength of the primer, EDTA should be the last irrigant used before rinsing the canal with sterile water, saline, or chlorhexidine.

After drying the canal, a self-etch primer (sulfonic acid–terminated functional monomer, 2-hydroxyethyl methacrylate [HEMA], water, and polymerization initiator) is used to condition the canal walls and prepare them for bonding to the

resin sealant (resin matrix of bisphenol A-glycidyl methacrylate [Bis-GMA], ethoxylated Bis-GMA, urethane dimethacrylate [UDMA], and hydrophilic difunctional methacrylates and fillers [70%] of calcium hydroxide, barium sulfate, barium glass, bismuth oxychloride, and silica). Two or three drops are placed in the canal with a pipette, a syringe, or a paper point that wicks the material to the working length. The excess primer is removed, the resin sealer is dispensed onto a mixing slab, and the viscosity is adjusted with the thinning resin. The sealer is applied with a paper point, Resilon point, or lentulo spiral. The canal is then obturated by lateral compaction, warm vertical compaction, or thermoplastic injection. The sealer takes approximately 25 minutes to set, so it is recommended that the coronal surface of the material be light cured for 40 seconds.

When using the System B (SybronEndo) for warm vertical compaction, the temperature setting should be 150°C at a power of 10. With the Obtura II thermoplasticized injection system (Obtura Spartan), the temperature settings vary depending on the needle tip employed. For the 25-gauge needle, a 160°C setting is selected; for the 23-gauge needle, a 140°C setting is used; and for the 20-gauge needle, the setting that is recommended is 120°C to 130°C.

Resilon appears to be comparable to gutta-percha in its ability to seal the radicular space.[22] Investigators evaluated coronal leakage of Resilon, using *Streptococcus mutans* and *E. faecalis* in roots that were filled by lateral and vertical compaction techniques with gutta-percha and AH-26 or Resilon and Epiphany sealer.[355] Resilon showed significantly less coronal leakage when compared with gutta-percha. In another study, investigators used a dog model to assess the ability of Resilon or gutta-percha and AH-26 to prevent apical periodontitis in teeth inoculated with microorganisms. Results indicated periapical inflammation in 18 of 22 roots (82%) obturated with gutta-percha and AH-26, whereas the Resilon group exhibited periapical inflammation in only 4 of 21 roots (19%).[356] Another study demonstrated that teeth filled with Resilon were more resistant to fracture than roots filled with gutta-percha and AH-26 sealer.[387] More recent evidence suggests that Resilon does not strengthen roots.[147,416]

Resilon appears to be biocompatible; implantation in the subcutaneous tissues of rats demonstrated fibrous encapsulation and negligible inflammation at 60 days.[41] One retrospective study compared the success and failure rates between obturation with gutta-percha and Kerr Pulp Canal Sealer and obturation with Resilon or Epiphany, with recall examination between 12 and 25 months. Statistical analysis indicated that the results were indistinguishable.[83] Another study demonstrated that 82 randomly selected clinical cases treated with Resilon produced success rates at 1 year that were comparable to cases treated with gutta-percha.[82] A recent review of the use of Resilon as a root-filling material reported that Resilon cannot be considered yet as an evidence-based replacement for the current gold-standard gutta-percha, due to the lack of long-term clinical outcome studies to demonstrate its clinical superiority over contemporary gutta-percha obturation techniques.[354]

Custom Cones

When the apical foramen is excessively large or the prepared root canal system is large, a custom cone may need to be fabricated (Fig. 7-26). This permits the adaptation of the cone to the canal walls, reduces the potential for extrusion of the core

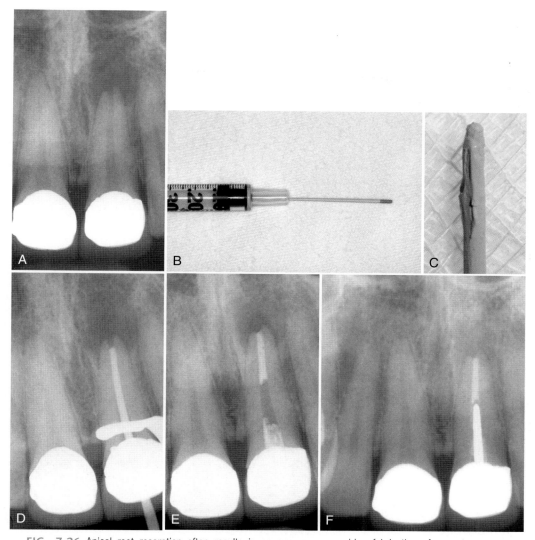

FIG. 7-26 Apical root resorption often results in an open apex requiring fabrication of a custom cone. A, Pretreatment radiograph of the maxillary left central incisor with pulp necrosis and chronic apical periodontitis. Apical root resorption is present. B, In fabricating a custom master cone a gutta-percha point is fit several millimeters short before softening in solvent and tamping into place. C, Softening the apical 2 to 3 mm in chloroform that has been placed in a tuberculin syringe. D, The completed custom cone represents an impression of the apical portion of the canal. E, The posttreatment radiograph with post space prepared. F, A 1-year follow-up radiograph demonstrating osseous regeneration.

material, and may improve the resultant seal.[28,194] The technique involves selection of a master cone and fitting that cone 2 to 4 mm short of the prepared length with frictional resistance. The cone is grasped with locking cotton pliers or a hemostat so that it can be placed into the canal in the same spatial relationship each time. The cone is removed and the tip is softened in chloroform, eucalyptol, or halothane for 1 or 2 seconds, depending on the clinical requirements. Only the outer superficial portion of the cone is softened. The central core of the cone should remain semi-rigid. The cone is then placed into the canal to the working length. The process can be repeated until an adequate impression of the canal is obtained at the prepared length. A radiograph is exposed to verify proper fit and position. An alternative to solvents is softening with heat.[196]

Large root canal systems may necessitate custom fabrication of a large master cone before canal adaptation. This may be accomplished by heating two, or more, large gutta-percha cones and rolling the mass between two glass slabs until an appropriate size is obtained (Fig. 7-27). A spatula may also be used to shape the cone.

METHODS OF OBTURATION

To date, little evidence exists to support one method of obturation as being superior to another based on outcome assessment investigations.[13,264] The prospective Toronto studies have suggested that warm vertical compaction may be superior to lateral compaction[92]; however, definitive evidence is lacking.[286]

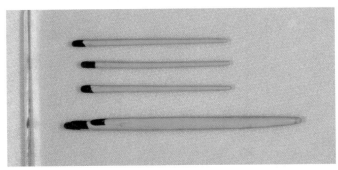

FIG. 7-27 For large canals, several gutta-percha points can be heated and rolled together, using a spatula or two glass slabs.

Lateral Compaction

Lateral compaction is a common method for obturation (Fig. 7-28).[59] The technique can be used in most clinical situations and provides for predictable length control during compaction.[136] A disadvantage is that the technique may not fill canal irregularities[427] as well as warm vertical compaction or other thermoplastic techniques.[424] The procedure can be accomplished with any of the acceptable sealers.

After root canal system preparation, a standard cone is selected that has a diameter consistent with the prepared canal diameter at the working length. Standard cones generally have less taper when compared with nonstandard cones and will permit deeper spreader penetration which will result in a better-quality resultant seal.[288] An alternative is to adapt an appropriately tapered nonstandard cone by cutting small

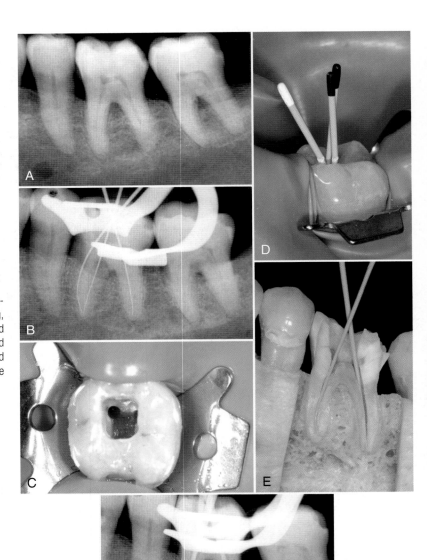

FIG. 7-28 Left first mandibular molar. A, Pretreatment radiograph. B, Working length radiograph. C, Coronal access opening, demonstrating the prepared mesiobuccal canal. D, Standardized master cones with coronal reference marked. E, Standard master cones fit to length as they exhibit minimal taper and permit deeper penetration of the spreader. F, Master cone radiograph.

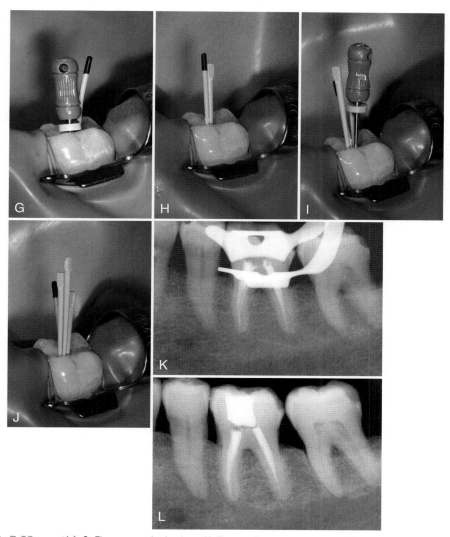

FIG. 7-28, cont'd **G,** Finger spreader in place. **H,** Fine-medium accessory cone placed in the space created by the spreader. **I,** Finger spreader placed in preparation, creating space for additional accessory cones. **J,** Additional cones are placed until the spreader does not penetrate past the coronal one third of the canal. The cones are then removed at the orifice with heat, and the coronal mass is vertically compacted with a plugger. **K,** Interim radiograph may be exposed to assess the quality of obturation. **L,** Posttreatment radiograph demonstrating adequate length, density, and taper. The gutta-percha is removed to the level of the orifice, and a coronal seal has been established with an adequate provisional restoration.

increments from the tip. This "master cone" is measured and grasped with forceps so that the distance from the tip of the cone to the reference point on the forceps is equal to the prepared length. A reference point on the cone can be made by pinching the cone. The cone is placed in the canal, and if an appropriate size is selected, there will be resistance to displacement or "tug back." If the cone is loose it can be adapted by removing small increments from the tip. If the master cone fails to go to the prepared length a smaller cone can be selected. Devices are available to cut cones accurately at a predetermined length (Tip Snip; SybronEndo). When the cone extends beyond the prepared length a larger cone must be adapted or the existing cone shortened until there is resistance to displacement at the corrected working length.

The master cone placement is confirmed with a radiograph. The canal is irrigated and dried with paper points. Sealer is applied to the canal walls, and a spreader is prefitted so as to allow it to be inserted to within 1 to 2 mm of the working length. Appropriately sized accessory points are also selected to closely match the size of the spreader. The correlation between spreader size and nonstandard cones is variable,[53,437] and in small curved canals there does not appear to be a difference in the quality of obturation with nonstandard cones when compared with standard cones.[169,395]

Finger spreaders provide better tactile sensation and are less likely to induce fractures in the root when compared with the more traditional D-11T hand spreader.[88,223,224] In addition to the type of spreader, forces applied, and amount of dentin removed, spreader size may be a factor in root fracture, with large sizes inducing more stress.[294] Spreaders made from nickel-titanium are available and provide increased flexibility,[35] reduced stress,[109] and provide deeper penetration when

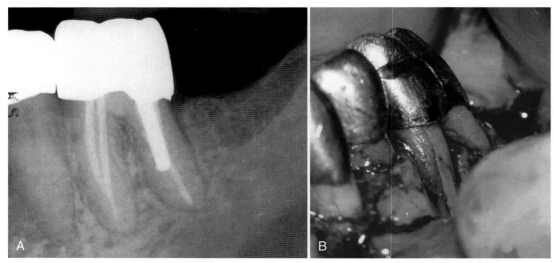

FIG. 7-29 Vertical root fractures can occur with excessive compaction forces. **A,** Follow-up radiograph of a mandibular left first molar. A deep isolated periodontal probing defect was associated with the buccal aspect of the mesiobuccal root. **B,** Flap reflection revealed a vertical root fracture.

compared with stainless steel instruments.[189,341,417] The spreader should fit to within 1 to 2 mm of the prepared length, and when introduced into the canal with the master cone in place, it should be within 2 mm of the working length.[7] There appears to be a correlation between the establishment of a higher quality seal and the depth of spreader penetration.[7,352]

After the spreader has been placed to its maximum depth, it is removed by rotating it back and forth as it is withdrawn. An accessory cone is placed in the space vacated by the spreader. The process is repeated until the spreader no longer goes beyond the coronal one third of the canal. The excess gutta-percha is removed with heat and the coronal mass is compacted with an appropriate unheated plugger. Only light pressure is required during lateral compaction because the gutta-percha is not condensed, and because as little as 1.5 kg of pressure is capable of fracturing a root (Fig. 7-29). In addition to the force applied, investigators have noted that removal of excessive amounts of dentin during preparation is a significant factor in root fracture.[415]

A disadvantage to lateral compaction is that the process does not produce a homogeneous mass. The accessory and master cones are laminated and remain separate. It is envisaged that the space between each of the cones is filled with sealer to aid in establishment of a water-tight seal.

The excess gutta-percha in the chamber is then seared off and vertically compacted with a heated plugger at the orifice or approximately 1 mm below the orifice in posterior teeth. Warm vertical compaction of the coronal gutta-percha enhances the seal.[429] In anterior teeth, the desired level is the cemento-enamel junction on the facial surface to avoid aesthetic issues if the dentin should become stained. An alternative to lateral compaction with finger spreaders is ultrasonics.[21] For example, one study found that the technique produced adequate obturation and a 93% clinical success rate.[436]

Another study used ultrasonic-energized files in a warm lateral compaction technique and reported that the amount of gutta-percha, by weight, increased by 33% with two applications of ultrasonics when compared with lateral compaction.[98] Unfortunately, investigators found that the mean internal

temperature rise was 29°C at the 6-mm level, with external heat generation exceeding the safe limit of 10°C.

Warm Vertical Compaction

Schilder introduced warm vertical compaction of gutta-percha as a method of obturating the radicular space in three dimensions.[339] Preparation requirements for the technique include preparing a root canal system with a continuously tapering funnel and keeping the apical foramen as small as possible.

The armamentarium includes a variety of pluggers and a heat source. Schilder pluggers come in a variety of sizes (#8 = 0.4 mm, # 8½ = 0.5 mm, etc., for sizes #9, #9½, #10, #10½, #11, #11½, #12) with increasing diameter. The instruments are marked vertically at 5-mm intervals. Various ISO standardized instruments are also available (Fig. 7-30).

The technique involves fitting a master cone short of the prepared working length (0.5 to 2 mm) with resistance to displacement (Fig. 7-31). This ensures that the cone diameter is larger than the prepared canal at the terminus. Nonstandard cones that closely replicate the canal taper are best because they permit the development of hydraulic pressure during compaction. After the adaptation of the master cone, it is removed and sealer is applied to the cone and the walls of the prepared canal. The cone is placed in the canal and the coronal portion is removed with a heated instrument. A heated spreader or plugger is used to remove portions of the coronal gutta-percha in successive increments and soften the remaining material in the canal. The Touch 'n Heat (SybronEndo) (Fig. 7-32), DownPak (Hu-Friedy, Chicago, Illinois), and System B (SybronEndo) (Fig. 7-33) are alternatives to applying heat with a flame-heated instrument because they permit improved temperature control. A plugger is inserted into the canal and the gutta-percha is compacted, forcing the plasticized material apically. The process is repeated until the apical portion has been reached. The coronal canal space is back-filled using small preheated pieces of gutta-percha. The sectional method consists of placing 3- to 4-mm sections of gutta-percha approximating the size of the canal into the root, applying heat, and compacting the mass with a plugger.

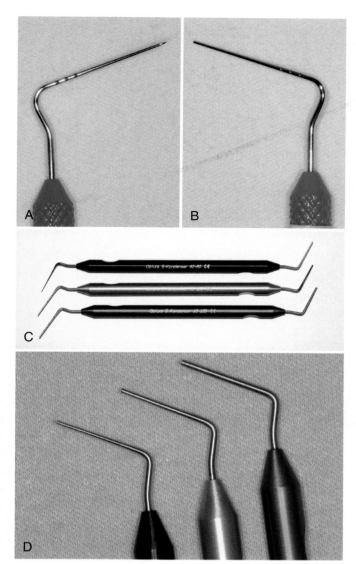

FIG. 7-30 Various pluggers are manufactured for compacting warm gutta-percha. **A,** ISO standard spreader. **B,** ISO standard plugger. **C,** Obtura S Kondensers. **D,** Closeup of Obtura S-Kondensers. (**C** courtesy Obtura Spartan, Algonquin, Illinois.)

One study measured temperature changes in a root canal system with warm vertical compaction.[40] The maximal temperatures occurred coronally and decreased apically. The authors reported that the maximal temperature in the canal was 118°C 8 mm from the apex. At 0 to 2 mm from the apical terminus, the maximal temperature had decreased to 44°C. Another study compared root surface temperatures for warm vertical obturation using the System B heat source, the Touch 'n Heat device, and a flame-heated carrier in maxillary and mandibular incisors and premolars 2 mm below the cemento-enamel junction. System B and the Touch 'n Heat produced a surface temperature rise that was less than 10°C for all maxillary incisors and premolar teeth. The Touch 'n Heat produced a greater than 10°C rise in mandibular incisors. The flame-heated carrier produced temperature changes greater than 10°C in all experimental teeth. Because the critical level of root surface heat required to produce irreversible bone damage is believed to be greater than 10°C the findings suggest that warm vertical compaction with the System B should not damage supporting periodontal structures; however, caution should be exercised with the Touch 'n Heat and flame-heated carriers.[219] The flame-heated spreader has no heat controls and the Touch 'n Heat controls only send heat to the tip and receive no feedback from the tip based on clinical conditions. The System B has a computer built in which allows it to receive feedback from the tip and adjust the tip temperature based on the clinical conditions, which allow the tip to remain at the dialed-in temperature.

The potential for vertical root fracture is also present with warm vertical compaction.[39] The forces developed appear to be equal to lateral compaction. Investigators compared warm vertical compaction and lateral compaction as a function of time. Results indicated that the forces developed with the two techniques were not significantly different. In a follow-up study, the mean value for wedging with warm vertical compaction was 0.65 ± 0.07 kg, whereas for lateral compaction it was 0.8 ± 0.1 kg.

Warm thermoplastic techniques have the advantage of producing movement of the plasticized gutta-percha within the obturated root canal system, resulting in a more homogeneous mass of gutta-percha, and filling irregularities and accessory canals better than lateral compaction.[105,421] This was illustrated in a study that reported a correlation between the quality of adaptation and the depth of heat application and canal size. Heat application close to the apical extent of the preparation produced the best results, and adaptation was better in small canals when compared with wide canals.[420] However, thermoplasticized techniques resulted in more extrusion of obturating materials.[213] There appeared to be no consistent differences between the techniques in sealing the canal space.[421]

Advantages of warm vertical compaction include filling of canal irregularities and accessory canals. Disadvantages include a slight risk of vertical root fracture because of compaction forces, less length control than with lateral compaction, and the potential for extrusion of material into the periradicular tissues. Warm vertical compaction is also difficult in more curved root canal systems, where the rigid pluggers may be unable to penetrate to the necessary depth. Occasionally, the canals have to be enlarged and tapered more to enable rigid carriers to penetrate within 4 to 5 mm of the apex. Additional removal of root canal dentin can weaken the root, making it more susceptible to root fracture.

Continuous Wave Compaction Technique

A variation of warm vertical compaction is the continuous wave compaction technique.[55] The increasing use of nickel-titanium rotary preparation techniques and the fabrication of greater taper standard cones have resulted in more clinicians using thermoplasticizing techniques. The manufacturing of gutta-percha cones to mimic the tapered preparation permits the application of greater hydraulic force during compaction when appropriately tapered pluggers are used. The continuous wave compaction technique employs the System B connected to 0.04, 0.06, 0.08, 0.10, or 0.12 tapered stainless steel dead-soft pluggers (see Fig. 7-33). The 0.06 tapered plugger also approximates the fine nonstandard gutta-percha cone, the 0.08 plugger the fine-medium cone, the 0.10 plugger the medium cone, and the 0.12 plugger the medium-large cone. Pluggers consistent with the ProFile GT instruments (DENTSPLY Tulsa

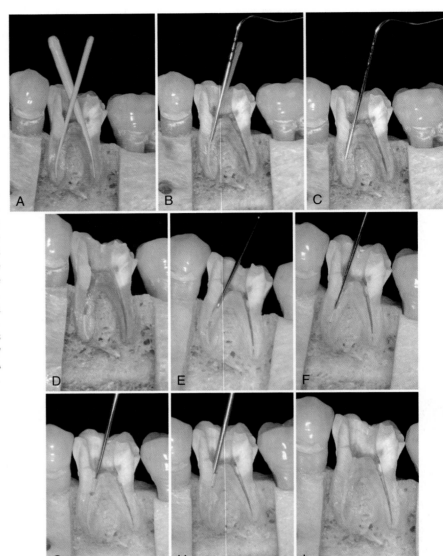

FIG. 7-31 Warm vertical compaction of gutta-percha employs heat and various condensers. **A,** Non-standard cones are selected and fit short of the prepared length because they more closely replicate the prepared canal. **B,** Heated pluggers or spreaders are used to apply heat to the master cone and remove the excess coronal material. **C,** A room temperature plugger is used to compact the heated gutta-percha. **D,** Apical compaction is complete. **E,** A gutta-percha segment is placed in the canal, and heat is applied. **F,** The heated segment is compacted. **G,** The process is repeated for the coronal portion of the canal by placing and heating a segment of gutta-percha. **H,** A plugger is again used to compact the heated material. **I,** Completed obturation.

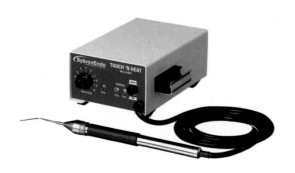

FIG. 7-32 The Touch 'n Heat unit. (Courtesy SybronEndo, Orange, Calif.)

Dental Specialties), and Autofit gutta-percha cones (Sybron-Endo) are also available.

The electric heat source permits a variable temperature setting. The recommended temperature setting for the System B unit is 200°C. One study evaluated internal and external temperature changes with the System B unit with varied tips and temperature settings of 200°C, 250°C, and 300°C. At 6 mm from the apex, the System B unit set at 300°C with a fine-medium plugger produced the highest mean internal temperature (74°C). However, the authors noted that the external temperature setting never exceeded the critical 10°C rise at the PDL with any temperature setting or tip configuration.[375] This was confirmed in another study that measured temperature changes 2 mm apical to the cementoenamel junction and 1.5 mm from the apex. Results indicated that temperature changes apically were negligible. The mean change near the cementoenamel junction was 4.1°C.[398]

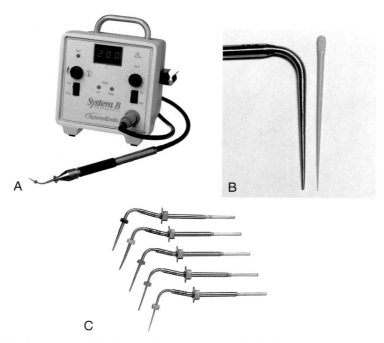

FIG. 7-33 Continuous wave obturation uses the System B unit. **A,** The System B unit. **B,** System B plugger with a nonstandard cone of similar taper. **C,** System B pluggers. (Courtesy SybronEndo, Orange, Calif.)

Another study reported that obturation temperature elevations produced during obturation with System B were significantly less than with traditional warm vertical compaction. An elevation of external root surface temperature by more than 10°C was noted with vertical compaction.[357] Investigators measured the root surface temperatures while using the System B heat source at various temperature settings from 250°C to 600°C. Results indicated that the highest temperature occurred 5 mm from the apex, and this was the only site that exceeded the 10°C rise. On the basis of this study, a temperature setting of 250°C or greater may be potentially hazardous.[101] For example, investigators using a thermocouple and simultaneous infrared analysis of temperatures found that the root surface temperature averaged 13.9°C, whereas the infrared technology indicated a 28.4°C rise at the same sites.[246]

After selecting an appropriate master cone, a plugger is prefitted to within 5 to 7 mm of the prepared length (Fig. 7-34). Placing the plugger deeper into the canal may enhance the flow of gutta-percha according to one investigator.[5] The point of plugger binding should be noted because once the instrument reaches this point the hydraulic forces on the gutta-percha will decrease and recompaction forces on the root will increase. There appears to be a correlation between the depth of the heated plugger relative to the working length and the quality of obturation and filling of canal irregularities.[46,190,424] Increasing the temperature settings does not seem to increase the effectiveness of obturation.[190]

The System B unit is set to 200°C in the touch mode. The plugger is inserted into the canal orifice and activated to remove excess coronal material. Compaction is initiated by placing a cold plugger against the gutta-percha at the canal orifice. Firm pressure is applied and heat is activated with the device. The plugger is moved rapidly (1 to 2 s) to within 3 mm of the binding point (Fig. 7-35). The heat is inactivated while firm pressure is maintained on the plugger for 5 to 10 seconds.

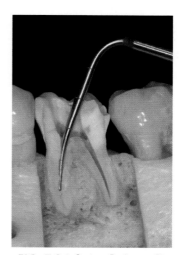

FIG. 7-34 System B plugger fit.

After the gutta-percha mass has cooled, a one-second application of heat separates the plugger from the gutta-percha and it is removed. The pluggers are designed to heat from the tip to their shank, which decreases the potential for dislodging the compacted mass and prevents a second application of heat to the material. Confirmation that the apical mass of gutta-percha is still present in the canal can be established with hand pluggers and/or radiographs. Two hand instruments are manufactured with tip diameters of 0.4 and 0.9 mm and 0.7 and 1.4 mm. It should be noted that with the continuous wave technique the heat source is placed only to within 5 to 7 mm from the tip of the gutta-percha; the apical portion of the gutta-percha remains essentially a single-cone technique as the heat transfer does not take place in the apical 2 to 5 mm of the gutta-percha.[145]

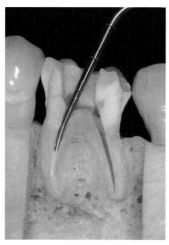

FIG. 7-35 System B activation and compaction.

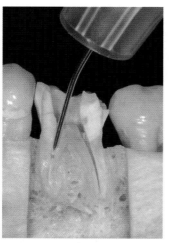

FIG. 7-36 Backfill by the Obtura II thermoplastic injection technique.

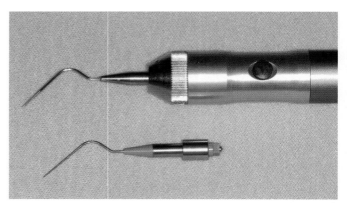

FIG. 7-37 Endotec II device (Medidenta) for warm lateral compaction.

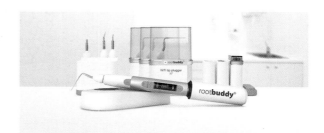

FIG. 7-38 The Rootbuddy device (previously the DownPak device) for heat softening and vibrating gutta percha. (Courtesy Nikinc Dental, Eindhoven, The Netherlands.)

In ovoid canals, where the canal configuration may prevent the generation of hydraulic forces, an accessory cone can be placed alongside the master cone before compaction. With type II canals, the master cones are placed in both canals before compaction. A hand plugger is used to stabilize the cone in one canal while the other is being obturated.

Filling the space left by the plugger may be accomplished by a thermoplastic injection technique (Obtura or Ultrafil 3D [Coltène/Whaledent], Calamus [DENTSPLY Tulsa Dental Specialties], Elements [SybronEndo], or HotShot [Discus Dental, Los Angeles, California]) (Fig. 7-36)[187] or by fitting an accessory cone into the space with sealer, heating it, and compacting by short applications of heat and vertical pressure.

Warm Lateral Compaction

Warm lateral compaction of gutta-percha provides for predictable length control, which is an advantage over thermoplastic techniques. The Endotec II device (Medidenta, Las Vegas, Nevada) provides the clinician with the ability to employ length control while incorporating a warm gutta-percha technique (Fig. 7-37). Investigators demonstrated that the Endotec II produced a fusion of the gutta-percha into a solid homogeneous mass.[182] One study evaluated three thermoplasticized filling techniques and lateral compaction, using a bacterial metabolite model, and found the Endotec to be superior to lateral compaction alone, lateral thermocompaction, and the Ultrafil 3D.[197] The use of warm lateral compaction with the Endotec demonstrated an increased weight of gutta-percha mass, by 14.63%, when compared with traditional lateral compaction.[227] Another study found a 24% increase in weight with warm lateral compaction when using the System B device.[260] Using the Endotec II, one investigation reported a statistically significantly better ability of warm vertical and warm lateral compaction techniques, versus cold lateral compaction, to reproduce artificially produced canal irregularities in a split-tooth model.[81] Another group of investigators used the Endo-Twinn (Hu-Friedy), an instrument for warm lateral compaction, in a similar experiment. The EndoTwinn instrument also possesses the ability to vibrate the electronically heated tip. They reported that warm lateral compaction, using both heat and vibration, and warm vertical compaction of gutta-percha provided statistically better replication of defects than cold lateral compaction.[211] Hu-Friedy introduced the DownPak* (Fig. 7-38), a variation of the original EndoTwinn that can be used with either warm lateral or warm vertical compaction techniques. Other investigators compared the stress generated with lateral compaction and warm lateral compaction, using the Endotec II, and found that the warm lateral compaction technique created less stress during obturation.[242] An additional concern is the heat generated by the technique. Evaluation of the effects of warm lateral and warm vertical compaction on periodontal tissues demonstrated that neither technique produced heat-related damage.[69]

---

*Downpak products and service are now supplied by Nikinc Dental, Eindhoven, The Netherlands. It's new name is RootBuddy.

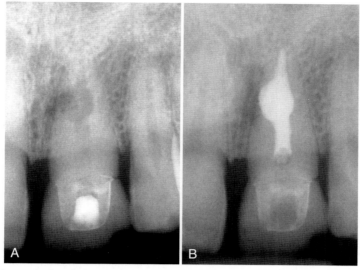

FIG. 7-39 Thermoplastic techniques are often used in cases with significant canal irregularities. **A**, A pretreatment radiograph of a maxillary central incisor exhibiting internal resorption. **B**, Posttreatment radiograph demonstrates a dense obturation of the resorptive defect with gutta-percha.

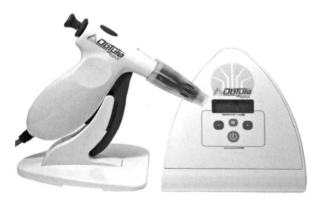

FIG. 7-40 Obtura III Max System. (Courtesy Kerr, Orange, CA.)

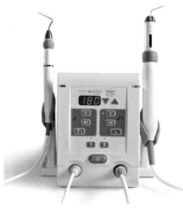

FIG. 7-41 The Calamus thermoplastic unit for heating and injecting gutta-percha. (Courtesy DENTSPLY Tulsa Dental Specialties, Tulsa, Okla.)

The warm lateral compaction technique involves adapting a master cone in the same manner as with traditional lateral compaction. An appropriate-size Endotec II tip is selected. Endotec II tips are available in various taper and tip diameters. The sizes consist of #0.02/20 and #0.02/40. The device is activated and the tip is inserted beside the master cone to within 2 to 4 mm of the apex, using light pressure. The tip is rotated for 5 to 8 seconds and removed. An unheated spreader can be placed in the channel created to ensure adaptation and then an accessory cone is placed. The process is continued until the canal is filled.

Thermoplastic Injection Techniques

Heating of gutta-percha outside the tooth and injecting the material into the canal is an additional variation of the thermoplastic technique (Fig. 7-39). The Obtura III (Fig. 7-40), Calamus (Fig. 7-41), Elements (Fig. 7-42), HotShot (Fig. 7-43), and Ultrafil 3D (Fig. 7-44) are available devices. The Obtura system heats the gutta-percha to 160°C, whereas the Ultrafil 3D system employs a low-temperature gutta-percha that is heated to 90°C.

Obtura III

The Obtura III system (Obtura Spartan) consists of a hand-held "gun" that contains a chamber surrounded by a heating element into which pellets of gutta-percha are loaded (see Fig. 7-40). Silver needles (varying gauges of 20, 23, and 25) are attached to deliver the thermoplasticized material to the canal. The control unit allows the operator to adjust the temperature and thus the viscosity of the gutta-percha. At 6 mm from the apex a study found that the highest internal temperature with the Obtura system was 27°C.[375]

Canal preparation is similar for other obturation techniques. The apical terminus should be as small as possible to prevent extrusion of gutta-percha. The technique requires the use of sealer, and once the canal is dried, the canal walls are coated with sealer, using the last file used to length or a paper point. Gutta-percha is preheated in the gun, and the needle is positioned in the canal so that it reaches within 3 to 5 mm of the apical preparation. Gutta-percha is then gradually, passively injected by squeezing the trigger of the "gun." The needle

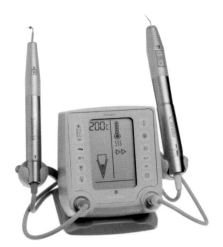

FIG. 7-42 The Elements obturation unit for injecting and compacting gutta-percha. (Courtesy Kerr, Orange, CA.)

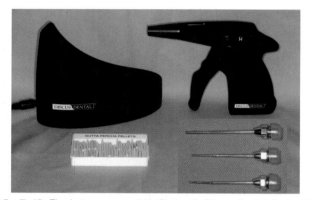

FIG. 7-43 The battery-powered HotShot unit (Discus Dental) for heating and injecting gutta-percha.

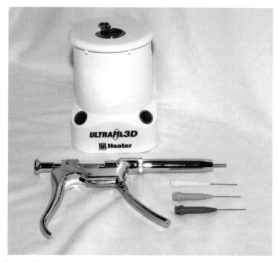

FIG. 7-44 The Ultrafil 3D system consists of an injection syringe, gutta-percha cannulas, and heating unit (Coltène/Whaledent).

backs out of the canal as the apical portion is filled. Pluggers dipped in alcohol are used to compact the gutta-percha. A segmental technique may also be used, in which 3- to 4-mm segments of gutta-percha are sequentially injected and compacted. In either case, compaction should continue until the gutta-percha cools and solidifies to compensate for the contraction that takes place on cooling.

The difficulties with this system include lack of length control. Both overextension and underextension are common results. To overcome this drawback, a hybrid technique may be used, in which the clinician begins filling the canal by the lateral compaction technique. When the master cone and several accessory cones have been placed so that the mass is firmly lodged in the apical portion of the canal, a hot plugger is introduced, searing the points off approximately 4 to 5 mm from the apex. Light vertical compaction is applied to restore the integrity of the apical plug of gutta-percha. The remainder of the canal is then filled with thermoplasticized gutta-percha injected as previously described.

Investigators studied, at 3, 6, and 12 months post treatment, the success rate of 236 teeth obturated with the Obtura system. Results indicated that 96% of the cases were successful, with the highest success rate being in teeth filled flush with the apex (97%) when compared with overextensions (93%) and filling short (93%).[377] Another study compared lateral compaction with Thermafil (DENTSPLY Tulsa Dental Specialties) and Obtura in root canal models and found that the Obtura produced the best adaptation to the canal walls.[408] Other investigators found that continuous wave obturation with the Obtura backfill initially produced a better bacterial seal when compared with lateral compaction, using bilaterally matched teeth and an anaerobic bacterial leakage model.[182]

Ultrafil 3D

Ultrafil 3D (Coltène/Whaledent) is a thermoplastic gutta-percha injection technique involving gutta-percha cannulas, a heating unit, and an injection syringe (see Fig. 7-44). The system employs three types of gutta-percha cannulas. The Regular Set is a low-viscosity material that requires 30 minutes to set. The Firm Set is also a low-viscosity material but differs in that it sets in 4 minutes. The manufacturer recommends compaction after the initial set with both materials. Endoset has a higher viscosity and does not flow as well. It is recommended for techniques employing compaction and sets in 2 minutes. The heater is preset at 90°C and does not require adjustment.

Each cannula has a 22-gauge stainless steel needle that measures 21 mm in length. The needles can be precurved. Cannulas can be disinfected but are not designed for heat sterilization procedures. Heating time varies, but for a cold unit it takes 10 to 15 minutes. In a warm heater the recommended time is 3 minutes. After removing the cannula from the heater the needle should be placed on the hot part of the heater for several seconds. The gutta-percha remains able to flow for 45 to 60 seconds depending on the viscosity.

Calamus

The Calamus flow obturation delivery system (DENTSPLY Tulsa Dental Specialties) is a thermoplastic device equipped with a cartridge system with 20- and 23-gauge needles (see Fig. 7-41). The unit permits control of temperature and also the flow rate. Pluggers are also available for use with the system. The 360-degree activation switch allows great tactile sensation during use.

Elements

The Elements obturation unit (SybronEndo) consists of a System B heat source and plugger as well as a handpiece extruder for delivering thermoplastic gutta-percha or RealSeal from a disposable cartridge (see Fig. 7-42). The cartridges come with 20-, 23-, and 25-gauge needles for gutta-percha and 20- and 23-gauges for RealSeal.

HotShot

The HotShot delivery system (Discus Dental [now part of Philips Oral Healthcare]) is a cordless thermoplastic device that has a heating range from 150°C to 230°C (see Fig. 7-43). The unit is cordless and can be used with either gutta-percha or Resilon. Needles are available in 20, 23, and 25 gauges.

Carrier-Based Gutta-Percha

Thermafil, Profile GT Obturators, GT Series X Obturators, and ProTaper Universal Obturators

Thermafil (DENTSPLY Tulsa Dental Specialties) was introduced as a gutta-percha obturation material with a solid core (Fig. 7-45). Originally manufactured with a metal core and a coating of gutta-percha, the carrier was heated over an open flame. The technique was popular because the central core provided a rigid mechanism to facilitate the placement of the gutta-percha. Advantages included ease of placement and the pliable properties of the gutta-percha. Disadvantages were that the metallic core made placement of a post challenging and retreatment procedures were difficult. In addition, the gutta-percha was often stripped from the carrier, leaving the

carrier as the obturating material in the apical area of the canal. Reports have stated that carrier-based systems result in minimal gaps and voids in the resulting obturation mass.[441] Other reports have stated that there was no difference in healing rates between carrier-based systems and lateral compaction of gutta-percha.[157]

Changes in the carrier systems include the development of a plastic core coated with α-phase gutta-percha (Fig. 7-46) and a heating device that controls the temperature (Fig. 7-47). Obturators are designed to correspond to the ISO standard file sizes, variable tapered nickel titanium rotary files, and the ProFile GT and GT Series X nickel-titanium rotary files (DENTSPLY Tulsa Dental Specialties) (see Fig. 7-46). Size verifiers are available to aid in selection of the appropriate carrier and should fit passively at the corrected working length (see Fig. 7-45).

As with all techniques, a sealer is required. Grossman formulation sealers and resin sealers consistent with AH-26 and AH Plus are acceptable; however, Tubli-Seal and Wach's paste are not recommended.

Removal of the smear layer is strongly recommended (see Chapters 5 and 7) and has been shown to enhance the seal with Thermafil.[29] After drying the canal a light coat of sealer is applied and a carrier is marked, set to the predetermined length. This is accomplished by using the millimeter calibration markings on the carrier shaft. Markings are made at 18, 19, 20, 22, 24, 27, and 29 mm. Gutta-percha on the shaft that may be obscuring the calibration rings can be removed with a surgical blade or knife. The carrier is disinfected with 5.25% NaOCl for 1 minute and rinsed in 70% alcohol.

The carrier is then placed in the heating device. When the carrier is heated to the appropriate temperature, the clinician

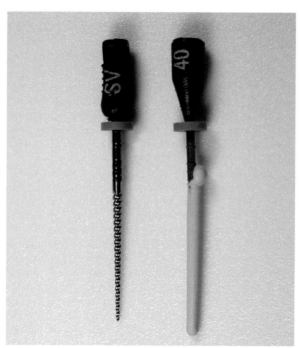

FIG. 7-45 Thermafil carrier and size verifier (DENTSPLY Tulsa Dental Specialties).

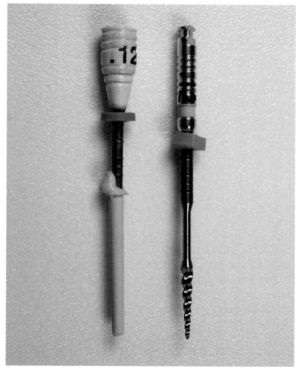

FIG. 7-46 GT obturator and instrument (DENTSPLY Tulsa Dental Specialties).

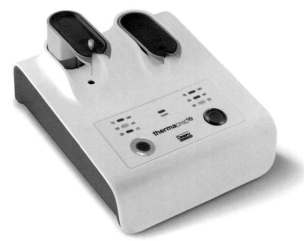

FIG. 7-47 The Thermafil oven with carrier in place (Thermaprep2 oven. Courtesy DENTSPLY Maillefer, Ballaigues, Switzerland.)

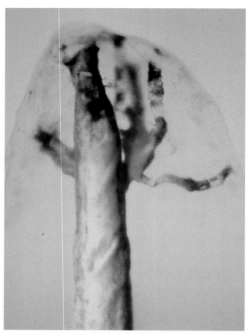

FIG. 7-49 Apical obturation of accessory canals by the Thermafil technique. (Courtesy DENTSPLY Tulsa Dental Specialties, Tulsa, Okla.)

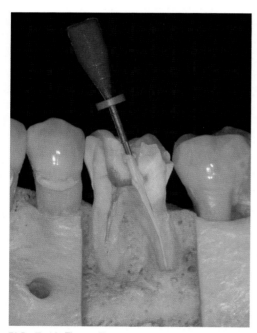

FIG. 7-48 Thermafil carrier placed in the distal canal.

has approximately 10 seconds to retrieve it and insert it into the canal (Fig. 7-48). This is accomplished without rotation or twisting. Evidence suggests that the insertion rate affects the obturation. The fill length and obturation of irregularities increase with increasing insertion rates.[225] A rapid insertion rate enhances obturation.[225]

The position of the carrier is verified radiographically. The gutta-percha is allowed 2 to 4 minutes to cool before resecting the coronal portion of the carrier, which can be several millimeters above the canal orifice. This is accomplished by applying stabilizing pressure to the carrier and cutting the device with an inverted cone, round bur, or a specially designed Prepi bur (DENTSPLY Tulsa Dental Specialties). Heated instruments are not recommended for this process because this may result in displacement.

Vertical compaction of the coronal gutta-percha can then be accomplished. When necessary, gutta-percha can be added, heat softened, and compacted. An advantage to this technique is the potential for movement of gutta-percha into lateral and accessory canals (Fig. 7-49)[419]; however, extrusion of material beyond the apical extent of the preparation is a disadvantage.[78,85,213]

Pro-Post drills (DENTSPLY Tulsa Dental Specialties) are recommended if post space is required for restoration of the tooth. The unique eccentric cutting tip keeps the instrument centered in the canal while friction softens and removes the gutta-percha and plastic carrier.

When retreatment is necessary the plastic carrier has a groove along its length to provide an access point for placement of a file. Chloroform and hand files can be used to remove the gutta-percha surrounding the carrier. Rotary #.04 and #.06 nickel-titanium files may also be used to remove the obturation materials. Retreatment rotary nickel-titanium files are available in three different sizes to facilitate removal of gutta-percha and the carrier.

The plastic carriers are composed of two nontoxic materials. Sizes #20 to #40 are manufactured from a liquid crystal plastic. Sizes #40 to #90 are composed of polysulfone polymer. Both have similar physical characteristics, with the polysulfone carriers being susceptible to dissolution in chloroform.

GuttaCore (DENTSPLY Tulsa Dental Specialties), the latest generation of core carriers, uses cross-linked gutta-percha as the carrier of the outer thermoplasticized gutta-percha. This makes retreatment simpler as the clinician can simply drill through the carrier to gain access into the canal space. A recent in vitro study comparing the time required to remove Gutta-Core, Thermafil Plus and thermoplasticized gutta-percha from moderately curved root canals with ProTaper retreatment files reported that GuttaCore was removed in significantly less time when compared with the other two techniques.[26]

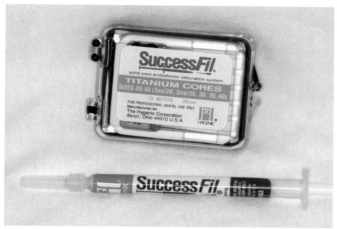

FIG. 7-50 SuccessFil is an additional carrier system (Coltène/Whaledent).

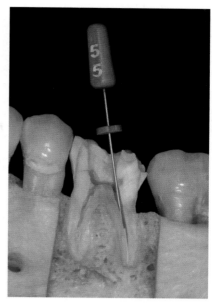

FIG. 7-52 SimpliFill fitted to 1 to 3 mm from the prepared length.

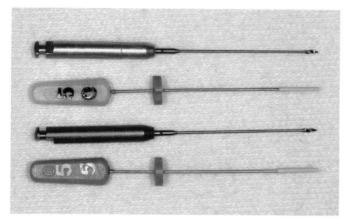

FIG. 7-51 SimpliFill carrier (SybronEndo) and LightSpeed file (LightSpeed Technology, San Antonio, Texas).

SuccessFil

SuccessFil (Coltène/Whaledent) is a carrier-based system associated with Ultrafil 3D (Fig. 7-50); however, the gutta-percha used in this technique comes in a syringe. Carriers (titanium or radiopaque plastic) are inserted into the syringe to the measured length of the canal. The gutta-percha is expressed on the carrier, with the amount and shape determined by the rate of withdrawal from the syringe. Sealer is lightly coated on the canal walls, and the carrier with gutta-percha is placed in the canal to the prepared length. The gutta-percha can be compacted around the carrier with various pluggers depending on the canal morphology. This is followed by severing of the carrier slightly above the orifice with a bur.

SimpliFill

SimpliFill (SybronEndo) is gutta-percha or Resilon manufactured for use after canal preparation with LightSpeed instruments (Fig. 7-51). The carrier has an apical plug with 5 mm of gutta-percha. The technique involves fitting a carrier that is consistent with the master apical rotary file (SybronEndo) to within 1 to 3 mm of the prepared length (Fig. 7-52). The apical gutta-percha plug can be modified by clipping the end in 1-mm increments to obtain an appropriate fit if the plug is too small.

Once the cone is fitted it is withdrawn and sealer is applied to the canal walls. AH Plus is recommended. The SimpliFill carrier is slowly advanced to the prepared length. This may require firm pressure. With the plug at the corrected working length the handle is quickly rotated a minimum of four complete terms in a counterclockwise direction to separate the shaft from the apical gutta-percha. The coronal space can then be filled with gutta-percha, using lateral compaction or the warm thermoplastic technique. When using lateral compaction it is recommended that the first cone be the same size as the SimpliFill carrier. This sectional technique is efficient, and leakage potential is similar to that of other common techniques.[324]

Thermomechanical Compaction

McSpadden introduced an instrument, the McSpadden Compactor, with flutes similar to a Hedström file but in reverse. When activated in a slow-speed handpiece, the instrument would generate friction, soften the gutta-percha, and move it apically. Rotary compactors similar in design have been developed and advocated. To increase flexibility, the instrument is available in nickel-titanium.

The technique requires fitting a master cone short of the prepared length and applying sealer. A compactor is selected on the basis of the size of the canal and inserted alongside the gutta-percha cone 3 to 4 mm from the prepared length. The handpiece is activated, and the friction of the rotating bur heats the gutta-percha. The pliable mass is compacted apically and laterally as the device is withdrawn from the canal.

Advantages include simplicity of the armamentarium, the ability to fill canal irregularities,[161,198,232,331,332] and time. Disadvantages include possible extrusion of material, instrument fracture,[270] gouging of the canal walls, the inability to use the technique in curved canals, and possible excessive heat generation.[27,124,159,245,332,333] Microseal condensers (SybronEndo) and the Gutta Condenser (DENTSPLY Tulsa Dental Specialties) are variations of this product.

Solvent Techniques

Gutta-percha can be plasticized with solvents, such as chloroform, eucalyptol, or xylol. Disadvantages include shrinkage caused by evaporation, voids, the inability to achieve predictable length control of the obturating material, and irritation of periradicular tissues. The Callahan and Johnston technique involved dissolving gutta-percha in chloroform and placing the mixture into the canal with a syringe.[60] A gutta-percha cone was then softened by immersion in this mixture and placed into the canal and the mass solidified as the solvent evaporated. Unfortunately, shrinkage occurred with the evaporation process.[299] Obturation techniques using solvents have been abandoned and replaced with materials and methods that exhibit minimum shrinkage.

Pastes

Pastes fulfill some of the criteria outlined by Grossman[149] and can adapt to the complex internal canal anatomy; however, the flow characteristic can result in extrusion or incomplete obturation. The inability to control the material is a distinct disadvantage, and when extrusion occurs it can be corrected only by surgical intervention. In addition, pastes are sometimes used as a substitute for complete cleaning and shaping procedures, and the addition of paraformaldehyde results in severe toxicity.

Immediate Obturation

Apical barriers may be necessary in cases with immature apical development, cases with external apical root resorption, and cases where instrumentation extends beyond the confines of the root. Dentin chips, calcium hydroxide, demineralized dentin, lyophilized bone, tricalcium phosphate, hydroxyapatite, and collagen have been advocated for placement as a barrier in canals exhibiting an open apex. The barriers are designed to permit obturation without extrusion of materials into the periradicular tissues but are often incomplete and do not seal the canal.[320]

Dentin chips appear to confine materials to the canal space during instrumentation/obturation and may encourage development of a biologic seal.[115,320] Enhanced healing, minimal inflammation, and apical cementum deposition have been noted histologically.[275] A concern with this technique is contamination of the dentin with bacteria or other nonhost materials, because investigators found that infected dentin adversely affected healing.[173]

Calcium hydroxide has also been extensively used as a common apical barrier. Calcium hydroxide has been shown to induce an apical barrier in apexification procedures. Calcifications similar to dentin plugs have been noted at the apical foramen.[295] Calcium hydroxide has the advantage of being free of bacterial contamination and may provide a better, although imperfect, apical seal.[406]

Immature teeth exhibiting pulp necrosis or teeth with apical resorption traditionally were treated with calcium hydroxide to establish an apical barrier (apexification) before obturation. Studies have demonstrated that teeth treated with calcium hydroxide for prolonged periods are more susceptible to fracture.[11,316] Immediate obturation is an alternative to apexification. An apical barrier material should confine obturation materials to the canal space[115] and enhance healing by inducing cementum and bone formation.[172,275,295] Mineral trioxide aggregate (MTA) (ProRoot MTA; DENTSPLY Tulsa

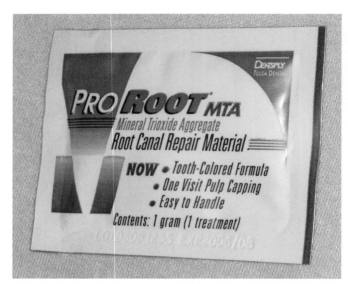

FIG. 7-53 Mineral trioxide aggregate is available as ProRoot MTA. This material is advocated for use in apexification, repair of root perforations, repair of root resorption, root-end fillings, and pulp capping. (Courtesy DENTSPLY Tulsa Dental Specialties, Tulsa, Okla.)

Dental Specialties) has been successfully employed as an apical barrier material before obturation (Fig. 7-53).[350]

After cleaning and shaping procedures, the root canal system is dried and a small increment of MTA is placed to the radiographic apex and the location verified through a radiograph. If the material is overextended, it can be easily irrigated out with sterile saline. If it is short of the radiographic apex, it can be compacted with prefitted pluggers to move it to the radiographic apex. The material is compacted into the apical portion of the root to form a barrier. After the material sets, any thermoplasticized technique can be used to backfill with gutta-percha without concern of overextension (Fig. 7-54). Other investigators have reported that hand compaction of MTA provided better adaptation to the canal walls with fewer voids when compared with ultrasonic placement.[9] Another investigation reported that ultrasonic placement of a 4-mm apical plug of MTA improved the seal[430] and that placement of a composite resin as the obturation material enhanced the seal and strengthened the root.[216]

Mineral trioxide aggregate is sterile, biocompatible, and capable of inducing hard tissue formation.[112,174] The technique has been shown to be clinically successful and can be accomplished quickly, eliminating the need for numerous patient visits and possible coronal recontamination during the many months required for apexification.[73,87,138]

Clinical evidence supports this technique. In a study comparing calcium hydroxide with mineral trioxide aggregate in 15 children, each having paired immature teeth with necrotic pulps, two teeth treated with $Ca(OH)_2$ exhibited pathosis on recall examination, whereas all the teeth treated with MTA were clinically and radiographically successful.[114] A prospective clinical study found the success rate of MTA barriers and immediate obturation in 43 cases to be 81%.[358] In another study, 85% of 20 teeth with immature apical development were considered healed and 5% were considered healing after immediate barrier placement.[171] The time required for healing is

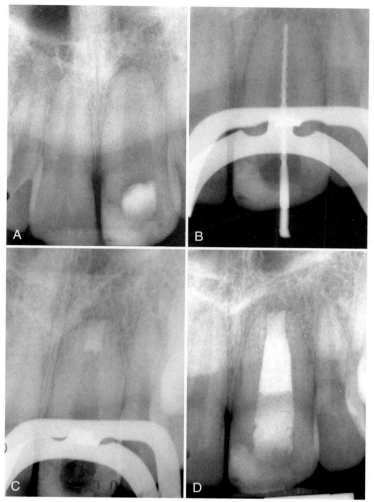

FIG. 7-54 Immediate obturation employs a barrier technique to prevent extrusion when the apex is open. This case involves a maxillary left central incisor with pulp necrosis caused by trauma. **A,** Pretreatment radiograph demonstrates a large canal with an open apex. **B,** Working length is established and the canal is prepared. **C,** Mineral trioxide plug is placed. **D,** The canal is obturated with gutta-percha.

comparable to traditional apexification with Ca(OH)$_2$ and treatment time is reduced.[298]

Another option for treating immature teeth with pulp necrosis involves regenerative endodontic techniques (see Chapter 10).[160,184,391,414] Advantages include continued increasing thickness of the canal walls, continued apical root development, and apical closure.[351] The technique involves copious irrigation, minimal canal preparation, and the use of an antibiotic paste as an interim medication. At a subsequent visit, bleeding is induced in the canal by placing a file beyond the root apex. When the bleeding comes within 3 mm of the canal orifice, the clot is lined with a resorbable membrane and then covered with MTA. When the MTA is set, a definitive restoration can be placed to ensure a coronal seal.[17]

CORONAL ORIFICE SEAL

No matter which technique is used to obturate the canals, coronal microleakage can occur within a short time through seemingly well-obturated canals,[68,389] potentially causing infection of the periapical area. Early research efforts focused on the quality of the seal in the apical part of the root canal system to prevent percolation of apical fluids. However, contemporary research efforts have identified the greater importance of maintaining a coronal seal to prevent bacterial leakage.[185] Leakage studies indicate that the coronal seal can be enhanced by the application of supplemental restorative materials over the canal orifice[293,407,418] and by placing a definitive coronal restoration as soon as is feasible.[305]

Cavit (3M ESPE) has traditionally been advocated as an acceptable material. One study demonstrated that placement of 3.5 mm of Cavit or Super EBA cement (Bosworth, Skokie, Illinois) decreased bacterial leakage by 85% and 65%, respectively, when compared with unsealed controls, which all leaked at 45 days.[293] In an animal study in which the access openings were left open for 8 months, placing a dentin-bonded composite resin or IRM in the orifice decreased periapical inflammation from 89% for teeth without orifice plugs to 39% with plugs.[428] Another study demonstrated in a dog model that MTA placed in the orifice decreased inflammation in teeth inoculated with bacteria.[235]

Another method to retard leakage through the obturated canal, should failure of the coronal restoration occur, is to cover the floor of the pulp chamber with a lining of bonded material after removal of excess gutta-percha and sealer to the canal orifice.[31,71,221] This results in the formation of a hybrid layer with microtags of resin in the tubules. A resin-modified glass ionomer cement is placed approximately 1 mm thick over the floor of the pulp chamber and polymerized with a curing light. Alternatively, a self-etching dentin adhesive and a flowable resin composite may be used. Investigators found that this procedure resulted in none of the experimental canals showing bacterial leakage at 60 days.[72] A material with a different color than dentin may be used for identification, in case subsequent placement of a post is required.

REFERENCES

1. Aguirre AM, el-Deeb ME, Aguirre R: The effect of ultrasonics on sealer distribution and sealing of root canals, *J Endod* 23:759, 1997.
2. Ainley JE: Fluorometric assay of the apical seal of root canal fillings, *Oral Surg Oral Med Oral Pathol* 29:753, 1970.
3. Aktener BO, Cengiz T, Pişkin B: The penetration of smear material into dentinal tubules during instrumentation with surface-active reagents: a scanning electron microscopic study, *J Endod* 15:588, 1989.
4. al-Khatib ZZ, Baum RH, Morse DR, et al: The antimicrobial effect of various endodontic sealers, *Oral Surg Oral Med Oral Pathol* 70:784, 1990.
5. Alicia Karr N, Baumgartner JC, Marshall JG: A comparison of gutta-percha and Resilon in the obturation of lateral grooves and depressions, *J Endod* 33:749, 2007.
6. Allan NA, Walton RC, Schaeffer MA: Setting times for endodontic sealers under clinical usage and in vitro conditions, *J Endod* 27:421, 2001.
7. Allison DA, Michelich RJ, Walton RE: The influence of master cone adaptation on the quality of the apical seal, *J Endod* 7:61, 1981.
8. American Association of Endodontists: *Guide to clinical endodontics*, ed 5, Chicago, 2013, The Association.
9. Aminoshariae A, Hartwell GR, Moon PC: Placement of mineral trioxide aggregate using two different techniques, *J Endod* 29:679, 2003.
10. Anderson AC, Hellwig E, Vespermann R, et al: Comprehensive analysis of secondary dental root canal infections: a combination of culture and culture-independent approaches reveals new insights, *PLoS One* 7:e49576, 2012.
11. Andreasen JO, Farik B, Munksgaard EC: Long-term calcium hydroxide as a root canal dressing may increase risk of root fracture, *Dent Traumatol* 18:134, 2002.
12. Anonymous: FDA explains status of N2 material, *J Am Dent Assoc* 123:236, 1992.
13. Aqrabawi JA: Outcome of endodontic treatment of teeth filled using lateral condensation versus vertical compaction (Schilder's technique), *J Contemp Dent Pract* 7:17, 2006.
14. Augsburger RA, Peters DD: Radiographic evaluation of extruded obturation materials, *J Endod* 16:492, 1990.
15. Babb BR, Loushine RJ, Bryan TE, et al: Bonding of self-adhesive (self-etching) root canal sealers to radicular dentin, *J Endod* 35:578, 2009.
16. Ballal NV, Kumar SR, Laxmikanth HK, et al: Comparative evaluation of different chelators in removal of calcium hydroxide preparations from root canals, *Aust Dent J* 57:344, 2012.
17. Banchs F, Trope M: Revascularization of immature permanent teeth with apical periodontitis: new treatment protocol? *J Endod* 30:196, 2004.
18. Barkhordar RA: Evaluation of antimicrobial activity in vitro of ten root canal sealers on *Streptococcus sanguis* and *Streptococcus mutans*, *Oral Surg Oral Med Oral Pathol* 68:770, 1989.
19. Barkhordar RA, Watanabe LG, Marshall GW, et al: Removal of intracanal smear by doxycycline in vitro, *Oral Surg Oral Med Oral Pathol Oral Radiol Endod* 84:420, 1997.

20. Barthel CR, Zimmer S, Trope M: Relationship of radiologic and histologic signs of inflammation in human root-filled teeth, *J Endod* 30:75, 2004.
21. Baumgardner KR, Krell KV: Ultrasonic condensation of gutta-percha: an in vitro dye penetration and scanning electron microscopic study, *J Endod* 16:253, 1990.
22. Baumgartner G, Zehnder M, Paqué F: *Enterococcus faecalis* type strain leakage through root canals filled with gutta-percha/AH Plus or Resilon/Epiphany, *J Endod* 33:45, 2007.
23. Baumgartner JC, Brown CM, Mader CL, et al: A scanning electron microscopic evaluation of root canal debridement using saline, sodium hypochlorite, and citric acid, *J Endod* 10:525, 1984.
24. Baumgartner JC, Cuenin PR: Efficacy of several concentrations of sodium hypochlorite for root canal irrigation, *J Endod* 18:605, 1992.
25. Baumgartner JC, Mader CL: A scanning electron microscopic evaluation of four root canal irrigation regimens, *J Endod* 13:147, 1987.
26. Beasley RT, Williamson AE, Justman BC, et al: Time required to remove GuttaCore, Thermafil plus, and thermoplasticized gutta-percha from moderately curved root canals with ProTaper files, *J Endod* 39:125, 2013.
27. Beatty RG, Vertucci FJ, Hojjatie B: Thermomechanical compaction of gutta-percha: effect of speed and duration, *Int Endod J* 21:367, 1988.
28. Beatty RG, Zakariasen KL: Apical leakage associated with three obturation techniques in large and small root canals, *Int Endod J* 17:67, 1984.
29. Behrend GD, Cutler CW, Gutmann JL: An in-vitro study of smear layer removal and microbial leakage along root-canal fillings, *Int Endod J* 29:99, 1996.
30. Belli S, Ozcan E, Derinbay O, et al: A comparative evaluation of sealing ability of a new, self-etching, dual-curable sealer: hybrid root SEAL (MetaSEAL), *Oral Surg Oral Med Oral Pathol Oral Radiol Endod* 106:45, 2008.
31. Belli S, Zhang Y, Pereira PN, et al: Adhesive sealing of the pulp chamber, *J Endod* 27:521, 2001.
32. Bender IB: Factors influencing the radiographic appearance of bony lesions, *J Endod* 23:5, 1997.
33. Bergenholtz G, Spångberg L: Controversies in endodontics, *Crit Rev Oral Biol Med* 15:99, 2004.
34. Bergmans L, Moisiadis P, De Munck J, et al: Effect of polymerization shrinkage on the sealing capacity of resin fillers for endodontic use, *J Adhes Dent* 7:321, 2005.
35. Berry KA, Loushine RJ, Primack PD, et al: Nickel-titanium versus stainless-steel finger spreaders in curved canals, *J Endod* 24:752, 1998.
36. Beyer-Olsen EM, Ørstavik D: Radiopacity of root canal sealers, *Oral Surg Oral Med Oral Pathol* 51:320, 1981.
37. Blasković-Subat V, Maricić B, Sutalo J: Asymmetry of the root canal foramen, *Int Endod J* 25:158, 1992.
38. Block RM, Lewis RD, Hirsch J, et al: Systemic distribution of N2 paste containing ^{14}C paraformaldehyde following root canal therapy in dogs, *Oral Surg Oral Med Oral Pathol* 50:350, 1980.
39. Blum JY, Esber S, Micallef JP: Analysis of forces developed during obturations: comparison of three gutta-percha techniques, *J Endod* 23:340, 1997.

40. Blum JY, Parahy E, Machtou P: Warm vertical compaction sequences in relation to gutta-percha temperature, *J Endod* 23:307, 1997.
41. Bodrumlu E, Muglali M, Sumer M, et al: The response of subcutaneous connective tissue to a new endodontic filling material, *J Biomed Mater Res B Appl Biomater* 84:463, 2008.
42. Boiesen J, Brodin P: Neurotoxic effect of two root canal sealers with calcium hydroxide on rat phrenic nerve in vitro, *Endod Dent Traumatol* 7:242, 1991.
43. Bolles JA, He J, Svoboda KK, et al: Comparison of Vibringe, EndoActivator, and needle irrigation on sealer penetration in extracted human teeth, *J Endod* 39:708, 2013.
44. Borges RP, Sousa-Neto MD, Versiani MA, et al: Changes in the surface of four calcium silicate-containing endodontic materials and an epoxy resin-based sealer after a solubility test, *Int Endod J* 45:419, 2012.
45. Bouillaguet S, Wataha JC, Tay FR, et al: Initial in vitro biological response to contemporary endodontic sealers, *J Endod* 32:989, 2006.
46. Bowman CJ, Baumgartner JC: Gutta-percha obturation of lateral grooves and depressions, *J Endod* 28:220, 2002.
47. Brackett MG, Martin R, Sword J, et al: Comparison of seal after obturation techniques using a polydimethylsiloxane-based root canal sealer, *J Endod* 32:1188, 2006.
48. Brady JM, del Rio CE: Corrosion of endodontic silver cones in humans: a scanning electron microscope and x-ray microprobe study, *J Endod* 1:205, 1975.
49. Brännström M: Smear layer: pathological and treatment considerations, *Oper Dent Suppl* 3:35, 1984.
50. Briseño BM, Willershausen B: Root canal sealer cytotoxicity on human gingival fibroblasts. I. Zinc oxide–eugenol-based sealers, *J Endod* 16:383, 1990.
51. Briseño BM, Willershausen B: Root canal sealer cytotoxicity on human gingival fibroblasts. II. Silicone- and resin-based sealers, *J Endod* 17:537, 1991.
52. Briseño BM, Willerhausen B: Root canal sealer toxicity on human gingival fibroblasts. III. Calcium hydroxide–based sealers, *J Endod* 18:110, 1992.
53. Briseño Marroquin B, Wolter D, Willershausen-Zonnchen B: Dimensional variability of nonstandardized greater taper finger spreaders with matching gutta-percha points, *Int Endod J* 34:23, 2001.
54. Brodin P, Roed A, Aars H, et al: Neurotoxic effects of root filling materials on rat phrenic nerve in vitro, *J Dent Res* 61:1020, 1982.
55. Buchanan L: Continuous wave of condensation technique, *Endod Prac* 1:7, 1998.
56. Burch JG, Hulen S: The relationship of the apical foramen to the anatomic apex of the tooth root, *Oral Surg Oral Med Oral Pathol Oral Radiol Endod* 34:262, 1972.
57. Byström A, Sundqvist G: Bacteriologic evaluation of the efficacy of mechanical root canal instrumentation in endodontic therapy, *Scand J Dent Res* 89:321, 1981.
58. Byström A, Sundqvist G: The antibacterial action of sodium hypochlorite and EDTA in 60 cases of endodontic therapy, *Int Endod J* 18:35, 1985.
59. Cailleteau JG, Mullaney TP: Prevalence of teaching apical patency and various instrumentation and obturation

techniques in United States dental schools, *J Endod* 23:394, 1997.

60. Callahan JR: Rosin solution for the sealing of the dental tubuli as an adjuvant in the filling of root canals, *J Allied Dent Soc* 9:110, 1914.
61. Camps J, About I: Cytotoxicity testing of endodontic sealers: a new method, *J Endod* 29:583, 2003.
62. Çalt S, Serper A: Smear layer removal by EGTA, *J Endod* 26:459, 2000.
63. Cameron JA: The synergistic relationship between ultrasound and sodium hypochlorite: a scanning electron microscope evaluation, *J Endod* 13:541, 1987.
64. Camilleri J: Evaluation of selected properties of mineral trioxide aggregate sealer cement, *J Endod* 35:1412, 2009.
65. Camilleri J, Pitt Ford TR: Mineral trioxide aggregate: a review of the constituents and biological properties of the material, *Int Endod J* 39:747, 2006.
66. Candeiro GT, Correia FC, Duarte MA, et al: Evaluation of radiopacity, pH, release of calcium ions, and flow of a bioceramic root canal sealer, *J Endod* 38:842, 2012.
67. Card SJ, Sigurdsson A, Ørstavik D, et al: The effectiveness of increased apical enlargement in reducing intracanal bacteria, *J Endod* 28:779, 2002.
68. Carratù P, Amato M, Riccitiello F, et al: Evaluation of leakage of bacteria and endotoxins in teeth treated endodontically by two different techniques, *J Endod* 28:272, 2002.
69. Castelli WA, Caffesse RG, Pameijer CH, et al: Periodontium response to a root canal condensing device (Endotec), *Oral Surg Oral Med Oral Pathol* 71:333, 1991.
70. Chailertvanitkul P, Saunders WP, MacKenzie D: The effect of smear layer on microbial coronal leakage of gutta-percha root fillings, *Int Endod J* 29:242, 1996.
71. Chailertvanitkul P, Saunders WP, MacKenzie D: Coronal leakage in teeth root-filled with gutta-percha and two different sealers after long-term storage, *Endod Dent Traumatol* 13:82, 1997.
72. Chailertvanitkul P, Saunders WP, Saunders EM, MacKenzie D: An evaluation of microbial coronal leakage in the restored pulp chamber of root-canal treated multirooted teeth, *Int Endod J* 30:318, 1997.
73. Chala S, Abouqal R, Rida S: Apexification of immature teeth with calcium hydroxide or mineral trioxide aggregate: systematic review and meta-analysis, *Oral Surg Oral Med Oral Pathol Oral Radiol Endod* 112:e36, 2011.
74. Chen SC, Chueh LH, Hsiao CK, et al: An epidemiologic study of tooth retention after nonsurgical endodontic treatment in a large population in Taiwan, *J Endod* 33:226, 2007.
75. Chogle S, Mickel AK, Huffaker SK, et al: An in vitro assessment of iodoform gutta-percha, *J Endod* 31:814, 2005.
76. Chugal NM, Clive JM, Spångberg LS: Endodontic treatment outcome: effect of the permanent restoration, *Oral Surg Oral Med Oral Pathol Oral Radiol Endod* 104:576, 2007.
77. Clark-Holke D, Drake D, Walton R, et al: Bacterial penetration through canals of endodontically treated teeth in the presence or absence of the smear layer, *J Dent* 31:275, 2003.
78. Clinton K, Van Himel T: Comparison of a warm gutta-percha obturation technique and lateral condensation, *J Endod* 27:692, 2001.
79. Cobankara FK, Adanr N, Belli S: Evaluation of the influence of smear layer on the apical and coronal sealing ability of two sealers, *J Endod* 30:406, 2004.
80. Cohler CM, Newton CW, Patterson SS, et al: Studies of Sargenti's technique of endodontic treatment: short-term response in monkeys, *J Endod* 6:473, 1980.
81. Collins J, Walker MP, Kulild J, et al: A comparison of three gutta-percha obturation techniques to replicate canal irregularities, *J Endod* 32:762, 2006.
82. Conner DA, Caplan DJ, Teixeira FB, et al: Clinical outcome of teeth treated endodontically with a nonstandardized protocol and root filled with Resilon, *J Endod* 33:1290, 2007.
83. Cotton TP, Schindler WG, Schwartz SA, et al: A retrospective study comparing clinical outcomes after obturation with Resilon/Epiphany or gutta-percha/Kerr sealer, *J Endod* 34:789, 2008.
84. Cunningham WT, Martin H: A scanning electron microscope evaluation of root canal debridement with the endosonic ultrasonic synergistic system, *Oral Surg Oral Med Oral Pathol* 53:527, 1982.
85. Da Silva D, Endal U, Reynaud A, et al: A comparative study of lateral condensation, heat-softened gutta-percha, and a modified master cone heat-softened backfilling technique, *Int Endod J* 35:1005, 2002.
86. Dai L, Khechen K, Khan S, et al: The effect of QMix, an experimental antibacterial root canal irrigant, on removal of canal wall smear layer and debris, *J Endod* 37:80, 2011.
87. Damle SG, Bhattal H, Loomba A: Apexification of anterior teeth: a comparative evaluation of mineral trioxide aggregate and calcium hydroxide paste, *J Clin Pediatr Dent* 36:263, 2012.
88. Dang DA, Walton RE: Vertical root fracture and root distortion: effect of spreader design, *J Endod* 15:294, 1989.
89. Darvell BW, Wu RC: "MTA"—a hydraulic silicate cement: review update and setting reaction, *Dent Mater* 27:407, 2011.
90. Davis MC, Walton RE, Rivera EM: Sealer distribution in coronal dentin, *J Endod* 28:464, 2002.
91. de Chevigny C, Dao TT, Basrani BR, et al: Treatment outcome in endodontics: the Toronto study—phase 4: initial treatment, *J Endod* 34:258, 2008.
92. de Chevigny C, Dao TT, Basrani BR, et al: Treatment outcome in endodontics: the Toronto study—phases 3 and 4: orthograde retreatment, *J Endod* 34:131, 2008.
93. de Deus G, Gurgel Filho ED, Ferreira CM, et al: [Intratubular penetration of root canal sealers], *Pesquisa Odontologica Brasileira [Braz Oral Res]* 16:332, 2002.
94. de Deus GA, Gurgel-Filho ED, Maniglia-Ferreira C, et al: The influence of filling technique on depth of tubule penetration by root canal sealer: a study using light microscopy and digital image processing, *Aust Endod J* 30:23, 2004.
95. de Lucena JM, Decker EM, Walter C, et al: Antimicrobial effectiveness of intracanal medicaments on *Enterococcus faecalis*: chlorhexidine versus octenidine, *Int Endod J* 46:53, 2013.
96. De Moor RJ, De Bruyne MA: The long-term sealing ability of AH 26 and AH Plus used with three gutta-percha obturation techniques, *Quintessence Int* 35:326, 2004.
97. de Paula-Silva FW, Santamaria M Jr, Leonardo MR, et al: Cone-beam computerized tomographic, radiographic, and histologic evaluation of periapical repair in dogs' post-endodontic treatment, *Oral Surg Oral Med Oral Pathol Oral Radiol Endod* 108:796, 2009.
98. Deitch AK, Liewehr FR, West LA, et al: A comparison of fill density obtained by supplementing cold lateral condensation with ultrasonic condensation, *J Endod* 28:665, 2002.
99. Delivanis PD, Mattison GD, Mendel RW: The survivability of F43 strain of *Streptococcus sanguis* in root canals filled with gutta-percha and Procosol cement, *J Endod* 9:407, 1983.
100. Desai S, Chandler N: Calcium hydroxide-based root canal sealers: a review, *J Endod* 35:475, 2009.
101. Diamond A, Carrel R: The smear layer: a review of restorative progress, *J Pedod* 8:219, 1984.
102. Dow PR, Ingle JI: Isotope determination of root canal failure, *Oral Surg Oral Med Oral Pathol* 8:1100, 1955.
103. Dr. Witte: The filling of a root canal with Portland cement. In: German Quarterly for Dentistry; Journal of the Central Association of German Dentists. Ed. Dr. Robert Baume. Arthur Felix Publisher 18:153, 1878.
104. Drake DR, Wiemann AH, Rivera EM, et al: Bacterial retention in canal walls in vitro: effect of smear layer, *J Endod* 20:78, 1994.
105. DuLac KA, Nielsen CJ, Tomazic TJ, et al: Comparison of the obturation of lateral canals by six techniques, *J Endod* 25:376, 1999.
106. Dummer PM, Kelly T, Meghji A, et al: An in vitro study of the quality of root fillings in teeth obturated by lateral condensation of gutta-percha or Thermafil obturators, *Int Endod J* 26:99, 1993.
107. Dummer PM, Lyle L, Rawle J, et al: A laboratory study of root fillings in teeth obturated by lateral condensation of gutta-percha or Thermafil obturators, *Int Endod J* 27:32, 1994.
108. Dummer PM, McGinn JH, Rees DG: The position and topography of the apical canal constriction and apical foramen, *Int Endod J* 17:192, 1984.
109. Dwan JJ, Glickman GN: 2-D photoelastic stress analysis of NiTi and stainless steel finger spreaders during lateral compaction, *J Endod* 21:221, 1995.
110. Ebert J, Pawlick H, Petschelt A: Relation between dye penetration and radiographic assessment of root canal fillings in vitro, *Int Endod J* 29:198, 1996.
111. Economides N, Liolios E, Kolokuris I, et al: Long-term evaluation of the influence of smear layer removal on the sealing ability of different sealers, *J Endod* 25:123, 1999.
112. Economides N, Pantelidou O, Kokkas A, et al: Short-term periradicular tissue response to mineral trioxide aggregate (MTA) as root-end filling material, *Int Endod J* 36:44, 2003.
113. Editorial Board of the Journal of Endodontics: Wanted: a base of evidence, *J Endod* 33:1401, 2007.
114. El-Meligy OA, Avery DR: Comparison of apexification with mineral trioxide aggregate and calcium hydroxide, *Pediatr Dent* 28:248, 2006.
115. ElDeeb ME, Thuc-Quyen NT, Jensen JR: The dentinal plug: its effect on confining substances to the canal and on the apical seal, *J Endod* 9:355, 1983.
116. Eldeniz AU, Mustafa K, Ørstavik D, et al: Cytotoxicity of new resin-, calcium hydroxide- and silicone-based root canal sealers on fibroblasts derived from human gingiva and L929 cell lines, *Int Endod J* 40:329, 2007.
117. Erişen R, Yücel T, Küçükay S: Endomethasone root canal filling material in the mandibular canal: a case report, *Oral Surg Oral Med Oral Pathol* 68:343, 1989.
118. Estrela C, Bueno MR, Leles CR, et al: Accuracy of cone beam computed tomography and panoramic and periapical radiography for detection of apical periodontitis, *J Endod* 34:273, 2008.
119. Fabricius L, Dahlén G, Sundqvist G, et al: Influence of residual bacteria on periapical tissue healing after chemomechanical treatment and root filling of experimentally infected monkey teeth, *Eur J Oral Sci* 114:278, 2006.
120. Farzaneh M, Abitbol S, Friedman S: Treatment outcome in endodontics: the Toronto Study. Phases I and II: orthograde retreatment, *J Endod* 30:627, 2004.
121. Farzaneh M, Abitbol S, Lawrence HP, et al: Treatment outcome in endodontics—the Toronto Study. Phase II: initial treatment, *J Endod* 30:302, 2004.
122. Felippe WT, Ruschel MF, Felippe GS, et al: SEM evaluation of the apical external root surface of teeth with chronic periapical lesion, *Aust Endod J* 35:153, 2009.
123. Figini L, Lodi G, Gorni F, et al: Single versus multiple visits for endodontic treatment of permanent teeth: a Cochrane systematic review, *J Endod* 34:1041, 2008.
124. Fors U, Jonasson E, Berquist A, et al: Measurements of the root surface temperature during thermo-mechanical root canal filling in vitro, *Int Endod J* 18:199, 1985.
125. Fransen JN, He J, Glickman GN, et al: Comparative assessment of Activ GP/glass ionomer sealer, Resilon/Epiphany, and gutta-percha/AH Plus obturation: a bacterial leakage study, *J Endod* 34:725, 2008.
126. Friedman CE, Sandrik JL, Heuer MA, et al: Composition and physical properties of gutta-percha endodontic filling materials, *J Endod* 3:304, 1977.
127. Friedman S, Abitbol S, Lawrence HP: Treatment outcome in endodontics: the Toronto Study. Phase 1: initial treatment, *J Endod* 29:787, 2003.

128. Friedman S, Löst C, Zarrabian M, et al: Evaluation of success and failure after endodontic therapy using a glass ionomer cement sealer, *J Endod* 21:384, 1995.

129. Friedman S, Torneck CD, Komorowski R, et al: In vivo model for assessing the functional efficacy of endodontic filling materials and techniques, *J Endod* 23:557, 1997.

130. Gandolfi MG, Parrilli AP, Fini M, et al: 3D micro-CT analysis of the interface voids associated with Thermafil root fillings used with AH Plus or a flowable MTA sealer, *Int Endod J* 46:253, 2013.

131. Gandolfi MG, Taddei P, Tinti A, et al: Apatite-forming ability (bioactivity) of ProRoot MTA, *Int Endod J* 43:917, 2010.

132. Gençoğlu N, Samani S, Gunday M: Dentinal wall adaptation of thermoplasticized gutta-percha in the absence or presence of smear layer: a scanning electron microscopic study, *J Endod* 19:558, 1993.

133. Gettleman BH, Messer HH, ElDeeb ME: Adhesion of sealer cements to dentin with and without the smear layer, *J Endod* 17:15, 1991.

134. Geurtsen W: Biocompatibility of root canal filling materials, *Aust Endod J* 27:12, 2001.

135. Ghoneim AG, Lutfy RA, Sabet NE, et al: Resistance to fracture of roots obturated with novel canal-filling systems, *J Endod* 37:1590, 2011.

136. Gilhooly RM, Hayes SJ, Bryant ST, et al: Comparison of lateral condensation and thermomechanically compacted warm alpha-phase gutta-percha with a single cone for obturating curved root canals, *Oral Surg Oral Med Oral Pathol Oral Radiol Endod* 91:89, 2001.

137. Gillen BM, Looney SW, Gu LS, et al: Impact of the quality of coronal restoration versus the quality of root canal fillings on success of root canal treatment: a systematic review and meta-analysis, *J Endod* 37:895, 2011.

138. Giuliani V, Baccetti T, Pace R, et al: The use of MTA in teeth with necrotic pulps and open apices, *Dent Traumatol* 18:217, 2002.

139. Givol N, Rosen E, Bjørndal L, et al: Medico-legal aspects of altered sensation following endodontic treatment: a retrospective case series, *Oral Surg Oral Med Oral Pathol Oral Radiol Endod* 112:126, 2011.

140. Goldberg F, Gurfinkel J, Spielberg C: Microscopic study of standardized gutta-percha points, *Oral Surg Oral Med Oral Pathol* 47:275, 1979.

141. Gomes-Filho JE, Moreira JV, Watanabe S, et al: Sealability of MTA and calcium hydroxide containing sealers, *J Appl Oral Sci* 20:347, 2012.

142. Gomes-Filho JE, Watanabe S, Bernabé PF, et al: A mineral trioxide aggregate sealer stimulated mineralization, *J Endod* 35:256, 2009.

143. Gomes-Filho JE, Watanabe S, Lodi CS, et al: Rat tissue reaction to MTA FILLAPEX®, *Dent Traumatol* 28:452, 2012.

144. Goodman A, Schilder H, Aldrich W: The thermomechanical properties of gutta-percha. Part II. The history and molecular chemistry of gutta-percha, *Oral Surg Oral Med Oral Pathol* 37:954, 1974.

145. Goodman A, Schilder H, Aldrich W: The thermomechanical properties of gutta-percha. Part IV. A thermal profile of the warm gutta-percha packing procedure, *Oral Surg Oral Med Oral Pathol* 51:544, 1981.

146. Granchi D, Stea S, Ciapetti G, et al: Endodontic cements induce alterations in the cell cycle of in vitro cultured osteoblasts, *Oral Surg Oral Med Oral Pathol Oral Radiol Endod* 79:359, 1995.

147. Grande NM, Plotino G, Lavorgna L, et al: Influence of different root canal-filling materials on the mechanical properties of root canal dentin, *J Endod* 33:859, 2007.

148. Grossman L: An improved root canal cement, *J Am Dent Assoc* 56:381, 1958.

149. Grossman L: *Endodontics*, ed 11. Philadelphia, 1988, Lea & Febiger.

150. Guignes P, Faure J, Maurette A: Relationship between endodontic preparations and human dentin permeability measured in situ, *J Endod* 22:60, 1996.

151. Gutiérrez JH, Aguayo P: Apical foraminal openings in human teeth: number and location, *Oral Surg Oral Med Oral Pathol Oral Radiol Endod* 79:769, 1995.

152. Gutiérrez JH, Brizuela C, Villota E: Human teeth with periapical pathosis after overinstrumentation and overfilling of the root canals: a scanning electron microscopic study, *Int Endod J* 32:40, 1999.

153. Gutmann JH, Hovland EJ: Problems in root canal obturation. In Gutmann J, Dumsha T, Lovdahl P, Hovland E, editors: *Problem Solving in Endodontics*, ed 2, St. Louis, MO, 1997, Mosby, pp 92–116.

154. Gutmann JL: Clinical, radiographic, and histologic perspectives on success and failure in endodontics, *Dent Clin North Am* 36:379, 1992.

155. Gutmann JL: Adaptation of injected thermoplasticized gutta-percha in the absence of the dentinal smear layer, *Int Endod J* 26:87, 1993.

156. Haapasalo HK, Sirén EK, Waltimo TM, et al: Inactivation of local root canal medicaments by dentine: an in vitro study, *Int Endod J* 33:126, 2000.

157. Hale R, Gatti R, Glickman GN, et al: Comparative analysis of carrier-based obturation and lateral compaction: a retrospective clinical outcomes study, *Int J Dent* 2012:954675, 2012.

158. Hall MC, Clement DJ, Dove SB, et al: A comparison of sealer placement techniques in curved canals, *J Endod* 22:638, 1996.

159. Hardie EM: Further studies on heat generation during obturation techniques involving thermally softened gutta-percha, *Int Endod J* 20:122, 1987.

160. Hargreaves KM, Giesler T, Henry M, et al: Regeneration potential of the young permanent tooth: what does the future hold? *J Endod* 34:S51, 2008.

161. Harris GZ, Dickey DJ, Lemon RR, et al: Apical seal: McSpadden vs lateral condensation, *J Endod* 8:273, 1982.

162. Hatton EH: Changes produced in the pulp and periapical regions, and their relationship to pulp-canal treatment and to systemic disease, *Dental Cosmos* 66:1183, 1924.

163. Hauman CH, Love RM: Biocompatibility of dental materials used in contemporary endodontic therapy: a review. Part 2. Root-canal-filling materials, *Int Endod J* 36:147, 2003.

164. Haznedaroğlu F, Ersev H: Tetracycline HCl solution as a root canal irrigant, *J Endod* 27:738, 2001.

165. Heard F, Walton RE: Scanning electron microscope study comparing four root canal preparation techniques in small curved canals, *Int Endod J* 30:323, 1997.

166. Heeren TJ, Levitan ME: Effect of canal preparation on fill length in straight root canals obturated with RealSeal 1 and Thermafil Plus, *J Endod* 38:1380, 2012.

167. Heling I: The antimicrobial effect within dentinal tubules of four root canal sealers, *J Endod* 22:257, 1996.

168. Heling I, Gorfil C, Slutzky H, et al: Endodontic failure caused by inadequate restorative procedures: review and treatment recommendations, *J Prosthet Dent* 87:674, 2002.

169. Hembrough MW, Steiman HR, Belanger KK: Lateral condensation in canals prepared with nickel titanium rotary instruments: an evaluation of the use of three different master cones, *J Endod* 28:516, 2002.

170. Herrera DR, Santos ZT, Tay LY, et al: Efficacy of different final irrigant activation protocols on smear layer removal by EDTA and citric acid, *Microsc Res Tech* 76:364, 2013.

171. Holden DT, Schwartz SA, Kirkpatrick TC, et al: Clinical outcomes of artificial root-end barriers with mineral trioxide aggregate in teeth with immature apices, *J Endod* 34:812, 2008.

172. Holland GR: Periapical response to apical plugs of dentin and calcium hydroxide in ferret canines, *J Endod* 10:71, 1984.

173. Holland R, de Souza V, Murata SS, et al: Healing process of dog dental pulp after pulpotomy and pulp covering with mineral trioxide aggregate or Portland cement, *Braz Dent J* 12:109, 2001.

174. Holland R, de Souza V, Nery MJ, et al: Reaction of dogs' teeth to root canal filling with mineral trioxide aggregate or a glass ionomer sealer, *J Endod* 25:728, 1999.

175. Hottel TL, el-Refai NY, Jones JJ: A comparison of the effects of three chelating agents on the root canals of extracted human teeth, *J Endod* 25:716, 1999.

176. Hugh CL, Walton RE, Facer SR: Evaluation of intracanal sealer distribution with 5 different obturation techniques, *Quintessence Int* 36:721, 2005.

177. Hülsmann M, Heckendorff M, Lennon A: Chelating agents in root canal treatment: mode of action and indications for their use, *Int Endod J* 36:810, 2003.

178. Hunter W: The role of sepsis and antisepsis in medicine, *Lancet* 79, 1911.

179. Ingle JI, Beveridge E, Glick D, et al: The Washington Study. In: Ingle I, Taintor JF, editors. *Endodontics*, Philadelphia, 1994, Lea & Febiger, pp 1–53.

180. Iqbal MK, Johansson AA, Akeel RF, et al: A retrospective analysis of factors associated with the periapical status of restored, endodontically treated teeth, *Int J Prosthodont* 16:31, 2003.

181. Iqbal MK, Ku J: Instrumentation and obturation of the apical third of root canals: addressing the forgotten dimension, *Compend Contin Educ Dent* 28:314, 2007.

182. Jacobsen EL, BeGole EA: A comparison of four root canal obturation methods employing gutta-percha: a computerized analysis of the internal structure, *Endod Dent Traumatol* 8:206, 1992.

183. Jasper E: Adaptation and tolerance of silver point canal filling, *J Dent Res* 4:355, 1941.

184. Jeeruphan T, Jantarat J, Yanpiset K, et al: Mahidol study 1: comparison of radiographic and survival outcomes of immature teeth treated with either regenerative endodontic or apexification methods: a retrospective study, *J Endod* 38:1330, 2012.

185. Jenkins S, Kulild J, Williams K, et al: Sealing ability of three materials in the orifice of root canal systems obturated with gutta-percha, *J Endod* 32:225, 2006.

186. Jia ET: Self-etching primer adhesive and method of use thereof. *United States Patent & Trademark Office*. Patent Number 7,226,900, June 5, 2007.

187. Johnson BT, Bond MS: Leakage associated with single or multiple increment backfill with the Obtura II gutta-percha system, *J Endod* 25:613, 1999.

188. Johnson WT, Zakariasen KL: Spectrophotometric analysis of microleakage in the fine curved canals found in the mesial roots of mandibular molars, *Oral Surg Oral Med Oral Pathol* 56:305, 1983.

189. Joyce AP, Loushine RJ, West LA, et al: Photoelastic comparison of stress induced by using stainless-steel versus nickel-titanium spreaders in vitro, *J Endod* 24:714, 1998.

190. Jung IY, Lee SB, Kim ES, et al: Effect of different temperatures and penetration depths of a System B plugger in the filling of artificially created oval canals, *Oral Surg Oral Med Oral Pathol Oral Radiol Endod* 96:453, 2003.

191. Kakehashi S, Stanley HR, Fitzgerald RJ: The effects of surgical exposures of dental pulps in germfree and conventional laboratory rats, *J South Calif Dent Assoc* 34:449, 1966.

192. Kazemi RB, Safavi KE, Spångberg LS: Dimensional changes of endodontic sealers, *Oral Surg Oral Med Oral Pathol* 76:766, 1993.

193. Keane HC: *A century of service to dentistry*, Philadelphia, 1944, SS White Dental Manufacturing.

194. Keane KM, Harrington GW: The use of a chloroform-softened gutta-percha master cone and its effect on the apical seal, *J Endod* 10:57, 1984.

195. Keinan D, Moshonov J, Smidt A: Is endodontic re-treatment mandatory for every relatively old temporary restoration? A narrative review, *J Am Dent Assoc* 142:391, 2011.

196. Kerezoudis NP, Valavanis D, Prountzos F: A method of adapting gutta-percha master cones for obturation of open apex cases using heat, *Int Endod J* 32:53, 1999.

197. Kersten HW: Evaluation of three thermoplasticized gutta-percha filling techniques using a leakage model in vitro, *Int Endod J* 21:353, 1988.

198. Kersten HW, Fransman R, Thoden van Velzen SK: Thermomechanical compaction of gutta-percha. I. A comparison of several compaction procedures, *Int Endod J* 19:125, 1986.

199. Kersten HW, Wesselink PR, Thoden van Velzen SK: The diagnostic reliability of the buccal radiograph after root canal filling, *Int Endod J* 20:20, 1987.

200. Kim YK, Grandini S, Ames JM, et al: Critical review on methacrylate resin-based root canal sealers. *J Endod* 36:383, 2010.

201. Kim YK, Mai S, Haycock JR, et al: The self-etching potential of Realseal vs RealSeal SE, *J Endod* 35:1264, 2009.

202. Kleier DJ, Averbach RE: Painful dysesthesia of the inferior alveolar nerve following use of a paraformaldehyde-containing root canal sealer, *Endod Dent Traumatol* 4:46, 1988.

203. Koch CRE, Thorpe BLT: *A history of dentistry*, vols. 2 and 3, Fort Wayne, IN, 1909, National Art Publishing Company.

204. Koch MJ: Formaldehyde release from root-canal sealers: influence of method, *Int Endod J* 32:10, 1999.

205. Kokkas AB, Boutsioukis A, Vassiliadis LP, et al: The influence of the smear layer on dentinal tubule penetration depth by three different root canal sealers: an in vitro study, *J Endod* 30:100, 2004.

206. Kontakiotis EG, Tzanetakis GN, Loizides AL: A 12-month longitudinal in vitro leakage study on a new silicon-based root canal filling material (Gutta-Flow), *Oral Surg Oral Med Oral Pathol Oral Radiol Endod* 103:854, 2007.

207. Kontakiotis EP: pH of root canal sealers containing calcium hydroxide, *Int Endod J* 29:202, 1996.

208. Kouvas V, Liolios E, Vassiliadis L, et al: Influence of smear layer on depth of penetration of three endodontic sealers: an SEM study, *Endod Dent Traumatol* 14:191, 1998.

209. Krastl G, Allgayer N, Lenherr P, et al: Tooth discoloration induced by endodontic materials: a literature review, *Dent Traumatol* 29:2, 2013.

210. Krell KV, Johnson RJ, Madison S: Irrigation patterns during ultrasonic canal instrumentation. I. K-type files, *J Endod* 14:65, 1988.

211. Kulild J, Lee C, Dryden J, et al: A comparison of 5 gutta-percha obturation techniques to replicate canal defects, *Oral Surg Oral Med Oral Pathol Oral Radiol Endod* 103:e28, 2007.

212. Kuttler Y: Microscopic investigation of root apexes, *J Am Dent Assoc* 50:544, 1955.

213. Kytridou V, Gutmann JL, Nunn MH: Adaptation and sealability of two contemporary obturation techniques in the absence of the dentinal smear layer, *Int Endod J* 32:464, 1999.

214. Langeland K: Root canal sealants and pastes, *Dent Clin North Am* 18:309, 1974.

215. Langeland K, Olsson B, Pascon EA: Biological evaluation of Hydron, *J Endod* 7:196, 1981.

216. Lawley GR, Schindler WG, Walker WA, III, et al: Evaluation of ultrasonically placed MTA and fracture resistance with intracanal composite resin in a model of apexification, *J Endod* 30:167, 2004.

217. Lawson MS, Loushine B, Mai S, et al: Resistance of a 4-META-containing, methacrylate-based sealer to dislocation in root canals, *J Endod* 34:833, 2008.

218. Lazarski MP, Walker WA, III, Flores CM, et al: Epidemiological evaluation of the outcomes of nonsurgical root canal treatment in a large cohort of insured dental patients, *J Endod* 27:791, 2001.

219. Lee FS, Van Cura JE, BeGole E: A comparison of root surface temperatures using different obturation heat sources, *J Endod* 24:617, 1998.

220. Leiendecker AP, Qi YP, Sawyer AN, et al: Effects of calcium silicate-based materials on collagen matrix integrity of mineralized dentin, *J Endod* 38:829, 2012.

221. Leonard JE, Gutmann JL, Guo IY: Apical and coronal seal of roots obturated with a dentine bonding agent and resin, *Int Endod J* 29:76, 1996.

222. Leonardo MR, Bezerra da Silva LA, Filho MT, et al: Release of formaldehyde by 4 endodontic sealers, *Oral Surg Oral Med Oral Pathol Oral Radiol Endod* 88:221, 1999.

223. Lertchirakarn V, Palamara JE, Messer HH: Load and strain during lateral condensation and vertical root fracture, *J Endod* 25:99, 1999.

224. Lertchirakarn V, Palamara JE, Messer HH: Patterns of vertical root fracture: factors affecting stress distribution in the root canal, *J Endod* 29:523, 2003.

225. Levitan ME, Himel VT, Luckey JB: The effect of insertion rates on fill length and adaptation of a thermoplasticized gutta-percha technique, *J Endod* 29:505, 2003.

226. Liang YH, Li G, Shemesh H, et al: The association between complete absence of post-treatment periapical lesion and quality of root canal filling, *Clin Oral Investig* 16:1619, 2012.

227. Liewehr FR, Kulild JC, Primack PD: Improved density of gutta-percha after warm lateral condensation, *J Endod* 19:489, 1993.

228. Lim TS, Wee TY, Choi MY, et al: Light and scanning electron microscopic evaluation of Glyde File Prep in smear layer removal, *Int Endod J* 36:336, 2003.

229. Loest C, Trope M, Friedman S: Follow-up of root canals obturated with glass ionomer and epoxy resin root canal sealer, *J Endod* 19:201, 1993.

230. Lohbauer U, Gambarini G, Ebert J, et al: Calcium release and pH-characteristics of calcium hydroxide plus points, *Int Endod J* 38:683, 2005.

231. Loushine BA, Bryan TE, Looney SW, et al: Setting properties and cytotoxicity evaluation of a premixed bioceramic root canal sealer, *J Endod* 37:673, 2011.

232. Lugassy AA, Yee F: Root canal obturation with gutta-percha: a scanning electron microscope comparison of vertical compaction and automated thermatic condensation, *J Endod* 8:120, 1982.

233. Lui JN, Sae-Lim V, Song KP, et al: In vitro antimicrobial effect of chlorhexidine-impregnated gutta percha points on *Enterococcus faecalis*, *Int Endod J* 37:105, 2004.

234. Lynch CD, Burke FM, Ní Ríordáin R, et al: The influence of coronal restoration type on the survival of endodontically treated teeth, *Eur J Prosthodont Restor Dent* 12:171, 2004.

235. Mah T, Basrani B, Santos JM, et al: Periapical inflammation affecting coronally-inoculated dog teeth with root fillings augmented by white MTA orifice plugs, *J Endod* 29:442, 2003.

236. Mai S, Kim YK, Arola DD, et al: Differential aggressiveness of ethylenediamine tetraacetic acid in causing canal wall erosion in the presence of sodium hypochlorite, *J Dent* 38:201, 2010.

237. Mai S, Kim YK, Hiraishi N, et al: Evaluation of the true self-etching potential of a fourth generation self-adhesive methacrylate resin-based sealer, *J Endod* 35:870, 2009.

238. Malkhassian G, Manzur AJ, Legner M, et al: Antibacterial efficacy of MTAD final rinse and two percent chlorhexidine gel medication in teeth with apical periodontitis: a randomized double-blinded clinical trial, *J Endod* 35:1483, 2009.

239. Malueg LA, Wilcox LR, Johnson W: Examination of external apical root resorption with scanning electron microscopy, *Oral Surg Oral Med Oral Pathol Oral Radiol Endod* 82:89, 1996.

240. Manzur A, González AM, Pozos A, et al: Bacterial quantification in teeth with apical periodontitis related to instrumentation and different intracanal medications: a randomized clinical trial, *J Endod* 33:114, 2007.

241. Marquis VL, Dao T, Farzaneh M, et al: Treatment outcome in endodontics: the Toronto Study. Phase III: initial treatment, *J Endod* 32:299, 2006.

242. Martin H, Fischer E: Photoelastic stress comparison of warm (Endotec) versus cold lateral condensation techniques, *Oral Surg Oral Med Oral Pathol* 70:325, 1990.

243. Mayne JR, Shapiro S, Abramson II: An evaluation of standardized gutta-percha points. I. Reliability and validity of standardization, *Oral Surg Oral Med Oral Pathol* 31:250, 1971.

244. McComb D, Smith DC: A preliminary scanning electron microscopic study of root canals after endodontic procedures, *J Endod* 1:238, 1975.

245. McCullagh JJ, Biagioni PA, Lamey PJ, et al: Thermographic assessment of root canal obturation using thermomechanical compaction, *Int Endod J* 30:191, 1997.

246. McCullagh JJ, Setchell DJ, Gulabivala K, et al: A comparison of thermocouple and infrared thermographic analysis of temperature rise on the root surface during the continuous wave of condensation technique, *Int Endod J* 33:326, 2000.

247. Melker KB, Vertucci FJ, Rojas MF, et al: Antimicrobial efficacy of medicated root canal filling materials, *J Endod* 32:148, 2006.

248. Messing JJ: An investigation of the sealing properties of some root filling materials, *J Br Endod Soc* 4:18, 1970.

249. Mickel AK, Nguyen TH, Chogle S: Antimicrobial activity of endodontic sealers on *Enterococcus faecalis*, *J Endod* 29:257, 2003.

250. Mjör IA, Smith MR, Ferrari M, et al: The structure of dentine in the apical region of human teeth, *Int Endod J* 34:346, 2001.

251. Mohammadi Z, Dummer PM: Properties and applications of calcium hydroxide in endodontics and dental traumatology, *Int Endod J* 44:697, 2011.

252. Molander A, Warfvinge J, Reit C, et al: Clinical and radiographic evaluation of one- and two-visit endodontic treatment of asymptomatic necrotic teeth with apical periodontitis: a randomized clinical trial, *J Endod* 33:1145, 2007.

253. Möller ÅJ, Fabricius L, Dahlén G, et al: Influence on periapical tissues of indigenous oral bacteria and necrotic pulp tissue in monkeys, *Scand J Dent Res* 89:475, 1981.

254. Morgan LA, Baumgartner JC: Demineralization of resected root-ends with methylene blue dye, *Oral Surg Oral Med Oral Pathol Oral Radiol Endod* 84:74, 1997.

255. Morgental RD, Vier-Pelisser FV, Oliveira SD, et al: Antibacterial activity of two MTA-based root canal sealers, *Int Endod J* 44:1128, 2011.

256. Nagas E, Uyanik MO, Eymirli A, et al: Dentin moisture conditions affect the adhesion of root canal sealers, *J Endod* 38:240, 2012.

257. Nair PN: Abusing technology? Culture-difficult microbes and microbial remnants, *Oral Surg Oral Med Oral Pathol Oral Radiol Endod* 104:569, 2007.

258. Nair PN, Henry S, Cano V, et al: Microbial status of apical root canal system of human mandibular first molars with primary apical periodontitis after "one-visit" endodontic treatment, *Oral Surg Oral Med Oral Pathol Oral Radiol Endod* 99:231, 2005.

259. Naito T: Better success rate for root canal therapy when treatment includes obturation short of the apex, *Evid Based Dent* 6:45, 2005.

260. Nelson EA, Liewehr FR, West LA: Increased density of gutta-percha using a controlled heat instrument with lateral condensation, *J Endod* 26:748, 2000.

261. Newton CW, Patterson SS, Kafrawy AH: Studies of Sargenti's technique of endodontic treatment: six-month and one-year responses, *J Endod* 6:509, 1980.

262. Ng YL, Mann V, Gulabivala K: A prospective study of the factors affecting outcomes of nonsurgical root canal treatment: part 1: periapical health, *Int Endod J* 44:583, 2011.

263. Ng YL, Mann V, Gulabivala K: A prospective study of the factors affecting outcomes of non-surgical root canal treatment: part 2: tooth survival, *Int Endod J* 44:610, 2011.

264. Ng YL, Mann V, Rahbaran S, et al: Outcome of primary root canal treatment: systematic review of the literature. 1. Effects of study characteristics on probability of success, *Int Endod J* 40:921, 2007.

265. Ng YL, Mann V, Rahbaran S, et al: Outcome of primary root canal treatment: systematic review of the literature. 2. Influence of clinical factors, *Int Endod J* 41:6, 2008.

266. Nygaard-Østby B: Chelation in root canal cleansing and widening of root canals, *Odontol Tidskr* 65:3, 1957.

267. Okşan T, Aktener BO, Sen BH, et al: The penetration of root canal sealers into dentinal tubules: a scanning electron microscopic study, *Int Endod J* 26:301, 1993.

268. Oliver CM, Abbott PV: Correlation between clinical success and apical dye penetration, *Int Endod J* 34:637, 2001.

269. Onay EO, Ungor M, Unver S, et al: An in vitro evaluation of the apical sealing ability of new polymeric endodontic filling systems, *Oral Surg Oral Med Oral Pathol Oral Radiol Endod* 108:49, 2009.

270. O'Neill KJ, Pitts DL, Harrington GW: Evaluation of the apical seal produced by the McSpadden compactor and the lateral condensation with a chloroform-softened primary cone, *J Endod* 9:190, 1983.

271. Ordinola-Zapata R, Bramante CM, Minotti PG, et al: Antimicrobial activity of triantibiotic paste, 2% chlorhexidine gel, and calcium hydroxide on an intraoral-infected dentin biofilm model, *J Endod* 39:115, 2013.

272. Ørstavik D, Haapasalo M: Disinfection by endodontic irrigants and dressings of experimentally infected dentinal tubules, *Endod Dent Traumatol* 6:142, 1990.

273. Ørstavik D, Nordahl I, Tibballs JE: Dimensional change following setting of root canal sealer materials, *Dent Mater* 17:512, 2001.

274. Oswald RJ, Cohn SA: Systemic distribution of lead from root canal fillings, *J Endod* 1:59, 1975.

275. Oswald RJ, Friedman CE: Periapical response to dentin filings: a pilot study, *Oral Surg Oral Med Oral Pathol* 49:344, 1980.

276. Ozok AR, van der Sluis LW, Wu MK, et al: Sealing ability of a new polydimethylsiloxane-based root canal filling material, *J Endod* 34:204, 2008.

277. Pallares A, Faus V, Glickman GN: The adaptation of mechanically softened gutta-percha to the canal walls in the presence or absence of smear layer: a scanning electron microscopic study, *Int Endod J* 28:266, 1995.

278. Pameijer CH, Zmener O: Resin materials for root canal obturation, *Dent Clin North Am* 54:325, 2010.

279. Parirokh M, Torabinejad M: Mineral trioxide aggregate: a comprehensive literature review. I. Chemical, physical, and antibacterial properties, *J Endod* 36:16, 2010.

280. Parirokh M, Torabinejad M: Mineral trioxide aggregate: a comprehensive literature review. III. Clinical applications, drawbacks, and mechanism of action, *J Endod* 36:400, 2010.

281. Pashley DH: Smear layer: overview of structure and function, *Proc Finn Dent Soc* 88:215, 1992.

282. Pashley EL, Birdsong NL, Bowman K, et al: Cytotoxic effects of NaOCl on vital tissue, *J Endod* 11:525, 1985.

283. Patel S, Dawood A, Whaites E, et al: New dimensions in endodontic imaging: part 1. Conventional and alternative radiographic systems, *Int Endod J* 42:447, 2009.

284. Patel S, Wilson R, Dawood A, et al: The detection of periapical pathosis using digital periapical radiography and cone beam computed tomography—part 2: a 1-year post-treatment follow-up, *Int Endod J* 45:711, 2012.

285. Penesis VA, Fitzgerald PI, Fayad MI, et al: Outcome of one-visit and two-visit endodontic treatment of necrotic teeth with apical periodontitis: a randomized controlled trial with one-year evaluation, *J Endod* 34:251, 2008.

286. Peng L, Ye L, Tan H, et al: Outcome of root canal obturation by warm gutta-percha versus cold lateral condensation: a meta-analysis, *J Endod* 33:106, 2007.

287. Perez F, Rochd T, Lodter JP, et al: In vitro study of the penetration of three bacterial strains into root dentine, *Oral Surg Oral Med Oral Pathol* 76:97, 1993.

288. Pérez Heredia M, Clavero González J, Ferrer Luque CM, et al: Apical seal comparison of low-temperature thermoplasticized gutta-percha technique and lateral condensation with two different master cones, *Med Oral Patol Oral Cir Bucal* 12:E175, 2007.

289. Perry SG: Preparing and filling the roots of teeth, *Dental Cosmos* 25:185, 1883.

290. Peters DD: Two-year in vitro solubility evaluation of four gutta-percha sealer obturation techniques, *J Endod* 12:139, 1986.

291. Peters LB, van Winkelhoff AJ, Buijs JF, et al: Effects of instrumentation, irrigation and dressing with calcium hydroxide on infection in pulpless teeth with periapical bone lesions, *Int Endod J* 35:13, 2002.

292. Peters LB, Wesselink PR: Periapical healing of endodontically treated teeth in one and two visits obturated in the presence or absence of detectable microorganisms, *Int Endod J* 35:660, 2002.

293. Pisano DM, DiFiore PM, McClanahan SB, et al: Intraorifice sealing of gutta-percha obturated root canals to prevent coronal microleakage, *J Endod* 24:659, 1998.

294. Piskin B, Aydin B, Sarikanat M: The effect of spreader size on fracture resistance of maxillary incisor roots, *Int Endod J* 41:54, 2008.

295. Pitts DL, Jones JE, Oswald RJ: A histological comparison of calcium hydroxide plugs and dentin plugs used for the control of gutta-percha root canal filling material, *J Endod* 10:283, 1984.

296. Pommel L, Jacquot B, Camps J: Lack of correlation among three methods for evaluation of apical leakage, *J Endod* 27:347, 2001.

297. Portenier I, Haapasalo H, Rye A, et al: Inactivation of root canal medicaments by dentine, hydroxylapatite and bovine serum albumin, *Int Endod J* 34:184, 2001.

298. Pradhan DP, Chawla HS, Gauba K, et al: Comparative evaluation of endodontic management of teeth with unformed apices with mineral trioxide aggregate and calcium hydroxide, *J Dent Child (Chic)* 73:79, 2006.

299. Price WA: Report of laboratory investigations on the physical properties of root canal filling materials and the efficiency of root canal fillings blocking infection from sterile tooth structure, *J Natl Dent Assoc* 5:1260, 1918.

300. Qian W, Shen Y, Haapasalo M: Quantitative analysis of the effect of irrigant solution sequences on dentin erosion, *J Endod* 37:1437, 2011.

301. Rached-Junior FJ, Souza-Gabriel AE, Alfredo E, et al: Bond strength of Epiphany sealer prepared with resinous solvent, *J Endod* 35:251, 2009.

302. Radovic I, Monticelli F, Goracci C, et al: Self-adhesive resin cements: a literature review, *J Adhes Dent* 10:251, 2008.

303. Raina R, Loushine RJ, Weller RN, et al: Evaluation of the quality of the apical seal in Resilon/Epiphany and gutta-percha/AH Plus-filled root canals by using a fluid filtration approach, *J Endod* 33:944, 2007.

304. Rasimick BJ, Shah RP, Musikant BL, et al: Radiopacity of endodontic materials on film and a digital sensor, *J Endod* 33:1098, 2007.

305. Ray HA, Trope M: Periapical status of endodontically treated teeth in relation to the technical quality of the root filling and the coronal restoration, *Int Endod J* 28:12, 1995.

306. Rechenberg DK, De-Deus G, Zehnder M: Potential systematic error in laboratory experiments on microbial leakage through filled root canals: review of published articles, *Int Endod J* 44:183, 2011.

307. Rechenberg DK, Thurnheer T, Zehnder M: Potential systematic error in laboratory experiments on microbial leakage through filled root canals: an experimental study, *Int Endod J* 44:827, 2011.

308. Rickert U, Dixon C: The control of root surgery, Transactions of the 8th International Dental Congress, Section IIIA, No. 9.20:1458, 1933.

309. Ricucci D: Apical limit of root canal instrumentation and obturation. Part 1. Literature review, *Int Endo J* 31:384, 1998.

310. Ricucci D, Bergenholtz G: Bacterial status in root-filled teeth exposed to the oral environment by loss of restoration and fracture or caries—a histobacteriological study of treated cases, *Int Endod J* 36:787, 2003.

311. Ricucci D, Grondahl K, Bergenholtz G: Periapical status of root-filled teeth exposed to the oral environment by loss of restoration or caries, *Oral Surg Oral Med Oral Pathol Oral Radiol Endod* 90:354, 2000.

312. Ricucci D, Langeland K: Apical limit of root canal instrumentation and obturation. 2. A histological study, *Int Endod J* 31:394, 1998.

313. Ricucci D, Siqueira JF Jr: Fate of the tissue in lateral canals and apical ramifications in response to pathologic conditions and treatment procedures, *J Endod* 36:1, 2010.

314. Ricucci D, Siqueira JF Jr: Recurrent apical periodontitis and late endodontic treatment failure related to coronal leakage: a case report, *J Endod* 37:1171, 2011.

315. Rôças IN, Siqueira JF. Identification of bacteria enduring endodontic treatment procedures by a combined reverse transcriptase–polymerase chain reaction and reverse-capture checkerboard approach, *J Endod* 36:45, 2010.

316. Rosenberg B, Murray PE, Namerow K: The effect of calcium hydroxide root filling on dentin fracture strength, *Dent Traumatol* 23:26, 2007.

317. Rosenow EC: Studies on elective localization: focal infection with special reference to oral sepsis, *J Dent Res* 1:205, 1919.

318. Sabeti MA, Nekofar M, Motahhary P, et al: Healing of apical periodontitis after endodontic treatment with and without obturation in dogs, *J Endod* 32:628, 2006.

319. Sabins RA, Johnson JD, Hellstein JW: A comparison of the cleaning efficacy of short-term sonic and ultrasonic passive irrigation after hand instrumentation in molar root canals, *J Endod* 29:674, 2003.

320. Safavi K, Horsted P, Pascon EA, et al: Biological evaluation of the apical dentin chip plug, *J Endod* 11:18, 1985.

321. Safavi KE, Dowden WE, Langeland K: Influence of delayed coronal permanent restoration on endodontic prognosis, *Endod Dent Traumatol* 3:187, 1987.

322. Salehrabi R, Rotstein I: Endodontic treatment outcomes in a large patient population in the USA: an epidemiological study, *J Endod* 30:846, 2004.

323. Salles LP, Gomes-Cornélio AL, Guimarães FC, et al: Mineral trioxide aggregate-based endodontic sealer stimulates hydroxyapatite nucleation in human osteoblast-like cell culture, *J Endod* 38:971, 2012.

324. Santos MD, Walker WA, III, Carnes DL, Jr: Evaluation of apical seal in straight canals after obturation using the Lightspeed sectional method, *J Endod* 25:609, 1999.

325. Sargenti A: *Endodontic course for the general practitioner*, ed 3. Bruxelles, Belgium, 1965, EES.

326. Sargenti A: The endodontic debate ends? *CDS Rev* 70:28, 1977.

327. Sargenti A: The Sargenti N-2 method, *Dent Surv* 54:55, 1978.

328. Sathorn C, Parashos P, Messer HH: Effectiveness of single- versus multiple-visit endodontic treatment of teeth with apical periodontitis: a systematic review and meta-analysis, *Int Endod J* 38:347, 2005.

329. Sathorn C, Parashos P, Messer HH: How useful is root canal culturing in predicting treatment outcome? *J Endod* 33:220, 2007.

330. Sathorn C, Parashos P, Messer H: Antibacterial efficacy of calcium hydroxide intracanal dressing: a systematic review and meta-analysis, *Int Endod J* 40:2, 2007.

331. Saunders EM: The effect of variation in thermomechanical compaction techniques upon the quality of the apical seal, *Int Endod J* 22:163, 1989.

332. Saunders EM: In vivo findings associated with heat generation during thermomechanical compaction of gutta-percha. 1. Temperature levels at the external surface of the root, *Int Endod J* 23:263, 1990.

333. Saunders EM: In vivo findings associated with heat generation during thermomechanical compaction of gutta-percha. 2. Histological response to temperature elevation on the external surface of the root, *Int Endod J* 23:268, 1990.

334. Sawyer AN, Nikonov SY, Pancio AK, et al: Effects of calcium silicate-based materials on the flexural properties of dentin, *J Endod* 38:680, 2012.

335. Scarfe WC, Levin MD, Gane D, et al: Use of cone beam computed tomography in endodontics, *Int J Dent* 2009:634567, 2009.

336. Scarparo RK, Haddad D, Acasigua GA, et al: Mineral trioxide aggregate-based sealer: analysis of tissue reactions to a new endodontic material, *J Endod* 36:1174, 2010.

337. Scelza MF, Teixeira AM, Scelza P: Decalcifying effect of EDTA-T, 10% citric acid, and 17% EDTA on root canal dentin, *Oral Surg Oral Med Oral Pathol Oral Radiol Endod* 95:234, 2003.

338. Schaeffer MA, White RR, Walton RE: Determining the optimal obturation length: a meta-analysis of literature, *J Endod* 31:271, 2005.

339. Schilder H: Filling root canals in three dimensions, *Dent Clin North Am* Nov:723, 1967.

340. Schilder H, Goodman A, Aldrich W: The thermomechanical properties of gutta-percha. V. Volume changes in bulk gutta-percha as a function of temperature and its relationship to molecular phase transformation, *Oral Surg Oral Med Oral Pathol* 59:285, 1985.

341. Schmidt KJ, Walker TL, Johnson JD, et al: Comparison of nickel–titanium and stainless-steel spreader penetration and accessory cone fit in curved canals, *J Endod* 26:42, 2000.

342. Segura JJ, Calvo JR, Guerrero JM, et al: The disodium salt of EDTA inhibits the binding of vasoactive intestinal peptide to macrophage membranes: endodontic implications, *J Endod* 22:337, 1996.

343. Seltzer S: *Endodontology: biologic considerations in endodontic practice*, ed 2. Philadelphia; 1988, Lea & Febiger.

344. Seltzer S, Green DB, Weiner N, et al: A scanning electron microscope examination of silver cones removed from endodontically treated teeth, *Oral Surg Oral Med Oral Pathol* 33:589, 1972.

345. Sen BH, Ertürk O, Pişkin B: The effect of different concentrations of EDTA on instrumented root canal walls, *Oral Surg Oral Med Oral Pathol Oral Radiol Endod* 108:622, 2009.

346. Sen BH, Piskin B, Demirci T: Observation of bacteria and fungi in infected root canals and dentinal tubules by SEM, *Endod Dent Traumatol* 11:6, 1995.

347. Sen BH, Wesselink PR, Türkün M: The smear layer: a phenomenon in root canal therapy, *Int Endod J* 28:141, 1995.

348. Serper A, Uçer O, Onur R, et al: Comparative neurotoxic effects of root canal filling materials on rat sciatic nerve, *J Endod* 24:592, 1998.

349. Shabahang S, Pouresmail M, Torabinejad M: In vitro antimicrobial efficacy of MTAD and sodium hypochlorite, *J Endod* 29:450, 2003.

350. Shabahang S, Torabinejad M: Treatment of teeth with open apices using mineral trioxide aggregate, *Pract Periodontics Aesthet Dent* 12:315, 2000.

351. Shah N, Logani A, Bhaskar U, et al: Efficacy of revascularization to induce apexification/apexogensis in infected, nonvital, immature teeth: a pilot clinical study, *J Endod* 34:919, 2008.

352. Shahi S, Zand V, Oskoee SS, et al: An in vitro study of the effect of spreader penetration depth on apical microleakage, *J Oral Sci* 49:283, 2007.

353. Shahravan A, Haghdoost AA, Adl A, et al: Effect of smear layer on sealing ability of canal obturation: a systematic review and meta-analysis, *J Endod* 33:96, 2007.

354. Shanahan DJ, Duncan HF: Root canal filling using Resilon: a review, *Br Dent J* 211:81, 2011.

355. Shipper G, Ørstavik D, Teixeira FB, et al: An evaluation of microbial leakage in roots filled with a thermoplastic synthetic polymer-based root canal filling material (Resilon), *J Endod* 30:342, 2004.

356. Shipper G, Teixeira FB, Arnold RR, et al: Periapical inflammation after coronal microbial inoculation of dog roots filled with gutta-percha or Resilon, *J Endod* 31:91, 2005.

357. Silver GK, Love RM, Purton DG: Comparison of two vertical condensation obturation techniques: Touch 'n Heat modified and System B, *Int Endod J* 32:287, 1999.

358. Simon S, Rilliard F, Berdal A, et al: The use of mineral trioxide aggregate in one-visit apexification treatment: a prospective study, *Int Endod J* 40:186, 2007.

359. Siqueira JF Jr, da Silva CH, Cerqueira M das D, et al: Effectiveness of four chemical solutions in eliminating *Bacillus subtilis* spores on gutta-percha cones, *Endod Dent Traumatol* 14:124, 1998.

360. Siqueira JF Jr, Guimarães-Pinto T, Rôças IN: Effects of chemomechanical preparation with 2.5% sodium hypochlorite and intracanal medication with calcium hydroxide on cultivable bacteria in infected root canals, *J Endod* 33:800, 2007.

361. Siqueira JF Jr, Paiva SS, Rôças IN: Reduction in the cultivable bacterial populations in infected root canals by a chlorhexidine-based antimicrobial protocol, *J Endod* 33:541, 2007.

362. Siqueira JF, Rôças IN: Diversity of endodontic microbiota revisited, *J Dent Res* 88:969, 2009.

363. Sjögren U, Figdor D, Persson S, et al: Influence of infection at the time of root filling on the outcome of endodontic treatment of teeth with apical periodontitis, *Int Endod J* 30:297, 1997.

364. Sjögren U, Hagglund B, Sundqvist G, et al: Factors affecting the long-term results of endodontic treatment, *J Endod* 16:498, 1990.

365. Sonat B, Dalat D, Gunhan O: Periapical tissue reaction to root fillings with Sealapex, *Int Endod J* 23:46, 1990.

366. Southard DW, Rooney TP: Effective one-visit therapy for the acute periapical abscess, *J Endod* 10:580, 1984.

367. Spångberg L: Biological effects of root canal filling materials. 7. Reaction of bony tissue to implanted root canal filling material in guinea pigs, *Odontologisk Tidskrift* 77:133, 1969.

368. Spångberg LS, Barbosa SV, Lavigne GD: AH 26 releases formaldehyde, *J Endod* 19:596, 1993.

369. Stamos DE, Gutmann JL, Gettleman BH: In vivo evaluation of root canal sealer distribution, *J Endod* 21:177, 1995.

370. Stevens RW, Strother JM, McClanahan SB: Leakage and sealer penetration in smear-free dentin after a final rinse with 95% ethanol, *J Endod* 32:785, 2006.

371. Stewart GG: A scanning electron microscopic study of the cleansing effectiveness of three irrigating modalities on the tubular structure of dentin, *J Endod* 24:485, 1998.

372. Su Y, Wang C, Ye L: Healing rate and post-obturation pain of single- versus multiple-visit endodontic treatment for infected root canals: a systematic review, *J Endod* 37:125, 2011.

373. Susini G, Pommel L, About I, et al: Lack of correlation between ex vivo apical dye penetration and presence of apical radiolucencies, *Oral Surg Oral Med Oral Pathol Oral Radiol Endod* 102:e19, 2006.

374. Swartz DB, Skidmore AE, Griffin JA Jr: Twenty years of endodontic success and failure, *J Endod* 9:198, 1983.

375. Reference deleted in proofs.

376. Tagger M, Tagger E, Kfir A: Release of calcium and hydroxyl ions from set endodontic sealers containing calcium hydroxide, *J Endod* 14:588, 1988.

377. Tani-Ishii N, Teranaka T: Clinical and radiographic evaluation of root-canal obturation with Obtura II, *J Endod* 29:739, 2003.

378. Tanomaru JM, Tanomaru-Filho M, Hotta J, et al: Antimicrobial activity of endodontic sealers based on calcium hydroxide and MTA, *Acta Odontol Latinoam* 21:147, 2008.

379. Tanomaru-Filho M, Jorge EG, Guerreiro Tanomaru JM, et al: Radiopacity evaluation of new root canal filling materials by digitalization of images, *J Endod* 33:249, 2007.

380. Tanomaru-Filho M, Leonardo MR, Silva LA, et al: Inflammatory response to different endodontic irrigating solutions, *Int Endod J* 35:735, 2002.

381. Tatsuta CT, Morgan LA, Baumgartner JC, et al: Effect of calcium hydroxide and four irrigation regimens on instrumented and uninstrumented canal wall topography, *J Endod* 25:93, 1999.

382. Tay FR, Loushine RJ, Monticelli F, et al: Effectiveness of resin-coated gutta-percha cones and a dual-cured, hydrophilic methacrylate resin-based sealer in obturating root canals, *J Endod* 31:659, 2005.

383. Tay FR, Pashley DH: Monoblocks in root canals: a hypothetical or a tangible goal, *J Endod* 33:391, 2007.

384. Tay FR, Pashley DH, Rueggeberg FA, et al: Calcium phosphate phase transformation produced by the interaction of the portland cement component of white mineral trioxide aggregate with a phosphate-containing fluid, *J Endod* 33:1347, 2007.

385. Tay KC, Loushine BA, Oxford C, et al: In vitro evaluation of a Ceramicrete-based root-end filling material, *J Endod* 33:1438, 2007.

386. Taylor JK, Jeansonne BG, Lemon RR: Coronal leakage: effects of smear layer, obturation technique, and sealer, *J Endod* 23:508, 1997.

387. Teixeira FB, Teixeira EC, Thompson JY, et al: Fracture resistance of endodontically treated roots using a new type of filling material, *J Am Dent Assoc* 135:646, 2004.

388. Tewary S, Luzzo J, Hartwell G: Endodontic radiography: who is reading the digital radiograph?, *J Endod* 37:919, 2011.

389. Torabinejad M, Ung B, Kettering JD: In vitro bacterial penetration of coronally unsealed endodontically treated teeth, *J Endod* 16:566, 1990.

390. Tronstad L, Barnett F, Flax M: Solubility and biocompatibility of calcium hydroxide–containing root canal sealers, *Endod Dent Traumatol* 4:152, 1988.

391. Trope M: Treatment of the immature tooth with a non-vital pulp and apical periodontitis, *Dent Clin North Am* 54:313, 2010.

392. Trope M, Chow E, Nissan R: In vitro endotoxin penetration of coronally unsealed endodontically treated teeth, *Endod Dent Traumatol* 11:90, 1995.

393. Uranga A, Blum JY, Esber S, et al: A comparative study of four coronal obturation materials in endodontic treatment, *J Endod* 25:178, 1999.

394. van der Burgt TP, Mullaney TP, Plasschaert AJ: Tooth discoloration induced by endodontic sealers, *Oral Surg Oral Med Oral Pathol* 61:84, 1986.

395. VanGheluwe J, Wilcox LR: Lateral condensation of small, curved root canals: comparison of two types of accessory cones, *J Endod* 22:540, 1996.

396. Vasiliadis L, Kodonas K, Economides N, et al: Short- and long-term sealing ability of Gutta-flow and AH-Plus using an ex vivo fluid transport model, *Int Endod J* 43:377, 2010.

397. Vera J, Siqueira JF Jr, Ricucci D, et al: One- versus two-visit endodontic treatment of teeth with apical periodontitis: a histobacteriologic study, *J Endod* 38:1040, 2012.

398. Venturi M, Pasquantonio G, Falconi M, et al: Temperature change within gutta-percha induced by the System-B Heat Source, *Int Endod J* 35:740, 2002.

399. on der Fehr F, Nygaard-Østby B: Effect of EDTAC and sulfuric acid on root canal dentine, *Oral Surg Oral Med Oral Pathol* 16:199, 1963.

400. Walker TL, del Rio CE: Histological evaluation of ultrasonic debridement comparing sodium hypochlorite and water, *J Endod* 17:66, 1991.

401. Waltimo T, Trope M, Haapasalo M, et al: Clinical efficacy of treatment procedures in endodontic infection control and one year follow-up of periapical healing, *J Endod* 31:863, 2005.

402. Walton RE: Histologic evaluation of different methods of enlarging the pulp canal space, *J Endod* 2:304, 1976.

403. Wang CS, Arnold RR, Trope M, et al: Clinical efficiency of 2% chlorhexidine gel in reducing intracanal bacteria, *J Endod* 33:1283, 2007.

404. Washington JT, Schneiderman E, Spears R, et al: Biocompatibility and osteogenic potential of new generation endodontic materials established by using primary osteoblasts, *J Endod* 37:1166, 2011.

405. Weinberger BW: *An introduction to the history of dentistry*, St. Louis, MO, 1948, Mosby.

406. Weisenseel JA Jr, Hicks ML, Pelleu GB Jr: Calcium hydroxide as an apical barrier, *J Endod* 13:1, 1987.

407. Welch JD, Anderson RW, Pashley DH, et al: An assessment of the ability of various materials to seal furcation canals in molar teeth, *J Endod* 22:608, 1996.

408. Weller RN, Kimbrough WF, Anderson RW: A comparison of thermoplastic obturation techniques: adaptation to the canal walls, *J Endod* 23:703, 1997.

409. Wennberg A, Ørstavik D: Adhesion of root canal sealers to bovine dentine and gutta-percha, *Int Endod J* 23:13, 1990.

410. White RR, Goldman M, Lin PS: The influence of the smeared layer upon dentinal tubule penetration by plastic filling materials, *J Endod* 10:558, 1984.

411. White RR, Goldman M, Lin PS: The influence of the smeared layer upon dentinal tubule penetration by endodontic filling materials. Part II, *J Endod* 13:369, 1987.

412. Whitworth J: Methods of filling root canals: principles and practices, *Endo Topics* 12:2, 2005.

413. Wiemann AH, Wilcox LR: In vitro evaluation of four methods of sealer placement, *J Endod* 17:444, 1991.

414. Wigler R, Kaufman AY, Lin S, et al: Revascularization: a treatment for permanent teeth with necrotic pulp and incomplete root development, *J Endod* 39:319, 2013.

415. Wilcox LR, Roskelley C, Sutton T: The relationship of root canal enlargement to finger-spreader induced vertical root fracture, *J Endod* 23:533, 1997.

416. Williams C, Loushine RJ, Weller RN, et al: A comparison of cohesive strength and stiffness of Resilon and gutta-percha, *J Endod* 32:553, 2006.

417. Wilson BL, Baumgartner JC: Comparison of spreader penetration during lateral compaction of .04 and .02 tapered gutta-percha, *J Endod* 29:828, 2003.

418. Wolanek GA, Loushine RJ, Weller RN, et al: In vitro bacterial penetration of endodontically treated teeth coronally sealed with a dentin bonding agent, *J Endod* 27:354, 2001.

419. Wolcott J, Himel VT, Powell W, et al: Effect of two obturation techniques on the filling of lateral canals and the main canal, *J Endod* 23:632, 1997.

420. Wu MK, Fan B, Wesselink PR: Leakage along apical root fillings in curved root canals. I. Effects of apical transportation on seal of root fillings, *J Endod* 26:210, 2000.

421. Wu MK, Kašt'aková A, Wesselink PR: Quality of cold and warm gutta-percha fillings in oval canals in mandibular premolars, *Int Endod J* 34:485, 2001.

422. Wu MK, Ozok AR, Wesselink PR: Sealer distribution in root canals obturated by three techniques, *Int Endod J* 33:340, 2000.

423. Wu MK, Shemesh H, Wesselink PR: Limitations of previously published systematic reviews evaluating the outcome of endodontic treatment, *Int Endod J* 42:656, 2009.

424. Wu MK, van der Sluis LW, Wesselink PR: A preliminary study of the percentage of gutta-percha–filled area in the apical canal filled with vertically compacted warm gutta-percha, *Int Endod J* 35:527, 2002.

425. Wu MK, van der Sluis LW, Wesselink PR: The capability of two hand instrumentation techniques to remove the inner layer of dentine in oval canals, *Int Endod J* 36:218, 2003.

426. Wu MK, Wesselink PR: Endodontic leakage studies reconsidered. I. Methodology, application and relevance, *Int Endod J* 26:37, 1993.

427. Wu MK, Wesselink PR: A primary observation on the preparation and obturation of oval canals, *Int Endod J* 34:137, 2001.

428. Yamauchi S, Shipper G, Buttke T, et al: Effect of orifice plugs on periapical inflammation in dogs, *J Endod* 32:524, 2006.

429. Yared GM, Dagher FB, Machtou P: Influence of the removal of coronal gutta-percha on the seal of root canal obturations, *J Endod* 23:146, 1997.

430. Yeung P, Liewehr FR, Moon PC: A quantitative comparison of the fill density of MTA produced by two placement techniques, *J Endod* 32:456, 2006.

431. Youngson CC, Nattress BR, Manogue M, et al: In vitro radiographic representation of the extent of voids within obturated root canals, *Int Endod J* 28:77, 1995.

432. Zhang H, Shen Y, Ruse ND, et al: Antibacterial activity of endodontic sealers by modified direct contact test against *Enterococcus faecalis*, *J Endod* 35:1051, 2009.

433. Zhang K, Tay FR, Kim YK, et al: The effect of initial irrigation with two different sodium hypochlorite concentrations on the erosion of instrumented radicular dentin, *Dent Mater* 26:514, 2010.

434. Zhang W, Li Z, Peng B. Effects of iRoot SP on mineralization-related genes expression in MG63 cells, *J Endod* 36:1978, 2010.

435. Zielinski TM, Baumgartner JC, Marshall JG: An evaluation of Guttaflow and gutta-percha in the filling of lateral grooves and depressions, *J Endod* 34:295, 2008.

436. Zmener O, Banegas G: Clinical experience of root canal filling by ultrasonic condensation of gutta-percha, *Endod Dent Traumatol* 15:57, 1999.

437. Zmener O, Hilu R, Scavo R: Compatibility between standardized endodontic finger spreaders and accessory gutta-percha cones, *Endod Dent Traumatol* 12:237, 1996.

438. Zmener O, Martinez Lalis R, Pameijer CH, et al: Reaction of rat subcutaneous connective tissue to a mineral trioxide aggregate-based and a zinc oxide and eugenol sealer, *J Endod* 38:1233, 2012.

439. Zmener O, Pameijer CH: Clinical and radiographic evaluation of a resin-based root canal sealer: 10-year recall data, *Int J Dent* 2012:763248, 2012.

440. Zmener O, Pameijer CH, Serrano SA, et al: Significance of moist root canal dentin with the use of methacrylate-based endodontic sealers: an in vitro coronal dye leakage study, *J Endod* 34:76, 2008.

441. Zogheib C, Naaman A, Sigurdsson A, et al: Comparative micro-computed tomographic evaluation of two carrier-based obturation systems, *Clin Oral Investig* 17:1879, 2013.

PART **II**

The Advanced Science of Endodontics

CHAPTER 8

Nonsurgical Retreatment

ROBERT S. RODA | BRADLEY H. GETTLEMAN

CHAPTER OUTLINE

Nonsurgical root canal therapy has become a routine procedure in modern dentistry. Technical and scientific advances in endodontics have resulted in the retention of millions of teeth that would otherwise be lost. Even as advances in surgical and prosthetic restorative care have made tooth replacement less onerous than in the past, it is universally accepted that a natural tooth with a good prognosis is a superior choice to loss and replacement.

Unfortunately, not all treatments result in optimum long-term healing. Given the large numbers of treatments performed, the very small rate of unsuccessful outcomes translates into relatively large numbers of patients requiring further treatment. Dental clinicians should be able to diagnose persistent or reintroduced endodontic disease and be aware of the options for treatment. If they wish to approach treating these teeth, they should have the appropriate armamentarium and be capable of performing these specialized techniques at the highest level (Fig. 8-1). Also, clinicians must always have a scientifically sound, evidence-based rationale for every treatment decision that is made so that they may best serve the patients who entrust them with their care. The purpose of this chapter is to provide information to allow the reader to maximize the likelihood of success in the treatment of persistent endodontic disease.

ETIOLOGY OF POSTTREATMENT DISEASE

In the past, undesirable outcomes of endodontic therapy were described as failures. Clinicians quote failure rates based on published success/failure studies. Using the words *success* and *failure* may be a holdover from a time when clinicians felt they needed to congratulate themselves on their successes and blame themselves for the failures of their treatment endeavors. This thought process does not reflect reality and can be potentially destructive. There are many instances in which treatments performed at the highest level of clinical competence result in an undesirable outcome, and there are other instances in which a procedure is performed well below a scientifically acceptable standard and yet provides long-term success.[203] We must begin to dissect the science from emotion and ego, and this separation may start with nomenclature. Friedman stated that "most patients can relate to the concept of disease-treatment-healing, whereas failure, apart from being a negative and relative term, does not imply the necessity to pursue treatment."[64] He has suggested using the term *posttreatment disease* to describe those cases that would previously have been referred to as treatment failures. This will be the term used in the remainder of this chapter to describe persistent or reintroduced endodontic disease.

Almost 16 million root canal procedures were performed in 1999,[29] and, with success rates varying between 86% and 98%,[65,66] it has been shown to be a reliable treatment option. Conversely, the incidence of posttreatment disease, although small, translates into a large number of cases where further treatment is needed. When faced with such a situation, the clinician must determine the etiology of the persistent pathosis and devise a rationale and strategy for treatment.

There are many causes for "failure" of initial endodontic therapy that have been described in the endodontic literature (Fig. 8-2). These include iatrogenic procedural errors such as poor access cavity design, untreated canals (both major and accessory),[266] canals that are poorly cleaned and obturated,[37,112] complications of instrumentation (ledges, perforations, or separated instruments),[231] and overextensions of root-filling materials.[164] Coronal leakage[131,147,196,236,248] has also been blamed for posttreatment disease, as has persistent intracanal and extracanal infection[166,216,232] and radicular cysts.[162] These etiologies may be obvious at the time of diagnosing the diseased, root-filled tooth, or they may remain uncertain until the completion of successful therapy. Occasionally, the cause of posttreatment disease may take years to become discernible or may ultimately never be known. The most important causative factors for the clinician, however, are those related to treatment planning and determination of prognosis.

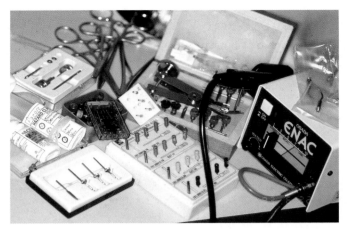

FIG. 8-1 Some of the armamentarium needed to perform retreatment at the highest level.

To treatment plan effectively, the clinician may place the etiologic factors into four groups[231] (Fig. 8-3):

1. Persistent or reintroduced intraradicular microorganisms
2. Extraradicular infection
3. Foreign body reaction
4. True cysts

Persistent or Reintroduced Intraradicular Microorganisms

When the root canal space and dentinal tubules are contaminated with microorganisms or their by-products and if these pathogens are allowed to contact the periradicular tissues, apical periodontitis ensues. As stated earlier, inadequate cleaning, shaping, obturation, and final restoration of an endodontically diseased tooth can lead to posttreatment disease. If initial endodontic therapy does not render the canal

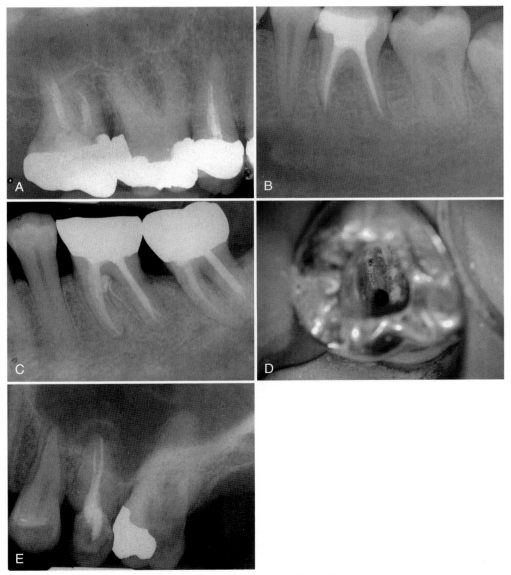

FIG. 8-2 Clinical presentations of posttreatment disease. **A,** Canals that are poorly cleaned, shaped, and obturated. **B,** Mesial canal with apical transport, ledge, and zip perforation. **C,** Strip perforation of the mesial root. **D,** Missed MB2 canal in an upper molar. **E,** Suspected coronal leakage of bacteria and a separated file.

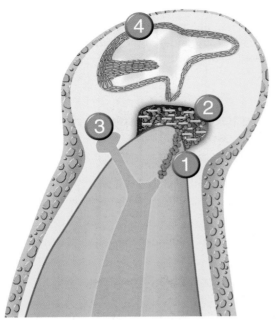

FIG. 8-3 The causes of posttreatment disease. *(1)* Intraradicular microorganisms. *(2)* Extraradicular infection. *(3)* Foreign body reaction. *(4)* True cysts. (Redrawn with permission from Sundqvist G, Figdor D. In Orstavik D, Pitt-Ford TR, editors: *Essential Endodontology*, London, 1998, Blackwell Science, p 260.)

space free of bacteria, if the obturation does not adequately entomb those that may remain, or if new microorganisms are allowed to reenter the cleaned and sealed canal space, then posttreatment disease can and usually does occur. In fact, it has been asserted that persistent or reintroduced microorganisms are the major cause of posttreatment disease.[163] Many iatrogenic treatment complications, such as creation of a ledge or separation of an instrument, result in persistence of bacteria in the canal system. It is not the complication itself, however, that results in persistent disease; rather, it is the inability to remove or entomb the microorganisms present that creates the pathologic state. While infected root canals of endodontically untreated teeth generally contain a polymicrobial, predominantly anaerobic flora,[230] cultures of infected, previously root-filled teeth produce very few or even a single species (see also Chapter 14). The infecting flora are predominantly gram positive, not anaerobic, and a commonly isolated species is *Enterococcus faecalis*,[71,182] which has been shown to be resistant to canal disinfection regimens.[16,33] Interestingly, if the previous root canal treatment is done so poorly that the canal space contains no obturating material in the apical half of the root canal space, its flora is more typical of the untreated necrotic infected pulp than that of classic "failed" root canal therapy.[231] Though posttreatment disease has been primarily blamed on bacteria in the root canal system, certain fungi, notably *Candida albicans*, are found frequently in persistent endodontic infections and may be responsible for the recalcitrant lesion.[214]

Extraradicular Infection

Occasionally bacterial cells can invade the periradicular tissues either by direct spread of infection from the root canal space via contaminated periodontal pockets that communicate with the apical area,[212] extrusion of infected dentin chips,[99] or by contamination with overextended, infected endodontic instruments.[257] Usually, the host response will destroy these organisms, but some microorganisms are able to resist the immune defenses and persist in the periradicular tissues, sometimes by producing an extracellular matrix or protective plaque.[249] It has also been shown[166,216,232] that two species of microorganisms, *Actinomyces israelii* and *Propionibacterium propionicum*, can exist in the periapical tissues and may prevent healing after root canal therapy.

Foreign Body Reaction

Occasionally, persistent endodontic disease occurs in the absence of discernible microorganisms and has been attributed to the presence of foreign material in the periradicular area. Several materials have been associated with inflammatory responses, including lentil beans[211] and cellulose fibers from paper points.[125] In the seemingly endless debate about which endodontic obturation technique is superior, there has been much discussion about the effect of overextended root canal filling materials upon apical healing. Outcomes assessments generally show that filling material extrusion (root filling flush to the radiographic apex or gross overextension) leads to a lower incidence of healing (see also Chapter 7).[63,215] Many of these cases involved not only overextension but also inadequate canal preparation and compaction of the root filling whereby persistent bacteria remaining in the canal space could leak out. Gutta-percha and sealers are usually well tolerated by the apical tissues, and if the tissues have not been inoculated with microorganisms by vigorous overinstrumentation, then healing in the presence of overextended filling materials can still occur.[63,70,137]

True Cysts

Cysts form in the periradicular tissues when nests of epithelial cells, retained from tooth development, begin to proliferate due to the chronic presence of inflammatory mediators. These epithelial cell rests of Malassez are the source of the epithelium that lines cystic walls, and cyst formation may be an attempt to help separate the inflammatory stimulus from the surrounding bone.[181] The incidence of periapical cysts has been reported to be 15% to 42% of all periapical lesions,[162,224] and determining whether a periapical radiolucency is a cyst or the more common periapical granuloma cannot be done with available radiographic methods.[23] There are two types of periapical cysts: the periapical true cyst and the periapical pocket cyst. True cysts have a contained cavity or lumen within a continuous epithelial lining and are therefore isolated from the tooth, whereas with pocket cysts, the lumen is open to the root canal of the affected tooth. True cysts, due to their self-sustaining nature, probably do not heal following nonsurgical endodontic therapy[112,165] and usually require surgical enucleation (Fig. 8-4).

When a patient presents with posttreatment disease, clinical decision making depends on determining the cause of the persistent disease and then making an assessment of how best to treat the pathologic condition. The following section presents a rationale and methods for performing endodontic diagnosis that offer the greatest likelihood of a successful outcome.

DIAGNOSIS OF POSTTREATMENT DISEASE

It has been stated that "there may be different ways of treating a disease; however, there can be but one correct diagnosis."[9]

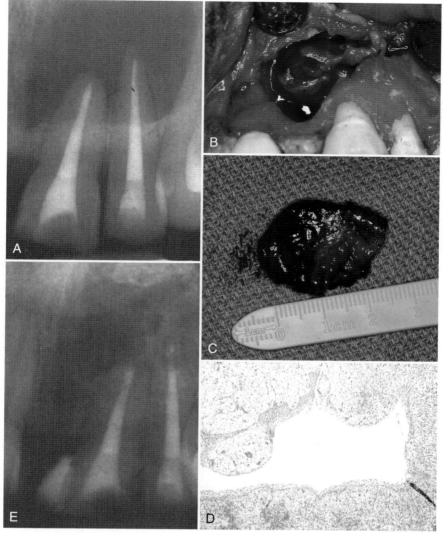

FIG. 8-4 A, Apparently good nonsurgical retreatment with large persistent lesion. B, Surgical exposure of apical lesion in situ. C, Large lesion removed in toto. D, Histopathologic section confirming cystic nature of the lesion. E, A 4-year post-operative film showing apical scar formation due to the large size of the lesion. The teeth were asymptomatic and in function.

The proper diagnosis is probably the most important portion of any endodontic procedure (see also Chapter 1). This is not as bold of a statement as one may first suspect when consideration is given to what the patient may undergo if treatment is performed based on an incorrect diagnosis (Fig. 8-5). To make a correct diagnosis, the clinician must rule out nonodontogenic etiology, perform all of the appropriate tests, properly interpret the patient's responses to these tests, derive at a definitive diagnosis, and decide on treatment options. When performing a diagnosis in endodontic cases where there is no history of previous endodontic therapy, both a pulpal and periradicular diagnoses are necessary. In cases of persistent disease, the diagnosis may not be as straightforward as the clinician may be dealing with partially treated pulp canals, missed canals, and many other types of problems associated with the previous treatment. These must be included in the diagnostic description for each case.

Endodontic diagnosis was thoroughly discussed in Chapter 1, and the reader is referred there for further details on these procedures. The diagnostic method requires collecting subjective information, developing objective findings, and using these to arrive at a diagnosis and plan of treatment.

The subjective information is collected by questioning the patient and then actively listening to the responses. Of particular interest in cases of suspected posttreatment disease is whether the patient recalls the use of aseptic techniques during the previous endodontic therapy. If a rubber dam was not used, for example, and this can be confirmed with a call to the previous clinician, nonsurgical retreatment will almost certainly be necessary because the canals can be assumed to be contaminated regardless of how aesthetically pleasing the previously filled case may appear on the radiograph. The diagnostician should be careful to avoid or to minimize communicating to the patient any negative feelings he or she has toward the

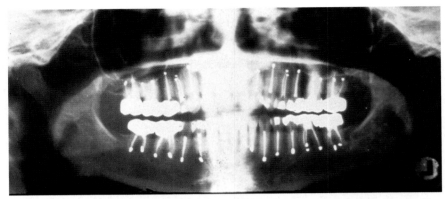

FIG. 8-5 This patient was misdiagnosed for years and underwent unnecessary endodontic therapy. The actual cause of the patient's complaint was nondental pain. (Courtesy Dr. Ramesh Kuba.)

previous treatment, however bad it may seem. This approach allows the patient to become more comfortable with the current clinician and the proposed corrective treatment. An irate patient is an irate patient, and negativity will color the patient's emotional state, level of trust, and ability to accept current or future treatment plans. If the patient asks a direct question about the previous treatment, an honest answer is necessary, but avoid the temptation to imply superiority by disparaging the former clinician. To state the situation honestly and correctly without being inflammatory, use a sentence such as "Well, it may be that your previous dentist (endodontist) had some difficulty with that tooth. Let's see if we can figure out what could have been the problem."

Following a thorough review of the patient's health history, the next step is to gather all of the objective information needed to obtain an accurate diagnosis. This information will include the clinical and radiographic examination. The clinical examination should include a visual extraoral and intraoral examination, and a thorough periodontal evaluation. Visual examination is greatly aided by magnification and illumination, which can allow the clinician to identify significant conditions invisible to the naked eye, such as fine fractures on root surfaces (Fig. 8-6). Exposed dentin from recession and narrow based probing defects may be the result of an endodontic infection draining through the sulcus; however, they sometimes indicate vertical root fracture.[40] The presence of occlusal wear facets indicates the presence of occlusal trauma that may complicate diagnosis and treatment outcome by predisposing the tooth to fracture,[90] and it has been associated with posttreatment disease.[113] Further information on diagnosis and management of cracks and fractures is provided in Chapter 21.

Radiographic assessment is obligatory. Even though radiographs may be a critical aid to the clinician, they should never be the sole support for a conclusive diagnosis. They are only one piece of the puzzle in determining endodontic etiology.[58] In cases with previous endodontic therapy, radiographs are useful in evaluation of caries, defective restorations, periodontal health, the quality of the obturation, existence of missed canals, impediments to instrumentation, periradicular pathosis, perforations, fractures,[238] resorption, and canal anatomy. Radiographs should be properly exposed and have a sharp, clear image. They should include the tooth and surrounding tissues, and multiple angulated films should be used to determine endodontic etiologies using the buccal object moves most

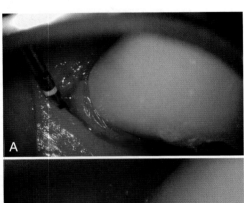

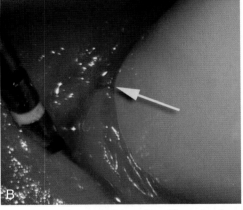

FIG. 8-6 A, Buccal aspect of a premolar with posttreatment disease. **B,** Higher magnification reveals a vertical fracture.

rule (Fig. 8-7).[80] Bitewing radiographs are useful for determining periodontal bone height and looking for caries or fractures. All sinus tracts should be traced with a cone of gutta-percha followed by a radiograph to localize their origin.[111]

Cone beam computed tomography (CBCT) has been introduced into endodontics, and its usefulness in the management of endodontic retreatment is unquestioned. It has provided a quantum leap in our ability to determine the causes of posttreatment apical periodontitis by giving the clinician, for the first time, the ability to easily, safely, and inexpensively visualize the tooth and surrounding structures in three dimensions (3D). CBCT use in endodontics is discussed in detail in Chapter 2, but when faced with a tooth needing retreatment, it is especially helpful. The CBCT allows the clinician to determine the true size, extent, and position of periapical and resorptive lesions

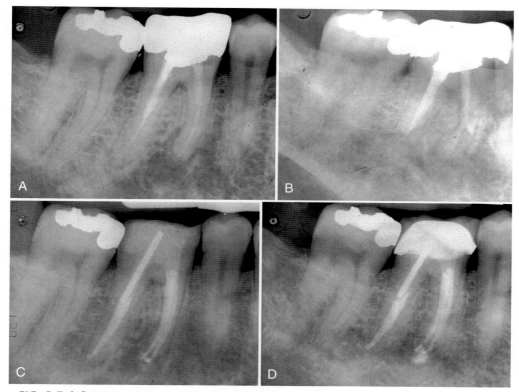

FIG. 8-7 **A,** Posttreatment disease. Previous endodontic therapy performed 3 years previously. **B,** Distal angle radiograph reveals asymmetry indicating the presence of an untreated mesiobuccal canal. **C,** Immediate postobturation film showing treated MB canal. **D,** A 14-month postoperative view. The patient was asymptomatic.

and gives added information about tooth fractures, missed canals, root canal anatomy, and the nature of the alveolar bone topography around teeth.[42] CBCT technology has greatly enhanced presurgical diagnosis and treatment planning, because the relationship of adjacent anatomic structures such as the maxillary sinus and inferior alveolar nerve to the root apices can be clearly visualized. This helps the clinician to decide on when to perform endodontic retreatment surgically or nonsurgically. CBCT is more accurate than periapical radiography in the diagnosis of apical periodontitis, and it can reveal the details of the lesions and adjacent structures, thus providing enhanced clinical diagnosis and treatment planning.[42,175,176]

There are many manufacturers and brands of CBCT machines on the market today, but the most useful ones for endodontic retreatment are those that produce the clearest image with the highest resolution.[155] These would be the small field of view (FOV) machines that image a small volume and use the smallest picture element (voxel) dimensions available. Radiation exposure to the patient with these machines is in the range of 23 to 488 µSv,[142] which is very small, but the "as low as reasonably achievable" (ALARA) principle applies, so its use in every diagnostic case cannot be encouraged. In a joint position statement in 2010, the American Association of Endodontists and the American Association of Oral and Maxillofacial Radiologists stated that "CBCT should only be used when the question for which imaging is required cannot be answered adequately by lower dose conventional dental radiography or alternate imaging modalities."[1] When managing posttreatment disease, however, almost every case will benefit from the use of three-dimensional imaging.

One major cause of posttreatment apical periodontitis is untreated canals, and the CBCT gives an unprecedented ability to discover those (Fig. 8-8). In one study, endodontist evaluators failed to identify at least 1 root canal system in approximately 4 of 10 teeth when using images obtained by conventional digital radiography compared with images from cone-beam computed tomography.[152]

Avoiding treatment, which will lead to a predictable failure, is beneficial for both the clinician and the patient. The ability to obtain 3D images of teeth will help the clinician to avoid these mishaps. The diagnosis of root fractures frequently frustrates the clinician, as a definitive diagnosis is often difficult and treating these teeth has a high likelihood of a poor outcome. Although visualizing root fractures in teeth with root fillings is still not predictable using CBCT,[45,50,96,122] the patterns of bone loss indicative of root fracture can sometimes be seen,[275] and this helps the clinician to infer their presence. The prognosis for the treatment of root resorption is directly related to the extent of the resorption, and this usually cannot be determined accurately using conventional radiography. Using small FOV CBCT, however, the extent of the lesions and the prognosis can be determined,[54] usually saving the patient from an exploratory procedure that may be doomed to fail (Fig. 8-9).

Though most clinicians believe that CBCT is not necessary for every patient treated, there are many retreatment situations where the additional information gained (relative to conventional radiography) is extremely valuable. In the future, specific protocols for use will be developed; but for now, the authors recommend that clinicians use their best judgment on when to use this new technology.

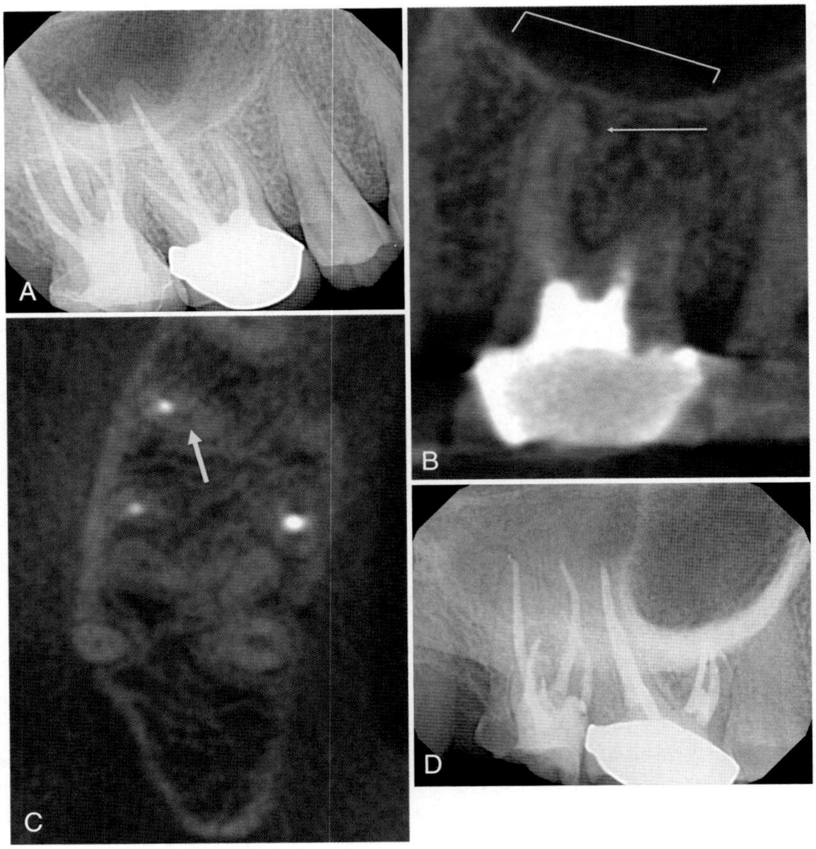

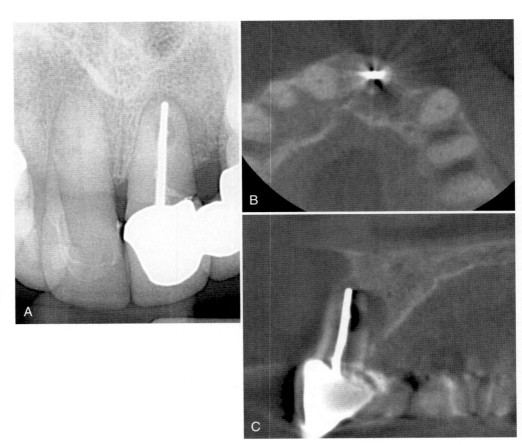

FIG. 8-8 **A,** Preoperative radiograph of symptomatic tooth #3. **B,** Sagittal slice of tooth #3 showing periodontal ligament thickening and associated sinus mucosal thickening. **C,** Axial slice showing untreated MB2 canal *(arrow).* **D,** Treated case.

FIG. 8-9 **A,** Preoperative radiograph showing suspected small area of resorption associated with an endodontically treated tooth filled with a silver cone. **B,** Axial slice showing how beam hardening artifact from the metallic root filling obscures the image. **C,** Sagittal view showing very large palatally oriented external root resorption. The prognosis for retention of this tooth was poor, and the patient elected to extract it.

Comparative testing is the next procedure performed to collect objective information about the pulpal and periradicular status. Most useful are the periradicular tests that include percussion, bite, and palpation.[256] These allow the diagnostician to begin developing a sense of the status of the periradicular tissues. These tests are of great importance anytime an endodontic diagnosis is needed. However, they are of even greater importance when evaluating teeth that have been previously treated with endodontic therapy due to the lack of significant and consistent evidence that can be gained from pulp vitality tests in these cases. If a tooth exhibits percussion tenderness, it may be due to persistent endodontic disease, but recent trauma or occlusal trauma may also cause this finding,[90] as can periodontal disease.[256]

Pulp vitality tests are often of little value when examining teeth with previous endodontic therapy. However, if the patient's chief complaint reveals the need for these tests, they must be performed because it is possible that the pain may be referred from a nearby vital tooth and not from the root canal–treated tooth. When there is vital tissue remaining in the canals of a previously root-filled tooth, either by way of a completely missed canal or from an improperly cleaned canal, patients may complain of sensitivity to heat or cold.[90] Pulp vitality tests should then be performed to assess the situation. They are also useful in testing adjacent and opposing nonendodontically treated teeth to rule out those as etiologies for poorly localized pain. Once the tissue is removed from the pulp chamber after root canal therapy, the results of these tests should almost always be negative, even with radicular pulp remaining. Thus, a negative response with previously treated teeth is not necessarily conclusive; whereas a positive response usually means there is responsive pulp tissue remaining in the tooth.[90] Care is always warranted in interpreting pulp test results, however, as false positive and negative results may occur.[204] As with cold tests, the same limits apply to heat tests as far as the reasons for false results and accuracy relative to retreatment cases.

The remaining pulp vitality tests—electric pulp test, test cavity, and direct mechanical dentin stimulation—are of even lesser value than thermal testing when evaluating teeth that have already received endodontic therapy. These are usually precluded by the existing restoration or endodontic therapy.

When all diagnostic information is collected, a diagnosis must be developed. It is important to record the diagnosis in the patient's record so that anyone reading the record can discern the clinician's rationale for treatment. The pulpal diagnosis will usually be recorded as previous endodontic treatment, but the periradicular diagnosis will vary depending on the clinical picture presented. In the case of previous endodontic treatment, however, a brief note about the suspected etiology of the persistent disease is warranted.

TREATMENT PLANNING

Once the diagnosis is complete, the cause of the persistent disease will usually become apparent. At this point in the clinical process, information must be given to the patient by the clinician as to what treatment options are available and the likely outcomes of each choice. The patient is then allowed to make a decision based on his or her own perceptions of the options, not by the clinician's opinion as to what is "best" for the patient. The reader is reminded, however, that if the cause of the posttreatment condition remains unknown despite thorough diagnostic workup, then any decision results in an empirical "trial and error" type of treatment. This approach should be avoided if possible, and prior to definitive treatment, consultation with an endodontist or other colleague is in order. This consultation may be as simple as a brief conversation or even referral of the patient, but a second opinion is extremely useful in these situations. In most instances due to the interdisciplinary nature of modern dentistry, consultation with other clinicians who are treating the patient becomes a necessity to enhance the potential for successful treatment outcomes.

Occasionally, a patient will have persistent symptoms that mimic posttreatment disease, but these symptoms are actually the result of nonendodontic conditions such as occlusal trauma, concurrent periodontal disease, or nondental pain conditions. Appropriate diagnostic procedures should allow the clinician to sift through these options and treat accordingly.

The patient harboring true endodontic posttreatment disease has four basic options for treatment, which are as follows:

1. Do nothing
2. Extract the tooth
3. Nonsurgical retreatment
4. Surgical retreatment

The first option is to do nothing with the condition and allow it to take its course (Fig. 8-10). This approach is sometimes a useful, short-term option if the etiology of the

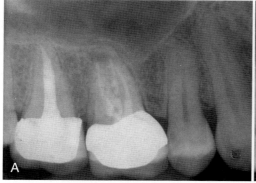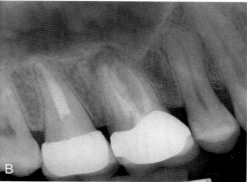

FIG. 8-10 A, Radiograph indicating presence of asymptomatic persistent apical periodontitis 7 years after initial treatment. The patient elected no treatment at that time. **B,** The 6-year follow-up. Lesion has enlarged, and the tooth has become symptomatic.

condition remains unknown and the clinician feels that another diagnostic sampling would help with diagnosis. Even though most clinicians would find this approach to be a less than desirable long-term course of action, the decision belongs to the patient. The clinician is bound, however, to ensure that the patient has complete information about what will happen if nothing is done. The events in the progression of the disease and a reasonable timeline are necessary, and the conversation needs to be thoroughly documented in the patient record to avoid possible subsequent accusations of abandonment. The question of whether the clinician is required to follow up with the patient or dismiss the patient from the practice is one that each clinician must make based on the clinician's experience, judgment, and knowledge of the patient.

Extraction of the tooth is usually considered a viable option. Advances in both prosthetic reconstruction techniques and dental implantology have made extraction and replacement a more desirable option in certain cases where previously "heroic" (read "expensive with an unknown prognosis") methods were needed to "save" the tooth. This alternative, however, provides results that are inferior, more expensive, and much more time consuming than preserving the natural tooth. The average titanium root-form implant restoration can take up to 6 months to finish, not counting preimplant site preparation, which can add months more. Despite published long-term success rates for dental implants,[4] postimplant disease does occur[4,85,86] (Fig. 8-11) and can leave the patient with few

options. The cost of implant treatment is high and usually not covered under dental benefit plans, so the net financial impact on the patient is large. Implant aesthetics can be inferior to that of natural teeth in the aesthetic zone of the mouth, and some patients are just not candidates for implant procedures.[4] Fixed partial dentures are another replacement alternative with a long history of successful use, but negative outcomes are also possible. Most concerning to the endodontist is the likelihood that retainer fabrication procedures will result in endodontic disease of the abutment teeth,[154] which may potentially occur at a rate of up to 10%[150,253] (Fig. 8-12). Removable partial dentures are a less desirable option to the patient because they are generally less comfortable, usually require a long period of patient adaptation, and frequently result in damage to adjacent oral tissues (tooth, gingiva, and mucosa) if not meticulously cleaned. Due to these factors, patient compliance with removable dentures is relatively low, and their use is declining. Occasionally, a patient will choose to have a tooth extracted and not pursue replacement. This decision is usually disastrous for the patient, but there are a few situations where this choice is a reasonable alternative. Diseased maxillary second molars with no opposing tooth, or with an opposing tooth in class I or class III occlusion that articulates with another tooth, may be extracted without concern for future inappropriate movement of the remaining teeth, which can be so occlusally and periodontally damaging. In most instances, however, removal of a tooth will result in the need for replacement, and unless the tooth is hopelessly nonrestorable, retaining the tooth with endodontic procedures is better for the patient.

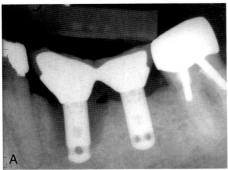

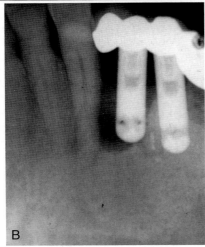

FIG. 8-11 **A,** Classic peri-implantitis. The implant needed removal. **B,** Another peri-implantitis. Note the endodontically treated root tip apical to the implant that may have contributed to the persistent disease. Perhaps apicoectomy should have been performed.

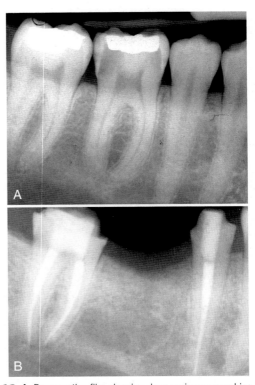

FIG. 8-12 **A,** Preoperative film showing deep caries approaching the pulp. The patient's holistic dentist advised extraction and replacement rather than endodontic therapy to retain the tooth. **B,** Fixed partial denture fabrication procedures resulted in irreversible pulpitis on both abutments requiring endodontic therapy.

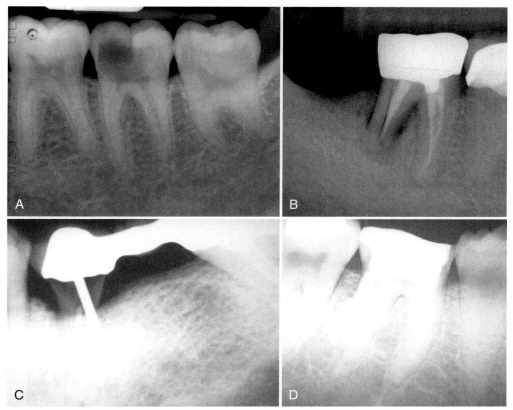

FIG. 8-13 **A,** Deep caries approaching the furcation and the biologic width. Necessary crown-lengthening surgery would open the furcation to bacterial invasion and persistent periodontal disease. **B,** Distal root vertical fracture resulting in a split root. **C,** Severe caries and post perforation. Inadequate root structure remaining to restore. **D,** Multiple distal root perforations so weaken the root as to make it nonrestorable. Note that cases A, B, and D could have resective endodontic surgery such as hemisection, but long-term prognosis is poorer than for extraction and replacement.[31,128]

Various situations may render a tooth nonrestorable (Fig. 8-13); however, the line of demarcation between restorable and nonrestorable is a movable one, depending on who is evaluating the tooth. There are several widely agreed upon situations that render a tooth nonrestorable. These include extensive caries or coronal fracture approaching or entering the furcation or the biologic width. This situation may render preprosthetic periodontal procedures ineffective (leaving a furcation involvement or poor crown-to-root ratio, for example) or, worse, removes bone that would otherwise be useful for implant procedures. Terminal periodontal disease (extensive pocketing or mobility) or root fracture[39] generally result in loss of the tooth despite all efforts at treatment. If the patient has a life-threatening endodontic infection with extensive trismus, most oral surgeons are going to extract the tooth rather than allow less aggressive management. Some previously root-filled teeth may have endured procedural complications, such as a nonretrievable separated instrument or irreparable ledge formation. In combination with the proximity to vital anatomic structures, such as the inferior alveolar canal, endodontic retreatment, either surgical or nonsurgical, may not be feasible and extraction may be the only option. These situations are, fortunately, quite rare, and in most instances, teeth presenting with posttreatment disease can be retained with endodontic procedures.

Once the decision has been made to retain the tooth, there are several choices for treatment. These can be grouped together into either nonsurgical or surgical endodontic treatments. The surgical options can be further broken down into periradicular curettage, apical root resection (with or without root filling), root amputation or hemisection, and intentional replantation (extraction/replantation).[89,170] Occasionally, a situation arises that will require both nonsurgical and surgical types of treatment to effect healing. The American Association of Endodontists has published guidelines that may help the clinician with clinical decision making.[7] However, the choice of which option to undertake will be determined by the clinician's experience, knowledge, patient considerations, and the preoperative diagnosis. If the etiology of the posttreatment disease can be made known, the choices become more obvious. In a previous section, four basic etiologies were presented. If the suspected etiology is in the first group, which is persistent or reintroduced microorganisms, then several choices are available. However, if the cause of the posttreatment disease is persistent extraradicular infection, foreign body reaction, or the presence of a true cyst, then nonsurgical root canal therapy has little likelihood of allowing healing to occur, and surgical methods should be employed.[231] The problem for the clinician is that in most instances, it cannot be determined which of these etiologies exist, so the treatment becomes more empirical.

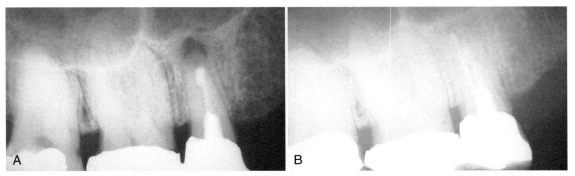

FIG. 8-14 **A,** Posttreatment disease following apical surgery. Off-center positioning of the root filling indicates the presence of a second, untreated canal. **B,** One year following nonsurgical retreatment showing complete healing.

The choice of nonsurgical retreatment versus apical surgery becomes the focus of the decision in most instances. Outcomes assessment studies provide some help in making this decision. The reported healing rates of nonsurgical retreatment range between 74% to 98%,[66,222,136,221,208] but with apical surgery alone, only 59% heal completely.[63] When apical surgery is preceded by orthograde retreatment, however, the incidence of complete healing rises to 80%.[63] In general, nonsurgical retreatment will be the preferred choice, because it seems to provide the most benefit with the lowest risk. It has the greatest likelihood of eliminating the most common cause of posttreatment disease, which is intraradicular infection. Nonsurgical retreatment is usually less invasive than surgery and has a less traumatic postoperative course. There is less likelihood of incurring damage to adjacent vital structures such as nerves, adjacent teeth, and sinus cavities. However, nonsurgical retreatment may be more costly than surgical treatment, especially if large restorations must be sacrificed during disassembly procedures prior to the retreatment. In addition, the amount of time needed for retreatment is usually longer than surgical intervention. There are times when the clinician may not be able to achieve the complete elimination of microorganisms from the canal space, and complete obturation may not be possible. Apical surgery is chosen, therefore, when nonsurgical retreatment is not possible or when the risk-to-benefit ratio of nonsurgical retreatment is outweighed by that of surgery.[64,144]

There are many factors to consider when deciding whether to retreat surgically or nonsurgically (see also Chapter 9). The patient must be fully aware of the proposed treatment and the alternatives, and he or she must be motivated to follow through with all treatment including the final restoration. The patient must have adequate time to undergo the required procedures. If he or she does not, then apical surgery alone may be indicated although the patient must be made aware of the potentially compromised nature of the treatment. Clinicians must be armed with the best equipment and knowledge available, and critical self-evaluation should allow experienced clinicians to know what they can treat and what they cannot. The tooth must be restorable and retreatable. Attempting nonsurgical retreatment on teeth where there is little likelihood of improving the previous treatment provides little benefit to the patient. Thus, in disease situations where there is an apparently adequate root filling and no evidence of coronal leakage, surgery may be indicated. If the previous treatment falls below any acceptable standard and there is no evidence of apical periodontitis, then there is no indication for any treatment unless a new coronal restoration is planned. In that case, conservative retreatment is indicated, and the reported success rates are very high.[63,66] If there has been a previous procedural complication, such as a ledge that cannot be bypassed or a separated instrument that cannot be removed, then surgery may become a better option. Most times, however, it is still prudent to attempt the retreatment because ledges or separated instruments that appear impenetrable on diagnostic films can frequently be bypassed. Even if they cannot, nonsurgical retreatment can enhance the success of subsequent apical surgery as noted previously. The clinician must be careful not to worsen the situation by overly vigorous attempts to treat the previous complication, as root perforation, worsening of a ledge, or another separated instrument may be the result. Previous failed apical surgery should be retreated nonsurgically and then followed up because many surgical failures are due to poorly cleaned and filled canal systems[187] (Fig. 8-14). In many instances, performing the surgery a second time can be avoided altogether. If there is evidence of root fracture (narrow-based probing defect or a "J"-shaped radiolucency encompassing the root apex and progressing in a coronal direction[237] (Fig. 8-15), then nonsurgical retreatment would be unlikely to improve that situation. Apical exploratory surgery may be necessary, which could result in root resection or even extraction of the tooth.

Each case should be approached as a unique set of considerations that need to be reviewed and interpreted prior to selecting a treatment method. Once the selected option is undertaken, however, the prudent clinician is always watchful, as additional pieces of information can be discovered during treatment that may modify previous decisions.

NONSURGICAL ENDODONTIC RETREATMENT

The primary difference between nonsurgical management of primary endodontic disease and that of posttreatment disease is the need to regain access to the apical area of the root canal space in the previously treated tooth. After that, all of the principles of endodontic therapy apply to the completion of the retreatment case. Coronal access needs to be completed, all previous root-filling materials need to be removed, canal obstructions must be managed, and impediments to achieving full working length must be overcome. Only then can cleaning

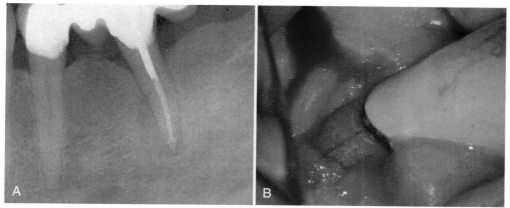

FIG. 8-15 **A,** "J"-shaped radiolucency possibly indicating root fracture. **B,** Exploratory surgery confirms presence of vertical root fracture.

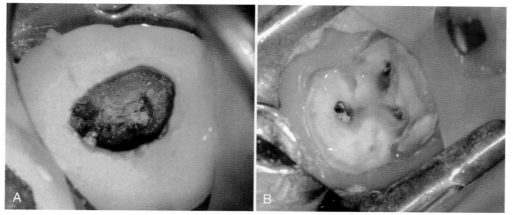

FIG. 8-16 **A,** Limited visibility and access with crown present. **B,** Enhanced visibility and access with crown off. Note that isolation was achieved by using a Silker-Glickman clamp and sealing putty.

and shaping procedures be instituted that will allow for effective obturation and case completion. The remainder of this chapter is devoted to these topics in the order that they generally present themselves to the clinician treating the previously root-filled tooth.

Coronal Access Cavity Preparation

Retreatment access has been called coronal disassembly[187,188] because of the frequent need to take apart or remove the previous coronal and radicular restoration. Following initial endodontic therapy, most teeth require and receive a full coverage restoration, and many times that restoration is supported by a post and core. Coronal-radicular access for retreatment is much more complicated in these cases when compared with endodontically treated teeth that have been minimally restored. The goal of the access preparation is to establish straight-line access to the root canal system while conserving as much tooth structure as possible. The ideal access preparation allows for instruments to enter the canals without being deflected by the access cavity walls. This is reasonably easy to achieve when the tooth is completely intact and a pulp chamber is present, because surface and internal anatomic landmarks can guide the search for the canals. Unfortunately, when endodontic retreatment is necessary, the tooth structure has almost always been

altered and is commonly quite misrepresentative of the original anatomy of the tooth.

When presented with a tooth in need of retreatment that has a full coverage restoration, the decision for the clinician becomes whether to attempt to preserve the restoration or to plan its replacement. This decision is made simpler if there is a defect or caries associated with the restoration or if the treatment plan calls for a new crown. The old one is simply removed and replaced later in the treatment sequence (Fig. 8-16). When the crown is considered to be satisfactory, the decision becomes more complex. If the restoration is maintained, the cost for replacement can be avoided, isolation is easier, the occlusion is preserved, and the aesthetics will be minimally changed. Even if the crown requires replacement, the clinician may elect to retain it during the endodontic retreatment to allow for better isolation with the rubber dam. Unfortunately, retreatment may be more difficult with the crown in place, as this could lead to an increased chance for an iatrogenic mishap due to restricted visibility. In addition, removal of canal obstructions, such as posts, will be more difficult, and there is an increased chance the clinician may miss something important such as hidden recurrent caries, a fracture, or an additional canal. To preserve the restoration, two approaches can be taken: access through the crown or crown removal and replacement when retreatment is completed. The simplest choice is to prepare an access cavity through the existing crown, although there is a significant risk of damaging the restoration resulting in the need to replace it.[160] This risk must be communicated to the patient prior to instituting therapy. If the clinician decides to access through the existing restoration, there are several choices of access burs to use, depending on what material the preparation will be cut through. If the access will be primarily cut through metal (amalgam alloy or cast metal) or composite resin, carbide fissure burs such as the #1556 are usually chosen. With many restorations, it is advisable to consider using a combination of burs to achieve access. For example, when a porcelain fused to metal crown is encountered, a round diamond is used to cut through the porcelain layer. Once the metal substructure is encountered an end-cutting bur, such as the Transmetal bur (Dentsply Maillefer, Ballaigues, Switzerland) or the Great White bur (SS White, Piscataway, NJ) can be used to cut through to and remove the core material efficiently. An important consideration for the clinician is the potential for porcelain fracture, which may occur during the preparation or possibly at a later date after completion of the treatment. This damage is especially common with porcelain jacket crowns. Restorations fabricated completely of porcelain are becoming more and more popular, thus creating added concern due to the increased likelihood of crack formation during access. Porcelain is a glass, and drilling through this material will create many microfractures, which in turn, may weaken the structure of the restoration, making it more prone to future failure.[94] Copious coolant water spray and the use of diamond burs are recommended during access through porcelain to minimize occurrence of this event.[235] In a novel approach, Sabourin and colleagues[189] recently showed that, compared with the use of drills, air abrasion produced almost no defects in the porcelain structure of all ceramic crowns when used for endodontic access. It was, however, significantly more time consuming to access through the crown this way.

If the decision is made to remove the crown for reuse, the visibility is increased, allowing for much easier removal of canal obstructions and a decrease in the potential for operator error; however, rubber dam clamp placement and tooth isolation may become a bigger problem. Also, despite all of the varying techniques and armamentaria available for removal of an existing restoration, the procedure remains unpredictable and many times can also result in damage to the restoration or the inability to remove it at all.

The clinician must decide how to remove the crown. If the crown is of no value, even as a temporary, then the clinician can take the easiest road and simply cut it off. However, if the crown is to be preserved, then a more conservative approach must be used. Two considerations, which may influence the decision about removal of a crown or bridge, are what material the restoration is made of and what is it cemented with. Conservative removal efforts are difficult with traditional, all-metal restorations cemented with nonbonded cements. This situation has been even more of a concern lately due to the increasing popularity of tooth-colored restorations, mainly different types of porcelain or porcelain fused to metal (PFM) restorations, which are being bonded to the tooth. These restorations are less likely to withstand the stresses of removal than those fabricated entirely of metal, and restorations that are bonded are much more difficult to remove due to the adhesive strengths of bonding agents. Each new generation of bonding agent is

stronger than the previous, making removal increasingly more difficult as cosmetic dentistry advances.

Many devices have been developed specifically for the conservative removal of crowns. Some of the more commonly used devices are forceps that have been designed specifically for crown removal such as the K.Y. Pliers (GC America, Alsip, IL) (Fig. 8-17), which use small replaceable rubber tips and emery powder to enable a firm grasp of the crown without damaging it. Other instruments of this type include the Wynman Crown Gripper (Integra Miltex, York, PA), the Trial Crown Remover (Hu-Friedy, Chicago, IL), and the Trident Crown Placer/Remover (CK Dental, Orange, CA). Unfortunately, a crown that has been cemented with long-term cement or has been bonded to the tooth will usually not be removed with one of these instruments. There are also forceps designed specifically to engage the margins of the crown while using an adjacent tooth as a fulcrum. Squeezing the handles together will cause the crown to be elevated off of the tooth. The Roydent Bridge Remover (Roydent, Rochester Hills, MI) works in this fashion and can be effective in crown removal, but care must be taken to avoid damage to fine, fragile margins, especially on porcelain crowns. Another type of instrument can be engaged under the margin, and a subsequent impact delivered at this site will dislodge the restoration. The Easy Pneumatic Crown and Bridge Remover (Dent Corp, White Plains, NY) and the Coronaflex (KaVo, Lake Zurich, IL) create this impact from compressed air, whereas the Morrell Remover (Henry Schein, Melville, NY) applies the force manually using a sliding weighted handle. The ATD Automatic Crown & Bridge Remover (J. Morita, Irvine, CA) uses vibrations to break the crown-to-preparation bond, and the Crown-A-Matic (Peerless International, N. Easton MA) delivers a shock impulse to loosen the crown. As mentioned earlier, crown margin damage may result, as can inadvertent extraction of the tooth if the periodontium is compromised[183] (Fig. 8-17, E). A different approach to conservative crown removal involves drilling a small hole through the crown to allow a device to thread a screw through the hole. This approach creates a lifting force that separates the crown and the tooth. The instruments that work in this manner are the Metalift (Classic Practice Resources, Baton Rouge, LA), the Kline Crown Remover (Brassler, Savannah, GA), and the Higa Bridge Remover (Higa Manufacturing, West Vancouver, BC, Canada). Although very effective on metal crowns, these instruments may cause damage to porcelain occlusal surfaces on PFM restorations, and their use in both anterior teeth and in all porcelain restorations is generally precluded.

Another interesting technique designed to remove a crown without causing damage is performed using the Richwil Crown & Bridge Remover (Almore, Portland OR). This material is a water-soluble resin, which is softened using warm water (Fig. 8-18). The small block of material is placed on the crown to be removed, and the patient bites into this material until the resin cools and hardens at which point the patient opens his or her mouth, generating enough force to pull the crown off. The clinician must be careful to avoid using this technique when the opposing tooth is extensively restored, because the opposing restoration may inadvertently be removed during the procedure. None of these techniques works in every case, and they may produce damage to the restoration being removed or possibly others. These are, however, methods that are available and may work while permitting reuse of the restoration.

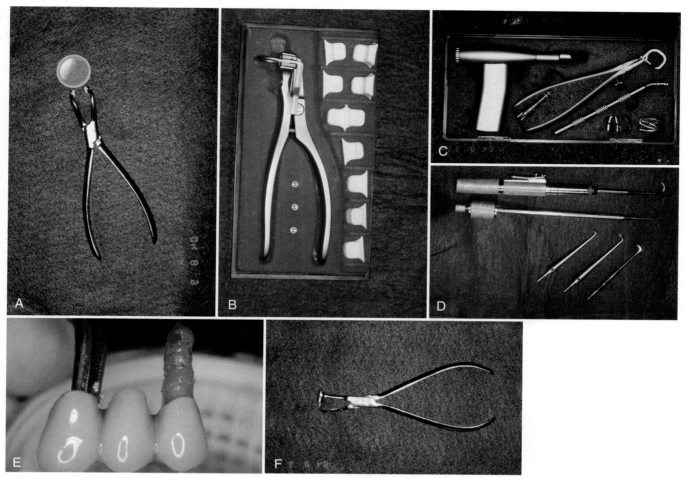

FIG. 8-17 **A,** KY Pliers (GC America) and supplied emery powder. **B,** Roydent Bridge Remover (Roydent). **C,** CoronaFlex Kit (KaVo). **D,** *(top)* Crown-A-Matic (Peerless International); *(bottom)* Morrell Crown Remover (Henry Schein) with interchangeable tips. **E,** Tooth inadvertently extracted using a crown/bridge remover. Endodontic therapy was performed in hand and the tooth was replanted, a procedure known as unintentional replantation. **F,** Kline Crown Remover (Brasseler USA).

Post Removal

Once the access is prepared, it is common to encounter a post, as posts are frequently used in the restoration of endodontically treated teeth. The clinician may encounter many different types of posts during retreatment (Fig. 8-19). They can be classified into two categories: prefabricated posts and custom cast posts. Historically, cast posts were more commonly used than prefabricated posts; however, since the 1990s, cast posts have become much less popular.[201] The main reason for this decrease is the convenience of placing the prefabricated post immediately after post preparation as opposed to waiting for a laboratory to fabricate the casting. There is also less likelihood of the interappointment contamination that frequently occurs with temporary post/core/crowns that are needed for cast/custom post and core fabrication. Prefabricated posts come in a variety of shapes, designs, and materials. The shapes can be subclassified into two groups: parallel sided or tapered. The design of posts also can be subclassified into active (threaded), passive, vented, fluted, and acid-etched groups. There are also many materials that have been used to fabricate posts, such as stainless steel, gold, titanium, ceramic, zirconium, and

fiber-reinforced composite posts. Cast posts, which are fabricated in a laboratory, will always be made up of precious or nonprecious metal alloys. These posts also come in a variety shapes and configurations because they are custom manufactured for each root in which they are placed. Most of these have some degree of taper, and many will be cast in one piece with the core included.

In addition to the shape, design, and material of posts, there are two more very important factors that will have some influence on the clinician's ability to remove them. These factors are the adhesive material used to cement the post and the location in the arch of the tooth that requires post removal.

The same concerns regarding cements that were discussed in the section on crown removal apply to post removal. The main consideration is whether the post was cemented with traditional cement or bonded with a composite resin and dentin-bonding agent. Several post systems on the market today, such as the ProPost (Dentsply, York, PA), use acid-etched metal posts that are bonded into the canal with cements, such as Panavia (Kuraray America, New York, NY) or C&B Metabond (Parkell, Edgewood, NY). Removal of these posts is

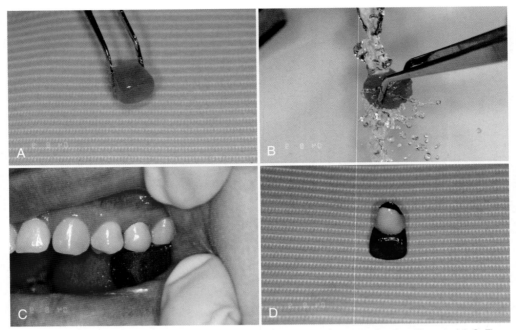

FIG. 8-18 **A,** Richwil Crown and Bridge Remover (Almore). **B,** Using hot water to soften the material. **C,** The remover is placed on the restoration to be removed and the patient bites into the material. **D,** Image showing the removed crown adhering to the material.

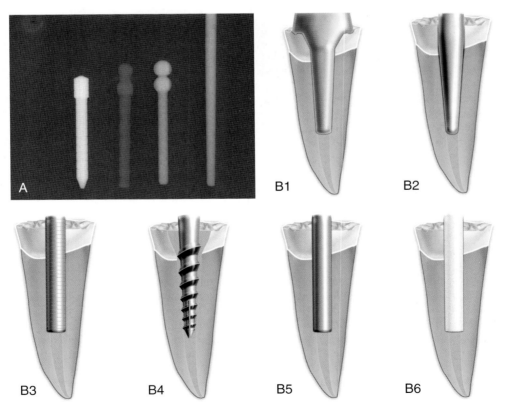

FIG. 8-19 **A,** Relative radiopacities of post materials: *left* to *right*—stainless steel, fiber post, titanium post, gutta-percha. **B,** Diagrammatic representation of post types: *(B1)* custom cast, *(B2)* tapered, *(B3)* parallel, *(B4)* active, *(B5)* passive/metal, and *(B6)* passive/nonmetal. (Diagrams courtesy DENTSPLY Endodontics.)

extremely difficult and occasionally impossible, regardless of which technique is used.[84] One study has shown that heat generation with ultrasonic vibration may help to decrease retention of resin cemented posts,[73] but concern for heat-generated periodontal ligament damage may preclude this technique.[201]

With regard to location, the more posterior in the arch, the more difficult the post is to remove. This predicament is a result of accessibility. The more accessible the tooth is, the easier the post is to remove because the clinician will have more techniques and instruments available to use.[2] Also, the more anterior the tooth is, the less the opposing occlusion will interfere with post removal.

Post Removal Techniques

After initial access and after the post to be removed has been located, the clinician is faced with the decision of how to remove it. Many techniques have been developed for the sole purpose of post removal. Regardless of which technique is chosen, there is one simple yet extremely important rule to follow: it is not only what is removed but what is left behind that is important. This rule applies to the removal of all intra-canal obstructions. The reason for this rule is to make sure that the remaining tooth, after removal of the obstruction, can be restored predictably with a good long-term prognosis. For example, there is little use in successfully removing a post and leaving behind a root that is eggshell thin and prone to fracture (Fig. 8-20).

The first step in post removal is to expose it properly by removing all adjacent restorative materials. With preformed posts, the bulk of the core material around the post and within the chamber can be removed with a high-speed handpiece using cylindrical or tapered carbide or diamond burs. When the majority of the restorative material is removed, a less aggressive instrument, such as a tapered bur in a slow-speed handpiece or a tapered, midsized ultrasonic tip, should be used to remove the last of the embedding core material. This process is greatly facilitated by use of magnification and illumination. Once there is minimal restorative material remaining, a smaller-sized ultrasonic instrument should be used to minimize the risk of removing unnecessary tooth structure or thinning of the post. The more post that is left, the more options for removal, and the more tooth structure that is left, the more options for restoration. At this point, a high-speed bur is too

risky to use. When the core is cast in one piece with the post, a high-speed instrument can perform this process to generate a shape that can facilitate removal.

Once the post is well isolated and freed from all restorative materials, the clinician can begin the retrieval process. There are many instruments and kits on the market that can be used to remove posts; however, prior to using one, the retention of the post should be reduced. The clinician can usually continue to use the same medium-sized ultrasonic tip that was used to get to this point. Using this instrument at the interface between the post and the tooth (the cement line) and constantly moving it around the circumference of the post will disrupt the cement structure along the post/canal wall interface and decrease post retention facilitating removal,[19,32,119] although the effects of ultrasonic vibration may be minimal in reducing retention of well-fitted, long, large-diameter titanium posts.[20] Titanium has a lower modulus of elasticity than stainless steel, so it may dampen the ultrasonic vibrations, which may decrease the effectiveness of the ultrasonic; however, one study failed to duplicate this effect.[98] Nonetheless, care should be taken not to push the ultrasonic tip against the post with too much force, as this will dampen the ultrasonic wave and actually reduce the effectiveness of this technique. Taking away a small amount of the dentin around the coronal aspect of the post is not critical at this time, as this will aid in the reduction of post retention without unduly weakening the root. If the root is thin, however, and the amount of space between the cement line and the root surface is restricted, the size of the tip that can be used may be limited. Unfortunately, the smaller tips are not only less effective for post removal, but they are also more prone to breakage. At this point, the ultrasonic handpiece should be used with copious air-water spray as a coolant. Due to the heat that can be generated from this procedure, the tip should be removed from the access every 10 to 15 seconds to allow the use of an air/water syringe not only to clean the area of debris but also to reduce the temperature produced that could potentially cause damage to the periradicular tissues.[201,274] If a rubber dam is in place, the area around the post may be flooded with a solvent such as chloroform prior to activating the ultrasonic instrument, as this will help dissolve the cement around the post. Using a solvent in conjunction with removal of cemented obstructions may prove beneficial because the ultrasonic energy produced will set up shock waves in the solvent and make it penetrate

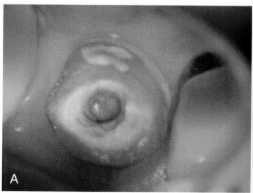
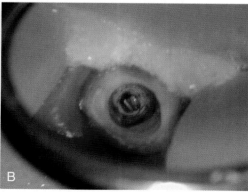

FIG. 8-20 A, Broken post (incisal view before excavation). **B,** Root has been so thinned and weakened by excavation procedures that restorability is questionable.

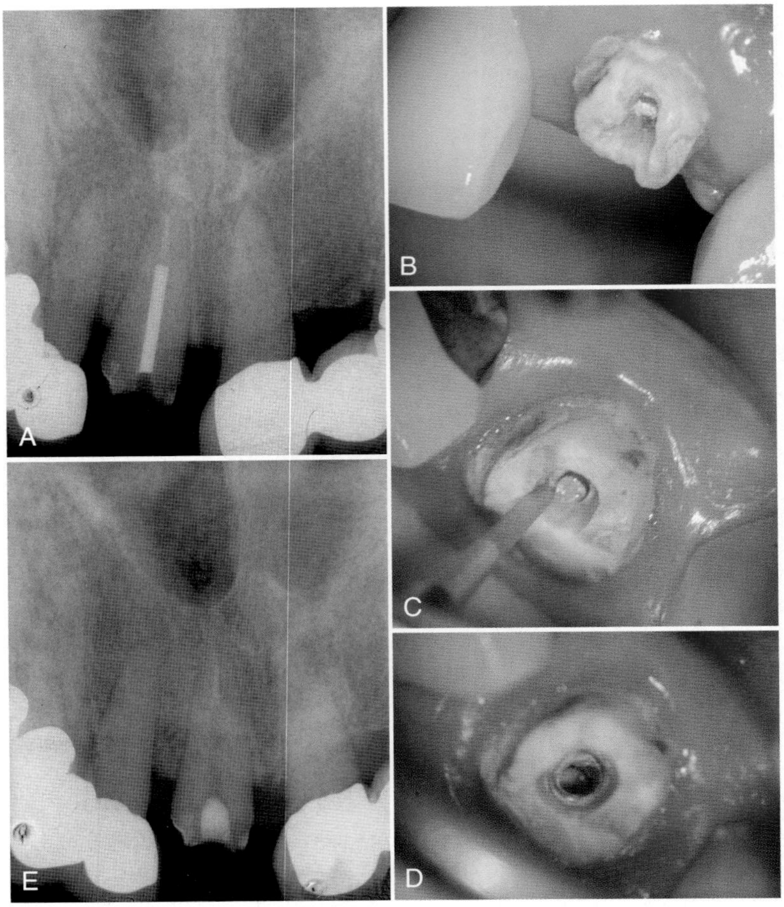

FIG. 8-21 **A,** Radiograph of fractured post. **B,** Fractured post, labial view. **C,** Ultrasonic troughing. **D,** Post removed by ultrasonic alone. **E,** Check film confirming complete post removal.

deeper into the canal space, exerting a faster solvent action on the cement.[78]

Using an ultrasonic instrument in this fashion is not simply helpful in reducing post retention; this may also prove to be all that is needed to remove the post. Many times, after judicious use of the ultrasonic instrument, the post will loosen and actually spin out of the preparation, completing post removal (Fig. 8-21). In addition, if post removal cannot be accomplished in this manner, the resulting post exposure will be very beneficial in contributing to the predictable use of other techniques, as many of the instruments to be discussed involve using a trephine bur to shape the coronal end of the post. Ultrasonic exposure will facilitate this process. Another instrument to consider for exposing and loosening a post is the Roto-Pro bur (Ellman International, Hicksville, NY) (Fig. 8-22). There are three shapes available, all of which are six-sided, noncutting tapered burs that are used in a high-speed handpiece around the circumference of the post. The vibrations created when the noncutting flutes come in contact with the post decrease the retention of the post, facilitating its removal.

If retention reduction does not remove the post, some form of vice is needed to pull the post from its preparation. Many post removal kits are available on the market today with varying degrees of effectiveness. One such device is the Gonon Post Removing System (Thomas Extracteur De Pivots, FFDM-Pneumat, Bourge, France), which is a very effective instrument for removing parallel or tapered, nonactive preformed posts.[145,191] This kit utilizes a hollow trephine bur that is

aligned with the long axis of the post and placed over its newly exposed end. The trephine then cuts in an apical direction, shaving off the post's outer layer not only to remove tooth structure adjacent to the post but also to reduce the circumference of the post to a specific size and shape. This procedure is necessary to allow a specific, matched-size extraction mandrel to create or tap a thread onto the exposed milled portion of the post. Once the extraction mandrel with its associated washer/bumpers (Fig. 8-23) is attached to the post, the extraction forceps or vice is applied to the tooth and post. Turning the screw on the handle of the vice applies a coronal force in a similar fashion as a corkscrew removes a cork from a bottle of wine. This method is effective because all the force is applied to the bond between the tooth and the post, ideally in the long axis of the root. The main problem with this technique is the size of the vice that can make access in the molar region and between crowded lower incisors difficult. Also, if the extraction force applied is not directed in the long axis of the root, root fracture may occur.[35]

The Thomas Screw Post Removal Kit (Thomas Extracteur De Pivots, FFDM-Pneumat) (Fig. 8-24) is an instrument designed specifically for the removal of active or screw posts. The trephine burs are identical to those used with the Gonon Post Removal System, although the extraction mandrels are threaded in the opposite direction. The mandrels are reverse threaded to enable them to tap onto the screw post in a counterclockwise direction so that continued torquing force while creating the thread will unscrew the post.

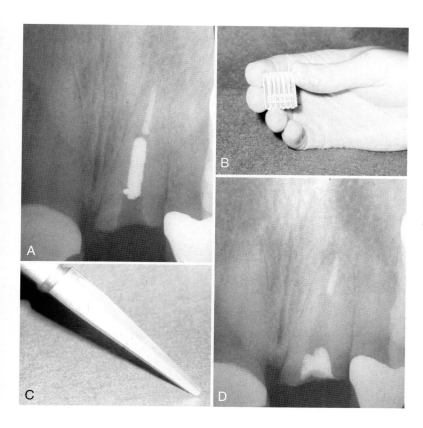

FIG. 8-22 **A,** Radiograph of fractured post. **B,** Roto-Pro Kit. **C,** Roto-Pro Bur. **D,** Post removed by vibration of the instrument alone.

The Ruddle Post Removal System (Sybron Dental Specialties)[187] (Fig. 8-25) and the Universal Post Remover (Thomas Extracteur De Pivots, FFDM-Pneumat) were designed to combine the properties of both the Gonon and Thomas kits. Both of these very similar kits are useful not only for removing parallel or tapered passive types of posts but also for removing screw posts. They can even be adapted to remove large separated instruments in the coronal straight portion of a large canal. These kits also use a trephine bur to machine the post to a specific size that will dictate which mandrel to use. These mandrels tap in the counterclockwise direction so that the same taps can be used for both passive and active posts. Once the mandrel is tapped onto the post, the extraction jaws, or vice, can be applied and activated, enabling removal of passive posts, or the tap is continuously rotated counterclockwise to unthread screw-type posts.

Another device that works in a similar fashion as the Gonon and the Ruddle Post Removal System is the JS Post Extractor (Roydent Dental Products). The biggest advantage of this kit is the size, as this is the smallest of the kits that work using a pulling action, which may help in cases where access is difficult. However, this kit does have one disadvantage: it does not have as large of a variety of trephine burs and extraction mandrels as some of the others. Therefore, the size of the post may be a limiting factor.

Another post removal device is the Post Puller, also known as the Eggler Post Remover (Automaton-Vertriebs-Gesellschaft, Germany)[228] (Fig. 8-26). This device works in a similar manner as some of the others; however, there are no trephine burs or extraction mandrels. The design of this instrument enables it to be used more efficiently with the crown removed. In addition, the design also allows this instrument to be used for cases in which the post and core are cast as one unit. This device consists of two sets of jaws that work independently of one another. With this device, both the post and the tooth are reduced to allow attachment of the post puller. Because there are no trephine burs, this reduction is done with a high-speed handpiece and bur. Next, the first set of jaws are attached to the post while the second set of jaws push away from the tooth in line with the long axis of the tooth removing the post from the canal.[228] Care must be taken to align the pulling forces of this instrument with the long axis of the root to prevent fracture,[35] and also, this technique is not recommended for the removal of screw posts. In a survey of the Australian and New Zealand Academy of Endodontists, this was the most commonly used technique for post removal.[34] However, in a survey of the American Association of Endodontists, this was one of the least used techniques.[229] Clearly, techniques that are common in one country are not always that common in another.

The increased popularity of cosmetic dentistry has created an impetus toward the use of tooth-colored posts that are fabricated from ceramic, zirconium, or various types of fiber-reinforced composite. Unfortunately, as with all posts, cosmetic posts also will need to be removed periodically. Neither the use of the Gonon Kit nor ultrasonic instruments allows for removal of fiber posts, whereas the use of a high-speed bur to channel down through the post may result in a high rate of root perforation.[178,201] The use of the Largo Bur (Dentsply)[75] and the Peeso drill[178] to remove these posts has been advocated, and most of the post manufacturers have removal burs in the kit.[47] These manufacturers' removal kits have been shown to be more efficient at removing their own fiber posts than the use of diamond burs and ultrasonics.[138] In addition, a new bur, the

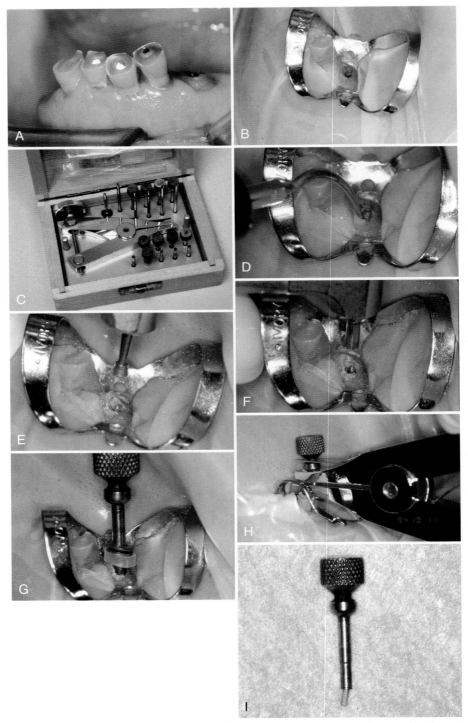

FIG. 8-23 Gonon post removal technique. **A,** Fractured post in a lower incisor. **B,** Tooth isolated with a rubber dam. **C,** Gonon Kit. **D,** Ultrasonic exposure of the post. **E,** Domer bur creating a shape that the trephine bur can engage. **F,** Trephine bur milling the post. **G,** Extraction device tapping a thread onto the post. Note the three bumpers needed to protect the tooth from the vice. **H,** Vice applied. Turning the screw on the vice opens the jaws, creating the extraction force. **I,** Post removed.

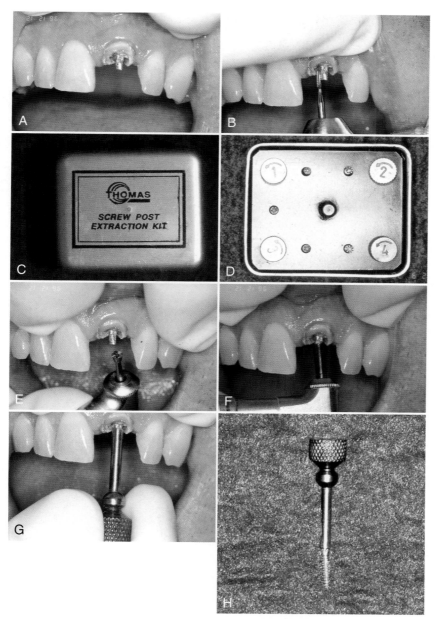

FIG. 8-24 Thomas screw post removal technique. **A,** Broken screw post. **B,** Head of post being contoured to a roughly cylindrical shape. **C** and **D,** Thomas Post Removal Kit. **E,** Domer bur creating a shape that the trephine bur can engage. **F,** Trephine bur milling the post. **G,** Application of counterclockwise rotational force using the wrench. **H,** Post removed.

GyroTip (MTI Precision Products, Lakewood, NJ), has been designed for the specific purpose of removing fiber-reinforced composite posts (Fig. 8-27). These drills consist of a heat-generating tip designed to soften the matrix that binds the fibers within the fiber-reinforced post. The fibers within the post are parallel, which assists the axial travel of the drill through the center of the post. The fluted zone of the drill allows the fibers to be safely removed, creating access to the root canal filling. Above the fluted zone, a layer of plasma-bonded silica carbide reduces the heat generation that would otherwise occur if a smooth carbide surface were rotating in contact with enamel or dentin. This abrasive zone also provides for a straight-line access preparation and facilitates the placement of a new post. Ceramic and zirconium posts are usually impossible to retrieve. They are more fragile than metal posts, and though ceramic posts may be removed by grinding them away with a bur (a procedure with a high risk of root perforation), zirconium has a hardness approaching that of diamond and cannot be removed by this method.[201]

Regardless of the post type or retrieval method used, once the post has been removed, the final step in exposing the underlying root filling material is to ensure that none of the post cement remains in the apical extent of the post space. This step can be easily accomplished by visualizing the cement using magnification and illumination and then using a straight ultrasonic tip to expose the underlying canal filling.

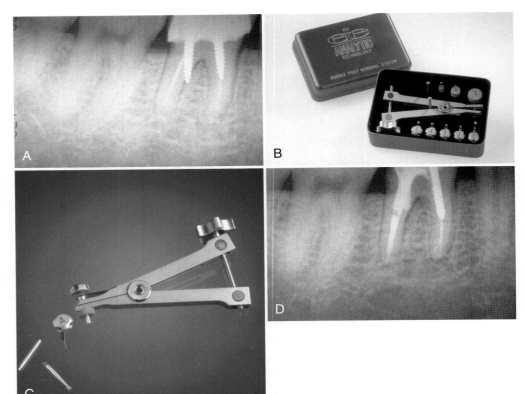

FIG. 8-25 **A,** Perforated post requiring removal. **B** and **C,** Ruddle postremoval kit. **D,** Post removed and perforation repaired. (B and C, Courtesy Kerr, Orange, CA.)

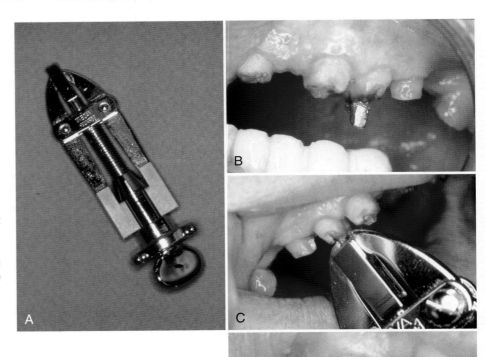

FIG. 8-26 **A,** Eggler Post Remover. **B,** Post has been contoured with a high-speed bur. **C,** Eggler Post Remover grasping the post. **D,** Elevating the post. (Reprinted with permission form Stamos DE, Gutmann JL: Revisiting the post puller, *J Endod* 17:467, 1991.)

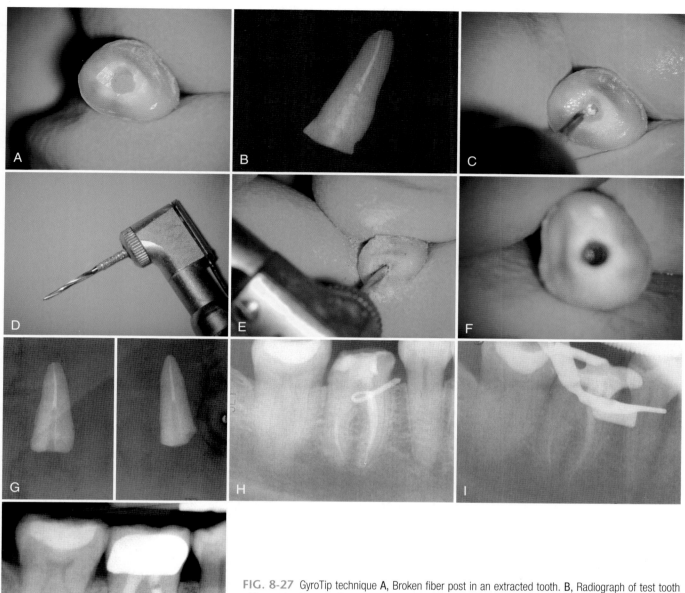

FIG. 8-27 GyroTip technique **A,** Broken fiber post in an extracted tooth. **B,** Radiograph of test tooth with post in place. **C,** Creating a pilot hole. **D,** GyroTip instrument. **E,** GyroTip cutting through the fiber post. Note alignment with long axis of post. **F** and **G,** Post removed. **H,** Clinical case showing fiber post perforation into furcation area. **I,** Post removed with the GyroTip. **J,** The 1-year follow-up of MTA repair.

Potential Complications of Post Removal

As with many dental procedures, post removal has risks. These risks include fracture of the tooth, leaving the tooth nonrestorable, root perforation, post breakage, and inability to remove the post.[229] An additional concern is ultrasonically generated heat damage to the periodontium.[201]

Even though there may still be some who feel posts strengthen teeth, it is widely accepted that they do not.[201] Actually, it has been shown that post preparation alone weakens teeth.[250] Therefore, it seems obvious that any additional work, which may require removal of further tooth structure, will further weaken the tooth, increasing the likelihood of fracture. An in vitro study showed that cracks can form in radicular dentin during post removal using both the Gonon Kit and ultrasonics, but there was no significant difference between these two groups, and teeth with posts that were not removed.[6] The authors speculated that the potential for vertical root fracture might increase; however, the clinical significance of this

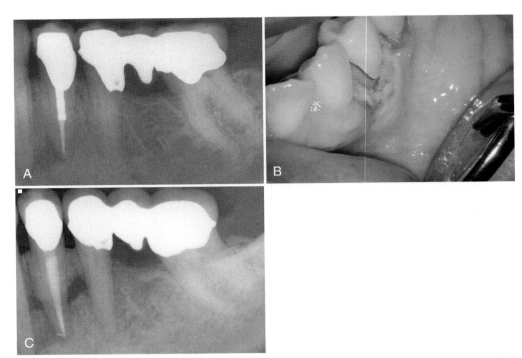

FIG. 8-28 Tissue damage from heat generated by ultrasonic application to a post during removal. The ultrasonic tip was applied to the post for no more than 5 minutes at high power with the assistant applying a constant water spray. **A,** Preoperative radiograph. **B,** and **C,** These images were taken 1 month after the retreatment. Note sloughing bone visible on Fig. 8-28, *C,* The tooth was lost 1 month later. (Reprinted with permission form Schwartz RS, Robbins JW: Post placement and restoration of endodontically treated teeth: a literature review, *J Endod* 30:289, 2004.)

remains unknown. A more recent study, however, concluded that the incidence of root fracture during post removal was extremely low and that with good case selection, post removal is, in fact, a predictable procedure.[2] If, however, post removal would also leave the remaining tooth structure in a state that may not be predictably restored with a good prognosis and if this situation can be predicted ahead of time, surgery may be the preferred treatment option.

Perforation is an additional possible complication that can happen during post removal, especially if the post is removed by simply attempting to drill it out with high-speed burs.[178] If perforation occurs, the clinician should repair it immediately, as the prognosis will worsen as the time between perforation and repair lengthens.[24,206] Once a perforation occurs, the clinician must reconsider the prognosis and determine whether the tooth should be salvaged. Terminating the procedure and pursuing a different treatment option could be considered at this point. Extraction and replacement with an implant or a fixed prosthesis was a treatment option prior to initiating the retreatment, and some may consider this treatment the best option once a perforation has occurred. However, with the development of mineral trioxide aggregate (Pro-Root MTA, Dentsply, York, PA), perforations can be repaired with a favorable prognosis.[184] The techniques and materials for perforation repair will be discussed in detail in a later section of this chapter.

Another complication is separation of the post, causing removal of the coronal segment leaving a small portion of the post with even less accessibility. This separation will decrease the likelihood of removal and occurs more frequently when attempting to retrieve titanium posts.[201]

The use of ultrasonic energy for prolonged periods of time can generate excessive amounts of heat. The heat generated can cause damage to the surrounding periodontium.[78,201] This damage may be as serious as both tooth and permanent bone loss (Fig. 8-28). For this reason, stopping periodically to cool off the area with a water spray is necessary. This will be discussed in detail in a later section.

If the clinician is unable to remove the post, he or she will be faced with a decision of what to do. This decision is based on whether the post is being removed for restorative purposes or due to the persistence of disease. If the reason is for restorative purposes and the clinician can adequately restore the tooth with the existing post or post segment, then he or she should do so. If the tooth cannot be properly restored without removal of the post and placement of a new post, then extraction and replacement with an implant or fixed prosthesis will be needed. If the reason for post removal is the persistence of disease, the tooth should be treated surgically and restored as well as possible.

Regaining Access to the Apical Area

Once the coronal-radicular access is made and all posts and obstructing restorations have been removed, then the clinician must regain access to the apical area by removing the previous root-filling materials (Fig. 8-29). This part of nonsurgical retreatment is complicated by the large variety of types of root fillings used. Today, the majority of root fillings are performed using gutta-percha in various forms; however, many other materials have been and are still being used. Silver points were popular until the 1970s and various types of pastes are, unfortunately, still in use. The authors have seen cases of definitive root filling with phenol-soaked paper points and sometimes no root filling at all. New materials, such as Resilon (Resilon Research LLC), a soft polyester material that is bonded into the canal space, are coming on the market all the time. Though all root-filling materials have their advocates and their critics, the only certainty is that all will have some incidence of persistent disease and will need retreatment.

During the diagnostic phase, it is important to ascertain the nature of the root filling to minimize surprises when attempting retreatment. Sometimes this is readily apparent, but, in other instances, this determination may require contacting the previous clinician to discover what type of root filling was used. Occasionally, this information cannot be determined until canal entry, so extreme caution should be used when performing access so as not to possibly remove parts of the root filling that may be useful in its removal, such as the core material in solid core obturators.

Gutta-Percha Removal

One of the great advantages of using gutta-percha for root filling is its relative ease of removal. When the canal contains gutta-percha and sealer or a chloropercha filling, it is relatively

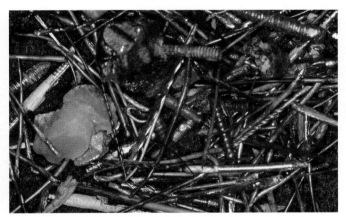

FIG. 8-29 Accumulation of materials removed from retreated teeth in a 3-month period.

easy to remove this material using a combination of heat, solvents, and mechanical instrumentation.[69,187] Upon access, it is usually relatively easy to find the treated canal orifices with the visible pink gutta-percha material inside. Initial probing with an endodontic explorer into the material can help rule out the possibility that there is a solid core carrier. If there is a plastic carrier, then heat should not be used to remove the coronal gutta-percha (more on this later). If there is no carrier, heat is applied using an endodontic heat carrier that has been heated to a cherry red glow in a torch. Unfortunately, the carrier begins to cool upon removal from the flame, so many endodontists are now using a heat source, such as the Touch 'n Heat (SybronEndo, Orange, CA) (Fig. 8-30, A), to provide constant, consistent heat application to soften the gutta-percha in the coronal portion of the canal.[141] Care must be exercised, however, not to overheat the root, which can cause damage to the periodontal ligament.[132,193,194] Thus, the heat should be applied in a short burst to allow the instrument to penetrate the gutta-percha mass, followed by cooling, which will cause the material to adhere to the heat carrier facilitating its removal (Fig. 8-30, B). After removing as much gutta-percha as possible with the heated instrument, then remove any remaining coronal material with small Gates-Glidden drills, taking care not to over enlarge the cervical portion of the canal. However, because the previously treated tooth may have had an underprepared cervical third of the canals, these drills can also be used to flare the coronal aspect in an anticurvature direction to facilitate enhanced straight line access to the apical one third of the canal and to create a reservoir for potential solvent use.[149] Again, probe the canal, this time using a #10 or #15 K-file. It is sometimes possible to remove or bypass the existing cones of gutta-percha if the canal has been poorly obturated, thus eliminating the need for solvents.[223] If that is not possible, then a gutta-percha solvent must be used to remove the remaining material in the apical portion of the canal.

Several solvents have been recommended to dissolve and remove gutta-percha for retreatment (Fig. 8-31) including chloroform,[153] methylchloroform,[259] eucalyptol,[273] halothane,[105,127] rectified turpentine,[120] and xylene.[93] All of the solvents have some level of toxicity,[14,38] so their use should be avoided if possible; however, a solvent is usually needed to

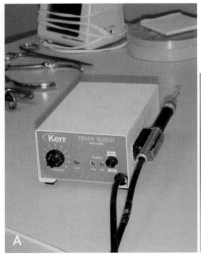
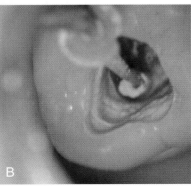

FIG. 8-30 A, Touch 'n Heat instrument. B, Gutta-percha adhering to the Touch 'n Heat tip as it cools.

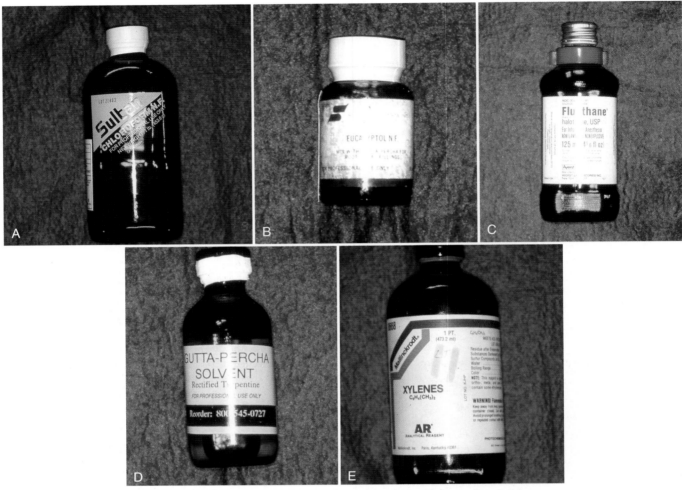

FIG. 8-31 **A,** Chloroform. **B,** Eucalyptol. **C,** Halothane. **D,** Rectified turpentine. **E,** Xylenes.

remove well-condensed gutta-percha. The most popular solvent is chloroform because it dissolves the gutta-percha rapidly and has a long history of clinical use. In 1976, the U.S. Food and Drug Administration (FDA) banned the use of chloroform in drugs and cosmetics due to a report of suspected carcinogenicity.[251] There was no associated ban on its use in dentistry[153]; however, the report did result in the search for alternatives, some of which are listed earlier. When used carefully, chloroform is regarded as a safe and effective endodontic solvent.[38,153] All of the others generally have been reported to be less effective or have some other drawback that limits their use. Xylene and eucalyptol dissolve gutta-percha slowly and only approach the effectiveness of chloroform when heated.[269] Rectified turpentine has a higher level of toxicity than chloroform,[14] and it produces a very pungent odor in the operatory. Halothane has been shown to be as effective a solvent as chloroform in several studies,[105,127] but a more recent study indicated that the time for removal of the root filling was longer than when using chloroform.[263] The increased cost and volatility of halothane and the potential for idiosyncratic hepatic necrosis make it less desirable to use as a gutta-percha solvent.[38] Although methylchloroform is less toxic than chloroform, it is also less effective as a solvent for gutta-percha.[259] Both halothane and chloroform have been shown to affect the chemical composition of dentin[51,121] and may affect bonding strengths of

adhesive cements to the altered dentin.[52] The clinical significance of these effects remains unknown, however. The evidence for the carcinogenicity of chloroform in humans is suspect,[153] but with careful use, its toxicity may be eliminated as a risk factor to both the patient[38] and the personnel in the operatory.[5] As such, its continued use as a gutta-percha solvent is recommended.

Using an irrigating syringe, the selected solvent is introduced into the coronal portions of the canals, which will then act as a reservoir for the solvent. Then, small hand files (sizes #15 and 20) are used to penetrate the remaining root filling and increase the surface area of the gutta-percha to enhance its dissolution. This procedure can be facilitated by using precurved, rigid files such as the C+ file (Dentsply Maillefer) (Fig. 8-32), which can penetrate the gutta-percha mass more efficiently than the more flexible types of K-files. The newly introduced C+ file is a stainless steel, end-cutting hand file that is twisted from a square blank. The secret to its stiffness is that the taper varies along the shaft, giving it the rigidity and strength to cut through well-condensed gutta-percha efficiently. The gutta-percha must be removed carefully, however, to avoid overextending the resultant mixture of gutta-percha and solvent beyond the confines of the canal to minimize the risk of severe postoperative pain.[141] Electronic apex locators are accurate in treatment and nonretreatment situations[123]; however, they seem

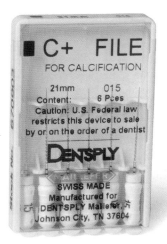

FIG. 8-32 C+ files. These rigid instruments remove gutta-percha more efficiently than more flexible types of K-files. (Courtesy Dentsply Maillefer, Ballaigues, Switzerland.)

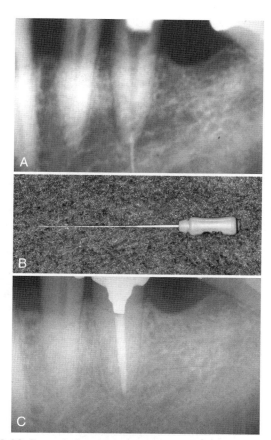

FIG. 8-33 Removal of overextended gutta-percha **A,** Preoperative radiograph showing overextended filling material. **B,** A small Hedstrom file pierces the overextended material and retrieves it. **C,** The 18-month reevaluation. The tooth is asymptomatic.

to misread the working length frequently when gutta-percha is initially being removed. This clinical observation may be due to the file being covered with chloropercha that may affect its conductivity. It has been shown that apex locators may be less accurate in retreatment situations[258]; however, in this study the error was that readings indicated a working length that was too short. In a more recent study, an apex locator built into a rotary handpiece indicated working lengths that were too long in simulated retreatment situations.[252] It is recommended that a radiograph be made to gain a preliminary measurement when the estimated length is approached in order to avoid overextending root-filling materials into the periodontium. Well into the retreatment, after the root fillings have been thoroughly removed, the apex locator will regain its accuracy if a clean file is used. Once the working length is reached, progressively larger diameter hand files are rotated in a passive, nonbinding, clockwise reaming fashion to remove the bulk of the remaining gutta-percha until the files come out of the canal clean (i.e., with no pink material on them). The solvent should be replenished frequently, and when the last loose fitting instrument is removed clean, the canal is flooded with the solvent, which then acts as an irrigant. The solvent is then removed with paper points. The wicking action of the absorbent points[187] will remove much of the remaining film of gutta-percha and sealer that remains adhered to the canal walls and in the irregularities of the canal system.[265] Verification of the cleanliness of canals after gutta-percha removal is not improved by merely using a microscope[12]; however, using kinked small files, the clinician should probe the canal wall looking for irregularities that may harbor the last remnants of gutta-percha. These irregularities can usually be felt rather than seen and should be cleaned using this method.[141]

It should be noted that there exists a glass ionomer based endodontic sealer (Ketac-Endo, ESPE, Seefeld, Germany) that is used in conjunction with gutta-per cha.[180] This sealer is virtually insoluble in both chloroform and halothane,[261] and it must be retreated by removing the gutta-percha and then by using ultrasonics to debride the canal walls. Canal cleanliness can approach that of other gutta-percha retreatment cases, but it is difficult and time consuming to achieve this result.[67,159]

Overextended gutta-percha removal can be attempted by inserting a new Hedstrom file into the extruded apical fragment of root filling using a gentle clockwise rotation to a depth of 0.5 to 1 mm beyond the apical constriction, which may engage the overextended obturation. The file is then slowly and firmly withdrawn with no rotation, removing the overextended material[156] (Fig. 8-33). This technique works frequently, but care must be taken not to force the instrument apically, which furthers the extrusion of the gutta-percha; in addition, the file may separate. The overextended apical fragment should not be softened with solvent, as this application can decrease the likelihood of the Hedstrom file getting a solid purchase of the apical extrusion.[227]

Using rotary systems to remove gutta-percha in the canals has been advocated due to enhanced efficiency and effectiveness in removing gutta-percha from treated root canals.[187] This has generally been borne out in the literature. Several types of mechanical rotary systems are available for gutta-percha removal, including rotary file systems such as the ProFile (Dentsply) (Fig. 8-34), a mechanical push-pull, quarter-turn file system; the Canal Finder (Endo Technique Co., Tustin CA); and dedicated gutta-percha removal instruments, such as the GPX (Brasseler USA), the ProTaper Universal retreatment files (Dentsply) (Fig. 8-35), and the Mtwo R (Sweden and Martina, Due Carrare, Italy). These engine-driven instruments mechanically chop up the gutta-percha and sealer

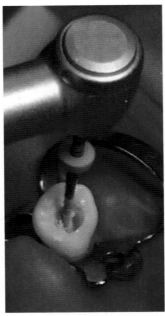

FIG. 8-34 Nickel-titanium rotary Profile thermoplasticizing and removing gutta-percha. Optimum rotary speed is 1500 rpm.

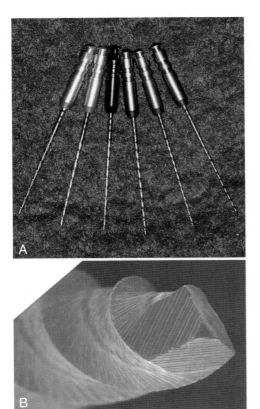

FIG. 8-35 Rotary gutta-percha removal instruments. **A,** Brasseler GPX instruments. **B,** ProTaper Universal retreatment file has a cutting tip for enhanced penetration of the root-filling materials.

while thermoplasticizing the root filling mass via frictional heat to aid in removal. A survey of Australian dentists showed that 54% of the respondents who perform endodontic retreatment used rotary instrumentation to remove gutta-percha either always (15%) or sometimes (39%) with an increased likelihood of rotary gutta-percha removal if the clinician had more experience with the use of these instruments.[173] In vitro studies have generally shown these systems to be efficient in that they typically need less time to remove the bulk of the gutta-percha filling material than is needed for hand removal,[13,59,77,103,104,190,242] although in two studies, they were slower to remove the root filling than hand filing.[15,108] Assessments of canal cleanliness and extruded apical debris generally indicated that there were no overall differences between hand and mechanical gutta-percha removal.[15,59,103,104,109,168,190,218,242,277] In one study using Quantec SC instruments (Kyocera Tycom Corporation, Irvine, CA), however, it was found that hand files with solvent cleaned canals more effectively.[22] This finding has been repeated using the ProTaper retreatment files[92]; however, in another study in the same journal issue, ProTaper retreatment files were found to leave canals cleaner than hand files.[77] Clearly, this is an area where further research is warranted. It is recommended that after rotary gutta-percha removal, subsequent hand instrumentation is needed to remove the residual obturating materials completely from the canal. In several studies of mechanical gutta-percha removal, either the mechanical instruments or the tooth root fractured.[13,22,27,104,108,242] However, this result was reported to occur less frequently when the instrument rotary speed was increased from 350 to 1500 rpm,[27] and one study showed no separation or other canal defects when using dedicated retreatment files, the Pro-Taper Universal and Mtwo R instruments.[220] The dedicated retreatment files have end-cutting tips to enhance penetration and removal of the root filling mass, thus increasing their efficiency[239] (Fig. 8-35, *B*). This, in combination with flute design and techniques advocated, may be the reason for the potential reduced risk of separation. Although the mechanical gutta-percha removal systems may provide an enhanced efficiency, the increased risk of instrument separation, further complicating retreatment, may outweigh this benefit. Dedicated retreatment files may reduce this risk.

Engine-driven instruments can also help with the removal of residual root-filling materials after the bulk of the gutta-percha has been removed. A new instrument, the Self-Adjusting File (SAF; ReDent, Ra'anana, Israel), has been recommended for removal of the root-filling residue that remains after root-filling removal. When the Self-Adjusting Files were used after rotary retreatment files, reduction of canal residues were 66%, 68%, and 81% in the coronal, apical, and middle thirds of the canal, respectively, when compared with using ProTaper Universal retreatment files alone.[3] Another study compared the use of ProTaper Retreatment files followed by F1 and F2 ProTaper instruments with the use of a #25 .06 Profile followed by the Self-Adjusting File for their effectiveness in removing gutta-percha-based root fillings.[219] With the use of high-resolution micro-CT and an arbitrarily selected threshold of less than 0.5% residue remaining as effectively cleaned, none of the ProTaper group cases met this threshold, whereas 57% of the cases in the ProFile/SAF group met the threshold. Unfortunately, in both of the previously mentioned studies, none of the retreatment methods rendered all of the treated canals completely free of all root-filling residue.

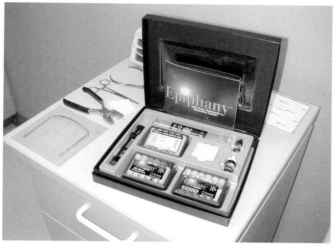

FIG. 8-36 Epiphany Obturation System using Resilon material.

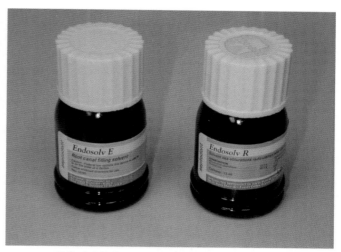

FIG. 8-37 Endosolv-E *(left)* and Endosolv-R *(right)*.

Use of the Nd:YAG laser to remove gutta-percha from root-filled teeth has been investigated in vitro.[254] The time taken to remove the gutta-percha was within the range of other studies of mechanical gutta-percha removal, and the addition of solvents did not improve the performance of the laser. As in most other studies, gutta-percha, in varying amounts, was left in the canals after laser removal. Root surface temperatures did increase, however, and without further investigation proving safety and efficacy, laser gutta-percha removal cannot be recommended at this time.

Resilon (Resilon Research LLC) (Fig. 8-36) is a thermoplastic polyester polymer that is bonded into the canal space using an unfilled resin bonding system (Epiphany, SybroEndo, Orange, CA). It is also marketed as RealSeal (SybroEndo). It has been advocated as a root canal obturating material to replace traditional gutta-percha and sealer due to its apparent, enhanced sealing ability[210] and potential to strengthen root resistance to fracture as a result of internal bonding.[241] Resin-bonded obturation systems have been advocated in the past[135]; however, the difficulty to retreat canals filled with this obturating material has prevented its widespread use. The Resilon polymer itself is reported by the manufacturer to be soluble in chloroform and may be removed by heat application, a behavior that is similar to gutta-percha. Studies have shown that the polycaprolactone polymer of the Resilon is removed easily and leaves canal walls cleaner than removal of gutta-percha and AH+ sealer,[44,46,56,199] although this finding has been disputed. Hassanloo and colleagues found that there was less residue on the walls when removing gutta-percha/AH+ if the materials were allowed to set for a longer period.[97] This finding has been corroborated[199,240] and indicates that there may be a temporal effect, which introduces a methodological bias in these studies. There may also be a problem with removal of the unfilled Epiphany resin sealer, especially because the sealer tags have been shown to penetrate deep into dentinal tubules[210] and presumably also into anatomic ramifications of the canal that need cleaning during retreatment. More research into this interesting material and technique is warranted, especially to determine the best technique for retreatment. After the Resilon core has been removed using heat and chloroform, the authors would recommend the use of a resin solvent such as Endosolv-R (Septodont,

Paris, France) (Fig. 8-37) to attempt elimination of the unfilled resin sealer prior to instrumentation.

Managing Solid Core Obturators

Solid core canal obturation systems, such as Thermafil, Dens-Fil, and the GT Obturator (DENTSPLY Tulsa Dental Specialties, Tulsa, OK), have become popular since their introduction several years ago (see also Chapter 7). After cleaning and shaping procedures are completed, the clinician, using this technique, heats a solid core obturator (alpha-phase gutta-percha surrounding a core that is attached to a handle) in an oven and places the carrier in the canal. The solid core carries the gutta-percha down in the canal and condenses it while the material is cooling. This system provides a rapid and simple technique for warm gutta-percha endodontic obturation; however, as with any obturating material, retreatment will be necessary occasionally.

Retreatment of solid core materials is considered to be more complex and difficult than is the case with removal of gutta-percha alone due to the presence of the solid carrier within the mass of gutta-percha. The nature of the carrier will determine the method used and complexity of the retrieval. Three types of carriers are found in these systems: metal (stainless steel or titanium), plastic, and modified gutta-percha. The plastic carriers are smooth sided, as are some brands of metal carriers; however, most metal carriers are fluted and resemble endodontic hand files with a layer of gutta-percha on the outside. The fluted metal carriers present an exceptional challenge to the retreating clinician because many times they are improperly inserted and either wedged or screwed into the canal to make up for inadequate canal shaping or the lack of skilled use of the size verifying techniques available. This makes them especially difficult to remove. Once the carrier has been placed, it is cut off in the pulp chamber using a bur and the tooth is restored. The level at which the metal carrier is severed is important in its retrieval. If it is cut down to the level of the canal orifice, retrieval is difficult,[141] so the prudent clinician plans for retrievability by severing the handle from the carrier leaving 2 to 3 mm of carrier exposed in the access above the pulp chamber floor to allow easier removal if retreatment is ever needed. Unfortunately, this is not always the case. Some clinicians place a nick in the midcanal level of the carrier to

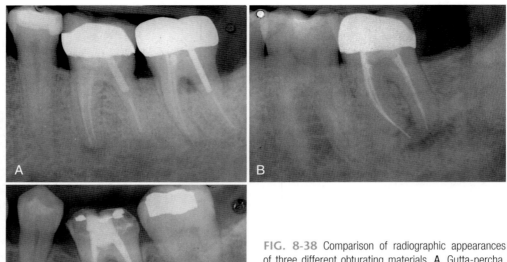

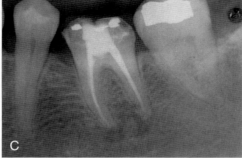

FIG. 8-38 Comparison of radiographic appearances of three different obturating materials. **A,** Gutta-percha. **B,** Stainless steel Thermafil carrier (note the subtle fluting effect in the fill). **C,** Plastic Thermafil carrier.

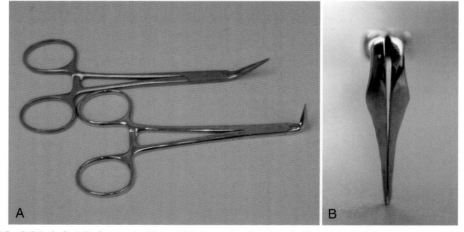

FIG. 8-39 **A,** Steiglitz forceps in 45- and 90-degree head angles. **B,** Tips of the Steiglitz forceps ground to a thinner contour to create the "modified" instrument. This allows deeper penetration into the tooth to enhance removal of obstructions. (*B,* Courtesy Dr. Daniel Erickson.)

allow the clinician to rotate the carrier handle and sever the obturator deep in the canal. This technique is used to allow creation of a post space; however, the rotational force used to create the "twist off" apical plug can engage the flutes of a metal carrier, increasing the complexity of removal if retreatment is needed.[276]

It is advantageous to determine prior to initiating treatment if there is a solid core obturation in the root-filled tooth. The preoperative radiograph may show this because the stainless steel carriers will exhibit a fluting effect on the radiograph (Fig. 8-38); however, the titanium carriers rarely are distinguishable from gutta-percha, and the plastic ones never are. Unfortunately, in most instances, the clinician finds that he or she is dealing with a carrier-based obturator after initial access to the pulp chamber. This is why, as stated in an earlier section,

careful access and probing of the root-filling material is necessary when entering a canal. If there is a carrier, it will be detected as either a metallic structure embedded in the gutta-percha mass or a black or gray spot indicating a plastic or modified gutta-percha carrier. Occasionally, the carrier may be found embedded in the coronal core material, so careful excavation with small burs and straight, tapered ultrasonic tips may be necessary to preserve the carrier intact to help with removal.[141]

Removal of a metal carrier is accomplished with initial use of heat application to the carrier that can soften the gutta-percha surrounding it, facilitating its removal with Peet silver point forceps (Silvermans, New York, NY) or modified Steiglitz forceps (Union Broach, York, PA)[141,187,262,264] (Fig. 8-39). Often, there is not enough of the carrier remaining in the access to

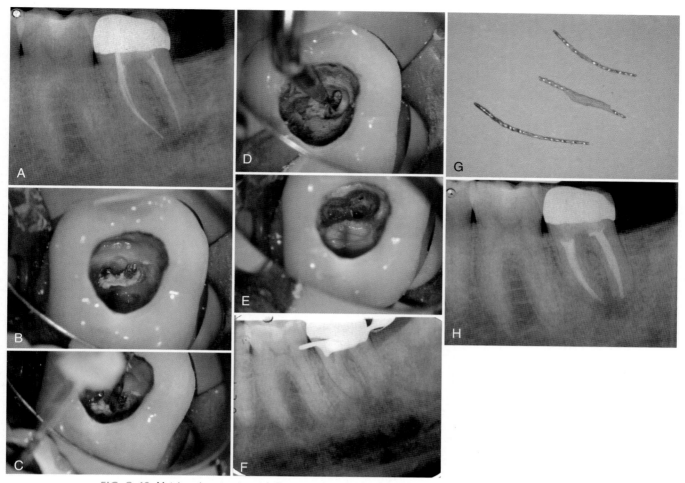

FIG. 8-40 Metal carrier retreatment **A,** Preoperative radiograph. **B,** Metal carriers exposed by careful excavation of gutta-percha. **C,** Use of the Touch 'n Heat instrument to heat the carriers and soften the gutta-percha. This allowed removal of one of the carriers using modified Steiglitz forceps. The other could not be removed using heat or solvents. **D,** Ultrasonic troughing around the carrier to facilitate grasping it with forceps. **E** and **F,** Carriers removed and confirmed with a radiograph. **G,** Metal carriers showing gutta-percha still adhering to them. **H,** Final obturation of the tooth.

grasp with forceps, so removal will require solvent application and removal of the surrounding coronal gutta-percha using small hand instruments, usually followed by ultrasonic excavation around the carrier and removing it like a separated instrument[141,187] (Fig. 8-40), as described in a later section of this chapter. Care should be exercised to avoid excessive heat generation during this procedure. This is also the case if the metal carrier has been sectioned for post space preparation. The metal carrier has been shown to be much more difficult to remove than plastic ones,[62,276] frequently resulting in nonretrieval. Fortunately, their use in endodontic therapy has been declining.

Removal of plastic carriers is similar to removal of gutta-percha root fillings, except that, in general, heat should be avoided to minimize the likelihood of damaging the carrier.[141] The older Thermafil plastic carriers were made of two different materials depending on their size. In the smaller sizes (up to size #40), the material used was Vectra, which is insoluble in available solvents, whereas the larger sizes used polysulfone, which is soluble in chloroform.[174] Solvents, on the other hand,

seem not to affect the newer GT plastic carriers, so their use can be recommended[21] (Fig. 8-41). The access is flooded with a solvent, such as chloroform, and the gutta-percha surrounding the carrier is removed with hand files in a larger to smaller sequence (#25, 20, 15, etc.) each file progressively penetrating deeper around the carrier. The solvent should be replenished frequently, and when a #08 file can penetrate to the apical extent of the carrier and there is little remaining gutta-percha, a larger Hedstrom file is inserted into the canal alongside the plastic carrier and gently turned clockwise to engage the flutes. When the file is withdrawn, it invariably brings the carrier with it, and the rest of the gutta-percha and sealer removal proceeds as described earlier. Care must be taken to avoid overstressing the Hedstrom file. It should not be "screwed" into the canal, or the file or the carrier may separate.[21] Occasionally, grasping pliers will be needed to remove the carrier if it is accessible[110,187] after the gutta-percha has been removed. Another potential problem with retrieval is present if the carrier has been overextended beyond the apical foramen during the previous root canal treatment. This overextension may make it

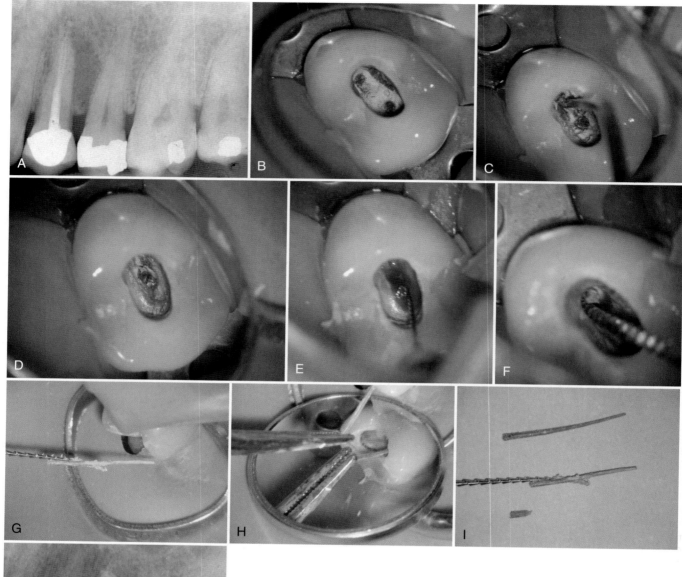

FIG. 8-41 Plastic carrier retreatment **A,** Preoperative radiograph. At this stage, the nature of the root filling is unknown. **B,** Plastic carriers visible in the access as two black spots in the gutta-percha mass. **C,** Gutta-percha in the chamber is carefully removed from the carriers. **D,** Carrier is exposed. **E,** chloroform solvent is placed into the chamber and a small file is worked alongside the carriers to remove the gutta-percha. **F** and **G,** A Hedstrom file is gently screwed into the canal alongside the carrier, and it is withdrawn upon removal. **H,** A hemostat removes the other carrier. **I,** Plastic carriers removed. **J,** Final obturation with Resilon and Epiphany sealer.

prone to separation and unable to be retrieved, potentially resulting in the need for apical surgery.[107]

A technique for plastic carrier removal has been described using a System B HeatSource (SybronEndo) to soften the gutta-percha surrounding the carrier without melting the carrier itself.[267] The temperature is set at 225° C, and the heat plugger is placed buccal and lingual to the carrier after which #50-55 Flex-R hand files are placed around the carrier and braided to engage the carrier and remove it. This technique has been shown to require significantly less time to remove the carrier compared with using solvent[267]; however, concerns regarding heat generation in the periradicular tissues have been raised,[139] with the authors concluding that caution should be exercised when using this technique. When other techniques have been unsuccessful and the plastic carrier has been sectioned apical to the orifice resulting in limited access, the clinician may attempt to retrieve the carrier by placing a heated System B tip directly into it. As apical pressure is maintained, the heat is

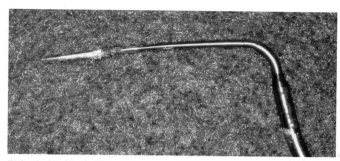

FIG. 8-42 Plastic Thermafil carrier adhering to a System B heat plugger.

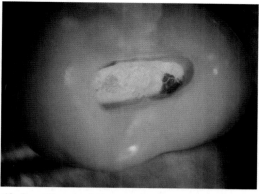

FIG. 8-43 Two different solid core carriers in an endodontic access preparation upon initial exposure. GuttaCore is on the left and a plastic carrier Thermafil Plus is on the right. Note the lighter gray color of the new modified gutta-percha core compared with the plastic carrier.

turned off. This allows the plastic carrier to adhere to the tip while cooling and may result in its removal upon withdrawal of the heat tip (Fig. 8-42).

Rotary instruments have been advocated for use in removal of plastic carriers and gutta-percha, and one study showed that removal of plastic carriers was successful in all but one of the teeth obturated with them.[13] Unfortunately, root fracture occurred in the lone specimen that did not have a successful retrieval, and two instances of rotary instrument fracture also occurred in the study. As with gutta-percha removal, the clinician must carefully weigh the risks of rotary carrier removal against the perceived benefits.[186]

Modified gutta-percha has been introduced as a core material for solid core obturation. This obturation system is called GuttaCore (DENTSPLY Tulsa Dental Specialties) and, at first glance, it appears similar to plastic carrier based systems. With GuttaCore, however, the carrier is fabricated from cross-linked gutta-percha rather than plastic. The cross-linking connects the polymer chains, which changes the material and gives the carrier different properties than the plastic carriers. The gutta-percha surrounding the carrier is alpha-phase gutta-percha, which is identical to that which encompasses the plastic carrier based systems.

To understand how to effectively remove this type of filling material, one must understand how it is used. Obturation with GuttaCore is performed in a similar manner as obturation with Plastic Thermafil. The obturator is heated in a proprietary oven and then gently placed into the canal. Although it is flexible, the modified gutta-percha carrier is much more brittle than the plastic carrier and too much insertion force will cause the shank to collapse and the handle can break off prior to full insertion. Thus, it is difficult to wedge these obturators into underprepared canals and usually, in that instance, a short fill will result. This forces the operator either to accept a short fill or, ideally to enlarge the canal preparation prior to inserting the obturator, but in either case, retrieval of the root filling during retreatment is made easier by not having the carrier wedged into the canal.

While performing initial obturation, when it is time to section the carrier, the clinician will experience another difference from plastic carriers. Although the use of a heat-generating Prepi bur (DENTSPLY Tulsa Dental Specialties) or a System B Heat Source (SybronEndo) has been shown to produce predictably reliable results in terms of sectioning plastic carriers at the desired level, heat has virtually no effect on the GuttaCore carrier, and the authors found using heat to section the carrier to be unsuccessful. The modified gutta-percha core will not melt, even when probed with a Touch 'n Heat (SybronEndo) tip at full power.

Because of the brittleness of the modified gutta-percha carrier, GuttaCore will separate by simply bending the carrier away from the access cavity wall. The material has little ability to resist even the smallest of lateral forces without separation, so simply pushing down laterally on the carrier handle will separate the carrier handle from the canal fill. This has implications for retreatment because this separation method generally results in the carrier being separated at or near the canal orifice level, leaving little or nothing to grasp with forceps when attempting to remove the carrier.

Removal of the GuttaCore obturators is directly affected by the properties of the modified gutta-percha carrier, so it is somewhat different from the approach taken to remove plastic carriers. For this reason, it is imperative that clinicians who discover a solid core, nonmetallic obturator while disassembling a tooth for nonsurgical retreatment can discern what type of core they are trying to remove. There are two ways to do this. First, the color of the plastic carrier is black, whereas the color of the modified gutta-percha carrier was originally gray (Fig. 8-43); however, the manufacturer recently changed the color of the carrier to pink. Second, because the GuttaCore carrier is heat resistant, the clinician can lightly touch the coronal extent of the unknown carrier to see if it melts (plastic carrier) or if it does not (modified gutta-percha carrier). Once the nature of the carrier is determined, then the clinician can proceed with removal. If it is plastic, then the methods of removal described previously can be used, but if it is a GuttaCore carrier, then a different approach will be needed.

The use of heat and solvents, which are two of the most common methods for endodontic retreatment, have no effect on the GuttaCore carrier. To date the authors are unaware of any known solvents or chair side heat sources that can soften the cross-linked gutta-percha carrier. Also, the use of hemostats or other grasping pliers have shown inconsistent results. When straight-line access can be achieved, and a few millimeters of the carrier is able to be grasped, removal may be accomplished; however, due to the brittleness of the GuttaCore carrier, often the carrier will separate at the apical extent of the grasping forceps. In spite of those concerns, the authors have found that GuttaCore can be removed easily with predictable results using a variety of hand, rotary, and retreatment instruments. One study found that when using ProTaper retreatment files, GuttaCore was more efficiently removed from moderately curved canals than either thermoplasticized gutta-percha or plastic carrier obturation.[17] However, the authors' experience shows that upon removal of the segment of the carrier within the canal, any overextended tip of the carrier will separate, remaining in the periapical tissues. This potentially contaminated foreign material becomes difficult and many times impossible to remove. If this occurs, and postretreatment apical periodontitis persists or recurs after initial resolution, then apical surgery or extraction will be necessary.

Another approach is to treat the carrier like some hard paste fills that the clinician is unable to find a solvent for. Using this approach, the clinician will find that using ultrasonic instruments in a similar fashion as they are used to remove pastes to be helpful. Once a proper access preparation has been created, GuttaCore can be safely and easily removed with the use of ultrasonic instruments in the straight coronal portion of the canal. Upon reaching the canal curvature, the authors recommend using hand files or rotary files with safe noncutting tips to avoid perforation or excessive thinning of canal walls.

Once the carrier has been removed, the remaining gutta-percha and sealer must be removed from the canal, and like removal of root-filling materials described previously, there is no technique that completely removes all materials from the canal system. Canal cleaning may be even more difficult when removing carrier-based obturations because the more highly processed gutta-percha used with these carriers may be more difficult to remove than other forms of the material. Wilcox and Juhlin described a sticky film of gutta-percha and sealer adhering to the canal walls upon removal of metal carrier obturators and found more of it than if the canals had been obturated with lateral condensation.[264] Their findings have not been corroborated, however, and other studies have shown no difference in residual debris remaining after carrier-based removal.[62,110,276] It is important to remove as much of the residual gutta-percha and sealer from the pulpal anatomic spaces as possible, so flooding the canal with solvent and "wicking" it out with paper points is also recommended for carrier based retreatment.[187]

Paste Retreatment

Various pastes have been used as root canal obturating materials, especially outside of North America. Because of the wide variety of paste compounds used in endodontics, it is impossible to categorize them all. The individual clinician who is using it formulates most pastes, so the ultimate composition of a paste found in a tooth with persistent disease is generally indiscernible. Many of the pastes used, such as N2 or RC2B, contain formaldehyde and heavy metal oxides and so are toxic and potentially present a danger to the patient's health, both local and systemic, if overextended beyond the confines of the root canal system.[25,172] None has the potential to seal the canal effectively,[91] and many render a tooth impossible to retreat,[200] so their use is strongly discouraged. On radiographic examination, they can usually be discerned due to their lack of radiopacity, the presence of voids, and they usually show evidence of inadequate canal shaping and poor length control (Fig. 8-44). When a paste fill is suspected or found in a tooth, a telephone call to the previous treating dentist should be made, if possible, to find out the exact formulation of the paste because this information may help in its removal.

For purposes of retreatment, paste fills can be categorized as soft or hard, and all should be considered potentially toxic.

Great care should be exercised when removing the paste to avoid overextension, potentially severe postoperative pain,[87] and possible paresthesia/dysesthesia from the paste's potential neurotoxicity.[28,207] Soft pastes are generally easy to remove using crown down instrumentation with copious sodium hypochlorite irrigation to minimize extrusion.[141] Greater difficulty arises when the paste is set hard.[200] Because the nature of the paste remains unknown, removing it becomes an empirical process. Following access preparation and coronal orifice exposure, the paste is probed with an endodontic explorer and files. If hard and impenetrable, then the coronal paste can be removed with burs[69] or a straight, tapered ultrasonic tip in the easily accessible straight portions of the canal using magnification and illumination.[187] Once the canal curvature is reached, further use of this method will result in damage to the canal walls and possible perforation. Precurved, small hand files are inserted to probe the apical area. Many times the density of the paste filling material decreases in the apical extent of the fill so that penetration to the apex may be possible.[187] If not, a solvent must be used to attempt to soften the remaining paste. The choice of solvent is usually made by trial and error starting with chloroform. If that does not soften the material in a reasonable amount of time and does not allow penetration with small files, then the chloroform is wicked out of the canal and another solvent is chosen. There are two frequently used solvents for paste fills: Endosolv-E and Endosolv-R (Septodont, Paris, France) (see Fig. 8-37). The Endosolv-E is selected if the paste contains zinc oxide and eugenol, and the Endosolv-R is chosen for resin-based pastes. The obvious problem is that the nature of the paste is usually unknown at the time of removal, so contacting the previous clinician, if possible, can help with this choice. Otherwise, the choice is just a guess. The chosen solvent should be placed in the access, and attempts should be made to penetrate the paste with hand or ultrasonic files; however, care must be taken to avoid creating a ledge or other defect in the canal that may preclude successful retreatment. The progress is frequently slow,[72] and the clinician may elect to leave some solvent in the canals between appointments to soften the paste.[187] Care should be taken in the choice of temporary restoration because the solvent left in the canal may also soften the temporary, potentially leading to breakdown of the interappointment seal.[158]

Ultrasonically activated files have been advocated for use in penetrating hard-set pastes in the curved apical segments of canals[117,126] (Fig. 8-45). The ultrasonic energy breaks up the paste, and the irrigation floats the fragments in a coronal direction until the apical terminus is reached.[69] This technique is reported to be time consuming, and care must be exercised to avoid instrument separation, perforations, or alteration of canal morphology. On occasion despite all best efforts, the paste cannot be removed from the tooth, so apical surgery or extraction should be considered in these cases.[87]

Biocalex 6.9 (currently known as Endocal 10) (Fig. 8-46) is a hard-setting calcium oxide paste that has been popular in Europe since the 1980s but is now being used in North America since its recent FDA approval.[83] The paste seems to seal well, but there is an unacceptably high incidence of root fracture due to the large amount of expansion on setting.[83] Retreatment will be complicated by the hard setting nature of this material; however, as it is a calcium oxide paste, ethylenediaminetetraacetic acid (EDTA) may soften it, facilitating its removal. Because EDTA also softens dentin, care must be taken not to

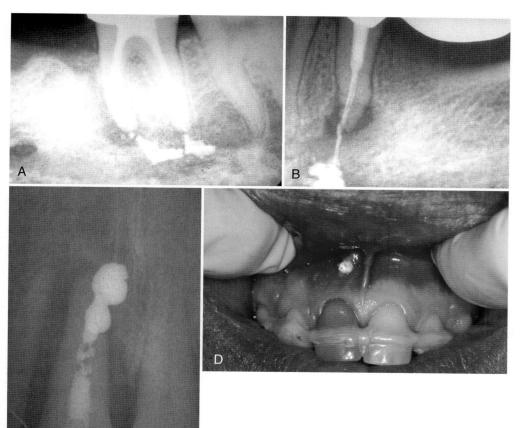

FIG. 8-44 Example of poor length control with paste root fillings **A,** Over-extended paste filling into the inferior alveolar canal. **B,** Overextended paste filling into the mental foramen. **C,** Over-extended paste filling extending through a perforation in an upper central incisor. **D,** Clinical appearance of the case in Fig. 8-41, *C.* Note the material extending out through a sinus tract.

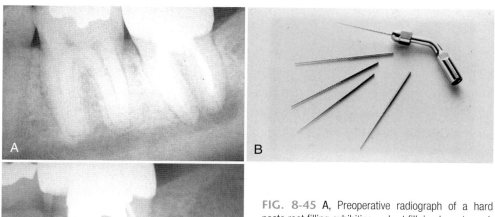

FIG. 8-45 **A,** Preoperative radiograph of a hard paste root filling exhibiting a short fill, inadequate seal, and periapical radiolucency. Note the proximity of the inferior alveolar canal. **B,** Ultrasonic files like this were used to break up the hard paste in the apical third of the canal allowing removal. **C,** A 17-month postoperative follow-up. The patient is asymptomatic and has no paresthesia.

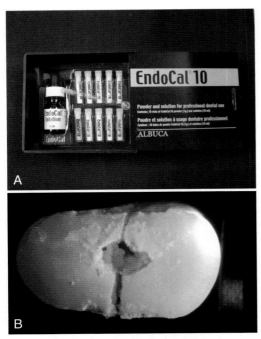

FIG. 8-46 **A,** Endocal 10 (formerly known as Biocalyx). **B,** Split root in a case filled with Endocal 10. (Courtesy Dr. Rob Goldberg.)

gouge or ledge the canal walls during retreatment, and root fractures must be suspected as a potential complicating factor in the outcome.

Silver Point Removal

Historically, the use of silver points for endodontic therapy has been extremely popular and quite successful, because of their ease of handling and placement, ductility, radiopacity, and that silver appears to have some antibacterial activity.[202] However, the use of silver points has dramatically diminished, so presently they are considered a deviation from the standard of care.[274] The main reason for this change is because they corrode over time (Fig. 8-47), and the apical seal may be lost.[26] Also, silver points do not produce an acceptable three-dimensional seal of the canal system; rather, they simply produce a plug in the apical constriction while not sealing the accessory canals that are frequently present[143,198] (Fig. 8-48). The corrosion of silver points occurs when they come in contact with tissue fluids and certain chemicals used in endodontics, including sodium hypochlorite and some sealers.[88] This corrosion produces chemicals such as silver sulfide, silver sulfate, silver carbonate, and silver amine hydrate,[205] which have been shown to be cytotoxic in tissue culture.[202] Corrosion occurs mainly at the apical and coronal portions of the points indicating that leakage is responsible.[205] Gutta-percha root-filling techniques

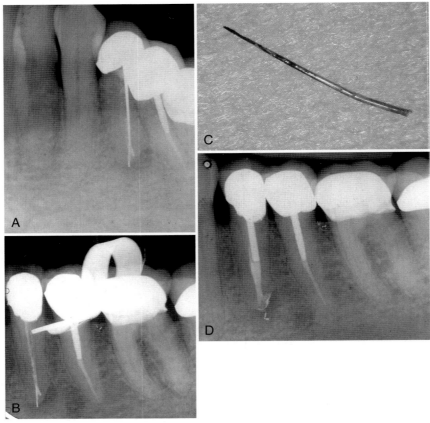

FIG. 8-47 **A,** Persistent disease in a silver point filled tooth. **B,** Silver point removed. Note the radiopaque material in the apical portion of the canal system. This represents corrosion products remaining in the canal and a possible separated apical segment of the cone. **C,** Removed silver point showing black corrosion products adhering to the apical one half. **D,** Crown-down instrumentation prevents extrusion of most of the corrosion products into the periradicular tissues.

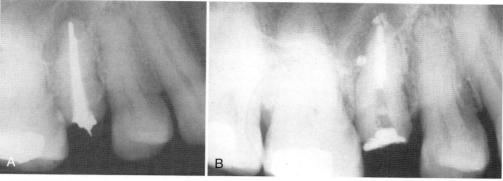

FIG. 8-48 A, Preoperative view of a silver point case with persistent disease. Note that the periapical radiolu-cency extends coronally on the distal aspect of the root end, indicating the presence of an unfilled lateral canal. B, Postobturation radiograph showing the cleaned and filled distal canal branch.

do not suffer from these disadvantages and have replaced the use of silver points in endodontics. Due to this decrease in use since the late 1980s, the quantity of cases the clinician will come across that will require silver point removal has also decreased. Nevertheless, there are still occasions when their removal will be necessary.

Many of the same techniques described for removing sepa-rated instruments in the following section apply to the removal of silver points. Silver points have a minimal taper and are smoothed sided, and corrosion may loosen the cone within the preparation. Therefore, the clinician should encounter a much easier time removing them than would be the case with sepa-rated instruments, which may be mechanically engaged into canals. Silver point canal preparation techniques produced a milled, round preparation in the apical 2 to 3 mm of the canal and, coronal to that, the clinician will frequently find space between the round silver point and the flared canal walls that can usually be negotiated with hand files facilitating point removal.[187]

The first step in removal of silver points is to establish proper access. Frequently, the coronal portion of the cone is embedded in the core material. This material must be carefully removed with burs and ultrasonics, taking care not to remove any of the silver point within the access cavity preparation. The more of the silver point the clinician has to work with, the more predictable will be its removal. Once proper access is established, the clinician should flood the access preparation with a solvent, such as chloroform, to soften or dissolve the cement, enabling easier removal. An endodontic explorer or small file may be used to carry the solvent down along the silver point to dissolve as much of the cement as possible. The chamber can be rinsed and dried, and this step may be repeated because fresh solvent enhances the efficiency of cement removal. At this point, the easiest technique, which is also predictable, is to grasp the exposed end of the silver point with Stieglitz pliers (Henry Schein) (see Fig. 8-39) or other appro-priate forceps and gently pull it out of the access cavity prepa-ration. If too much extraction force is needed, however, the point may separate, so slow force application is advised. The clinician will need a variety of sizes and angles of forceps avail-able to deal with the variety of cases that will need to be treated. Occasionally, the forceps may not get a good purchase on the silver cone and will slip off. In these instances, gripping the cone with the forceps and then gripping the forceps in a hemostat or needle driver to increase the squeezing force of

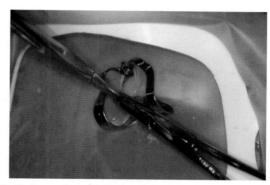

FIG. 8-49 Removal of a highly retentive silver point using a needle driver to squeeze the tips of the Steiglitz forceps. This applies increased gripping force to aid in removal.

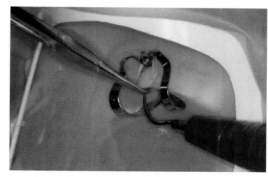

FIG. 8-50 Application of indirect ultrasonic energy to a silver point by placing the ultrasonic tip against forceps that are holding the silver point.

the forceps will allow removal of the cone[141] (Fig. 8-49). If the silver point is held tight by the frictional fit in the preparation, indirect ultrasonics may be employed to loosen it. The silver point is retained in a pair of forceps and ultrasonic energy is applied to the forceps, not the point (Fig. 8-50). This transmits energy down the cone and may loosen it. If there is not much of the silver point exposed in the chamber, the clinician can attempt to remove it using the Caufield silver point retrievers (Integra Miltex). This instrument is a spoon with a groove in the tip (Fig. 8-51) that can engage the exposed end of the silver point so it may be elevated from the canal or possibly elevated to the point where it may be grasped by forceps.[141] The

Caufield silver point retrievers are available in three sizes: 25, 35, and 50.

If the silver point cannot be dislodged by the forgoing techniques, the clinician should consider using Hedstrom files to remove the silver point. The Hedstrom file technique requires at least some coronal length of canal space around the silver point to be negotiated first.[140] The sealer is dissolved as previously mentioned, and then files are negotiated as far apically as possibly in two to three areas around the silver point. If only one space can be negotiated, this technique may still be effective. The spaces surrounding the silver point are carefully instrumented to size 15, and then small Hedstrom files are gently screwed in as far as possible apically. They should not be screwed in too tightly so as to prevent breakage. The flute design of Hedstrom file allows for much better engagement into the silver point compared with other file designs. The files are then twisted together and pulled out through the access (Fig. 8-52). If the first attempt fails, this technique may be repeated, possibly using larger Hedstrom files. If this technique does not completely remove the silver point from the canal, it may still be dislodged to the point where it can be grasped by forceps and removed.

If the clinician needs to expose more of the silver point to enable removal, the use of trephine burs and microtubes or ultrasonics may be necessary.[69] Trephine burs are used in the same manner as described for separated instrument removal; however, the clinician must be more careful when using ultrasonic instruments for retrieval of silver points. When using ultrasonics for post removal, or separated instrument removal, the tip of the ultrasonic instrument can be placed at the interface between the obstruction and the canal wall. Although applying the ultrasonic energy directly to a post or file may prove beneficial in vibrating them loose, silver points are much softer, and if ultrasonic instruments are applied directly to them, the portion in contact may be shredded leaving a smaller segment to work with because elemental silver rapidly erodes during mechanical manipulation.[187] The ultrasonic instrument is used on tooth structure circumferentially around the silver point. This is a delicate process requiring a microscope or other powerful source of magnification. The energy supplied by the careful use of the ultrasonic instrument can safely expose silver points as well as break up the cement around them.

In many cases, a silver point may have been sectioned deep in the canal to allow post space preparation. In these cases, where the most coronal portion of the silver point is well below the orifice, the use of Gates-Glidden burs to obtain straight-line access to the most coronal extent of the point may be necessary. The burs should be used in a brushlike manner, cutting on the outstroke while applying gentle pressure in an anticurvature direction to decrease the risk of root perforation. Following this step, techniques that involve the use of an end-cutting trephine bur to remove tooth structure around the point and then use of an extraction device to remove it may be employed (Fig. 8-53). There are many kits that use these principals with slight variations from one another, including the Endo Extractor (Brasseler USA),[226] the Masserann Kit (Medidenta International, Woodside, NY), and the Extractor System (Roydent, Johnson City, TN) (Fig. 8-54). Additional techniques, which are effective for removing silver points, include the S.I.R. (Separated Instrument Retrieval) System (Vista Dental Products, Racine, WI), the use of a dental injection needle with a 0.14-mm wire, the use of stainless-steel tubing with a Hedstrom file,[187] and the Instrument Removal System (Dentsply Tulsa Dental Specialties).

These kits are not only effective in the removal of silver points but also in the removal of separated instruments, and because of this common approach to removing both during endodontic retreatment, these techniques will be discussed

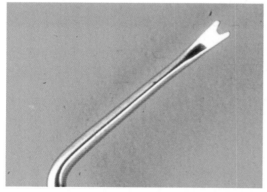

FIG. 8-51 Caufield elevator tip, useful for gripping and elevating silver points that are protruding a small amount into the pulp chamber.

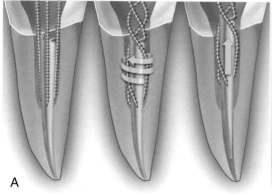
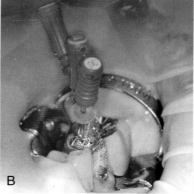
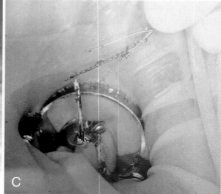

FIG. 8-52 **A,** Diagram illustrating the braiding of Hedstrom files around a silver point. By twisting the braided files, a gripping force is applied, which aids in removal of the obstruction. **B,** Small files being braided around a silver point. **C,** Pulling coronally with the braided files removes the silver point.

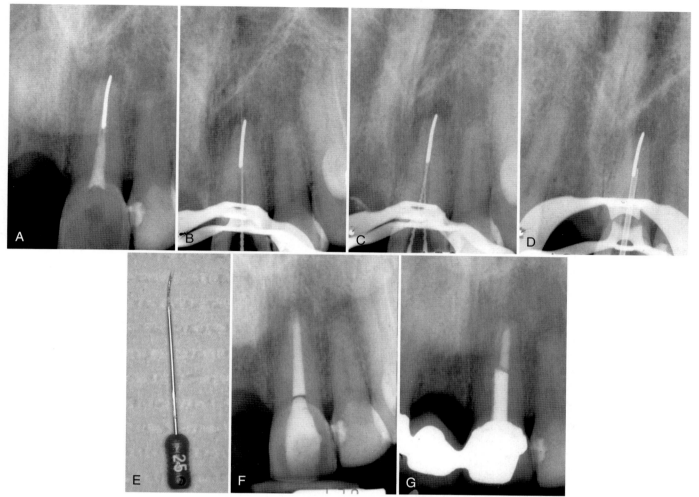

FIG. 8-53 Twist-off silver point case **A,** Preoperative radiograph showing apical periodontitis and a split silver cone ("twist-off") obturation technique. **B,** The cone was initially bypassed but could not be loosened. **C,** The braided Hedstrom file technique was attempted but was unsuccessful. **D,** A Brasseler Endo Extractor tube is cemented to the cone with cyanoacrylate cement. **E,** The silver point is removed. **F,** Immediate postobturation radiograph. **G,** The 1-year follow-up showing apical healing. (Reprinted with permission from Gutmann JL, Dumsha TC, Lovdahl PE, Hovland EJ, editors: *Problem solving in endodontics,* ed 3, St. Louis, 1997, Mosby, pp 180-81.)

in detail in the following section on separated instrument removal.

After the silver point is removed, it is important that subsequent instrumentation procedures be performed in a crown-down manner to minimize extrusion of the silver corrosion products into the periradicular tissues to decrease the occurrence of painful acute flare-ups. This goal is complicated by the fact that ledges are frequently encountered at the level of the apical extent of the silver point due to the type of milled preparation that was frequently used in this technique. Managing ledges will be discussed in a following section of this chapter.

Occasionally, the apical portion of a silver point will separate upon the removal attempt. If it cannot be bypassed or removed, then the case should be completed and followed carefully (Fig. 8-55). Apical surgery or extraction could be necessary in the future (Fig. 8-56).

Removal of Separated Instruments

Causes of Instrument Separation

Occasionally during nonsurgical root canal therapy, an instrument will separate in a canal system blocking access to the apical canal terminus. This instrument is usually some type of file or reamer but can include Gates-Glidden or Peeso drills, lentulo spiral paste fillers, thermomechanical gutta-percha compactors, or the tips of hand instruments, such as explorers or gutta-percha spreaders. During retreatment, it may be obvious after completing the diagnostic phase that there is a separated instrument in the canal system or it may only become apparent after removal of the root-filling materials (Fig. 8-57). It is useful, therefore, to expose a check radiograph after removal of the root filling to see if there is any metallic obstruction in the canal. Regardless of which type of instruments the clinician uses, whether stainless steel or nickel-titanium, and

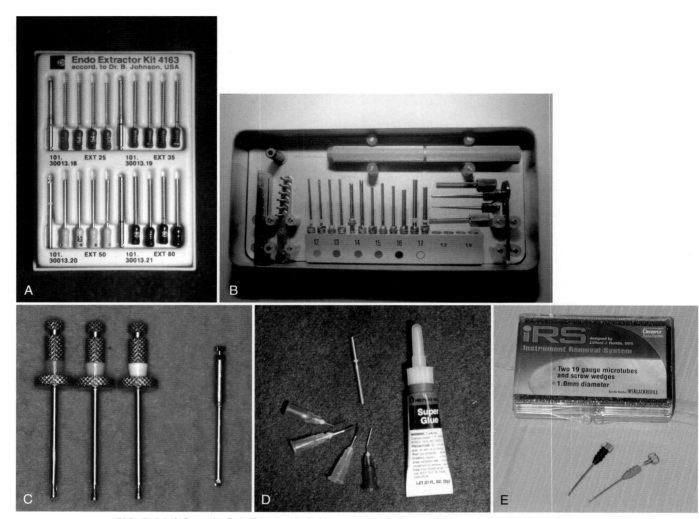

FIG. 8-54 **A,** Brasseler Endo Extractor Kit. **B,** Masserann Kit. **C,** Roydent Extractor System. **D,** Separated Instrument Retrieval System (SIR). **E,** Instrument Removal System (IRS). (*B,* Courtesy Dr. Daniel Erickson.)

how they are used, by hand or engine driven, the potential for separation exists. The incidence of hand instrument separation has been reported to be 0.25%,[114] and for rotary instruments it ranges from 1.68% to 2.4%.[114,268] The most common causes for file separation are improper use, limitations in physical properties, inadequate access, root canal anatomy, and possibly manufacturing defects.

A common cause for instrument separation is improper use. Included in this category are overuse and not discarding an instrument and replacing it with a new one when needed. The following is a list of guidelines for when to discard and replace instruments[79]:

1. Flaws, such as shiny areas or unwinding, are detected on the flutes.
2. Excessive use has caused instrument bending or crimping (common with smaller-sized instruments). A major concern with nickel-titanium instruments is that they tend to fracture without warning; as a result, constant monitoring of usage is critical.
3. Excessive bending or precurving has been necessary.
4. Accidental bending occurs during file use.
5. The file kinks instead of curving.

6. Corrosion is noted on the instrument.
7. Compacting instruments have defective tips or have been excessively heated.[79]

Another type of improper use is to apply too much apical pressure during instrumentation,[247] especially when using rotary nickel-titanium files. This pressure can lead to deflection of the instrument within the canal system or increased frictional binding against the canal walls that can overstress the metal, resulting in separation. Regardless of which type of files the clinician uses, they should never be used in a dry canal, as attempting to instrument a dry canal will cause excessive frictional stresses on an instrument.[247] Continual lubrication of the canal with either irrigating solutions or lubricants is required,[79] as this will reduce the frictional resistance as well as increase the efficiency of the instrument. All files have flutes that have the ability to build up with dentin shavings, which will decrease the efficiency of the instrument leading to greater frictional forces and ultimately separation. Therefore, files should be periodically removed and cleaned during the instrumentation process.

Inadequate access cavity preparations can lead to many problems, one of which is excessive or unnecessary force

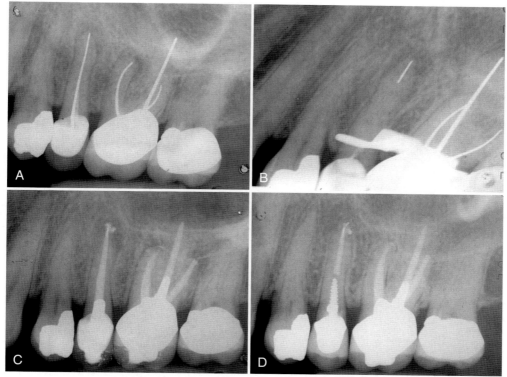

FIG. 8-55 Case illustrating healing despite inability to remove a separated silver point A, Preoperative radiograph showing persistent disease in an upper premolar and molar. B, Working film showing the separated cone that could not be retrieved despite extensive clinical efforts. C, Final obturation after a two-appointment procedure using a calcium hydroxide interappointment medicament. D, The 4-year follow-up showing apical healing.

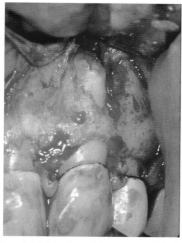

FIG. 8-56 If silver point retreatment is unsuccessful, then apical surgery may be needed. Note the silver point visible on the resected root end. If the point cannot be pulled out in a retrograde direction, then ultrasonic root-end preparation may be complicated by its presence, and root-end preparation using rotary burs may be necessary.

applied to the instrument if it is not allowed to enter the canal freely without interference from the access cavity walls. If the file is in contact with the access cavity wall during instrumentation, the chance for separation is greatly increased. Inadequately enlarged access preparations also increase the number and severity of curvatures that the file must negotiate. This underprepared access can lead to the creation of an iatrogenic "S" curve that can overstress the instrument. This situation is especially hazardous when using rotary instrumentation because traversing an "S" curve greatly stresses the rotating file, leading to separation (Fig. 8-58).

Anatomy, such as abrupt curvatures or anatomic ledges, increases the likelihood of instrument fracture. When the file's progress is hindered, it is natural to try to force it further. This approach will rarely result in the file advancing along the naturally occurring path and indeed may result in file separation, perforation, or ledge creation. Some clinicians would like to blame instrument separation on manufacturing defects; however, this has never been shown to be of clinical relevance and is quite rare.[247]

The best treatment for the separated instrument is prevention. If proper techniques for cleaning and shaping of the root canal system are followed, file separation should be an infrequent occurrence. Nevertheless, an occasional event may take place. When instrument separation occurs, a radiograph should be taken immediately.[247] This radiograph will not only confirm the separation, it will give the clinician information that may aid in removal, such as location, size of the file segment, root canal anatomy, and, ultimately, the possibility of removal. The patient should be advised of the accident as well as its effect on the prognosis.[41] In addition, when a file separates, as with other procedural accidents, detailed documentation is necessary for medical-legal considerations,[247] and the remaining segment of the file should not be discarded but, rather, placed in a coin envelope and kept in the patients record.[41,274]

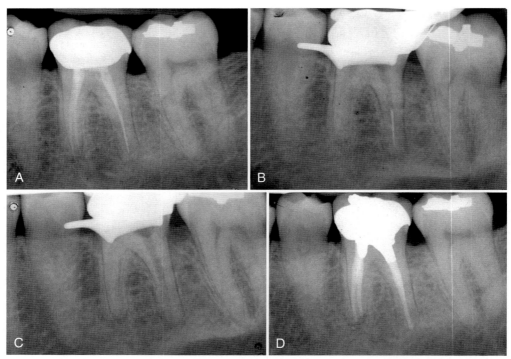

FIG. 8-57 **A,** Preoperative radiograph of a tooth with symptomatic posttreatment disease. **B,** Although not readily apparent on the preoperative film, there is a separated nickel-titanium instrument in the distal canal. **C,** Check film showing that ultrasonics has removed the separated file. **D,** A 13-month recall film. The patient was asymptomatic.

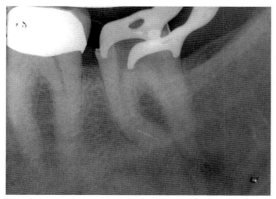

FIG. 8-58 Complicated canal anatomy can increase stress on rotary instruments, leading to separation such as in this "S"-shaped canal.

Prognosis

A separated instrument does not necessarily mean surgery or loss of the tooth. Actually, the prognosis may not be reduced at all depending on what stage of instrumentation the separation occurs, the preoperative status of the pulp and periradicular tissues, and whether or not the file can be removed or bypassed.[225] The presence of a separated instrument in the canal in itself does not predispose the case to posttreatment disease. Rather, it is the presence of any necrotic, infected pulp tissue that remains in the apical canal space that determines the prognosis. The outcome is better if the canal was instrumented to the later stages of preparation when the separation occurs.[247] If the preoperative pulp was vital and noninfected (irreversible pulpitis, for example), and there was no apical

periodontitis, the presence of the separated instrument should not affect the prognosis.[43] If the file can be removed without excessive over enlargement of the canal or causing an additional iatrogenic mishap, such as a perforation, the prognosis will not be affected. Bypassing the instrument and incorporating it into the obturation should also have no effect on the prognosis. However, if the instrument cannot be removed or bypassed in a tooth with a necrotic, infected pulp and apical periodontitis, the prognosis will be uncertain. These cases should be followed closely and, if symptoms persist, apical surgery or extraction should be considered.[247,271]

The potential to remove a separated instrument depends on many factors that should be considered during the diagnostic workup. The location of the separated instrument is critical. If the separated instrument extends into the straight, coronal portion of the canal, retrieval is likely. If, however, the instrument has separated deep in the canal and the entire broken segment is apical to the canal curvature, then orthograde removal will not be possible and attempts to do so could lead to a much higher rate of iatrogenic complication.[209,223] If there is persistent disease and the file cannot be bypassed safely, either apical surgery or extraction will be necessary. Because of the need to enlarge the coronal radicular access, root curvatures, external root concavities, and root thickness all will be important factors to consider when deciding which treatment option will provide the best chance of long-term success. Teeth with thin roots and deep external root concavities have a greater likelihood of being perforated during the coronal radicular access, so surgery should be considered as an alternative to orthograde instrument retrieval. The type of material the separated instrument is made of will affect the chances of removal. Nickel-titanium files tend to shatter when ultrasonic

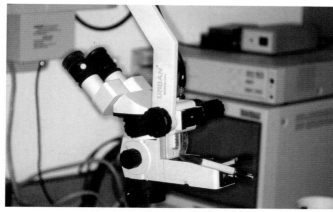

FIG. 8-59 The surgical operating microscope is not only invaluable in helping to remove separated instruments, but it is in fact a necessary tool for these procedures.

energy is applied to them, hindering removal, whereas stainless steel instruments are more robust and more easily removed with ultrasonics.[187]

Removal Techniques

Many different instruments and techniques will be discussed in this section, all of which are important to include in the armamentarium for separated instrument removal. None, however, is more important than the operating microscope (Fig. 8-59). This instrument will not only increase visibility by the use of magnification and light, but it will also increase the efficiency and safety of almost all of the techniques to be discussed. The use of a headlamp and magnifying loupes will help with the removal of many canal impediments. However, the use of the operating microscope has caused a quantum leap in visualization due to the enhanced lighting and magnification that it offers,[124] and many of the techniques to be described should not even be attempted without the use of this valuable tool.[234]

Once the patient has been advised of the treatment options and the decision has been made to attempt removal, the clinician's first choice in treatment will be based on the location of the instrument. If the file is clinically visible in the coronal access and can be grasped with an instrument, such as a hemostat or Stieglitz Pliers (Sullivan-Schein, Port Washington, NY) (see Fig. 8-39), then these should be used to obtain a firm hold of the file and extract it out through the access cavity preparation. Many sizes and angles of forceps are available, and almost all are necessary in order to have the ability to remove obstructions from the many different angles and levels of accessibility presented to the clinician. These will work well if the object is loose fitting within the canal and if the clinician has good access. However, establishing a firm purchase can sometimes be difficult without removing excessive tooth structure. Once a purchase onto the file has been achieved, it is best to pull it from the canal with a slight counterclockwise action. This action will unscrew the flutes that are engaged in the dentin as the file is being removed. This is the easiest technique for removal of a separated file; however, unfortunately, many files separate at a point where these forceps cannot be used.

Frequently, a file will separate at a point deeper in the canal where visibility is difficult. To remove separated root canal

instruments predictably, the clinician must create straight-line coronal radicular access. Either removing the crown or creating a large access cavity preparation establishes adequate coronal access to allow the use of the appropriate instruments. Straight-line radicular access can be created with the use of modified Gates-Glidden drills. These drills may be ground down or sectioned with a bur at their maximum cross-sectional diameter. This process will create a circumferential staging platform to facilitate ultrasonic use (Fig. 8-60).[187] One study showed that use of similarly modified Lightspeed nickel-titanium rotary instruments (Lightspeed Technology Inc, San Antonio, TX) created a staging platform that was more centered in curved canals than the Gates-Glidden drills.[115]

Ultrasonic instruments have been shown to be very effective for the removal of canal obstructions.[36,161,187] The ultrasonic tip is placed on the staging platform between the exposed end of the file and the canal wall and is vibrated around the obstruction in a counterclockwise direction that applies an unscrewing force to the file as it is being vibrated. This technique will help with removing instruments that have a clockwise cutting action. If the file had a counterclockwise cutting action (such as the hand GT files), then a clockwise rotation will be needed. The energy applied will aid in loosening the file, and occasionally, the file will appear to jump out of the canal. It is prudent to cover the orifices of the adjacent open canals with cotton or paper points to prevent the removed file fragment from falling into them, causing further case complication[187] (Fig. 8-61). Many sizes and angles of ultrasonic tips are available for this purpose, but in general, the deeper in the canal the obstruction is, the longer and thinner an ultrasonic tip must be. It should be remembered that long, thin tips must be used on very low power settings to prevent tip breakage (Fig. 8-62). Occasionally, if the separated instrument can be bypassed, the use of ultrasonic files can loosen it. Care must be taken, however, to avoid ultrasonic file separation or root perforation.[102] As mentioned previously, nickel-titanium instruments often break into fragments when subject to the energy supplied by an ultrasonic instrument. Clinicians may be tempted to use this information to their advantage by applying the tip of the ultrasonic directly onto nickel-titanium files. Occasionally, this method may work; however, the chance of pushing the separated file further into the canal or beyond the apical foramen may increase the risk of this technique.

If the direct application of ultrasonic energy does not loosen the separated instrument sufficiently to remove it, the fragment must be grabbed and retrieved. This is accomplished with a variety of techniques most using some variant of a microtube. The staging platform is further reduced by ultrasonics until enough of the separated instrument is exposed to retrieve (about 2 to 3 mm).[187] This reduction must be done carefully to avoid root perforation. One relatively simple microtube technique is to use a short piece of stainless-steel tubing that is pushed over the exposed end of the object. A small Hedstrom file is then pushed between the tube and the end of the object using a clockwise turning motion that produces a good mechanical lock between the separated instrument, the tube, and the Hedstrom file. The three connected objects can then be removed by pulling them in a coronal direction[233] (Fig. 8-63).

Another technique is to use a 25-gauge dental injection needle along with a 0.14-mm-diameter steel ligature wire. The needle is cut to remove the beveled end as well as the opposite

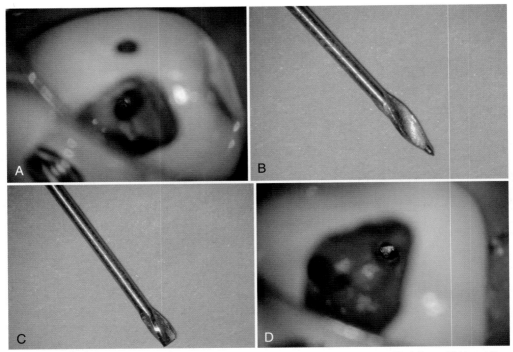

FIG. 8-60 **A,** Separated instrument in the mesiobuccal canal of a molar. **B,** Unmodified Gates-Glidden drill. **C,** Modified instrument. The tip has been ground off to the maximum diameter of the cutting head. **D,** Staging platform created in the straight coronal section of the canal. Note the enhanced visibility and the triangular cross section of this rotary instrument.

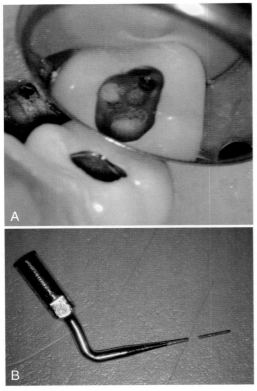

FIG. 8-61 **A,** Cotton pellets protecting the orifices of the other canals when ultrasonic obstruction removal is needed. **B,** Ultrasonic tip separated during excavation around separated instrument. If the adjacent canals were not protected, further unnecessary complication could result.

end so it no longer extends beyond the hub. Both ends of the wire are then passed through the needle from the injection end until they slide out of the hub end, creating a wire loop that extends from the injection end of the needle. Once the loop has passed around the object to be retrieved, a small hemostat is used to pull the wire loop up and tighten it around the obstruction and then the complete assembly is withdrawn from the canal.[185] Occasionally, a larger diameter tube and thinner (0.11-mm) ligature wire will facilitate assembly of this extractor (Fig. 8-64).

Another effective technique, especially in cases where access or obtaining an adequate purchase on the file is difficult, is to use an end-cutting trephine bur to remove tooth structure around the file and then use an extraction device to remove it. There are many kits that use these principals with slight variations from one another, including the Endo Extractor (Brasseler USA), the Masserann Kit (Medidenta International), and the Extractor System (Roydent) (see Fig. 8-54).

The Endo Extractor kit includes a cyanoacrylate adhesive, which is used to bond a hollow tube to the exposed end of the file for removal. This kit also includes four sizes of trephine burs and extractors. The most important factor in using this kit is the snugness of fit between the extractor tube and the obstruction. It has been shown that, even with only 1 millimeter of overlap between the extractor tube and the obstruction, if there is a snug fit, the bond created with the cyanoacrylate may be strong enough to remove many obstructions. However, the recommended amount of overlap between the tube and the obstruction is 2 millimeters. The time needed for the adhesive to set to ensure adequate bond strength for removal is 5 minutes for a snug fit and 10

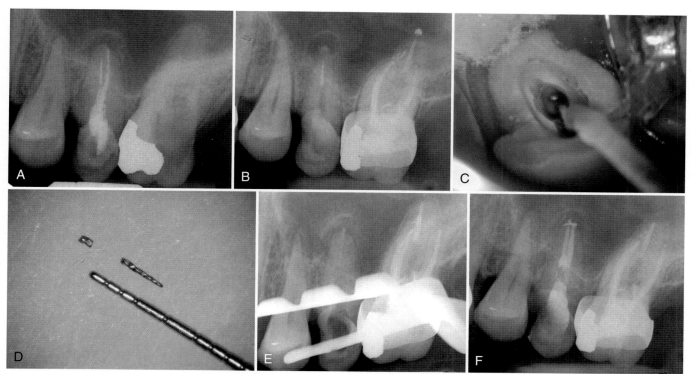

FIG. 8-62 **A**, Preoperative radiograph showing a separated file in the palatal canal, potential coronal leakage, and apical periodontitis. **B**, Check film showing the separated instrument after gutta-percha removal. **C**, Photograph showing the separated instrument in the palatal canal and a paper point in the buccal canal to protect it. **D**, Separated nickel-titanium file removed. Note that it is in two pieces, a result typical when applying ultrasonic energy to nickel-titanium. **E**, Check film showing that the file has been completely removed. **F**, Final canal obturation.

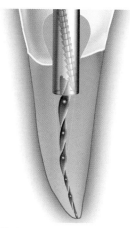

FIG. 8-63 Tube and Hedstrom file removal technique. The tube is slipped over the obstruction and a Hedstrom file is gently screwed into the space between the tube and the obstruction. Pulling the tube and Hedstrom file together can withdraw the obstruction. (Diagram courtesy DENTSPLY Tulsa Dental Specialties, Tulsa, OK.)

minutes for a loose fit.[76,226] One disadvantage of this instrument is that the trephine burs are much larger than their International Standards Organization ISO equivalents, so the manufacturer has also added a separate smaller trephine bur, which is sold separately from the kit. This bur corresponds better with the smaller extractors and removes less dentin

that can decrease the likelihood of weakening the root leading to fracture.[61] Another disadvantage is that the burs cut aggressively when new but dull rather quickly. When new, this aggressive cutting may lead to perforation, or even separation of the obstruction. Therefore, great care is needed when using this instrument (Fig. 8-65). Once the separated instrument has been removed, the extractors may be reused, either by using the debonding agent that is included in the kit to remove the embedded instrument from the extractor tube or by simply cutting the extraction device with a bur beyond the extent that the separated instrument has penetrated.

The Masserann technique has also been recommended for the removal of separated instruments.[151] This technique is similar to the Endo Extractor in that it uses trephine burs and a specific extraction device. This kit comes with a convenient gauge that aids in predicting the size of the bur and the extractor to be used, and it contains many sizes of trephine burs. In addition, the trephine burs with this kit cut in a counterclockwise direction that provides an unscrewing force on separated files. The extraction mandrels have an internal stylus that wedges the file against the internal wall of the mandrel allowing the obstruction to be removed. Although effective, this technique may require removal of an excessive amount of radicular dentin,[69] leading to root weakening and the risk of perforation[272]; therefore, this instrument must be used with caution.

The Extractor System from Roydent comes with only one bur and three extraction devices. The bur is very conservative

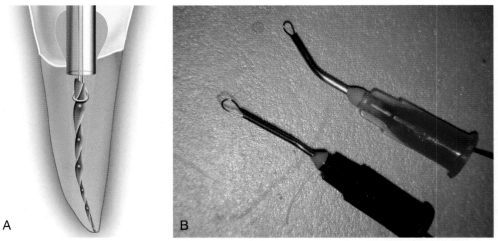

FIG. 8-64 **A**, Diagram illustrating the wire loop and tube method of obstruction removal The wire loop is carefully placed around the obstruction, tightened, and then removed. **B**, Larger diameter tubes and smaller diameter (0.11-mm) ligature wire enhances the efficiency of this technique. (*A*, Diagram courtesy DENTSPLY Tulsa Dental Specialties, Tulsa, OK.)

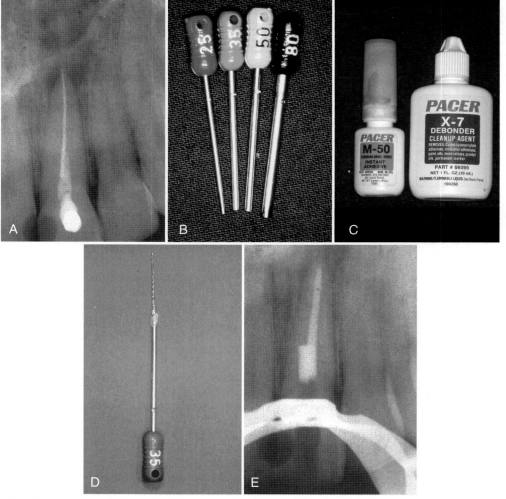

FIG. 8-65 **A**, Separated file wedged into an upper incisor. **B**, Brasseler Endo Extractor tubes. **C**, Cyanoacrylate cement and debonding agent. **D**, Separated file pulled out by the bonded tube. **E**, Final obturation. Note the excessive amount of tooth structure removal by the trephine bur that was needed to bond the tube.

and removes a minimal amount of tooth structure, enabling access to the obstruction. The extractor tubes are also quite small and, therefore, will only work for the removal of small obstructions. The extractor surrounds the obstruction with six prongs that can be tightened onto the object, enabling removal. This works in the same way a drill chuck tightens onto a drill bit (Fig. 8-66). The disadvantages of this kit are the lack of variety of instruments, the possibility of separating the obstruction with the bur, and the potential problem of breakage of the prongs in the extractor if they are submitted to bending rather than applying strict tensile force during removal.

Two techniques have been designed specifically for removing instruments in conjunction with the operating microscope:

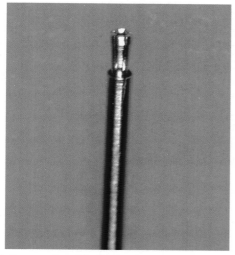

FIG. 8-66 Close-up view of the Roydent Extractor tip. The tip is placed over the separated instrument and tightened to grasp the obstruction.

the Cancellier instrument and the Mounce extractor (Sybron-Endo) (Fig. 8-67). The Cancellier instrument works in a similar manner to the Brasseler Endo Extractor in that it is used in conjunction with cyanoacrylate adhesive to bond onto the separated end of the instrument. Unlike the Brasseler extractors, the Cancellier extractors are attached to a handle that enables them to be used without blocking visibility when using the operating microscope. The Brasseler extractors are finger instruments that interfere with the line of sight the microscope requires. There are no trephine burs in the Cancellier kit; rather, it is used in conjunction with ultrasonic exposure of the separated instrument. Four sizes of extractor tubes are available, each of which corresponds to specific file sizes. The Mounce extractors are also hand instruments that enable use with the operating microscope. These instruments are similar to a ball burnisher with slots cut into the ball end. These slots are cut at various angles and are designed to slide onto the broken end of the file. Cyanoacrylate is used to bond the extractor to the file allowing removal. This instrument can be used when the separated file is lying against the canal wall; however, the ball tip is relatively large and is only useful in retrieving instruments that are in the most accessible coronal portion of the canal.

Another device designed specifically for the purpose of separated file removal is the Instrument Removal System (DENTSPLY Tulsa Dental Specialties) (see Fig. 8-54). This kit consists of two different sizes of extraction devices that are tubes with a 45-degree bevel on the end and a side cutout window. Each tube has a corresponding internal stylus or screw wedge. Prior to use of this instrument, 2 to 3 mm of the obstruction is exposed by troughing around it with an ultrasonic instrument. Once the file is exposed, the appropriate size microtube is selected and slid into place over the obstruction. Once in place, the screw wedge is turned counterclockwise to engage and displace the head of the obstruction through the

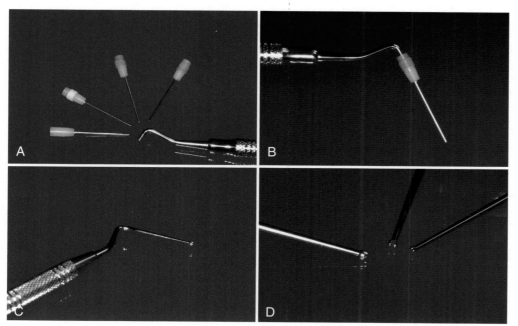

FIG. 8-67 **A,** The Cancellier Kit with four tube sizes available. **B,** The Cancellier instrument is used with super glue to bond the obstruction but its design allows for greater visibility during use. **C,** The Mounce instrument. **D,** Varying tip sizes for the Mounce instrument.

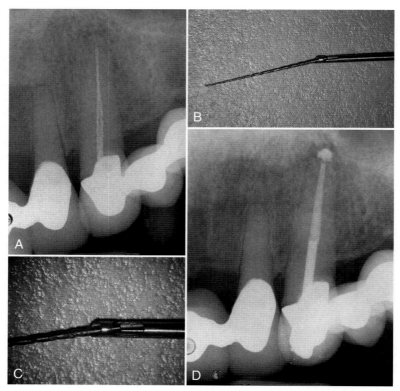

FIG. 8-68 **A**, Preoperative radiograph showing two separated instruments in one tooth. **B**, IRS instrument with a removed file. **C**, Note that large size files are difficult to push through the cutout window. **D**, Postoperative radiograph.

side window. The assembly is then removed.[187] This instrument is useful in the straight portion of the canal, but it is difficult to force large-diameter separated files through the cutout window, hampering their removal (Fig. 8-68).

The S.I.R. (Separated Instrument Retrieval) System (Vista Dental Products) (see Fig. 8-54) is another microtube method of separated instrument retrieval. Like the Cancellier instrument, it utilizes extractor tubes bonded onto an obstruction, enabling removal. Once the obstruction is exposed using ultrasonics or the trephine burs from one of the other kits described, the bendable dead-soft tubes are bonded onto it. Once the adhesive is set, the obstruction is removed through the access cavity preparation. Included in this kit are the necessary bonding agent, a bottle of accelerator, five different sizes of tubes, assorted fulcrum props, and a hemostat. The accelerator causes the bonding agent to set almost instantaneously. The ability to bend these tubes allows for access in most areas of the mouth. A hemostat allows the clinician to establish a firm purchase onto the tube, creating the ability to lever the bonded obstruction out of the canal. A vinyl, autoclavable instrument prop provides protection for the next most anterior tooth, which is to be used as a fulcrum; however, if the clinician has access to grasp the extractor with his or her fingers to remove the extractor/obstruction unit, the hemostat may not be necessary.

Heat Generation During Retreatment Procedures

There are many procedures in endodontic therapy that can generate heat, but perhaps the area with the greatest risk of

heat related tissue damage occurs during nonsurgical retreatment. Use of heat to soften canal filling materials to aid in their removal[132,139] and use of ultrasonics to dislodge posts[192] and separated instruments[95,146] can potentially generate enough heat to raise the temperature of the external root surface by 10° C or more. Temperature elevations of the periodontal ligament in excess of 10° C can cause damage to the attachment apparatus.[11,53,194,195]

The greatest danger of heat-related damage occurs with the use of ultrasonic energy to dislodge foreign objects in the canal space in order to gain access to the apical portion. As described earlier, this has recently become an extremely important and useful part of the clinician's armamentarium due to the ability of ultrasonic energy application to conserve tooth structure while removing the obstruction. These instruments have allowed clinicians to perform predictable retreatment when surgery would have been previously indicated. As with most instruments used in dentistry, however, these devices must be used with caution as in vitro research and clinical case reports imply that they have the potential to damage the tooth attachment apparatus due to the heat generated during use.[30,78,201] One in vitro study has showed that ultrasonic vibration for post removal without coolant can cause root surface temperature increases approaching 10° C in as little as 15 seconds.[48] Thermal damage to the periradicular tissues may be so serious as to result in both tooth loss and permanent bone loss (see Fig. 8-28). This is not to say that ultrasound energy should be avoided for the removal of canal obstructions because it is many times the only way to reach the apical area of the canal.

The factors that may contribute to a heat-induced injury are the length of the post, post diameter, post material, and type of luting cement. Studies need to be done to establish heat reduction protocols based on these variables. Some have proposed that the dentin thickness between the outer surface of the post and the root surface may affect root surface temperature rise,[81,82] and one study showed this.[192] However, a more recent study has shown that the dentin thickness is statistically insignificant as a factor in root surface temperature rise.[101] One possible mitigating factor would be the effect of the periradicular blood supply, which could act as a heat sink dissipating the generated thermal energy and thus helping to prevent injury. This may be why the effect of seemingly similar conditions of ultrasonic application can have such differing results on different patients. Clearly, more in vivo research is needed in this area.

It has become accepted that the heat-induced damage to periradicular tissues during the usage of ultrasound energy for post removal is time dependent.[30,106] Studies have advised cooling of the ultrasonic tips can greatly reduce heat buildup[30,106] despite reducing the efficiency of debonding resin bonded posts.[48,73] The amount of time the clinician can use these instruments safely is difficult to determine, as specific protocols that are evidence based using in vivo research have yet to be established. Therefore, the authors feel any specific recommendations regarding rest intervals between usage of ultrasound energy, ways of monitoring heat buildup, or duration of consistent activation cannot be made based on the available research at the time of publication. However, the authors do feel strongly with regard to several recommendations for the use of ultrasound energy during the removal of canal obstructions, and they are as follows:

- Use ultrasonic tips with water ports whenever possible.
- If your ultrasound device does not have tips with water ports, have your assistant use a continuous coolant air/water spray during usage.[55]
- Take frequent breaks to let the tooth cool down.
- Avoid using the ultrasound on the high power setting.[55]

Prudent clinicians must take extreme care when applying ultrasound energy to a canal obstruction, as it has been shown that even with the use of water coolant, the temperature of root surfaces can increase rapidly.[48,192] Thus, until evidence-based heat reduction protocols are developed, caution is required when using instruments that can generate heat in the periodontal ligament.

Management of Canal Impediments

Following removal of all root-filling materials, further progress to the apical constriction may be prevented by the presence of a block or a ledge in the apical portion of the canal. Most of these impediments are iatrogenic mishaps resulting from vigorous instrumentation short of the appropriate working length and failure to confirm apical patency regularly during instrumentation. A blocked canal contains residual pulp tissue (sometimes necrotic, often fibrosed or calcified) and packed dentinal "mud" in the apical several millimeters of the canal system.[187] This debris is frequently infected, resulting in persistent disease, and must be removed if possible. A ledge is the result of placing non-precurved, end-cutting instruments into curved canals and filing with too much apical pressure.[79,116] It is a type of canal transportation that results in a canal irregularity on the outside of the canal curvature that is difficult or impossible to bypass. The canal space apical to the ledge is not thoroughly cleaned and sealed, so ledges frequently result in

posttreatment disease. The best treatment for blocked and ledged canals, as with all iatrogenic problems, is prevention. If the clinician is careful and attentive during the instrumentation process, the chance for an impediment to develop is minimized. When the clinician becomes careless or hurried, problems occur. The strategies for preventing blocks and ledges are found in Chapter 19.

During the treatment-planning phase, blocks and ledges may be detectible on radiographs as a root filling short of the ideal working length, and the patient should be warned that they might prove impenetrable and require future apical surgery or extraction.[68] This should not deter the clinician from choosing nonsurgical retreatment, however. In one study, 74% of teeth showing short root fillings were successfully negotiated to adequate length, with the authors stating that presence of a short fill should not be considered a technical contraindication to retreatment.[57] The clinical encounter usually occurs after removal of the previous root-filling material when apical advancement of small files is impeded. At this point, the clinician may be unaware of which type of impediment exists, but a common approach to management is helpful in the early stages of the process. The coronal portion of the canal should be enlarged to enhance tactile sensation and remove cervical and middle third obstructions in the canal space. The canal should be flooded with irrigant, and instrumentation to the level of the impediment should be accomplished using non-end-cutting rotary files, such as the Lightspeed (Lightspeed Endodontics, San Antonio, TX), the Profile or GT instruments (Dentsply, York, PA), or the K-3 instrument (Sybron Endodontics, Orange, CA), in a crown-down manner. This procedure will enlarge and flare the canal space coronal to the impediment while minimizing the likelihood of worsening any ledge present.

At this point, the impediment should be gently probed with a precurved #8 or #10 file to determine if there are any "sticky" spots that could be the entrance to a blocked canal. A directional rubber stop should be used so that the clinician knows in which direction the tip of the instrument is pointing, which helps in visualizing the three-dimensional layout of the canal system. Frequently, evacuating the irrigant and using a lubricant, such as RC Prep (Premier, Plymouth Meeting, PA) or Pro-Lube (Dentsply), will enhance the ability to place the small file into the apical canal segment. If repeated, gentle apical pressure or "pecking" of the hand file against the blockage results in some resistance when withdrawing the instrument on the outstroke ("stickiness"), then the clinician should continue to peck at the "sticky" spot until further apical advancement is accomplished.[187] This is frequently a slow and tedious process. The endeavor can be made more efficient by using precurved stiff files such as the C+ file (Maillefer, Baillagues, Switzerland), but there is a risk of deviating from the original canal path, creating a ledge, and ultimately a false canal leading to zip perforation.[79] It is prudent to make a working radiograph when some apical progress has been made to confirm the placement of the instrument into the suspected apical extent of the canal. The clinician should resist the urge to rotate the file excessively. If the tip of a small instrument is tightly bound in the blocked segment of the canal and the tip has been worked by pecking, it is prone to fracture in the apical area further complicating the case.[187] The separated file tip is frequently irretrievable, and surgery or extraction may be the result. Dropping down to the next smaller size file and using a gentle reciprocal rotational motion ("twiddling") will aid in

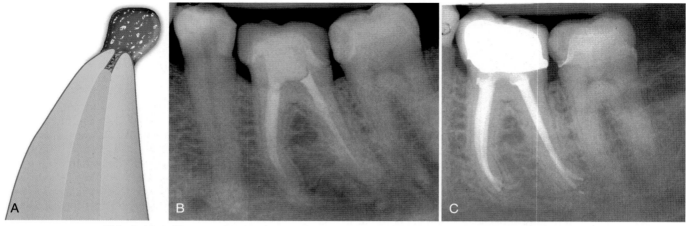

FIG. 8-69 **A,** Diagrammatic representation of a canal block. Fibrotic or calcified pulp and debris that is potentially infected remains in the apical segment of the canal when the canal is instrumented short of the apical constriction. **B,** Preoperative radiograph showing obturation short of ideal length. The patient was symptomatic and the canals were blocked. **C,** The 3-month posttreatment. Treatment took a total of 3.5 hours over three appointments due to the time-consuming nature of bypassing blocked canals. (*A,* Diagram courtesy DENTSPLY Tulsa Dental Specialties, Tulsa, OK.)

advancement through the blocked canal. Frequently, as apical progress is being made, the clinician will be using an electronic apex locator to gauge the proximity of the apical constriction. Unfortunately, the apex locator is sometimes not able to give an accurate reading in a blocked canal, and because of the continued "sticky" feel that occurs even as the instrument bypasses the foramen and penetrates apical tissues, an overextension may result. To prevent this complication with its attendant risk of a painful postoperative flare-up, when the estimated working length is reached, a working length radiograph is necessary.[149] Once apical working length is achieved, apical patency should be confirmed, and gentle, short amplitude 1- to 2-mm push pull strokes should be made until the file can pass freely to the apical constriction (Fig. 8-69).

If, after a reasonable amount of time, no sticky spot can be found, the clinician must consider the possible presence of a ledge despite possibly not detecting it on the preoperative radiograph. The main problem with ledges is that instruments will invariably find their way to the ledge while finding the original canal is many times impossible. They feel like a hard brick wall, short of length when encountered, and care must be used to prevent worsening the ledge by indiscriminately burrowing into it.[255] To manage a ledge, the tip of a small #08 or #10 file has a small bend placed in it 1 to 2 mm from the end,[116,247] so the tip of the file forms an approximately 45-degree angle with the shaft of the instrument. The directional stop is oriented to the bend, and the file is carefully negotiated to the level of the ledge. Because ledges form mainly on the outside of curvatures, the directional stop (and thus the bent tip of the file) is turned in the direction of the suspected apical curvature away from the ledge (Fig. 8-70). The file tip is slowly scraped along the internal wall of the canal curve slightly coronal to the level of the ledge[247] in an effort to find another sticky spot. This spot will be the entrance to the apical canal segment, and gentle reciprocal rotation will usually allow the file to be negotiated to the canal terminus. Confirm with a radiograph. Once the ledge has been bypassed, short amplitude push-pull and rotational forces keeping the file tip apical to the ledge will be needed to clean and enlarge the apical canal space. When the

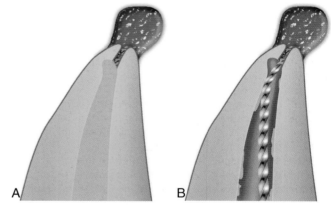

FIG. 8-70 **A,** Diagrammatic representation of a ledged canal. Potentially infected debris remaining in the apical segment can result in posttreatment disease. **B,** Attempting to bypass the ledge with a small file having a 45-degree bend in the tip. Note that the opening to the apical canal segment is on the inside of the canal curvature and coronal to the level of the ledge. (Diagrams courtesy DENTSPLY Tulsa Dental Specialties, Tulsa, OK.)

file can be easily negotiated around the ledge, anticurvature filing will enable the clinician to blend the ledge into the canal preparation (Fig. 8-71). Many times this cannot be completely accomplished,[255] but as long as the apical segment can be cleaned and obturated, the prognosis should not be adversely affected.

The use of Greater Taper (GT) NiTi hand files (DENTSPLY Tulsa Dental Specialties) for the blending of ledges has been advocated.[187] The advantage these instruments have is that they are non-end cutting, and their rate of taper is two to six times that of conventional 0.02 tapered files, so they can do the work of multiple 0.02 tapered hand files. Once the ledge has been bypassed and the canal can be negotiated with a conventional size #15 or 20 K-file, a GT hand file is selected. The K-file creates a pilot hole so that the tip of the GT file can passively follow this glide path beyond the ledge. The GT file must have

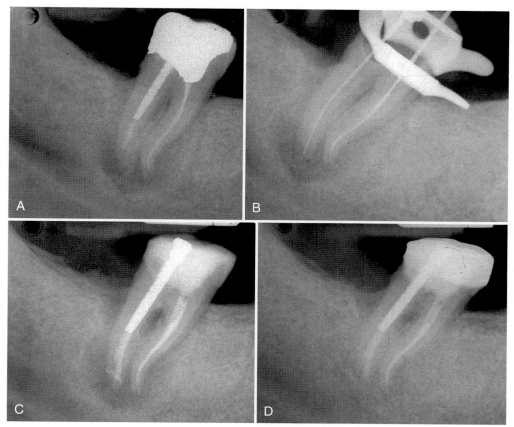

FIG. 8-71 **A,** Preoperative radiograph showing a distal canal ledge with a small amount of sealer that has entered the apical segment. The ledge prevented proper cleaning and sealing of the canal system resulting in posttreatment disease. **B,** The ledge has been bypassed. The attempt is made to blend the ledge into the contour of the prepared canal wall. **C,** Final obturation showing the filled ledge and apical segment. **D,** A 13-month recall showing healing. The patient was then directed to have a definitive coronal restoration placed.

a tip diameter of 0.2 mm (#20) and a taper that will vary depending on the requirements of the preparation. The largest taper that will enter the apical segment is used; however, these instruments must be precurved, which presents a challenge because they are made from nickel-titanium alloy. To precurve this superelastic shape memory alloy, a file-bending tool, such as the Endo Bender Pliers (SybronEndo), is needed. The pliers grasp the tip of the instrument, and the file is overcurved between 180 and 270 degrees to plastically deform the alloy. At this time, the appropriate tapered GT file is then carried into the canal, and the rubber stop is oriented so that the instruments precurved, working end can bypass and move apical to the ledge. The GT file is then worked to length, and the ledge is either reduced or eliminated (Fig. 8-72).

If the canal blockage or ledge cannot be negotiated, then the canal space coronal to the impediment should be cleaned, shaped, obturated, and coronally sealed. The patient must be informed of this complication, the guarded prognosis, and the need for regular reevaluation (Fig. 8-73). If symptoms of posttreatment disease arise subsequently, apical surgery or extraction will be needed.[187,247]

Finishing the Retreatment

After regaining the apical extent of the canal system, routine endodontic procedures are instituted to complete the retreatment. Any missed canals must be found using magnification,

micro-excavation techniques and, most important, the knowledge of canal anatomy that is discussed in another section of this text (Fig. 8-74). One cannot find a canal unless one suspects it is there. Cleaning and shaping procedures must focus on a crown-down approach to minimize extrusion of irritants into the periradicular tissues and also must emphasize enlargement of the apical portion of the preparation to ensure complete removal of apical debris. These aims are best accomplished using technique hybridization during instrumentation and keeping the goals of the retreatment procedure in mind. These matters are covered in detail in Chapter 6. Canal disinfection procedures are, however, paramount after the completion of cleaning and shaping. Because the primary cause of posttreatment disease is usually microbial[64,163] and these microbes (i.e., *Enterococcus faecalis*) are frequently resistant to traditional canal disinfection regimens,[16] every effort must be made to eliminate these organisms from the canal system. This effort is complicated by the fact that no instrumentation regimen can predictably remove the entire previous root filling from the canal space after retreatment.[12] This leaves areas where microbes can reside underneath fragments of root-filling materials and remain protected from standard antimicrobial canal irrigants such, as sodium hypochlorite. Whether the canal space can be adequately disinfected when completing treatment in one visit or whether an interappointment medicament such as calcium hydroxide is needed is still a matter of debate, and the reader

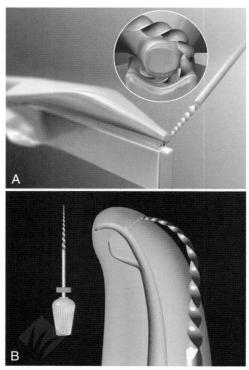

FIG. 8-72 **A,** Endobender Pliers (SybronEndo) used to overbend a nickel-titanium Hand GT file. **B,** GT hand file can hold a bend to allow it to bypass ledges. (Images courtesy Dr. Steve Buchanan.)

is directed to the appropriate chapter of this text for details of the problem. It is important to keep in mind, however, that teeth that require retreatment also require the highest level of disinfection possible to ensure the most favorable outcome.

REPAIR OF PERFORATIONS

Occasionally posttreatment endodontic disease will be the result of root perforation.[112] Root perforations are created pathologically by resorption and caries, and iatrogenically during root canal therapy (zip, strip, and furcation perforations) or its aftermath (e.g., post preparation perforation)[184] (Fig. 8-75). When they are present, perforations may usually be found during the diagnostic phase as areas where the root-filling materials or possibly restorative materials such as posts are found to radiographically leave the confines of the presumed canal space and approach or cross the radiographic interface between the dentin and the periodontal ligament. Angled radiographs are of paramount importance in determining whether a perforation exists and locating which surface or surfaces of the root have been perforated. This information is necessary when deciding upon treatment options. Frequently, cervical and occasionally midroot perforations are associated with epithelial downgrowth and subsequent periodontal defects, so thorough periodontal assessment is required[148,206] (Fig. 8-76). If there were no evidence of posttreatment disease associated with the defect or tooth, then no treatment would be indicated. If, however, there is evidence of periradicular periodontitis, repair may be instituted in one of two ways,

FIG. 8-73 **A,** Preoperative radiograph showing mesial canal blockages and potential distal root ledging with accompanying posttreatment disease. **B,** Final film showing mesial blockages bypassed but inability to negotiate beyond the distal ledge. The patient elected to pursue no further treatment at this time. **C,** One-year recall. Despite not achieving all of the aims of conventional endodontic therapy, periradicular healing is apparent. The patient is asymptomatic and will now begin the final restoration with the knowledge that apical surgery may be needed in the future.

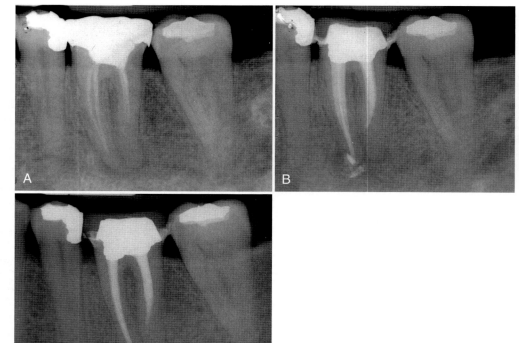

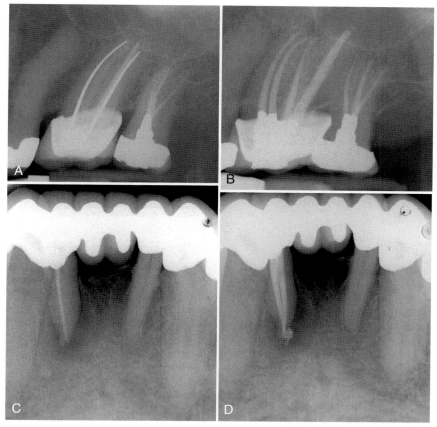

FIG. 8-74 Frequently missed canals that may result in posttreatment disease **A,** Missed second mesiobuccal canal (MB2) in an upper molar. **B,** Final obturation showing cleaned, shaped, and filled MB2 canal. **C,** Missed lingual canal on a lower incisor results in posttreatment disease. **D,** Immediate postoperative film showing management of the missed canal.

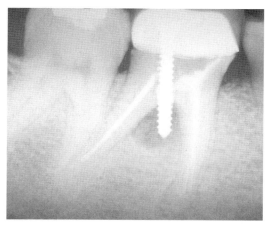

FIG. 8-75 Furcal post perforation resulting in persistent infection and furcal bone loss.

either nonsurgically by approaching the defect internally through the tooth or surgically by using an external approach through the periradicular tissues.[184] In general, if all other factors are considered equal, internal nonsurgical perforation repair will be the preferred method, as it is usually less invasive, produces less destruction of periradicular tissues via the surgical access wound needed, and usually enhances isolation from microbes and disinfection. If, however, the defect is readily accessible surgically and disassembly of the existing restorations would impose an unacceptably high cost and long treatment time to the patient, surgical repair should be selected. If a longstanding defect has a periodontal lesion that has formed around it, surgery perhaps with guided tissue regeneration will usually be needed. However, in most of these cases, nonsurgical retreatment and internal perforation repair prior to surgery will be beneficial to the treatment outcome. A multidisciplinary approach will be required, usually in consultation with the restorative dentist, a periodontist, and perhaps an orthodontist.[187,260]

Factors that affect the prognosis of perforation repair include location of perforation, time delay before perforation repair, ability to seal the defect, and previous contamination with microorganisms.[129,206,213] In general, the more apical the perforation site, the more favorable is the prognosis; however, the converse is true for the repair procedure itself. The difficulty of the repair will be determined by the level at which the perforation occurred. If the defect is in the furcal floor of a multirooted tooth or in the coronal one third of a straight canal (access perforation), it is considered to be easily accessible. If it is in the middle one third of the canal (strip or post perforations), difficulty increases, and in the apical one third of the canal (instrumentation errors), predictable repair is most challenging and, frequently, apical surgery will be needed.

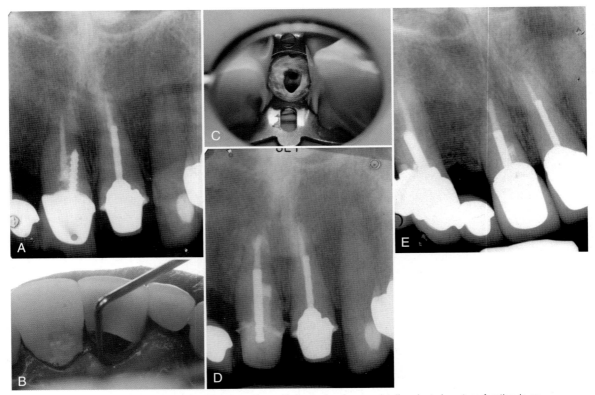

FIG. 8-76 A, Mesially angulated preoperative radiograph showing a palatally oriented post perforation in an upper incisor. **B,** An 8-mm narrow-based probing defect on the mesiopalatal corner of the tooth. **C,** Following coronal disassembly, the true canal can be seen lying in a facial direction relative to the palatal post preparation. **D,** The perforation was repaired with an external matrix of Colla-Cote and MTA. Subsequently, in conjunction with a periodontist, periodontal flap surgery was used to remove periodontal disease etiology from the longstanding pocket, and guided tissue regeneration procedures were instituted. **E,** The 3-year reevaluation. The tooth is asymptomatic, and the mesiopalatal probing depth is 4 mm.

Immediate repair is better than delayed repair, as delay can cause breakdown of the periodontium, resulting in endo-perio lesions that are difficult to manage,[118,212] and elimination of microbial contamination of the defect and sealing it properly is critical to success. Many materials have been advocated for the repair of perforations in the past; however, none provided predictable healing after treatment. Commonly used materials include amalgam, Super EBA cement (Bosworth, Skokie, IL), various bonded composite materials, and, more recently, mineral trioxide aggregate (Pro-Root MTA, DENT-SPLY Tulsa Dental Specialties)[187] (Fig. 8-77).

Since the recent introduction of mineral trioxide aggregate for perforation repair, the choice of which repair material to use is more clear.[148,184] MTA has many advantages over other restoratives when being used for perforation repair. This material seals well,[167,270] even when the cavity preparation is contaminated with blood.[243] It is very biocompatible,[171,179,244,246] rarely eliciting any response from the periradicular tissues, and a cementum-like material has been consistently shown to grow directly on the material after placement.[100,179] MTA has also been shown to have a high degree of clinically favorable long-term outcomes when used as a perforation repair material.[148,184] The main disadvantage of MTA is the long time required for setting,[245] which makes this material inappropriate for transgingival defects such as those associated with cervical

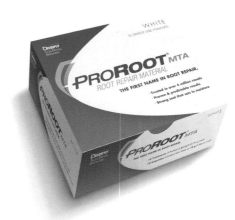

FIG. 8-77 ProRoot MTA is a medical grade of Portland cement that has had the arsenic removed so that it can be used in the human body. It is the material of choice for endodontic perforation repair. (Courtesy DENTSPLY Tulsa Dental Specialties, Tulsa, OK.)

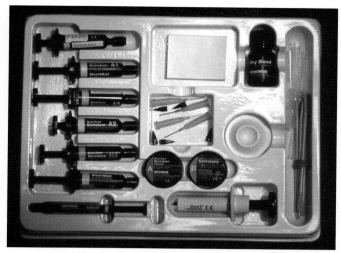

FIG. 8-78 Geristore Kit. This and other resin-ionomers have been advocated for cervical perforation repair due to good biocompatibility and the shorter more controlled setting times that make them useful for transgingival root fillings.

resorption. If the material is in contact with oral fluids, it will wash out of the defect prior to setting, so a more rapid setting resin-ionomer such as Geristore (Den-Mat, Lompoc, CA) is recommended for lesions that cross the gingival margin[18,49,197] (Fig. 8-78). MTA is available in the original gray-colored formulation and a newer, more aesthetic off-white color for treatments in the aesthetic zone of the mouth, although there is little research on the differences between the two formulations. Their sealing ability seems comparable,[60] but questions remain as to whether white MTA exhibits the same biocompatibility[177] and will have the same long-term success as the older variety.

If the perforation is to be repaired nonsurgically through the tooth, coronal-radicular access to the defect is prepared as stated previously (Fig. 8-79). First, the root canals are located and preliminarily instrumented to create enough coronal shape to allow them to be protected from blockage by the repair material. The defect is cleaned and sometimes enlarged with the use of ultrasonics or appropriate rotary drills such as the Gates-Glidden to remove any potentially contaminated dentin surrounding the perforation. Use of a disinfectant irrigating solution such as sodium hypochlorite should be considered if the perforation is not so large as to allow the irrigant to significantly damage the periradicular tissues. If the perforation is large, then sterile saline should be used as an irrigant, and disinfection of the margins of the defect is performed using mechanical dentin removal. Arens and Torabinejad have advocated the use of copious flushing of the defect with 2.5% hypochlorite,[10] but in light of the potential severe complications of hypochlorite overextension through a perforation,[74] extreme care should be used. After the defect has been cleaned, vigorous bleeding may result. Hemostasis should be undertaken using collagen (Colla-Cote, Integra Life Sciences, Plainsboro, NJ) (Fig. 8-79, *B*), calcium sulfate (Capset, Lifecore Biomedical, Chaska, MN), or calcium hydroxide[187]; however, astringents such as ferric sulfate should be avoided, as the coagulum they leave behind may promote bacterial growth and may compromise the seal of the repair.[134]

When the bleeding has been controlled, some easily removable material should be placed over the entrances to the deeper portion of the canals to prevent the repair material from blocking reaccess to the apical terminus. The canals may be protected with cotton, gutta-percha cones, paper points, or shredded collagen. The use of severed files is not recommended, as removal of the files after placement of the repair material is difficult because the material tends to lock into the instrument's flutes (Fig. 8-79, *F*). After protecting the canals, the perforation site is inspected to determine if an external matrix is needed to ensure a proper contour of the restoration.[133] If the surrounding bone is closely adapted to the defect margins, minimal to no matrix material will be necessary; however, if the perforation is associated with a large osseous defect, this must be filled with an external matrix to minimize overcontouring of the repair restoration. The matrix material should be a biocompatible, usually absorbable material such as collagen, freeze-dried demineralized bone allograft (FDDB), hydroxyapatite, Gelfoam, or calcium sulfate.[184,187] Care must be exercised so that the external matrix material is not condensed so forcefully that it damages adjacent vital structures, such as the mental nerve or the floor of the sinus.

Following the preparation of the defect, the repair material is placed. It may be carried in a small syringe or amalgam carrier, and it is condensed with pluggers or microspatulas. In the case of MTA in an accessible defect, the butt end of paper points make an excellent condenser because they can wick some of the water out of the material giving it a firmer consistency, aiding condensation. When the MTA has been positioned, a moist cotton pellet is placed over it to hydrate the material and the tooth is sealed to allow the MTA to set. Upon reentry, the material should be set hard and well retained in the perforation site[217] (see Fig. 8-79, *F*). If there is an overextension of the material beyond the normal external root contour, it seems not to affect the prognosis of the repair.[10,184]

If the perforation is deeper in the canal, the objectives and principles of repair as just outlined all apply, except that access to the defect is more complicated (Fig. 8-80). Protecting the canal from blockage is somewhat more difficult, and placement of the repair material requires the enhanced vision that is provided by the surgical operating microscope. Ideally, the canal should be fully shaped prior to the repair attempt,[187] and a canal patency protector should be placed apical to the defect. In some of these instances, the canal can be protected by using a severed file, notwithstanding the previous warning, because not only can it protect the canal from blockage, but it can also be used as an indirect carrier for transmitting ultrasonic energy to the MTA, causing it to "slump" into the defect when direct condensation is impossible. The file is placed into the canal to a level well below the defect, and the MTA is carried to place. Once condensation has been performed as well as possible, the coronal extent of the file is touched with an ultrasonic tip to vibrate the MTA into the defect. After this is accomplished, the file must be vigorously instrumented in a short 1- to 2-mm amplitude push-pull motion to free it from the placed MTA so that it can be easily removed after the material is set[187] (Fig. 8-81). There is some evidence that ultrasonic placement of MTA may enhance the seal against bacteria in an apexification model,[130] although other researchers have not agreed with this conclusion and found poorer canal wall adaptation when filling the apical extent of canals using ultrasonic condensation compared with hand filling.[8] Further study of ultrasonic MTA placement is warranted, but clinical observation suggests that this method has merit.

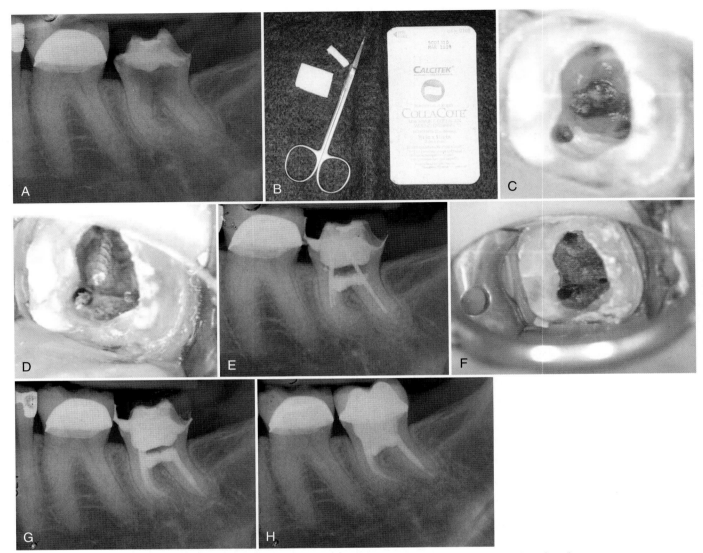

FIG. 8-79 A, Large furcal perforation created during an attempt at endodontic access. **B,** Colla-Cote (Integra Life Sciences, Plainsboro, NJ) to be used as an external matrix material to recreate the external root contour. **C,** Canals have been found, preliminarily instrumented, and the external matrix has been placed. **D,** Canals are protected from being blocked using large endodontic files cut off above the orifice. MTA has been placed into the defect. **E,** Radiograph showing the initial repair with MTA recreating the vault of the furcation. **F,** On the second appointment, the blocking files are removed with difficulty because the MTA has flowed into the flutes and set. At this time, endodontic therapy is completed as normal. **G,** Postobturation radiograph. Note the radiolucency in the furcal vault, which represents the Colla-Cote external matrix material. **H,** The 19-month reevaluation. The patient is asymptomatic, and there is evidence of healing in the furcal vault area.

If the perforation is in the apical portion of the canal, it is usually due to a procedural accident during instrumentation of a curved canal and is invariably accompanied by a block or ledge. This type of perforation is the most difficult to repair, because repair not only involves cleaning and sealing the defect but also finding, cleaning, and filling the apical canal segment. All of the aforementioned techniques for managing blocks and ledges are required to find and clean the apical canal segment. When this has been accomplished, the decision is made as to whether the canal should be filled with MTA or with gutta-percha and sealer. The MTA is undoubtedly more effective in sealing the canal (especially if it cannot be dried) and is much more biocompatible, but carrying it predictably to the apical extent of a curved canal is problematic. If a holding file is placed in the apical canal segment to anticipate eventual gutta-percha placement after the MTA repair material is set, then the presence of the file precludes consistent extension of the MTA into the apical end of the defect, even when ultrasonically vibrated. If a holding file is not placed, the MTA will also flow into the prepared apical segment, which may not be completely three-dimensionally obturated. In general, whichever choice is made, the outcome will be unpredictable, so the patient must be advised that regular reevaluation is necessary and apical surgery or extraction may ultimately be needed.

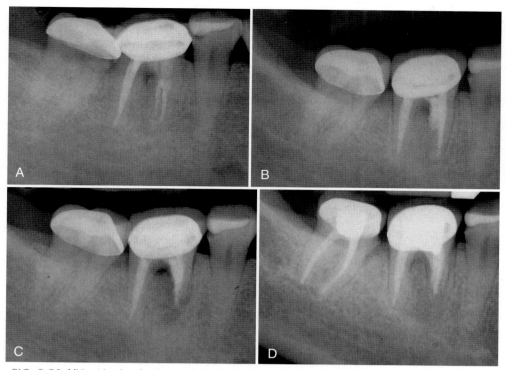

FIG. 8-80 Midroot level perforation repair. **A,** Preoperative film showing mesial strip perforation with bone loss. **B,** Nonsurgical internal repair with inability to negotiate canals to the apical terminus and MTA overextension into the furca. **C,** Apical and perforation repair surgery performed. **D,** he 1-year follow-up showing complete healing.

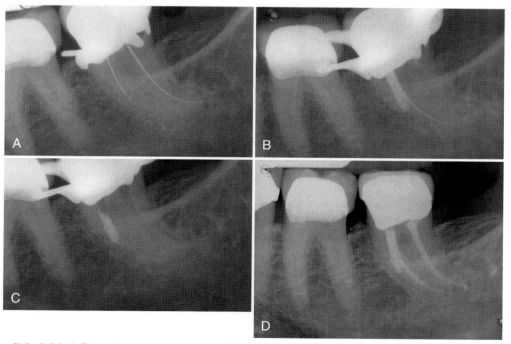

FIG. 8-81 **A,** This patient was in extreme pain following initial endodontic instrumentation by her dentist. Midroot level perforation found on access. **B,** The original canal was found and protected with an endodontic file. MTA was vibrated using ultrasonic energy applied to the file, and it flowed into the defect. Then the file was moved in a push-pull manner to dislodge it from the MTA prior to closure. Note that the defect was intentionally enlarged to allow for more predictable application of the MTA. **C,** On the second appointment, the file was withdrawn easily because it was detached from the MTA repair material. The endodontic therapy could then be concluded as normal. The patient has been asymptomatic since the end of the first appointment. **D,** The 27-month follow-up showing complete healing.

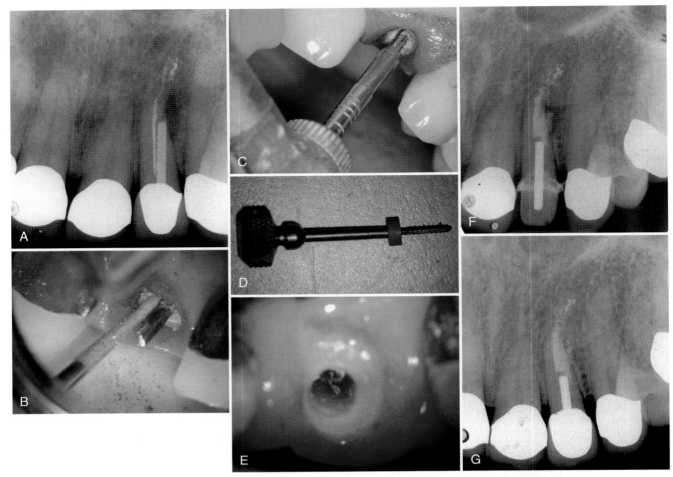

FIG. 8-82 A, Preoperative radiograph showing mid-root level post perforation and associated periradicular periodontitis. **B,** The crown was removed and ultrasonic energy was applied to the post. **C,** Using the trephine bur from the Ruddle Post Removal kit to mill the endo of the post. **D,** The screw post is removed using the wrench from the Ruddle kit. **E,** After removal of the post and gutta-percha, a plastic solid core carrier is found in the canal and removed using the techniques described in this chapter. **F,** Postoperative radiograph showing MTA perforation repair, canal seal with gutta-percha, and post and core fabrication. **G,** The 13-month recall showing healing around the perforation repair site.

PROGNOSIS OF RETREATMENT

When the proper diagnosis has been made and all of the technical aspects of retreatment are carefully performed, orthograde retreatment can be highly successful (Fig. 8-82). The prognosis depends to a large extent on whether apical periodontitis exists prior to retreatment.[169] In a systematic review of outcomes studies,[66] Friedman and Mor reported that in the absence of prior apical periodontitis, the incidence of healed cases after both initial treatment and orthograde retreatment ranges from 92% to 98% up to 10 years after treatment. When prior apical periodontitis is present, the incidence of healing drops to 74% to 86% regardless of whether initial treatment or orthograde retreatment was performed. The authors stated that this "similar potential to heal after initial treatment and orthograde retreatment challenges the historic perception of the latter having a poorer prognosis than the former."[66]

Unfortunately, these numbers mean that the desired outcome will not occur in potentially one quarter of retreatment cases. Many techniques and devices for endodontic retreatment have been mentioned here to aid the clinician. However, none of this will guarantee success. Even when strict endodontic principles and fundamentals are followed, the result may be persistent posttreatment disease. When healing does not occur, the clinician is faced with the decision of what to do next. The choice is between four treatment options: observation, endodontic surgery, extraction-replantation, or extraction.

Many times a tooth that has persistent apical periodontitis may remain in asymptomatic function for an extended period of time, a state that has been referred to as functional retention of the tooth.[66] If the patient's goal of treatment is not necessarily complete healing of the tooth, but simply to retain it in function and without pain, then regular evaluation by the clinician is warranted. If signs and symptoms of worsening infection such as progressive enlargement of a periapical

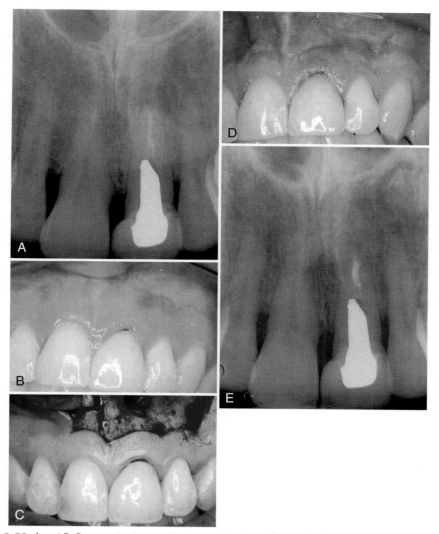

FIG. 8-83 **A** and **B**, Preoperative images showing posttreatment disease in the upper left central incisor and a large custom cast post. The patient elected to leave the post and perform surgery rather than risk damage to his new crown. **C**, Submarginal rectangular flap design. **D**, The 3-week follow-up showing excellent soft tissue healing. **E**, The 18-month follow-up showing excellent healing of the periradicular tissues.

radiolucency, pain, periodontal pocket formation, or sinus tract eruption occur, then further treatment may be needed. However, many teeth classified early on as uncertain healing may indeed be retained for many years.[157]

Endodontic surgery (Fig. 8-83) is a very predictable procedure[66,89] that can be performed on most teeth; however, there are some anatomic and medical concerns regarding treatment planning for this procedure, which are covered in detail in another chapter. Extraction-replantation (Fig. 8-84), also referred to as intentional replantation,[170] is another treatment option. This involves extraction of the tooth and performing the apicoectomy and root-end filling while the tooth is out of the patient's mouth, followed by replantation and splinting if indicated. This procedure is also discussed in detail in Chapter 9. Extraction and replacement should be the treatment of last resort to be selected only when the tooth has been shown to be nonrepairable. If the decision is made to extract

the tooth, usually replacement will be necessary to prevent shifting of the dentition with its attendant problems. Replacement can be with an implant, a fixed partial denture, or a removable partial denture.

SUMMARY

Posttreatment endodontic disease does not preclude saving the involved tooth. In fact, the majority of these teeth can be returned to health and long-term function by current retreatment procedures. In most instances the retreatment option provides the greatest advantage to the patient because there is no replacement that functions as well as a natural tooth. Armed with the information in the preceding section, appropriate armamentaria, and the desire to do what is best for the patient, the clinician will provide the foundation for long-term restorative success.

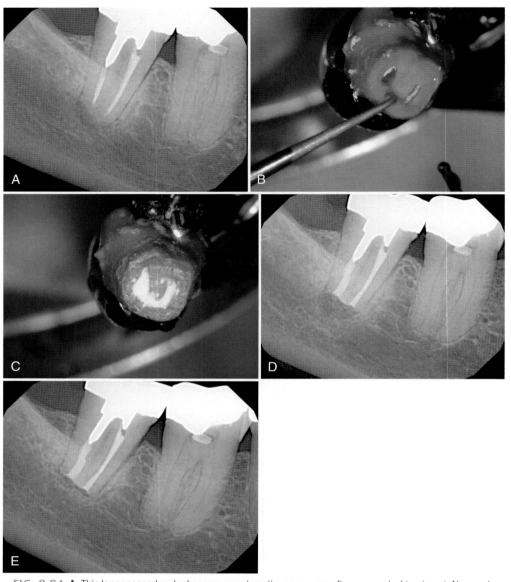

FIG. 8-84 **A,** This lower second molar became symptomatic many years after nonsurgical treatment. Nonsurgical retreatment had a guarded prognosis due to the large multiroot cast custom post and core. Surgery was precluded by the poor access and proximity of the inferior alveolar canal. **B,** Ultrasonic root end preparation is made in the extracted tooth. **C,** A white MTA retrograde filling was placed. Note the C-shape. **D,** Immediate postimplantation radiograph. **E,** The 7-month reevaluation showing apical healing. The patient was asymptomatic.

REFERENCES

1. AAE/AAOMR: *Use of cone-beam-computed tomography in endodontics,* 2009.
2. Abbott PV: Incidence of root fractures and methods used for post removal, *Int Endod J* 35:63, 2002.
3. Abramovitz I, Relles-Bonar S, Baransi B, Kfir A: The effectiveness of a self-adjusting file to remove residual gutta-percha after retreatment with rotary files, *Int Endod J* 45:386, 2012.
4. ADA Council on Scientific Affairs: Dental endosseous implants: an update, *J Am Dent Assoc* 135:92, 2004.
5. Allard U, Andersson L: Exposure of dental personnel to chloroform in root-filling procedures, *Endod Dent Traumatol* 8:155, 1992.
6. Altshul JH, Marshall G, Morgan LA, Baumgartner JC: Comparison of dentinal crack incidence and of post removal time resulting from post removal by ultrasonic or mechanical force, *J Endod* 23:683, 1997.
7. American Association of Endodontists: *Guide to clinical endodontics,* Chicago, 2004, American Association of Endodontists.
8. Aminoshariae A, Hartwell GR, Moon PC: Placement of mineral trioxide aggregate using two different techniques, *J Endod* 29:679, 2003.
9. Amsterdam M: Periodontal prosthesis: twenty-five years in retrospect, *Alpha Omegan* 67:8, 1974.
10. Arens DE, Torabinejad M: Repair of furcal perforations with mineral trioxide aggregate: two case reports, *Oral Surg Oral Med Oral Pathol Oral Radiol Endod* 82:84, 1996.
11. Atrizadeh F, Kennedy J, Zander H: Ankylosis of teeth following thermal injury, *J Periodontal Res* 6:159, 1971.
12. Baldassari-Cruz LA, Wilcox LR: Effectiveness of gutta-percha removal with and without the microscope, *J Endod* 25:627, 1999.
13. Baratto Filho F, Ferreira EL, Fariniuk LF: Efficiency of the 0.04 taper ProFile during the re-treatment of gutta-percha-filled root canals, *Int Endod J* 35:651, 2002.
14. Barbosa SV, Burkard DH, Spångberg LS: Cytotoxic effects of gutta-percha solvents, *J Endod* 20:6, 1994.

15. Barrieshi-Nusair KM: Gutta-percha retreatment: effectiveness of nickel-titanium rotary instruments versus stainless steel hand files, *J Endod* 28:454, 2002.

16. Basrani B, Tjaderhane L, Santos JM, et al: Efficacy of chlorhexidine- and calcium hydroxide-containing medicaments against *Enterocaucus faecalis* in vitro, *Oral Surg* 96:618, 2003.

17. Beasley RT, Williamson AE, Justman BC, Qian F: Time required to remove GuttaCore, Thermafil Plus, and Thermoplasticized gutta-percha from moderately curved root canals with ProTaper files, *J Endod* 39:125, 2013.

18. Behnia A, Strassler HE, Campbell R: Repairing iatrogenic root perforations, *J Am Dent Assoc* 131:196, 2000.

19. Berbert A, Filho MT, Ueno AH, et al: The influence of ultrasound in removing intraradicular posts, *Int Endod J* 28:100, 1995.

20. Bergeron BE, Murchison DF, Schindler WG, Walker WA 3rd: Effect of ultrasonic vibration and various sealer and cement combinations on titanium post removal, *J Endod* 27:13, 2001.

21. Bertrand MF, Pellegrino JC, Rocca JP, et al: Removal of Thermafil root canal filling material, *J Endod* 23:54, 1997.

22. Betti LV, Bramante CM: Quantec SC rotary instruments versus hand files for gutta-percha removal in root canal retreatment, *Int Endod J* 34:514, 2001.

23. Bhaskar SN: Periapical lesion: types, incidence, and clinical features, *Oral Surg* 21:657, 1966.

24. Bhaskar SN, Rappaport HM: Histologic evaluation of endodontic procedures in dogs, *Oral Surg Oral Med Oral Pathol* 31:526, 1971.

25. Block RM, Lewis RD, Hirsch J, et al: Systemic distribution of N2 paste containing 14C paraformaldehyde following root canal therapy in dogs, *Oral Surg Oral Med Oral Pathol* 50:350, 1980.

26. Brady JM, del Rio CE: Corrosion of endodontic silver cones in humans: a scanning electron microscope and X-ray microprobe study, *J Endod* 1:205, 1975.

27. Bramante CM, Betti LV: Efficacy of Quantec rotary instruments for gutta-percha removal, *Int Endod J* 33:463, 2000.

28. Brodin P: Neurotoxic and analgesic effects of root canal cements and pulp-protecting dental materials, *Endod Dent Traumatol* 4:1, 1988.

29. Brown LJ, Nash KD, Johns BA, Warren M: *The economics of endodontics*, Chicago, 2003, American Association of Endodontists.

30. Budd JC, Gekelman D, White JM: Temperature rise of the post and on the root surface during ultrasonic post removal, *Int Endod J* 38:705, 2005.

31. Buhler H: Evaluation of root-resected teeth: results after 10 years, *J Periodontol* 59:805, 1988.

32. Buoncristiani J, Seto BG, Caputo AA: Evaluation of ultrasonic and sonic instruments for intraradicular post removal, *J Endod* 20:486, 1994.

33. Bystrom A, Claesson R, Sundqvist G: The antibacterial effect of camphorated paramonochlorophenol, camphorated phenol and calcium hydroxide in the treatment of infected root canals, *Endod Dent Traumatol* 1:170, 1985.

34. Castrisos T, Abbott PV: A survey of methods used for post removal in specialist endodontic practice, *Int Endod J* 35:172, 2002.

35. Castrisos TV, Palamara JE, Abbott PV: Measurement of strain on tooth roots during post removal with the Eggler post remover, *Int Endod J* 35:337, 2002.

36. Chenail BL, Teplitsky PE: Orthograde ultrasonic retrieval of root canal obstructions, *J Endod* 13:186, 1987.

37. Chugal NM, Clive JM, Spangberg LS: Endodontic infection: some biologic and treatment factors associated with outcome, *Oral Surg Oral Med Oral Pathol Oral Radiol Endod* 96:81, 2003.

38. Chutich MJ, Kaminski EJ, Miller DA, Lautenschlager EP: Risk assessment of the toxicity of solvents of gutta-percha used in endodontic retreatment, *J Endod* 24:213, 1998.

39. Cohen AS, Brown DC: Orofacial dental pain emergencies: endodontic diagnosis and management. In Cohen S, Burns RC, editors: *Pathways of the pulp*, ed 8, St. Louis, 2002, Mosby, p 31.

40. Cohen S, Liewehr F: Diagnostic procedures. In Cohen S, Burns RC, editors: *Pathways of the pulp*, ed 8, St. Louis, 2002, Mosby, p 3.

41. Cohen S, Schwartz S: Endodontic complications and the law, *J Endod* 13:191, 1987.

42. Cotton TP, Geisler TM, Holden DT, et al: Endodontic applications of cone-beam volumetric tomography, *J Endod* 33:1121, 2007.

43. Crump MC, Natkin E: Relationship of broken root canal instruments to endodontic case prognosis: a clinical investigation, *J Am Dent Assoc* 80:1341, 1970.

44. Cunha RS, De Martin AS, Barros PP, et al: In vitro evaluation of the cleansing working time and analysis of the amount of gutta-percha or Resilon remnants in the root canal walls after instrumentation for endodontic retreatment, *J Endod* 33:1426, 2007.

45. da Silveira PF, Vizzotto MB, Liedke GS, et al: Detection of vertical root fractures by conventional radiographic examination and cone beam computed tomography: an in vitro analysis, *Dent Traumatol* 29:41, 2013.

46. de Oliveira DP, Barbizam JV, Trope M, Teixeira FB: Comparison between gutta-percha and resilon removal using two different techniques in endodontic retreatment, *J Endod* 32:362, 2006.

47. de Rijk WG: Removal of fiber posts from endodontically treated teeth, *Am J Dent* 13:19B, 2000.

48. Dominici JT, Clark S, Scheetz J, Eleazer PD: Analysis of heat generation using ultrasonic vibration for post removal, *J Endod* 31:301, 2005.

49. Dragoo MR: Resin-ionomer and hybrid-ionomer cements: part II, human clinical and histologic wound healing responses in specific periodontal lesions, *Int J Periodontics Restorative Dent* 17:75, 1997.

50. Edlund M, Nair MK, Nair UP: Detection of vertical root fractures by using cone-beam computed tomography: a clinical study, *J Endod* 37:768, 2011.

51. Erdemir A, Eldeniz AU, Belli S: Effect g-percha solvents on mineral contents of human root dentin using ICP-AES technique, *J Endod* 30:54, 2004.

52. Erdemir A, Eldeniz AU, Belli S, Pashley DH: Effects of solvents on bonding to root canal dentin [abstract], *J Dent Res (Spec Iss A)* 81:241, 2002.

53. Eriksson AR, Albrektsson T: Temperature threshold levels for heat-induced bone tissue injury: a vital-microscopic study in the rabbit, *J Prosthet Dent* 50: 101, 1983.

54. Estrela C, Bueno MR, De Alencar AH, et al: Method to evaluate inflammatory root resorption by using cone beam computed tomography, *J Endod* 35:1491, 2009.

55. Ettrich CA, Labossiere PE, Pitts DL, Johnson JD: An investigation of the heat induced during ultrasonic post removal, *J Endod* 33:1222, 2007.

56. Ezzie E, Fleury A, Solomon E, et al: Efficacy of retreatment techniques for a resin-based root canal obturation material, *J Endod* 32:341, 2006.

57. Farzaneh M, Abitbol S, Friedman S: Treatment outcome in endodontics: the Toronto study. Phases I and II: orthograde retreatment, *J Endod* 30:627, 2004.

58. Fava LR, Dummer PM: Periapical radiographic techniques during endodontic diagnosis and treatment, *Int Endod J* 30:250, 1997.

59. Ferreira JJ, Rhodes JS, Ford TR: The efficacy of gutta-percha removal using ProFiles, *Int Endod J* 34:267, 2001.

60. Ferris DM, Baumgartner JC: Perforation repair comparing two types of mineral trioxide aggregate, *J Endod* 30:422, 2004.

61. Fors UG, Berg JO: Endodontic treatment of root canals obstructed by foreign objects, *Int Endod J* 19:2, 1986.

62. Frajlich SR, Goldberg F, Massone EJ, et al: Comparative study of retreatment of Thermafil and lateral condensation endodontic fillings, *Int Endod J* 31:354, 1998.

63. Friedman S: Treatment outcome and prognosis of endodontic therapy. In Orstavik D, Pitt-Ford TR, editors: *Essential endodontology: prevention and treatment of apical periodontitis*, London, 1998, Blackwell Science, p 367.

64. Friedman S: Orthograde retreatment. In Walton RE, Torabinejad M, editors: *Principles and practice of endodontics*, ed 3, Philadelphia, 2002, Saunders, p 345.

65. Friedman S, Abitbol S, Lawrence HP: Treatment outcome in endodontics: the Toronto study. Phase 1: Initial treatment, *J Endod* 29:787, 2003.

66. Friedman S, Mor C: The success of endodontic therapy: healing and functionality, *Calif Dent Assoc J* 32:493, 2004.

67. Friedman S, Moshonov J, Trope M: Efficacy of removing glass ionomer cement, zinc oxide eugenol, and epoxy resin sealers from retreated root canals, *Oral Surg Oral Med Oral Pathol* 73:609, 1992.

68. Friedman S, Stabholz A: Endodontic retreatment—case selection and technique. Part 1: criteria for case selection, *J Endod* 12:28, 1986.

69. Friedman S, Stabholz A, Tamse A: Endodontic retreatment—case selection and technique. 3. Retreatment techniques, *J Endod* 16:543, 1990.

70. Fristad I, Molven O, Halse A: Nonsurgically retreated root-filled teeth: radiographic findings after 20-27 years, *Int Endod J* 37:12, 2004.

71. Fukushima H, Yamamoto K, Hirohata K, et al: Localization and identification of root canal bacteria in clinically asymptomatic periapical pathosis, *J Endod* 16:534, 1990.

72. Gambrel MG, Hartwell GR, Moon PC, Cardon JW: The effect of endodontic solutions on resorcinol-formalin paste in teeth, *J Endod* 31:25, 2005.

73. Garrido ADB, Fonseca TS, Alfredo E, et al: Influence of ultrasound, with and without water spray cooling, on removal of posts cemented with resin or zinc phosphate cements, *J Endod* 30:173, 2004.

74. Gernhardt CR, Eppendorf K, Kozlowski A, Brandt M: Toxicity of concentrated sodium hypochlorite used as an endodontic irrigant, *Int Endod J* 37:272, 2004.

75. Gesi A, Magnolfi S, Goracci C, Ferrari M: Comparison of two techniques for removing fiber posts, *J Endod* 29:580, 2003.

76. Gettleman BH, Spriggs KA, ElDeeb ME, Messer HH: Removal of canal obstructions with the Endo Extractor, *J Endod* 17:608, 1991.

77. Giuliani V, Cocchetti R, Pagavino G: Efficacy of ProTaper universal retreatment files in removing filling materials during root canal retreatment, *J Endod* 34:1381, 2008.

78. Glick DH, Frank AL: Removal of silver points and fractured posts by ultrasonics, *J Pros Dent* 55:212, 1986.

79. Glickman GN, Dumsha TC: Problems in canal cleaning and shaping. In Gutmann JL, Dumsha TC, Lovdahl PE, Hovland EJ, editors: *Problem solving in endodontics: prevention, identification, and management*, ed 3, St. Louis, 1997, Mosby, p 91.

80. Glickman GN, Pileggi R: Preparation for treatment. In Cohen S, Burns RC, editors: *Pathways of the pulp*, ed 8, St. Louis, 2002, Mosby, p 103.

81. Gluskin AH, Peters CI, Wong RDM, Ruddle CJ: Retreatment of non-healing endodontic therapy and management of mishaps. In Ingle JI, Bakland LK, Baumgartner JC, editors: *Endodontics*, ed 6, Hamilton, 2008, BC Decker, p 1088.

82. Gluskin AH, Ruddle CJ, Zinman EJ: Thermal injury through intraradicular heat transfer using ultrasonic devices: precautions and practical preventive strategies, *J Am Dent Assoc* 136:1286, 2005.

83. Goldberg RA, Kuttler S, Dorn SO: The properties of Endocal 10 and its potential impact on the structural integrity of the root, *J Endod* 30:159, 2004.

84. Gomes AP, Kubo CH, Santos RA, et al: The influence of ultrasound on the retention of cast posts cemented with different agents, *Int Endod J* 34:93, 2001.

85. Goodacre CJ, Bernal G, Rungcharassaeng K, Kan JY: Clinical complications with implants and implant prostheses, *J Prosthet Dent* 90:121, 2003.

86. Goodacre CJ, Kan JY, Rungcharassaeng K: Clinical complications of osseointegrated implants, *J Prosthet Dent* 81:537, 1999.

87. Gound TG, Marx D, Schwandt NA: Incidence of flare-ups and evaluation of quality after retreatment of resorcinol-formaldehyde resin ("Russian Red Cement") endodontic therapy, *J Endod* 29:624, 2003.

88. Gutierrez JH, Villena F, Gigoux C, Mujica F: Microscope and scanning electron microscope examination of silver points corrosion caused by endodontic materials, *J Endod* 8:301, 1982.

89. Gutmann JL, Harrison JW: *Surgical endodontics*, ed 2, St. Louis, 1994, Ishiyaku EuroAmerica, p 468.

90. Gutmann JL, Lovdahl PE: Problems in the assessment of success and failure, quality assurance, and their integration into endodontic treatment planning. In Gutmann JL, Dumsha TC, Lovdahl PE, Hovland EJ, editors: *Problem solving in endodontics. Prevention, identification, and management*, ed 3, St. Louis, 1997, Mosby, p 1.

91. Gutmann JL, Witherspoon DE: Obturation of the cleaned and shaped root canal system. In Cohen S, Burns RC, editors: *Pathways of the pulp*, St. Louis, 2002, Mosby, p 293.

92. Hammad M, Qualtrough A, Silikas N: Three-dimensional evaluation of effectiveness of hand and rotary instrumentation for retreatment of canals filled with different materials, *J Endod* 34:1370, 2008.

93. Hansen MG: Relative efficiency of solvents used in endodontics, *J Endod* 24:38, 1998.

94. Haselton DR, Lloyd PM, Johnson WT: A comparison of the effects of two burs on endodontic access in all-ceramic high lucite crowns, *Oral Surg Oral Med Oral Pathol Oral Radiol Endod* 89:486, 2000.

95. Hashem AA: Ultrasonic vibration: temperature rise on external root surface during broken instrument removal, *J Endod* 33:1070, 2007.

96. Hassan B, Metska ME, Ozok AR, et al: Detection of vertical root fractures in endodontically treated teeth by a cone beam computed tomography scan, *J Endod* 35:719, 2009.

97. Hassanloo A, Watson P, Finer Y, Friedman S: Retreatment efficacy of the Epiphany soft resin obturation system, *Int Endod J* 40:633, 2007.

98. Hauman CHJ, Chandler NP, Purton DG: Factors influencing the removal of posts, *Int Endod J* 36:687, 2003.

99. Holland R, De Souza V, Nery MJ, et al: Tissue reactions following apical plugging of the root canal with infected dentin chips: a histologic study in dogs' teeth, *Oral Surg Oral Med Oral Pathol* 49:366, 1980.

100. Holland R, Filho JA, de Souza V, et al: Mineral trioxide aggregate repair of lateral root perforations, *J Endod* 27:281, 2001.

101. Horan BB, Tordik PA, Imamura G, Goodell GG: Effect of dentin thickness on root surface temperature of teeth undergoing ultrasonic removal of posts, *J Endod* 34:453, 2008.

102. Hulsmann M: Removal of fractured instruments using a combined automated/ultrasonic technique, *J Endod* 20:144, 1994.

103. Hulsmann M, Bluhm V: Efficacy, cleaning ability and safety of different rotary NiTi instruments in root canal retreatment, *Int Endod J* 37:468, 2004.

104. Hulsmann M, Stotz S: Efficacy, cleaning ability and safety of different devices for gutta- percha removal in root canal retreatment, *Int Endod J* 30:227, 1997.

105. Hunter KR, Doblecki W, Pelleu GB Jr: Halothane and eucalyptol as alternatives to chloroform for softening gutta-percha, *J Endod* 17:310, 1991.

106. Huttula AS, Tordik PA, Imamura G, et al: The effect of ultrasonic post instrumentation on root surface temperature, *J Endod* 32:1085, 2006.

107. Ibarrola JL, Knowles KI, Ludlow MO: Retrievability of Thermafil plastic cores using organic solvents, *J Endod* 19:417, 1993.

108. Imura N, Kato AS, Hata GI, et al: A comparison of the relative efficacies of four hand and rotary instrumentation techniques during endodontic retreatment, *Int Endod J* 33:361, 2000.

109. Imura N, Zuolo ML, Ferreira MO, Novo NF: Effectiveness of the Canal Finder and hand instrumentation in removal of gutta-percha root fillings during root canal retreatment, *Int Endod J* 29:382, 1996.

110. Imura N, Zuolo ML, Kherlakian D: Comparison of endodontic retreatment of laterally condensed gutta-percha and Thermafil with plastic carriers, *J Endod* 19:609, 1993.

111. Ingle JI, Heithersay GS, Hartwell GR, et al: Endodontic diagnostic procedures. In Ingle JI, Bakland LK, editors: *Endodontics*, ed 5, Hamilton, 2002, BC Decker, p 203.

112. Ingle JI, Simon JH, Machtou P, Bogaerts P: Outcome of endodontic treatment and retreatment. In Ingle JI, Bakland LK, editors: *Endodontics*, ed 5, Hamilton, 2002, BC Decker, p 747.

113. Iqbal MK, Johansson AA, Akeel RF, et al: A retrospective analysis of factors associated with the periapical status of restored, endodontically treated teeth, *Int J Prosthodont* 16:31, 2003.

114. Iqbal MK, Kohli MR, Kim JS: A retrospective clinical study of incidence of root canal instrument separation in an endodontics graduate program: a PennEndo database study, *J Endod* 32:1048, 2006.

115. Iqbal MK, Rafailov H, Kratchman SI, Karabucak B: A comparison of three methods for preparing centered platforms around separated instruments in curved canals, *J Endod* 32:48, 2006.

116. Jafarzadeh H, Abbott PV: Ledge formation: review of a great challenge in endodontics, *J Endod* 33:1155, 2007.

117. Jeng HW, ElDeeb ME: Removal of hard paste fillings from the root canal by ultrasonic instrumentation [published erratum appears in *J Endod* 13:565, 1987], *J Endod* 13:295, 1987.

118. Jew RC, Weine FS, Keene JJ Jr, Smulson MH: A histologic evaluation of periodontal tissues adjacent to root perforations filled with Cavit, *Oral Surg Oral Med Oral Pathol* 54:124, 1982.

119. Johnson WT, Leary JM, Boyer DB: Effect of ultrasonic vibration on post removal in extracted human premolar teeth, *J Endod* 17:496, 1996.

120. Kaplowitz GJ: Using rectified turpentine oil in endodontic retreatment, *J Endod* 22:621, 1996.

121. Kaufman D, Mor C, Stabholz A, Rotstein I: Effect of gutta-percha solvents on calcium and phosphorus levels of cut human dentin, *J Endod* 23:614, 1997.

122. Khedmat S, Rouhi N, Drage N, et al: Evaluation of three imaging techniques for the detection of vertical root fractures in the absence and presence of gutta-percha root fillings, *Int Endod J* 45:1004, 2012.

123. Kim E, Lee SJ: Electronic apex locator, *Dent Clin North Am* 48:35, 2004.

124. Koch K: The microscope. Its effect on your practice, *Dent Clin North Am* 41:619, 1997.

125. Koppang HS, Koppang R, Solheim T, et al: Cellulose fibers from endodontic paper points as an etiological factor in postendodontic periapical granulomas and cysts, *J Endod* 15:369, 1989.

126. Krell KV, Neo J: The use of ultrasonic endodontic instrumentation in the re-treatment of a paste-filled endodontic tooth, *Oral Surg Oral Med Oral Pathol* 60:100, 1985.

127. Ladley RW, Campbell AD, Hicks ML, Li SH: Effectiveness of halothane used with ultrasonic or hand instrumentation to remove gutta-percha from the root canal, *J Endod* 17:221, 1991.

128. Langer B, Stein SD, Wagenberg B: An evaluation of root resections: a ten-year study, *J Periodontol* 52:719, 1981.

129. Lantz B, Persson PA: Periodontal tissue reactions after root perforations in dog's teeth: a histologic study, *Odontologisk Tidskrift* 75:209, 1967.

130. Lawley GR, Schindler WG, Walker WA, Kolodrubetz D: Evaluation of ultrasonically placed MTA and fracture resistance with intracanal composite resin in a model of apexification, *J Endod* 30:167, 2004.

131. Lazarski MP, Walker WA 3rd, Flores CM, et al: Epidemiological evaluation of the outcomes of nonsurgical root canal treatment in a large cohort of insured dental patients, *J Endod* 27:791, 2001.

132. Lee FS, Van Cura JE, BeGole E: A comparison of root surface temperatures using different obturation heat sources, *J Endod* 24:617, 1998.

133. Lemon RR: Nonsurgical repair of perforation defects: internal matrix concept, *Dent Clin North Am* 36:439, 1992.

134. Lemon RR, Steele PJ, Jeansonne BG: Ferric sulfate hemostasis: effect on osseous wound healing: left in situ for maximum exposure, *J Endod* 19:170, 1993.

135. Leonard JE, Gutmann JL, Guo IY: Apical and coronal seal of roots obturated with a dentine bonding agent and resin, *Int Endod J* 29:76, 1996.

136. Li H, Zhai F, Zhang R, Hou B: Evaluation of microsurgery with SuperEBA as root-end filling material for treating post-treatment endodontic disease: a 2-year retrospective study, *J Endod* 40:345, 2014.

137. Lin LM, Skribner JE, Gaengler P: Factors associated with endodontic treatment failures, *J Endod* 18:625, 1992.

138. Lindemann M, Yaman P, Dennison JB, Herrero AA: Comparison of the efficiency and effectiveness of various techniques for removal of fiber posts, *J Endod* 31:520, 2005.

139. Lipski M, Wozniak K: In vitro infrared thermographic assessment of root surface temperature rises during thermafil retreatment using system B, *J Endod* 29:413, 2003.

140. Lovdahl PE: Endodontic retreatment, *Dent Clin North Am* 36:473, 1992.

141. Lovdahl PE, Gutmann JL: Problems in nonsurgical root canal retreatment. In Gutmann JL, Dumsha TC, Lovdahl PE, Hovland EJ, editors: *Problem solving in endodontics. Prevention, identification, and management*, ed 3, St. Louis, 1997, Mosby, p 157.

142. Ludlow JB: Dose and risk in dental diagnostic imaging: with emphasis on dosimetry of CBCT, *Kor J Oral and Maxillofac Rad* 39:175, 2009.

143. Luks S: Gutta percha vs. silver points in the practice of endodontics, *NY State Dent J* 31:341, 1965.

144. Maalouf EM, Gutmann JL: Biological perspectives on the non-surgical endodontic management of periradicular pathosis, *Int Endod J* 27:154, 1994.

145. Machtou P, Sarfati P, Cohen AG: Post removal prior to retreatment, *J Endod* 15:552, 1989.

146. Madarati AA, Qualtrough AJ, Watts DC: Factors affecting temperature rise on the external root surface during ultrasonic retrieval of intracanal separated files, *J Endod* 34:1089, 2008.

147. Madison S, Swanson K, Chiles SA: An evaluation of coronal microleakage in endodontically treated teeth. Part II. Sealer types, *J Endod* 13:109, 1987.

148. Main C, Mirzayan N, Shabahang S, Torabinejad M: Repair of root perforations using mineral trioxide aggregate: a long-term study, *J Endod* 30:80, 2004.

149. Mandel E, Friedman S: Endodontic retreatment: a rational approach to root canal reinstrumentation, *J Endod* 18:565, 1992.

150. Martin JA, Bader JD: Five-year treatment outcomes for teeth with large amalgams and crowns, *Oper Dent* 22:72, 1997.

151. Masserann J: Entfernen metallischer Fragmente aus Wurzelkanalen (Removal of metal fragments from the root canal), *J Br Endod Soc* 5:55, 1971.

152. Matherne RP, Angelopoulos C, Kulild JC, Tira D: Use of cone-beam computed tomography to identify root canal systems in vitro, *J Endod* 34:87, 2008.

153. McDonald MN, Vire DE: Chloroform in the endodontic operatory, *J Endod* 18:301, 1992.

154. Messer HH: Permanent restorations and the dental pulp. In Hargreaves KM, Goodis HE, editors: *Seltzer and*

Bender's dental pulp, Chicago, 2002, Quintessence Books, p 345.

155. Metska ME, Aartman IH, Wesselink PR, Ozok AR: Detection of vertical root fractures in vivo in endodontically treated teeth by cone-beam computed tomography scans, *J Endod* 38:1344, 2012.

156. Metzger Z, Ben-Amar A: Removal of overextended gutta-percha root canal fillings in endodontic failure cases, *J Endod* 21:287, 1995.

157. Molven O, Halse A, Fristad I, MacDonald-Jankowski D: Periapical changes following root-canal treatment observed 20-27 years postoperatively, *Int Endod J* 35:784, 2002.

158. Moshonov J, Peretz B, Ben-Zvi K, et al: Effect of gutta-percha solvents on surface microhardness of IRM fillings, *J Endod* 26:142, 2000.

159. Moshonov J, Trope M, Friedman S: Retreatment efficacy 3 months after obturation using glass ionomer cement, zinc oxide-eugenol, and epoxy resin sealers, *J Endod* 20:90, 1994.

160. Mulvay PG, Abbott PV: The effect of endodontic access cavity preparation and subsequent restorative procedures on molar crown retention, *Aust Dent J* 41:134, 1996.

161. Nagai O, Tani N, Kayaba Y, et al: Ultrasonic removal of broken instruments in root canals, *Int Endod J* 19:298, 1986.

162. Nair PN: New perspectives on radicular cysts: do they heal? *Int Endod J* 31:155, 1998.

163. Nair PN, Sjogren U, Krey G, et al: Intraradicular bacteria and fungi in root-filled, asymptomatic human teeth with therapy-resistant periapical lesions: a long-term light and electron microscopic follow-up study, *J Endod* 16:580, 1990.

164. Nair PN, Sjogren U, Krey G, Sundqvist G: Therapy-resistant foreign body giant cell granuloma at the periapex of a root-filled human tooth, *J Endod* 16:589, 1990.

165. Nair PN, Sjogren U, Schumacher E, Sundqvist G: Radicular cyst affecting a root-filled human tooth: a long-term post-treatment follow-up, *Int Endod J* 26:225, 1993.

166. Nair PNR, Schroeder HE: Periapical actinomycosis, *J Endod* 10:567, 1984.

167. Nakata TT, Bae KS, Baumgartner JC: Perforation repair comparing mineral trioxide aggregate and amalgam using an anaerobic bacterial leakage model, *J Endod* 24:184, 1998.

168. Nearing MV, Glickman GN: Comparative efficacy of various rotary instrumentation systems for gutta-percha removal [Abstract], *J Endod* 24:295, 1999.

169. Ng YL, Mann V, Gulabivala K: Outcome of secondary root canal treatment: a systematic review of the literature, *Int Endod J* 41:1026, 2008.

170. Niemczyk SP: Re-inventing intentional replantation: a modification of the technique, *Pract Proced Aesthet Dent* 13:433, 2001.

171. Osorio RM, Hefti A, Vertucci FJ, Shawley AL: Cytotoxicity of endodontic materials, *J Endod* 24:91, 1998.

172. Ozgoz M, Yagiz H, Cicek Y, Tezel A: Gingival necrosis following the use of a paraformaldehyde-containing paste: a case report, *Int Endod J* 37:157, 2004.

173. Parashos P, Messer HH: Questionnaire survey on the use of rotary nickel-titanium endodontic instruments by Australian dentists, *Int Endod J* 37:249, 2004.

174. Parker H, Glickman GN: Solubility of plastic Thermafil carriers, *J Dent Res* 72:188, 1993.

175. Patel S: New dimensions in endodontic imaging: part 2. Cone beam computed tomography, *Int Endod J* 42:463, 2009.

176. Patel S, Dawood A, Ford TP, Whaites E: The potential applications of cone beam computed tomography in the management of endodontic problems, *Int Endod J* 40:818, 2007.

177. Perez AL, Spears R, Gutmann JL, Opperman LA: Osteoblasts and MG-63 osteosarcoma cells behave differently when in contact with ProRoot MTA and White MTA, *Int Endod J* 36:564, 2003.

178. Peters SB, Canby FL, Miller DA: Removal of a carbon-fiber post system [abstract PR35], *J Endod* 22:215, 1996.

179. Pitt-Ford TR, Torabinejad M, McKendry DJ, et al: Use of mineral trioxide aggregate for repair of furcal perforations, *Oral Surg Oral Med Oral Pathol* 79:756, 1995.

180. Ray H, Seltzer S: A new glass ionomer root canal sealer, *J Endod* 17:598, 1991.

181. Regezi JA, Sciubba JJ: Cysts of the oral region. In Regezi JA, Sciubba JJ, editors: *Oral pathology: clinical pathologic correlations*, ed 3, Philadelphia, 1999, Saunders, p 288.

182. Rocas IN, Siqueira JFJ, Santos KR: Association of enterococcus faecalis with different forms of periradicular diseases, *J Endod* 30:315, 2004.

183. Roda R: Clinical showcase—unintentional replantation: a technique to avoid, *J Can Dent Assoc* 72:133, 2006.

184. Roda RS: Root perforation repair: surgical and nonsurgical management, *Pract Proced Aesthet Dent* 13:467, 2001.

185. Roig-Greene JL: The retrieval of foreign objects from root canals: a simple aid, *J Endod* 9:394, 1983.

186. Royzenblat A, Goodell GG: Comparison of removal times of Thermafil plastic obturators using ProFile rotary instruments at different rotational speeds in moderately curved canals, *J Endod* 33:256, 2007.

187. Ruddle CJ: Non-surgical endodontic retreatment. In Cohen S, Burns RC, editors: *Pathways of the pulp*, ed 8, St. Louis, 2002, Mosby, p 875.

188. Ruddle CJ: Nonsurgical retreatment, *J Endod* 30:827, 2004.

189. Sabourin CR, Flinn BD, Pitts DL, et al: A novel method for creating endodontic access preparations through all-ceramic restorations: air abrasion and its effect relative to diamond and carbide bur use, *J Endod* 31:616, 2005.

190. Sae-Lim V, Rajamanickam I, Lim BK, Lee HL: Effectiveness of ProFile .04 taper rotary instruments in endodontic retreatment, *J Endod* 26:100, 2000.

191. Sakkal S, Gauthier G, Milot P, Lemian L: A clinical appraisal of the Gonon post-pulling system, *J Can Dent Assoc–Journal de l Association Dentaire Canadienne* 60:537, 1994.

192. Satterthwaite JD, Stokes AN, Frankel NT: Potential for temperature change during application of ultrasonic vibration to intra-radicular posts, *Eur J Prosthodont Restor Dent* 11:51, 2003.

193. Saunders EM: In vivo findings associated with heat generation during thermomechanical compaction of gutta-percha. 1. Temperature levels at the external surface of the root, *Int Endod J* 23:263, 1990.

194. Saunders EM: In vivo findings associated with heat generation during thermomechanical compaction of gutta-percha. 2. Histological response to temperature elevation on the external surface of the root, *Int Endod J* 23:268, 1990.

195. Saunders EM, Saunders WP: The heat generated on the external root surface during post space preparation, *Int Endod J* 22:169, 1989.

196. Saunders WP, Saunders EM: Coronal leakage as a cause of failure in root-canal therapy: a review, *Endod Dent Traumatol* 10:105, 1994.

197. Scherer W, Dragoo MR: New subgingival restorative procedures with Geristore resin ionomer, *Pract Periodontics Aesthet Dent* 7:1, 1995.

198. Schilder H: Filling root canals in three dimensions, *Dent Clin North Am* Nov:723, 1967.

199. Schirrmeister JF, Meyer KM, Hermanns P, et al: Effectiveness of hand and rotary instrumentation for removing a new synthetic polymer-based root canal obturation material (Epiphany) during retreatment, *Int Endod J* 39:150, 2006.

200. Schwandt NW, Gound TG: Resorcinol-formaldehyde resin "Russian Red" endodontic therapy, *J Endod* 29:435, 2003.

201. Schwartz RS, Robbins JW: Post placement and restoration of endodontically treated teeth: a literature review, *J Endod* 30:289, 2004.

202. Seltzer S: *Endodontology: biologic considerations in endodontic procedures*, ed 2, Philadelphia, 1988, Lea & Febiger, p x.

203. Seltzer S, Bender IB: Cognitive dissonance in endodontics, *Oral Surg Oral Med Oral Pathol* 20:505, 1965.

204. Seltzer S, Bender IB, Ziontz BA: The dynamics of pulp inflammation: correlations between diagnostic data and actual histologic findings in the pulp, *Oral Surg* 16:846, 1963.

205. Seltzer S, Green DB, Weiner N, DeRenzis F: A scanning electron microscope examination of silver cones removed from endodontically treated teeth, *Oral Surg Oral Med Oral Pathol* 33:589, 1972.

206. Seltzer S, Sinai I, August D: Periodontal effects of root perforations before and during endodontic procedures, *J Dent Res* 49:332, 1970.

207. Serper A, Ucer O, Onur R, Etikan I: Comparative neurotoxic effects of root canal filling materials on rat sciatic nerve, *J Endod* 24:592, 1998.

208. Setzer FC, Kohli MR, Shah SB, et al: Outcome of endodontic surgery: a meta-analysis of the literature—Part 2: comparison of endodontic microsurgical techniques with and without the use of higher magnification, *J Endod* 38:1, 2012.

209. Shen Y, Peng B, Cheung GS: Factors associated with the removal of fractured NiTi instruments from root canal systems, *Oral Surg Oral Med Oral Pathol Oral Radiol Endod* 98:605, 2004.

210. Shipper G, Orstavik D, Teixeira FB, Trope M: An evaluation of microbial leakage in roots filled with a thermoplastic synthetic polymer-based root canal filling material (Resilon), *J Endod* 30:342, 2004.

211. Simon JH, Chimenti RA, Mintz GA: Clinical significance of the pulse granuloma, *J Endod* 8:116, 1982.

212. Simon JH, Glick DH, Frank AL: The relationship of endodontic-periodontic lesions, *J Periodontol* 43:202, 1972.

213. Sinai IH: Endodontic perforations: their prognosis and treatment, *J Am Dent Assoc* 95:90, 1977.

214. Siqueira JF, Sen BH: Fungi in endodontic infections, *Oral Surg Oral Med Oral Pathol Oral Radiol Endod* 97:632, 2004.

215. Sjogren U, Hagglund B, Sundqvist G, Wing K: Factors affecting the long-term results of endodontic treatment, *J Endod* 16:498, 1990.

216. Sjogren U, Happonen RP, Kahnberg KE, Sundqvist G: Survival of Arachnia propionica in periapical tissue, *Int Endod J* 21:277, 1988.

217. Sluyk SR, Moon PC, Hartwell GR: Evaluation of setting properties and retention characteristics of mineral trioxide aggregate when used as a furcation perforation repair material, *J Endod* 24:768, 1998.

218. So MV, Saran C, Magro ML, et al: Efficacy of ProTaper retreatment system in root canals filled with gutta-percha and two endodontic sealers, *J Endod* 34:1223, 2008.

219. Solomonov M, Paque F, Kaya S, et al: Self-adjusting files in retreatment: a high-resolution micro-computed tomography study, *J Endod* 38:1283, 2012.

220. Somma F, Cammarota G, Plotino G, et al: The effectiveness of manual and mechanical instrumentation for the retreatment of three different root canal filling materials, *J Endod* 34:466, 2008.

221. Song M, Chung W, Lee SJ, Kim E: Long-term outcome of the cases classified as successes based on short-term follow-up in endodontic microsurgery, *J Endod* 38:1192, 2012.

222. Song M, Nam T, Shin SJ, Kim E: Comparison of clinical outcomes of endodontic microsurgery: 1 year versus long-term follow-up, *J Endod* 40:490, 2014.

223. Souter NJ, Messer HH: Complications associated with fractured file removal using an ultrasonic technique, *J Endod* 31:450, 2005.

224. Spatafore CM, Griffin JA Jr, Keyes GG, et al: Periapical biopsy report: an analysis of over a 10-year period, *J Endod* 16:239, 1990.

225. Spili P, Parashos P, Messer HH: The impact of instrument fracture on outcome of endodontic treatment, *J Endod* 31:845, 2005.

226. Spriggs K, Gettleman B, Messer HH: Evaluation of a new method for silver point removal, *J Endod* 16:335, 1990.

227. Stabholz A, Friedman S: Endodontic retreatment—case selection and technique. Part 2: treatment planning for retreatment, *J Endod* 14:607, 1988.

228. Stamos DE, Gutmann JL: Revisiting the post puller, *J Endod* 17:466, 1991.

229. Stamos DE, Gutmann JL: Survey of endodontic retreatment methods used to remove intraradicular posts, *J Endod* 19:366, 1993.

230. Sundqvist G: Ecology of the root canal flora, *J Endod* 18:427, 1992.

231. Sundqvist G, Figdor D: Endodontic treatment of apical periodontitis. In Orstavik D, Pitt-Ford TR, editors: *Essential endodontology: prevention and treatment of apical periodontitis*, London, 1998, Blackwell Science, p 242.

232. Sundqvist G, Reuterving CO: Isolation of *Actinomyces israelii* from periapical lesion, *J Endod* 6:602, 1980.

233. Suter B: A new method for retrieving silver points and separated instruments from root canals, *J Endod* 24:446, 1998.

234. Suter B, Lussi A, Sequeira P: Probability of removing fractured instruments from root canals, *Int Endod J* 38:112, 2005.

235. Sutherland JK, Teplitsky PE, Moulding MB: Endodontic access of all-ceramic crowns, *J Prosthodont Res* 61:146, 1989.

236. Swanson K, Madison S: An evaluation of coronal microleakage in endodontically treated teeth. Part I. Time periods, *J Endod* 13:56, 1987.

237. Tamse A, Fuss Z, Lustig J, Kaplavi J: An evaluation of endodontically treated vertically fractured teeth, *J Endod* 25:506, 1999.

238. Tamse A, Kaffe I, Lustig J, et al: Radiographic features of vertically fractured endodontically treated mesial roots of mandibular molars, *Oral Surg Oral Med Oral Pathol Oral Radiol Endod* 101:797, 2006.

239. Tasdemir T, Er K, Yildirim T, Celik D: Efficacy of three rotary NiTi instruments in removing gutta-percha from root canals, *Int Endod J* 41:191, 2008.

240. Tasdemir T, Yildirim T, Celik D: Comparative study of removal of current endodontic fillings, *J Endod* 34:326, 2008.

241. Teixeira FB, Teixeira EC, Thompson JY, Trope M: Fracture resistance of roots endodontically treated with a new resin filling material, *J Am Dent Assoc* 135:646, 2004.

242. Teplitsky PE, Rayner D, Chin I, Markowsky R: Gutta percha removal utilizing GPX instrumentation, *J Can Dent Assoc–Journal de l Association Dentaire Canadienne* 58:53, 1992.

243. Torabinejad M, Higa RK, McKendry DJ, Pitt Ford TR: Dye leakage of four root end filling materials: effects of blood contamination, *J Endod* 20:159, 1994.

244. Torabinejad M, Hong C, Pitt Ford TR: Tissue reaction to implanted super-EBA and Mineral trioxide aggregate in the mandible of guinea pigs: a preliminary report, *J Endod* 21:569, 1995.

245. Torabinejad M, Hong CU, McDonald F, Pitt Ford TR: Physical and chemical properties of a new root-end filling material, *J Endod* 21:349, 1995.

246. Torabinejad M, Hong CU, Pitt Ford TR, Kettering JD: Cytotoxicity of four root end filling materials, *J Endod* 21:489, 1995.

247. Torabinejad M, Lemon RR: Procedural accidents. In Walton RE, Torabinejad M, editors: *Principles and practice of endodontics*, ed 3, Philadelphia, 2002, Saunders, p 310.

248. Torabinejad M, Ung B, Kettering JD: In vitro bacterial penetration of coronally unsealed endodontically treated teeth, *J Endod* 16:566, 1990.

249. Tronstad L, Barnett F, Cervone F: Periapical bacterial plaque in teeth refractory to endodontic treatment, *Endod Dent Traumatol* 6:73, 1990.

250. Trope M, Maltz DO, Tronstad L: Resistance to fracture of restored endodontically treated teeth, *Endod Dent Traumatol* 1:108, 1985.

251. United States Drug Administration: *Chloroform used as an ingredient (active or inactive) in drug products. Federal Register No. 26845*. Washington DC, 1976, US Government Printing Office.

252. Uzun O, Topuz O, Tinaz C, et al: Accuracy of two root canal length measurement devices integrated into rotary endodontic motors when removing gutta-percha from root-filled teeth, *Int Endod J* 41:725, 2008.

253. Valderhaug J, Jokstad A, Ambjornsen E, Norheim PW: Assessment of the periapical and clinical status of crowned teeth over 25 years, *J Dent* 25:97, 1997.

254. Viducic D, Jukic S, Karlovic Z, et al: Removal of gutta-percha from root canals using an Nd:YAG laser, *Int Endod J* 36:670, 2003.

255. Walton RE, Rivera EM: Cleaning s. In Walton RE, Torabinjad M, editors: *Principles and practice of endodontics*, ed 3, Philadelphia, 2002, Saunders, p 206.

256. Walton RE, Torabinejad M: Diagnosis and treatment planning. In Walton RE, Torabinejad M, editors: *Principles and practice of endodontics*, ed 3, Philadelphia, 2002, Saunders, p 49.

257. Weiger R, Manncke B, Werner H, Lost C: Microbial flora of sinus tracts and root canals of non-vital teeth, *Endod Dent Traumatol* 11:15, 1995.

258. Welk AR, Baumgartner JC, Marshall JG: An in vivo comparison of two frequency-based electronic apex locators, *J Endod* 29:497, 2003.

259. Wennberg A, Orstavik D: Evaluation of alternatives to chloroform in endodontic practice, *Endod Dent Traumatol* 5:234, 1989.

260. White C, Bryant N: Combined therapy of mineral trioxide aggregate and guided tissue regeneration in the treatment of external root resorption and an associated osseous defect, *J Periodontol* 73:1517, 2002.

261. Whitworth JM, Boursin EM: Dissolution of root canal sealer cements in volatile solvents, *Int Endod J* 33:19, 2000.

262. Wilcox LR: Thermafil retreatment with and without chloroform solvent, *J Endod* 19:563, 1993.

263. Wilcox LR: Endodontic retreatment with halothane versus chloroform solvent, *J Endod* 21:305, 1995.

264. Wilcox LR, Juhlin JJ: Endodontic retreatment of Thermafil versus laterally condensed gutta-percha, *J Endod* 20:115, 1994.

265. Wilcox LR, Krell KV, Madison S, Rittman B: Endodontic retreatment: evaluation of gutta-percha and sealer removal and canal reinstrumentation, *J Endod* 13:453, 1987.

266. Wolcott J, Ishley D, Kennedy W, et al: A 5 yr clinical investigation of second mesiobuccal canals in endodontically treated and retreated maxillary molars, *J Endod* 31:262, 2005.

267. Wolcott JF, Himel VT, Hicks ML: Thermafil retreatment using a new "System B" technique or a solvent, *J Endod* 25:761, 1999.

268. Wolcott S, Wolcott J, Ishley D, et al: Separation incidence of protaper rotary instruments: a large cohort clinical evaluation, *J Endod* 32:1139, 2006.

269. Wourms DJ, Campbell AD, Hicks ML, Pelleu GB Jr: Alternative solvents to chloroform for gutta-percha removal, *J Endod* 16:224, 1990.

270. Yatsushiro JD, Baumgartner JC, Tinkle JS: Longitudinal study of the microleakage of two root-end filling materials using a fluid conductive system, *J Endod* 24:716, 1998.

271. Yeo JF, Loh FC: Retrograde removal of fractured endodontic instruments, *Ann Acad Med Singapore* 18:594, 1989.

272. Yoldas O, Oztunc H, Tinaz C, Alparslan N: Perforation risks associated with the use of Masserann endodontic kit drills in mandibular molars, *Oral Surg Oral Med Oral Pathol Oral Radiol Endod* 97:513, 2004.

273. Zakariasen KL, Brayton SM, Collinson DM: Efficient and effective root canal retreatment without chloroform, *J Can Dent Assoc–Journal de l Association Dentaire Canadienne* 56:509, 1990.

274. Zinman EJ: Records and legal responsibilities. In Cohen S, Burns RC, editors: *Pathways of the pulp*, ed 8, St. Louis, 2002, Mosby, p 365.

275. Zou X, Liu D, Yue L, Wu M: The ability of cone-beam computerized tomography to detect vertical root fractures in endodontically treated and nonendodontically treated teeth: a report of 3 cases, *Oral Surg Oral Med Oral Pathol Oral Radiol Endod* 111:797, 2011.

276. Zuolo ML, Imura N, Ferreira MO: Endodontic retreatment of thermafil or lateral condensation obturations in post space prepared teeth, *J Endod* 20:9, 1994.

277. Zuolo ML, Kherlakian N, Imura N: Effectiveness of nickel titanium rotary and hand instrumentation in endodontic retreatment [Abstract], *J Endod* 22:209, 1996.

CHAPTER 9

Periradicular Surgery

BRADFORD R. JOHNSON | MOHAMED I. FAYAD*

CHAPTER OUTLINE

*The authors would like to acknowledge the contributions of David Witherspoon for his involvement with previous editions.

Although nonsurgical endodontic treatment is a highly predictable option in most cases, surgery may be indicated for teeth with persistent periradicular pathoses that have not responded to nonsurgical approaches. Surgical root canal therapy, including root-end resection, has been practiced since at least the mid-1800s.[211] In 1906, Schamberg[473] described using radiographs to assist diagnosis and the use of surgical burs to perform a rapid osteotomy and root-end "ablation."

Perhaps the single most important development in dental practice in the early 20th century was the introduction of safe, effective local anesthesia, which allowed for more meticulous and comfortable surgical treatment. Formal recognition of endodontics as a specialty in 1963 ushered in a new era of basic and clinical research focused on the prevention and treatment of pulpal and periradicular pathosis.

Since the 1990s, periradicular surgery has continued to evolve into a precise, biologically based adjunct to nonsurgical root canal therapy. The parallel development of new instruments and materials, along with a better understanding of the biology of wound healing, has made surgical treatment a viable alternative to extraction and tooth replacement, rather than a treatment of last resort.

Periradicular surgery, when indicated, should be considered an extension of nonsurgical treatment, because the underlying etiology of the disease process and the objectives of treatment are the same: prevention or elimination of apical periodontitis. Surgical root canal treatment should not be considered as somehow separate from nonsurgical treatment, although the instruments and techniques are obviously quite different. Surgical treatment accounts for about 3% to 10% of the typical endodontic specialty practice.[1,75,374] A web-based survey found that 91% of active endodontists perform some type of root-end surgery, and almost all are using a dental operating microscope and ultrasonics.[115] Endodontists perform almost 78% of surgical root canal treatments; general dentists and other specialists perform 15.5% and 6.6%, respectively.[242] Although appropriately trained general dentists and other dental specialists may perform periradicular surgery, individuals with advanced training in endodontics have developed most of the current periradicular surgery techniques and science presented in this chapter. We believe that endodontists must continue to include periradicular surgery as a routine part of clinical endodontic practice and not abrogate this treatment option to others, who may not possess the same background, skills, or values.[343,424,439] When patient preferences and quality of life measures are considered, patients can be expected to place high value on endodontic treatment and the retention of a natural tooth.[153,180]

INDICATIONS FOR PERIRADICULAR SURGERY

Etiology of Persistent Periradicular Disease

The first and arguably most important step in treatment decision making is attempting to determine the cause of persistent periradicular disease. Treatment then is directed at eliminating the etiology, which most often is the presence of bacteria and other microbial irritants in the root canal space.[492] Nonsurgical retreatment, when possible, often is the first choice for attempting to correct obvious deficiencies in the previous treatment (see Chapter 8).[564] However, microorganisms can survive even in apparently well-treated teeth in dentinal tubules, canal irregularities, deltas, and isthmus areas.[275,307,568] If residual microorganisms remain completely entombed in the root canal system, periradicular healing should occur. Sealing off all potential routes of microbial escape from the root canal system is the goal of both nonsurgical and surgical treatment. When microorganisms of sufficient pathogenicity and number gain access to the periradicular tissues, pathosis develops.

Enterococcus faecalis is commonly isolated from failing root canal–treated teeth and is known to be especially difficult to eliminate with standard instrumentation and irrigation techniques.[510] Unlike primary endodontic infections, which predominantly are associated with mixed anaerobic microbiota, it has been commonly accepted that treatment failures are more frequently associated with one or two microorganisms.[492] However, research using more sophisticated techniques (16S ribosomal RNA gene clone library analysis) has determined that multiple, previously uncultivated phylotypes can be identified in the majority of teeth with persistent apical periodontitis.[464] Fungi and viruses have also emerged as potential causes of root canal failure and may play either a primary or secondary role in persistent periradicular pathosis.[369,399,462,575]

Established extraradicular colonies of microorganisms also may be a reason for failure of some teeth to respond to nonsurgical treatment. When microorganisms are able to arrange in an extraradicular biofilm, they may be particularly resistant to elimination by host defense mechanisms and antimicrobial agents.[490] Persistent extraradicular root surface colonization cannot be diagnosed by noninvasive methods but may be suspected in well-treated cases that are refractory to nonsurgical treatment.[166,218,465,495,511] Although the presence of extraradicular microbial colonies has been somewhat controversial, studies using DNA-DNA hybridization techniques have confirmed the persistence of microorganisms in the periradicular tissues of some root canal–treated teeth.[187,509]

Overextended filling materials may contribute to treatment failure, presumably as a result of a chronic inflammatory response.[369] Although this is possible and even likely with certain toxic materials (e.g., pastes containing formaldehyde[376]), the role of relatively inert materials such as gutta-percha and set sealer is less clear, and these materials probably become a significant contributing factor only if microorganisms are present. If the root apex is close to the buccal cortical plate, apical fenestration may occur, leading to persistent symptoms, especially tenderness to palpation over the root apex.[72] Some have suggested that overextension of filling materials may contribute to endodontic failure because certain dental materials may induce periodontal ligament (PDL) cell apoptosis.[467] This specific interaction between filling materials and periradicular tissues is not fully understood and deserves further research. The poorer prognosis often reported with overextended root canal fillings also may be related simply to lack of an adequate apical seal and subsequent egress of microorganisms from the root canal space. Regardless, minor overextension of filling material is rarely a sole indication for surgery except when symptoms or periradicular pathosis develops. Significant overextension of filling material, especially when important anatomic areas and possibly toxic materials are involved, is an indication for referral to an endodontist or oral surgeon for evaluation and, possibly, treatment.

The presence of periradicular cholesterol crystals may interfere with healing after nonsurgical root canal treatment.[365]

Although relatively uncommon, true periradicular cysts (completely enclosed, epithelium-lined cavities) may not be expected to resolve after nonsurgical treatment.[364] As with other extraradicular causes of failure, surgery is indicated, because definitive diagnosis and treatment require an excisional biopsy and removal of the periradicular tissue.

Vertical root fractures are a significant cause of failure and may be difficult to diagnose in the early stages.[90] Exploratory surgery often is required to confirm a root fracture. Cone-beam computed tomography (CBCT) is a promising tool for noninvasive diagnosis of root fractures[155,165] and is discussed in greater detail later in this chapter and in Chapter 2. Although several promising approaches to the management of vertical root fractures have been proposed,[226,268,506] the prognosis generally is believed to be poor. Extraction usually is the treatment of choice, especially if appropriate tooth replacement options are available (see Chapter 21). Root amputation or hemisection may be considered in a multirooted tooth if the remaining tooth structure is uninvolved and sufficient periodontal support is present.

The relationship between systemic disease and periradicular healing is not completely understood. The possible influence of certain systemic medications on wound healing is discussed later in the chapter. Compromised host healing capacity may be a contributing factor in delayed healing and failure of some root canal–treated teeth. For example, complete healing after nonsurgical root canal treatment is less likely in diabetic patients with preoperative periradicular pathosis.[78,175] Patients undergoing immunosuppressive therapy may be at greater risk for delayed healing, treatment failure, or acute exacerbation of a subclinical infection, although two studies involving subgroups of immunocompromised patients (bone marrow transplant and acquired immunodeficiency syndrome [AIDS]) did not find these patients to be at higher risk for complications related to endodontic treatment.[197,406]

Rationale for Surgical Treatment

Although nonsurgical retreatment generally is believed to be the preferred first approach in the management of persistent apical periodontitis,[77,492,510,564] periradicular surgery is indicated when nonsurgical retreatment is impractical or unlikely to improve on the previous result (see Chapter 8). In particular, a surgical approach may be the first choice for managing teeth with long posts or irretrievable separated instruments, nonnegotiable ledges and canal blockages or transportation, hard cement filling materials, failure of previous nonsurgical retreatment, and suspected vertical root fracture, or when a biopsy is indicated (Figs. 9-1 to 9-4). Even when surgical treatment is the likely definitive approach, nonsurgical therapy before the procedure may be recommended to help reduce the number of microorganisms in the root canal system and ensure a more favorable long-term prognosis.[230] On the other hand, surgery may be the first choice even if a tooth can be treated nonsurgically if the risks and costs of retreatment are considered excessive. For example, disassembling a recently restored bridge abutment tooth to allow endodontic retreatment may be technically possible but not economically feasible. One study found that endodontic microsurgery may be the most cost-effective option for management of persistent periapical disease, compared to nonsurgical retreatment, extraction and placement of a fixed partial denture, and extraction and placement of a single tooth implant.[284] Case-specific variables and clinical

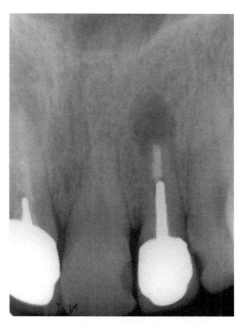

FIG. 9-1 Previously treated maxillary lateral incisor with persistent periradicular disease. Nonsurgical retreatment is possible but would involve disassembly of an otherwise adequate coronal restoration. Periradicular surgery is a reasonable option.

judgment are key elements in the decision-making process, as current evidence supports the contention that the prognosis for surgical treatment is approximately the same as that for nonsurgical retreatment.[127,128,135,293,468,577]

Clinical Decision Making

Clinical decision making is a process that combines the best available evidence, clinical judgment, and patient preferences. Treatment choices are always made under conditions of at least some uncertainty. Surgical root canal treatment rarely is the only possible choice. Clinicians and patients must weigh the relative benefits, risks, and costs of two or more acceptable alternatives. Patients and clinicians can be expected to hold different attitudes about the value of potential treatment outcomes.[269] In a prognosis study of single-tooth dental implants, Gibbard and Zarb[193] reported that factors considered significant by health care professionals may not be important to patients. Even among groups of dentists and dental specialists, the threshold for treatment varies widely and treatment recommendations may depend more on personal values and experience than objective analysis of treatment costs, prognosis, risks, and alternatives.[56,343,439]

Shared decision making, in which the patient and clinician consider outcome probabilities and patient preferences and agree on the appropriate treatment, is preferable to a clinician-directed treatment decision.[46,179] Such a two-way exchange allows the clinician to provide the best available current evidence and case-specific clinical judgment while encouraging a decision that considers the patient's personal values and preferences. This decision-making model has been shown to increase patient knowledge about and satisfaction with the treatment choice.[262,386,387] In general, most patients prefer to be actively involved in the decision-making process but want to leave the specifics of the treatment to the clinician.[179] That is, the risks,

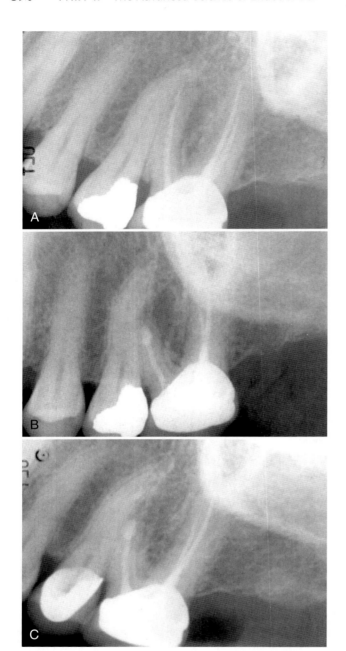

FIG. 9-2 **A,** Previously treated maxillary first molar with periradicular disease and obvious transportation of the main mesiobuccal (MB-1) canal. Nonsurgical retreatment is unlikely to correct this iatrogenic condition, and surgery is the preferred choice. **B,** Immediate postsurgery radiograph. The root-end preparation and fill was extended from the MB-1 canal in a palatal direction to include the isthmus area and the second (MB-2) canal. **C,** One-year follow-up examination: the tooth is asymptomatic, and periradicular healing is apparent radiographically. Although surgery was the first-choice treatment in this case and the outcome was favorable, a good argument could be made for nonsurgical retreatment before surgery to ensure disinfection of the canal and to attempt to locate a MB-2 canal.

benefits, and costs of treatment alternatives are important to patients, but the details of the procedure usually are not. Shared decision making is particularly relevant in light of the current trend in some areas to recommend implants as an alternative to root canal treatment.

Comparative probabilities for a successful outcome after surgical root canal treatment, nonsurgical retreatment, or extraction and replacement with a fixed prosthesis or implant are difficult to project. Many treatment variables are complex and not easily quantified, such as the affected location in the mouth, bone quality, practitioner's skill, possible influence of systemic disease on healing, periodontal support, bulk of the remaining tooth structure and resistance to fracture, quality of the coronal restoration, patient susceptibility to recurrent caries, materials used, and other factors. In addition, the definition of success varies considerably and is inconsistent from study to study.

Boioli and colleagues[66] performed a meta-analysis of implant studies and reported a 93% survival rate at 5 years. The 5- to 10-year success rate for implant retention routinely is reported to be 90% to 97%, depending on the location in the mouth and other variables.[302,309] Surgical root canal treatment was previously reported to have a lower success rate than implant placement.[230,546] However, most of these older studies would be considered weak by today's evidence-based standards and, more important, do not reflect the use of many of the newer surgical materials and techniques. With careful case selection, surgical skill, and the use of materials and techniques described later in this chapter, many studies have demonstrated success rates over 90% for surgical root canal treatment.[326,448,500,501,546,609] von Arx reported that the 5-year success for teeth receiving endodontic microsurgery was 8% less than observed at 1 year.[566] A similar study found an 85% success rate after 10 years.[500] A systematic review and meta-analysis comparing traditional root-end surgery to modern endodontic microsurgery (ultrasonic root-end preparation; root-end filling with IRM, Super EBA, or MTA; and high power [> ×10] magnification and illumination) found that the outcome for endodontic microsurgery using current materials and techniques was 94%, compared to 59% success with traditional root-end surgery.[483]

In broad terms and under ideal conditions, the prognoses for nonsurgical retreatment, surgical treatment, and implant placement should be roughly equal. The choice of treatment should be based on the best available evidence, case-specific clinical judgment, and the patient's preferences. As a stronger evidence base continues to develop, we predict that algorithms encompassing multiple patient and treatment variables will be devised to assist clinical decision making.

GENERAL BIOLOGIC PRINCIPLES OF WOUND HEALING

Wound healing varies from region to region in the body and depends on several factors, including the type of tissue, the type of wound, and the type of healing. In periradicular surgery, the tissues include free and attached gingiva, the alveolar mucosa, periosteum, bone, the periodontal ligament, and cementum. The wound may be intentional surgical trauma, which includes incision, blunt dissection, and excision (surgical), or pathologic or traumatic wounds. Healing occurs by primary or secondary intention.[212]

An incisional blunt dissectional wound, for example, can be considered to heal typically by primary intention, whereas a dissectional wound involving the resected root surface and osseous crypt heals by secondary intention. An important concept of the wound healing process in general is the difference between regeneration and repair. The goal of all surgical

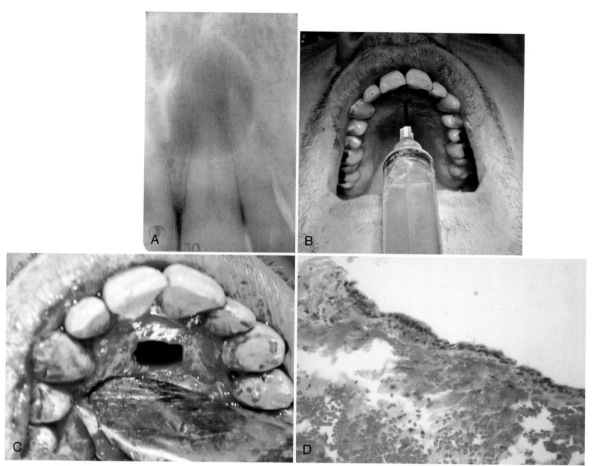

FIG. 9-3 **A**, Indication for surgery (biopsy): large radiolucent lesion in the area of the maxillary left central and lateral incisors was detected on routine radiographic examination. All anterior teeth responded within normal limits to pulp vitality testing. **B**, After administration of a local anesthetic but before surgery, the lesion was aspirated with a large-gauge needle to rule out a vascular lesion. **C**, Buccal and palatal flaps were reflected. The lesion was directly accessible from the palate. An excisional biopsy was performed, and the sample was submitted for evaluation. **D**, Light microscopic section of the biopsy specimen; the lesion was diagnosed as a nasopalatine duct cyst. (×400.) (Courtesy Dr. Vince Penesis.)

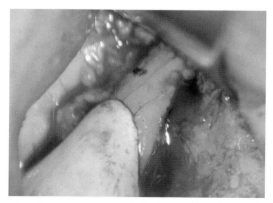

FIG. 9-4 Exploratory surgery was indicated to rule out or confirm a root fracture. Magnification and staining with methylene blue dye confirmed the presence of multiple root fractures. The tooth was subsequently extracted. (Courtesy Dr. Martin Rogers.)

procedures should be *regeneration,* which returns the tissues to their normal microarchitecture and function, rather than *repair,* a healing outcome in which tissues do not return to normal architecture and function. Repair typically results in the formation of scar tissue.

The wounding process varies, depending on the types of tissue and injury. However, all wounds progress through three broad, overlapping phases in the process of healing; these are the inflammatory phase, the proliferative phase, and the maturation phase.[240,570] Although these phases can be identified in healing tissue, none of them has a clear beginning or end. Furthermore, in a wound such as an endodontic surgical site, which involves more than one tissue type, these phases progress at different rates in each type of tissue.

SOFT-TISSUE WOUND HEALING

Inflammatory Phase

Broadly speaking, the inflammatory phase of healing is similar for all tissues.[543] This phase can be broken down further into clot formation, early inflammation, and late inflammation.

Clot Formation

Clot formation begins with three events: (1) blood vessel contraction is initiated by platelet degranulation of serotonin, which acts on the endothelial cell and increases the permeability of the vessel, allowing a protein-rich exudate to enter the wound site; (2) a plug composed of platelets forms, primarily through intravascular platelet aggregation; (3) both the extrinsic and intrinsic clotting mechanisms are activated. Several other events occur simultaneously, including activation of the kinin, complement, and fibrinolytic systems and the generation of plasmin.[34,247,521] These events stabilize hemostasis, begin the production of a number of mitogens and chemoattractants, and initiate the process of wound decontamination. The result is a coagulum consisting of widely spaced, haphazardly arranged fibrin strands with serum exudate, erythrocytes, tissue debris, and inflammatory cells. Compression of the surgical flap with sterile iced gauze immediately after surgery is designed to minimize the thickness of the fibrin clot and thereby accelerate optimal wound healing.

Early Inflammation: Polymorphonuclear Neutrophil (PMN) Organization

As a result of production of chemoattractants by the various components of the clot, polymorphonuclear neutrophils (PMNs) begin to enter the wound site within 6 hours of clot stabilization. The number of PMNs increases steadily, peaking at about 24 to 48 hours after the injury. Three key steps mark PMN migration into the wound site: (1) *pavementing,* in which the red blood cells undertake intravascular agglutination, allowing the PMNs to adhere to the endothelial cells; (2) *emigration,* in which the PMNs actively pass through the vascular wall; and (3) *migration,* in which the PMNs use ameboid motion, under the influence of the various chemotactic mediators, to move into the injured tissues.[212]

The principal role of the PMNs is wound decontamination by means of phagocytosis of bacteria. The high number of PMNs in the wound site is relatively short lived; the number drops rapidly after the third day.

Late Inflammation: Macrophage Organization

About the time the PMN population is declining (48 to 96 hours after injury), macrophages begin to enter the wound site. They reach a peak concentration by approximately the third or fourth day. These cells, which are derived from circulating monocytes, leave the bloodstream under the influence of the chemoattractants in the wound site. The monocytes subsequently evolve into macrophages. Macrophages have a much longer life span than PMNs; they remain in the wound until healing is complete. Similar to PMNs, macrophages play a major role in wound decontamination through phagocytosis and digestion of microorganisms and tissue debris.

Macrophages are considerably more bioactive than PMNs and can secrete a vast array of cytokines. A key action of many of these bioactive substances is initiation of the proliferative phase of wound healing, which is accomplished by prompting the formation of granulation tissue. Two other major functions of macrophages are ingestion and processing of antigens for presentation to T lymphocytes, which enter the wound after the macrophages. Unlike PMNs, macrophages play an essential role in the regulation of wound healing.[109,224] A reduction in the number of macrophages in the wound site delays healing, because the wound does not progress to the next phase. For example, the age-related reduction in healing potential appears to be partly the result of loss of estrogen regulation of macrophages in healing tissues.[33]

Proliferative Phase

The proliferative phase is characterized by the formation of granulation tissue in the wound. Two key cell types, fibroblasts and endothelial cells, have a primary role in the formation of granulation tissue. Granulation tissue is a fragile structure composed of an extracellular matrix of fibrin, fibronectin, glycosaminoglycans, proliferating endothelial cells, new capillaries, and fibroblasts mixed with inflammatory macrophages and lymphocytes. Epithelial cells also are active during this phase of soft-tissue healing and are responsible for initial wound closure. Guided tissue regeneration (GTR) procedures are based on control of the epithelial cell growth rate during this phase.

Fibroblasts: Fibroplasia

Undifferentiated mesenchymal stem cells in the perivascular tissue and fibroblasts in the adjacent connective tissue migrate into the wound site on the third day after injury and achieve their peak numbers by approximately the seventh day. This action is stimulated by a combination of cytokines (e.g., fibroblast growth factor [FGF], insulin-like growth factor–1 [IGF-1], and 2-15 platelet-derived growth factor [PDGF]), which are produced initially by platelets and subsequently by macrophages and lymphocytes. As the number of macrophages declines and the fibroblast population increases, the tissue in the wound transforms from a *granulomatous* tissue to a *granulation* tissue.

Fibroblasts are the crucial reconstructive cell in the progression of wound healing, because they produce most of the structural proteins forming the extracellular matrix (e.g., collagen). Collagen is first detected in the wound about the third day after injury. The fibroblasts produce type III collagen initially and then, as the wound matures, type I collagen. As this network of collagen fibers is laid down, endothelial and smooth muscle cells begin to migrate into the wound. Subsequently, as wound healing progresses, the collagen fibers become organized by cross-linking. Regularly aligned bundles of collagen begin to orient so as to resist stress in the healing wound.[108,286,413,516]

A focused type of fibroblast, known as a *myofibroblast,* plays a significant role in wound contraction, particularly in incisional-type wounds.[316,524] Myofibroblasts align themselves parallel with the wound surface and then contract, drawing the wound edges together. These cells are eliminated by apoptosis after wound closure.[137,138]

Endothelial Cells: Angiogenesis

Capillary buds originate from the vessels at the periphery of the wound and extend into the wound proper. This occurs concurrently with fibroblast proliferation and can begin as early as 48 to 72 hours after injury. Without angiogenesis, the wound would not have the blood supply needed for further active healing. The capillary sprouts eventually join to form a network of capillary loops (*capillary plexuses*) throughout the wound.

In addition to a low oxygen concentration in the wound proper,[198,289] several factors have been identified as potent stimulators of angiogenesis, including vascular endothelial growth factor (VEGF), basic fibroblast growth factor (bFGF), acidic FGF (aFGF), transforming growth factor–alpha

(TGF-alpha) and transforming growth factor–beta (TGF-beta), epidermal growth factor (EGF), interleukin-1 (IL-1), and tumor necrosis factor–alpha (TNF-alpha),[145] as well as lactic acid.[248,258,503] All of these have been shown to stimulate new vessel development.

Epithelium

The first step in epithelial healing is the formation of an epithelial seal on the surface of the fibrin clot. This process begins at the edge of the wound, where the basal and suprabasal prickle cells rapidly undergo mitosis. The cells then migrate across the fibrin clot at a remarkable rate (0.5 to 1 mm per day). This monolayer of epithelial cells continues to migrate by contact guidance along the fibrin scaffold of the clot below. Migration stops as a result of contact inhibition of the epithelial cells from the opposing wound edge. Once the epithelium from both sides of the wound is in contact, an epithelial seal is achieved. In wounds healing by primary intention, formation of an epithelial seal typically takes 21 to 28 hours after reapproximation of the wound margins.[222]

Maturation Phase

Under ideal conditions, maturation of the wound begins 5 to 7 days after injury. A reduction in fibroblasts, vascular channels, and extracellular fluids marks the transition to this phase of healing. During the early stages of wound maturation, the wound matrix is chiefly composed of fibronectin and hyaluronic acid. As the tensile strength of the wound increases, significant upregulation of collagen fibrogenesis occurs. Collagen remodeling ensues, with the formation of larger collagen bundles and alteration of intermolecular cross-linking. The result is a conversion of granulation tissue to fibrous connective tissue and a decreased parallelism of collagen to the plane of the wound. Aggregated collagen fibril bundles increase the tensile strength of the wound. As healing progresses in the wound, the collagen gradually reorganizes; this requires degradation and reaggregation of the collagen. The degradation of collagen is controlled by a variety of collagenase enzymes. Remodeling results in a gradual reduction in the cellularity and vascularity of the reparative tissue; the degree to which this occurs determines the extent of scar tissue formation. Active remodeling of scar tissue can continue very slowly for life.[138,247]

Maturation of the epithelial layer quickly follows formation of the epithelial seal. The monolayer of cells forming the epithelial seal differentiates and undergoes mitosis and maturation to form a definitive layer of stratified squamous epithelium. In this way an epithelial barrier is formed that protects the underlying wound from further invasion by oral microbes. The epithelial barrier typically forms by 36 to 42 hours after suturing of the wound and is characterized by a significant increase in wound strength.[222]

HARD-TISSUE HEALING: EXCISIONAL DENTOALVEOLAR WOUND

The inflammatory and proliferative phases of healing for hard tissue are similar to those for soft tissue. A clot forms in the bony crypt, and an inflammatory process ensues that involves PMNs initially and macrophages subsequently. This is followed by the formation of granulation tissue with an angiogenic component. However, the maturation phase of hard-tissue healing differs markedly from that for soft tissues, primarily because of the tissues involved: cortical bone, cancellous bone, alveolar bone proper, endosteum, periodontal ligament, cementum, dentin, and inner mucoperiosteal tissue.

Osteoblasts: Osteogenesis

The healing of an excisional osseous wound that is approximately 1 cm in diameter is similar to that of a fractured long bone. It progresses from hematoma to inflammation, eradication of nonvital debris, proliferation of granulation tissue, callus formation, conversion of woven bone to lamellar bone and, finally, remodeling of the united bone ends. The coagulum that initially forms delays healing and must be removed to allow wound healing to progress.

A major difference between soft- and hard-tissue wound healing is found in the role of the osteoclast. Functionally, osteoclasts act as organizational units to debride necrotic bone from the wound margin, much as macrophages remove tissue debris from the clot. Granulation tissue begins to proliferate from the severed periodontal ligament by 2 to 4 days after root-end resection.[223] This tissue rapidly encapsulates the root end. Simultaneously, endosteal proliferation into the coagulum occurs from the deep surface of the bony wound edge. The coagulum in the bony crypt is quickly converted into a mass of granulation tissue. In addition to those already discussed, several cell types migrate into the coagulum, including osteoprogenitor cells, preosteoblasts, and osteoblasts. These cells begin the formation of woven bone within the mass of granulation tissue. New bone formation is apparent about 6 days after surgery.[223]

Bone formation can be categorized into two types, each having several phases. The phases differ, depending on which type of formation is involved. One type of bone formation is a matrix vesicle–based process, and the other type is based on osteoid secretion. In both processes, osteoblasts produce the bone matrix. They secrete a collagen-rich ground substance that is essential for mineralization. Osteoblasts also cause calcium and phosphorus to precipitate from the blood.

In the formation of woven bone, which occurs by the matrix vesicle–based process, osteoblasts produce matrix vesicles through exocytosis (the release of substances contained in a vesicle within a cell by a process in which the membrane surrounding the vesicle unites with the membrane forming the outer wall of the cell) of their plasma membranes. As hydroxyapatite crystals accrue in the vesicles, they become enlarged and eventually rupture. This process begins with the deposition and growth of hydroxyapatite crystals in the pore regions. The crystals then amalgamate to form structures known as *spherulites*. Union of the separate spherulites results in mineralization.

The formation of lamellar bone does not require the production of matrix vesicles; rather, it proceeds by the osteoblast secretion process. Osteoblasts secrete an organic matrix composed of longitudinally arranged collagen matrix fibrils (mainly type I collagen). Mineralization occurs by mineral deposition directly along the collagen fibrils.[239,240] This stage has been associated with a rise in pH, most likely because of the enzyme alkaline phosphatase, which is secreted by osteoblasts and other cells and plays an important role in mineralization. The exact role of alkaline phosphatase during mineralization is unclear. The balance of evidence favors a positive catalytic role.[19,20] Some hypothesize[71,70,552,553] that alkaline phosphatase promotes mineralization through a combination of mechanisms involving various cells, extracellular matrix proteins, and elements. The interaction of alkaline phosphatase and phosphoproteins in both bone and dentin appears to be especially critical to the mineralization process.[71,72,557,558]

Inhibitor molecules, such as pyrophosphate and acidic non-collagenous bone proteins, regulate mineralization. Several growth factors also have been identified as key components in the production of osseous tissue. These include TGF-beta, bone morphogenetic protein (BMP), PDGF, FGF, and IGF.[97,191,476,513] One clinical study demonstrated that the addition of autologous platelet concentrate to the surgical site decreased postsurgical pain and may accelerate the healing process.[134]

Three to 4 weeks after surgery, an excisional osseous wound is 75% to 80% filled with trabeculae surrounded by intensely active osteoid and osteoblastic cells. A reforming periosteum can be seen on the outer surface of the wound; it is highly cellular and has more fibrous connective tissue oriented parallel to the plane of the former cortical plate. At 8 weeks after surgery, the trabeculae are larger and denser and the osteoblasts are less active; these cells occupy about 80% of the original wound. Also, fewer osteoid cells are associated with the maturing trabeculae. The overlying periosteum has reformed and is in contact with the newly developed bone. The osseous defect typically is filled with bone tissue by 16 weeks after surgery. However, the cortical plate has not yet totally reformed. Maturation and remodeling of the osseous tissue continues for several more months.[223]

Local healing is also influenced systemically by the endocrine system and its three general categories of hormones: polypeptide regulators (parathyroid hormone, calcitonin, insulin, and growth hormone), steroid hormones (vitamin D_3, glucocorticoids, and the sex hormones), and thyroid hormones.[219]

Cementoblasts: Cementogenesis

During regeneration of the periradicular tissues, cementum forms over the surface of surgically resected root ends.[114] The exact spatial and temporal sequences of events leading to this formation of new cementum remains undefined; however, cementogenesis is important, because cementum is relatively resistant to resorption (osteoclasts have little affinity for attaching to cementum).

Cementogenesis begins 10 to 12 days after root-end resection. Cementoblasts develop at the root periphery and proceed centrally toward the root canal.[24] Considerable evidence indicates that the cells that regulate cementogenesis are derived from ectomesenchymal cells in the tooth germ proper rather than from bone or other surrounding tissues. The migration and attachment of precementoblasts to the root surface dentin is monitored by mediators from within the dentin itself.[140,210] Cementum covers the resected root end in approximately 28 days. Newly formed PDL fibers show a functional realignment that involves reorientation of fibers perpendicular to the plane of the resected root end, extending from the newly formed cementum to the woven bone trabeculae. This occurs about 8 weeks after surgery.[212,319,320]

SYSTEMIC MEDICATIONS AND WOUND HEALING

Bisphosphonates

Bisphosphonates are commonly used for the treatment of osteopenia, osteoporosis, Paget's disease of bone, multiple myeloma, and metastatic bone, breast, and prostate cancer. The potential association between bisphosphonate use and osteonecrosis of the jaw was first reported in 2003.[332,351] The current preferred term for this condition is antiresorptive agent–induced osteonecrosis of the jaw (ARONJ)[229] or medication-related osteonecrosis of the jaw (MRONJ). The change in terminology reflects the finding that, in addition to bisphosphonates, other antiresorptive agents can increase the risk for osteonecrosis of the jaw (e.g., denosumab). ARONJ can occur spontaneously but is more commonly associated with dental procedures that involve bone trauma. Patient variables that increase the risk for ARONJ include age (over 65 years old), chronic use of corticosteroids, use of bisphosphonates for more than 2 years, smoking, diabetes, and obesity.[278,334,340,583] It is important to note that the risk for ARONJ with commonly prescribed oral bisphosphonates appears to be very low, whereas the overall benefits of this drug class for reducing morbidity and mortality related to hip, vertebral, and other bone fractures are significant.[229] The estimated incidence for ARONJ in patients taking oral bisphosphonates ranges from zero to 1 in 2260 cases, although dental extractions may quadruple the risk of developing ARONJ.[7,340] A reasonable upper estimate of the risk of developing ARONJ in a patient who does not have cancer is about 0.1%.[229] One clinical study reported a much higher 4% risk for developing ARONJ in patients taking a specific oral bisphosphonate (alendronate sodium),[479] although this was a retrospective study using an electronic patient record at a dental school and may not have adequately controlled for other relevant variables. The majority of ARONJ cases have been reported in patients taking IV bisphosphonates (e.g., zoledronic acid and pamidronate). According to one report, approximately 20% of patients taking IV bisphosphonates may develop ARONJ.[7,340] A systematic review found that there was a strong association between cancer and risk of ARONJ, with the prevalence ranging from 0.7% to 13.3%.[352] Interestingly, this same review found that the higher-quality studies reported the highest prevalence of ARONJ in cancer patients.

Conservative and timely management of apical periodontitis is essential to reduce the risk of ARONJ in patients taking bisphosphonates. Because periapical pathosis may exacerbate or increase the risk for ARONJ, the "no treatment" option is not a viable choice. The potential risk for ARONJ should be thoroughly discussed with all patients that are taking bisphosphonates, as well as treatment options. Nonsurgical retreatment should usually be considered the first choice, especially for patients with a history of IV bisphosphonate use or other risk factors. Even so, surgical treatment may be indicated to manage chronic or acute apical periodontitis. When the only viable treatment options for the management of persistent periradicular inflammation are surgical root canal therapy or extraction, the question of which option is more or less likely to lead to ARONJ in at-risk patients remains unanswered. In general, the procedure that could most predictably eliminate the periradicular inflammation with the least amount of surgical trauma would be preferred. Conservative surgical technique, primary tissue closure, and use of chlorhexidine mouth rinses preoperatively and during the healing stage are recommended.[229] There is some limited evidence to support the use of prophylactic antibiotics and chlorhexidine mouth rinse to decrease the risk of ARONJ for patients undergoing surgical dental treatment.[229] Because bisphosphonates have a substantial half-life when incorporated into bone, discontinuation of bisphosphonates prior to dental treatment is unlikely to provide any measurable benefit and may place the patient at greater risk for complications that the drug is intended to prevent.

The possibility of predicting which patients may be at greater risk for ARONJ based on serum levels of C-terminal cross-linking telopeptide of type I collagen (CTX) has been suggested based on clinical observations.[333] This observation may provide a useful clue for future risk assessment but requires additional refinement and validation prior to widespread acceptance. In fact, one study found that although serum CTX levels were lower in patients taking bisphosphonates (as expected), there was no association between lower CTX levels and increased risk of ARONJ.[208] This same study found that patients taking a once-a-year dose of 5 mg zoledronic acid were at no greater risk for ARONJ than a control group (1 case in 5903 patients). Once ARONJ develops, treatment options are limited. A possible treatment strategy proposed in a series of case reports is the use of teriparatide, an anabolic drug that stimulates osteoblast formation and is used for the management of osteoporosis (see also Chapter 3).[505]

Glucocorticoids

Glucocorticoid therapy has been shown to induce rapid bone loss within the first 3 months of treatment. Even inhaled steroids have been implicated as a cause of bone loss. Bone formation is inhibited partly through a decrease in osteoblast life span and function, a reduction in the mineral apposition rate, and a prolonged mineralization lag time. Biochemical markers of bone formation (i.e., osteocalcin and bone-specific alkaline phosphatase) are suppressed. In addition to this primary suppressive effect, glucocorticoids cause accelerated bone resorption. The number and activity of osteoclasts increase during early glucocorticoid exposure. With continued use of glucocorticoids, the rapid rate of osteoclast-mediated bone resorption slows, but suppression of bone formation continues as the overriding skeletal activity.[272] Bone loss therefore is progressive, because bone resorption chronically exceeds bone formation.

The adverse effects of glucocorticoids on bone are mediated by sex steroid deficiency and expression of locally produced growth factors and related proteins, such as reduced production of IGF-1 and alterations in IGF-binding proteins in osteoblasts. The direct effect on calcium metabolism through alteration of vitamin D metabolism leads to a state of secondary hyperparathyroidism.[447,581,582]

Nonsteroidal Anti-inflammatory Drugs (NSAIDs)

Bone homeostasis is regulated by many factors, including prostaglandins (PGs).[267] PGs are important to both normal and pathologic bone turnover. PGs modulate osteoblast proliferation and differentiated functions.[426,427] The levels of prostaglandins E (PGE) and F (PGF) are elevated in the early phase of fracture healing, and administration of PGE_2 has increased the rate of osseous repair in several animal studies.[272] NSAID inhibition of the enzyme cyclooxygenase (COX), which is involved in the synthesis of PGs, is the same mechanism by which NSAIDs control pain. By inhibiting the COX enzymes and the subsequent production of prostaglandins, NSAIDs accomplish the desired anti-inflammatory effects—but also prevent the increased production of PGs required for bone healing. In vitro studies using animal models have shown that NSAIDs inhibit osteoblast proliferation and stimulate protein synthesis.[235] These drugs also have been shown to delay fracture healing and to affect bone formation adversely in animals and humans.[15,192] In one study, the use of NSAIDs reduced the amount of bony ingrowth into an orthopedic implant.[220]

In other studies, NSAIDs reduced bone resorption associated with experimentally induced periapical lesions,[18,390] and systemic NSAIDs may play a positive role in maintaining bone height around endosseous titanium dental implants.[257] Additional research is needed to clarify the specific influence of NSAIDs on healing after periradicular surgery.

Cyclooxygenase-2 (COX-2) Inhibitors

Although both COX-1 and COX-2 have been identified in osteoblasts, the different roles of the two cyclooxygenases in bone formation remain unclear. A study using COX-1 and COX-2 knockout mice compared the roles of the two enzymes in fracture healing. COX-2 was shown to have an essential role in both endochondral and intramembranous bone formation during wound healing. COX-2 knockout mice showed a persistent delay in cartilage tissue ossification. No difference in fracture healing was observed between the COX-1 knockout mice and the wild-type control used in this study.[603] Additional studies have shown a persistent delay in healing with COX-2 NSAIDs[202,203]; however, this difference in effect was not apparent clinically in a study examining the healing of spinal fusion wounds.[182]

PREOPERATIVE EVALUATION OF MEDICALLY COMPLEX PATIENTS

The preoperative assessment must take into account both the type of procedure planned and the type of patient (i.e., physical health and psychological status). Healthy patients clearly can be expected to tolerate surgical procedures better than medically complex patients (see Chapters 3 and 26). Clinicians should anticipate and prepare for the inevitability of treating more medically complex patients as the population ages. It is beyond the scope of this brief section to cover all possible medical considerations; rather, the most common issues that may require modification of an endodontic surgical treatment plan are presented. Relatively few absolute contraindications to periradicular surgery exist for patients well enough to seek care in an ambulatory dental office. Nonetheless, if any question arises about a patient's ability to tolerate a surgical procedure, medical consultation is advised. A thorough medical history and assessment of vital signs are required parts of the presurgical evaluation.

The American Society of Anesthesiologists (ASA) has developed a widely used system for establishing surgical risk. Patients categorized as ASA 1 are healthy and usually require no modification of the surgical treatment plan. Patients classified as ASA 4 or ASA 5 are not treated in a dental office; these individuals have significant medical problems that take priority over dental considerations. Patients considered ASA 2 or ASA 3 are commonly seen on an outpatient basis and may require medical consultation and modification of the surgical treatment plan. Patients in the ASA 2 and ASA 3 categories have mild to moderate systemic disease and often are undergoing treatment with one or more prescription medications. The ASA classification system should only be used as a general guide because, when used alone, the ASA system is not a reliable predictor of operative risk.[201] In addition, even experienced anesthesiologists exhibit differences of opinion when using the ASA system to classify patients.[227,395] The patient's psychological status and anticipated procedural stress should be considered in addition to the ASA classification of physical health. A stress reduction protocol may be helpful for patients who report moderate dental anxiety with concurrent mild to moderate systemic disease (see Chapter 28).

Surgical procedures typically require a larger amount of local anesthetic with a vasoconstrictor than nonsurgical root canal treatment. An essential part of the presurgical evaluation is an assessment of the patient's cardiovascular status and tolerance for local anesthetics that contain epinephrine. In particular, patients with advanced cardiovascular disease, geriatric patients, and patients taking certain medications may have a reduced tolerance for local anesthetics containing a vasoconstrictor (see Chapters 3 and 4). Treatment-induced stress associated with surgical procedures can cause a significant increase in heart rate and systolic blood pressure when compared to nonsurgical root canal therapy.[189] The use of local anesthetics with vasoconstrictors was addressed in the seventh report of the Joint National Committee on Prevention, Detection, Evaluation, and Treatment of High Blood Pressure (JNC 7).[231] An updated version of this report (JNC 8) was issued in 2013. In patients with cardiovascular disease, 0.036 to 0.054 mg of epinephrine (approximately two to three cartridges of local anesthetic with 1 : 100,000 epinephrine) should be safe for most patients except those with severe cardiovascular disease or other specific risk factors.[38,231,594] Local anesthetics with vasoconstrictors should be avoided or used with extreme caution in patients with the following cardiovascular conditions: severe or poorly controlled hypertension, arrhythmias that are refractory to treatment, myocardial infarction within the past month, stroke within the past 6 months, coronary artery bypass graft within the past 3 months, and uncontrolled congestive heart failure.[311] Patients unable to tolerate vasoconstrictors may not be good candidates for periradicular surgery, because a local anesthetic with a vasoconstrictor is essential for obtaining adequate hemostasis and visibility during this type of procedure. Surgery can be performed using only local anesthetics without vasoconstrictors, but this is not recommended.

The potential for multiple drug interactions is increasing because of the aging population and the introduction of many new drugs. Many elderly patients have diminished liver and kidney function and therefore cannot metabolize and excrete drugs as efficiently as younger, healthy patients. The potential for drug interactions and decreased metabolism and excretion of drugs should be considered even for commonly used agents such as local anesthetics and analgesics.

A transient bacteremia is a virtual certainty with periradicular surgery; therefore, patients at high risk for bacterial endocarditis should receive appropriate antibiotic prophylaxis as recommended by the American Heart Association. New guidelines for prevention of infective endocarditis were published in 2007 and represent a significant change from previous American Heart Association guidelines.[588] For example, antibiotic prophylaxis is no longer recommended for patients with a history of mitral valve prolapse (with or without regurgitation), rheumatic heart disease, bicuspid valve disease, aortic stenosis, and certain congenital heart conditions. Antibiotic

prophylaxis is now only recommended for patients with valvular disease associated with the highest risk of adverse outcomes from infective endocarditis. For patients in the highest risk category, antibiotic prophylaxis is recommended for dental procedures that involve manipulation of gingival tissues or the periapical region of teeth or perforation of the oral mucosa. For all other patients with valvular disease, the risks associated with routine antibiotic prophylaxis are greater than the potential benefits.[588] Although these guidelines represent the best available current evidence, practitioners should be aware that a recent study from England found a significant increase in cases of infective endocarditis after widespread adoption of the new guidelines in 2008. However, the authors point out that their data do not establish a causal relationship and recommend adherence to the current guidelines at this time (Dayer MJ, et al. Lancet 2014).

New clinical practice guidelines for the management of patients with prosthetic joints were co-developed by the American Association of Orthopaedic Surgeons and the American Dental Association in December 2012.[578] The working group conducted a systematic review and presented three recommendations. Recommendation 1 states that "the practitioner might consider discontinuing the practice of routinely prescribing prophylactic antibiotics for patients with hip and knee prosthetic joint implants undergoing dental procedures." The level of evidence to support this recommendation was classified as "limited," but that was the highest level of evidence assigned to any of the three recommendations. Two case-control studies provide evidence for this recommendation.[51,498] In recommendation 2, the group was unable to recommend for or against the use of topical antimicrobial agents (grade of recommendation = inconclusive). Recommendation 3 was a consensus recommendation to support the maintenance of appropriate oral hygiene (grade of recommendation = consensus). A recent American Dental Association Council on Scientific Affairs report added further clarification by concluding that: "In general, for patients with prosthetic joint implants, prophylactic antibiotics are not recommended prior to dental procedures to prevent prosthetic joint infection." (Sollecito TP, et al. JADA 2015).

Management of patients undergoing anticoagulant therapy depends on the type of anticoagulant, the reason for anticoagulant therapy, and the type of oral surgery planned. Warfarin (Coumadin), a commonly prescribed anticoagulant used to treat or prevent thromboembolisms, blocks the formation of prothrombin and other clotting factors. The international normalized ratio (INR) value is the accepted standard for measuring prothrombin time (PT). The desired therapeutic range for the INR usually is 2 to 3.5, depending on the underlying medical indication for anticoagulant therapy. Limited oral surgery procedures, such as simple forceps extraction of one to three teeth, may be performed safely on patients with INR values within the normal therapeutic range.[8,89,255,478] Periradicular surgery, however, may present a greater challenge for hemostasis, even for patients well maintained within the therapeutic range. The clear field visibility normally required for proper surgical management of the root end may not be possible in patients undergoing anticoagulant therapy. The patient's physician must be consulted for assistance in developing an appropriate treatment plan. Some patients may be able to tolerate discontinuation of warfarin therapy 2 days before a planned surgical procedure, which allows the INR to drift downward.

In a prospective cohort study, Russo and colleagues[461] reported that suspension of warfarin 2 days before a surgical procedure resulted in no bleeding problems and no thromboembolic events. They found that the average time spent at an INR below 2 (critical value) was 28 hours and that 90% of the patients returned to the desired therapeutic INR value within 7 days. However, this strategy may place certain patients at greater risk for a thromboembolic event; therefore, discontinuation of anticoagulant therapy would not be recommended.

In general, patients undergoing anticoagulant therapy should present minimal risk for significant bleeding during or after oral surgery, and local measures to control bleeding should be adequate.[88,569] In a review prepared for the American Dental Association Council on Scientific Affairs and Division of Science, Jeske and Suchko[260] recommended against routine discontinuation of anticoagulant therapy before dental procedures, including surgical procedures. Regardless of the management approach selected, consultation with the patient's physician and an INR test on the day of surgery are strongly recommended. A retrospective study of an urban dental school population found that INR values for 43% of patients taking warfarin were not within the recommended therapeutic range.[266] To underscore the challenge of maintaining anticoagulation levels within an appropriate therapeutic range, warfarin has been implicated in more emergency hospital admissions than any other medication.[83]

Hospitalization and conversion to heparin therapy may be considered in special cases, but the patient, physician, and surgeon must carefully weigh the potential risks against the expected outcome and benefits. A new category of heparin anticoagulant, low-molecular-weight heparins (LMWHs), allows patient self-administration and may be an alternative for patients who need to maintain a high level of anticoagulation but want to reduce the cost and time required for traditional heparin conversion therapy.

Novel oral anticoagulant drugs (NOACs) have recently emerged as an alternative to warfarin for most indications (e.g., previous stroke, atrial fibrillation, and deep vein thrombosis) *except* mechanical heart valves. Examples include: apixaban (Eliquis), dabigatran (Pradaxa), edoxaban (Lixiana), and rivaroxaban (Xarelto). NOACs have fewer interactions with foods and other drugs, and there is no need for routine blood work monitoring. However, although NOACs are known to prolong prothrombin time (PT) by inhibiting factor X to Xa conversion, there is currently no reliable test to accurately measure level of anticoagulation. Medical consultation may be indicated to help evaluate the relative benefits and risks of discontinuing NOAC drugs for one or two days prior to endodontic surgery.

Low-dose aspirin therapy is known to increase bleeding time by irreversibly inhibiting platelet aggregation. A common practice has been to advise patients to discontinue aspirin therapy for 7 to 10 days before oral surgery.[28] At low-dose therapeutic levels (less than 100 mg per day), aspirin may increase bleeding time and complicate surgical procedures. However, Ardekian and colleagues[28] concluded that low-dose aspirin therapy should *not* be discontinued before surgical procedures and that bleeding could be controlled by local measures. Higher-dose therapy may create a greater risk of bleeding during or after surgery.

Although a patient undergoing aspirin therapy may not be at high risk for significant bleeding during or after surgery, a concern in periradicular surgery is the visibility problems created by oozing blood. The clinician should consult the patient's physician about the medical reason for aspirin therapy and should weigh the risks and benefits of discontinuing aspirin before the proposed surgery. It should be possible to perform periradicular surgery without discontinuing aspirin therapy if necessary, but visibility during the procedure may be compromised, which may adversely affect the prognosis.

Herbs, dietary supplements, and vitamins can contribute to bleeding problems during surgery, and patients often fail to report use of these substances in the preoperative evaluation.[385] In a survey of surgical patients, approximately one third reported using a nonprescription medication that might inhibit coagulation or interact with anesthetics.[384] In particular, ginkgo biloba, ginger, garlic, ginseng, feverfew, and vitamin E inhibit platelet aggregation and can increase the risk of bleeding.[96] Ingredients in over-the-counter (OTC) weight loss products can potentiate the effect of epinephrine and increase cardiac stress, although the most obvious example of this phenomenon, ephedra, has been removed from the U.S. market by a Food and Drug Administration (FDA) order.

Patients with inherited or acquired bleeding disorders are also at risk for excessive bleeding during and after periradicular surgery. Impaired liver function associated with past or current alcohol or drug abuse may also predispose a patient to excessive bleeding during surgery. A thorough medical history and patient interview should help identify these patients and, in consultation with the patient's physician, allow for any necessary treatment modifications.

Many other medical conditions, such as recent myocardial infarction, stroke, cardiac arrhythmias, diabetes, radiation therapy for head and neck cancer, immunocompromising conditions, seizure disorders, adrenal suppression, liver or kidney disease, and pregnancy may require modification of the treatment plan. However, these conditions usually present more general problems that are not unique to a surgical procedure. The value of a thorough medical history and patient interview cannot be overemphasized.

ANATOMIC CONSIDERATIONS

Evaluating the access to the surgical site is one of the most important steps in case selection for periradicular surgery. Anatomic studies can provide some guidance, but individual variation is great, and there is no substitute for a complete clinical examination. A small oral opening, active facial muscles, shallow vestibule, and thick buccal alveolar bone all can significantly increase the difficulty of the procedure, even in cases that appear straightforward on radiographic examination.

Posterior Mandible

The primary anatomic structure of concern for periradicular surgery in the posterior mandible is the neurovascular bundle that courses through the mandibular canal and exits through the mental foramen. The relationship among the mandibular canal, the mental foramen, and the root apices of mandibular teeth has been well studied; however, anthropometric averages have limited value in the treatment of individual patients. An understanding of the typical anatomic relationships is important, but even more important is an evaluation of the individual patient to develop a case-specific risk assessment.

The depth of the vestibular fornix generally is a good predictor of the possible difficulty involved in obtaining surgical

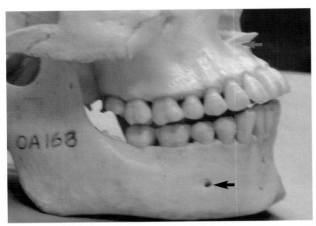

FIG. 9-5 Lateral view of the skull showing the anterior nasal spine and the proximity of the maxillary anterior root apices to the floor of the nose *(red arrow)*, as well as the typical location of the mental foramen *(black arrow)*.

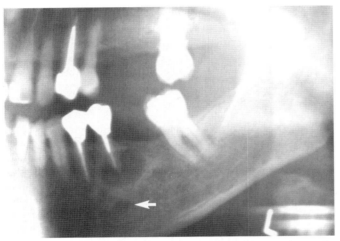

FIG. 9-6 Preoperative evaluation of a mandibular left second premolar included a panoramic radiograph to help locate the mental foramen *(white arrow)*, which was not visible on a standard periapical radiograph.

access to the mandibular posterior teeth.[305] A shallow vestibule usually portends thicker alveolar bone and more difficult access to the root end.

The mental foramen, another key anatomic structure, usually is located between and apical to the mandibular first and second premolars[118,356]; however, this varies considerably, and the practitioner must examine each patient carefully to determine its location (Figs. 9-5 and 9-6). Vertical location of the mental foramen may vary even more than horizontal location. Moiseiwitsch[356] found that the average location was 16 mm inferior to the cementoenamel junction (CEJ) of the second premolar, although the range was 8 to 21 mm, which would place approximately 20% of the foramina at or coronal to the root apex. Fortunately, the mental foramen usually is easily visualized with standard periapical and panoramic radiographs. A vertically positioned periapical radiograph often may be more useful than a horizontally positioned one, especially in individuals with longer roots. Also, the mental foramen usually can be palpated.

When a vertical releasing incision is indicated, it typically is made at the mesial line angle of the mandibular canine. This location is always mesial to the mental foramen, because the foramen is located in the area ranging from the apex of the mandibular first premolar to slightly distal to the second premolar. The nerve bundle exits from the foramen in a distal direction. An alternative technique for gaining access to mandibular posterior teeth involves a distal releasing incision between the mandibular first and second molars.[355] This approach may be especially useful for access to the mandibular second premolar and first molar. Care must be taken to avoid the facial artery as it crosses the level of the inferior vestibular fornix near the mandibular first molar. Inadvertent contact with the facial artery is unlikely if the incision is not extended beyond the depth of the vestibule.

Regardless of the approach selected, it obviously is important to avoid making an incision in the immediate vicinity of the mental foramen. The mental nerve is encased in a relatively tough sheath, and permanent damage can be avoided if careful blunt dissection is used in the area. A misguided vertical releasing incision, however, may sever the nerve, causing permanent injury. Trauma to the nerve from blunt dissection in this area or from pressure from a misplaced retractor may cause temporary paresthesia but is much less likely to do permanent injury. (Documentation and management of nerve injuries are discussed later in the chapter.)

The borders of the mandibular canal often are more difficult to visualize with conventional radiographic techniques. A parallel periapical radiograph, either horizontally or vertically positioned, usually can provide a reasonably accurate image of the relationship between the superior border of the mandibular canal and the root apices. However, the mandibular canal sometimes cannot be readily visualized. Such cases should be approached with extreme caution, because an increased risk of paresthesia secondary to nerve injury may be an unacceptable risk for many patients. Cone-beam computed tomography (CBCT) imaging can be very useful for identifying the location of the mandibular canal and determining its relationship to the root apices (see Chapter 2).[68,285,556]

In the buccolingual dimension, the mandibular canal commonly follows a curving pathway from the buccal half of the mandible near the distal root of the second molar to the lingual half of the mandible near the first molar, then curving back to the buccal near the second premolar as it exits the mental foramen.[136] The average vertical distance from the superior border of the mandibular canal to the distal root apex of the mandibular second molar is approximately 3.5 mm; this increases gradually to approximately 6.2 mm for the mesial root of the mandibular first molar and to 4.7 mm for the second premolar.[136,312] This relationship typically provides a greater margin of safety for surgery on the mandibular first molar compared with the second premolar and especially the second molar. Surgery on the mandibular second molar may be further complicated by relatively thick overlying buccal bone, lingual inclination of the roots, and a more buccal location of the mandibular canal. This is not to say that periradicular surgery should not be performed on mandibular second molars; rather, it points out that the relative risks and benefits must be carefully considered. Often the most prudent choice for a mandibular second molar is an intentional replantation procedure or extraction and placement of an implant.

Posterior Maxilla

The primary anatomic structure of concern in the posterior maxilla is the maxillary sinus. CBCT allows for a more precise preoperative three-dimensional evaluation of the relationship between the roots of maxillary posterior teeth and the sinus.[69,79] Perforation of the sinus during surgery is fairly common, with a reported incidence of about 10% to 50% of cases.[157,177,456] Even without periradicular pathosis, the distance between the root apices of the maxillary posterior teeth and the maxillary sinus sometimes is less than 1 mm.[225] An inflammatory periradicular lesion often increases the likelihood of sinus exposure during surgery. Fortunately, perforation of the maxillary sinus rarely results in long-term postoperative problems.[225] In a report of 146 cases of sinus exposure during periradicular surgery, Watzek and colleagues[579] found no difference in healing compared with similar surgical procedures without sinus exposure. The sinus membrane usually regenerates, and a thin layer of new bone often forms over the root end, although osseous regeneration is less predictable.[50,157,579] The general rule of placing a vertical releasing incision at least one tooth mesial and distal to the surgical site is especially important when sinus perforation is possible, because the exposure site should be completely covered with the mucoperiosteal flap to provide primary closure.

If the maxillary sinus is entered during surgery, special care must be taken to prevent infected root fragments and debris from entering the sinus. The most commonly used root resection technique involves grinding the root apex with a high-speed drill for approximately 3 mm in an apical to coronal direction; therefore, an opening could allow infected debris into the sinus. A sinus opening can be temporarily occluded with a material such as Telfa gauze, although the gauze should be secured so as to prevent inadvertent displacement into the sinus. A suture can be placed through the packing material to prevent displacement and aid retrieval. Jerome and Hill[259] suggested securing the apical root segment by drilling a small hole in the root tip and threading a piece of suture material through the hole. The root is then resected at the appropriate level, and the root-end fragment is removed in one piece. If a root fragment or other foreign object is displaced into the sinus, it should be removed. An orascope or endoscope may be useful for visualizing the foreign object, but referral for evaluation and surgical removal may be indicated if the fragment cannot be located and removed.

The palatal roots of maxillary molars present a special challenge for surgical access. Palatal roots may be reached from either a buccal (transantral) or palatal approach. Wallace[572] described a transantral approach in which a buccal flap is reflected, the buccal roots are resected, the osteotomy access into the sinus is enlarged to approximately 1 by 1.5 cm, and the palatal root tip is resected, ultrasonically prepared, and filled. The sinus may be packed with moist gauze to catch debris, and it should be irrigated with sterile saline upon completion of the surgery. In some cases, careful reflection and retraction of the sinus membrane may be possible, allowing access to the palatal root end without direct invasion of the sinus.[16] Many who have tried this approach find it more challenging than it might initially seem. The enhanced illumination and magnification provided by a dental operating microscope, endoscope, or orascope are essential aids in this type of surgery.[40]

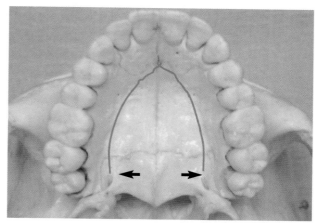

FIG. 9-7 Palatal view showing the position of the greater palatine foramen *(arrows)*. The approximate location of the anterior palatine artery is marked in red.

A palatal approach to the palatal root of maxillary molars may seem more direct than a transantral approach, but it can present certain difficulties. Visibility in the surgical field is reduced and manipulation of instruments is more difficult than with most routine buccal approaches. Patients with a deep, vertical palatal vault are better candidates for this approach than individuals with a wide, shallow palate. A sinus tract or a large lesion on the palatal root may allow easier access and better visualization of the palatal root, because only limited bone removal would be required. The position of the anterior palatine artery must be carefully considered when the incision is made and the flap reflected. This artery emerges from the greater palatine foramen distal to the maxillary second molar at the junction of the vertical section of the alveolar process and the flat portion of the palate and continues anteriorly (Fig. 9-7). A vertical releasing incision can be placed between the maxillary first premolar and canine, where the artery is relatively narrow and branches off into smaller arteries. If needed, a short distal vertical releasing incision may be made distal to the second molar, but it should not approach the junction of the alveolar process and roof of the palate. If the anterior palatine artery is severed, local clamping and pressure may not stop the hemorrhage, and ligation of the external carotid artery may be necessary. Because of the palatal vault's concave shape, repositioning the flap may be challenging. An acrylic surgical stent may be fabricated before surgery to assist repositioning of the flap and to help prevent pooling of blood under the flap.

Anterior Maxilla and Mandible

Periradicular surgery on anterior teeth generally involves fewer anatomic hazards and potential complications than in posterior teeth. Nonetheless, access to the root apex in some patients may be unexpectedly difficult because of long roots, a shallow vestibule, or lingual inclination of the roots. As shown in Figure 9-5, the root apices of maxillary central and lateral incisors can be quite close to the floor of the nose and the bony anterior nasal spine. Figure 9-8 demonstrates isolation and protection of the nasopalatine neurovascular bundle during maxillary anterior surgery. The average maxillary canine is about 26 mm long and usually presents no difficulty for surgical access; however, the combination of a shallow vestibule and

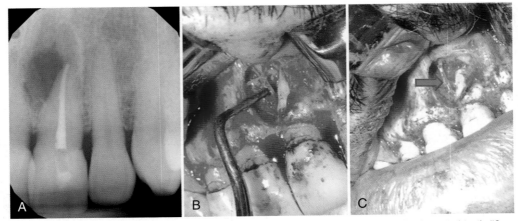

FIG. 9-8 **A,** Radiograph demonstrating periradicular radiolucency associated with previously treated tooth #9. **B-C,** After full thickness flap reflection, the nasopalatine neurovascular bundle was identified (**B**), protected, and isolated (*arrow* in **C**) during curettage of cystic lesion. (Courtesy Dr. Tim Rogers.)

a longer than average root length could complicate access to the root apex area. In such cases, the creation of an osteotomy apical to the root end may be impossible. An alternative approach for long-rooted teeth and root tips in the vicinity of critical anatomic structures is to enter the bone and resect the root at a level approximately 3 mm coronal to the apex. After the root tip is removed, the area apical to the root can be inspected and curetted as needed.

Periradicular surgery on mandibular incisors often is more challenging than expected. The combination of lingual root inclination, a shallow vestibule, and a prominent mental protuberance all can increase the degree of difficulty, as can proximity to adjacent roots and the need for perpendicular root-end resection and preparation to include a possible missed lingual canal.

CONE-BEAM COMPUTED TOMOGRAPHY

Radiographic examination is an essential component in all aspects of endodontic treatment from diagnosis and treatment planning to assessing outcome (see also Chapter 2). Information gained from conventional films and digital periapical radiographs is limited by the fact that the three-dimensional anatomy of the area is compressed into a two-dimensional image. As a result of superimposition, periapical radiographs reveal limited aspects of the three-dimensional anatomy. In addition, there may also be geometric distortion of the anatomic structures imaged. These problems may be overcome using small volume cone-beam computed tomography (CBCT) imaging techniques, which can produce three-dimensional images of individual teeth and the surrounding tissues. CBCT may be particularly useful in diagnosis and treatment planning for periradicular surgery[112,163,249,318] (Fig. 9-9). The term *cone-beam computed tomography* is often used interchangeably with *cone-beam volumetric tomography* (CBVT).

Differences Between CT and CBCT Imaging

The benefits of three-dimensional medical computer tomography (CT) imaging are already well established in certain dental specialties. Current CT scanners have a linear array of multiple detectors, allowing multiple slices to be taken simultaneously, resulting in faster scan times and often less radiation exposure to the patient.[507] The slices of data are then "stacked" and can be reformatted to obtain three-dimensional images. The high-radiation dose, cost, availability, poor resolution, and difficulty in interpretation have resulted in limited use of CT imaging in endodontics. These issues may be addressed by cone-beam innovations in CBCT technology.

In 2000, the Food and Drug Administration approved the first CBCT unit for dental use in the United States. Cone-beam technology uses a cone-shaped beam of radiation to acquire a volume in a single 360-degree rotation, similar to panoramic radiography. The volume of acquired images by a CBCT is composed of voxels. Essentially, a voxel is a 3D pixel. Because the data are captured in a volume as opposed to slices, all the voxels are isotropic, which enables objects within the volume to be accurately measured in different directions. Unlike the CBCT voxel, a medical CT voxel is not a perfect cube, and measurements made in multiple planes are not accurate. In addition to increased accuracy and higher resolution, CBCT offers significant scan-time reduction, radiation dose reduction, and reduced cost for the patient.[472,595,606] CBCT systems can be classified into two categories: limited (dental or regional) CBCT or full (ortho or facial) CBCT. The field of view (FOV) of limited CBCT ranges in diameter from 40 to 100 mm, whereas the FOV of full CBCT ranges from 100 to 200 mm.[112] Another difference between the limited CBCT and full CBCT is that a voxel is generally smaller for the limited version (0.1 to 0.2 mm versus 0.3 to 0.4 mm). Thus, limited CBCT systems offer higher resolution and are better suited for endodontic applications. Limited volume CBCT scanners capture small volumes of data that can include just two or three individual teeth. The most important and clinically useful feature of CBCT technology is the highly sophisticated software that allows the huge volume of data collected to be reconstructed. Tomographic slices, as thin as one voxel, may be displayed in a number of ways. One option, for example, is for the images to be displayed in the three orthogonal planes—axial, sagittal and coronal—simultaneously. The axial and proximal (sagittal in the anterior, coronal in the posterior) views are of particular value, because they are generally not seen with conventional periapical radiography. The ability to reduce or eliminate

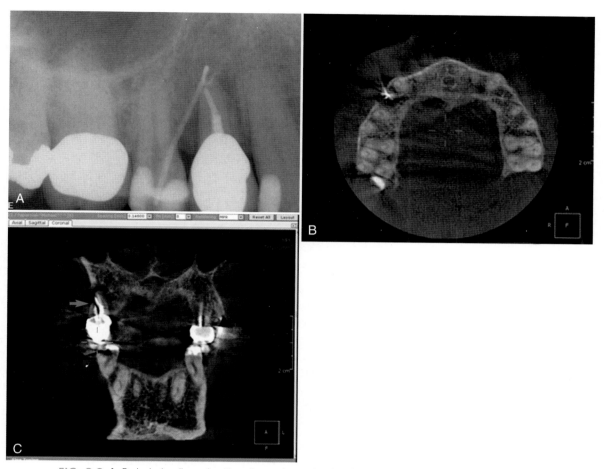

FIG. 9-9 **A,** Periapical radiograph with gutta percha tracing the sinus tract to tooth #5. Periodontal probings were WNL. This tooth was initially referred for exploratory surgery to rule out root fracture. CBCT confirmed root fracture and the treatment plan was changed to extraction with possible bone graft and guided tissue regeneration for ridge augmentation prior to implant placement. **B,** Axial CBCT view demonstrating extent of lesion. **C,** Coronal CBCT view demonstrating root fracture *(red arrow)* and perforation of buccal cortical plate in area of root fracture but intact bone in the cervical area.

superimposition of the surrounding structures makes CBCT superior to conventional periapical radiography.[314]

Scan times are typically 10 to 40 s, although the actual exposure time is significantly less (2 to 5 s) as scans involve a number (up to 360) of separate, small, individual exposures rather than one continuous exposure. With medical CT scanners, the scanning and exposure times for the skull can be significantly longer. Most CBCT scanners are much smaller than medical CT scanners, taking up about the same space as a dental panoramic machine. They are also significantly less expensive than medical CT scanners. With the help of viewer software, the clinician is able to scroll through the entire volume and simultaneously view axial, coronal, and sagittal 2D sections that range from 0.125 to 2 mm thick. Comparing the radiation dose of different CBCT scanners with medical CT scanners may be confusing because different units of radiation dose are often used. There are three basic measurement units in radiation dosimetry: the radiation absorbed dose (D), the equivalent dose (H), and the effective dose (E). The *radiation absorbed dose* is defined as the measure of the amount of energy absorbed from the radiation beam per unit mass of tissue and is measured in joules per kilogram. The *equivalent dose* is

defined as a measure that indicates the radiobiologic effectiveness of different types of radiation and thus provides a common unit. The *effective dose* is calculated by multiplying the equivalent dose by different tissue weighting factors, which converts all doses to an equivalent whole-body dose and allows doses from different investigations of different parts of the body to be compared. The unit remains as the Sievert (Sv) and can be used to estimate the damage from radiation to an exposed population. The reported effective doses from CBCT scanners vary but can be almost as low as those from panoramic dental x-ray units and considerably less than that from medical CT scanners.[398] The higher effective doses from particular models of CBCT scanners is in part due to the larger size of the field of view used as well as the type of image receptor employed. The small volume scanners capture information from a small region of the jaw, approximately the same area as a periapical radiograph. The effective dose has been reported to be in the same range as 2 to 3 standard periapical radiograph exposures, whereas the effective dose for a full mouth series of periapical radiographs has been reported to be similar to the effective dose of a large volume CBCT scan.[124,194] If multiple teeth in different quadrants require endodontic evaluation or treatment, a large volume CBCT scan with a large field of view may be more appropriate. If endodontic information is required from multiple teeth in one jaw, a large volume CBCT scan with the field of view only limited to the jaw of interest could be the investigation of choice. This has the advantage of reducing the effective dosage from the full large volume CBCT scan by up to 65%.[321]

Potential Applications of CBCT in the Management of Endodontic Posttreatment Disease

Clinical radiographic examinations are usually limited to two-dimensional views captured using radiographic film or digital sensors. Crucial information related to the true three-dimensional anatomy of teeth and adjacent structures is obscured. Even with paralleling techniques, distortion and superimposition of dental structures in periapical views is unavoidable. A major reported advantage of CBCT is the accuracy of measurements in all dimensions.[331] The ability to view thin sagittal, coronal, and axial slices effectively eliminates the problem of superimposition of anatomic structures. For example, roots of maxillary posterior teeth and surrounding tissues can be viewed without superimposition of the zygomatic buttress, alveolar bone, maxillary sinus, and other roots (Fig. 9-10). CBCT enables clinicians to detect changes in apical bone density at an earlier stage when compared to conventional periapical radiographs and therefore has the potential to detect previously undiagnosed periradicular pathoses.[163,314,371] CBCT may also prove to be a useful tool for noninvasive differentiation of periapical cysts and granulomas,[489] a previously unattainable goal using conventional radiographic imaging.

Three-dimensional imaging allows for clear identification of the anatomic relationship of the root apices to important neighboring anatomic structures such as the mandibular canal, mental foramen, and maxillary sinus (Fig. 9-11). Velvart and colleagues reported that the relationship of the inferior alveolar canal to the root apices could be determined in every case when utilizing medical CT, but in less than 40% of cases when using conventional radiography.[556] It is likely that similar results could be achieved with CBCT using considerably less radiation. Rigolone and coworkers concluded that CBCT may play an important role in periapical microsurgery of palatal roots of maxillary first molars.[442] The distance between the cortical plate and the palatal root apex could be measured using CBCT and the presence of the maxillary sinus between the roots could be assessed. Additional information such as the thickness of the cortical plate, cancellous bone pattern, fenestrations, and inclination of the roots can be obtained prior to surgical entry.[371] Root morphology (shape, size, curvature, and number of canals) can be visualized in three dimensions. Unidentified (and untreated) canals in root-filled teeth can be routinely visualized in axial slices. CBCT has been used to determine the location and extent of invasive external root resorptive defects.[398]

One of the most useful potential applications of CBCT may be the assessment of endodontic treatment outcomes, both nonsurgical and surgical. When compared to two-dimensional film and digital images, CBCT is dimensionally precise and can detect smaller changes in bone density.[331]

It is worth remembering that CBCT still uses ionizing radiation and is not without risk. It is essential that patient exposure is kept as low as reasonably practical and that justifiable selection criteria for CBCT use are developed. CBCT may be indicated when it is determined that the additional information obtained is likely to result in a more accurate diagnosis and enhanced patient safety.

PATIENT PREPARATION FOR SURGERY

Informed-Consent Issues Specific to Surgery

The general principles of informed consent discussed in Chapter 29 form the basis for informed consent for periradicular surgery. The patient must be thoroughly advised of the benefits, risks, and other treatment options and must be given an opportunity to ask questions. The main consent issues specific to surgical procedures are closely related to the anatomic considerations discussed in the previous section. That is, major neurovascular bundles may be traumatized, and a sinus exposure may occur. Paresthesia after mandibular posterior surgery is uncommon but should be discussed with the patient because this potential complication is a risk some patients may be unwilling to assume. Postoperative swelling, bruising, bleeding, and infections are possible complications that typically are self-limiting or readily manageable. Although the incidence of serious complications related to surgical procedures is very low, patients should be advised of any risks unique to their situation. Prompt attention to any surgical complications and thorough follow-up are essential from a medical-legal standpoint.

Premedication: NSAIDs, Antibiotics, Chlorhexidine, and Conscious Sedation

Administration of an NSAID, either before or up to 30 minutes after surgery, enhances postoperative analgesia.[494] NSAIDs generally have proved more effective in the management of postoperative oral surgery pain than placebo or acetaminophen and codeine combinations.[9,41,143] The combination of preoperative administration of an NSAID and use of a long-acting local anesthetic may be particularly helpful for reducing postoperative pain.[144] Many types of NSAIDs are available, but ibuprofen remains the usual standard for comparison. Ibuprofen (400 mg) provides analgesia approximately equal to that obtained with morphine (10 mg) and significantly greater than that from codeine (60 mg), tramadol (100 mg), or acetaminophen (1000 mg).[346] The analgesic effectiveness of ibuprofen tends to level off at about the 400-mg level (*ceiling effect*), although a slight increase in analgesic potential may be expected in doses up to 800 mg. (See Chapter 4 for further discussion of analgesics.)

The value of antibiotic prophylaxis before or after oral surgery is controversial, and the current best available evidence does not support the routine use of prophylactic antibiotics for periradicular surgery.[11] For most patients, the risks of indiscriminate antibiotic therapy are believed to be greater than the potential benefits.[526] The incidence of infection after oral surgery in healthy patients is very low. Peterson reported that only 1% of patients developed infections after third molar extractions.[355] A systematic review of the use of antibiotics to prevent complications after placement of dental implants found that evidence was lacking either to recommend or discourage the use of antibiotics for this purpose.[162] However, the

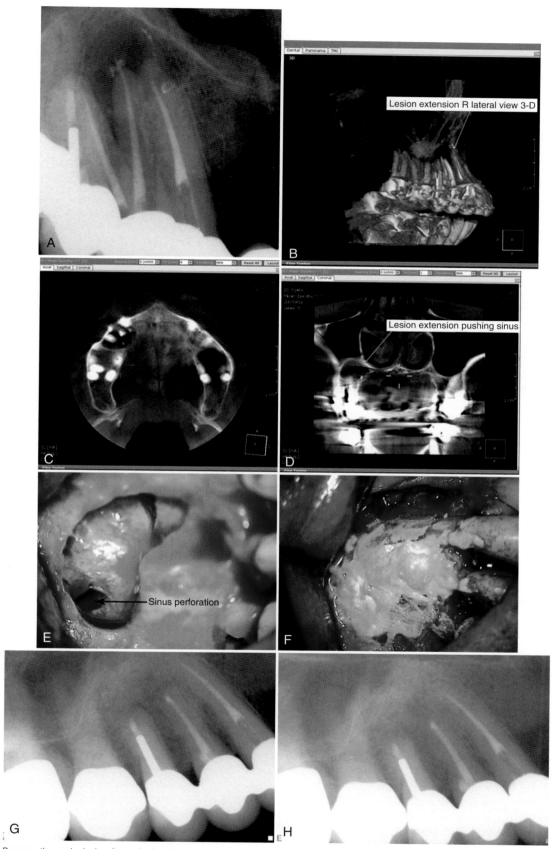

FIG. 9-10 **A,** Preoperative periapical radiograph showing large radiolucency associated with teeth #4, 5, and 6. **B,** CBCT reconstruction *(lateral view).* Rotation of the 3D volume on a computer monitor demonstrated that intact bone was present around the apex of tooth #6 and the lesion was associated only with #4 and 5 (this could not be detected with multiple angled periapical radiographs). **C,** Axial CBCT view demonstrating facial-palatal extent of the lesion. **D,** Coronal CBCT view showing displacement of the sinus membrane (a finding that suggests a sinus membrane perforation will be detected during surgery). **E,** Clinical image after surgical access removal of granulation tissue, and root-end resection (note sinus perforation [*arrow*]). **F,** Placement of bone graft and Capset. **G,** Immediate postoperative radiograph. **H,** Two-year follow-up radiograph demonstrating good healing.

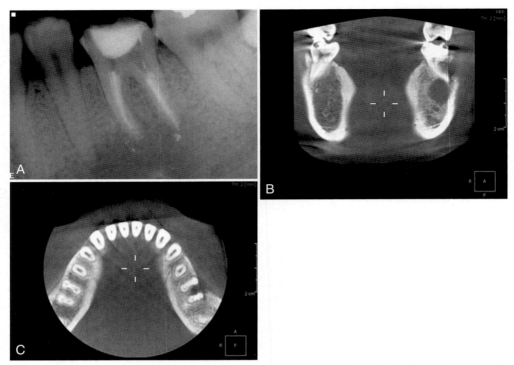

FIG. 9-11 A, Periapical radiograph demonstrating persistent periradicular pathosis following nonsurgical retreatment of tooth #19. The extension of the lesion in the vicinity of the mandibular canal and possible involvement of tooth #20 was uncertain based on interpretation of periapical and panoramic radiographs. Tooth #20 responded WNL to pulp vitality test. **B,** Coronal CBCT demonstrates that the periradicular lesion does not extend apical or lingual to the mandibular canal. **C,** Axial CBCT view demonstrating perforation of the buccal cortical plate and extension into, but not through, the furcation of #19 and presence of intact bone around #20.

use of prophylactic antibiotics for more invasive procedures, such as orthognathic surgery, has significantly reduced the risk of postoperative infection and complications.[146] Although routine use of prophylactic antibiotics for periradicular surgery is not currently recommended, clinical judgment is important in determining exceptions to the general rule. For example, immunocompromised patients may be good candidates for prophylactic antibiotic coverage. Certain categories of medically complex patients also may benefit from antibiotic coverage. Diabetic patients have shown impaired healing capacity after nonsurgical root canal treatment,[78,175] and a like pattern of delayed or impaired healing may emerge in studies of surgical outcomes. The global problems associated with overprescription of antibiotics are significant and should prompt due caution in the decision on whether to use these drugs prophylactically.

Chlorhexidine gluconate (0.12%) often is recommended as a mouth rinse to reduce the number of surface microorganisms in the surgical field, and its use may be continued during the postoperative healing stage.[7,281,545] Although no solid evidence supports this practice in periradicular surgery, the use of chlorhexidine follows from the general surgical principle of surface disinfection before incision and opening into a body cavity. In addition, chlorhexidine has proved to be a safe, effective adjunct in the treatment of periodontitis, and short-term use (i.e., several days) poses little or no risk. Chlorhexidine may be useful for reducing the risk of postoperative infection after oral surgery,[67,598] although the evidence in this area is

conflicting. Postoperative use of chlorhexidine mouth rinse can reduce bacterial growth on sutures and wound margins,[389] but it may interfere with fibroblast reattachment to the root surface.[14] A useful empirical regimen is to have the patient rinse for 30 seconds twice a day beginning 1 or 2 days before surgery and continuing until the sutures are removed.

Conscious sedation, either by an orally administered sedative or by nitrous oxide/oxygen inhalation analgesia, may be useful for patients who are anxious about the surgical procedure or dental treatment in general. Benzodiazepines with a short half-life are particularly useful because they generally have a wide margin of safety, good absorption after oral administration, and limited residual sedative effects. When these drugs are used in sedative-hypnotic doses, the blood pressure, pulse, and respiration must be monitored, and states differ in their requirement for additional training or certification of staff members who do this monitoring. With oral conscious sedation, pulse oximetry should be used to monitor the pulse and blood oxygen saturation during the surgery.[84] As with all orally administered drugs, the dosage cannot be closely titrated; therefore, the effect of the agent varies somewhat. A typical protocol is a single dose at bedtime the evening before the procedure and a second dose 1 hour before the start of surgery. The patient should not drive to or from the office and should have a responsible adult for assistance as needed. In appropriate doses, benzodiazepines and similar drugs may allow for a more relaxed patient and thus a less stressful surgical experience for both patient and surgeon.

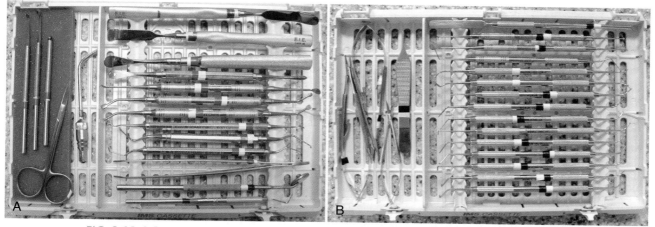

FIG. 9-12 **A,** Basic tray setup for initial surgical access. Surgical instruments shown are distributed by Hu-Friedy ([HF] Chicago), CK Dental Specialities ([CKDS] Orange, CA), EIE ([EIE]), and G. Hartzell & Son ([GHS]). *Left to right* (left section of tray): Small round micromirror (CKDS); medium oval micromirror (CKDS); handle for microscalpel (CKDS); scissors (S18 [HF]); surgical suction tip (GHS). *Top to bottom* (main section of tray): Carr #1 retractor (EIE); Carr #2 retractor (EIE); TRH-1 retractor (HF); periosteal elevator (HF); Ruddle R elevator (EIE); Ruddle L elevator (EIE); Jacquette curette (SJ 34/35 [HF]); spoon curette (CL 84 [HF]); scaler (7/8 [HF]); surgical forceps (TP 5061 [HF]); mouth mirror (HF); periodontal probe (HF). **B,** Instrument tray for root-end filling and suturing. *Left to right* (left section of tray): Two Castroviejo needle holders (Roydent Dental Products, Rochester Hills, MI); Castroviejo scissors (S31 [HF]); micro–tissue forceps (TP 5042 [HF]). *Top to bottom* (main section of tray): Cement spatula (HF); Feinstein super plugger (F1L); microexplorer (CX-1 [EIE]); endoexplorer (DG-16 [EIE]); right Super-EBA Placing & Plugging instrument (MRFR [HF]); left Super-EBA Placing & Plugging instrument (MRFL [HF]); small anterior microburnisher and plugger (HF); small left microburnisher and plugger (HF); small right microburnisher and plugger (HF); medium anterior microburnisher and plugger (HF); medium left microburnisher and plugger (HF); medium right microburnisher and plugger (HF); large anterior microburnisher and plugger (HF); large left microburnisher and plugger (HF); large right microburnisher and plugger (HF).

INSTRUMENTS AND OPERATORY SETUP

The development of microsurgical techniques and new materials has changed the typical surgical instrument tray dramatically. Instruments have been designed to take full advantage of the increased visibility obtained with dental operating microscopes, endoscopes, and orascopes. Better visualization of the surgical site would have limited value without microsurgical instruments, such as ultrasonic tips for root-end preparation and micromirrors for inspecting the root end. Figure 9-12 shows a typical basic surgery tray arrangement. This setup is not a definitive guide to surgical armamentarium but rather an adequate, efficient starting point for most periradicular surgical procedures. Although the number of instruments can easily be doubled or even tripled, the ease of locating a specific instrument is inversely proportional to the number of instruments on a tray. Specialized instruments can be kept readily available in separate sterilized bags or trays and opened as needed. A skilled surgeon can use a wide variety of instruments (Figs. 9-12 to 9-24) to achieve excellent results.

Periradicular surgery can be performed without the benefit of enhanced magnification and illumination; however, those who use microscopes, endoscopes, and orascopes report dramatically improved visualization and control of the surgical site.[39,92,280,350] Studies reporting the highest surgical success rates and those cited previously in this chapter all involved some form of enhanced magnification and illumination as part of the standard operating protocol. A systematic review and meta-analysis found that the outcome for endodontic surgery performed with high magnification and illumination (micro-

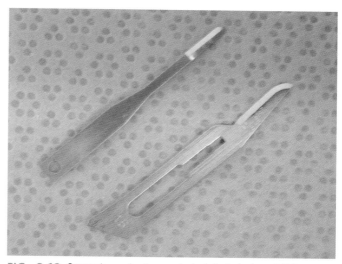

FIG. 9-13 Comparison of microsurgical scalpel *(top)* to #15C surgical blade. Microsurgical scalpels are particularly useful for the intrasulcular incision and for delicate dissection of the interproximal papillae.

scope or endoscope) was significantly higher than surgery performed with loupes only or no magnification.[482]

LOCAL ANESTHESIA FOR SURGERY

Local anesthesia for surgical root canal procedures differs from that for nonsurgical root canal treatment primarily in the need

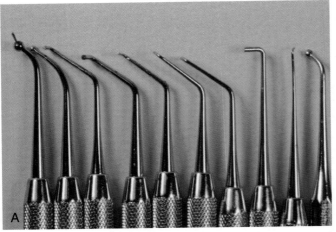

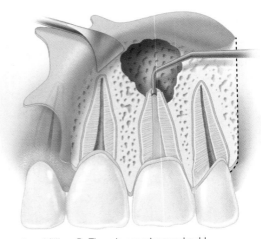

FIG. 9-14 **A,** Microcondensers in assorted shapes and sizes for root-end filling. **B,** The microcondenser should be selected to fit the root-end preparation.

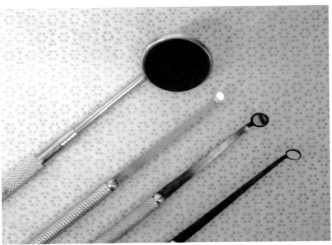

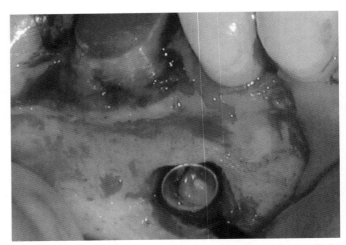

FIG. 9-15 Comparison of standard #5 mouth mirror *(top)* to diamond-coated micromirrors (CK Dental Specialties).

FIG. 9-16 Micromirror used to inspect resected mesial root of a mandibular first molar.

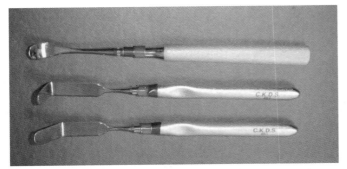

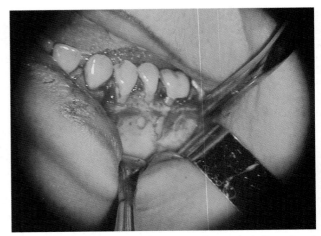

FIG. 9-17 Retractors used in periradicular surgery. *Top to bottom,* EHR-1, ER-2, and ER-1 (equivalent to Carr #2 and #1 retractors) (CK Dental Specialties).

FIG. 9-18 Retractors positioned to expose the surgical site and protect adjacent soft tissues from injury. Care must be taken to rest the retractors only on bone, not on the reflected soft-tissue flap or on the neurovascular bundle as it exits the mental foramen.

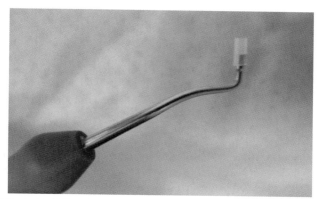

FIG. 9-19 Teflon sleeve and plugger specially designed for placement of MTA (DENTSPLY Tulsa Dental Specialties).

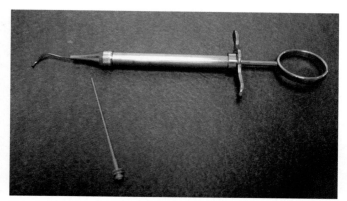

FIG. 9-20 Messing gun–type syringe (CK Dental Specialties) can be used for placement of various root-end filling materials.

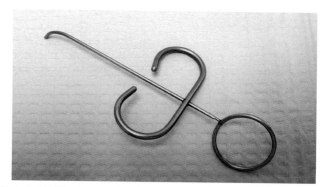

FIG. 9-21 Another delivery system designed specifically for MTA placement (Roydent). Kit includes a variety of tips for use in different areas of the mouth and a single-use Teflon plunger.

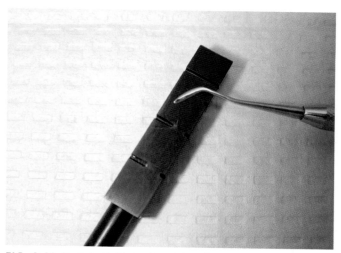

FIG. 9-22 Hard plastic block with notches of varying shapes and sizes (G. Hartzell & Son). MTA is mixed on a glass slab to the consistency of wet sand and then packed into a notch. The applicator instrument is used to transfer the preformed plug of MTA from the block to the root end.

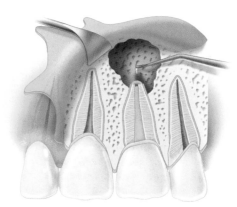

FIG. 9-23 Placement of a root-end filling.

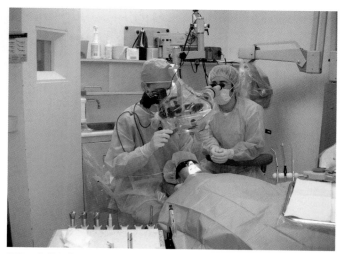

FIG. 9-24 Surgeon, assistant, and patient positioned for initiation of surgery. The patient should be given tinted goggles or some other form of eye protection before the procedure begins.

for localized hemostasis in addition to profound local anesthesia. In fact, use of a local anesthetic with a vasoconstrictor may be the single most important local measure to help control hemorrhage and provide a clear surgical field. Otherwise, the same regional block and local infiltration techniques used for nonsurgical treatment (see Chapter 4) are used for surgical root canal procedures. Infiltration of the surgical site with a local anesthetic containing 1:50,000 epinephrine is the technique of choice to obtain vasoconstriction and hemostasis.[280] The local anesthetic is first slowly deposited in the buccal root apex area of the alveolar mucosa at the surgical site and extended two or three teeth on either side of the site. Usually palatal or lingual infiltration is also required, although this requires a much smaller amount of local anesthetic than the primary buccal infiltration. After the injections for anesthesia, the surgeon should wait at least 10 minutes before making the first incision.

Long-acting local anesthetics (e.g., 0.5% bupivacaine with 1 : 200,000 epinephrine) have been shown to reduce postoperative pain and analgesic use after surgical removal of impacted third molars.[125,204] However, use of a local anesthetic with 1 : 200,000 epinephrine may result in greater blood loss during surgery.[234,493] To maximize postoperative analgesia and minimize intraoperative bleeding, a local anesthetic can be used with higher epinephrine concentrations (1 : 100,000 or 1 : 50,000) for the primary surgical anesthesia and supplemented with one cartridge of long-acting local anesthetic immediately after surgery. Long-lasting local anesthetics are particularly beneficial in mandibular surgery but much less so for surgery in the maxillary arch.

Every effort must be made to ensure profound local anesthesia before surgery begins. Usually a minimum of 10 to 20 minutes is required from the time of injection to the start of surgery to ensure both profound local anesthesia and adequate vasoconstriction for hemostasis. The patient should be asked about the usual signs of soft-tissue anesthesia, and a sharp explorer can be used to test the surgical area for sensation. Even when the surgeon pays careful attention to local anesthetic technique, a patient sometimes has inadequate anesthesia or loss of anesthesia during the surgical procedure. Providing supplemental infiltration anesthesia is difficult after a full-thickness flap has been reflected. A supplemental block injection may be useful for mandibular teeth and maxillary posterior teeth. In the maxillary anterior area, a palatal approach to the anterior middle superior nerve may be helpful. The key to this approach is slow injection of approximately 1 mL of local anesthetic in the area of the first and second maxillary premolars midway between the gingival crest and the palatal midline. An intraosseous injection also may be used to regain lost anesthesia, but even when it is effective, the area of local anesthesia often is smaller than desired for a surgical procedure. As a last resort, the procedure can be terminated short of completion and the patient can be rescheduled for surgery under sedation or general anesthesia.

SURGICAL ACCESS

The goals of periradicular surgery are to access the affected area, remove the diseased tissue, evaluate the root circumference and root canal system, and place a biocompatible seal in the form of a root-end filling that can stimulate regeneration of the periodontium. The formation of new cementum on the surgically exposed root surface and on the root-end filling material is essential to regeneration of the periodontium.

Successful endodontic surgery requires the surgeon to use several conceptual elements in planning the procedure. A vision of the immediate postoperative surgical end point (i.e., replacement of the reflected tissues) is essential for designing each phase of the surgery. Visualization of a three-dimensional image of the surgical procedure allows the surgeon to anticipate and prepare for unusual circumstances. In surgical root canal treatment, once a procedure is started, it must

be completed uninterrupted within a limited time; this is a paramount difference between nonsurgical and surgical root canal treatment. For this reason, it is absolutely essential that the surgeon plan the procedure thoroughly and include alternative plans of action that anticipate unusual findings during the process of discovery.

Several general principles are important for designing the access to a diseased region: (1) the surgeon must have a thorough knowledge of the anatomic structures in relation to each other, including tooth anatomy; (2) the surgeon must be able to visualize the three-dimensional nature of the structures in the soft and hard tissue (this reduces unnecessary tissue damage); (3) the trauma of the surgical procedure itself must be minimized, which includes the preservation of tooth and supporting structures; (4) the tissue and instruments must be manipulated within a limited space with the aim of removing diseased tissues and retaining healthy tissues.

Soft-Tissue Access

In designing the soft-tissue access window to the diseased tissue, the surgeon must take into consideration various anatomic features, such as frenum-muscle attachments, the width of attached gingiva, papillary height and width, bone eminence, and crown margins. The supraperiosteal blood vessels of the attached gingiva extend from the alveolar mucosa and run parallel to the long axis of the teeth, lying in the reticular layer superficial to the periosteum.[172] A vertical, rather than an angled, releasing incision severs fewer vessels,[325] reducing the possibility of hemorrhage. Also, the blood supply to the tissue coronal to the incision is not compromised,[477] which prevents localized ischemia and sloughing of these tissues. Ultimately, the result is less bleeding during the procedure and enhanced healing. For these reasons, an angled releasing incision is contraindicated in periradicular surgery.

Vertical Incision

The general principles for placement of a vertical relieving incision are as follows:

1. The incision should be made parallel to the supraperiosteal vessels in the attached gingiva and submucosa (Fig. 9-25).
2. No cuts should be made across frenum and muscle attachments.
3. Frenum and muscle attachments should not be located in the reflected tissue, if possible.
4. The incision should be placed directly over healthy bone.

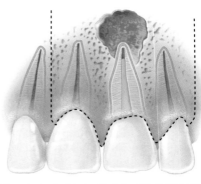

FIG. 9-25 Intrasulcular incision with two vertical releasing incisions (rectangular flap).

5. The incision should not be placed superior to a bony eminence.
6. The dental papilla should be included or excluded but not dissected.
7. The incision should extend from the depth of the vestibular sulcus to the midpoint between the dental papilla and the horizontal aspect of the buccal gingival sulcus.

Horizontal Incision

Three types of horizontal incisions can be used to gain access to a surgical site in hard tissue:

- *An intrasulcular incision that includes the dental papilla.* This incision extends from the gingival sulcus through the PDL fibers and terminates at the crestal bone of the alveolar bone proper. The incision then passes in a buccolingual direction adjacent to each tooth of the dental papilla and includes the midcol region of each dental papilla. Thus, the entire dental papilla is completely mobilized.

- *An intrasulcular incision that excludes the dental papilla (papillary-based incision, Fig. 9-26).* This technique consists of a shallow first incision at the base of the papilla and a second incision directed to the crestal bone.

- *An incision made in the attached gingiva (a submarginal or Ochsenbein-Luebke flap).*[322] With this technique, at least 2 mm of attached gingiva must be retained to prevent mucogingival degeneration.[296] Consequently, the incision must be placed at least 2 mm from the depth of the gingival sulcus. Extensive periodontal probing should be done to establish the depth of the gingival sulcus before the incision is made. The average width of the attached gingiva is 2.1 to 5.1 mm in the maxilla and 1.8 to 3.8 mm in the mandible.[10,199,341,563] It is widest over the central and lateral incisors, narrows over the canine and the first premolar, and then widens over the second premolar and the first molar. These variances were similar for both the maxilla and mandible.[517] Overall, this incision technique has a narrow margin of safety. It generally is recommended for use in the maxilla, especially where the aesthetics of existing crown margins are a concern.

Studies have compared the incision techniques that include and exclude the dental papilla in patients with healthy marginal periodontal conditions.[554,555,557] These researchers found that the papilla base incision resulted in rapid, recession-free healing. In contrast, complete mobilization of the papilla led to a marked loss of papilla height. The authors suggested that use of the papilla base incision in aesthetically sensitive regions could help prevent papilla recession and surgical cleft, or double papilla.

Flap Design

Combinations of vertical and horizontal incisions are used to achieve various flap designs (Figs. 9-27 and 9-28). The full mucoperiosteal and limited mucoperiosteal are the two major categories of flap design used during periradicular surgery, the main differentiating feature being the position of the horizontal incision. In each case the entire body of soft tissue is reflected as one unit and includes the alveolar mucosa, the gingival tissues, and the periosteum. The number and position of the vertical relaxing incisions therefore governs the major variation in design:

1. Full mucoperiosteal (intrasulcular incision including the dental papilla or papillary based) (Figs 9-27 and 9-28):
   a. Triangular: one vertical relieving incision
   b. Rectangular: two vertical relieving incisions
   c. Trapezoidal: two angled vertical relieving incisions
   d. Horizontal: no vertical relieving incision
2. Limited mucoperiosteal (Figs 9-29 and 9-30):
   a. Curve submarginal (semilunar)
   b. Freeform rectilinear submarginal (Ochsenbein-Luebke)

Tissue Reflection

Elevation and reflection of the entire mucoperiosteal complex, maintaining the microvasculature in the body of the tissue flap, increases hemostatic control during surgery. Tissue reflection should begin from the vertical releasing incision at the junction

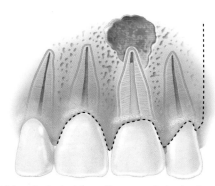

FIG. 9-27 Intrasulcular incision with one vertical releasing incision (triangular flap).

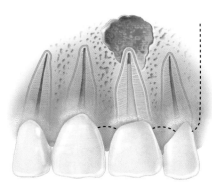

FIG. 9-26 Papillary-based incision with one vertical releasing incision.

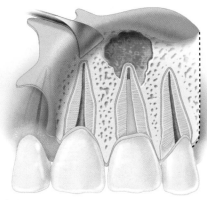

FIG. 9-28 Reflection of the triangular flap to expose the root-end area.

of the submucosa and the attached gingiva (Figs. 9-31 and 9-32). By initiating the reflection process at this point, damage to the delicate supracrestal root-attached fibers is avoided. Using a flap reflection technique that reduces reflective tissue forces in the intrasulcular incisional wound and avoids curettage of the root surface conserves the root-attached tissues and helps prevent apical down-growth of epithelium and loss of soft-tissue attachment.[222] Force should be applied such that the periosteum and superficial tissues are reflected as a complete unit. Using a gentle rocking motion, the surgeon initially should reflect the tissue in a horizontal direction.[213] The underlying bone of the cortical plate is irregular, and it is critical to avoid damaging the fragile tissues during elevation.

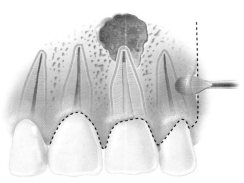

FIG. 9-31 Elevator placed in the vertical incision for the first step in undermining flap reflection.

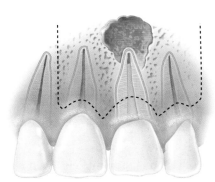

FIG. 9-29 Submarginal (Ochsenbein-Luebke) flap.

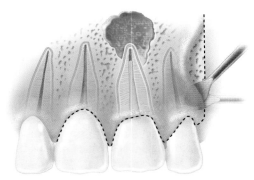

FIG. 9-32 Continuation of reflection of full-thickness flap.

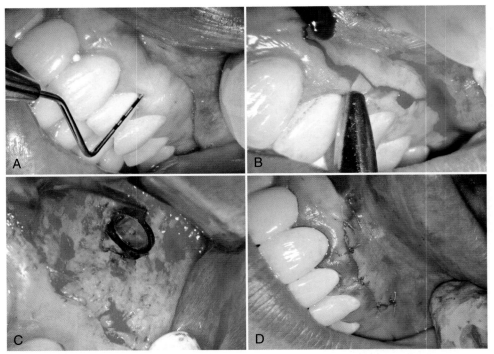

FIG. 9-30 Clinical case involving a submarginal incision and flap. **A,** Periodontal probing of the entire area was performed before this type of flap was selected and the incision started. A submarginal incision often is used in aesthetic anterior areas of the mouth where postoperative gingival recession might expose the crown margins. **B,** The incision should be at least 2 mm apical to the depth of the sulcus. **C,** With the flap reflected, osteotomy and root-end resection were performed. Methylene blue dye was placed to mark the outline of the root end and to help identify cracks or fractures before root-end cavity preparation and filling. **D,** The flap was repositioned and sutured with 5-0 Tevdek. (Courtesy Dr. Martin Rogers.)

The operator should take great care not to slip during the tissue reflection process by using an appropriate instrument stabilized with adequate finger support. Slipping can result not only in puncture of the immediate overlying tissue but also damage to the surrounding structures.

As space permits, the elevator should be directed coronally, undermining the attached gingiva. As the interdental papilla is approached, a narrower instrument may be required to undermine and gently elevate the tissue in this region, to avoid crushing the delicate free gingival tissues. This process should be continued gradually until the osseous tissues overlying the diseased tooth structure have been adequately exposed. Generally, elevation of the flap 0.75 cm apical to the estimated apex of the root should allow adequate space to perform the surgical procedure.

No single instrument is essential for the flap elevation procedure, because every instrument has both advantages and disadvantages. Surgeons should familiarize themselves with the various instruments available.

Tissue Retraction

After the tissue is reflected, it must be retracted to provide adequate access for bone removal and root-end procedures. The main goals of tissue retraction are to provide a clear view of the bony surgical site and to prevent further soft-tissue trauma. Accidental crushing of the soft tissues leads to more postoperative swelling and ecchymoses.[222,223]

The general principles of retraction are as follows: (1) retractors should rest on solid cortical bone; (2) firm but light pressure should be used; (3) tearing, puncturing, and crushing of the soft tissue should be avoided; (4) sterile physiologic saline should be used periodically to maintain hydration of the reflected tissue; and (5) the retractor should be large enough to protect the retracted soft tissue during surgical treatment (e.g., prevent it from becoming entangled in the bone bur). No one retractor suffices for all surgical procedures, therefore the surgeon should have a selection of retractors available for the various situations that arise during surgery. If difficulty is encountered in stabilizing the retractor, a small groove can be cut into the cortical plate to support it.

Hard-Tissue Access

Two biologic principles govern the removal of bone for hard-tissue access to diseased root ends: (1) healthy hard tissue must be preserved, and (2) heat generation during the process must be minimized.

Temperature increases above normal body temperature in osseous tissues are detrimental. Heating osseous tissue to 117° to 122°F (47° to 50°C) for 1 minute significantly reduces bone formation and is associated with irreversible cellular damage and fatty cell infiltration.[161,338] Two critical factors determine the degree of injury: how high the temperature increases and how long it remains elevated. As the temperature rises above 104°F (40°C), blood flow initially increases. It stagnates at 198°F (46°C) applied for 2 minutes. Heating osseous tissue to 133°F (56°C) deactivates alkaline phosphatase.[422,423] Studies using animal bone have shown that at temperatures above 109°F (42.5°C), for every 1°C elevation in temperature, the exposure time for the same biologic effect decreases by a factor of approximately 2.[158-161] Temperatures above 117°F (47°C) maintained for 1 minute produce effects similar to those at 118°F (48°C) applied for 30 seconds. This correlation means that the decisive exposure time declines quickly as the temperature increases. Temperatures above 127°F (53°C) applied for less than 1 second can adversely affect osteogenesis.[158-161]

Several factors determine the amount of heat generated during bone removal, including the shape and composition of the bur, the rotational speed, the use of coolant, and the pressure applied during cutting.

The round bur has the best shape for removing osseous tissue, and it should be used with a gentle brushstroke action.[519] This type of bur also readily allows access of coolant to the actual cutting surfaces. Studies comparing the heat generated with round and fissure burs found more favorable results with the round burs.[85,111,216,338,360] Cutting with round burs produced a wound site with less inflammation, which is more favorable for rapid wound healing. Although fissure-type burs cut efficiently on the sides, the tip of the bur is very inefficient because it allows no coolant access. The net result is increased inflammation and a reduced healing response.

Use of a diamond bur to remove osseous tissue is inefficient and retards ultimate wound healing. Because of its larger surface area, more of a diamond bur is in contact with the bone tissue. As a result, less coolant reaches the cutting surface, and the bur has a greater tendency to become clogged with residual bone fragments. The net effect is greater heat generation, increased inflammation, and reduced healing.[85,586]

Use of a coolant during bone cutting is essential. If an appropriate irrigant is not used, temperatures can exceed those known to impair bone healing[274]; histologically, healing can be delayed up to 3 weeks.[169] It also is critical that the coolant reach the cutting surface. Temperatures can rise above 212°F (100°C) when excess pressure is applied during cutting; this burrows the bur into the bone, where little or no irrigant can reach the cutting tip,[519] hence the recommendation for a gentle brushstroke technique.[213] Favorable results are obtained with these provided the surgeon follows the basic tenet of minimizing heat generation: using a round fluted bur with coolant and a brushstroke technique. A high-speed handpiece that exhausts air from the base rather than the cutting end is recommended to reduce the risk of air embolism (Fig. 9-33).

PERIRADICULAR CURETTAGE AND BIOPSY

Most periradicular lesions originate in the pulp and can be classified histopathologically as granulomas or

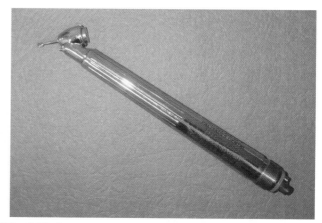

FIG. 9-33 Surgical handpiece with 45-degree angle head and rear air exhaust (Impact Air 45).

cysts.[53,58,292,295,297,359,367,382,488] Histologically, such lesions consist mainly of granulation tissue associated with angiogenesis, fibroblasts, connective tissue fibers, and inflammatory cells. Foreign material, cholesterol clefts,[365,370] and stimulated strands of epithelium also may be present. The stimulated epithelium can form into a stratified, squamous epithelium–lined cystic cavity.[366] These periradicular lesions (granulomas and cysts) are inflammatory lesions that develop in response to irritation caused by intraradicular and extraradicular microorganisms associated with the root canal system[363,368] or by foreign materials forced into the periradicular tissues.[600]

An important aspect of periradicular surgery is the removal of diseased tissue associated with the root apex. Because a large portion of this tissue is reactionary, the focus of surgical root canal treatment is removal of the irritant or diseased tissues. Histologically, an inflammatory periradicular lesion is similar to healing granulation tissue. If the irritant can be readily identified and successfully eliminated, it is not always necessary to completely curette all the inflamed periradicular tissues during surgery.[306] This is especially true when complete removal might result in injury to neural or vascular tissues. In addition to removing diseased tissue, periradicular curettage provides visibility and accessibility to facilitate treatment of the apical root canal system or removal of foreign materials in the periradicular tissues.

The need for a histopathologic assessment of all tissues removed from the body cannot be overstated. Although only a small percentage of periradicular lesions are associated with pathoses other than a periradicular cyst or granuloma, all lesions must be diagnosed definitively because of the potential gravity of the few rare diseases associated with periradicular lesions.[12,121,185,383,409]

The technical aspect of removing soft tissue from the bony crypt varies among surgeons and clinical settings. Various bone and periodontal curettes are available for this purpose, and no one instrument suffices for all cases. Regardless of the instrument selected, the basic principles are the same. A sharp instrument is always preferable to a blunt instrument. The soft-tissue lesion first should be peeled away from the osseous crypt, starting at the lateral borders. This can be accomplished efficiently by using the curette with the concave surface facing the internal wall of the osseous crypt. Once the soft-tissue lesion has been separated from the osseous crypt to the point where the crypt changes its convexity, the curette can be used in a scraping manner to remove the remainder of the lesion from the medial wall of the osseous defect.

LOCALIZED HEMOSTASIS

Localized hemostasis during periradicular surgery is essential to successful management of the resected root end. Appropriate hemostasis during surgery minimizes surgical time, surgical blood loss, and postoperative hemorrhage and swelling.[213] The hemostatic agents used during endodontic surgery are intended to control bleeding from small blood vessels or capillaries. Localized hemorrhage control not only enhances visibility and assessment of the root structure, but it also ensures the appropriate environment for placement of the current root-end filling materials and minimizes root-end filling contamination.

Many hemostatic agents have been advocated for use during surgery, and the action of these agents, their ability to control bleeding, and their effect on healing vary considerably. They generally aid coagulation by inducing rapid development of an occlusive clot, either by exerting a physical tamponade action or by enhancing the clotting mechanism and vasoconstriction (or both). No one local hemostatic agent is ideal; each has disadvantages. Therefore, further investigation is indicated to find the ideal local hemostatic agent.

Preoperative Considerations

A thorough review of the patient's body systems and medical history increases the likelihood of detecting an undiagnosed condition that might affect hemostasis during periradicular surgery. Review of the patient's medications, both prescribed and over-the-counter (OTC) drugs, is essential. Many OTC drugs can affect the clotting mechanism. The patient's vital signs (i.e., blood pressure, heart rate, and respiratory rate) should be assessed. Vital signs also can be used to monitor anxious patients. An increase in blood pressure and heart rate above a patient's known normal values indicates increased stress or poorly controlled hypertension. Easing the patient's anxiety before surgery reduces the possible hemostatic-potentiating effect of elevated cardiac output during surgery.[156] Anxiety and stress can be alleviated with planning, sedation, and profound local anesthesia.

Local Hemostatic Agents
Collagen-Based Materials
Various collagen-based hemostatic agents are available for use as local hemostatic agents. The principal differences are in the microstructure and density of the collagen. Collagen can act as a mild allergen, but the problem of allergenization and unwanted tissue reaction does not occur when highly purified animal collagen is used.[49] The mechanisms by which collagen products help achieve hemostasis involves stimulation of platelet adhesion, platelet aggregation and release reaction,[270,271] activation of factor XII (Hageman factor),[335,336] and mechanical tamponade by the structure that forms at the collagen-blood wound interface. Collagen shows minimal interference in the wound healing process, with a limited foreign body reaction.[215] It does not increase the incidence of infection and only slightly delays early bone repair.[246] Osseous regeneration in the presence of collagen typically proceeds uneventfully, without a foreign body reaction.[168]

Collagen-based materials can be difficult to apply to the bony crypt because they adhere to wet surfaces, particularly instruments and gloves.[466] Several collagen-based products are commercially available. They include CollaCote (Integra Life Sciences, Plainsboro, NJ) (Fig. 9-34, A), CollaStat (American Medical Products Corp, Eatontown, NJ), Hemocollagene (Septodont, United Kingdom) and Instat (Ethicon, Somerville, NJ). These materials act in essentially similar ways, and the surgical area undergoes a similar healing pattern.[485,504] Overall, studies of wound healing with collagen-based hemostatic agents have shown favorable results.

Surgicel
Surgicel (Ethicon) is a chemically sterilized material prepared through oxidation of regenerated alpha cellulose (oxycellulose). The basic element of Surgicel is polyanhydroglucuronic acid, which is spun into threads and then woven into gauze. Surgicel has a pH of 3. If the material is maintained in the wound for up to 120 days, a pH this low could retard healing.[408]

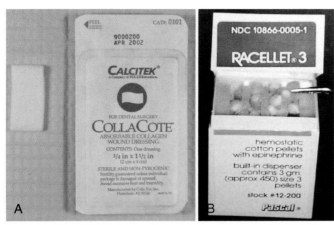

FIG. 9-34 A, Absorbable collagen (CollaCote) is a convenient, biocompatible packing material for localized hemostasis. **B,** Cotton pellets impregnated with racemic epinephrine (Racellet) also may be used for localized hemostasis.

It is primarily a physical hemostatic agent, which acts as a barrier to blood and then becomes a sticky mass that serves as an artificial coagulum. It does not enhance the clotting cascade through adhesion or aggregation of platelets. Surgicel is retained in the surgical wound,[373] and healing is retarded, with little evidence of resorption of the material at 120 days.[57] Use of Surgicel in extraction sockets resulted in greater postoperative pain compared with a control in a split mouth–designed study.[408]

Gelfoam

Gelfoam (Pharmacia, Peapack, NJ) is a gelatin-based sponge that is water insoluble and biologically resorbable. It stimulates the intrinsic clotting pathway by promoting platelet disintegration and the subsequent release of thromboplastin and thrombin.[164] The initial reaction to Gelfoam in the surgical site is a decrease in the rate of healing. Extraction sockets containing Gelfoam showed a greater inflammatory cell infiltrate, marked reduction in bone ingrowth, and a foreign body reaction at 8 days.[74] However, these effects were transitory and did not impair long-term bone healing.[392]

Bone Wax

Historically, bone wax has been advocated for controlling both hemostasis and debris in the bony crypt during periradicular surgery.[480] It is a nonabsorbable product composed of 88% beeswax and 12% isopropyl palmitate. Healing with bone wax is best described as poor. The bony crypt typically contains fibrous connective tissue and has no bony or hematopoietic tissue. Bone wax retards bone healing and predisposes the surgical site to infection[117,378] by producing a chronic inflammatory foreign body reaction[35] and impairing the clearance of bacteria.[263] The use of bone wax can no longer be recommended because it impairs healing and several good alternatives are available.[589]

Ferric Sulfate

Ferric sulfate (Cut-Trol, Ichthys Enterprises, Mobile, AL), a necrotizing agent with an extremely low pH, is one of the few products investigated for use in periradicular surgery. In studies using a rabbit model, Lemon and colleagues[301] and

Jeansonne and colleagues[256] reported hemostatic control for 5 minutes and near normal healing with only a mild foreign body reaction, provided the surgical wound was adequately curetted and irrigated with saline. Failure to remove ferric sulfate from the surgical wound site resulted in severely impaired healing, a foreign body–type reaction, and, in some cases, abscess formation. The possibility of acute inflammation and necrosis of the surrounding soft tissue with careless use of this solution should not be underestimated.[298] A similar product, Monsel's solution (ferric subsulfate), has been used to control local hemostasis in dermatologic procedures. However, the popularity of this solution has declined because application to wound sites has resulted in tissue necrosis for up to 2 weeks,[130] differences in the degree of epidermal maturation, and tattoo formation.[536]

Calcium Sulfate

Calcium sulfate has been used as a substitute bone graft material to fill bone defects since the late 1800s. The presence of calcium sulfate in an osseous wound does not inhibit bone formation.[574] It is gradually removed from the site of implantation regardless of whether new bone has formed.[110] Use of calcium sulfate during periradicular surgery does not significantly affect healing, and deposition of cementum and osseous healing proceed normally.[27] As a hemostatic agent, calcium sulfate acts as a physical barrier. The material is placed in the bony crypt, allowed to set, and then partly carved away to allow access to the root end.[283] The remaining material lines the crypt walls, preventing bleeding. When the root-end filling has been placed and all extraneous root-end filling material removed, the residual calcium sulfate can be removed or left in situ.

Epinephrine Pellets

Epinephrine, a sympathomimetic-amine vasoconstrictor, is frequently used to control hemorrhage during oral surgery.[82,283] All granulation tissue should be removed from the root apex area prior to placement of the epinephrine pellet to assure direct contact with bone.[282] Vasoconstrictive amines exert their effects by binding to and interacting with adrenergic receptors in various body tissues. When epinephrine is bound to alpha$_1$- and alpha$_2$-adrenergic receptors, a powerful vasoconstricting effect results. Racemic epinephrine cotton pellets (Racellet #3; Pascal Co., Bellevue, WA) contain an average of 0.55 mg of racemic epinephrine hydrochloride per pellet, half of which is the pharmacologically active L-form. Racellets (see Fig. 9-31, *B*) provide good localized hemostasis in periradicular surgery.[558]

Two concerns arise with the use of Racellets in the surgical site: the cardiovascular impact of the additional epinephrine and the retention of cotton fibers in the wound, resulting in impaired wound healing.[213,265] A study by Vickers and coworkers[558] examined the cardiovascular effects of epinephrine pellets and concluded that no evidence existed of cardiovascular changes (blood pressure and pulse) compared with saline-saturated pellet controls. These authors hypothesized that the vasoconstrictive effect on the capillaries is localized and immediate and that little or no systemic uptake of epinephrine occurred.

Although the cardiovascular effect appears to be of little concern, retention of cotton fibers in the surgical site could result in inflammation and impaired wound healing. Therefore, due diligence on the part of the surgeon is paramount when epinephrine pellets are used. Each pellet applied during surgery must be accounted for, and the bony crypt should be lightly curetted to remove any embedded cotton fibers before the wound is closed. The retention of cotton fibers in the crypt can be eliminated by substituting CollaCote saturated with 10 drops of 2.25% racepinephrine inhalation solution.[567] As previously noted, CollaCote is biocompatible and does not interfere with wound healing.

Cautery/Electrosurgery

Cautery stops the flow of blood through coagulation of blood and tissue protein, leaving an eschar that the body attempts to slough.[537] The effect of cautery in the bony crypt during periradicular surgery has not been studied to date. However, the effect of electrosurgery on alveolar bone has been studied in periodontal surgery. Tissue destruction was greater in areas exposed to electrosurgery and healing was delayed compared with surgical sites not exposed to electrosurgery. Twelve hours after surgery, a more extensive inflammatory reaction and greater destruction of periosteum were noted with electrosurgery.[36] At 24 hours, many empty lacunae were observed in the bone associated with electrosurgery, and this necrosis was even more extensive by 48 hours. At 96 hours the electrosurgical connective tissue wounds were still lined by coagulum, whereas the scalpel wound was beginning to repair.[381] The detrimental effect of applying heat to bone is proportional to both temperature and the duration of application.

MANAGEMENT OF THE ROOT END

Management of the resected root end during periradicular surgery is critical to the overall success of a case. The aim of surgery should be to create an environment conducive to regeneration of the periodontium—that is, healing and regeneration of the alveolar bone, periodontal ligament, and cementum overlying the root end and root-end filling material. The key to regeneration is the presence of appropriate inducible cell types, growth factors, and specific substances necessary for mineralization. Failure to create an environment conducive to this process results in tissue repair rather than regeneration and possibly less than ideal healing.

Determination of the Need for Root-End Resection and Filling

The basis for periradicular surgery is twofold. The first objective is to remove the etiologic factor; the second is to prevent recontamination of the periradicular tissues once the etiologic agent has been removed.

Etiologic factors typically can be categorized as intraradicular or extraradicular bacteria,[254,287,367,491,540,541,559,580] intraradicular or extraradicular chemical substances, or extraradicular physical factors.[370,496,497] The etiology cannot always be determined with complete certainty; frequently, a number of factors are involved.[98] However, most cases involve some form of bacterial participation (e.g., bacteria within apical ramifications). The only definitive means of eradicating such an irritant is physical removal through root-end resection. The rationale for root-end resection in such cases is to establish access to and remove the diseased tissues. This ensures that the optimum environment for wound healing is established.

As mentioned, the second objective of periradicular surgery is to prevent recontamination of the tissues after removal of the etiologic agent. It follows, then, that if the remainder of the canal system cannot be verified to be irritant free, a root-end filling should be placed to seal any remaining irritants within the canal system, thus preventing recontamination of the periradicular tissues.

Root-End Resection

Two main principles dictate the extent of the root-end resection. First, the cause (or causes) of an ongoing disease process must be removed; this includes removal of the diseased tissue and, when indicated, reduction of an apically fenestrated root. Second, adequate room must be provided for inspection and management of the root end.

The anatomy of each tooth root is complex (see Chapter 5). The surgeon must understand the anatomy of the apical third of the root to determine the extent of a root-end resection. Approximately 75% of teeth have canal aberrations (e.g., accessory or lateral canals) in the apical 3 mm of the tooth.[131,481] An apical resection of approximately 3 mm should include most accessory and lateral canals and thus eliminate most residual microorganisms and irritants (Fig. 9-35). When roots with more than one main canal are resected, isthmus tissue may be present, and the preparation should be modified to include the isthmus area (Fig. 9-36).

If the root apex is close to the buccal cortical plate, apical fenestration can occur, leading to persistent symptoms, especially tenderness to palpation over the root apex.[72] Reduction of an apically fenestrated root apex below the level of the surrounding cortical bone allows remodeling of the bone over the tooth structure. The buccal root of the maxillary first premolar often is closest to the buccal cortical plate.

The surgeon's convenience as a rationale for root-end resection depends on the individual case and the surgeon's abilities. The basic principle of the dental surgeon's convenience should be modified by the desire to minimize the trauma of the surgical procedure itself, including the preservation of tooth and supporting structures. Access to and visibility of the periradicular root structures historically has determined the extent of root-end resection. The surgeon must be able to inspect the

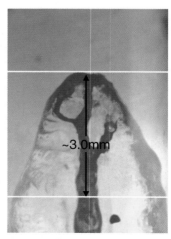

FIG. 9-35 Cleared section of a typical single-canal root that was injected with dye to demonstrate apical accessory canals. Most of the apical ramifications can be eliminated with a 3-mm resection.

resected root end, prepare a root-end cavity, and place a root-end filling. Enhanced visualization equipment (e.g., microscopes, endoscopes, and orascopes) have reduced the need to resect large amounts of the root to gain adequate visualization and access.[91,94,228,280,440,441,448,486] In some cases part of the root must be resected to gain access to the entire soft-tissue lesion, an additional palatally positioned root (e.g., maxillary premolars), or foreign material in the periradicular tissues.

A major consideration in determining the extent of root-end resection is the presence of anatomic structures such as the mental foramen or mandibular canal.[355,410-412] The surgeon should position the resection of the root to avoid possible damage to these structures.

Angle of Resection

Enhanced magnification and illumination techniques have eliminated the need to create a beveled root surface in most cases.[94,441] From a biologic perspective, the most appropriate angle of root-end resection is perpendicular to the long axis of the tooth (Figs. 9-37 and 9-38). The rationale for a perpendicular root-end resection is based on several anatomic parameters. First, a perpendicular resection approximately 3 mm from the anatomic apex is more likely to include all the apical ramifications in that region of the tooth.[339] Second, as the angle of resection increases, the number of dentinal tubules that communicate with the periradicular region and the root canal system increases significantly; therefore, the probability that irritants from within the canal system will gain access to the healing tissues also rises as the resection angle increases.[181,523] Third, extending the root-end cavity preparation beyond the coronal extent of the root surface is simpler if the root-end resection is perpendicular to the long axis of the tooth.[195] Finally, with a perpendicular root-end resection, the stress forces exerted in the apical region are more evenly distributed; this may reduce the propagation of apical fractures and provide a better environment for apical healing.[470]

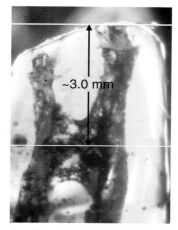

FIG. 9-36 Cleared section of a mesiobuccal (MB) root in a maxillary first molar. Root resection at the recommended 3-mm level exposes isthmus tissue connecting the MB-1 and MB-2 canals.

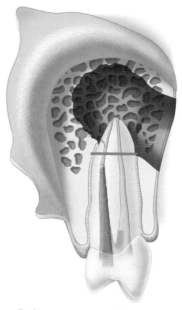

FIG. 9-38 Perpendicular or near perpendicular root-end resection *(green line)* can be achieved with the use of microsurgical instruments and enhanced magnification and illumination.

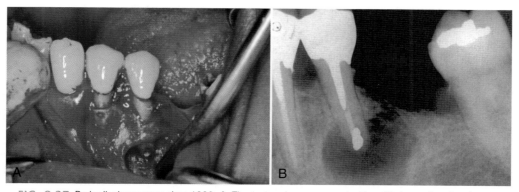

FIG. 9-37 Periradicular surgery circa 1990. **A,** The root end was prepared with a 45-degree bevel and rotary bur microhandpiece. Amalgam was a commonly used root-end filling material at this time. **B,** Immediate postoperative radiograph of a mandibular second premolar with amalgam root-end filling. Although many teeth treated this way healed successfully, newer materials and techniques described in this chapter are currently recommended.

Root-End Surface Preparation

As with all phases of endodontic surgery, the goal is to produce a resected root end with optimum conditions for the growth of cementum and subsequent regeneration of the periodontal ligament across the resected root end. Two important aspects of this process are the surface topography of the resected root end and chemical treatment of the resected root end. Healthy cementum on the root end is required for successful regeneration of periodontal tissues.[22] A number of substances found in cementum stimulate the migration, growth, and attachment of periodontal fibroblasts. Cementum extracts also activate fibroblast, protein, and collagen synthesis, which is necessary to reestablish a functional periodontal ligament.[52,471,562]

Resected Root-End Surface Topography

The conventional axiom for surface preparation of the resected root end has been to produce a smooth, flat root surface without sharp edges or spurs of root structure that might serve as irritants during the healing process. However, little information exists on whether smooth root ends heal differently or more quickly than rough root ends after root-end resection. A study investigating the effect of the surface topography of resected root ends on human PDL fibroblast attachment found no significant difference in fibroblast attachment to the root ends prepared with various instruments.[584] However, with a smooth resected root-end surface, the surgeon is better able to detect surface cracks and anatomic variations.[357] Given that human PDL fibroblast attachment to a smooth surface was not impaired, it would seem appropriate to produce as smooth a surface as possible to facilitate inspection of the resected root end. A smooth root end therefore should be considered advantageous.

Different types of burs tend to produce different patterns on the resected root surface.[212] Several studies have compared the root-end surface after resection.[357,377,585] Generally, crosscut fissure burs in both high-speed and low-speed handpieces produced the roughest and most irregular surfaces. Morgan and Marshall[357] compared the surface topography of root-end resection with a #57 straight fissure bur (Midwest Dental Products, Des Plains, IL), a Lindeman bone bur (Brasseler USA, Savannah, GA), and the Multi-Purpose bur (Dentsply Maillefer, Ballaigues, Switzerland), then finished with a either a multifluted carbide finishing bur (Brasseler USA) or an ultra-fine diamond finishing bur (Brasseler). The Multi-Purpose bur produced the smoothest, most uniplanar resected root-end surface with the least amount of shattering. Regardless of the type of bur used, smearing and shredding of the gutta-percha across the root face occurred only when the handpiece was moved across the root face in reverse direction in relation to the bur's direction of rotation.[585] Burs that produce a smooth surface also tend to cut with less vibration and chatter, resulting in greater patient comfort.

Root-End Conditioning

Root surface conditioning removes the smear layer and provides a surface conducive to mechanical adhesion and cellular mechanisms for growth and attachment. It exposes the collagenous matrix of dentin and retains biologically active substances, such as growth factors, in the dentin proper. Experimental studies have shown that demineralized dentin can induce the development of bonelike mineralized tissue.[42,43,241,550,597] Some contend that root surface conditioning produces a biocompatible surface conducive to periodontal

cell colonization without compromising the vitality of the adjacent periodontium.

Three solutions have been advocated for root surface modification: citric acid, tetracycline, and ethylenediamine tetraacetic acid (EDTA). All three solutions have enhanced fibroblast attachment to the root surface in vitro. However, citric acid is the only solution tested in an endodontic surgical application.

Citric acid traditionally has been the solution of choice. Periodontists have used an aqueous solution of citric acid (pH 1) for 2 to 3 minutes to etch diseased root surfaces to facilitate formation, new attachment, and cementogenesis.[434-438] Craig and Harrison[114] examined the effect of citric acid demineralization of resected root ends on periradicular healing. They found that 1- or 2-minute applications of 50% citric acid (pH 1) resulted in demineralized root ends and earlier complete healing than in the nondemineralized root ends. However, the periodontal literature has questioned the benefit of etching dentin surfaces with low pH agents. At a low pH, adjacent vital periodontal tissues may be compromised. Also, extended application (3 minutes) has been shown to discourage alveolar bone growth.[60,62]

EDTA, a solution with a neutral pH that endodontists have used as a canal irrigant, has been shown to be equally effective at exposing collagen fibers on dentin surfaces.[64] Unlike the lower pH solution, EDTA does not adversely affect the surrounding tissues.[63]

A series of studies that examined the effect of EDTA and citric and phosphoric acids in a periodontal application showed that application of 15% to 24% EDTA for approximately 2 minutes produces the optimum root surface.[59,61,64] These researchers concluded that EDTA, at neutral pH, was able to selectively remove mineral from a dentin surface, exposing a collagenous matrix. Citric and phosphoric acids, which have a low pH, appeared not only to remove the mineral component but also to denature the collagenous matrix.

Tetracycline has been shown to remove the dentin smear layer, leaving clean, open tubules, with application times as short as 30 seconds.[327] A histologic evaluation of new attachment in periodontally diseased human roots treated with tetracycline hydrochloride showed a trend for greater connective tissue attachment after tetracycline treatment of roots.[13] Studies comparing the effect of a 3-minute application of either EDTA (pH 7.3) or tetracycline HCl (pH 1.8) showed no significant difference in the treated tooth surfaces.[37] However, EDTA has been shown to be more favorable to human PDL cell attachment.[601]

Although the root surface conditioning effects of citric acid, EDTA, and tetracycline are well documented in the periodontal literature, this treatment has not translated into significant gains in periodontal attachment in periodontally diseased teeth.[330] Currently only citric acid has been assessed as a root-end conditioning agent. In an animal model, citric acid was shown to enhance periradicular healing. Nonetheless, its effect and the effect of other root-end conditioning agents on the outcome of human periradicular surgery have not been established. Based on periodontal research, it would appear that if a root surface conditioning agent were to be used during periradicular surgery, EDTA might be the most appropriate solution. However, the manufacturer (personnel communication, Dr. Torabinejad) has advised against the use of EDTA when mineral trioxide aggregate (MTA) is used as a root-end filling material, because it may interfere with the hard tissue–producing effect of MTA.

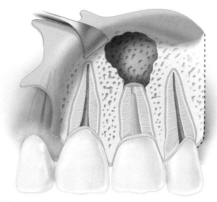

FIG. 9-39 Diagram of a perpendicular root-end preparation and 3-mm deep cavity preparation along the long axis of the root.

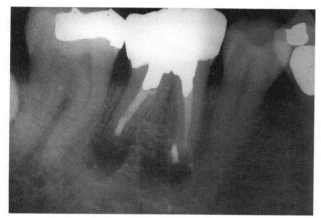

FIG. 9-40 Error in root-end cavity preparation: ultrasonic preparation did not follow the long axis of the mesial root and therefore did not allow for proper sealing of this root. Healing is unlikely.

ROOT-END CAVITY PREPARATION

The root-end cavity preparation is a crucial step in the establishment of an apical seal. The goal is to make a cavity in the resected root end that is dimensionally sufficient for placement of a root-end filling material and at the same time avoid unnecessary damage to the root-end structures. The ideal preparation is a class I cavity prepared along the long axis of the tooth to a depth of at least 3 mm (Figs. 9-39 and 9-40). The surgical procedure is most likely to be successful if the remaining canal system has been thoroughly cleaned and shaped to eliminate microorganisms and irritants.[178,449] Traditionally, a microhandpiece with a rotating bur has been used for this purpose. However, with the advent of ultrasonic tips designed specifically for this purpose (Fig. 9-41), root-end preparations now are most often performed with the ultrasonic technique.[91] Clinical evidence is emerging to support the benefit of an ultrasonic root-end preparation when compared to traditional bur preparation, especially in molar surgery.[132]

Ultrasonic root-end preparation techniques have several advantages over the microhandpiece method. Less osseous tissue must be removed to gain proper access to the resected root end. Also, the surgeon is better able to produce a more conservative preparation that follows the long axis of the tooth and remains centered in the canal. The risk of root-end

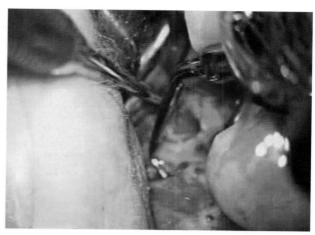

FIG. 9-41 Ultrasonic tip in use. Preparation along the long axis of the root is possible using tips designed for each area of the mouth. In this case, the tip is properly positioned for root-end cavity preparation of a maxillary first premolar but is dangerously close to the lip because of improper retraction. Heat generated by an ultrasonic tip can cause a thermal burn, which may result in scar tissue formation.

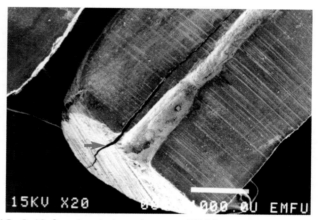

FIG. 9-42 Scanning electron microscope (SEM) image of a root end prepared in vitro with an ultrasonic device at high-power setting. A distinct fracture line can be seen (red arrow). Root-end preparation with ultrasonic devices should be done at low power and with water coolant.

perforation is reduced, partly because of enhanced manipulation of the instrument. In addition, ultrasonic root-end techniques produce a more consistent, deeper cavity preparation that requires less beveling of the root.[95,304,347,592] Ultrasonic apical preparation generates significantly less smear layer compared with burs alone[205]; root-end preparation with a bur produces a heavy smear layer at all levels of preparation.[214]

The major concern with ultrasonic root-end preparation is the potential for creating root fractures as a result of the ultrasonic vibration (Fig. 9-42).

Ultrasonic Root-End Preparation and Apical Fractures

Several studies have investigated the fracture-inducing potential of ultrasonic root-end preparation techniques. This is possibly the most controversial question that arises in relation to the use of ultrasonic root-end preparation tips. Three types of root-end fractures have been described: intracanal fractures (originating from the root canal system and extending into the dentin), extracanal fractures (originating on the root surface and extending into the dentin), and communicating fractures (extending from the root surface to the root canal system).[425] This classification system is not universally used in studies of root-end cavity preparation; therefore, it is difficult to establish the significance, if any, of one type of fracture over another. When a strain gauge was used to measure root deformation, ultrasonic root-end preparation was shown to produce significantly greater strain, on average, than that generated by a microhandpiece. However, this did not translate into an increase in cracks observed on the resected surface of roots after root-end cavity preparation.[48,303,375,425] Several other in vitro studies that used different models to assess root-end fractures conversely concluded that ultrasonic root-end preparation does induce apical fractures.[2,184,299,354,469] Thus, the degree to which apical fractures are induced during ultrasonic root-end cavity preparation is difficult to determine from in vitro studies.

On the other hand, in an in vivo study[358] and cadaver-based studies[86,207] designed to replicate the clinical scenario, root fractures were not attributed to ultrasonic use. In these studies ultrasonic root-end preparation did not induce a significant number of root-end fractures. Several explanations may account for the differences observed in these studies. The surrounding tissues in cadaver and clinical subjects may disperse the ultrasonic energy away from the root tip. Thermal energy produced during ultrasonic preparation may have been controlled more adequately in some studies than in others. The power setting used on the ultrasonic unit may have been in the low range; a low power setting has been shown to produce fewer fractures in an in vitro setting[176,299] and therefore is recommended for clinical use.

Significance of Ultrasonic Tip Design

Different types of ultrasonic tips are available for root-end preparation (Figs. 9-43 and 9-44), including tips of varying lengths and diameters constructed of stainless steel. These tips are left uncoated or are coated with diamond or zirconium nitride. Tips with a curvature of 70 degrees or greater are more susceptible to fracture under continuous loading, and fracture typically occurs at the bend.[573] Coating of ultrasonic tips undoubtedly improves the cutting efficiency compared with uncoated stainless steel tips; this translates into significantly less time required to prepare a root-end cavity.[200,405] In the coated tips, the diamond coating appears to be the most aggressive and requires the least amount of time to produce a root-end cavity preparation.[253] Furthermore, the type of tip (i.e., stainless steel, diamond coated, or zirconium nitride coated) appears to have little effect on the number or types of fractures that can be induced in the root end during root-end preparation.[76,200,253,375,425] The cavity walls of root-end preparations formed by stainless steel tips typically have cleaner canal walls than those formed by coated root-end preparation tips. Stainless steel tips appear to produce less superficial debris and smear layer. Coated root-end preparation instruments typically produce a heavily abraded, debris-covered cavity wall surface.[76,610] However, overall the quality of the coated-tip preparation has been suggested to be superior.[405]

Temperature Changes Induced by Ultrasonic Instruments

The importance of heat generation and temperature changes has already been discussed. All ultrasonic surgical tips should have an irrigation port. Use of an ultrasonic instrument in the periradicular tissues without adequate irrigation results in an extreme temperature increase in the tissues, although this specific effect has not been demonstrated during root-end preparation. Scaling without irrigation can increase the temperature in dentin as much as 95° F (35° C) above the baseline temperature[290]; such an increase can injure pulpal and periodontal tissues.[380]

Bonded Root-End Fillings

Root-end cavity preparation for bonded root-end filling materials requires a change in the standard root-end cavity preparation technique. A shallow, scalloped preparation of the entire root surface should be made using a round or oval bur; the preparation should be at least 1 mm at the deepest concavity.[26,453] An ultrasonic preparation can be made into the root

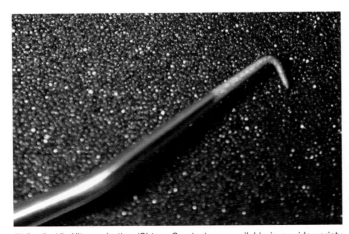

FIG. 9-43 Ultrasonic tips (Obtura Spartan) are available in a wide variety of configurations for use in different areas of the mouth. Most new tips have a special coating (zirconium nitride or diamond) that improves cutting efficiency.

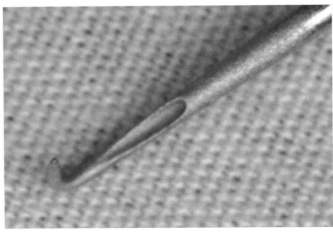

FIG. 9-44 Ultrasonic tip with diamond coating and irrigation port (DENTSPLY Tulsa Dental Specialties).

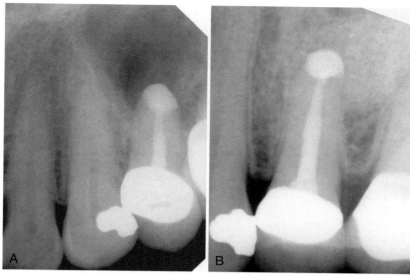

FIG. 9-45 **A,** Immediate postoperative radiograph of a bonded root-end filling in a maxillary first premolar. **B,** Follow-up radiograph at 20 months showing good periradicular healing.

canal system, but this may not be necessary. The root-end filling material is placed in a dome fashion and bonded to the entirety of the resected root end (Fig. 9-45).

ROOT-END FILLING MATERIALS

The ideal root-end filling material seals the contents of the root canal system within the canal, preventing egress of any bacteria, bacterial by-products, or toxic material into the surrounding periradicular tissues. The material should be nonresorbable, biocompatible, and dimensionally stable over time. It should be able to induce regeneration of the PDL complex, specifically cementogenesis over the root-end filling itself. Finally, the handling properties and working time should be such that the endodontic surgeon can place a root-end filling with sufficient ease.

Many materials have been used as root-end fillings, including gutta-percha, polycarboxylate cements, silver cones, amalgam, Cavit (3M ESPE, St. Paul, MN) zinc phosphate cement, gold foil, and titanium screws. However, this section focuses on root-end filling materials discussed in the literature within the past 10 years that are in common clinical use. These materials are zinc oxide–eugenol cements (IRM and Super-EBA), glass ionomer cement, Diaket, composite resins (Retroplast), resin–glass ionomer hybrids (Geristore), and mineral trioxide aggregate (ProRoot-MTA), and bioceramics.

Zinc Oxide–Eugenol (ZOE) Cements

Zinc oxide powder and eugenol liquid can be mixed to form a paste that is compacted into a cavity preparation. Use of this material dates back to the 1870s. Eugenol is released from ZOE mixtures, although this declines exponentially with time and is directly proportional to the liquid-powder ratio.[243] When ZOE comes in contact with water, it undergoes surface hydrolysis, producing zinc hydroxide and eugenol. This reaction continues until all the ZOE in contact with the free water is converted to zinc hydroxide.[243-245] Eugenol can have a number of effects on mammalian cells, depending on the concentration and length of exposure. These effects include cell respiration

depression, macrophage and fibroblast cytotoxicity, depressed vasoconstrictor response, inhibition of prostaglandin, and suppressing or enhancing effects on the immune response.[139,349,561] Other materials have been added to the basic ZOE mixture in an effort to increase the strength and radiopacity and reduce the solubility of the final material. Commercially available ZOE materials include intermediate restorative material (IRM; Dentsply Caulk, Milford, DE) and Super-EBA (Bosworth Company, Skokie, IL).

Intermediate Restorative Material (IRM)

IRM consists of a powder containing greater than 75% zinc oxide and approximately 20% polymethacrylate mixed in equal parts with a liquid that contains greater than 99% eugenol and less than 1% acetic acid. IRM seals better than amalgam and is not affected by the liquid-powder ratio or root-end conditioning agents.[116,407] IRM appears to be tolerated in the periradicular tissue, but it has no dental hard-tissue regenerative capacity. The response is similar to that seen with other ZOE-based materials.[221,329,417-420] In vitro, IRM prevents adherence of enamel matrix proteins.[463]

Super-EBA

Super-EBA consists of a powder containing 60% zinc oxide, 34% aluminum oxide, and 6% natural resins. It is mixed in equal parts with a liquid that contains 37.5% eugenol and 62.5% o-methoxybenzoic acid. Super-EBA is available in two forms, fast set and regular set. Other than the setting time, the properties of the two forms appear to be the same.[593] Super-EBA has radiopacity[484] and sealing effects similar to those of IRM and is less leaky than amalgam.[232,388] The leakage pattern of Super-EBA does not appear to be affected by root-end conditioning or finishing techniques.[174,469] When Super-EBA and IRM were finished with a carbide finishing bur in a high-speed handpiece, marginal adaptation was better than with ball burnishing, which was equal to burnishing with a moistened cotton pellet.[170] The environment of the periradicular wound may affect the long-term stability of Super-EBA, which has been shown to disintegrate over time in an acid pH environment.[30]

Biologically, Super-EBA is well tolerated in the periradicular tissues when used as a root-end filling. However, it has no capacity to regenerate cementum. Bone healing has been demonstrated at 12 weeks, with some fibrous tissue persisting. Super-EBA root-end fillings show a basophilic-stained line adjacent to the filling material, which may indicate hard-tissue formation.[404,418,419,542] Collagen fibers appear to grow into the cracks of the material,[396] but the significance of this is unknown. Super-EBA has limited antibacterial effect.[101] The cytotoxicity of Super-EBA is similar to that of amalgam and IRM.[102,605] The incidence of persistent disease after endodontic surgery in which Super-EBA was used as a root-end filling material ranges from 4% to 20%. In comparative studies in which amalgam was also used as a root-end filling material, use of Super-EBA always resulted in less persistent disease. The follow-up period for these studies ranged from 0.5 to 4.6 years.[147,326,397,448,518,565]

Glass-Ionomer Cements

Glass-ionomer cement (GIC) consists of aqueous polymeric acids, such as polyacrylic acid, plus basic glass powders, such as calcium aluminosilicate. GIC sets by a neutralization reaction of aluminosilicate, which is chelated with carboxylate groups to cross-link the polyacids; a substantial amount of the glass remains unreacted and acts as reinforcing filler. Glass-ionomer cements can be either light or chemically cured. Silver has been incorporated into GIC to improve the physical properties, including compressive and tensile strength and creep resistance. Both forms of GIC have been suggested as an alternative root-end filling material.[44,415,416]

The seal and marginal adaptation of light-cured GIC are superior to those with chemical-cured GIC. The seal achieved with GIC generally is better than that with amalgam and similar to that with IRM.[105,106,252,444,520,591] Long-term surface changes can occur in silver-GIC that may affect the stability of silver-GIC in the periradicular tissues.[55] Glass-ionomer cements are susceptible to attack by moisture during the initial setting period, resulting in increased solubility and decreased bond strength.[188,508,596] Contamination with moisture and blood adversely affected the outcome when GIC was used as a root-end filling material; this occurred significantly more often in unsuccessful cases.[602] The cytotoxicity of chemical- and light-cured GIC does not differ significantly from that of Super-EBA or amalgam.[102,394] The tissue response to GIC is considerably more favorable than to amalgam and similar to that with ZOE-based materials.[100,104,133,416] In a comparative clinical study using amalgam or GIC for root-end filling, healing was evaluated clinically and radiographically after 1 and 5 years.[261,602] No difference was seen in healing capacity between the two materials. The overall success rate in both groups was 90% at 1 year and 85% at 5 years. This study showed that the 5-year follow-up result can be predicted in more than 95% of the cases at the 1-year follow-up. These authors concluded that GIC is a valid alternative to amalgam for use as an apical sealant after root-end resection and that it provides equally good long-term clinical results.[261,602]

Diaket

Diaket (ESPE GmbH, Seefeld, Germany) a polyvinyl resin initially intended for use as a root canal sealer, has been advocated for use as a root-end filling material.[587] It is a powder consisting of approximately 98% zinc oxide and 2% bismuth phosphate mixed with a liquid consisting of 2.2-dihydroxy-5.5

dichlorodiphenylmethane, propionylacetophenone, triethanolamine, caproic acid copolymers of vinyl acetate, and vinyl chloride vinyl isobutylether. Leakage studies comparing Diaket to other commonly used root-end filling materials have shown it to have a superior sealing ability.[190,264,313,571] Its sealing ability has not been directly compared to that of MTA. When Diaket was used as a root canal sealer, biocompatibility studies showed that it was cytotoxic in cell culture[276] and generated long-term chronic inflammation in osseous[502] and subcutaneous tissues.[393] However, when mixed at the thicker consistency advocated for use as a root-end filling material, Diaket has shown good biocompatibility with osseous tissues.[379,587] Histologically, a unique tissue barrier has been observed to form across the Diaket at the resected root end, the nature of which is unknown. This tissue resembles an osteoid or cementoid type of matrix with a close approximation of periodontal tissue fibers, suggesting a regenerative response to the root-end filling material.[587] In animal studies Diaket has shown a better healing response than resected gutta-percha in uninfected teeth[590] and a healing response similar to that with MTA. However, no cementum formation was evident.[433] This material is no longer available in the United States.

Composite Resins and Resin-Ionomer Hybrids

Composite resin materials have some desirable properties and may be considered for use as root-end filling materials. Generally, when assessed for sealability, composite resins perform well in invitro studies. Composite resins also tend to leak less than amalgam, Super-EBA, IRM, and GICs.[126,344,345,520] However, blood contamination during the bonding process reduces bond strength and increases leakage.[353,560] Marginal adaptation varies, depending on the conditions and the bonding agents.[17] Certain components of composite resins and dentin-bonding agents can have a cytotoxic effect on cells; this effect varies, depending on the agent and its concentration.[80,217,428,429,514] Studies have shown that once the composite resin sets, cells can grow on its surface.[328,362,402,604] The healing response of the periradicular tissues to composite resins in general appears to be very diverse, ranging from poor to good[25,542]; this may depend on the type of material used. Two composite resin–based materials, Retroplast (Retroplast Trading, Rørvig, Denmark) and Geristore (Den-Mat, Santa Maria, CA), have been advocated for use as root-end filling materials.

Retroplast

Retroplast is a dentin-bonding composite resin system developed in 1984 specifically for use as a root-end filling material. The formulation was changed in 1990, when the silver was replaced with ytterbium trifluoride and ferric oxide. Retroplast is a two-paste system that forms a dual-cure composite resin when mixed. Paste A is composed of Bis-GMA/TEGDMA 1:1, benzoyl peroxide N,N-di-(2-hyydroxyethyl)-p-toluidine, and butylated hydroxytoluene (BHT). This is mixed in equal parts with paste B, which is composed of resin ytterbium trifluoride aerosil ferric oxide. A Gluma-based dentin bonding agent is used to adhere the material to the root-end surface. The working time is $1\frac{1}{2}$ to 2 minutes, and the radiopacity (due to the ytterbium trifluoride content) is equivalent to 6 mm of aluminum.

Only limited information is available on the physical and chemical properties of Retroplast, although a number of human clinical studies have been published.[22,25,361,451-455,457-460] In all cases the material appeared to be well tolerated and promoted a good healing response. There is evidence that Retroplast promotes hard-tissue formation at the root apex, and some have suggested that this is a form of cementum. In a limited number of case reports, Retroplast root-end fillings have demonstrated regeneration of the periodontium with a cementum layer over the root-end restoration.[22,453,454] The healing response in these cases showed deposition of minimal cementum and the insertion of new Sharpey's fibers. The PDL fibers also entered the newly formed adjacent alveolar bone, indicating that tissue regeneration, including cementogenesis, may occur on composite material, consequently forming a biologic closure of the root canal.[25] In an investigation of 388 cases comparing root-end fillings of Retroplast or amalgam, radiographic healing after 1 year was as follows: with Retroplast, 74% showed complete healing, 4% showed fibrous healing, 15% were uncertain, and 7% were failures; with amalgam, 59% showed complete healing, 3% showed fibrous healing, 30% were uncertain, and 8% were failures.[453] Complete healing occurred significantly more often after root-end filling with Retroplast. The number of immediate postoperative complications did not differ significantly between the composite and the amalgam groups. A more recent clinical study of 351 cases reported a complete healing rate of 80% to 89%.[459] A 10-year follow-up of 34 of these cases showed complete healing in 33 of the cases.[458]

Resin-Ionomer Suspension (Geristore) and Compomer (Dyract)

The resin-ionomer suspension and compomer group of materials attempts to combine the various properties of composite resins and glass ionomers. Geristore and Dyract (Dentsply, Tulsa, OK) have been investigated for use as root-end filling materials, although the available published literature on both is limited. These two materials require light activation and resin-dentin bonding agents to attach to the tooth.

Geristore has been recommended both as a root-end filling material[93] and for use in restoring subgingival surface defects such as root surface caries, external root resorption lesions, iatrogenic root perforations, and subgingival oblique fractured roots. Clinical evaluation of Geristore as a restorative material for root caries and cervical erosions showed it to be an acceptable material.[183,372,475,548] When it is used for surgical repair of root perforations and as an adjunct to guided tissue regeneration, the results have been favorable in isolated case reports.[3,4,47,440,487] Geristore's dual-curing paste/paste formulation is a hydrophilic Bis-GMA with long-term fluoride release. Light activation for 40 seconds cures the material to approximately 4 mm. However, the top layer is harder until the material achieves uniform hardness at 1 day after activation.[512] In vitro leakage assessment of Geristore and Dyract indicates that the materials leak less than root-end fillings made of IRM, amalgam, or Super-EBA.[65,209] Geristore has a leakage pattern similar to that of MTA.[474] An acid pH significantly reduces dye leakage of Geristore.[446] These materials are less sensitive to moisture than conventional glass-ionomer cement; however, dry environments produce stronger bonds.[99] The effect of blood contamination during the bonding phase in a clinical scenario is unknown. Geristore appears to have the potential to allow regeneration of the periradicular tissue. In one study, PDL and gingival fibroblasts attached to Geristore, and the attachment improved with time and cell proliferation.[87] Studies

investigating epithelial and connective tissue adherence to Geristore found clinical and histologic evidence of cellular attachment when the material was placed in subgingival cavities.[150,151,475] However, the healing response in the periradicular region is best described as unpredictable. In a study in dogs, 10 of the 18 root end–filled teeth developed abscesses. The author attributed this to the technical difficulty of placing Geristore root-end filling. However, a small number of specimens developed cementum on the root-end fillings. The cemental covering was never greater than 25% of the root-end filling surface, which was considerably less than the amount of cementum developed on both white and gray MTA.[315]

Mineral Trioxide Aggregate (MTA)

MTA (ProRoot MTA; DENTSPLY Tulsa Dental Specialties), a material developed specifically as a root-end filling,[529] has undergone numerous in vitro and in vivo investigations comparing its various properties to Super-EBA, IRM, and amalgam. In vitro sealing ability and biocompatibility studies comparing root-end filling materials have shown MTA to be superior to other commonly used materials.[277,300,527,530,531,533-535] When various in vitro leakage models were used, MTA prevented leakage as well as composite resin and GIC.[6,129,171,591] However, the setting and subsequent leakage of MTA are not affected by the presence of blood.[527] Torabinejad and colleagues[535] developed the original product (gray MTA). The main constituents of this material are calcium silicate ($CaSiO_4$), bismuth oxide (Bi_2O_3), calcium carbonate ($CaCO_3$), calcium sulfate ($CaSO_4$), and calcium aluminate ($CaAl_2O_4$). Hydration of the powder produces a colloidal gel that solidifies into a hard structure consisting of discrete crystals in an amorphous matrix. The crystals are composed of calcium oxide, and the amorphous region is composed of 33% calcium, 49% phosphate, 2% carbon, 3% chloride, and 6% silica.[529] In a study comparing the setting time, compressive strength, radiopacity, and solubility of MTA to those of amalgam, Super-EBA, and IRM, MTA was found to be less radiopaque than amalgam but more radiopaque than Super-EBA and IRM.[529] MTA had the longest setting time (2 hours, 45 minutes) and the lowest compressive strength at 24 hours after mixing (40 MPa), although compressive strength increased to 67 MPa at 21 days after mixing. The solubility of MTA after setting was similar to that of amalgam and Super-EBA. Initially MTA has a pH of 10.2, which rises to 12.5 3 hours after mixing.[529] The pH has been reported to be approximately 9.5 at 168 hours after mixing.[152] MTA is less cytotoxic than amalgam, Super-EBA, or IRM root-end fillings.[531] Endodontic surgery studies in dogs and monkeys have reported less periradicular inflammation and cementum deposition immediately adjacent to the root-end filling material.[27,173,236,528,532] Holland and colleagues[236,237] theorized that the tricalcium oxide in MTA reacts with tissue fluids to form calcium hydroxide, resulting in hard-tissue formation.

The importance of the presence of cementum-like tissue adjacent to MTA cannot be understated. Cementum deposition is essential to regeneration of the periodontal apparatus.[310] Augmentation of new cementum across the root end and root-end restoration is essential for ideal healing of the periodontium. A layer would also enhance the integrity of the apical barrier, making it more resistant to penetration by microorganisms; in effect, establishing a biologic barrier.[22] This is seen most frequently in sections where MTA was used as the filling material. MTA appears to be able to induce cementoblastic cells to produce hard tissue. Cementogenesis in the presence of MTA has been evaluated by assessment of the expression of osteocalcin (OCN), cell growth, and the morphology of cementoblast-like cells.[522] Scanning electron microscope (SEM) analysis indicated that cementoblasts could attach to and grow on MTA. In addition, strong expression of the OCN gene was seen after application of MTA. MTA can also increase the production of both proinflammatory and anti-inflammatory cytokines from osteoblasts. The clinical significance of this reaction is not known. The effect of MTA on periradicular tissues probably is partly due to these reactions.

In a human outcomes assessment study comparing ProRoot MTA to IRM, the rate of persistent disease with MTA was 16% at 12 months and 8% at 24 months.[103] The rate of persistent disease with IRM was 24% at 12 months and 13% at 24 months. These authors concluded that the use of MTA as a root-end filling material resulted in a high success rate that was not significantly better than that obtained with IRM. A prospective clinical trial using MTA as a root-end filling material along with current microsurgical techniques reported 89% clinical success, with follow-up time ranging from 4 to 72 months.[468]

A variation of the original formula of gray MTA has been introduced. This material, which is a white cream color, is often called white MTA. The chemical composition of white MTA is very similar to that of the original. White and gray ProRoot-MTA materials differ by less than 6% in any one component. Both are fine powders with a mean particle size of approximately 10 μm (the range in particle size is approximately 0.1 to 100 μm). The radiopacity of both materials is equivalent to approximately 3.04 mm of aluminum.[45] When white MTA was implanted in the subcutaneous connective tissue of rats, the results were similar to those reported for gray MTA.[238] One study compared the tissue reaction evoked by the two materials when used as root-end fillings in canines.[315] The only statistically significant difference observed was for the presence of macrophages or multinucleated giant cells adjacent to material. Gray MTA had more samples with mild to moderate infiltration of macrophages or multinucleated giant cells, and white MTA had more samples with no macrophages and/or multinucleated giant cells adjacent to the material. All other parameters assessed were essentially the same.

Bioceramics

Bioceramics are a relatively new and potentially promising addition to the group of materials available for root-end filling. In vitro testing of EndoSequence Root Repair Material (ERRM; Brasseler, Savannah, GA) demonstrates biocompatibility and antimicrobial activity that is similar to MTA.[107,122,317,323] ERRM is composed of calcium silicates, monobasic calcium phosphate, and zirconium oxide.[107] The material is hydrophilic, radiopaque, and has high pH. ERRM is available as a putty and a syringable paste. Because this is a relatively new material, long-term clinical studies are not yet available.

Overview of Root-End Filling Materials

Many different materials have been advocated for use as root-end filling materials, and each has specific advantages and disadvantages. However, from the biologic perspective of regeneration of the periradicular tissues, MTA, followed by Retroplast, appears to have a clear advantage over the other available materials. Bioceramic materials may join this group, but require more clinical testing. Retroplast and other composite

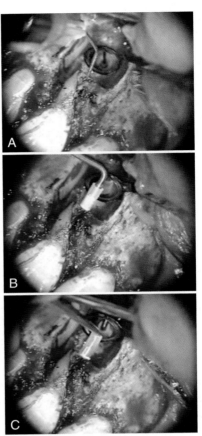

FIG. 9-46 **A,** Stropko syringe used to dry a root-end preparation before placement of the root-end filling material. **B,** Clinical use of an MTA delivery system (Dentsply Tulsa Dental). The device is loaded with MTA and placed over the root-end preparation. **C,** Pressing the plugger into the sleeve delivers the filling material to the root-end cavity preparation. The filling material then is compacted with microcondensers, and additional filling material is placed as needed.

resin–based filling materials require meticulous hemostasis and a dry surgical field for optimum results. The most commonly cited disadvantage of MTA is its handling properties. Even when properly prepared, MTA is more difficult to place in the root-end cavity than most other materials. Several devices have been modified or developed specifically for use with MTA (see Figs. 9-19 to 9-23 and 9-46). Typical clinical cases showing the surgical procedures described in the previous sections are presented in Figures 9-47 to 9-49.

CLOSURE OF THE SURGICAL SITE AND SELECTION OF SUTURE MATERIAL

Closure of the Surgical Site

The surgical site should be closed only after careful visual and radiographic inspection of the area. Before suturing, a radiograph should be taken with the flap held loosely in place to detect any foreign objects in the crypt or adhering to the flap. This image is also important for confirming the depth and density of the root-end filling. The osteotomy site then is gently curetted and irrigated with sterile saline or water to remove any remnants of hemostatic agents and packing

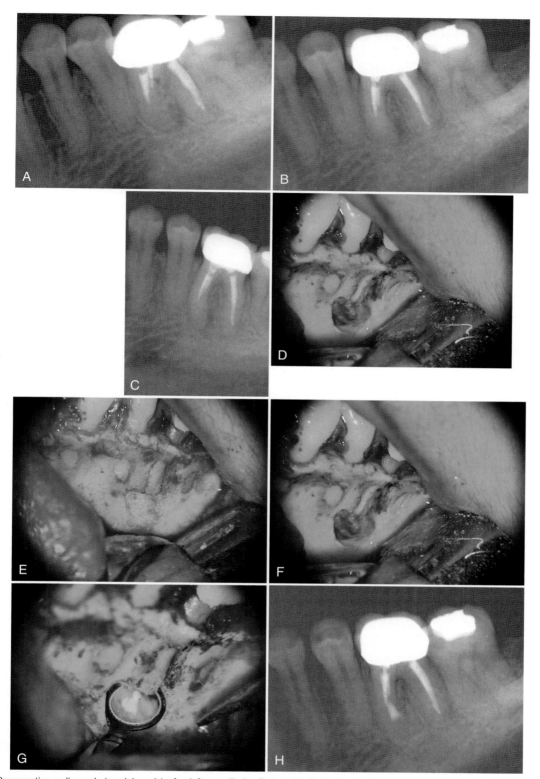

FIG. 9-47 A, Preoperative radiograph (mesial angle) of a left mandibular first molar. Periradicular disease and symptoms had persisted after nonsurgical retreatment by an endodontic resident. The mesial canals were completely obstructed at the midroot level. The preoperative evaluation included three periapical radiographs, two different horizontal angulations, and one vertically positioned radiograph. B, Straight view preoperative radiograph. C, Vertical periapical view preoperative radiograph. D, Osteotomy and root resection perpendicular to the long axis of the root were performed; a partial bony dehiscence over the mesial root can be seen. E, Racellets were packed into the bony crypt to establish hemostasis. F, The Racellets were removed (one usually is left in the deepest part of the crypt during root-end preparation and filling), and the root end was beveled perpendicular to the long axis of the root. Methylene blue dye can be useful for identifying the root outline and locating any cracks. Ultrasonic root-end preparation was completed to a depth of 3 mm, connecting the MB and ML canals. G, MTA root-end filling was placed and inspected. The bony crypt was then gently curetted to initiate bleeding and to remove any remnants of hemostatic materials. The flap was repositioned, and a radiograph was taken. H, An immediate postoperative radiograph confirmed the depth and density of the root-end filling and the absence of any foreign objects. Note that calcium sulfate and bone grafting material was placed in the osseous defect and over the root because of the large buccal dehiscence, although this is not routinely required in these cases. (Courtesy Dr. Vince Penesis.)

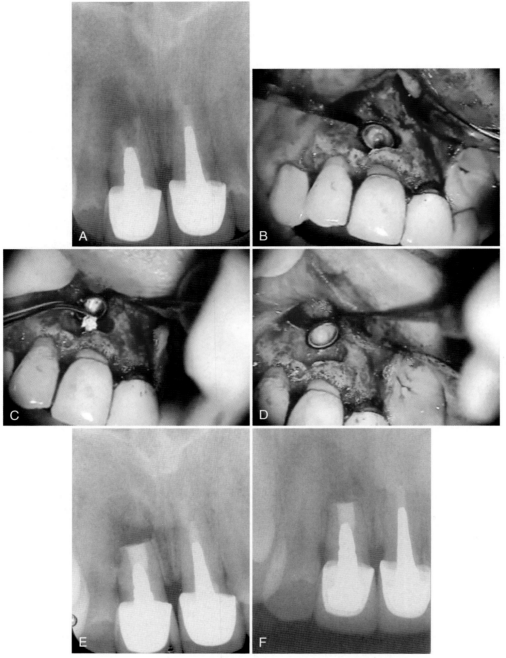

FIG. 9-48 A, Preoperative radiograph of a maxillary left central incisor showing evidence of previous surgery but no apparent root-end filling. Because of the short root length and inadequate band of keratinized gingiva, an intrasulcular incision and full-thickness triangular mucoperiosteal flap design were selected. **B,** The root was minimally resected, and the root-end cavity was prepared ultrasonically. **C,** MTA was placed and condensed into the root-end cavity preparation. **D,** The root-end filling was inspected before the flap was repositioned and sutured. **E,** Immediate postoperative radiograph. **F,** The 6-month follow-up radiograph showed good initial periradicular healing. (Courtesy Dr. Shawn Velez.)

materials. Some bleeding is encouraged at this point, because the blood clot forms the initial scaffold for subsequent healing and repair. If indicated, grafting materials or barriers may be placed at this time. Slight undermining of the unreflected soft tissue adjacent to the flap facilitates the placement of sutures. The flap is then repositioned and gently compressed with a

piece of chilled, sterile moist cotton gauze to express excess blood and tissue fluids.

For the common flap designs discussed in this chapter, the corners are first identified and sutured in place with a single interrupted suture. Interrupted sutures are initially passed through the free portion of the flap approximately 2 to 3 mm

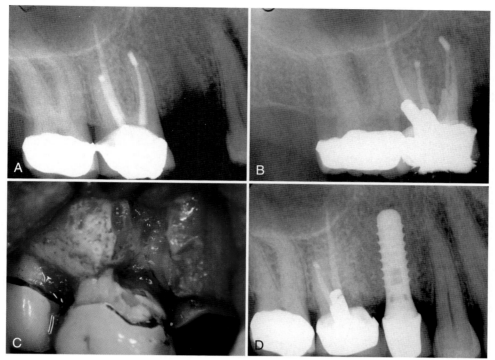

FIG. 9-49 **A,** A maxillary right first molar that was sensitive to percussion and tender to palpation over the MB root. Periodontal probing revealed a deep, narrow bony defect on the facial aspect of the MB root. The presence of a vertical root fracture was confirmed visually using magnification and methylene blue dye. The maxillary right second premolar had been recently extracted because of a vertical root fracture. **B,** A bonded amalgam core buildup was placed in the DB and P canals, and Geristore was placed in the MB canal system. **C,** The MB root was resected, and methylene blue dye was used to help define the extent of the fracture. **D,** At the 3-year follow-up visit, a new crown had been fabricated for the molar, and the premolar had been replaced with an implant.

from the edge and then connected to the attached tissue. The suture is secured with a simple surgeon's knot, which is positioned away from the incision line. The center of the flap then is located and sutured with either an interrupted or a sling suture. A continuous locking suture technique may be used to close a submarginal (Ochsenbein-Luebke) flap.[288] The primary advantage of a continuous suture technique is the ease of suture removal compared with multiple interrupted sutures. The disadvantages are possible difficulty with precise control of tension in each area, and the fact that the entire suture may loosen if one suture pulls through the flap. A sling suture is commonly used for the central tooth in the surgical site to close a full-thickness intrasulcular (rectangular or triangular) flap. The tension on this type of suture can be varied slightly to allow some control of the apicocoronal positioning of the flap. Interrupted sutures then are placed as needed.

When suturing is complete, chilled, sterile moist cotton gauze is again placed over the flap and pressure is applied for 5 minutes. Pressure to the area provides stability for the initial fibrin stage of clot formation and reduces the possibility of excessive postoperative bleeding and hematoma formation under the flap. The iced gauze also supports hemostasis. Final inspection of the area should confirm that all soft-tissue margins have been closely approximated and bleeding has been controlled. An additional injection of long-acting local anesthetic may be administered at this time, although care must be taken not to inject it directly under the newly repositioned flap.

The patient is given a cold compress and instructed to hold it on the face in the surgical area, on for 20 minutes and then off for 20 minutes, for the rest of the day. The patient also is given verbal and written postoperative instructions, including after-hours contact information (Fig. 9-50). The patient should sit in an upright position for approximately 15 minutes and the surgical site should be inspected one more time before the patient is discharged.

Selection of the Suture Material

The properties of an ideal suture material for periradicular surgery include pliability for ease of handling and knot tying, a smooth surface that discourages bacterial growth and wicking of oral fluids, and a reasonable cost. Suture material in size 5-0 is most commonly used, although some clinicians prefer slightly larger (4-0) or smaller (6-0) suture. Sutures smaller than 6-0 tend to cut through the relatively fragile oral tissues when tied with the tension required to approximate the wound margins. Silk suture material has been commonly used in dental surgery for decades and is both inexpensive and easy to handle. However, silk tends to support bacterial growth and allows for a wicking effect around the sutures. For these reasons, other materials are preferable to silk.[92]

Resorbable suture materials (plain gut and chromic gut) are not routinely used for periradicular surgery, although this material may be indicated if the patient will be unavailable for the regular suture removal appointment (48 to 96 hours after

---

Care of Your Mouth After Endodontic Surgery

1.) Apply an ice pack to your face next to the surgery area (on for 20 minutes and off for 20 minutes) for the next 5 to 6 hours to help decrease postoperative swelling. Swelling is usually greatest the day after surgery and may be at its worst 2 or 3 days after surgery.

2.) Take all medications as directed. Approximately 45 minutes should be allowed for you to feel the effect of pain medication.

3.) Clean your mouth as usual (brushing, flossing, etc.) in all areas except the surgical site. Modify cleaning procedures of the teeth in the area of the surgical site to keep from disturbing the area. Do not rinse vigorously during the first 24 hours following surgery. Continue using the prescribed mouth rinse twice a day until after you return to have the sutures removed.

4.) Minor oozing of blood from the surgical site may occur in the first 24 hours after surgery. This will produce a pink tinge in the saliva and is not a cause for concern. However, if bleeding is excessive, please contact our office. You may apply pressure to the area with a tea bag or moist cotton gauze.

5.) Sutures have been placed and will need to be removed at your next appointment. Please do not lift or pull on your lip to examine the surgical site during the first 2 to 3 days because this may disturb the healing process.

6.) A soft diet is recommended for the first 2 or 3 days. Try to avoid foods that are hot, spicy, or hard to chew. It is very important that you drink plenty of fluids (nonalcoholic). This will help your mouth heal.

7.) Avoid cigarettes and all other tobacco products.

8.) A slight increase in body temperature may occur during the first 24 hours following surgery. This is normal. Infection after endodontic surgery is not typical but can occur. If an infection develops, it usually occurs 2 to 3 days after the surgery. Signs of an infection include sudden increase in pain or swelling, feverish feeling, sore glands in the neck area, and a general flulike feeling. If you think an infection has developed, please contact the office immediately.

If you have any questions, please contact the office during normal office hours at 312-XXX-5555. If you are experiencing problems after office hours, you may contact Dr. _____ at: 312-XXX-1212.

FIG. 9-50 Example of postoperative instructions. Written instructions provide an essential reference for the patient, because verbal instructions often are difficult to remember after surgery. The instructions may be modified as needed; it is important to provide instructions that the patient can understand. For example, the readability of these instructions is at approximately the eighth grade level using the Flesch-Kincaid Grade Level scale.

surgery) or if the suture will be used in areas of the mouth where access is difficult. The primary problem with resorbable suture materials is the variable rate of resorption—that is, sutures may weaken and dissolve too soon or, more commonly, remain in the incision area for longer than desired. Gut suture materials are packed in isopropyl alcohol. The handling properties of gut sutures can be improved by immersion in sterile water for 3 to 5 minutes before use.[430]

Suture materials with a smooth Teflon or polybutilate coating (e.g., Tevdec and Ethibond, respectively) are particularly well suited for use in periradicular surgery. Synthetic monofilament suture materials (e.g., Supramid and Monocryl) are also commonly used. These materials are easy to handle and do not promote bacterial growth or wicking of oral fluids to the same extent as silk. Gortex (expanded PTEE-Teflon) sutures have many desirable properties but are more expensive than the previously mentioned materials.

Tissue adhesives such as cyanoacrylate and fibrin glues may hold promise for wound closure after periradicular surgery.[113,196,403,599] Although the currently available research is insufficient to recommend these adhesives as a routine replacement for more traditional suture materials, future applications in periradicular surgery are possible.

GUIDED TISSUE REGENERATION AND ENDODONTIC SURGERY

The amount and location of bone adjacent to the root structures affect the prognosis of periradicular surgery. Kim and Kratchman[282] propose a six-category classification system to assist in predicting surgical prognosis and determining the need for bone grafting and barrier techniques. Class A (no lesion), class B (small periapical lesion), and class C (large periapical lesion without periodontal communication) all represent situations that are favorable for healing without supplemental grafting or barriers. Class D (similar to class C with independent periodontal pocketing), class E (endodontic-periodontal communication to the apex), and class F (apical lesion with complete loss of buccal bone) represent situations with a more guarded prognosis and usually require concurrent use of bone grafting and barrier techniques. Figs. 9-51 to 9-63 are examples of cases that required guided tissue regeneration (GTR).

An apicomarginal defect[141] or a localized bony defect distinguished by a total deficiency of alveolar bone over the entire root length has a significant adverse effect on the outcome, reducing the rate of complete healing by approximately 20%

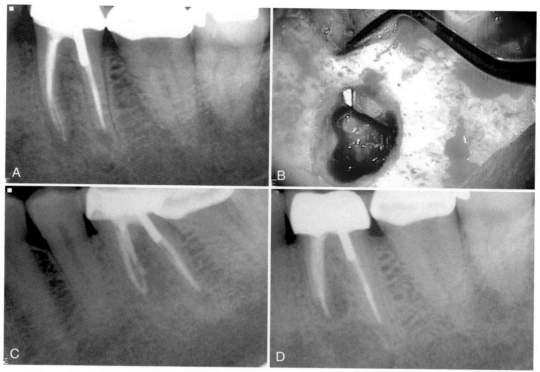

FIG. 9-51 **A,** Preoperative periapical radiograph of tooth #19. **B,** Clinical image demonstrating periodontal defect along the facial aspect of the mesial root. **C,** Immediate postsurgical radiograph. The mesial root end was prepared with ultrasonics and filled with MTA. A mixture of DFDBA and Capse was placed for guided tissue regeneration. **D,** One-year follow-up radiograph demonstrating good healing. Periodontal probings were WNL.

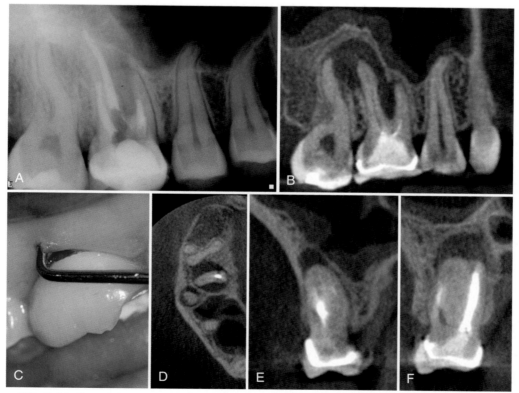

FIG. 9-52 (Case 1): **A,** Periapical radiograph of tooth #3. Retreatment RCT was attempted, but MB1 and MB2 were blocked. **B,** Sagittal view demonstrating the extent of the periapical lesion. **C,** Clinical view of periodontal probing to the apex. **D,** Axial view of the apical one third demonstrating the close proximity of the periapical defect to the MB root of tooth #2 (#2 responded WNL to pulp vitality testing). **E, F,** Coronal views of the MB and DB/P roots, respectively.

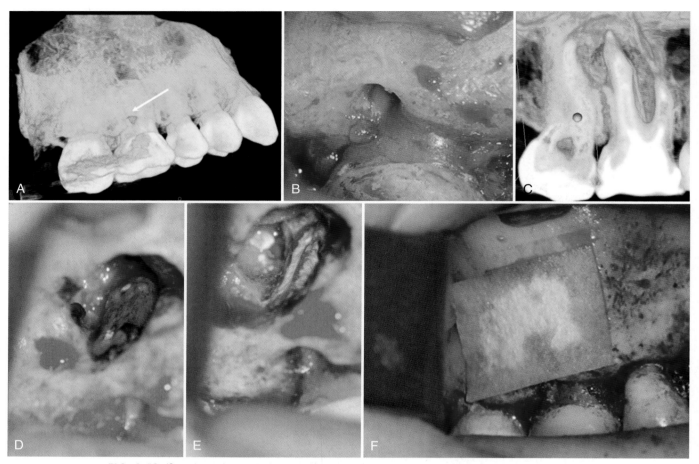

FIG. 9-53 (Case 1, continued): **A,** A 3D reconstruction of the tooth #3 area demonstrating the furcation periodontal defect. **B,** After flap reflection, clinical view demonstrating the periodontal defect. **C,** A 3D reconstruction with the buccal plate cropped to visualize the extent of the periradicular defect. **D, E,** DB and P root resection, root-end preparation, root-end filling with MTA. **F,** Periradicular defect grafted with Puros allograft (Zimmer Dental, Carlsbad, CA) and CopiOs pericardium membrane (Zimmer Dental).

or more when compared to teeth with an isolated endodontic-only lesion.[233,279,499] The presence of a periradicular lesion 15 mm or greater in diameter also has been linked to a poorer prognosis.[233] Advanced periodontitis with deep pocket formation has been associated with chronic periradicular inflammation after endodontic surgery and subsequent failure of the root-end surgery.[450] The cause of failure has been identified as in-growth of nonosteogenic tissues into the periradicular surgical site and down-growth of epithelial tissue along the root surface. Successful treatment may depend more on controlling epithelial proliferation than root-end management. Guided tissue regeneration techniques have been advocated for use in such cases.[206,547]

The basic principle of guided tissue and bone regeneration is that different types of cells repopulate a wound at different rates during healing. The soft-tissue cells are considerably more motile than the hard-tissue cells, therefore they tend to migrate into the wound more quickly during healing. A barrier interposed between the gingival tissue and the exposed root surfaces and supporting alveolar bone prevents colonization of the exposed root surface by gingival cells. This encourages selective repopulation of the root surface by PDL cells. The use of an absorbable barrier theoretically would allow PDL cells and

other cells with osteogenic potential to repopulate the defect, resulting in new connective tissue attachment and bone formation. Dahlin and coworkers[119,120] demonstrated that in monkeys, a significant increase in osseous healing occurs when membranes are used in through-and-through bone defects in periradicular surgery of the lateral maxillary incisors. The use of resorbable guided tissue regeneration (GTR) membranes in endodontic surgery with buccal apicomarginal type defects also has been shown to enhance regeneration of the periodontium and surrounding bone in dogs.[149] This type of matrix barrier promoted greater amounts of connective tissue and alveolar bone and minimized the formation of junctional epithelium.

Several case reports have discussed the use of guided tissue regeneration techniques in conjunction with endodontic surgery.[5,32,81,123,154,273,337,414,421,432,515,544,549,607] These studies largely have reported favorable outcomes in cases involving large periradicular lesions, through-and-through bone defects, and repair of a surgical perforation or loss of the buccal cortical plate adjacent to the root.

Pecora and colleagues[400] compared the healing of 20 large periradicular defects (greater than 10 mm diameter) with and without the use of resorbable membrane. They reported that

Text continued on p. 434

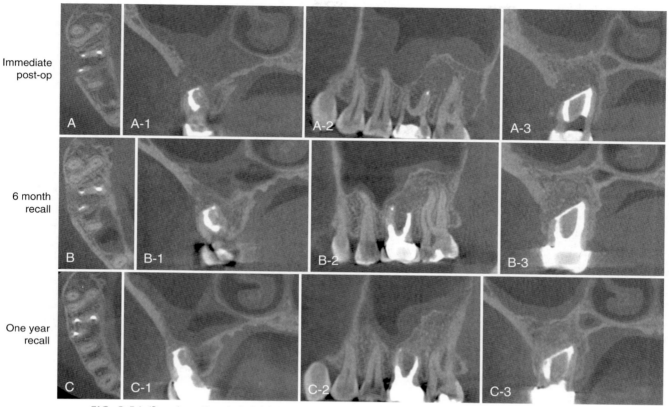

FIG. 9-54 (Case 1, continued): **A,** Axial view of immediate postoperative CBCT scan, A-1 coronal view of MB root, A-2 sagittal view and A-3 coronal view of DB and palatal roots. **B,** A 6-month recall, axial view, B-1 coronal view of MB root, B-2 sagittal view, and B-3 coronal view of DB and palatal roots. **C,** A 1-year recall, axial view, C-1 coronal view of MB root, C-2 sagittal view, and C-3 coronal view of DB and palatal roots.

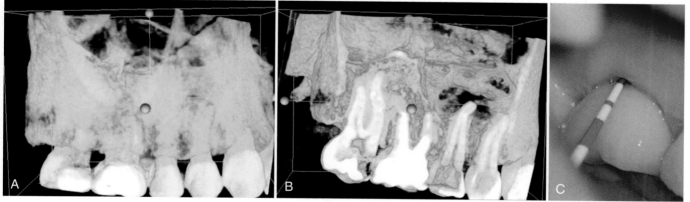

FIG. 9-55 (Case 1, 1-year recall): **A, B,** A 3D reconstruction of 1-year recall. **C,** Clinical picture showing resolution of the periodontal defect.

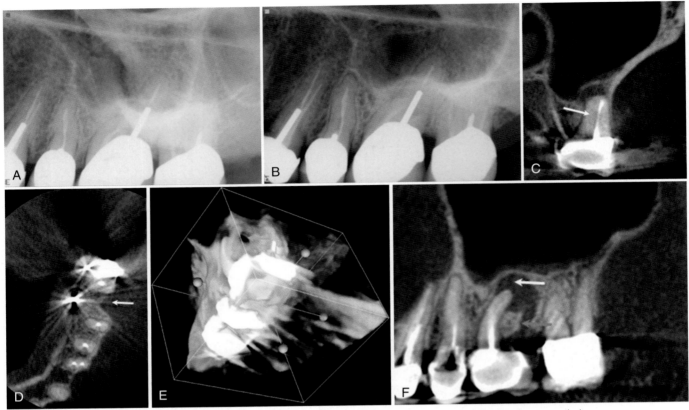

FIG. 9-56 (Case 2, tooth #14): **A, B,** Periapical radiographs of tooth #14, mesial and distal angles, respectively. **C,** Coronal view of the MB root demonstrating a missed MB2 canal *(arrow).* **D,** Axial view showing a previous DB root amputation site *(arrow)* that was not obvious in the periapical radiograph. **E,** A 3D reconstruction demonstrating a crestal defect. **F,** Sagittal view demonstrating the crestal defect *(red arrow)* communicating with the periapical lesion *(white arrow),* elevation of the floor of the maxillary sinus but no evidence of sinus perforation.

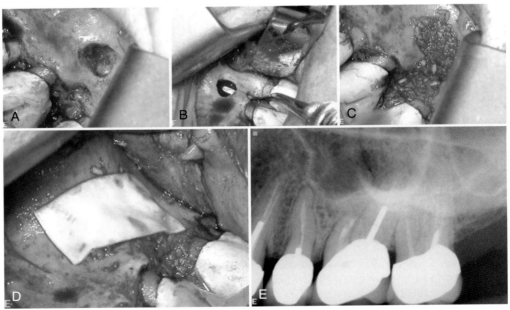

FIG.9-57 (Case 2, continued): **A,** Clinical view after flap reflection demonstrating both crestal and periapical lesions. **B,** Communication between both defects. **C,** Both defects grafted with EnCore Combination Allograft (Osteogenics Biomedical, Lubbock, TX). **D,** CopiOs pericardium membrane (Zimmer Dental, Carlsbad, CA). **E,** Immediate postoperative radiograph.

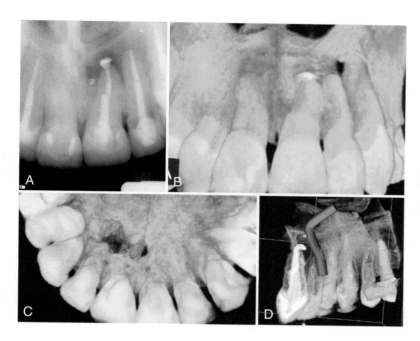

FIG. 9-58 (Case 3): **A,** Periapical radiograph of maxillary anterior region demonstrating a periapical lesion associated with tooth #9. **B,** CBCT reconstruction demonstrating the intact buccal cortical plate. **C,** Palatal view of the 3D reconstruction demonstrating perforation of the palatal plate. **D,** A 3D reconstruction showing the nasopalatine bundle.

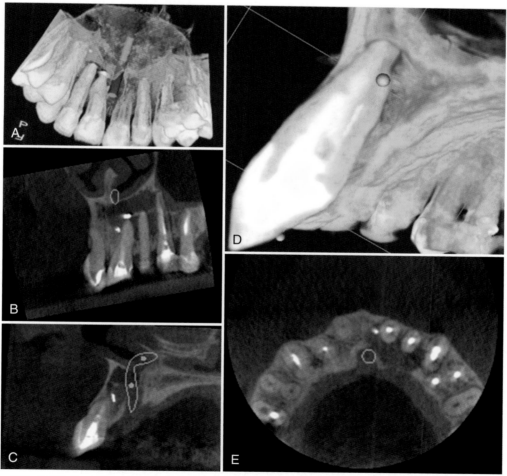

FIG. 9-59 (Case 3, continued): **A,** Palatal view CBCT reconstruction showing the exit of the nasopalatine neurovascular bundle from the incisive canal. **B,** Sagittal view demonstrating the periapical radiolucency involving teeth #9, 10, and 11. **C,** Coronal view the exit of the nasopalatine bundle from incisive canal. **D,** A 3D reconstruction demonstrating the periapical lesion extension to tooth #11. **E,** Axial view demonstrating the extension of the lesion, palatal plate perforation, and relation of the nasopalatine bundle to the periapical lesion.

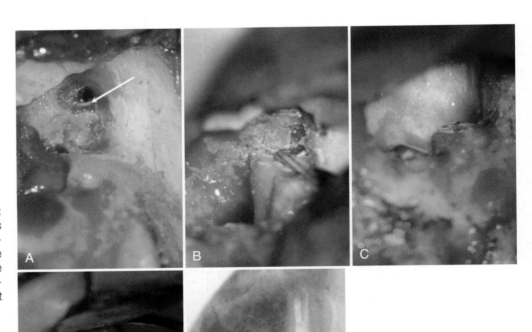

FIG. 9-60 (Case 3, continued): A, B, Clinical pictures before and after flap reflection showing the intact buccal plate. C, Periapical defect after degranulation showing the apices of teeth #9 and 10 prior to resection. D, Palatal bone perforation with palatal mucosa evident *(circle)*. E, F, Clinical pictures of the nasopalatine bundle intact after degranulation.

FIG. 9-61 (Case 3, continued): A, B, Lateral wall of the maxillary sinus distal to tooth #11. C, CopiOs membrane placed palatally to cover the palatal mucosa. D, CopiOs membrane covering the Puros allografting material. E, Through-and-through defect immediate postoperative radiograph.

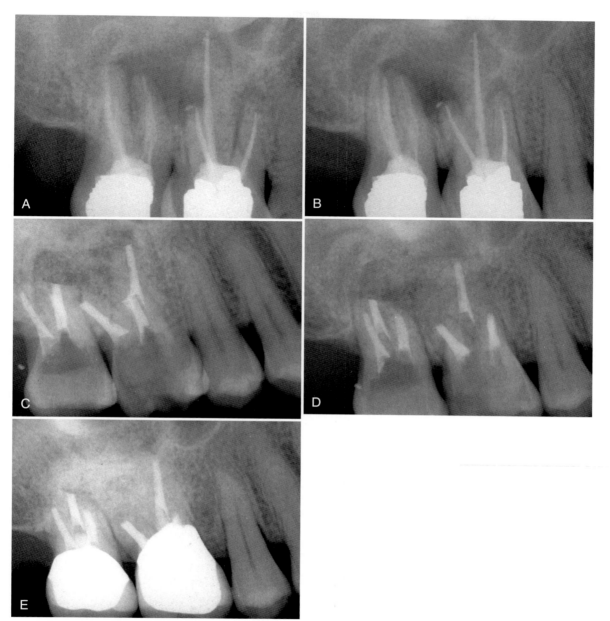

FIG. 9-62 **A,** Preoperative angled radiograph of maxillary right first and second molars. Both teeth had been treated previously, and the patient has reported a history of pain in the area for the past 5 years. The treatment plan included nonsurgical retreatment followed by periradicular surgery with bone grafting and guided tissue regeneration (GTR). **B,** Preoperative straight-on radiograph of the maxillary right first and second molars. **C,** Immediate postoperative radiograph showing root-end resections and fillings. The root ends were prepared with ultrasonics, conditioned with 17% ethylenediaminetetraacetic acid (EDTA), filled with Diaket, and smoothed with a superfine diamond finishing bur. The crypt was packed with BioOss xenograft material, and a Guidor resorbable membrane was placed. **D,** Immediate postoperative radiograph (straight on view). **E,** A 4-year follow-up radiograph. The patient was asymptomatic, and all objective findings were within normal limits. The teeth were restored with porcelain fused to metal crowns.

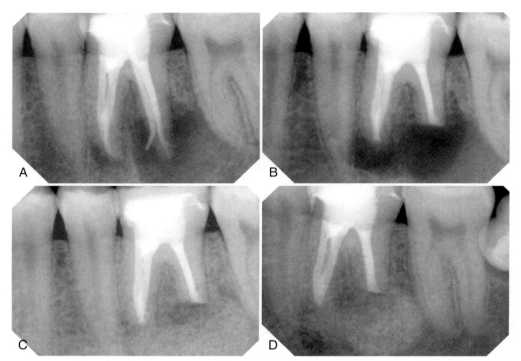

FIG. 9-63 **A,** Preoperative radiograph of a mandibular left first molar. Gutta-percha was inserted into the buccal sulcus and traced to the apex of the distal root. Nonsurgical root canal treatment had been performed 12 months earlier. **B,** Root-end resection and MTA root-end fillings (M and D roots). **C,** Immediate postoperative radiograph. BioOss xenograft material was placed. **D,** The 19-month follow-up radiograph showed good periradicular healing.

at 12 months after surgery, the sites in which membranes had been used had healed more quickly and that the quality and quantity of the regenerated bone was superior. One study evaluated periradicular and periodontal healing in cases involving apicomarginal defects when guided tissue regeneration (Bio-Oss and Bio-Gide membrane; Osteohealth Co., Shirley, NY) was performed in conjunction with periradicular surgery. At 12 months after surgery, 86% were considered healed clinically and radiographically. It was concluded that GTR should be considered as an adjunct to periradicular surgery in cases of apicomarginal defects.[142] However, use of a resorbable membrane when a standard apical osteotomy is performed and the buccal bone over the remainder of the root is intact has no beneficial effect on healing.[186]

Several different types of membranes are available. They can be grouped into two broad categories, nonresorbable and resorbable (Table 9-1). Resorbable membranes are generally better suited for endodontic uses because a second surgical procedure is not required to remove the membrane.

Membranes frequently require support so that the membrane does not collapse into the defect itself. Support for the membrane may be provided by using either a titanium-tented membrane or a graft material. Graft materials have two main functions: to act as a mechanical substructure that supports the membrane and the overlying soft tissues and to serve as a biologic component that enhances bone formation. Bone graft materials (Table 9-2) can be categorized as osteoconductive or osteoinductive. An osteoconductive material provides a framework into which bone can grow. The pore size of the material is similar to that of normal bone, and the material eventually is absorbed and remodeled. An osteoinductive

material stimulates the production of new bone cells such that healing occurs more quickly. The bone morphogenic protein (BMP) family has been investigated extensively for use in this role. A combination of osetoconductive and osteoinductive materials also can be used for bone grafts.

The use of GTR techniques raises several additional issues that should be discussed with the patient before surgery. These include the cost of the additional material, the origin of the material (synthetic, animal, or human), the need to manage the wound for a longer period, and potential postoperative complications related specifically to these techniques and materials. Discussion of the composition of the materials to be used is very important, because some patients may have concerns based on religious or ethical grounds. The surgeon must discuss all the ramifications of using these materials with the patient before beginning the procedure, because it is not always possible to predict before surgery when grafting materials may be needed.

If GTR techniques are to be used during periradicular surgery, a resorbable membrane should be chosen and a protocol should be followed (Figs. 9-62 and 9-63):

1. The membrane is extended to cover 2 to 3 mm of bone peripheral to the margins of the crypt; it should be supported with a bone substitute graft material so that it does not collapse into the crypt or onto underlying tooth structures.
2. Tissue closure techniques should ensure total tissue coverage of the membrane. The traditional postoperative compression is eliminated, because this would collapse the membrane onto the underlying structures.
3. Smoking is contraindicated with GTR techniques because it consistently has been shown to affect the outcome adversely.[73,324,445,525,538,539]

TABLE 9-1

Examples of Membrane Materials

Composition	Trade Name/Manufacturer
Nonresorbable	
Polytetrafluoroethylene	Gortex (WL Gore & Associates Inc, Flagstaff, AZ)
	TefGen FD (Lifecore Biomedical, Chaska, MN)
	Bicon Barrier Membrane (Bicon, Boston, MA)
	Cytoflex (Unicare Biomedical, Laguna Hills, CA)
Resorbable	
Laminar bone	Lambone (Pacific Coast Tissues Bank, Los Angeles, CA)
Polylactic acid	Guidor* This product was used extensively in early research with very favorable results (Guidor USA)
	Atrisorb (CollaGenex Pharmaceuticals, Newtown, PA)
Polyglactic acid	Vicyl Mesh (Ethicon, Somerville, NJ)
Polylactic acid, polyglycolic acid, and trimethylene carbonate	Resolut (WL Gore & Associates Inc, Flagstaff, AZ)
Collagen	Biomend (Zimmer Dental, Carlsbad, CA)
	Bio-Guide (Osteohealth, Shirley, NY)
	Bicon Resorbable Collagen Membrane (Bicon, Boston, MA)

*No longer available.

TABLE 9-2

Examples of Bone Graft Materials

Graft Type	Description	Product/Manufacturer or Source
Autogenous graft	Obtained from patient's own body	Ramus, chin, iliac crest
Allograft	Demineralized freeze-dried human bone (DFDBA)	Osteofil (Regeneration Technologies, Alachua, FL)
		Grafton (Osteotech, Eatontown, NJ)
		Dynagraft (GenSci, Toronto, Ontario, Canada)
		Opteform (Exactech, Gainesville, FL)
		Puros (Zimmer Dental, Carlsbad CA)
		MTF DeMin Bone (DENTSPLY Friadent CeraMed, Lakewood, CO)
Xenograft	Inorganic bovine/porcine bone particles	BioOss (Osteohealth, Shirley, NY)
		OsteoGraf (DENTSPLY Friadent CeraMed, Lakewood, CO)
Ceramic/synthetic grafts	Calcium sulfate, calcium phosphate/hydroxyapatite, bioactive glass	CapSet (Lifecore Biomedical, Chaska, MN)
		OsteoSet (Wright Medical Technology, Arlington, TN)
		HTR (Bioplant HTR, Kerr Corporation, West Collins, CA)
		Biogran (3i, Palm Beach Gardens, FL)
		Norian SRS (Synthes, West Chester, PA)
		NovaBone-C/M (NovaBone Products, LLC, Sales and Manufacturing, Alachua, FL)
		PerioGlas (NovaBone Products, LLC, Sales and Manufacturing, Alachua, FL)
Bioactive proteins	Bone morphogenic proteins (BMP)	Experimental
Combination graft	Allograft, xenograft, or ceramic/synthetic grafts plus bioactive protein	PepGen P15 (DENTSPLY Friadent CeraMed, Lakewood, CO)

Ridge Preservation

With the growing use of dental implants for the replacement of missing teeth, clinicians should be aware of ridge preservation strategies, even if they do not place implants.[308] As an example, ridge preservation should be considered when a tooth is determined to have a vertical root fracture during an exploratory surgical procedure and is extracted. In this situation, there is often a complete absence of the buccal bony plate, and simple extraction of the tooth would predispose the patient to a loss of ridge height and width, thereby complicating future implant placement. GTR with graft and barrier placement (as previously described) at the time of extraction may be indicated to create a more favorable site for future implant placement.[31,251,342,608] An atraumatic extraction technique is desirable, as one of the goals is to preserve the maximum amount of existing bone. Periotomes are particularly useful for this type of bone-preserving extraction technique.

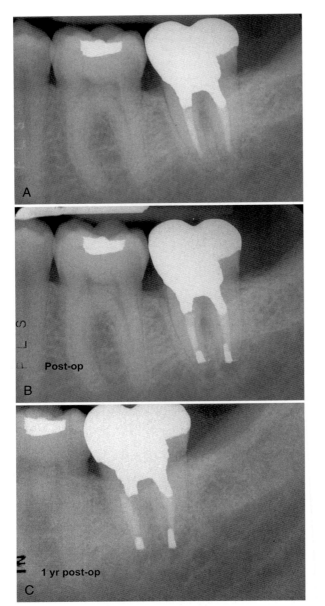

FIG. 9-64 Intentional replantation. **A,** Preoperative radiograph of a mandibular left second molar. The tooth was persistently sensitive to percussion and biting after nonsurgical retreatment. **B,** Radiograph of the tooth immediately after extraction, root-end preparation and filling, and replantation. **C,** At the 1-year follow-up visit, the tooth was asymptomatic and showed good periradicular healing. (Courtesy Dr. Matt Davis.)

INTENTIONAL REPLANTATION

Intentional replantation may be an option when surgical access is limited or presents unacceptable risks. Mandibular second molars are a common example for this technique because of the typically thick overlying buccal bone, shallow vestibular depth, and proximity of the root apices to the mandibular canal (Fig. 9-64). However, any tooth that can be atraumatically removed in one piece is a potential candidate for intentional replantation. Contraindications include teeth with flared or moderately curved roots and the presence of periodontal disease. Vertical root fracture has often been considered a

contraindication,[401] although some investigators have demonstrated moderate success using a dentin-bonded resin and intentional replantation for the treatment of teeth with root fractures.[226,268,506] The prognosis was generally better for incisors and for teeth with fractures less than two thirds of the root length. Clinical success after 1 year was about 89% and decreased to 59% at 5 years.[226]

The tooth should be extracted with minimal trauma to the tooth and socket. Ideally, elevators are not used and the root surface is not engaged with the forceps. All instruments and materials for root-end preparation and filling should be arranged before extraction to minimize extraoral working time. The root surface must be kept moist by wrapping the root with gauze soaked in a physiologic solution, such as Hank's Balanced Salt Solution. After root-end preparation and filling (as described previously in this chapter), the tooth is replanted and the buccal bone is compressed. The patient may be instructed to bite on a cotton roll or other semisolid object to help position the tooth properly in the socket. Occlusal adjustment is indicated to minimize traumatic forces on the tooth during the initial stage of healing. A splint may be applied, but this is often not necessary. The patient should eat a soft diet and avoid sticky foods, candy, and chewing gum for at least 7 to 10 days. Based on clinical observations and several animal model studies, the prognosis for successful healing after replantation is most closely related to avoiding trauma to the PDL and cementum during extraction and minimizing extraoral time.[21,23,391]

POSTOPERATIVE CARE

As previously noted, NSAIDs generally are the preferred class of drugs for managing postoperative pain (also see Chapter 4).[9,41,54,143] Ibuprofen (400 to 800 mg) or an equivalent NSAID typically is given before or immediately after surgery and can be continued for several days postoperatively as needed. When additional pain relief is required, a narcotic such as codeine, hydrocodone, or tramadol may be added to the standard NSAID regimen. This strategy may result in a synergistic effect, and therefore greater pain relief, than would be expected with the separate analgesic value of each drug.[148] A useful short-term approach to the management of moderate to severe pain is a "by the clock" alternating schedule of an NSAID and an acetaminophen/narcotic combination.[250,348] Pain after periradicular surgery typically is only mild to moderate. Postoperative pain usually is managed quite well with NSAIDs only, especially when the previously recommended strategy of preoperative NSAID therapy and a long-acting local anesthetic is combined with a minimally traumatic surgical approach.

Sutures commonly are removed 2 to 4 days after surgery.[92,213] This recommendation is based on the current understanding of wound healing and the desire to remove any potential irritants from the incision area as soon as possible. Local anesthesia is rarely required, although application of a topical anesthetic may be helpful, especially to releasing incisions in nonkeratinized mucosa. Sharp suture scissors or a #12 scalpel blade can be used to cut the sutures before they are removed with cotton pliers or tissue forceps. A transient bacteremia can be expected after suture removal, even when a preprocedural chlorhexidine mouth rinse is used.[79] Antibiotic coverage should be considered only for patients at high risk of developing bacterial endocarditis.

If healing is progressing normally at the suture removal appointment, the patient does not need to be seen again in the office until the first scheduled recall examination, typically 3 to 12 months after surgery. However, phone contact with the patient approximately 7 to 10 days after suture removal is recommended to confirm the absence of problems. Patients with questionable healing at the suture removal appointment should be reevaluated in the office in 7 to 10 days or sooner if necessary.

MANAGEMENT OF SURGICAL COMPLICATIONS

Although serious postoperative surgical complications are rare, the clinician should be prepared to respond to patient concerns and recognize when additional treatment may be necessary. Careful case evaluation, adherence to a minimally traumatic surgical technique, and proper patient management, as described previously in this chapter, should result in a low incidence of postoperative complications. Even so, some patients experience mild to moderate postoperative pain, swelling, ecchymosis, or infection. In a prospective study of 82 patients undergoing endodontic surgical treatment, Tsesis and coworkers[545] reported that 76.4% were pain free 1 day after surgery and 64.7% did not report any swelling. Only 4% of the patients in this study experienced moderate pain, and this sequela was closely related to the presence of presurgical symptoms. Postoperative pain typically peaks the day of surgery, and swelling reaches its maximum 1 to 2 days after surgery.[294] As previously noted, good evidence supports the use of prophylactic NSAID therapy and a long-acting local anesthetic to reduce the magnitude and duration of postoperative pain.

Patients should be advised that some postoperative oozing of blood is normal, but significant bleeding is uncommon and may require attention. Most bleeding can be controlled by applying steady pressure for 20 to 30 minutes, typically with a piece of moist cotton gauze or a tea bag. Bleeding that persists requires attention by the clinician. Pressure to the area and injection of a local anesthetic containing 1 : 50,000 epinephrine are reasonable first steps. If bleeding continues, it may be necessary to remove the sutures and search for a small severed blood vessel. When located, the blood vessel can be crushed or cauterized to control bleeding. Cauterization may be performed with a heat source commonly used for warm obturation techniques. Local hemostatic agents, as previously described, may also be used. Occasionally, a patient may require hospitalization and surgical intervention to control bleeding, but this is an extremely rare event. Extraoral ecchymosis (Fig. 9-65) occurs when blood seeps through the interstitial tissues; although it may be alarming to the patient and clinician, this condition is self-limiting and does not affect the prognosis.[281] Moist heat applied to the area may be helpful, although complete resolution of the discoloration may take up to 2 weeks. Heat should not be applied to the face during the first 24 hours after surgery.

Sinus exposure during surgical root canal procedures on maxillary posterior teeth is not uncommon. Postoperative antibiotics and decongestants are often recommended[16,29,281,568]; however, this practice is controversial, and no evidence supports the routine use of antibiotics and decongestants in these cases. Walton[576] makes a persuasive argument that antibiotics are not routinely indicated for the management of sinus

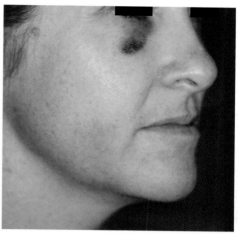

FIG. 9-65 Postoperative ecchymosis can be alarming to the patient but resolves spontaneously within 7 to 14 days.

exposures during periradicular surgery when primary closure of the oral-antral communication is possible. Further support for this position is provided by other clinicians who have observed excellent healing and minimal complications after sinus exposure during periradicular surgery.[291,456,579] Clinical judgment should guide the use of antibiotics and decongestants on a case-by-case basis until more conclusive evidence on this practice is available.

No reliable data are available to provide an accurate estimate of the likelihood of paresthesia after surgical root canal treatment. The incidence of paresthesia after third molar removal is estimated to be 1% to 4.4%[443]; however, most reported cases of paresthesia after third molar extraction involved the lingual nerve, which is rarely encountered in mandibular periradicular surgery. The incidence of damage to the inferior alveolar nerve after third molar surgery is approximately 1.3%, with only about 25% of these cases resulting in permanent injury.[551] Unless the nerve is resected during surgery, most patients can be expected to return to normal sensation within 3 to 4 months. If the paresthesia does not show signs of resolving within 10 to 12 weeks, referral and evaluation for possible neuromicrosurgical repair should be considered.[167,431] Robinson and Williams[443] presented a useful method for charting and documenting paresthesias. The area of altered sensation is determined by pinching the skin or mucosa with cotton pliers; alternatively, a pinprick can be applied with a sharp instrument. The area of paresthesia is noted with a series of marks on a diagram of the face and mouth. This method provides a graphic and chronologic record of the paresthesia.

SUMMARY

Periradicular surgery today bears little resemblance to the surgical procedures commonly performed as recently as the 1990s. Enhanced magnification and illumination, microsurgical instruments, ultrasonics, new materials for hemostasis, root-end filling, and GTR, and a greater understanding of the biology of wound healing and the etiology of persistent periradicular disease all have contributed to the rapid evolution of periradicular surgery. With proper case selection and operator skill, periradicular surgery can be considered a predictable, cost-effective alternative to extraction and tooth replacement.

REFERENCES

1. Abbott PV: Analysis of a referral-based endodontic practice: part 2. Treatment provided, *J Endod* 20:253, 1994.

2. Abedi HR, Van Mierlo BL, Wilder-Smith P, Torabinejad M: Effects of ultrasonic root-end cavity preparation on the root apex, *Oral Surg Oral Med Oral Pathol Oral Radiol Endod* 80:207, 1995.

3. Abitbol T, Santi E, Scherer W: Use of a resin-ionomer in guided tissue regeneration: case reports, *Am J Dent* 8:267, 1995.

4. Abitbol T, Santi E, Scherer W, Palat M: Using a resin-ionomer in guided tissue regenerative procedures: technique and application–case reports, *Periodontal Clin Investig* 18:17, 1996.

5. Abramowitz PN, Rankow H, Trope M: Multidisciplinary approach to apical surgery in conjunction with the loss of buccal cortical plate, *Oral Surg Oral Med Oral Pathol* 77:502, 1994.

6. Adamo HL, Buruiana R, Schertzer L, Boylan RJ: A comparison of MTA, Super-EBA, composite and amalgam as root-end filling materials using a bacterial microleakage model, *Int Endod J* 32:197, 1999.

7. Affairs RotCoS: Dental management of patients receiving oral bisphosphonate therapy—expert panel recommendations, American Dental Association.

8. Aframian DJ, Lalla RV, Peterson DE: Management of dental patients taking common hemostasis-altering medications, *Oral Surg Oral Med Oral Pathol Oral Radiol Endod* 103 (suppl S45):e1, 2007.

9. Ahlstrom U, Bakshi R, Nilsson P, Wahlander L: The analgesic efficacy of diclofenac dispersible and ibuprofen in postoperative pain after dental extraction, *Eur J Clin Pharmacol* 44:587, 1993.

10. Ainamo J, Loe H: Anatomical characteristics of gingiva: a clinical and microscopic study of the free and attached gingiva, *J Periodontol* 37:5, 1966.

11. Ainsworth G: Preoperative clindamycin prophylaxis does not prevent postoperative infections in endodontic surgery, *Evid Based Dent* 7:72, 2006.

12. Al-Bayaty HF, Murti PR, Thomson ER, Deen M: Painful, rapidly growing mass of the mandible, *Oral Surg Oral Med Oral Pathol Oral Radiol Endod* 95:7, 2003.

13. Alger FA, Solt CW, Vuddhakanok S, Miles K: The histologic evaluation of new attachment in periodontally diseased human roots treated with tetracycline-hydrochloride and fibronectin, *J Periodontol* 61:447, 1990.

14. Alleyn CD, O'Neal RB, Strong SL, et al: The effect of chlorhexidine treatment of root surfaces on the attachment of human gingival fibroblasts in vitro, *J Periodontol* 62:434, 1991.

15. Altman RD, Latta LL, Keer R, et al: Effect of nonsteroidal antiinflammatory drugs on fracture healing: a laboratory study in rats, *J Orthopaed Trauma* 9:392, 1995.

16. Altonen M: Transantral, subperiosteal resection of the palatal root of maxillary molars, *Int J Oral Surg* 4:277, 1975.

17. Ambus C, Munksgaard EC: Dentin bonding agents and composite retrograde root filling, *Am J Dent* 6:35, 1993.

18. Anan H, Akamine A, Hara Y, et al: A histochemical study of bone remodeling during experimental apical periodontitis in rats, *J Endod* 17:332, 1991.

19. Anderson HC: Mechanism of mineral formation in bone, *Lab Invest* 60:320, 1989.

20. Anderson HC: Molecular biology of matrix vesicles, *Clin Orthop Relat Res* May (314):266, 1995.

21. Andreasen JO, Borum MK, Jacobsen HL, Andreasen FM: Replantation of 400 avulsed permanent incisors. 4. Factors related to periodontal ligament healing, *Endod Dent Traumatol* 11:76, 1995.

22. Andreasen JO, Munksgaard EC, Fredebo L, Rud J: Periodontal tissue regeneration including cementogenesis adjacent to dentin-bonded retrograde composite fillings in humans, *J Endod* 19:151, 1993.

23. Andreasen JO, Pitt Ford TR: A radiographic study of the effect of various retrograde fillings on periapical healing after replantation, *Endod Dent Traumatol* 10:276, 1994.

24. Andreasen JO, Rud J: Correlation between histology and radiography in the assessment of healing after endodontic surgery, *Int J Oral Surg* 1:161, 1972.

25. Andreasen JO, Rud J, Munksgaard EC: [Retrograde root obturations using resin and a dentin bonding agent: a preliminary histologic study of tissue reactions in monkeys], *Tandlaegebladet* 93:195, 1989.

26. *Retroplast*, Rønne, Denmark, 2004, Retroplast Trading.

27. Apaydin ES, Shabahang S, Torabinejad M: Hard-tissue healing after application of fresh or set MTA as root-end-filling material, *J Endod* 30:21, 2004.

28. Ardekian L, Gaspar R, Peled M, et al: Does low-dose aspirin therapy complicate oral surgical procedures? *J Am Dent Assoc* 131:331, 2000.

29. Arens D: Surgical endodontics. In Cohen S, Burns RC, editors: *Pathways of the pulp*, ed 4, St. Louis, 1987, Mosby.

30. Arnold JW, Rueggeberg FA, Anderson RW, et al: The disintegration of superEBA cement in solutions with adjusted pH and osmolarity, *J Endod* 23:663, 1997.

31. Artzi Z, Tal H, Dayan D: Porous bovine bone mineral in healing of human extraction sockets. Part 1: histomorphometric evaluations at 9 months, *J Periodontol* 71:1015, 2000.

32. Artzi Z, Wasersprung N, Weinreb M, et al: Effect of guided tissue regeneration on newly formed bone and cementum in periapical tissue healing after endodontic surgery: an in vivo study in the cat, *J Endod* 38:163, 2012.

33. Ashcroft GS, Mills SJ, Lei K, et al: Estrogen modulates cutaneous wound healing by downregulating macrophage migration inhibitory factor, *J Clin Invest* 111:1309, 2003.

34. Aukhil I: Biology of wound healing, *Periodontology* 22:44, 2000.

35. Aurelio J, Chenail B, Gerstein H: Foreign-body reaction to bone wax: report of a case, *Oral Surg Oral Med Oral Pathol* 58:98, 1984.

36. Azzi R, Kenney EB, Tsao TF, Carranza FA Jr: The effect of electrosurgery on alveolar bone, *J Periodontol* 54:96, 1983.

37. Babay N: Comparative SEM study on the effect of root conditioning with EDTA or tetracycline HCl on periodontally involved root surfaces, *Indian J Dent Res* 11:53, 2000.

38. Bader JD, Bonito AJ, Shugars DA: Cardiovascular effects of Epinephrine on hypertensive dental patients: evidence report/technology assessment number 48. In *AHRQ Publication No. 02-E006*. Rockville, MD, July 2002, Agency for Healthcare Research and Quality.

39. Bahcall J, Barss J: Orascopic visualization technique for conventional and surgical endodontics, *Int Endod J* 36:441, 2003.

40. Bahcall JK, DiFiore PM, Poulakidas TK: An endoscopic technique for endodontic surgery, *J Endod* 25:132, 1999.

41. Bakshi R, Frenkel G, Dietlein G, et al: A placebo-controlled comparative evaluation of diclofenac dispersible versus ibuprofen in postoperative pain after third molar surgery, *J Clin Pharmacol* 34:225, 1994.

42. Bang G, Urist MR: Bone induction in excavation chambers in matrix of decalcified dentin, *Arch Surg* 94:781, 1967.

43. Bang G, Urist MR: Recalcification of decalcified dentin in the living animal, *J Dent Res* 46:722, 1967.

44. Barkhordar RA, Pelzner RB, Stark MM: Use of glass ionomers as retrofilling materials, *Oral Surg Oral Med Oral Pathol* 67:734, 1989.

45. Barnes D, Adachi E, Iwamoto C, et al: Testing of the White Version of ProRoot® MTA Root Canal Repair Material1, DENTSPLY Tulsa Dental, Tulsa, Oklahoma, 2002.

46. Barry MJ: Health decision aids to facilitate shared decision making in office practice, *Ann Intern Med* 136:127, 2002.

47. Behnia A, Strassler HE, Campbell R: Repairing iatrogenic root perforations, *J Am Dent Assoc* 131:196, 2000.

48. Beling KL, Marshall JG, Morgan LA, Baumgartner JC: Evaluation for cracks associated with ultrasonic root-end preparation of gutta-percha filled canals, *J Endod* 23:323, 1997.

49. Bell E, Ehrlich HP, Sher S, et al: Development and use of a living skin equivalent, *Plast Reconstr Surg* 67:386, 1981.

50. Benninger MS, Sebek BA, Levine HL: Mucosal regeneration of the maxillary sinus after surgery, *Otolaryngol Head Neck Surg* 101:33, 1989.

51. Berbari EF, Osmon DR, Carr A, et al: Dental procedures as risk factors for prosthetic hip or knee infection: a hospital-based prospective case-control study, *Clin Infect Dis* 50:8, 2010.

52. Berry JE, Zhao M, Jin Q, et al: Exploring the origins of cementoblasts and their trigger factors, *Connect Tissue Res* 44:97, 2003.

53. Bhaskar SN: Bone lesions of endodontic origin, *Dent Clin North Am* Nov:521, 1967.

54. Biddle C: Meta-analysis of the effectiveness of nonsteroidal anti-inflammatory drugs in a standardized pain model, *AANA J* 70:111, 2002.

55. Biggs JT, Benenati FW, Powell SE: Ten-year in vitro assessment of the surface status of three retrofilling materials, *J Endod* 21:521, 1995.

56. Bigras BR, Johnson BR, BeGole EA, Wenckus CS: Differences in clinical decision making: a comparison between specialists and general dentists, *Oral Surg Oral Med Oral Pathol Oral Radiol Endod* 106:963, 2008.

57. Bjorenson JE, Grove HF, List MG Sr, et al: Effects of hemostatic agents on the pH of body fluids, *J Endod* 12:289, 1986.

58. Block RM, Bushell A, Rodrigues H, Langeland K: A histopathologic, histobacteriologic, and radiographic study of periapical endodontic surgical specimens, *Oral Surg Oral Med Oral Pathol* 42:656, 1976.

59. Blomlof J: Root cementum appearance in healthy monkeys and periodontitis-prone patients after different etching modalities, *J Clin Periodontol* 23:12, 1996.

60. Blomlof J, Jansson L, Blomlof L, Lindskog S: Long-time etching at low pH jeopardizes periodontal healing, *J Clin Periodontol* 22:459, 1995.

61. Blomlof J, Jansson L, Blomlof L, Lindskog S: Root surface etching at neutral pH promotes periodontal healing, *J Clin Periodontol* 23:50, 1996.

62. Blomlof J, Lindskog S: Periodontal tissue-vitality after different etching modalities, *J Clin Periodontol* 22:464, 1995.

63. Blomlof J, Lindskog S: Root surface texture and early cell and tissue colonization after different etching modalities, *Eur J Oral Sci* 103:17, 1995.

64. Blomlof JP, Blomlof LB, Lindskog SF: Smear removal and collagen exposure after non-surgical root planing followed by etching with an EDTA gel preparation, *J Periodontol* 67:841, 1996.

65. Bohsali K, Pertot WJ, Hosseini B, Camps J: Sealing ability of super EBA and Dyract as root-end fillings: a study in vitro, *Int Endod J* 31:338, 1998.

66. Boioli LT, Penaud J, Miller N: A meta-analytic, quantitative assessment of osseointegration establishment and evolution of submerged and non-submerged endosseous titanium oral implants, *Clin Oral Implants Res* 12:579, 2001.

67. Bonine FL: Effect of chlorhexidine rinse on the incidence of dry socket in impacted mandibular third molar extraction sites, *Oral Surg Oral Med Oral Pathol Oral Radiol Endod* 79:154, 1995.

68. Bornstein MM, Lauber R, Sendi P, von Arx T: Comparison of periapical radiography and limited cone-beam computed tomography in mandibular molars for analysis of anatomical landmarks before apical surgery, *J Endod* 37:151, 2011.

69. Bornstein MM, Wasmer J, Sendi P, et al: Characteristics and dimensions of the Schneiderian membrane and apical bone in maxillary molars referred for apical surgery: a comparative radiographic analysis using limited cone beam computed tomography, *J Endod* 38:51, 2012.

70. Boskey AL: Matrix proteins and mineralization: an overview, *Connect Tissue Res* 35:357, 1996.

71. Boskey AL: Biomineralization: an overview, *Connect Tissue Res* 44:5, 2003.

72. Boucher Y, Sobel M, Sauveur G: Persistent pain related to root canal filling and apical fenestration: a case report, *J Endod* 26:242, 2000.

73. Bowers GM, Schallhorn RG, McClain PK, et al: Factors influencing the outcome of regenerative therapy in mandibular Class II furcations: part I, *J Periodontol* 74:1255, 2003.

74. Boyes-Varley JG, Cleaton-Jones PE, Lownie JF: Effect of a topical drug combination on the early healing of extraction sockets in the vervet monkey, *Int J Oral Maxillofac Surg* 17:138, 1988.

75. Boykin MJ, Gilbert GH, Tilashalski KR, Shelton BJ: Incidence of endodontic treatment: a 48-month prospective study, *J Endod* 29:806, 2003.

76. Brent PD, Morgan LA, Marshall JG, Baumgartner JC: Evaluation of diamond-coated ultrasonic instruments for root-end preparation, *J Endod* 25:672, 1999.

77. Briggs PF, Scott BJ: Evidence-based dentistry: endodontic failure–how should it be managed? *Br Dent J* 183:159, 1997.

78. Britto LR, Katz J, Guelmann M, Heft M: Periradicular radiographic assessment in diabetic and control individuals, *Oral Surg Oral Med Oral Pathol Oral Radiol Endod* 96:449, 2003.

79. Brown AR, Papasian CJ, Shultz P, et al: Bacteremia and intraoral suture removal: can an antimicrobial rinse help? *J Am Dent Assoc* 129:1455, 1998.

80. Bruce GR, McDonald NJ, Sydiskis RJ: Cytotoxicity of retrofill materials, *J Endod* 19:288, 1993.

81. Brugnami F, Mellonig JT: Treatment of a large periapical lesion with loss of labial cortical plate using GTR: a case report, *Int J Periodontics Restorative Dent* 19:243, 1999.

82. Buckley JA, Ciancio SG, McMullen JA: Efficacy of epinephrine concentration in local anesthesia during periodontal surgery, *J Periodontol* 55:653, 1984.

83. Budnitz DS, Lovegrove MC, Shehab N, Richards CL: Emergency hospitalizations for adverse drug events in older Americans, *N Engl J Med* 365:2002, 2011.

84. Byrne BE, Tibbetts LS: Conscious sedation and agents for the control of anxiety. In Ciancio SG, editor: *ADA guide to dental therapeutics*, ed 3, Chicago, 2003, American Dental Association, p 17.

85. Calderwood RG, Hera SS, Davis JR, Waite DE: A comparison of the healing rate of bone after the production of defects by various rotary instruments, *J Dent Res* 43:207, 1964.

86. Calzonetti KJ, Iwanowski T, Komorowski R, Friedman S: Ultrasonic root end cavity preparation assessed by an in situ impression technique, *Oral Surg Oral Med Oral Pathol Oral Radiol Endod* 85:210, 1998.

87. Camp MA, Jeansonne BG, Lallier T: Adhesion of human fibroblasts to root-end-filling materials, *J Endod* 29:602, 2003.

88. Campbell JH, Alvarado F, Murray RA: Anticoagulation and minor oral surgery: should the anticoagulation regimen be altered? *J Oral Maxillofac Surg* 58:131, 2000.

89. Cannon PD, Dharmar VT: Minor oral surgical procedures in patients on oral anticoagulants: a controlled study, *Aust Dent J* 48:115, 2003.

90. Caplan DJ, Weintraub JA: Factors related to loss of root canal filled teeth, *J Public Health Dent* 57:31, 1997.

91. Carr G: Advanced techniques and visual enhancement for endodontic surgery, *End Rep* 7:6, 1992.

92. Carr G, Bentkover SK: Surgical endodontics. In Cohen S, Burns RC, editors: *Pathways of the pulp*, ed 7, St. Louis, 1994, Mosby.

93. Carr G, Bentkover SK: Surgical endodontics. In Cohen S, Burns RC, editors: *Pathways of the pulp*, ed 7, St. Louis, 1998, Mosby, p 608.

94. Carr GB: Microscopes in endodontics, *J Calif Dent Assoc* 20:55, 1992.

95. Carr GB: Ultrasonic root end preparation, *Dent Clin North Am* 41:541, 1997.

96. Chang LK, Whitaker DC: The impact of herbal medicines on dermatologic surgery, *Dermatol Surg* 27:759, 2001.

97. Cheng H, Jiang W, Phillips FM, et al: Osteogenic activity of the fourteen types of human bone morphogenetic proteins (BMPs), *J Bone Joint Surg Am* 85-A:1544, 2003.

98. Cheung GS: Endodontic failures: changing the approach, *Int Dent J* 46:131, 1996.

99. Cho E, Kopel H, White SN: Moisture susceptibility of resin-modified glass-ionomer materials [see comment], *Quintessence Int* 26:351, 1995.

100. Chong BS, Ford TR, Kariyawasam SP: Tissue response to potential root-end filling materials in infected root canals, *Int Endod J* 30:102, 1997.

101. Chong BS, Owadally ID, Pitt Ford TR, Wilson RF: Antibacterial activity of potential retrograde root filling materials, *Endod Dent Traumatol* 10:66, 1994.

102. Chong BS, Owadally ID, Pitt Ford TR, Wilson RF: Cytotoxicity of potential retrograde root-filling materials, *Endod Dent Traumatol* 10:129, 1994.

103. Chong BS, Pitt Ford TR, Hudson MB: A prospective clinical study of mineral trioxide aggregate and IRM when used as root-end filling materials in endodontic surgery, *Int Endod J* 36:520, 2003.

104. Chong BS, Pitt Ford TR, Kariyawasam SP: Short-term tissue response to potential root-end filling materials in infected root canals, *Int Endod J* 30:240, 1997.

105. Chong BS, Pitt Ford TR, Watson TF: Light-cured glass ionomer cement as a retrograde root seal, *Int Endod J* 26:218, 1993.

106. Chong BS, Pitt Ford TR, Watson TF, Wilson RF: Sealing ability of potential retrograde root filling materials, *Endod Dent Traumatol* 11:264, 1995.

107. Ciasca M, Aminoshariae A, Jin G, et al: A comparison of the cytotoxicity and proinflammatory cytokine production of EndoSequence root repair material and ProRoot mineral trioxide aggregate in human osteoblast cell culture using reverse-transcriptase polymerase chain reaction, *J Endod* 38:486, 2012.

108. Clark RA: Regulation of fibroplasia in cutaneous wound repair, *Am J Med Sci* 306:42, 1993.

109. Clark RA, Stone RD, Leung DY, et al: Role of macrophages in wound healing, *Surg Forum* 27:16, 1976.

110. Clokie CM, Moghadam H, Jackson MT, Sandor GK: Closure of critical sized defects with allogenic and alloplastic bone substitutes, *J Craniofac Surg* 13:111, 2002.

111. Costich ER, Youngblood PJ, Walden JM: A study of the effects of high-speed rotary instruments on bone repair in dogs, *Oral Surg Oral Med Oral Pathol* 17:563, 1964.

112. Cotton TP, Geisler TM, Holden DT, et al: Endodontic applications of cone-beam volumetric tomography, *J Endod* 33:1121, 2007.

113. Coulthard P, Worthington H, Esposito M, et al: Tissue adhesives for closure of surgical incisions, *Cochrane Database Syst Rev* CD004287, 2004.

114. Craig KR, Harrison JW: Wound healing following demineralization of resected root ends in periradicular surgery, *J Endod* 19:339, 1993.

115. Creasy JE, Mines P, Sweet M: Surgical trends among endodontists: the results of a web-based survey, *J Endod* 35:30, 2009.

116. Crooks WG, Anderson RW, Powell BJ, Kimbrough WF: Longitudinal evaluation of the seal of IRM root end fillings, *J Endod* 20:250, 1994.

117. Culliford AT, Cunningham JN Jr, Zeff RH, et al: Sternal and costochondral infections following open-heart surgery: a review of 2,594 cases, *J Thorac Cardiovasc Surg* 72:714, 1976.

118. Cutright B, Quillopa N, Schubert W: An anthropometric analysis of the key foramina for maxillofacial surgery, *J Oral Maxillofac Surg* 61:354, 2003.

119. Dahlin C, Gottow J, Linde A, Nyman S: Healing of maxillary and mandibular bone defects using a membrane technique: an experimental study in monkeys, *Scand J Plast Reconstr Surg Hand Surg* 24:13, 1990.

120. Dahlin C, Linde A, Gottlow J, Nyman S: Healing of bone defects by guided tissue regeneration, *Plast Reconstr Surg* 81:672, 1988.

121. Dahlkemper P, Wolcott JF, Pringle GA, Hicks ML: Periapical central giant cell granuloma: a potential endodontic misdiagnosis [see comment][erratum appears in *Oral Surg Oral Med Oral Pathol Oral Radiol Endod* 92:2-3, 2001; PMID: 11458236], *Oral Surg Oral Med Oral Pathol Oral Radiol Endod* 90:739, 2000.

122. Damas BA, Wheater MA, Bringas JS, Hoen MM: Cytotoxicity comparison of mineral trioxide aggregates and EndoSequence bioceramic root repair materials, *J Endod* 37:372, 2011.

123. Danesh-Meyer MJ: Guided tissue regeneration in the management of severe periodontal-endodontic lesions, *N Z Dent J* 95:7, 1999.

124. Danforth RA, Clark DE: Effective dose from radiation absorbed during a panoramic examination with a new generation machine, *Oral Surg Oral Med Oral Pathol Oral Radiol Endod* 89:236, 2000.

125. Danielsson K, Evers H, Holmlund A, et al: Long-acting local anaesthetics in oral surgery: clinical evaluation of bupivacaine and etidocaine for mandibular nerve block, *Int J Oral Maxillofac Surg* 15:119, 1986.

126. Danin J, Linder L, Sund ML, et al: Quantitative radioactive analysis of microleakage of four different retrograde fillings, *Int Endod J* 25:183, 1992.

127. Danin J, Linder LE, Lundqvist G, et al: Outcomes of periradicular surgery in cases with apical pathosis and untreated canals, *Oral Surg Oral Med Oral Pathol Oral Radiol Endod* 87:227, 1999.

128. Danin J, Stromberg T, Forsgren H, et al: Clinical management of nonhealing periradicular pathosis: surgery versus endodontic retreatment, *Oral Surg Oral Med Oral Pathol Oral Radiol Endod* 82:213, 1996.

129. Daoudi MF, Saunders WP: In vitro evaluation of furcal perforation repair using mineral trioxide aggregate or resin modified glass ionomer cement with and without the use of the operating microscope, *J Endod* 28:512, 2002.

130. Davis JR, Steinbronn KK, Graham AR, Dawson BV: Effects of Monsel's solution in uterine cervix, *Am J Clin Pathol* 82:332, 1984.

131. De Deus QD: Frequency, location, and direction of the lateral, secondary, and accessory canals, *J Endod* 1:361, 1975.

132. de Lange J, Putters T, Baas EM, van Ingen JM: Ultrasonic root-end preparation in apical surgery: a prospective randomized study, *Oral Surg Oral Med Oral Pathol Oral Radiol Endod* 104:841, 2007.

133. DeGrood ME, Oguntebi BR, Cunningham CJ, Pink R: A comparison of tissue reactions to Ketac-Fil and amalgam, *J Endod* 21:65, 1995.

134. Del Fabbro M, Ceresoli V, Lolato A, Taschieri S: Effect of platelet concentrate on quality of life after periradicular surgery: a randomized clinical study, *J Endod* 38:733, 2012.

135. Del Fabbro M, Taschieri S, Testori T, et al: Surgical versus non-surgical endodontic re-treatment for periradicular lesions, *Cochrane Database Syst Rev* CD005511, 2007.

136. Denio D, Torabinejad M, Bakland LK: Anatomical relationship of the mandibular canal to its surrounding structures in mature mandibles, *J Endod* 18:161, 1992.

137. Desmouliere A, Gabbiani G: Myofibroblast differentiation during fibrosis, *Exp Nephrol* 3:134, 1995.

138. Desmouliere A, Redard M, Darby I, Gabbiani G: Apoptosis mediates the decrease in cellularity during the transition between granulation tissue and scar, *Am J Pathol* 146:56, 1995.

139. Dewhirst FE: Structure-activity relationships for inhibition of prostaglandin cyclooxygenase by phenolic compounds, *Prostaglandins* 20:209, 1980.

140. Diekwisch TG: The developmental biology of cementum, *J Dev Biol* 45:695, 2001.

141. Dietrich T, Zunker P, Dietrich D, Bernimoulin JP: Apicomarginal defects in periradicular surgery: classification and diagnostic aspects, *Oral Surg Oral Med Oral Pathol Oral Radiol Endod* 94:233, 2002.

142. Dietrich T, Zunker P, Dietrich D, Bernimoulin JP: Periapical and periodontal healing after osseous grafting and guided tissue regeneration treatment of apicomarginal defects in periradicular surgery: results after 12 months, *Oral Surg Oral Med Oral Pathol Oral Radiol Endod* 95:474, 2003.

143. Dionne RA, Snyder J, Hargreaves KM: Analgesic efficacy of flurbiprofen in comparison with acetaminophen, acetaminophen plus codeine, and placebo after impacted third molar removal, *J Oral Maxillofac Surg* 52:919, 1994.

144. Dionne RA, Wirdzek PR, Fox PC, Dubner R: Suppression of postoperative pain by the combination of a nonsteroidal anti-inflammatory drug, flurbiprofen, and a long-acting local anesthetic, etidocaine, *J Am Dent Assoc* 108:598, 1984.

145. Distler JH, Hirth A, Kurowska-Stolarska M, et al: Angiogenic and angiostatic factors in the molecular control of angiogenesis, *Q J Nucl Med* 47:149, 2003.

146. Dodson T, Halperin L: Prophylactic antibiotics reduce complications of orthognathic surgery, *Evid Based Dent* 2:66, 2000.

147. Dorn SO, Gartner AH: Retrograde filling materials: a retrospective success-failure study of amalgam, EBA, and IRM, *J Endod* 16:391, 1990.

148. Doroschak AM, Bowles WR, Hargreaves KM: Evaluation of the combination of flurbiprofen and tramadol for management of endodontic pain, *J Endod* 25:660, 1999.

149. Douthitt JC, Gutmann JL, Witherspoon DE: Histologic assessment of healing after the use of a bioresorbable membrane in the management of buccal bone loss concomitant with periradicular surgery, *J Endod* 27:404, 2001.

150. Dragoo MR: Resin-ionomer and hybrid-ionomer cements: part I. Comparison of three materials for the treatment of subgingival root lesions, *Int J Periodontics Restorative Dent* 16:594, 1996.

151. Dragoo MR: Resin-ionomer and hybrid-ionomer cements: part II, human clinical and histologic wound healing responses in specific periodontal lesions, *Int J Periodontics Restorative Dent* 17:75, 1997.

152. Duarte MA, Demarchi AC, Yamashita JC, et al: pH and calcium ion release of 2 root-end filling materials, *Oral Surg Oral Med Oral Pathol Oral Radiol Endod* 95:345, 2003.

153. Dugas NN, Lawrence HP, Teplitsky P, Friedman S: Quality of life and satisfaction outcomes of endodontic treatment, *J Endod* 28:819, 2002.

154. Duggins LD, Clay JR, Himel VT, Dean JW: A combined endodontic retrofill and periodontal guided tissue regeneration technique for the repair of molar endodontic furcation perforations: report of a case, *Quintessence Int* 25:109, 1994.

155. Edlund M, Nair MK, Nair UP: Detection of vertical root fractures by using cone-beam computed tomography: a clinical study, *J Endod* 37:768, 2011.

156. Enqvist B, von Konow L, Bystedt H: Pre- and perioperative suggestion in maxillofacial surgery: effects on blood loss and recovery, *Int J Clin Exp Hypn* 43:284, 1995.

157. Ericson S, Finne K, Persson G: Results of apicoectomy of maxillary canines, premolars and molars with special reference to oroantral communication as a prognostic factor, *Int J Oral Surg* 3:386, 1974.

158. Eriksson A, Albrektsson T, Grane B, McQueen D: Thermal injury to bone: a vital-microscopic description of heat effects, *Int J Oral Surg* 11:115, 1982.

159. Eriksson AR, Albrektsson T: Temperature threshold levels for heat-induced bone tissue injury: a vital-microscopic study in the rabbit, *J Prosthet Dent* 50:101, 1983.

160. Eriksson AR, Albrektsson T, Albrektsson B: Heat caused by drilling cortical bone: temperature measured in vivo in patients and animals, *Acta Orthop Scand* 55:629, 1984.

161. Eriksson RA, Albrektsson T, Magnusson B: Assessment of bone viability after heat trauma: a histological, histochemical and vital microscopic study in the rabbit, *Scand J Plast Reconstr Surg* 18:261, 1984.

162. Esposito M, Coulthard P, Oliver R, et al: Antibiotics to prevent complications following dental implant treatment, *Cochrane Database Syst Rev* CD004152, 2003.

163. Estrela C, Bueno MR, Leles CR, et al: Accuracy of cone beam computed tomography and panoramic and periapical radiography for detection of apical periodontitis, *J Endod* 34:273, 2008.

164. Evans BE: Local hemostatic agents, *N Y J Dent* 47:109, 1977.

165. Fayad MI, Ashkenaz PJ, Johnson BR: Different representations of vertical root fractures detected by cone-beam volumetric tomography: a case series report, *J Endod* 38:1435, 2012.

166. Ferreira FB, Ferreira AL, Gomes BP, Souza-Filho FJ: Resolution of persistent periapical infection by endodontic surgery, *Int Endod J* 37:61, 2004.

167. Fielding AF, Rachiele DP, Frazier G: Lingual nerve paresthesia following third molar surgery: a retrospective clinical study, *Oral Surg Oral Med Oral Pathol Oral Radiol Endod* 84:345, 1997.

168. Finn MD, Schow SR, Schneiderman ED: Osseous regeneration in the presence of four common hemostatic agents, *J Oral Maxillofac Surg* 50:608, 1992.

169. Fister J, Gross BD: A histologic evaluation of bone response to bur cutting with and without water coolant, *Oral Surg Oral Med Oral Pathol* 49:105, 1980.

170. Fitzpatrick EL, Steiman HR: Scanning electron microscopic evaluation of finishing techniques on IRM and EBA retrofillings, *J Endod* 23:423, 1997.

171. Fogel HM, Peikoff MD: Microleakage of root-end filling materials [erratum appears in *J Endod* 27:634, 2001], *J Endod* 27:456, 2001.

172. Folke LE, Stallard RE: Periodontal microcirculation as revealed by plastic microspheres, *J Periodontal Res* 2:53, 1967.

173. Ford TR, Torabinejad M, McKendry DJ, et al: Use of mineral trioxide aggregate for repair of furcal perforations, *Oral Surg Oral Med Oral Pathol Oral Radiol Endod* 79:756, 1995.

174. Forte SG, Hauser MJ, Hahn C, Hartwell GR: Microleakage of super-EBA with and without finishing as determined by the fluid filtration method, *J Endod* 24:799, 1998.

175. Fouad AF, Burleson J: The effect of diabetes mellitus on endodontic treatment outcome: data from an electronic patient record, *J Am Dent Assoc* 134:43, 2003.

176. Frank RJ, Antrim DD, Bakland LK: Effect of retrograde cavity preparations on root apexes, *Endod Dent Traumatol* 12:100, 1996.

177. Freedman A, Horowitz I: Complications after apicoectomy in maxillary premolar and molar teeth, *Int J Oral Maxillofac Surg* 28:192, 1999.

178. Friedman S: Management of post-treatment endodontic disease: a current concept of case selection, *Aust Endod J* 26:104, 2000.

179. Frosch DL, Kaplan RM: Shared decision making in clinical medicine: past research and future directions, *Am J Prev Med* 17:285, 1999.

180. Fyffe HE, Kay EJ: Assessment of dental health state utilities, *Community Dent Oral Epidemiol* 20:269, 1992.

181. Gagliani M, Taschieri S, Molinari R: Ultrasonic root-end preparation: influence of cutting angle on the apical seal, *J Endod* 24:726, 1998.

182. Gajraj NM: The effect of cyclooxygenase-2 inhibitors on bone healing, *Reg Anesth Pain Med* 28:456, 2003.

183. Galan D: Clinical application of Geristore glass-ionomer restorative in older dentitions, *J Esthet Dent* 3:221, 1991.

184. Gallagher CS, Mourino AP: Root-end induction, *J Am Dent Assoc* 98:578, 1979.

185. Garlock JA, Pringle GA, Hicks ML: The odontogenic keratocyst: a potential endodontic misdiagnosis, *Oral Surg Oral Med Oral Pathol Oral Radiol Endod* 85:452, 1998.

186. Garrett K, Kerr M, Hartwell G, et al: The effect of a bioresorbable matrix barrier in endodontic surgery on the rate of periapical healing: an in vivo study, *J Endod* 28:503, 2002.

187. Gatti JJ, Dobeck JM, Smith C, et al: Bacteria of asymptomatic periradicular endodontic lesions identified by DNA-DNA hybridization, *Endod Dent Traumatol* 16:197, 2000.

188. Gemalmaz D, Yoruc B, Ozcan M, Alkumru HN: Effect of early water contact on solubility of glass ionomer luting cements, *J Prosthet Dent* 80:474, 1998.

189. Georgelin-Gurgel M, Diemer F, Nicolas E, Hennequin M: Surgical and nonsurgical endodontic treatment-induced stress, *J Endod* 35:19, 2009.

190. Gerhards F, Wagner W: Sealing ability of five different retrograde filling materials, *J Endod* 22:463, 1996.

191. Gerstenfeld LC, Cullinane DM, Barnes GL, et al: Fracture healing as a post-natal developmental process: molecular, spatial, and temporal aspects of its regulation, *J Cell Biochem* 88:873, 2003.

192. Giannoudis PV, MacDonald DA, Matthews SJ, et al: Nonunion of the femoral diaphysis: the influence of reaming and non-steroidal anti-inflammatory drugs [see comment], *J Bone Joint Surg Br* 82:655, 2000.

193. Gibbard LL, Zarb G: A 5-year prospective study of implant-supported single-tooth replacements, *J Can Dent Assoc* 68:110, 2002.

194. Gibbs SJ: Effective dose equivalent and effective dose: comparison for common projections in oral and maxillofacial radiology, *Oral Surg Oral Med Oral Pathol Oral Radiol Endod* 90:538, 2000.

195. Gilheany PA, Figdor D, Tyas MJ: Apical dentin permeability and microleakage associated with root end resection and retrograde filling, *J Endod* 20:22, 1994.

196. Giray CB, Atasever A, Durgun B, Araz K: Clinical and electron microscope comparison of silk sutures and n-butyl-2-cyanoacrylate in human mucosa, *Aust Dent J* 42:255, 1997.

197. Glick M, Abel SN, Muzyka BC, DeLorenzo M: Dental complications after treating patients with AIDS, *J Am Dent Assoc* 125:296, 1994.

198. Glowacki J: Angiogenesis in fracture repair, *Clin Orthop Relat Res* Oct:S82, 1998.

199. Goaslind GD, Robertson PB, Mahan CJ, et al: Thickness of facial gingiva, *J Periodontol* 48:768, 1977.

200. Gondim E Jr, Figueiredo Almeida de Gomes BP, Ferraz CC, et al: Effect of sonic and ultrasonic retrograde cavity preparation on the integrity of root apices of freshly extracted human teeth: scanning electron microscopy analysis, *J Endod* 28:646, 2002.

201. Goodchild J, Glick M: A different approach to medical risk assessment, *Endod Topics* 4:1, 2003.

202. Goodman S, Ma T, Trindade M, et al: COX-2 selective NSAID decreases bone ingrowth in vivo, *J Orthop Res* 20:1164, 2002.

203. Goodman SB, Ma T, Genovese M, Lane Smith R: COX-2 selective inhibitors and bone, *Intl J Immunopathol Pharmacol* 16:201, 2003.

204. Gordon SM, Dionne RA, Brahim J, et al: Blockade of peripheral neuronal barrage reduces postoperative pain, *Pain* 70:209, 1997.

205. Gorman MC, Steiman HR, Gartner AH: Scanning electron microscopic evaluation of root-end preparations, *J Endod* 21:113, 1995.

206. Goyal B, Tewari S, Duhan J, Sehgal PK: Comparative evaluation of platelet-rich plasma and guided tissue regeneration membrane in the healing of apicomarginal defects: a clinical study, *J Endod* 37:773, 2011.

207. Gray GJ, Hatton JF, Holtzmann DJ, et al: Quality of root-end preparations using ultrasonic and rotary instrumentation in cadavers, *J Endod* 26:281, 2000.

208. Grbic JT, Landesberg R, Lin SQ, et al: Incidence of osteonecrosis of the jaw in women with postmenopausal osteoporosis in the health outcomes and reduced incidence with zoledronic acid once yearly pivotal fracture trial, *J Am Dent Assoc* 139:32, 2008.

209. Greer BD, West LA, Liewehr FR, Pashley DH: Sealing ability of Dyract, Geristore, iRM, and super-EBA as root-end filling materials, *J Endod* 27:441, 2001.

210. Grzesik WJ, Narayanan AS: Cementum and periodontal wound healing and regeneration, *Crit Rev Oral Biol Med* 13:474, 2002.

211. Gutmann JL: Perspectives on root-end resection, *J Hist Dent* 47:135, 1999.

212. Gutmann JL, Harrison JW: *Surgical endodontics*, London, 1991, Blackwell Scientific Publications, p 468.

213. Gutmann JL, Harrison JW: *Surgical endodontics*, ed 1, St. Louis, 1994, Ishiyaku EuroAmerica, p 468.

214. Gutmann JL, Saunders WP, Nguyen L, et al: Ultrasonic root-end preparation. Part 1. SEM analysis, *Int Endod J* 27:318, 1994.

215. Haasch GC, Gerstein H, Austin BP: Effects of two hemostatic agents on osseous healing, *J Endod* 15:310, 1989.

216. Hall RM: The effect of high-speed bone cutting without the use of water coolant, *Oral Surg Oral Med Oral Pathol* 20:150, 1965.

217. Hanks CT, Wataha JC, Parsell RR, Strawn SE: Delineation of cytotoxic concentrations of two dentin bonding agents in vitro, *J Endod* 18:589, 1992.

218. Happonen RP: Periapical actinomycosis: a follow-up study of 16 surgically treated cases, *Endod Dent Traumatol* 2:205, 1986.

219. Harada S, Rodan GA: Control of osteoblast function and regulation of bone mass, *Nature* 423:349, 2003.

220. Harder AT, An YH: The mechanisms of the inhibitory effects of nonsteroidal anti-inflammatory drugs on bone healing: a concise review, *J Clin Pharmacol* 43:807, 2003.

221. Harrison JW, Johnson SA: Excisional wound healing following the use of IRM as a root-end filling material, *J Endod* 23:19, 1997.

222. Harrison JW, Jurosky KA: Wound healing in the tissues of the periodontium following periradicular surgery. I. The incisional wound, *J Endod* 17:425, 1991.

223. Harrison JW, Jurosky KA: Wound healing in the tissues of the periodontium following periradicular surgery. 2. The dissectional wound, *J Endod* 17:544, 1991.

224. Hart J: Inflammation. 1: Its role in the healing of acute wounds, *J Wound Care* 11:205, 2002.

225. Hauman CH, Chandler NP, Tong DC: Endodontic implications of the maxillary sinus: a review, *Int Endod J* 35:127, 2002.

226. Hayashi M, Kinomoto Y, Takeshige F, Ebisu S: Prognosis of intentional replantation of vertically fractured roots reconstructed with dentin-bonded resin, *J Endod* 30:145, 2004.

227. Haynes SR, Lawler PG: An assessment of the consistency of ASA physical status classification allocation, *Anaesthesia* 50:195, 1995.

228. Held SA, Kao YH, Wells DW: Endoscope: an endodontic application, *J Endod* 22:327, 1996.

229. Hellstein JW, Adler RA, Edwards B, et al: Managing the care of patients receiving antiresorptive therapy for prevention and treatment of osteoporosis: executive summary of recommendations from the American Dental Association Council on Scientific Affairs, *J Am Dent Assoc* 142:1243, 2011.

230. Hepworth MJ, Friedman S: Treatment outcome of surgical and non-surgical management of endodontic failures, *J Can Dent Assoc* 63:364, 1997.

231. Herman WW, Konzelman JL Jr, Prisant LM: New national guidelines on hypertension: a summary for dentistry, *J Am Dent Assoc* 135:576, 2004.

232. Higa RK, Torabinejad M, McKendry DJ, McMillan PJ: The effect of storage time on the degree of dye leakage of root-end filling materials, *Int Endod J* 27:252, 1994.

233. Hirsch JM, Ahlstrom U, Henrikson PA, et al: Periapical surgery, *Int J Oral Surg* 8:173, 1979.

234. Hlava GL, Reinhardt RA, Kalkwarf KL: Etidocaine HCl local anesthetic for periodontal flap surgery, *J Periodontol* 55:364, 1984.

235. Ho ML, Chang JK, Chuang LY, et al: Effects of nonsteroidal anti-inflammatory drugs and prostaglandins on osteoblastic functions, *Biochem Pharmacol* 58:983, 1999.

236. Holland R, de Souza V, Nery MJ, et al: Reaction of dogs' teeth to root canal filling with mineral trioxide aggregate or a glass ionomer sealer, *J Endod* 25:728, 1999.

237. Holland R, de Souza V, Nery MJ, et al: Reaction of rat connective tissue to implanted dentin tubes filled with mineral trioxide aggregate or calcium hydroxide, *J Endod* 25:161, 1999.

238. Holland R, Souza V, Nery MJ, et al: Reaction of rat connective tissue to implanted dentin tubes filled with a white mineral trioxide aggregate, *Braz Dent J* 13:23, 2002.

239. Hollinger J: Factors for osseous repair and delivery: part II, *J Craniofac Surg* 4:135, 1993.

240. Hollinger J, Wong ME: The integrated processes of hard tissue regeneration with special emphasis on fracture healing, *Oral Surg Oral Med Oral Pathol Oral Radiol Endod* 82:594, 1996.

241. Huggins CB, Urist MR: Dentin matrix transformation: rapid induction of alkaline phosphatase and cartilage, *Science* 167:896, 1970.

242. Hull TE, Robertson PB, Steiner JC, del Aguila MA: Patterns of endodontic care for a Washington state population, *J Endod* 29:553, 2003.

243. Hume WR: An analysis of the release and the diffusion through dentin of eugenol from zinc oxide-eugenol mixtures, *J Dent Res* 63:881, 1984.

244. Hume WR: Effect of eugenol on respiration and division in human pulp, mouse fibroblasts, and liver cells in vitro, *J Dent Res* 63:1262, 1984.

245. Hume WR: In vitro studies on the local pharmacodynamics, pharmacology and toxicology of eugenol and zinc oxide-eugenol, *Int Endod J* 21:130, 1988.

246. Hunt LM, Benoit PW: Evaluation of a microcrystalline collagen preparation in extraction wounds, *J Oral Surg* 34:407, 1976.

247. Hunt TK, Hopf H, Hussain Z: Physiology of wound healing, *Adv Skin Wound Care* 13:6, 2000.

248. Hunt TK, Knighton DR, Thakral KK, et al: Studies on inflammation and wound healing: angiogenesis and collagen synthesis stimulated in vivo by resident and activated wound macrophages, *Surgery* 96:48, 1984.

249. Huumonen S, Kvist T, Grondahl K, Molander A: Diagnostic value of computed tomography in re-treatment of root fillings in maxillary molars, *Int Endod J* 39:827, 2006.

250. Huynh MP, Yagiela JA: Current concepts in acute pain management, *J Calif Dent Assoc* 31:419, 2003.

251. Iasella JM, Greenwell H, Miller RL, et al: Ridge preservation with freeze-dried bone allograft and a collagen membrane compared to extraction alone for implant site development: a clinical and histologic study in humans, *J Periodontol* 74:990, 2003.

252. Inoue S, Yoshimura M, Tinkle JS, Marshall FJ: A 24-week study of the microleakage of four retrofilling materials using a fluid filtration method, *J Endod* 17:369, 1991.

253. Ishikawa H, Sawada N, Kobayashi C, Suda H: Evaluation of root-end cavity preparation using ultrasonic retrotips, *Int Endod J* 36:586, 2003.

254. Iwu C, MacFarlane TW, MacKenzie D, Stenhouse D: The microbiology of periapical granulomas, *Oral Surg Oral Med Oral Pathol* 69:502, 1990.

255. Jafri SM: Periprocedural thromboprophylaxis in patients receiving chronic anticoagulation therapy, *Am Heart J* 147:3, 2004.

256. Jeansonne BG, Boggs WS, Lemon RR: Ferric sulfate hemostasis: effect on osseous wound healing. II. With curettage and irrigation, *J Endod* 19:174, 1993.

257. Jeffcoat MK, Reddy MS, Wang IC, et al: The effect of systemic flurbiprofen on bone supporting dental implants, *J Am Dent Assoc* 126:305, 1995.

258. Jensen JA, Hunt TK, Scheuenstuhl H, Banda MJ: Effect of lactate, pyruvate, and pH on secretion of angiogenesis and mitogenesis factors by macrophages, *Lab Invest* 54:574, 1986.

259. Jerome CE, Hill AV: Preventing root tip loss in the maxillary sinus during endodontic surgery, *J Endod* 21:422, 1995.

260. Jeske AH, Suchko GD: Lack of a scientific basis for routine discontinuation of oral anticoagulation therapy before dental treatment, *J Am Dent Assoc* 134:1492, 2003.

261. Jesslen P, Zetterqvist L, Heimdahl A: Long-term results of amalgam versus glass ionomer cement as apical sealant after apicectomy, *Oral Surg Oral Med Oral Pathol Oral Radiol Endod* 79:101, 1995.

262. Johnson BR, Schwartz A, Goldberg J, Koerber A: A chairside aid for shared decision making in dentistry: a randomized controlled trial, *J Dent Educ* 70:133, 2006.

263. Johnson P, Fromm D: Effects of bone wax on bacterial clearance, *Surgery* 89:206, 1981.

264. Kadohiro G: A comparative study of the sealing quality of zinc-free amalgam and Diaket when used as a retrograde filling material, *Hawaii Dent J* 15:8, 1984.

265. Kalbermatten DF, Kalbermatten NT, Hertel R: Cotton-induced pseudotumor of the femur, *Skeletal Radiol* 30:415, 2001.

266. Kassab MM, Radmer TW, Glore JW, et al: A retrospective review of clinical international normalized ratio results and their implications, *J Am Dent Assoc* 142:1252, 2011.

267. Kawaguchi H, Pilbeam CC, Harrison JR, Raisz LG: The role of prostaglandins in the regulation of bone metabolism, *Clin Orthop Relat Res* (Apr)313:36, 1995.

268. Kawai K, Masaka N: Vertical root fracture treated by bonding fragments and rotational replantation, *Dent Traumatol* 18:42, 2002.

269. Kay EJ, Nuttall NM, Knill-Jones R: Restorative treatment thresholds and agreement in treatment decision-making, *Community Dent Oral Epidemiol* 20:265, 1992.

270. Kay WW, Kurylo E, Chong G, Bharadwaj B: Inhibition and enhancement of platelet aggregation by collagen derivatives, *J Biomed Mater Res* 11:365, 1977.

271. Kay WW, Swanson R, Chong G, et al: Binding of collagen by canine blood platelets, *Thromb Haemost* 37:309, 1977.

272. Keller J: Effects of indomethacin and local prostaglandin E2 on fracture healing in rabbits, *Danish Med Bull* 43:317, 1996.

273. Kellert M, Chalfin H, Solomon C: Guided tissue regeneration: an adjunct to endodontic surgery, *J Am Dent Assoc* 125:1229, 1994.

274. Kerawala CJ, Martin IC, Allan W, Williams ED: The effects of operator technique and bur design on temperature during osseous preparation for osteosynthesis self-tapping screws, *Oral Surg Oral Med Oral Pathol Oral Radiol Endod* 88:145, 1999.

275. Kersten HW, Wesselink PR, Thoden van Velzen SK: The diagnostic reliability of the buccal radiograph after root canal filling, *Int Endod J* 20:20, 1987.

276. Kettering JD, Torabinejad M: Cytotoxicity of root canal sealers: a study using HeLa cells and fibroblasts, *Int Endod J* 17:60, 1984.

277. Kettering JD, Torabinejad M: Investigation of mutagenicity of mineral trioxide aggregate and other commonly used root-end filling materials, *J Endod* 21:537, 1995.

278. Khamaisi M, Regev E, Yarom N, et al: Possible association between diabetes and bisphosphonate-related jaw osteonecrosis, *J Clin Endocrinol Metab* 92:1172, 2007.

279. Kim E, Song JS, Jung IY, et al: Prospective clinical study evaluating endodontic microsurgery outcomes for cases with lesions of endodontic origin compared with cases

with lesions of combined periodontal-endodontic origin, *J Endod* 34:546, 2008.

280. Kim S: Principles of endodontic microsurgery, *Dent Clin North Am* 41:481, 1997.

281. Kim S: Endodontic microsurgery. In Cohen S, Burns RC, editors: *Pathways of the pulp*, ed 8, St. Louis, 2002, Mosby.

282. Kim S, Kratchman S: Modern endodontic surgery concepts and practice: a review, *J Endod* 32:601, 2006.

283. Kim S, Rethnam S: Hemostasis in endodontic microsurgery, *Dent Clin North Am* 41:499, 1997.

284. Kim SG, Solomon C: Cost-effectiveness of endodontic molar retreatment compared with fixed partial dentures and single-tooth implant alternatives, *J Endod* 37:321, 2011.

285. Kim TS, Caruso JM, Christensen H, Torabinejad M: A comparison of cone-beam computed tomography and direct measurement in the examination of the mandibular canal and adjacent structures, *J Endod* 36:1191, 2010.

286. Kirsner RS, Eaglstein WH: The wound healing process, *Dermatol Clin* 11:629, 1993.

287. Kiryu T, Hoshino E, Iwaku M: Bacteria invading periapical cementum, *J Endod* 20:169, 1994.

288. Kleier DJ: The continuous locking suture technique, *J Endod* 27:624, 2001.

289. Knighton DR, Hunt TK, Scheuenstuhl H, et al: Oxygen tension regulates the expression of angiogenesis factor by macrophages, *Science* 221:1283, 1983.

290. Kocher T, Plagmann HC: Heat propagation in dentin during instrumentation with different sonic scaler tips, *Quintessence Int* 27:259, 1996.

291. Kretzschmar D: In reply, *Oral Surg Oral Med Oral Pathol Oral Radiol Endod* 97:3, 2004.

292. Kuc I, Peters E, Pan J: Comparison of clinical and histologic diagnoses in periapical lesions, *Oral Surg Oral Med Oral Pathol Oral Radiol Endod* 89:333, 2000.

293. Kvist T, Reit C: Results of endodontic retreatment: a randomized clinical study comparing surgical and nonsurgical procedures, *J Endod* 25:814, 1999.

294. Kvist T, Reit C: Postoperative discomfort associated with surgical and nonsurgical endodontic retreatment, *Endod Dent Traumatol* 16:71, 2000.

295. Lalonde ER, Luebke RG: The frequency and distribution of periapical cysts and granulomas: an evaluation of 800 specimens, *Oral Surg Oral Med Oral Pathol* 25:861, 1968.

296. Lang NP, Loe H: The relationship between the width of keratinized gingiva and gingival health, *J Periodontol* 43:623, 1972.

297. Langeland K, Block RM, Grossman LI: A histopathologic and histobacteriologic study of 35 periapical endodontic surgical specimens, *J Endod* 3:8, 1977.

298. Larson PO: Topical hemostatic agents for dermatologic surgery [see comment], *J Dermatol Surg Oncol* 14:623, 1988.

299. Layton CA, Marshall JG, Morgan LA, Baumgartner JC: Evaluation of cracks associated with ultrasonic root-end preparation, *J Endod* 22:157, 1996.

300. Lee SJ, Monsef M, Torabinejad M: Sealing ability of a mineral trioxide aggregate for repair of lateral root perforations, *J Endod* 19:541, 1993.

301. Lemon RR, Steele PJ, Jeansonne BG: Ferric sulfate hemostasis: effect on osseous wound healing. Left in situ for maximum exposure, *J Endod* 19:170, 1993.

302. Leonhardt A, Grondahl K, Bergstrom C, Lekholm U: Long-term follow-up of osseointegrated titanium implants using clinical, radiographic and microbiological parameters, *Clin Oral Implants Res* 13:127, 2002.

303. Lin CP, Chou HG, Chen RS, et al: Root deformation during root-end preparation, *J Endod* 25:668, 1999.

304. Lin CP, Chou HG, Kuo JC, Lan WH: The quality of ultrasonic root-end preparation: a quantitative study, *J Endod* 24:666, 1998.

305. Lin L, Skribner J, Shovlin F, Langeland K: Periapical surgery of mandibular posterior teeth: anatomical and surgical considerations, *J Endod* 9:496, 1983.

306. Lin LM, Gaengler P, Langeland K: Periradicular curettage, *Int Endod J* 29:220, 1996.

307. Lin LM, Pascon EA, Skribner J, et al: Clinical, radiographic, and histologic study of endodontic treatment failures, *Oral Surg Oral Med Oral Pathol* 71:603, 1991.

308. Lin S, Cohenca N, Muska EA, Front E: Ridge preservation in cases requiring tooth extraction during endodontic surgery: a case report, *Int Endod J* 41:448, 2008.

309. Lindh T, Gunne J, Tillberg A, Molin M: A meta-analysis of implants in partial edentulism, *Clin Oral Implants Res* 9:80, 1998.

310. Lindskog S, Blomlof L, Hammarstrom L: Repair of periodontal tissues in vivo and in vitro, *J Clin Periodontol* 10:188, 1983.

311. Little JW, Falace DA, Miller CS, Rhodus NL: *Dental management of the medically compromised patient*, ed 6, St. Louis, 2002, Mosby.

312. Littner MM, Kaffe I, Tamse A, Dicapua P: Relationship between the apices of the lower molars and mandibular canal: a radiographic study, *Oral Surg Oral Med Oral Pathol* 62:595, 1986.

313. Lloyd A, Gutmann J, Dummer P, Newcombe R: Microleakage of Diaket and amalgam in root-end cavities prepared using MicroMega sonic retro-prep tips, *Int Endod J* 30:196, 1997.

314. Lofthag-Hansen S, Huumonen S, Grondahl K, Grondahl HG: Limited cone-beam CT and intraoral radiography for the diagnosis of periapical pathology, *Oral Surg Oral Med Oral Pathol Oral Radiol Endod* 103:114, 2007.

315. Loftus D: Assessment of MTA, White MTA, Diaket, and Geristore when used as surgical root-end fillings in dogs. In *Endodontics 1*, Dallas, 2003, Baylor College of Dentistry, the Texas A&M University System Health Science Center.

316. Lorena D, Uchio K, Costa AM, Desmouliere A: Normal scarring: importance of myofibroblasts, *Wound Repair Regen* 10:86, 2002.

317. Lovato KF, Sedgley CM: Antibacterial activity of endosequence root repair material and proroot MTA against clinical isolates of *Enterococcus faecalis*, *J Endod* 37:1542, 2011.

318. Low KM, Dula K, Burgin W, von Arx T: Comparison of periapical radiography and limited cone-beam tomography in posterior maxillary teeth referred for apical surgery, *J Endod* 34:557, 2008.

319. Lowenguth RA, Blieden TM: Periodontal regeneration: root surface demineralization, *Periodontology* 1:54, 2000.

320. Lowenguth RA, Polson AM, Caton JG: Oriented cell and fiber attachment systems in vivo, *J Periodontol* 64:330, 1993.

321. Ludlow JB, Davies-Ludlow LE, Brooks SL, Howerton WB: Dosimetry of 3 CBCT devices for oral and maxillofacial radiology: CB Mercuray, NewTom 3G and i-CAT, *Dentomaxillofac Radiol* 35:219, 2006.

322. Luebke RG: Surgical endodontics, *Dent Clin North Am* 18:379, 1974.

323. Ma J, Shen Y, Stojicic S, Haapasalo M: Biocompatibility of two novel root repair materials, *J Endod* 37:793, 2011.

324. Machtei EE, Oettinger-Barak O, Peled M: Guided tissue regeneration in smokers: effect of aggressive anti-infective therapy in Class II furcation defects, *J Periodontol* 74:579, 2003.

325. Macphee TC, Cowley G: *Essentials of periodontology and periodontics*, ed 3, Oxford, 1981, Blackwell Scientific Publications, p 273.

326. Maddalone M, Gagliani M: Periapical endodontic surgery: a 3-year follow-up study, *Int Endod J* 36:193, 2003.

327. Madison S, Hokett SD: The effects of different tetracyclines on the dentin root surface of instrumented, periodontally involved human teeth: a comparative scanning electron microscope study, *J Periodontol* 68:739, 1997.

328. Maeda H, Hashiguchi I, Nakamuta H, et al: Histological study of periapical tissue healing in the rat molar after retrofilling with various materials, *J Endod* 25:38, 1999.

329. Maher WP, Johnson RL, Hess J, Steiman HR: Biocompatibility of retrograde filling materials in the ferret canine: amalgam and IRM, *Oral Surg Oral Med Oral Pathol* 73:738, 1992.

330. Mariotti A: Efficacy of chemical root surface modifiers in the treatment of periodontal disease: a systematic review, *Ann Periodontol* 8:205, 2003.

331. Marmulla R, Wortche R, Muhling J, Hassfeld S: Geometric accuracy of the NewTom 9000 Cone Beam CT, *Dentomaxillofac Radiol* 34:28, 2005.

332. Marx RE: Pamidronate (Aredia) and zoledronate (Zometa) induced avascular necrosis of the jaws: a growing epidemic, *J Oral Maxillofac Surg* 61:1115, 2003.

333. Marx RE, Cillo JE Jr, Ulloa JJ: Oral bisphosphonate-induced osteonecrosis: risk factors, prediction of risk using serum CTX testing, prevention, and treatment, *J Oral Maxillofac Surg* 65:2397, 2007.

334. Marx RE, Sawatari Y, Fortin M, Broumand V: Bisphosphonate-induced exposed bone (osteonecrosis/osteopetrosis) of the jaws: risk factors, recognition, prevention, and treatment, *J Oral Maxillofac Surg* 63:1567, 2005.

335. Mason RG, Read MS: Some effects of a microcrystalline collagen preparation on blood, *Haemostasis* 3:31, 1974.

336. Mason RG, Read MS: Effects of collagen and artificial surfaces on platelets that influence blood coagulation, *Thromb Res* 7:471, 1975.

337. Mastromihalis N, Goldstein S, Greenberg M, Friedman S: Applications for guided bone regeneration in endodontic surgery, *N Y State Dent J* 65:30, 1999.

338. Matthews LS, Hirsch C: Temperatures measured in human cortical bone when drilling, *J Bone Joint Surg Am* 54:297, 1972.

339. Mauger MJ, Schindler WG, Walker WA 3rd: An evaluation of canal morphology at different levels of root resection in mandibular incisors, *J Endod* 24:607, 1998.

340. Mavrokokki T, Cheng A, Stein B, Goss A: Nature and frequency of bisphosphonate-associated osteonecrosis of the jaws in Australia, *J Oral Maxillofac Surg* 65:415, 2007.

341. Mazeland GR: Longitudinal aspects of gingival width, *J Periodontal Res* 15:429, 1980.

342. McAllister BS, Haghighat K: Bone augmentation techniques, *J Periodontol* 78:377, 2007.

343. McCaul LK, McHugh S, Saunders WP: The influence of specialty training and experience on decision making in endodontic diagnosis and treatment planning, *Int Endod J* 34:594, 2001.

344. McDonald NJ, Dumsha TC: A comparative retrofill leakage study utilizing a dentin bonding material, *J Endod* 13:224, 1987.

345. McDonald NJ, Dumsha TC: Evaluation of the retrograde apical seal using dentine bonding materials, *Int Endod J* 23:156, 1990.

346. McQuay H, Moore R: *An evidence-based resource for pain relief*. Oxford, 1998, Oxford University Press.

347. Mehlhaff DS, Marshall JG, Baumgartner JC: Comparison of ultrasonic and high-speed-bur root-end preparations using bilaterally matched teeth, *J Endod* 23:448, 1997.

348. Mehlisch DR: The efficacy of combination analgesic therapy in relieving dental pain, *J Am Dent Assoc* 133:861, 2002.

349. Meryon SD, Riches DW: A comparison of the in vitro cytotoxicity of four restorative materials assessed by changes in enzyme levels in two cell types, *J Biomed Mater Res* 16:519, 1982.

350. Michaelides PL: Use of the operating microscope in dentistry [erratum appears in *J Calif Dent Assoc* 24:9, 1996], *J Calif Dent Assoc* 24:45, 1996.

351. Migliorati CA: Bisphosphonates and oral cavity avascular bone necrosis, *J Clin Oncol* 21:4253, 2003.

352. Migliorati CA, Woo SB, Hewson I, et al: A systematic review of bisphosphonate osteonecrosis (BON) in cancer, *Support Care Cancer* 18:1099, 2010.

353. Miles DA, Anderson RW, Pashley DH: Evaluation of the bond strength of dentin bonding agents used to seal resected root apices, *J Endod* 20:538, 1994.

354. Min MM, Brown CE Jr, Legan JJ, Kafrawy AH: In vitro evaluation of effects of ultrasonic root-end preparation on resected root surfaces, *J Endod* 23:624, 1997.

355. Moiseiwitsch JR: Avoiding the mental foramen during periapical surgery, *J Endod* 21:340, 1995.

356. Moiseiwitsch JR: Position of the mental foramen in a North American, white population, *Oral Surg Oral Med Oral Pathol Oral Radiol Endod* 85:457, 1998.

357. Morgan LA, Marshall JG: The topography of root ends resected with fissure burs and refined with two types of finishing burs, *Oral Surg Oral Med Oral Pathol Oral Radiol Endod* 85:585, 1998.

358. Morgan LA, Marshall JG: A scanning electron microscopic study of in vivo ultrasonic root-end preparations, *J Endod* 25:567, 1999.

359. Mortensen H, Winther JE, Birn H: Periapical granulomas and cysts: an investigation of 1,600 cases, *Scand J Dent Res* 78:241, 1970.

360. Moss RW: Histopathologic reaction of bone to surgical cutting, *Oral Surg Oral Med Oral Pathol* 17:405, 1964.

361. Munksgaard EC, Rud J, Asmussen E: [Retrograde root obturations employing composite and a dentin bonding agent: adaptions of the filling materials and bond strength], *Tandlaegebladet* 93:157, 1989.

362. Murray PE, Hafez AA, Windsor LJ, et al: Comparison of pulp responses following restoration of exposed and non-exposed cavities, *J Dent* 30:213, 2002.

363. Nair PN: Apical periodontitis: a dynamic encounter between root canal infection and host response, *Periodontology 2000* 13:121, 1997.

364. Nair PN: New perspectives on radicular cysts: do they heal? *Int Endod J* 31:155, 1998.

365. Nair PN: Cholesterol as an aetiological agent in endodontic failures: a review, *Aust Endod J* 25:19, 1999.

366. Nair PN, Pajarola G, Luder HU: Ciliated epithelium-lined radicular cysts, *Oral Surg Oral Med Oral Pathol Oral Radiol Endod* 94:485, 2002.

367. Nair PN, Sjogren U, Figdor D, Sundqvist G: Persistent periapical radiolucencies of root-filled human teeth, failed endodontic treatments, and periapical scars, *Oral Surg Oral Med Oral Pathol Oral Radiol Endod* 87:617, 1999.

368. Nair PN, Sjogren U, Krey G, et al: Intraradicular bacteria and fungi in root-filled, asymptomatic human teeth with therapy-resistant periapical lesions: a long-term light and electron microscopic follow-up study, *J Endod* 16:580, 1990.

369. Nair PN, Sjogren U, Krey G, Sundqvist G: Therapy-resistant foreign body giant cell granuloma at the periapex of a root-filled human tooth, *J Endod* 16:589, 1990.

370. Nair PN, Sjogren U, Sundqvist G: Cholesterol crystals as an etiological factor in non-resolving chronic inflammation: an experimental study in guinea pigs, *Eur J Oral Sci* 106:644, 1998.

371. Nakata K, Naitoh M, Izumi M, et al: Effectiveness of dental computed tomography in diagnostic imaging of periradicular lesion of each root of a multirooted tooth: a case report, *J Endod* 32:583, 2006.

372. Nakazawa Y, Mitsui K, Hirai Y, et al: Histo-pathological study of a glass-ionomer/resin (Geristore) restoration system, *Bull Tokyo Dent Coll* 35:197, 1994.

373. Nappi JF, Lehman JA Jr: The effects of Surgicel on bone formation, *Cleft Palate J* 17:291, 1980.

374. Nash KD, Brown LJ, Hicks ML: Private practicing endodontists: production of endodontic services and implications for workforce policy, *J Endod* 28:699, 2002.

375. Navarre SW, Steiman HR: Root-end fracture during retropreparation: a comparison between zirconium nitride-coated and stainless steel microsurgical ultrasonic instruments, *J Endod* 28:330, 2002.

376. Neaverth EJ: Disabling complications following inadvertent overextension of a root canal filling material, *J Endod* 15:135, 1989.

377. Nedderman TA, Hartwell GR, Protell FR: A comparison of root surfaces following apical root resection with various burs: scanning electron microscopic evaluation, *J Endod* 14:423, 1988.

378. Nelson DR, Buxton TB, Luu QN, Rissing JP: The promotional effect of bone wax on experimental Staphylococcus aureus osteomyelitis [see comment], *J Thorac Cardiovasc Surg* 99:977, 1990.

379. Nencka D, Walia H, Austin BP: Histological evaluation of the biocompatability of Diaket, *J Dent Res* 74:101, 1995.

380. Nicoll BK, Peters RJ: Heat generation during ultrasonic instrumentation of dentin as affected by different irrigation methods, *J Periodontol* 69:884, 1998.

381. Nixon KC, Adkins KF, Keys DW: Histological evaluation of effects produced in alveolar bone following gingival incision with an electrosurgical scalpel, *J Periodontol* 46:40, 1975.

382. Nobuhara WK, del Rio CE: Incidence of periradicular pathoses in endodontic treatment failures, *J Endod* 19:315, 1993.

383. Nohl FS, Gulabivala K: Odontogenic keratocyst as periradicular radiolucency in the anterior mandible: two case reports, *Oral Surg Oral Med Oral Pathol Oral Radiol Endod* 81:103, 1996.

384. Norred CL: Complementary and alternative medicine use by surgical patients, *AOM J* 76:1013, 2002.

385. Norred CL, Brinker F: Potential coagulation effects of preoperative complementary and alternative medicines, *Altern Ther Health Med* 7:58, 2001.

386. O'Connor AM, Bennett C, Stacey D, et al: Do patient decision aids meet effectiveness criteria of the international patient decision aid standards collaboration? A systematic review and meta-analysis, *Med Decis Making* 27:554, 2007.

387. O'Connor AM, Stacey D, Rovner D, et al: Decision aids for people facing health treatment or screening decisions, *Cochrane Database Syst Rev* CD001431, 2001.

388. O'Connor RP, Hutter JW, Roahen JO: Leakage of amalgam and Super-EBA root-end fillings using two preparation techniques and surgical microscopy, *J Endod* 21:74, 1995.

389. O'Neal RB, Alleyn CD: Suture materials and techniques, *Curr Opin Periodontol* 4:89, 1997.

390. Oguntebi BR, Barker BF, Anderson DM, Sakumura J: The effect of indomethacin on experimental dental periapical lesions in rats, *J Endod* 15:117, 1989.

391. Oikarinen KS, Stoltze K, Andreasen JO: Influence of conventional forceps extraction and extraction with an extrusion instrument on cementoblast loss and external root resorption of replanted monkey incisors, *J Periodontol Res* 31:337, 1996.

392. Olson RA, Roberts DL, Osbon DB: A comparative study of polylactic acid, Gelfoam, and Surgicel in healing extraction sites, *Oral Surg Oral Med Oral Pathol* 53:441, 1982.

393. Olsson B, Wennberg A: Early tissue reaction to endodontic filling materials, *Endod Dent Traumatol* 1:138, 1985.

394. Osorio RM, Hefti A, Vertucci FJ, Shawley AL: Cytotoxicity of endodontic materials, *J Endod* 24:91, 1998.

395. Owens WD, Felts JA, Spitznagel EL Jr: ASA physical status classifications: a study of consistency of ratings, *Anesthesiology* 49:239, 1978.

396. Oynick J, Oynick T: A study of a new material for retrograde fillings, *J Endod* 4:203, 1978.

397. Pantschev A, Carlsson AP, Andersson L: Retrograde root filling with EBA cement or amalgam: a comparative clinical study, *Oral Surg Oral Med Oral Pathol* 78:101, 1994.

398. Patel S, Dawood A: The use of cone beam computed tomography in the management of external cervical resorption lesions, *Int Endod J* 40:730, 2007.

399. Peciuliene V, Reynaud AH, Balciuniene I, Haapasalo M: Isolation of yeasts and enteric bacteria in root-filled teeth with chronic apical periodontitis, *Int Endod J* 34:429, 2001.

400. Pecora G, Kim S, Celletti R, Davarpanah M: The guided tissue regeneration principle in endodontic surgery: one-year postoperative results of large periapical lesions, *Int Endod J* 28:41, 1995.

401. Peer M: Intentional replantation: a "last resort" treatment or a conventional treatment procedure? Nine case reports, *Dent Traumatol* 20:48, 2004.

402. Peltola M, Salo T, Oikarinen K: Toxic effects of various retrograde root filling materials on gingival fibroblasts and rat sarcoma cells, *Endod Dent Traumatol* 8:120, 1992.

403. Perez M, Fernandez I, Marquez D, Bretana RM: Use of N-butyl-2-cyanoacrylate in oral surgery: biological and clinical evaluation, *Artif Organs* 24:241, 2000.

404. Pertot WJ, Stephan G, Tardieu C, Proust JP: Comparison of the intraosseous biocompatibility of Dyract and Super EBA, *J Endod* 23:315, 1997.

405. Peters CI, Peters OA, Barbakow F: An in vitro study comparing root-end cavities prepared by diamond-coated and stainless steel ultrasonic retrotips, *Int Endod J* 34:142, 2001.

406. Peters E, Monopoli M, Woo SB, Sonis S: Assessment of the need for treatment of postendodontic asymptomatic periapical radiolucencies in bone marrow transplant recipients, *Oral Surg Oral Med Oral Pathol* 76:45, 1993.

407. Peters LB, Harrison JW: A comparison of leakage of filling materials in demineralized and non-demineralized resected root ends under vacuum and non-vacuum conditions, *Int Endod J* 25:273, 1992.

408. Petersen JK, Krogsgaard J, Nielsen KM, Norgaard EB: A comparison between 2 absorbable hemostatic agents: gelatin sponge (Spongostan) and oxidized regenerated cellulose (Surgicel), *Int J Oral Surg* 13:406, 1984.

409. Philipsen HP, Srisuwan T, Reichart PA: Adenomatoid odontogenic tumor mimicking a periapical (radicular) cyst: a case report, *Oral Surg Oral Med Oral Pathol Oral Radiol Endod* 94:246, 2002.

410. Phillips JL, Weller RN, Kulild JC: The mental foramen: 1. Size, orientation, and positional relationship to the mandibular second premolar, *J Endod* 16:221, 1990.

411. Phillips JL, Weller RN, Kulild JC: The mental foramen: 2. Radiographic position in relation to the mandibular second premolar, *J Endod* 18:271, 1992.

412. Phillips JL, Weller RN, Kulild JC: The mental foramen: 3. Size and position on panoramic radiographs, *J Endod* 18:383, 1992.

413. Phillips SJ: Physiology of wound healing and surgical wound care, *ASAIO J* 46:S2, 2000.

414. Pinto VS, Zuolo ML, Mellonig JT: Guided bone regeneration in the treatment of a large periapical lesion: a case report, *Pract Periodontics Aesthet Dent* 7:76, 1995.

415. Pissiotis E, Sapounas G, Spangberg LS: Silver glass ionomer cement as a retrograde filling material: a study in vitro, *J Endod* 17:225, 1991.

416. Pissiotis E, Spangberg L: Reaction of bony tissue to implanted silver glass ionomer and a reinforced zinc oxide-eugenol cement, *Oral Surg Oral Med Oral Pathol Oral Radiol Endod* 89:623, 2000.

417. Pitt Ford TR, Andreasen JO, Dorn SO, Kariyawasam SP: Effect of IRM root end fillings on healing after replantation, *J Endod* 20:381, 1994.

418. Pitt Ford TR, Andreasen JO, Dorn SO, Kariyawasam SP: Effect of super-EBA as a root end filling on healing after replantation, *J Endod* 21:13, 1995.

419. Pitt Ford TR, Andreasen JO, Dorn SO, Kariyawasam SP: Effect of various zinc oxide materials as root-end fillings on healing after replantation, *Int Endod J* 28:273, 1995.

420. Pitt Ford TR, Andreasen JO, Dorn SO, Kariyawasam SP: Effect of various sealers with gutta-percha as root-end fillings on healing after replantation, *Endod Dent Traumatol* 12:33, 1996.

421. Pompa DG: Guided tissue repair of complete buccal dehiscences associated with periapical defects: a clinical retrospective study, *J Am Dent Assoc* 128:989, 1997.

422. Posen S: Alkaline phosphatase, *Ann Intern Med* 67:183, 1967.

423. Posen S, Neale FC, Brudenell-Woods J, Birkett DJ: Continuous determination of enzyme activity during heat inactivation, *Lancet* 1:264, 1966.

424. Rahbaran S, Gilthorpe MS, Harrison SD, Gulabivala K: Comparison of clinical outcome of periapical surgery in endodontic and oral surgery units of a teaching dental hospital: a retrospective study, *Oral Surg Oral Med Oral Pathol Oral Radiol Endod* 91:700, 2001.

425. Rainwater A, Jeansonne BG, Sarkar N: Effects of ultrasonic root-end preparation on microcrack formation and leakage, *J Endod* 26:72, 2000.

426. Raisz LG: Bone cell biology: new approaches and unanswered questions, *J Bone Miner Res* 8:S457, 1993.

427. Raisz LG, Pilbeam CC, Fall PM: Prostaglandins: mechanisms of action and regulation of production in bone, *Osteoporos Int* 3:136, 1993.

428. Rakich DR, Wataha JC, Lefebvre CA, Weller RN: Effects of dentin bonding agents on macrophage mitochondrial activity, *J Endod* 24:528, 1998.

429. Rakich DR, Wataha JC, Lefebvre CA, Weller RN: Effect of dentin bonding agents on the secretion of inflammatory mediators from macrophages, *J Endod* 25:114, 1999.

430. Rakusin H, Harrison JW, Marker VA: Alteration of the manipulative properties of plain gut suture material by hydration, *J Endod* 14:121, 1988.

431. Ramadas Y, Sealey CM: Third molar removal and nerve injury, *N Z Dent J* 97:25, 2001.

432. Rankow HJ, Krasner PR: Endodontic applications of guided tissue regeneration in endodontic surgery, *Oral Health* 86:33, 1996.

433. Regan JD, Gutmann JL, Witherspoon DE: Comparison of Diaket and MTA when used as root-end filling materials to support regeneration of the periradicular tissues, *Int Endod J* 35:840, 2002.

434. Register AA: Bone and cementum induction by dentin, demineralized in situ, *J Periodontol* 44:49, 1973.

435. Register AA: Induced reattachment in periodontic-endodontic lesions by root demineralization in situ, *Oral Surg Oral Med Oral Pathol* 45:774, 1978.

436. Register AA, Burdick FA: Accelerated reattachment with cementogenesis to dentin, demineralized in situ. I. Optimum range, *J Periodontol* 46:646, 1975.

437. Register AA, Burdick FA: Accelerated reattachment with cementogenesis to dentin, demineralized in situ. II. Defect repair, *J Periodontol* 47:497, 1976.

438. Register AA, Scopp IW, Kassouny DY, Pfau FR, Peskin D: Human bone induction by allogeneic dentin matrix, *J Periodontol* 43:459, 1972.

439. Reit C, Kvist T: Endodontic retreatment behaviour: the influence of disease concepts and personal values, *Int Endod J* 31:358, 1998.

440. Resillez-Urioste F, Sanandajt K, Davidson RM: Use of a resin-ionomer in the treatment of mechanical root perforation: report of a case, *Quintessence Int* 29:115, 1998.

441. Reuben HL, Apotheker H: Apical surgery with the dental microscope, *Oral Surg Oral Med Oral Pathol* 57:433, 1984.

442. Rigolone M, Pasqualini D, Bianchi L, et al: Vestibular surgical access to the palatine root of the superior first molar: "low-dose cone-beam" CT analysis of the pathway and its anatomic variations, *J Endod* 29:773, 2003.

443. Robinson RC, Williams CW: Documentation method for inferior alveolar and lingual nerve paresthesias, *Oral Surg Oral Med Oral Pathol* 62:128, 1986.

444. Rosales JI, Vallecillo M, Osorio R, et al: An in vitro comparison of micro leakage in three glass ionomer cements used as retrograde filling materials, *Int Dent J* 46:15, 1996.

445. Rosenberg ES, Cutler SA: The effect of cigarette smoking on the long-term success of guided tissue regeneration: a preliminary study, *Ann R Australas Coll Dent Surg* 12:89, 1994.

446. Roy CO, Jeansonne BG, Gerrets TF: Effect of an acid environment on leakage of root-end filling materials, *J Endod* 27:7, 2001.

447. Rubin MR, Bilezikian JP: Clinical review 151: The role of parathyroid hormone in the pathogenesis of glucocorticoid-induced osteoporosis: a re-examination of the evidence, *J Clin Endocrinol Metab* 87:4033, 2002.

448. Rubinstein RA, Kim S: Long-term follow-up of cases considered healed one year after apical microsurgery, *J Endod* 28:378, 2002.

449. Rud J, Andreasen JO: A study of failures after endodontic surgery by radiographic, histologic and stereomicroscopic methods, *Int J Oral Surg* 1:311, 1972.

450. Rud J, Andreasen JO, Jensen JF: A multivariate analysis of the influence of various factors upon healing after endodontic surgery, *Int J Oral Surg* 1:258, 1972.

451. Rud J, Andreasen JO, Rud V: [Retrograde root filling utilizing resin and a dentin bonding agent: frequency of healing when compared to retrograde amalgam], *Tandlaegebladet* 93:267, 1989.

452. Rud J, Munksgaard EC: [Retrograde root canal filling using resin and a dentin bonding agent: analysis of failures], *Tandlaegebladet* 93:343, 1989.

453. Rud J, Munksgaard EC, Andreasen JO, Rud V: Retrograde root filling with composite and a dentin-bonding agent. 2, *Endod Dent Traumatol* 7:126, 1991.

454. Rud J, Munksgaard EC, Andreasen JO, et al: Retrograde root filling with composite and a dentin-bonding agent. 1, *Endod Dent Traumatol* 7:118, 1991.

455. Rud J, Munksgaard EC, Rud V: [Retrograde root canal filling using resin and a dentin bonding agent: operative procedures], *Tandlaegebladet* 93:401, 1989.

456. Rud J, Rud V: Surgical endodontics of upper molars: relation to the maxillary sinus and operation in acute state of infection, *J Endod* 24:260, 1998.

457. Rud J, Rud V, Munksgaard EC: [Retrograde root filling utilizing resin and a dentin bonding agent: indication and applications], *Tandlaegebladet* 93:223, 1989.

458. Rud J, Rud V, Munksgaard EC: Long-term evaluation of retrograde root filling with dentin-bonded resin composite, *J Endod* 22:90, 1996.

459. Rud J, Rud V, Munksgaard EC: Retrograde root filling with dentin-bonded modified resin composite, *J Endod* 22:477, 1996.

460. Rud J, Rud V, Munksgaard EC: Effect of root canal contents on healing of teeth with dentin-bonded resin composite retrograde seal, *J Endod* 23:535, 1997.

461. Russo G, Corso LD, Biasiolo A, et al: Simple and safe method to prepare patients with prosthetic heart valves for surgical dental procedures, *Clin Appl Thromb Hemost* 6:90, 2000.

462. Sabeti M, Simon JH, Nowzari H, Slots J: Cytomegalovirus and Epstein-Barr virus active infection in periapical lesions of teeth with intact crowns, *J Endod* 29:321, 2003.

463. Safavi K, Kazemi R, Watkins D: Adherence of enamel matrix derivatives on root-end filling materials, *J Endod* 25:710, 1999.

464. Sakamoto M, Siqueira JF Jr, Rocas IN, Benno Y: Molecular analysis of the root canal microbiota associated with endodontic treatment failures, *Oral Microbiol Immunol* 23:275, 2008.

465. Sakellariou PL: Periapical actinomycosis: report of a case and review of the literature, *Endod Dent Traumatol* 12:151, 1996.

466. Sammonds JH: *Drug evaluations*, ed 6, Chicago, 1986, American Medical Association, p 658.

467. Satchell PG, Gutmann JL, Witherspoon DE: Apoptosis: an introduction for the endodontist, *Int Endod J* 36:237, 2003.

468. Saunders WP: A prospective clinical study of periradicular surgery using mineral trioxide aggregate as a root-end filling, *J Endod* 34:660, 2008.

469. Saunders WP, Saunders EM, Gutmann JL: Ultrasonic root-end preparation, Part 2. Microleakage of EBA root-end fillings, *Int Endod J* 27:325, 1994.

470. Sauveur G, Boccara E, Colon P, et al: A photoelastimetric analysis of stress induced by root-end resection, *J Endod* 24:740, 1998.

471. Saygin NE, Giannobile WV, Somerman MJ: Molecular and cell biology of cementum, *Periodontology* 24:73, 2000.

472. Scarfe WC, Farman AG, Sukovic P: Clinical applications of cone-beam computed tomography in dental practice, *J Can Dent Assoc* 72:75, 2006.

473. Schamberg M: The surgical treatment of chronic alveolar abscess, *Dent Cosmos* 48:15, 1906.

474. Scheerer SQ, Steiman HR, Cohen J: A comparative evaluation of three root-end filling materials: an in vitro leakage study using *Prevotella nigrescens*, *J Endod* 27:40, 2001.

475. Scherer W, Dragoo MR: New subgingival restorative procedures with Geristore resin ionomer, *Pract Periodontics Aesthet Dent* 7:1, 1995.

476. Schilephake H: Bone growth factors in maxillofacial skeletal reconstruction, *Int J Oral Maxillofac Surg* 31:469, 2002.

477. Sciubba JJ, Waterhouse JP, Meyer J: A fine structural comparison of the healing of incisional wounds of mucosa and skin, *J Oral Pathol* 7:214, 1978.

478. Scully C, Wolff A: Oral surgery in patients on anticoagulant therapy, *Oral Surg Oral Med Oral Pathol Oral Radiol Endod* 94:57, 2002.

479. Sedghizadeh PP, Stanley K, Caligiuri M, et al: Oral bisphosphonate use and the prevalence of osteonecrosis of the jaw: an institutional inquiry, *J Am Dent Assoc* 140:61, 2009.

480. Selden HS: Bone wax as an effective hemostat in periapical surgery, *Oral Surg Oral Med Oral Pathol* 29:262, 1970.

481. Seltzer S, Soltanoff W, Bender IB, Ziontz M: Biologic aspects of endodontics. 1. Histological observations of the anatomy and morphology of root apices and surroundings, *Oral Surg Oral Med Oral Pathol* 22:375, 1966.

482. Setzer FC, Kohli MR, Shah SB, et al: Outcome of endodontic surgery: a meta-analysis of the literature—Part 2: Comparison of endodontic microsurgical techniques with and without the use of higher magnification, *J Endod* 38:1, 2012.

483. Setzer FC, Shah SB, Kohli MR, et al: Outcome of endodontic surgery: a meta-analysis of the literature–part 1: Comparison of traditional root-end surgery and endodontic microsurgery, *J Endod* 36:1757, 2010.

484. Shah PM, Chong BS, Sidhu SK, Ford TR: Radiopacity of potential root-end filling materials, *Oral Surg Oral Med Oral Pathol Oral Radiol Endod* 81:476, 1996.

485. Shaw N: Textured collagen, a hemostatic agent: a pilot study, *Oral Surg Oral Med Oral Pathol* 72:642, 1991.

486. Shulman BB, Leung A: Endoscopic surgery: an alternative technique, *Dent Today* 15:42, 1996.

487. Shuman IE: Repair of a root perforation with a resin-ionomer using an intentional replantation technique, *General Dent* 47:392, 1999.

488. Simon JH: Incidence of periapical cysts in relation to the root canal, *J Endod* 6:845, 1980.

489. Simon JH, Enciso R, Malfaz JM, et al: Differential diagnosis of large periapical lesions using cone-beam computed tomography measurements and biopsy, *J Endod* 32:833, 2006.

490. Siqueira JF Jr, Lopes HP: Bacteria on the apical root surfaces of untreated teeth with periradicular lesions: a scanning electron microscopy study, *Int Endod J* 34:216, 2001.

491. Siqueira JF Jr, Rocas IN: Polymerase chain reaction-based analysis of microorganisms associated with failed endodontic treatment, *Oral Surg Oral Med Oral Pathol Oral Radiol Endod* 97:85, 2004.

492. Siqueira Junior JF Jr: Aetiology of root canal treatment failure: why well-treated teeth can fail, *Int Endod J* 34:1, 2001.

493. Sisk AL, Dionne RA, Wirdzek PR: Evaluation of etidocaine hydrochloride for local anesthesia and postoperative pain control in oral surgery, *J Oral Maxillofac Surg* 42:84, 1984.

494. Sisk AL, Mosley RO, Martin RP: Comparison of preoperative and postoperative diflunisal for suppression

of postoperative pain, *J Oral Maxillofac Surg* 47:464, 1989.

495. Sjogren U, Happonen RP, Kahnberg KE, Sundqvist G: Survival of *Arachnia propionica* in periapical tissue, *Int Endod J* 21:277, 1988.

496. Sjogren U, Ohlin A, Sundqvist G, Lerner UH: Gutta-percha-stimulated mouse macrophages release factors that activate the bone resorptive system of mouse calvarial bone, *Eur J Oral Sci* 106:872, 1998.

497. Sjogren U, Sundqvist G, Nair PN: Tissue reaction to gutta-percha particles of various sizes when implanted subcutaneously in guinea pigs, *Eur J Oral Sci* 103:313, 1995.

498. Skaar DD, O'Connor H, Hodges JS, Michalowicz BS: Dental procedures and subsequent prosthetic joint infections: findings from the Medicare Current Beneficiary Survey, *J Am Dent Assoc* 142:1343, 2011.

499. Skoglund A, Persson G: A follow-up study of apicoectomized teeth with total loss of the buccal bone plate, *Oral Surg Oral Med Oral Pathol* 59:78, 1985.

500. Song M, Chung W, Lee SJ, Kim E: Long-term outcome of the cases classified as successes based on short-term follow-up in endodontic microsurgery, *J Endod* 38:1192, 2012.

501. Song M, Kim E: A prospective randomized controlled study of mineral trioxide aggregate and super ethoxy-benzoic acid as root-end filling materials in endodontic microsurgery, *J Endod* 38:875, 2012.

502. Spangberg L: Biological effects of root canal filling materials. 7. Reaction of bony tissue to implanted root canal filling material in guinea pigs, *Odontologisk Tidskrift* 77:133, 1969.

503. Spector JA, Mehrara BJ, Greenwald JA, et al: Osteoblast expression of vascular endothelial growth factor is modulated by the extracellular microenvironment, *Am J Physiol Cell Physiol* 280:C72, 2001.

504. Stein MD, Salkin LM, Freedman AL, Glushko V: Collagen sponge as a topical hemostatic agent in mucogingival surgery, *J Periodontol* 56:35, 1985.

505. Subramanian G, Cohen HV, Quek SY: A model for the pathogenesis of bisphosphonate-associated osteonecrosis of the jaw and teriparatide's potential role in its resolution, *Oral Surg Oral Med Oral Pathol Oral Radiol Endod* 112:744, 2011.

506. Sugaya T, Kawanami M, Noguchi H, et al: Periodontal healing after bonding treatment of vertical root fracture, *Dent Traumatol* 17:174, 2001.

507. Sukovic P: Cone beam computed tomography in craniofacial imaging, *Orthod Craniofac Res* 6 (suppl 1):31, 2003.

508. Suliman AA, Schulein TM, Boyer DB, Kohout FJ: Effects of etching and rinsing times and salivary contamination on etched glass-ionomer cement bonded to resin composites, *Dent Mater* 5:171, 1989.

509. Sunde PT, Tronstad L, Eribe ER, et al: Assessment of periradicular microbiota by DNA-DNA hybridization, *Endod Dent Traumatol* 16:191, 2000.

510. Sundqvist G, Figdor D, Persson S, Sjogren U: Microbiologic analysis of teeth with failed endodontic treatment and the outcome of conservative re-treatment, *Oral Surg Oral Med Oral Pathol Oral Radiol Endod* 85:86, 1998.

511. Sundqvist G, Reuterving CO: Isolation of *Actinomyces israelii* from periapical lesion, *J Endod* 6:602, 1980.

512. Swift EJ Jr, Pawlus MA, Vargas MA, Fortin D: Depth of cure of resin-modified glass ionomers, *Dent Mater* 11:196, 1995.

513. Sykaras N, Opperman LA: Bone morphogenetic proteins (BMPs): how do they function and what can they offer the clinician? *J Oral Sci* 45:57, 2003.

514. Tai KW, Chang YC: Cytotoxicity evaluation of perforation repair materials on human periodontal ligament cells in vitro, *J Endod* 26:395, 2000.

515. Taschieri S, Corbella S, Tsesis I, et al: Effect of guided tissue regeneration on the outcome of surgical endodontic treatment of through-and-through lesions: a retrospective

study at 4-year follow-up, *Oral Maxillofac Surg* 15:153, 2011.

516. Taub DD, Oppenheim JJ: Chemokines, inflammation and the immune system, *Therapeutic Immunology* 1:229, 1994.

517. Tenenbaum H, Tenenbaum M: A clinical study of the width of the attached gingiva in the deciduous, transitional and permanent dentitions, *J Clin Periodontol* 13:270, 1986.

518. Testori T, Capelli M, Milani S, Weinstein RL: Success and failure in periradicular surgery: a longitudinal retrospective analysis, *Oral Surg Oral Med Oral Pathol Oral Radiol Endod* 87:493, 1999.

519. Tetsch P: Development of raised temperature after osteotomies, *J Maxillofac Oral Surg* 2:141, 1974.

520. Thirawat J, Edmunds DH: Sealing ability of materials used as retrograde root fillings in endodontic surgery, *Int Endod J* 22:295, 1989.

521. Thomas S: Platelet membrane glycoproteins in haemostasis, *Clin Lab* 48:247, 2002.

522. Thomson TS, Berry JE, Somerman MJ, Kirkwood KL: Cementoblasts maintain expression of osteocalcin in the presence of mineral trioxide aggregate, *J Endod* 29:407, 2003.

523. Tidmarsh BG, Arrowsmith MG: Dentinal tubules at the root ends of apicected teeth: a scanning electron microscopic study, *Int Endod J* 22:184, 1989.

524. Tomasek JJ, Gabbiani G, Hinz B, et al: Myofibroblasts and mechano-regulation of connective tissue remodeling, *Nat Rev Mol Cell Biol* 3:349, 2002.

525. Tonetti MS, Pini-Prato G, Cortellini P: Effect of cigarette smoking on periodontal healing following GTR in infrabony defects: a preliminary retrospective study, *J Clin Periodontol* 22:229, 1995.

526. Tong DC, Rothwell BR: Antibiotic prophylaxis in dentistry: a review and practice recommendations, *J Am Dent Assoc* 131:366, 2000.

527. Torabinejad M, Higa RK, McKendry DJ, Pitt Ford TR: Dye leakage of four root end filling materials: effects of blood contamination, *J Endod* 20:159, 1994.

528. Torabinejad M, Hong CU, Lee SJ, et al: Investigation of mineral trioxide aggregate for root-end filling in dogs, *J Endod* 21:603, 1995.

529. Torabinejad M, Hong CU, McDonald F, Pitt Ford TR: Physical and chemical properties of a new root-end filling material, *J Endod* 21:349, 1995.

530. Torabinejad M, Hong CU, Pitt Ford TR, Kaiyawasam SP: Tissue reaction to implanted super-EBA and mineral trioxide aggregate in the mandible of guinea pigs: a preliminary report, *J Endod* 21:569, 1995.

531. Torabinejad M, Hong CU, Pitt Ford TR, Kettering JD: Cytotoxicity of four root end filling materials, *J Endod* 21:489, 1995.

532. Torabinejad M, Pitt Ford TR, McKendry DJ, et al: Histologic assessment of mineral trioxide aggregate as a root-end filling in monkeys, *J Endod* 23:225, 1997.

533. Torabinejad M, Rastegar AF, Kettering JD, Pitt Ford TR: Bacterial leakage of mineral trioxide aggregate as a root-end filling material, *J Endod* 21:109, 1995.

534. Torabinejad M, Smith PW, Kettering JD, Pitt Ford TR: Comparative investigation of marginal adaptation of mineral trioxide aggregate and other commonly used root-end filling materials, *J Endod* 21:295, 1995.

535. Torabinejad M, Watson TF, Pitt Ford TR: Sealing ability of a mineral trioxide aggregate when used as a root end filling material, *J Endod* 19:591, 1993.

536. Traub EF, Tennen JS: Permanent pigmentation following the application of iron salts, *JAMA* 106:1711, 1936.

537. Trent CS: Electrocautery versus epinephrine-injection tonsillectomy [see comment], *Ear Nose Throat J* 72:520, 1993.

538. Trombelli L, Kim CK, Zimmerman GJ, Wikesjo UM: Retrospective analysis of factors related to clinical outcome of guided tissue regeneration procedures in intrabony defects, *J Clin Periodontol* 24:366, 1997.

539. Trombelli L, Scabbia A: Healing response of gingival recession defects following guided tissue regeneration procedures in smokers and non-smokers, *J Clin Periodontol* 24:529, 1997.

540. Tronstad L, Barnett F, Cervone F: Periapical bacterial plaque in teeth refractory to endodontic treatment, *Endod Dent Traumatol* 6:73, 1990.

541. Tronstad L, Kreshtool D, Barnett F: Microbiological monitoring and results of treatment of extraradicular endodontic infection, *Endod Dent Traumatol* 6:129, 1990.

542. Trope M, Lost C, Schmitz HJ, Friedman S: Healing of apical periodontitis in dogs after apicoectomy and retrofilling with various filling materials, *Oral Surg Oral Med Oral Pathol Oral Radiol Endod* 81:221, 1996.

543. Trowbridge HO, Emling RC: *Inflammation: a review of the process*, ed 5, Chicago, 1997, Quintessence Books, p 1.

544. Tseng CC, Harn WM, Chen YH: A new approach to the treatment of true-combined endodontic-periodontic lesions by the guided tissue regeneration technique, *J Endod* 22:693, 1996.

545. Tsesis I, Fuss Z, Lin S, et al: Analysis of postoperative symptoms following surgical endodontic treatment, *Quintessence Int* 34:756, 2003.

546. Tsesis I, Rosen E, Schwartz-Arad D, Fuss Z: Retrospective evaluation of surgical endodontic treatment: traditional versus modern technique, *J Endod* 32:412, 2006.

547. Tsesis I, Rosen E, Tamse A, et al: Effect of guided tissue regeneration on the outcome of surgical endodontic treatment: a systematic review and meta-analysis, *J Endod* 37:1039, 2011.

548. Tyas MJ: Clinical evaluation of five adhesive systems, *Am J Dent* 7:77, 1994.

549. Uchin RA: Use of a bioresorbable guided tissue membrane as an adjunct to bony regeneration in cases requiring endodontic surgical intervention, *J Endod* 22:94, 1996.

550. Urist MR: Bone histogenesis and morphogenesis in implants of demineralized enamel and dentin, *J Oral Surg* 29:88, 1971.

551. Valmaseda-Castellon E, Berini-Aytes L, Gay-Escoda C: Inferior alveolar nerve damage after lower third molar surgical extraction: a prospective study of 1117 surgical extractions, *Oral Surg Oral Med Oral Pathol Oral Radiol Endod* 92:377, 2001.

552. Veis A: Mineral-matrix interactions in bone and dentin, *J Bone Miner Res* 8:S493, 1993.

553. Veis A, Sfeir C, Wu CB: Phosphorylation of the proteins of the extracellular matrix of mineralized tissues by casein kinase-like activity, *Crit Rev Oral Biol Med* 8:360, 1997.

554. Velvart P: Papilla base incision: a new approach to recession-free healing of the interdental papilla after endodontic surgery, *Int Endod J* 35:453, 2002.

555. Velvart P, Ebner-Zimmermann U, Ebner JP: Comparison of long-term papilla healing following sulcular full thickness flap and papilla base flap in endodontic surgery, *Int Endod J* 37:687, 2004.

556. Velvart P, Hecker H, Tillinger G: Detection of the apical lesion and the mandibular canal in conventional radiography and computed tomography, *Oral Surg Oral Med Oral Pathol Oral Radiol Endod* 92:682, 2001.

557. Velvart P, Peters CI: Soft tissue management in endodontic surgery, *J Endod* 31:4, 2005.

558. Vickers FJ, Baumgartner JC, Marshall G: Hemostatic efficacy and cardiovascular effects of agents used during endodontic surgery, *J Endod* 28:322, 2002.

559. Vigil GV, Wayman BE, Dazey SE, et al: Identification and antibiotic sensitivity of bacteria isolated from periapical lesions, *J Endod* 23:110, 1997.

560. Vignaroli PA, Anderson RW, Pashley DH: Longitudinal evaluation of the microleakage of dentin bonding agents used to seal resected root apices, *J Endod* 21:509, 1995.

561. Vishteh A, Thomas I, Imamura T: Eugenol modulation of the immune response in mice, *Immunopharmacology* 12:187, 1986.

562. Viswanathan HL, Berry JE, Foster BL, et al: Amelogenin: a potential regulator of cementum-associated genes, *J Periodontol* 74:1423, 2003.

563. Voigt JP, Goran ML, Flesher RM: The width of lingual mandibular attached gingiva, *J Periodontol* 49:77, 1978.

564. von Arx T: Failed root canals: the case for apicoectomy (periradicular surgery), *J Oral Maxillofac Surg* 63:832, 2005.

565. von Arx T, Gerber C, Hardt N: Periradicular surgery of molars: a prospective clinical study with a one-year follow-up, *Int Endod J* 34:520, 2001.

566. von Arx T, Jensen SS, Hanni S, Friedman S: Five-year longitudinal assessment of the prognosis of apical microsurgery, *J Endod* 38:570, 2012.

567. Vy C: Cardiovascular effects and efficacy of hemostatic agent in periradicular surgery, *J Endod* 30:379, 2004.

568. Wada M, Takase T, Nakanuma K, et al: Clinical study of refractory apical periodontitis treated by apicectomy. Part 1. Root canal morphology of resected apex, *Int Endod J* 31:53, 1998.

569. Wahl MJ: Dental surgery in anticoagulated patients, *Arch Intern Med* 158:1610, 1998.

570. Waldorf H, Fewkes J: Wound healing, *Adv Dermatol* 10:77, 1995.

571. Walia HD, Newlin S, Austin BP: Electrochemical analysis of retrofilling microleakage in extracted human teeth, *J Dent Res* 74:101, 1995.

572. Wallace JA: Transantral endodontic surgery, *Oral Surg Oral Med Oral Pathol Oral Radiol Endod* 82:80, 1996.

573. Walmsley AD, Lumley PJ, Johnson WT, Walton RE: Breakage of ultrasonic root-end preparation tips, *J Endod* 22:287, 1996.

574. Walsh WR, Morberg P, Yu Y, et al: Response of a calcium sulfate bone graft substitute in a confined cancellous defect, *Clin Orthop Relat Res* 406:2003.

575. Waltimo T, Kuusinen M, Jarvensivu A, et al: Examination on *Candida* spp. in refractory periapical granulomas, *Int Endod J* 36:643, 2003.

576. Walton RE: Iatrogenic maxillary sinus exposure during maxillary posterior root-end surgery, *Oral Surg Oral Med Oral Pathol Oral Radiol Endod* 97:3; author reply 3, 2004.

577. Wang N, Knight K, Dao T, Friedman S: Treatment outcome in endodontics—The Toronto Study. Phases I and II: apical surgery, *J Endod* 30:751, 2004.

578. Watters W 3rd, Rethman MP, Hanson NB, et al: Prevention of orthopaedic implant infection in patients undergoing dental procedures, *J Am Acad Orthop Surg* 21:180, 2013.

579. Watzek G, Bernhart T, Ulm C: Complications of sinus perforations and their management in endodontics, *Dent Clin North Am* 41:563, 1997.

580. Wayman BE, Murata SM, Almeida RJ, Fowler CB: A bacteriological and histological evaluation of 58 periapical lesions, *J Endod* 18:152, 1992.

581. Weinstein RS, Chen JR, Powers CC, et al: Promotion of osteoclast survival and antagonism of bisphosphonate-induced osteoclast apoptosis by glucocorticoids, *J Clin Investig* 109:1041, 2002.

582. Weinstein RS, Jilka RL, Parfitt AM, Manolagas SC: Inhibition of osteoblastogenesis and promotion of apoptosis of osteoblasts and osteocytes by glucocorticoids. Potential mechanisms of their deleterious effects on bone, *J Clin Investig* 102:274, 1998.

583. Wessel JH, Dodson TB, Zavras AI: Zoledronate, smoking, and obesity are strong risk factors for osteonecrosis of the jaw: a case-control study, *J Oral Maxillofac Surg* 66:625, 2008.

584. Weston GD, Moule AJ, Bartold PM: A comparison in vitro of fibroblast attachment to resected root-ends, *Int Endod J* 32:444, 1999.

585. Weston GD, Moule AJ, Bartold PM: A scanning electron microscopic evaluation of root surfaces and the gutta-percha interface following root-end resection in vitro, *Int Endod J* 32:450, 1999.

586. Wiggins KL, Malkin S: Drilling of bone, *J Biomech* 9:553, 1976.

587. Williams SS, Gutmann JL: Periradicular healing in response to Diaket root-end filling material with and without tricalcium phosphate, *Int Endod J* 29:84, 1996.

588. Wilson W, Taubert KA, Gewitz M, et al: Prevention of infective endocarditis: guidelines from the American Heart Association: a guideline from the American Heart Association Rheumatic Fever, Endocarditis and Kawasaki Disease Committee, Council on Cardiovascular Disease in the Young, and the Council on Clinical Cardiology, Council on Cardiovascular Surgery and Anesthesia, and the Quality of Care and Outcomes Research Interdisciplinary Working Group, *J Am Dent Assoc* 138:739, 2007.

589. Witherspoon DE, Gutmann JL: Haemostasis in periradicular surgery, *Int Endod J* 29:135, 1996.

590. Witherspoon DE, Gutmann JL: Analysis of the healing response to gutta-percha and Diaket when used as root-end filling materials in periradicular surgery, *Int Endod J* 33:37, 2000.

591. Wu MK, Kontakiotis EG, Wesselink PR: Long-term seal provided by some root-end filling materials, *J Endod* 24:557, 1998.

592. Wuchenich G, Meadows D, Torabinejad M: A comparison between two root end preparation techniques in human cadavers, *J Endod* 20:279, 1994.

593. Yaccino JM, Walker WA 3rd, Carnes DL Jr, Schindler WG: Longitudinal microleakage evaluation of Super-EBA as a root-end sealing material, *J Endod* 25:552, 1999.

594. Yagiela JA: Injectable and topical local anesthetics. In Ciancio SG, editors: *ADA guide to dental therapeutics*, ed 3, Chicago, 2003, American Dental Association, p 1.

595. Yajima A, Otonari-Yamamoto M, Sano T, et al: Cone-beam CT (CB Throne) applied to dentomaxillofacial region, *Bull Tokyo Dent Coll* 47:133, 2006.

596. Yao K, Chien M, Kohara O, et al: Effect of water isolation and early finishing on hardness of glass ionomer cements, *J Osaka Dent Univ* 24:141, 1990.

597. Yeomans JD, Urist MR: Bone induction by decalcified dentine implanted into oral, osseous and muscle tissues, *Arch Oral Biol* 12:999, 1967.

598. Young MP, Korachi M, Carter DH, et al: The effects of an immediately pre-surgical chlorhexidine oral rinse on the bacterial contaminants of bone debris collected during dental implant surgery, *Clin Oral Implants Res* 13:20, 2002.

599. Yucel EA, Oral O, Olgac V, Oral CK: Effects of fibrin glue on wound healing in oral cavity, *J Dent* 31:569, 2003.

600. Yusuf H: The significance of the presence of foreign material periapically as a cause of failure of root treatment, *Oral Surg Oral Med Oral Pathol* 54:566, 1982.

601. Zaman KU, Sugaya T, Hongo O, Kato H: A study of attached and oriented human periodontal ligament cells to periodontally diseased cementum and dentin after demineralizing with neutral and low pH etching solution, *J Periodontol* 71:1094, 2000.

602. Zetterqvist L, Hall G, Holmlund A: Apicectomy: a comparative clinical study of amalgam and glass ionomer cement as apical sealants, *Oral Surg Oral Med Oral Pathol* 71:489, 1991.

603. Zhang X, Schwarz EM, Young DA, et al: Cyclooxygenase-2 regulates mesenchymal cell differentiation into the osteoblast lineage and is critically involved in bone repair [erratum appears in *J Clin Invest* 110:1211, 2002], *J Clin Investi* 109:1405, 2002.

604. Zhu Q, Haglund R, Safavi KE, Spangberg LS: Adhesion of human osteoblasts on root-end filling materials, *J Endod* 26:404, 2000.

605. Zhu Q, Safavi KE, Spangberg LS: Cytotoxic evaluation of root-end filling materials in cultures of human osteoblast-like cells and periodontal ligament cells, *J Endod* 25:410, 1999.

606. Ziegler CM, Woertche R, Brief J, Hassfeld S: Clinical indications for digital volume tomography in oral and maxillofacial surgery, *Dentomaxillofac Radiol* 31:126, 2002.

607. Zubery Y, Kozlovsky A: Two approaches to the treatment of true combined periodontal-endodontal lesions, *J Endod* 19:414, 1993.

608. Zubillaga G, Von Hagen S, Simon BI, Deasy MJ: Changes in alveolar bone height and width following post-extraction ridge augmentation using a fixed bioabsorbable membrane and demineralized freeze-dried bone osteoinductive graft, *J Periodontol* 74:965, 2003.

609. Zuolo ML, Ferreira MO, Gutmann JL: Prognosis in periradicular surgery: a clinical prospective study, *Int Endod J* 33:91, 2000.

610. Zuolo ML, Perin FR, Ferreira MO, de Faria FP: Ultrasonic root-end preparation with smooth and diamond-coated tips, *Endod Dent Traumatol* 15:265, 1999.

CHAPTER 10

Regenerative Endodontics

ANIBAL DIOGENES | STÉPHANE SIMON | ALAN S. LAW

OVERVIEW OF REGENERATIVE DENTISTRY

Advancements in tissue engineering are dramatically changing medicine and dentistry. Tissue engineering is an interdisciplinary field that applies the principles of engineering and the life sciences to restoring, maintaining, or replacing biologic function.[127] It involves the interplay among stem cells, growth factors, and scaffolds (biologic matrices). It has become increasingly clear that the intentional manipulation of these three factors can lead to the regeneration of tissue function that would not otherwise occur if repair had taken place without intervention.[54] This relatively young field was first applied to medicine with many examples of regenerative medicine approaches used in the clinical practice.[125,188,240] Although the inclusion of tissue engineering in dentistry is more recent, it is also fundamentally changing the way clinicians are treating patients while providing a fertile research field that fosters future advancements and therapies.

Most of the history of dentistry is marked by the evolution of dental materials and techniques tailored to the replacement of lost or diseased tissues with inert materials. This prosthetic replacement of missing dental tissues has prevailed in dentistry since the primordial examples of dental treatments in ancient civilizations.[136,145,238] In contrast, the goal of regenerative dentistry is to induce biologic replacement of dental tissues and their supporting structures. The potential for regenerative dentistry is in large part due to advancements in biologic therapies that apply principles of tissue engineering with the spatial and temporal assembly of stem cells, growth factors, and scaffolds to achieve the functional regeneration of a missing tissue.

Pioneering work supporting the concept of regenerating dental tissues was reported in the 1960s when Dr. B.W. Hermann described the application of calcium hydroxide $(Ca[OH]_2)$ for vital pulp therapy[219] and Professor Nygaard-Østby evaluated a revascularization method for reestablishing a pulp-dentin complex in permanent teeth with pulpal necrosis (discussed later).[172,173] The scope and clinical application of regenerative dental procedures have advanced to now include guided tissue or bone regeneration (GTR, GBR) procedures and distraction osteogenesis,[32,133,175] the application of platelet-rich plasma for bone augmentation,[85] Emdogain for regeneration of periodontal tissues and pulp,[7,45] recombinant human bone morphogenic protein (rhBMP) for augmentation of bone,[4,151] and clinical trials on the use of fibroblast growth factor 2 (FGF-2) for periodontal tissue regeneration.[253] The potential of regenerative procedures in endodontics has been emphasized by elegant studies demonstrating the regeneration of pulp, dentin, and enamel using scaffold materials and stem cells.[81,107,210,265] Thus, regenerative dental procedures are emerging as a vital, evolving field of dental care, creating a paradigm shift in many dental specialties, including endodontics.[152] This chapter reviews the current status of regenerative endodontic procedures with an emphasis on biologic principles and the advantages and limitations of currently available clinical procedures.

Overview of Regenerative Endodontics

The developing dentition is at risk for pulpal necrosis due to trauma, caries, and developmental dental anomalies such as dens evaginatus.[13,16,122,144,220,225,260] Loss of an immature permanent tooth in young patients with mixed dentition can be devastating, leading to loss of function, malocclusion, and inadequate maxillofacial development. These teeth were traditionally treated with apexification procedures using either long-term calcium hydroxide treatment[53,52] or immediate placement of a mineral trioxide aggregate (MTA) apical plug.[247] Although these treatments often resolve the signs and symptoms of pathosis, they provide little to no benefit for continued root development.[33] Thus, immature teeth treated with these procedures are considered in a state of arrested development, and no further root growth, normal pulpal nociception, and immune defense should be expected.

Regenerative endodontic procedures (REPS) have been defined as biologically based procedures designed to replace damaged structures such as dentin, root structures, and cells of the pulp-dentin complex.[152] This new treatment modality has emerged as an alternative that, in addition to healing apical periodontitis, aims to promote normal pulpal physiologic functions. These include continued root development, immune competency, and normal nociception, as seen in some published cases.[62] Thus, the ultimate goal of these procedures is to regenerate the components and normal function of the pulp-dentin complex.

Regenerative endodontics is founded on the seminal work of Dr. Nygaard-Østby, completed in the 1960s. He hypothesized that a blood clot could be the first step in the healing of a damaged dental pulp, similar to the role of the blood clot in the healing process observed in other areas (e.g., alveolar bone following extraction).[171] To test the hypothesis that the presence of a blood clot within a root canal system promotes healing, mature teeth diagnosed with either vital or necrotic pulp received pulp space debridement followed by foraminal enlargement, medicament dressing for the necrotic cases, evoked intracanal bleeding, and a kloroperka obturation placed coronal to the formed blood clot. Patients (n = 17) were followed for various time periods (17 days to 3.5 years), and then the treated tooth was extracted and the newly formed tissues were histologically examined. The outcomes were similar for all teeth: (1) resolution of symptoms of inflammation related to foraminal enlargement and over-instrumentation in as early as 17 days; (2) resolution of signs and symptoms of pathosis for the necrotic cases; and, in certain cases, (3) radiographic evidence of apical closure. For the histologic analysis, it was observed that there was ingrowth of connective tissue into the canal space and varied levels of mineralized tissue found along the canal walls as well as "islands" of mineralized tissue embedded within the newly formed tissue (Fig. 10-1). Because dental pulp is a type of connective tissue with a rich supply of fibroblasts, this general finding was quite promising. However, the inclusion of undesired cell types (e.g., cementoblasts) and the lack of desired cell types (e.g., odontoblasts) indicate that this protocol did not lead to complete histologic regeneration of dental pulp. Despite its shortcomings, this pioneer study laid the foundation for the subsequent studies in the field of regenerative endodontics.

In 1966, a study was published reporting that disinfection could be established primarily with inter-appointment medication with polyantibiotic mixes (three different formulations used in five cases).[196] The investigators did not purposely evoke intracanal bleeding in this study, but instrumented canals short of what they thought to be vital tissue, determined by visualization of tissue and pain sensation upon instrumentation. Signs and symptoms of disease and continued root development were resolved for all reported cases. The study represented the first reported case in which polyantibiotic pastes were used in immature necrotic teeth for disinfection and to promote root development. Five years later, another study was published that included the use of antibiotics in the disinfection protocol and the intentional promotion of intracanal bleeding.[173] Resolution of symptoms and continued root development was a common finding. However, the histology of the extracted teeth demonstrated that connective tissue was formed in 28 out of 35 teeth, whereas cellular cementum was formed in 18 out of 35 teeth. Again, these protocols generated acceptable clinical outcomes (e.g., healing of apical periodontitis, lack of symptoms, etc.) with only partial evidence of dental pulp phenotype. Collectively, these findings laid the foundation for contemporary regenerative endodontics, demonstrating that repair could take place following root canal disinfection in immature teeth.

The first case report of a "contemporary" regenerative endodontic procedure occurred in 2001.[62] Since then, there has been an exponential increase in published cases reporting unprecedented clinical outcomes such as resolution of signs and symptoms of apical periodontitis, continued root development, and, in certain cases, normal nociceptive responses to vitality testing.[62] Despite the lack of randomized clinical trials, these published clinical observations support the hypothesis that patients with otherwise limited treatment options benefit from these procedures. Importantly, the field of regenerative endodontics has seen a dramatic increase in knowledge gained from translational basic science studies evaluating the interplay of the tissue engineering components (stem cells, growth factors, and scaffolds) applied to the clinical need and challenges.

PRECLINICAL STUDIES ON REGENERATIVE ENDODONTICS

Applying the principles of tissue engineering to the development of regenerative endodontic procedures requires research on the correct spatial assembly of distinct stem cells, growth factors/morphogens, and scaffolds to form a functional pulp-dentin complex.[95,107,127,161] In this section, we review each of these critical components in turn.

Stem Cells

Stem cells are defined as a distinct subpopulation of undifferentiated cells with self-renewal and differentiation potential. They can be classified as pluripotent or multipotent cells. Pluripotent stem cells have the capacity of becoming specialized cells and belong to all three germ layers. Embryonic stem cells are the best example of pluripotent cells. There is a significant body of research on embryonic stem cells, but ethical, legal, and medical (tissue-rejection) issues can render these cell types unsuitable for clinical applications.[152] True pluripotent stem cells can only be found in the developing embryo, and the harvesting of these cells requires destruction of the embryo, hence the legal and ethical concerns with such practice. Dr. Yamanka and colleagues reported the groundbreaking finding that somatic cells can be transformed into pluripotent stem cells—namely, induced pluripotent stem cells (iPSC).[177] The use of iPSCs does not have the same legal and ethical concerns as the use of embryonic stem cells, but iPSCs share the lack of control over their uninhibited proliferation and differentiation of embryonic stem cells. These cells tend to form teratomas after implanted into a host, a true testament of their high proliferative and differentiation capacities, but this makes them unsuitable for immediate common clinical practice.[177,221] On the other hand, all adult mesenchymal stem cells are more restricted in their capacity to differentiate, only forming tissues of mesenchymal origin, and therefore are classified as multipotent.[40] These cells can be found compartmentalized within tissues in "stem cell niches." The mesenchymal tissues (e.g.,

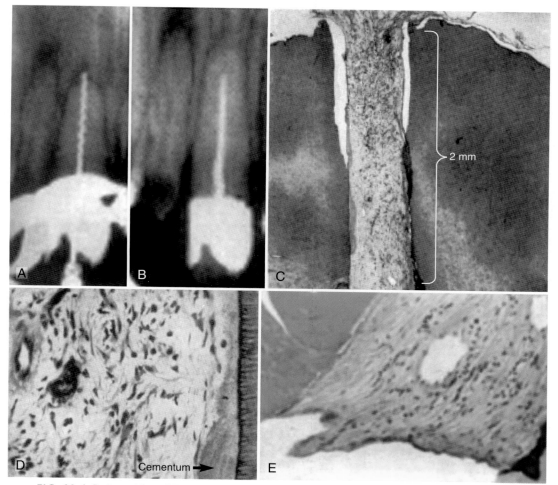

FIG. 10-1 Radiographic and histologic findings from a central incisor with a necrotic pulp, from Nygaard-Østby. **A,** Evidence of a file going beyond the apex. There is also evidence of a radiolucency in the apical area. **B,** Second radiograph at 14 months, taken shortly before tooth was extracted, showing the short fill. **C,** Histologic section of same tooth, showing fibrous connective tissue has grown into the apical 2 mm of the tooth. **D,** Higher magnification *(upper right)* shows evidence of what appears to be cementum deposition on the canal wall and fibrous connective tissue in the pulp space. **E,** Evidence of collagen bundles in the canal space. (From Nygaard-Østby B: The role of the blood clot in endodontic therapy: an experimental histologic study, *Acta Odontol Scand* 19:323, 1961.)

bone, dental pulp, periodontal ligament, etc.) appear to have an enriched population of adult stem cells.[40] These cells were first found in bone marrow decades ago and were characterized as self-renewing and plastic-adherent, and they formed cell colonies with a fibroblastic appearance.[79,80] They were initially called stromal stem cells but later received the now widely accepted name *mesenchymal stem cells (MSCs)*.[40] Most stem cells found in the orofacial region are MSCs.[66]

Different populations of adult stem cells have been identified in tissue compartments in the oral region. These include stem cells of the apical papilla (SCAP), inflammatory periapical progenitor cells (iPAPCs), dental follicle stem cells (DFSCs), dental pulp stem cells (DPSCs), periodontal ligament stem cells (PDLSCs), bone marrow stem cells (BMSCs), tooth germ progenitor cells (TGPCs), salivary gland stem cells (SGSCs), stem cells from human exfoliated deciduous teeth (SHED), oral epithelial stem cells (OESCs), gingival-derived mesenchymal stem cells (GMSCs), and periosteal derived stem cells

(PSCs) (Fig. 10-2).[66,132] Although stem cells have been identified in most oral tissues, the stem cells more likely to be involved in REPS are localized around the periapical region. These include SCAP, PDLSCs, BMSCs, iPAPCs, and DPSCs (if vital pulp is still present apically).

The apical papilla and its residing stem cells (SCAP) were first characterized in 2006.[223] The apical papilla (Fig. 10-3) is a dense reservoir of undifferentiated MSCs with great proliferative and odontogenic differentiation capacity.[104,197] Importantly, SCAP are regulated by Hertwig's epithelial root sheath through a series of complex epithelial-mesenchymal interactions that dictate root development and shape.[249] Further, the close proximity of the apical papilla to the apices of teeth in continuum with the root canal space makes this rich source of stem cells readily available for regenerative endodontic therapeutics. The IPAPCs represent another important potential source of stem cells for regenerative endodontics in teeth with well-established apical periodontitis.[132,141] Lastly, stem cells of the periodontal

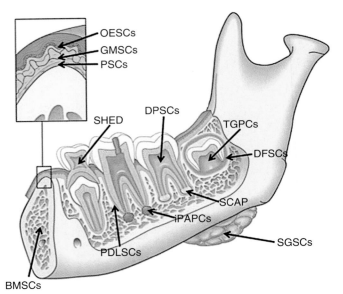

FIG. 10-2 Schematic drawing illustrating potential sources of postnatal stem cells in the oral environment. Cell types include tooth germ progenitor cells (TGPCS); dental follicle stem cells (DFSCS); salivary gland stem cells (SGSCS); stem cells of the apical papilla (SCAP); dental pulp stem cells (DPSCS); inflamed periapical progenitor cells (IPAPCS); stem cells from human exfoliated deciduous teeth (SHED); periodontal ligament stem cells (PDLSCS), bone marrow stem cells (BMSCS) and, as illustrated in the inset, oral epithelial stem cells (OESCS); gingival-derived mesenchymal stem cells (GMSCS); and periosteal stem cells (PSCS). (From Hargreaves KM, Diogenes A, Teixeira FB: Treatment options: biologic basis of regenerative endodontic procedures, *J Endod* 39:s30, 2013.)

ligament (PDL) and bone marrow should be also considered as stem cells sources for regenerative procedures because the action of mechanical disruption of the apical tissue (evoked bleeding) could also trigger the release of these cells, albeit their relative abundance is thought to be significantly less than SCAP and IPAPCs. In 2011, a study was conducted to evaluate the presence of mesenchymal stem cells following the evoked-bleeding step in regenerative procedures.[135] It was found that there is a substantial influx of mesenchymal stem cells into root canals during regenerative procedures resulting in an increase greater than 700-fold in the expression of MSC markers (Fig. 10-4). In addition, the cells could be harvested from clinical samples and examined under confocal microscopy (Fig. 10-5). This was the first demonstration that REPs are stem cell-based therapies.[62] Although this study did not evaluate whether the MSCs detected in REPs are derived from the apical papilla, it was assumed that these cells were SCAP because the evoked bleeding step lacerated the apical papilla. However, these MSCs are a heterogeneous population of cells that could come from any of the periradicular tissues after the mechanical step of evoking bleeding into the root canal system.

The delivery of substantial concentrations of MSCs into the root canal space, despite advanced apical periodontitis or abscess, points to an impressive survival capacity of these cells. In these clinical presentations, low oxygen tension, low pH, and a high concentration of endotoxins and inflammatory mediators are expected.[70,111,129,211] Indeed, the finding of high concentrations of the immune cell marker CD14 in those clinical samples indicates that there was still a substantial chronic inflammatory exudate present at the apical region of those teeth. These findings raise the question of how MSCs such as SCAP can survive during apical periodontitis where a complex microflora, an array of inflammatory mediators, immune cells, and presumably low oxygen tension are commonly encountered. The biologic reason for this apparent resilient survival,

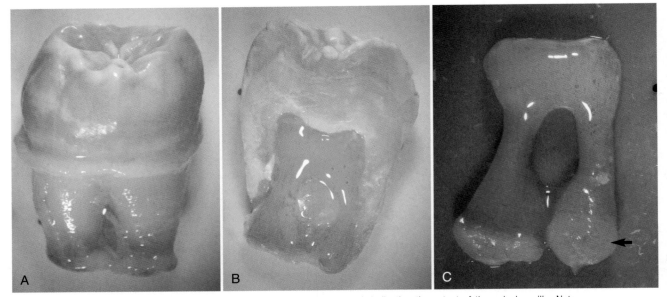

FIG. 10-3 A-C, Dissection of an immature permanent tooth indicating the extent of the apical papilla. Note that this structure is likely lacerated during the evoked bleeding step of revascularization cases and thus cells from this structure, including mesenchymal stem cells of the apical papilla (SCAP), are likely to be delivered into the root canal space. Arrow in C denotes junction of apical papilla and dental pulp. (Courtesy Dr. Michael Henry.)

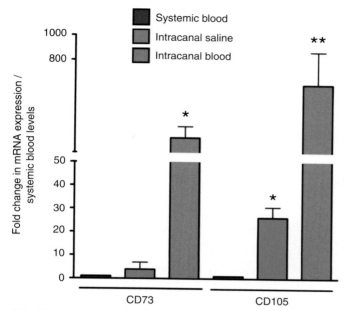

FIG. 10-4 Evoked-bleeding step in endodontic regenerative procedures in immature teeth with open apices leads to significant increase in expression of undifferentiated mesenchymal stem cell markers in the root canal space. Systemic blood, saline irrigation, and intracanal blood samples were collected during second visit of regenerative procedures. Real-time RT-PCR was performed by using RNA isolated from each sample as template, with validated specific primers for target genes and 18S ribosomal RNA endogenous control. Expression of mesenchymal stem cell markers CD73 and CD105 was upregulated after the evoked-bleeding step in regenerative procedures. Data were normalized to the housekeeping gene 18S levels and presented as mean ± standard deviation fold increase in relation to systemic blood levels for each gene and analyzed with one-way analysis of variance with Bonferroni post hoc test (n = 8; *$P < .05$; **$P < .01$; n.s., not statistically significant). (From Lovelace TW, Henry MA, Hargreaves KM, Diogenes A: Evaluation of the delivery of mesenchymal stem cells into the root canal space of necrotic immature teeth after clinical regenerative endodontic procedure, *J Endod* 37:133, 2011.)

despite challenging conditions, may be explained by the relatively low density of blood vessels in the apical papilla in comparison to the adjacent dental pulp, whereas the dental follicle surrounding the apical papilla is highly vascularized and may act as a capillary bed to supply nutrients to SCAP.[62] Indeed, the apical papilla was found to remain vital despite complete pulpal necrosis and advanced apical periodontitis in an animal model of endodontic infection.[169] Further, it has been demonstrated that hypoxic environments enhance the proliferation, survival, and angiogenic potential of dental stem cells.[5,19,57,106,201] Interestingly, similar enhancing effects were observed when dental stem cells were exposed to bacterial by-products such as endotoxin.[1] Thus, it appears that SCAP and surrounding stem cells are equipped to survive and maintain their potential for differentiation in adverse conditions such as apical periodontitis and apical abscesses. Nonetheless, stem cells delivered into root canals after bleeding is evoked from the periradicular tissues are likely from various apical sources or niches.

The dental pulp can be viewed as a core of innervated and vascularized loose connective tissue surrounded by a layer of odontoblasts. The major cell type of this core region

is the fibroblast. Together with blood vessels, lymphatics, and neurons, this core tissue is embedded in an extracellular matrix consisting of collagen and other fiber types (see also Chapter 12). Dental pulp stem cells (DPSCs) can be found throughout the dental pulp but are known to accumulate in the perivascular region and the cell-rich zone of Hohl adjacent to the odontoblastic layer.[75,205] Thus, DPSCs from both sources are thought to be active participants in the process of reparative dentinogenesis.

Dental pulp stem cells are recruited to the site of injury following a gradient of chemotactic agents released by resident immune cells and from the damaged dentin.[2,227] The reparative dentin formed by these cells is distinct from the primary, secondary, and reactionary dentin that has been lost.[8,159,259] It is often called "osteodentin" when found to be disorganized, atubular, and having cellular inclusions. This process of cellular repair is enhanced by bioactive materials (e.g., MTA and Biodentine). These materials increase the inherent mineralizing potential of the dental pulp when used in both indirect and direct pulp applications.[187] However, the process of tertiary dentinogenesis requires a vital pulp and the resolution of the etiology (e.g., caries or trauma). This process becomes disrupted when the pulp succumbs to injury, resulting in liquefaction necrosis of the dental pulp. Regeneration in this case is only possible with the recruitment or delivery of autologous stem cells to the canal space following adequate disinfection.[62]

Odontoblasts are one of the most specialized cells of the pulp dentin complex with dentinogenic, immunogenic, and possibly sensorial functions.[34,67,226] Odontoblasts in the intact pulp-dentin complex are easily identified based on their location and distinct morphologic characteristics (i.e., columnar polarized cell body with cellular projections into the dentinal tubules). However, it is far more challenging to identify and characterize an odontoblast-like cell, mainly because these cells lack a primary odontoblast morphology and unique markers that could be used for identification.[102] Indeed, many markers used for the identification of odontoblast-like cells are also expressed in other mineralizing cell types such as osteoblasts. For example, both odontoblasts-like cells and osteoblasts are similar in the formation of mineralized nodules and in the expression of several proteins such as dentin sialoprotein (DSP), although DSP levels are nearly 400 times greater in odontoblasts than in osteoblasts.[244] Measuring only one or two characteristics of a cell might not conclusively identify whether the cell is a true odontoblast. Even among odontoblasts, the phenotype varies in cells located in the apical (squamous shape) versus coronal (tall columnar) pulpal tissue. Importantly, molecular studies have identified many of the genes selectively expressed in odontoblasts.[134,178-180] Lastly, an intermediate filament protein called nestin has been shown to be preferentially expressed in odontoblasts or odontoblast-like cells when in the active secretory function. Nestin expression could be used in conjunction with other markers to better identify odontoblast-like cells.[3,4] This knowledge is expected to aid future studies characterizing the conditions necessary for mesenchymal cells of multiple origins to differentiate into odontoblast-like cells. It is likely that definitive cellular identification depends on both the morphology of the cell and an assessment of the expression of multiple genes.

At least five different types of postnatal mesenchymal stem cells, in addition to DPSCs, have been reported to differentiate

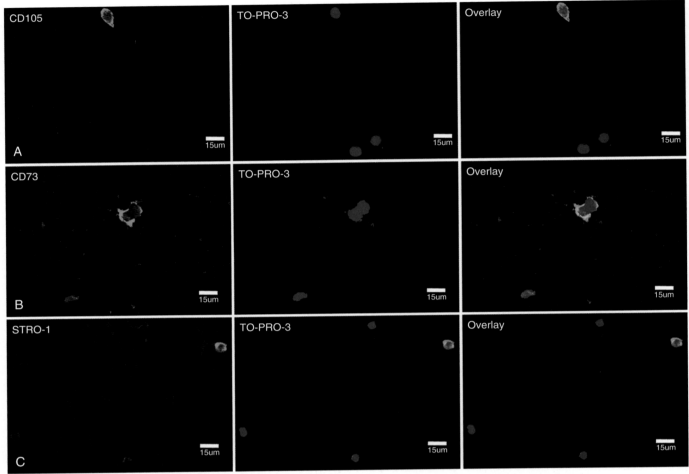

FIG. 10-5 Mesenchymal stem cells were delivered into root canal spaces during regenerative procedures in immature teeth with open apices. Cells collected from intracanal blood samples after the evoked-bleeding step or from systemic blood were stained with antibodies against CD105, CD73, or Stro-1 and evaluated with a laser-scanning confocal microscope. Cells in intracanal blood samples collected after the evoked-bleeding step showed expression of mesenchymal stem cell marker (**A**) and CD105 (green in **A**), CD73 (green in **B**), and STRO-1 (green in **C**), whereas nuclei appear blue as stained with TO-PRO-3. (From Lovelace TW, Henry MA, Hargreaves KM, Diogenes A: Evaluation of the delivery of mesenchymal stem cells into the root canal space of necrotic immature teeth after clinical regenerative endodontic procedure, *J Endod* 37:133, 2011.)

into odontoblast-like cells, including SHED,[147] SCAP,[124,125] IPAPCs,[132] DFPC,[149] and BMMSC.[22] One study demonstrated that over-instrumentation into the periradicular tissues followed by bleeding into the canal space results in a robust influx of cells with mesenchymal stem cell markers in fully mature teeth, similar to that seen in immature teeth.[135] Thus, it appears that MSCs from the apical region can be delivered into the root canal spaces in both immature and mature teeth. However, there is growing evidence that MSCs have decreased proliferative and differentiation potential with aging.[117,132,162] Further research is required to elucidate the age limit for the use of autologous dental-derived stem cells, but these findings suggest that regenerative procedures may be applicable to mature fully formed teeth in adults. In fact, in a proof-of-concept case report, resolution of apical periodontitis followed by narrowing of the canal space and apical closure was seen in two fully mature teeth in adult patients treated with regenerative endodontic procedures.[182] Thus, more research and development

is required to make regenerative procedures more predictable for immature teeth, and these procedures may transition to be applicable to fully formed teeth.

Growth Factors/Morphogens

Dentine is composed of collagen fibers (90%, collagen type I) and noncollagenous matrix molecules (proteoglycans, phosphoproteins, and phospholipids). The collagen fibers act as a grid or matrix, and this structure behaves as a scaffold upon which mineralization can occur. Dentine phosphoprotein (DPP) and dentine sialoprotein (DSP) are the most abundant dentine-specific proteins among the noncollagenous proteins of organic matrix.[38] DSP resembles other sialoproteins such as bone sialoprotein, but its precise function is still unclear; it may have a role in matrix mineralization.[92] Both DSP and DPP make up part of the small integrin-binding, ligand N-linked glycoproteins (SIBLINGS), which include dentine matrix acidic phosphoprotein 1 (DMP-1), bone sialoprotein,

TABLE 10-1

List of Growth Factors Found into the Mineralized Dentin Matrix

Growth Factors in Dentin Matrix	
Transforming growth factor beta-1 (TGFβ-1)	Cassidy et al., 1997[42]
Transforming growth factor beta-2 (TGFβ-2)	Cassidy et al., 1997[42]
Transforming growth factor beta-2 (TGFβ-3)	Cassidy et al., 1997[42]
Bone morphogenic protein –2 (BMP-2)	Thomadakis et al., 1999[230]
Bone morphogenic protein –4 (BMP-4)	About et al., 2000[4]
Bone morphogenic protein –7 (BMP-7)	Thomadakis et al., 1999[230]
Insulin growth factor-1 (IGF-I)	Finkleman et al., 1990[74]
Insulin growth factor-2 (IGF-II)	Finkleman et al., 1990[74]
Hepatocyte growth factor (HGF)	Tomson et al., 2013[232]
Vascular endothelial growth factor (VEGF)	Roberts-Clark and Smith, 2000[194]
Adrenomedullin (ADM)	Musson et al., 2010[155]

osteopontin, osteocalcin, and osteonectin. These proteins are only a small part of the whole cocktail of noncollagenous proteins that form components of the dentine.[87]

Research on dentine structure and composition has highlighted that the matrix contains some components that may be important in regulating tissue due to their bioactive properties. For this reason, dentine is today considered a reservoir of growth factors and cytokines.[212] These growth factors/cytokines are secreted by the odontoblasts during primary dentinogenesis, becoming sequestered and "fossilized" into the dentine after biomineralization (Table 10-1). However, they may become solubilized by demineralization of the matrix, bacterial acid (caries decay), chemical treatment (EDTA rinsing solution, calcium hydroxide or acid etching for bonded restorations), or restorative materials such as mineral trioxide aggregate and Biodentine.[213,231]

These growth factors and their receptors have been shown to be present at the enamel organ-dental papilla interface by immunohistochemistry and in situ hybridization during tooth development and have been implicated in odontoblast differentiation:

- Growth hormone (GH) plays a paracrine or autocrine role in dental development.[263]
- IGF-1 and -2 (of the family of IGF: insulin-like growth factor).[25,42,112]
- TGFβ-1, -2, and -3[56,228] and BMP-2, -4, and -6[239] play a role in the polarization and the differentiation of odontoblasts.[25] Notably in adult pulp, TGFβ-1 plays an important role in the regulation of the inflammatory response and tissue regenerative processes.[131]

The dental pulp has well recognized regenerative potential observed in the process of reparative dentinogenesis.[153,212] In this process, dentin-derived growth factors are thought to play a key role to be deciphered into the regulation of progenitor cell recruitment, cell proliferation, and differentiation of new dentine-secreting cells.[153,212] Indeed, the differentiation of new odontoblast-like cells has also been reported following pulp capping with basic fibroblast growth factor (FGF), TGF-β1,[131] and BMP-7.[86]

The sequestration of these growth factors in the dentine matrix and their subsequent "fossilization" during the mineralization process appears key to the pulp healing process where their release from the matrix may be responsible for various signaling events. These growth factors are extremely potent and have a variety of cell signaling properties. However, their precise localization in the dentine[214] and their various biologic roles remain to be elucidated.

It is possible to imagine opportunities for therapeutic stimulation, inducing a targeted release of these proteins. For example, treatment of dentin with EDTA solution has been shown to dissolve the mineral phase, liberating growth factors that orchestrate the stimulation of progenitors or stem cell differentiation.[216-218] Etching with orthophosphoric acid, used for conditioning the dentine in bonding procedures, also promotes demineralization of the dentine and liberation of biologic factors.[64,72] For a long time, calcium hydroxide has been used as a protective lining, especially beneath amalgams fillings, or as a canal disinfection medication. It has been shown to have the ability to release bioactive components from the dentine, including growth factors.[91] Unlike dentin-etching acids, which only have brief contact with the dentine, calcium hydroxide remains in place beneath restorations or in canals allowing for a gentle and continued dissolution, thus releasing growth factors; its action is prolonged and potentially controllable depending on the form of the product. Lastly, calcium hydroxide, a by-product of the use of MTA and Biodentine, appears to underlie release of bioactive dentin-derived growth factors by these two bioactive materials.[231] Thus, clinicians may take advantage of potent growth factors stored within dentin with the use of chemical treatments and materials that promote the release of these factors.

Morphogens

It is also important to clearly keep in mind that a second level of regulation exists during dental development (and thus during pulp regeneration process)—transcription factors. Notably, Msx1 is expressed in polarized preodontoblasts, whereas Msx2 is present in mature odontoblasts.[25] Protein and transcripts for Msx1 have been identified in the pulp mesenchyme at early stages of tooth development and their concentrations decreased at the bell stage.[49] The expression of these transcription factors is under the control of growth factors, and they can ultimately have broad-ranging effects. Significantly, BMP4 upregulates Msx1 and Msx2 expression. In turn, transcription factors regulate further growth factor expression; for example, Msx1 upregulates BMP4 synthesis in the mesenchyme, and Msx2 regulates Runx2 and osteocalcin gene expression during odontogenesis.[30,31]

Growth factors and transcription factors are central to the cascade of molecular and cellular events during tooth development and are responsible for many of the temporospatial morphologic changes observed in the developing tooth germ. For these reasons, they are also likely involved in the regeneration process.

It is also important to consider the nature of the signaling process between the injurious agent and the pulp cells. Bacteria and their toxins are key candidates in the direct stimulation of pulp cells.[65] Lipopolysaccharides (LPS) and other bacterial toxins initiate intrapulpal inflammatory processes by activation of Toll-like receptors (e.g., TLR4 activation by LPS).[65,226,242] Importantly, both progenitor and dental stem cells have been shown to express these receptors.[34,35] Thus, stem cells within the dental pulp or periradicular tissues are equipped to detect microorganisms. Exposure of these cells to microbial antigens has been shown to directly modulate the proliferation and differentiation potential of these cells.[34,46,139,213,237] Lastly, cytokines commonly found in the inflammatory milieu (including that of the dental pulp) have a profound effect on stem cells. For example, it has been shown that TNF-alpha stimulates differentiation of dental pulp cells toward an odontoblastic phenotype via MAP kinase pathway activation and p38 phosphorylation.[183,209] Therefore, stem cell fate within the dental pulp is ultimately dictated by a complex cascade of intracellular signaling pathways activated by agents released from microorganisms, dentin, and immune cells.

Interestingly, morphogens are not only naturally occurring factors found within teeth. Several growth factors have also been evaluated for their ability to trigger the differentiation of selected mesenchymal stem cell populations into odontoblast-like cells (Table 10-2). Interestingly, several case studies have

reported that patients taking long-term corticosteroids often present with dramatic reduction of the radiographic size of the pulp chamber and up to a fivefold increase in the thickness of the predentin layer.[164,165,248] Although these were medically complex patients (e.g., those experiencing renal failure) taking multiple drugs, the use of corticosteroids appeared to be associated with the observed increased activity of human odontoblasts. Further, these unexpected "side-effects" were also observed in a retrospective study evaluating the association of pulp calcifications and the long-term use of statins.[186] These incidental effects of commonly prescribed medications were further evaluated in translational studies that have extended this general observation by demonstrating that the application of dexamethasone or statins greatly increased the differentiation of human dental pulp cells into odontoblast-like cells.[102,176] This was particularly evident when dexamethasone was combined with 1,25-dihydroxyvitamin D_3.[102] Merely changing the composition of growth factors completely altered the differentiation of these cells, with the same population of cells able to express markers of odontoblasts, chondrocytes, or adipocytes, depending on their exposure to different combinations of growth factors.[244] Such findings emphasize the importance of growth factors in guiding the differentiation of these cells. Other studies have evaluated growth factors administered alone or in various combinations for promoting differentiation of odontoblast-like cells.

TABLE 10-2

Effects of Selected Growth Factors on the Differentiation of Odontoblast-Like Cells

Growth Factors	Cell Source	Phenotype	Condition	Authors
Dexamethasone	Human dental pulp	Odontoblast-like	In vitro × 8 weeks	Huang et al., 2006[102]
Dexamethasone and Vitamin D_3	Human dental pulp	Odontoblast-like	In vitro × 8 weeks	Huang et al., 2006[102]
Dexamethasone and Ascorbate-2-phosphate and β-Glycerophosphate	Human or rat dental pulp	Odontoblast-like	In vitro × 3 weeks	Wei et al., 2007[244] Zhang et al., 2005[266]
Insulin and Indomethacin and 3-Isobatyl-1-methylxanthine (IMBX)	Human dental pulp	Adipocyte	In vitro × 19 days	Wei et al., 2007[244]
Dexamethasone and Insulin and Ascorbate-2-phosphate and Sodium pyruvate and TGF-β1	Human dental pulp	Chondrocyte	In vitro × 8 weeks	Wei et al., 2007[130]
Growth/differentiation factor 11 (Gdf11)	Dental pulp	Odontoblast-like	In vitro/in vivo 10 days	Nakashima et al., 2004[75]
Simvastatin (statins)	Human dental pulp	Odontoblast-like	In vitro/in vivo	Okamoto et al., 2009[88]
LIM mineralization protein 1 (LMP-1)	Human dental pulp	Odontoblast-like	In vitro/in vivo	Wang et al., 2007[129]
Bone morphogenetic proteins	Dental pulp	Odontoblast-like	In vitro	Saito et al., 2004[99] Sloan et al., 2000[107] Chen et al., 2008[19]
TGF-β1-3	Rat/monkey dental pulp	Odontoblast-like	In vitro	Sloan et al., 1999[109]
Demineralized dentin	Human or rodent pulp	Odontoblast-like	In vitro/in vivo	Smith et al., 1990[111] Smith et al., 2001[110] Tziafas, 2004[123]
Nerve growth factor (NGF)	Immortalized apical papilla	Odontoblast-like	In vitro	Arany et al., 2009[11]
Fibroblast growth factor 2	Human dental pulp	Odontoblast-like	In vitro	He et al., 2008[43]
Dentin matrix protein 1	Rat dental pulp	Odontoblast-like	In vivo	Almushayt et al., 2006[1]

Several of the approaches using compounds later found to have growth factor–like effects have immediate clinical implications. First, it is unlikely that a single growth factor will result in maximal differentiation, so combinations of growth factors may be required for evaluation in clinical trials. Related to this point, many of the studied growth factors (e.g., dexamethasone, insulin) are drugs already approved for human use in other medical/dental applications. Second, the demonstration that statins promote the differentiation of an odontoblast-like phenotype suggests that patients clinically taking statins may also have narrowing of the pulp chamber space, similar to the findings previously described for corticosteroids. This would be an important future area of research. Third, clinicians have long used demineralized human bone to augment healing after surgical procedures.[190] Demineralized human bone is thought to contain a natural combination of appropriate growth factors and scaffolds, thereby providing an appropriate environment for osteoblast differentiation or function. Extending this concept, several research groups have demonstrated that demineralized human dentin has significant benefit for promoting the differentiation of odontoblast-like cells. Importantly, translational studies in regenerative endodontics have demonstrated that irrigation of dentin with 17% EDTA increases the survival of stem cells[105,142] and odontoblastic differentiation,[81,142] possibly due to the release of bioactive molecules from dentin.[215] Collectively these findings suggest that EDTA irrigation of the dentinal walls as part of an REP could improve clinical outcomes.

Scaffolds

An important component of tissue engineering is a physical scaffold.[160,245] Tissues are organized as three-dimensional structures, and appropriate scaffolding is necessary to (1) provide a spatially correct position of cell location and (2) regulate differentiation, proliferation, or metabolism while promoting nutrient and gaseous exchanges. Extracellular matrix molecules are known to control the differentiation of stem cells,[189,254] and an appropriate scaffold might selectively bind and localize cells, contain growth factors,[251,252] and undergo biodegradation over time.[261] Thus, a scaffold is far more than a simple lattice to contain cells, but instead can be viewed as the blueprint of the engineered tissue.

Scaffolds can be classified as either natural or synthetic. Examples of natural scaffolds include collagen,[103,159] glycosaminoglycans, hyaluronic acid (HA), demineralized or native dentin matrix,[24,93,158,236,255] and fibrin.[82] On the other hand, examples of synthetic scaffolds include poly-L-lactic acid (PLLA),[60] polyglycolic acid (PGA), polylactic-coglycolic acid (PLGA),[68] polyepsilon caprolactone,[256] hydroxyapatite/tricalcium phosphate,[11] bioceramics, and hydrogels such as self-assembly peptide hydrogels.[71,140] The great majority of currently published regenerative endodontic procedures involve evoked bleeding and the formation of a blood clot to serve as a scaffold.[62] Although it is relatively straightforward as it does not require ex vivo manipulation, this simplistic approach is not without challenges. The blood clot is often difficult to achieve, and it does not have many of the properties of the ideal scaffold. These properties include easy delivery, adequate mechanical properties, controllable biodegradation, and incorporation of growth factors.[82] In addition, the blood clot contains a great number of hematopoietic cells that eventually undergo cell death, releasing their toxic intracellular enzymes

into the microenvironment, which may be detrimental to stem cell survival.

Another approach for creating a scaffold involves the use of autologous platelet-rich plasma (PRP). It requires minimal ex vivo manipulation, being fairly easy to prepare in a dental setting. PRP is rich in growth factors, degrades over time, and forms a three-dimensional fibrin matrix.[17,18,109,174] Platelet rich fibrin (PRF) is an alternative to PRP, as it has a three-dimensional architecture conducive with stem cell proliferation and differentiation and contains bioactive molecules.[58,61] These autologous scaffolds have been used successfully in regenerative cases.[21,222,264,267] However, it should be emphasized that, despite their reported use, there are some drawbacks to their clinical use: the process requires collection of intravenous blood that can be challenging in children, the diversity and concentration of growth factors within PRP and PRF preparations are not controllable,[20,116,241] and they lack temporal degradation control and the mechanical strength to support a coronal restoration. Thus, despite some desirable characteristics, other scaffold alternatives to PRP and PRF should be carefully considered.

Hydrogels are a class of scaffolds composed of three-dimensional hydrophilic polymers that absorb water or tissue fluids up to several times their weight.[73,250] These water-swollen materials are easily injectable in their colloidal form, undergoing gelation by chemical (e.g., changes in pH and osmolarity) or physical (e.g., temperature change) cues. These materials are highly tunable, biocompatible, and can be designed to resemble naturally occurring extracellular matrices.[250] They are of particular interest for regenerative endodontics because they can be easily injected into narrow root canal spaces and can be modified to deliver chemotactic and angiogenic agents to drive stem cell homing and supportive angiogenesis.[62,89] Hydrogels made of self-assembly peptides (e.g., Puramatrix)[43] show great potential to be used in endodontic tissue engineering because their sequence includes short peptide sequences, similar to those naturally occurring in tissues, enhancing cell attachment and proliferation.[84]

Delivery System

Even with selection of the appropriate cell source, growth factors, and scaffold, the resultant mixture must be delivered in a spatially appropriate fashion into the space of the root canal system. For example, nearly all cells of the body are within 0.1 to 1 mm of a blood vessel in order to maintain adequate diffusion of oxygen and nutrients.[90,98] This represents a challenge still to be overcome in the currently performed regenerative endodontic procedures that recruit stem cells[135] to a canal space devoid of lateral vascularity and several millimeters away from apical blood vessels. If one were to inject cells, in a cell-based approach, along the entire coronal-apical extent of a root canal system, the majority of cells would be expected to succumb to tissue hypoxia. Interestingly, it has been demonstrated that under hypoxic conditions, stem cells proliferate faster and release greater levels of angiogenic factors such as vascular endothelial growth factor 1 (VEGF) that promote targeted angiogenesis into the engineered space.[19] Thus, an alternative approach would be to inject a scaffold with chemotactic factors into the root canal. This approach is called cell homing, as cells are attracted to the scaffold along with supportive blood vessels in a progressive manner[121]; instead of being abruptly delivered to an avascular space (i.e., similar to

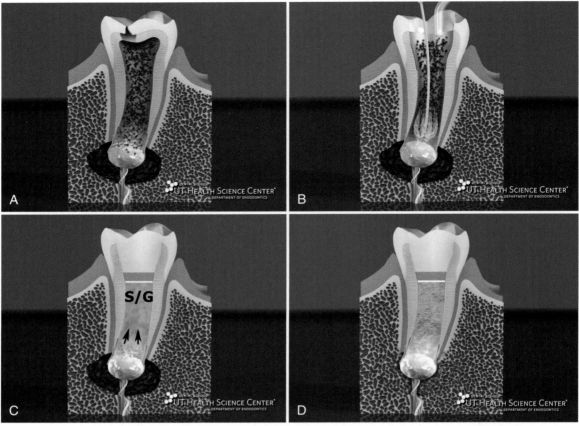

FIG. 10-6 Schematic drawing illustrating bioengineering using a cell homing approach. An immature premolar with a necrotic pulp and apical lesion (panel A) is disinfected (panel B), followed by placement of a biodegradable scaffold (s) containing growth factors and chemotactic factors (g) to allow progressive proliferation and migration of apical stem cells into the canal space (panel C) leading to the population of the canal space with stem cells concomitantly with vascular supply and tissue organization (panel D). (From Diogenes A, Henry MA, Teixeira FB, Hargreaves KM: An update on clinical regenerative endodontics, *Endod Topics* 28:2, 2013.)

the current revascularization procedures), the cell-homing approach can be applied in a cell-free[83] (no cells implanted along the chemotactic factors, see Fig. 10-6) or cell-based approach (cells are delivered in the chemotactic-containing scaffold).[152] Because dental pulp can be approximated as a loose connective tissue core surrounded by a layer of odontoblasts, the spatial arrangement of cells and growth factors within the scaffold may be particularly important to promote odontogenesis without having complete calcification of the root canal system. Complete recapitulation of the pulp-dentin complex architecture requires additional research effort.

Translational Studies

Several elegant studies in regenerative endodontics have used various translational methodologies including evaluation of clinical samples,[135] organotypic root canal models,[142,235] tooth slice models,[60,88,102] whole tooth culture, and animal models.[81,119,121,162,229,243] These studies have been crucial to provide a strong scientific foundation for the field of regenerative endodontics while allowing for clinical treatment protocol optimization and the development of new treatment strategies such as inclusion of scaffold and growth factors in regenerative procedures.[71,157]

One study demonstrated that new dentin and pulplike tissue could be generated in human root segments implanted subcutaneously in immune-compromised mice.[130] In this study, root segments had one of the openings sealed with MTA to mimic the coronal restoration of regenerative endodontic cases. The canal space was filled with either SCAP or DPSCs in a PLGA-based scaffold. The implants were harvested 3 months later and processed for immunohistochemical analysis. The results indicated that there was a dramatic circumferential apposition of dentin-like material along the dentinal walls. The new mineralized tissue was lined with polarized cells expressing odontoblastic markers. In addition, the dentin-like tissue was largely atubular and displayed cellular inclusions similar to the histologic presentation of osteodentin. Importantly, the cells from the engineered pulp were positive for human mitochondria, demonstrating that they originated from the implanted human stem cells and not from the host (mouse). Lastly, the root segments that were implanted without stem cells had only connective tissue that did not resemble a pulplike tissue, nor did it have mineralized tissues and odontoblast-like cells. Thus, a pulp-dentin complex could be engineered in human roots implanted subcutaneously in immune-deficient mice.

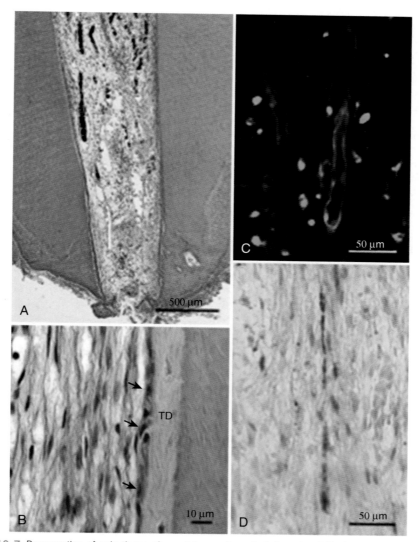

FIG. 10-7 Regeneration of pulp tissue after autologous transplantation of mobilized dental pulp stem cells (MDPSCs) with G-CSF in pulpectomized teeth of young dogs on day 14. **A-B,** Regenerated pulp tissue. **B,** Odontoblastic cells *(black arrows)* lining to newly formed osteodentin/tubular dentin (TD) along with the dentin. **C,** Immunohistochemical staining of BS-1 lectin. **D,** Immunohistochemical staining of PGP9.5. (From Nakashima M, Iohara K: Mobilized dental pulp stem cells for pulp regeneration, *J Endod* 40:S29, 2014.)

Nakashima and colleagues accomplished complete pulpal regeneration in dogs.[107] In this elegant study, dental pulp was removed via a sterile pulpectomy procedure, followed by placement of sorted CD105+ DPSCs in a collagen gel to the mid-root. The remaining coronal part of the canal was back-filled with the collagen gel containing the chemotactic factor stromal derived factor 1 (SDF-1). Subsequent histology demonstrated the formation of new pulp tissue with innervation, vascularization, and odontoblast-like cells lining the dentinal walls. In addition, the engineered pulp had protein and RNA expression similar to the native dental pulp.[107]

In another important study, mobilized DPSCs were generated by selecting DPSCs that migrated toward a concentration gradient of granulocyte-colony stimulating factor (G-CSF).[108,150,163] These selected cells were implanted in a collagen gel into pulpectomized root canals.[108] Complete pulpal regeneration was observed, with evidence of new dentin formation, blood vessels, and innervation in the engineered tissue

(Fig. 10-7). The impressive results of this cell-based approach have laid the foundation for the use of this technology in emerging clinical trials.[163]

It is noteworthy that all of the demonstrations of pulp regeneration in animal models were in root canals without any history of infection and pulpal necrosis.[107,108,130,159,200] Previously infected root canals must be adequately disinfected in order to suppress chronic inflammation that is detrimental to regeneration.[48] However, many irrigants and medicaments have detrimental effects on stem cell survival and differentiation.[63] Several studies using organotypic root canal models and animal models evaluated the combination and concentrations of irrigants and medicaments that allowed for stem cell proliferation and differentiation.[81,142,235] Thus, adequate disinfection and resolution of inflammation appears to be a limiting factor in complete pulpal regeneration, despite exciting results from current advances in dental pulp tissue engineering.

Summary of Basic Research on Regenerative Endodontics

Regeneration of a functional pulp-dentin complex relies on the foundation of tissue engineering and can be viewed as a function of the spatially correct delivery of appropriate stem cells and growth factors embedded within a scaffold. Although considerable research has used in vitro cell-culture methods to identify key factors regulating the differentiation of odontoblast-like cells, emerging studies conducted in animal models are promising for regeneration of this pulp tissue. Preclinical studies involving surgical placement of a human tooth filled with a human stem cell/growth factor/scaffold combination into immunocompromised mice[119,130] have permitted histologic analysis of neovascularization as well as the differentiation and mineralization activity of newly formed odontoblasts. The use of human cells in a mouse model permits histologic confirmation that the resulting odontoblast-like cells were of human origin. These novel findings provide strong evidence that either human SCAP or DPSC cell sources, on a PLGA scaffold, were able to regenerate a vascularized tissue that had histologic evidence of odontoblast-like cell differentiation and the spatially appropriate formation of dentin-like material onto the root canal walls. Although no specific growth factors were added to this mixture, it is important to note that the root canal walls were treated with 17% EDTA, an irrigant known to expose endogenous growth-factor proteins embedded in the dentinal walls.[268] This and other related studies provide strong impetus for clinical translational research evaluating various potential regenerative endodontic therapies.

CLINICAL STUDIES ON REGENERATIVE ENDODONTICS

To date, most case reports, case series, and retrospective studies published in regenerative endodontic have not fully incorporated the tissue-engineering concepts described. Instead, most of these reports present cases with variations of revascularization techniques.[62] These procedures were initially performed empirically with a strong focus on disinfection and the intentional bleeding into the root canal. However, it became obvious that these were in fact stem-cell based procedures with all three components of the tissue engineering triad present: stem cells,[135] growth factors,[26] and scaffolds.[23,234] Important preclinical studies previously described in this chapter have provided the foundational framework for a paradigm shift. This shift represents a clear departure from the traditional "disinfect the canals at all cost" to "disinfect while creating a microenvironment conducive for tissue engineering." Varied terminologies have been given to these procedures, including *revascularization*,[23] *revitalization*,[234] and *maturogenesis*.[6,101,115] Of these terms, the most popularly used has been *revascularization*. This term is largely based on the trauma literature observation that immature teeth could become *revascularized* after trauma. However, *revascularization* is a term better used for the reestablishment of the vascularity of an ischemic tissue, such as the dental pulp of an avulsed tooth. From this perspective, a focus on revascularization would ignore the potential importance of growth factors and scaffolds that are required for histologic recapitulation of the pulp-dentin complex. Although we appreciate that angiogenesis and the establishment of a functional blood supply are key requirements in the

maintenance and maturation of a regenerating tissue, it is noteworthy that some of the published cases report positive responses to pulp sensitivity tests such as cold or electric pulp tests.[62] This is evidence that a space that was previously vacant (debrided root canal) may become populated with an innervated tissue supported by vascularity. Taken together, the core concepts of tissue engineering distinguish a regenerative treatment philosophy from a revascularization philosophy derived from certain trauma cases (which only occur in a low percentage of replanted teeth). Lastly, a number of procedures have been performed with intentional manipulation of the principles of tissue engineering such as use of autologous platelet-rich plasma (PRP),[234] platelet-rich fibrin (PRF),[208] and exogenous growth factors and scaffolds.[157] Thus, instead of using different terms for each variant of these procedures, we will refer to them simply as regenerative endodontic procedures (REPS), which include past, present, and future procedures that aim for the functional regeneration of the pulp dentin–complex.

Clinical Procedures Related to Regenerative Endodontics

Clinicians face several challenges when presented with an incompletely formed root in need of endodontic treatment.[62] Because the apex is not fully developed and often has a blunderbuss shape, cleaning and shaping of the apical portion of the root canal system can be difficult. The process is further complicated by the presence of thin, fragile dentinal walls that may be prone to fracture during instrumentation or obturation. In addition, the open apex increases the risk of extruding material into the periradicular tissues. Traditionally, an immature tooth with an open apex is treated by apexification, which involves creating an apical barrier to prevent extrusion. In many cases, this entails an involved, long-term treatment with $Ca(OH)_2$, resulting in the formation of a hard-tissue apical barrier.[50-52,78,77,96,97,247] However, a disadvantage of the traditional apexification procedures is that the short-term[195] or long-term[14,15,257,258] use of $Ca(OH)_2$ has the potential to reduce root strength.[14,257,258] This finding is consistent with a large case series using the traditional apexification protocol; it showed that a major reason for tooth loss following apexification was root fracture.[53] In a retrospective study, the use of calcium hydroxide in apexification procedures resulted in the fracture of 23% of the teeth treated during the follow-up period of up to 18 months.[110] The advent of one-step apexification, by the creation of artificial barriers using materials such as MTA,[146,181,233] has greatly decreased the number of appointments and time to completion. Importantly, one-step apexification has been shown to have as high a success rate as apexification with calcium hydroxide in resolving apical periodontitis (both symptoms and radiographic presentation).[247] However, apexification procedures do not generally result in further root development. A primary advantage of regenerative endodontic procedures in these cases is the greater likelihood there will be an increase in root length and root wall thickness, in addition to the possibility that the patient will regain vitality responses.

There have been numerous published cases of regenerative endodontic procedures. Investigators and clinicians have used a variety of medicaments to disinfect the canal space.[62] Approximately 51% of the cases included the use of a triple antibiotic paste (a 1:1:1 mixture of ciprofloxacin/

metronidazole/minocycline), whereas 37% used $Ca(OH)_2$ as an intracanal medicament.[62]

The development of the triple antibiotic paste was led in large part by Hoshino and colleagues.[100,202] They demonstrated the effectiveness of combinations of antibiotics (and in particular the high efficacy of the combination of ciprofloxacin, metronidazole, and minocycline) in eradicating bacteria from the infected dentin of root canals.[202] Astute practitioners realized that the triple antibiotic paste could be a valuable adjunct for revascularization procedures, because it could be used to create an environment favorable for the ingrowth of vasculature and regenerative cells by reducing or eradicating bacteria in the canal space of teeth with necrotic pulps and incompletely formed apices. The efficacy of the triple antibiotic paste in disinfecting necrotic root canal systems has been demonstrated in a preclinical model.[246] In this dog study, 60 teeth were accessed and infected by sealing dental plaque and sterile saline on a cotton pellet into the pulp chamber for 6 weeks. By the end of this period, each premolar was radiographically confirmed to have apical periodontitis. The canals were then sampled at three time points: before and after irrigation with 1.25% NaOCl, and 2 weeks after the delivery of the triple antibiotic paste into the root canal system using a Lentulo spiral. Before irrigation, all of the teeth had positive cultures for anaerobic bacteria, with a mean colony-forming unit (CFU) count of $1.7 \times 10.^8$ After irrigation with 1.25% NaOCl, 10% of the teeth sampled cultured bacteria free. The mean CFU count was 1.4×10^4, or an approximate 10,000-fold reduction in viable bacteria. After dressing with the triple antibiotic paste for 2 weeks, 70% of the teeth sampled cultured bacteria free. The mean CFU count was only 26, which is about another 1000-fold drop in bacteria. These findings were confirmed in another related dog study.[229] This study provides strong support for the effectiveness of triple antibiotic paste in disinfection of immature teeth with apical periodontitis.

As stated previously, calcium hydroxide has been the second most used intracanal medicament in published cases. This application represents a new use of a long established intracanal medicament in endodontics. Although $Ca(OH)_2$ appears to be less effective against some intracanal bacterial species than antibiotic paste formulations,[199] its use is associated with lower cytotoxicity to stem cells,[126,198] release of important bioactive growth factors from the treated dentin,[94] and greater survival and proliferation of stem cells in the presence of the conditioned dentin.[167] Also, the relatively short-term use of this medicament in regenerative procedures does not appear sufficient to reduce fracture resistance.[258] Another factor to consider when choosing an intracanal medicament is the ability to remove the medicament from the canal space. One study that addressed this question incorporated radioactive tracers in both calcium hydroxide paste (Ultracal, Ultradent, Inc.) and triple antibiotic paste (Champs Pharmacy, San Antonio, TX).[28] The radiolabeled medicaments were placed in extracted teeth with standardized root canals. After 28 days of incubation, canal spaces were irrigated with a standardized protocol using different techniques. Surprisingly, greater than 80% of the triple antibiotic paste could not be removed from the tooth (Fig. 10-8), and it was found not in the canal lumen, but greater than 350 μm into the dentinal tubules. In contrast, greater than 80% of calcium hydroxide was removed (see Fig. 10-8) with the remaining medicament present superficially within dentin.[28] This is an important finding, given that drugs

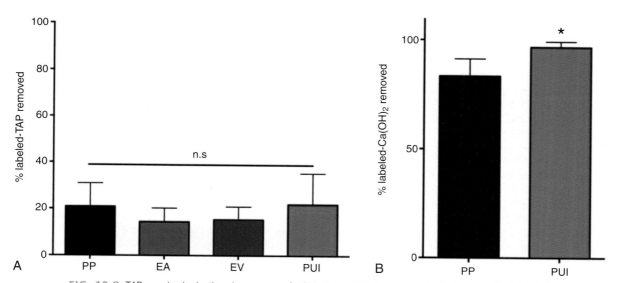

FIG. 10-8 TAP remains in dentin, whereas most $Ca(OH)_2$ is eliminated after endodontic irrigation. Radiolabeled TAP or $Ca(OH)_2$ was placed within canals of standardized root segments and incubated for 28 days at 37° C. The canals were flushed with standardized volumes of EDTA and saline using either positive pressure with a side-vented needle (PP) or positive pressure with ultrasonic activation of irrigants (PUI). There was no difference in labeled TAP removal among groups with only approximately 20% of the medicament being removed by the irrigation protocols **(A)**. In contrast, > 80% of $Ca(OH)_2$ was removed, with more efficient removal observed in canals irrigated with PUI **(B)**. Data are presented as the mean percentage of total radiolabeled medicament removal ± standard error of the mean. *P < .05 tested by the Student t test (n = 12/group). (Modified with permission from Berkhoff JA, Chen PB, Teixeira FB, Diogenes A: Evaluation of triple antibiotic paste removal by different irrigation procedures, J Endod 40:1172, 2014.)

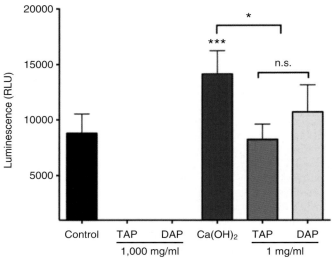

FIG. 10-9 Dentin conditioning for 7 days with medicaments used in REPs has a profound effect on SCAP survival. Standardized dentin disks were treated for 7 days with TAP or double antibiotic paste (DAP) (concentrations of 1000 mg/mL or 1 mg/mL), Ca(OH)$_2$ (Ultracal), or sterile saline (control). SCAP in a Matrigel scaffold (BD Biosciences, Bedford, MA) was seeded into the lumen of the disks after the medicaments were removed and cultured for 7 days. Cell viability (survival) was determined using a luminescent assay. SCAP culture on dentin treated with TAP or DAP at the concentration of 1000 mg/mL resulted in no viable cells. Conversely, dentin conditioning with TAP or DAP at the concentration of 1 mg/mL supported cell viability with no difference from untreated dentin disks (control). Greater survival and proliferation were detected in the group treated with Ca(OH)$_2$. Data are presented as mean ± standard deviation of relative luminescence units ($n = 12$/group). *$P < .05$. ***$P < .001$. n.s., no statistical difference as tested by 1-way analysis of variance. (From Althumairy RI, Teixeira FB, Diogenes A: Effect of dentin conditioning with intracanal medicaments on survival of stem cells of apical papilla, *J Endod* 40:521, 2014.)

remaining within dentin are likely to have an effect on the fate of stem cells in contact with the treated dentin. One study revealed that triple antibiotic paste (TAP), when used at concentrations typically used in case reports (1 g/mL) and removed with standardized irrigation protocol, resulted in no SCAP survival.[9] In contrast, dentin treated with calcium hydroxide promoted SCAP survival and proliferation, and dentin treated with TAP at a 1 mg/mL had no effect on SCAP survival (Fig. 10-9). Thus, clinicians must carefully evaluate the advantages and disadvantages of each intracanal medicament while observing the ideal therapeutic concentration.[63]

Regardless of the intracanal medicament used, regenerative endodontic procedures have common features. Most of these published procedures reported minimal to no instrumentation.[62] This might be due, at least in part, to the concern of further weakening fragile dentinal walls and the difficulty of mechanically debriding canals of such large diameters. Because of the lack of mechanical debridement, clinicians relied on copious irrigation for maximum antimicrobial and tissue dissolution effects.[62] Canals were then medicated for a period that varied from days to several weeks. At the second visit, if signs and symptoms of disease had subsided, the medicament was removed, the canal was dried, and intracanal bleeding was evoked in most, but not all, cases.[62] In most cases, a coronal

plug of MTA was placed over the blood clot or a collagen-based internal matrix, followed by a bonded coronal restoration. Each of these steps will be discussed later in light of the current American Association of Endodontists (AAE) considerations for REPs.

Overview of Clinical Regenerative Endodontic Procedures (REPS)

To date, most published clinical studies on REPS are composed of case reports and case series, with only one retrospective cohort study[110] and one prospective randomized clinical trial[157] on regenerative endodontics treatment available; no randomized controlled clinical trials have been published. Although case series do not provide definitive evidence to support a given treatment modality, they do have the advantage of being conducted on actual patients and thus provide a higher level of evidence than do preclinical studies. Although techniques for regenerative endodontics have varied in published case reports and case series,[62] there have been some consistent features worth noting. Nearly all reported cases involve patients 8 to 18 years old and teeth with immature apices with the exception of two published cases performed in mature, fully formed teeth.[182] Thus, the patient age appears to be an important factor in case selection because some studies suggest that younger patients have a greater healing capacity or stem cell regenerative potential.[10,12,55,128,154] Another important factor related to age is the stage of root development, because the large diameter of the immature (open) apex may foster the ingrowth of tissue into the root canal space and may indicate a rich source of mesenchymal stem cells of the apical papilla (SCAP; see Fig. 10-3).[104,197,224] These tissues are likely lacerated during the evoked bleeding step and constitute a likely source of mesenchymal stem cells delivered into the root canal space.[135] Another consistent finding reported in nearly every case is the lack of instrumentation of the dentinal walls related to concerns about the potential fracture of these thin, incompletely developed roots. The lack of instrumentation would be expected to have the benefit of avoiding generation of a smear layer that could occlude the dentinal walls or tubules. On the other hand, the lack of instrumentation could result in remaining bacterial biofilms within dentinal tubes. This is an issue that has not been evaluated in many cases, but the lack of canal wall instrumentation (and subsequent identification of bacteria in the apical dentin) has been suggested as a reason for failure of a regeneration case.[183] Nonetheless, these procedures are marked by robust disinfection protocols. Sodium hypochlorite, either alone or in combination with other irrigants, has been used to disinfect the canal space in most cases. In a majority of cases, a combination of triple antibiotic (minocycline, metronidazole, and ciprofloxacin) was left in the canal space for a period of days to weeks, so the disinfection protocol was primarily a chemical method rather than the chemomechanical approach used in conventional nonsurgical endodontic therapy.[62] In most cases, a blood clot formed in the canal.[62] The formation of a blood clot might serve as a protein scaffold, permitting the three-dimensional ingrowth of tissue.

Nearly all of these reports noted continued thickening of the root walls and subsequent apical closure. Examples of increased root length and thickening of root walls following regenerative endodontic procedures are seen in Figs. 10-10 through 10-13. Because of the lack of histology in most clinical

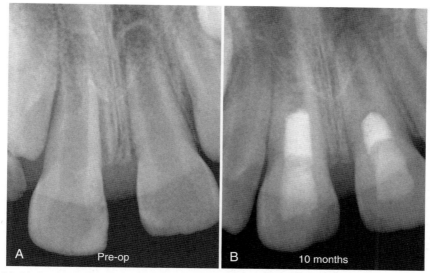

FIG. 10-10 Revascularization case illustrating treatment delivered to a 9-year-old male patient with a diagnosis of pulpal necrosis secondary to trauma, with a class 3 fracture in tooth #8 and a class 2 fracture in tooth #9 (A). The patient reported moderate to severe pain in both teeth. The teeth were isolated, accessed, and irrigated with 5% sodium hypochlorite, followed by placement of a mixture of ciprofloxacin, metronidazole, and minocycline for 55 days. Upon recall, the teeth were isolated, and the triple antibiotic paste was removed by irrigation. Bleeding was established in tooth #9 but not in tooth #8, where CollaCote was placed prior to mineral trioxide aggregate (MTA). The root canal systems were sealed with white MTA and a composite restoration (B). (Courtesy Dr. Alan Law.)

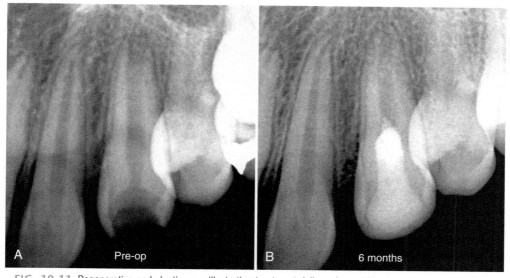

FIG. 10-11 Regenerative endodontic case illustrating treatment delivered to a 13-year-old female patient with a diagnosis of pulpal necrosis secondary to caries, with an unspecified prior history of trauma (A). The tooth was isolated, accessed, and irrigated with 5% sodium hypochlorite, followed by placement of a mixture of ciprofloxacin, metronidazole, and minocycline for 21 days. Upon recall, the tooth was isolated, and the triple antibiotic paste was removed by irrigation. Bleeding was established in both teeth, and the root canal system was sealed with white mineral trioxide aggregate and a composite restoration (B). (Courtesy Dr. Alan Law.)

cases, it should be recognized that radiographic findings of continued root wall thickness do not necessarily indicate that dentin was formed. Based on histologic results from preclinical studies, it is possible that the radiographic appearance of increased root wall thickness might be due to the ingrowth of cementum, bone, or a dentin-like material. Histologic evidence from human extracted teeth following REPS suggests that regenerated pulp tissue may be in the canal space,[123,206] and that the mineralized tissue along the dentinal walls appears to be cementum-like or osteodentin.[143,207] It should also be noted that in some of the case reports,[11,118] although the teeth were nonresponsive to pulp testing, the authors suggested that vital tissue was identified in the apical portion of the canal space. In these cases, necrotic tissue was removed until bleeding was

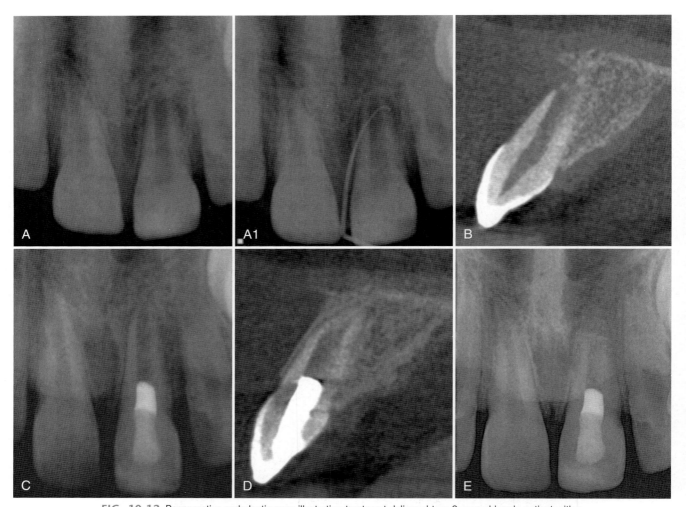

FIG. 10-12 Regenerative endodontic case illustrating treatment delivered to a 9-year-old male patient with a diagnosis of pulpal necrosis secondary to trauma and periradicular chronic apical abscess on tooth #9 seen on preoperative periapical radiograph (**A**) and CBCT (**B**). The patient was asymptomatic and has draining facial sinus tract. The tooth was treated with a regenerative procedure using double antibiotic paste (DAP), a mixture of ciprofloxacin and metronidazole for 1 month. At the second appointment, the sinus tract had resolved. Then, the tooth was isolated, and the double antibiotic paste was removed by irrigation with 20 mL 17% EDTA. Intracanal bleeding was evoked from the apical tissues using a precurved #25 hand-file extending approximately 2 mm beyond the root apex. A Collaplug barrier was placed at the midroot level, then covered with 3 mm white MTA. Fuji II LC glass ionomer was used as a coronal seal of the MTA. The access was then restored with a composite resin and polished (**C**). At the 1-year follow-up, the patient was asymptomatic, responsive to electrical pulp test (EPT), periodontal probings were no greater than 3 mm, and the tooth exhibited grade I mobility without coronal discoloration. Importantly, there was appreciable root maturation in addition to resolution of apical radiolucency seen on CBCT (**D**) and periapical radiograph (**E**). (Courtesy Dr. Obadah Austah.)

observed, then the canals were disinfected with antibiotic paste or Ca(OH)$_2$.[62] One could argue that by leaving vital pulp tissue in the apical segment of the canal, the resulting progression of root formation is more similar to apexogenesis than revascularization. Although the biologic process may differ between the revascularization and apexogenesis cases presented in these case reports, the goals of the procedures are similarly advantageous and significant. In both procedures, there is healing of the periradicular tissues and a progression of root development in a tooth that would otherwise have had a progression of pulpal and periradicular pathosis.

A retrospective study has compared the radiographic changes in 48 revascularization cases to 40 control cases.[33]

Although published revascularization cases have been treated with varying clinical protocols, they can be grouped by method of canal disinfection—namely, triple antibiotic paste, Ca(OH)$_2$ treatment, or formocresol treatment. This study applied a mathematical image-correction procedure that permitted the comparison of nonstandardized radiographs with subsequent statistical analysis of radiographic outcomes. The percentage change in root dimensions was first compared in two negative control groups (nonsurgical root canal treatment [NSRCT] and MTA apexification) predicted to have little to no change in root dimensions. This provides an internal test that the mathematical analysis was appropriate. The results indicate that these two negative control groups had minimal measured changes in root

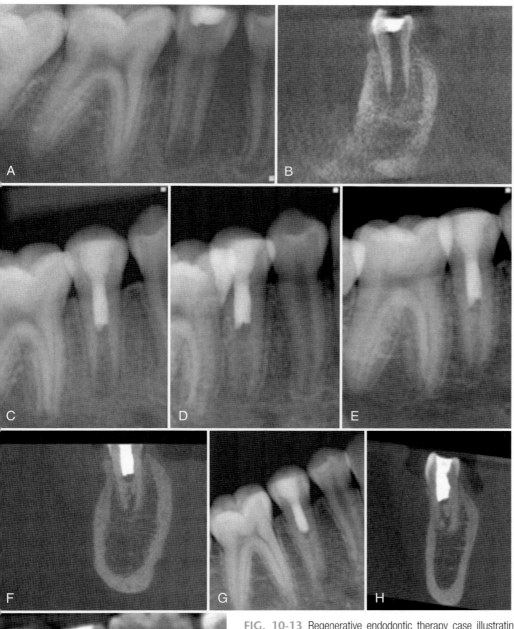

FIG. 10-13 Regenerative endodontic therapy case illustrating treatment delivered to a 9-year-old female patient with a diagnosis of previously initiated endodontic therapy (pulpectomy) due to pain from pulpal inflammation on #29. Bilateral examination revealed presence of a talon cusp (dens evaginatus), which may have been the etiology of pulpal inflammation on #29. Radiographic examination revealed large periapical radiolucency on a periapical radiograph (A) and CBCT (B). The tooth was treated with a regenerative procedure using double antibiotic paste as an intracanal medicament for 48 days. On the second visit, the tooth was isolated, and the double antibiotic paste removed by saline irrigation followed by a final rinse with 17% EDTA. The canal was dried and bleeding was evoked followed by placement of an internal matrix of Collaplug 3 to 4 mm below the CEJ. Mineral trioxide aggregate (MTA) was then placed over it and the tooth was restored with Fuji II LC and Build It. There was complete resolution of apical radiolucency on 1-month recall (C), appreciable root development at 5-month recall (D), and complete root maturation seen at 1-year recall on both perirapical radiograph and CBCT (E and F, respectively). Greater root maturation is observed at 2.5-year recall periapical radiograph (G) and CBCT (H and I). In addition, the tooth responded to EPT on the 1- and 2.5-year recall visits. (Courtesy Dr. Nikita Ruparel.)

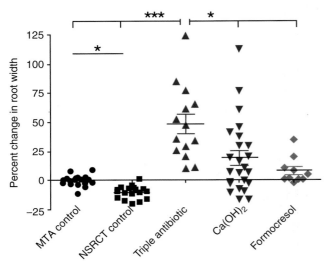

FIG. 10-14 Retrospective analysis of the percentage of change in root length from preoperative image to postoperative image, measured from the cementoenamel junction (CEJ) to the root apex in 40 control patients and in 48 patients following a revascularization procedure. ***$P < 0.001$ versus mineral trioxide aggregate (MTA) apexification control group (n = 20) and NSRCT control group (n = 20). $P < 0.05$ versus MTA control group only. Median values for each group are depicted by horizontal line, and individual cases are indicated by the corresponding symbol. (From Bose R, Nummikoski P, Hargreaves K: A retrospective evaluation of radiographic outcomes in immature teeth with necrotic root canal systems treated with regenerative endodontic procedures, *J Endod* 35:1343, 2009.)

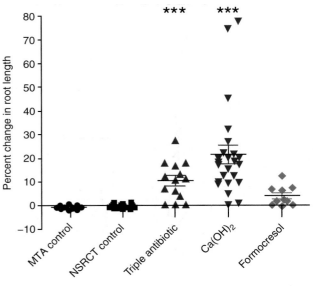

FIG. 10-15 Retrospective analysis of the percentage of change in dentinal wall thickness from preoperative image to postoperative image, measured at the apical third of the root (position of apical third defined in the preoperative image) in 40 control patients and in 48 patients following a revascularization procedure. ***$P < 0.001$ versus mineral trioxide aggregate (MTA) apexification control group and NSRCT control group. $P < 0.05$ versus NSRCT control group only. $P < 0.05$ versus calcium hydroxide (Ca[OH]$_2$) and formocresol groups. $P < 0.05$ versus NSRCT control group only. (From Bose R, Nummikoski P, Hargreaves K: A retrospective evaluation of radiographic outcomes in immature teeth with necrotic root canal systems treated with regenerative endodontic procedures, *J Endod* 35:1343, 2009.)

width (Fig. 10-14) or root length (Fig. 10-15), with the anticipated finding that instrumentation with files of greater taper resulted in a slight but detectable loss of apical root wall width. The results indicated that revascularization treatment with either the triple antibiotic paste or Ca(OH)$_2$ medicament produced significantly greater increases in root length compared with either the MTA or NSRCT control groups. Also, treatment with the triple antibiotic paste produced significantly greater increases in root wall thickness compared with the MTA and NSRCT control groups. Treatment with Ca(OH)$_2$ resulted in significantly greater changes in root wall thickness compared with the NSRCT group, but no differences were observed between these medicaments and the MTA apexification group. Finally, the triple antibiotic paste produced significantly greater differences in root wall thickness compared with either the Ca(OH)$_2$ or formocresol groups. In general, the formocresol group showed the smallest improvement in root length and wall thickness. Secondary analyses indicated that a 12- to 18-month recall is probably the minimal time to judge radiographic evidence of root development, although later time points (36 months) often demonstrate continued root development. Jeeruphan and colleagues (2012) used a similar method to measure changes in root length and width following apexification versus revascularization.[110] They reported that teeth treated with revascularization showed a significantly greater percentage increase in root length (14.9%) compared with teeth treated by either MTA apexification (6.1%) or calcium hydroxide apexification. They also reported that the revascularization protocol produced significantly greater percentage increases in root width (28.2%) compared with teeth treated

by either MTA apexification (0.0%) or calcium hydroxide apexification. In addition to measuring changes in root dimensions, the authors reported survival (defined as retention of the tooth in the arch at the time of the postoperative recall) rate of 100% at an average of 14 months after revascularization treatment. This compared favorably with survival rates of 95% for MTA apexification and 77% for calcium hydroxide apexification. Although prospective randomized clinical trials with standardized radiographic assessment are clearly required, the results of this retrospective study are consistent with a robust outcome of revascularization procedures, particularly when medicated with either a triple antibiotic paste or a Ca(OH)$_2$ medicament. The demonstration of continued root development does not reveal whether this radiopaque material is dentin, cementum, or bone, so given the known reliance of stem cells on an appropriate scaffold and growth factor combination, this will be an important focus for future research efforts.

Example of a Revascularization Protocol

Based on current research, several factors can be reviewed when considering a protocol for revascularization treatment. The first issue is case selection; the best available evidence indicates that this treatment should be considered for the incompletely developed permanent tooth that has an open apex and is negative to pulpal responsiveness testing. Although the ultimate goal of this approach may include a tissue engineering–based method of pulpal regeneration in the fully developed permanent tooth, it should be recognized that current revascularization protocols have not been developed or evaluated for these more challenging cases. Informed consent should include the number of appointments (at least two), the possible adverse effects (primarily potential staining of the crown), the potential lack of response to treatment and alternative treatments, and possible posttreatment symptoms. Because the canal space will not be accessible following revascularization, teeth requiring retention in the canal space for the restoration are not good candidates for REPs. Clinical staining of the crown and any root structure above the gingival margin appears to be due to the presence of minocycline.[120,185,191] This outcome can be minimized by using a delivery system that restricts the drug below the cementoenamel junction (CEJ).[191] When it does occur, it can often be reduced or eliminated by a walking bleach method with sodium perborate. The use of mineral trioxide aggregate (MTA; ProRoot, Dentsply Tulsa Dental, Tulsa, OK), in both gray and white form variants,[27,36,39] may also cause tooth discoloration, which can also be reduced or eliminated by a walking bleach technique.[36] Alternative treatments that should be discussed with the patient and guardian would include MTA apexification, no treatment, or extraction.

At the first appointment (Fig. 10-16, *A-E*), the treatment alternatives, risks, and potential benefits should be described to the patient and guardian after collecting clinical information and establishing pulpal and apical diagnoses. Following informed consent, the tooth is anesthetized, isolated, and accessed. Minimal instrumentation should be accomplished, but the use of a small file to "scout" the root canal system and determine working length is important. If sensation is experienced within the canal system, this may suggest that some residual vital pulp tissue remains.[59] The root canal system should be copiously and slowly irrigated. Because of its proven efficacy as a canal disinfectant and a tissue dissolution agent, sodium hypochlorite (NaOCl) has been the irrigant of choice in most of the revascularization case reports.[62] However, studies have demonstrated that NaOCl is cytotoxic to stem cells.[62,142,235] Importantly, a minimally deleterious effect was seen with the use of 1.5% NaOCl followed by 17% EDTA. Thus, a lower concentration (1.5%) of NaOCl should be considered as the standard irrigant for REPs. Moreover, the use of chlorhexidine should be limited or avoided because it does not have tissue dissolution capability and has also been shown to be cytotoxic to stem cells.[235] Because canal disinfection relies considerably on chemical irrigants, it is important to place the needle into the apical third and irrigate using needles with a closed end and side-port vents (e.g., Max-I-Probe needles), together with a slow rate of infusion, to help to reduce any irrigants passing through the open apex.

The root canal system is then dried with sterile paper points, and the antimicrobial medicament is delivered into the root canal space. The best available evidence would support the use of either a triple antibiotic paste or Ca(OH)$_2$. Triple antibiotic paste (TAP) and Ca(OH)$_2$ have been shown to be effective (see Figs. 10-9 and 10-10). The TAP has the advantage of being a very effective antibiotic combination against endodontic microorganisms[203]; its efficacy is supported by its use in most published cases.[62] This combination is not approved by the U.S. Food and Drug Administration (FDA), however, and carries a potential for minocycline staining of the crown. In addition, triple antibiotic paste has been shown to be cytotoxic to stem cells. It is important to note that Ruparel and colleagues

(2012)[197] have shown that higher TAP at concentrations used in many published case reports has a profound detrimental effect on stem cell survival. Importantly, it had minimal to no deleterious effect when used at the concentrations of 0.1 or 1 mg/mL, whereas these concentrations are several orders of magnitude greater than those required to eliminate bacteria from infected dentin.[203] In addition, the same report showed that all concentrations of calcium hydroxide promoted stem cell survival. Moreover, TAP has an indirect detrimental effect on stem cell survival, as cells do not survive when in contact with dentin previously treated with TAP at the concentration of 1 g/mL.[167] This effect is largely avoided if TAP is used at the lower concentration of 1 mg/mL.[167] Thus, The use of TAP at the concentration of 1 mg/mL or calcium hydroxide pastes as intracanal medicaments seems warranted; however, further investigation is needed to determine appropriate formulations and lower concentrations of antibiotic pastes, if necessary, to be used. When performing REPs on teeth in aesthetic areas, practitioners should consider eliminating minocycline from the antibiotic paste, sealing the coronal dentin with a dentin bonding agent or composite,[120] or using calcium hydroxide paste. After antimicrobial medicament is placed, the tooth is then sealed with a sterile sponge and a temporary filling (e.g., Cavit), and the patient is discharged for 3 to 4 weeks.

At the second appointment (see Fig. 10-16, *F-M*), the patient is evaluated for resolution of any signs or symptoms of an acute infection (\swelling, sinus tract pain, etc.) that may have been present at the first appointment. The antimicrobial treatment is repeated if resolution has not occurred.[47,113] In most reported cases, the acute signs and symptoms resolved after treatment with the intracanal medicament.[62] Because revascularization-induced bleeding will be evoked at this appointment, the tooth should not be treated with a local anesthetic containing a vasoconstrictor. Instead, 3% mepivacaine can be used, which will facilitate the ability to trigger bleeding into the root canal system.[185] Following isolation and reestablishment of coronal access, the tooth should be copiously and slowly irrigated, possibly together with gentle agitation with a small hand file to remove the antimicrobial medicament. When choosing an irrigant at the second appointment, it is worth considering that irrigants such as NaOCl and chlorhexidine may be cytotoxic to stem cells either directly[69] or indirectly after dentin has been exposed to the irrigants.[69,142,235] It has been demonstrated that exposure of dentin to 5% to 6% sodium hypochlorite leads to decreased stem cell survival and odontoblastic differentiation.[81,142,235] This indirect effect is likely related to various deleterious effects of sodium hypochlorite on the dentin matrix leading to reduced cell attachment[192] and a decrease in dentin matrix–derived growth factors such as TGF-β1.[268] Thus, it is prudent to avoid sodium hypochlorite on the second visit. Instead, irrigation with 17% EDTA may be advantageous because it has been shown to release growth factors from dentin[26,268] and promote stem cell survival and differentiation.[142] In addition, Galler and colleagues (2011), using dentin cylinders transplanted into immunocompromised mice, showed that dental pulp stem cells seeded onto EDTA-conditioned dentin differentiated into odontoblast-like cells and had cellular processes extending into the dentin.[81] On the other hand, stem cells differentiated into osteoclasts/odontoclasts caused resorption on the dentinal walls if dentin was previously treated with sodium hypochlorite. Thus, the use of 17% EDTA as the last irrigant promotes

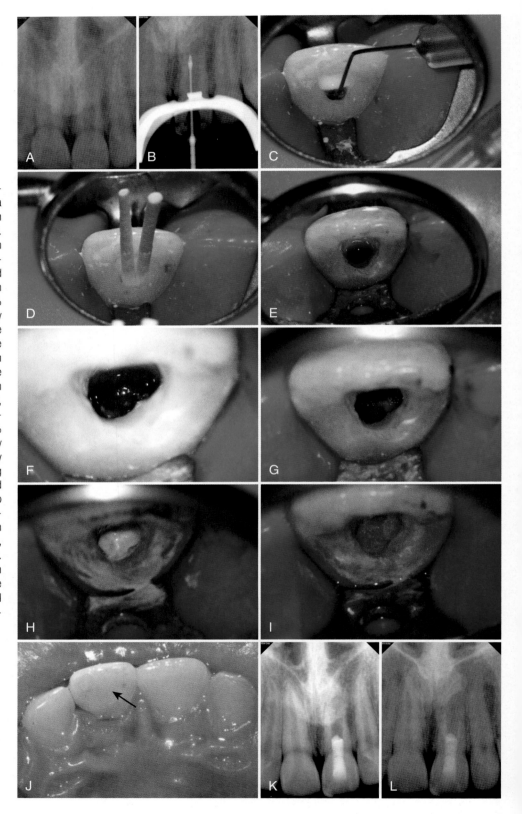

FIG. 10-16 Example of a revascularization case. Treatment was delivered to a 12-year-old boy who suffered trauma on tooth# 9 2 years prior to the appointment. First appointment: Clinical examination revealed a pain upon percussion and palpation (A). A working length file was placed into the root canal system (B). The tooth was slowly irrigated with 20 mL of 1.5% sodium hypochlorite (NaOCl) followed by 20 mL of saline using a Max-I-Probe needle inserted to the apical third (C). The canals were dried and medicated with calcium hydroxide paste (Ultracal) (D). The patient returned asymptomatic 1 month later. The tooth was isolated, accessed, and the medicament removed by slow irrigation with 1.5% NaOCl followed by 17% EDTA. After the canal was adequately dried, intracanal bleeding was achieved by lacerating the apical tissues (E). CollaPlug as seen in access (F). CollaPlug was placed below the CEJ (G) to serve as a matrix to position the white mineral trioxide aggregate coronal to the blood clot (H). The tooth was then sealed with a layer of Fuji IX (I), etched and restored with a composite (J). A final radiograph was taken (K). The tooth responded to electrical pulp tested at the 1-year recall, and it demonstrated apical closure and moderate dentinal wall thickening (L). (Courtesy Dr. Anibal Diogenes.)

the attachment, proliferation, and odontoblastic differentiation of stem cells.

After drying the canal system with sterile paper points, a file is placed a few millimeters beyond the apical foramen, and the apical tissue is lacerated with bleeding up to 3 mm from the CEJ. A small piece of Colla-Plug (Zimmer Dental, Carlsbad, CA) may be inserted into the root canal system to serve as a resorbable matrix to restrict excessive apical positioning of the MTA. About 3 mm of MTA is then placed. MTA has been used in many of the case reports and may have advantages over other materials because it creates a bacteria-tight seal, is biocompatible, and has conductive and inductive properties.[118,148,166,170] However, the use of MTA, including white MTA, has been associated with tooth discoloration; thus, its use should be avoided in aesthetic areas. Biodentin is a bioactive material with desirable handling characteristics and less susceptibility to staining.[124] Although this material is relatively new, there have been encouraging studies demonstrating that it induces stem cell proliferation and odontoblastic differentiation.[137,138,262] Indeed, the use of Biodentine in pulpotomies and direct pulp capping cases is associated with an adequate dentin bridge and continued root development.[29,59,204] Thus, MTA and Biodentine appear suitable to be used in regenerative endodontic procedures.

In addition to follow-up visits in the first several months after REPs to assess for signs of healing, a 12- to 18-month recall should be considered as a reasonable time point to radiographically assess apical healing and root development.[33]

Box 10-1 summarizes the steps in a regenerative endodontic procedure. Importantly, these considerations are based on the best available evidence and are likely to change as the field progresses.

Clinical Measures of Treatment Outcome

The goal of conventional endodontic therapy is to maintain or restore the health of periradicular tissues by preventing or healing apical periodontitis. The goals of regenerative procedures extend beyond the goals of conventional endodontic therapy and include continued root development and reestablishment of pulpal vitality. As mentioned earlier, contemporary regenerative endodontic procedures are being modified and evolving toward accomplishing these additional objectives, which are not achievable with conventional nonsurgical root canal therapy. Accordingly, the definition of success for regenerative endodontic procedures has not been fully determined. Also, assessments of clinical outcomes of REPs are not always easily achievable. Although the resolution of signs and symptoms of disease can be easily assessed by a clinical and radiographic examination, evidence of root development and vitality responses are more challenging.

It is well established that the primary goal of endodontics is the prevention and healing of pulpal and periradicular inflammation (i.e., resolution of signs and symptoms of disease). Immature teeth with pulpal necrosis have been traditionally treated with apexification procedures.[78] A retrospective study reported a success rate of 93.5% for apexification procedures performed in one visit and 90.5% for those performed in two-visit appointments.[247] Another retrospective study reported that apexification procedures resulted in complete healing of apical periodontitis in 85% of the treated teeth.[99] For teeth treated with regenerative procedures, the healing of apical periodontitis has been reported to vary from 90%[114,157]

BOX 10-1

Treatment Procedures for Regenerative Endodontics

First Treatment Visit for Regenerative Endodontics

1. Informed consent, including explanation of risks and alternative treatments or no treatment.
2. After ascertaining adequate local anesthesia, rubber dam isolation is obtained.
3. The root canal systems are accessed and working length is determined (radiograph of a file loosely positioned at 1 mm from root end).
4. The root canal systems are slowly irrigated first with 1.5% NaOCl (20 mL/canal, 5 min) and then irrigated with saline (20 mL/canal, 5 min), with irrigating needle positioned about 1 mm from root end.
5. Canals are dried with paper points.
6. Calcium hydroxide or an antibiotic paste or solution (combined total of 0.1 to 1 mg/mL) is delivered to canal system.
7. Access is temporarily restored.

Final (Second) Treatment Visit for Regenerative Endodontics (Typically 2 to 4 Weeks after the First Visit)

1. A clinical exam is first performed to ensure that that there is no moderate to severe sensitivity to palpation and percussion. If such sensitivity is observed, or a sinus tract or swelling is noted, then the treatment provided at the first visit is repeated.
2. After ascertaining adequate local anesthesia with 3% mepivacaine (no epinephrine), rubber dam isolation is obtained.
3. The root canal systems are accessed; the intracanal medicament is removed by irrigating with 17% ethylenediaminetetraacetic acid (EDTA) (30 mL/canal, 5 min) and then a final flush with saline (5 mL/canal, 1 min).
4. The canals are dried with paper points.
5. Bleeding is induced by rotating a precurved K-file size #25 at 2 mm past the apical foramen with the goal of having the whole canal filled with blood to the level of the cementoenamel junction.
6. Once a blood clot is formed, a premeasured piece of Collaplug (Zimmer Dental Inc., Warsaw, IN) is carefully placed on top of the blood clot to serve as an internal matrix for the placement of approximately 3 mm of white MTA (Dentsply, Tulsa, OK) or Biodentin (Septodont).
7. A (3- to 4-mm) layer of glass ionomer layer (e.g., Fuji IX, GC America, Alsip, IL, or other) is flowed gently over the bioactive coronal barrier and light cured for 40 secs.
8. A bonded reinforced composite resin restoration (e.g., Z-100, 3M, St Paul, MN, or other) is placed over the glass ionomer.
9. The case needs to be followed-up at 3 months, 6 months, and yearly after that for a total of 4 years.

---

to 100%.[44,110,156] Most of these studies did not directly compare apexification to regenerative endodontic procedures with the exception of one prospective clinical trial[157] and one retrospective study.[110] Thus, the success rate for both apexification and regenerative endodontic procedures are similarly high (i.e., above 90%) based on most current evidence. Nonetheless, larger randomized clinical trials with adequate follow-up periods are warranted to provide greater insight in the long-term outcome for both apexification and regenerative procedures.

Continued root development is another desirable outcome of regenerative endodontic procedures. Most published cases of regenerative endodontics report continued root development or apical closure.[62] It is important to note that there were highly varied treatment protocols in the case reports and case series.[62] In addition, the reports of continued root development are often subjective, without an attempt to quantify root development. This shortcoming is due, at least in part, to the difficulty in acquiring standardized radiographs in young patients undergoing rapid cranioskeletal development. A study reported the methodology to perform computational digital correction and the quantification of root length and width on nonstandardized regenerative endodontics radiographs.[33] Studies that have used this methodology to quantify root development have collectively reported that apexification procedures did not promote any root development, whereas regenerative procedures allowed mean increases in root width of 25% to 35.5%[33,110,114] and in root length of 11.3% to 14.9%.[33,110,114] This methodology has been modified to measure changes in radiographic root area (RRA).[76] Regenerative endodontic procedures resulted in a 31.6% increase in RRA, whereas apexification procedures, as with the other studies, had no effect.[76] Thus, regenerative endodontic procedures allowed continued root development not seen with other treatment alternatives.

Although achieving regeneration of pulp tissue continues to be a preferred objective, an alternative acceptable outcome— retention of a tooth with healed apical tissue—could be considered satisfactory. A retrospective study by Jeeruphan and colleagues[110] compared survival rates (defined as retention of the tooth in the arch at the time of the postoperative recall) of teeth that underwent revascularization procedures versus teeth that underwent calcium hydroxide or MTA apexification. They reported a 100% survival rate for revascularization-treated teeth versus 95% for MTA apexification cases and 77.2% for calcium hydroxide apexification cases.[110] Survival of teeth treated with these procedures is noteworthy, because premature loss of these permanent teeth would likely have led to a loss of alveolar bone and compromised future replacement of the tooth. Retention of a tooth following a revascularization procedure, even in the absence of continued root development, would potentially allow for implant placement (if necessary) following alveolar bone growth[37,184] and should be considered an acceptable outcome for patients, parents, and practitioners.

Vitality responses have been reported in approximately 50% of the published cases.[62] Responses to electric pulp tester (EPT) are more commonly reported than cold responses. These responses to vitality testing (with either cold or EPT), as well as the lack of signs and symptoms of pathosis, suggest the presence of functioning tissue in the canal space. Vitality responses, in addition to continued root development, are a desirable outcome because "normal" nociception is protective and suggest immune-competence of the vascularized tissue. However, the lack of responses should not be interpreted as failure because there have been several reports of cases demonstrating healing of apical periodontitis and appreciable root development in the absence of a positive response to vitality testing. Although vitality response is a desirable outcome because it suggests a "functional regeneration," its presence likely depends on several factors, including the depth level of coronal restoration placement and the degree of intracanal mineralization. Thus, from a clinical perspective, the ideal clinical outcome is an asymptomatic tooth that does not require retreatment and demonstrates continued root development and perhaps vitality responses.

It is worth noting that the published revascularization cases have shown increased root wall thickness that is limited to the midroot and apical root.[62] There has been no demonstration of increased root thickness in the cervical area, an area shown to be prone to fracture in immature teeth with a history of trauma and subsequent endodontic treatment. Future clinical studies should focus on not only on making these procedures more predictable, but extending regeneration into the cervical area, potentially strengthening this area and decreasing the risk of root fracture.

SUMMARY

The field of regenerative endodontics is rapidly advancing. This progress is based on the principles of tissue engineering —namely, the spatial delivery of appropriate cells, scaffolds, and growth factors. Similar to most rapidly developing fields, the preclinical area of research has outpaced translational clinical studies. Preclinical studies have identified several mesenchymal stem cell sources capable of differentiating into odontoblast-like cells, as well as candidate scaffolds and growth factors capable of guiding this development. The initial preclinical animal studies indicate that using all three components of the tissue engineering triad (stem cells, growth factors, and scaffolds) can result in complete regeneration of the pulp-dentin complex. There is a delicate balance between disinfection of the root canal system and the interplay of these three components that warrants more research. It is likely that this combined approach of in vitro and in vivo preclinical research will greatly advance our understanding of the conditions necessary to regenerate a functional pulp-dentin complex.

The translational nature of regenerative endodontic research is allowing for changes to take place in the clinical practice in a relatively short time. This cross-talk between basic and clinical sciences is largely fueled by the realization that all three components of the tissue engineering triad are already present in revascularization procedures: stem cells, scaffold (blood clot), and growth factors (from dentin and blood). Preclinical studies that evaluated the effect of irrigants[81,142,235] and medicaments[167,197] on the survival of stem cells, release of growth factors from dentin,[231,268] and odontoblastic differentiation[41,81] are shaping the future generations of regenerative procedures. Further, the incorporation of other scaffolds such as PRP, PRF, and gelatin sponges has been used in the clinical practice with encouraging results.[123,143,157,208,234] Discussion about the requirements of an appropriate scaffold and growth factor was begun in the 1960s by Nygaard-Østby,[173] who had no access to our contemporary instruments, materials, and knowledge base of tissue engineering. Although clinical revascularization procedures do not constitute the ideal regenerative treatment, it is important to note that they do generate a scaffold (fibrin) and growth factors (from platelets and access to proteins embedded in the dentinal walls), and the clinical outcome results in continued radiographic root development of the immature permanent tooth with a diagnosis of pulpal necrosis. Thus, REPs provide a treatment of high value in cases with an otherwise poor prognosis. Histologic analyses of REPs conducted in patients[123,143,171,206] or animals[168,193,243] suggest that the increase in root dimensions is often due to deposition of cementum-like material, osteodentin, dentin, or bone.

Future clinical research will likely focus on further translating basic research findings into improved regenerative procedures. For example, the formation of a cementum-like material on the dentinal walls may lead to studies evaluating benefits of REPs for overall tooth resistance to fracture. In addition, it is clear that the multipotent nature of many mesenchymal stem cell types could contribute to the finding of cementum deposition. Controlled differentiation of stem cells into odontoblasts is an important area of research and amenable to tissue-engineering concepts. The development of delivery systems that permit structural reinforcement of the cervical area (or, ideally, the pulp chamber) might provide clinical opportunities to regenerate lost tooth structure, thereby permitting natural teeth to be retained instead of possible fracture or extraction. Finally, the ultimate and long-term goal for regenerative endodontic procedures should be to treat the fully formed permanent tooth. Although this situation is more complex than the immature tooth with an open apex and a ready source of stem cells, it provides the unique potential of saving the natural dentition while restoring the sensory, immunologic, and defensive properties of the pulp-dentin complex.

REFERENCES

1. Abe S, Imaizumi M, Mikami Y, et al: Oral bacterial extracts facilitate early osteogenic/dentinogenic differentiation in human dental pulp-derived cells, *Oral Surg Oral Med Oral Pathol Oral Radiol Endod* 109:149, 2010.

2. About I: Dentin regeneration in vitro: the pivotal role of supportive cells, *Adv Dent Res* 23:320, 2011.

3. About I, Bottero MJ, de Denato P, et al: Human dentin production in vitro, *Exp Cell Res* 258:33, 2000.

4. About I, Laurent-Maquin D, Lendahl U, Mitsiadis TA: Nestin expression in embryonic and adult human teeth under normal and pathological conditions, *Am J Pathol* 157:287, 2000.

5. Agata H, Kagami H, Watanabe N, Ueda M: Effect of ischemic culture conditions on the survival and differentiation of porcine dental pulp-derived cells, *Differentiation* 76:981, 2008.

6. Aggarwal V, Miglani S, Singla M: Conventional apexification and revascularization induced maturogenesis of two non-vital, immature teeth in same patient: 24 months follow up of a case, *J Conserv Dent* 15:68, 2012.

7. Al-Hezaimi K, Al-Tayar BA, Bajuaifer YS, et al: A hybrid approach to direct pulp capping by using emdogain with a capping material, *J Endod* 37:667, 2011.

8. Al-Hezaimi K, Salameh Z, Al-Fouzan K, et al: Histomorphometric and micro-computed tomography analysis of pulpal response to three different pulp capping materials, *J Endod* 37:507, 2011.

9. Althumairy RI, Teixeira FB, Diogenes A: Effect of dentin conditioning with intracanal medicaments on survival of stem cells of apical papilla, *J Endod* 40:521, 2014.

10. Amler MH: The age factor in human extraction wound healing, *J Oral Surg* 35:193, 1977.

11. Ando Y, Honda MJ, Ohshima H, et al: The induction of dentin bridge-like structures by constructs of subcultured dental pulp-derived cells and porous HA/TCP in porcine teeth, *Nagoya J Med Sci* 71:51, 2009.

12. Andreasen JO, Andreasen FM, Mejare I, Cvek M: Healing of 400 intra-alveolar root fractures. 1. Effect of pre-injury and injury factors such as sex, age, stage of root development, fracture type, location of fracture and severity of dislocation, *Dent Traumatol* 20:192, 2004.

13. Andreasen JO, Borum MK, Jacobsen HL, Andreasen FM: Replantation of 400 avulsed permanent incisors. 2. Factors related to pulpal healing, *Endod Dent Traumatol* 11:59, 1995.

14. Andreasen JO, Farik B, Munksgaard EC: Long-term calcium hydroxide as a root canal dressing may increase risk of root fracture, *Dent Traumatol* 18:134, 2002.

15. Andreasen JO, Munksgaard EC, Bakland LK: Comparison of fracture resistance in root canals of immature sheep teeth after filling with calcium hydroxide or MTA, *Dent Traumatol* 22:154, 2006.

16. Andreasen JO, Ravn JJ: Epidemiology of traumatic dental injuries to primary and permanent teeth in a Danish population sample, *Int J Oral Surg* 1:235, 1972.

17. Anitua E, Andia I, Ardanza B, et al: Autologous platelets as a source of proteins for healing and tissue regeneration, *Thromb Haemost* 91:4, 2004.

18. Anitua E, Sanchez M, Nurden AT, et al: New insights into and novel applications for platelet-rich fibrin therapies, *Trends Biotechnol* 24:227, 2006.

19. Aranha AM, Zhang Z, Neiva KG, et al: Hypoxia enhances the angiogenic potential of human dental pulp cells, *J Endod* 36:1633, 2010.

20. Astudillo P, Rios S, Pastenes L, et al: Increased adipogenesis of osteoporotic human-mesenchymal stem cells (MSCs) characterizes by impaired leptin action, *J Cell Biochem* 103:1054, 2008.

21. Bajek A, Czerwinski M, Olkowska J, Gurtowska N, Kloskowski T, Drewa T: Does aging of mesenchymal stem cells limit their potential application in clinical practice? *Aging Clin Exp Res* 24:404, 2012.

22. Baksh D, Song L, Tuan RS: Adult mesenchymal stem cells: characterization, differentiation, and application in cell and gene therapy, *J Cell Mol Med* 8:301, 2004.

23. Banchs F, Trope M: Revascularization of immature permanent teeth with apical periodontitis: new treatment protocol? *J Endod* 30:196, 2004.

24. Bang G, Nordenram A, Anneroth G: Allogenic demineralized dentin implants in jaw defects of Java monkeys, *Int J Oral Surg* 1:126, 1972.

25. Begue-Kirn C, Smith AJ, Loriot M, et al: Comparative analysis of TGF beta s, BMPs, IGF1, msxs, fibronectin, osteonectin and bone sialoprotein gene expression during normal and in vitro-induced odontoblast differentiation, *Int J Dev Biol* 38:405, 1994.

26. Begue-Kirn C, Smith AJ, Ruch JV, et al: Effects of dentin proteins, transforming growth factor beta 1 (TGF beta 1) and bone morphogenetic protein 2 (BMP2) on the differentiation of odontoblast in vitro, *Int J Dev Biol* 36:491, 1992.

27. Belobrov I, Parashos P: Treatment of tooth discoloration after the use of white mineral trioxide aggregate, *J Endod* 37:1017, 2011.

28. Berkhoff JA, Chen PB, Teixeira FB, Diogenes A: Evaluation of triple antibiotic paste removal by different irrigation procedures, *J Endod* 40:1172, 2014.

29. Bhat SS, Hegde SK, Adhikari F, Bhat VS: Direct pulp capping in an immature incisor using a new bioactive material, *Contemp Clin Dent* 5:393, 2014.

30. Bidder M, Latifi T, Towler DA: Reciprocal temporospatial patterns of Msx2 and Osteocalcin gene expression during murine odontogenesis, *J Bone Miner Res* 13:609, 1998.

31. Blin-Wakkach C, Lezot F, Ghoul-Mazgar S, et al: Endogenous Msx1 antisense transcript: in vivo and in vitro evidences, structure, and potential involvement in skeleton development in mammals, *Proc Natl Acad Sci U S A* 98:7336, 2001.

32. Blond-Elguindi S, Goldberg ME: Kinetic characterization of early immunoreactive intermediates during the refolding of guanidine-unfolded Escherichia coli tryptophan synthase beta 2 subunits, *Biochemistry* 29:2409, 1990.

33. Bose R, Nummikoski P, Hargreaves K: A retrospective evaluation of radiographic outcomes in immature teeth with necrotic root canal systems treated with regenerative endodontic procedures, *J Endod* 35:1343, 2009.

34. Botero TM, Shelburne CE, Holland GR, et al: TLR4 mediates LPS-induced VEGF expression in odontoblasts, *J Endod* 32:951, 2006.

35. Botero TM, Son JS, Vodopyanov D, Hasegawa M, et al: MAPK signaling is required for LPS-induced VEGF in pulp stem cells, *J Dent Res* 89:264, 2010.

36. Boutsioukis C, Noula G, Lambrianidis T: Ex vivo study of the efficiency of two techniques for the removal of mineral trioxide aggregate used as a root canal filling material, *J Endod* 34:1239, 2008.

37. Bryant SR: The effects of age, jaw site, and bone condition on oral implant outcomes, *Int J Prosthodont* 11:470, 1998.

38. Butler WT: Dentin matrix proteins, *Eur J Oral Sci* 106 (suppl 1):204, 1998.

39. Camilleri J: Color stability of white mineral trioxide aggregate in contact with hypochlorite solution, *J Endod* 40:436, 2014.

40. Caplan AI: Mesenchymal stem cells, *J Orthop Res* 9:641, 1991.

41. Casagrande L, Demarco FF, Zhang Z, et al: Dentin-derived BMP-2 and odontoblast differentiation, *J Dent Res* 89:603, 2010.

42. Cassidy N, Fahey M, Prime SS, Smith AJ: Comparative analysis of transforming growth factor-beta isoforms 1-3 in human and rabbit dentine matrices, *Arch Oral Biol* 42:219, 1997.

43. Cavalcanti BN, Zeitlin BD, Nor JE: A hydrogel scaffold that maintains viability and supports differentiation of dental pulp stem cells, *Dent Mater* 29:97, 2013.

44. Cehreli ZC, Isbitiren B, Sara S, Erbas G: Regenerative endodontic treatment (revascularization) of immature necrotic molars medicated with calcium hydroxide: a case series, *J Endod* 37:1327, 2011.

45. Chang SW, Lee SY, Ann HJ, et al: Effects of calcium silicate endodontic cements on biocompatibility and mineralization-inducing potentials in human dental pulp cells, *J Endod* 40:1194, 2014.

46. Choi BD, Jeong SJ, Wang G, et al: Temporal induction of secretory leukocyte protease inhibitor (SLPI) in odontoblasts by lipopolysaccharide and wound infection, *J Endod* 35:997, 2009.

47. Chueh LH, Ho YC, Kuo TC, et al: Regenerative endodontic treatment for necrotic immature permanent teeth, *J Endod* 35:160, 2009.

48. Cooper PR, Takahashi Y, Graham LW, et al: Inflammation-regeneration interplay in the dentine-pulp complex, *J Dent* 38:687, 2010.

49. Coudert AE, Pibouin L, Vi-Fane B, et al: Expression and regulation of the Msx1 natural antisense transcript during development, *Nucleic Acids Res* 33:5208, 2005.

50. Cvek M: Treatment of non-vital permanent incisors with calcium hydroxide. I. Follow-up of periapical repair and apical closure of immature roots, *Odontol Revy* 23:27, 1972.

51. Cvek M: Clinical procedures promoting apical closure and arrest of external root resorption in non-vital permanent incisors, *Trans Int Conf Endod* 5:30, 1973.

52. Cvek M: Treatment of non-vital permanent incisors with calcium hydroxide. IV. Periodontal healing and closure of the root canal in the coronal fragment of teeth with intra-alveolar fracture and vital apical fragment: a follow-up, *Odontol Revy* 25:239, 1974.

53. Cvek M: Prognosis of luxated non-vital maxillary incisors treated with calcium hydroxide and filled with gutta-percha: a retrospective clinical study, *Endod Dent Traumatol* 8:45, 1992.

54. d'Aquino R, De Rosa A, Laino G, et al: Human dental pulp stem cells: from biology to clinical applications, *J Exp Zool B Mol Dev Evol* 312B:408, 2009.

55. D'Ippolito G, Schiller PC, Ricordi C, et al: Age-related osteogenic potential of mesenchymal stromal stem cells from human vertebral bone marrow, *J Bone Miner Res* 14:1115, 1999.

56. D'Souza RN, Happonen RP, Ritter NM, Butler WT: Temporal and spatial patterns of transforming growth factor-beta 1 expression in developing rat molars, *Arch Oral Biol* 35:957, 1990.

57. Dai Y, He H, Wise GE, Yao S: Hypoxia promotes growth of stem cells in dental follicle cell populations, *J Biomed Sci Eng* 4:454, 2011.

58. De Barros S, Dehez S, Arnaud E, et al: Aging-related decrease of human ASC angiogenic potential is reversed by hypoxia preconditioning through ROS production, *Mol Ther* 21:399, 2013.

59. De Rossi A, Silva LA, Gaton-Hernandez P, et al: Comparison of pulpal responses to pulpotomy and pulp capping with biodentine and mineral trioxide aggregate in dogs, *J Endod* 40:1362, 2014.

60. Demarco FF, Casagrande L, Zhang Z, et al: Effects of morphogen and scaffold porogen on the differentiation of dental pulp stem cells, *J Endod* 36:1805, 2010.

61. Diderich KE, Nicolaije C, Priemel M, et al: Bone fragility and decline in stem cells in prematurely aging DNA repair deficient trichothiodystrophy mice, *Age (Dordr)* 34:845, 2012.

62. Diogenes A, Henry MA, Teixeira FB, Hargreaves KM: An update on clinical regenerative endodontics, *Endod Topics* 28:2, 2013.

63. Diogenes AR, Ruparel NB, Teixeira FB, Hargreaves KM: Translational science in disinfection for regenerative endodontics, *J Endod* 40:S52, 2014.

64. Duque C, Hebling J, Smith AJ, et al: Reactionary dentinogenesis after applying restorative materials and bioactive dentin matrix molecules as liners in deep cavities prepared in nonhuman primate teeth, *J Oral Rehabil* 33:452, 2006.

65. Durand SH, Flacher V, Romeas A, et al: Lipoteichoic acid increases TLR and functional chemokine expression while reducing dentin formation in in vitro differentiated human odontoblasts, *J Immunol* 176:2880, 2006.

66. Egusa H, Sonoyama W, Nishimura M, et al: Stem cells in dentistry—part I: stem cell sources, *J Prosthodont Res* 56:151, 2012.

67. El Karim IA, Linden GJ, Curtis TM, et al: Human odontoblasts express functional thermo-sensitive TRP channels: implications for dentin sensitivity, *Pain* 152:2211, 2011.

68. El-Backly RM, Massoud AG, El-Badry AM, et al: Regeneration of dentine/pulp-like tissue using a dental pulp stem cell/poly(lactic-co-glycolic) acid scaffold construct in New Zealand white rabbits, *Aust Endod J* 34:52, 2008.

69. Essner MD, Javed A, Eleazer PD: Effect of sodium hypochlorite on human pulp cells: an in vitro study, *Oral Surg Oral Med Oral Pathol Oral Radiol Endod* 112:662, 2011.

70. Fang Y, Hu J: Toll-like receptor and its roles in myocardial ischemic/reperfusion injury, *Med Sci Monit* 17:RA100, 2011.

71. Fanton d'Andon M, Quellard N, Fernandez B, et al: Leptospira Interrogans induces fibrosis in the mouse kidney through Inos-dependent, TLR- and NLR-independent signaling pathways, *PLoS Negl Trop Dis* 8:e2664, 2014.

72. Ferracane JL, Cooper PR, Smith AJ: Can interaction of materials with the dentin-pulp complex contribute to dentin regeneration? *Odontology* 98:2, 2010.

73. Fichman G, Gazit E: Self-assembly of short peptides to form hydrogels: design of building blocks, physical properties and technological applications, *Acta Biomater* 10:1671, 2014.

74. Finkelman RD, Mohan S, Jennings JC, et al: Quantitation of growth factors IGF-I, SGF/IGF-II, and TGF-beta in human dentin, *J Bone Miner Res* 5:717, 1990.

75. Fitzgerald M, Chiego DJ Jr, Heys DR: Autoradiographic analysis of odontoblast replacement following pulp exposure in primate teeth, *Arch Oral Biol* 35:707, 1990.

76. Flake NM, Gibbs JL, Diogenes A, et al: A standardized novel method to measure radiographic root changes after endodontic therapy in immature teeth, *J Endod* 40:46, 2014.

77. Frank AL: Therapy for the divergent pulpless tooth by continued apical formation, *J Am Dent Assoc* 72:87, 1966.

78. Frank AL: Apexification: therapy for the divergent pulpless tooth, *Shikai Tenbo* 61:729, 1983.

79. Friedenstein AJ, Chailakhyan RK, Latsinik NV, et al: Stromal cells responsible for transferring the microenvironment of the hemopoietic tissues: cloning in vitro and retransplantation in vivo, *Transplantation* 17:331, 1974.

80. Friedenstein AJ, Deriglasova UF, Kulagina NN, et al: Precursors for fibroblasts in different populations of hematopoietic cells as detected by the in vitro colony assay method, *Exp Hematol* 2:83, 1974.

81. Galler KM, D'Souza RN, Federlin M, et al: Dentin conditioning codetermines cell fate in regenerative endodontics, *J Endod* 37:1536, 2011.

82. Galler KM, D'Souza RN, Hartgerink JD, Schmalz G: Scaffolds for dental pulp tissue engineering, *Adv Dent Res* 23:333, 2011.

83. Galler KM, Eidt A, Schmalz G: Cell-free approaches for dental pulp tissue engineering, *J Endod* 40:S41, 2014.

84. Garcia-Irigoyen O, Carotti S, Latasa MU, et al: Matrix metalloproteinase-10 expression is induced during hepatic injury and plays a fundamental role in liver tissue repair, *Liver Int* 34:e257, 2014.

85. Goldberg M, Six N, Decup F, et al: Mineralization of the dental pulp: contributions of tissue engineering to tomorrow's therapeutics in odontology, *Pathol Biol (Paris)* 50:194, 2002.

86. Goldberg M, Six N, Decup F, et al: Application of bioactive molecules in pulp-capping situations, *Adv Dent Res* 15:91, 2001.

87. Goldberg M, Smith AJ: Cells and extracellular matrices of dentin and pulp: a biological basis for repair and tissue engineering, *Crit Rev Oral Biol Med* 15:13, 2004.

88. Goncalves SB, Dong Z, Bramante CM, et al: Tooth slice-based models for the study of human dental pulp angiogenesis, *J Endod* 33:811, 2007.

89. Gonzalez-Ramos M, Calleros L, Lopez-Ongil S, et al: HSP70 increases extracellular matrix production by human vascular smooth muscle through TGF-beta1 up-regulation, *Int J Biochem Cell Biol* 45:232, 2013.

90. Gould TR: Ultrastructural characteristics of progenitor cell populations in the periodontal ligament, *J Dent Res* 62:873, 1983.

91. Graham L, Cooper PR, Cassidy N, et al: The effect of calcium hydroxide on solubilisation of bio-active dentine matrix components, *Biomaterials* 27:2865, 2006.

92. Gu K, Chang S, Ritchie HH, et al: Molecular cloning of a human dentin sialophosphoprotein gene, *Eur J Oral Sci* 108:35, 2000.

93. Guo W, He Y, Zhang X, et al: The use of dentin matrix scaffold and dental follicle cells for dentin regeneration, *Biomaterials* 30:6708, 2009.

94. Habich C, Baumgart K, Kolb H, Burkart V: The receptor for heat shock protein 60 on macrophages is saturable, specific, and distinct from receptors for other heat shock proteins, *J Immunol* 168:569, 2002.

95. Hargreaves KM, Giesler T, Henry M, Wang Y: Regeneration potential of the young permanent tooth: what does the future hold? *J Endod* 34:S51, 2008.

96. Heithersay GS: Stimulation of root formation in incompletely developed pulpless teeth, *Oral Surg Oral Med Oral Pathol* 29:620, 1970.

97. Heithersay GS: Calcium hydroxide in the treatment of pulpless teeth with associated pathology, *J Br Endod Soc* 8:74, 1975.

98. Helmlinger G, Yuan F, Dellian M, Jain RK: Interstitial pH and pO2 gradients in solid tumors in vivo: high-resolution measurements reveal a lack of correlation, *Nat Med* 3:177, 1997.

99. Holden DT, Schwartz SA, Kirkpatrick TC, Schindler WG: Clinical outcomes of artificial root-end barriers with mineral trioxide aggregate in teeth with immature apices, *J Endod* 34:812, 2008.

100. Hoshino E, Kurihara-Ando N, Sato I, et al: In-vitro antibacterial susceptibility of bacteria taken from infected root dentine to a mixture of ciprofloxacin, metronidazole and minocycline, *Int Endod J* 29:125, 1996.

101. Huang GT: A paradigm shift in endodontic management of immature teeth: conservation of stem cells for regeneration, *J Dent* 36:379, 2008.

102. Huang GT, Shagramanova K, Chan SW: Formation of odontoblast-like cells from cultured human dental pulp cells on dentin in vitro, *J Endod* 32:1066, 2006.

103. Huang GT, Sonoyama W, Chen J, Park SH: In vitro characterization of human dental pulp cells: various isolation methods and culturing environments, *Cell Tissue Res* 324:225, 2006.

104. Huang GT, Sonoyama W, Liu Y, et al: The hidden treasure in apical papilla: the potential role in pulp/dentin regeneration and bioroot engineering, *J Endod* 34:645, 2008.

105. Hugle T, Geurts J, Nuesch C, et al: Aging and osteoarthritis: an inevitable encounter? *J Aging Res* 2012:950192, 2012.

106. Iida K, Takeda-Kawaguchi T, Tezuka Y, et al: Hypoxia enhances colony formation and proliferation but inhibits differentiation of human dental pulp cells, *Arch Oral Biol* 55:648, 2010.

107. Iohara K, Imabayashi K, Ishizaka R, et al: Complete pulp regeneration after pulpectomy by transplantation of CD105+ stem cells with stromal cell-derived factor-1, *Tissue Eng Part A* 17:1911, 2011.

108. Iohara K, Murakami M, Takeuchi N, et al: A novel combinatorial therapy with pulp stem cells and granulocyte colony-stimulating factor for total pulp regeneration, *Stem Cells Transl Med* 2:521, 2013.

109. Ito K, Yamada Y, Nagasaka T, et al: Osteogenic potential of injectable tissue-engineered bone: a comparison among autogenous bone, bone substitute (Bio-oss), platelet-rich plasma, and tissue-engineered bone with respect to their mechanical properties and histological findings, *J Biomed Mater Res A* 73:63, 2005.

110. Jeeruphan T, Jantarat J, Yanpiset K, et al: Mahidol study 1: comparison of radiographic and survival outcomes of immature teeth treated with either regenerative endodontic or apexification methods: a retrospective study, *J Endod* 38:1330, 2012.

111. Jiang HW, Zhang W, Ren BP, et al: Expression of toll like receptor 4 in normal human odontoblasts and dental pulp tissue, *J Endod* 32:747, 2006.

112. Joseph BK, Savage NW, Daley TJ, Young WG: In situ hybridization evidence for a paracrine/autocrine role for insulin-like growth factor-I in tooth development, *Growth Factors* 13:11, 1996.

113. Jung IY, Lee SJ, Hargreaves KM: Biologically based treatment of immature permanent teeth with pulpal necrosis: a case series, *Tex Dent J* 129:601, 2012.

114. Kahler B, Mistry S, Moule A, et al: Revascularization outcomes: a prospective analysis of 16 consecutive cases, *J Endod* 40:333, 2014.

115. Kalaskar RR, Kalaskar AR: Maturogenesis of non-vital immature permanent teeth, *Contemp Clin Dent* 4:268, 2013.

116. Kang XQ, Zang WJ, Bao LJ, et al: Differentiating characterization of human umbilical cord blood-derived mesenchymal stem cells in vitro, *Cell Biol Int* 30:569, 2006.

117. Kellner M, Steindorff MM, Strempel JF, et al: Differences of isolated dental stem cells dependent on donor age and consequences for autologous tooth replacement, *Arch Oral Biol* 59:559, 2014.

118. Kelsh RM, McKeown-Longo PJ: Topographical changes in extracellular matrix: activation of TLR4 signaling and solid tumor progression, *Trends Cancer Res* 9:1, 2013.

119. Khan MM, Gandhi C, Chauhan N, et al: Alternatively-spliced extra domain A of fibronectin promotes acute inflammation and brain injury after cerebral ischemia in mice, *Stroke* 43:1376, 2012.

120. Kim JH, Kim Y, Shin SJ, et al: Tooth discoloration of immature permanent incisor associated with triple antibiotic therapy: a case report, *J Endod* 36:1086, 2010.

121. Kim JY, Xin X, Moioli EK, et al: Regeneration of dental-pulp-like tissue by chemotaxis-induced cell homing, *Tissue Eng Part A* 16:3023, 2010.

122. Kling M, Cvek M, Mejare I: Rate and predictability of pulp revascularization in therapeutically reimplanted permanent incisors, *Endod Dent Traumatol* 2:83, 1986.

123. Klyn SL, Kirkpatrick TC, Rutledge RE: In vitro comparisons of debris removal of the EndoActivator system, the F file, ultrasonic irrigation, and NaOCl irrigation alone after hand-rotary instrumentation in human mandibular molars, *J Endod* 36:1367, 2010.

124. Koubi G, Colon P, Franquin JC, et al: Clinical evaluation of the performance and safety of a new dentine substitute, biodentine, in the restoration of posterior teeth: a prospective study, *Clin Oral Investig* 17:243, 2013.

125. Kuroda R, Matsumoto T, Niikura T, et al: Local transplantation of granulocyte colony stimulating factor-mobilized CD34+ cells for patients with femoral and tibial nonunion: pilot clinical trial, *Stem Cells Transl Med* 3:128, 2014.

126. Labban N, Yassen GH, Windsor LJ, Platt JA: The direct cytotoxic effects of medicaments used in endodontic regeneration on human dental pulp cells, *Dent Traumatol*, 2014.

127. Langer R, Vacanti JP: Tissue engineering, *Science* 260:920, 1993.

128. Lei L, Liao W, Sheng P, et al: Biological character of human adipose-derived adult stem cells and influence of donor age on cell replication in culture, *Sci China C Life Sci* 50:320, 2007.

129. Leites AB, Baldissera EZ, Silva AF, et al: Histologic response and tenascin and fibronectin expression after pulp capping in pig primary teeth with mineral trioxide aggregate or calcium hydroxide, *Oper Dent* 36:448, 2011.

130. Li J, Lee DS, Madrenas J: Evolving Bacterial Envelopes and Plasticity of TLR2-Dependent Responses: Basic Research and Translational Opportunities. *Front Immunol* 4:347, 2013.

131. Li Z, Jiang CM, An S, et al: Immunomodulatory properties of dental tissue-derived mesenchymal stem cells, *Oral Dis* 20:25, 2014.

132. Liao J, Al Shahrani M, Al-Habib M, et al: Cells isolated from inflamed periapical tissue express mesenchymal stem cell markers and are highly osteogenic, *J Endod* 37:1217, 2011.

133. Lin ZM, Qin W, Zhang NH, et al: Adenovirus-mediated recombinant human bone morphogenetic protein-7 expression promotes differentiation of human dental pulp cells, *J Endod* 33:930, 2007.

134. Liu J, Jin T, Chang S, et al: Matrix and TGF-beta-related gene expression during human dental pulp stem cell (DPSC) mineralization, *In Vitro Cell Dev Biol Anim* 43:120, 2007.

135. Lovelace TW, Henry MA, Hargreaves KM, Diogenes A: Evaluation of the delivery of mesenchymal stem cells into the root canal space of necrotic immature teeth after clinical regenerative endodontic procedure, *J Endod* 37:133, 2011.

136. Lucas K, Maes M: Role of the toll like receptor (TLR) radical cycle in chronic inflammation: possible treatments targeting the TLR4 pathway, *Mol Neurobiol* 48:190, 2013.

137. Luo Z, Kohli MR, Yu Q, et al: Biodentine induces human dental pulp stem cell differentiation through mitogen-activated protein kinase and calcium-/calmodulin-dependent protein kinase II pathways, *J Endod* 40:937, 2014.

138. Luo Z, Li D, Kohli MR, et al: Effect of biodentine on the proliferation, migration and adhesion of human dental pulp stem cells, *J Dent* 42:490, 2014.

139. Magloire H, Bouvier M, Joffre A: Odontoblast response under carious lesions, *Proc Finn Dent Soc* 88 (Suppl 1):257, 1992.

140. Mariappan MM, DeSilva K, Sorice GP, et al: Combined acute hyperglycemic and hyperinsulinemic clamp induced profibrotic and proinflammatory responses in the kidney, *Am J Physiol Cell Physiol* 306:C202, 2014.

141. Marrelli M, Paduano F, Tatullo M: Cells isolated from human periapical cysts express mesenchymal stem cell-like properties, *Int J Biol Sci* 9:1070, 2013.

142. Martin DE, De Almeida JF, Henry MA, et al: Concentration-dependent effect of sodium hypochlorite on stem cells of apical papilla survival and differentiation, *J Endod* 40:51, 2014.

143. Martin G, Ricucci D, Gibbs JL, Lin LM: Histological findings of revascularized/revitalized immature permanent molar with apical periodontitis using platelet-rich plasma, *J Endod* 39:138, 2013.

144. McCulloch KJ, Mills CM, Greenfeld RS, Coil JM: Dens evaginatus: review of the literature and report of several clinical cases, *J Can Dent Assoc* 64:104, 1998.

145. McFadden JP, Puangpet P, Basketter DA, et al: Why does allergic contact dermatitis exist? *Br J Dermatol* 168:692, 2013.

146. Mente J, Hage N, Pfefferle T, et al: Mineral trioxide aggregate apical plugs in teeth with open apical foramina: a retrospective analysis of treatment outcome, *J Endod* 35:1354, 2009.

147. Miura M, Gronthos S, Zhao M, et al: SHED: stem cells from human exfoliated deciduous teeth, *Proc Natl Acad Sci U S A* 100:5807, 2003.

148. Moghaddame-Jafari S, Mantellini MG, Botero TM, et al: Effect of ProRoot MTA on pulp cell apoptosis and proliferation in vitro, *J Endod* 31:387, 2005.

149. Morsczeck C, Gotz W, Schierholz J, et al: Isolation of precursor cells (PCs) from human dental follicle of wisdom teeth, *Matrix Biol* 24:155, 2005.

150. Murakami M, Horibe H, Iohara K, et al: The use of granulocyte-colony stimulating factor induced mobilization for isolation of dental pulp stem cells with high regenerative potential, *Biomaterials* 34:9036, 2013.

151. Murray PE, About I, Lumley PJ, et al: Human odontoblast cell numbers after dental injury, *J Dent* 28:277, 2000.

152. Murray PE, Garcia-Godoy F, Hargreaves KM: Regenerative endodontics: a review of current status and a call for action, *J Endod* 33:377, 2007.

153. Murray PE, Smith AJ, Windsor LJ, Mjor IA: Remaining dentine thickness and human pulp responses, *Int Endod J* 36:33, 2003.

154. Murray PE, Stanley HR, Matthews JB, et al: Age-related odontometric changes of human teeth, *Oral Surg Oral Med Oral Pathol Oral Radiol Endod* 93:474, 2002.

155. Musson DS, McLachlan JL, Sloan AJ, et al: Adrenomedullin is expressed during rodent dental tissue development and promotes cell growth and mineralization, *Biol Cell* 102:145, 2010.

156. Nagata JY, Gomes BP, Rocha Lima TF, et al: Traumatized immature teeth treated with 2 protocols of pulp revascularization, *J Endod* 40:606, 2014.

157. Nagy MM, Tawfik HE, Hashem AA, Abu-Seida AM: Regenerative potential of immature permanent teeth with necrotic pulps after different regenerative protocols, *J Endod* 40:192, 2014.

158. Nakashima M: Dentin induction by implants of autolyzed antigen-extracted allogeneic dentin on amputated pulps of dogs, *Endod Dent Traumatol* 5:279, 1989.

159. Nakashima M: Induction of dentin formation on canine amputated pulp by recombinant human bone morphogenetic proteins (BMP)-2 and -4, *J Dent Res* 73:1515, 1994.

160. Nakashima M: Tissue engineering in endodontics, *Aust Endod J* 31:111, 2005.

161. Nakashima M, Akamine A: The application of tissue engineering to regeneration of pulp and dentin in endodontics, *J Endod* 31:711, 2005.

162. Nakashima M, Iohara K: Regeneration of dental pulp by stem cells, *Adv Dent Res* 23:313, 2011.

163. Nakashima M, Iohara K: Mobilized dental pulp stem cells for pulp regeneration: initiation of clinical trial, *J Endod* 40:S26, 2014.

164. Nasstrom K: Dentin formation after corticosteroid treatment: a clinical study and an experimental study on rats, *Swed Dent J Suppl* 115:1, 1996.

165. Nasstrom K, Forsberg B, Petersson A, Westesson PL: Narrowing of the dental pulp chamber in patients with renal diseases, *Oral Surg Oral Med Oral Pathol* 59:242, 1985.

166. Natale LC, Rodrigues MC, Xavier TA, et al: Ion release and mechanical properties of calcium silicate and calcium hydroxide materials used for pulp capping, *Int Endod J*, 2014.

167. Netea MG, Van der Graaf C, Van der Meer JW, Kullberg BJ: Recognition of fungal pathogens by Toll-like receptors, *Eur J Clin Microbiol Infect Dis* 23:672, 2004.

168. Nevins A, Finkelstein F, Laporta R, Borden BG: Induction of hard tissue into pulpless open-apex teeth using collagen-calcium phosphate gel, *J Endod* 4:76, 1978.

169. Nowak UM, Newkirk MM: Rheumatoid factors: good or bad for you? *Int Arch Allergy Immunol* 138:180, 2005.

170. Nowicka A, Lipski M, Parafiniuk M, et al: Response of human dental pulp capped with biodentine and mineral trioxide aggregate, *J Endod* 39:743, 2013.

171. Nyggard-Østby: The role of the blood clot in endodontictherapy: an experimental histological study, *Acta Odontol Scand* 79:333, 1961.

172. Nygaard-Østby B: Mortal or vital treatment of the inflamed pulp? *SSO Schweiz Monatsschr Zahnheilkd* 76:545, 1966.

173. Nygaard-Østby B, Hjortdal O: Tissue formation in the root canal following pulp removal, *Scand J Dent Res* 79:333, 1971.

174. Ogino Y, Ayukawa Y, Kukita T, Koyano K: The contribution of platelet-derived growth factor, transforming growth factor-beta1, and insulin-like growth factor-I in platelet-rich plasma to the proliferation of osteoblast-like cells, *Oral Surg Oral Med Oral Pathol Oral Radiol Endod* 101:724, 2006.

175. Oh SY, Choi JS, Kim EJ, et al: The role of macrophage migration inhibitory factor in ocular surface disease pathogenesis after chemical burn in the murine eye, *Mol Vis* 16:2402, 2010.

176. Okamoto Y, Sonoyama W, Ono M, et al: Simvastatin induces the odontogenic differentiation of human dental pulp stem cells in vitro and in vivo, *J Endod* 35:367, 2009.

177. Okita K, Ichisaka T, Yamanaka S: Generation of germline-competent induced pluripotent stem cells, *Nature* 448:313, 2007.

178. Paakkonen V, Bleicher F, Carrouel F, et al: General expression profiles of human native odontoblasts and pulp-derived cultured odontoblast-like cells are similar but reveal differential neuropeptide expression levels, *Arch Oral Biol* 54:55, 2009.

179. Paakkonen V, Tjaderhane L: High-throughput gene and protein expression analysis in pulp biologic research: review, *J Endod* 36:179, 2010.

180. Paakkonen V, Vuoristo JT, Salo T, Tjaderhane L: Comparative gene expression profile analysis between native human odontoblasts and pulp tissue, *Int Endod J* 41:117, 2008.

181. Parirokh M, Torabinejad M: Mineral trioxide aggregate: a comprehensive literature review—part III: clinical applications, drawbacks, and mechanism of action, *J Endod* 36:400, 2010.

182. Paryani K, Kim SG: Regenerative endodontic treatment of permanent teeth after completion of root development: a report of 2 cases, *J Endod* 39:929, 2013.

183. Paula-Silva FW, Ghosh A, Silva LA, Kapila YL: TNF-alpha promotes an odontoblastic phenotype in dental pulp cells, *J Dent Res* 88:339, 2009.

184. Percinoto C, Vieira AE, Barbieri CM, et al: Use of dental implants in children: a literature review, *Quintessence Int* 32:381, 2001.

185. Petrino JA, Boda KK, Shambarger S, et al: Challenges in regenerative endodontics: a case series, *J Endod* 36:536, 2010.

186. Pettiette MT, Zhong S, Moretti AJ, Khan AA: Potential correlation between statins and pulp chamber calcification, *J Endod* 39:1119, 2013.

187. Poole JA, Romberger DJ: Immunological and inflammatory responses to organic dust in agriculture, *Curr Opin Allergy Clin Immunol* 12:126, 2012.

188. Pruksakorn D, Khamwaen N, Pothacharoen P, et al: Chondrogenic properties of primary human chondrocytes culture in hyaluronic acid treated gelatin scaffold, *J Med Assoc Thai* 92:483, 2009.

189. Ravindran S, Huang CC, George A: Extracellular matrix of dental pulp stem cells: applications in pulp tissue engineering using somatic MSCs, *Front Physiol* 4:395, 2014.

190. Reddi AH: Role of morphogenetic proteins in skeletal tissue engineering and regeneration, *Nat Biotechnol* 16:247, 1998.

191. Reynolds K, Johnson JD, Cohenca N: Pulp revascularization of necrotic bilateral bicuspids using a modified novel technique to eliminate potential coronal discolouration: a case report, *Int Endod J* 42:84, 2009.

192. Ring KC, Murray PE, Namerow KN, et al: The comparison of the effect of endodontic irrigation on cell adherence to root canal dentin, *J Endod* 34:1474, 2008.

193. Ritter AL, Ritter AV, Murrah V, et al: Pulp revascularization of replanted immature dog teeth after treatment with minocycline and doxycycline assessed by laser Doppler flowmetry, radiography, and histology, *Dent Traumatol* 20:75, 2004.

194. Roberts-Clark DJ, Smith AJ: Angiogenic growth factors in human dentine matrix, *Arch Oral Biol* 45:1013, 2000.

195. Rosenberg B, Murray PE, Namerow K: The effect of calcium hydroxide root filling on dentin fracture strength, *Dent Traumatol* 23:26, 2007.

196. Rule DC, Winter GB: Root growth and apical repair subsequent to pulpal necrosis in children, *Br Dent J* 120:586, 1966.

197. Ruparel NB, de Almeida JF, Henry MA, Diogenes A: Characterization of a stem cell of apical papilla cell line: effect of passage on cellular phenotype, *J Endod* 39:357, 2013.

198. Ruparel NB, Teixeira FB, Ferraz CC, Diogenes A: Direct effect of intracanal medicaments on survival of stem cells of the apical papilla, *J Endod* 38:1372, 2012.

199. Sabrah AH, Yassen GH, Gregory RL: Effectiveness of antibiotic medicaments against biofilm formation of Enterococcus faecalis and Porphyromonas gingivalis, *J Endod* 39:1385, 2013.

200. Sakai VT, Zhang Z, Dong Z, et al: SHED differentiate into functional odontoblasts and endothelium, *J Dent Res* 89:791, 2010.

201. Sakdee JB, White RR, Pagonis TC, Hauschka PV: Hypoxia-amplified proliferation of human dental pulp cells, *J Endod* 35:818, 2009.

202. Sato I, Ando-Kurihara N, Kota K, et al: Sterilization of infected root-canal dentine by topical application of a mixture of ciprofloxacin, metronidazole and minocycline in situ, *Int Endod J* 29:118, 1996.

203. Sato T, Hoshino E, Uematsu H, Noda T: In vitro antimicrobial susceptibility to combinations of drugs on bacteria from carious and endodontic lesions of human deciduous teeth, *Oral Microbiol Immunol* 8:172, 1993.

204. Shayegan A, Jurysta C, Atash R, et al: Biodentine used as a pulp-capping agent in primary pig teeth, *Pediatr Dent* 34:e202, 2012.

205. Shi S, Gronthos S: Perivascular niche of postnatal mesenchymal stem cells in human bone marrow and dental pulp, *J Bone Miner Res* 18:696, 2003.

206. Shimizu E, Jong G, Partridge N, et al: Histologic observation of a human immature permanent tooth with irreversible pulpitis after revascularization/regeneration procedure, *J Endod* 38:1293, 2012.

207. Shimizu E, Ricucci D, Albert J, et al: Clinical, radiographic, and histological observation of a human immature permanent tooth with chronic apical abscess after revitalization treatment, *J Endod* 39:1078, 2013.

208. Shivashankar VY, Johns DA, Vidyanath S, Kumar MR: Platelet rich fibrin in the revitalization of tooth with necrotic pulp and open apex, *J Conserv Dent* 15:395, 2012.

209. Simon S, Smith AJ, Berdal A, et al: The MAP kinase pathway is involved in odontoblast stimulation via p38 phosphorylation, *J Endod* 36:256, 2010.

210. Simon SI, Hu Y, Vestweber D, Smith CW: Neutrophil tethering on E-selectin activates beta 2 integrin binding to ICAM-1 through a mitogen-activated protein kinase signal transduction pathway, *J Immunol* 164:4348, 2000.

211. Sirisinha S: Insight into the mechanisms regulating immune homeostasis in health and disease, *Asian Pac J Allergy Immunol* 29:1, 2011.

212. Smith AJ, Lesot H: Induction and regulation of crown dentinogenesis: embryonic events as a template for dental tissue repair? *Crit Rev Oral Biol Med* 12:425, 2001.

213. Smith AJ, Lumley PJ, Tomson PL, Cooper PR: Dental regeneration and materials: a partnership, *Clin Oral Investig* 12:103, 2008.

214. Smith AJ, Matthews JB, Hall RC: Transforming growth factor-beta1 (TGF-beta1) in dentine matrix: ligand activation and receptor expression, *Eur J Oral Sci* 106 (suppl 1):179, 1998.

215. Smith AJ, Smith JG, Shelton RM, Cooper PR: Harnessing the natural regenerative potential of the dental pulp, *Dent Clin North Am* 56:589, 2012.

216. Smith AJ, Tobias RS, Cassidy N, et al: Odontoblast stimulation in ferrets by dentine matrix components, *Arch Oral Biol* 39:13, 1994.

217. Smith AJ, Tobias RS, Murray PE: Transdentinal stimulation of reactionary dentinogenesis in ferrets by dentine matrix components, *J Dent* 29:341, 2001.

218. Smith AJ, Tobias RS, Plant CG, et al: In vivo morphogenetic activity of dentine matrix proteins, *J Biol Buccale* 18:123, 1990.

219. Smith HS: Activated microglia in nociception, *Pain Physician* 13:295, 2010.

220. Sobhi MB, Rana MJ, Ibrahim M, et al: Frequency of dens evaginatus of permanent anterior teeth, *J Coll Physicians Surg Pak* 14:88, 2004.

221. Sobieszczyk ME, Lingappa JR, McElrath MJ: Host genetic polymorphisms associated with innate immune factors and HIV-1, *Curr Opin HIV AIDS* 6:427, 2011.

222. Sokolova IB, Sergeev IV, Anisimov SV, et al: Effect of transplantation of mesenchymal stem cells on the density of pial microvascular network in rats of different age, *Bull Exp Biol Med* 154:548, 2013.

223. Sonoyama W, Liu Y, Fang D, et al: Mesenchymal stem cell-mediated functional tooth regeneration in swine, *PloS one* 1:e79, 2006.

224. Sonoyama W, Liu Y, Yamaza T, et al: Characterization of the apical papilla and its residing stem cells from human immature permanent teeth: a pilot study, *J Endod* 34:166, 2008.

225. Soriano EP, Caldas Ade F Jr, Diniz De Carvalho MV, Amorim Filho Hde A: Prevalence and risk factors related to traumatic dental injuries in Brazilian schoolchildren, *Dent Traumatol* 23:232, 2007.

226. Staquet MJ, Durand SH, Colomb E, et al: Different roles of odontoblasts and fibroblasts in immunity, *J Dent Res* 87:256, 2008.

227. Tecles O, Laurent P, Aubut V, About I: Human tooth culture: a study model for reparative dentinogenesis and direct pulp capping materials biocompatibility, *J Biomed Mater Res B Appl Biomater* 85:180, 2008.

228. Thesleff I, Vaahtokari A: The role of growth factors in determination and differentiation of the odontoblastic cell lineage, *Proc Finn Dent Soc* 88 (suppl 1):357, 1992.

229. Thibodeau B, Teixeira F, Yamauchi M, et al: Pulp revascularization of immature dog teeth with apical periodontitis, *J Endod* 33:680, 2007.

230. Thomadakis G, Ramoshebi LN, Crooks J, et al: Immunolocalization of bone morphogenetic protein-2 and -3 and osteogenic protein-1 during murine tooth root morphogenesis and in other craniofacial structures, *Eur J Oral Sci* 107:368, 1999.

231. Tomson PL, Grover LM, Lumley PJ, et al: Dissolution of bio-active dentine matrix components by mineral trioxide aggregate, *J Dent* 35:636, 2007.

232. Tomson PL, Lumley PJ, Alexander MY, et al: Hepatocyte growth factor is sequestered in dentine matrix and promotes regeneration-associated events in dental pulp cells, *Cytokine* 61:622, 2013.

233. Torabinejad M, Chivian N: Clinical applications of mineral trioxide aggregate, *J Endod* 25:197, 1999.

234. Torabinejad M, Turman M: Revitalization of tooth with necrotic pulp and open apex by using platelet-rich plasma: a case report, *J Endod* 37:265, 2011.

235. Trevino EG, Patwardhan AN, Henry MA, et al: Effect of irrigants on the survival of human stem cells of the apical papilla in a platelet-rich plasma scaffold in human root tips, *J Endod* 37:1109, 2011.

236. Tziafas D, Kolokuris I: Inductive influences of demineralized dentin and bone matrix on pulp cells: an approach of secondary dentinogenesis, *J Dent Res* 69:75, 1990.

237. Tziafas D, Smith AJ, Lesot H: Designing new treatment strategies in vital pulp therapy, *J Dent* 28:77, 2000.

238. Unterholzner L: The interferon response to intracellular DNA: why so many receptors? *Immunobiology* 218:1312, 2013.

239. Vainio S, Karavanova I, Jowett A, Thesleff I: Identification of BMP-4 as a signal mediating secondary induction between epithelial and mesenchymal tissues during early tooth development, *Cell* 75:45, 1993.

240. Vangsness CT Jr, Farr J 2nd, Boyd J, et al: Adult human mesenchymal stem cells delivered via intra-articular injection to the knee following partial medial meniscectomy: a randomized, double-blind, controlled study, *J Bone Joint Surg Am* 96:90, 2014.

241. Viccica G, Francucci CM, Marcocci C: The role of PPARgamma for the osteoblastic differentiation, *J Endocrinol Invest* 33:9, 2010.

242. Wadachi R, Hargreaves KM: Trigeminal nociceptors express TLR-4 and CD14: a mechanism for pain due to infection, *J Dent Res* 85:49, 2006.

243. Wang X, Thibodeau B, Trope M, et al: Histologic characterization of regenerated tissues in canal space after the revitalization/revascularization procedure of immature dog teeth with apical periodontitis, *J Endod* 36:56, 2010.

244. Wei X, Ling J, Wu L, et al: Expression of mineralization markers in dental pulp cells, *J Endod* 33:703, 2007.

245. Wiesmann HP, Joos U, Meyer U: Biological and biophysical principles in extracorporal bone tissue engineering: part II, *Int J Oral Maxillofac Surg* 33:523, 2004.

246. Windley W 3rd, Teixeira F, Levin L, et al: Disinfection of immature teeth with a triple antibiotic paste, *J Endod* 31:439, 2005.

247. Witherspoon DE, Small JC, Regan JD, Nunn M: Retrospective analysis of open apex teeth obturated with mineral trioxide aggregate, *J Endod* 34:1171, 2008.

248. Wysocki GP, Daley TD, Ulan RA: Predentin changes in patients with chronic renal failure, *Oral Surg Oral Med Oral Pathol* 56:167, 1983.

249. Xu L, Tang L, Jin F, et al: The apical region of developing tooth root constitutes a complex and maintains the ability to generate root and periodontium-like tissues, *J Periodontal Res* 44:275, 2009.

250. Xu X, Jha AK, Harrington DA, et al: Hyaluronic acid-based hydrogels: from a natural polysaccharide to complex networks, *Soft Matter* 8:3280, 2012.

251. Yamada Y, Ueda M, Hibi H, Nagasaka T: Translational research for injectable tissue-engineered bone regeneration using mesenchymal stem cells and platelet-rich plasma: from basic research to clinical case study, *Cell Transplant* 13:343, 2004.

252. Yamada Y, Ueda M, Naiki T, et al: Autogenous injectable bone for regeneration with mesenchymal stem cells and platelet-rich plasma: tissue-engineered bone regeneration, *Tissue Eng* 10:955, 2004.

253. Yamagishi VT, Torneck CD, Friedman S, et al: Blockade of TLR2 inhibits porphyromonas gingivalis suppression of mineralized matrix formation by human dental pulp stem cells, *J Endod* 37:812, 2011.

254. Yamamura T: Differentiation of pulpal cells and inductive influences of various matrices with reference to pulpal wound healing, *J Dent Res* 64 Spec No:530, 1985.

255. Yang B, Chen G, Li J, et al: Tooth root regeneration using dental follicle cell sheets in combination with a dentin matrix-based scaffold, *Biomaterials* 33:2449, 2012.

256. Yang X, Yang F, Walboomers XF, et al: The performance of dental pulp stem cells on nanofibrous PCL/gelatin/nHA scaffolds, *J Biomed Mater Res A* 93:247, 2010.

257. Yassen GH, Platt JA: The effect of nonsetting calcium hydroxide on root fracture and mechanical properties of radicular dentine: a systematic review, *Int Endod J* 46:112, 2013.

258. Yassen GH, Vail MM, Chu TG, Platt JA: The effect of medicaments used in endodontic regeneration on root fracture and microhardness of radicular dentine, *Int Endod J* 46:688, 2013.

259. Yildirim S, Can A, Arican M, et al: Characterization of dental pulp defect and repair in a canine model, *Am J Dent* 24:331, 2011.

260. Yip WK: The prevalence of dens evaginatus, *Oral Surg Oral Med Oral Pathol* 38:80, 1974.

261. Young CS, Terada S, Vacanti JP, et al: Tissue engineering of complex tooth structures on biodegradable polymer scaffolds, *J Dent Res* 81:695, 2002.

262. Zanini M, Sautier JM, Berdal A, Simon S: Biodentine induces immortalized murine pulp cell differentiation into odontoblast-like cells and stimulates biomineralization, *J Endod* 38:1220, 2012.

263. Zhang CZ, Li H, Young WG, et al: Evidence for a local action of growth hormone in embryonic tooth development in the rat, *Growth Factors* 14:131, 1997.

264. Zhang J, An Y, Gao LN, et al: The effect of aging on the pluripotential capacity and regenerative potential of human periodontal ligament stem cells, *Biomaterials* 33:6974, 2012.

265. Zhang T, Kurita-Ochiai T, Hashizume T, et al: Aggregatibacter actinomycetemcomitans accelerates atherosclerosis with an increase in atherogenic factors in spontaneously hyperlipidemic mice, *FEMS Immunol Med Microbiol* 59:143, 2010.

266. Zhang W, Walboomers XF, Jansen JA: The formation of tertiary dentin after pulp capping with a calcium phosphate cement, loaded with PLGA microparticles containing TGF-beta1, *J Biomed Mater Res A* 85:439, 2008.

267. Zhang X, Tamasi J, Lu X, et al: Epidermal growth factor receptor plays an anabolic role in bone metabolism in vivo, *J Bone Miner Res* 26:1022, 2011.

268. Zhao S, Sloan AJ, Murray PE, et al: Ultrastructural localisation of TGF-beta exposure in dentine by chemical treatment, *Histochem J* 32:489, 2000.

CHAPTER 11

Evaluation of Outcomes

YUAN-LING NG | KISHOR GULABIVALA

CHAPTER OUTLINE

CONTEXT OF EVALUATING ENDODONTIC OUTCOMES

The development of medical and dental practices has been guided by prevailing philosophies and consensus of expert opinions. The foundations of modern endodontics were shaken when Billings[97] brought the apparent relationship between oral sepsis and bacterial endocarditis to the attention of dentistry and medicine. He had strengthened the concept further from Miller[134] who had coined the term *focus of infection* to highlight a possible link between "mouth germs" and systemic disease. The disastrous consequences of the focal infection era were sealed when Hunter[96] delivered his famous address at McGill University. Fears of fatal oral sepsis from deficient root canal treatments led to widespread extraction of pulpless teeth. Endodontics virtually disappeared from many dental schools, whereas in some areas, treatment was restricted to anterior teeth. The focal infection theory reigned for about 50 years[83] until around 1940.

The discipline of endodontics was rescued by individual, diligent practitioners in Europe and USA who meticulously recorded their treatments, as well as their outcomes, to demonstrate the effectiveness of the procedures in controlling root canal infection. It was through these individual endeavors of merit that the reputation of endodontic procedures was restored and the discipline granted its specialist status in 1952 in the United States.[59]

Toward the 1990s, the improvements in general health and longer survival of Western populations as well as their teeth, coupled with the rising costs of health care for longer-living individuals, prompted a host of reevaluations of the altered economic burdens on society. Among them, the *cost-effectiveness of treatment procedures* for management of diseases loomed large. Thus began the era of evidence-based medicine and dentistry, with its emphasis on costs, benefits, and outcomes of treatment. Attempts to pool outcome data for greater power brought with it the realization that studies originating from different centers varied in diverse ways, leading to very heterogeneous data that challenged formal attempts at drawing definitive conclusions. Characterization of data types and its quality prompted calls for standardization of approaches in measuring outcomes to enable more meaningful pooling.

Because of the better established science of evidence assessment, a modern revisitation of the "focal infection era"[94] did not lead to the same threat to the endodontic discipline that was evident at the beginning of the 20th century. In fact, it was suggested as an opportunity to secure research funding for assessing and managing the importance of dental care on systemic health.

Interestingly, the modern threat to endodontics was posed by the cost-economic pressures exerted on treatment planning decisions centering on the question of whether to "save the tooth" or extract it with replacement by an implant-supported crown.[238] Once again, the science of evidence-based practice has helped to avert irrational treatment recommendations leaning toward extraction of savable teeth.[54,100,103]

Types of Disease and Their Treatment

The statement, "Endodontists provide endodontic treatment to manage endodontic disease" is a gross oversimplification that masks important subtleties in recognition of the nature of the diseases and how best to address them. Endodontists manage inflammation of the specialized connective tissues within and surrounding the teeth; more specifically, they deal with inflammation that generally commences in the pulp tissue and progresses to the periradicular tissues via portals of communication that convey the neurovascular supply. Incipient or established pulpitis may be managed by vital pulp therapy when judged reversible, largely because a sufficient body of pulp tissue remains healthy and unaffected. More advanced pulpitis that approaches the foramina into the periodontal ligament may require root canal treatment. When pulpal inflammation, necrosis, or infection encroaches on the apical periodontal ligament, root canal treatment is required. Apical periodontitis that persists despite technically adequate root canal treatment may require root canal retreatment, periradicular surgery, or extraction to manage the source of the persistent disease. *Endodontic treatment* is therefore a collective and nonspecific term for a range of procedures directed at managing the spread of pulpal inflammation or infection. Endodontic treatment encompasses the following procedures:

1. Vital pulp therapy (indirect pulp therapy, direct pulp capping, pulpotomy, regenerative pulp therapy)
2. Nonsurgical root canal treatment
3. Nonsurgical root canal retreatment
4. Surgical retreatment

The ideal outcome for endodontic treatment consists of controlled reduction of inflammation, accompanied by healing through regeneration, although sometimes repair may follow instead. Unfortunately, none of the involved tissues are within the direct sight of the clinician, hidden as they are by their housings of hard tooth structure or alveolar bone and their gingival/mucosal coverings. Consequently, surrogate measures must be employed to evaluate the presence or absence of the disease process and its resolution. The evaluation process is further complicated by the lack of direct correlation between measures of the disease process and its clinical manifestation.

WHAT ARE SURROGATE OUTCOME MEASURES?

Signs of acute inflammation are classically described in the "triple response" exhibited by mechanically injured skin, which includes altered color (redness), texture/contour (swelling), and sensation (pain), which are directly accessible and viewable. These changes have a direct correlation with histopathologic and molecular alterations. Chronic inflammation does not necessarily exhibit the same highly visible signs and symptoms of its histopathologic character. When hidden from view, as are pulpal and periradicular tissues, the task of recognizing the presence or absence of chronic inflammation is even more challenging. The clinician is therefore left with indirect or associated (proxy) changes by which to judge the presence or absence of disease; these are called "surrogate" measures. Some of these may have to be inferred through associations, some may be directly visualized, and others are only indirectly "viewable" through various imaging techniques (such as radiography). The process therefore calls upon the clinician to assimilate various sources of information to form a judgment about the presence or absence of disease.

Types of Outcome Measures

In its broadest sense, an outcome measure for a treatment intervention may constitute any consistently anticipated and measurable consequence of the treatment. The prepared shape of the root canal system, bacterial load reduction, and technical quality of the root filling may all be regarded as outcome measures by this definition. But the ultimate *clinical* measure of a treatment outcome is assessing the prevention and resolution of disease.

The outcome of endodontic treatment may be assessed in four dimensions as in other medical disciplines.[9] The first dimension is physical/physiologic and related to presence or absence of pulpal/periapical health/disease, pain, and function. The second dimension assesses longevity or tooth survival. The third dimension relates to economics and assesses direct and indirect costs. Finally, the fourth dimension examines psychologic aspects involving perceptions of oral health–related quality of life (OHRQoL) and aesthetics.

WHAT IS THE PURPOSE OF EVALUATING OUTCOMES?

Apart from the importance of developing a solid foundation of evidence-based practice, it is important to evaluate treatment outcomes for a number of reasons.

Effectiveness of Procedures

First, treatment procedures must be effective. Otherwise, there is no reason to recommend them to patients as a treatment option. The patient must be properly informed as to the risks, benefits, and potential outcomes of the offered treatment. The availability of pooled outcome data and consensus guidelines offers both patients and endodontists reassurance and confidence in the validity and predictability of the offered procedure. However, the pooled average outcome data may not pertain if the clinician does not have the requisite experience, skill, and personal outcomes matching at least these average figures of performance. Personal outcome data offer the patient more precise measures for comparison and expectation. It also aids practitioners in refining their technique and knowledge to further improve their outcomes and, ultimately, to help improve the overall pooled data.[34] The treating clinician must assess his or her own personal outcome data and personal expectation of success. If the clinician is uncertain of a result or feels that the outcome could be enhanced by treatment from another clinician, then referral to someone else more qualified is paramount.

Factors Affecting Outcomes

Pooling data (that is preferably homogeneous) offers the potential to evaluate and prioritize the factors that exert a dominant influence on outcomes. In this way, protocols for treatment may be improved in a progressive fashion, bringing about the perfect meld of technical, clinical, and biologic insight necessary for the highest performance and most predictable outcome. Evaluation of factors affecting treatment outcomes arguably provides the strongest influence for making changes that will improve the clinical outcomes. Weighing the relative importance of individual factors should help to identify the key biologic factors at play and how best to manage them from a clinical or technical perspective.

Value for Prognostication

Prognostication, which could be defined as the prediction, projection, prophesizing, or foretelling the likely outcome of treatment, is not often well defined in endodontics. The overall prognosis of a tooth depends on the interaction among three individual and often independent variables, including endodontic, periodontal, and restorative prognoses. Each has a set of subsidiary factors that must be considered to derive an overall prognosis. Finally, the tooth in question must be considered from a strategic perspective, relative to its position in the dental arch and the contribution it makes in the dynamic occlusion.

A deeper analysis of the factors affecting outcomes as prognostic indicators is merited in order to clarify the degree of complexity inherent in the problem. A comparison may be made with the randomized controlled trial of a drug as a treatment intervention. The drug therapy is delivered as a clearly prescribed and standardized dose regimen delivered by specified timings to effect an anticipated blood or target tissue concentration for a specified duration. Data recording is confined to compliance with the prescription and possibly checking of actual blood levels achieved as well as the final outcome effect.

In stark contrast, a surgical intervention, regardless of any standardization of the described procedural protocol, is subject to enormous variation in its delivery dependent on interpretation and execution of the protocol by each operator. To add to the levels of complexity and variation, surgical protocols are often multistep, sequential procedures, each prospective step dependent on the previous for its efficacy. Even characterizing and accurately recording any variations in treatment protocols becomes a challenge because many aspects and steps must be documented. This leads to the next challenge, that of demonstrating compliance with the accuracy of such complex data gathering. Furthermore, it becomes important from an analytic perspective to not only consider the effect of individual steps (factors) alone but also any interactive effect between the multiple steps inherent in the procedure. Even when such comprehensive prospective outcome data are available, utilizing these data to individually calculate the prognosis in a particular scenario may be challenging. Clinically, there may be two distinct ways to estimate prognosis: (1) to apply heuristic principles and intuitively gauge the effect of dominant factors or, at the other end of the extreme, (2) to mathematically input comprehensive data into an algorithmic model to calculate the estimated outcome. An even more sophisticated approach may be to use mathematical modeling to calculate iterations on variations within the system. At present, the evidence base is insufficient to allow such a sophisticated approach.

It therefore follows that evaluating outcomes and the factors that affect them are fundamental to the creation of a suitable data foundation for future application to endodontic prognostication. The endodontic treatment option is in competition with other alternative therapies and therefore, for the discipline to survive and thrive, a suitable blend of efficacy, efficiency, utility, predictability, and cost-effectiveness data must be generated for its principal therapies. Achievement of such

a goal will require a diligent and conscientious collection of data from many sources. Analyses of such powerful datasets will ultimately yield proper insight into outcomes of the procedures we use. Coupled with biologic insight of the problem, it will become possible to derive new therapeutic solutions necessary to deliver them.

OUTCOME MEASURES FOR ENDODONTIC TREATMENT

Before determining the success or failure of an endodontic procedure, the parameters as to what is considered a success or a failure have to be discussed. These are termed the *outcome measures* of the procedures.

Outcome Measures for Vital Pulp Therapy Procedures

The techniques used to maintain the vitality and health of pulps in teeth with extensive caries or those with traumatic/mechanical exposures include (1) indirect pulp capping with one-step or stepwise caries excavation; (2) direct pulp capping of exposed pulps; and (3) partial/full pulpotomy procedures for more extensively involved pulps. The surrogate outcome measures adopted in studies include (1) clinical success (pulp sensitivity to cold test and absence of pain, soft-tissue swelling, sinus tract, periradicular radiolucency, or pathologic root resorption), (2) patient satisfaction, (3) adverse events (pain, swelling, tooth fracture), and (4) tooth extraction.[89,136] Although not providing a specific follow-up strategy, the quality guidelines of the European Society of Endodontology[61] suggests "initial review at no longer than 6 months and thereafter at further regular intervals." They also provide the criteria for judging the favorable outcome of vital pulp therapy (Table 11-1). There are substantial differences in the criteria adopted

TABLE 11-1

Criteria for Assessing the Outcome of Pulp Therapy

Quality Guidelines for Endodontic Treatment: Consensus Report of the European Society of Endodontology (2006)	Guidelines on Pulp Therapy for Primary and Immature Permanent Teeth (The American Academy of Paediatric Dentistry 2014)
1. Normal response to pulp sensitivity tests (when feasible)	1. Tooth vitality maintained
2. Absence of pain and other symptoms	2. Absence of posttreatment signs or symptoms such as sensitivity, pain, or swelling
3. Radiologic evidence of dentinal bridge formation	3. Occurrence of pulp healing and reparative dentin formation
4. Radiologic evidence of continued root formation in immature teeth	4. Absence of radiographic evidence of internal or external root resorption, periapical radiolucency, abnormal calcification, or other pathologic changes
5. Absence of clinical and radiographic signs of internal root resorption and apical periodontitis	5. Teeth with immature roots should show continued root development and apexogenesis

in published clinical studies on outcomes of vital pulp therapy[89,136] with few studies adopting all of the criteria. The frequency of radiologic review adopted in published studies also varies substantially, with some recommending the first review at 1 month followed by subsequent 3 monthly reviews.[172,242] The relative benefit of acquired information versus unnecessary radiation to patients has been questioned.[66] An initial assessment at 6 to 12 weeks, followed by a review 6 and 12 months after treatment, seems to have been accepted and is recommended. Some studies reported up to 10 years follow-up on case series demonstrating lower success rates, inferring the possibility of slow spread of pulpal inflammation and late failures. The conclusion is that longer follow-up periods are merited.

The process at each review consists of obtaining a history of symptoms, coupled with an examination to determine the presence or absence of tenderness to palpation of adjacent soft tissues, tenderness to pressure and percussion of the tooth, signs of radiographic pulpal, and periapical changes, and responses to pulp tests. The accuracy of pulp tests may be limited in pulpotomized teeth because of the distance of the remaining pulp tissue from the tooth's surface. In the case of pulp capping and pulpotomy, additional tests include radiographic verification of the presence of the calcific barrier (Fig. 11-1) and its integrity by removal of the dressing and direct probing. Although an initial examination at 6 weeks has been suggested, this can be modified for the radiographic assessment. If there is no evidence of complete bridge formation, the treatment is considered failed and root canal treatment should be considered. In addition, in the case of incompletely formed roots there should be radiographic evidence of continued root development (Fig. 11-2).

Outcome Measures for Nonsurgical Root Canal Treatment and Retreatment

Root canal treatment may be employed either to prevent or resolve periapical disease. Given that periapical lesions develop as a result of *interaction* between bacteria (and their by-products) and the host defenses, it is clear that prevention or resolution

of the disease process depends on preventing or terminating this interaction.

Prevention of apical periodontitis applies to the clinical situation where it is judged that the pulp is irreversibly inflamed, necrotic, or infected to the extent that vital pulp therapy would not resolve the problem, which therefore requires pulpectomy. The implication is that the procedure demands asepsis as a prime requirement. The precise technical details of the protocol may not be so important, as long as they are focused on effective and aseptic removal of the pulp tissue. This is validated by the high chance of retaining periapical health (judged by conventional radiography), regardless of the clinical protocol used.[153]

Once the periapical lesion has become established, the challenge is a different one because the purpose now is to remove the bacterial biofilm and effect switching-off the periapical host response. The challenge seems to be greater still if the periapical lesion is larger as it is associated with a more diverse infection. A number of approaches (protocols) have been used to achieve this general aim. The periapical healing process that occurs after root canal treatment is less clear. Nevertheless,

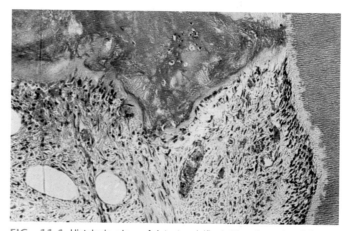

FIG. 11-1 Histologic view of intact calcific bridge formation following pulpotomy.

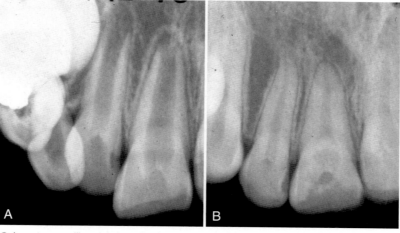

FIG. 11-2 Immature maxillary right lateral and central incisors (A) showing continued root development following pulpotomies (B).

ideal healing would eventually result in regeneration and the formation of cementum over the apical termini, isolating the root canal system from the periapex (Fig. 11-3); but this is not an inevitable result. Incomplete removal of the infection will reduce but not eliminate the periradicular inflammatory reaction, and in fact this is generally what happens.[147] This implies that residual infection in the apical anatomy is typical following completion of root canal treatment and that an ongoing interaction continues between the residual infection, root filling material, and host defenses, which plays a definitive role in determining the final healing outcome.

The culture test has been used during root canal treatment as an interim measure of the efficacy of the chemomechanical procedure; however, it has fallen out of favor in contemporary practice for a variety of reasons.[139] The outcome measures that quantitate healing subsequent to root canal treatment are the absence of clinical signs and symptoms of persistent periapical disease.[17,18] The definitive outcome measure (in conjunction with the absence of signs and symptoms), however, is periapical healing, because the treatment is aimed at resolution of periapical disease (Fig. 11-4).[152] Clinical judgment of the outcome of treatment is based on the absence of signs of infection and inflammation, such as pain, tenderness to pressure/percussion of the tooth, tenderness to palpation of the related soft tissues, absence of swelling and sinus tract, and radiographic demonstration of reduction in the size of the periapical lesion (if sufficient time has lapsed), with a completely normal development of the periodontal ligament space. Although the majority of periapical lesions heal within 1 year, healing may continue for up to 4 years or longer.[229]

Absence of signs and symptoms of periapical disease with radiographic evidence of a persistent periapical radiolucency may indicate either fibrous repair (Fig. 11-5) or persistent chronic inflammation or infection. Only time and acute exacerbation would identify the latter, whereas the former should remain asymptomatic.

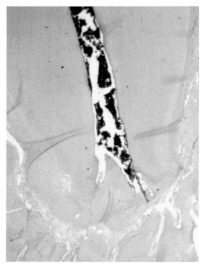

FIG. 11-3 Low-power view of healing by cementum formation when Sealpex is used (black particles are residual Sealapex and root filling material). (Courtesy Prof. M. Tagger.)

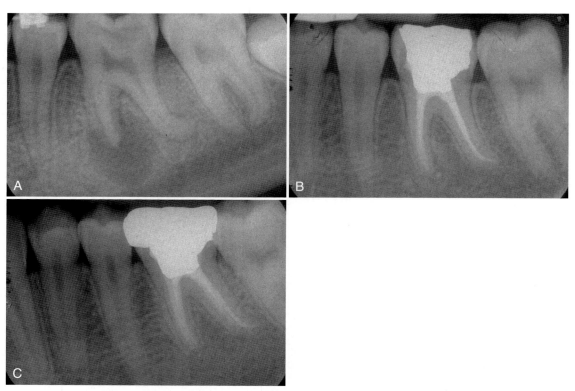

FIG. 11-4 Resolution of periapical disease after root canal treatment of the mandibular left molar with preoperative periapical radiolucency associated with mesial and distal roots (A), delayed healing caused by extruded filling material from the distal canal (B), and nearing complete healing as extruded material is resorbed (C).

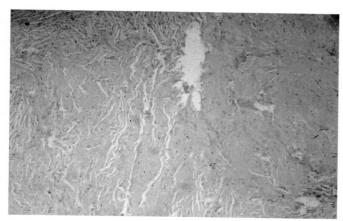

FIG. 11-5 Histologic view of fibrous periapical healing.

Longevity measures include survival of the root canal fillings or treatment[118,228,236] and tooth retention or survival.[111,149,190] The term *functional retention* was coined by Friedman in 2004[69] to mean retention of the tooth in the absence of signs and symptoms regardless of the radiographic presence of a lesion. The term *functionality* should further and more specifically cover the functional utility of the tooth—that is, some patients may complain that despite the absence of specific signs and symptoms of infection or inflammation, they find it impossible to use the tooth because it "feels" weak.

Modern definitions of health embrace a broader spectrum of measures including psychological well-being.[116] Instruments to assess these aspects have been developed in general medicine and adapted for application to dentistry, such as the Oral Health Related Quality of Life instrument.[55,87,115] There is no definitive instrument for measuring these aspects in endodontics as yet. Studies published so far have mainly adapted versions of the Oral Health Impact Profile (OHIP).

The periapical status of root-treated teeth has traditionally been assessed using two-dimensional conventional radiographic imaging. The use and limitations of two-dimensional radiographic images for assessing treatment outcome has been reviewed thoroughly and reported to suffer from low sensitivity, particularly in the posterior parts of the mouth.[98] The development of digital imaging technology[80] brought the possibility of image manipulation, including digital subtraction,[50,158,243,259] densitometric analysis,[156] correction of gray values,[32] and the manipulation of brightness and contrast.[75] However, none of these approaches has addressed the main deficiencies of accurately elucidating and quantitating the actual existence or progression of periapical bone loss.

Cone-beam computed tomography (CBCT), a new three-dimensional imaging technique requiring only 8% of the effective dose of conventional computed tomography,[119] has been proposed as a means of overcoming the problem of superimposition of tissue layers and structures. The diagnostic values of periapical radiography and cone-beam computed tomography were compared on dogs' teeth using histology as the comparative method of determining apical periodontitis 180 days after root canal treatment.[44] CBCT was found to be significantly more accurate in detecting minor bone lesions compared with two-dimensional radiology.[44,174] Other evidence to support the superior sensitivity of CBCT is available from studies using a

variety of simulated defects created in bone in pig[226] or human[165,221] jaws. Although the validity of clinical outcome data derived using conventional radiographic techniques has been questioned,[256] the *routine use* of CBCT is not recommended[62,91,197] owing to its higher radiation dosage.[5,91] The use of CBCT, which may be more sensitive for detection of periapical healing,[114,167] may give lower healing rates and longer durations to complete healing.

Many studies consider the treatment successful only when both radiographic and clinical criteria are satisfied.[69] It has been documented that a small proportion of cases present with persistent symptoms despite complete radiographic resolution of the periapical lesion.[176] Comparison of success rates estimated with or without clinical examination revealed no[93] or only a very small difference (1%).[150]

The widely accepted definition for endodontic success and failure by Strindberg[229] embraces both radiographic and clinical findings (Table 11-2). Friedman and Mor[69] preferred the terms *healed, healing,* and *diseased* instead of *success* and *failure* because of the potential of the latter to confuse patients. The "healed" category corresponds to "success" as defined by Strindberg,[229] whereas "healing" corresponds to "success" as defined by Bender and colleagues[17,18] (see Table 11-2).

The long duration of the periapical healing process coupled with the reduced recall rates at longer follow-up periods has provided opportunity for setting the thresholds of success at either complete healing or partial healing (reduced lesion size). The success criteria used for complete resolution have been described either as "strict"[152] or "stringent,"[69] whereas the criteria established for reduction in periapical radiolucency size has been described as either "loose"[152] or "lenient."[69] The frequency of adoption of these two thresholds has been similar in previous studies; the expected success rates using "strict" criteria would be expected to be lower than those based on "loose" criteria. The literature finds the difference to vary from 4% to 48%.[153]

A periapical index (PAI) consisting of five points on the scale was devised for measuring the periapical status and used in some studies.[157,159] However, the studies only reported the increase or decrease in mean scores for the clinical factors under investigation coupled with the proportion of successful cases. This approach precluded direct comparison of their data with studies reporting conventional dichotomized outcomes. Other studies using the index dichotomized the scores into "healthy" (PAI 1 or 2) or "diseased" (PAI 3 to 5) categories,[160] thus allowing the data to be compared directly with the more traditionally used binary outcomes of success or failure. In this system of designation, given that the PAI score 2 represents periodontal ligament widening, it effectively signals adoption of the "loose" threshold. The longitudinal follow-up[86] of 14 cases presenting with widened apical periodontal ligament (PAI score at 2) for 10 years revealed unfavorable future healing in only a small proportion of the cases (28%, 4/14).

Outcome Measures for Periapical Surgery

Nonsurgical root canal treatment alone may fail to resolve apical periodontitis in a small proportion of cases because it may not allow access to the infection or resolution of the cause of the infection (i.e., root fracture or crestal bone

TABLE 11-2

Criteria for Determination of Periapical Status

Strindberg (1956)	Bender et al. (1966, a and b)	Friedman & Mor (2004)
Success	**Success**	**Healed**
Clinical: No symptoms *Radiographic:* The contours, width, and structure of the periodontal margin were normal OR The periodontal contours were widened mainly around the excess filling	*Clinical:* Absence of pain/swelling; disappearance of fistula; no loss of function; no evidence of tissue destruction *Radiographic:* An eliminated or arrested area of rarefaction after a posttreatment interval of 6 months to 2 years	*Clinical:* Normal presentation *Radiographic:* Normal presentation
Failure		**Diseased**
Clinical: Presence of symptoms *Radiographic:* A decrease in the periradicular rarefaction OR Unchanged periradicular rarefaction OR An appearance of new rarefaction or an increase in the initial rarefaction		Radiolucency has emerged or persisted without change, even when the clinical presentation is normal OR Clinical signs or symptoms are present, even if the radiographic presentation is normal
Uncertain		**Healing**
Radiographic: There were ambiguous or technically unsatisfactory control radiographs that could not, for some reason, be repeated OR The tooth was extracted prior to the 3-year follow-up owing to the unsuccessful treatment of another root of the tooth		*Clinical:* Normal presentation *Radiographic:* Reduced radiolucency

communication to the periapical infection). Where the cause is microbial persistence, the infection may be localized intra-radicularly (in the apical canal anatomy [Fig. 11-6] or in the apical dentinal tubules [Fig. 11-7] or extraradicularly [Fig. 11-8]). In these instances, a surgical approach to the periapex may be required in addition to the nonsurgical approach to removing such microbes (see Fig. 11-7).

The success of periapical surgery has been assessed with the same clinical and radiographic criteria as for nonsurgical root canal treatment. However, the radiographic criteria for successful periapical healing are different from those for nonsurgical root canal treatment[140,186] (Table 11-3; Figs. 11-9, 11-10, and 11-11). Moreover, periodontal attachment loss in the form of marginal gingival recession is an additional criterion for measuring the outcome of periapical surgery.

Now that the parameters have been discussed as to the variables that need to be considered when assessing healing or nonhealing outcomes, the following discussion will describe the expected outcomes of the various endodontic procedures.

OUTCOMES OF VITAL PULP THERAPY PROCEDURES

The vital pulp therapy procedures discussed in this chapter include those for managing extensive caries with a high risk of pulpal exposure or pulps exposed through caries or traumatic injuries.

Indirect Pulp Capping (One-Step versus Stepwise Excavation)

The most conservative management for extensive caries is indirect pulp capping using either the one-step or the stepwise excavation approach. The stepwise excavation approach with initial partial caries removal was advocated to reduce the risk of pulpal exposure and is generally considered to be associated with poorer outcomes. The clinical outcomes of the one-step or stepwise approaches have been compared in three randomized controlled trials on permanent teeth with deep caries.[19,113,121,122] Stepwise excavation was found to be associated with a lower rate of pulp exposure and higher chance of long-term clinical success than the one-step excavation approach[19,113] (Table 11-4). Maltz and colleagues,[121,122] however, found the contrary, and they attributed the low long-term clinical success rate of the stepwise approach to patients being noncompliant in returning for scheduled completion of treatment. Interestingly, comparison of the cost-effectiveness of the one-step versus the stepwise excavation techniques using health-economic modeling involving simulated treatment of a molar tooth with deep caries in a 15-year-old patient revealed the one-step procedure to accrue lower long-term costs as well as longer tooth retention and pulp vitality.[200]

Meta-analyses of data from studies[19,20,65,81,89,113,120-122,141] listed in Table 11-4 revealed that the weighted pooled success rate for indirect pulp capping using the one-step approach (81.7%; 95% confidence interval [CI]: 72.7%, 90.6%)

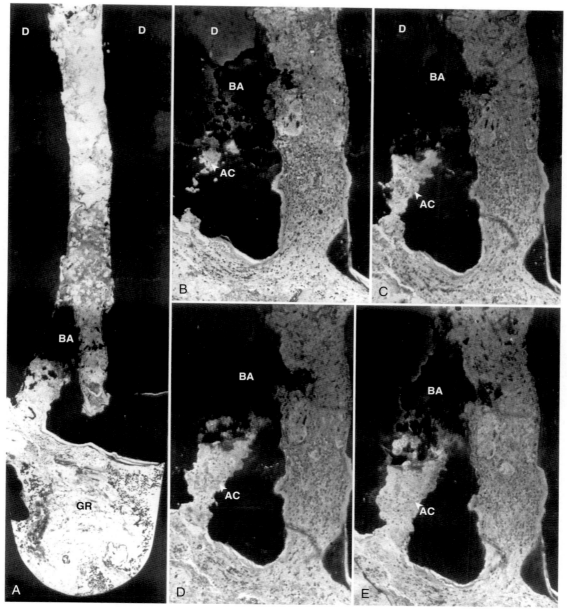

FIG. 11-6 Axial sections through the surgically removed apical portion of the root with a therapy-resistant periapical lesion (GR). Note the cluster of bacteria (BA) visible in the root canal. Parts B–E show serial semithin sections taken at varying distances from the section plane of (A) to reveal the emerging (B) and gradually widening (C–E) profiles of an accessory root canal (AC). Note that the accessory canal is clogged with bacteria (BA). Original magnification: A ×52; B–E ×62. (From Nair PN, Sjogren U, Krey G, Sundqvist G: Therapy-resistant foreign body giant cell granuloma at the periapex of a root-filled human tooth, *J Endod* 16:589, 1990.)

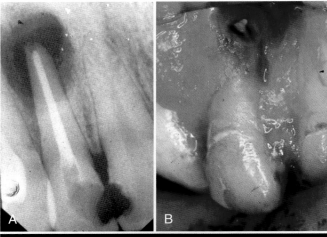

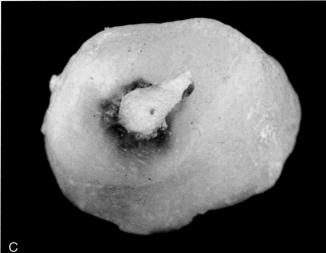

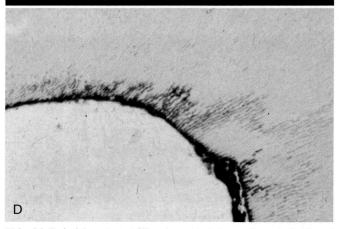

FIG. 11-7 A, Adequate root filling demonstrated on radiograph. **B,** View of the periapical surgery and root resection of the tooth shown in **(A)** shows stained root dentine. **C,** Resected root showing stained/infected dentine. **D,** Histologic view of the root end shown in **(C)** showing infected dentinal tubules (S).

TABLE 11-3

Classification of Periapical Healing Following Apical Surgery

Rud et al. (1972) and Molven et al. (1987)

Complete Healing

Reformation of a Periodontal Space with

Normal width and lamina dura to be followed around the apex
Slight increase in width of apical periodontal space but less than twice the width of noninvolved parts of the root
Tiny defect in the lamina dura (maximum 1 mm) adjacent to the root filling

Complete Bone Repair with

Bone bordering the apical area does not have the same density as surrounding noninvolved bone
No apical periodontal space can be discerned

Incomplete Healing (Scar Tissue)

The Rarefaction Has Decreased in Size or Remained Stationary with

Bone structure recognized within the rarefaction
The irregular periphery of the rarefaction and demarcation by a compact bone border
The rarefaction located asymmetrically around the apex
Angular connection between the rarefaction and the periodontal space

An Isolated Scar Tissue in the Bone with Findings Above

Uncertain Healing

The Rarefaction Has Decreased in Size with

The size larger than twice the width of the periodontal space
Lamina-dura like bone structures around the border
A circular or semicircular periphery
Symmetric location around the apex as a funnel-shaped extension of the periodontal space
Bone structure discernible within the bony cavity
A collar-shaped increase in width of lamina dura coronal to the radiolucency

Unsatisfactory Healing (Failures)

The rarefaction has enlarged or is unchanged
If a case still demonstrated "uncertain healing" 4 years postoperatively, the treatment should be considered a failure[186]

(Fig. 11-12) was similar to that for the stepwise approach (81.9%; 95% CI: 72.1%, 91.7%) (Fig. 11-13).

Calcium hydroxide cement was the preferred lining material for the pulpal surface, whereas zinc oxide–eugenol–based cement was the preferred base material in most studies. Recently, resin-modified-glass-ionomer liner has also been used, but the type of lining material did not influence the outcome (see Table 11-4). The age of patients, presence of preoperative pain, and pulpal exposure during excavation were significant negative prognostic factors.[19]

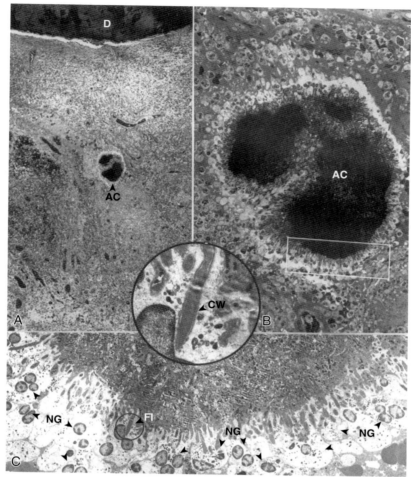

FIG. 11-8 Actinomyces in the body of a human periapical granuloma. The colony (AC in B) is magnified in B. The rectangular area demarcated in B is magnified in C. Note the starburst appearance of the colony with needle-like peripheral filaments surrounded by few layers of neutrophilic granulocytes (NG), some of which contain phagocytosed bacteria. A dividing peripheral filament (FI) is magnified in the inset. Note the typical Gram-positive wall (CW): D = dentine. Original magnification: A ×60; B ×430; C ×1680; inset ×6700. (From Nair PR, Schroeder H: Periapical actinomycosis, *J Endod* 10:567, 1984.)

Direct Pulp Capping

Direct pulp capping is performed on teeth with pulp exposures caused by caries, caries excavation, or traumatic injuries. Most studies investigating the clinical outcome of direct pulp capping on permanent teeth had excluded teeth with signs and symptoms of irreversible pulpitis and apical pathosis (Table 11-5). Saline, sodium hypochlorite, and chlorhexidine have been reportedly used to irrigate the exposed pulp and to achieve hemostasis. Calcium hydroxide paste and mineral trioxide aggregate (MTA) were the commonly used capping materials (see Table 11-5).

A meta-analysis of data from studies* listed in Table 11-5 revealed the weighted pooled success rate to be 70.1% (95% CI: 59.9%, 80.2%) (Fig. 11-14). The patient's age and sex;

tooth location and type; pulp exposure type, size, and its location; and the restoration type, size, and quality did not have a significant influence on success. Although the outcome of direct pulp capping of teeth with immature versus mature apices has not been systematically compared in individual studies, indirect comparison of pooled data from different studies[1] revealed that teeth with immature roots were associated with significantly more successful outcomes.

The type of capping material was another significant prognostic factor,[90,197,207] with MTA performing superiorly to calcium hydroxide in a randomized controlled trial[90] and in a systematic review.[1]

Pulpotomy

Earlier studies on the outcome of *partial pulpotomy* (specifying varying degrees of coronal pulp removal) had only included teeth with vital traumatic pulp exposures; however, more recent studies have also included teeth with carious pulp exposures. Teeth with spontaneous or severe pain and signs and

---

*Please see the following references: 12, 19, 21, 64, 65, 72, 88, 90, 92, 128, 132, 133, 193, 207, and 254.

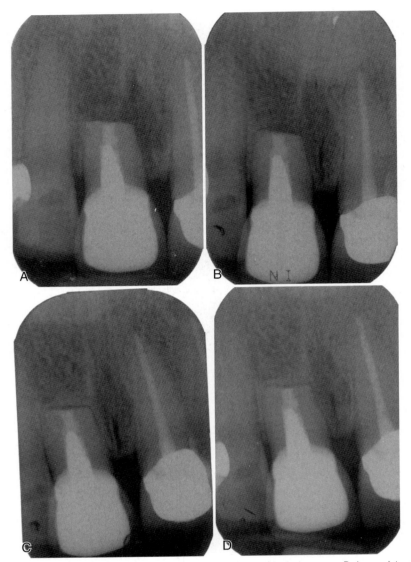

FIG. 11-9 **A,** A maxillary right central incisor having undergone periapical surgery. **B,** Incomplete periapical healing at 1 year postoperatively. Complete healing at 3 (**C**) and 4 years (**D**) postoperatively.

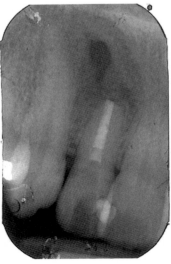

FIG. 11-10 Example of incomplete healing with isolated scar tissue.

symptoms of apical pathosis were excluded (Table 11-6). On the other hand, the outcomes of *full pulpotomies* (completely removing the coronal pulp and retaining the radicular pulp) had only been investigated in teeth with carious exposures (Table 11-7). Saline irrigation has been preferred for achieving hemostasis, whereas calcium hydroxide and more recently MTA were the preferred pulp capping materials (see Table 11-6).

A meta-analysis of data from studies listed in Tables 11-6[10,11,19,40,71,125,131,177] and 11-7[6,30,31,52,58,126,187,192,235,251,255] revealed the weighted pooled success rate to be 79.3% (95% CI: 66.7%, 91.8%) for partial pulpotomies (Fig. 11-15) and 82.4% (95% CI: 69.3%, 95.4%) for full pulpotomies (Fig. 11-16).

The effects of potential prognostic factors for pulpotomy have not been explored systematically except for the pulp capping material. Randomized controlled trials revealed that MTA achieved similar outcomes in partial[177] or full pulpotomies[58] when compared with calcium hydroxide.

Text continued on p. 495

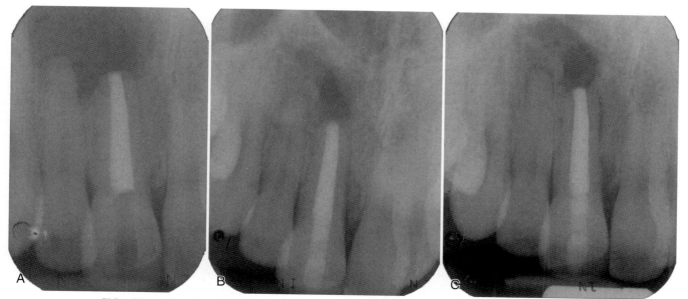

FIG. 11-11 Example of uncertain healing. Periapical radiographs of a maxillary left central incisor taken immediately after periapical surgery (A), at 2 years postoperatively (B), and at 3 years postoperatively (C).

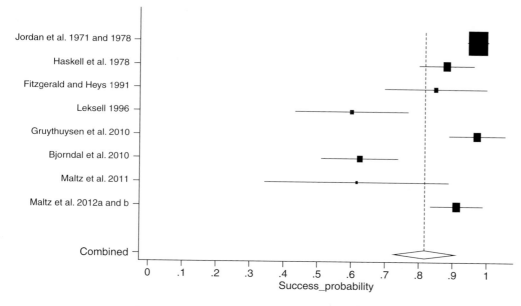

FIG. 11-12 Forest plot showing individual study and weighted pooled probabilities of success for one-step indirect pulp capping.

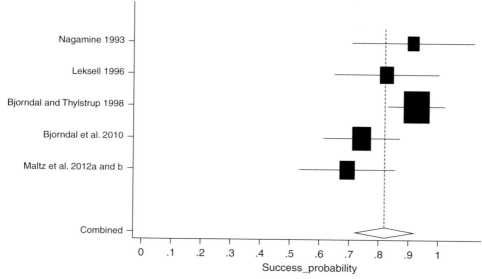

FIG. 11-13 Forest plot showing individual study and weighted pooled probabilities of success for stepwise indirect pulp capping.

TABLE 11-4

Studies Investigating the Clinical/Radiographic Outcome of Indirect Pulp Capping of Permanent Teeth

Study	Study Design	Type of Indirect Pulp Capping	No. of Teeth	Success (%)	Age	Pretreatment Status	Capping Material	Criteria for Success	Duration after Treatment	Notes
More, 1967	Case series	Stepwise	8	8 (100%)	11 to 18	Carious Vital Apical pathosis	1st visit: ZOE. 2nd visit: CH/Amal	Vital/asymptomatic/intact PDL	6 to 36 mo	
Jordan et al., 1971 (in Hayashi et al., 2011) and 1978	Case series	1-step	243	236 (97.1%)	8 to 37	Deep caries without pulpitis	CH, CH + cresatin, or ZOE/ZOE + amalgam	Vital/asymptomatic/intact PDL	Not given	24 teeth were followed up for 11 yr, 11 remained vital with no evidence of pathosis
Sawusch, 1982 (in Hayashi et al., 2011)	CCT	Stepwise	48	48 (100%)	14 or younger	Deep caries without pulpitis	CH (Dycal versus improved Dycal)/ZOE or ZnP04	Clinical	6 mo	
Fitzgerald & Heys, 1991	Case series	1-step	46	39 (84.8%)	20 to 60	Deep caries Vital	CH (Dycal versus Life)	Asymptomatic	1 yr	The brand of CH did not have significant effect
Nagamine, 1993 (in Hayashi et al., 2011)	CCT	Stepwise	23	21 (91.3%)	17 to 46	Deep caries without pulpitis	Polycarboxylate cement with tannin-fluoride versus hydraulic temporary sealing material/GIC	Vital	3 mo	
Leksell, 1996	RCT	Stepwise	57	47 (82.5%)	6 to 16	Not given	CH/ZOE then CH/GIC	Asymptomatic/intact PDL	1 to 11 yr (mean = 43 mo)	47/57 without exposure; duration of CH dressing had no significant influence on exposure 42/70 without exposure
		1-step	70	42 (60.0%)						

Study	Study type	Treatment	N	Success	Age	Criteria	CH/temporary filling	Outcome	Follow-up	Comments
Bjorndal & Thylstrup, 1998	Case series	Stepwise	94	87 (92.6%)	Not given	Deep caries	CH/temporary filling	Absence of perforation, asymptomatic	1 yr	88/94 without exposure
Bjorndal et al., 2010	RCT	Stepwise 1-step	143 149	106 (74.1%) 93 (62.4%)	29 (25-38)	Deep caries Only provoked pain Vital	CH/GIC	Vital/intact PDL	1 yr	Stepwise better than complete; preoperative pain, older patients reduce success
Gruythuysen et al., 2010	Case series	1-step	34	33 (97.1%)	Up to 18	Carious (> 2/3) No spontaneous, persistent pain No apical pathosis	GIC	Survive/ asymptomatic/ intact PDL/no resorption	3 yr	
Maltz et al., 2011	Case series	1-step	26	16 (61.5%)		Vital Deep caries	CH/ZOE then composite	Vital	10 yr	
Maltz et al., 2012 (a and b)	RCT (multicenter)	1-step Stepwise	112 101	111 (18 mo) 102 (91.7%) (3 yr) 87 (18 mo) 70 (69.3%) (3 yr)	≥ 6	Vital Carious (> 1/2) No spontaneous, persistent pain No apical pathosis	GIC/amalgam or composite CH/ZOE then GIC/ amalgam or composite	Vital/intact PDL Vital/intact PDL	18 mo, 3 yr (clinical and radiographic outcome)	Indirect pulp capping was associated with significantly higher success rate than stepwise, regardless of duration after treatment; the low success rate of stepwise was attributed to patients not returning for completion of treatment

TABLE 11-5

Studies Investigating the Clinical/Radiographic Outcome of Direct Pulp Capping of Permanent Teeth

Study	Study Design	No. of Teeth	Success (%)	Age (year)	Pretreatment Status	Hemostasis	Capping Material	Base/Restorative Material	Criteria for Success	Duration after Treatment	Notes
Weiss, 1966	Case series	160	141 (88.0%)	16 to 67	Not given	Not given	CH + cresatin	ZOE	Vital/asymptomatic/intact PDL	3 yr	
Shovelton et al., 1971	RCT	154 (1-step) 53 (2-step)	115 (74.7%) 33 (64.7%)	15 to 44	Carious or traumatic exposure Vital Asymptomatic Molar/premolar	Saline	Corticosteroid + antibiotic, glycyrrhetinic acid + antibiotics, ZOE, or CH	ZOE/amalgam	Vital/asymptomatic/intact PDL	24 mo	There was no significant difference in success rates among the various capping materials
Haskell et al., 1978	Case series	133	117 (88.0%)	8 to 74	Carious exposure Asymptomatic	Not given	CH or penicillin	ZOE	Vital/asymptomatic/intact PDL	> 5 yr	5- to 22-year survival Success rate was not affected by age and tooth type
Gillien & Schuman, 1985	Case series	17	13 (76.4%)	6 to 9	Carious exposure	Not given	CH	Base material not given/amalgam or crown	Asymptomatic/intact PDL	6 to 12 mo	
Horsted et al., 1985	Case series	510	485 (95.1%)	Not given	Exposure during cavity preparation or caries removal No periapical pathosis No pain	2% chloramine or 0.2% CHX	CH	ZOE	Vital/asymptomatic/intact PDL	5 yr	Type of exposure and tooth type had no significant effects Older age had lower survival
Fitzgerald & Heys, 1991	Case series	8	6 (75.0%)	20 to 60	Vital Exposure during caries removal	Sterile cotton pellets	CH	ZnPO$_4$/amalgam or composite	Asymptomatic	12 mo	The brand of setting CH paste did not have significant effect

Study	Design	N	Success	Age	Clinical condition	Irrigant	Material	Restoration	Outcome	Follow-up	Comments
Matsuo et al., 1996	Case series	44	36 (81.2%)	20 to 69	Carious exposure No intense pain	10% NaOCl and 3% H_2O_2	CH	ZOE/GIC	Vital/ asymptomatic/ intact PDL	3 yr	
Santucci, 1999	Case series	29	15 (51.7%)	Not given	Exposure due to caries, or its removal Sensitive to cold or sweat with no other pain No periapical pathosis	Not given	CH	Composite or cast gold restoration	Asymptomatic	4.5 yr	
Barthel et al., 2000	Case series	123	29 (23.6%)	10 to 70	Carious exposure	3% H_2O_2	CH/$ZnPO_4$ or other materials	Not given	Vital/ asymptomatic/ intact PDL	5 to 10 yr	Age, tooth type, site of exposure had no significant effects Immediate placement of permanent restoration had significantly higher success rate
Farsi et al., 2006	Case series	30	28 (93.3%)	9 to 12	Deep caries Potential exposure Reversible pulpitis Intact PDL	Saline	MTA	ZOE/composite	Vital/ asymptomatic/ intact PDL/ continuous root development	2 yr	
Bogen et al., 2008	Case series	49	48 (98.0%)	7 to 45	Carious exposure (.25 to 2.5 mm) Reversible pulpitis	5.25/6% NaOCl	MTA	Composite	Dentine Vital/ bridge/ asymptomatic/ root development/ intact PDL	1 to 9 yr	
Bjorndal et al., 2010	RCT	22	7 (31.8%)	25 to 38	Exposure during caries removal Only provoked pain Vital	Saline	CH	GIC	Vital/intact PDL	1 yr	

Continued

TABLE 11-5

Studies Investigating the Clinical/Radiographic Outcome of Direct Pulp Capping of Permanent Teeth—cont'd

Study	Study Design	No. of Teeth	Success (%)	Age (year)	Pretreatment Status	Hemostasis	Capping Material	Base/Restorative Material	Criteria for Success	Duration after Treatment	Notes
Mente et al., 2010	Case series	122	86 (70.5%)	8 to 78	Carious or mechanical exposure	0.12% CHX	MTA or CH	GIC/composite or crown	Vital/no clinical or radiographic evidence of apical pathosis	12 to 18 mo	Use of MTA for capping and immediate placement of permanent restoration had significantly higher success rate; Age; sex; tooth location and type; exposure site and type; restoration type, size, and quality did not have significant effects
Miles et al., 2010	Case series	51	23 (45.1%)	21 to 85	Carious exposure	2.5% NaOCl	MTA	GIC/composite or amalgam	Vital/asymptomatic/intact PDL	12 to 27 mo	
Hilton et al., 2013	RCT	126 144	81 (64.3%) 116 (80.6%)	9 to 90 8 to 89	Carious, traumatic, mechanical exposure	5.25% NaOCl	CH MTA	GIC	Vital/intact PDL/ no resorption/ not requiring extraction or root canal treatment	2 yr	MTA was associated with significantly higher success rate than CH; Patient, dentist, tooth, pulp exposure, and pulp capping characteristics did not have significant influence on the results

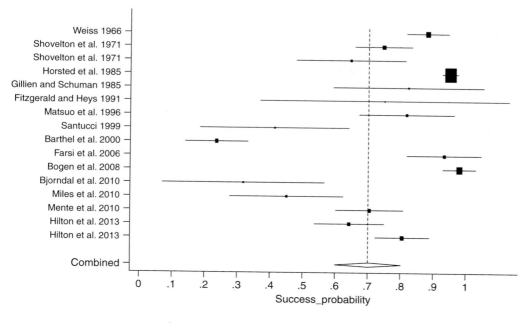

FIG. 11-14 Forest plot showing individual study and weighted pooled probabilities of success for direct pulp capping.

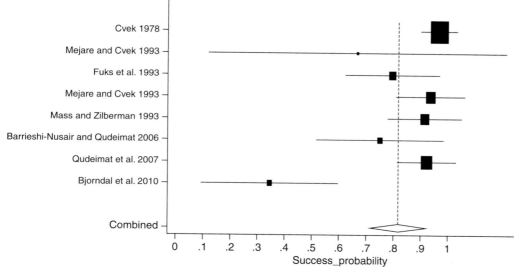

FIG. 11-15 Forest plot showing individual study and weighted pooled probabilities of success for partial pulpotomy.

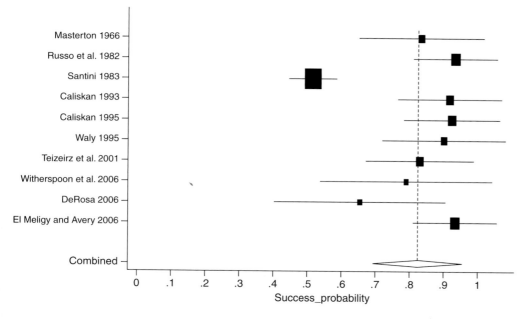

FIG. 11-16 Forest plot showing individual study and weighted pooled probabilities of success for full pulpotomy.

TABLE 11-6

Studies Investigating the Clinical/Radiographic Outcome of Partial Pulpotomy of Permanent Teeth

Author	No. of Teeth	Success (%)	Age	Pretreatment Status	Exposure Size	Hemostasis	Pulp Dressing Material	Base/ Restorative Material	Criteria for Success	Duration after Treatment	Notes
Cvek, 1978	60	58 (96.7%)	Not given	Traumatic exposure Vital Bleeding wound	0.5 to 4.0 mm	Saline	1st visit: nonsetting CH 2nd visit: setting CH	1st visit: ZOE 2nd visit: Composite	EPT/asymptomatic/ intact PDL/ continued root development/ hard tissue barrier	14 to 60 mo	Size and duration of exposure, root maturity did not affect outcome
Baratieri et al., 1989	26	26 (100%)	12 to 44	Exposure due to caries or caries removal Pulp tissue bleeding without signs of degeneration	Not given	Calcium hydroxide solution	CH powder then hard set CH cement	Zinc oxide cement	Asymptomatic/vital	1 to 2 yr	
Fuks et al., 1993	44	35 (79.5%)	Not given	Traumatic exposure Vital Bleeding wound	Not given	Saline	CH	ZOE	Asymptomatic/ bridge/root development/ vital	0.5 to 4 yr	
Mass & Zilberman, 1993	35	32 (91.4%)	7.5 to 25	Molar Deep caries Asymptomatic No apical pathosis	Less than 1 to 2 mm in diameter; 2 to 3 mm deep	Saline	CH	ZOE/ amalgam or crown	Asymptomatic/ intact PDL/root development	1 to 2 yr	

Study	N	Success (n, %)	Age	Diagnosis	Exposure/Depth	Irrigant	Material	Restoration	Outcome measure	Follow-up	Notes
Mejare & Cvek, 1993	31 (2-step) 6 (1-step)	29 (93.5%) 4 (66.7%)	Not given	Carious exposure Asymptomatic No apical pathosis	N/A	Saline	CH	ZOE	Asymptomatic/ intact PDL/root development	24 to 140 mo	
Barrieshi-Nusair & Qudeimat, 2006	28	21 (75.0%)	7.2 to 13.1	Carious exposure Molar Reversible pulpitis No apical pathosis	2 to 4 mm deep	Saline	MTA	GIC/amalgam or crown	Vital/asymptomatic/ intact PCL/root development	1 to 2 yr	
Qudeimat et al., 2007*	23 28	21 (91.3%) 26 (92.9%)	6.8 to 13.3	Carious exposure Molar	2 to 4 mm deep	Saline	CH MTA	GIC/amalgam or crown	Absence of signs and symptoms/ intact PDL/root development	24.5 to 45.6 mo	There was no significant difference in outcome between CH and MTA
Bjorndal et al., 2010*	29	10 (34.5%)	25 to 38	Deep caries Only provoked pain Vital Expose during removal	Not given	Saline	CH	GIC	Vital/intact PDL	1 yr	

NB: All the studies were case series except those labeled with *.
Qudeimat et al. (2007) is a randomized controlled trial comparing calcium hydroxide versus MTA as pulp dressing material.
Bjørndal et al. (2010) is a randomized controlled trial comparing the outcomes of 1-step versus stepwise indirect pulp capping for teeth without exposure, and direct pulp capping versus partial pulpotomy for teeth with exposure during caries removal.

TABLE 11-7

Studies Investigating the Clinical/Radiographic Outcome of Full Pulpotomy of Permanent Teeth

Author	No. of Teeth	Success (%)	Age	Pretreatment Status	Hemostasis	Capping Material	Base/Restorative Material	Criteria for Success	Duration after Treatment	Notes
Masterson, 1966	30	25 (83.3%)	6 to 39	Not given	Not given	CH	Not given	Vital/asymptomatic	1 to 70 mo	
Russo et al., 1982	30	28 (93.3%)	9 to 28	Carious exposure No apical pathosis	Not given	CH	Not given	Intact PDL	8 w	
Santini, 1983	373	192 (51.4%)	Not given	Carious exposure or near exposure Symptomatic	Cotton wool pellet	CH or CH + Ledermix	ZOE	Vital/bridge/asymptomatic	6 mo	Sex and medicament had no significant effect Poor healing was associated with age < 7.5
Caliskan, 1993	24	22 (91.7%)	10 to 22	Hyperplastic pulpitis	Saline	CH	ZOE/Amalgam or composite	Vital/asymptomatic/ dentine bridge/ intact PDL	1 to 4 yr	
Caliskan, 1995	26	24 (92.3%)	10 to 24	Carious exposure Asymptomatic Apical pathosis	Saline	CH	ZOE	Asymptomatic/bridge/ root development/ vital	16 to 72 mo	
Waly, 1995	20	18 (90.0%)		Carious exposure Molar		CH-glutaraldehyde CH	Not given	Not given	5 yr	
Teizeira et al., 2001	41	34 (82.9%)	6 to 16	Deep caries or exposed pulp With or without apical pathosis	Not given	CH	GIC	Vital/asymptomatic/ dentine bridge/ intact PDL	24 to 32 w	
DeRosa, 2006	26	17 (65.4%)		Not given		CH	Amalgam	Asymptomatic	14 to 88 mo	
El Meligy & Avery, 2006	15 15	13 (86.7%) 15 (100%)	6 to 12	Carious or traumatized teeth Immature apex No apical pathosis Saline		CH MTA	ZOE/Amalgam or composite	Asymptomatic/intact PDL/no resorption/ root development	1 yr	
Witherspoon et al., 2006	19	15 (79.0%)	7 to 16	Carious or traumatic exposure Irreversible pulpitis	6% NaOCl	MTA	Not given	Vital/asymptomatic/ intact PDL/root development	1 yr	
Asgary & Ehsani, 2009	12	12 (100%)	14 to 62	Carious Irreversible pulpitis	Saline	NEC	Permanent rest	Asymptomatic/intact PDL	13 to 20 mo	

NB: All the studies were case series except El Meligy & Avery (2006), which was a randomized controlled trial comparing calcium hydroxide and MTA as pulp dressing material.

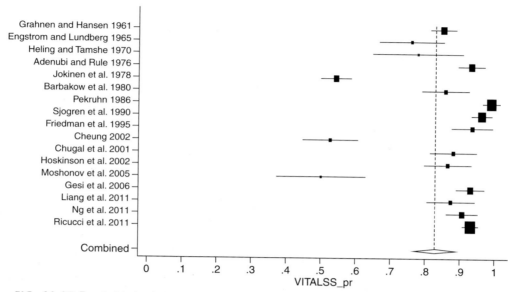

FIG. 11-17 Forest plot showing results of pooled and individual study's probability of maintained periapical health for preoperatively vital teeth undergoing root canal treatment (pooled probability = 0.83; 95% confidence interval: 0.77, 0.89).

Summary of Prognostic Factors for Vital Pulp Therapy

In summary, vital pulp therapy performed under guideline standards with optimal coronal seal achieved promising long-term success in teeth with carious, mechanical, or traumatic exposures of healthy pulps.

The most important factors affecting the outcome of vital pulp therapy are preexisting health of the pulp, adequate removal of infected hard or soft tissues, careful operative technique to avoid damage to residual tissues, and elimination of microbial leakage around the final restoration. It can be difficult to gauge the health of the residual pulp as it is a matter of subjective assessment and relies on experience in pulp diagnosis. The degree of pulp bleeding upon exposure is a more reliable tool to judge the status of the pulp than the preoperative clinical signs and symptoms. Continued bleeding after 10 minutes, even after rinsing with sodium hypochlorite solution, may suggest that the residual pulp was still heavily inflamed and a complete pulpectomy may be a more effective treatment modality. Removal of infected tissue is a matter of subjective experience but may be aided by various dyes. The final factor relies on the correct choice of restorative material and its adequate manipulation to prevent leakage.

Factors such as age and health of the patient, size and nature (carious or traumatic) of pulp exposure, and its duration of exposure to the oral environment (up to 48 hours) do not in themselves compromise outcomes of vital pulp therapy.

OUTCOMES OF NONSURGICAL ROOT CANAL TREATMENT

In contrast to other areas of endodontics, the number of studies and extent of investigation of nonsurgical root canal treatment is more comprehensive, yielding a much greater insight even though the quality and scope of the research does not always reach the highest levels.

A systematic review and meta-analysis of the factors affecting primary root canal treatment outcome conducted by the authors revealed the following: the mean success rate was 83% when vital pulpectomy was performed (Fig. 11-17), which reduced to 72% when the root canal treatment procedure was used to eradicate the established infection associated with a periapical lesion (Fig. 11-18).

Factors Affecting Periapical Health or Healing Following Root Canal Treatment

The factors influencing the maintenance of periapical health or periapical healing of preexisting lesions following root canal treatment may be broadly classified into patient factors (age, sex, general health, tooth anatomy, preoperative pulpal and periapical status), treatment factors (operator variables, canal enlargement, irrigation, medication, culture test, and obturation), and restorative factors. Some factors had a profound impact on success rates, whereas others showed a negligible effect. Patient factors characterizing the nature of the disease showed the most significant effect (periapical status), whereas most of the treatment factors were found to exert a less significant effect; the exceptions were the apical extent of root canal treatment relative to the root canal terminus. In addition, the quality of the postoperative restorative care also exerted a profound influence on outcome of treatment.

Patient Factors

Patient's age and sex consistently had no significant effect on outcome, whereas some specific health conditions (diabetes,[54,67] compromised immune response[123]) apparently had a significant influence. The evidence for the effect of host immune response characterized by the general health of the patient is, however, weak. Emerging evidence indicates that the host response measured by polymorphisms of various genes involved in periapical healing may have an effect on outcomes[142,183,212,213] (Table 11-8). The importance of the host

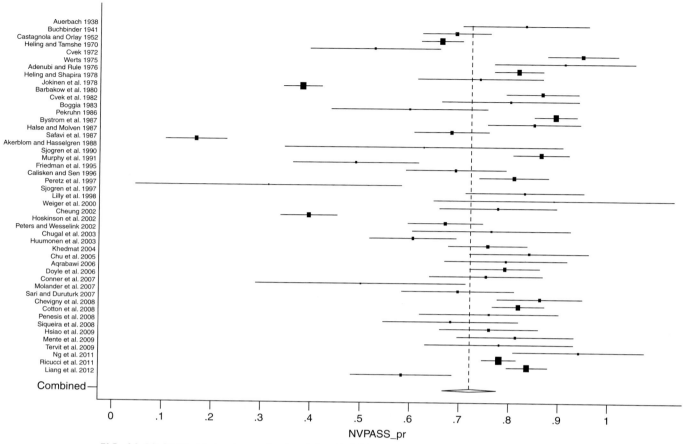

FIG. 11-18 Forest plot showing results of pooled and individual study's probability of periapical health for teeth associated with nonvital pulps and periapical radiolucencies undergoing root canal treatment (pooled probability = 0.72; 95% confidence interval: 0.67, 0.78).

TABLE 11-8

Type of Genes Investigated in Studies on SNPs and Periapical Healing

Study	Gene Function	Genes	Findings
Siqueira et al., 2009	Interleukin 1 Fcγ receptor	IL-1α, IL-1β FcγRIIa, FcγRIIIb	No significant association Significant association
Morsani et al., 2011	Interleukin	IL-1β	Significant association
Siqueira et al., 2011	Fcγ receptor	FcγRIIIa	No significant association
Rôças et al., 2014	Pattern recognition receptors	CD14, TLR4	No significant association

response to maintenance of periapical health or periapical healing was also supported by the statistically significant clustering effect of multiple teeth within the same patient in a prospective study.[150]

The widespread perception that single-rooted teeth with less complicated anatomy should benefit with more predictable and favorable outcomes proves to be untrue. Having accounted for potential confounding factors such as the presence of periapical disease, tooth type does not seem to exert a strong influence on success rates. This would appear to be counterintuitive but may be explained by the logical inference that canal complexities in the apical anatomy probably play a more dominant role than other complexities such as the number and curvature of canals.

The presence and size of a periapical lesion seem to have the most negative effect on periapical health/healing; it therefore follows that these factors must be accounted for when analyzing the influence of any other factor. The profound change in success rates once a periapical lesion becomes established is interesting, as it is correlated with the establishment of infection in the apical canal anatomy. This seems to suggest that once the apical canal complexities become infected, it may be much more difficult to eradicate the infection. The negative influence of large periapical lesions has a reasonable biologic explanation: the diversity of bacteria (by number of species and their relative abundance) is greater in teeth with larger periapical lesions.[230] An endodontic infection is more likely to persist in canals with a higher number of bacteria present preoperatively.[27] In addition, larger lesions may represent longer-standing root canal infections that may have penetrated deeper into dentinal tubules and accessory anatomy in the complex canal system[206] where mechanical and chemical decontamination procedures may not be so effective. Larger lesions may also represent cystic transformation.[145] Finally, the host response may also play a part, as patients with larger lesions may innately respond less favorably to residual bacteria.[147] This speculation may crystallize into distinct questions for further biologic research into the nature of interactions among host, bacterial infection, and treatment intervention.

Most of the other investigated preoperative factors (pain, tooth tenderness to percussion, soft tissue tenderness to palpation, soft tissue swelling and sinus tract, periodontal probing defect of endodontic origin, root resorption) are in fact different clinical manifestations of periapical disease.[254] They may therefore act as surrogate measures or complement "presence and size of periapical lesion" in measuring the effect of severity of periapical disease within a broad continuous spectrum. Of these, only presence of preoperative pain,[68] sinus tract,[150] swelling,[150] and apical resorption[229] have been found to be significant prognostic factors that have been associated with significantly reduced success rates in root canal treatment.

The biologic explanation for the negative impact of sinus tract and swelling, either in the acute or chronic form, on periapical healing is interesting, as both represent suppuration and the proliferation of microbiota into the periapical tissues, with the inference being that the host tissues must have become locally overwhelmed. The precise reasons for reduced success rates under these conditions remain unclear but must somehow be related to the nature of the host-microbial interaction.

Treatment Factors
Operator
Although the impact of operator qualification and skill has not been specifically investigated, systematic review has shown that the involved clinicians may be grouped into undergraduate students, general practitioners, postgraduate students, and specialists. Studies show a clear trend in superior outcomes by greater experience and training. Clearly technical skills play an important role, but this is difficult and often impossible to quantify. In addition, the technical abilities must be augmented by the overall understanding of the biologic issues and the quest for superior treatment by the operator. If clinicians do not feel they can do optimal treatment, it is incumbent upon them to refer the patient to a more qualified practitioner.

Isolation
The use of rubber dams in modern root canal treatment is widely accepted, and the justification seems almost empirical. One study on retreatment[244] analyzed the influence of rubber dam use compared to cotton roll isolation and found significantly higher success rates with the former approach. Another study reported a significantly higher success rate of root canal–treated teeth[76] when a rubber dam was employed during post placement compared to when it was not. Perhaps as a consequence, the principal justification for rubber dam use is based

on medicolegal implications of root canal instrument ingestion or aspiration by the patient.[61]

Magnification and Illumination
Endodontists have repeatedly reinforced the value of magnification and illumination during root canal treatment,[166] but a systematic review failed to draw any objective conclusions on their influence as no article was identified in the current literature that satisfied their inclusion criteria.[46] A prospective study investigated this factor,[150] but researchers found only an insignificant influence on the final outcome. Use of a microscope may sometimes assist location of the second mesiobuccal canal in maxillary molars, but this only made a small difference to the success rates associated with mesiobuccal roots, when a periapical lesion was present.[150] The true benefit of a microscope can only be verified through a randomized controlled trial. However, canal negotiation with less tooth structure removal and fewer procedural accidents is favorable and seems intuitively more consistent with the use of superior magnification and illumination.

Mechanical Preparation: Size, Taper, Extent, and Procedural Errors
The root canal system may be mechanically prepared to a requisite size and taper[199] using a variety of instruments of different cutting designs, tips, tapers, and materials of construction. Their efficacy is often tested in laboratory studies, and the instruments and their utility may have well-characterized properties.[95] Investigation of the influence of type of instrument used for canal enlargement has been undertaken in one nonrandomized prospective study, but the outcome is likely subjective because of many factors, including the protocol adopted for teaching technical skills.[150] In this study, the better success rates for hand or rotary NiTi instruments compared with stainless steel instruments[150] were attributable to the fact that tactile skills training was achieved through a preliminary focus on the use of stainless steel files to develop tactile sensitivity and consistency. Only on demonstration of this competency did the trainees progress to NiTi instruments. More important, such senior students may also have had a better understanding of the biologic rationale for root canal treatment. The ability to gain and maintain apical patency as well as to avoid procedural errors was better instilled in the senior students, whereas in selected cases, NiTi instruments appear capable of achieving the same in primary root canal treatment undertaken by undergraduates.[175]

A key tenet of the European Society of Endodontology (ESE)[61] guidelines is that root canal debridement must be extended to the terminus of the canal system, which is expressed variously as extension to the "apical constriction," or to "0.5 to 2 mm from the radiographic apex," or to the "cementodentinal junction." This guideline is broadly supported by the fact that outcome of treatment is compromised by canal obstruction or failure to achieve patency to the canal terminus.[150,216,229] Ng and colleagues[150] reported a twofold reduction in the success of treatment when the patency to the canal terminus was not achieved. It could be speculated that the lack of mechanical negotiability of canals may be due to the presence of obstructions caused by "denticles," tertiary dentine, acute branching or a fine plexus of apical canals, or dentine/organic debris.

The continued debate on the optimal size of apical preparation remains topical in the absence of definitive evidence; the findings from relevant in vitro and clinical studies have been previously reviewed.[15] So far, four clinical outcome studies have considered this issue or have systematically investigated the effect of apical size of canal preparation on treatment outcome.[93,102,150,188,223,229] One randomized controlled trial revealed that enlargement of the canal to three sizes larger than the first apical binding file was adequate[188] (the mean final size was ISO #30). The observational studies[95,150,229] had not designed their investigation with apical canal size as their principal focus and neither had they found a statistically significant influence from this factor; nevertheless, they all reported the same inverse trend of decreasing success rates with an increase in size of apical preparation. It was speculated that canal preparation to larger apical sizes may compromise treatment success by generation of more apical dentine debris, which in the absence of an adequate irrigation regimen serves to block apical canal exits that may still be contaminated with bacteria. Continued generation of dentine debris, in the absence of sufficient irrigation, may lead to what is termed *dentine mud*, which ultimately creates a blockage. The impatient or neophyte clinician fails to resist the temptation to force the instrument back to length, resulting in the classically described procedural errors of apical transportation, canal straightening, and perforation. An alternative mechanism is required to explain the higher failures in initially large canals; it is likely that immature roots present a different debridement challenge, where the canal shape is not amenable to planing of the main portions of the canal by conventional instruments. Perhaps an intracanal brush may be a more suitable cleaning device in such teeth. The findings from these studies therefore do not concur with views that more effective bacterial debridement may be achieved with larger apical preparations.[33,164,184]

The issue of apical preparation size should be considered together with that of the size and taper of the rest of the canal preparation. Again, there is a paucity of sufficient direct evidence for the influence of degree of canal taper on root canal treatment outcome. The ESE guidelines[63] recommend only that canal preparation should be tapered from crown to apex without stipulating any particular degree of taper. Three studies have analyzed the influence of canal preparation taper on primary treatment and retreatment outcome, although again, none had focused their investigation primarily on this factor.[93,150,220] Smith and coworkers,[220] using loose criteria for determination of success, found that a "flared" preparation (wide taper) resulted in a significantly higher success rate compared with a "conical" preparation (narrow taper); the exact degree of taper was not reported and the effects of other treatment and nontreatment parameters were not controlled. In contrast, Hoskinson and associates[93] and Ng and colleagues,[150] using strict criteria, did not find any significant difference in treatment outcome between narrow (.05) and wide (.10) canal tapers. The controlled use of stainless steel instruments in a step-back technique may create .05 (1 mm step-back) or .10 (0.5 mm step-back) tapers, although, of course, uncontrolled use of such instruments may generate a variety of shapes. Ng and colleagues[150] also compared these (.05 and .10) preparation tapers with .02, .04, .06, and .08 tapers (generally achieved by using greater taper nickel-titanium instruments) and found no significant effect on treatment outcome. They cautioned that their investigation of the influence of canal preparation taper without randomization

could be influenced by the initial size of the canal, the type of instrument used, and operator experience.

Triangulation of the data on the effects of canal preparation size and taper on treatment outcome may intuitively lead to the conclusion that as far as current best evidence indicates, it is not necessary to over-enlarge the canal to achieve periapical healing. An apical preparation size of ISO 30 with a .05 taper for stainless steel instrumentation or .06 taper for NiTi instrumentation is sufficient. Precisely what biologic and hydrodynamic mechanisms underpin such sufficiency is more difficult to define based on available evidence. Although a number of laboratory studies[4,84,112] have investigated the interaction between canal dimensions and irrigation or obturation dynamics, the precise physical, chemical, or biologic mechanisms that ultimately enable periapical healing remain unknown, although collaborations with fluid dynamics specialists[84] and (micro) biologists[82] may ultimately yield a clearer picture.

Procedural errors during root canal preparation include canal blockage, ledge formation, apical zipping and transportation, straightening of canal curvature, tooth or root perforation at the pulp chamber or radicular level, and separation of instruments. Instrument separation during treatment has been found to reduce the success rate significantly[150,229]; however, the reported prevalence of instrument separation was low (0.5% to 0.9%) in these studies, precluding an analysis of causative factors. A case-control study[225] revealed no significant difference in success rates between periapically involved teeth with or without retained separated instruments. The stage of canal debridement at which instrument separation occurred and the justification for their retention may have implications on the outcome. The coronoapical location of a separated instrument and whether the instrument was successfully bypassed were found to have no effect on treatment outcome.

Irrigant

Different chemical agents have been used as irrigants for root canal treatment, singly or in various combinations, both in clinical practice and in the studies reviewed. They have included water, saline and solutions of local anesthetic, sodium hypochlorite, iodine, chloramine, sulfuric acid, EDTA, hydrogen peroxide, organic acid, Savlon, urea peroxide, and Biosept (a quaternary ammonium compound).[153] Most of the studies had used sodium hypochlorite as an irrigant[153] regardless of whether it was primary treatment or retreatment. This is consistent with the ESE guidelines[61] for irrigation, which recommend a solution possessing disinfectant and tissue-dissolving properties.

One prospective study[150] systematically investigated the effect of the irrigant on the success rates of root canal retreatment, which, although not a randomized controlled trial, revealed interesting new findings on the effects of irrigants. Even though a higher concentration of sodium hypochlorite made negligible difference to treatment outcome, the additional use of other specific irrigants had a significant influence on success rates.[150] The finding of a lack of improvement in periapical healing with the use of a higher concentration NaOCl solution is consistent with previous clinical/microbiologic findings.[29,41] Comparing 0.5% to 5.0% NaOCl solution for irrigation, it was found that the concentration of solution, per se, did not appear to increase the proportion of teeth rendered culture-negative[29] or associated with greater periapical healing.[41] As iodine and sodium hypochlorite are both halogen-releasing agents and attack common key protein groups,[129] the finding that the additional use of 10% povidone-iodine for irrigation had no additional influence on treatment success was as expected. Surprisingly, however, the additional use of 0.2% chlorhexidine solution for irrigation was found to reduce the success of treatment significantly.[150] This finding was in complete contrast to previous reports[211,252] on its equivalent or superior in vivo antibacterial efficacy when compared with sodium hypochlorite solution. The use of chlorhexidine as a final irrigant following sodium hypochlorite irrigation had been recommended[107] and was justified on several grounds, including its substantivity in root dentin (i.e., prolonged antibacterial effect),[185] relative lack of toxicity,[117] and broadspectrum efficacy.[130] Not until recently has alternate irrigation with sodium hypochlorite and chlorhexidine solution raised serious concerns because of their interaction product. The interaction product is thought to be an insoluble precipitate containing para-chloroaniline, which is cytotoxic and carcinogenic.[14,24] Apart from mutually depleting the active moiety in the two solutions for bacterial inactivation, the precipitate may cause persistent irritation to the periapical tissue and block dentinal tubules and accessory anatomy, possibly explaining the observed lower success rate when chlorhexidine was used as an additional irrigant.

Ng and associates[150] also found that the additional use of EDTA had a profound effect on improving radiographically observed periapical healing associated with root canal treatment (OR = 1.5 [1.1, 2.0]). In contrast, the observed synergistic effect of sodium hypochlorite and EDTA had been previously demonstrated in terms of bacterial load reduction[26] but not periapical healing. The long-term (≥ 2 years) outcome of their cases stratified by canal disinfection protocols[25] did not support their microbiologic findings. Their reported success rate for alternate irrigation with sodium hypochlorite and EDTA solutions (67%) was low when compared to the success rate for irrigation using saline (91%), 0.5% sodium hypochlorite (92%), or 5% sodium hypochlorite (86%) solutions.[162] The reported outcome data were unexpected, as preobturation negative bacterial culture was achieved in all cases. Given the complexity of their study design (clinical and microbiologic), their sample size was restricted to 11 to 15 teeth per group, limiting their outcome data. The synergistic effect of the two disinfectants has been attributed to the chelating properties of the sodium salts of EDTA, and their roles have been reviewed by Zehnder.[261] EDTA solution assists negotiation of narrow or sclerosed canals by demineralization of root dentine and helps in the removal of compacted debris from noninstrumented canal anatomy. It may also facilitate deeper penetration of sodium hypochlorite solution into dentine by opening dentinal tubules and removing the smear layer from the instrumented surface. Lastly, it may help detach or break up biofilms adhering to root canal walls.[85]

Medicament

Most previous treatment outcome studies have not standardized the type of root canal medicament used in the interappointment period, but the use of several different medicaments has been reported. The list was consistent with that recommended in the ESE guidelines for a medicament with disinfectant properties and included calcium hydroxide, creosote, and iodine solutions.[153] However, there is an absence of studies investigating the influence of this factor on treatment outcome.

The use of a mixture of calcium hydroxide and chlorhexidine has been tested based on the speculation that the mixture would be more effective against *E. faecalis*.[13,78,198]

Root Canal Bacterial Culture Results Prior to Obturation

In the past, in various centers of endodontic excellence, completion of root canal treatment by obturation would only be acceptable after a negative culture test was obtained from the canal, confirming the absence of bacteria in the part of the root canal system that could be sampled.[23,70,143] This practice has fallen out of clinical favor because of the perceived predictability and good prognosis of root canal treatment without microbiologic sampling. Sampling procedures are considered lengthy, difficult, often inaccurate, requiring laboratory support and having low benefit-to-cost ratio.[138,139] A preobturation negative culture result may increase treatment success twofold (Fig. 11-19). One large study[201] helped contribute to the demise of the canal-culture test; however, even this study showed a 10% difference in success in favor of the negative culture test when periapical disease was present. The outcome is even worse when a positive culture test result combines with the presence of a periapical lesion.

Numerous studies* have evaluated the effect of different stages of root canal treatment on the intraradicular microbiota, both qualitatively and quantitatively (Table 11-9). Some studies merely report positive culture tests, whereas others have identified and quantified intraradicular microbiota before and after various stages of treatment.

The effect of the "mechanical preparation" of the canal(s) on the microbiota has been tested using only water or saline as the irrigant. Taken collectively, the studies show that negative cultures were achieved on a weighted pooled average in 31% of the cases (range 0 to 79%). When sodium hypochlorite (concentration range 0.5% to 5%) irrigation supplemented the "mechanical preparation," the frequency of negative cultures immediately increased to a weighted pooled average of 52% (range 13% to 95%) (see Table 11-9).

Most studies report culture reversals during the interappointment period when active antibacterial dressing is not used in the root canal system between appointments. The reversals are due to regrowth of residual bacteria or recontamination by bacteria from coronal restoration leakage. When active interappointment antibacterial dressing is used, negative cultures in the subsequent visit were achieved on average in 71% of cases (range 25% to 100%) (see Table 11-9).

Effect of Persistent Bacteria on Root Canal Treatment Outcome

The bacteria present in preobturation cultures have included *Enterococcus, Streptococcus, Staphylococcus, Lactobacillus, Veillonella, Pseudomonas, Fusobacterium* species, and yeasts. Studies have been variable as to the relationship between individual species and treatment failure. Although the overall failure rate for cases with positive cultures was 31%, teeth testing positive for *Enterococcus* species had a failure rate of 55%, and teeth with positive cultures for *Streptococcus* species had 90%

Text continued on p. 504

---

*Please see the following references: 2, 7, 10, 16, 26-29, 33, 37, 41, 42, 60, 77, 79, 99, 104, 108, 110, 124, 137, 154, 161, 163, 168, 169, 173, 179, 181, 208, 209, 210, 214, 215, 217, 227, 248, 252, 257, and 258.

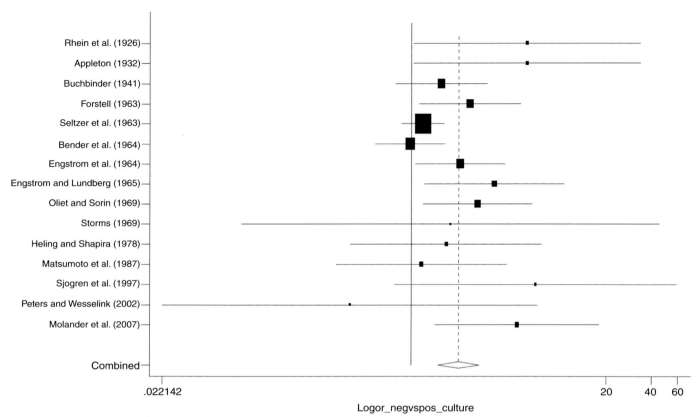

FIG. 11-19 Forest plot showing pooled and individual study's odds ratio (OR) for periapical health of teeth undergoing root canal treatment with preobturation negative versus positive culture test results (pooled OR = 2.1; 95% CI: 1.5, 2.9).

TABLE 11-9

Summary of Studies Evaluating the Effect of Root Canal Treatment Procedures on Bacterial Presence by Culture

			Percentage of Samples with Bacterial Presence		
Study	Year	Sample Size	At Baseline	After Preparation ± Irrigation	Next Visit (after Dressing+/–)
Auerbach	1953	60 teeth	93% (56/60)	Chlorinated soda (double strength): 22% (12/56)	—
Ingle & Zeldow	1958	89 teeth	73% (65/89)	H_2O: 70% (62/89) Some initially –ve became +ve after treatment	—
Stewart et al.	1961	77 teeth	100% (77/77)	0.5% NaOCl + Gly-oxide: 2% (1/44) 0.5% NaOCl + 3% H_2O_2: 9% (3/33)	No dressing: 0.5% NaOCl + Gly-oxide: 34% (15/44) 0.5% NaOCl + 3% H_2O_2: 39% (17/33)
Nicholls	1962	155 teeth	100% (155/155)	Alkaline chloramine: 53% (39/74) H_2O_2 and 2% NaOCl: 50% (30/60) H_2O and 2% NaOCl: 71% (15/21)	—
Grahnén & Krasse	1963	97 teeth	77% (75/97)	NaCl: 72% (23/32) Biocept: 66% (21/32) Nebacin: 36% (12/33) Some initially –ve became +ve after Tx	No dressing: NaCl: 47% (15/32) Biocept: 47% (15/32) Nebacin: 18% (6/33)

TABLE 11-9

Summary of Studies Evaluating the Effect of Root Canal Treatment Procedures on Bacterial Presence by Culture—cont'd

Study	Year	Sample Size	Percentage of Samples with Bacterial Presence		
			At Baseline	After Preparation ± Irrigation	Next Visit (after Dressing+/−)
Engström	1964	223 teeth (untreated or retreated)	60% (134/223)	Biosept or Iodophor, plus alcohol, chloroform, and 0.5% NaOCl: No data	5% I$_2$ in 10% IKI: 2nd visit: 43% (58/134); 3rd visit: 22% (29/134); 4th visit: 8% (9/134); 5th visit: 3% (4/134); 6th visit: 2% (3/134); 7th visit: 16% (22/134)
Olgart	1969	207 teeth	72% (149/207)	H$_2$O$_2$ and 0.5% NaOCl or H$_2$O$_2$ and 1% NaOCl: 43% (88/207)	No dressing: 34% (70/207)
Bence et al.	1973	33 teeth	100% (33/33)	Pre-irritation: 1st file: 93%, enlargement with #3: 14%, #4: 11%, #5: 21% (32% of instruments showed +ve culture, regardless of size) 5.25% NaOCl: 48-hr culture: 4% dentine, 10% pp 5-day culture: 8% dentine, 26% pp	No dressing: 8% dentine, 12% pp samples of teeth with negative culture after irrigation
Akpata	1976	20 extracted teeth	100% (20/20)	NaCl: 65% (13/20)	38% CMCP: 20% (2/10) When PP sample −ve, crushed tooth yielded −ve culture; When PP +ve, crushed teeth yielded +ve or −ve cultures
Cvek et al.	1976	108 teeth	NaCl group: 53% (18/34) 0.5% NaOCl group: 63% (29/46) 5% NaOCl group: 79% (22/28)	NaCl: 83% (15/18) 0.5% NaOCl: 59% (17/29) 5% NaOCl: 68% (15/22)	—
Byström & Sundqvist	1981	15 teeth	100% (15/15)	Saline: 100% (15/15)	No dressing: 47% (7/15) (5th visit) Where initial bacteria load high, difficult to eliminate
Byström & Sundqvist	1983	15 teeth	100% (15/15)	0.5% NaOCl: 87% (13/15)	No dressing: 20% (3/15) (5th visit)
Byström & Sundqvist	1985	60 teeth	100% (60/60)	0.5% NaOCl: No data 5% NaOCl: No data 5% NaOCl + 15% EDTA: No data	No dressing: 0.5% NaOCl: 12/20 (2nd visit); 8/20 (3rd visit) 5% NaOCl: 10/20 (2nd visit); 6/20 (3rd visit) 5% NaOCl + 15% EDTA: 11/20 (2nd visit); 3/20 (3rd visit)
Byström et al.	1985	65 teeth	100% (65/65)	0.5% NaOCl: No data 5.0% NaOCl: No data	CH: 0/35 (1 month), 1/35 (2-4 days) CP/CMCP (2 wks): 10/30
Sjögren & Sundqvist	1987	31 teeth	100% (31/31)	0.5% NaOCl plus ultrasonic debridement: No data	No dressing: 29% (9/31) at 2nd visit; 23% (7/31) at 3rd visit

Continued

TABLE 11-9

Summary of Studies Evaluating the Effect of Root Canal Treatment Procedures on Bacterial Presence by Culture—cont'd

Study	Year	Sample Size	Percentage of Samples with Bacterial Presence		
			At Baseline	After Preparation ± Irrigation	Next Visit (after Dressing+/−)
Koontongkaew et al.	1988	15 teeth	100% (15/15)	3% H_2O_2/5.25% NaOCl: No data	**CMCP:** 1-day dressing: 40% (2/5); 3-day dressing: 20% (1/5); 7-day dressing 10% (1/10) **No dressing:** 60% (3/5) after 1 day, 20% (1/5) after 3 or 7 days
Reit & Dahlén	1988	35 teeth	91% (32/35)	**0.5% NaOCl:** No data	**CH:** After 14 days: 23% (8/35); after 21 days: 26% (9/35)
Molander et al.	1990	25 teeth	96% (24/25)	**0.04% iodine:** No data	**Clindamycin:** After 14 days: 16% (4/25); after 21 days: 24% (6/25)
Sjögren et al.	1991	30 teeth	100% (30/30)	**0.5% NaOCl:** 50% (15/30)	**CH:** 10 min: 50% (6/12) at 1 wk later 7 day: 0% (0/18) (none after 1-5 wks later without dressing)
Ørstavik et al.	1991	23 teeth	96% (22/23)	**NaCl** irrigation and enlarged to: #20-25: 87% (20/23) further to #35-80: No data	**CH:** 34% (8/23); #35/40: 40% (6/15) #>40: 25% (2/8)
Yared & Bou Dagher	1994	60 teeth	100% (60/60)	**1% NaOCl:** Enlarged to #25: 73% (22/30) Enlarged to #40: 23% (7/30)	**CH:** 0% (0/60)
Gomes et al..	1996	42 root canals: Untreated (n = 15) Retreated (n = 27)	95% (40/42)	**2.5% NaOCl:** No data	**Empty canal** (7-10 days): 73% (29/40)
Sjögren et al.	1997	55 teeth (single canal)	100% (55/55)	**0.5% NaOCl:** 40% (22/55)	—
Dalton et al.	1998	46 teeth	100% (46/46)	**NaCl + NiTi files:** 68% (15/22); **NaCl + K-files:** 75% (18/24)	—
Reit et al.	1999	50 teeth	84% (42/50)	Enlarged to #35 (curved) or #50 (straight) with **0.5% NaOCl:** No data	**5% IKI** (5-7 days): 44% (22/50) **Empty** (7 days): 44% (22/50)
Peciuliene et al.	2000	25 teeth	80% (20/25);	**2.5% NaOCl and 17% EDTA:** No data	**Medication unknown:** 28% (7/25)
Shuping et al.	2000	42 teeth	98% (41/42)	**1.25% NaOCl:** 38% (16/42)	**CH:** 8% (3/40)
Lana et al.	2001	31 teeth	87% (27/31)	**2.5% NaOCl:** No data	**CH:** 13% (4/31) **Empty for 7 days:** 23% (7/31)
Peciuliene et al.	2001	40 teeth	83% (33/40)	**2.5% NaOCl and 17% EDTA:** 30% (10/33)	**CH (10-14 days):** 25% (5/20) **IKI: 2% I_2 in 4% KI (10 min):** 5% (1/20)
Peters et al.	2002	42 teeth	Instrumentation to #20: 100% (42/42)	**Enlarged to #35 with 2% NaOCl:** 23% (10/42)	**CH (4 weeks):** 71% (15/21); further irrigation: 43% (9/21)

TABLE 11-9

Summary of Studies Evaluating the Effect of Root Canal Treatment Procedures on Bacterial Presence by Culture—cont'd

Study	Year	Sample Size	Percentage of Samples with Bacterial Presence		
			At Baseline	After Preparation ± Irrigation	Next Visit (after Dressing+/−)
Card et al.	2002	40 mandibular teeth/canals	95% (38/40)	**1% NaOCl** Profile instrumentation (.04 taper): 0/13 of cuspids and bicuspids, 5/27 of mesiobuccal canals Further LightSpeed instrumentation to size 57.5-65: 3/27 mesiobuccal canals of molars Only 1/16 of those mesiobuccal canals with detectable communication with the mesiolingual canals had +ve culture after the first preparation using ProFile instruments	No data
Kvist et al.	2004	96 teeth	98% (94/96)	**0.5% NaOCl:** 63% (60/96)	**CH** (7 days): 36% (16/44) **IPI** (10 min): 29% (15/52)
Chu et al.	2006	88 canals	99% (87/88)	**0.5% NaOCl:** No data	**CH, Septomixine forte, or Ledermix:** 36% (32/88) Exposure of pulp, tooth type, acute versus chronic condition, size of lesion, and type of medication had no significant effect
Paquette et al.	2007	22 teeth (single canal)	100% (22/22)	**2.5% NaOCl:** 68% (15/22)	**2% CHX:** 45% (10/22)
Siqueira et al.	2007a	11 teeth (single root)	100% (11/11)	**2.5% NaOCl:** 55% (6/11)	**CH/CPMC:** 9% (1/11)
Siqueira et al.	2007b	11 teeth (single root)	100% (11/11)	**2.5% NaOCl:** 45% (5/11)	**CH:** 18% (2/11)
Vianna et al.	2007	24 teeth (single root)	100% (24/24)	**Saline + 2% CHX gel:** 33% (8/24)	**2% CHX, CH or mixture:** 54% (13/24) Type of medication had no significant effect
Wang et al.	2007	43 canals	91% (39/43)	**Saline + 2% CHX gel:** 8% (4/39)	**2% CHX + CH:** 8% (3/36) Size of apical preparation (40 versus 60) had no significant effect.
Markvart et al.	2012	24 teeth	88% (21/24)	**2.5% NaOCl:** 63% (15/24)	**17% EDTA irrigation and 10 min 5% IKI medication:** 50% (12/24) Box preparation (#60): 67% (8/12) Cone preparation (#25-30): 33% (4/12)
Xavier et al.	2013	48 teeth (single canal)	100% (40/40)	**1% NaOCl:** 75% (9/12) **2% CHX:** 75% (9/12)	**CH:** 75% (18/24)

NaOCl, sodium hypochlorite; CH, calcium hydroxide; CP, camphorated phenol; CMCP, camphorated monochlorophenol; PP, paper point sample; r culture, culture test before obturation.

failures.[70] In another study, good-quality root canal treatment on 54 teeth with asymptomatic periapical disease gave an overall success rate of 74%, but teeth with positive cultures for *Enterococcus faecalis* achieved a success rate of only 66%.[231] The success rate for teeth with no bacteria was 80%, whereas that for teeth with bacteria in the canal before obturation was 33%. These associations cannot be regarded as direct cause-and-effect associations, but they further emphasize the need to determine a relationship between microbial diversity and treatment outcome.

A monkey-model study[63] used a four- or five-strain infection to test the effect of debridement and obturation procedures on outcome. When bacteria remained after chemomechanical debridement, 79% of the root canals were associated with non-healed periapical lesions, compared with 28% when no bacteria were found to remain. Combinations of several residual bacterial species were more frequently related to nonhealed lesions than were single strains. When no bacteria remained at the end of chemomechanical debridement, healing occurred independently of the quality of the root filling. In contrast, when bacteria remained in the canal system, there was a greater correlation with nonhealing associated with poor-quality root fillings than in technically well-performed fillings. In root canals where bacteria were found after removal of the root filling, 97% had not healed, compared with 18% for those root canal systems with no bacteria detected upon removal of root filling. The study emphasizes the importance of reducing bacteria below detection limits before permanent root filling in order to achieve optimal healing conditions for the periapical tissues. It also reinforces the view that obturation does indeed play a role when residual infection is present.

Regardless of the technique used for obtaining a sample for a canal culture, the presence of a negative culture seems to have a positive impact on treatment outcome. The association of specific species with treatment failure is not well established but the identity of the small group of species isolated from positive cultures is relatively constant and may hold answers to treatment resistance and failure. However, it is important to understand that there are many other factors that can influence root canal treatment outcome.

Root Filling Material and Technique

The interrelationship among the core root filling material, sealer (for filling the gaps between the core material and canal surface), and technique for their placement complicates the investigation of the effect of obturation and technique on treatment outcome. In previous studies on treatment outcome, the most commonly used core root filling material was gutta-percha with various types of sealer or gutta-percha softened in chloroform (chloropercha).[153] The sealers used may be classified into zinc oxide–eugenol–based, glass ionomer–based, and resin-based types.[153] Materials such as Resilon, SmartSeal, and MTA have been adopted but have not significantly penetrated the market, except for the use of MTA in surgical repairs or repairs for immature apices. In any case, there is no evidence to show that the nature of root filling material and the technique used for placement has any significant influence on treatment outcome.

Apical Extent of Root Filling

Of the many intraoperative factors associated with success and failure of root canal treatment, the apical extent of the root canal filling material has been the most frequently and thoroughly investigated. In these previous studies, the apical extent of root fillings has been classified into three categories for statistical analyses: more than 2 mm short of radiographic apex (short), 0 to 2 mm within the radiographic apex (flush), and extended beyond the radiographic apex (long).[153] The apical extent of root filling was found to have a significant influence on the success rates of treatment, regardless of the periapical status.[150,153] Flush root fillings were associated with the highest success rates, whereas long root fillings were associated with the lowest success rates.

Most previous retrospective studies could not distinguish between the effects of apical extent of instrumentation versus the apical extent of obturation; however, the London Eastman study[150] was able to separate the effect of these two factors and found them both to independently and significantly affect periapical healing. The factors correlated with each other, consistent with the fact that canals are normally filled to the same extent as canal preparation.

Extrusion of cleaning, medication, or filling materials beyond the apical terminus into the surrounding tissues may result in delayed healing or even treatment failure due to a foreign body reaction.[105,146,218,260] Magnesium and silicon from the talc-contaminated extruded gutta-percha were found to induce a foreign body reaction, resulting in treatment failure.[146] An animal study has shown that large pieces of subcutaneously implanted gutta-percha in guinea pigs were well encapsulated in collagenous capsules, but fine particles of gutta-percha induced an intense, localized tissue response.[218] The inference that perhaps extrusion of large pieces of gutta-percha may not impact on periapical healing was not supported by data from previous studies.[150,153] The discrepancy may possibly be accounted for by bacterial contamination of the extruded gutta-percha in the clinical data.

The radiographic evidence of "sealer puffs" extruding through the main apical foramina and lateral/accessory canals has been pursued with vigor by some endodontists based on the undaunted belief of its value as "good practice." Their perception is that this represents a measure of root canal system cleanliness, and they ardently argue that healing would follow, albeit with some delay. The published evidence on the effects of sealer extrusion into the periapical tissues has been contradictory. Friedman and colleagues[68] found that extrusion of a glass ionomer-based sealer significantly reduced success rates. In contrast, Ng and associates[150] reported that extrusion of a zinc oxide–eugenol based–sealer had no significant effect on periapical healing. The discrepancy may be attributed to the difference in sealer type and the duration of treatment follow-up. The radiographic assessment of the presence or resorption of sealer may be complicated by the radiolucent property of its basic components and the insufficient sensitivity of the radiographic method used to detect small traces of it.[150] It is possible that, in some cases, the radiographic disappearance of extruded sealer may simply be due to resorption of the radio opaque additive, barium sulfate, or its uptake by macrophages, still resident in the vicinity.[146]

Extruded glass ionomer–based[68] zinc oxide–eugenol–based,[98] silicone-based[98] sealers or endomethasone[22] were not found to be resorbed/absorbed by periapical tissues after 1 year. Traces of calcium hydroxide–based sealer (Sealapex) could still be detected after 3 years.[194] In the latter study, treatments were carried out on primary molar teeth and the canals were obturated with Sealapex without gutta-percha. With longer duration of follow-up, complete resorption of extruded zinc oxide–eugenol–based sealers (Procosol, Roth Elite)[8] and a resin-based sealer (AH Plus, Dentsply/DeTrey, Konstanz, Germany)[194] was demonstrated in 69% and 45% of the cases after 4 and 5 years, respectively. Ng and associates[150] advanced two explanations for the difference between the effect of extruded core gutta-percha and the zinc oxide–eugenol sealer: the latter is antibacterial and may kill residual microorganisms, whereas it is also more soluble and readily removed by host cells compared to gutta-percha.

Quality of Root Filling

Another much investigated parameter of obturation in retrospective studies has been the radiographic measure of the "quality of root filling." The rationale for complete obturation of the root canal system is to prevent recontamination by colonization from the residual infection or newly invading bacteria. Both are supposedly prevented by a "tight" seal with the canal wall and an absence of voids within the body of the material. Quality of root filling may therefore be regarded either as poor root-filling technique or as a surrogate measure of the quality of the entire root canal treatment, because good obturation relies on properly executed preliminary steps in canal preparation. A systematic review[153] reported that the criteria for judging the quality of root fillings have not been well defined in previous studies.[43,93,216] An unsatisfactory root filling has been defined as "inadequate seal," "poor apical seal," or "radiographic presence of voids." Nevertheless, satisfactory root fillings were found to be associated with significantly higher success rates than unsatisfactory root fillings.[153]

Acute Exacerbation During Treatment

The causes for interappointment "flare-up" or pain have not been precisely determined, and several hypothetical mechanisms involving chemical, mechanical, or microbial injury to the periradicular tissues, as well as psychological influences, have been suggested as contributory to postpreparation pain or swelling.[202,203] Although these factors have not been specifically studied in the context of periapical healing, acute "flare-ups" during treatment were not found to be significantly associated with periapical healing in two studies.[102,216] In contrast, the London Eastman study[150] found that pain or swelling occurred in 15% of cases after chemomechanical debridement and was found to significantly reduce success as measured by periapical healing. This interesting finding may be explained by the hypothesis that "flare-ups" were caused by extrusion of contaminated material during canal preparation. Such material may elicit a foreign body reaction or (transient) extraradicular infection, resulting in treatment failure in a proportion of such cases. Alternatively, acute symptoms may be the result of incomplete chemomechanical debridement at the first appointment, leading to a shift in canal microbial ecology favoring the growth of more virulent microorganisms, leading to further postpreparation pain and treatment failure. The exact biologic mechanisms of failure in these cases remain obscure and warrant further investigation.

Number of Treatment Visits

The number of treatment visits for completing root canal treatment and its effect on periapical healing remains an ongoing controversy. Generally, the argument for single-visit treatment centers around better patient acceptability and cost-effectiveness versus the preference of multiple-visit treatments based on biologic rationale.[224] The premise for multiple-visit treatments has been that primary debridement is not completely effective in eliminating all the adherent bacterial biofilm[147] and the residual bacteria may multiply and recolonize the canal system.[25,29] Therefore, the proponents consider it desirable to use the interappointment period to dress the canal with a long-lasting or slow-release antibacterial agent capable of destroying or incapacitating residual bacteria, as well as to take the opportunity to gauge the initial periapical response before root filling. Calcium hydroxide has served in this capacity for many years because of its ability to dissolve organic tissue, kill bacteria, detoxify antigenic material, and act as a slow-release agent because of its low solubility-product in an aqueous environment. However, its antibacterial ability has come under close scrutiny, with advocates suggesting that the material is not suitable for this purpose.[195] A final resolution to this debate is awaited based on robust clinical evidence. Most of the published randomized controlled trials found no significant influence of healing attributable to number of treatment visits, but they all lacked robust statistical power.

The debate about the merits of single- or multiple-visit treatments will continue unabated given the respective strengths of the motivational drivers among the opposing groups. The issue may only be resolved by properly documented, large randomized controlled trials (which are currently unavailable) because undocumented variables (i.e., operator skill, biologic or technical case complexity, and patient compliance) would continue to bias the outcome.

Post Root Canal Treatment Restorative Factors
Effect of Quality and Type of Restoration

The placement of a coronal restoration after root canal obturation is the final step in the management of teeth undergoing root canal treatment. It has been shown to have a major influence on endodontic outcomes. Teeth with satisfactory coronal restorations were found to have significantly better periapical healing compared with those with unsatisfactory restorations (OR = 3.31; 95% CI: 1.07, 10.30).[153] The term *satisfactory restorations* has been defined as a restoration with no evidence of marginal discrepancy, discoloration, or recurrent caries with absence of a history of decementation.[93,182]

Given that one of the roles of coronal restorations is to prevent postoperative root canal reinfection via coronal leakage, the criteria for unsatisfactory restoration given by Hoskinson and colleagues[93] could not infer coronal leakage when the inner core was still intact. Consequently, the London Eastman study[150] adopted a different classification and definition for unsatisfactory restorations in order to illustrate obvious and potential coronal leakage more accurately. The two groups of unsatisfactory restorations were defined as those with (1) obvious signs of exposed root filling and (2) potential leakage indicated by marginal defects and history of de-cementation. It is perhaps this strategy that contributed to the finding of a profound effect (OR = 10.7; 95% CI: 3.7, 31.5) of coronal leakage on the endodontic outcome.

A number of investigations have been performed based on comparisons between the types of post root canal treatment restorations, including permanent versus temporary restorations,[43,68,150] crown versus acrylic restorations,[43,68,150,216] presence versus absence of posts,[68,150] and nonabutment versus abutment.[150,216] Teeth that had been permanently restored were associated with significantly higher success rates than their temporarily restored counterparts in some studies[43,68] but not in others.[38,150] The type of permanent restoration[43,68,150,216] was found to have no significant influence on the outcome of treatment.

It has often been recommended that it would be wise to provide a subseal over the root filling in case of loss of a permanent or temporary restoration; the subseal would be glass ionomer (GIC) or zinc oxide–eugenol cement.[196] The placement of a GIC or zinc oxide–eugenol (IRM) cement lining coronal to the gutta-percha filling and underneath the permanent core in order to provide an additional antibacterial coronal seal was found in a prospective study to have no beneficial effect on treatment success.[150]

In summary, the preceding findings overall support the ESE guidelines[61] that an adequate restoration should be placed after root canal treatment to prevent subsequent bacterial recontamination. Therefore, the provision of a good-quality coronal restoration, regardless of type, should be considered the final part of the root canal treatment procedure following obturation.

Use of Root Treated Teeth as Abutments for Prostheses and Occlusal Contacts

Mechanical stress on restorations is a function of the role of individual teeth in the occlusal scheme. The pattern of occlusal loading both in static and dynamic occlusion is dictated by whether the teeth are involved as single units or abutments (bridge/denture) and whether they have holding or guiding contacts. It is reasonable to expect that bridge and denture abutments may be placed under unfavorable loads, as may last-standing teeth in the dental arch.[127] These teeth may therefore be expected to have lower success rates because of a potential increase in the development of cracks and fractures due to fatigue. This observation has been confirmed for teeth

functioning as bridge abutments compared with those restored as individual units following root canal treatment.[216]

Summary of Factors Influencing Periapical Healing Following Nonsurgical Root Canal Treatment

The following factors are considered as having a major impact on periapical health subsequent to root canal treatment:

◆ Presence (Fig. 11-20) and size (Fig. 11-21) of periapical lesion
◆ Patency at the canal terminus (achieving patency significantly increased the chance of success twofold)[150]
◆ Apical extent of chemomechanical preparation in relation to the radiographic apex (Fig. 11-22)
◆ Outcome of intraoperative culture test (see Fig. 11-19)
◆ Iatrogenic perforation (if present, reduces the odds of success by 30%)[150]
◆ Quality of root canal treatment judged by the radiographic appearance of the root filling (Fig. 11-23)
◆ Quality of the final coronal restoration (Fig. 11-24)

The following factors are considered as having minimal impact on root canal treatment outcome:

◆ Age of patient
◆ Gender of patient
◆ Tooth morphologic type
◆ Specific root canal treatment protocol and technique (preparation, irrigation, and obturation material and technique)

Contemporary improvements in mechanical and chemical canal preparation have not resulted in an increase in the success rate for root canal treatment over the past century (Fig. 11-25). This observation may be explained by the currently available techniques not being effective in eliminating the infection in the apical canal anatomy.

It is notable that all factors that have a strong influence on periapical health after root canal treatment are associated

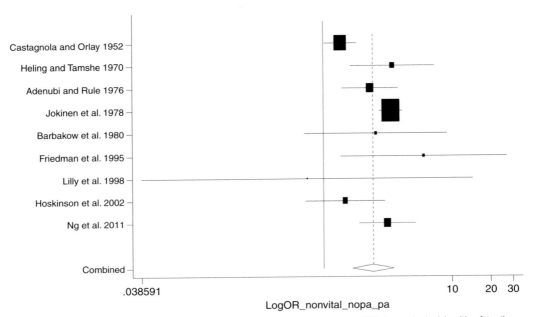

FIG. 11-20 Forest plot showing pooled and individual study's odds ratio (OR) for periapical health of teeth undergoing root canal treatment with preoperative nonvital pulps and absence of periapical radiolucencies versus teeth with nonvital pulps and presence of periapical radiolucencies (pooled OR = 2.4; 95% CI: 1.7, 3.5).

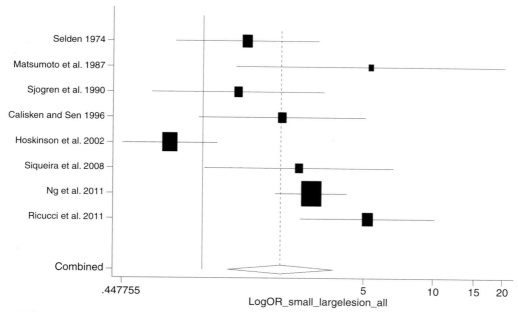

FIG. 11-21 Forest plot showing pooled and individual study's odds ratio (OR) for periapical health of teeth undergoing root canal treatment with preoperative large (> 5 mm) versus small (< 5 mm) periapical radiolucencies (pooled OR = 2.2; 95% CI: 1.3, 3.7).

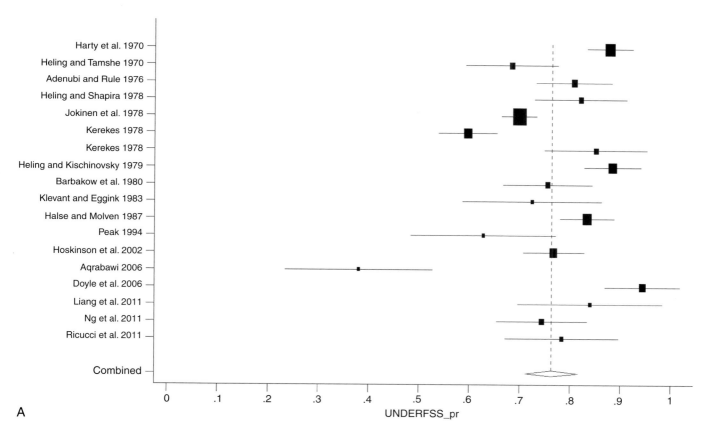

FIG. 11-22 Forest plot showing pooled and individual study's probability of periapical health for teeth undergoing root canal treatment with underextended (0.76 [0.71, 0.82]) (**A**), flush (0.81 [0.76, 0.86]) (**B**), or overextended (0.66 [0.56, 0.75]) (**C**) root fillings.

Continued

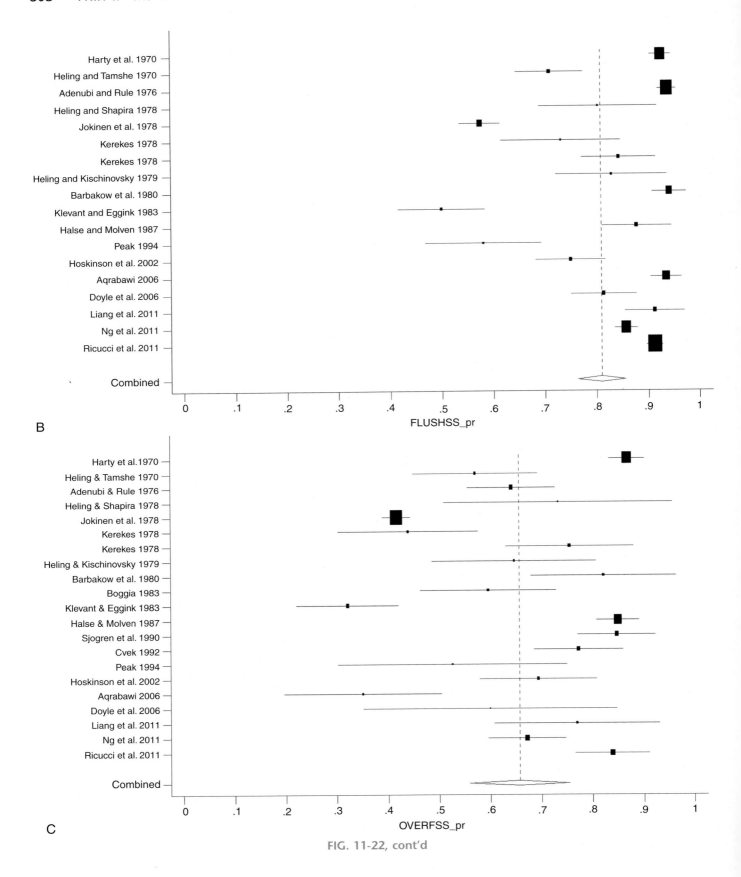

FIG. 11-22, cont'd

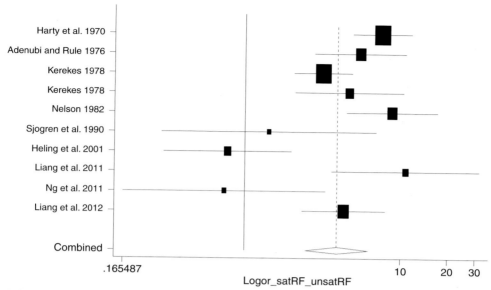

FIG. 11-23 Forest plot showing pooled and individual study's odds ratio (OR) of periapical health for teeth undergoing root canal treatment with good quality versus suboptimal quality root filling (pooled OR = 3.9; 95% CI: 2.5, 6.2).

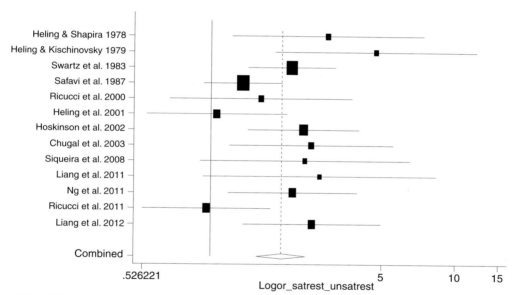

FIG. 11-24 Forest plot showing pooled and individual study's odds ratio (OR) of periapical health for teeth undergoing root canal treatment with satisfactory versus unsatisfactory coronal restoration at follow-up (pooled OR = 1.9; 95% CI: 1.5, 2.5).

in some way with a persistent root canal infection. Further improvements in root canal treatment outcomes may therefore be achieved by understanding the nature of the root canal infection (especially apically) and the manner in which the microbiota is altered or eliminated during root canal treatment.

Factors Affecting Tooth Survival Following Root Canal Treatment

A systematic review and meta-analysis has shown that 93% of endodontically treated teeth survive at 2 years postoperatively; but this survival reduced to 88% at 10 years following

treatment (Fig. 11-26). The most common reasons for such tooth loss were due to problems of endodontic origin, tooth/ root fracture, or restoration failure.[149,151] Consistent with the studies on periapical healing, the considerations affecting the survival of endodontically treated teeth may be divided into patient, intraoperative, and restorative factors.

Patient Factors

Ng and colleagues[151] found that teeth in patients suffering from diabetes or receiving systemic steroid therapy had a higher chance of being extracted after root canal treatment. The negative influence of diabetes on tooth survival is consistent with

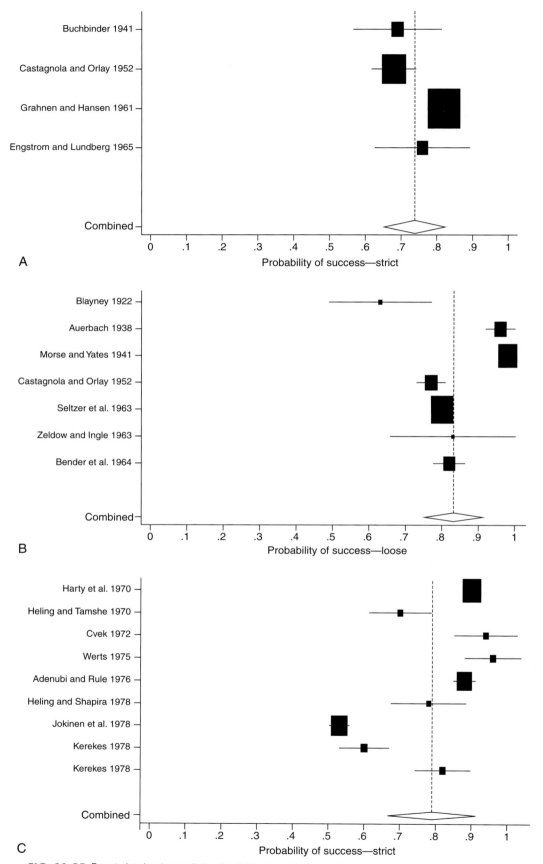

FIG. 11-25 Forest plot showing pooled and individual study's probability of periapical health for teeth undergoing root canal treatment by "decade of publication" and "criteria for success."

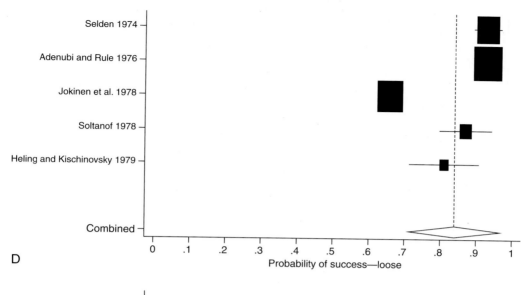

D

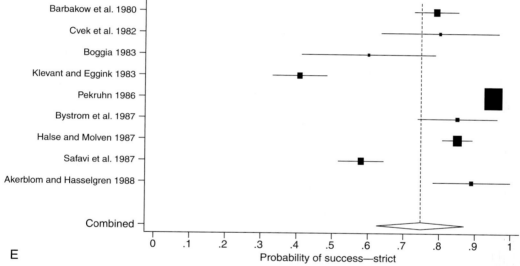

E

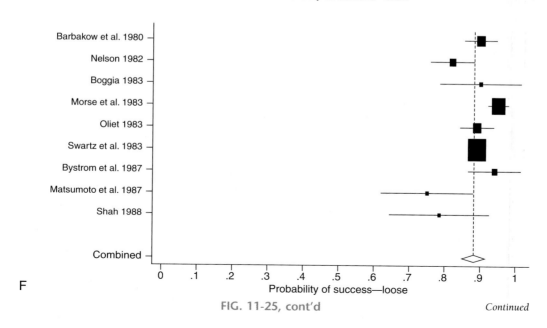

F

FIG. 11-25, cont'd

Continued

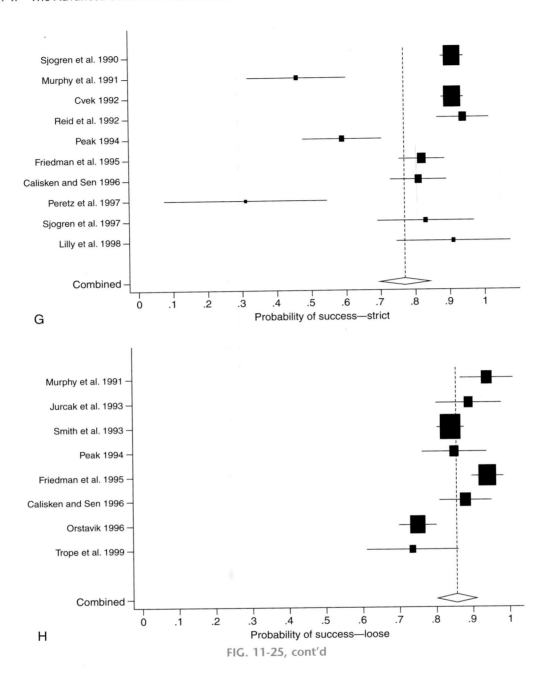

FIG. 11-25, cont'd

the report by Mindiola and associates,[135] whereas the influence of steroid therapy had never been reported previously. It may be argued that patients with diabetes are more susceptible to periodontal disease[74] or have a lower success rate of root canal treatment[67] because of being immunologically compromised. However, the researchers reported that over 50% of such teeth were extracted due to persistent pain. Some of these observations may be explained by the presence of neuropathy, a debilitating painful complication of diabetes.[57] It is interesting to note that systemic steroid therapy is often prescribed to control such chronic pain.[39,51,101]

Tooth Morphologic Type and Location
Tooth types (i.e., location within the arch) may vary with respect to their susceptibility to tooth fracture, a common

reason for tooth loss after endodontic treatment. Ng and coworkers[149] found that tooth type had a significant influence on survival. Maxillary premolars and mandibular molars were found to have the highest frequency of extraction, with tooth fracture being the most common reason. The observation is consistent with previous reports on fracture incidence of maxillary premolars and mandibular molars.[56,109] The factors "proximal contacts" and "terminal (last standing) teeth" were found to affect tooth survival considerably,[149,151] but they were significantly correlated with molar teeth. Most of the extractions of terminal teeth or teeth with one or fewer proximal contacts were due to tooth fracture.[151] The observation may be explained by the unfavorable distribution of occlusal forces and higher nonaxial stress on terminal teeth and those with fewer than two proximal contacts. Other possible reasons for

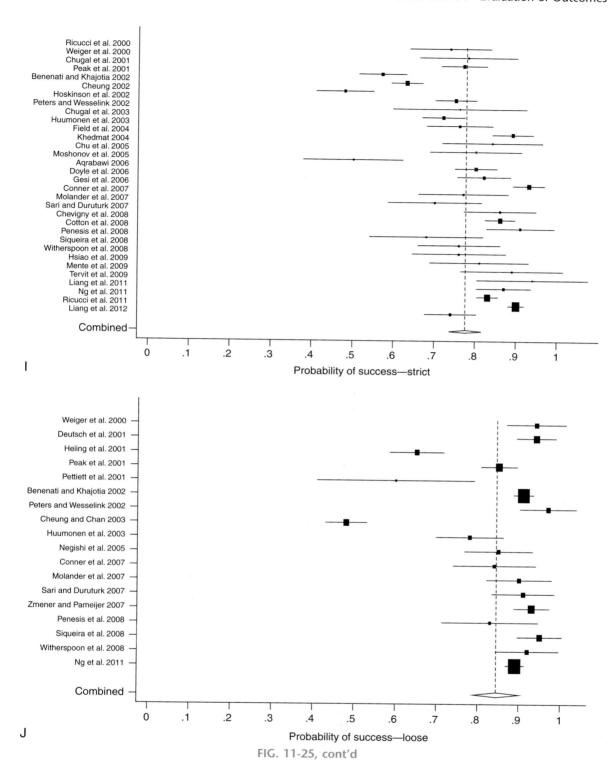

FIG. 11-25, cont'd

their higher rate of loss are (1) failure of root canal treatment in a terminal tooth may be accepted more willingly because of little perceived aesthetic value and (2) clinicians may be less likely to offer further treatment on terminal molar teeth due to difficult access. Therefore, when restoring molar teeth, the favorable distribution of occlusal forces must be considered, especially on teeth with one or fewer adjacent teeth or on terminal teeth.

Preoperative Conditions of Teeth

The presence of preoperative periapical lesions, which is the most significant prognostic factor for periapical healing, was found to have no significant influence on tooth survival.[151] On the other hand, the presence of preoperative periodontal probing defects of endodontic origin, preoperative pain, and preoperative sinus tracts were found to reduce tooth survival.[151] These observations are consistent with a previous

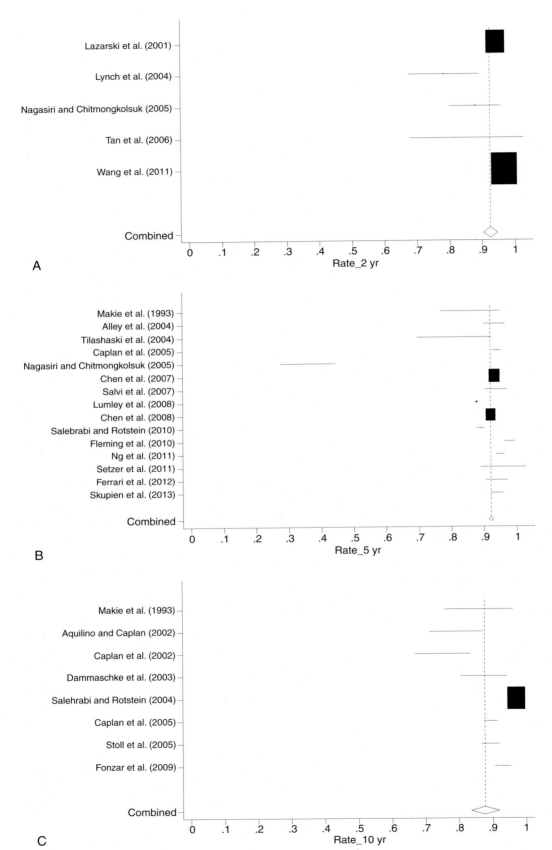

FIG. 11-26 Forest plot showing pooled and individual study's probability of 2-year (pooled probability = 0.93; 95% CI: 0.90, 0.95) **(A)**, 5-year (pooled probability = 0.92; 95% CI: 0.91, 0.93) **(B)**, and 10-year (pooled probability = 0.88; 95% CI: 0.84, 0.92) **(C)** survival of teeth undergoing root canal treatment.

report that the mere presence of a persistent periapical lesion was not a sufficient reason for dentists and patients to opt for further treatment, either retreatment or extraction.[180] The negative impact of preoperative pain on survival outcome highlights the importance of accurate pain diagnosis. In some instances, the pain may have been of nonendodontic origin and therefore would persist after treatment.[176] In other instances, preoperative pain of endodontic origin may persist following treatment, as a result of peripheral or central sensitization. Therefore, effective pain diagnosis and management for patients presenting with preoperative pain are crucial.

The presence of preoperative cervical resorption and perforation was also found to significantly reduce tooth survival.[151] This was as expected because tooth fracture and reinfection due to leakage through the resorption and perforating defects are likely sequelae in such cases. In the presence of reinfection, clinicians are more inclined to suggest extraction due to the intuitive perception of poor long-term prognosis of such teeth.

Treatment Factors

Considering all of the intraoperative factors, the "lack of patency at apical foramen" and the "extrusion of gutta-percha root filling" were found to be the most significant intraoperative factors in reducing tooth survival.[151] In the presence of persistent problems and knowing that the treatment objective of cleaning to the canal terminus could not be achieved, patients and dentists may be more likely to opt for extraction sooner than later.

Restorative Factors

Protection of teeth with crowns or cast restorations has not been shown to influence periapical healing; however, the placement of good cores had a positive effect on endodontic outcome. In contrast, placement of crowns or cast restorations was found to improve tooth survival.[149,151,189] This suggests that crowns and cast restorations help prevent tooth fracture, whereas the mere placement of a satisfactory core is sufficient to prevent reinfection after endodontic treatment. Unfortunately, the study was not able to investigate the interrelationship between tooth morphologic type, the extent of tooth tissue loss after treatment, or the type of final restoration. Although the clinical inference from these findings is that cast restorations should preferably be placed on all teeth after root canal treatment, this is probably a gross exaggeration of the true need. On the basis of laboratory[178] and clinical findings,[144] posterior teeth with compromised marginal ridges (mesial or distal), together with heavy occlusal loading evidenced by faceting, may benefit from full coverage restorations. The restoration design should attempt to preserve as much remaining tooth tissue as possible; the implication is that the so-called nonaesthetic but technically demanding partial veneer onlays and partial coverage crowns would be the restorations of choice for root-treated teeth. In anterior teeth, the missing tooth tissue may often be adequately replaced with composite restorative materials. A crown is only indicated when tooth structure or aesthetics become compromised.

The use of cast post and cores for retention of restorations have also been found to reduce tooth survival.[149,151] It may be speculated that the presence of a post has different effects on anterior versus posterior teeth as they are subjected to different directions and amount of occlusal force. It has been reported that only 12% of the extracted teeth with cast post and cores

were incisors or canines. Therefore, the inference is that the use of such retention should be particularly avoided in premolar and molar teeth. Alternative treatment options should be considered for molar or premolar teeth lacking sufficient tooth structure.

Ng and colleagues[151] observed that teeth functioning as prosthetic abutments had poorer survival rates; however, the number of teeth (n = 94) in the study that functioned as abutments was too small a sample to be considered statistically significant. As previously described, the explanation may reside in the excessive and unfavorable distribution of occlusal stresses on abutment teeth. If possible, root-treated teeth should be avoided as abutments for prostheses or in provision of occlusal guidance in excursive movements.

Summary of Factors Influencing the Survival of Teeth Following Root Canal Treatment

The following conditions have been found to significantly improve tooth survival following root canal treatment:

- Nonmolar teeth (Fig. 11-27)
- Teeth with both mesial and distal adjacent teeth (Fig. 11-28)
- Teeth not located as the distal-most tooth in the arch[151]
- Teeth (molar) with cast restorations after treatment (Fig. 11-29)
- Teeth not requiring cast post and core for support and retention of restoration[111,151]
- Teeth not functioning as abutments for fixed prosthesis[3,111,191,151]
- Absence of preoperative deep periodontal probing defects, pain, sinus tract, or perforation[151]
- Achievement of patency at canal terminus and absence of root-filling extrusion during treatment[151]

In addition, it is important to ensure favorable distribution of occlusal forces when designing restorations for endodontically treated teeth.

Impact of Root Canal Treatment on Quality of Life

The impact of root canal treatment on the oral health–related quality of life of patients has been evaluated using the short form (OHIP-14) or modified version (OHIP-17) of the Oral Health Impact Profile (OHIP-14)[219] (Table 11-10). The distinctly positive impact of root canal treatment was apparent, regardless of cultural background of the patient group or the measure used.[55,73,87,115] As expected, physical pain, psychological discomfort (feeling tense), and disability (difficulty in relaxing) were the most improved domains following treatment.

OUTCOME OF NONSURGICAL RETREATMENT

When root canal treatment fails to resolve periapical disease, it is often considered appropriate to retreat the tooth using conventional approaches first, especially when the previous treatment is technically deficient (Fig. 11-30). This requires removal of the previous root-filling material and any other material placed for restorative reasons. Correction of any procedural errors may also be required, if possible. All materials must be removed in their entirety to ensure delivery of

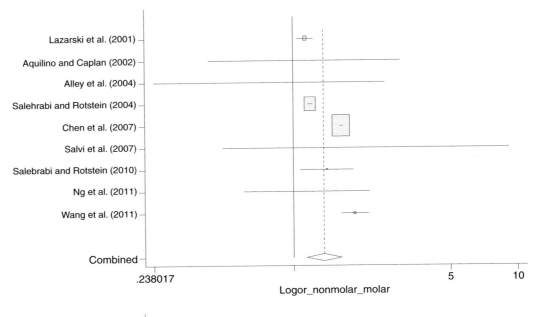

FIG. 11-27 Forest plot showing pooled and individual study's odds ratio (OR) of survival probability for nonmolar versus molar teeth (pooled OR = 1.4; 95% CI: 1.1, 1.6).

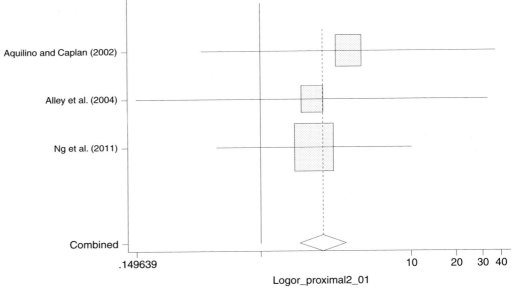

FIG. 11-28 Forest plot showing pooled and individual study's odds ratio (OR) of survival probability for teeth with both mesial and distal contacts present versus absent (pooled OR = 2.6; 95% CI: 1.8, 3.7).

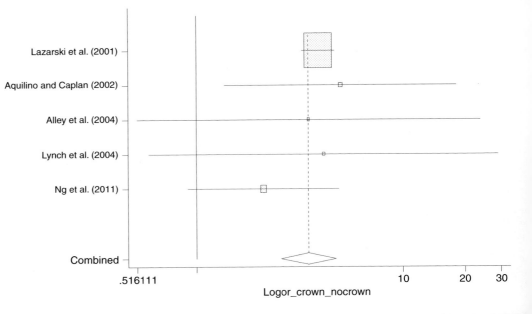

FIG. 11-29 Forest plot showing pooled and individual study's odds ratio (OR) of survival probability for teeth restored with cast versus plastic restoration (pooled OR = 3.5; 95% CI: 2.6, 4.7).

TABLE 11-10

The OHIP-14 and Modified Oral Health Impact Profile Instrument (OHIP-17) (Dugas et al., 2002)

OHIP #	Item Question
OHIP1	Have you had trouble pronouncing words because of your teeth and mouth?
OHIP2	Have you felt that your sense of taste has worsened because of your teeth or mouth?
OHIP3	Have you had painful aching in your mouth?
OHIP4	Have you found it uncomfortable to eat any foods because of your teeth or mouth?
OHIP5*	Have you had to alter the temperature of the foods that you eat because of your teeth or mouth?
OHIP6	Have you been self-conscious because of your teeth or mouth?
OHIP7	Have you felt tense because of your teeth or mouth?
OHIP8	Has your diet been unsatisfactory because of your teeth or mouth?
OHIP9	Have you had to interrupt meals because of your teeth or mouth?
OHIP10	Have you found it difficult to relax because of your teeth or mouth?
OHIP11*	Have you found it difficult to fall asleep because of your teeth or mouth?
OHIP12*	Have you ever been awakened by problems with your teeth or mouth?
OHIP13	Have you been embarrassed because of your teeth or mouth?
OHIP14	Have you been irritable with other people because of your teeth or mouth?
OHIP15	Have you had difficulty doing your usual jobs because of problems with your teeth or mouth?
OHIP16	Have you felt that life in general was less satisfying because of your teeth or mouth?
OHIP17	Have you been totally unable to function because of your teeth or mouth?

OHIP-14 contains all the items except those with an asterisk (*).

antibacterial agents to all surfaces of the root canal dentin (see Fig. 11-30). The periapical healing rates of root canal retreatment are generally perceived to be lower compared to primary treatment for the following reasons:

- Obstructed access to the apical infection
- A potentially more resistant microbiota

The outcomes from a range of studies show that the mean weighted success rate of nonsurgical root canal retreatment is 66% (Figs. 11-31 and 11-32), which is about 6% lower than in the case of primary treatment on teeth with apical periodontitis.[148,150] However, it has also been shown that the survival rate of teeth having undergone nonsurgical root canal retreatment may be similar to that for primary root canal treatment.[151]

The factors affecting outcomes of periapical health and tooth survival following root canal retreatment are otherwise identical to those affecting primary root canal treatment. Of the potential prognostic factors unique to retreatment cases, the most significant factor influencing the outcome of treatment is the ability to remove or bypass preexisting root-filling material or separated instruments during retreatment. This is understandable because it would have a direct impact on the ability to achieve canal patency and canal disinfection at the apical terminus.[150]

OUTCOME OF SURGICAL RETREATMENT

Factors Affecting Periapical Health or Healing Following Periapical Surgery and Root-End Filling

There are a number of published systematic reviews on the prognostic factors for periapical surgery with apical filling.[45,47,48,155,204,205,239-241,250] The major limitations of this pooled data include the variable length of time for evaluating success following treatment as well as the radiographic criteria used to assess healing. An unpublished meta-analysis[130] of data from the studies listed in Table 11-11 reveals that the weighted pooled probability of success from periapical surgery with retrograde restorations, based on complete radiographic healing, is 67.5% (95% CI: 62.9%, 72.0%) (Fig. 11-33). The trend shows higher success rates reported in more recent studies. This observation is consistent with the much higher pooled success rate of 92% (95% CI: 86%, 95%) revealed in the meta-analysis of prospective outcome data of surgical endodontic treatments performed by a "modern" technique (using magnification, root-end resection with minimal or no bevel, retrograde cavity preparation with ultrasonic tips, and modern retrograde root canal filling materials).[240,241] In congruence with these findings, Setzer and colleagues reported that the pooled success rate of treatment using a microsurgical approach (94%; 95% CI: 89%, 98%) was more favorable than traditional root-end surgery (59%; 95% CI: 55%, 63%).[205] However, the studies included in the latter meta-analysis differed in design, case selection, duration after treatment, and the provision of preoperative nonsurgical treatment, which may bias the higher success rate of the contemporary treatment.

The unpublished meta-analysis[130] stratified by duration following treatment reveals that the pooled probability of success based on complete healing plateaued after 2 years postoperatively, being 51% (95% CI: 42%, 60%) after 6 months, 68% (95% CI: 63%, 73%) after 12 months, 76% (95% CI: 67%, 84%) after 24 months, 74% (95% CI: 52%, 95%) after 48 months, and 74% (95% CI: 66%, 82%) after more than 48 months. It is therefore advisable to follow up on cases that have undergone periapical surgery for a minimum period of 2 years and up to 4 years as suggested in quality guidelines.[61]

The factors having a major impact on outcome of periapical surgery with retrograde cavities and fillings in teeth with preoperative periapical radiolucencies revealed in the (as yet) unpublished meta-analyses[130] of data from studies listed in Table 11-11 are as follows:

- Small (≤ 5 mm) versus large (> 5 mm) periapical lesion (risk ratio = 1.2; 95% CI: 1.1, 1.3)
- Periapical lesion involving one versus both cortical plates (risk ratio = 1.2; 95% CI: 1.0, 1.5)
- Absence versus presence of previous surgery (risk ratio = 1.2; 95% CI: 1.1, 1.3)

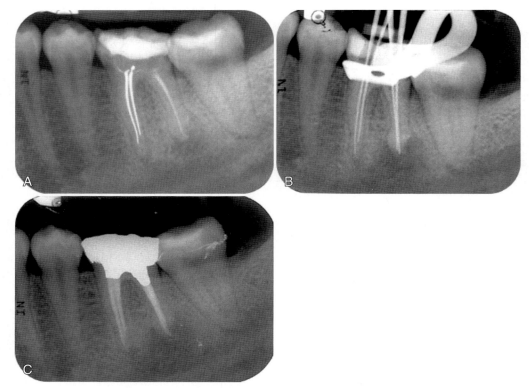

FIG. 11-30 Tooth with technically deficient root canal treatment (**A**); having undergone (**B** and **C**) root canal retreatment.

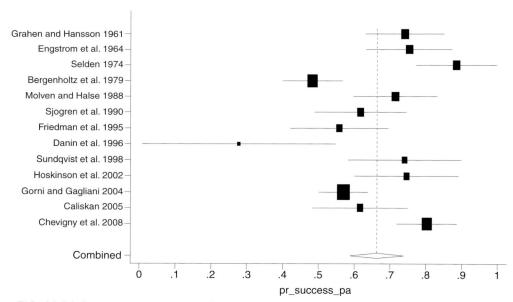

FIG. 11-31 Forest plot showing pooled and individual study's probability of complete periapical healing following root canal retreatment.

- Using magnification versus without the use of magnification during surgery (risk ratio = 1.5; 95% CI: 1.3, 1.8)
- Root-end resection with minimum versus obvious bevel (risk ratio = 1.3; 95% CI: 1.2, 1.4)
- Use of ultrasonic tip versus bur for retro-cavity preparation (risk ratio = 1.3; 95% CI: 1.2, 1.4)
- Use of retro-filling material with mineral trioxide aggregate (MTA) cement, super ethoxybenzoic acid (EBA) cement, or

intermediate restorative material (IRM) versus amalgam; the use of MTA resulted in a similar outcome to SuperEBA (risk ratio = 1.0; 95% CI: 0.99, 1.1) or IRM (risk ratio = 1.1; 95% CI: 0.98, 1.1); SuperEBA and IRM were associated with significantly higher chances of success than amalgam (risk ratio = 1.2; 95% CI: 1.1, 1.3) as the retro-filling material

The preoperative presence of signs or symptoms (risk ratio = 1.2; 95% CI: 1.1, 1.3),[249] periodontal status (risk ratio = 2.1;

TABLE 11-11

Studies Investigating Periapical Healing Following Apical Surgery

Author	Design	Examination	Type of Radiograph	Radiographic Criteria for Success	Sample Size			Duration after Treatment (months)
					Patients	Teeth	Roots	
Harty et al., 1970	Retrospective	C & R	Pa	Other		169		6-60
Nordendram, 1970	Prospective	C & R	Pa	Rud et al., 1972	66	66		6-24
Rud et al., 1972	Prospective	R	Pa	Rud et al., 1972		237		12-180
Finne et al., 1977	Prospective	C & R	Pa	Persson, 1973	156	218		36
Hirsch et al., 1979	Prospective	C & R	Pa	Rud et al., 1972	467	467		6-36
Ioannides & Borstlap, 1983	Retrospective	C & R	Pa	Other	50	50	45	6-60
Allen et al., 1989	Retrospective	C & R	Pa	Rud et al., 1972		175		12-60
Amagasa et al., 1989	Prospective	C & R	Pa	Other	42	64		12-90
Dorn & Gartner, 1990	Retrospective	R	Pa	Other		488		6-120
Grung et al., 1990	Prospective	C & R	Pa	Rud et al., 1972		161		12-96
Lustmann et al., 1991	Retrospective	C & R	Pa	Rud et al., 1972			123	6-96
Rapp et al., 1991	Retrospective	R	Pa	Rud et al., 1972	331	226		6-24
Rud et al., 1991	Retrospective	C & R	Pa	Rud et al., 1972	388	388		12
Waikakul et al., 1991	Prospective	C & R	Pa	Other	34	62		6-24
Pantschev et al., 1994	Prospective	C & R	Pa	Persson, 1973	79	103		36
Jesselen et al., 1995	Prospective	C & R	Pa	Other	67	82		12-60
Rud et al., 1996	Prospective	R	Pa	Rud et al., 1972			347	12-48
Sumi et al., 1996	Retrospective	C & R	Pa	Other	86	157		6-36
Jansson et al., 1997	Retrospective	C & R	Pa	Other	59	59		11-16
Testori et al., 1999	Retrospective	R	Pa	Rud et al., 1972	130	181	302	12-72
Von Arx & Kurt, 1999	Prospective	C & R	Pa	Von Arx & Kurt, 1999	38	43		12
Zuolo et al., 2000	Prospective	C & R	Pa	Molven et al., 1987	106	102		12-48
Pecora et al., 2001	RCT	R	Pa	Rud et al., 1972	20	20		6
Penarrocha et al., 2001	Retrospective	R	Pa	Von Arx & Kurt, 1999	30	31	71	12
Rahbaran et al., 2001	Retrospective	C & R	Pa	Other	154	154		48-108
Rud et al., 2001	Prospective	C & R	Pa	Rud et al., 1972		520	834	6-150
Von Arx et al., 2001	Prospective	C & R	Pa	Other	24	25	39	12
Jensen et al., 2002	RCT	C & R	Pa	Rud et al., 1972		122		
Rubinstein & Kim, 2002	Prospective	C & R	Pa	Rud et al., 1972	52	59	59	68
Tobon et al., 2002	RCT	R	Pa	Rud et al., 1972	25	26		12
Vallecillo et al., 2002	Prospective	R	Pa	Other	29	29		12
Chong et al., 2003	RCT	C & R	Pa	Molven et al., 1987	86	86		12-24
Maddalone & Gagliani, 2003	Prospective	C & R	Pa	Molven et al., 1987	79	120		3-36
Schwartz-Arad et al., 2003	Prospective	R	Pa	Other	101	122		6-45
Platt et al., 2004	RCT	C & R	Pa	Molven et al., 1987	28	34		12
Gagliani et al., 2005	Prospective	C & R	Pa	Rud et al., 1972	164	168	231	60
Lindeboom et al., 2005	RCT	C & R	Pa	Rud et al., 1972	100	100		12
Marti-Bowen et al., 2005	Retrospective	C & R	DPT	Von Arx & Kurt, 1999	52	71	95	6-12
Taschieri et al., 2005	Prospective	C & R	Pa	Rud et al., 1972	32	46		12
Taschieri et al., 2007	Prospective	C & R	Pa	Molven et al., 1987	28	28		12
Tsesis et al., 2006	Retrospective	C & R	Pa	Rud et al., 1972	71	88		6-48
Marin-Botero et al., 2006	RCT	C & R	Pa	Rud et al., 1972	30	30		12

Continued

TABLE 11-11

Studies Investigating Periapical Healing Following Apical Surgery—cont'd

Author	Design	Examination	Type of Radiograph	Radiographic Criteria for Success	Sample Size			Duration after Treatment (months)
					Patients	Teeth	Roots	
Taschieri et al., 2006	RCT	C & R	Pa	Molven et al., 1987	53	71		12
De Lange et al., 2007	RCT	C & R	Pa	Rud et al., 1972	290	290		12
Leco-Berrocal et al., 2007	Prospective	R	Pa and DPT	Other	45	45		6-24
Penarrocha et al., 2007	Prospective	C & R	Pa	Von Arx & Kurt, 1999	235	333	384	6-144
Taschieri et al., 2007a	Prospective	C & R	Pa	Molven et al., 1987	17	27		12
Taschieri et al., 2007b	Prospective	C & R	Pa	Molven et al., 1987	41	59		12
Von Arx et al., 2007	Prospective	C & R	Pa	Rud et al., 1972	200	177		12
Walivaara et al., 2007	Prospective	C & R	Pa	Rud et al., 1972	54	55		12
Garcia et al., 2008	Prospective	C & R	DPT	Von Arx & Kurt, 1999	92	106	129	6-12
Kim et al., 2008	Prospective	C & R	Pa	Molven et al., 1987		148		24
Penarrocha et al., 2008	Prospective	C & R	DPT	Von Arx & Kurt, 1999	278	278		12
Taschieri et al., 2008b	Prospective	C & R	Pa	Molven et al., 1987	27	31		12
Taschieri et al., 2008a	RCT	C & R	Pa	Molven et al., 1987	61	100		25
Christiansen et al., 2009	RCT	C & R	Pa	Molven et al., 1987		25		12
Dominiak et al., 2009	Retrospective	C & R	Pa	Other	106	106		12
Ortega-Sanchez et al., 2009	Retrospective	C & R	DPT	Von Arx & Kurt, 1999	30	30	37	
Pantschev et al., 2009	Retrospective	C & R	Pa	Other		147		12
Waalivaara et al., 2009	RCT	C & R	Pa	Molven et al., 1987	131	147		12
Barone et al., 2010	Prospective	C & R	Pa	PAI		129		48-120
Garcia-Mira et al., 2010	Retrospective	C & R	DPT	Von Arx & Kurt, 1999	75	87		12
Taschieri et al., 2010	Retrospective	C & R	Pa	Molven et al., 1987	76	112		48
Von Arx et al., 2010	Prospective	C & R	Pa	Rud et al., 1972		339		12
Goyal et al., 2011	RCT	C & R	Pa	Rud et al., 1972	25	25		12
Penarrocha et al., 2011	Retrospective	C & R	DPT	Von Arx & Kurt, 1999	150	178	178	12
Song et al., 2011a	Retrospective	C & R	Pa	Molven et al., 1987		441		3-12
Song et al., 2011b	Prospective	C & R	Pa	Molven et al., 1987	42	42		12
Taschieri et al., 2011	Retrospective	C & R	Pa	Molven et al., 1987	33	43		12-48
Waalivaara et al., 2011	RCT	C & R	Pa	Molven et al., 1987	153	194		12-21
Penarrocha et al., 2012	Prospective	C & R	DPT	Von Arx & Kurt, 1999	23	31		12-19
Song & Kim, 2012	RCT	C & R	Pa	Molven et al., 1987	192	192		12
Von Arx et al., 2012	Prospective	C & R	Pa	Rud et al., 1972		170		12-60
Kreisler et al., 2013	Prospective	C & R	Pa	Rud et al., 1972	255	281		6-12
Penarrocha et al., 2013	Retrospective	C & R	Pa and DPT	Von Arx & Kurt	96	139		6-12
Song et al., 2013a	Prospective	C & R	Pa	Molven et al., 1987		344		12-120
Song et al., 2013b	Prospective	C & R	Pa	Molven et al., 1987		135		12
Song et al., 2014	Retrospective	C & R	Pa	Rud et al., 1972		115		12-96
Taschieri et al., 2013	Retrospective	C & R	Pa	Molven et al., 1987		86		6-12
Villa-Machado et al., 2013	Retrospective	C & R	Pa	PAI	154	171		12-192
Li et al., 2014	Retrospective	C & R	Pa	Molven et al., 1987	82	101		48

RCT, randomized controlled trial; C, clinical; R, radiographic; Pa, periapical; DPT, dental pantomogram; PAI, periapical index.

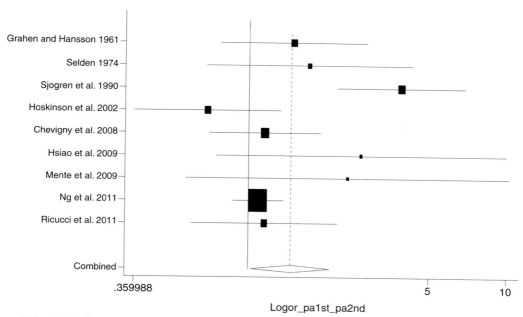

FIG. 11-32 Forest plot showing pooled and individual study's odds ratio of periapical health for teeth with preoperative periapical radiolucency undergoing primary root canal treatment versus root canal retreatment (pooled OR = 1.5; 95% CI: 1.0, 2.1).

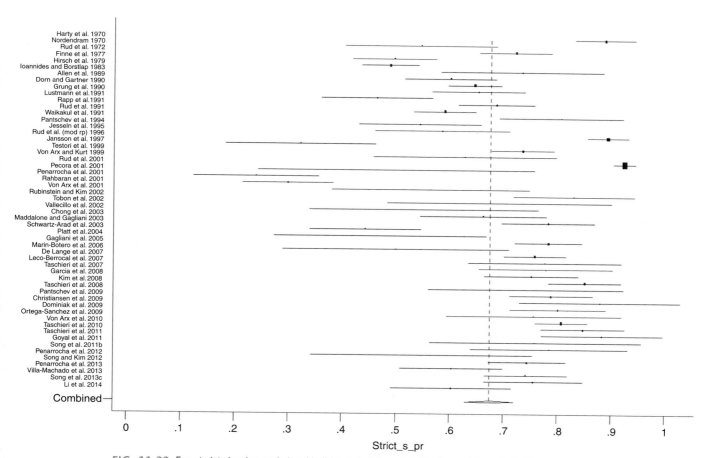

FIG. 11-33 Forest plot showing pooled and individual study's probability of complete periapical healing following apical surgery.

95% CI: 1.1, 3.8),[222] and quality of the coronal restoration (risk ratio = 1.6; 95% CI: 1.2, 2.1)[249] have also been revealed as significant prognostic factors by individual studies.

The following factors have minimal effect on surgical retreatment[43]:

◆ Age of patient
◆ Gender of patient
◆ General health of patient
◆ Tooth type
◆ Quality of the preexisting root canal filling, as judged radiographically
◆ Histologic diagnosis of the biopsied periapical lesion (cyst or granuloma)

The use of guided periodontal tissue regenerative membrane or grafting material has been advocated for cases with through-and-through defects (missing buccal and palatal cortical plates), but there are conflicting reports as to their benefits.[53,162,170,232-234,237,249] The unpublished meta-analyses[130] of data from these studies did not reveal a significant influence of such approaches on the periapical healing outcome.

Factors Affecting Periodontal Incisional Wound Healing

Periodontal attachment level after periapical surgery is an additional physical outcome measure compared to nonsurgical root canal treatment. Studies have compared the effect of different soft tissue incision techniques (intrasulcular with or without involving interproximal papilla, submarginal, papilla-base, etc.).[106,245-247] As expected, all concluded that negligible marginal recession could be achieved by adopting a flap design that avoided reflection of the interproximal papilla.

The improvement in outcomes of periapical surgery has been attributed to modern surgical techniques plus greater biologic awareness of clinicians.[205,250] In addition, and perhaps even more important, case selection may be more critical in excluding potential failures, inferring that prognostication may have improved.

Factors Affecting Tooth Survival Following Periapical Surgery and Root-End Filling

Unlike nonsurgical root canal treatment, the outcome measure of tooth survival had only been adopted by one study[253] on surgical cases at the time of this writing. The reported median survival time for first-time surgery was 92.1 months (95% CI: 40.9, 143.4) and that for resurgery was 39.1 months (95% CI: 6.1, 72.1).[253] The failure events, however, included tooth extraction and clinical and radiographic signs of periapical disease after treatment.

Impact of Periapical Surgery on Quality of Life

The impact of periapical surgery on the patient's quality of life has only been evaluated using a questionnaire including three domains: physical function (chewing, talking, sleeping, daily routine, and work), physical pain, and other physical symptoms (swelling, bleeding, nausea, bad taste/breath).[49] It was concluded that the papilla-base incision flap design resulted in a lower impact on physical pain and other symptoms within the first week postoperation. The impact on physical pain has also been explored by two other studies[35,36]; both reported the postoperative pain was of relatively short duration, with the intensity peaking at 3 to 5 hours postoperatively and progressively decreasing with time with no significant influencing factors identified.

CONCLUDING REMARKS

The procedures used to maintain pulp vitality and for prevention and treatment of periapical disease are able to achieve excellent outcomes. The outcome data and potential prognostic factors should be considered during treatment options appraisal and planning. Despite the fact that most important prognostic factors are beyond the control of clinicians, optimal outcomes for individual cases may still be achieved by performing the procedure to guideline standards. From a health and economic perspective, conventional root canal treatment is a highly cost-effective treatment as a first-line intervention to extend the life of the tooth with a preoperative periapical lesion.[103,171] If a root canal treatment subsequently fails, nonsurgical and surgical retreatments are also more cost-effective than replacement with a prosthesis.[103,171] Ultimately, all sources of evidence must be assessed for biasing influences based on the local cultures, expertise, treatment predilection, and funding sources.

REFERENCES

1. Aguilar P, Linsuwanont P: Vital pulp therapy in vital permanent teeth with cariously exposed pulp: a systematic review, *J Endod* 37:581, 2011.
2. Akpata ES: Effect of endodontic procedures on the population of viable microorganisms in the infected root canal, *J Endod* 2:369, 1976.
3. Alley BS, Kitchens GG, Alley LW, Eleazer PD: A comparison of survival of teeth following endodontic treatment performed by general dentists or by specialists, *Oral Surg Oral Med Oral Pathol Oral Radiol Endod* 98:115, 2004.
4. Allison DA, Weber CR, Walton RE: The influence of the method of canal preparation on the quality of apical and coronal obturation, *J Endod* 5:298, 1979.
5. Arai Y, Honda K, Iwai K, Shinoda K: Practical model "3DX" of limited cone-beam X-ray CT for dental use, *Cars 2001: Computer Assisted Radiology and Surgery* 1230:671, 2001.
6. Asgary S, Ehsani S: Permanent molar pulpotomy with a new endodontic cement: a case series, *J Conserv Dent* 12:31, 2009.
7. Auerbach M: Antibiotics vs. instrumentation in endodontics, *N Y State Dent J* 19:225, 1953.
8. Augsburger RA, Peters DD: Radiographic evaluation of extruded obturation materials, *J Endod* 16:492, 1990.
9. Bader JD, Shugars DA: Variation, treatment outcomes, and practice guidelines in dental practice, *J Dent Edu* 59:61, 1995.
10. Baratieri LN, Monteiro S Jr, Caldeira de Andrada MA: Pulp curettage: surgical technique, *Quintessence Int* 20:285, 1989.
11. Barrieshi-Nusair KM, Qudeimat MA: A prospective clinical study of mineral trioxide aggregate for partial pulpotomy in cariously exposed permanent teeth, *J Endod* 32:731, 2006.
12. Barthel CR, Rosenkranz B, Leuenberg A, Roulet JF: Pulp capping of carious exposures: treatment outcome after 5 and 10 years: a retrospective study, *J Endod* 26:525, 2000.
13. Basrani B, Tjaderhane L, Santos JM, et al: Efficacy of chlorhexidine- and calcium hydroxide-containing medicaments against Enterococcus faecalis in vitro, *Oral Surg Oral Med Oral Pathol Oral Radiol Endod* 96:618, 2003.
14. Basrani BR, Manek S, Sodhi RN, et al: Interaction between sodium hypochlorite and chlorhexidine gluconate, *J Endod* 33:966, 2007.
15. Baugh D, Wallace J: The role of apical instrumentation in root canal treatment: a review of the literature, *J Endod* 31:333, 2005.
16. Bence R, Madonia JV, Weine FS, Smulson MH: A microbiologic evaluation of endodontic instrumentation in pulpless teeth, *Oral Surg Oral Med Oral Pathol* 35:676, 1973.

17. Bender IB, Seltzer S, Soltanof W: Endodontic success: a reappraisal of criteria, 1, *Oral Surg Oral Med Oral Pathol Oral Radiol Endod* 22:780, 1966.

18. Bender IB, Seltzer S, Soltanof W: Endodontic success: a reappraisal of criteria. 2, *Oral Surg Oral Med Oral Pathol Oral Radiol Endod* 22:790, 1966.

19. Bjorndal L, Reit C, Bruun G, et al: Treatment of deep caries lesions in adults: randomized clinical trials comparing stepwise vs. direct complete excavation, and direct pulp capping vs. partial pulpotomy, *Eur J Oral Sci* 118:290, 2010.

20. Bjorndal L, Thylstrup A: A practice-based study on stepwise excavation of deep carious lesions in permanent teeth: a 1-year follow-up study, *Community Dent Oral Epidemiol* 26:122, 1998.

21. Bogen G, Kim JS, Bakland LK: Direct pulp capping with mineral trioxide aggregate: an observational study, *J Am Dent Assoc* 139:305; quiz 305, 2008.

22. Boggia R: A single-visit treatment of septic root canals using periapically extruded endomethasone, *Br Dent J* 155:300, 1983.

23. Buchbinder M, Wald A: An improved method of culturing root canals, *J Am Dent Assoc* 26:1697, 1939.

24. Bui TB, Baumgartner JC, Mitchell JC: Evaluation of the interaction between sodium hypochlorite and chlorhexidine gluconate and its effect on root dentin, *J Endod* 34:181, 2008.

25. Bystrom A: *Evaluation of endodontic treatment of teeth with apical periodontitis*, Sweden, 1986, University of Umeå.

26. Bystrom A, Claesson R, Sundqvist G: The antibacterial effect of camphorated paramonochlorophenol, camphorated phenol and calcium hydroxide in the treatment of infected root canals, *Endod Dent Traumatol* 1:170, 1985.

27. Bystrom A, Sundqvist G: Bacteriologic evaluation of the efficacy of mechanical root canal instrumentation in endodontic therapy, *Scand J Dent Res* 89:321, 1981.

28. Bystrom A, Sundqvist G: Bacteriologic evaluation of the effect of 0.5 percent sodium hypochlorite in endodontic therapy, *Oral Surg Oral Med Oral Pathol* 55:307, 1983.

29. Bystrom A, Sundqvist G: The antibacterial action of sodium hypochlorite and EDTA in 60 cases of endodontic therapy, *Int Endod J* 18:35, 1985.

30. Caliskan MK: Success of pulpotomy in the management of hyperplastic pulpitis, *Int Endod J* 26:142, 1993.

31. Caliskan MK: Pulpotomy of carious vital teeth with periapical involvement, *Int Endod J* 28:172, 1995.

32. Camps J, Pommel L, Bukiet F: Evaluation of periapical lesion healing by correction of gray values, *J Endod* 30:762, 2004.

33. Card SJ, Sigurdsson A, Orstavik D, Trope M: The effectiveness of increased apical enlargement in reducing intracanal bacteria, *J Endod* 28:779, 2002.

34. Chambers D: Outcomes-based practice: how outcomes-based practices get better, *Dental Economics* 3:34, 2001.

35. Chong BS, Pitt Ford TR: Postoperative pain after root-end resection and filling, *Oral Surg Oral Med Oral Pathol Oral Radiol Endod* 100:762, 2005.

36. Christiansen R, Kirkevang LL, Horsted-Bindslev P, Wenzel A: Patient discomfort following periapical surgery, *Oral Surg Oral Med Oral Pathol Oral Radiol Endod* 105:245, 2008.

37. Chu FC, Leung WK, Tsang PC, et al: Identification of cultivable microorganisms from root canals with apical periodontitis following two-visit endodontic treatment with antibiotics/steroid or calcium hydroxide dressings, *J Endod* 32:17, 2006.

38. Chugal NM, Clive JM, Spangberg LS: Endodontic treatment outcome: effect of the permanent restoration, *Oral Surg Oral Med Oral Pathol Oral Radiol Endod* 104:576, 2007.

39. Colman I, Friedman BW, Brown MD, et al: Parenteral dexamethasone for acute severe migraine headache: meta-analysis of randomised controlled trials for preventing recurrence, *BMJ* 336:13591, 2008.

40. Cvek M: A clinical report on partial pulpotomy and capping with calcium hydroxide in permanent incisors with complicated crown fracture, *J Endod* 4:232, 1978.

41. Cvek M, Hollender L, Nord CE: Treatment of non-vital permanent incisors with calcium hydroxide. VI. A clinical, microbiological and radiological evaluation of treatment in one sitting of teeth with mature or immature root, *Odontol Revy* 27:93, 1976.

42. Dalton BC, Orstavik D, Phillips C, et al: Bacterial reduction with nickel-titanium rotary instrumentation, *J Endod* 24:763, 1998.

43. de Chevigny C, Dao TT, Basrani BR, et al: Treatment outcome in endodontics: the Toronto study–phase 4: initial treatment, *J Endod* 34:258, 2008.

44. de Paula-Silva FW, Wu MK, Leonardo MR, et al: Accuracy of periapical radiography and cone-beam computed tomography scans in diagnosing apical periodontitis using histopathological findings as a gold standard, *J Endod* 35:10092, 2009.

45. Del Fabbro M, Taschieri S: Endodontic therapy using magnification devices: a systematic review, *J Dent* 38:269, 2010.

46. Del Fabbro M, Taschieri S, Lodi G, et al: Magnification devices for endodontic therapy, *Cochrane Database Syst Rev* CD005969, 2009.

47. Del Fabbro M, Taschieri S, Lodi G, et al: *Magnification devices for endodontic therapy*, Cochrane Database of Systematic Reviews, 2009, John Wiley & Sons.

48. Del Fabbro M, Taschieri S, Testori T, et al: *Surgical versus non-surgical endodontic re-treatment for periradicular lesions*. Cochrane Database of Systematic Reviews, 2007, John Wiley & Sons.

49. Del Fabbro M, Taschieri S, Weinstein R: Quality of life after microscopic periradicular surgery using two different incision techniques: a randomized clinical study, *Int Endod J* 42:360, 2009.

50. Delano EO, Tyndall D, Ludlow JB, et al: Quantitative radiographic follow-up of apical surgery: a radiometric and histologic correlation, *J Endod* 24:420, 1998.

51. DePalma MJ, Slipman CW: Evidence-informed management of chronic low back pain with epidural steroid injections, *Spine J* 8:45, 2008.

52. DeRosa TA: A retrospective evaluation of pulpotomy as an alternative to extraction, *Gen Dent* 54:37, 2006.

53. Dominiak M, Lysiak-Drwal K, Gedrange T, et al: Efficacy of healing process of bone defects after apicectomy: results after 6 and 12 months, *J Physiol Pharmacol* 60(suppl 8):51, 2009.

54. Doyle SL, Hodges JS, Pesun IJ, et al: Retrospective cross sectional comparison of initial nonsurgical endodontic treatment and single-tooth implants, *J Endod* 32:822, 2006.

55. Dugas NN, Lawrence HP, Teplitsky P, Friedman S: Quality of life and satisfaction outcomes of endodontic treatment, *J Endod* 28:819, 2002.

56. Eakle WS, Maxwell EH, Braly BV: Fractures of posterior teeth in adults, *J Am Dent Assoc* 112:215, 1986.

57. Edwards JL, Vincent AM, Cheng HT, Feldman EL: Diabetic neuropathy: mechanisms to management, *Pharmacol Ther* 120:1, 2008.

58. El-Meligy OA, Avery DR: Comparison of mineral trioxide aggregate and calcium hydroxide as pulpotomy agents in young permanent teeth (apexogenesis), *Pediatr Dent* 28:399, 2006.

59. American Association of Endodontists, "Evolution of the Root Canal", Source: www.aae.org/uploadedfiles/news_room/press_releases/rcawendodontictimeline.pdf (accessed June 2015).

60. Engström B: The significance of enterococci in root canal treatment, *Odontol Revy* 15:87, 1964.

61. European Society of Endodontology: Quality guidelines for endodontic treatment: consensus report of the European Society of Endodontology, *Int Endod J* 39:921, 2006.

62. European Society of Endodontology, Patel S, Durack C, et al: European Society of Endodontology position statement: the use of CBCT in endodontics, *Int Endod J* 47:502, 2014.

63. Fabricius L, Dahlen G, Sundqvist G, et al: Influence of residual bacteria on periapical tissue healing after chemomechanical treatment and root filling of experimentally infected monkey teeth, *Eur J Oral Sci* 114:278, 2006.

64. Farsi N, Alamoudi N, Balto K, Al Mushayt A: Clinical assessment of mineral trioxide aggregate (MTA) as direct pulp capping in young permanent teeth, *J Clin Pediatr Dent* 31:72, 2006.

65. Fitzgerald M, Heys RJ: A clinical and histological evaluation of conservative pulpal therapy in human teeth, *Oper Dent* 16:101, 1991.

66. Ford TP: Frequency of radiological review in pulp studies, *Int Endod J* 41:931, 2008.

67. Fouad AF, Burleson J: The effect of diabetes mellitus on endodontic treatment outcome: data from an electronic patient record, *J Am Dent Assoc* 134:43; quiz 117, 2003.

68. Friedman S, Lost C, Zarrabian M, Trope M: Evaluation of success and failure after endodontic therapy using a glass ionomer cement sealer, *J Endod* 21:384, 1995.

69. Friedman S, Mor C: The success of endodontic therapy—healing and functionality, *J Calif Dent Assoc* 32:493, 2004.

70. Frostell G: Clinical significance of the root canal culture, pp. 112-122, Transactions of Third International Conference of Endodontics, 1963.

71. Fuks AB, Gavra S, Chosack A: Long-term followup of traumatized incisors treated by partial pulpotomy, *Pediatr Dent* 15:334, 1993.

72. Gallien GS Jr, Schuman NJ: Local versus general anesthesia: a study of pulpal response in the treatment of cariously exposed teeth, *J Am Dent Assoc* 111:599, 1985.

73. Gatten DL, Riedy CA, Hong SK, et al: Quality of life of endodontically treated versus implant treated patients: a University-based qualitative research study, *J Endod* 37:903, 2011.

74. Genco RJ, Loe H: The role of systemic conditions and disorders in periodontal disease, *Periodontol 2000* 2:98, 1993.

75. Gesi A, Hakeberg M, Warfvinge J, Bergenholtz G: Incidence of periapical lesions and clinical symptoms after pulpectomy—a clinical and radiographic evaluation of 1- versus 2-session treatment, *Oral Surg Oral Med Oral Pathol Oral Radiol Endod* 101:379, 2006.

76. Goldfein J, Speirs C, Finkelman M, Amato R: Rubber dam use during post placement influences the success of root canal-treated teeth, *J Endod* 39:14814, 2013.

77. Gomes BP, Lilley JD, Drucker DB: Variations in the susceptibilities of components of the endodontic microflora to biomechanical procedures, *Int Endod J* 29:235, 1996.

78. Gomes BP, Souza SF, Ferraz CC, et al: Effectiveness of 2% chlorhexidine gel and calcium hydroxide against Enterococcus faecalis in bovine root dentine in vitro, *Int Endod J* 36:267, 2003.

79. Grahnen H, Krasse B: The effect of instrumentation and flushing of non-vital teeth in endodontic therapy, *Odontol Rev* 14:167, 1963.

80. Gratt BM, Sickles EA, Gould RG, et al: Xeroradiography of dental structures. IV. Image properties of a dedicated intraoral system, *Oral Surg Oral Med Oral Pathol* 50:572, 1980.

81. Gruythuysen RJ, van Strijp AJ, Wu MK: Long-term survival of indirect pulp treatment performed in primary and permanent teeth with clinically diagnosed deep carious lesions, *J Endod* 36:14903, 2010.

82. Gulabivala K: *Species richness of gram-positive coccoid morphotypes isolated from untreated and treated root canals of teeth associated with periapical disease*, London, 2004, University of London.

83. Gulabivala K, Ng Y: Endodontology. In Wilson N, editor: *Clinical dental medicine 2020*, New Malden, Surrey, 2009, Quintessence, pp 147-182.

84. Gulabivala K, Ng YL, Gilbertson M, Eames I: The fluid mechanics of root canal irrigation, *Physiol Meas* 31:R49, 2010.

85. Gulabivala K, Patel B, Evans G, Ng YL: Effects of mechanical and chemical procedures on root canal surfaces, *Endodontic Topics* 10:103, 2005.

86. Halse A, Molven O: Increased width of the apical periodontal membrane space in endodontically treated teeth may represent favourable healing, *Int Endod J* 37:552, 2004.

87. Hamasha AA, Hatiwsh A: Quality of life and satisfaction of patients after nonsurgical primary root canal treatment provided by undergraduate students, graduate students and endodontic specialists, *Int Endod J* 46:11319, 2013.

88. Haskell EW, Stanley HR, Chellemi J, Stringfellow H: Direct pulp capping treatment: a long-term follow-up, *J Am Dent Assoc* 97:607, 1978.

89. Hayashi M, Fujitani M, Yamaki C, Momoi Y: Ways of enhancing pulp preservation by stepwise excavation—a systematic review, *J Dent* 39:95, 2011.

90. Hilton TJ, Ferracane JL, Mancl L: Northwest Practice-based Research Collaborative in Evidence-based Dentistry (NWP): Comparison of CaOH with MTA for direct pulp capping: a PBRN randomized clinical trial, *J Dent Res* 92:16SS, 2013.

91. Holroyd J, Gulson A: *The radiation protection implications of the use of cone beam computed tomography (CBCT) in dentistry: what you need to know*, London, 2009, Health Protection Agency.

92. Horsted P, Sandergaard B, Thylstrup A, et al: A retrospective study of direct pulp capping with calcium hydroxide compounds, *Endod Dent Traumatol* 1:29, 1985.

93. Hoskinson SE, Ng YL, Hoskinson AE, et al: A retrospective comparison of outcome of root canal treatment using two different protocols, *Oral Surg Oral Med Oral Pathol Oral Radiol Endod* 93:705, 2002.

94. Hughes R: Focal infection revisited, *Rheumatology* 33:370, 1994.

95. Hülsmann M, Peters OA, Dummer PM: Mechanical preparation of root canals: shaping goals, techniques and means, *Endodontic Topics* 10:30, 2005.

96. Hunter W: The role of sepsis and antisepsis in medicine, *Lancet* 1:79, 1911.

97. Hunter W: Chronic sepsis as a cause of mental disorder, *Br J Psychiatr* 73:549, 1927.

98. Huumonen S, Lenander-Lumikari M, Sigurdsson A, Orstavik D: Healing of apical periodontitis after endodontic treatment: a comparison between a silicone-based and a zinc oxide-eugenol-based sealer, *Int Endod J* 36:296, 2003.

99. Ingle J, Zeldow B: An evaluation of mechanical instrumentation and the negative culture in endodontic therapy, *J Am Dent Assoc* (1939) 57:471, 1958.

100. Iqbal MK, Kim S: For teeth requiring endodontic treatment, what are the differences in outcomes of restored endodontically treated teeth compared to implant-supported restorations? *Int J Oral Maxillofac Implants* 22:96, 2006.

101. Kalichman L, Hunter DJ: Diagnosis and conservative management of degenerative lumbar spondylolisthesis, *Eur Spine J* 17:327, 2008.

102. Kerekes K, Tronstad L: Long-term results of endodontic treatment performed with a standardized technique, *J Endod* 5:83, 1979.

103. Kim SG, Solomon C: Cost-effectiveness of endodontic molar retreatment compared with fixed partial dentures and single-tooth implant alternatives, *J Endod* 37:321, 2011.

104. Koontongkaew S, Silapichit R, Thaweboon B: Clinical and laboratory assessments of camphorated monochlorophenol in endodontic therapy, *Oral Surg Oral Med Oral Pathol* 65:757, 1988.

105. Koppang HS, Koppang R, Stolen SO: Identification of common foreign material in postendodontic granulomas and cysts, *J Dent Assoc S Afr* 47:210, 1992.

106. Kreisler M, Gockel R, Schmidt I, et al: Clinical evaluation of a modified marginal sulcular incision technique in endodontic surgery, *Oral Surg Oral Med Oral Pathol Oral Radiol Endod* 108:e22, 2009.

107. Kuruvilla JR, Kamath MP: Antimicrobial activity of 2.5% sodium hypochlorite and 0.2% chlorhexidine gluconate separately and combined, as endodontic irrigants, *J Endod* 24:472, 1998.

108. Kvist T, Molander A, Dahlen G, Reit C: Microbiological evaluation of one- and two-visit endodontic treatment of teeth with apical periodontitis: a randomized, clinical trial, *J Endod* 30:572, 2004.

109. Lagouvardos P, Sourai P, Douvitsas G: Coronal fractures in posterior teeth, *Oper Dent* 14:28, 1989.

110. Lana MA, Ribeiro-Sobrinho AP, Stehling R, et al: Microorganisms isolated from root canals presenting necrotic pulp and their drug susceptibility in vitro, *Oral Microbiol Immunol* 16:100, 2001.

111. Lazarski MP, Walker WA 3rd, Flores CM, et al: Epidemiological evaluation of the outcomes of nonsurgical root canal treatment in a large cohort of insured dental patients, *J Endod* 27:791, 2001.

112. Lee SJ, Wu MK, Wesselink PR: The efficacy of ultrasonic irrigation to remove artificially placed dentine debris from different-sized simulated plastic root canals, *Int Endod J* 37:607, 2004.

113. Leksell E, Ridell K, Cvek M, Mejare I: Pulp exposure after stepwise versus direct complete excavation of deep carious lesions in young posterior permanent teeth, *Endod Dent Traumatol* 12:192, 1996.

114. Liang YH, Li G, Wesselink PR, Wu MK: Endodontic outcome predictors identified with periapical radiographs and cone-beam computed tomography scans, *J Endod* 37:326, 2011.

115. Liu P, McGrath C, Cheung GS: Improvement in oral health-related quality of life after endodontic treatment: a prospective longitudinal study, *J Endod* 40:805, 2014.

116. Locker D: Concepts of health, disease and quality of life. In Slade GD, editor: *Measuring oral health and quality of life*, Chapel Hill, North Carolina, 1997, University of North Carolina, pp 11-23.

117. Loe H: Does chlorhexidine have a place in the prophylaxis of dental diseases? *J Periodontal Res Suppl* 12:93, 1973.

118. Lumley PJ, Lucarotti PS, Burke FJ: Ten-year outcome of root fillings in the General Dental Services in England and Wales, *Int Endod J* 41:577, 2008.

119. Mah JK, Danforth RA, Bumann A, Hatcher D: Radiation absorbed in maxillofacial imaging with a new dental computed tomography device, *Oral Surg Oral Med Oral Pathol Oral Radiol Endod* 96:508, 2003.

120. Maltz M: Does incomplete caries removal increase restoration failure? *J Dent Res* 90:541; author reply 542, 2011.

121. Maltz M, Garcia R, Jardim JJ, et al: Randomized trial of partial vs. stepwise caries removal: 3-year follow-up, *J Dent Res* 91:10261, 2012.

122. Maltz M, Henz SL, de Oliveira EF, Jardim JJ: Conventional caries removal and sealed caries in permanent teeth: a microbiological evaluation, *J Dent* 40:776, 2012.

123. Marending M, Peters OA, Zehnder M: Factors affecting the outcome of orthograde root canal therapy in a general dentistry hospital practice, *Oral Surg Oral Med Oral Pathol Oral Radiol Endod* 99:119, 2005.

124. Markvart M, Dahlen G, Reit CE, Bjorndal L: The antimicrobial effect of apical box versus apical cone preparation using iodine potassium iodide as root canal dressing: a pilot study, *Acta Odontol Scand* 71:786, 2013.

125. Mass E, Zilberman U: Clinical and radiographic evaluation of partial pulpotomy in carious exposure of permanent molars, *Pediatr Dent* 15:257, 1993.

126. Masterton JB: The healing of wounds of the dental pulp: an investigation of the nature of the scar tissue and of the phenomena leading to its formation, *Dent Pract Dent Rec* 16:325, 1966.

127. Matsumoto M, Goto T: Lateral force distribution in partial denture design, *J Dent Res* 49:359, 1970.

128. Matsuo T, Nakanishi T, Shimizu H, Ebisu S: A clinical study of direct pulp capping applied to carious-exposed pulps, *J Endod* 22:551, 1996.

129. McDonnell G, Russell AD: Antiseptics and disinfectants: activity, action, and resistance, *Clinical Microbiol Rev* 12:147, 1999.

130. Mehta D, Gulabivala K, Ng Y-L: Personal communication. *Outcome of periapical surgery*, unpublished manuscript, 2014.

131. Mejare I, Cvek M: Partial pulpotomy in young permanent teeth with deep carious lesions, *Endod Dent Traumatol* 9:238, 1993.

132. Mente J, Geletneky B, Ohle M, et al: Mineral trioxide aggregate or calcium hydroxide direct pulp capping: an analysis of the clinical treatment outcome, *J Endod* 36:806, 2010.

133. Miles JP, Gluskin AH, Chambers D, Peters OA: Pulp capping with mineral trioxide aggregate (MTA): a retrospective analysis of carious pulp exposures treated by undergraduate dental students, *Oper Dent* 35:20, 2010.

134. Miller WD: An introduction to the study of the bacterio-pathology of the dental pulp, *The Dental Cosmos* 36:505-528, 1894.

135. Mindiola MJ, Mickel AK, Sami C, et al: Endodontic treatment in an American Indian population: a 10-year retrospective study, *J Endod* 32:828, 2006.

136. Miyashita H, Worthington HV, Qualtrough A, Plasschaert A: Pulp management for caries in adults: maintaining pulp vitality (review), *Cochrane Database Syst Rev*, 2007.

137. Molander A, Reit C, Dahlen G: Microbiological evaluation of clindamycin as a root canal dressing in teeth with apical periodontitis, *Int Endod J* 23:113, 1990.

138. Molander A, Reit C, Dahlen G: Microbiological root canal sampling: diffusion of a technology, *Int Endod J* 29:163, 1996.

139. Molander A, Reit C, Dahlen G: Reasons for dentists' acceptance or rejection of microbiological root canal sampling, *Int Endod J* 29:168, 1996.

140. Molven O, Halse A, Grung B: Observer strategy and the radiographic classification of healing after endodontic surgery, *Int J Oral Maxillofac Surg* 16:432, 1987.

141. Moore DL: Conservative treatment of teeth with vital pulps and periapical lesions: a preliminary report, *J Prosthet Dent* 18:476, 1967.

142. Morsani JM, Aminoshariae A, Han YW, et al: Genetic predisposition to persistent apical periodontitis, *J Endod* 37:455, 2011.

143. Morse F, Yates M: Follow up studies of root-filled teeth in relation to bacteriologic findings, *J Am Dent Assoc* 28:956, 1941.

144. Nagasiri R, Chitmongkolsuk S: Long-term survival of endodontically treated molars without crown coverage: a retrospective cohort study, *J Prosthet Dent* 93:164, 2005.

145. Nair PN: On the causes of persistent apical periodontitis: a review, *Int Endod J* 39:249, 2006.

146. Nair PN, Sjogren U, Krey G, Sundqvist G: Therapy-resistant foreign body giant cell granuloma at the periapex of a root-filled human tooth, *J Endod* 16:589, 1990.

147. Nair PNR, Henry S, Cano V, Vera J: Microbial status of apical root canal system of human mandibular first molars with primary apical periodontitis after "one-visit" endodontic treatment, *Oral Surg Oral Med Oral Pathol Oral Radiol Endod* 99:231, 2005.

148. Ng YL, Mann V, Gulabivala K: Outcome of secondary root canal treatment: a systematic review of the literature, *Int Endod J* 41:10266, 2008.

149. Ng YL, Mann V, Gulabivala K: Tooth survival following non-surgical root canal treatment: a systematic review of the literature, *Int Endod J* 43:171, 2010.

150. Ng YL, Mann V, Gulabivala K: A prospective study of the factors affecting outcomes of nonsurgical root canal treatment: part 1: periapical health, *Int Endod J* 44:583, 2011.

151. Ng YL, Mann V, Gulabivala K: A prospective study of the factors affecting outcomes of non-surgical root canal treatment: part 2: tooth survival, *Int Endod J* 44:610, 2011.

152. Ng YL, Mann V, Rahbaran S, et al: Outcome of primary root canal treatment: systematic review of the literature. Part 1. Effects of study characteristics on probability of success, *Int Endod J* 40:921, 2007.

153. Ng YL, Mann V, Rahbaran S, et al: Outcome of primary root canal treatment: systematic review of the literature. Part 2. Influence of clinical factors, *Int Endod J* 41:6, 2008.

154. Nicholls E: The efficacy of cleansing of the root canal, *Br Dent J* 112:167, 1962.

155. Niederman R, Theodosopoulou JN: A systematic review of in vivo retrograde obturation materials, *Int Endod J* 36:577, 2003.

156. Orstavik D: Radiographic evaluation of apical periodontitis and endodontic treatment results: a computer approach, *Int Dent J* 41:89, 1991.

157. Orstavik D: Time-course and risk analyses of the development and healing of chronic apical periodontitis in man, *Int Endod J* 29:150, 1996.

158. Orstavik D, Farrants G, Wahl T, Kerekes K: Image analysis of endodontic radiographs: digital subtraction and quantitative densitometry, *Endod Dent Traumatol* 6:6, 1990.

159. Orstavik D, Horsted-Bindslev P: A comparison of endodontic treatment results at two dental schools, *Int Endod J* 26:348, 1993.

160. Orstavik D, Kerekes K, Eriksen HM: Clinical performance of three endodontic sealers, *Endod Dent Traumatol* 3:178, 1987.

161. Orstavik D, Kerekes K, Molven O: Effects of extensive apical reaming and calcium hydroxide dressing on bacterial infection during treatment of apical periodontitis: a pilot study, *Int Endod J* 24:1, 1991.

162. Pantchev A, Nohlert E, Tegelberg A: Endodontic surgery with and without inserts of bioactive glass PerioGlas: a clinical and radiographic follow-up, *Oral Maxillofac Surg* 13:21, 2009.

163. Paquette L, Legner M, Fillery ED, Friedman S: Antibacterial efficacy of chlorhexidine gluconate intracanal medication in vivo, *J Endod* 33:788, 2007.

164. Parris J, Wilcox L, Walton R: Effectiveness of apical clearing: histological and radiographical evaluation, *J Endod* 20:219, 1994.

165. Patel S, Dawood A, Mannocci F, et al: Detection of periapical bone defects in human jaws using cone beam computed tomography and intraoral radiography, *Int Endod J* 42:507, 2009.

166. Patel S, Rhodes J: A practical guide to endodontic access cavity preparation in molar teeth, *Br Dent J* 203:133, 2007.

167. Patel S, Wilson R, Dawood A, et al: The detection of periapical pathosis using digital periapical radiography and cone beam computed tomography—part 2: a 1-year post-treatment follow-up, *Int Endod J* 45:711, 2012.

168. Peciuliene V, Balciuniene I, Eriksen HM, Haapasalo M: Isolation of Enterococcus faecalis in previously root-filled canals in a Lithuanian population, *J Endod* 26:593, 2000.

169. Peciuliene V, Reynaud AH, Balciuniene I, Haapasalo M: Isolation of yeasts and enteric bacteria in root-filled teeth with chronic apical periodontitis, *Int Endod J* 34:429, 2001.

170. Pecora G, De Leonardis D, Ibrahim N, et al: The use of calcium sulphate in the surgical treatment of a 'through and through' periradicular lesion, *Int Endod J* 34:189, 2001.

171. Pennington MW, Vernazza CR, Shackley P, et al: Evaluation of the cost-effectiveness of root canal treatment using conventional approaches versus replacement with an implant, *Int Endod J* 42:874, 2009.

172. Percinoto C, de Castro AM, Pinto LM: Clinical and radiographic evaluation of pulpotomies employing calcium hydroxide and trioxide mineral aggregate, *Gen Dent* 54:258, 2006.

173. Peters LB, van Winkelhoff AJ, Buijs JF, Wesselink PR: Effects of instrumentation, irrigation and dressing with calcium hydroxide on infection in pulpless teeth with periapical bone lesions, *Int Endod J* 35:13, 2002.

174. Petersson A, Axelsson S, Davidson T, et al: Radiological diagnosis of periapical bone tissue lesions in endodontics: a systematic review, *Int Endod J* 45:783, 2012.

175. Pettiette MT, Delano EO, Trope M: Evaluation of success rate of endodontic treatment performed by students with stainless-steel K-files and nickel-titanium hand files, *J Endod* 27:124, 2001.

176. Polycarpou N, Ng YL, Canavan D, et al: Prevalence of persistent pain after endodontic treatment and factors affecting its occurrence in cases with complete radiographic healing, *Int Endod J* 38:169, 2005.

177. Qudeimat MA, Barrieshi-Nusair KM, Owais AI: Calcium hydroxide vs mineral trioxide aggregates for partial pulpotomy of permanent molars with deep caries, *Eur Arch Paediatr Dent* 8:99, 2007.

178. Reeh ES, Messer HH, Douglas WH: Reduction in tooth stiffness as a result of endodontic and restorative procedures, *J Endod* 15:512, 1989.

179. Reit C, Dahlen G: Decision making analysis of endodontic treatment strategies in teeth with apical periodontitis, *Int Endod J* 21:291, 1988.

180. Reit C, Grondahl HG: Endodontic retreatment decision making among a group of general practitioners, *Scand J Dent Res* 96:112, 1988.

181. Reit C, Molander A, Dahlen G: The diagnostic accuracy of microbiologic root canal sampling and the influence of antimicrobial dressings, *Endod Dent Traumatol* 15:278, 1999.

182. Ricucci D, Russo J, Rutberg M, et al: A prospective cohort study of endodontic treatments of 1,369 root canals: results after 5 years, *Oral Surg Oral Med Oral Pathol Oral Radiol Endod* 112:825, 2011.

183. Rocas IN, Siqueira JF Jr, Del Aguila CA, et al: Polymorphism of the CD14 and TLR4 genes and post-treatment apical periodontitis, *J Endod* 40:168, 2014.

184. Rollison S, Barnett F, Stevens RH: Efficacy of bacterial removal from instrumented root canals in vitro related to instrumentation technique and size, *Oral Surg Oral Med Oral Pathol Oral Radiol Endod* 94:366, 2002.

185. Rosenthal S, Spangberg L, Safavi K: Chlorhexidine substantivity in root canal dentin, *Oral Surg Oral Med Oral Pathol Oral Radiol Endod* 98:488, 2004.

186. Rud J, Andreasen JO: A study of failures after endodontic surgery by radiographic, histologic and stereomicroscopic methods, *Int J Oral Surg* 1:311, 1972.

187. Russo MC, Holland R, de Souza V: Radiographic and histological evaluation of the treatment of inflamed dental pulps, *Int Endod J* 15:137, 1982.

188. Saini HR, Tewari S, Sangwan P, et al: Effect of different apical preparation sizes on outcome of primary endodontic treatment: a randomized controlled trial, *J Endod* 38:1309, 2012.

189. Salehrabi R, Rotstein I: Endodontic treatment outcomes in a large patient population in the USA: an epidemiological study, *J Endod* 30:846, 2004.

190. Salehrabi R, Rotstein I: Epidemiologic evaluation of the outcomes of orthograde endodontic retreatment, *J Endod* 36:790, 2010.

191. Salvi GE, Siegrist Guldener BE, Amstad T, et al: Clinical evaluation of root filled teeth restored with or without post-and-core systems in a specialist practice setting, *Int Endod J* 40:209, 2007.

192. Santini A: Assessment of the pulpotomy technique in human first permanent mandibular molars. Use of two direct inspection criteria, *Br Dent J* 155:151, 1983.

193. Santucci PJ: Dycal versus Nd:YAG laser and Vitrebond for direct pulp capping in permanent teeth, *J Clin Laser Med Surg* 17:69, 1999.

194. Sari S, Okte Z: Success rate of Sealapex in root canal treatment for primary teeth: 3-year follow-up, *Oral Surg Oral Med Oral Pathol Oral Radiol Endod* 105:e93, 2008.

195. Sathorn C, Parashos P, Messer H: Antibacterial efficacy of calcium hydroxide intracanal dressing: a systematic review and meta-analysis, *Int Endod J* 40:2, 2007.

196. Saunders WP, Saunders EM: Coronal leakage as a cause of failure in root-canal therapy: a review, *Endod Dent Traumatol* 10:105, 1994.

197. Scarfe W: Use of cone-beam computed tomography in endodontics Joint Position Statement of the American Association of Endodontists and the American Academy of Oral and Maxillofacial Radiology, *Oral Surgery Oral Medicine Oral Pathology Oral Radiol Endodontol* 111:234, 2011.

198. Schafer E, Bossmann K: Antimicrobial efficacy of chlorhexidine and two calcium hydroxide formulations against *Enterococcus faecalis*, *J Endod* 31:53, 2005.

199. Schilder H: Cleaning and shaping the root canal, *Dent Clin North Am* 18:269, 1974.

200. Schwendicke F, Stolpe M, Meyer-Lueckel H, et al: Cost-effectiveness of one- and two-step incomplete and complete excavations, *J Dent Res* 92:880, 2013.

201. Seltzer S, Bender IB, Turkenkopf S: Factors affecting successful repair after root canal therapy, *J Am Dent Assoc* 67:651, 1963.

202. Seltzer S, Naidorf IJ: Flare-ups in endodontics: I. Etiological factors, *J Endod* 11:472, 1985.

203. Seltzer S, Naidorf IJ: Flare-ups in endodontics: II. Therapeutic measures, *J Endod* 11:559, 1985.

204. Setzer FC, Kohli MR, Shah SB, et al: Outcome of endodontic surgery: A meta-analysis of the literature. Part 2: Comparison of endodontic microsurgical techniques with and without the use of higher magnification, *J Endod* 38:1, 2012.

205. Setzer FC, Shah SB, Kohli MR, et al: Outcome of endodontic surgery: a meta-analysis of the literature. Part 1: Comparison of traditional root-end surgery and endodontic microsurgery, *J Endod* 36:17575, 2010.

206. Shovelton D: The presence and distribution of microorganisms within non-vital teeth, *Br Dent J* 117:101, 1964.

207. Shovelton DS, Friend LA, Kirk EE, Rowe AH: The efficacy of pulp capping materials: a comparative trial, *Br Dent J* 130:385, 1971.

208. Shuping GB, Orstavik D, Sigurdsson A, Trope M: Reduction of intracanal bacteria using nickel-titanium rotary instrumentation and various medications, *J Endod* 26:751, 2000.

209. Siqueira JF Jr, Guimaraes-Pinto T, Rocas IN: Effects of chemomechanical preparation with 2.5% sodium hypochlorite and intracanal medication with calcium hydroxide on cultivable bacteria in infected root canals, *J Endod* 33:800, 2007.

210. Siqueira JF Jr, Magalhaes KM, Rocas IN: Bacterial reduction in infected root canals treated with 2.5% NaOCl as an irrigant and calcium hydroxide/camphorated paramonochlorophenol paste as an intracanal dressing, *J Endod* 33:667, 2007.

211. Siqueira JF Jr, Rocas IN, Paiva SS, et al: Bacteriologic investigation of the effects of sodium hypochlorite and chlorhexidine during the endodontic treatment of teeth with apical periodontitis, *Oral Surg Oral Med Oral Pathol Oral Radiol Endod* 104:122, 2007.

212. Siqueira JF Jr, Rocas IN, Provenzano JC, et al: Relationship between Fcgamma receptor and interleukin-1 gene polymorphisms and post-treatment apical periodontitis, *J Endod* 35:11862, 2009.

213. Siqueira JF Jr, Rocas IN, Provenzano JC, Guilherme BP: Polymorphism of the FcgammaRIIIa gene and post-treatment apical periodontitis, *J Endod* 37:13458, 2011.

214. Sjogren U, Figdor D, Persson S, Sundqvist G: Influence of infection at the time of root filling on the outcome of endodontic treatment of teeth with apical periodontitis, *Int Endod J* 30:297, 1997.

215. Sjogren U, Figdor D, Spangberg L, Sundqvist G: The antimicrobial effect of calcium hydroxide as a short-term intracanal dressing, *Int Endod J* 24:119, 1991.

216. Sjogren U, Hagglund B, Sundqvist G, Wing K: Factors affecting the long-term results of endodontic treatment, *J Endod* 16:498, 1990.

217. Sjogren U, Sundqvist G: Bacteriologic evaluation of ultrasonic root canal instrumentation, *Oral Surg Oral Med Oral Pathol* 63:366, 1987.

218. Sjogren U, Sundqvist G, Nair PN: Tissue reaction to gutta-percha particles of various sizes when implanted subcutaneously in guinea pigs, *Eur J Oral Sci* 103:313, 1995.

219. Slade GD: Derivation and validation of a short-form oral health impact profile, *Community Dent Oral Epidemiol* 25:284, 1997.

220. Smith CS, Setchell DJ, Harty FJ: Factors influencing the success of conventional root canal therapy—a five-year retrospective study, *Int Endod J* 26:321, 1993.

221. Sogur E, Baksi BG, Grondahl HG, et al: Detectability of chemically induced periapical lesions by limited cone beam computed tomography, intra-oral digital and conventional film radiography, *Dentomaxillofac Radiol* 38:458, 2009.

222. Song M, Kim SG, Lee SJ, et al: Prognostic factors of clinical outcomes in endodontic microsurgery: a prospective study, *J Endod* 39:14917, 2013.

223. Souza RA, Dantas JC, Brandao PM, et al: Apical third enlargement of the root canal and its relationship with the repair of periapical lesions, *Eur J Dent* 6:385, 2012.

224. Spangberg LS: Evidence-based endodontics: the one-visit treatment idea, *Oral Surg Oral Med Oral Pathol Oral Radiol Endod* 91:617, 2001.

225. Spili P, Parashos P, Messer HH: The impact of instrument fracture on outcome of endodontic treatment, *J Endod* 31:845, 2005.

226. Stavropoulos A, Wenzel A: Accuracy of cone beam dental CT, intraoral digital and conventional film radiography for the detection of periapical lesions: an ex vivo study in pig jaws, *Clin Oral Investig* 11:101, 2007.

227. Stewart GG, Cobe H, Rappaport H: Study of new medicament in chemomechanical preparation of infected root canals, *J Am Dent Assoc* 63:33, 1961.

228. Stoll R, Betke K, Stachniss V: The influence of different factors on the survival of root canal fillings: a 10-year retrospective study, *J Endod* 31:783, 2005.

229. Strindberg LZ: The dependence of the results of pulp therapy on certain factors: an analytic study based on radiographic and clinical follow-up examinations, *Mauritzon*, 1956.

230. Sundqvist G: *Bacteriological studies of necrotic dental pulps*, Sweden, 1976, University of Umeå.

231. Sundqvist G, Figdor D, Persson S, Sjogren U: Microbiologic analysis of teeth with failed endodontic treatment and the outcome of conservative re-treatment, *Oral Surg Oral Med Oral Pathol Oral Radiol Endod* 85:86, 1998.

232. Taschieri S, Corbella S, Tsesis I, et al: Effect of guided tissue regeneration on the outcome of surgical endodontic treatment of through-and-through lesions: a retrospective study at 4-year follow-up, *Oral Maxillofac Surg* 15:153, 2011.

233. Taschieri S, Del Fabbro M, Testori T, et al: Efficacy of guided tissue regeneration in the management of through-and-through lesions following surgical endodontics: a preliminary study, *Int J Periodontics Restorative Dent* 28:265, 2008.

234. Taschieri S, Del Fabbro M, Testori T, Weinstein R: Efficacy of xenogeneic bone grafting with guided tissue regeneration in the management of bone defects after surgical endodontics, *J Oral Maxillofac Surg* 65:11217, 2007.

235. Teixeira LS, Demarco FF, Coppola MC, Bonow ML: Clinical and radiographic evaluation of pulpotomies performed under intrapulpal injection of anaesthetic solution, *Int Endod J* 34:440, 2001.

236. Tickle M, Milsom K, Qualtrough A, et al: The failure rate of NHS funded molar endodontic treatment delivered in general dental practice, *Br Dent J* 204:E8; discussion 254, 2008.

237. Tobón SI, Arismendi JA, Marín ML, et al: Comparison between a conventional technique and two bone regeneration techniques in periradicular surgery, *Int Endod J* 35:635, 2002.

238. Torabinejad M, Goodacre CJ: Endodontic or dental implant therapy, *J Amer Dent Assoc* 137:973, 2006.

239. Tsesis I, Rosen E, Tamse A, et al: Effect of guided tissue regeneration on the outcome of surgical endodontic treatment: a systematic review and meta-analysis, *J Endod* 37:10395, 2011.

240. Tsesis I, Rosen E, Taschieri S, et al: Outcomes of surgical endodontic treatment performed by a modern technique: an updated meta-analysis of the literature, *J Endod* 39:332, 2013.

241. Tsesis I, Taivishevsky V, Kfir A, Rosen E: Outcome of surgical endodontic treatment performed by a modern technique: a meta-analysis of literature, *J Endod* 35:1505, 2009.

242. Tuna D, Olmez A: Clinical long-term evaluation of MTA as a direct pulp capping material in primary teeth, *Int Endod J* 41:273, 2008.

243. Tyndall DA, Kapa SF, Bagnell CP: Digital subtraction radiography for detecting cortical and cancellous bone changes in the periapical region, *J Endod* 16:173, 1990.

244. Van Nieuwenhuysen JP, Aouar M, D'Hoore W: Retreatment or radiographic monitoring in endodontics, *Int Endod J* 27:75, 1994.

245. Velvart P: Papilla base incision: a new approach to recession-free healing of the interdental papilla after endodontic surgery, *Int Endod J* 35:453, 2002.

246. Velvart P, Ebner-Zimmermann U, Ebner JP: Comparison of papilla healing following sulcular full-thickness flap and papilla base flap in endodontic surgery, *Int Endod J* 36:653, 2003.

247. Velvart P, Ebner-Zimmermann U, Ebner JP: Comparison of long-term papilla healing following sulcular full thickness flap and papilla base flap in endodontic surgery, *Int Endod J* 37:687, 2004.

248. Vianna ME, Horz HP, Conrads G, et al: Effect of root canal procedures on endotoxins and endodontic pathogens, *Oral Microbiol Immunol* 22:411, 2007.

249. Villa-Machado PA, Botero-Ramírez X, Tobón-Arroyave SI: Retrospective follow-up assessment of prognostic variables associated with the outcome of periradicular surgery, *Int Endod J* 46:1063, 2013.

250. Von Arx T, Peñarrocha M, Jensen S: Prognostic factors in apical surgery with root-end filling: A meta-analysis, *J Endod* 36:957, 2010.

251. Waly NG: A five-year comparative study of calcium hydroxide-glutaraldehyde pulpotomies versus calcium hydroxide pulpotomies in young permanent molars, *Egypt Dent J* 41:993, 1995.

252. Wang CS, Arnold RR, Trope M, Teixeira FB: Clinical efficiency of 2% chlorhexidine gel in reducing intracanal bacteria, *J Endod* 33:1283, 2007.

253. Wang Q, Cheung GS, Ng RP: Survival of surgical endodontic treatment performed in a dental teaching hospital: a cohort study, *Int Endod J* 37:764, 2004.

254. Weiss M: Pulp capping in older patients, *N Y State Dent J* 32:451, 1966.

255. Witherspoon DE, Small JC, Harris GZ: Mineral trioxide aggregate pulpotomies: a case series outcomes assessment, *J Am Dent Assoc* 137:610, 2006.

256. Wu MK, Shemesh H, Wesselink PR: Limitations of previously published systematic reviews evaluating the outcome of endodontic treatment, *Int Endod J* 42:656, 2009.

257. Xavier AC, Martinho FC, Chung A, et al: One-visit versus two-visit root canal treatment: effectiveness in the removal of endotoxins and cultivable bacteria, *J Endod* 39:959, 2013.

258. Yared GM, Dagher FE: Influence of apical enlargement on bacterial infection during treatment of apical periodontitis, *J Endod* 20:535, 1994.

259. Yoshioka T, Kobayashi C, Suda H, Sasaki T: An observation of the healing process of periapical lesions by digital subtraction radiography, *J Endod* 28:589, 2002.

260. Yusuf H: The significance of the presence of foreign material periapically as a cause of failure of root treatment, *Oral Surg Oral Med Oral Pathol* 54:566, 1982.

261. Zehnder M: Root canal irrigants, *J Endod* 32:389, 2006.

FIGURE AND TABLE REFERENCES

Adenubi JO, Rule DC: Success rate for root fillings in young patients: a retrospective analysis of treated cases, *Br Dent J* 141:237, 1976.

Akerblom A, Hasselgren G: The prognosis for endodontic treatment of obliterated root canals, *J Endod* 14:565, 1988.

Akpata ES: Effect of endodontic procedures on the population of viable microorganisms in the infected root canal, *J Endod* 2:369, 1976.

Allen RK, Newton CW, Brown CE Jr: A statistical analysis of surgical and nonsurgical endodontic retreatment cases, *J Endod* 15:261, 1989.

Alley BS, Kitchens GG, Alley LW, Eleazer PD: A comparison of survival of teeth following endodontic treatment performed by general dentists or by specialists, *Oral Surg Oral Med Oral Pathol Oral Radiol Endod* 98:115, 2004.

Amagasa T, Nagase M, Sato T, Shioda S: Apicoectomy with retrograde gutta-percha root filling, *Oral Surg Oral Med Oral Pathol* 68:339, 1989.

American Academy of Pediatric Dentistry 2014 Pulp Therapy Subcommittee, Clinical Affairs Committee: *American Academy of Pediatric Dentistry (AAPD) guideline on pulp therapy for primary and immature permanent teeth reference manual*, vol 36, no 6, Chicago, 2014, AAPD, p. 242, www.aapd.org/media/Policies_Guidelines/G_Pulp.pdf. Accessed April 19, 2015.

Appleton JLT: A note on the clinical value of bacteriologically controlling the treatment of periapical infection, *Dental Cosmos* 74:798, 1932.

Aqrabawi J: Management of endodontic failures: case selection and treatment modalities, *Gen Dent* 53:63, 2005.

Aqrabawi JA: Outcome of endodontic treatment of teeth filled using lateral condensation versus vertical compaction (Schilder's technique), *J Contemp Dent Pract* 7:17, 2006.

Aquilino SA, Caplan DJ: Relationship between crown placement and the survival of endodontically treated teeth, *J Prosthet Dent* 87:256, 2002.

Asgary S, Ehsani S: Permanent molar pulpotomy with a new endodontic cement: A case series, *J Conserv Dent* 12:31, 2009.

Auerbach M: Antibiotics vs. instrumentation in endodontics, *N Y State Dent J* 19:225, 1953.

Auerbach MB: Clinical approach to the problem of pulp canal therapy, *J Am Dent Assoc* 25:939, 1938.

Baratieri LN, Monteiro S Jr, Caldeira de Andrada MA: Pulp curettage: surgical technique, *Quintessence Int* 20:285, 1989.

Barbakow FH, Cleaton-Jones P, Friedman D: An evaluation of 566 cases of root canal therapy in general dental practice. 2. Postoperative observations, *J Endod* 6:485, 1980.

Barone C, Dao TT, Basrani BB, et al: Treatment outcome in endodontics: the Toronto study—phases 3, 4, and 5: apical surgery, *J Endod* 36:28, 2010.

Barrieshi-Nusair KM, Qudeimat MA: A prospective clinical study of mineral trioxide aggregate for partial pulpotomy in cariously exposed permanent teeth, *J Endod* 32:731, 2006.

Barthel CR, Rosenkranz B, Leuenberg A, Roulet JF: Pulp capping of carious exposures: treatment outcome after 5 and 10 years: a retrospective study, *J Endod* 26:525, 2000.

Bence R, Madonia JV, Weine FS, Smulson MH: A microbiologic evaluation of endodontic instrumentation in pulpless teeth, *Oral Surg Oral Med Oral Pathol* 35:676, 1973.

Bender IB, Seltzer S, Soltanof W: Endodontic success: a reappraisal of criteria 1, *Oral Surg Oral Med Oral Pathol Oral Radiol Endod* 22:780, 1966.

Bender IB, Seltzer S, Soltanof W: Endodontic success: a reappraisal of criteria 2, *Oral Surg Oral Med Oral Pathol Oral Radiol Endod* 22:790, 1966.

Bender IB, Seltzer S, Turkenkopf S: To culture or not to culture? *Oral Surg Oral Med Oral Pathol* 18:527, 1964.

Benenati FW, Khajotia SS: A radiographic recall evaluation of 894 endodontic cases treated in a dental school setting, *J Endod* 28:391, 2002.

Bergenholtz G, Lekholm U, Milthon R, Engstrom B: Influence of apical overinstrumentation and overfilling on re-treated root canals, *J Endod* 5:310, 1979.

Bjorndal L, Reit C, Bruun G, et al: Treatment of deep caries lesions in adults: randomized clinical trials comparing stepwise vs. direct complete excavation, and direct pulp capping vs. partial pulpotomy, *Eur J Oral Sci* 118:290, 2010.

Bjorndal L, Thylstrup A: A practice-based study on stepwise excavation of deep carious lesions in permanent teeth: a 1-year follow-up study, *Community Dent Oral Epidemiol* 26:122, 1998.

Blayney JR: The clinical results of pulp treatment, *J Natl Dent Assoc* 9:198, 1922.

Bogen G, Kim JS, Bakland LK: Direct pulp capping with mineral trioxide aggregate: an observational study, *J Am Dent Assoc* 139:305; quiz 305, 2008.

Boggia R: A single-visit treatment of septic root canals using periapically extruded endomethasone, *Br Dent J* 155:300, 1983.

Buchbinder M: A statistical comparison of cultured and non-cultured root canal cases, *J Dent Res* 20:93, 1941.

Bystrom A, Claesson R, Sundqvist G: The antibacterial effect of camphorated paramonochlorophenol, camphorated phenol and calcium hydroxide in the treatment of infected root canals, *Endod Dent Traumatol* 1:170, 1985.

Bystrom A, Happonen RP, Sjogren U, Sundqvist G: Healing of periapical lesions of pulpless teeth after endodontic treatment with controlled asepsis, *Endod Dent Traumatol* 3:58, 1987.

Bystrom A, Sundqvist G: Bacteriologic evaluation of the efficacy of mechanical root canal instrumentation in endodontic therapy, *Scand J Dent Res* 89:321, 1981.

Bystrom A, Sundqvist G: Bacteriologic evaluation of the effect of 0.5 percent sodium hypochlorite in endodontic therapy, *Oral Surg Oral Med Oral Pathol* 55:307, 1983.

Bystrom A, Sundqvist G: The antibacterial action of sodium hypochlorite and EDTA in 60 cases of endodontic therapy, *Int Endod J* 18:35, 1985.

Caliskan MK: Success of pulpotomy in the management of hyperplastic pulpitis, *Int Endod J* 26:142, 1993.

Caliskan MK: Pulpotomy of carious vital teeth with periapical involvement, *Int Endod J* 28:172, 1995.

Çaliskan MK: Nonsurgical retreatment of teeth with periapical lesions previously managed by either endodontic or surgical intervention, *Oral Surg Oral Med Oral Pathol Oral Radiol Endod* 100:242, 2005.

Çaliskan MK, Şen BH: Endodontic treatment of teeth with apical periodontitis using calcium hydroxide: a long-term study, *Endod Dent Traumatol* 12:215, 1996.

Caplan DJ, Cai J, Yin G, White BA: Root canal filled versus non-root canal filled teeth: a retrospective comparison of survival times, *J Public Health Dent* 65:90, 2005.

Caplan DJ, Kolker J, Rivera EM, Walton RE: Relationship between number of proximal contacts and survival of root canal treated teeth, *Int Endod J* 35:193, 2002.

Card SJ, Sigurdsson A, Orstavik D, Trope M: The effectiveness of increased apical enlargement in reducing intracanal bacteria, *J Endod* 28:779, 2002.

Castagnola L, Orlay HG: Treatment of gangrene of the pulp by the Walkhoff method, *Br Dent J* 19:93, 1952.

Chen SC, Chueh LH, Hsiao CK, et al: An epidemiologic study of tooth retention after nonsurgical endodontic treatment in a large population in Taiwan, *J Endod* 33:226, 2007.

Chen S-C, Chueb L-H, Hsiao CK, et al: First untoward events and reasons for tooth extraction after nonsurgical endodontic treatment in Taiwan, *J Endod* 34:671, 2008.

Cheung GS: Survival of first-time nonsurgical root canal treatment performed in a dental teaching hospital, *Oral Surg Oral Med Oral Pathol Oral Radiol Endod* 93:596, 2002.

Cheung GS, Chan TK: Long-term survival of primary root canal treatment carried out in a dental teaching hospital, *Int Endod J* 36:117, 2003.

Chong BS, Pitt Ford TR, Hudson MB: A prospective clinical study of Mineral Trioxide Aggregate and IRM when used as root-end filling materials in endodontic surgery, *Int Endod J* 36:520, 2003.

Christiansen R, Kirkevang LL, Horsted-Bindslev P, Wenzel A: Randomized clinical trial of root-end resection followed by root-end filling with mineral trioxide aggregate or smoothing of the orthograde gutta-percha root filling—1-year follow-up, *Int Endod J* 42:105, 2009.

Chu FC, Leung WK, Tsang PC, et al: Identification of cultivable microorganisms from root canals with apical periodontitis following two-visit endodontic treatment with antibiotics/steroid or calcium hydroxide dressings, *J Endod* 32:17, 2006.

Chu FC, Tsang CS, Chow TW, Samaranayake LP: Identification of cultivable microorganisms from primary endodontic infections with exposed and unexposed pulp space, *J Endod* 31:424, 2005.

Chugal NM, Clive JM, Spångberg LSW: A prognostic model for assessment of the outcome of endodontic treatment: effect of biologic and diagnostic variables, *Oral Surg Oral Med Oral Pathol Oral Radiol Endod* 91:342, 2001.

Chugal NM, Clive JM, Spångberg LS: Endodontic infection: some biologic and treatment factors associated with outcome, *Oral Surg Oral Med Oral Pathol Oral Radiol Endod* 96:81, 2003.

Conner DA, Caplan DJ, Teixeira FB, Trope M: Clinical outcome of teeth treated endodontically with a nonstandardized protocol and root filled with resilon, *J Endod* 33:1290, 2007.

Cotton TP, Schindler WG, Schwartz SA, et al: A retrospective study comparing clinical outcomes after obturation with Resilon/Epiphany or Gutta-Percha/Kerr sealer, *J Endod* 34:789, 2008.

Cvek M: Treatment of non-vital permanent incisors with calcium hydroxide, *Odontol Revy* 23:27, 1972.

Cvek M: A clinical report on partial pulpotomy and capping with calcium hydroxide in permanent incisors with complicated crown fracture, *J Endod* 4:232, 1978.

Cvek M: Prognosis of luxated non-vital maxillary incisors treated with calcium hydroxide and filled with gutta-percha: a retrospective clinical study, *Endod Dent Traumatol* 8:45, 1992.

Cvek M, Granath L, Lundberg M: Failures and healing in endodontically treated non-vital anterior teeth with posttraumatically reduced pulpal lumen, *Acta Odontol Scandi* 40:223, 1982.

Cvek M, Hollender L, Nord CE: Treatment of non-vital permanent incisors with calcium hydroxide. VI: A clinical, microbiological and radiological evaluation of treatment in one sitting of teeth with mature or immature root, *Odontol Revy* 27:93, 1976.

Dalton BC, Orstavik D, Phillips C, et al: Bacterial reduction with nickel-titanium rotary instrumentation, *J Endod* 24:763, 1998.

Dammaschke T, Steven D, Kaup M, Ott KH: Long-term survival of root-canal-treated teeth: a retrospective study over 10 years, *J Endod* 29:638, 2003.

Danin J, Strömberg T, Forsgren H, et al: Clinical management of nonhealing periradicular pathosis: surgery versus endodontic retreatment, *Oral Surg Oral Med Oral Pathol Oral Radiol Endod* 82:213, 1996.

de Chevigny C, Dao TT, Basrani BR, et al: Treatment outcome in endodontics: the Toronto study–phase 4: initial treatment, *J Endod* 34:258, 2008.

de Lange J, Putters T, Baas EM, van Ingen JM: Ultrasonic root-end preparation in apical surgery: a prospective randomized study, *Oral Surg Oral Med Oral Pathol Oral Radiol Endod* 104:841, 2007.

DeRosa TA: A retrospective evaluation of pulpotomy as an alternative to extraction, *Gen Dent* 54:37, 2006.

Deutsch AS, Musikant BL, Cohen BI, Kase D: A study of one visit treatment using EZ-Fill root canal sealer, *Endod Prac* 4:29, 2001.

Dominiak M, Lysiak-Drwal K, Gedrange T, et al: Efficacy of healing process of bone defects after apicectomy: results after 6 and 12 months, *J Physiol Pharmacol* 60 (suppl 8):51, 2009.

Dorn SO, Gartner AH: Retrograde filling materials: a retrospective success-failure study of amalgam, EBA, and IRM, *J Endod* 16:391, 1990.

Doyle SL, Hodges JS, Pesun IJ, et al: Retrospective cross sectional comparison of initial nonsurgical endodontic treatment and single-tooth implants, *J Endod* 32:822, 2006.

Dugas NN, Lawrence HP, Teplitsky P, Friedman S: Quality of life and satisfaction outcomes of endodontic treatment, *J Endod* 28:819, 2002.

El-Meligy OA, Avery DR: Comparison of mineral trioxide aggregate and calcium hydroxide as pulpotomy agents in young permanent teeth (apexogenesis), *Pediatr Dent* 28:399, 2006.

Engström B: The significance of enterococci in root canal treatment, *Odontol Revy* 15:87, 1964.

Engström B, Lundberg M: The correlation between positive culture and the prognosis of root canal therapy after pulpectomy, *Odontol Revy* 16:193, 1965.

Engström B, Segerstad LHA, Ramstrom G, Frostell G: Correlation of positive cultures with the prognosis for root canal treatment, *Odontol Revy* 15:257, 1964.

European Society of Endodontology: Quality guidelines for endodontic treatment: consensus report of the European Society of Endodontology, *Int Endod J* 39:921, 2006.

Farsi N, Alamoudi N, Balto K, Al Mushayt A: Clinical assessment of mineral trioxide aggregate (MTA) as direct pulp capping in young permanent teeth, *J Clin Pediatr Dent* 31:72, 2006.

Ferrari M, Vichi A, Fadda GM, et al: A randomized controlled trial of endodontically treated and restored premolars, *J Dent Res* 91:72S, 2012.

Field JW, Gutmann JL, Solomon ES, Rakusin H: A clinical radiographic retrospective assessment of the success rate of single-visit root canal treatment, *Int Endod J* 37:70, 2004.

Finne K, Nord PG, Persson G, Lennartsson B: Retrograde root filling with amalgam and cavit, *Oral Surg Oral Med Oral Pathol* 43:621, 1977.

Fitzgerald M, Heys RJ: A clinical and histological evaluation of conservative pulpal therapy in human teeth, *Oper Dent* 16:101, 1991.

Fleming CH, Litaker MS, Alley LW, Eleazer PD: Comparison of classic endodontic techniques versus contemporary techniques on endodontic treatment success, *J Endod* 36:414, 2010.

Fonzar F, Fonzar A, Buttolo P, et al: The prognosis of root canal therapy: a 10-year retrospective cohort study on 411 patients with 1175 endodontically treated teeth, *Eur J Oral Implantol* 2:201, 2009.

Friedman S, Lost C, Zarrabian M, Trope M: Evaluation of success and failure after endodontic therapy using a glass ionomer cement sealer, *J Endod* 21:384, 1995.

Friedman S, Mor C: The success of endodontic therapy—healing and functionality, *J Calif Dent Assoc* 32:493, 2004.

Frostell G: Clinical significance of the root canal culture, *Transactions of 3rd Int Conferences of Endodontics* 112, 1963.

Fuks AB, Gavra S, Chosack A: Long-term followup of traumatized incisors treated by partial pulpotomy, *Pediatr Dent* 15:334, 1993.

Gagliani MM, Gorni FG, Strohmenger L: Periapical resurgery versus periapical surgery: a 5-year longitudinal comparison, *Int Endod J* 2005 38:320.

Gallien GS Jr, Schuman NJ: Local versus general anesthesia: a study of pulpal response in the treatment of cariously exposed teeth, *J Am Dent Assoc* 111:599, 1985.

Garcia B, Penarrocha M, Martí E, et al: Periapical surgery in maxillary premolars and molars: Analysis in terms of the distance between the lesion and the maxillary sinus, *J Oral Maxillofac Surg* 66:1212, 2008.

García-Mira B, Ortega-Sánchez B, Peñarrocha-Diago M, Peñarrocha-Diago M: Ostectomy versus osteotomy with repositioning of the vestibular cortical in periapical surgery of mandibular molars: a preliminary study, *Medicina Oral, Patología Oral y Cirugía Bucal* 15:e628, 2010.

Gesi A, Hakeberg M, Warfvinge J, Bergenholtz G: Incidence of periapical lesions and clinical symptoms after pulpectomy—a clinical and radiographic evaluation of 1- versus 2-session treatment, *Oral Surg Oral Med Oral Pathol Oral Radiol Endod* 101:379, 2006.

Gomes BP, Lilley JD, Drucker DB: Variations in the susceptibilities of components of the endodontic microflora to biomechanical procedures, *Int Endod J* 29:235, 1996.

Gorni FGM, Gagliani MM: The outcome of endodontic retreatment: a 2-yr follow-up, *J Endod* 30:1, 2004.

Goyal B, Tewari S, Duhan J, Sehgal PK: Comparative evaluation of platelet-rich plasma and guided tissue regeneration membrane in the healing of apicomarginal defects: a clinical study, *J Endod* 37:773, 2011.

Grahnén H, Hansson L: The prognosis of pulp and root canal therapy, *Odontol Revy* 12:146, 1961.

Grahnen H, Krasse B: The effect of instrumentation and flushing of non-vital teeth in endodontic therapy, *Odontol Rev* 14:167, 1963.

Grung B, Molven O, Halse A: Periapical surgery in a Norwegian county hospital: Follow-up findings of 477 teeth, *J Endod* 16:411, 1990.

Gruythuysen RJ, van Strijp AJ, Wu MK: Long-term survival of indirect pulp treatment performed in primary and permanent teeth with clinically diagnosed deep carious lesions, *J Endod* 36:1490, 2010.

Halse A, Molven O: Overextended gutta-percha and Kloroperka N-Ø root canal fillings: radiographic findings after 10–17 years, *Acta Odontol Scandi* 45:171, 1987.

Harty FJ, Parkins BJ, Wengraf AM: Success rate in root canal therapy: a retrospective study on conventional cases, *Br Dent J* 128:65, 1970.

Haskell EW, Stanley HR, Chellemi J, Stringfellow H: Direct pulp capping treatment: a long-term follow-up, *J Am Dent Assoc* 97:607, 1978.

Hayashi M, Fujitani M, Yamaki C, Momoi Y: Ways of enhancing pulp preservation by stepwise excavation—a systematic review, *J Dent* 39:95, 2011.

Heling B, Kischinovsky D: Factors affecting successful endodontic therapy, *J Br Endod Soc* 12:83, 1979.

Heling B, Shapira J: Roentgenologic and clinical evaluation of endodontically treated teeth, with or without negative culture, *Quintessence Int* 11:79, 1978.

Heling B, Tamshe A: Evaluation of the success of endodontically treated teeth, *Oral Surg Oral Med Oral Pathol* 30:533, 1970.

Heling I, Bialla-Shenkman S, Turetzky A, et al: The outcome of teeth with periapical periodontitis treated with nonsurgical endodontic treatment: a computerized morphometric study, *Quintessence Int* 32:397, 2001.

Hilton TJ, Ferracane JL, Mancl L, Northwest Practice-based Research Collaborative in Evidence-based Dentistry (NWP):

Comparison of CaOH with MTA for direct pulp capping: a PBRN randomized clinical trial, *J Dent Res* 92:16S, 2013.

Hirsch J-M, Ahlström U, Henrikson P-Å, et al: Periapical surgery, *Int J Oral Surg* 8:173, 1979.

Horsted P, Sandergaard B, Thylstrup A, et al: A retrospective study of direct pulp capping with calcium hydroxide compounds, *Endod Dent Traumatol* 1:29, 1985.

Hoskinson SE, Ng YL, Hoskinson AE, et al: A retrospective comparison of outcome of root canal treatment using two different protocols, *Oral Surg Oral Med Oral Pathol Oral Radiol Endod* 93:705, 2002.

Hsiao A, Glickman G, He J: A retrospective clinical and radiographic study on healing of periradicular lesions in patients taking oral bisphosphonates, *J Endod* 35:1525, 2009.

Huumonen S, Lenander-Lumikari M, Sigurdsson A, Orstavik D: Healing of apical periodontitis after endodontic treatment: a comparison between a silicone-based and a zinc oxide-eugenol-based sealer, *Int Endod J* 36:296, 2003.

Ingle J, Zeldow B: An evaluation of mechanical instrumentation and the negative culture in endodontic therapy, *J Am Dent Assoc* (1939) 57:471, 1958.

Ioannides C, Borstlap WA: Apicoectomy on molars: a clinical and radiographical study, *Int J Oral Surg* 12:73, 1983.

Jansson L, Sandstedt P, Låftman A-C, Skoglund A: Relationship between apical and marginal healing in periradicular surgery, *Oral Surg Oral Med Oral Pathol Oral Radiol Endod* 83:596, 1997.

Jensen S, Nattestad A, Egdø P, et al: A prospective, randomized, comparative clinical study of resin composite and glass ionomer cement for retrograde root filling, *Clin Oral Investig* 6:236, 2002.

Jesslén P, Zetterqvist L, Heimdahl A: Long-term results of amalgam versus glass ionomer cement as apical sealant after apicectomy, *Oral Surg Oral Med Oral Pathol Oral Radiol Endod* 79:101, 1995.

Jokinen MA, Kotilainen R, Poikkeus P, et al: Clinical and radiographic study of pulpectomy and root canal therapy, *Scand J Dent Res* 86:366, 1978.

Jordan RE, Suzuki M: Conservative treatment of deep carious lesions, *J Can Dent Assoc* 37:337, 1971.

Jordan RE, Suzuki M, Skinner DH: Indirect pulp-capping of carious teeth with periapical lesions, *J Am Dent Assoc* 97:37, 1978.

Jurcak JJ, Bellizzi R, Loushine RJ: Successful single-visit endodontics during Operation Desert Shield, *J Endod* 19:412, 1993.

Kerekes K: Radiographic assessment of an endodontic treatment method, *J Endod* 4:210, 1978.

Khedmat S: Evaluation of endodontic treatment failure of teeth with periapical radiolucent areas and factors affecting it, *J Dent*, Tehran University of Medical Sciences 1:34, 2004.

Kim E, Song J-S, Jung I-Y, et al: Prospective clinical study evaluating endodontic microsurgery outcomes for cases with lesions of endodontic origin compared with cases with lesions of combined periodontal–endodontic origin, *J Endod* 34:546, 2008.

Klevant FJH, Eggink CO: The effect of canal preparation on periapical disease, *Int Endod J* 16:68, 1983.

Koontongkaew S, Silapichit R, Thaweboon B: Clinical and laboratory assessments of camphorated monochlorophenol in endodontic therapy, *Oral Surg Oral Med Oral Pathol* 65:757, 1988.

Kreisler M, Gockel R, Aubell-Falkenberg S, et al: Clinical outcome in periradicular surgery: effect of patient- and tooth-related factors—a multicenter study, *Quintessence Int* 44:53, 2013.

Kvist T, Molander A, Dahlen G, Reit C: Microbiological evaluation of one- and two-visit endodontic treatment of teeth with apical periodontitis: a randomized, clinical trial, *J Endod* 30:572, 2004.

Lana MA, Ribeiro-Sobrinho AP, Stehling R, et al: Microorganisms isolated from root canals presenting necrotic pulp and their drug susceptibility in vitro, *Oral Microbiol Immunol* 16:100, 2001.

Lazarski MP, Walker WA 3rd, Flores CM, et al: Epidemiological evaluation of the outcomes of nonsurgical root canal treatment in a large cohort of insured dental patients, *J Endod* 27:791, 2001.

Leco-Berrocal MI, Martinez Gonzalez JM, Donado Rodriguez M: Clinical and radiological course in apicoectomies with the Erbium:YAG laser, *Medicina Oral, Patología Oral y Cirugía Bucal* 12:E65, 2007.

Leksell E, Ridell K, Cvek M, Mejare I: Pulp exposure after stepwise versus direct complete excavation of deep carious lesions in young posterior permanent teeth, *Endod Dent Traumatol* 12:192, 1996.

Li H, Zhai F, Zhang R, Hou B: Evaluation of microsurgery with SuperEBA as root-end filling material for treating post-treatment endodontic disease: a 2-year retrospective study, *J Endod* 40:345, 2014.

Liang YH, Li G, Wesselink PR, Wu MK: Endodontic outcome predictors identified with periapical radiographs and cone-beam computed tomography scans, *J Endod* 37:326, 2011.

Liang YH, Yuan M, Li G, et al: The ability of cone-beam computed tomography to detect simulated buccal and lingual recesses in root canals, *Int Endod J* 45:724, 2012.

Lilly JP, Cox D, Arcuri M, Krell KV: An evaluation of root canal treatment in patients who have received irradiation to the mandible and maxilla, *Oral Surg Oral Med Oral Pathol Oral Radiol Endod* 86:224, 1998.

Lindeboom JAH, Frenken J, Kroon FHM, van den Akker HP: A comparative prospective randomized clinical study of MTA and IRM as root-end filling materials in single-rooted teeth in endodontic surgery, *Oral Surg Oral Med Oral Pathol Oral Radiol Endod* 100:495, 2005.

Lumley PJ, Lucarotti PS, Burke FJ: Ten-year outcome of root fillings in the General Dental Services in England and Wales, *Int Endod J* 41:577, 2008.

Lustmann J, Friedman S, Shaharabany V: Relation of pre- and intraoperative factors to prognosis of posterior apical surgery, *J Endod* 17:239, 1991.

Lynch CD, Burke FM, Ní Ríordáin R, Hannigan A: The influence of coronal restoration type on the survival of endodontically treated teeth, *Eur J Prosthodont Restor Dent* 12:171, 2004.

Mackie IC, Worthington HV, Hill FJ: A follow-up study of incisor teeth which had been treated by apical closure and root filling, *Br Dent J* 175:99, 1993.

Maddalone M, Gagliani M: Periapical endodontic surgery: a 3-year follow-up study, *Int Endod J* 36:193, 2003.

Maltz M, Alves LS, Jardim JJ, et al: Incomplete caries removal in deep lesions: a 10-year prospective study, *Am J Dent* 24:211, 2011.

Maltz M, Garcia R, Jardim JJ, et al: Randomized trial of partial vs. stepwise caries removal: 3-year follow-up, *J Dent Res* 91:1026, 2012.

Maltz M, Henz SL, de Oliveira EF, Jardim JJ: Conventional caries removal and sealed caries in permanent teeth: a microbiological evaluation, *J Dent* 40:776, 2012.

Marín-Botero ML, Domínguez-Mejía JS, Arismendi-Echavarría JA, et al: Healing response of apicomarginal defects to two guided tissue regeneration techniques in periradicular surgery: A double-blind, randomized-clinical trial, *Int Endod J* 39:368, 2006.

Markvart M, Dahlén G, Reit CE, Bjørndal L: The antimicrobial effect of apical box versus apical cone preparation using iodine potassium iodide as root canal dressing: a pilot study, *Acta Odontol Scand* 71:786, 2013.

Marti-Bowen E, Penarrocha-Diago M, Garcia-Mira B: Periapical surgery using the ultrasound technique and silver amalgam retrograde filling. A study of 71 teeth with 100 canals, *Medicina Oral, Patología Oral y Cirugia Bucal* 10:E67, 2005.

Mass E, Zilberman U: Clinical and radiographic evaluation of partial pulpotomy in carious exposure of permanent molars, *Pediatr Dent* 15:257, 1993.

Masterton JB: The healing of wounds of the dental pulp: an investigation of the nature of the scar tissue and of the phenomena leading to its formation, *Dent Pract Dent Rec* 16:325, 1966.

Matsumoto T, Nagai T, Ida K, et al: Factors affecting successful prognosis of root canal treatment, *J Endod* 13:239, 1987.

Matsuo T, Nakanishi T, Shimizu H, Ebisu S: A clinical study of direct pulp capping applied to carious-exposed pulps, *J Endod* 22:551, 1996.

Mejare I, Cvek M: Partial pulpotomy in young permanent teeth with deep carious lesions, *Endod Dent Traumatol* 9:238, 1993.

Mente J, Geletneky B, Ohle M, et al: Mineral trioxide aggregate or calcium hydroxide direct pulp capping: an analysis of the clinical treatment outcome, *J Endod* 36:806, 2010.

Mente J, Hage N, Pfefferle T, et al: Mineral trioxide aggregate apical plugs in teeth with open apical foramina: a retrospective analysis of treatment outcome, *J Endod* 35:1354, 2009.

Miles JP, Gluskin AH, Chambers D, Peters OA: Pulp capping with mineral trioxide aggregate (MTA): a retrospective analysis of carious pulp exposures treated by undergraduate dental students, *Oper Dent* 35:20, 2010.

Molander A, Reit C, Dahlen G: Microbiological evaluation of clindamycin as a root canal dressing in teeth with apical periodontitis, *Int Endod J* 23:113, 1990.

Molander A, Warfvinge J, Reit C, Kvist T: Clinical and radiographic evaluation of one- and two-visit endodontic treatment of asymptomatic necrotic teeth with apical periodontitis: a randomized clinical trial, *J Endod* 33:1145, 2007.

Molven O, Halse A: Success rates for gutta-percha and Kloropercha N-Ø root fillings made by undergraduate students: radiographic findings after 10-17 years, *Int Endod J* 21:243, 1998.

Molven O, Halse A, Grung B: Observer strategy and the radiographic classification of healing after endodontic surgery, *Int J Oral Maxillofac Surg* 16:432, 1987.

Moore DL: Conservative treatment of teeth with vital pulps and periapical lesions: a preliminary report, *J Prosthet Dent* 18:476, 1967.

Morsani JM, Aminoshariae A, Han YW, et al: Genetic predisposition to persistent apical periodontitis, *J Endod* 37:455, 2011.

Morse DR, Esposito JV, Pike C, Furst ML: A radiographic evaluation of the periapical status of teeth treated by the gutta-percha-eucapercha endodontic method: a one-year follow-up study of 458 root canals. Part I, *Oral Surg Oral Med Oral Pathol* 55:607, 1983a.

Morse DR, Esposito JV, Pike C, Furst ML: radiographic evaluation of the periapical status of teeth treated by the gutta-percha-eucapercha endodontic method: a one-year follow-up study of 458 root canals. Part II, *Oral Surg Oral Med Oral Pathol* 56:89, 1983b.

Morse DR, Esposito JV, Pike C, Furst ML: A radiographic evaluation of the periapical status of teeth treated by the gutta-percha-eucapercha endodontic method: a one-year follow-up study of 458 root canals. Part III, *Oral Surg Oral Med Oral Pathol* 56:190, 1983c.

Morse F, Yates M: Follow up studies of root-filled teeth in relation to bacteriologic findings, *J Am Dent Assoc* 28:956, 1941.

Moshonov J, Slutzky-Goldberg I, Gottlieb A, Peretz B: The effect of the distance between post and residual gutta-percha on the clinical outcome of endodontic treatment, *J Endod* 31:177, 2005.

Murphy WK, Kaugars GE, Collett WK, Dodds RN: Healing of periapical radiolucencies after nonsurgical endodontic therapy, *Oral Surg Oral Med Oral Pathol* 71:620, 1991.

Nagamine M: Studies on treatment of deep caries lesions utilizing polycarboxylate cement combined with tanninfluoride preparation, *J Okayama Dent Soc* 12:1, 1993 [Japanese].

Nagasiri R, Chitmongkolsuk S: Long-term survival of endodontically treated molars without crown coverage: a retrospective cohort study, *J Prosthet Dent* 93:164, 2005.

Negishi J, Kawanami M, Ogami E: Risk analysis of failure of root canal treatment for teeth with inaccessible apical constriction, *J Dent* 33:399, 2005.

Nelson IA: Endodontics in general practice: a retrospective study, *Int Endod J* 15:168, 1982.

Ng YL, Mann V, Gulabivala K: A prospective study of the factors affecting outcomes of nonsurgical root canal treatment: part 1: periapical health, *Int Endod J* 44:583, 2011.

Ng YL, Mann V, Gulabivala K: A prospective study of the factors affecting outcomes of non-surgical root canal treatment: part 2: tooth survival, *Int Endod J* 44:610, 2011.

Nicholls E: The efficacy of cleansing of the root canal, *Br Dent J* 112:167, 1962.

Nordenram A: Biobond for retrograde root filling in apicoectomy, *Eur J Oral Sci* 78:251, 1970.

Olgart LG: Bacteriological sampling from root canals directly after chemo-mechanical treatment: a clinical and bacteriological study, *Acta Odontol Scand* 27:91, 1969.

Oliet S: Single-visit endodontics: a clinical study, *J Endod* 9:147, 1983.

Oliet S, Sorin SM: Evaluation of clinical results based upon culturing root canals, *J Br Endod Soc* 3:3, 1969.

Orstavik D: Time-course and risk analyses of the development and healing of chronic apical periodontitis in man, *Int Endod J* 29:150, 1996.

Orstavik D, Kerekes K, Molven O: Effects of extensive apical reaming and calcium hydroxide dressing on bacterial infection during treatment of apical periodontitis: a pilot study, *Int Endod J* 24:1, 1991.

Ortega-Sánchez B, Peñarrocha-Diago M, Rubio-Martínez LA, Vera-Sempere JF: Radiographic morphometric study of 37 periapical lesions in 30 patients: validation of success criteria, *J Oral Maxillofac Surg* 67:846, 2009.

Pantchev A, Nohlert E, Tegelberg A: Endodontic surgery with and without inserts of bioactive glass PerioGlas: a clinical and radiographic follow-up, *Oral Maxillofac Surg* 13:21, 2009.

Pantschev A, Carlsson AP, Andersson L: Retrograde root filling with EBA cement or amalgam: a comparative clinical study, *Oral Surg Oral Med Oral Pathol* 78:101, 1994.

Paquette L, Legner M, Fillery ED, Friedman S: Antibacterial efficacy of chlorhexidine gluconate intracanal medication in vivo, *J Endod* 33:788, 2007.

Peak JD: The success of endodontic treatment in general dental practice: a retrospective clinical and radiographic study, *Prim Dent Care* 1:9, 1994.

Peak JD, Hayes SJ, Bryant ST, Dummer PM: The outcome of root canal treatment. A retrospective study within the armed forces (Royal Air Force), *Br Dent J* 190:140, 2001.

Peciuliene V, Balciuniene I, Eriksen HM, Haapasalo M: Isolation of *Enterococcus faecalis* in previously root-filled canals in a Lithuanian population, *J Endod* 26:593, 2000.

Peciuliene V, Reynaud AH, Balciuniene I, Haapasalo M: Isolation of yeasts and enteric bacteria in root-filled teeth with chronic apical periodontitis, *Int Endod J* 34:429, 2001.

Pecora G, De Leonardis D, Ibrahim N, et al: The use of calcium sulphate in the surgical treatment of a 'through and through' periradicular lesion, *Int Endod J* 34:189, 2001.

Pekruhn RB: The incidence of failure following single-visit endodontic therapy, *J Endod* 12:68, 1986.

Peñarrocha M, Carrillo C, Peñarrocha M, et al: Symptoms before periapical surgery related to histologic diagnosis and postoperative healing at 12 months for 178 periapical lesions, *J Oral Maxillofac Surg* 69:e31, 2011.

Peñarrocha M, Martí E, García B, Gay C: Relationship of periapical lesion radiologic size, apical resection, and retrograde filling with the prognosis of periapical surgery, *J Maxillofac Oral Surg* 65:1526, 2007.

Peñarrocha-Diago M, Maestre-Ferrín L, Peñarrocha-Oltra D, et al: Influence of hemostatic agents upon the outcome of periapical surgery: dressings with anesthetic and vasoconstrictor or aluminum chloride, *Medicina Oral, Patologia Oral y Cirugia Bucal* 18:e272, 2013.

Peñarrocha Diago M, Ortega Sánchez B, García Mira B, et al: Evaluation of healing criteria for success after periapical surgery, *Medicina Oral, Patologia Oral y Cirugia Bucal* 13:143, 2008.

Penarrocha-Diago MA, Ortega-Sanchez B, Garcia-Mira B, et al: A prospective clinical study of polycarboxylate cement in periapical surgery, *Medicina Oral, Patologia Oral y Cirugia Bucal* 17:e276, 2012.

Peñarrocha Diago M, Sanchis Bielsa JM, Gay Escoda C: Periapical surgery of 31 lower molars based on the ultrasound technique and retrograde filling with silver amalgam, *Medicina Oral* 6:376, 2001.

Penesis VA, Fitzgerald PI, Fayad MI, et al: Outcome of one-visit and two-visit endodontic treatment of necrotic teeth with apical periodontitis: a randomized controlled trial with one-year evaluation, *J Endod* 34:251, 2008.

Peretz B, Yakir O, Fuks AB: Follow up after root canal treatment of young permanent molars, *J Clin Pediatr Dent* 21:237, 1997.

Persson G: Periapical surgery of molars, *Int J Oral Surg* 11:96, 1982.

Peters LB, van Winkelhoff AJ, Buijs JF, Wesselink PR: Effects of instrumentation, irrigation and dressing with calcium hydroxide on infection in pulpless teeth with periapical bone lesions, *Int Endod J* 35:13, 2002.

Peters LB, Wesselink PR: Periapical healing of endodontically treated teeth in one and two visits obturated in the presence or absence of detectable microorganisms, *Int Endod J* 35:660, 2002.

Pettiette MT, Delano EO, Trope M: Evaluation of success rate of endodontic treatment performed by students with stainless-steel K-files and nickel-titanium hand files, *J Endod* 27:124, 2001.

Platt AS, Wannfors K: The effectiveness of compomer as a root-end filling: a clinical investigation, *Oral Surg Oral Med Oral Pathol Oral Radiol Endod* 97:508, 2004.

Qudeimat MA, Barrieshi-Nusair KM, Owais AI: Calcium hydroxide vs mineral trioxide aggregates for partial pulpotomy of permanent molars with deep caries, *Eur Arch Paediatr Dent* 8:99, 2007.

Rahbaran S, Gilthorpe MS, Harrison SD, Gulabivala K: Comparison of clinical outcome of periapical surgery in endodontic and oral surgery units of a teaching dental hospital: a retrospective study, *Oral Surg Oral Med Oral Pathol Oral Radiol Endod* 91:700, 2001.

Rapp EL, Brown CE Jr, Newton CW: An analysis of success and failure of apicoectomies, *J Endod* 17:508, 1991.

Reid RJ, Abbott PV, McNamara JR, Heithersay GS: A five-year study of hydron root canal fillings, *Int Endod J* 25:213, 1992.

Reit C, Dahlen G: Decision making analysis of endodontic treatment strategies in teeth with apical periodontitis, *Int Endod J* 21:291, 1988.

Reit C, Molander A, Dahlen G: The diagnostic accuracy of microbiologic root canal sampling and the influence of antimicrobial dressings, *Endod Dent Traumatol* 15:278, 1999.

Rhein ML, Krasnow F, Gies WJ: A prolonged study of the electrolytic treatment of dental focal infection: a preliminary report, *Dent Cosmos* 68:971, 1926.

Ricucci D, Grondahl K, Bergenholtz G: Periapical status of root-filled teeth exposed to the oral environment by loss of restoration or caries, *Oral Surg Oral Med Oral Pathol Oral Radiol Endod* 90:354, 2000.

Ricucci D, Russo J, Rutberg M, et al: A prospective cohort study of endodontic treatments of 1,369 root canals: results after 5 years, *Oral Surg Oral Med Oral Pathol Oral Radiol Endod* 112:825, 2011.

Rocas IN, Siqueira JF Jr, Del Aguila CA, et al: Polymorphism of the CD14 and TLR4 genes and post-treatment apical periodontitis, *J Endod* 40:168, 2014.

Rubinstein RA, Kim S: Long-term follow-up of cases considered healed one year after apical microsurgery, *J Endod* 28:378, 2002.

Rud J, Andreasen JO: A study of failures after endodontic surgery by radiographic, histologic and stereomicroscopic methods, *Int J Oral Surg* 1:311, 1972.

Rud J, Munksgaard EC, Andreasen JO, Rud V: Retrograde root filling with composite and a dentin-bonding agent. 2, *Endod Dent Traumatol* 7:126, 1991.

Rud J, Rud V, Munksgaard EC: Long-term evaluation of retrograde root filling with dentin-bonded resin composite, *J Endod* 22:90, 1996.

Rud J, Rud V, Munksgaard EC: Periapical healing of mandibular molars after root-end sealing with dentine-bonded composite, *Int Endod J* 34:285, 2001.

Russo MC, Holland R, de Souza V: Radiographic and histological evaluation of the treatment of inflamed dental pulps, *Int Endod J* 15:137, 1982.

Safavi KE, Dowden WE, Langeland K: Influence of delayed coronal permanent restoration on endodontic prognosis, *Endod Dent Traumatol* 3:187, 1987.

Salehrabi R, Rotstein I: Endodontic treatment outcomes in a large patient population in the USA: an epidemiological study, *J Endod* 30:846, 2004.

Salehrabi R, Rotstein I: Epidemiologic evaluation of the outcomes of orthograde endodontic retreatment, *J Endod* 36:790, 2010.

Salvi GE, Siegrist Guldener BE, Amstad T, et al: Clinical evaluation of root filled teeth restored with or without post-and-core systems in a specialist practice setting, *Int Endod J* 40:209, 2007.

Santini A: Assessment of the pulpotomy technique in human first permanent mandibular molars: use of two direct inspection criteria, *Br Dent J* 155:151, 1983.

Santucci PJ: Dycal versus Nd:YAG laser and Vitrebond for direct pulp capping in permanent teeth, *J Clin Laser Med Surg* 17:69, 1999.

Sari S, Duruturk L: Radiographic evaluation of periapical healing of permanent teeth with periapical lesions after extrusion of AH Plus sealer, *Oral Surg Oral Med Oral Pathol Oral Radiol Endod* 104:e54, 2007.

Sawusch RH: Direct and indirect pulp capping with two new products, *J Am Dent Assoc* 104:459, 1982.

Schwartz-Arad D, Yarom N, Lustig JP, Kaffe I: A retrospective radiographic study of root-end surgery with amalgam and intermediate restorative material, *Oral Surg Oral Med Oral Pathol Oral Radiol Endod* 96:472, 2003.

Selden HS: Pulpoperiapical disease: diagnosis and healing: a clinical endodontic study, *Oral Surg* 27:271, 1974.

Seltzer S, Bender IB, Turkenkopf S: Factors affecting successful repair after root canal therapy, *J Am Dent Assoc* 67:651, 1963.

Setzer FC, Boyer KR, Jeppson JR, et al: Long-term prognosis of endodontically treated teeth: a retrospective analysis of preoperative factors in molars, *J Endod* 37:21, 2011.

Shah N: Non-surgical management of periapical lesions: a prospective study, *Oral Surg Oral Med Oral Pathol* 66:365, 1988.

Shovelton DS, Friend LA, Kirk EE, Rowe AH: The efficacy of pulp capping materials: a comparative trial, *Br Dent J* 130:385, 1971.

Shuping GB, Orstavik D, Sigurdsson A, Trope M: Reduction of intracanal bacteria using nickel-titanium rotary instrumentation and various medications, *J Endod* 26:751, 2000.

Siqueira JF Jr, Guimaraes-Pinto T, Rocas IN: Effects of chemomechanical preparation with 2.5% sodium hypochlorite and intracanal medication with calcium hydroxide on cultivable bacteria in infected root canals, *J Endod* 33:800, 2007.

Siqueira JF Jr, Magalhaes KM, Rocas IN: Bacterial reduction in infected root canals treated with 2.5% NaOCl as an irrigant and calcium hydroxide/camphorated paramonochlorophenol paste as an intracanal dressing, *J Endod* 33:667, 2007.

Siqueira JF Jr, Rocas IN, Paiva SS, et al: Bacteriologic investigation of the effects of sodium hypochlorite and chlorhexidine during the endodontic treatment of teeth with apical periodontitis, *Oral Surg Oral Med Oral Pathol Oral Radiol Endod* 104:122, 2007.

Siqueira JF Jr, Rocas IN, Provenzano JC, et al: Relationship between Fcgamma receptor and interleukin-1 gene polymorphisms and post-treatment apical periodontitis, *J Endod* 35:1186, 2009.

Siqueira JF Jr, Rocas IN, Provenzano JC, Guilherme BP: Polymorphism of the FcgammaRIIIa gene and post-treatment apical periodontitis, *J Endod* 37:1345, 2011.

Siqueira JF Jr, Rôcas IN, Riche FN, Provenzano JC: Clinical outcome of the endodontic treatment of teeth with apical periodontitis using an antimicrobial protocol, *Oral Surg Oral Med Oral Pathol Oral Radiol Endod* 106:757, 2008.

Sjogren U, Figdor D, Persson S, Sundqvist G: Influence of infection at the time of root filling on the outcome of endodontic treatment of teeth with apical periodontitis, *Int Endod J* 30:297, 1997.

Sjogren U, Figdor D, Spangberg L, Sundqvist G: The antimicrobial effect of calcium hydroxide as a short-term intracanal dressing, *Int Endod J* 24:119, 1991.

Sjogren U, Hagglund B, Sundqvist G, Wing K: Factors affecting the long-term results of endodontic treatment, *J Endod* 16:498, 1990.

Sjogren U, Sundqvist G: Bacteriologic evaluation of ultrasonic root canal instrumentation, *Oral Surg Oral Med Oral Pathol* 63:366, 1987.

Skupien JA, Opdam N, Winnen R, et al: A practice-based study on the survival of restored endodontically treated teeth, *J Endod* 39:1335, 2013.

Smith CS, Setchell DJ, Harty FJ: Factors influencing the success of conventional root canal therapy—a five-year retrospective study, *Int Endod J* 26:321, 1993.

Soltanoff W: A comparative study of the single-visit and the multiple-visit endodontic procedure, *J Endod* 4:278, 1978.

Song M, Jung IY, Lee SJ, et al: Prognostic factors for clinical outcomes in endodontic microsurgery: a retrospective study, *J Endod* 37:927, 2011. Erratum in *J Endod* 37:1595, 2011a.

Song M, Kim E: A prospective randomized controlled study of mineral trioxide aggregate and super ethoxy–benzoic acid as root-end filling materials in endodontic microsurgery, *J Endod* 38:875, 2012.

Song M, Kim SG, Lee SJ, et al: Prognostic factors of clinical outcomes in endodontic microsurgery: a prospective study, *J Endod* 39:1491, 2013a.

Song M, Kim SG, Shin SJ, et al: The influence of bone tissue deficiency on the outcome of endodontic microsurgery: a prospective study, *J Endod* 39:1341, 2013b.

Song M, Nam T, Shin S-J, Kim E: Comparison of clinical outcomes of endodontic microsurgery: 1 year versus long-term follow-up, *J Endod* 40:490, 2014.

Song M, Shin SJ, Kim E: Outcomes of endodontic micro-resurgery: a prospective clinical study, *J Endod* 37:316, 2011b.

Stewart GG, Cobe H, Rappaport H: Study of new medicament in chemomechanical preparation of infected root canals, *J Am Dent Assoc* 63:33, 1961.

Stoll R, Betke K, Stachniss V: The influence of different factors on the survival of root canal fillings: a 10-year retrospective study, *J Endod* 31:783, 2005.

Storms JL: Factors that influence the success of endodontic treatment, *J Can Dent Assoc (Tor)* 35:83, 1969.

Strindberg LZ: *The dependence of the results of pulp therapy on certain factors: an analytic study based on radiographic and clinical follow-up examinations*, 1956, Mauritzon.

Sumi Y, Hattori H, Hayashi K, Ueda M: Ultrasonic root-end preparation: clinical and radiographic evaluation of results, *J Oral Maxillofac Surg* 54:590, 1996.

Sundqvist G, Figdor D, Persson S, Sjogren U: Microbiologic analysis of teeth with failed endodontic treatment and the outcome of conservative re-treatment, *Oral Surg Oral Med Oral Pathol Oral Radiol Endod* 85:86, 1998.

Swartz DB, Skidmore AE, Griffin JA: Twenty years of endodontic success and failure, *J Endod* 9:198, 1983.

Tan L, Chen NN, Poon CY, Wong HB: Survival of root filled cracked teeth in a tertiary institution, *Int Endod J* 2006 39:886.

Taschieri S, Corbella S, Tsesis I, et al: Effect of guided tissue regeneration on the outcome of surgical endodontic treatment of through-and-through lesions: a retrospective study at 4-year follow-up, *Oral Maxillofac Surg* 15:153, 2011.

Taschieri S, Del Fabbro M, Testori T, et al: Endodontic surgery with ultrasonic retrotips: one-year follow-up, *Oral Surg Oral Med Oral Pathol Oral Radiol Endod* 100:380, 2005.

Taschieri S, Del Fabbro M, Testori T, et al: Endodontic surgery using 2 different magnification devices: preliminary results of a randomized controlled study, *J Oral Maxillofac Surg* 64:235, 2006.

Taschieri S, Del Fabbro M, Testori T, et al: Efficacy of guided tissue regeneration in the management of through-and-through lesions following surgical endodontics: a preliminary study, *Int J Periodontics Restorative Dent* 28:265, 2008b.

Taschieri S, Del Fabbro M, Testori T, Weinstein R: Endoscopic periradicular surgery: a prospective clinical study, *Br J Oral Maxillofac Surg* 45:242, 2007.

Taschieri S, Del Fabbro M, Testori T, Weinstein RL: Endodontic reoperation using an endoscope and microsurgical instruments: one year follow-up, *Br J Oral Maxillofac Surg* 45:582, 2007a.

Taschieri S, Del Fabbro M, Testori T, Weinstein R: Efficacy of xenogeneic bone grafting with guided tissue regeneration in the management of bone defects after surgical endodontics, *J Oral Maxillofac Surg* 65:1121, 2007b.

Taschieri S, Del Fabbro M, Testori T, Weinstein R: Microscope versus endoscope in root-end management: a randomized controlled study, *Int J Oral Maxillofac Surg* 37:1022, 2008a, doi:10.1016/j.ijom.2008.07.001. Epub Aug 22, 2008.

Taschieri S, Machtou P, Rosano G, et al: The influence of previous non-surgical re-treatment on the outcome of endodontic surgery, *Minerva Stomatol* 59:625, 2010.

Taschieri S, Weinstein T, Tsesis I, et al: Magnifying loupes versus surgical microscope in endodontic surgery: a four-year retrospective study, *Aust Endod J* 39:78, 2013.

Teixeira LS, Demarco FF, Coppola MC, Bonow ML: Clinical and radiographic evaluation of pulpotomies performed under intrapulpal injection of anaesthetic solution, *Int Endod J* 34:440, 2001.

Tervit C, Paquette L, Torneck CD, et al: Proportion of healed teeth with apical periodontitis medicated with two percent chlorhexidine gluconate liquid: a case-series study, *J Endod* 35:1182, 2009.

Testori T, Capelli M, Milani S, Weinstein RL: Success and failure in periradicular surgery: a longitudinal retrospective analysis, *Oral Surg Oral Med Oral Pathol Oral Radiol Endod* 87:493, 1999.

Tilashalski KR, Gilbert GH, Boykin MJ, Shelton BJ: Root canal treatment in a population-based adult sample: status of teeth after endodontic treatment, *J Endod* 30:577, 2004.

Tobón SI, Arismendi JA, Marín ML, et al: Comparison between a conventional technique and two bone regeneration techniques in periradicular surgery, *Int Endod J* 35:635, 2002.

Trope M, Delano EO, Orstavik D: Endodontic treatment of teeth with apical periodontitis: single vs. multivisit treatment, *J Endod* 25:345, 1999.

Tsesis I, Rosen E, Schwartz-Arad D, Fuss Z: Retrospective evaluation of surgical endodontic treatment: traditional versus modern technique, *J Endod* 32:412, 2006.

Vallecillo Capilla M, Muñoz Soto E, Reyes Botella C, et al: Periapical surgery of 29 teeth: a comparison of conventional technique, microsaw and ultrasound, *Med Oral* 7:46, 50, 2002.

Vianna ME, Horz HP, Conrads G, et al: Effect of root canal procedures on endotoxins and endodontic pathogens, *Oral Microbiol Immunol* 22:411, 2007.

Villa-Machado PA, Botero-Ramírez X, Tobón-Arroyave SI: Retrospective follow-up assessment of prognostic variables associated with the outcome of periradicular surgery, *Int Endod J* 46:1063, 2013.

von Arx T, Gerber C, Hardt N: Periradicular surgery of molars: a prospective clinical study with a one-year follow-up, *Int Endod J* 34:520, 2001.

von Arx T, Jensen SS, Hanni S: Clinical and radiographic assessment of various predictors for healing outcome 1 year after periapical surgery, *J Endod* 33:123, 2007.

von Arx T, Jensen SS, Hanni S, Friedman S: Five-year longitudinal assessment of the prognosis of apical microsurgery, *J Endod* 38:570, 2012.

von Arx T, Kurt B: Root-end cavity preparation after apicoectomy using a new type of sonic and diamond-surfaced retrotip: a 1-year follow-up study, *J Oral Maxillofac Surg* 57:656, 1999.

Von Arx T, Peñarrocha M, Jensen S: Prognostic factors in apical surgery with root-end filling: a meta-analysis, *J Endod* 36:957, 2010.

Waikakul A, Punwutikorn J: Clinical study of retrograde filling with gold leaf: comparison with amalgam, *Oral Surg Oral Med Oral Pathol* 71:228, 1991.

Wälivaara DÅ, Abrahamsson P, Fogelin M, Isaksson S: Super-EBA and IRM as root-end fillings in periapical surgery with ultrasonic preparation: a prospective randomized clinical study of 206 consecutive teeth, *Oral Surg Oral Med Oral Pathol Oral Radiol Endod* 112:258, 2011.

Wälivaara DA, Abrahamsson P, Isaksson S, et al: Prospective study of periapically infected teeth treated with periapical surgery including ultrasonic preparation and retrograde intermediate restorative material root-end fillings, *J Oral Maxillofac Surg* 65:931, 2007.

Wälivaara DA, Abrahamsson P, Sämfors KA, Isaksson S: Periapical surgery using ultrasonic preparation and thermoplasticized gutta-percha with AH Plus sealer or IRM as retrograde root-end fillings in 160 consecutive teeth: a prospective randomized clinical study, *Oral Surg Oral Med Oral Pathol Oral Radiol Endod* 108:784, 2009.

Waly NG: A five-year comparative study of calcium hydroxide-glutaraldehyde pulpotomies versus calcium hydroxide pulpotomies in young permanent molars, *Egypt Dent J* 41:993, 1995.

Wang CH, Chueh LH, Chen SC, et al: Impact of diabetes mellitus, hypertension, and coronary artery disease on tooth extraction after nonsurgical endodontic treatment, *J Endod* 37:1, 2011.

Wang CS, Arnold RR, Trope M, Teixeira FB: Clinical efficiency of 2% chlorhexidine gel in reducing intracanal bacteria, *J Endod* 33:1283, 2007.

Weiger R, Rosendahl R, Löst C: Influence of calcium hydroxide intracanal dressings on the prognosis of teeth with endodontically induced periapical lesions, *Int Endod J* 33:219, 2000.

Weiss M: Pulp capping in older patients, *N Y State Dent J* 32:451, 1966.

Werts R: Endodontic treatment: a five-year follow-up, *Dent Survey* 51:29, 1975.

Witherspoon DE, Small JC, Harris GZ: Mineral trioxide aggregate pulpotomies: a case series outcomes assessment, *J Am Dent Assoc* 137:610, 2006.

Witherspoon DE, Small JC, Regan JD, Nunn M: Retrospective analysis of open apex teeth obturated with mineral trioxide aggregate, *J Endod* 34:1171, 2008.

Xavier AC, Martinho FC, Chung A. et al: One-visit versus two-visit root canal treatment: effectiveness in the removal of endotoxins and cultivable bacteria, *J Endod* 39:959, 2013.

Yared GM, Dagher FE: Influence of apical enlargement on bacterial infection during treatment of apical periodontitis, *J Endod* 20:535, 1994.

Zeldow BI, Ingle JI: Correlation of the positive culture to the prognosis of endodontically treated teeth: a clinical study, *J Am Dent Assoc* 66:9, 1963.

Zmener O, Pameijer CH: Clinical and radiographical evaluation of a resin-based root canal sealer: a 5-year follow-up, *J Endod* 33:676, 2007.

Zuolo ML, Ferreira MO, Gutmann JL: Prognosis in periradicular surgery: a clinical prospective study, *Int Endod J* 33:91, 2000.

CHAPTER 12

Structure and Functions of the Dentin-Pulp Complex

INGE FRISTAD | ELLEN BERGGREEN[1]

CHAPTER OUTLINE

MORPHOLOGIC ZONES OF THE PULP

The Pulp-Dentin Complex

The dental pulp and dentin function as a unit, and the odontoblasts represent a crucial element in this system. The odontoblasts are located in the periphery of the pulp tissue, with extensions into the inner part of dentin. Dentin would not exist unless produced by odontoblasts, and the dental pulp is dependent on the protection provided by the dentin and enamel. Likewise, integrated dynamics of the pulp-dentin complex imply that impacts on dentin may affect the pulpal components and that disturbances in the dental pulp will in turn affect the quantity and quality of the dentin produced.

---

[1]The authors acknowledge the outstanding work of Drs. Henry Trowbridge, Syngcuk Kim, Hideaki Suda, David H. Pashley, and Fredrik R. Liewehr in previous editions of this text. The present chapter is built on their foundational work.

Odontoblast Layer

The outermost stratum of cells of the healthy pulp is the odontoblast layer (Figs. 12-1 and 12-2). This layer is located immediately subjacent to the predentin. The odontoblast processes, however, pass on through the predentin into the inner part of dentin. Consequently, the odontoblast layer is actually composed of the cell bodies of odontoblasts. In addition, capillaries, nerve fibers, and dendritic cells may be found among the odontoblasts.

In the coronal portion of a young pulp that is actively secreting collagen, the odontoblasts assume a tall columnar form.[62] The odontoblasts vary in height; consequently, their nuclei are not all at the same level and are aligned in a staggered array, often described as a palisade appearance. This organization makes the layers appear to be three to five cells in thickness even though there is only one actual layer of odontoblasts. Between adjacent odontoblasts there are small intercellular

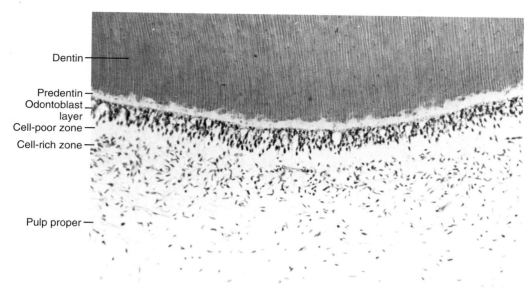

FIG. 12-1 Morphologic zones of the mature pulp.

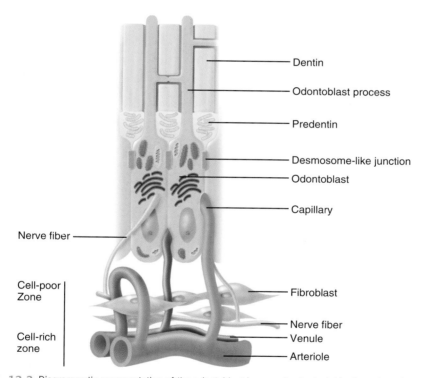

FIG. 12-2 Diagrammatic representation of the odontoblast layer and subodontoblastic region of the pulp.

spaces approximately 30 to 40 nm in width. Odontoblast cell bodies are connected by tight and gap junctional complexes.[29,62,160] Gap junctions are formed by connexin proteins[113] that permit cell-to-cell passage of signal molecules.

The odontoblast layer in the coronal pulp contains more cells per unit area than in the radicular pulp.[240] Whereas the odontoblasts of the mature coronal pulp are usually columnar, those in the midportion of the radicular pulp are more cuboidal (Fig. 12-3).[62] Near the apical foramen, the odontoblasts appear as a squamous layer of flattened cells. Because fewer dentinal tubules per unit area are present in the root than in the crown of the tooth, the odontoblast cell bodies are less crowded and

are able to spread out laterally.[240] During maturation and aging, there is a continued ongoing crowding in the odontoblast layer, particularly in the coronal pulp, due to narrowing of the pulp space. Apoptosis of odontoblasts seems to adjust for this limited space during development.[252]

There is a series of specialized cell-to-cell junctions (i.e., junctional complexes), including desmosomes (i.e., zonula adherens), gap junctions (i.e., nexuses), and tight junctions (i.e., zonula occludens) that connect adjacent odontoblasts. Spot desmosomes located in the apical part of odontoblast cell bodies mechanically join odontoblasts together. The numerous gap junctions provide permeable pathways through which

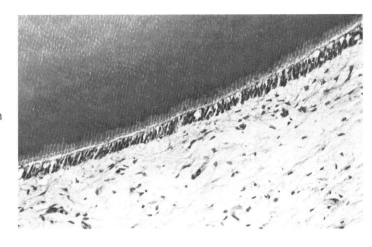

FIG. 12-3 Low columnar odontoblasts of the radicular pulp. The cell-rich zone is inconspicuous.

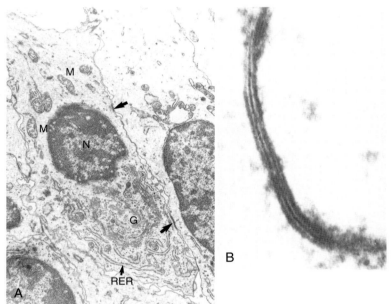

FIG. 12-4 **A,** Electron micrograph of a mouse molar odontoblast demonstrating gap junctions *(arrows),* nucleus (N), mitochondria (M), Golgi complex (G), and rough endoplasmic reticulum (RER). **B,** High magnification of a section fixed and stained with lanthanum nitrate to demonstrate a typical gap junction. (Courtesy Dr. Charles F. Cox, School of Dentistry, University of Alabama.)

signal molecules can pass between cells (Fig. 12-4) to synchronize secretory activity that produces relatively uniform predentin layers (see Fig. 12-2). These junctions are most numerous during the formation of primary dentin. Gap junctions and desmosomes have also been observed joining odontoblasts to the processes of fibroblasts in the subodontoblastic area. Tight junctions are found mainly in the apical part of odontoblasts in young teeth. These structures consist of linear ridges and grooves that close off the intercellular space. However, tracer studies suggest direct passage of small elements from subodontoblastic capillaries to predentin and dentin between the odontoblasts.[352] It appears that tight junctions determine the permeability of the odontoblast layer when dentin is covered by enamel or cementum by restricting the passage of molecules, ions, and fluid between the extracellular compartments of the pulp and predentin.[29] During cavity preparation, these junctions are disrupted, thereby increasing dentin permeability.[375,376]

Cell-Poor Zone

Immediately subjacent to the odontoblast layer in the coronal pulp, there is often a narrow zone approximately 40 μm in width that is relatively free of cells (see Fig. 12-1) and hence is called the *cell-free layer of Weil.* It is traversed by blood capillaries, unmyelinated nerve fibers and the slender cytoplasmic processes of fibroblasts (see Fig. 12-2). The presence or absence of the cell-poor zone depends on the functional status of the pulp.[62] It may not be apparent in young pulps, where dentin forms rapidly, or in older pulps, where reparative dentin is being produced.

Cell-Rich Zone

In the subodontoblastic area, there is a stratum containing a relatively high proportion of fibroblasts compared with the more central region of the pulp (see Fig. 12-1). It is much more prominent in the coronal pulp than in the radicular pulp. Besides fibroblasts, the cell-rich zone may include a variable number of immune cells like macrophages and dendritic cells, but also undifferentiated mesenchymal stem cells.

On the basis of evidence obtained in rat molar teeth, it has been suggested[126] that the cell-rich zone forms as a result of peripheral migration of cells populating the central regions of the pulp, commencing at about the time of tooth eruption. Migration of immunocompetent cells out of and into the cell-rich zone has been demonstrated as a result of antigenic challenge.[421] Although cell division within the cell-rich zone is rare in normal pulps, the death of the odontoblasts triggers a great increase in the rate of mitosis. Because odontoblasts are postmitotic cells, irreversibly injured odontoblasts are replaced by cells that migrate from the cell-rich zone onto the inner surface of the dentin.[98] This mitotic activity is probably the first step in the formation of a new odontoblast layer.[73,256,258,339] Studies implicate stem cells as a source for these replacement odontoblasts.[346]

Pulp Proper

The pulp proper is the central mass of the pulp (see Fig. 12-1). It consists of loose connective tissue and contains the larger blood vessels and nerves. The most prominent cell in this zone is the fibroblast.

CELLS OF THE PULP

Odontoblast

Because odontoblasts are responsible for dentinogenesis, both during tooth development and aging, the odontoblast is the most characteristic and specialized cell of the dentin-pulp complex. During dentinogenesis, the odontoblasts form dentin and the dentinal tubules, and their presence within the tubules makes dentin a living responsive tissue.

Dentinogenesis, osteogenesis, and cementogenesis are in many respects quite similar, and odontoblasts, osteoblasts, and cementoblasts have many characteristics in common. Each of these cells produces a matrix composed of collagen fibrils, noncollagenous proteins, and proteoglycans that are capable of undergoing mineralization. The ultrastructural characteristics of odontoblasts, osteoblasts, and cementoblasts are likewise similar in that each exhibits a highly ordered rough endoplasmic reticulum (RER), a prominent Golgi complex, secretory granules, and numerous mitochondria. In addition, these cells are rich in RNA, and their nuclei contain one or more prominent nucleoli. These are the general characteristics of protein-secreting cells.

The most significant differences among odontoblasts, osteoblasts, and cementoblasts are their morphologic characteristics and the anatomic relationship between the cells and the mineralized structures they produce. Whereas osteoblasts and cementoblasts are polygonal to cuboidal in form, the fully developed odontoblast of the coronal pulp is a tall columnar cell.[62,240] In bone and cementum, some of the osteoblasts and cementoblasts become entrapped in the matrix as osteocytes or cementocytes, respectively. The odontoblast, on the other hand, leaves behind a cellular process to form the dentinal tubule, and the cell body resides outside the mineralized tissue. Lateral branches between the major odontoblast processes interconnect[178,253] through canaliculi, just as osteocytes and cementocytes are linked through the canaliculi in bone and cementum. This provides a pathway for intercellular communication and circulation of fluid and metabolites through the mineralized matrix.

The ultrastructural features of the odontoblast have been the subject of numerous investigations. The cell body of the active odontoblast has a large nucleus that may contain up to four nucleoli (Fig. 12-5). The nucleus is situated at the basal end of the cell and is contained within a nuclear envelope. A well-developed Golgi complex, centrally located in the supranuclear cytoplasm, consists of an assembly of smooth-walled vesicles and cisternae. Numerous mitochondria are evenly distributed throughout the cell body. RER is particularly prominent, consisting of closely stacked cisternae forming parallel arrays that are dispersed diffusely within the cytoplasm. Numerous ribosomes closely associated with the membranes of the cisternae mark the sites of protein synthesis. Within the lumen of the cisternae, filamentous material (probably representing newly synthesized protein) can be observed.

The odontoblast appears to synthesize mainly type I collagen,[208,401] although small amounts of type V collagen have been found in the extracellular matrix (ECM). In addition to proteoglycans[38,83,123] and collagen,[208,220] the odontoblast secretes dentin sialoprotein[40] and phosphophoryn,[40,69] a highly phosphorylated phosphoprotein involved in extracellular mineralization.[40,77] Phosphophoryn is unique to dentin and is not found in any other mesenchymal cell types.[77] The odontoblast also secretes both acid phosphatase and alkaline phosphatase. The latter enzyme is closely linked to mineralization, but the precise role of alkaline phosphatase in dentinogenesis is not completely understood. Acid phosphatase, a lysosomal enzyme, may be involved in digesting material that has been resorbed from predentin matrix.[87]

In contrast to the active odontoblast, the resting or inactive odontoblast has a decreased number of organelles and may become progressively shorter.[62,240] These changes can begin with the completion of root development and eruption when dentin production shifts from primary to secondary dentin.

Direct actions of odontoblasts on dental nerves and vice versa have been proposed based on the excitability of odontoblasts, the differential expression of receptors for neuropeptides on odontoblasts (Fig. 12-6), the demonstration of the thermosensitive transient receptor potential (TRP) ion channels, and the finding that all nine voltage-gated sodium channels are variably expressed on odontoblasts in developing, mature, and aging rat teeth.[52,71,107,221,231,232] In addition, a possible function of odontoblast in immune regulation has been proposed by the finding of innate immune components in the odontoblast layer.[382] Hence, the odontoblasts should be capable of recognizing and differentially responding to bacterial components, thereby serving immune and pulp-dentine barrier functions.

Odontoblast Process

A dentinal tubule forms around each of the major odontoblastic processes. The odontoblast process occupies most of the space within the tubule and coordinates the formation of peritubular dentin.

Microtubules and microfilaments are the principal ultrastructural components of the odontoblast process and its lateral branches.[110,158] Microtubules extend from the cell body out into the process.[110,151] These straight structures follow a course that is parallel with the long axis of the cell and impart the impression of rigidity. Although their precise role is unknown, theories as to their functional significance suggest that they may be involved in cytoplasmic extension, transport of materials, or the provision of a structural framework. Occasionally, mitochondria can be found in the process where it passes through the predentin.

The plasma membrane of the odontoblast process closely approximates the wall of the dentinal tubule. Localized

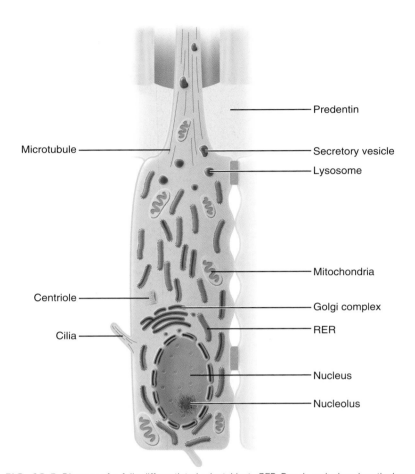

FIG. 12-5 Diagram of a fully differentiated odontoblast. *RER,* Rough endoplasmic reticulum.

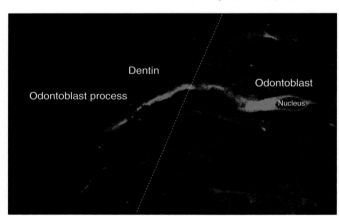

FIG. 12-6 Confocal microscopic image showing an odontoblast with its process expressing neurokinin 2 receptor. Neurokinin 2 has affinity to all the neuropeptides of the neurokinin family. The dotted line represents the border of the predentin. (From Fristad I, Vandevska-Radunovic V, Fjeld K, et al: NK1, NK2, NK3 and CGRP1 receptors identified in rat oral soft tissues, and in bone and dental hard tissue cells, *Cell Tissue Res* 311:383-391, 2003.)

constrictions in the process occasionally produce relatively large spaces between the tubule wall and the process. Such spaces may contain collagen fibrils and fine granular material that presumably represents ground substance (see also The Pulpal Interstitium and Ground Substance in this chapter). The peritubular dentin matrix within the tubule is lined by an electron-dense limiting membrane called the *lamina limitans.*[260,354,398] A narrow space separates the limiting membrane from the plasma membrane of the odontoblast process, except for the areas where the process is constricted.

In restoring a tooth, the removal of enamel and dentin often disrupts odontoblasts.[41,45,73,80,202,257] It would be of considerable clinical importance to establish the extent of the odontoblast processes in human teeth, because with this knowledge, the clinician would be in a better position to estimate the impact of the restorative procedure on the underlying odontoblasts. However, the extent to which the process penetrates into dentin has been a matter of considerable controversy. It has long been thought that the process is present throughout the full thickness of dentin. Although ultrastructural studies using transmission electron microscopy have described the process as being limited to the inner third of the dentin,[48,111,354,398] it should be noted that this could possibly be the result of shrinkage occurring during fixation and dehydration. Other studies employing scanning electron microscopy have described the process extending further into the tubule, often as far as the dentoenamel junction (DEJ),[130,179,337,412] but it has been suggested that what has been observed in scanning electron micrographs is actually the lamina limitans.[354,355,398]

In an attempt to resolve this issue, monoclonal antibodies directed against microtubules were used to demonstrate tubulin in the microtubules of the process. Immunoreactivity was observed throughout the dentinal tubule, suggesting that the process extends throughout the thickness of dentin.[337]

However, a study employing confocal microscopy found that odontoblast processes in rat molars do not extend to the outer dentin or DEJ, except during the early stages of tooth development.[48] It is likely that the walls of tubules contain many proteins originally derived from odontoblasts that no longer remain at that site. Because dentin matrix has no turnover, these antigens remain fixed in place. From a clinical perspective, it is important to remember that these processes in the tubules represent appendages from living odontoblasts in the pulp, which explains why the dentin must be considered a vital tissue, the destruction of which will affect the pulp.

The odontoblast is considered to be a fixed postmitotic cell in that once it has fully differentiated, it apparently cannot undergo further cell division. If this is indeed the case, the life span of the odontoblast coincides with the life span of the viable pulp. However, its metabolic activity can be dynamically altered (described under the heading Pulpal Repair).

Relationship of Odontoblast Structure to Secretory Function

Studies using radiolabeled chemicals have shed a great deal of light on the functional significance of the cytoplasmic organelles of the active odontoblast.[401,400] In experimental animals, intraperitoneal injection of a collagen precursor (e.g., ^{3}H-proline) is followed by autoradiographic labeling of the odontoblasts and predentin matrix[401] (Fig. 12-7). Rapid incorporation of the isotope in the RER soon leads to labeling of the Golgi complex in the area where the procollagen is packed and concentrated into secretory vesicles. Radiolabeled vesicles can then be followed along their migration pathway until they reach the base of the odontoblast process. Here they fuse with the cell membrane and release their tropocollagen molecules into the predentin matrix by the process of exocytosis.

It is now known that collagen fibrils precipitate from a solution of secreted tropocollagen and that the aggregation of fibrils occurs on the outer surface of the odontoblast plasma membrane. Fibrils are released into the predentin and increase in thickness as they approach the mineralized matrix. Whereas

fibrils at the base of the odontoblast process are approximately 15 nm in diameter, fibrils in the region of the calcification front have attained a diameter of about 50 nm.

Similar tracer studies[400] have elucidated the pathway of synthesis, transport, and secretion of the predentin proteoglycans. The protein moiety of these molecules is synthesized by the RER of the odontoblast, whereas sulfation and addition of the glycosaminoglycan (GAG) moieties to the protein molecules take place in the Golgi complex. Secretory vesicles then transport the proteoglycans to the base of the odontoblast process, where they are secreted into the predentin matrix. Proteoglycans, principally chondroitin sulfate, accumulate near the calcification front. The role of the proteoglycans is speculative, but mounting evidence suggests that they act as inhibitors of calcification by binding calcium. It appears that just before calcification, the proteoglycans are removed, probably by lysosomal enzymes secreted by the odontoblasts.[84]

Pulp Fibroblast

Fibroblasts are the most numerous cells of the pulp. They appear to be tissue-specific cells capable of giving rise to cells that are committed to differentiation (e.g., odontoblast-like cells) if given the proper signal. These cells synthesize types I and III collagen, as well as proteoglycans and GAGs. Thus, they produce and maintain the matrix proteins of the ECM. Because they are also able to phagocytose and digest collagen, fibroblasts are responsible for collagen turnover in the pulp.

Although distributed throughout the pulp, fibroblasts are particularly abundant in the cell-rich zone. The early differentiating fibroblasts are polygonal and appear to be widely separated and evenly distributed within the ground substance. Cell-to-cell contacts are established between the multiple processes that extend out from each of the cells. Many of these contacts take the form of gap junctions that provide for electronic coupling or chemical signaling from one cell to another. In terms of ultrastructure, the organelles of the immature fibroblasts are generally in a rudimentary stage of development, with an inconspicuous Golgi complex, numerous free ribosomes, and sparse RER. As they mature, the cells become stellate in form, and the Golgi complex enlarges, the RER proliferates, secretory vesicles appear, and the fibroblasts take on the characteristic appearance of protein-secreting cells. In addition, collagen fibrils accumulate along the outer surface of the cell body. With an increase in the number of blood vessels, nerves, and collagen fibers, there is a relative decrease in the number of fibroblasts in the pulp.

Many fibroblasts of the pulp are characterized by being relatively undifferentiated. A more modern term for undifferentiated cells is *stem cells*. Many pulpal cells do seem to remain in a relatively undifferentiated modality, compared with fibroblasts of most other connective tissues.[136] This perception has been supported by the observation of large numbers of reticulin-like fibers in the pulp. Reticulin fibers have an affinity for silver stains and are similar to the argyrophilic fibers of the pulp. However, in a careful review, it appears that actual reticulin fibers may not be present in the pulp; instead the previously described fibers are actually *argyrophilic collagen fibers*.[15] The fibers apparently acquire a GAG sheath, and it is this sheath that is impregnated by silver stains. In the young pulp, the nonargyrophilic collagen fibers are sparse, but they progressively increase in number as the pulp ages.

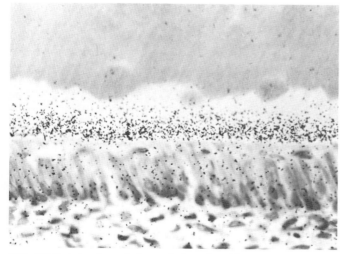

FIG. 12-7 Autoradiograph demonstrating odontoblasts and predentin in a developing rat molar 1 hour after intraperitoneal injection of ^{3}H-proline.

Many experimental models have been developed to study wound healing in the pulp, particularly dentinal bridge formation after pulp exposure or pulpotomy. One study[98] demonstrated that mitotic activity preceding the differentiation of replacement odontoblasts appears to occur primarily among perivascular fibroblasts.

Pulpal fibroblasts seem to take active part in signaling pathways in the dental pulp. For example, fibroblast growth and synthesis are stimulated by neuropeptides; in turn, fibroblasts produce nerve growth factor (NGF) and proinflammatory cytokines during inflammation.[31,408,413] NGF plays an important role not only in tooth development but also in regulating neuronal and possibly odontoblast responses to injury via activation of similar neurotrophin receptors expressed on both cell types (see also Plasticity of Intradental Nerve Fibers in this chapter).[408]

Macrophage

Macrophages are monocytes that have left the bloodstream, entered the tissues, and differentiated into various subpopulations. The different subpopulations can be studied by their antigenic properties in immunohistochemical studies. Many are found in close proximity to blood vessels. A major subpopulation of macrophages is active in endocytosis and phagocytosis (Fig. 12-8). Because of their mobility and phagocytic activity, they are able to act as scavengers, removing extravasated red blood cells, dead cells, and foreign bodies from the tissue. Ingested material is destroyed by the action of lysosomal enzymes. Another subset of macrophages participates in immune reactions by processing antigen and presenting it to memory T cells.[281] The processed antigen is bound to class II major histocompatibility complex (MHC) molecules on the macrophage, where it can interact with specific receptors present on naive or memory T cells.[133] Such interactions are essential for T cell–dependent immunity. Similar to fibroblasts, macrophages take an active part in the signaling pathways in the pulp. When activated by the appropriate inflammatory stimuli, macrophages are capable of producing a large variety of soluble factors, including interleukin 1, tumor necrosis factor, growth factors, and other cytokines. One study showed that a subset of macrophages express lymphatic markers, indicating a link between macrophages and lymphatic function and development.[19]

Dendritic Cell

Dendritic cells are accessory cells of the immune system. Similar cells are found in the epidermis and mucous membranes, where they are called *Langerhans cells*.[173,280] Dendritic cells are primarily found in lymphoid tissues, but they are also widely distributed in connective tissues, including the pulp[319] (Fig. 12-9). These cells are termed *antigen-presenting cells* and are characterized by dendritic cytoplasmic processes and the presence of class II MHC complexes on their cell surface (Fig. 12-10). In the normal pulp they are mostly located in the periphery of the coronal pulp close to the predentin, but they migrate centrally in the pulp after antigenic challenge.[421] They are known to play a central role in the induction of T cell–dependent immunity. Like antigen-presenting macrophages, dendritic cells engulf protein antigens and then present an assembly of peptide fragments of the antigens and MHC class II molecules. It is this assembly that T cells can recognize. Then the assembly binds to a T-cell receptor and T-cell activation

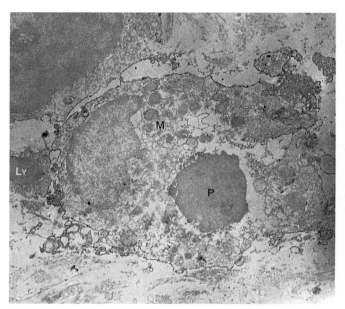

FIG. 12-8 Immunoelectron micrograph of an HLA-DR+ matured macrophage (M) in the human pulp, showing a phagosome (P). *Ly,* lymphocyte.

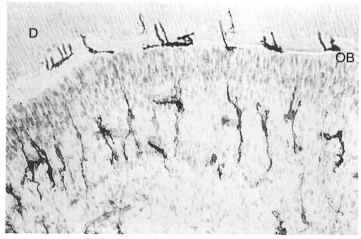

FIG. 12-9 Class II antigen-expressing dendritic cells in the pulp and dentin border zone in normal human pulp, as demonstrated by immunocytochemistry. *D,* dentin; *OB,* odontoblastic layer.

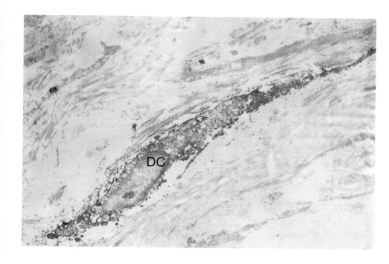

FIG. 12-10 Immunoelectron micrograph of a dendritic-like cell (DC) in the human pulp, showing a dendritic profile with a relatively small number of lysosomal structures.

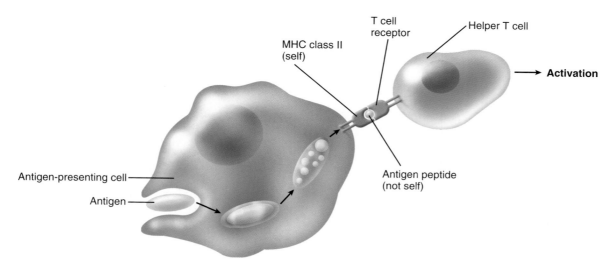

FIG. 12-11 Function of MHC class II molecule-expressing cells. They act as antigen-presenting cells that are essential for the induction of helper T cell–dependent immune responses.

occurs (Fig. 12-11). Fig. 12-12 shows a cell-to-cell contact between a dendritic-like cell and a lymphocyte.

Lymphocyte

Hahn and colleagues[133] reported finding T lymphocytes in normal pulps from human teeth. T8 (suppressor) lymphocytes were the predominant T-lymphocyte subset present in these samples. Lymphocytes have also been observed in the pulps of impacted teeth.[201] The presence of macrophages, dendritic cells, and T lymphocytes indicates that the pulp is well equipped with cells required for the initiation of immune responses.[173,319] B lymphocytes are scarcely found in the normal uninflamed pulp.

Mast Cell

Mast cells are widely distributed in connective tissues, where they occur in small groups in relation to blood vessels. Mast cells are seldom found in the normal pulp tissue, although they are routinely found in chronically inflamed pulps.[319] The mast cell has been the subject of considerable attention because of its dramatic role in inflammatory reactions. The granules of mast cells contain heparin, an anticoagulant, and histamine,

an important inflammatory mediator, as well as many other chemical factors.

METABOLISM

The metabolic activity of the pulp has been studied by measuring the rate of oxygen consumption and the production of carbon dioxide or lactic acid.[26,95,96,97,135,320] An investigation employed an oxygen-sensitive microelectrode inserted into a rat incisor pulp with a micromanipulator.[418] The authors reported that odontoblasts consumed O_2 at the rate of 3.2 ± 0.2 ml/min/100 g of pulp tissue.[418]

Because of the relatively sparse cellular composition of the pulp, the rate of oxygen consumption is low in comparison with that of most other tissues. During active dentinogenesis, metabolic activity is much higher than after the crown is completed. As would be anticipated, the greatest metabolic activity is found in the region of the odontoblast layer, and the lowest is found in the central pulp, where most of the nerves and blood vessels are located.[25]

In addition to the usual glycolytic pathway, the pulp has the ability to produce energy through a phosphogluconate (i.e.,

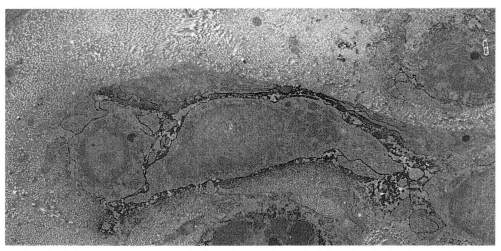

FIG. 12-12 Immunoelectron micrograph of a cell resembling a dendritic cell and a lymphocyte. They show cell-to-cell contact.

pentose phosphate) shunt type of carbohydrate metabolism,[97] a metabolic pathway that permits tissues to function under varying degrees of ischemia. This could explain how the pulp manages to withstand periods of low perfusion resulting from vasoconstriction induced by epinephrine-containing infiltration anesthesia.[190]

Several commonly used dental materials (e.g., eugenol, zinc oxide and eugenol, calcium hydroxide, silver amalgam) inhibit oxygen consumption by pulp tissue, indicating that these agents may be capable of depressing the metabolic activity of pulpal cells.[96,172] One study[135] found that application of orthodontic force to human premolars for 3 days resulted in a 27% reduction in respiratory activity in the pulp. This study utilized carbon-14-labeled succinic acid in the medium. As cells metabolize succinic acid, they produce $^{14}CO_2$ that can be trapped and quantitated by a liquid scintillation counter.[135] This technique requires only a few milligrams of tissue.

THE PULPAL INTERSTITIUM AND GROUND SUBSTANCE

The interstitium consists of the interstitial fluid and the interstitial (extracellular) matrix and occupies the extracellular and extravascular space. It is amorphous and generally regarded as a gel rather than a solid. Its constituents are similar in all tissues, but their relative amount varies. The major structural component of the interstitium is collagen (Fig. 12-13). The network of collagen fibers also supports the other components of the interstitium, the proteoglycans, hyaluronan, and elastic fibers. The two former components represent the glycosaminoglycans of the interstitial matrix.

Because of its content of polyanionic polysaccharides, the interstitium is responsible for the water-holding properties of connective tissues and acts as a molecular sieve in regulating the diffusion of substances through this space. The magnitude of the excluded volume has important consequences because the effective protein concentration in the interstitium is higher than the value that would be estimated from fluid volume per se.[404]

Connective tissue consists of cells and fibers, both embedded in ground substance or ECM. Cells that produce

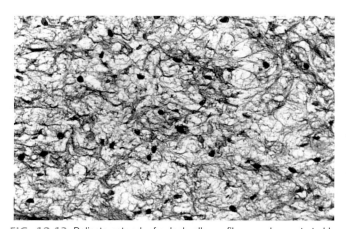

FIG. 12-13 Delicate network of pulpal collagen fibers as demonstrated by the Pearson silver impregnation method.

connective tissue fibers also synthesize the major constituents of the ECM. Whereas the fibers and cells have recognizable shapes, the ECM is described as being amorphous. It is generally regarded as a gel rather than a solid. Because of its content of polyanionic polysaccharides, the ECM is responsible for the water-holding properties of connective tissues.[404]

Nearly all proteins of the ECM are glycoproteins.[237] Proteoglycans are an important subclass of glycoproteins.[123] These molecules support cells, provide tissue turgor, and mediate a variety of cell interactions. They have in common the presence of GAG chains and a protein core to which the chains are linked. Except for heparan sulfate and heparin, the chains are composed of disaccharides. The primary function of GAG chains is to act as adhesive molecules that can bond to cell surfaces and other matrix molecules.

Fibronectin is a major surface glycoprotein that, together with collagen, forms an integrated fibrillary network that influences adhesion, motility, growth, and differentiation of cells. Laminin, an important component of basement membranes, binds to type IV collagen and cell surface receptors.[118] Tenascin is another substrate adhesion glycoprotein.

In the pulp, the principal proteoglycans include hyaluronic acid dermatan sulfate, heparan sulfate, and chondroitin sulfate.[130] The proteoglycan content of pulp tissue decreases approximately 50% with tooth eruption.[220] During active dentinogenesis, chondroitin sulfate is the principal proteoglycan, particularly in the odontoblast and predentin layer, where it is somehow involved with mineralization; with tooth eruption, hyaluronic acid and dermatan sulfate increase, and chondroitin sulfate decreases greatly.

The consistency of a connective tissue (e.g., the pulp) is largely determined by the proteoglycan components of the ground substance. The long GAG chains of the proteoglycan molecules form relatively rigid coils constituting a network that holds water, thus forming a characteristic gel. Hyaluronic acid in particular has a strong affinity for water and is a major component of ground substance in tissues with a large fluid content, such as Wharton's jelly of the umbilical cord. The water content of the young pulp is very high (approximately 90%), so the ground substance forms a cushion capable of protecting cells and vascular components of the tooth.

Ground substance also acts as a molecular sieve in that it excludes large proteins. Cell metabolites, nutrients, and wastes pass through the ground substance between cells and blood vessels. In some ways, ground substance can be likened to an ion exchange resin, because the polyanionic chains of the GAGs bind cations. In addition, osmotic pressures can be altered by excluding osmotically active molecules. Thus, proteoglycans can regulate the dispersion of interstitial matrix solutes, colloids, and water, and (in large measure) they determine the physical characteristics of a tissue, such as the pulp.

Degradation of ground substance can occur in certain inflammatory lesions that have a high concentration of macrophage lysosomal enzymes. Proteolytic enzymes, hyaluronidases, and chondroitin sulfatases of lysosomal and bacterial origin are examples of the hydrolytic enzymes that can attack components of the ground substance. The pathways of inflammation and infection are strongly influenced by the state of polymerization of the ground substance components.

Hyaluronan

Another major structural component of the interstitial matrix is hyaluronan. It is an unbranched, random-coil molecule from repeating nonsulfated disaccharide units and is found in the interstitium as free molecules or bound to cells, possibly via the connection to fibronectin.[205] Its large molecular weight together with its protein structure accounts for its unique properties. It has a high viscosity even at low concentration, exhibits exclusion properties, and has a strong affinity for water.

Hyaluronan is one of several types of GAGs in the pulp.[219,237] The hyaluronan receptor-1 is expressed on lymphatic vessels and also on immune cells in the dental pulp.[19] Hyaluronan is removed from the tissue by the lymphatics and metabolized in the lymph nodes[101] and by endothelial cells in the liver.[134,298]

Elastic Fibers

Elastic fibers constitute an elastin core and a surrounding microfibrillar network and provide elasticity to the tissue.[289] The amount of elastin in the interstitial matrix in most tissue is small. There is no evidence for elastic fibers in the matrix in the pulp.[134,298]

The Inflamed Interstitium

Hyaluronidases, and chondroitin sulfatases of lysosomal and bacterial origin, are examples of the hydrolytic enzymes that can attack components of the interstitium. During infection and inflammation, the physical properties of the pulp tissue may then be altered due to production of such degrading enzymes.[145,318] In addition to their own damaging effect, they may also pave the way for the deleterious effects of bacterial toxins, increasing the magnitude of the damage.[177]

The pathways of inflammation and infection are strongly influenced by the particular composition of the interstitium in every tissue and its degradation by either host or microbial enzymes.

CONNECTIVE TISSUE FIBERS OF THE PULP

Two types of structural proteins are found in the pulp: collagen and elastin. Elastin fibers are confined to the walls of arterioles and, unlike collagen, are not a part of the ECM.

A single collagen molecule, referred to as *tropocollagen*, consists of three polypeptide chains, designated as either alpha-1 or alpha-2 depending on their amino acid composition and sequence. In the human pulp, the amount of collagen is reported to be 26% to 32% of dry weight in premolars and molars.[378] Type I and type III collagen represent the major subtypes of collagen in the pulp, and type I is found in thick striated fibrils throughout the pulp tissue.[206,336] The different combinations and linkages of chains making up the tropocollagen molecule have allowed collagen fibers and fibrils to be classified into a number of types:

- Type I collagen is found in skin, tendon, bone, dentin, and pulp.
- Type II collagen is found in cartilage.
- Type III collagen is found in most unmineralized connective tissues. It is a fetal form found in the dental papilla and the mature pulp. In bovine pulp, it constitutes 45% of the total pulp collagen during all stages of development.[378]
- Types IV and VII collagen are components of basement membranes.
- Type V collagen is a constituent of interstitial tissues.
- Type VI collagen is a heterotrimer of three distinct chains, alpha 2 (VI) and alpha 3 (VI), and is widely distributed in low concentrations in soft tissues at interfibrillar filaments.

Type I collagen is synthesized by odontoblasts and osteoblasts; fibroblasts synthesize types I, III, V, and VII collagen.

In collagen synthesis, the protein portion of the molecule is formed by the polyribosomes of the RER of connective tissue cells. The proline and lysine residues of the polypeptide chains are hydroxylated in the cisternae of the RER, and the chains are assembled into a triple-helix configuration in the smooth endoplasmic reticulum. The product of this assembly is termed *procollagen*, and it has a terminal unit of amino acids known as the *telopeptide of the procollagen molecule.* When these molecules reach the Golgi complex, they are glycosylated and packaged in secretory vesicles. The vesicles are transported to the plasma membrane and secreted by way of exocytosis into the extracellular milieu, thus releasing the procollagen. Here the terminal telopeptide is cleaved by a hydrolytic enzyme, and the tropocollagen molecules begin aggregating to form collagen fibrils. It is believed that the GAGs somehow mediate aggregation of tropocollagen. The conversion of soluble collagen into

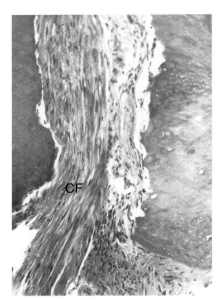

FIG. 12-14 Dense bundles of collagen fibers (CF) in the apical pulp.

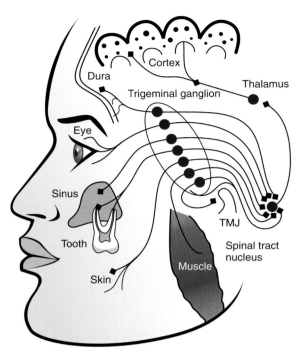

FIG. 12-15 Schematic drawing illustrating the convergence of sensory information from teeth to higher brain centers.

insoluble fibers occurs as a result of cross-linking of tropocollagen molecules. The presence of collagen fibers passing from the dentin matrix between odontoblasts into the dental pulp has been reported in fully erupted teeth.[28] Larger collagen fiber bundles are much more numerous in the radicular pulp than in the coronal pulp. The highest concentration of these larger fiber bundles is usually found near the apex (Fig. 12-14). Pulpectomy procedures should engage the pulp with a barbed broach in the region of the apex, as it generally affords the best opportunity to remove this tissue intact.[366]

THE TRIGEMINAL SYSTEM

Innervation

Pain is a subjective phenomenon involving not only sensory physiologic responses, but also emotional, conceptual, and motivational aspects of behavior. The existence of peripheral "nociceptive" (pain-detecting) sensory neurons forms the basis for pain, and pain sensations of varying qualities and intensities are evoked by activation of the intradental nerves innervating teeth. Noxious stimuli in teeth are transmitted in primary afferent neurons located in the trigeminal ganglion via second-order neurons in the brain stem to the brain (Fig. 12-15; see also Chapter 17 and later in this chapter). Transmission of sensory information consists of a cascade of events involving input, processing, and sensing,[329] so the control of dental pain should be based on an understanding of the origin of pain signals and the complex modulation that may take place locally and at higher levels. The sensory system of the pulp appears to be well suited for signaling potential damage to the tooth. The tooth is innervated by a large number of myelinated and unmyelinated axons. The number of axons entering a human premolar may reach 2000 or more, and each axon can arborize to form multiple points of innervation.[90,170,169]

Regardless of the nature of the sensory stimulus (i.e., thermal, mechanical, chemical, electric [e.g., pulp tester]), almost all afferent impulses generated from pulp tissue result in the sensation of pain. However, when the pulp is weakly stimulated by an electric pulp tester under carefully controlled experimental conditions, a nonpainful sensation (i.e., prepain) has been reported.[247] Thus, not all afferent neurons that innervate the pulp are nociceptors. The innervation of the pulp includes both *afferent neurons*, which conduct sensory impulses, and *autonomic or efferent neurons*,[163] which provide neurogenic modulation of the microcirculation, inflammatory reactions,[148] and perhaps regulate dentinogenesis.[46]

The sympathetic innervation of teeth derives from the superior cervical ganglion (SCG).[8,301] Postganglionic sympathetic nerves travel with the internal carotid nerve, join the trigeminal nerve at the ganglion, and supply teeth and supporting structures via the maxillary and mandibular division of the trigeminal nerve.[239] Sympathetic fibers appear with blood vessels at the time the vascular system is established in the dental papilla.[104] In the adult tooth pulp, sympathetic fibers form plexuses, usually around pulpal arterioles (Fig. 12-16). Stimulation of these fibers results in constriction of the arterioles and a decrease in blood flow.[1,82] The sympathetic neuron terminals contain the classic neurotransmitter, norepinephrine (NE), and neuropeptide Y (NPY) (see Neuropeptides later in this chapter). NPY is synthesized in sympathetic neurons and supplied to terminals by axonal transport. By contrast, NE is mainly produced locally in the terminals. Compared with the sensory nerves, these fibers are most often located in deeper parts of the pulp proper, but fibers have also been found in close relation to odontoblasts.[1,164]

The presence of parasympathetic cholinergic nerves in dental tissues has been and is still controversial, although it has been concluded that there is absence of parasympathetic vasodilation in the cat dental pulp.[286,323] It has been reported that the neuropeptide vasoactive intestinal polypeptide (VIP) is localized in the parasympathetic neurons.[225,226] The origin of VIP-containing fibers in the pulp is uncertain insofar as no form of surgical denervation has resulted in complete loss of these fibers from the dental pulp.[390]

Sensory nerve fibers are usually classified according to their diameter, conduction velocity, and function as shown in Table 12-1. The pulp contains two types of sensory nerve fibers: myelinated (A fibers) and unmyelinated (C fibers). It has been shown that there is some functional overlap between pulpal A and C fibers, as both fiber types can be nociceptors.[163,169,170,246,267] The A fibers include both A-beta and A-delta fibers. The A-beta fibers may be slightly more sensitive to stimulation than the A-delta fibers, but functionally these fibers are grouped together in the dental pulp, because both innervate the dentinal tubules, and both are stimulated by dentinal fluid movement (Fig. 12-17). Approximately 90% of the A fibers in dental pulp are A-delta fibers.[246] Table 12-2 summarizes the principal characteristics of the main sensory fibers.

During the bell stage of tooth development, "pioneer" nerve fibers enter the dental papilla following the path of blood vessels.[104] Although only unmyelinated fibers are observed in the dental papilla, a proportion of these fibers are probably A fibers that have lost or not developed their myelin sheath. Myelinated fibers are the last major structures to appear in the developing human dental pulp.[11] The number of nerve fibers gradually increases, and branching occurs as the fibers approach dentin. During the bell stage, very few fibers enter the predentin.[104]

The sensory nerves of the pulp arise from the trigeminal nerve and pass into the radicular pulp in bundles by way of

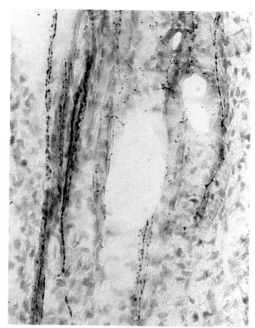

FIG. 12-16 Histologic section, immunohistologically stained for neuropeptide Y (NPY), shows the distribution of sympathetic nerves in the root pulp of a rat molar. NPY fibers are seen associated with blood vessels. (Courtesy Dr. Inge Fristad, Department of Clinical Dentistry, University of Bergen.)

TABLE 12-1

Classification of Nerve Fibers

Type of Fiber	Function	Diameter (µm)	Conduction Velocity (m/sec)
A-alpha	Motor, proprioception	12-20	70-120
A-beta	Pressure, touch	5-12	30-70
A-gamma	Motor, to muscle spindles	3-6	15-30
A-delta	Pain, temperature, touch	1-5	6-30
B	Preganglionic autonomic	< 3	3-15
C dorsal root	Pain	0.4-1	0.5-2
Sympathetic	Postganglionic sympathetic	0.3-1.3	0.7-2.3

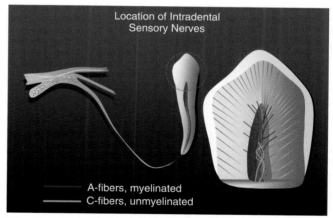

FIG. 12-17 Schematic drawing illustrating the location of A and C fibers in the dental pulp. Myelinated A fibers are located in the periphery of the pulp, penetrating the inner part of dentin. Unmyelinated C fibers are located in the deeper part of the pulp proper.

TABLE 12-2

Characteristics of Sensory Fibers

Fiber	Myelination	Location of Terminals	Pain Characteristics	Stimulation Threshold
A-delta	Yes	Principally in region of pulp-dentin junction	Sharp, pricking	Relatively low
C	No	Probably distributed throughout pulp	Burning, aching, less bearable than A-delta fiber sensations	Relatively high, usually associated with tissue injury

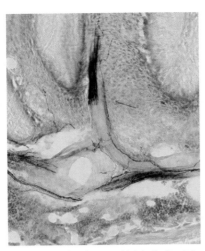

FIG. 12-18 Histologic section, immunohistologically stained for calcitonin gene-related peptide (CGRP), shows distribution of sensory nerves in the apical area of a rat molar. Nerve fibers are seen associated with blood vessels and enter the dental pulp in nerve bundles. (Courtesy Dr. Inge Fristad, Department of Clinical Dentistry, University of Bergen.)

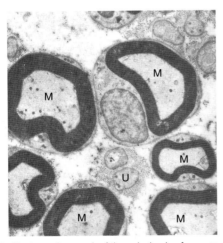

FIG. 12-19 Electron micrograph of the apical pulp of a young canine tooth, showing in cross section myelinated nerve axons (M) within Schwann cells. Smaller, unmyelinated axons (U) are enclosed singly and in groups by Schwann cells. (Courtesy Dr. David C. Johnsen, School of Dentistry, Case Western Reserve University.)

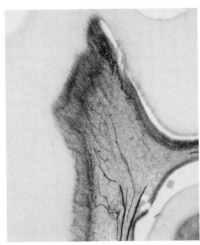

FIG. 12-20 Histologic section, immunohistologically stained for calcitonin gene-related peptide (CGRP), shows the distribution of sensory nerves in a rat molar. Nerves enter the coronal pulp in bundles and ramify in a network beneath the odontoblasts (i.e., plexus of Raschkow), before entering between the odontoblasts and the inner part of dentin.

patients have difficulty identifying the inflamed tooth until the inflammation reaches the periradicular tissue, which is highly innervated with proprioceptors. This is discussed in greater detail in Chapter 17.

In the human premolar, the number of unmyelinated axons entering the tooth at the apex reached a maximal number shortly after tooth eruption.[170] At this stage, an average of 1800 unmyelinated axons and more than 400 myelinated axons were found, although in some teeth fewer than 100 myelinated axons were present. Five years after eruption, the number of A fibers gradually increased to more than 700. The relatively late appearance of A fibers in the pulp may help to explain why the electric pulp test tends to be unreliable in young teeth, as A fibers are more easily electrically stimulated than C fibers.[108]

A quantitative study of axons 1 to 2 mm coronal to the root apex of fully developed human canine and incisor teeth[170] reported a mean of about 360 myelinated axons in canines and incisors, whereas there were 1600 to 2200 unmyelinated axons. However, this does not reflect the actual number of neurons supporting a single tooth, because multiple branching of the axons may occur in the peripheral tissues. Overall, approximately 80% of the axons were unmyelinated fibers.[169,170]

The nerve bundles pass upward through the radicular pulp together with blood vessels (see Fig. 12-18). Once they reach the coronal pulp, they fan out beneath the cell-rich zone, branch into smaller bundles, and finally ramify into a plexus of single-nerve axons known as the *plexus of Raschkow* (Fig. 12-20). Full development of this plexus does not occur until the final stages of root formation.[90] It has been estimated that each axon entering the pulp sends at least eight branches to the plexus of Raschkow. There is prolific branching of the fibers in the plexus, producing a tremendous overlap of receptor fields.[143,267,268,269,273] It is in the plexus that the A fibers emerge from their encircling Schwann cells and branch repeatedly to form the subodontoblastic plexus. Finally, terminal axons pass between the odontoblasts as free nerve endings (Figs. 12-21 and 12-22). The extent to which dentin is innervated has been the subject of numerous investigations.[42,45,46,49,90,215] With the exception of the innervation of

the foramen in close association with arterioles and venules (Fig. 12-18). Each of the nerves entering the pulp is invested within Schwann cells, and the A fibers acquire their myelin sheath from these cells. With the completion of root development, the myelinated fibers appear grouped in bundles in the central region of the pulp (Fig. 12-19). Most of the unmyelinated C fibers entering the pulp are located within these fiber bundles; the remainder is situated toward the periphery of the pulp (see Fig. 12-17).[307] It should be noted that single neurons have been reported to innervate the pulps of multiple teeth in animal studies.[155] Assuming a similar innervation pattern in humans, this finding may partially explain why patients often have difficulty localizing pulpal pain to a specific tooth. An alternative explanation to this clinical observation is that the pulp has a relatively low density of proprioceptors, and thus

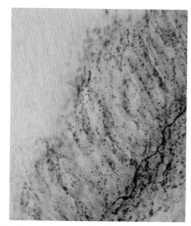

FIG. 12-21 Detailed histologic section, immunohistologically stained for calcitonin gene-related peptide (CGRP), shows the distribution of sensory nerves in the odontoblast layer of a rat molar. (Courtesy Dr. Inge Fristad, Department of Clinical Dentistry, University of Bergen.)

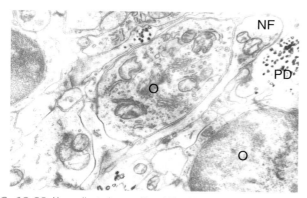

FIG. 12-22 Unmyelinated nerve fiber (NF) without a Schwann cell covering located between adjacent odontoblasts (O) overlying pulp horn of a mouse molar tooth. Predentin (PD) can be seen at upper right. Within the nerve, there are longitudinally oriented fine neurofilaments, microvesicles, and mitochondria. (From Corpron RE, Avery JK: The ultrastructure of intradental nerves in developing mouse molars, *Anat Rec* 175:585, 1973.)

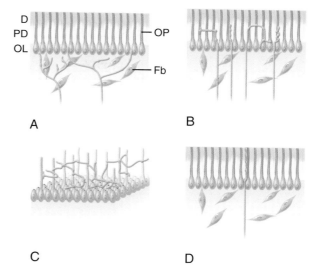

FIG. 12-23 Schematic drawing showing distribution of nerve fibers in the dentin-pulp border zone. **A,** Fibers running from the subodontoblastic plexus to the odontoblast layer. *D,* dentin; *Fb,* fibroblast; *OL,* odontoblast layer; *OP,* odontoblast process; *PD,* predentin. **B,** Fibers extending into the dentinal tubules in the predentin. **C,** Complex fibers that branch extensively in the predentin. **D,** Intratubular fibers extending into the dentin.

dentinal tubules, discussed later in this chapter, the bulk of dentin is devoid of sensory nerve fibers. This offers an explanation as to why pain-producing agents (e.g., potassium chloride) do not always elicit pain when applied to exposed dentin. Similarly, application of topical anesthetic solutions to dentin does not decrease its sensitivity. A high concentration of lidocaine solution is needed to block the response of intradental nerves to mechanical stimulation of the dentin.[4]

One investigator[131] studied the distribution and organization of nerve fibers in the dentin-pulp border zone of human teeth. On the basis of their location and pattern of branching, several types of nerve endings were described (Fig. 12-23). Some fibers were found running from the subodontoblastic nerve plexus toward the odontoblast layer. However, these fibers do not reach the predentin; they terminate in extracellular spaces in the cell-rich zone, the cell-poor zone, or the odontoblast layer. Other fibers extend into the predentin and run through a dentinal tubule in close association with an odontoblast process. Most of these intratubular fibers extend

into the dentinal tubules for only a few micrometers, but a few may penetrate as far as 100 µm (see Fig. 12-20). The area covered by a single such terminal complex often reaches thousands of square micrometers.[131,268]

Intratubular nerve endings are most numerous in the area of the pulp horns, where as many as 40% of the tubules may contain fibers.[46,215] The number of intratubular fibers decreases in other parts of the dentin, and in root dentin only about 1% of dentinal tubules contain fibers. This notion has been challenged in a study that stained pulps for protein gene-product 9.5, a specific marker for nerves.[230] In that study, root dentin appeared to be as well innervated as coronal dentin. The anatomic relationship between the odontoblast processes and sensory nerve endings has led to much speculation as to the functional relationships between these structures, if any.[45] When present, nerve fibers lie in a groove or gutter along the surface of the odontoblast process, and toward their terminal ends, they twist around the process like a corkscrew. The cell membranes of the odontoblast process and the nerve fiber are closely approximated and run closely parallel for the length of their proximity, but they are not synaptically linked.[160]

Although it may be tempting to speculate that the odontoblasts and their associated nerve axons are functionally interrelated and that together they play a role in dentin sensitivity, there is a paucity of evidence supporting this hypothesis. If the odontoblast were acting as a classic receptor cell,* it would have chemical, electric, or mechanical communication with the adjacent nerve fiber. However, researchers have been unable to find classical anatomic structures (e.g., synaptic junctions) that could functionally couple odontoblasts and

*A receptor cell is a non–nerve cell capable of exciting adjacent afferent nerve fibers. Synaptic junctions connect receptor cells to afferent nerves.

nerve fibers together. With regard to the membrane properties of odontoblasts, it has been reported that the membrane potential of the odontoblast is low (−24 to −30 mV),[198,227] and that the cell does not respond to electric stimulation.[198,406] It would appear that the odontoblast does not possess the properties of an excitable cell. Further, the sensitivity of dentin is not diminished after disruption of the odontoblast layer.[37,216] It is still possible that odontoblasts could modulate neuronal function via alteration in sodium channel activity or the release of paracrine factors that diffuse to the closely approximated nerve terminal.

Another study showed that a reduction in pulpal blood flow, induced by stimulation of sympathetic fibers leading to the pulp, results in depressed excitability of pulpal A fibers.[82] The excitability of C fibers is less affected than that of A fibers by a reduction in blood flow.[365]

Of clinical interest is the evidence that nerve fibers of the pulp may be resistant to necrosis[85,255] because their cell bodies are found in ganglia outside the pulp. Because nerve bundles in general are more resistant to autolysis than other tissue elements, even in degenerating pulps, C fibers might still be able to respond to noxious stimulation. It may be that C fibers remain excitable even after blood flow has been compromised in the diseased pulp, as C fibers are often able to function in the presence of hypoxia.[365] This may explain why instrumentation of the root canals of apparently nonvital teeth sometimes elicits pain. On the other hand, histologic studies on nonvital teeth failed to demonstrate high levels of innervation, leading to the suggestion that pain may be due to the transfer of noxious chemicals to terminals located in periapical tissues.[255]

Steps and Mechanisms in Pain Perception

When activated by a stimulus sufficient to cause tissue damage or release of inflammatory mediators, nerve endings in the pulp and periradicular tissues begin to send bursts of messages to the central nervous system (CNS) that may eventually be perceived as pain. The anatomic pathway for this transmission of information has been fairly well established, and it is tempting to view the perception of pain of orofacial origin as a simple graded response to the intensity of the stimulus. However, researchers have come to realize that the pain system is a complex, multilevel system that begins with the *detection* of tissue-damaging stimuli in the periphery, the *processing* of that input at the level of the medullary spinal cord, and the *perception* of what is felt as pain in higher brain regions such as the cerebral cortex (Fig. 12-24). After a noxious stimulus is detected in the periphery, there is ample opportunity for a great deal of endogenous and possibly exogenous modification of the message prior to its ultimate perception. The clinician deals with all three levels of the pain system in diagnosing and treating odontalgia, and a practitioner with a basic understanding of each level will be able to recognize therapeutic opportunities and apply effective pain control methods.

Detection: The First Step in Pain Perception

Various types of peripheral neurons are found in the trigeminal system, including large-diameter, heavily myelinated Aα, Aβ, and Aγ fibers associated with motor, proprioception, touch, pressure, and muscle spindle stretch functions. But it is the

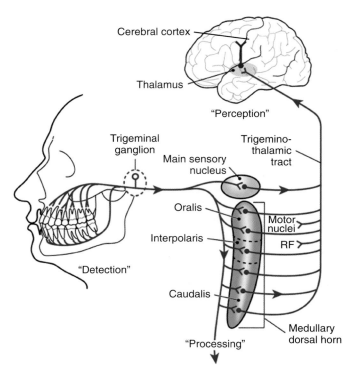

FIG. 12-24 Schematic diagram of the pathway of transmission of nociceptive information from the orofacial region. The trigeminal pain system is a complex multilevel system that begins with the *detection* of tissue damaging stimuli in the periphery, the *processing* of that input at the level of the medullary spinal cord, and the final *perception* of what is felt as pain in the cerebral cortex. There is growing appreciation for the concept that once a noxious stimulus is detected in the periphery, there is the opportunity for a great deal of modification of the message prior to ultimate perception.

smaller, less myelinated Aδ and yet smaller and unmyelinated C fibers that conduct information likely to be perceived as pain. These two classes of pain-sensing nerve fibers, or *nociceptors*, are both found in the tooth pulp, but there are three to eight times more unmyelinated C fibers than Aδ fibers.[41,45,170,371] It should be noted that this classification system is based purely on the size and myelination of the neurons and does not necessarily indicate function. For example, another class of pulpal C fibers are the postganglionic sympathetic efferents found in association with blood vessels, where they regulate pulpal blood flow[2,187,299,300] and may also influence the activity of peripheral nociceptors (for reviews, see Perl[296] or Hargreaves[137]). Because most pulpal sensory fibers are nociceptive, their terminal branches are free nerve endings, and physiologic stimulation by any modality (temperature, hyperosmotic fluids) results in the perception of pure pain, which can be difficult for patients to localize. Under experimental conditions, electrical stimulation can result in a *prepain* sensation that is also difficult to localize. Once inflammation has extended to the periodontal ligament, which is well endowed with Aβ discriminative touch receptors, localization of pain is more predictable with light mechanical stimuli such as the percussion test.

In the normal uninflamed pulp and periradicular tissues, a noxious stimulus causes depolarization of nociceptors sufficient to generate action potentials by means of the opening of voltage-gated sodium channels (Na_v). After generation of an action potential, not only is information sent to the CNS, but also in an *antidromic* fashion (i.e., in the reverse direction of the impulse) in which proinflammatory neuropeptides such as substance P (SP), calcitonin gene-related peptide (CGRP), neurokinins, and the classic neurotransmitter, glutamate, are released from afferent terminals in the pulp and periradicular tissues.

Neuropeptides

Of immense importance in pulp biology is the presence of neuropeptides in pulpal nerves.[42,46,49,349] Pulpal nerve fibers contain neuropeptides such as calcitonin gene–related peptide (CGRP) (see Figs. 12-18, 12-20, and 12-21),[41] substance P (SP),[268,285] neuropeptide Y (see Fig. 12-16), neurokinin A (NKA),[12] and VIP.[228,389] In rat molars, the largest group of intradental sensory fibers contains CGRP. Some of these fibers also contain other peptides, such as SP and NKA.[42,45] Release of these peptides can be triggered by numerous stimuli, including tissue injury,[12] complement activation, antigen-antibody reactions,[280] or antidromic stimulation of the inferior alveolar nerve.[285,282] Once released, vasoactive peptides produce vascular changes that are similar to those evoked by histamine and bradykinin (i.e., vasodilation).[282] In addition to their neurovascular properties, SP and CGRP contribute to inflammation and promote wound healing.[31,369] The release of CGRP can be modified by sympathetic agonists and antagonists,[115,138] offering the promise of using such agonists to treat dental pain. This latter point is important because clinicians use sympathetic agonists every day—the vasoconstrictors present in local anesthetic solutions may have direct effects on inhibiting dental nerve activity. Local anesthetic reduction in pain may be due to the actions of both the local anesthetic and the vasoconstrictor.[137,138] In cats, capsaicin acutely activates and chronically blocks the TRPV1-expressing classes of C and A-delta nociceptors in the pulp.[163] In addition, the chronic application of capsaicin ointment to skin has been shown to relieve pain in patients, suggesting that clinical trials evaluating chronic application of capsaicin for treating pulpal or periradicular pain may be of value.

Antidromic stimulation of nerves (i.e., toward the peripheral terminals) simply means that the afferent barrage goes in the opposite direction of the orthograde stimulation (toward the CNS). Normally, sensory nerves are stimulated at their peripheral terminations, and their action potentials then travel toward the brain. In antidromic nerve stimulation, the sensory nerve is usually cut. The peripheral end of the nerve is then electrically stimulated. This causes an action potential to travel backward toward the periphery, which causes release of neuropeptides in the pulp.[285] All branches of the nerve also depolarize and release neuropeptides (the so-called axon reflex).[322]

It has been reported[246,285] that mechanical stimulation of dentin produces vasodilation within the pulp, presumably by causing the release of neuropeptides from intradental sensory fibers (neurogenic inflammation).[285] Electric stimulation of the tooth has a similar effect.[152] The pulpal concentrations of CGRP, SP, and NKA are elevated in painful human teeth over healthy control teeth extracted for orthodontic reasons.[12] These peptides are also elevated in pulps beneath advancing carious lesions.[310,311]

Pulp Testing

The electric pulp tester delivers a current sufficient to overcome the resistance of enamel and dentin and stimulate the sensory A fibers at the dentin-pulp border zone. Smaller C fibers of the pulp do not respond to the conventional pulp tester because significantly more current is needed to stimulate them.[267] Bender and associates[17] found that in anterior teeth, the optimal placement site of the electrode is the incisal edge, as the response threshold is lowest at that location and increases as the electrode is moved toward the cervical region of the tooth.

Cold tests using carbon dioxide (CO_2) snow or liquid refrigerants and heat tests employing heated gutta-percha or hot water activate hydrodynamic forces within the dentinal tubules, which in turn excite the intradental A fibers. C fibers are generally not activated by these tests unless they produce injury to the pulp. It has been shown that cold tests do not injure the pulp.[108] Heat tests have a greater potential to produce injury, but if the tests are used properly, injury is not likely.

Sensitivity of Dentin

The mechanisms underlying dentin sensitivity have been a subject of interest for many years. How are stimuli relayed from the peripheral dentin to the sensory terminals located in the region of the dentin-pulp border zone? Converging evidence indicates that movement of fluid in the dentinal tubules is the basic event in the arousal of dentinal pain.[35,37,263,385,387] It now appears that pain-producing stimuli, such as heat, cold, air blasts, and probing with the tip of an explorer, have in common the ability to displace fluid in the tubules.[35,246] This is referred to as the *hydrodynamic mechanism of dentin sensitivity*. The hydrodynamic theory suggests that dentinal pain associated with stimulation of a sensitive tooth ultimately involves mechanotransduction. Classical mechanotransducers have been recognized on pulpal afferents, providing a mechanistic support to this theory.[149] Thus, fluid movement in the dentinal tubules is translated into electric signals by receptors located in the axon terminals innervating dentinal tubules. Using single-fiber recording techniques, a positive correlation was found between the degree of pressure change and the number of nerve impulses leaving the pulp (Figs. 12-25 and 12-26).[246,266,384] Thus, the outward fluid movements (negative pressure) produce a much stronger nerve response than inward movements.[246,388]

In experiments on humans, brief application of heat or cold to the outer surface of premolar teeth evoked a painful response before the heat or cold could have produced temperature changes capable of activating sensory receptors in the underlying pulp.[266,372] The evoked pain was of short duration: 1 or 2 seconds. The thermal diffusivity of dentin is relatively low, yet the response of the tooth to thermal stimulation is rapid, often less than 1 second. Evidence suggests that thermal stimulation of the tooth results in a rapid movement of fluid into the dentinal tubules. This results in activation of the sensory nerve terminal in the underlying pulp. Presumably, heat expands the fluid within the tubules faster than it expands dentin, causing the fluid to flow toward the pulp, whereas cold causes the fluid to contract more rapidly than dentin, producing an outward flow. It is speculated that the rapid movement of fluid across the cell membrane of the axon terminal activates a mechanosensitive receptor, similar to how fluid movement activates hair cells in the cochlea of the ear. All axon terminals have membrane channels through which charged ions pass, and this initial receptor current, if sufficient, can trigger voltage-gated sodium channels to depolarize the cell, leading

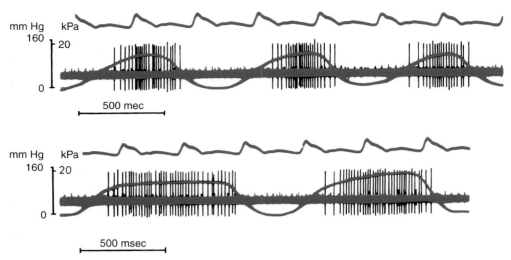

FIG. 12-25 Response of a single dog pulp nerve fiber to repeated hydrostatic pressure stimulation pulses. Lower solid wavy line of each recording indicates the stimulation pressure applied to the pulp. Upper line (kPa) is the femoral artery blood pressure curve recorded to indicate the relative changes in the pulse pressure and the heart cycle. (Modified from Närhi M: Activation of dental pulp nerves of the cat and the dog with hydrostatic pressure, *Proc Finn Dent Soc* 74[suppl 5]:1, 1978.)

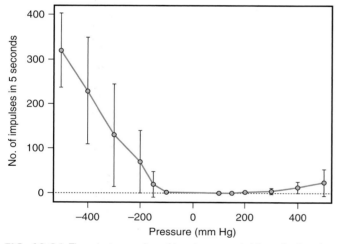

FIG. 12-26 The average number of impulses recorded from dentine after application of pressure stimuli to the dentine. More impulses are recorded after application of negative pressure (outward fluid flow) than after positive pressure (inward fluid flow). (From Vongsavan N, Matthews B: The relationship between the discharge of intradental nerves and the rate of fluid flow through dentine in the cat, *Arch Oral Biol.* 52:643, 2007.)

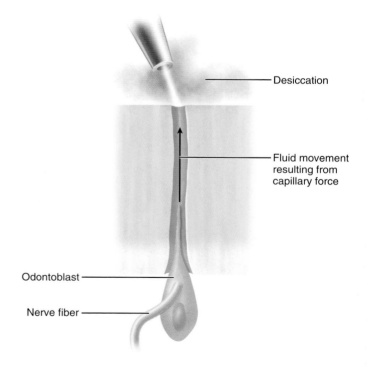

FIG. 12-27 Diagram illustrating movement of fluid in the dentinal tubules resulting from the dehydrating effect of a blast of air from an air syringe.

to a barrage of impulses to the brain. Some ion channels are activated by voltage, some by chemicals, and some by mechanical pressure.[246,263,268] In the case of pulpal nerve fibers that are activated by hydrodynamic forces, pressure would be transduced, gating mechanosensitive ion channels.

The dentinal tubule is a capillary tube with an exceedingly small diameter.*[111] The physical properties of capillarity are significant because fluid force increases as the diameter is

reduced. If fluid is removed from the outer end of exposed dentinal tubules by dehydrating the dentinal surface with an air blast or absorbent paper, capillary forces produce a rapid outward movement of fluid in the tubule (Fig. 12-27). According to Brännström,[35] desiccation of dentin can theoretically cause dentinal fluid to flow outward at a rate of 2 to 3 mm/sec. In addition to air blasts, dehydrating solutions containing hyperosmotic concentrations of sucrose or calcium chloride can produce pain if applied to exposed dentin.

---

*To appreciate fully the dimensions of dentin tubules, understand that the diameter of the tubules (about 1 μm) is much smaller than that of red blood cells (about 7 μm). The thickness of coronal dentin is about 3 mm, so each tubule is 3000 μm long but only 1 μm in diameter. Thus, each tubule is 3000 diameters long.

Investigators have shown that it is the A fibers rather than the C fibers that are activated by hydrodynamic stimuli (e.g., heat, cold, air blasts) applied to exposed dentin.[265,273] However, if heat is applied long enough to increase the temperature of the dentin-pulp border by several degrees Celsius, then C fibers may respond, particularly if the heat produces injury. It seems that the A fibers are mainly activated by a rapid displacement of the tubular contents.[263] Slow heating of the tooth produced no response until the temperature reached 111° F (43.8° C), at which time C fibers were activated, presumably because of heat-induced injury to the pulp. These C fibers are called *polymodal nociceptors* because they contain numerous receptors that confer the ability to detect and respond to many different types of stimuli.[268,269] Capsaicin, the pungent active ingredient in hot peppers, is known to simulate C fibers and a subset of A-delta fibers.[163] Capsaicin activates a receptor termed the "transient receptor potential, subtype vanilloid 1" or TRPV1.[58] The TRPV1 receptor is expressed primarily on a major subclass of nociceptors and responds to heat (> 110° F [> 43° C]), certain inflammatory mediators, and acid (pH < 6). Thus TRPV1 has been considered a molecular integrator of polymodal noxious stimuli.[277] The ability of the TRPV1 antagonist, capsazepine, to inhibit acid-, heat-, and capsaicin-activated trigeminal neurons[222] has led to the development of new drugs (i.e., TRPV1 antagonists) for the treatment of pulpal pain. Eugenol is known to activate and ultimately desensitize TRPV1, and this may explain the anodyne action of zinc oxide eugenol temporary restorations.[415]

It has also been shown that pain-producing stimuli are more readily transmitted from the dentin surface when the exposed tubule apertures are open[157,171] and the fluid within the tubules is free to flow outward.[171,246,387] For example, acid treatment of exposed dentin to remove the smear layer opens the tubule orifices and makes the dentin much more responsive to stimuli such as air blasts and probing.[157,269]

Perhaps the most difficult phenomenon to explain is dentinal pain associated with light probing of dentin. Even light pressure of an explorer tip can produce strong forces.* These forces have been shown to mechanically compress dentin and close open tubule orifices with a smear layer that causes sufficient displacement of fluid to excite the sensory receptors in the underlying pulp (Fig. 12-28).[54,55] Considering the density of the tubules in which hydrodynamic forces would be generated by probing, multiple nerve endings would be simultaneously stimulated when a dental explorer is scratched across dentin. Another newly suggested explanation is that the nerves innervating teeth are special in nature and that low-threshold mechanoreceptors are signaling nociceptive input in teeth.[103] Similar low-threshold mechanoreceptors convey tactile sensation in skin. The authors used the term low-threshold "algoneurons" for these nerves. This theory is not in conflict with the hydrodynamic theory but may help to explain the sensation of pain felt after weak mechanical stimuli like air puffs and water spray.

Another example of the effect of strong hydraulic forces that are created within the dentinal tubules is the phenomenon of odontoblast displacement. In this reaction, the nuclei and cell

*A force of 44 cM (44 g) applied to an explorer having a tip 40 µm in diameter would produce a pressure of 2437 MPa on the dentin.[54] This is far in excess of the compressive strength of dentin, listed as 245MPa, as evidenced by the shallow grooves lined by smear layers created in dentin using this force.[55]

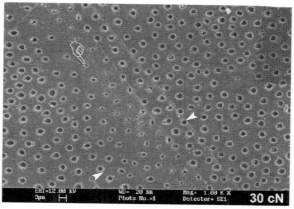

FIG. 12-28 Scanning electron micrograph of a shallow groove *(between white arrowheads)* created in polished dentin by a dental explorer tine under a force of 30 g (30 cN). Note the partial occlusion of the tubules by smeared matrix. (From Camps J, Salomon JP, Meerbeek BV, et al: Dentin deformation after scratching with clinically relevant forces, *Arch Oral Biol* 48:527, 2003.)

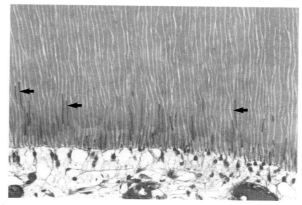

FIG. 12-29 Odontoblasts *(arrows)* displaced upward into the dentinal tubules.

bodies of odontoblasts are displaced upward in the dentinal tubules, presumably by a rapid movement of fluid in the tubules produced when exposed dentin is desiccated, as with the use of an air syringe or cavity-drying agents (Fig. 12-29).[79,202] Such cellular displacement results in the destruction of odontoblasts, because cells thus affected soon undergo autolysis and disappear from the tubules. Displaced odontoblasts may eventually be replaced by stem cells that migrate from the cell-rich zone of the pulp, as discussed later in the chapter.

The hydrodynamic theory can also be applied to an understanding of the mechanism responsible for hypersensitive dentin.[36,37] There is controversy regarding whether exposed dentin is simply sensitive or becomes truly hypersensitive.[268,269,273] Growing evidence indicates that new sodium channels responsible for activating nerves are expressed in nerve tissue exposed to inflammation.[119,137,308] An increase in the density of sodium channels or their sensitivity may contribute to dentinal hypersensitivity. Hypersensitive dentin is also associated with the exposure of dentin normally covered by cementum or enamel. The thin layer of cementum is frequently lost as gingival recession exposes cementum to the oral environment. Cementum is subsequently worn away by brushing, flossing, or using toothpicks. Once exposed, the dentin may respond to the same stimuli to which any exposed dentin surface responds (e.g., mechanical pressure, dehydrating agents). Although the dentin may at first be very sensitive, within a few weeks the sensitivity usually subsides. This desensitization is thought to occur as a result of gradual occlusion of the tubules by mineral deposits, thus reducing hydrodynamic forces. In addition, deposition of reparative dentin over the pulpal ends of the exposed tubules probably also reduces sensitivity, because reparative dentin is less innervated by sensory nerve fibers.[44] However, some hypersensitive dentin does not spontaneously desensitize, so hypersensitivity may be caused by either inflammatory changes in the pulp or mechanical changes in the patency of dentinal tubules.

Currently, the treatment of hypersensitive teeth is directed toward reducing the functional diameter of the dentinal tubules to limit fluid movement. Four possible treatment modalities[287,373,389] can accomplish this objective:

1. Formation of a smear layer on the sensitive dentin by burnishing the exposed root surface[157,268,269]
2. Application of agents, such as oxalate compounds, that form insoluble precipitates within the tubules[157,292]
3. Application of agents such as hydroxyethyl methacrylate (HEMA) with or without glutaraldehyde that are thought to occlude tubules with precipitated plasma proteins in dentinal fluid[325]
4. Application of dentin bonding agents to seal off the tubules[303]

Dentin sensitivity can be modified by laser irradiation, but clinicians must be concerned about its effect on the pulp.[346,357]

Peripheral Sensitization

Following repeated noxious stimuli, both A and polymodal C fiber nociceptors undergo a process of sensitization manifested by three obvious changes in response patterns. First, firing thresholds may decrease, so that previously non-noxious stimuli may trigger discharges, contributing to the sensation of pain (allodynia). Second, after-discharges may occur, so that noxious stimuli may produce an even greater increase in the perceived intensity of pain (hyperalgesia). And third, firing may occur spontaneously, contributing to the development of spontaneous pain. These changes are often seen in endodontic pain patients and may be explained in part by the effects of chemical mediators released into inflamed pulp and periradicular tissues. Such mediators include substances produced from damaged tissues, agents of vascular origin, and peptides released from the nerve fibers themselves (Table 12-3). Other mechanisms of peripheral sensitization are listed in Box 12-1.

Hyperalgesia and Allodynia

Three characteristics of hyperalgesia are (1) spontaneous pain, (2) a decreased pain threshold, and (3) an increased response to a painful stimulus.[137] The peripheral mechanisms for these symptoms include a decrease in firing threshold, an increase in responsiveness to noxious stimuli, and development of spontaneous discharges of nociceptors. All three of these characteristics can be seen in patients experiencing inflammatory pain of pulpal origin (Table 12-4). It is recognized that hyperalgesia can be produced by sustained inflammation, as in the case of sunburned skin. Clinical observation has shown that the sensitivity of dentin often increases when the underlying pulp becomes acutely inflamed, and the tooth may be more difficult to anesthetize. This is due in part to the upregulation of tetrodotoxin-resistant (TTX-resistant) sodium channels in

---

BOX 12-1

Peripheral Mechanisms Contributing to Hyperalgesia and Allodynia

Mechanism

- Composition and concentration of inflammatory mediators[142]
- Changes in afferent fiber: activation and sensitization[199,243,324]
- Changes in afferent fiber: sprouting[51]
- Changes in afferent fiber: proteins[51,119,409]
- Tissue pressure[264,265]
- Tissue temperature[250]
- Sympathetic primary afferent fiber interactions[166,210,295]
- Aβ fiber plasticity[272]

Modified from Hargreaves KM, Swift JQ, Roszkowski MT, et al: Pharmacology of peripheral neuropeptide and inflammatory mediator release, *Oral Surg Oral Med Oral Pathol* 78:503, 1994.

TABLE 12-3

Effect of Inflammatory Mediators on Nociceptive Afferent Fibers

Mediator	Effect on Nociceptors	Effect on Human Volunteers
Potassium[174]	Activate	++
Protons[218,343]	Activate	++
Serotonin[16,174]	Activate	++
Bradykinin[16,174,211]	Activate	+++
Histamine[174]	Activate	+
Tumor necrosis factor-α	Activate	?
Prostaglandins[27]	Sensitize	±
Leukotrienes[27,229]	Sensitize	±
Nerve growth factor[213,297]	Sensitize	++
Substance P[132]	Sensitize	±
Interleukin 1[99]	Sensitize (?)	?

+, Positive; ++, very positive; +++, extremely positive; ±, equivalent; ?, unknown.
Modified from Fields H: *Pain,* New York, 1987, McGraw-Hill.

TABLE 12-4

Signs of Hyperalgesia and Allodynia and Endodontic Diagnostic Tests

Signs of Hyperalgesia	Related Diagnostic Tests or Symptoms
Spontaneous pain	Spontaneous pain
Reduced pain threshold	Percussion test, palpation test, throbbing pain
Increased response to painful stimuli	Increased response to pulp test (electric or thermal test)

From Hargreaves KM, Swift JQ, Roszkowski MT, et al: Pharmacology of peripheral neuropeptide and inflammatory mediator release, *Oral Surg Oral Med Oral Pathol* 78:503, 1994.

inflamed neural tissue.[119,137] NGF seems to play an important role in hyperalgesia. NGF regulates chronic inflammatory hyperalgesia by controlling gene expression in sensory neurons,[274] including genes involved in inflammatory hyperalgesia in the dental pulp.[74] Although a precise explanation for hyperalgesia is lacking, apparently localized elevations in tissue pressure and inflammatory mediators that accompany acute inflammation play an important role.[151,154,344,362,379] Clinically, we know that when the pulp chamber of a painful tooth with an abscessed pulp is opened, drainage of exudate soon produces a reduction in the level of pain. This suggests that mechanical stimuli may contribute substantially to pain during inflammatory hyperalgesia.

From a clinical point of view, *thermal allodynia* is the term that best describes a patient whose chief complaint is "I have pain when I drink cold beverages." *Mechanical allodynia* is involved when the chief complaint is "It now hurts when I bite on this tooth." These previously non-noxious stimuli now cause the perception of pain. Hyperalgesia is manifested in endodontic pain patients when noxious stimuli (e.g., refrigerant sprays or carbon dioxide snow used in the cold test) produce much more pain than they would in teeth with normal pulp tissues. Spontaneous pain involves episodes of pain that seem to be unprovoked. All these changes can be partly explained by sensitization of peripheral nerve endings in the pulp and periradicular tissues.

Many silent nerve fibers are present in the normal pulp[268,269] and are termed *silent* because they are not excited by ordinary external stimuli. Once they are sensitized through pulpal inflammation, they begin to respond to hydrodynamic stimuli.[46,268,269,273] This phenomenon may provide an additional mechanism for dentin hypersensitivity. The molecular mechanisms of this activation are not known in detail but involve upregulation of numerous genes and their products.[12,45,119]

Inflammatory Mediators

Among the best characterized of the inflammatory mediators are the prostaglandins (PGs), which are derived from arachidonic acid via the action of the cyclooxygenase (COX) enzyme systems. The human COX enzyme is known to exist in at least two forms, COX-1 and COX-2. COX-1 is constitutively expressed and produces PGs that are involved in basic housekeeping functions such as cytoprotection in the stomach, regulation of blood flow in the kidneys, and the formation of thromboxane A_2. The formation of thromboxane A_2 can ultimately lead to platelet aggregation; therefore, inhibition of thromboxane A_2 should decrease platelet aggregation. COX-2 is inducible, synthesized in inflamed tissues (including dental pulp),[262] and is important in the production of the proinflammatory PGs as well as the vasodilating prostacyclin (PGI_2). Although they do not produce pain if applied alone, PGs are known to sensitize peripheral nociceptors, which increases the algogenic (pain-producing) properties of serotonin and bradykinin.[76,124] The exact mechanism by which PGs increase neuronal excitability is not clear, but there is a growing body of evidence to suggest that they activate the PG E receptor subtypes EP2 and EP3 in the trigeminal system[293] and exert their effects by regulating the activity of certain ion channels,[394] including voltage-gated sodium channels (for a review, see England[86]). For example, application of prostaglandin E_2 (PGE_2) to isolated dorsal root ganglion neuronal somata more than doubles the responsiveness of certain sodium channels

found predominantly on nociceptors—channels thought to be relatively resistant to lidocaine.[9,120] When administered to rats before an inflammatory insult, ibuprofen, a nonselective COX inhibitor, has been shown to block the increased expression of $Na_v1.7$ and $Na_v1.8$.[127,128] Therefore, if the concentrations of PGs in inflamed pulp and periradicular tissues can be decreased with nonsteroidal antiinflammatory drugs (NSAIDs) or corticosteroids, postoperative pain may be relieved; in addition, more profound local anesthesia may be achieved in patients with hyperalgesia of pulpal origin.[140,161,254] It is interesting to note that sensory neurons themselves are a source of PGs; during inflammation, the levels of PGE_2 appear to increase in dorsal root ganglia and spinal cord, suggesting that NSAIDs also have a central site of action (discussed in Chapter 4).[235,405]

Bradykinin (BK) is a proinflammatory mediator derived from circulating plasma proteins and also causes direct activation of nociceptive neurons, resulting in pain. Increased levels of BK have been demonstrated in the inflamed dental pulp,[207] and the presence of growth factors associated with inflammation (e.g., nerve growth factor) have been reported to cause an increase in the expression of mRNA encoding B1 and B2 receptors in primary cultures of rat trigeminal ganglia,[363] as well as other receptors such as TRPV1 and TRPA1.[74,168] The *transient receptor potential subtype V1* (TRPV1) is the "capsaicin receptor"; it plays a key role in mediating inflammatory pain. TRPA1 is expressed on capsaicin-sensitive neurons[74] and interacts with TRPV1.[314] Bradykinin likely increases the excitability of nociceptive neurons through its action on TRPV1 and TRPA1 (for review, see Tominaga et al[358]).

Cytokines are a diverse group of regulatory proteins synthesized and secreted by a variety of cell types, such as leukocytes, neurons, and glia. In particular, tumor necrosis factor α (TNF-α) and the interleukins IL-1β, IL-6, and IL-8 are thought to play a role in the neuroplastic changes that occur in nociceptors innervating inflamed tissues, leading to hyperalgesia.[197] Application of TNF-α rapidly sensitizes TRPV1,[183] contributing to activation of the capsaicin-sensitive class of nociceptors. All of the above are thought to exist in the inflamed pulp (for review, see Fouad[100]) and are thought to act at least in part by causing increased release of prostanoids.[347]

Painful Pulpitis

From the foregoing, it is apparent that pain associated with the stimulation of the A fibers does not necessarily signify that the pulp is inflamed or that tissue injury has occurred. Clinically, pain produced by A fibers in response to the hydrodynamic mechanism has a sharp or bright quality as contrasted with the dull, boring, or throbbing pain associated with C fibers. A fibers have a relatively low threshold of excitability to external stimuli,[246,267] and painful pulpitis is more likely to be associated with nociceptive C fiber activity indicative of pulpal tissue injury.[267-269,273] The clinician should carefully examine symptomatic teeth to rule out the possibility of hypersensitive dentin, cracked or leaky fillings, or fracture lines—each of which may initiate hydrodynamic forces—before establishing a diagnosis of reversible or irreversible pulpitis (see also Chapters 1 and 21).

Pain associated with an inflamed or degenerating pulp may be either provoked or spontaneous. The hyperalgesic pulp may demonstrate a lowered threshold of pain by responding to stimuli that usually do not evoke pain (allodynia), or the pain may be exaggerated and persist longer than normal (hyperalgesia).[6] On the other hand, the tooth may commence to ache spontaneously in the absence of any external stimulus.[137] Spontaneous, unprovoked pain generally indicates a pulp that is seriously damaged and generally will not respond to noninvasive therapy.

Plasticity of Intradental Nerve Fibers

It has become apparent that the innervation of the tooth is a dynamic process in which the number, size, and cytochemistry of nerve fibers can change because of aging,[102,224,349] tooth injury,[42,45,46,49] and dental caries.[310] For example, in rats, nerve fibers sprout into inflamed tissue surrounding sites of pulpal injury, and the content of CGRP and SP increases in these sprouting fibers.[42,45,46,49,53] When inflammation subsides, the number of sprouts decreases. Fig. 12-30 compares the normal distribution of CGRP-immunoreactive sensory fibers in an adult rat molar with those beneath a shallow cavity preparation. The innervational pattern in normal and inflamed teeth is governed by neuronal growth factors. Neurotrophic and target-derived factors regulate neuronal structure, survival, and function and are important for the maintenance of neuronal phenotype characteristics. During development, all dental fibers appear to require nerve growth factor (NGF) and express its receptor, TrkA, at some stages,[244] whereas in adult teeth the large trigeminal neurons are potentially dependent only on dental pulp–derived, glial cell line–derived neurotrophic factor

(GDNF); the smaller trigeminal neurons remain dependent on NGF.[200,305] This suggests that GDNF may function as a neurotrophic factor for the subset of larger neurons supporting the tooth, which apparently mediate mechanosensitive stimuli, whereas NGF is suggested to support neurons responsible for nociception.[259] NGF is the most extensively investigated among the trophic factors.[209] Binding of target-derived NGF is dependent on specific TrkA receptors located on the axonal surface, with subsequent internalization and transport to the cell body, where the effects are mediated.

Regulation of neural changes during inflammation seems to be a function of NGF expression.[47,53] NGF receptors are found on intradental sensory fibers and Schwann cells.[45] Evidence indicates that NGF is synthesized by fibroblasts in the coronal subodontoblastic zone (i.e., cell-rich zone), particularly in the tip of the pulp horn.[45] Maximal sprouting of CGRP- and SP-containing nerve fibers corresponds to areas of the pulp where there is increased production of NGF.[53] Fig. 12-31 shows the expression of NGF-mRNA in a pulp horn subjacent to cavity preparation.

It has been suggested that neuroimmune interactions take place in the dental pulp, because a coordinated increase of pulpal nerves and immune cells has been demonstrated.[173,319] In addition, recruitment of immunocompetent cells has been demonstrated in the dental pulp after electrical tooth stimulation.[66,106] Similar responses have been seen in periapical bone in rats with radicular pulpitis.[195] Neurogenic inflammation is generally thought to enhance healing, because denervated teeth show poorer healing following pulp exposures than innervated teeth.[42,50]

Another consideration in the neural response to inflammation is the possibility of a change in the distribution and activity of voltage-gated sodium channels. In particular, mice lacking the gene for $Na_v1.7$ show reduced painlike behaviors when treated with a variety of proinflammatory agents.[270] Also implicated in the altered firing characteristics of nociceptors innervating inflamed tissues are the sodium channels that are resistant to tetrodotoxin (TTX), the biotoxin found in the tetraodon pufferfish. The two main TTX-R sodium channels are $Na_v1.8$ and $Na_v1.9$, and both have been shown to be increased two- to fourfold in inflamed dental pulp collected

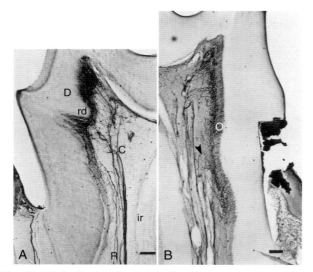

FIG. 12-30 **A,** Normal distribution of calcitonin gene–related peptide (CGRP)-immunoreactive sensory fibers in adult rat molar. Nerve fibers typically are unbranched in the root (R), avoid interradicular dentin (ir), and form many branches in coronal pulp (C) and dentin (D). Nerve distribution is often asymmetric, with endings concentrated near the most columnar odontoblasts (in this case on the left side of the crown). When reparative dentin (rd) forms, it alters conditions so that dentinal innervation is reduced (magnification ×75). **B,** Shallow class I cavity preparation on the cervical root of a rat molar was made 4 days earlier. Primary odontoblast (O) layer survived, and many new CGRP-immunoreactive terminal branches spread beneath and into the injured pulp and dentin. Terminal arbor can be seen branching *(arrowhead)* from a larger axon and growing into the injury site. Scale bar: 0.1 mm (magnification. *A,* ×45). (From Taylor PE, Byers MR and Redd PE: Sprouting of CGRP nerve fibers in response to dentin injury in rat molars. Brain Res 461:371-376, 1988.)

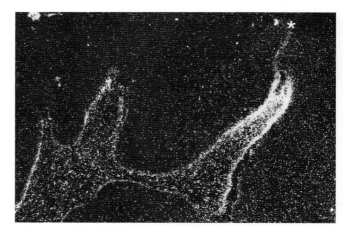

FIG. 12-31 NGF-mRNA is upregulated in the mesial pulp horn 6 hours after cavity preparation. (From Byers MR, Wheeler EF, and Bothwell M: Altered expression of NGF and p75 NGF-Receptor mRNA by fibroblasts of injured teeth precedes sensory nerve sprouting. Growth Factors 6:41-45, 1992.)

from patients with a diagnosis of irreversible pulpitis.[396,402] When exposed to PGE₂, neurons isolated from dorsal root ganglia cells have been shown to increase TTX-resistant sodium channel currents within minutes,[120] indicating an increased activation of existing channels, rather than de novo protein synthesis. These sodium channels are relatively resistant to lidocaine,[313] and this may explain the difficulty in achieving profound anesthesia in inflamed tissues (see also Chapter 4).[140]

Tissue Injury and Deafferentation

When a peripheral nerve is cut or crushed, an interruption of the afferent input to the CNS occurs, which is called *deafferentation*. It would be logical to assume that the result of deafferentation would be anesthesia of the formerly innervated area, but occasionally other symptoms may occur, which may surprisingly include pain. Following nerve injury, a dramatic shift in transcription of neuropeptides, receptors, and sodium channels has been documented. The bidirectional contact between the nerve cell and the peripheral target tissue is lost, and the neurons change into a state of either regeneration or neuronal cell death. The impact on neurons in the trigeminal ganglion is dependent on the injury site. A peripheral injury has less effect than a more centrally located one. However, even a small pulp exposure induces neuronal changes, both in the trigeminal ganglion and at the second-order neuronal level in the brain stem.[43,391] Because each single-rooted tooth contains about 2000 nerve fibers,[169,170] extirpation of the pulp is shown to cause both neurochemical and degenerative changes of their cell bodies in the gasserian (trigeminal) ganglion.[129,186,334] The central projection of these nerves to the spinal nucleus of the trigeminal nerve is also affected,[367] and there is evidence for transsynaptic changes[330,334] that are reflected in the sensory cortex. Even larger responses would be expected from tooth extraction, where both periodontal ligament and pulpal innervation are destroyed.

When an axon is severed peripherally, a complete degeneration of the cell bodies may not always occur.[392] Attempted regeneration by axonal sprouting may result in altered expression of various receptors, resulting in sensitivity to norepinephrine (via increased adrenergic receptor activity)[278] or acetylcholine (via increased cholinergic receptor activity),[72] sensitizing sensory neurons to autonomic activity. In addition, dorsal horn neurons, deprived of their normal sensory input, may begin to respond to other nearby afferents. Thus, normal inhibitory influences are reduced, and a widening of the sensory receptive field is produced, which can produce central sensitization (see Central Sensitization later in this chapter). *Phantom tooth pain* is another term often used synonymously with pain following deafferentation. Different reports suggest an incidence of persistent pain following pulpectomy to be in the range of 3% to 6%.[238,383]

Following tissue injury or tissue inflammation, extensive changes occur in the gene expression of sensory ganglion neurons and, by way of transsynaptic mechanisms, in their central projections.[45,268,269,334] One example is the upregulation of inducible gene transcription factors such as c-fos[43] and different subsets of sodium channels.[119] This is thought to result in alterations in threshold properties and the size of receptor fields. C-fos is not normally expressed in neurons in the brain stem, but chronic pulpitis causes prolonged increases in c-fos expression is some brain stem neurons (Fig. 12-32).[43]

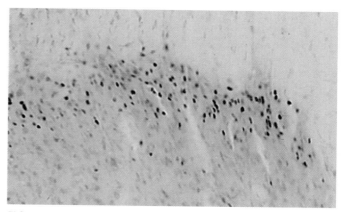

FIG. 12-32 The interstitial cells of the trigeminal tract of medullary dorsal horn express c-*fos* during chronic tooth pulp inflammation in rat. (Adapted from Byers MR, Chudler EH, Ladarola MJ: Chronic tooth pulp inflammation causes transient and persistent expression of Fos in dynorphin-rich regions of rat brainstem. Brain Res 861:191-207, 2000.)

If such changes also occur in humans, they may help to explain why certain patients may complain of vague, poorly described pain for months following endodontic treatment. If their pulpitis caused sprouting of periapical nerves,[49,50,53,195] these nerves may have taken part in transport of peripheral signaling molecules to the cell body by way of retrograde axoplasmic flow.[42,53] This could induce changes in the expression of many genes, resulting in central sensitization[6,41] that may require many months to correct.[351] Reports of nerve sprouting in human inflamed pulps have been confirmed in different studies.[310,312,319] Such reactions might contribute to increases in dentin sensitivity as well as expansion of receptive fields.[268,269,273] Sprouting of sympathetic fibers has also been reported,[147] but the timing appears to be different. The functional implications and how this relates to pain mechanisms are unknown, but it has been suggested that these reactions are involved in healing and nociception following pulpal inflammation.[115,147,148]

Processing: The Second Step in Pain Perception

The Medullary Dorsal Horn

After activation of peripheral nociceptors, nerve impulses in the form of action potentials convey information about the intensity (encoded by firing frequency), quality (encoded by type of neuron activated), and temporal features (encoded by onset, duration, and offset of depolarization) of the peripheral stimuli to the CNS. In the trigeminal pain system, these action potentials arrive at the trigeminal spinal tract nuclear complex located in the medulla.[141,214,329] Three distinct subnuclei can be found in this complex. Named for their anatomic position, they are the *subnuclei oralis, interpolaris,* and *caudalis* (see Fig. 12-24). Although the more rostral subnuclei (oralis and interpolaris) receive some nociceptive input from oral tissues,[70] most such input is received at the level of the subnucleus caudalis.[89,233,329] Because of its organizational similarity to the dorsal horn of the spinal cord (which receives nociceptive input from the somatosensory system), the subnucleus caudalis has been termed the *medullary dorsal horn.*

Components of the Medullary Dorsal Horn

The medullary dorsal horn relays information to higher centers in the brain and serves as the site of much potential processing of the signals from primary afferent sensory nerve fibers. Output from this region can be increased (hyperalgesia), decreased (analgesia), or misinterpreted (referred pain). Understanding the functional components involved in such processing not only helps explain some of these clinical phenomena but also allows evaluation of potential therapeutic modalities currently under investigation. Functional components include the central terminals of primary nociceptors (Aδ and C fiber afferents), the second-order projecting neurons, interneurons, the terminals of descending neurons, and glial[241] cells (for review, see Hargreaves[137]).

Primary afferent fibers (whose cell bodies are located in the trigeminal ganglion) transmit signals to projection neurons via the release of transmitters such as the excitatory amino acid, glutamate, and the neuropeptide, substance P. Receptors for these neurotransmitters are found on postsynaptic membranes and include the N-methyl-D-aspartate receptor (NMDA) and α-amino-3-hydroxy-5-methyl-4-isoxazolepropionic acid receptor (AMPA) classes of glutamate receptors and the neurokinin 1 (NK1) class of substance P receptors. Antagonists to these receptors have been shown to reduce hyperalgesia in animal studies.[59] In a human clinical trial using an oral surgery model, the AMPA/kainate antagonist, LY293558, was shown to be antihyperalgesic.[117] NK1 antagonists have shown promising results in animal studies, but in general, they have displayed limited analgesic efficacy in humans.[156]

The cell bodies of the second-order (projection) neurons in the trigeminal pain system are found in the medullary dorsal horn; their processes cross the midline and project rostrally to the thalamus via the trigeminothalamic tract (Fig. 12-33). From the thalamus, third-order neurons relay information to the cerebral cortex via a thalamocortical tract. Once signals have reached the cortex, the input may be perceived as pain. Evidence exists that referred pain is caused by convergence of afferent input from different areas onto the same projection neurons.

Approximately 50% of subnucleus caudalis neurons are estimated to receive convergence of sensory input from cutaneous and deep structures.[329] In one study of a cat, a single nucleus caudalis neuron received input from sensory neurons innervating the cornea, the skin overlying the maxilla, a maxillary premolar tooth, and a mandibular canine and premolar tooth on one side.[333] Subnuclei oralis and interpolaris also receive converging input from orofacial and muscle afferents.[332] This would explain the clinical observation of patients who perceive pain in a particular tooth that actually originates from either a different tooth or structure (see also Chapter 17). In such cases, anesthetizing the tooth suspected by the patient would afford no relief. However, if an anesthetic is delivered selectively to the suspected primary source of pain, the patient's discomfort should greatly diminish.[279] Likewise, if the source of a perceived toothache were located in a muscle of mastication, palpation of that muscle should aggravate the pain.[410]

In the medullary dorsal horn, local circuit interneurons have the potential to affect transmission of nociceptive input from primary afferents to projection neurons. Depending on the transmitter released, these neurons have the ability to enhance or diminish the signal. Typically, excitatory interneurons release glutamate or substance P, whereas inhibitory interneurons release the amino acid, glycine, or gamma amino butyric acid (GABA).[214,331]

The terminals of neurons that descend from brain structures such as the locus coeruleus and nucleus raphe magnus tend to inhibit nociceptive transmission at the level of the medullary dorsal horn.[14] These terminals release a variety of neuroeffective agents, including the endogenous opioid peptides (EOPs). The EOPs, similar in three-dimensional structure to many of the exogenous opiates from which their name derives, are released in response to nociceptive input and act to suppress the pain system. The EOPs likely are partly responsible for the placebo effect seen in pain control studies, because this effect can be reversed by administration of the opioid antagonist, naloxone.[139,212]

The final component of the medullary dorsal horn complex to be considered is the glial cell population. Historically considered to be solely supportive in function, they are now recognized to play an important role in the pain processing system.[302,397] Following nociceptive input from primary afferents, glia release cytokines such as TNF-α and IL-1, as well as certain PGs that may facilitate the activity of projection neurons. Glial modulating agents have been shown to be effective in experimental models of neuropathic pain,[348] and NSAIDs potentially could exert part of their analgesic mechanism by acting at this level.

Central Sensitization

Central sensitization can be defined as an increased responsiveness of central nociceptive neurons to peripheral stimulation that occurs in addition to *peripheral sensitization* of the primary afferent nociceptors. Central sensitization is thought to be a major cause of hyperalgesia and allodynia.[204] Clinical trials implicate central sensitization in patients reporting pain due to irreversible pulpitis. In one survey of nearly 1000 patients, 57% of patients with irreversible pulpitis reported mechanical allodynia (pain due to percussion).[288] This appears to be due at least in part to central sensitization, as both the ipsilateral (pulpitis) tooth and a contralateral (normal) tooth demonstrated mechanical allodynia to a force transducer.[185] Thus, central sensitization contributes to a spread of endodontic pain, and the clinical application of bite force transducers may provide a novel method for diagnosing pain mechanisms.[184,185]

Different studies shed light on the molecular mechanisms involved in central sensitization (for review, see Cousins and Power[63] and Hargreaves[137]), but the process is generally initiated by a barrage of nociceptive impulses from peripheral C fibers. The level and duration of pain prior to endodontic intervention have been cited in several studies as predictors of postoperative endodontic pain,[364,393] and this may be due to such a prolonged and intense input from C nociceptors. Any reduction of such a barrage should limit the occurrence of central sensitization and the development of pain of longer duration after tissue injury (including surgical and nonsurgical endodontic procedures). The use of long-acting local anesthetics following tonsillectomies and third molar extractions has been shown to provide pain relief far beyond the duration of the peripheral tissue anesthesia.[125,167]

A reduction in the chemical mediators of inflammation at the level of the medullary dorsal horn also should reduce sensitization of second-order neurons. Decreasing the synthesis of proinflammatory PGs, cytokines, nitric oxide, or the use of drugs that block the receptors of such agents probably will

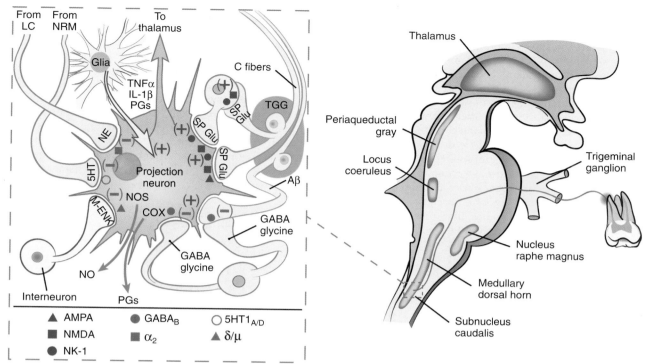

FIG. 12-33 Schematic diagram of the perception and modulation of orofacial pain. Activation of primary afferent fibers (in this example from an inflamed maxillary molar) leads to the entry of a nociceptive signal that is conveyed across a synapse in the subnucleus caudalis of the trigeminal spinal nucleus. The second-order neuron projects to the thalamus; the information is then relayed to the cortex. A great deal of processing of nociceptive input can occur at the level of the medullary dorsal horn (MDH). The *inset* depicts a typical wide dynamic range (WDR) projection neuron and its relationship with other components of the MDH. Primary afferent fibers release the excitatory amino acid, glutamate—which binds and activates either AMPA or NMDA receptors—and substance P—which activates NK-1 receptors on the WDR neuron or excitatory interneurons. Descending fibers from the locus coeruleus (LN) and nucleus raphe magnus (NRM) secrete serotonin (5HT) and norepinephrine (NE), respectively, which inhibit transmission. Release of γ amino butyric acid (GABA), the amino acid, glycine, and endogenous opioid peptides such as met-enkephalin (M-ENK) also inhibit transmission of nociceptive information. Projection neurons may have autocrine or paracrine effects by the synthesis and release of prostaglandins (PGs) and nitric oxide (NO) via the action of cyclooxygenase (COX) and nitric oxide synthase (NOS), respectively. Glial cells can modulate nociceptive processing by the release of cytokines such as tumor necrosis factor alpha (TNF-α) and interleukin 1 beta (IL-1β). The + sign indicates an excitatory action, whereas the – sign denotes an inhibitory action.

become accepted pharmacotherapy in the future. For example, application of an inflammatory agent to the tooth pulp of rat maxillary molars results in an increased receptive field of Aβ touch receptors on the face. This can be blocked by pretreatment with a glutamate NMDA receptor antagonist, indicating that such centrally acting drugs may offer highly efficacious means of treating odontogenic pain.[59] A similar investigation implicated nitric oxide synthesis at the level of the subnucleus caudalis in the development of tactile hypersensitivity following dental injury.[416] Reduction in nitric oxide synthase levels may also provide protection from central sensitization.[234,248]

Perception: Thalamus to Cortex

The final anatomic step in the trigeminal pain pathway relies on neurons that leave the thalamus and extend to the cerebral cortex (see Fig. 12-24). The patient actually perceives a stimulus as painful at the cortical level. It is interesting to note (but likely of no surprise to the experienced clinician) that a disproportionately large portion of the sensory cortex in humans is devoted to input from orofacial regions.[294]

It is becoming increasingly obvious that higher-order (i.e., cortical) perceptual processes have a profound effect on the ultimate state of pain the patient experiences (for a review, see Yaksh[411]). Memories of previous pain experiences provide a framework by which similar new experiences are judged and serve to shape the patient's response to a given stimulus. In the field of dentistry, the anxiety level of the patient at the time of treatment has been shown to affect not only the patient's response to pain experienced during treatment,[78,407] but also the tendency of the patient to recall the experience as painful or unpleasant even 18 months after treatment.[112] The clinician should do everything possible to control a patient's anxiety level prior to endodontic treatment (see also Chapter 28). One simple pretreatment method is to provide patients with positive written information regarding the control of pain during their endodontic treatment. In a placebo-controlled clinical trial, 437 endodontic patients were given one of five informative paragraphs to read prior to treatment. One of the paragraphs contained positive information about pain during treatment. Patients completed questionnaires following treatment that evaluated their dental anxiety and dental fear. Subjects given positive information were shown to be less fearful of pain during endodontic therapy.[381] Along with a positive and caring attitude, pharmacologic intervention may help reduce anxiety. Nitrous oxide has been shown to be effective in a dental setting,[75] but it may interfere with radiography procedures during endodontic therapy. In a placebo-controlled clinical trial in patients undergoing the extraction of impacted third molars, 0.25 mg of oral triazolam (a benzodiazepine) provided comparable anxiolysis to intravenous diazepam titrated to a typical clinical endpoint.[176] Of course, the patient so medicated must be provided transportation to and from the dental office, and the potential drug-drug interactions with other centrally acting agents such as opioids, barbiturates, and alcohol must be considered. One interaction that should be considered is the capacity of grapefruit juice to prolong the half-life of triazolam.[217] It has been shown that furanocoumarins in grapefruit juice inhibit cytochrome P450 3A4,[290] which is the enzyme responsible for the metabolism of triazolam in the liver. Patients should be told not to take oral triazolam with grapefruit juice.

VASCULAR SUPPLY

Blood from the dental artery enters the tooth by way of arterioles having diameters of 100 μm or less. These vessels pass through the apical foramen or foramina with nerve bundles. Smaller vessels may enter the pulp by way of lateral or accessory canals. They are richly innervated by autonomic and sensory nerves, and the regulation of blood flow seems to be dominated by neuronal control[2,20,188,283,359] (Fig. 12-34).

The arterioles course up through the central portion of the radicular pulp and give off branches that spread laterally toward the odontoblast layer, beneath which they ramify to form a capillary plexus[196] (Fig. 12-35). As the arterioles pass into the coronal pulp, they fan out toward the dentin, diminish in size, and give rise to a capillary network in the subodontoblastic region[351] (Fig. 12-36). This network provides the odontoblasts with a rich source of metabolites.

Capillary blood flow in the coronal portion of the pulp is nearly twice that in the root portion.[192] Moreover, blood flow in the region of the pulp horns is greater than in all other areas of the pulp.[249] In young teeth, capillaries commonly extend into the odontoblast layer, thus ensuring an adequate supply of nutrients for the metabolically active odontoblasts (Fig. 12-37). In the subodontoblastic capillaries, fenestrations are observed in the vessel wall.[306] These fenestrations are thought to promote rapid transport of fluid and metabolites from the capillaries to the adjacent odontoblasts. The average capillary density is about 1400/mm², which is greater than in most other tissues of the body.[386]

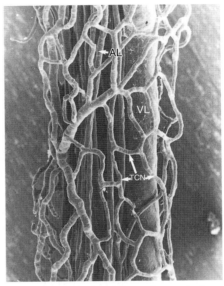

FIG. 12-35 High-power scanning electron micrograph of vascular network in the radicular pulp of a dog molar showing the configuration of the subodontoblastic terminal capillary network (TCN). Venules (VL) and arterioles (AL) are indicated. (Courtesy Dr. Y. Kishi, Kanagawa Dental College, Kanagawa, Japan.)

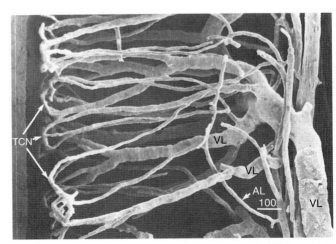

FIG. 12-36 Subodontoblastic terminal capillary network (TCN), arterioles (AL), and venules (VL) of young canine pulp. Dentin would be to the far left and the central pulp to the right. Scale bar: 100 μm. (From Takahashi K, Kishi Y, Kim S: A scanning electron microscopic study of the blood vessels of dog pulp using corrosion resin casts, *J Endod* 8:131, 1982.)

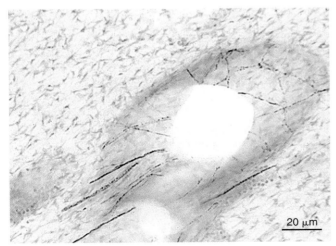

FIG. 12-34 Substance P–positive nerve fibers in the wall of pulpal blood vessels. (Courtesy Dr. K.J. Heyeraas.)

Blood passes from the capillary plexus, first into postcapillary venules (see Figs. 12-36 and 12-38) and then into larger venules.[196] Venules in the pulp have unusually thin walls, and the muscular layer is discontinuous,[68] which may facilitate the movement of fluid in or out of the vessel. The collecting venules become progressively larger as they course to the central region of the pulp. The largest venules have a diameter that may reach a maximum of 200 µm, considerably larger than the arterioles of the pulp.

The resting pulpal blood flow is relatively high, averaging 0.15 to 0.60 ml/min/g tissue,[245,360] and blood volume represents about 3% of pulpal wet weight,[30] approximately the same as in mammary tumor tissue.[403] As would be anticipated, pulpal blood flow is greater in the peripheral layer of the pulp (i.e., the subodontoblastic capillary plexus)[196] where the oxygen consumption has been shown to be higher than in the central pulp.[26]

Changes in pulpal blood flow can be measured through dentin using laser Doppler flowmeters. Sensitivity to movement requires that they are stabilized in an occlusal stent or a modified rubber dam clamp.[93,321] Because up to 80% of the Doppler signal originates from periodontal tissue, it is helpful to cover periodontal tissues with a black rubber dam.[144] Laser

Doppler flowmetry can be used to detect revascularization of traumatized teeth.[79,88] Although measurement of pulpal blood flow would be an ideal tool for determining pulp vitality, the use of laser Doppler and other techniques is limited due to sensitivity, specificity, reproducibility, and costs.

Regulation of Pulpal Blood Flow

Under normal physiologic conditions, pulpal vascular tone is controlled by neuronal, paracrine, and endocrine mechanisms that keep the blood vessels in a state of partial constriction. The pulpal blood flow is also influenced by vascular tone in neighboring tissues. Vasodilatation in these tissues has been shown to cause a drop in pulpal blood flow due to reduction in local arterial pressure of the teeth and thereby reduced pulpal perfusion pressure.[361] The "stealing" of dental perfusion pressure makes the dental pulp vulnerable in clinical situations with inflammatory processes in the adjacent tissues, as in gingivitis and periodontitis.

Neuronal regulation of blood flow is extensive in the pulp. There is little or no vasoconstrictor tone of sympathetic origin in the dental pulp during resting conditions,[165,359] but a neuronal vasodilator tone caused by release of sensory neuropeptides has been demonstrated (Fig. 12-39).[21,20]

There are α-adrenergic receptors in the pulp,[162] and stimulation of the cervical sympathetic trunk causes vasoconstriction and fall in pulpal blood flow that can be partially reversed by α-receptor blockade.[188,359] NPY, colocalized with norepinephrine in pulpal sympathetic nerve fibers, contributes also to vasoconstriction in the pulp.[81,194]

Increase in pulpal blood flow is observed after electrical tooth stimulation and is caused by the release of sensory neuropeptides followed by vasodilatation.[20,153,181] CGRP released from sensory nerve fibers is mainly responsible for the observed vasodilatation.[21,20]

Glutamate, present in CGRP negative sensory afferent nerve fibers in the pulp, also has a vasodilatory effect when applied in the pulp during experimental conditions.[419]

There is evidence for sympathetic modulation of sensory neuropeptide release in the dental pulp[138]; presynaptic adrenoceptors are found on the sensory nerve terminals and attenuate the release of vasodilators from the sensory nerves.[34,180]

Muscarinic receptors have been identified in the pulp,[32] and the parasympathetic neurotransmitter acetylcholine (ACh)

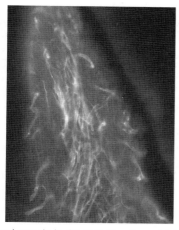

FIG. 12-37 Blood vessels in the pulp horn fan out into the odontoblast layer. (Courtesy Dr. S.R. Haug.)

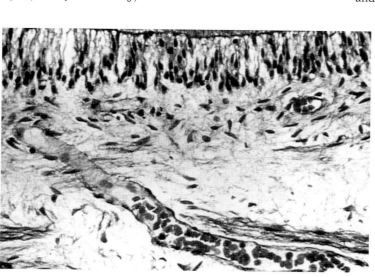

FIG. 12-38 Postcapillary venule draining blood from subodontoblastic capillary plexus.

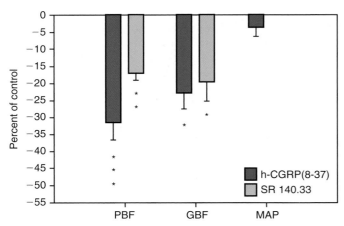

FIG. 12-39 Effect of antagonist infusion of h-CGRP(8-37) (calcitonin gene–related peptide inhibitor) and SR 140.33 (substance P inhibitor) on basal pulpal blood flow (PBF) and gingival blood flow (GBF). (From Berggreen E, Heyeraas KJ: Effect of the sensory neuropeptide antagonists h-CGRP[8-37] and SR 140.33 on pulpal and gingival blood flow in ferrets, *Arch Oral Biol* 45:537, 2000.)

causes vasodilatation and increases blood flow in the tissue.[417] The vasodilation evoked by acetylcholine has been demonstrated to be partly dependent on nitric oxide (NO) production.

VIP, which coexists with ACh in postganglionic neurons, is found in the dental pulp[105,377] and has been demonstrated to cause vasodilatation and increase in pulpal blood flow in cats.[283]

On the other hand, Sasano and coworkers[323] failed to demonstrate parasympathetic nerve-evoked vasodilatation in the cat dental pulp, leaving pulpal vascular responses to parasympathetic neurotransmitters with some uncertainty.

Local Control of Blood Flow

The microvascular bed in the dental pulp has the ability to regulate hemodynamics in response to local tissue demands. Endothelin-1 is located in the endothelium of pulpal vasculature,[57] and close intraarterial infusions of endothelin-1 reduce pulpal blood flow.[22,116,417] However, endothelin-1 does not seem to influence blood vessel vascular tone under basal, resting conditions.[22]

The endothelium in pulpal blood vessels modulates vascular tone by release of vasodilators such as prostacyclin and NO. A basal synthesis of NO provides a vasodilator tone on pulpal vessels.[20,223] The shear forces that blood flow exert on endothelial cells seem to regulate the release of NO.[73]

Adenosine is released from ischemic and hypoxic tissue and is probably important in the metabolic regulation of blood flow in periods of low pulpal oxygen tension. When applied from the extraluminal side of the vessel wall, adenosine mediates vasodilatation in pulpal vessels.[417]

Humoral Control of Blood Flow

Evidence for humoral control of pulpal blood flow exists and takes place when vasoactive substances transported by the bloodstream reach the receptors in the pulp tissue. Angiotensin II is produced by activation of the renin/angiotensin system and exerts a vasoconstrictive basal tone on pulpal blood vessels.[22] The angiotensin II receptors, AT1 and AT2, have been identified in the rat pulp.[341]

Similarly to the effect of norepinephrine released from sympathetic nerve fibers in the pulp, epinephrine released from the adrenal medulla will cause vasoconstriction due to activation of α-adrenergic receptors in the pulp. Another catecholamine, dihydroxyphenylalanine (DOPA), also induces vasoconstriction in pulpal arterioles when applied intraarterially.[417]

Fluid Drainage

Interstitial fluid, which accumulates in the tissue during normal conditions through net filtration out of the blood vessels or during inflammation where the net filtration is increased, must be removed in order to maintain normal fluid balance. In most tissues in the body, the lymphatic vessels drain excess fluid from the peripheral tissue and return it into the blood vessel system. In addition, the lymphatic system is important because it transports captured antigen and presents it in the lymph nodes. The existence of lymphatics in the pulp has been a matter of debate because it is difficult to distinguish between blood and lymphatic vessels by ordinary microscopic techniques without specific lymphatic markers.

Several specific lymphatic markers have now been applied, and contradictory conclusions have been drawn. One of the markers tested is vascular endothelial growth factor receptor (VEGFR-3) known to be expressed by lymphatic endothelial cells in adult tissue.[114,242] The receptor expression was reported in human and mouse pulp tissue, but to identify lymphatic vessels, use of more than one lymphatic marker is recommended. However, other studies have failed to demonstrate lymphatic markers in the pulp [114,242] and one study showed lymphatic vessel endothelium receptor-1 (LYVE-1) staining in immune cells in human pulp, but not in vascular structures (Fig. 12-40). Taken together it seems that the pulp is not supplied with draining lymphatic vessels.

Transcapillary Fluid Exchange

In all tissues in the body, the fluid transport between the blood vessels and the interstitial space is regulated by differences in colloid osmotic and hydrostatic pressures in the plasma and the interstitium, and by properties in the capillary membrane (Fig. 12-41). From the interstitium excess fluid is transported back to the blood circulation through the lymphatic system. The pulp seems to be an exception along with, for example, the brain and bone marrow, as lymphatic vessels are not detected in the tissue (see the previous section). During normal conditions, a steady state is achieved as the fluid filtered into the interstitial space equals the amount of fluid transported out of the same compartment. Using radioisotopes, the interstitial fluid volume in the pulp was measured and averaged 0.6 ± 0.03 ml/g wet weight,[30] demonstrating that as much as 60% of the extracellular fluid in dental pulp is located outside the vascular system. Measurements of interstitial fluid pressure in the pulp with the micropuncture method have given values that range from 6 to 10 mm Hg,[20,150] but higher values measured with different methods have also been reported.[39,380,385]

Colloid osmotic pressure (COP) measurements in interstitial fluid isolated from rat incisors have shown a relatively high pulpal COP, reaching 83% of plasma COP.[30] The high value may imply that the normal permeability of pulpal vessels to plasma proteins is relatively high or the drainage of plasma proteins is ineffective.

Because lymphatic vessels are lacking inside the pulp, excess interstitial fluid and proteins must be transported

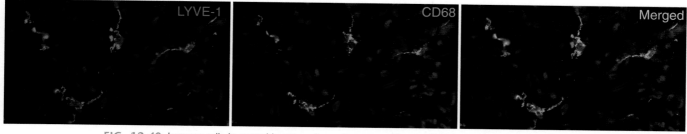

FIG. 12-40 Immune cells in normal human pulp are immunopositive to LYVE-1, known as a lymphatic vessel marker. The CD68+/LYVE-1+ cells derive from the monocytic lineage of cells. Immunostaining demonstrated the lack of LYVE-1+ lymphatic vessels in the pulp. (Courtesy Dr. A Virtej.)

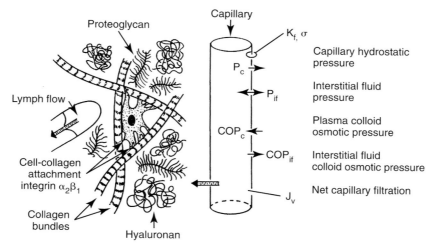

FIG. 12-41 Interstitial structure and pressures that govern transcapillary fluid transport. K_f, Capillary filtration coefficient; σ, capillary reflection coefficient for plasma proteins. (From Wiig H, Rubin K, Reed RK: New and active role of the interstitium in control of interstitial fluid pressure: potential therapeutic consequences, *Acta Anaesthesiol Scand* 47:111, 2003.)

out of the pulp by other transport routes in order to achieve a steady-state situation. Two possibilities exists: (1) transport of fluid in the interstitial compartment toward the apical part of the pulp and furthermore out of the apex, and (2) a combination of fluid reabsorption into pulpal blood vessels in addition to transport of protein-rich fluid toward the apex.

Circulation in the Inflamed Pulp

Inflammation in the pulp takes place in a low-compliance environment composed of rigid dentinal walls. *Compliance* is defined as the relationship between volume (V) and interstitial pressure (P) changes: $C = \Delta V / \Delta P$. Consequently, in the low-compliant pulp, an increase in blood or interstitial volume will lead to a relatively large increase in the hydrostatic pressure in the pulp. The acute vascular reactions to an inflammatory stimulus are vasodilatation and increased vascular permeability, both of which will increase pulp interstitial fluid pressure[151,154,359,379] and may tend to compress blood vessels and counteract a beneficial blood flow increase (Fig. 12-42).

Classical studies have demonstrated that an increase in intrapulpal tissue pressure promoted absorption of tissue fluid back into the circulation, thereby reducing the pressure.[151,154] This observation can explain why pulpal tissue pressure in inflamed pulps may persist in local regions for long observation periods,[362] contradicting the old concept of a wide,

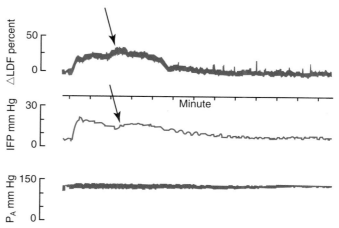

FIG. 12-42 Original simultaneous recordings of percent change in pulpal blood flow (ΔLDF%), interstitial fluid pressure (IFP), and systemic blood pressure (P_A mm Hg) in a cat during electrical tooth stimulation. Note that when IFP is first decreasing after an initial rise, the pulpal blood flow reaches its maximal level *(arrows)*, demonstrating compression of vessels in the first phase. (Courtesy Dr. K.J. Heyeraas.)

generalized collapse of pulpal venules and cessation of blood flow (pulpal strangulation theory).

The delivery of dental restorative procedures may lead to substantial increases or decreases in pulpal blood flow, depending on the precise procedure and time point sampled.[189] Vasoactive mediators are locally released upon an inflammatory insult, and in the pulp, prostaglandin E2, bradykinin, SP, and histamine have all been demonstrated to increase pulpal blood flow after application.[191,284] In contrast, serotonin (5-HT) is released primarily from the platelets, and given intraarterially, it has been shown to reduce pulpal blood flow.[193,417]

Acute inflammation in the dental pulp induces an immediate rise in blood flow and can reach a magnitude of up to nearly 200% of control flow followed by increased vascular permeability.[152,154]

A common outcome of pulpal inflammation is development of tissue necrosis. One study found circulatory dysfunction developed in the pulp after exposure to lipopolysaccharide (LPS) from gram-negative bacteria.[30]

In addition, the inflammatory cytokines IL-1 and TNF-α are elevated in the inflamed pulp. When the endothelium is exposed to endotoxin, it expresses cytokines, chemokines, and thromboxane A2. The latter has been demonstrated to be produced in the pulp exposed to LPS[281] and induces vasoconstriction. The set of changes in endothelial function have been called *endothelial perturbation* and were first described in endothelial cells exposed to endotoxin or to cytokines such as IL-1, TNF-α, and IL-6.[24,271] The activated endothelium also participates in procoagulant reactions that promote fibrin clot formation.[345] A reduced pulpal perfusion due to endothelial perturbation might be the consequence of bacterial infection impairing pulpal defense mechanisms and promoting necrosis. Downregulation of vascular endothelial growth factor (VEGF) expression in stromal cells and reduced microvessel density have been observed in human dental pulps with irreversible pulpitis.[10] VEGF is an essential proangiogenic factor, and the reduced microvessel density might also lead to reduced pulpal perfusion and contribute to development of pulpal necrosis.

Vascular Permeability

Increased vascular permeability takes place as a result of acute inflammation, and vascular leakage has been demonstrated in the pulp after release of inflammatory mediators such as prostaglandin, histamine, bradykinin, and the sensory neuropeptide, SP.[182,191,236]

LPS and lipoteichoic acid () from gram-negative and gram-positive bacteria, respectively, cause upregulation of VEGF in activated pulpal cells.[33,353] VEGF increases vascular permeability,[91,328] and it is likely that it also causes leakage in pulpal vessels. It is a potent agent, because its ability to enhance microvascular permeability is estimated to be 50,000 times higher than that of histamine.[335] Cytokines such as IL-1 and TNF-α are released into the pulp interstitial fluid during inflammation[30] and upregulate VEGF mRNA gene expression in pulpal fibroblasts.[60]

The resulting increased vascular permeability allows increased transport of proteins through the capillary vessel wall and results in increased COP in the tissue. In acute pulpitis induced by LPS, it has been shown that COP in the pulp can reach the level of plasma COP, meaning that a protein transport barrier between plasma and interstitium can be eliminated.[30]

Clinical Aspects

The influence of posture on pulpal blood flow has been observed in humans.[60] Significantly greater pulpal blood flow was measured when subjects changed from an upright to a supine position. The supine position increases venous return from all tissues below the level of the heart, thereby increasing cardiac output and producing a transient increase in systemic blood pressure. The increase in blood pressure stimulates baroreceptors that reflexively decrease sympathetic vasoconstriction to all vascular beds, thereby increasing peripheral blood flow.

Patients with pulpitis often report an inability to sleep at night because they are disturbed by throbbing tooth pain. In addition to the lack of distractions normally present during the day, the following mechanism may be operative in patients with inflamed pulps. When these patients lie down at the end of the day, their pulpal blood flow probably increases due to the cardiovascular postural responses described earlier. This may increase their already elevated pulpal tissue pressure,[151,154,344,362,379] which is then sufficient to activate sensitized pulpal nociceptors and initiate spontaneous pulpal pain. Thus, the "throbbing" sensation of toothache was previously considered as an effect of the pulsation in the pulp that follows heart contractions (systole), but a study investigating the rhythm of toothache and the patient pulse showed lack of synchrony between the two parameters.[251] The authors raised an alternative hypothesis: that the throbbing quality is not a primary sensation but rather an emergent property, or perception, whose "pacemaker" lies within the CNS causing intermittent increases in pulpal tissue pressure.

PULPAL REPAIR

The inherent healing potential of the dental pulp is well recognized. As in all other connective tissues, repair of tissue injury commences with débridement by macrophages, followed by proliferation of fibroblasts, capillary buds, and the formation of collagen. Local circulation is of critical importance in wound healing and repair. An adequate supply of blood is essential to transport immune cells into the area of pulpal injury and to dilute and remove deleterious agents from the area. It is also important to provide fibroblasts with nutrients from which to synthesize collagen. Unlike most tissues, the pulp has essentially no collateral circulation; for this reason, it is theoretically more vulnerable than most other tissues. In the case of severe injury, healing would be impaired in teeth with a limited blood supply. It seems reasonable to assume that the highly cellular pulp of a young tooth, with a wide-open apical foramen and rich blood supply, has a much better healing potential than an older tooth with a narrow foramen and a restricted blood supply.

Dentin can be classified as primary, secondary, or tertiary, depending on when it was formed. *Primary dentin* is the regular tubular dentin formed before eruption, including mantle dentin. *Secondary dentin* is the regular circumferential dentin formed after tooth eruption, whose tubules remain continuous with that of primary dentin. *Tertiary dentin* is the irregular dentin that is formed in response to abnormal stimuli, such as excess tooth wear, cavity preparation, restorative materials, and caries.[64,65] In the past, tertiary dentin has been called *irregular dentin, irritation dentin, reparative dentin,* and *replacement dentin.* Much of the confusion was caused by a lack of understanding of how tertiary dentin is formed.

If the original odontoblasts that made *secondary dentin* are responsible for focal tertiary dentin formation, that particular type of tertiary dentin is termed *reactionary dentin*.[339] Generally, the rate of formation of dentin is increased, but the tubules remain continuous with the secondary dentin.[342] However, if the provoking stimulus caused the destruction of the original odontoblasts, the new, less tubular, more irregular dentin formed by newly differentiated odontoblast-like cells is called *reparative dentin*. In this dentin the tubules are usually not continuous with those of secondary dentin. Initially, the newly formed cells tend to be cuboidal in shape, without the odontoblast process that is necessary to form dentinal tubules. They seem to form in response to the release of a host of growth factors that were bound to collagen during the formation of secondary dentin.[92,309,339] The loss of the continuous layer of odontoblasts exposes unmineralized predentin that is thought to contain both soluble and insoluble forms of TGF-β, insulin-like growth factor (IGF)-1 and IGF-2, bone morphogenetic proteins (BMPs), VEGF, and other growth factors that attract and cause proliferation and differentiation of mesenchymal stem cells to form reparative dentin and new blood vessels. During caries progression, bacterial acids may solubilize these growth factors from mineralized dentin, liberating them to diffuse to the pulp, where they could stimulate reactionary dentin formation. This is also thought to be the mechanism of action of calcium hydroxide during apexification treatment. Despite its high pH, calcium hydroxide has a slight demineralizing effect on dentin and has been shown to cause the release of TGF-β.[338] TGF-β and other growth factors stimulate and accelerate reparative dentinogenesis. Other researchers have attempted to apply growth factors to dentin to allow it to diffuse through the tubules to the pulp.[316,317,340] Although this has been successful, the remaining dentin thickness must be so thin that this approach may not be practical from a therapeutic perspective. Others have inserted deoxyribonucleic acid (DNA)-sequenced BMP-7 into retroviruses to transfect ferret pulpal fibroblasts to stimulate increased BMP-7 production. Although this was successful in normal pulps,[316] it was unsuccessful in inflamed pulps.[315] Specific amelogenin gene splice products, A+4 and A-4, adsorbed onto agarose beads and applied to pulp exposures, induced complete closure and mineralization of the root canal in rat molars.[122] The regulation of peritubular dentin formation is not well understood. Some have claimed that this is a passive process resulting in occlusion of the tubules over time, but it has also been claimed that this is a mechanism under odontoblast control. If odontoblasts could be stimulated to form excessive peritubular dentin by the application of an appropriate biologic signaling molecule to the floor of cavity preparations, then the tubules of the remaining dentin could be occluded, rendering this dentin impermeable and protecting the pulp from the inward diffusion of noxious substances that might leak around restorations.[291] These are examples of how molecular biology may be used in future restorative dentistry.

The term most commonly applied to irregularly formed dentin is *reparative dentin*, presumably because it frequently forms in response to injury and appears to be a component of the reparative process. It must be recognized, however, that this type of dentin has also been observed in the pulps of normal, unerupted teeth without any obvious injury.[276]

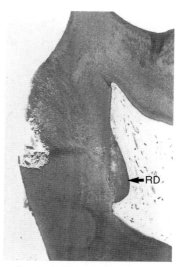

FIG. 12-43 Reparative dentin (RD) deposited in response to a carious lesion in the dentin. (From Trowbridge HO: Pathogenesis of pulpitis resulting from dental caries, *J Endod* 7:52, 1981.)

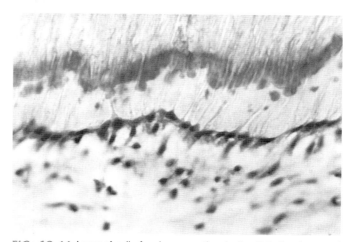

FIG. 12-44 Layer of cells forming reparative dentin. Note the decreased tubularity of reparative dentin compared with the developmental dentin above it.

It will be recalled that secondary dentin is deposited circumpulpally at a slow rate throughout the life of the vital tooth.[342] In contrast, when a carious lesion has invaded dentin, the pulp usually responds by depositing a layer of tertiary dentin over the dentinal tubules of the primary or secondary dentin that communicate with the carious lesion (Fig. 12-43). Similarly, when occlusal wear removes the overlying enamel and exposes the dentin to the oral environment, tertiary dentin is deposited on the pulpal surface of the exposed dentin. Thus, the formation of tertiary dentin allows the pulp to retreat behind a barrier of mineralized tissue.[370]

Compared with primary or secondary dentin, tertiary dentin tends to be less tubular, and the tubules tend to be more irregular with larger lumina. In some cases, particularly when the original odontoblasts are destroyed, no tubules are formed. The cells that form reparative dentin are often cuboidal and not as columnar as the primary odontoblasts of the coronal pulp (Fig. 12-44). The quality of tertiary dentin (i.e., the extent to which it resembles primary or secondary dentin) is quite

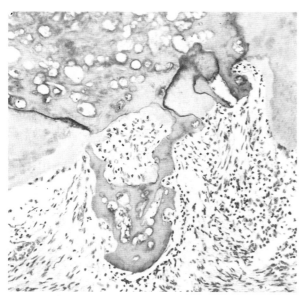

FIG. 12-45 Swiss-cheese type of reparative dentin. Note the numerous areas of soft-tissue inclusion and infiltration of inflammatory cells in the pulp.

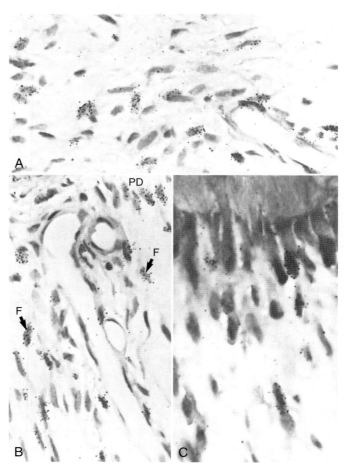

FIG. 12-46 Autoradiographs from dog molars illustrating uptake of ³H-thymidine by pulp cells preparing to undergo cell division after pulpotomy and pulp capping with calcium hydroxide. **A,** Two days after pulp capping. Fibroblasts, endothelial cells, and pericytes beneath the exposure site are labeled. **B,** By the fourth day, fibroblasts (F) and preodontoblasts adjacent to the predentin (PD) are labeled, which suggests that differentiation of pre-odontoblasts occurred within 2 days. **C,** Six days after pulp capping, new odontoblasts are labeled, and tubular dentin is being formed. (Titrated thymidine was injected 2 days after the pulp capping procedures in **B** and **C**.) (From Yamamura T, Shimono M, Koike H, et al: Differentiation and induction of undifferentiated mesenchymal cells in tooth and periodontal tissue during wound healing and regeneration, *Bull Tokyo Dent Coll* 21:181, 1980.)

variable. If irritation to the pulp is relatively mild, as in the case of a superficial carious lesion, then the tertiary dentin formed may resemble primary dentin in terms of tubularity and degree of mineralization. On the other hand, dentin deposited in response to a deep carious lesion may be relatively atubular and poorly mineralized, with many areas of interglobular dentin. The degree of irregularity of this dentin is probably determined by numerous factors, such as the amount of inflammation present, the extent of cellular injury, and the state of differentiation of the replacement odontoblasts.

The poorest quality of reparative dentin is usually observed in association with marked pulpal inflammation.[64,370] In fact, the dentin may be so poorly organized that areas of soft tissue are entrapped within the dentinal matrix. In histologic sections, these areas of soft-tissue entrapment impart a Swiss-cheese appearance to the dentin (Fig. 12-45). As the entrapped soft tissue degenerates, products of tissue degeneration are released that further contribute to the inflammatory stimuli assailing the pulp.[370]

It has been reported that trauma caused by cavity preparation that is too mild to result in the loss of primary odontoblasts does not lead to reparative dentin formation, even if the cavity preparation is relatively deep.[73] This has been confirmed both in rat teeth[258] and human teeth.[256] However, chronic pulpal inflammation associated with deep caries produces reparative dentin. This reparative dentin is formed by new odontoblast-like cells. For many years, it has been recognized that destruction of primary odontoblasts is soon followed by increased mitotic activity within fibroblasts of the subjacent cell-rich zone. It has been shown that the progeny of these dividing cells differentiate into functioning odontoblasts.[98] Investigators[414] have studied dentin bridge formation in healthy teeth of dogs and found that pulpal fibroblasts appeared to undergo dedifferentiation and revert to undifferentiated mesenchymal stem cells (Fig. 12-46). The similarity of primary odontoblasts to replacement odontoblasts was established by D'Souza and colleagues.[77] They were able to show that cells forming reparative dentin synthesize type I (but not type III) collagen, and they are immunopositive for dentin sialoprotein.

Destruction of primary odontoblasts can occur from cutting cavity preparations dry,[80,202] from bacterial products such as endotoxins shed from deep carious lesions,[18,395] or from mechanical exposure of pulps.[257] Such pulpal wounds do not heal if the tissue is inflamed.[64] Local fibroblast-like cells divide, and the new cells then redifferentiate in a new direction to become odontoblasts. Recalling the migratory potential of ectomesenchymal cells from which the pulpal fibroblasts are derived, it is not difficult to envision the differentiating odontoblasts moving from the subodontoblastic zone to the area of injury to constitute a new odontoblast layer. Activation of antigen-presenting dendritic cells by mild inflammatory processes may also promote osteoblast/odontoblast-like differentiation and expression of molecules implicated in mineralization.

Recognition of bacteria by specific odontoblast and fibroblast membrane receptors triggers an inflammatory and immune response within the pulp tissue that would also modulate the repair process.[121]

Although many animal studies have shown dentin bridge formation in healthy pulps following pulp capping with adhesive resins,[64] such procedures fail in normal human teeth.[61]

When small mechanical pulp exposures are inadvertently made in healthy teeth, the recommendation has been to place a small, calcium hydroxide–containing dressing on the wound. After setting, the surrounding dentin can be bonded using a no-rinse, self-etching primer adhesive.[175] Calcium silicate cements like mineral trioxide aggregate (MTA) have also been recognized to promote hard-tissue formation, and available information indicates that the dentin bridge formed under these cements is more dense and has fewer defects compared with calcium hydroxide–containing dressings.[3,5,261,368]

The formation of atubular "fibrodentin" is another potential product of newly differentiated odontoblasts, provided that a capillary plexus develops beneath the fibrodentin.[15] This is consistent with the observation made by other researchers[64,98] that the newly formed dentin bridge is composed first of a thin layer of atubular dentin on which a relatively thick layer of tubular dentin is deposited. The fibrodentin was lined by cells resembling mesenchymal cells, whereas the tubular dentin was associated with cells closely resembling odontoblasts.

Other researchers[342] studied reparative dentin formed in response to relatively traumatic experimental class V cavity preparations in human teeth. They found that seldom was reparative dentin formed until about the 30th postoperative day. The rate of dentin formation was 3.5 µm/day for the first 3 weeks after the onset of dentinogenesis, after which it decreased markedly. By postoperative day 132, dentin formation had nearly ceased. Assuming that most of the odontoblasts were destroyed during traumatic cavity preparation, as was likely in this experiment, the 30-day delay between cavity preparation and the onset of reparative dentin formation is thought to reflect the time required for the proliferation, migration, and differentiation of new replacement odontoblasts.

Does reparative dentin protect the pulp, or is it simply a form of scar tissue? To serve a protective function, it would have to provide a relatively impermeable barrier that would exclude irritants from the pulp and compensate for the loss of developmental dentin. The junction between developmental and reparative dentin has been studied using a dye diffusion technique, which demonstrated the presence of an atubular zone situated between secondary dentin and reparative dentin (Fig. 12-47).[94] In addition to a dramatic reduction in the number of tubules, the walls of the tubules along the junction were often thickened and occluded with material similar to peritubular matrix.[326] Taken together, these observations would indicate that the junctional zone between developmental and reparative dentin is an atubular zone of low permeability. Moreover, the accumulation of pulpal dendritic cells was reduced after reparative dentin formation, which may indicate the reduction of incoming bacterial antigens.[319]

One group[356] studied the effect of gold foil placement on human pulp and found that this was better tolerated in teeth in which reparative dentin had previously been deposited beneath the cavity than in teeth that lacked this deposit. It would thus appear that reparative dentin can protect the pulp,[18] but it must be emphasized that this is not always the

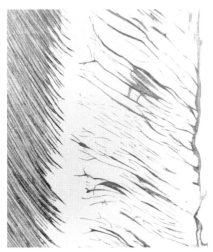

FIG. 12-47 Diffusion of dye from the pulp into reparative dentin. Note atubular zone between reparative dentin (RD) and primary dentin on the left. (From Fish EW: *Experimental investigation of the enamel, dentin, and dental pulp,* London, 1932, John Bale Sons & Danielson.)

case. It is well known that reparative dentin can be deposited in a pulp that is irreversibly injured and that its presence does not necessarily signify a favorable prognosis (see Fig. 12-45). The quality of the dentin formed, and hence its ability to protect the pulp, to a large extent reflects the environment of the cells producing the matrix. The presence of a single tunnel defect[64] through reparative dentin would circumvent the protective effect of atubular reparative dentin. Therefore, any clinical attempt at pulp therapy must include sealing dentin with bonding agent.

Periodontally diseased teeth have smaller root canal diameters than teeth that are periodontally healthy.[203] The root canals of such teeth are narrowed by the deposition of large quantities of reactionary dentin along the dentinal walls.[327] The decrease in root canal diameter with increasing age, in the absence of periodontal disease, is more likely to be the result of secondary dentin formation.

One study showed that in a rat model, frequent scaling and root planing resulted in reparative dentin formation along the pulpal wall subjacent to the instrumented root surface.[146] However, given that normal rat root dentin is only 100 µm thick, these procedures are probably more traumatic to the pulp in the rat model than in humans, where normal root dentin is more than 2000 µm thick.

Not uncommonly, the cellular elements of the pulp are largely replaced by fibrous connective tissue over a span of 5 decades. It appears that in some cases, the pulp responds to noxious stimuli by accumulating large fiber bundles of collagen, rather than by elaborating reparative dentin (Fig. 12-48). However, fibrosis and reparative dentin formation often go hand in hand, indicating that both are expressions of a reparative potential. In periodontally diseased teeth, the pulp tissue is found to be the site of an enhanced process of collagenous fibrosis associated with an inflammatory infiltrate.[56]

With the expanding knowledge of tooth regeneration and biologic mechanisms of functional dental tissue repair, current treatment strategies are beginning to give way to evolving fields such as tissue engineering and biomimetics. Pulpal stem cells in scaffolds have been shown to produce pulplike tissues with

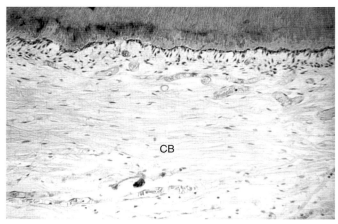

FIG. 12-48 Fibrosis of dental pulp showing replacement of pulp tissue by large collagen bundles (CB).

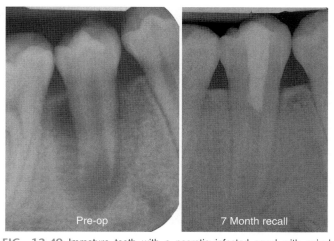

FIG. 12-49 Immature tooth with a necrotic infected canal with apical periodontitis. The canal is disinfected with copious irrigation with sodium hypochlorite and an antibiotic paste. Seven months after treatment, the patient is asymptomatic, and the apex shows healing of the apical periodontitis and some closure of the apex. (From Banchs F, Trope M: Revascularization of immature permanent teeth with apical periodontitis: new treatment protocol? *J Endod* 30:196, 2004.)

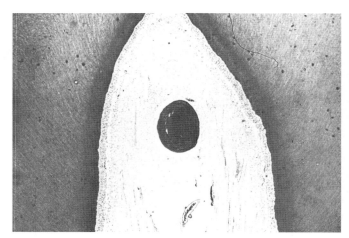

FIG. 12-50 Pulp stone with a smooth surface and concentric laminations in the pulp of a newly erupted premolar extracted in the course of orthodontic treatment.

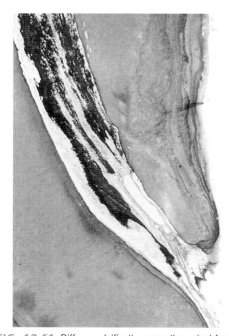

FIG. 12-51 Diffuse calcification near the apical foramen.

tubular-like dentin,[87] and in animal models, root perforations have been treated with scaffolds of collagen, pulpal stem cells, and dentin matrix protein 1, resulting in organized matrix similar to that of pulpal tissue.[304]

Studies investigating new possibilities for regeneration of the pulp/dentin complex are now frequently reported and are described in detail in Chapter 10. A first interesting case report, which has been followed up by others, has led to new strategies for treatment of necrotic immature roots (Fig. 12-49; see also Chapter 10).[13] In the future, the field of pulpal repair will probably develop rapidly, and new treatment strategies will appear.

PULPAL CALCIFICATIONS

Calcification of pulp tissue is a common occurrence. Although estimates of the incidence of this phenomenon vary widely, it is safe to say that one or more pulp calcifications are present in at least 50% of all teeth. In the coronal pulp, calcification usually takes the form of discrete, concentric pulp stones (Fig. 12-50), whereas in the radicular pulp, calcification tends to be diffuse (Fig. 12-51).[374] There is no clear evidence as to whether pulp calcification is a pathologic process related to various forms of injury or a natural phenomenon. The clinical significance of pulp calcification is that it may hinder root canal treatment.

Pulp stones (denticles) range in size from small, microscopic particles often seen in association with the wall of arterioles to accretions that occupy almost the entire pulp chamber (Fig. 12-52). The mineral phase of pulp calcifications has been shown to consist of typical carbonated hydroxyapatite.[374] Histologically, two types of stones are recognized: (1) those that are round or ovoid, with smooth surfaces and concentric laminations (see Fig. 12-50), and (2) those that assume no particular shape, lack laminations, and have rough surfaces (Fig. 12-53). Laminated stones appear to grow by the addition of collagen fibrils to their surface, whereas unlaminated stones develop by way of the mineralization of preformed collagen fiber bundles. In the latter type, the mineralization front seems to extend out along the coarse fibers, making the surface of the stones appear fuzzy (Fig. 12-54). Often these coarse fiber bundles appear to have undergone hyalinization, thus resembling old scar tissue.

Pulp stones may also form around epithelial cells (i.e., remnants of Hertwig's epithelial root sheath). Presumably the epithelial remnants induce adjacent mesenchymal stem cells to differentiate into odontoblasts. Characteristically these pulp stones are found near the root apex and contain dentinal tubules.

The cause of pulpal calcification is largely unknown. Calcification may occur around a nidus of degenerating cells, blood thrombi, or collagen fibers. Many authors believe that this represents a form of dystrophic calcification. In this type of calcification, calcium is deposited in tissues that are degenerating. Calcium phosphate crystals may be deposited within the cells themselves. Initially this takes place within the mitochondria because of the increased membrane permeability to calcium resulting from a failure to maintain active transport systems within the cell membranes. Thus, degenerating cells serving as a nidus may initiate calcification of a tissue. In the absence of obvious tissue degeneration, the cause of pulpal calcification is enigmatic. It is often difficult to assign the term *dystrophic calcification* to pulp stones because they so often occur in apparently healthy pulps, suggesting that functional stress need not be present for calcification to occur. Calcification in the mature pulp is often assumed to be related to the aging process, but in a study involving 52 impacted canines from patients between 11 and 76 years of age, there was a constant incidence of concentric denticles for all age groups, indicating no relation to aging.[276] Diffuse calcifications, on the other hand, increased in incidence to age 25 years; thereafter they remained constant in successive age groups.

At times, numerous concentric pulp stones with no apparent cause are seen in all the teeth of young individuals. In such cases, the appearance of pulp stones may be ascribed to individual biologic characteristics (e.g., tori, cutaneous nevi).[276]

Although soft-tissue collagen does not usually calcify, it is common to find calcification occurring in old hyalinized scar tissue in the skin. This may be due to the increase in the extent of cross-linking between collagen molecules (because increased cross-linkage is thought to enhance the tendency for collagen

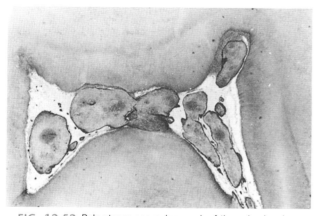

FIG. 12-52 Pulp stones occupying much of the pulp chamber.

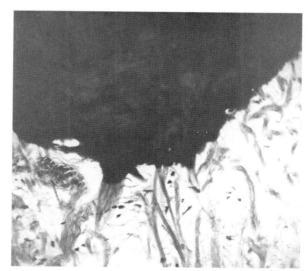

FIG. 12-54 High-power view of a pulp stone from Fig. 12-53, showing the relationship of mineralization fronts to collagen fibers.

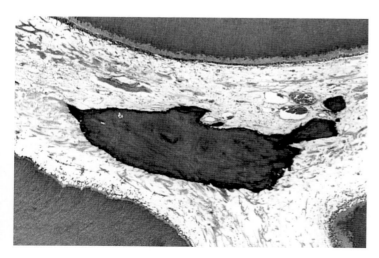

FIG. 12-53 Rough surface form of pulp stone. Note hyalinization of collagen fibers.

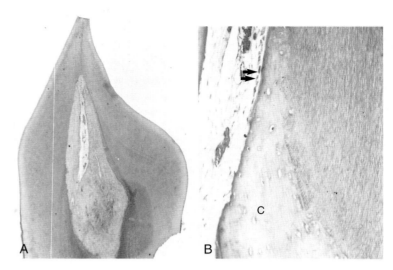

FIG. 12-55   A, Calcific metamorphosis of pulp tissue after luxation of tooth as a result of trauma. Note presence of soft-tissue inclusion. **B,** High-power view showing cementoblasts *(arrows)* lining cementum **(C),** which has been deposited on the dentin walls.

fibers to calcify). A relationship may exist between pathologic alterations in collagen molecules within the pulp and pulpal calcification.

Calcification replaces the cellular components of the pulp and may possibly hinder the blood supply, although concrete evidence for this strangulation theory is lacking. Idiopathic pulpal pain was classically attributed to the presence of pulp stones. Modern knowledge of mechanisms of nociceptor activation coupled with the observation that pulp stones are so frequently observed in teeth lacking a history of pain have largely discounted this hypothesis. Therefore, from a clinical perspective, it would be unlikely that a patient's unexplained pain symptoms are due to pulpal calcifications, no matter how dramatic they may appear on a radiograph.

Luxation of teeth as a result of trauma may result in calcific metamorphosis, a condition that can, in a matter of months or years, lead to partial or complete radiographic obliteration of the pulp chamber. The cause of radiographic obliteration is excessive deposition of mineralized tissue resembling cementum or, occasionally, bone on the dentin walls, also referred to as *internal ankylosis* (Fig. 12-55). Histologic examination invariably reveals the presence of some soft tissue, and cells resembling cementoblasts can be observed lining the mineralized tissue. This calcific metamorphosis of the pulp has also been reported in replanted teeth of the rat.[275]

Clinically, the crowns of teeth affected by calcific metamorphosis may show a yellowish hue compared with adjacent normal teeth. This condition usually occurs in teeth with incomplete root formation. Trauma results in disruption of blood vessels entering the tooth, thus producing pulpal infarction. The wide periapical foramen allows connective tissue from the periodontal ligament to proliferate and replace the infarcted tissue, bringing with it cementoprogenitor and osteoprogenitor cells capable of differentiating into either cementoblasts or osteoblasts or both.

When calcific metamorphosis is noted on a patient's radiograph, it is sometimes suggested that the tooth be treated endodontically because the pulp is expected to be secondarily infected, and endodontic therapy should be performed while the pulp canal is still large enough to instrument. In a classic study of luxated teeth, Andreasen[7] found that only 7% of the pulps that underwent calcific metamorphosis exhibited secondary infection. Because the success rate for nonsurgical endodontic therapy, not only in general[399] but also for obliterated teeth,[67] is considered high, prophylactic intervention does not seem to be warranted.

AGE CHANGES

Continued formation of secondary dentin throughout life gradually reduces the size of the pulp chamber and root canals, although the width of the cementodentinal junction appears to stay relatively the same.[109,342] In addition, certain regressive changes in the pulp appear to be related to the aging process (see also Chapter 26). There is a gradual decrease in the cellularity and a concomitant increase in the number and thickness of collagen fibers, particularly in the radicular pulp. The thick collagen fibers may serve as foci for pulpal calcification (see Fig. 12-53). The odontoblasts decrease in size and number, and they may disappear altogether in certain areas of the pulp, particularly on the pulpal floor over the bifurcation or trifurcation areas of multirooted teeth.

With age there is a progressive reduction in the number of nerves[102] and blood vessels.[23,25] Evidence also suggests that aging results in an increase in the resistance of pulp tissue to the action of proteolytic enzymes,[420] hyaluronidase, and sialidase,[25] suggesting an alteration of both collagen and proteoglycans in the pulps of older teeth. The main changes in dentin associated with aging are an increase in peritubular dentin, dentinal sclerosis, and the number of dead tracts.*[342] Dentinal sclerosis produces a gradual decrease in dentinal permeability as the dentinal tubules become progressively reduced in diameter.[350]

---

*The term *dead tract* refers to a group of dentinal tubules in which odontoblast processes are absent. Dead tracts are easily recognized in ground sections because the empty tubules refract transmitted light, and the tract appears black in contrast to the light color of normal dentin.

REFERENCES

1. Aars H, Brodin P, Anderson E: A study of cholinergic and β-adrenergic components in the regulation of blood flow in the tooth pulp and gingiva of man, *Acta Physiol Scand* 148:441, 1993.

2. Aars H, Gazelius B, Edwall L, Olgart L: Effects of autonomic reflexes on tooth pulp blood flow in man, *Acta Physiol Scand* 146:423, 1992.

3. Accorinte ML, Loguercio AD, Reis A, et al: Response of human dental pulp capped with MTA and calcium hydroxide powder, *Oper Dent* 33:488, 2008.

4. Amess TR, Matthews B: The effect of topical application of lidocaine to dentin in the cat on the response of intra-dental nerves to mechanical stimuli. In Shimono M, Maeda T, Suda H, Takahashi K, editors: *Proceedings of the international conference on dentin/pulp complex*, Tokyo, 1996, Quintessence Publishing.

5. Andelin WE, Shabahang S, Wright K, Torabinejad M: Identification of hard tissue after experimental pulp capping using dentin sialoprotein (DSP) as a marker, *J Endod* 29:646, 2003.

6. Anderson LC, Vakoula A, Veinote R: Inflammatory hypersensitivity in a rat model of trigeminal neuropathic pain, *Arch Oral Biol* 48:161, 2003.

7. Andreasen JO: Luxation of permanent teeth due to trauma: a clinical and radiographic follow-up study of 189 injured teeth, *Scand J Dent Res* 78:273, 1970.

8. Anneroth G, Norberg KA: Adrenergic vasoconstrictor innervation in the human dental pulp, *Acta Odontol Scand* 26:89, 1968.

9. Arbuckle JB, Docherty RJ: Expression of tetrodotoxin-resistant sodium channels in capsaicin-sensitive dorsal root ganglion neurons of adult rats, *Neurosci Lett* 185:70, 1995.

10. Artese L, Rubini C, Ferrero G, et al: Vascular endothelial growth factor (VEGF) expression in healthy and inflamed human dental pulps, *J Endod* 28:20, 2002.

11. Avery JK: Structural elements of the young normal human pulp, *Oral Surg Oral Med Oral Pathol* 32:113, 1971.

12. Awawden L, Lundy FT, Shaw C, et al: Quantitative analysis of substance P, neurokinin A, and calcitonin gene-related peptide in pulp tissue from painful and healthy human teeth, *Int Endod J* 36:30, 2002.

13. Banchs F, Trope M: Revascularization of immature permanent teeth with apical periodontitis: new treatment protocol? *J Endod* 30:196, 2004.

14. Basbaum AI, Fields HL: Endogenous pain control systems: brainstem spinal pathways and endorphin circuitry, *Ann Rev Neurosci* 7:309, 1984.

15. Baume LJ: The biology of pulp and dentine. In Myers HM, editor: *Monographs in oral science*, vol 8, Basel, 1980, S Karger AG.

16. Beck P, Handwerker H: Bradykinin and serotonin effects on various types of cutaneous nerve fibers, *Pflugers Arch* 347:209, 1974.

17. Bender IB, Landau MA, Fonseca S, Trowbridge HO: The optimum placement-site of the electrode in electric pulp testing of the 12 anterior teeth, *J Am Dent Assoc* 118:305, 1989.

18. Bergenholtz G: Evidence for bacterial causation of adverse pulpal responses in resin-based dental restorations, *Crit Rev Oral Biol Med* 11:467, 2000.

19. Berggreen E, Haug SR, Mkony LE, Bletsa A: Characterization of the dental lymphatic system and identification of cells immunopositive to specific lymphatic markers, *Eur J Oral Sci* 117:34, 2009.

20. Berggreen E, Heyeraas KJ: The role of sensory neuropeptides and nitric oxide on pulpal blood flow and tissue pressure in the ferret, *J Dent Res* 78:1535, 1999.

21. Berggreen E, Heyeraas KJ: Effect of the sensory neuropeptide antagonists h-CGRP(8) and SR 140.33 on pulpal and gingival blood flow in ferrets, *Arch Oral Biol* 45:537, 2000.

22. Berggreen E, Heyeraas KJ: Role of K+ATP channels, endothelin A receptors, and effect of angiotensin II on blood flow in oral tissues, *J Dent Res* 82:33,2003.

23. Bernick S, Nedelman C: Effect of aging on the human pulp, *J Endod* 1:88, 1975.

24. Bevilacqua MP, et al: Interleukin-1 activation of vascular endothelium. Effects on procoagulant activity and leukocyte adhesion, *Am J Pathol* 121:394, 1985.

25. Bhussary BR: Modification of the dental pulp organ during development and aging. In Finn SB, editor: *Biology of the dental pulp organ: a symposium*, Birmingham, 1968, University of Alabama Press.

26. Biesterfeld RC, Taintor JF, Marsh CL: The significance of alterations of pulpal respiration: a review of the literature, *J Oral Pathol* 8:129, 1979.

27. Bisgaard H, Kristensen J: Leukotriene B4 produces hyperalgesia in humans, *Prostaglandins* 30:791, 1985.

28. Bishop MA, Malhotra MP: An investigation of lymphatic vessels in the feline dental pulp, *Am J Anat* 187:247, 1990.

29. Bishop MA, Yoshida S: A permeability barrier to lanthanum and the presence of collagen between odontoblasts in pig molars, *J Anat* 181:29, 1992.

30. Bletsa A, et al: Cytokine signalling in rat pulp interstitial fluid and transcapillary fluid exchange during lipopolysaccharide-induced acute inflammation, *J Physiol* 573 (Pt 1):225, 2006.

31. Bongenhielm U, Haegerstrand A, Theodorsson E, Fried K: Effects of neuropeptides on growth of cultivated rat molar pulp fibroblasts, *Regul Pept* 60:2391, 1995.

32. Borda E, Furlan C, Orman B, et al: Nitric oxide synthase and PGE2 reciprocal interactions in rat dental pulp: cholinoceptor modulation, *J Endod* 33:142, 2007.

33. Botero TM, Shelburne CE, Holland GR, Hanks CT, et al: TLR4 mediates LPS-induced VEGF expression in odontoblasts, *J Endod* 32:951, 2006.

34. Bowles WR, Flores CM, Jackson DL, Hargreaves KM: beta 2-Adrenoceptor regulation of CGRP release from capsaicin-sensitive neurons, *J Dent Res* 82:308, 2003.

35. Brännström M: The transmission and control of dentinal pain. In Grossman LJ, editor: *Mechanisms and control of pain*, New York, 1979, Masson Publishing USA.

36. Brännström M: Communication between the oral cavity and the dental pulp associated with restorative treatment, *Oper Dent* 9:57, 1984.

37. Brännström M, Aström A: A study of the mechanism of pain elicited from the dentin, *J Dent Res* 43:619,1964.

38. Breschi L, Lopes M, Gobbi P, et al: Dentin proteoglycans: an immunocytochemical FEISEM study, *J Biomed Mater Res* 61:40, 2002.

39. Brown AC, Yankowitz D: Tooth pulp tissue pressure and hydraulic permeability, *Circ Res* 15:42, 1964.

40. Butler WT, D'Sousa RN, Bronckers AL, et al: Recent investigations on dentin specific proteins, *Proc Finn Dent Soc* 88(suppl 1):369, 1992.

41. Byers MR: Dynamic plasticity of dental sensory nerve structure and cytochemistry, *Arch Oral Biol* 39(suppl):13S, 1994.

42. Byers MR: Neuropeptide immunoreactivity in dental sensory nerves: variations related to primary odontoblast function and survival. In Shimono M, Takahashi K, editors: *Dentin/pulp complex*, Tokyo, 1996, Quintessence Publishing.

43. Byers MR, Chudler EH, Iadarola MJ: Chronic tooth pulp inflammation causes transient and persistent expression of Fos in dynorphin-rich regions of rat brainstem, *Brain Res* 861:191, 2000.

44. Byers MR, Narhi MV, Mecifi KB: Acute and chronic reactions of dental sensory nerve fibers to cavities and desiccation in rat molars, *Anat Rec* 221:872, 1988.

45. Byers MR, Narhi MVO: Dental injury models: experimental tools for understanding neuroinflammatory interactions and polymodal nociceptor functions, *Crit Rev Oral Biol Med* 10:4, 1999.

46. Byers MR, Närhi MVO: Nerve supply of the pulpodentin complex and response to injury. In Hargreaves K, Goodis H, editors: *Seltzer and Bender's dental pulp*, Chicago, 2002, Quintessence Publishing.

47. Byers MR, Schatteman GC, Bothwell MA: Multiple functions for NGF-receptor in developing, aging and injured rat teeth are suggested by epithelial, mesenchymal and neural immunoreactivity, *Development* 109:461, 1990.

48. Byers MR, Sugaya A: Odontoblast process in dentin revealed by fluorescent Di-I, *J Histochem Cytochem* 43:159, 1995.

49. Byers MR, Suzuki H, Maeda T: Dental neuroplasticity, neuro-pulpal interactions and nerve regeneration, *Microsc Res Tech* 60:503, 2003.

50. Byers MR, Taylor PE: Effect of sensory denervation on the response of rat molar pulp to exposure injury, *J Dent Res* 72:613, 1993.

51. Byers MR, Taylor PE, Khayat BG, et al: Effects of injury and inflammation on pulpal and periapical nerves, *J Endod* 16:78, 1990.

52. Byers MR, Westenbroek RE: Odontoblasts in developing, mature and ageing rat teeth have multiple phenotypes that variably express all nine voltage-gated sodium channels, *Arch Oral Biol* 56:1199, 2011.

53. Byers MR, Wheeler EF, Bothwell M: Altered expression of NGF and P75 NGF-receptor by fibroblasts of injured teeth precedes sensory nerve sprouting, *Growth Factors* 6:41, 1992.

54. Camps J, Pashley DH: In vivo sensitivity to air blasts and scratching of human root dentin, *J Periodontol* 74:1589, 2003.

55. Camps J, Salomon JP, Van Meerbeek B, et al: Dentin deformation after scratching with clinically-relevant forces, *Arch Oral Biol* 48:527, 2003.

56. Caraivan O, Manolea H, Corlan Puscu D, et al: Microscopic aspects of pulpal changes in patients with chronic marginal periodontitis, *Rom J Morphol Embryol* 53:725, 2012.

57. Casasco A, Calligaro A, Casasco M, et al: Immunohistochemical localization of endothelin-like immunoreactivity in human tooth germ and mature dental pulp, *Anat Embryol (Berl)* 183:515, 1991.

58. Chaudhary P, Martenson ME, Baumann TK: Vanilloid receptor expression and capsaicin excitation of rat dental primary afferent neurons, *J Dent Res* 80:1518, 2001.

59. Chiang CY, Park SJ, Kwan CL, et al: NMDA receptor mechanisms contribute to neuroplasticity induced in caudalis nociceptive neurons by tooth pulp stimulation, *J Neurophysiol* 80:2621, 1998.

60. Chu SC, et al: Induction of vascular endothelial growth factor gene expression by proinflammatory cytokines in human pulp and gingival fibroblasts, *J Endod* 30:704, 2004.

61. Costos CAS, Hebling J, Hanks CT: Current status of pulp capping with dentin adhesive systems: a review, *Dent Mater* 16:188, 2000.

62. Coure E: Ultrastructural changes during the life cycle of human odontoblasts, *Arch Oral Biol* 31:643, 1986.

63. Cousins M, Power I: Acute and postoperative pain. In Wall P, Melzack R, editors: *Textbook of pain*, Edinburgh, 2002, Churchill Livingstone, p 456.

64. Cox CF, Bogen G, Kopel HM, Ruby JP: Repair of pulpal injury by dental materials, Chap. 14. In Hargreaves K, Goodis H, editors: *Seltzer and Bender's dental pulp*, Chicago, 2002, Quintessence Publishing.

65. Cox CF, White KC, Ramus DL, et al: Reparative dentin: factors affecting its deposition, *Quintessence Int* 23:257, 1992.

66. Csillag M, Berggreen E, Fristad I, et al: Effect of electrical tooth stimulation on blood flow and immunocompetent cells in rat dental pulp after sympathectomy, *Acta Odontol Scand* 62:305, 2004.

67. Cvek M, Granath L, Lundberg M: Failures and healing in endodontically treated non-vital anterior teeth with posttraumatically reduced pulpal lumen, *Acta Odontol Scand* 40:223, 1982.

68. Dahl E, Major IA: The fine structure of the vessels in the human dental pulp, *Acta Odontol Scand* 31:223, 1973.

69. Dahl T, Sabsay B, Veis A: Type I collagen-phosphophoryn interactions: specificity of the monomer-monomer binding, *J Struct Biol* 123:162, 1998.

70. Dallel R, Clavelou P, Woda A: Effects of tractotomy on nociceptive reactions induced by tooth pulp stimulation in the rat, *Exp Neurol* 106:78, 1989.

71. Davidson RM: Neural form of voltage-dependent sodium current in human cultured dental pulp cells, *Arch Oral Biol* 39:613, 1994.

72. Diamond J: The effect of injecting acetylcholine into normal and regenerating nerves, *J Physiol (Lond)* 145:611, 1959.

73. Diamond RD, Stanley HR, Swerdlow H: Reparative dentin formation resulting from cavity preparation, *J Prosthet Dent* 16:1127, 1966.

74. Diogenes A, Akopian AN, Hargreaves KM: NGF upregulates TRPA1: implications for orofacial pain, *J Dent Res* 86:550, 2007.

75. Dionne R: Oral sedation, *Compend Contin Educ Dent* 19:868, 1998.

76. Dray A: Inflammatory mediators of pain, *Br J Anaesth* 75:125, 1995.

77. D'Souza RN, Bachman T, Baumgardner KR, et al: Characterization of cellular responses involved in reparative dentinogenesis in rat molars, *J Dent Res* 74:702, 1995.

78. Dworkin SF: Anxiety and performance in the dental environment: an experimental investigation, *J Am Soc Psychosom Dent Med* 14:88, 1967.

79. Ebihara A, Tokita Y, Izawa T, Suda H: Pulpal blood flow assessed by laser Doppler flowmetry in a tooth with a horizontal root fracture, *Oral Surg Oral Med Oral Path* 81:229, 1996.

80. Eda S, Saito T: Electron microscopy of cells displaced into the dentinal tubules due to dry cavity preparation, *J Oral Pathol* 7:326, 1978.

81. Edwall B, Gazelius B, Fazekas A, et al: Neuropeptide Y (NPY) and sympathetic control of blood flow in oral mucosa and dental pulp in the cat, *Acta Physiol Scand* 125:253, 1985.

82. Edwall L, Kindlová M: The effect of sympathetic nerve stimulation on the rate of disappearance of tracers from various oral tissues, *Acta Odontol Scand* 29:387, 1971.

83. Embery G: Glycosaminoglycans of human dental pulp, *J Biol Buccale* 4:229, 1976.

84. Embery G, Hall R, Waddington R, et al: Proteoglycans in dentinogenesis, *Crit Rev Oral Biol Med* 12:331, 2001.

85. England MC, Pellis EG, Michanowicz AE: Histopathologic study of the effect of pulpal disease upon nerve fibers of the human dental pulp, *Oral Surg Oral Med Oral Pathol* 38:783, 1974.

86. England S: Molecular basis of peripheral hyperalgesia. In Wood J, editor: *Molecular basis of pain induction*, ed 1, New York, 2000, Wiley-Liss, p 261.

87. Engström C, Linde A, Persliden B: Acid hydrolases in the odontoblast-predentin region of dentinogenically active teeth, *Scand J Dent Res* 84:76, 1976.

88. Evans D, Reid T, Strang R, Stirrups D: A comparison of laser Doppler flowmetry with other methods of assessing vitality in traumatized anterior teeth, *Endod Dent Traumatol* 15:284, 1999.

89. Fava L: A comparison of one versus two appointment endodontic therapy in teeth with non-vital pulps, *Int Endod J* 22:179, 1989.

90. Fearnhead RW: Innervation of dental tissues. In Miles AEW, editor: *Structural and chemical organization of the teeth*, vol 1, New York, 1967, Academic Press.

91. Ferrara N: Vascular endothelial growth factor, *Eur J Cancer* 32A:2413, 1996.

92. Finkelman RD, Mohan S, Jennings JC, et al: Quantitation of growth factors IGF-1, SGF/IGF-11 and TGF-b in human dentin, *J Bone Miner Res* 5:717, 1990.

93. Firestone AR, Wheatley AM, Thüer UW: Measurement of blood perfusion in the dental pulp with laser Doppler flowmetry, *Int J Microcirc Clin Exp* 17:298, 1997.

94. Fish WE: *An experimental investigation of enamel, dentine and the dental pulp*, London, 1932, John Bale, Sons & Danielson.

95. Fisher AK: Respiratory variations within the normal dental pulp, *J Dent Res* 46:424, 1967.

96. Fisher AK, Schumacher ER, Robinson NR, Sharbondy GP: Effects of dental drugs and materials on the rate of oxygen consumption in bovine dental pulp, *J Dent Res* 36:447, 1957.

97. Fisher AK, Walters VE: Anaerobic glycolysis in bovine dental pulp, *J Dent Res* 47:717, 1968.

98. Fitzgerald M, Chiego DJ, Heys DR: Autoradiographic analysis of odontoblast replacement following pulp exposure in primate teeth, *Arch Oral Biol* 35:707, 1990.

99. Follenfant R, Nakamura-Craig M, Henderson B, Higgs GA: Inhibition by neuropeptides of interleukin-1B-induced, prostaglandin-independent hyperalgesia, *Br J Pharmacol* 98:41, 1989.

100. Fouad A: Molecular mediators of pulpal inflammation. In Hargreaves KM, Goodis HE, editors: *Seltzer and Bender's dental pulp*, Chicago, 2002, Quintessence Publishing, p 247.

101. Fraser JR, Kimpton WG, Laurent TC, et al: Uptake and degradation of hyaluronan in lymphatic tissue, *Biochem J* 256:153, 1988.

102. Fried K: Changes in pulp nerves with aging. *Proc Finn Dent Soc* 88(suppl 1):517, 1992.

103. Fried K, Sessle BJ, Devor M: The paradox of pain from tooth pulp: low-threshold "algoneurons"? *Pain* 152:2685, 2011.

104. Fristad I, Heyeraas KJ, Kvinnsland I: Nerve fibres and cells immunoreactive to neurochemical markers in developing rat molars and supporting tissues, *Arch Oral Biol* 39:633, 1994.

105. Fristad I, Jacobsen EB, Kvinnsland IH: Coexpression of vasoactive intestinal polypeptide and substance P in reinnervating pulpal nerves and in trigeminal ganglion neurones after axotomy of the inferior alveolar nerve in the rat, *Arch Oral Biol* 43:183, 1998.

106. Fristad I, Kvinnsland IH, Jonsson R, Heyeraas KJ: Effect of intermittent long-lasting electrical tooth stimulation on pulpal blood flow and immunocompetent cells: a hemodynamic and immunohistochemical study in young rat molars, *Exp Neurol* 146:230, 1997.

107. Fristad I, Vandevska-Radunovic V, Fjeld K, et al: NK1, NK2, NK3 and CGRP1 receptors identified in rat oral soft tissues, and in bone and dental hard tissue cells, *Cell Tissue Res* 311:383, 2003.

108. Fuss Z, Trowbridge H, Bender IB, et al: Assessment of reliability of electrical and thermal pulp testing agents, *J Endod* 12:301, 1986.

109. Gani O, Visvisian C: Apical canal diameter in the first upper molar at various ages, *J Endod* 10:689, 1999.

110. Garant PR: The organization of microtubules within rat odontoblast processes revealed by perfusion fixation with glutaraldehyde, *Arch Oral Biol* 17:1047, 1972.

111. Garberoglio R, Brännström M: Scanning electron microscopic investigation of human dentinal tubules, *Arch Oral Biol* 21:355, 1976.

112. Gedney JJ, Logan H, Baron RS: Predictors of short-term and long-term memory of sensory and affective dimensions of pain, *J Pain* 4:47, 2003.

113. George CH, Kendall JM, Evans WH: Intracellular trafficking pathways on assembly of connexins into tight junctions, *J Biol Chem* 274:8678, 1999.

114. Gerli R, Secciani I, Sozio F, et al: Absence of lymphatic vessels in human dental pulp: a morphological study, *Eur J Oral Sci* 118:110, 2010.

115. Gibbs JL, Hargreaves KM: Neuropeptide Y Y1 receptor effects on pulpal nociceptors, *J Dent Res* 87:948, 2008.

116. Gilbert TM, Pashley DH, Anderson RW: Response of pulpal blood flow to intra-arterial infusion of endothelin, *J Endod* 18:228, 1992.

117. Gilron I, Max MB, Lee G, et al: Effects of the 2-amino-3-hydroxy-5-methyl-4-isoxazole-proprionic acid/ kainate antagonist LY293558 on spontaneous and evoked postoperative pain, *Clin Pharmacol Ther* 68:320, 2000.

118. Gloe T, Pohl U: Laminin binding conveys mechanosensing in endothelial cells, *News Physiol Sci* 17:166, 2002.

119. Gold M: Tetrodotoxin-resistant Na currents and inflammatory hyperalgesia, *Proc Natl Acad Sci U S A* 96:7645, 1999.

120. Gold MS, Reichling DB, Shuster MJ, Levine JD: Hyperalgesic agents increase a tetrodotoxin-resistant Na+ current in nociceptors, *Proc Natl Acad Sci U S A* 93:1108, 1996.

121. Goldberg M, Farges J-C, Lacerda-Pinheiro S, et al: Inflammatory and immunological aspects of dental pulp repair, *Pharmacol Res* 58:137, 2008.

122. Goldberg M, Six N, Decup F, et al: Bioactive molecules and the future of pulp therapy, *Am J Dent* 16:66, 2003.

123. Goldberg M, Takagi M: Dentine proteoglycans: composition, ultrastructure and functions, *Histochem J* 25:781, 1993.

124. Goodis H, Bowles W, Hargreaves K: Prostaglandin E2 enhances bradykinin-evoked iCGRP release in bovine dental pulp, *J Dent Res* 79:1604, 2000.

125. Gordon SM, Dionne RA, Brahim J, et al: Blockade of peripheral neuronal barrage reduces postoperative pain, *Pain* 70:209, 1997.

126. Gotjamanos T: Cellular organization in the subodontoblastic zone of the dental pulp. II. Period and mode of development of the cell-rich layer in rat molar pulps, *Arch Oral Biol* 14:1011, 1969.

127. Gould HJ, England JD, Soignier RD, et al: Ibuprofen blocks changes in Na,1.7 and 1.8 sodium channels associated with complete Freund's adjuvant-induced inflammation in rat, *J Pain* 5:270, 2004.

128. Gould HJ 3rd, Gould TN, Paul D, et al: Development of inflammatory hypersensitivity and augmentation of sodium channels in rat dorsal root ganglia, *Brain Res* 824:296, 1999.

129. Gregg JM, Dixon AD: Somatotopic organization of the trigeminal ganglion, *Arch Oral Biol* 18:487, 1973.

130. Grossman ES, Austin JC: Scanning electron microscope observations on the tubule content of freeze-fractured peripheral vervet monkey dentine (Cercopithecus pygerythrus), *Arch Oral Biol* 28:279, 1983.

131. Gunji T: Morphological research on the sensitivity of dentin, *Arch Histol Jpn* 45:45, 1982.

132. Hagermark O, Hokfelt T, Pernow B: Flare and itch produced by substance P in human skin, *J Invest Dermatol* 71:233, 1979.

133. Hahn C-L, Falkler WA Jr, Siegel MA: A study of T cells and B cells in pulpal pathosis, *J Endod* 15:20, 1989.

134. Hals E, Tonder KJ: Elastic pseudoelastic tissue in arterioles of the human and dog dental pulp, *Scand J Dent Res* 89:218, 1981.

135. Hamersky PA, Weimer AD, Taintor JF: The effect of orthodontic force application on the pulpal tissue respiration rate in the human premolar, *Am J Orthod* 77:368, 1980.

136. Han SS: The fine structure of cells and intercellular substances of the dental pulp. In Finn SB, editor: *Biology of the dental pulp organ*, Birmingham, 1968, University of Alabama Press, p 103.

137. Hargreaves KM: Pain mechanisms of the pulpodentin complex. In Hargreaves KM, Goodis HE, editors: *Seltzer and Bender's dental pulp*, Chicago, 2002, Quintessence Publishing Company, p 181.

138. Hargreaves KM, Bowles WR, Jackson DL: Intrinsic regulation of CGRP release by dental pulp sympathetic fibers, *J Dent Res* 82:398, 2003.

139. Hargreaves KM, Dionne RA, Mueller GP, et al: Naloxone, fentanyl, and diazepam modify plasma beta-endorphin levels during surgery, *Clin Pharmacol Ther* 40:165, 1986.

140. Hargreaves KM, Keiser K: Local anesthetic failure in endodontics: mechanisms and management, *Endod Topics* 1:26, 2002.

141. Hargreaves KM, Milam SB: Mechanisms of pain and analgesia. In Dionne R, Phero J, editors: *Management of pain and anxiety in dental practice*, New York, 2001, Elsevier, p 18.

142. Hargreaves KM, Swift JQ, Roszkowski MT, et al: Pharmacology of peripheral neuropeptide and inflammatory mediator release, *Oral Surg Oral Med Oral Pathol* 78:503, 1994.

143. Harris R, Griffin CJ: Fine structure of nerve endings in the human dental pulp, *Arch Oral Biol* 13:773, 1968.

144. Hartmann A, Azerad J, Boucher Y: Environmental effects on laser Doppler pulpal blood-flow measurements in man, *Arch Oral Biol* 41:333, 1996.

145. Hashioka K, Suzuki K, Yoshida T, et al: Relationship between clinical symptoms and enzyme-producing bacteria isolated from infected root canals, *J Endod*, 20:75, 1994.

146. Hattler AB, Listgarten MA: Pulpal response to root planing in a rat model, *J Endod* 10:471, 1984.

147. Haug SR, Heyeraas KJ: Effects of sympathectomy on experimentally induced pulpal inflammation and periapical lesions in rats, *Neuroscience* 120:827, 2003.

148. Haug SR, Heyeraas KJ: Modulation of dental inflammation by the sympathetic nervous system, *J Dent Res* 85:488, 2006.

149. Hermanstyne TO, Markowitz K, Fan L, Gold MS: Mechanotransducers in rat pulpal afferents, *J Dent Res* 87:834, 2008.

150. Heyeraas KJ: Pulpal hemodynamics and interstitial fluid pressure: balance of transmicrovascular fluid transport, *J Endod* 15:468, 1989.

151. Heyeraas KJ, Berggreen E: Interstitial fluid pressure in normal and inflamed pulp, *Crit Rev Oral Biol Med* 10:328, 1999.

152. Heyeraas KJ, Jacobsen EB, Fristad I: Vascular and immunoreactive nerve fiber reactions in the pulp after stimulation and denervation: proceedings of the International Conference, in Dentin/Pulp Complex. Shimono M, Maeda T, Suda H, Takahashi K, editors. Tokyo, 1996, Quintessence Publishing, p 162.

153. Heyeraas KJ, Kim S, Raab WH, et al: Effect of electrical tooth stimulation on blood flow, interstitial fluid pressure and substance P and CGRP-immunoreactive nerve fibers in the low compliant cat dental pulp, *Microvasc Res* 47:329, 1994.

154. Heyeraas KJ, Kvinnsland I: Tissue pressure and blood flow in pulpal inflammation, *Proc Finn Dent Soc* 88(suppl 1):393, 1992.

155. Hikiji A, Yamamoto H, Sunakawa M, Suda H: Increased blood flow and nerve firing in the cat canine tooth in response to stimulation of the second premolar pulp, *Arch Oral Biol* 45:53, 2000.

156. Hill R: NK1 (substance P) receptor antagonists—why are they not analgesic in humans? [see comment], *Trends Pharmacol Sci* 21:244, 2000.

157. Hirvonen T, Närhi M, Hakumäki M: The excitability of dog pulp nerves in relation to the condition of dentine surface, *J Endod* 10:294, 1984.

158. Holland GR: The extent of the odontoblast process in the cat, *Arch Anat* 121:133, 1976.

159. Holland GR: The odontoblast process: form and function, *J Dent Res* 64(special issue):499, 1985.

160. Holland GR: Morphological features of dentine and pulp related to dentine sensitivity, *Arch Oral Biol* 39(suppl):3S, 1994.

161. Ianiro SR, Jeansonne BG, McNeal SF, Eleazer PD: The effect of preoperative acetaminophen or a combination of acetaminophen and ibuprofen on the success of inferior alveolar nerve block for teeth with irreversible pulpitis, *J Endod* 33:11, 2007.

162. Ibricevic H, Heyeraas KJ, Pasic Juhas E, et al: Identification of alpha 2 adrenoceptors in the blood vessels of the dental pulp, *Int Endod J* 24:279, 1991.

163. Ikeda H, Tokita Y, Suda H: Capsaicin-sensitive A fibers in cat tooth pulp, *J Dent Res* 76:1341, 1997.

164. Inoue H, Kurosaka Y, Abe K: Autonomic nerve endings in the odontoblast/predentin border and predentin of the canine teeth of dogs, *J Endod* 18:149, 1992.

165. Jacobsen EB, Heyeraas KJ: Pulp interstitial fluid pressure and blood flow after denervation and electrical tooth stimulation in the ferret, *Arch Oral Biol* 42:407, 1997.

166. Janig W, Kollman W: The involvement of the sympathetic nervous system in pain, *Fortschr Arzneimittelforsch* 34:1066, 1984.

167. Jebeles JA, Reilly JS, Gutierrez JF, et al: Tonsillectomy and adenoidectomy pain reduction by local bupivacaine infiltration in children, *Int J Ped Otorhinolaryngology* 25:149, 1993.

168. Jeske NA, Diogenes A, Ruparel NB, et al: A-kinase anchoring protein mediates TRPV1 thermal hyperalgesia through PKA phosphorylation of TRPV1, *Pain* 138:604, 2008.

169. Johnsen D, Johns S: Quantitation of nerve fibers in the primary and permanent canine and incisor teeth in man, *Arch Oral Biol* 23:825, 1978.

170. Johnsen DC, Harshbarger J, Rymer HD: Quantitative assessment of neural development in human premolars, *Anat Rec* 205:421, 1983.

171. Johnson G, Brännström M: The sensitivity of dentin: changes in relation to conditions at exposed tubule apertures, *Acta Odontol Scand* 32:29, 1974.

172. Jones PA, Taintor JF, Adams AB: Comparative dental material cytotoxicity measured by depression of rat incisor pulp respiration, *J Endod* 5:48, 1979.

173. Jontell M, Okiji T, Dahlgren U, Bergenholtz G: Immune defense mechanisms of the dental pulp, *Crit Rev Oral Biol Med* 9:179, 1998.

174. Juan H, Lembeck F: Action of peptides and other analgesic agents on paravascular pain receptors of the isolated perfused rabbit ear, *Naunyn Schmiedebergs Arch Pharmacol* 283:151, 1974.

175. Katoh Y, Yamaguchi R, Shinkai K, et al: Clinicopathological study on pulp-irritation of adhesive resinous materials (report 3). Direct capping effects on exposed pulp of Macaca fascicularis, *Jpn J Conserv Dent* 40:163, 1997.

176. Kaufman E, Hargreaves KM, Dionne RA: Comparison of oral triazolam and nitrous oxide with placebo and intravenous diazepam for outpatient premedication, *Oral Surg Oral Med Oral Pathol* 75:156, 1993.

177. Kayaoglu G, Orstavik D: Virulence factors of Enterococcus faecalis: relationship to endodontic disease, *Crit Rev Oral Biol Med* 15:308, 2004.

178. Kaye H, Herold RC: Structure of human dentine. I. Phase contrast, polarization, interference, and bright field microscopic observations on the lateral branch system, *Arch Oral Biol* 11:355, 1966.

179. Kelley KW, Bergenholtz G, Cox CF: The extent of the odontoblast process in rhesus monkeys (Macaca mulatta) as observed by scanning electron microscopy, *Arch Oral Biol* 26:893, 1981.

180. Kerezoudis NP, Funato A, Edwall L, et al: Activation of sympathetic nerves exerts an inhibitory influence on afferent nerve-induced vasodilation unrelated to vasoconstriction in rat dental pulp, *Acta Physiol Scand* 147:27, 1993.

181. Kerezoudis NP, Olgart L, Edwall L: CGRP(8) reduces the duration but not the maximal increase of antidromic vasodilation in dental pulp and lip of the rat, *Acta Physiol Scand* 151:73, 1994.

182. Kerezoudis NP, Olgart L, Edwall L: Involvement of substance P but not nitric oxide or calcitonin gene-related peptide in neurogenic plasma extravasation in rat incisor pulp and lip, *Arch Oral Biol* 39:769, 1994.

183. Khan A, Diogenes A, Jeske N, et al: Tumor necrosis factor alpha enhances the sensitivity of trigeminal ganglion neurons to capsaicin, *Neuroscience* 155:503, 2008.

184. Khan AA, McCreary B, Owatz CB, et al: The development of a diagnostic instrument for the measurement of mechanical allodynia, *J Endod* 33:663, 2007.

185. Khan AA, Owatz CB, Schindler WG, et al: Measurement of mechanical allodynia and local anesthetic efficacy in patients with irreversible pulpitis and acute periradicular periodontitis, *J Endod* 33:796, 2007.

186. Khullar SM, Fristad I, Brodin P, Kvinnsland IH: Upregulation of growth associated protein 43 expression and neuronal co-expression with neuropeptide Y following inferior alveolar nerve axotomy in the rat, *J Peripher Nerv Syst* 3:79, 1998.

187. Kim S: Regulation of pulpal blood flow, *J Dent Res* 64(Spec No):590, 1985.

188. Kim S, Dorscher-Kim JE, Liu M: Microcirculation of the dental pulp and its autonomic control, *Proc Finn Dent Soc* 85:279, 1989.

189. Kim S, Dorscher-Kim JE, Liu M, et al: Functional alterations in pulpal microcirculation in response to various dental procedures and materials, *Proc Finn Dent Soc* 88(suppl 1):65, 1992.

190. Kim S, Edwall L, Trowbridge H, Chien S: Effects of local anesthetics on pulpal blood flow in dogs, *J Dent Res* 63:650, 1984.

191. Kim S, Liu M, Simchon S, et al: Effects of selected inflammatory mediators on blood flow and vascular permeability in the dental pulp, *Proc Finn Dent Soc* 88(suppl 1):387, 1992.

192. Kim S, Schuessler G, Chien S: Measurement of blood flow in the dental pulp of dogs with the 133xenon washout method, *Arch Oral Biol* 28:501, 1983.

193. Kim S, Trowbridge HO, Dorscher-Kim JE: The influence of 5-hydroxytryptamine (serotonin) on blood flow in the dog pulp, *J Dent Res* 65:682, 1986.

194. Kim SK, Ang L, Hsu YY, et al: Antagonistic effect of D-myo-inositol-1,2,6-trisphosphate (PP56) on neuropeptide Y-induced vasoconstriction in the feline dental pulp, *Arch Oral Biol* 41:791, 1996.

195. Kimberly CL, Byers BR: Inflammation of rat molar pulp and periodontium causes increased calcitonin-gene-related peptide and axonal sprouting, *Anat Rec* 222:289, 1988.

196. Kramer IRH: The distribution of blood vessels in the human dental pulp. In Finn SB, editor: *Biology of the dental pulp organ*, Birmingham, 1968, University of Alabama Press, p 361.

197. Kress M, Sommer C: Neuroimmunology and pain: peripheral effects of proinflammatory cytokines. In Brune K, Handwerker H, editors: *Hyperalgesia: molecular mechanisms and clinical implications*, Seattle, WA, 2003, IASP Press, p 57.

198. Kroeger DC, Gonzales F, Krivoy W: Transmembrane potentials of cultured mouse dental pulp cells, *Proc Soc Exp Biol Med* 108:134, 1961.

199. Kumazawa T, Mizumura K: Thin-fiber receptors responding to mechanical, chemical and thermal stimulation in the skeletal muscle of the dog, *Arch Physiol* 273:179, 1977.

200. Kvinnsland IH, Luukko K, Fristad I, et al: Glial cell line-derived neurotrophic factor (GDNF) from adult rat tooth serves a distinct population of large-sized trigeminal neurons, *Eur J Neurosci* 19:2089, 2004.

201. Langeland K, Langeland LK: Histologic study of 155 impacted teeth, *Odontol Tidskr* 73:527, 1965.

202. Langeland K, Langeland LK: Pulp reactions to cavity and crown preparations, *Aust Dent J* 15:261, 1970.

203. Lantelme RL, Handleman SL, Herbison RJ: Dentin formation in periodontally diseased teeth, *J Dent Res* 55:48, 1976.

204. Latremoliere A, Woolf CJ: Central sensitization: a generator of pain hypersensitivity by central neural plasticity, *J Pain* 10:895, 2009.

205. Laurent TC, et al: The catabolic fate of hyaluronic acid, *Connect Tissue Res* 15:33, 1986.

206. Lechner JH, Kalnitsky G: The presence of large amounts of type III collagen in bovine dental pulp and its significance with regard to the mechanism of dentinogenesis, *Arch Oral Biol* 26:265, 1981.

207. Lepinski AM, Hargreaves KM, Goodis HE, Bowles WR: Bradykinin levels in dental pulp by microdialysis, *J Endod* 26:744, 2000.

208. Lesot H, Osman M, Ruch JV: Immunofluorescent localization of collagens, fibronectin and laminin during terminal differentiation of odontoblasts, *Dev Biol* 82:371, 1981.

209. Levi-Montalcini R: The nerve growth factor: its mode of action on sensory and sympathetic nerve cells, *Harvey Lect* 60:217, 1966.

210. Levine J, Moskowitz M, Basbaum A: The contribution of neurogenic inflammation in experimental arthritis, *J Immunol* 135:843, 1985.

211. Levine J, Taiwo Y: Inflammatory pain. In Wall P, Melzack R, editors: *Textbook of pain*, Edinburgh, 1994, Churchill-Livingston.

212. Levine JD, Gordon NC, Fields HL: The mechanism of placebo analgesia, *Lancet* 2:654, 1978.

213. Lewin G, Rueff A, Mendell L: Peripheral and central mechanisms of NGF-induced hyperalgesia, *Eur J Neurosci* 6:1903, 1994.

214. Light A: *The initial processing of pain and its descending control: spinal and trigeminal systems*, Basel, 1992, Karger.

215. Lilja J: Innervation of different parts of the predentin and dentin in a young human premolar, *Acta Odontol Scand* 37:339, 1979.

216. Lilja J, Noredenvall K-J, Brännström M: Dentin sensitivity, odontoblasts and nerves under desiccated or infected experimental cavities, *Swed Dent J* 6:93, 1982.

217. Lilja JJ, Kivisto KT, Backman JT, Neuvonen PJ: Effect of grapefruit juice dose on grapefruit juice-triazolam interaction: repeated consumption prolongs triazolam half-life, *Eur J Clin Pharmacol* 56:411, 2000.

218. Lindahl O: Pain-a chemical explanation, *Acta Rheumatol Scand* 8:161, 1962.

219. Linde A: A study of the dental pulp glycosamino-glycans from permanent human teeth and rat and rabbit incisors, *Arch Oral Biol* 18:49, 1973.

220. Linde A: The extracellular matrix of the dental pulp and dentin, *J Dent Res* 64(special issue):523, 1985.

221. Linden GJ, Curtis TM, About I, et al: Human odontoblasts express functional thermo-sensitive TRP channels: implications for dentin sensitivity, *Pain* 152: 2211-2223, 2011.

222. Liu L, Simon SA: Capsaicin, acid and heat-evoked currents in rat trigeminal ganglion neurons: relationship to functional VR1 receptors, *Physiol Behav* 69:363, 2000.

223. Lohinai Z, Balla I, Marczis J, et al: Evidence for the role of nitric oxide in the circulation of the dental pulp, *J Dent Res* 74:1501, 1995.

224. Lohinai Z, Szekely AD, Benedek P, Csillag A: Nitric oxide synthetase containing nerves in the cat and dog dental pulps and gingiva, *Neurosci Lett* 227:91, 1997.

225. Lundberg JM, Änggård A, Fahrenkrug J, et al: Vasoactive intestinal polypeptide in cholinergic neurons of exocrine glands: functional significance of coexisting transmitters for vasodilation and secretion, *Proc Natl Acad Sci U S A* 77:1651, 1980.

226. Lundberg JM, Fried G, Fahrenkrug J, et al: Subcellular fractionation of cat submandibular gland: comparative studies on the distribution of acetylcholine and vasoactive intestinal polypeptide (VIP), *Neuroscience* 6:1001, 1981.

227. Lundgren T, Nannmark U, Linde A: Calcium ion activity and pH in the odontoblast-predentin region: ion-selective microelectrode measurements, *Calcif Tissue Int* 50:134, 1992.

228. Luthman J, Luthman D, Hökfelt T: Occurrence and distribution of different neurochemical markers in the human dental pulp, *Arch Oral Biol* 37:193, 1992.

229. Madison S, Whitsel EA, Suarez-Roca H, Maixner W: Sensitizing effects of leukotriene B4 on intradental primary afferents, *Pain* 49:99, 1992.

230. Maeda T, Honma S, Takano Y: Dense innervation of radicular human dental pulp as revealed by immunocytochemistry for protein gene-product 9.5, *Arch Oral Biol* 39:563, 1994.

231. Magloire H, Couble ML, Thivichon-Prince B, et al: Odontoblast: a mechano-sensory cell, *J Exp Zool (Mol Dev Evol)* 312B:416, 2009.

232. Magloire H, Maurin JC, Couble ML, et al: Topical review. Dental pain and odontoblasts: facts and hypotheses, *J Orofacial Pain* 24:335, 2010.

233. Maixner W, Dubner R, Kenshalo DR Jr, et al: Responses of monkey medullary dorsal horn neurons during the detection of noxious heat stimuli, *J Neurophysiol* 62:437, 1989.

234. Malmberg AB, Yaksh TL: Spinal nitric oxide synthesis inhibition blocks NMDA-induced thermal hyperalgesia and produces antinociception in the formalin test in rats, *Pain* 54:291, 1993.

235. Malmberg AB, Yaksh TL: Cyclooxygenase inhibition and the spinal release of prostaglandin E2 and amino acids evoked by paw formalin injection: a microdialysis study in unanesthetized rats, *J Neurosci* 15:2768, 1995.

236. Maltos KL, Menezes GB, Caliari MV, et al: Vascular and cellular responses to pro-inflammatory stimuli in rat dental pulp, *Arch Oral Biol* 49:443, 2004.

237. Mangkornkarn C, Steiner JC: In vivo and in vitro glycosaminoglycans from human dental pulp, *J Endod* 18:327, 1992.

238. Marbach JJ, Raphael KG: Phantom tooth pain: a new look at an old dilemma. *Pain Med* 1:68, 2000.

239. Marfurt CF, Zaleski EM, Adams CE, Welther CL: Sympathetic nerve fibers in rat orofacial and cerebral tissues as revealed by the HRP-WGA tracing technique: a light and electron microscopic study, *Brain Res* 366:373, 1986.

240. Marion D, Jean A, Hamel H, et al: Scanning electron microscopic study of odontoblasts and circumferential dentin in a human tooth, *Oral Surg Oral Med Oral Pathol* 72:473, 1991.

241. Marriott D, Wilkin GP, Coote PR, Wood JN: Eicosanoid synthesis by spinal cord astrocytes is evoked by substance P; possible implications for nociception and pain, *Adv Prostaglandin Thromboxane Leukot Res* 21B:739, 1991.

242. Martin A, Gasse H, Staszyk C: Absence of lymphatic vessels in the dog dental pulp: an immunohistochemical study, *J Anat* 217:609, 2010.

243. Martin H, Basbaum AI, Kwiat GC, et al: Leukotriene and prostaglandin sensitization of cutaneous high-threshold C- and A-delta mechanoreceptors in the hairy skin of rat hindlimbs, *Neuroscience* 22:651, 1987.

244. Matsuo S, Ichikawa H, Henderson TA, et al: trkA modulation of developing somatosensory neurons in oro-facial tissues: tooth pulp fibers are absent in trkA knockout mice, *Neuroscience* 105:747, 2001.

245. Matthews B, Andrew D: Microvascular architecture and exchange in teeth, *Microcirculation* 2:305, 1995.

246. Matthews B, Vongsavan N: Interactions between neural and hydrodynamic mechanisms in dentine and pulp, *Arch Oral Biol* 39(suppl 1):87S, 1994.

247. McGrath PA, Gracely RH, Dubner R, Heft MW: Non-pain and pain sensations evoked by tooth pulp stimulation, *Pain* 15:377, 1983.

248. Meller ST, Dykstra C, Gebhart GF: Production of endogenous nitric oxide and activation of soluble guanylate cyclase are required for N-methyl-D-aspartate-produced facilitation of the nociceptive tail-flick reflex, *Eur J Pharmacol* 214:93, 1992.

249. Meyer MW, Path MG: Blood flow in the dental pulp of dogs determined by hydrogen polarography and radioactive microsphere methods, *Arch Oral Biol* 24:601, 1979.

250. Meyer R, Campbell J: Myelinated nociceptive afferents account for the hyperalgesia that follows a burn to the hand, *Science* 213:1527, 1981.

251. Mirza AF, Mo J, Holt JL, et al: Is there a relationship between throbbing pain and arterial pulsations? *J Neurosci* 32:7572, 2012.

252. Mitsiadis TA, De Bari C, About I: Apoptosis in developmental and repair-related human tooth remodeling: a view from the inside, *Exp Cell Res* 314:869, 2008.

253. Mjör IA, Nordahl I: The density and branching of dentinal tubules in human teeth, *Arch Oral Biol* 41:401, 1996.

254. Modaresi J, Dianat O, Mozayeni MA: The efficacy comparison of ibuprofen, acetaminophen-codeine, and placebo premedication therapy on the depth of anesthesia during treatment of inflamed teeth, *Oral Surg Oral Med Oral Pathol* 102:399, 2006.

255. Mullaney TP, Howell RM, Petrich JD: Resistance of nerve fibers to pulpal necrosis, *Oral Surg* 30:690, 1970.

256. Murray PE, About I, Lumley PJ, et al: Human odontoblast cell numbers after dental injury, *J Dent* 28:277, 2000.

257. Murray PE, Hafez AA, Windsor LJ, et al: Comparison of pulp responses following restoration of exposed and non-exposed cavities, *J Dent* 30:213, 2002.

258. Murray PE, Lumley PJ, Ross HF, Smith AJ: Tooth slice organ culture for cytotoxicity assessment of dental materials, *Biomaterials* 21:1711, 2000.

259. Naftel JP, et al: Course and composition of the nerves that supply the mandibular teeth of the rat, *Anat Rec* 256:433, 1999.

260. Nagaoka S, Miyazaki Y, Liu HJ, et al: Bacterial invasion into dentinal tubules of human vital and nonvital teeth, *J Endod* 21:70, 1995.

261. Nair PN, et al: Histological, ultrastructural and quantitative investigations on the response of healthy human pulps to experimental capping with mineral trioxide aggregate: a randomized controlled trial, *Int Endod J* 41:128, 2008.

262. Nakanishi P, Shimizu H, Hosokawa Y, et al: An immunohistological study on cyclooxygenase-2 in human dental pulp, *J Endod* 27:385, 2001.

263. Närhi M: Activation of dental pulp nerves of the cat and the dog with hydrostatic pressure, *Proc Finn Dent Soc* 74(suppl 5):1, 1978.

264. Narhi M: The characteristics of intradental sensory units and their responses to stimulation, *J Dent Res* 64:564, 1985.

265. Narhi M, Jyväsjärvi E, Virtanen A, et al: Role of intradental A and C type nerve fibers in dental pain mechanisms, *Proc Finn Dent Soc* 88:507, 1992.

266. Närhi M, Jyväsjärvi E, Hirronen T: Activation of heat-sensitive nerve fibers in the dental pulp of the cat, *Pain* 14:317, 1982.

267. Närhi M, Virtanen A, Kuhta J, Huopaniemi T: Electrical stimulation of teeth with a pulp tester in the cat, *Scand J Dent Res* 87:32, 1979.

268. Närhi M, Yamamoto H, Ngassapa D: Function of intradental nociceptors in normal and inflamed teeth. In Shimono M, Maeda T, Suda H, Takahashi K, editors: *Dentin/pulp complex*, Tokyo, 1996, Quintessence Publishing, p 136.

269. Närhi M, Yamamoto H, Ngassapa D, Hirvonen T: The neurophysiological basis and the role of inflammatory reactions in dentine hypersensitivity, *Arch Oral Biol* 39(suppl):23S, 1994.

270. Nassar M, Stirling L, Forlani G, et al: Nociceptor-specific gene deletion reveals a major role for NAv 1.7 (PN1) in acute and inflammatory pain, *Proc Natl Acad Sci U S A* 101:12706, 2004.

271. Nawroth PP, Stern DM: Modulation of endothelial cell hemostatic properties by tumor necrosis factor, *J Exp Med* 163:740, 1986.

272. Neumann S, Doubell TP, Leslie T, Woolf CJ: Inflammatory pain hypersensitivity mediated by phenotype switch in myelinated primary sensory neurons, *Nature* 384:360, 1996.

273. Ngassapa D, Närhi M, Hirvonen T: The effect of serotonin (5-HT) and calcitonin gene-related peptide (CGRP) on the function of intradental nerves in the dog, *Proc Finn Dent Soc* 88(suppl 1):143, 1992.

274. Nicol GD, Vasko MR: Unraveling the story of NGF-mediated sensitization of nociceptive sensory neurons: ON or OFF the Trks? *Mol Interv* 7:26, 2007.

275. Nishioka M, Shiiya T, Ueno K, Suda H: Tooth replantation in germ-free and conventional rats, *Endod Dent Traumatol* 14:163, 1998.

276. Nitzan DW, Michaeli Y, Weinreb M, Azaz B: The effect of aging on tooth morphology: a study on impacted teeth, *Oral Surg Oral Med Oral Pathol* 61:54, 1986.

277. O'Neil RG, Brown RC: The vanilloid receptor family of calcium-permeable channels: molecular integrators of

microenvironmental stimuli, *News Physiol Sci* 18:226, 2003.

278. Ochoa JL, Torebjork E, Marchettini P, Sivak M: Mechanism of neuropathic pain: cumulative observations, new experiments, and further speculation. In Fields HL, Dubner R, Cervero F, editors: *Advances in pain research and therapy*, New York, 1985, Raven Press, p 431.

279. Okeson JP: Assessment of orofacial pain disorders. In Okeson JP, editors: *Orofacial pain: guidelines for assessment, diagnosis, and management*, Chicago, 1996, Quintessence Publishing, p 35.

280. Okiji T, Kawashima N, Kosaka T, et al: An immunohistochemical study of the distribution of immunocompetent cells, especially macrophages and Ia antigen-presenting cells of heterogeneous populations, in normal rat molar pulp, *J Dent Res* 71:1196, 1992.

281. Okiji T, Morita I, Sunada I, et al: Involvement of arachidonic acid metabolites in increases in vascular permeability in experimental dental pulpal inflammation in the rat, *Arch Oral Biol* 34:523, 1989.

282. Olgart L, Kerezoudis NP: Nerve-pulp interactions, *Arch Oral Biol* 39(suppl):47S, 1994.

283. Olgart LM, Edwall L, Gazelius B: Neurogenic mediators in control of pulpal blood flow, *J Endod* 15:409, 1989.

284. Olgart LM, Edwall L, Gazelius B: Involvement of afferent nerves in pulpal blood-flow reactions in response to clinical and experimental procedures in the cat, *Arch Oral Biol* 36:575, 1991.

285. Olgart LM, Gazelius B, Brodin E, Nilsson G: Release of substance P-like immunoreactivity from the dental pulp, *Acta Physiol Scand* 101:510, 1977.

286. Orchardson R, Cadden SW: An update on the physiology of the dentine-pulp complex, *Dent Update* 28:200, 208, 2001.

287. Orchardson R, Gillam DG: Managing dentin hypersensitivity, *J Am Dent Assoc* 137:990; quiz 1028, 2006.

288. Owatz CB, Khan AA, Schindler WG, et al: The incidence of mechanical allodynia in patients with irreversible pulpitis, *J Endod* 33:552, 2007.

289. Oxlund H, Manschot J, Viidik A: The role of elastin in the mechanical properties of skin, *J Biomech* 21:213, 1988.

290. Paine MF, Widmer WW, Hart HL, et al: A furanocoumarin-free grapefruit juice establishes furanocoumarins as the mediators of the grapefruit juice-felodipine interaction [erratum appears in *Am J Clin Nutr* 84:264, 2006], *Am J Clin Nutr* 83:1097, 2006.

291. Pashley DH: Dynamics of the pulpodentin complex, *Crit Rev Oral Biol Med* 7:104, 1996.

292. Pashley DH: Potential treatment modalities for dentin hypersensitivity—in office products. In Addy M, Orchardson R, editors: *Tooth wear and sensitivity*, London, 2000, Martin-Dunitz Publishers, p 351.

293. Patwardhan A, Cerka K, Vela J, Hargreaves KM: Trigeminal nociceptors express prostaglandin receptor subtypes EP2 and EP3, *J Dent Res* 87:262, 2008.

294. Penfield W, Rasmussen G: *The cerebral cortex of man*, New York, 1950, Macmillan.

295. Perl E: Causalgia, pathological pain and adrenergic receptors, *Proc Natl Acad Sci U S A* 96:7664, 1999.

296. Perl ER: Ideas about pain, a historical view [review] [140 refs], *Nature Revi Neuroscie* 8:71, 2007.

297. Petty B, Cornblath DR, Adornato BT, et al: The effect of systemically administered recombinant human nerve growth factor in healthy human subjects, *Ann Neurol* 36:244, 1994.

298. Poggi P, Casasco A, Marchetti C, et al: Ultrastructural localization of elastin-like immunoreactivity in the extracellular matrix around human small lymphatic vessels, *Lymphology* 28:189, 1995.

299. Pohto P: Sympathetic adrenergic innervation of permanent teeth in the monkey (*Macaca irus*), *Acta Odontol Scand* 30:117, 1972.

300. Pohto P, Antila R: Demonstration of adrenergic nerve fibres in human dental pulp by histochemical fluorescence method, *Acta Odontol Scand* 26:137, 1968.

301. Pohto P, Antila R: Innervation of blood vessels in the dental pulp, *Int Dent J* 22:228, 1972.

302. Pomonis JD, Rogers SD, Peters CM, et al: Expression and localization of endothelin receptors: implications for the involvement of peripheral glia in nociception, *J Neurosci* 21:999, 2001.

303. Prati C, Cervellati F, Sanasi V, Montebugnoli L: Treatment of cervical dentin hypersensitivity with resin adhesives: 4 week evaluation, *Arch Dent* 14:378, 2001.

304. Prescott RS, Alsanea R, Fayad MI, et al: In vivo generation of dental pulp-like tissue by using dental pulp stem cells, a collagen scaffold, and dentin matrix protein 1 after subcutaneous transplantation in mice, *J Endod* 34:421, 2008.

305. Qian XB, Naftel JP: Effects of neonatal exposure to anti-nerve growth factor on the number and size distribution of trigeminal neurones projecting to the molar dental pulp in rats, *Arch Oral Biol* 41:359, 1996.

306. Rapp R, el-Labban NG, Kramer IR, Wood D: Ultrastructure of fenestrated capillaries in human dental pulps, *Arch Oral Biol* 22:317, 1977.

307. Reader A, Foreman DW: An ultrastructural qualitative investigation of human intradental innervation, *J Endod* 7:493, 1981.

308. Renton T, Yiangou Y, Plumpton C, et al: Sodium channel Nav1.8 immunoreactivity in painful human dental pulp, *BMC Oral Health* 5:5, 2005.

309. Roberts-Clark D, Smith AJ: Angiogenic growth factors in human dentine matrix, *Arch Oral Biol* 42:1013, 2000.

310. Rodd HD, Boissonade FM: Innervation of human tooth pulp in relation to caries and dentition type, *J Dent Res* 80:389, Jan 2001.

311. Rodd HD, Boissonade FM: Comparative immunohistochemical analysis of the peptidergic innervation of human primary and permanent tooth pulp, *Arch Oral Biol* 47:375, 2002.

312. Rodd HD, Boissonade FM, Day PF: Pulpal status of hypomineralized permanent molars, *Pediatr Dent* 29:514, 2007.

313. Roy ML, Narahashi T: Differential properties of tetrodotoxin-sensitive and tetrodotoxin-resistant sodium channels in rat dorsal root ganglion neurons, *J Neurosci* 12:2104, 1992.

314. Ruparel NB, Patwardhan AM, Akopian A, Hargreaves KM: Homologous and heterologous desensitization of capsaicin and mustard oil responses utilize different cellular pathways in nociceptors, *Pain* 135:271, 2008.

315. Rutherford B: BMP-7 gene transfer into inflamed ferret-dental pulps, *Eur J Oral Sci* 109:422, 2001.

316. Rutherford B, Fitzgerald M: A new biological approach to vital pulp therapy, *Crit Rev Oral Biol Med* 6:218, 1995.

317. Rutherford RB, Spanberg L, Tucker M, et al: The time-course of the induction of reparative dentine formation in moneys by recombinant human osteogenic protein-1, *Arch Oral Biol* 39:833, 1994.

318. Sakamoto N, Nakajima T, Ikunaga K, et al: Identification of hyaluronidase activity in rabbit dental pulp, *J Dent Res* 60:850, 1981.

319. Sakurai K, Okiji T, Suda H: Co-increase of nerve fibers and HLA-DR- and/or factor XIIIa-expressing dendritic cells in dentinal caries-affected regions of the human dental pulp: an immunohistochemical study, *J Dent Res* 78:1596, 1999.

320. Sasaki S: Studies on the respiration of the dog tooth germ, *J Biochem (Tokyo)* 46:269, 1959.

321. Sasano T, Kuriwada S, Sanjo D: Arterial blood pressure regulation of pulpal blood flow as determined by laser Doppler, *J Dent Res* 68:791, 1989.

322. Sasano T, Kuriwada S, Shoji N, et al: Axon reflex vasodilatation in cat dental pulp elicited by noxious stimulation of the gingiva, *J Dent Res* 73:1797, 1994.

323. Sasano T, Shoji N, Kuriwada S, et al: Absence of parasympathetic vasodilatation in cat dental pulp, *J Dent Res* 74:1665, 1995.

324. Schaible H, Schmidt R: Discharge characteristics of receptors with fine afferents from normal and inflamed joints: influence of analgesics and prostaglandins, *Agents Actions* 19:99, 1986.

325. Schüpbach P, Lutz F, Finger WT: Closing of dentin tubules by Gluma desensitizer, *Eur J Oral Sci* 105:414, 1997.

326. Scott JN, Weber DF: Microscopy of the junctional region between human coronal primary and secondary dentin, *J Morphol* 154:133, 1977.

327. Seltzer S, Bender IB, Ziontz M: The interrelationship of pulp and periodontal disease, *Oral Surg* 16:1474, 1963.

328. Senger DR, Galli SJ, Dvorak AM, et al: Tumor cells secrete a vascular permeability factor that promotes accumulation of ascites fluid, *Science* 219:983, 1983.

329. Sessle BJ: Recent developments in pain research: central mechanisms of orofacial pain and its control, *J Endodon* 12:435, 1986.

330. Sessle BJ: The neurobiology of facial and dental pain: present knowledge, future directions, *J Dent Res* 66:962, 1987.

331. Sessle BJ: Acute and chronic craniofacial pain: brainstem mechanisms of nociceptive transmission and neuroplasticity, and their clinical correlates, *Crit Rev Oral Biol Med* 11:57, 2000.

332. Sessle BJ, Greenwood LF: Inputs to trigeminal brain stem neurones from facial, oral, tooth pulp and pharyngolaryngeal tissues: I. Responses to innocuous and noxious stimuli, *Brain Res* 117:211, 1976.

333. Sessle BJ, Hu JW, Amano N, Zhong G: Convergence of cutaneous, tooth pulp, visceral, neck and muscle afferents onto nociceptive and non-nociceptive neurones in trigeminal subnucleus caudalis (medullary dorsal horn) and its implications for referred pain, *Pain* 27:219, 1986.

334. Shortland PJ, Jacquin MF, De Maro JA, et al: Central projections of identified trigeminal primary afferents after molar pulp differentiation in adult rats, *Somatosens Mot Res* 12:227, 1995.

335. Shulman K, Rosen S, Tognazzi K, et al: Expression of vascular permeability factor (VPF/VEGF) is altered in many glomerular diseases, *J Am Soc Nephrol* 7:661, 1996.

336. Shuttleworth CA, Ward JL, Hirschmann PN: The presence of type III collagen in the developing tooth, *Biochim Biophys Acta* 535:348, 1978.

337. Sigal MJ, Pitaru S, Aubin JE, Ten Cate AR: A combined scanning electron microscopy and immunofluorescence study demonstrating that the odontoblast process extends to the dentinoenamel junction in human teeth, *Anat Rec* 210:453, 1984.

338. Smith AJ, Garde C, Cassidy N, et al: Solubilization of dentin extracellular matrix by calcium hydroxide, *J Dent Res* 74:829, 1995 (abstract).

339. Smith AJ, Sloan AJ, Matthews JB, et al: Reparative processes in dentine and pulp. In Addy M, Embery G, Edger WM, Orchardson R, editors: *Tooth wear and sensitivity: clinical advances in restorative dentistry*, 2000, Martin Dunitz.

340. Smith AJ, Tobias RS, Cassidy N, et al: Odontoblast stimulation in ferrets by dentine matrix components, *Arch Oral Biol* 39:13, 1994.

341. Souza PP, Fukada SY, Cunha FQ, et al: Regulation of angiotensin II receptors levels during rat induced pulpitis, *Regul Pept* 140:27, 2007.

342. Stanley HR, White CL, McCray L: The rate of tertiary (reparative) dentin formation in the human tooth, *Oral Surg* 21:180, 1966.

343. Steen KH, Reeh PW, Anton F, Handwerker HO: Protons selectively induce lasting excitation and sensitization to mechanical stimulation of nociceptors in rat skin in vitro, *J Neurosci* 21:86, 1992.

344. Stenvik A, Iverson J, Mjör IA: Tissue pressure and histology of normal and inflamed tooth pulps in Macaque monkeys, *Arch Oral Biol* 17:1501, 1972.

345. Stern D, Nawroth P, Handley D, Kisiel W: An endothelial cell-dependent pathway of coagulation, *Proc Natl Acad Sci U S A* 82:2523, 1985.

346. Sunakawa M, Tokita Y, Suda H: Pulsed Nd:YAG laser irradiation of the tooth pulp in the cat. II. Effect of scanning lasing, *Lasers Surg Med* 26:477, 2000.

347. Sundqvist G, Lerner UH: Bradykinin and thrombin synergistically potentiate interleukin 1 and tumour

necrosis factor induced prostanoid biosynthesis in human dental pulp fibroblasts, *Cytokine* 8:168, 1996.

348. Sweitzer SM, Schubert P, DeLeo JA: Propentofylline, a glial modulating agent, exhibits antiallodynic properties in a rat model of neuropathic pain, *J Pharmacol Exp Ther* 297:1210, 2001.

349. Swift ML, Byers MR: Effects of aging responses of nerve fibers to pulpal inflammation in rat molars analyzed by quantitative immunohistochemistry, *Arch Oral Biol* 37:901, 1992.

350. Tagami J, Hosoda H, Burrow MF, Nakajima M: Effect of aging and caries on dentin permeability, *Proc Finn Dent Soc* 88(suppl 1):149, 1992.

351. Takahashi K, Kishi Y, Kim S: A scanning electron microscope study of the blood vessels of dog pulp using corrosion resin casts, *J Endod* 8:131, 1982.

352. Tanaka T: The origin and localization of dentinal fluid in developing rat molar teeth studied with lanthanum as a tracer, *Arch Oral Biol* 25:153, 1980.

353. Telles PD, Hanks CT, Machado MA, Nör JE: Lipoteichoic acid up-regulates VEGF expression in macrophages and pulp cells, *J Dent Res* 82:466, 2003.

354. Thomas HF: The extent of the odontoblast process in human dentin, *J Dent Res* 58(D):2207, 1979.

355. Thomas HF, Payne RC: The ultrastructure of dentinal tubules from erupted human premolar teeth, *J Dent Res* 62:532, 1983.

356. Thomas JJ, Stanley HR, Gilmore HW: Effects of gold foil condensation on human dental pulp, *J Am Dent Assoc* 78:788, 1969.

357. Tokita Y, Sunakawa M, Suda H: Pulsed ND: YAG laser irradiation of the tooth pulp in the cat. I. Effect of spot lasing, *Lasers Surg Med* 26:477, 2000.

358. Tominaga M, Numazaki M, Iida T, et al: *Molecular mechanisms of TRPV1-mediated thermal hypersensitivity*, vol 30, p 37. Seattle, 2003, IASP Press.

359. Tönder KH, Naess G: Nervous control of blood flow in the dental pulp in dogs, *Acta Physiol Scand* 104:13, 1978.

360. Tönder KJ: Blood flow and vascular pressure in the dental pulp. Summary, *Acta Odontol Scand* 38:135, 1980.

361. Tönder KJ: Effect of vasodilating drugs on external carotid and pulpal blood flow in dogs: "stealing" of dental perfusion pressure, *Acta Physiol Scand* 97:75, 1976.

362. Tönder KJH, Kvinnsland I: Micropuncture measurements of interstitial fluid pressure in normal and inflamed dental pulp in cats, *J Endod* 9:105, 1983.

363. Tonioli M, Patel T, Diogenes A, et al: Effect of neurotrophic factors on bradykinin expression in rat trigeminal sensory neurons determined by real-time polymerase chain reaction, *J Endod* 30:263, 2004.

364. Torabinejad M, Cymerman JJ, Frankson M, et al: Effectiveness of various medications on postoperative pain following complete instrumentation, *J Endod* 20:345, 1994.

365. Torebjörk HE, Hanin RG: Perceptual changes accompanying controlled preferential blocking of A and C fiber responses in intact human skin nerves, *Exp Brain Res* 16:321, 1973.

366. Torneck CD: Dentin-pulp complex. In Ten Cate AR, editor: *Oral histology: development, structure, and function*, ed 5, St Louis, 1998, Mosby, p 150.

367. Torneck CD, Kwan CL, Hu JW: Inflammatory lesions of the tooth pulp induce changes in brainstem neurons of the rat trigeminal subnucleus oralis, *J Dent Res* 75:553, 1996.

368. Tran XV, Gorin C, Willig C, et al: Effect of a calcium-silicate-based restorative cement on pulp repair, *J Dent Res* 91:1166, 2012.

369. Trantor IR, Messer HH, Birner R: The effects of neuropeptides (calcitonin-gene-related peptide and substance P) on cultured human pulpal cells, *J Dent Res* 74:1066, 1995.

370. Trowbridge HO: Pathogenesis of pulpitis resulting from dental caries, *J Endod* 7:52, 1981.

371. Trowbridge HO: Review of dental pain–histology and physiology, *J Endod* 12:445, 1986.

372. Trowbridge HO, Franks M, Korostoff E, Emling R: Sensory response to thermal stimulation in human teeth, *J Endod* 6:405, 1980.

373. Trowbridge HO, Silver DR: Review of current approaches to in-office management of tooth hypersensitivity, *Dent Clin North Am* 16:561, 1990.

374. Trowbridge HO, Stewart JCB, Shapiro IM: Assessment of indurated, diffusely calcified human dental pulps. In *Proceedings of the International Conference on Dentin/Pulp Complex*, Tokyo, 1996, Quintessence Publishing, p 297.

375. Turner D, Marfurt C, Sattelburg C: Demonstration of physiological barrier between pulpal odontoblasts and its perturbation following routine restorative procedures: a horseradish peroxidase tracing study in the rat, *J Dent Res* 68:1262, 1989.

376. Turner DF: Immediate physiological response of odontoblasts, *Proc Finn Dent Soc* 88(suppl 1):55, 1992.

377. Uddman R, et al: Occurrence of VIP nerves in mammalian dental pulps, *Acta Odontol Scand* 38:325, 1980.

378. van Amerongen JP, Lemmens IG, Tonino GJ: The concentration, extractability and characterization of collagen in human dental pulp, *Arch Oral Biol*, 28:339, 1983.

379. Van Hassel HJ: Physiology of the human dental pulp, *Oral Surg Oral Med Oral Path* 32:126, 1971.

380. Van Hassel HJ, Brown AC: Effect of temperature changes on intrapulpal pressure and hydraulic permeability in dogs, *Arch Oral Biol* 14:301, 1969.

381. van Wijk AJ, Hoogstraten J: Reducing fear of pain associated with endodontic therapy, *Int Endod J* 39:384, 2006.

382. Veerayutthwilai O, Byers MR, Pham TT, et al: Differential regulation of immune responses by odontoblasts, *Oral Microbiol Immunol* 22:5, 2007.

383. Vickers ER, Cousins MJ: Neuropathic orofacial pain part 1: prevalence and pathophysiology, *Aust Endod J* 26:19, 2000.

384. Vongsavan N, Matthews B: The permeability of cat dentine in vivo and in vitro, *Arch Oral Biol* 36:641, 1991.

385. Vongsavan N, Matthews B: Fluid flow through cat dentine in vivo, *Arch Oral Biol* 37:175, 1992.

386. Vongsavan N, Matthews B: The vascularity of dental pulp in cats, *J Dent Res*, 71:1913, 1992.

387. Vongsavan N, Matthews B: The relation between fluid flow through dentine and the discharge of intradental nerves, *Arch Oral Biol* 39(suppl):140S, 1994.

388. Vongsavan N, Matthews B: The relationship between the discharge of intradental nerves and the rate of fluid flow through dentine in the cat, *Arch Oral Biol* 52:640, 2007.

389. Wakisaka S: Neuropeptides in the dental pulp: their distribution, origins and correlation, *J Endod* 16:67, 1990.

390. Wakisaka S, Ichikawa H, Akai M: Distribution and origins of peptide- and catecholamine-containing nerve fibres in the feline dental pulp and effects of cavity preparation on these nerve fibres, *J Osaka Univ Dent Sch* 26:17, 1986.

391. Wakisaka S, Sasaki Y, Ichikawa H, Matsuo S: Increase in c-fos-like immunoreactivity in the trigeminal nucleus complex after dental treatment, *Proc Finn Dent Soc* 88(suppl 1):551, 1992.

392. Wall PD: Alterations in the central nervous system after deafferentation: connectivity control. In Bonica JJ, Lindblom U, Iggo A, editors: *Advances in pain research and therapy*, vol 5, New York, 1983, Raven Press, p 677.

393. Walton R, Fouad A: Endodontic interappointment flare-ups: a prospective study of incidence and related factors, *J Endod* 18:172, 1992.

394. Wang C, Li GW, Huang LY: Prostaglandin E2 potentiation of P2X3 receptor mediated currents in dorsal root ganglion neurons, *Mol Pain* 3:22, 2007.

395. Warfvinge J, Dahlen G, Bergenholtz G: Dental pulp response to bacterial cell wall material, *J Dent Res* 64:1046, 1985.

396. Warren C, Mok L, Gordon S, et al: Quantification of neural protein in extirpated tooth pulp, *J Endod* 34:7, 2008.

397. Watkins LR, Milligan ED, Maier SF: Glial activation: a driving force for pathological pain, *Trends Neurosci* 24:450, 2001.

398. Weber DK, Zaki AL: Scanning and transmission electron microscopy of tubular structure presumed to be human odontoblast processes, *J Dent Res* 65:982, 1986.

399. Weiger R, Axmann-Kremar D, Lost C: Prognosis of conventional root canal treatment reconsidered, *Endodon Dent Traumatol* 14:1, 1998.

400. Weinstock A, Weinstock M, Leblond CP: Autoradiographic detection of 3H-fucose incorporation into glycoprotein by odontoblasts and its deposition at the site of the calcification front in dentin, *Calcif Tissue Res* 8:181, 1972.

401. Weinstock M, Leblond CP: Synthesis, migration and release of precursor collagen by odontoblasts as visualized by radioautography after 3H-proline administration, *J Cell Biol* 60:92, 1974.

402. Wells J, Bingham V, Rowland K, Hatton J: Expression of Na$_v$1.9 channels in human dental pulp and trigeminal ganglion, *J Endod* 33:1172, 2007.

403. Wiig H, Aukland K, Tenstad O: Isolation of interstitial fluid from rat mammary tumors by a centrifugation method, *Arch Physiol Heart Circ Physiol* 284:H416-H424, 2003.

404. Wiig H, Gyenge C, Iversen PO, et al: The role of the extracellular matrix in tissue distribution of macromolecules in normal and pathological tissues: potential therapeutic consequences, *Microcirculation* 15:283, 2008.

405. Willingale HL, Gardiner NJ, McLymont N, et al: Prostanoids synthesized by cyclo-oxygenase isoforms in rat spinal cord and their contribution to the development of neuronal hyperexcitability, *Br J Pharmacol* 122:1593, 1997.

406. Winter HF, Bishop JG, Dorman HL: Transmembrane potentials of odontoblasts, *J Dent Res* 42:594, 1963.

407. Wong M, Lytle WR: A comparison of anxiety levels associated with root canal therapy and oral surgery treatment, *J Endod* 17:461, 1991.

408. Woodnutt DA, Wager-Miller J, O'Neill PC, et al: Neurotrophin receptors and nerve growth factor are differentially expressed in adjacent nonneuronal cells of normal and injured tooth pulp, *Cell Tissue Res* 299:225, 2000.

409. Woolf C: Transcriptional and posttranslational plasticity and the generation of inflammatory pain, *Proc Natl Acad Sci U S A* 96:7723, 1999.

410. Wright EF: Referred craniofacial pain patterns in patients with temporomandibular disorder [see comment][erratum appears in *J Am Dent Assoc* 131:1553, 2000], *J Am Dent Assoc* 131:1307, 2000.

411. Yaksh TL: Central pharmacology of nociceptive transmission. In Wall P, Melzack R, editors: *Textbook of pain*, Edinburgh, 2002, Churchill Livingstone, p 285.

412. Yamada T, Nakamura K, Iwaku M, Fusayama T: The extent of the odontoblast process in normal and carious human dentin, *J Dent Res* 62:798, 1983.

413. Yamaguchi M, Kojima T, Kanekawa M, et al: Neuropeptides stimulate production of interleukin-1 beta, interleukin-6, and tumor necrosis factor-alpha in human dental pulp cells, *Inflamm Res* 53:199, 2004.

414. Yamamura T: Differentiation of pulpal wound healing, *J Dent Res* 64(special issue):530, 1985.

415. Yang BH, Piao ZG, Kim Y-B: Activation of vanilloid receptor 1 (VR1) by eugenol, *J Dent Res* 82:781, 2003.

416. Yonehara N, Amano K, Kamisaki Y: Involvement of the NMDA-nitric oxide pathway in the development of hypersensitivity to tactile stimulation in dental injured rats, *Jpn J Pharmacol* 90:145, 2002.

417. Yu CY, Boyd NM, Cringle SJ: An in vivo and in vitro comparison of the effects of vasoactive mediators on pulpal blood vessels in rat incisors, *Arch Oral Biol* 47:723, 2002.

418. Yu CY, Boyd NM, Cringle SJ, et al: Oxygen distribution and consumption in rat lower incisor pulp, *Arch Oral Biol* 47:529, 2002.

419. Zerari-Mailly F, Braud A, Davido N, et al: Glutamate control of pulpal blood flow in the incisor dental pulp of the rat, *Eur J Oral Sci* 120:402, 2012.

420. Zerlotti E: Histochemical study of the connective tissue of the dental pulp, *Arch Oral Biol* 9:149, 1964.

421. Zhang J, Kawashima N, Suda H, et al: The existence of CD11c+ sentinel and F4/80+ interstitial dendritic cells in dental pulp and their dynamics and functional properties, *Int Immunol* 18:1375, 2006.

CHAPTER 13

Pulpal Reactions to Caries and Dental Procedures

ASHRAF FOUAD | LINDA G. LEVIN

CHAPTER OUTLINE

The dental pulp is a dynamic tissue that responds to external stimuli in many ways. However, there are certain unique features about the dental pulp response that distinguish it from other connective tissues in the body. The pulp's exposure to dental caries, a prevalent chronic infectious disease, its encasement in an unyielding environment after complete tooth maturation, and the scarcity of collateral circulation render it susceptible to injury and complicate its regeneration. Moreover, the pulp is endowed with a rich neurovascular supply that regulates the effects of inflammation that may ultimately lead to rapid degeneration and necrosis. The treatment of dental caries and other tooth abnormalities involves removal of the enamel and dentin, the hardest tissues in the body, thus adding to the irritation of the pulp. This chapter discusses the response of the pulp to all of these variables and presents advances in our understanding of dental procedures and their effects on the pulp.

PULPAL REACTION TO CARIES

Dental caries is a localized, destructive, and progressive infection of dentin, which, if left unchecked, can result in pulpal necrosis and potential tooth loss. Both bacterial by-products and products from the dissolution of the organic and inorganic constituents of dentin mediate the effects of dental caries on the pulp. Three basic reactions tend to protect the pulp against caries: (1) a decrease in dentin permeability, (2) tertiary dentin formation, and (3) inflammatory and immune reactions.[133] These responses occur concomitantly, and their robustness is highly dependent on the aggressive nature of the advancing lesion as well as host responses such as the age of the patient (see also Chapter 26).

In the advancing infection front of the carious lesion, multiple intrinsic and extrinsic factors are released that stimulate nearby pulpal tissue. Bacterial proteolytic enzymes, toxins, and metabolic by-products have been thought to initiate pulpal reactions, yet the buffering capacity of dentin and dentinal fluid likely attenuate these deleterious effects. This protective function is significantly reduced when the remaining dentin thickness is minimal.[237] When relatively unhindered access to pulpal tissue is present, both bacterial metabolites and their cell wall components induce inflammation. In initial-to-moderate lesions, current evidence suggests that acidic by-products of the carious process act indirectly by degrading the dentin matrix and thereby liberating bioactive molecules previously sequestered during dentinogenesis. Once liberated, these molecules again assume their role in dentin formation, this time stimulatory for *tertiary* dentinogenesis.[238] This theory is

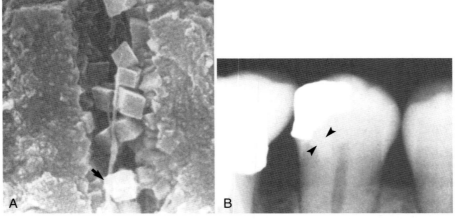

FIG. 13-1 **A,** Whitlockite crystals occlude the dentinal tubules in sclerotic dentin. **B,** Dentinal sclerosis is radiographically apparent beneath a deep class II lesion. (**A,** From Yoshiyama M, Masada J, Uchida A, Ishida H: Scanning electron microscopic characterization of sensitive vs. insensitive human radicular dentin, *J Dent Res* 68:1498, 1989.)

supported by the findings that demineralized dentin matrix implanted at the site of pulpal exposure can induce dentinogenesis.[266] Furthermore, placement of purified dentin matrix proteins on exposed dentin or exposed pulp stimulates tertiary dentin formation, indicating that these molecules can act directly or across intact dentin.[239,265] More information on growth factors embedded in dentin is reviewed in the chapter on regenerative endodontics (see Chapter 10).

Evidence offers several candidate molecules that stimulate reparative dentinogenesis. Heparin-binding growth factor, transforming growth factor (TGF)-β1, TGF-β3, insulin-like growth factors I and II, platelet-derived growth factor, bone morphogenetic protein-2 (BMP-2) and angiogenic growth factors have been shown to be embedded in dentin and stimulatory for dentinogenesis in vitro. The TGF-β superfamily in particular seems to be important in the signaling process for odontoblast differentiation from mesenchymal stem or progenitor cells as well as primary and tertiary dentinogenesis. As the predominant isoform, TGF-β1 is equally distributed in the soluble and insoluble fractions of dentin matrix.[41] During the carious dissolution of dentin, it is believed that the soluble pool of TGF-β1 can diffuse across intact dentin while the insoluble pool is immobilized on insoluble dentin matrix and serves to stimulate odontoblasts much like membrane-bound TGF-βs during odontogenesis.[237,240]

Despite the research interest in tertiary dentinogenesis, it is neither the first nor necessarily the most effective pulpally mediated defense against invading pathogens. A combination of an increased deposition of intratubular dentin and the direct deposition of mineral crystals into the narrowed dentin tubules to decrease dentin permeability is the first defense to caries and is called *dentin sclerosis*. It occurs by a combination of increased deposition of intratubular dentin and tubule occlusion by precipitated crystals. This results in an effective decrease in dentin permeability underneath the advancing carious lesion.[206] In vitro studies with cultured tooth slices implicate TGF-β1 as a central player in the increased deposition of intratubular dentin.[236] The deposition of whitlockite crystals in the tubular lumen most likely results from a similar stimulation of vital associated odontoblasts, possibly in combination with

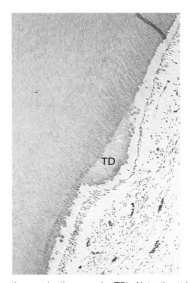

FIG. 13-2 Reactionary dentinogenesis (TD). Note the tubular morphology and the discontinuity of the tubules at the interface of secondary and reactionary dentin. Resident odontoblasts are still present.

precipitation of mineral released during the demineralization process[156,262] (Fig. 13-1).

The formation of tertiary dentin occurs over a longer period than does that of sclerotic dentin, and its resultant character is highly dependent on the stimulus. Mild stimuli activate resident quiescent odontoblasts whereupon they elaborate the organic matrix of dentin. This type of tertiary dentin is referred to as *reactionary dentin* and can be observed when initial dentin demineralization occurs beneath the noncavitated enamel lesion.[151] Mediators present during the carious process induce a focal upregulation of matrix production by resident odontoblasts. The resultant dentin is similar in morphology to physiologic dentin and may only be apparent due to a change in the direction of the new dentinal tubules (Fig. 13-2). In contrast, in aggressive lesions the carious process may prove cytocidal to subjacent odontoblasts and require repopulation of the

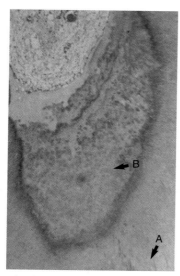

FIG. 13-3 Reparative dentin; the strong stimulus of the impinging infection is cytocidal for odontoblasts. The resultant dentin is irregular with soft tissue inclusions.

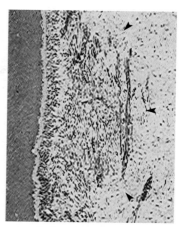

FIG. 13-4 The early pulpal response to caries is represented by a focal accumulation of chronic inflammatory cells. Note that peripheral to the inflammation the pulpal parenchyma is relatively unaffected.

disrupted odontoblast layer with differentiating progenitors. The organization and composition of the resultant matrix are a direct reflection of the differentiation state of the secretory cells. This accounts for the heterogeneity of *reparative dentin,* where the morphology can range from organized tubular dentin to more disorganized irregular *fibrodentin.* Fibrodentin, due to its irregular configuration and tissue inclusions, is more permeable than physiologic dentin[275] (Fig. 13-3).

Although dentin can provide a physical barrier against noxious stimuli, the pulpal immune response provides humoral and cellular challenges to invading pathogens. In the progressing carious lesion, the host immune response increases in intensity as the infection advances. It has been shown that titers of T-helper cells, B-lineage cells, neutrophils, and macrophages are directly proportional to lesion depth in human teeth.[118] The disintegration of large amounts of dentin, however, is not necessary to elicit a pulpal immune response. This is supported by the observation that a pulpal inflammatory response can be seen beneath noncavitated lesions and noncoalesced pits and fissures.[34]

The early inflammatory response to caries is characterized by the focal accumulation of chronic inflammatory cells (Fig. 13-4). This is mediated initially by odontoblasts and later by dendritic cells. As the most peripheral cell in the pulp, the odontoblast is positioned to encounter foreign antigens first and initiate the innate immune response. Pathogen detection in general is accomplished via specific receptors called pattern recognition receptors (PRRs).[120] These receptors recognize pathogen associated molecular patterns (PAMPs) on invading organisms and initiate a host defense through the activation of the NF-κB pathway.[101] One class of the PAMP recognition molecules is the Toll-like receptor family (TLRs). Odontoblasts have been shown to increase expression of certain TLRs in response to bacterial products. Under experimental conditions, odontoblasts expression of TLR3, 5, and 9 increased in response to lipoteichoic acid, whereas lipopolysaccharide increased TLR2 and 4 expression.[66,107,183] It was also shown that TGFβ-1 inhibits the expression of TLR2 and 4 by odontoblasts in response to gram-positive and gram-negative bacteria.[27,107]

Once the odontoblast TLR is stimulated by a pathogen, proinflammatory cytokines, chemokines, and antimicrobial peptides are elaborated by the odontoblast, resulting in recruitment and stimulation of immune effector cells as well as direct bacterial killing.[74,76,129]

Many cells produce chemokines at low levels constitutively. Unstimulated odontoblasts express genes coding for CCl2, CXCL12, and CXCL14, three genes known to code for factors chemotactic for immature dendritic cells.[42] They also produce CCL26, a natural antagonist for CCR1, CCR2, and CCR5 that are chemokines normally produced by monocytes and dendritic cells.[287] Stimulation with bacterial cell wall constituents has been shown to upregulate the expression of multiple chemokine genes including CXCL12, CCL2, CXCL9, CX3CL1, CCL8, CXCL10, CCL16, CCL5, CXCL2, CCL4, CXCL11, and CCL3, and nine chemokine receptor genes including CXCR4, CCR1, CCR5, CX3CR1, CCR10, and CXCR3, suggesting that odontoblasts sense pathogens and express factors that recruit immune effector cells[42,75,106,152] (Fig. 13-5). These data suggest a scenario whereby stimulated odontoblasts express high levels of chemokines such as IL-8 (CXCL8) that act in concert with the release of formerly sequestered growth factors from carious dentin that induce a focal increase in dendritic cell numbers with the additional release of chemotactic mediators.[77,240] The subsequent influx of immune effector cells is composed of lymphocytes, macrophages, and plasma cells. This cellular infiltrate is accompanied by localized capillary sprouting in response to angiogenic factors as well as co-aggregation of nerve fibers and human leukocyte antigen-DR (HLA-DR)-positive dendritic cells.[280,281]

As the carious lesion progresses, the density of the chronic inflammatory infiltrate as well as that of dendritic cells in the odontoblast region increases. Pulpal dendritic cells are responsible for antigen presentation and stimulation of T lymphocytes. In the uninflamed pulp they are scattered throughout the pulp. With caries progression they aggregate initially in the pulp and subodontoblastic regions, then extend into the odontoblast layer, and eventually migrate into the entrance to tubules beside the odontoblast process[282] (Fig. 13-6). Two distinct populations of dendritic cells have been identified in the dental pulp. CD11c+ is found in the pulp/dentin border and

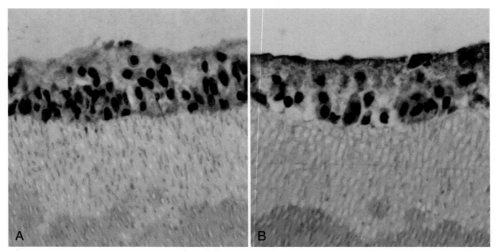

FIG. 13-5 Odontoblasts exposed to LPS in an in vitro culture model express IL-8, as evidenced by immunostaining with anti–IL-8 antibodies.

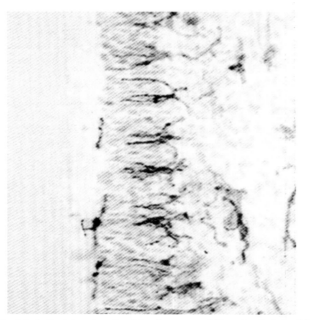

FIG. 13-6 Dental caries stimulates the accumulation of pulpal dendritic cells in and around the odontoblastic layer. (Reprinted with permission from Mats Jontell.)

subjacent to pits and fissures. F4/80+ dendritic cells are concentrated in the perivascular spaces in the subodontoblastic zone and inner pulp.[287] CD11c+ dendritic cells express Toll-like receptors 2 and 4 and are CD205 positive. F4/80+ dendritic cells have migratory ability. As they migrate from the central pulp they increase in size and become CD86 positive. The close spatial relationship between odontoblasts and dendritic cells under the carious lesion has led to speculation that dendritic cells may play a role in odontoblast differentiation or secretory activity in the immune defense and in dentinogenesis. Recent studies have demonstrated that pulp dendritic cell can migrate to regional lymph nodes, for antigen presentation.[24a] In vitro studies have suggested that the secretion of granulocyte-macrophage colony-stimulating factor

(GM-CSF) and osteopontin by dendritic cells and macrophages represents a mechanism whereby they contribute to odontoblast differentiation.[227] Pulpal Schwann cells have also been shown to produce molecules in response to caries, which indicates the acquisition of the ability for antigen presentation.

Evidence suggests that odontoblasts also play a role in the humoral immune response to caries. IgG, IgM, and IgA have been localized in the cytoplasm and cell processes of odontoblasts in human carious dentin, suggesting that these cells actively transport antibodies to the infection front.[189] In the incipient lesion, antibodies accumulate in the odontoblast layer and with lesion progression can be seen in the dentinal tubules. Eventually this leads to a focal concentration of antibodies beneath the advancing lesion.[188]

In the most advanced phase of carious destruction, the humoral immune response is accompanied by immunopathologic destruction of pulpal tissue. In animal studies where monkeys were hyperimmunized to bovine serum albumin (BSA), there was an observed increase in pulpal tissue destruction subsequent to antigenic challenge across freshly cut dentin.[20] The odontoblasts also appear to be involved in the production of innate antimicrobial molecules such as human beta defensing-2 (HBD2). Therefore, interleukin (IL)-1 and tumor necrosis factor (TNF)-alpha as well as bacterial lipopolysaccharide (LPS) were responsible for significant increases in HBD2 in response to caries.[106] In summary, it appears the odontoblasts play a central role in orchestrating local and chemotactic inflammatory responses to dental caries (Fig. 13-7).

Pulpal exposure in primary and immature permanent teeth can lead to a proliferative response or *hyperplastic pulpitis*. Exuberant inflammatory tissue proliferates through the exposure and forms a "pulp polyp" (Fig. 13-8). It is presumed that a rich blood supply allows this proliferative response. Conventional root canal therapy or progressive vital pulp therapy is indicated.

NEUROGENIC MEDIATORS

Neurogenic mediators are involved in the pulpal response to irritants and, like immune components, they can mediate pathology as well as the healing response (see also Chapter 12).

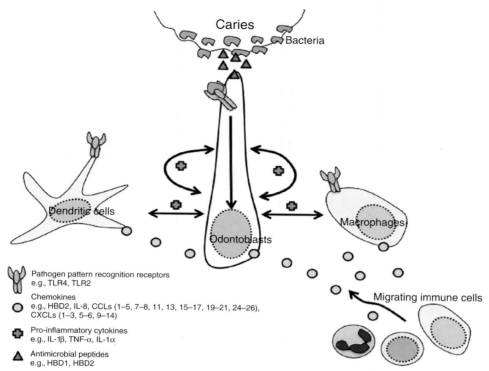

Caries
Bacteria

Macrophages

Dendritic cells

Odontoblasts

Pathogen pattern recognition receptors
e.g., TLR4, TLR2

Chemokines
e.g., HBD2, IL-8, CCLs (1–5, 7–8, 11, 13, 15–17, 19–21, 24–26),
CXCLs (1–3, 5–6, 9–14)

Pro-inflammatory cytokines
e.g., IL-1β, TNF-α, IL-1α

Antimicrobial peptides
e.g., HBD1, HBD2

Migrating immune cells

FIG. 13-7 Innate immunity in the odontoblast layer (ODL). Bacterial components from caries activate cytokine/chemokine release from odontoblasts, dendritic cells, or macrophages via Toll-like receptors (TLRs). Proinflammatory cytokines released from these cells act as autocrine and paracrine signals to amplify cytokine responses, including antimicrobial peptide, cytokine, and chemokine production. The release of chemokines creates a migration gradient for immune cells to ODL while antimicrobial peptides reduce bacterial load. (From Horst OV, Horst JA, Samudrala R, Dale BA: Caries induced cytokine network in the odontoblast layer of human teeth, *BMC Immunol* 12:9, Fig. 4C, 2011. Reprinted with permission.)

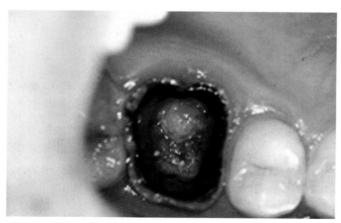

FIG. 13-8 A proliferative response to caries in a young tooth, typically referred to as proliferative pulpitis, hyperplastic pulpitis, or pulp polyp. (Courtesy Dr. Howard Strassler, University of Maryland, with permission.)

External stimulation of dentin causes the release of proinflammatory neuropeptides from pulpal afferent nerves.[36,130] Substance P (SP), calcitonin gene–related peptide (CGRP), neurokinin A (NKA), neurokinin Y, and vasoactive intestinal peptide are released and effect vascular events such as vasodilation and increased vascular permeability. This results in a net increase in tissue pressure that can progress to necrosis in

extreme and persistent circumstances. Stimulation of sympathetic nerves in response to the local release of mediators such as norepinephrine, neuropeptide Y, and adenosine triphosphate (ATP) has been shown to alter pulpal blood flow. Receptor field studies as well as anatomic studies have shown sprouting of afferent fibers in response to inflammation.[36]

Neuropeptides can act to modulate the pulpal immune response. It has been demonstrated that SP acts as a chemotactic and stimulatory agent for macrophages and T lymphocytes. The result of this stimulation is increased production of arachidonic acid metabolites, stimulation of lymphocytic mitosis, and production of cytokines. CGRP demonstrates immunosuppressive activity, which is evidenced by a diminution of class II antigen presentation and lymphocyte proliferation.

SP and CGRP are mitogenic for pulpal and odontoblast-like cells; thereby they initiate and propagate the pulpal healing response.[260] CGRP has been shown to stimulate the production of bone morphogenic protein by human pulpal cells. The result of this stimulation has been postulated to induce tertiary dentinogenesis.[38] Substance P appears to increase in the dental pulp and periodontal ligament as a result of acutely induced occlusal trauma,[45] which may be related to the pain associated with concussion traumatic injury.

It has been shown that there may be gender differences in CGRP release in the dental pulp.[29,159] In one study, serotonin (a peripheral pronociceptive mediator) induced a significant increase in capsaicin-evoked CGRP release in dental pulps obtained from female but not male patients.[159] This interplay of inflammatory mediators may explain some of the gender differences in clinical presentation with dental pain.

CORRELATION BETWEEN CLINICAL SYMPTOMS AND ACTUAL PULPAL INFLAMMATION

From a clinical perspective, it would be most helpful to the clinician to be able to diagnose pulpal conditions from a profile of symptoms with which a patient presents. If symptoms are not conclusive, a number of objective tests should aid the clinician in reaching a definitive diagnosis of the pulpal pathologic status. In actuality, combinations of subjective and objective findings are frequently insufficient in reaching definitive diagnosis of the status of the dental pulp. This is particularly true in cases of vital inflamed pulp, where it is difficult for the practitioner to determine clinically whether the inflammation is reversible or irreversible.

Many practitioners rely on painful symptoms to determine the status of the pulp. Several studies have examined this question in some detail. A number of classic studies were performed in which the subjective and objective clinical findings related to carious teeth were recorded prior to extracting the teeth and examining them histologically. The underlying hypothesis in these studies was that the more severe the clinical symptoms, the more intense pulpal inflammation and destruction was evident histologically. These studies showed that in the vital pulp, clinical symptoms generally did not correlate with gross histologic findings.[100,169,232] Furthermore, carious pulp exposure was associated with severe inflammatory response or liquefactive necrosis, regardless of symptoms (Fig. 13-9). These histologic changes ranged in extent from being present only at the site of the exposure to deep into the root canals.[232] In a few studies prolonged or spontaneous severe symptoms were associated with chronic partial, total pulpitis, or pulp necrosis.[64,232] However, in these as well as other studies it was common to find cases with evidence of severe inflammatory responses

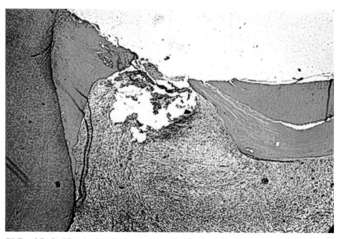

FIG. 13-9 Histologic photomicrograph of a molar with carious pulp exposure. The exposure had been capped but had failed and the patient presented with symptoms. The photomicrograph shows an area of necrosis and extensive inflammation throughout the coronal pulp. (Courtesy Dr. Larz Spangberg, University of Connecticut, with permission.)

including partial necrosis histologically, but with little or no clinical symptoms—the so-called painless pulpitis.[64,100,169,232] Moreover, the density of nerve fibers[224] and the vascularity[225] in inflamed pulp do not correlate with clinical symptoms in primary and permanent teeth. It has been reported that the incidence of painless pulpitis that leads to pulp necrosis and asymptomatic apical periodontitis is about 40% to 60% of all pulpitis cases.[168]

Objective clinical findings are essential for determining the vitality of the pulp and whether the inflammation has extended into the periapical tissues (see also Chapter 1). Lack of response to electric pulp testing generally indicates that the pulp has become necrotic.[221,232] Thermal pulp testing is valuable for reproducing a symptom of thermal sensitivity and allowing the practitioner to assess the reaction of the patient to a stimulus and the duration of the response. However, pulp testing cannot determine the degree of pulpal inflammation.[64,232] These studies show that irreversible pulpal inflammation can be diagnosed with some certainty only in cases where, in addition to being responsive to pulp testing, the pulp develops severe spontaneous symptoms. Pulp necrosis could be predictably diagnosed by a consistent negative response to pulp tests, preferably to both cold and electrical tests to avoid false responses.[210,211] Pulp necrosis could be verified by a test cavity or lack of hemorrhagic pulp tissue upon access preparation. It should be noted, however, that the latter sign should be assessed cautiously. Occasionally, the pulp space is very small, such as in older individuals with calcified canals, and hemorrhage upon access to the pulp may not be clinically appreciable. Conversely, cases with pulp necrosis and acute periapical infections may have hemorrhagic purulent drainage through the large pulp space upon access preparation, particularly after initial instrumentation.

The lack of correlation between the histologic status of the pulp and clinical symptoms may be explained by advances in the science of pulp biology. Studies have shown that numerous molecular mediators may act in synchrony to initiate, promote or modulate the inflammatory response in the dental pulp. The nature and quantity of these inflammatory mediators cannot be determined from histologic analysis, without the use of specialized staining techniques. Many of these molecular mediators tend to reduce the pain threshold, either directly by acting on peripheral nerve cells or by promoting the inflammatory process. Thus, a number of these mediators were shown to be elevated in human pulp diagnosed with painful pulpitis. These mediators include prostaglandins,[51,223] the vasoactive amine bradykinin,[150] tumor necrosis factor alpha,[139] neuropeptides such as substance P,[30] CGRP and neurokinin A,[13] and catecholamines.[185] In fact, it was even shown that when patients have painful pulpitis, the crevicular fluid related to the affected teeth has significantly increased neuropeptides compared to the levels in contralateral teeth.[13] In another study, trained volunteers stimulated an incisor with a constant current three fold the threshold value for 90 seconds.[12] This resulted in a significant increase in crevicular matrix metalloproteinase 8 (MMP-8), one of the collagenases involved in tissue destruction.

It has also been determined that peripheral opioid receptors are present in the dental pulp,[119] and these could play a role in why many cases with irreversible pulpitis are asymptomatic. As noted before, carious teeth are frequently not associated with significant symptoms. However, they still have a significant amount of inflammation. The pulp in teeth with mild to moderate caries has increased neuropeptide Y,[68] and its Y1 receptor,[69] compared to that in normal teeth. Neuropeptide Y is a neurotransmitter for the sympathetic nervous system and is thought to act as a modulator of neurogenic inflammation. Likewise, the levels of vasoactive intestinal peptide (VIP), although not its receptor VPAC1, seemed to increase in the pulp of moderately carious teeth.[67]

With the advances in molecular biology, efficient detection of hundreds of molecular mediators simultaneously by their gene expression has become a reality. Current research seeks to examine which genes are specifically expressed or upregulated in the pulp, in response to the carious lesion. In this regard, preliminary studies have shown that various cytokines and other inflammatory mediators are upregulated underneath a carious lesion in a manner that correlates with the depth of caries.[164] Several researchers have used gene microarrays to obtain an accurate mapping of candidate genes that show elevated expression in inflamed pulp and the odontoblastic cell layer.[165,194,195] In addition, research has revealed the differential expression of microRNAs (miRNAs) in the healthy and diseased dental pulp.[288] MiRNAs are noncoding RNA molecules that regulate gene expression in complex inflammatory responses and may eventually assist in clinical predictions of pulpal status. Therefore, more accurate chairside diagnostic methods are potentially feasible to develop, especially a method that involves sampling from crevicular fluid, dentinal fluid, or the pulp directly. For this reason, more research is needed to determine the key mediators that would predict survival or degeneration of the dental pulp in difficult diagnostic cases.

DENTIN HYPERSENSITIVITY AND ITS MANAGEMENT

Dentin hypersensitivity is a special situation in which a significant, chronic, pulpal pain arises, which does not seem to be associated with irreversible pulpal pathosis in the majority of cases. Dentin hypersensitivity is characterized by brief sharp pain arising from exposed dentin in response to stimuli, typically thermal, evaporative, tactile, osmotic, or chemical, that cannot be ascribed to any other form of dental defect or pathosis.[104] Facial root surfaces in canines, premolars, and molars are particularly affected, especially in areas of periodontal attachment loss. Dentin hypersensitivity may be related to excessive abrasion during tooth brushing, periodontal disease, or erosion from dietary or gastric acids,[2,3,47] and it may increase following scaling and root planing.[47,274] The dentin is hypersensitive, most likely due to the lack of protection by cementum, loss of smear layer by acidic dietary fluids, and the hydrodynamic movement of fluid in dentinal tubules.[4,33] The degree of inflammation in the pulp in cases of dentin hypersensitivity is not well characterized, because the condition is usually not severe enough to warrant tooth extraction or endodontic therapy. However, patent dentinal tubules are present in areas of hypersensitivity[284] (Fig. 13-10) and may result in increased irritation and localized reversible inflammation of the pulp at the sites involved.

The application of neural modulating agents such as potassium nitrate,[163] or tubule blocking agents such as strontium chloride, oxalates or dentin bonding agents (Fig. 13-11),[4,202] usually alleviates the condition, at least temporarily. However,

the placement of passive molecules or crystals may provide only temporary relief, thus there has been the need to provide biocompatible materials that bond to the root surface in order to provide a more lasting solution. One such material was a calcium sodium phosphosilicate bioactive glass,[157] which was developed into a commercial product (SootheRx, NovaMin Technology Inc., Alachua, FL). Another product uses a combination of a calcium oxalate and an acid-etched bonding material to seal the dentinal tubules (BisBlock, Bisco Inc., Schaumberg, IL). A concern has been raised that the acidic pH during etching may cause dissolution of the oxalate crystals, thus interfering with the effectiveness of the material.[279] However, one study found that BisBlock and two other products—Seal&Protect (Dentsply Professional, York, Pennsylvania) and Vivasens (Ivoclar Vivadent AG, Schaan, Liechtenstein)—were effective compared to placebo several weeks after treatment.[198] In the long term, the development of smear layer, such as from tooth brushing, dentin sclerosis, reactionary dentin, and the blockage of tubules with large endogenous macro molecules, is all thought to reduce the problem[203] (see animation from the online edition of this chapter). A practice-based, randomized clinical trial compared the effectiveness of non-desensitizing toothpaste (Colgate Cavity Protection Regular, Colgate-Palmolive, New York, New York), desensitizing toothpaste (Colgate Sensitive Fresh Stripe, Colgate-Palmolive), and a professionally applied desensitizing agent (Seal & Protect).[89] The findings showed a significant reduction of dentin hypersensitivity in the desensitizing therapies compared to the non-desensitizing group that was a much more significant reduction in the professionally applied desensitizing agent over a 6-month period.

PULPAL REACTIONS TO LOCAL ANESTHETICS

An intact pulpal blood flow is critical for maintaining the health of the dental pulp. Because the dental pulp is enclosed in a rigid chamber and is supplied by few arterioles through the apical foramina, it cannot benefit from collateral circulation or volumetric changes that compensate for changes in blood flow in other soft tissues. Furthermore, reduction in blood flow has the compounding effect of reducing the clearance of large molecular weight toxins or waste products,[201] thus causing irreversible pulpal pathosis. Vasoconstrictors are added to local anesthetics to enhance the duration of anesthesia. However, vasoconstrictors in local anesthetics could negatively impact the health of the pulp if they reduce blood flow, particularly if the pulp is inflamed preoperatively. Earlier studies have documented that vasoconstrictors in local anesthetics do reduce pulpal blood flow in experimental animals when administered by infiltration and nerve block[132] (Fig. 13-12), and that this effect was more severe with periodontal ligament injections[131] (Fig. 13-13). More recently, clinical trials were conducted in which subjects were given infiltration of different local anesthetics with or without epinephrine at a concentration of 1 : 100,000 and the pulpal blood flow was measured by laser Doppler flowmetry. In groups that received the epinephrine, there were consistently significant reductions in pulpal blood flow,[5,49,177] even if the infiltration was palatal to maxillary premolars.[213] Interestingly, in one study the reduction in pulpal blood flow with epinephrine infiltration was more than the reduction in gingival blood flow and did not return to baseline

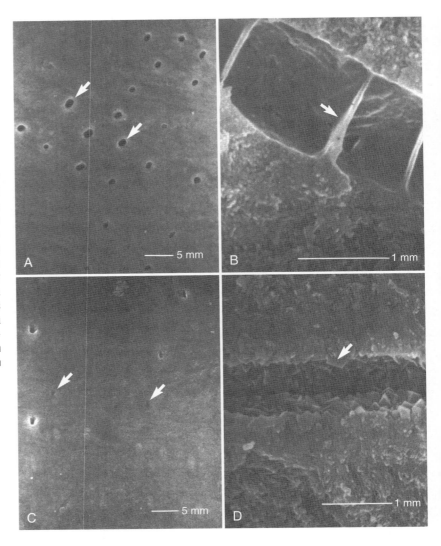

FIG. 13-10 SEM image of an exposed dentin surface of a hypersensitive area. **A,** A large proportion of dentinal tubules *(arrows)* are shown to be open. **B,** SEM image of a fractured dentinal tubule of a hypersensitive area. The lumen of the dentinal tubule is partitioned by membranous structures *(arrow).* **C,** SEM image of exposed dentin surface of a naturally desensitized area. The lumens of dentinal tubules *(arrows)* are mostly occluded, and the surface is extremely smooth. **D,** SEM image of a fractured dentinal tubule of a naturally desensitized area. Rhombohedral platelike crystals of from 0.1 to 0.3 μm *(arrow)* are present. (From Yoshiyama M, Masada J, Uchida A, Ishida H: Scanning electron microscopic characterization of sensitive vs. insensitive human radicular dentin, *J Dent Res* 68:1498, 1989. Reprinted with permission.)

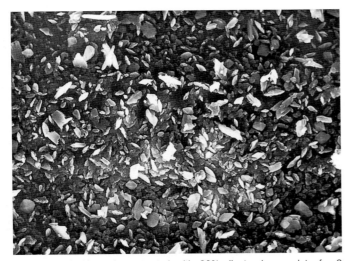

FIG. 13-11 Smear layer treated with 30% dipotassium oxalate for 2 minutes plus 3% monopotassium and monohydrogen oxalate for 2 minutes. Dentin surface is completely covered with calcium oxalate crystals (original magnification ×1900). (From Pashley DH, Galloway SE: The effects of oxalate treatment on the smear layer of ground surfaces of human dentine, *Arch Oral Biol* 30:731, 1985. Reprinted with permission.)

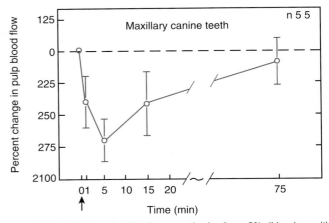

FIG. 13-12 Effects of infiltration anesthesia (i.e., 2% lidocaine with 1:100,000 epinephrine) on pulpal blood flow in the maxillary canine teeth of dogs. There is a drastic decrease in pulpal blood flow soon after the injection. Arrow indicates the time of injection. Bars depict standard deviation. (From Kim S, Edwall L, Trowbridge H, Chien S: Effects of local anesthetics on pulpal blood flow in dogs, *J Dent Res* 63:650, 1984. Reprinted with permission.)

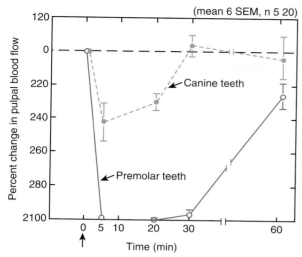

FIG. 13-13 Effects of ligamental injection (i.e., 2% lidocaine with 1 : 100,000 epinephrine) on pulpal blood flow in the mandibular canine and premolar teeth of dogs. Injection was given in the mesial and distal sulcus of premolar teeth. Injection caused total cessation of pulpal blood flow, which lasted about 30 minutes in the premolar teeth. Arrow indicates time of injection. (From Kim S: Ligamental injection: a physiological explanation of its efficacy, *J Endod* 12:486, 1986. Reprinted with permission.)

values after 1 hour of injection.[5] Similar reductions in pulpal blood flow were reported when inferior alveolar nerve block injections of lidocaine and 1 : 100,000 or 1 : 80,000 epinephrine were administered.[187] It is important to note a limitation of studies using laser Doppler flowmetry, which is that a large proportion of the signal measured may be from sources other than the dental pulp.[212,241] Thus, the monitoring of minor changes in pulpal blood flow must be interpreted with caution, particularly if the rubber dam or a similar barrier was not used.[99] Human studies on the effects of periodontal ligament or intraosseous injections on pulpal blood flow are not available, but from animal studies it is probable that these supplemental anesthetic techniques cause a more severe reduction or even transient cessation of pulpal blood flow.[133] It was also shown that intraosseous injection of Depo-Medrol™ (a corticosteroid) in patients with symptomatic irreversible pulpitis causes a significant reduction of prostaglandin E2 in the pulp 1 day after administration, indicating that this route of injection results in significant permeation into the pulpal tissues.[116] Taken together, these findings suggest that local anesthesia with vasoconstrictors may compromise the inflamed pulp's ability to recover from inflammation, particularly if it is severely inflamed, or if the tooth is subjected to extensive restorative procedures, and if the anesthetic is delivered via a periodontal ligament or an intraosseous route. However, it is important to realize that this hypothesis should be supported or refuted by prospective randomized clinical trials.

Intrapulpal anesthesia is often used as a last resort, when pulpal anesthesia is insufficient during root canal therapy. The effect of intrapulpal anesthesia on the pulp in these cases is not considered, as the pulp will be removed. However, occasionally a pulpotomy is performed to maintain pulpal vitality, such as in children where the tooth has an immature apex. One study has shown that intrapulpal anesthesia can be used in these cases, with no clinical differences on follow-up of over 24 weeks between the groups that did or did not receive intrapulpal anesthesia, and when given, in the groups where the anesthetic contained or did not contain epinephrine.[254]

PULPAL REACTIONS TO RESTORATIVE PROCEDURES

A large body of literature exists on the effects of restorative procedures on the dental pulp. This topic, understandably, has been important for practicing dentists for many years. Restorative procedures are performed primarily to treat an infectious disease, dental caries, which itself causes significant irritation of the pulp. They may also be performed to help restore missing teeth; correct developmental anomalies; address fractures, cracks, or failures of previous restorations; or a myriad of other abnormalities. One key requirement of a successful restorative procedure is to cause minimal additional irritation of the pulp so as not to interfere with normal pulpal healing. When pulp vitality is to be maintained during a restorative procedure, then a provisional diagnosis of reversible pulpitis rather than irreversible pulpitis must preexist. Therefore, it would be most desirable to perform a minimally traumatic restorative procedure, which would not potentially convert the diagnosis to irreversible pulpitis. As discussed previously, irreversible pulpitis may present clinically with severe spontaneous postoperative pain, but it may also be asymptomatic, leading to the asymptomatic demise of the pulp. The additive effects of restorative procedures are particularly critical in borderline cases, such as those of moderately symptomatic teeth with deep caries but no pulp exposure. There are still many factors whose influence on the response of the dental pulp to the cumulative effects of caries, microleakage, restorative procedures, and materials is not well understood. It is generally accepted that the effects of pulpal insults, be they from caries, restorative procedures, or trauma, are cumulative—that is, with each succeeding irritation, the pulp has a diminished capacity to remain vital. As a part of informed consent, the clinician is often faced with the task of outlining possible risks of restorative treatment. One study from a hospital in Hong Kong addressed the fate of pulps beneath single-unit metal-ceramic (MC) crowns or MC bridge abutments.[48] Patients who had received either treatment were invited to attend a recall appointment that involved both clinical and radiographic examinations. Researchers examined 122 teeth with preoperatively vital pulps treated with single-unit MC crowns and 77 treated as bridge abutments. The mean observation period was 14 years for the former and 15.6 years for the latter. Pulpal necrosis had occurred in 15.6% of the teeth treated with single-unit crowns, whereas 32.5% of the pulps in the bridge retainer groups had become necrotic. There was a significantly higher percentage of pulpal necrosis in anterior teeth that served as bridge abutments (54.5% of anterior abutment teeth examined). In general, however, the available evidence indicates that the effects of dental procedures on the pulp depend on the following factors.

The Degree of Inflammation of the Pulp Preoperatively

As stated previously, the dental pulp is compromised in its ability to respond to external irritants because it is enclosed in a noncompliant environment and because it lacks collateral circulation. Thus, the more severe the pulp is inflamed, the less will be its ability to respond to further irritation, such as in the form of restorative procedures.[147]

Most research studies designed to evaluate the effects of restorative procedures (or materials) on the pulp are conducted on human or experimental animal teeth with normal pulp. Furthermore, many of the animal research projects have been performed on anesthetized animals without the use of local anesthesia, which as stated previously, reduces pulpal blood flow. Therefore, the results of these studies may not reveal the true effects of these procedures when the carious lesion already causes inflammation of the pulp, and pulpal blood flow is reduced by local anesthetic with vasoconstrictors. A study that evaluated the response of the pulp to capping procedures as a function of duration of exposure showed that the pulp responds favorably to exposures for up to 24 hours after exposure, but not as favorably after longer periods of exposure to the oral environment.[58] It may be that the longer exposure periods lead to the formation of a bacterial biofilm, which is difficult for the pulpal immune responses to eliminate, or the extension of the infection so deep into the pulp as to preclude healing. This is relevant in cases of aseptic mechanical exposures or teeth where the pulp is exposed by traumatic injuries for a brief duration. In these cases, the pulp usually responds favorably to vital pulp therapy procedures.[6] Models of standardized pulpal inflammation with chronic caries are not commonly used in determining the effects of dental procedures. Older clinical studies show an unfavorable long-term outcome of capping cases with carious pulp exposures[17,108]; however, newer studies in which mineral trioxide aggregate (MTA) was used show more favorable results in these cases.[26,166,287a]

In the absence of severe spontaneous symptoms or pulp exposure, as indicated previously, the clinician currently cannot determine accurately the degree of preoperative pulpal inflammation. Thus, every effort should be made to minimize added irritation during restorative procedures, as it is possible that excessive irritation could convert the inflammatory status of the pulp from a reversible to an irreversible condition. In addition, the patient should always be advised of the possibility of pulpal degeneration and the importance of follow-up.

The Amount of Physical Irritation Caused by the Procedure

Physical irritation during restorative procedures such as from heat, desiccation, or vibration may adversely affect the dental pulp.

Heat

Restorative procedures such as cavity or crown preparation, or curing of resins during direct fabrication of provisional restorations,[255] may cause significant increases in pulpal temperatures. It has been shown using primate models that an intrapulpal temperature rise of 10° C causes irreversible pulp pathosis in 15%, and a 20° C rise caused pulp abscess formation in 60% of teeth evaluated.[285] A number of other older studies documented burns or severe inflammation in the pulp when cavity or crown preparations were performed without coolants (Figs. 13-14 to 13-16). However, a more recent study, in which gradual controlled heat application over a large area of the intact occlusal surface of human unanesthetized teeth was employed, failed to corroborate these earlier findings.[14]

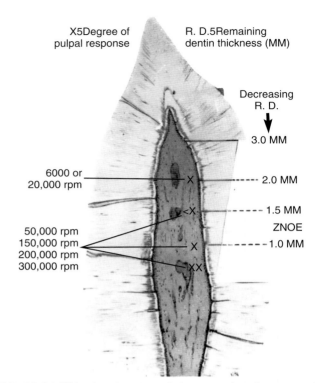

FIG. 13-14 With adequate water and air spray coolant, the same cutting tools, and a comparable remaining dentin thickness, the intensity of the pulpal response with high-speed techniques (i.e., decreasing force) is considerably less traumatic than with lower speed techniques (i.e., increasing force). (From Stanley HR, Swerdlow H: An approach to biologic variation in human pulpal studies, *J Prosthet Dent* 14:365, 1964. Reprinted with permission.)

In this study, an increase of intrapulpal temperature of about 11°C followed by a 2- to 3-month evaluation did not show any clinical or histologic changes in the pulp of any of the teeth evaluated. Heat increase in rat pulp tissue to 42° C in vitro raised heat shock protein-70, which is known to be tissue protective, and caused changes in alkaline phosphatase and gap junction proteins that were reversed to normalcy a few hours later.[8] By contrast in another study, heat applied in deep cavity preparations, prepared atraumatically in human teeth, caused histologic changes that were dependent on the proximity of the heat source to the pulp.[186] It was common in that study to see a loss of odontoblasts or their aspiration into the dentinal tubules. In cases where the cavity floor was less than 0.5 mm from the pulp, areas of coagulation necrosis could be seen, although the patients remained asymptomatic for the 1-month duration of the study. The measurement of heat in the tooth being prepared, in areas other than the site of tooth preparation, occasionally shows reduction in temperature,[91] presumably because of the poor conductive properties of dentin and the cooling effect of compressed air of the high-speed hand piece. Furthermore, cavity and crown preparations include a number of other irritating stimuli such as desiccation, severance of odontoblastic processes, vibration, and smearing of bacterial irritants onto the surface of dentin. Therefore, taken together, these findings suggest that the transient increase in temperature to levels relevant to modern dental procedures on its own may not be the culprit in inducing pulpal changes. Rather, the synergistic application of

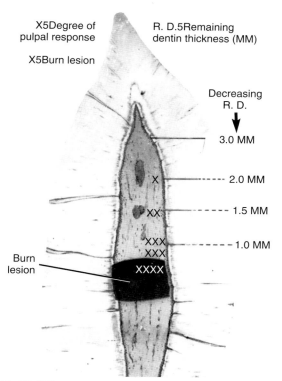

X5Degree of
pulpal response

X5Burn lesion

R. D.5Remaining
dentin thickness (MM)

Decreasing
R. D.

3.0 MM

X ----- 2.0 MM

XX ----- 1.5 MM

XXX ----- 1.0 MM
XXX

Burn
lesion

XXXX

FIG. 13-15 Without adequate water coolant, larger cutting tools (e.g., no. 37 diamond point) create typical burn lesions within the pulp when the remaining dentin thickness becomes less than 1.5 mm. (From Stanley HR, Swerdlow H: An approach to biologic variation in human pulpal studies, *J Prosthet Dent* 14:365, 1964. Reprinted with permission.)

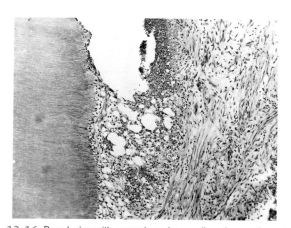

FIG. 13-16 Burn lesion with necrosis and expanding abscess formation in a 10-day specimen. Cavity preparation dry at 20,000 rpm with remaining dentin thickness is 0.23 mm. (From Swerdlow H, Stanley HR Jr: Reaction of the human dental pulp to cavity preparation. I. Effect of water spray at 20,000 rpm, *J Am Dent Assoc* 56:317, 1958. Reprinted with permission.)

excessive heat with other irritation factors and its proximity to the pulp may induce pathologic changes.

Desiccation

Desiccation during cavity and crown preparation has long been known to cause aspiration of odontoblastic nuclei into dentinal tubules and pulpal inflammation.[31] One study showed that as little as 30 seconds of continuous air drying of class V cavities

in human molars with uninflamed pulp caused significant displacement of odontoblastic nuclei, pulp inflammation, and even areas of necrosis related to the areas that were dried.[57] However, another study showed that the effects of desiccation are transient in that within 7 to 30 days there is autolysis of the aspirated cells and formation of reactionary dentin.[32] The pulp in cases with aspirated odontoblasts, following desiccation for 1 minute, was not sensitive to clinical scraping with an explorer. The sensitivity was restored with rehydration of the cavities and was increased in other cases where pulp inflammation was induced by microbial contamination.[154] In this study, despite the lack of sensitivity in desiccated cavities, neural elements were seen histologically to be pushed into the tubules like the odontoblastic nuclei. The disruption of the odontoblastic layer and peripheral neural elements in the pulp with desiccation was also observed in a rat model using axonal transport of radioactive protein.[37]

Biologic and Chemical irritation

Dental caries is clearly an infectious disease in which microorganisms and their virulence determinants constantly irritate the pulp, even at the early stages, long before pulp exposure.[34] However, despite the elimination of visible caries during cavity preparation, the cavity floor is undoubtedly left with some contamination by caries bacteria. Although the rubber dam should be used with any cavity preparation to prevent cavity contamination with salivary microorganisms, the use of water coolants allows the cavity to be contaminated with bacteria from water lines. Concerns about residual cavity contamination prompted some to use cavity disinfection with caustic chemicals. Chemicals such as hydrogen peroxide, sodium hypochlorite, or calcium hydroxide solutions have been proposed for this purpose, although they may exert a toxic effect.[54] An earlier study showed that the amounts of residual bacteria following adequate restoration are not significant.[170] Once dentin is exposed, there is a constant outward flow of dentinal fluid that minimizes the inward flow of any noxious agents.[275] This may aid in the reduction of irritation from residual microbial factors in dentinal tubules.

In contemporary practice, most chemical irritation during restorative procedures results from the application of etching agents, especially strong acids, in the form of total dentin etch, particularly if capping of exposed pulp is performed.[93,197] Etching is performed to remove the smear layer, promote physical adhesion of bonding agents to dentin by forming resin tags in the dentinal tubules, and permeate the newer unfilled resin primers into the unmineralized surface layer of collagen to form the so-called hybrid layer.

If the cavity is relatively superficial and is adequately sealed with a restorative resin, then etching of dentin is probably not detrimental to the pulp because of the narrow diameter of dentinal tubules and their low density in peripheral dentin.[28] In fact, one study documented that histologic evidence of bacteria in human cavities restored with composite was significantly less if the cavity had been etched with phosphoric acid than if it were etched with 17% EDTA or nonetched.[176] Pulpal inflammation in this study was not correlated with the etching treatments but with bacterial presence; thus, in cases of etching with phosphoric acid, if bacteria were also present, severe pulpal inflammation and necrosis could be seen.

Self-etching formulations have become popular because they eliminate the separate etching step involved in total-etch procedures. Some have speculated that the bonding of self-etching systems may be poorer than total-etch systems because of the weaker acidity of the acidic primers of self-etching systems when compared to that of total-etch systems.[28] However, studies have shown no significant differences between the two adhesive systems in postoperative sensitivity,[208] long-term in vivo degradation,[141] or long-term in vitro bond strength.[10] One clinical study showed no differences between the two systems with respect to bacterial leakage and the inflammatory response in the pulp.[181] The most important variable that affected the pulp in this study was the amount of bacterial leakage with either system.

Other factors that may contribute to pulpal irritation during resin placement from chemical/biologic irritants include unpolymerized monomer and polymerization shrinkage. Higher concentrations of monomeric resin components were shown to exert an inhibitory effect on T lymphocytes and spleen cells,[124] and monocytes/macrophages[149,216,217,231] in vitro. These components may leach directly into the pulp in deep cavities and cause chemical irritation.[59,110] Shrinkage during polymerization of composites may induce internal stresses on dentin and create voids that allow microleakage. Shrinkage of resins is estimated to range from 0.6% to 1.4%, and should be minimized during placement by incremental curing and possibly starting the restoration with flowable resins.[28]

In summary, the available evidence indicates that chemicals involved in modern restorative procedures may irritate the pulp if placed directly on an exposure, or if there is microbial leakage along the tooth/restoration interface.

The Proximity of the Restorative Procedures to the Dental Pulp and the Surface Area of Dentin Exposed

It has been known for several decades that as the carious lesion progresses toward the pulp, particularly when the remaining dentin thickness (RDT) is less than 0.5 mm, there is an increasingly severe pulpal reaction, with a greater likelihood of the pulp undergoing irreversible pathosis.[220] The diameter and density of dentinal tubules increase closer to the pulp (Fig. 13-17). Based on the dentinal tubule density at the DEJ (about 65,000/mm²) and the pulp (about 15,000/mm²),[84,88] it was

estimated that the area occupied by tubule lumina at the DEJ was 1% of the total surface area at the DEJ and 22% at the pulp.[203] Thus, it is not surprising that several studies have shown that pulpal inflammation in response to restorative procedures increases with the reduction in RDT.[159,175] One study examined the differential effects on the rat pulp of the preparation method, remaining dentin thickness, coolant, drill speed, conditioning with EDTA, and filling materials.[174] Subsequent to the cavity preparations a tooth slice was obtained and maintained ex vivo as an organ culture for up to 2 weeks. The results showed that the remaining dentin thickness was the most important factor in pulpal injury.

With the passage of time following cavity preparation, there is reduction in the permeability of RDT.[204] This may be due to rapid deposition of reactionary dentin, the migration of large proteins into the tubules, or the diminution of tubule diameter as dentin becomes more sclerotic. Using a primate model, it was shown that the basic rate of secondary dentin deposition was about 0.8 μm/day and that this rate increased to an average of 2.9 μm/day following restorative procedures. Interestingly, in this study dentin deposition was also more rapid next to shallow cavities than deep cavities[277]; however, another study showed that total reactionary dentin deposited was thicker in deeper and wider cavities.[173]

Clinically, it has been observed that postoperative sensitivity is common with many restorative procedures. Following resin composite restorations on patients, it was shown that postoperative sensitivity was related to the depth of the cavity, but not to the presence or absence of liners or bases.[268]

In addition to the depth or the width of a large cavity preparation, a crown preparation exposes more dentinal tubules to microbial or chemical irritation. During crown fabrication, there are added irritation factors such as length of time of the preparation, impression techniques, and the imperfect adaptation of temporary restorations, causing microleakage during the temporization period. Because of the precise engineering requirements of some restorations, some providers may be inclined to reduce the coolant during crown preparation steps such as finalizing the finishing lines. However, crown preparations without coolants have been shown to dramatically reduce pulpal blood flow in an animal model (Fig. 13-18).[133] There are few studies available on the direct effects of modern crown and bridge techniques on the

FIG. 13-17 Schematic of convergence of tubules toward the pulp. **A,** Periphery of the dentin. Most surface area is occupied by intertubular dentin (☆), with a few tubules surrounded by hypermineralized peritubular dentin (✪). **B,** Near the pulp, the increase in tubule diameter has occurred largely at the expense of the peritubular dentin. This substrate has high protein content. As the remaining dentin is made thinner (from **A** to **B**), the permeability of the dentin increases, because both the diameter and the density of dentinal tubules are increased. (From Bouillaguet S: Biological risks of resin-based materials to the dentin-pulp complex, *Crit Rev Oral Biol Med* 15:47, 2004. Reprinted with permission.)

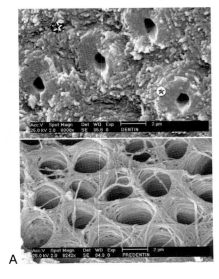

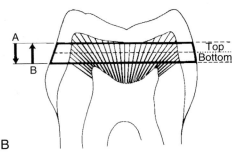

pulp. However, some long-term outcome studies have documented that the incidence of pulp necrosis following crown placement ranges from 10% to 50%.[48,79,269]

The Permeability of Dentin and the Odontoblastic Layer Between the Area Being Restored and the Pulp

The permeability of dentin plays an important role in the ingress of potential irritants to the pulp. It is clear from research done since the 1980s that dentin is not uniformly permeable

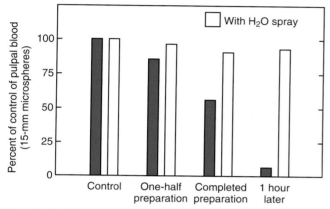

FIG. 13-18 Effects of crown preparation in dogs, with and without water and air spray (at 350,000 rpm), on pulpal blood flow. Tooth preparation without water and air spray caused a substantial decrease in pulpal blood flow, whereas that with water and air spray caused insignificant changes in the flow.

and that permeability depends on factors such as the location within the same tooth, the age of the patient, and the presence of pathologic conditions such as dental caries. Fundamentally, the permeability of dentin depends on the collective sum of the permeability of individual tubules at a particular site in the tooth. The tubular diameter increases from about 0.6 to 0.8 μm close to the DEJ to about 3 μm at the pulp.[200] Given that bacterial cells are about 0.5 to 1 μm in diameter, it is evident that in deep cavity preparations, particularly when total-etch procedures are employed, bacteria can migrate through the remaining dentin into the pulp.

With age the width of peritubular dentin increases, causing a reduction in tubular lumen or sclerosis. Caries causes demineralization in superficial dentin, which is associated with remineralization and the formation of caries crystals within the tubules of inner undemineralized dentin (Fig. 13-19). This causes a decrease in permeability in dentin subjacent to the carious lesion[202] and could be considered a protective mechanism, as it may delay the progress of the carious lesion.

It was shown that irritation from cavity preparation increased the permeability of the odontoblastic cell layer only at the site of the cavity preparation.[117,263] In addition to the physical barrier to permeability and the production of reactionary or reparative dentin, the odontoblastic layer may, in fact, contribute to the host response of the dental pulp by expressing important inflammatory mediators[152,196] or recognizing bacteria through Toll-like receptors.[22,66,74,123]

The Age of the Patient (see also Chapter 26)

Resting pulpal blood flow (PBF), as well as the changes in PBF in response to cold application, will decrease with age.[112] Age

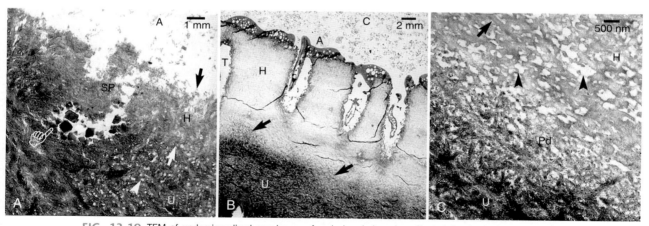

FIG. 13-19 TEM of undemineralized specimens of resin-bonded, caries-affected dentin. **A,** Stained TEM of undemineralized specimens following the application of the self-etch ABF system to caries-affected dentin. The hybrid layer (H; between arrows) was about 3 μm thick, and the underlying undemineralized dentin (U) was highly porous (arrowhead). The dentinal tubule was covered with a smear plug (SP) and was partially obliterated with large caries crystals (pointer). A, filled adhesive. **B,** Stained section of the total-etch single bond adhesive bonded to caries-affected dentin. A hybrid layer (H) between 15 and 19 μm thick could be seen, with a partially demineralized zone (open arrows) above the undemineralized caries affected dentin (U). T, dentinal tubule. C, composite. **C,** Higher magnification of the basal part of the unusually thick hybrid layer (H), shown in **(A).** Banded collagen fibrils (open arrow) were separated by unusually wide and porous interfibrillar spaces (open arrowheads). A partially demineralized zone (Pd) was present along the demineralization front. This zone was not seen in phosphoric-acid-etched sound dentin **(B).** U, undemineralized caries-affected dentin. (From Yoshiyama M, Tay FR, Doi J, et al: Bonding of self-etch and total-etch adhesives to carious dentin, *J Dent Res* 81:556, 2002. Reprinted with permission.)

may also be associated with reduction in pulpal neuropeptides.[85] However, studies show no differences between young and old pulp in the regenerative capacity of odontoblast-like cells and in the presence of cells positive for class II major histocompatibility complex, heat shock protein 25, or nestin, when subjected to cavity preparation.[128] An examination of young versus old normal human pulp showed that young pulp had increased expression of biologic factors related to cell differentiation, proliferation, and the immune response, whereas older pulp had increased factors related to apoptosis.[259] These analyses cannot translate to the pulp's ability to deal with irritation and its sequelae. Thus, the net result of the ability of the pulp to cope with external stimulation or irritation in humans with advancing age is not clear.

PULPAL REACTIONS TO RESTORATIVE MATERIALS

The effects of restorative materials on the dental pulp have been investigated and seem to relate directly to the permeability of the associated dentin. The degree of dentin permeability, however, is often variable and is governed by several factors including age and caries status.[251] The most important variable in dentin permeability to restorative materials is the thickness of dentin between the floor of the cavity preparation and the pulp.[1]

Given the importance of dentin permeability, there are direct pulpal effects of any given restorative material that are governed by the composition of the material and associated eluted or degraded products. Unbound components of resin materials and preparative agents such as acid etchants can affect the subjacent pulp by inducing an inflammatory response.[87,93,215] The indirect effects of desiccation or demineralization of dentin as well as the direct effects of the material itself when in contact with pulpal tissue mediate this inflammatory response. Studies have shown that the certain cytotoxic components of resin monomers (e.g., triethylene glycol dimethacrylate and 2-hydroxyethyl methacrylate) readily penetrate dentin.[81] Similarly, eugenol and components of Ledermix (triamcinolone and demeclocycline) have been shown to pass through dentin into the subjacent pulp.[109,111] In vivo data show that these chemicals have an effect on the pulp; however, the effect seems to be short lived and, in the absence of bacteria, it is reversible.[21]

The mechanisms whereby restorative materials exert an injurious effect on the dental pulp vary. Evidence exists that supports direct and, in some instances, prolonged cytotoxicity, stimulation of hypersensitivity reactions, or impairment of the host immune response to bacteria.[229] Some of the components of resin restorations are released at cytotoxic levels after polymerization is completed, leading to chronic stimulation and a resultant prolonged inflammatory response.[80] Furthermore, even subtoxic concentrations of certain agents are capable of eliciting allergic reactions in humans.[110] Primates hyperimmunized with BSA showed significant pulpal damage with repeated antigenic challenge in class V cavity preparations, suggesting a role for antigen-antibody complex–mediated hypersensitivity in tissue destruction.[24] In a separate study, exposure to dentin primers elicited a delayed-type hypersensitivity reaction in guinea pigs.[127] These studies taken together present a compelling argument for immune-mediated pulpal tissue damage subsequent to exposure to restorative materials. Foreign body reactions have also been described in pulps containing extruded globules of resin material.[114,115] Histologic examination of these pulps shows macrophages and giant cells surrounding the resin particles. Lastly, resin monomers have been shown to decrease the activity of immunocompetent cells in a dose-dependent manner in in vitro functional assays.[124] Although all of these effects are documented, their extent and therefore morbidity on the dental pulp is speculative and doubtless does not act solely to effect pulpal demise. As previously noted, most restorative materials are placed adjacent to pulps that are previously compromised by bacterial insult, and disease, debridement, and restoration of the tooth have cumulative effects on the dental pulp.

Although pulpal irritation is largely considered to be a negative sequela, the irritant potential of certain restorative materials is central to their usefulness in restorative dentistry. Calcium hydroxide is one of the oldest and most widely used medicaments for stimulation of dentinal bridge formation subsequent to microscopic or gross pulpal exposure. The low-grade pulpal irritation that it induces is important for dentinal bridge formation in exposures.[61,230] The degree of inflammation is dependent on the preparation of calcium hydroxide used. Aqueous suspensions of calcium hydroxide applied to exposed pulps cause superficial necrosis of pulpal tissue followed by low-grade inflammatory changes. Within 30 days the tissue subjacent to the necrotic zone has reorganized and resumed normal architecture. Hard-setting calcium hydroxide preparations as well as mineral trioxide aggregates are effective in eliciting dentinal bridge formation with a much smaller to nonexistent necrotic zone.[102] This is preferable in vital pulp therapies such as the Cvek pulpotomy, where maintenance of the maximum amount of vital pulp tissue is desirable and the extent of pulpal inflammation is minimal[60] (Fig. 13-20). The irritation potential of calcium hydroxide across intact dentin is dependent on factors such as the remaining dentin thickness and permeability. Application of calcium hydroxide to intact dentin appears to induce sclerosis by promoting crystal precipitation within the tubules accompanied by reductions in permeability.[172]

Although the irritation potential of calcium hydroxide plays a role in its effectiveness, the high pH of this material can liberate bioactive molecules from dentin. Numerous authors have demonstrated that dentin matrix proteins like TGF-β1 and adrenomedullin are liberated by both calcium hydroxide and mineral trioxide aggregate.[92,257] Once liberated they are able to facilitate hard tissue formation yet again. This offers another explanation for the ability of these materials to induce hard tissue formation in vivo. Acid etching or the use of chelating agents such as EDTA represent a common step in the placement of bonded restorations. The etching process removes mineral and exposes collagen fibrils. As with a high pH, sequestered bioactive molecules are released and can act on pulpal cells. These include growth factors and metalloproteinases, which can be inductive for healing but can also degrade the bond of the restoration.[205] EDTA has been shown to be even more effective at extracting noncollagenous proteins from dentin than either calcium hydroxide or MTA but less so than citric acid.[92,257]

Investigations into the pulpal response to glass-ionomer materials have shown that both the lowered pH of the material and the release of high concentrations of fluoride can inflict damage to pulp tissues.[126] In direct contact with pulpal cells, glass ionomers are toxic.[143] Direct pulp capping studies have

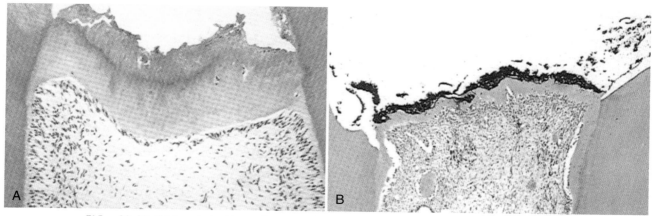

FIG. 13-20 Calcium hydroxide produces an inflammatory response that stimulates dentinal bridge formation. The dentin bridge forms lower in the tooth with calcium hydroxide paste (A) versus hard-setting calcium hydroxide (B).

shown it to be inferior to calcium hydroxide.[63,105] When applied to intact dentin and in the absence of bacteria, there is a transient inflammatory response and reparative dentin is formed.[55]

In addition to the direct chemical effects of restorative materials, there are indirect factors that contribute to pulpal irritation. The technique sensitivity of certain materials predisposes them to faulty bonds to tooth structure that can translate to dentin hypersensitivity, recurrent disease, and pulpal inflammation or necrosis. Much attention has been given to the interface created between resin-bonded materials and dentin. During the etching process, the more highly mineralized peritubular dentin is preferentially dissolved, leaving free collagen fibrils and opening lateral tubular branches.[93,94,171] Applied resin infiltrates the exposed collagen mesh, creating a layer 5 to 10 μm thick referred to as the hybrid layer.[178] This layer, along with the resin permeating exposed tubules, forms the bond between the resin and dentin. If the preparation is too dry, the collagen fibrils collapse and the resin cannot effectively permeate the mesh, which results in a defective bond. As the optimal degree of hydration of the preparation surface can vary from material to material, resin restoration placement is technique sensitive. This same principle is applicable to the practice of bonding fractured tooth fragments where the segment has become dehydrated while outside of the mouth. Current protocols recommend rehydration of the segment prior to bonding, thus increasing the mechanical and presumably the microbial seal.[78] This is particularly important with a complicated crown fracture where the pulpal protection by intact dentin is absent.

Some restorative materials rely on their medicinal properties as well as their ability to seal a cavity preparation. Materials containing zinc oxide and eugenol (ZOE) fall into this category. ZOE is used for a variety of purposes in dentistry largely because of its anesthetic and antiseptic properties. It has been shown to block transmission of action potentials in nerve fibers and to suppress nerve excitability in the pulp when applied to deep excavations.[261] In addition, ZOE has good adaptation to dentin and inhibits bacterial growth on cavity walls. These properties have made this a favored material for temporary fillings but not for long-term restorations, as ZOE temporaries have been shown to leak after only a few weeks in situ.[286]

DIRECT PULP CAPPING WITH MINERAL TRIOXIDE AGGREGATE

Direct capping of pulp exposures is indicated in pulps that were previously healthy and exposed by trauma or dental restorative procedures.[250] Although calcium hydroxide has historically been the preferred dressing agent on mechanically exposed pulps, the use of mineral trioxide aggregate (MTA) has been proposed, even on carious pulp exposures.[16,26,166] Prospective animal studies and human case reports have evaluated the ability of MTA to allow for the formation of a reparative dentin bridge and maintain continued pulp vitality.[73,83,137] Although the results are generally favorable, one concern is of tooth discoloration if the gray MTA formulation is used on anterior teeth.

In one clinical study, MTA was used as a pulp capping material for carious pulp exposures.[26] Forty patients, ages 7 to 45, who were diagnosed with reversible pulpitis had caries removed using a caries detection dye and sodium hypochlorite for hemostasis. The treatment was performed in two visits to allow the MTA to set up and to confirm pulp sensibility to pulp tests in the second visit. Success was determined radiographically, with subjective symptoms, pulp testing with cold, and continued root formation on immature teeth. Outcomes were measured over a period of up to 9 years postoperatively and showed an overall success of 97%, with all the teeth in the immature root group showing success. In another clinical study in which dentists and students participated in the treatment, pulp capping of carious pulp exposures was compared between MTA and calcium hydroxide.[166] At follow-up, 122 cases of patients with a mean age of 40 years were available. The success with MTA was 78% and that with calcium hydroxide was 60%, a difference that was statistically significant. More recently, the same group reported an update of their findings with a sample size of 229 teeth, which were evaluated from 24 to 123 months following treatment. The overall success rates were 80.5% of teeth in the MTA group (137/170) and 59% of teeth in the CH group (35/59), which was a statistically significant difference. The outcome was also significantly better in any group if the tooth was promptly restored. Within the parameters of these studies, it seems that white MTA is a suitable capping agent for pulp exposures of healthy or reversibly inflamed pulps, including cases with asymptomatic carious exposures. However, given that the prognosis of root canal therapy in this last category has been shown to be predictably high in many studies, the patient needs to be educated carefully of the options, and consent must be documented.

Other calcium silicate–based materials are gaining popularity as pulp capping agents and appear to have properties and effects similar to MTA.[11,184] Biodentine deserves special reference because in addition to the biocompatibility, it has physical properties that are similar to dentin.[39,142]

THE USE OF HEMOSTATIC AGENTS AND DISINFECTANTS ON DIRECT PULP EXPOSURES

There is still debate as to whether the outcome of pulp capping for exposure depends on the toxicity of medicaments and materials placed on vital pulp tissues, the ability of these materials to induce mineralization, or their ability to seal the cavity from further bacterial ingress. It is likely a combination of these factors, as was shown in the clinical trial with MTA mentioned before.[26] Another factor in the prognosis of direct pulp caps is the ability to control hemorrhage at the exposure site.[243] Given the difficulty in creating a bacteria-free operating environment during tooth preparation, the ideal hemostatic agent also would have the ability to kill bacteria.

One study compared the effects of two hemostatic/disinfectant agents on the healing of experimental pulp exposures created in human third molar teeth and capped with calcium hydroxide.[234] Pulp exposures were made in 45 maxillary wisdom teeth scheduled for extraction for orthodontic reasons. Teeth were randomly assigned to receive hard-setting calcium hydroxide pulp caps after a 30-second surface treatment with one of three agents: 0.9% saline, 2% chlorhexidine, or 5.25% sodium hypochlorite. Although the 7-day saline specimens showed slightly less inflammatory response, there were no statistically significant differences between the groups with respect to all dependent measures over the course of the study. Complete healing was seen in 88% of all specimens at 90 days.

The pulps in these teeth were previously uninjured, and the exposures were made in a clean environment. Therefore, it seems that a *mechanical* exposure of a healthy pulp created during cavity preparation could be disinfected with either 2% chlorhexidine or 5.25% sodium hypochlorite, capped with a hard-setting calcium hydroxide formulation, and expected to have a favorable prognosis for healing.

PULPAL REACTIONS TO LASER PROCEDURES

Numerous studies have been published on the effect of using lasers on enamel, dentin, and pulp (see also Chapter 8). Laser use on hard tissue has been a popular area of research because of the potential benefits of efficiency, reduced sensitivity, disinfection, and precision. Several types of laser technologies are available that depend on the wavelength, active medium, emission mode, delivery system, power output, and duration of application. The main types available in dentistry today are shown in Fig. 13-21. The CO_2 *laser* is historically the oldest type used on soft tissues and thus has been the most studied.

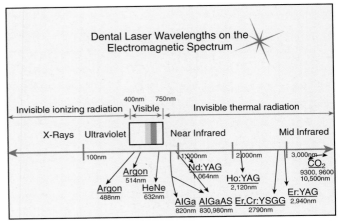

FIG. 13-21 Currently available dental wavelengths on the electromagnetic spectrum. Note all of the wavelengths are nonionizing. (From Coluzzi DJ: An overview of laser wavelengths used in dentistry, *Dent Clin North Am* 44:753, 2000. Reprinted with permission.)

It has the longest wavelength (10,600 nm). It cannot be delivered in an optic fiber, thus it must be used in a hollow-tube-like wave guide in continuous gated-pulse mode. This means that the operator does not feel a solid resistance when using this laser. *Er:YAG, Nd:YAG or Ho:YAG lasers* all have an active medium of a solid crystal of yttrium-aluminum-garnet, which is impregnated in erbium, neodymium, or holmium, respectively. Er:YAG has a wavelength of 2940 nm and is delivered using a solid optic fiber. It has a high affinity for water and hydroxyapatite, thus it can be used to remove caries and cut dentin with coolant. It can also be used on soft tissue. Ho:YAG laser has a wavelength of 2120 nm and has high affinity to water but not to tooth structure, thus it is used primarily for soft tissue surgery. Nd:YAG laser is also delivered fiberoptically, has a wavelength of 1064 nm, and has been used extensively in dentistry because it has a high affinity for water and pigmented tissues and offers good hemostasis; thus is used extensively in surgery.[52] In addition, there are some low-power output lasers such as *HeNe* (helium-neon) (632 nm), and *GaAlAs* (gallium-aluminum-arsenide) (diode; semiconductor) (720-904 nm) lasers, which have been used in laser Doppler flowmetry and in treating dentin hypersensitivity.[134]

To summarize the available data, a discussion of the application of lasers for two specific purposes follows.

Lasers in the Prevention, Diagnosis, and Treatment of Caries

Laser irradiation of deep susceptible pits and fissures may reduce the incidence of dental caries. Once caries develops, some lasers may be effective in removing the carious lesion and sparing undemineralized dentin, because of their differential absorption by water and hydroxyapatite. Furthermore, if caries exposes the pulp in young teeth, particularly those with immature apices, lasers may be able to effectively excise coronal infected pulp in pulpotomy, because of their hemostatic and antibacterial properties. All these potential uses prompted a large number of investigations on the effectiveness of lasers in these applications.

Some clinicians have proposed using lasers to enhance adhesion of pit and fissure sealants; however, this was shown to not

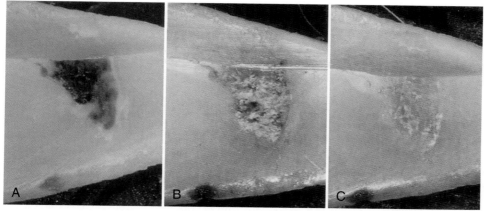

FIG. 13-22 **A,** Dental caries. **B,** Pulsed Nd:YAG ablation by-products (160 mJ, 10 Hz). **C,** Debris removed with acid etch and polishing. Enamel surface was faceted for reflection spectroscopy. (From Harris DM, White JM, Goodis H, et al: Selective ablation of surface enamel caries with a pulsed Nd:YAG dental laser, *Lasers Surg Med* 30:342, 2002. Reprinted with permission.)

add any advantage following acid etching—a necessity for adhesion.[160] Laser fluorescence is used by the DIAGNOdent and DIAGNOdent pen, which are laser devices that have been introduced for the diagnosis of noncavitated caries. Although these devices initially showed some promising results,[161] more recent work shows that they are best used as adjunctive devices to radiography and visual examination.[7,53,144]

Laser ablation of superficial carious lesions may be more conservative than bur preparation. A recent controlled clinical trial supports this tenet, when a free-running pulsed Nd:YAG laser was used to ablate superficial pit and fissure caries in third molars scheduled for extraction[98] (Fig. 13-22). In this study there were no histologic differences in the pulp response between the two groups.

From the perspective of the effects on the pulp, most laser applications that are employed in cutting or modifying cavities in dentin or acting directly on the pulp tissue are important. Earlier studies showed reduced permeability of dentin in vitro with a XeCl excimer laser (a laser with a relatively short wavelength of 308 nm in the ultraviolet range).[242] The apparent fusion of tubules in superficial layers of dentin was shown to occur with CO_2, Nd:YAG, and Er:YAG lasers in vitro.[278] The pulpal responses to Nd:YAG and CO_2 lasers were not favorable. It was shown that Nd:YAG and to a lesser degree CO_2 lasers may be associated with charring and significant inflammation in the pulp compared with the Er:YAG laser[256,278] (Fig. 13-23). More recently it was reported that water cooling was necessary for laser ablation as it is for high-speed bur preparations.[43] Studies have shown that the Er:YAG laser appears to induce similar responses in the pulp to those seen with high-speed bur preparations, at the level of light microscopy analysis.[72,252,253,278] However, the findings with electron microscopy were different: it was reported that while shallow cavities ablated in rat molars using Er:YAG lasers did not show changes from base-line using light microscopy, transmission electron microscopy showed disruption and degeneration of pulpal peripheral nerve endings and of myelin sheath in the immediate postoperative period (Fig. 13-24).[113] This may explain the reduced sensitivity that accompanies laser cavity preparations. Thus, in summary, it does not appear that the use of lasers provides predictable advantages

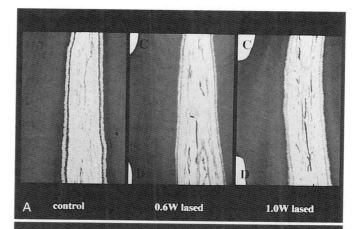
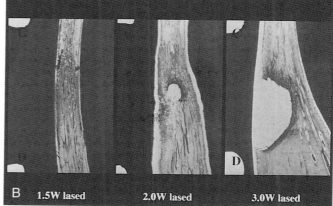

FIG. 13-23 **A, B,** Histopathologic picture of Nd:YAG laser specimen with an increasing power. There is direct relationship between the degree of pathologic changes and the increasing power of the laser. In fact, 1.5W and the greater power cause permanent damage to the pulp.

in cavity preparation compared with traditional methods at this time.

For pulpotomy procedures, such as in primary teeth, permanent teeth with immature apices, or pulps that are exposed due to fracture and treated promptly, the lasers, particularly

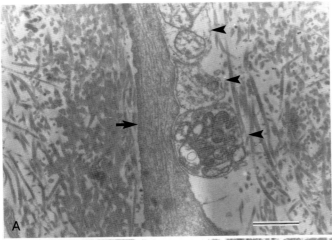

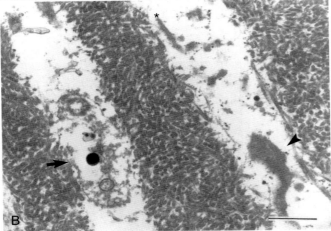

FIG. 13-24 **A,** Control; normal odontoblastic process *(arrow)* and a few nerve terminals *(arrowheads)* are seen in a dental tubule of rat upper first molar. **B,** Six hours after Er:YAG laser irradiation; disrupted cell membrane of a nerve terminal that contains some granular vesicles *(arrow)* and shrinkage of an odontoblastic process *(arrowhead)* are noted in dentinal tubules just under the ablated area. An asterisk indicates the irradiated side (TEM, ×13,700, bar = 1 μm). (From Inoue H, Izumi T, Ishikawa H, Watanabe K: Short-term histomorphological effects of Er:YAG laser irradiation to rat coronal dentin-pulp complex, *Oral Surg Oral Med Oral Pathol Oral Radiol Endod* 97:246, 2004. Reprinted with permission.)

CO_2 lasers, may be useful in achieving precise surgical excision of coronal pulp and immediate hemostasis. A controlled clinical study showed that CO_2 laser pulpotomy was comparable to traditional methods in experimental pulpotomies of primary teeth scheduled for extraction for orthodontic reasons.[70] However, an animal study in which CO_2 and Nd:YAG lasers were compared revealed poor response with both lasers compared with calcium hydroxide.[125] An animal study using the Er:YAG laser showed that the results are dependent on the power settings, in that lower energy delivered with this laser produced favorable results.[135]

Lasers in the Treatment of Dentin Hypersensitivity

Earlier studies have shown effectiveness ranging from 5% to 100% of low-output lasers on dentin hypersensitivity.[134] One author reported a reduction of hypersensitivity in 73% of mild cases, 19% of moderate cases, and 14% of severe cases after 4 months using a GaAlAs laser.[134] Low-output lasers do not have any effects on the morphology of enamel or dentin, but they are thought to cause a transient reduction in action potential mediated by pulpal C-fibers, but not Aδ-fibers,[276] although this finding was not consistent.[192] Nd:YAG lasers have also been used in dentin hypersensitivity. Because of the higher power output, these lasers cause superficial occlusion of dentinal tubules of up to 4 μm,[158] in addition to action potential blockage within the pulp in vitro or in experimental animals.[191,192] However, a placebo-controlled clinical trial has shown that both Nd:YAG and placebo caused a significant reduction in dentin hypersensitivity for up to 4 months postoperatively but were not different from each other.[153] More recent clinical trials show that although lasers are useful for managing hypersensitivity, they do not appear to be better than less costly and more readily available alternatives.[82,267]

Use of Lasers as a Protective Measure for Dentin, Under Traditional Cavity Preparation

One clinical study has proposed that if lasers are used to prepare cavities or used on prepared dentin after traditional cavity preparation with burs, this would protect the dentin, as its permeability and bacterial content may decrease. In this study, two patients were scheduled to have six teeth extracted during orthodontic treatment.[90] In the teeth that had laser irradiation (GaA1As laser, lambda = 660 nm, power of 30 mW and energy dose of 2 J/cm²) and were examined with transmission electron microscopy (TEM) after 28 days, the odontoblastic process had increased contact with the extracellular matrix, and the collagen fibrils appeared more organized than those of the control group (traditional bur preparation only). The study concluded that laser irradiation accelerates the recovery of the dental tissues in the predentin region.

PULPAL REACTIONS TO VITAL BLEACHING TECHNIQUES

Vital bleaching techniques employ strong oxidizing agents, namely 10% carbamide peroxide and hydrogen peroxide, to bleach enamel of teeth with vital pulp. There have been concerns about the potential for pulpal irritation during these procedures because of the long duration that the chemicals are in contact with the teeth, particularly if dentin with open tubules or cracks is present. Histologic or histochemical analysis of the pulp following bleaching for up to 2 weeks showed minor inflammatory changes in the pulp of the bleached teeth that were reversible.[9,86] One clinical report documented that if 16% carbamide peroxide was used, gingival irritation was evident; however, no changes in pulp vitality or in symptoms were noted. Even in patients who develop symptoms postoperatively, these tend to be reversible and could be prevented by treating the teeth with fluorides and by correcting restorative deficiencies preoperatively.[180] Clinical symptoms are likely to be due to increases in neuropeptides, such as substance P, in the pulp.[44] An earlier clinical trial showed that vital bleaching using 10% carbamide peroxide in a custom

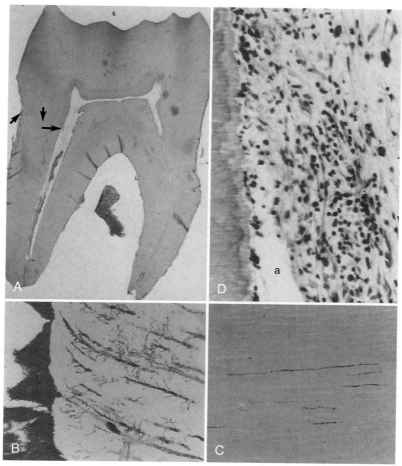

FIG. 13-25 Mandibular first molar of 49-year-old female, no pain. Clinically caries free. Calculus, periodontal disease, and bone loss from two thirds to three fourths of root. **A,** Note narrowness of pulp chamber seen throughout all serial sections (original magnification ×8.5). **B,** Bacterial plaque and adjacent dentinal tubules with bacteria (*oblique arrow* in **A**) (original magnification ×400). **C,** Farthest penetration of bacteria in dentinal tubules (*vertical arrow* in **A**) (original magnification ×400). **D,** Where dentinal tubules invaded by bacteria terminate in the pulp (*horizontal arrow* in A), a small but dense accumulation of lymphocytes and macrophages appears (*a,* artifact; pulp tissue torn away from dentin during processing) (original magnification ×400). (From Langeland K: Tissue response to dental caries, *Endod Dent Traumatol* 3:149, 1987. Reprinted with permission.)

tray for 6 weeks was safe for the pulp health for up to 10 years postoperatively, although the bleaching effectiveness may decline with time.[222] In one clinical study, premolars scheduled for orthodontic extraction had 38% H_2O_2 bleaching gel with and without a halogen light source applied. There were no histologic effects on the dental pulp at 2 to 15 days after bleaching.[136] When the study was performed on incisors with the same treatment for 45 minutes, areas of coagulation necrosis could be seen in the pulp.[56] Therefore, caution should be exercised when this caustic agent is used for extended bleaching.

PULPAL REACTIONS TO PERIODONTAL PROCEDURES

In an intact nontraumatized tooth, the dental pulp maintains its healthy existence throughout life because it is insulated from microbial irritation in the oral cavity (see also Chapter 17). Periodontal disease causes attachment loss, which exposes

the root surface to the oral cavity. Occasionally, pulpal inflammation secondary to severe periodontitis is observed.[148] Some reports have described bacterial infiltration through dentinal tubules of exposed root surface causing mild inflammatory changes in the pulp (Fig. 13-25).[146] However, in a case report of 25 teeth that were extracted in a patient with extensive periodontal disease, none of the pulp tissue had significant inflammatory changes.[258] It is much more common for pulp necrosis, or for failure of healing of periapical lesions, to present clinically with signs of periodontal disease than for periodontal disease to cause pulpal pathosis. Primary endodontic, secondary periodontal pathosis is particularly evident if a perforation occurs in the pulp chamber or coronal third of the root during endodontic treatment and is not promptly treated in cases of cracked teeth/vertical root fractures or in cases of congenital tooth defects such as palatal groove defects. Thus, it is more likely for microbial irritants to move outward from a necrotic pulp to cause periodontal breakdown than for them to move inward from a periodontal pocket to cause irreversible pathosis in the pulp. The reasons for this observation are not fully understood. However, if the assumption is that bacteria may migrate through patent dentinal tubules in these situations, as shown in Fig. 13-25, then it may be that the outward dentinal fluid flow in teeth with vital pulp contributes to the resistance to ingress of bacteria in sufficient amounts to cause a clinically significant disease process. Once the pulp degenerates, dentinal fluid flow no longer exists. Thus, microbial irritants from the pulp may promote pocket formation and periodontal bone loss,[121] and the prognosis of endodontic and periodontal treatment may be related,[122] as the microbial factors may pass across dentin more readily.

Periodontal scaling and root planing may result in removal of cementum and exposure of dentin to the oral cavity. Frequently, this treatment results in dentin hypersensitivity, as discussed previously. In theory, periodontal disease and its treatment should be associated with an increased incidence of pulpal pathosis. In an older study, investigators induced periodontal disease in a primate model using ligatures, and they compared the effects on the pulp of periodontal disease with or without scaling.[22] In teeth with periodontal disease, mild chronic inflammatory changes were observed in 29% of the teeth and could be seen in areas of the pulp related to bone loss. One of 40 teeth developed pulp necrosis. In teeth that received scaling, a similar percentage of 32% developed the same mild inflammation and none developed pulp necrosis. In a later clinical study,[23] 52 periodontitis patients who had 672 teeth with vital pulp were followed up and maintained every 3 to 6 months for 4 to 13 years (mean 8.7 years). Of those teeth, 255 were bridge abutments. The results showed a significantly higher chance of pulpal complications in teeth that were bridge abutments than in teeth that were not abutments (15% versus 3%; $P < 0.01$). Considering that both types of teeth had similar degrees of periodontal disease, the authors concluded that prosthodontic treatment is associated with pulpal involvement more frequently than periodontal disease and its treatment. Another histologic analysis of 46 teeth with varying degrees of periodontal disease and coronal restorations reached a similar conclusion.[62] Furthermore, two comprehensive reviews of the topic concluded that although the potential exists for periodontal disease and its treatment to cause pulpal pathosis, particularly if large lateral or accessory canals are exposed, this occurrence is rare.[97,226]

MECHANICAL IRRITANTS: ORTHODONTIC MOVEMENT

The most conspicuous pulpal change observed in response to orthodontic forces is hemodynamic. Both human and animal studies have confirmed that both lateral and intrusive forces increase pulpal blood flow.[145,182,190] Furthermore, blood flow alterations are not confined to the tooth in active movement. Observed increases in blood flow are seen in teeth adjacent to the focus of movement forces, implying that directed forces on one tooth could shunt blood to proximal vessels supplying other oral structures, including teeth. If orthodontic forces are extreme, circulatory interruptions can occur, resulting in pulpal necrosis.[35]

Biochemical, biologic, and histologic studies of the effects of orthodontic movement have confirmed that metabolic as well as inflammatory changes can result. The dental pulp tissue respiration rate is depressed after short-term application of orthodontic force.[95] Biochemical and molecular markers confirm that apoptosis and necrosis of pulpal cells is also increased subsequent to movement.[209] However, it was shown that the inflammatory mediators IL-1 alpha and TNF-alpha show a minor increase in the pulp during orthodontic movement, compared to the increase in periodontal tissues.[25] Histologic examination of pulps in teeth subjected to intrusive forces showed vascular congestion and dilatation as well as vacuolization of the odontoblastic layer.[245-247] Most if not all of these effects are due to circulatory changes, and the consensus is that they are transient provided that the movement forces are not excessive.[140] It was shown, however, that pulp necrosis of teeth that were undergoing orthodontic treatment, and had also been traumatized prior to that, is significantly increased compared to teeth that had either of these conditions but not the other, particularly in lateral incisors, and if the traumatized tooth had pulp canal obliteration.[18,19] As noted previously, substance P appears to increase in the dental pulp as a result of acutely induced occlusal trauma.[45] Also, CGRP increases under the influence of orthodontic forces.[46]

PULPAL REACTIONS TO ORTHODONTIC/ ORTHOGNATHIC SURGERY

It has been known for decades that osteotomies in the maxilla or mandible may cause disruption in the blood supply to teeth in the area of the surgery, with resultant inflammation or necrosis.[15,138,179,207] Occasionally, the teeth affected show postoperative manifestations common with traumatic injuries, such as pulp canal obliteration.[271] Animal studies have shown that if a safe distance of 5 to 10 mm is maintained between the site of the surgery and the teeth, minimal disruption occurs.[65,283] A number of studies have documented, using laser Doppler flowmetry, actual reduction in pulpal blood flow (PBF) immediately following maxillary Le Fort I osteotomy,[193,218,228] particularly if segmental osteotomy is performed.[71] In most cases, the blood flow is regained within months of the surgery. A modification of the Le Fort I osteotomy technique has been described in which the Le Fort I sectioning is combined with a horseshoe palatal osteotomy to spare any disruption to the descending palatine artery.[96] An examination of PBF of maxillary teeth using laser Doppler flowmetry as well as the responsiveness to electric pulp testing showed significant differences between the two surgical techniques in the postoperative recovery values (Fig. 13-26). In cases where the surgery did not disrupt the palatine artery, the PBF in the anterior teeth consistently increased without disruption in the postoperative period.

It should also be noted that, occasionally, teeth are traumatized during endotracheal intubation for surgery that requires general anesthesia, when the surgery itself is not related to the jaws or teeth.[235]

BIOMECHANICAL IRRITATION: PARAFUNCTIONAL HABITS

Occlusal loading of teeth affects deformation to varying degrees.[167] Whereas enamel is largely resistant to flexure, the underlying dentin demonstrates considerable elastic and viscoelastic characteristics. As a result, defects in enamel secondary to cracks, decay, or restorative preparation allow cuspal flexure with subsequent pulpal responses, presumably due to dentinal fluid flow secondary to compression and

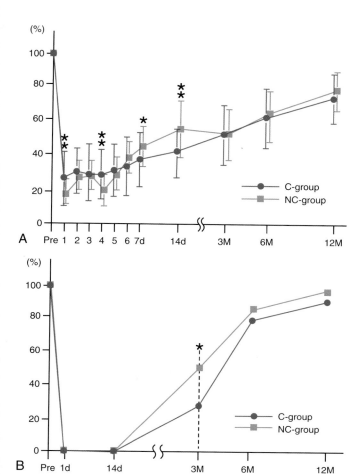

FIG. 13-26 **A,** The postoperative change of the mean pulpal blood flow in the upper incisors of the two groups (*Pre,* before the operation; *d,* day[s] after the operation; *M,* months after the operation; bars, SD; *, *P <* .05; **, *P <* .01). **B,** The postoperative change in the percentages of teeth (upper incisors) with positive pulpal sensitivity in the two groups (*Pre,* before the operation; *d,* day[s] after the operation; *M,* months after the operation; *, *P <* .05). (From Harada K, Sato M, Omura K: Blood-flow and neurosensory changes in the maxillary dental pulp after differing Le Fort I osteotomies, *Oral Surg Oral Med Oral Pathol Oral Radiol Endod* 97:12, 2004. Reprinted with permission.)

microleakage.[103] The magnitude of the pulpal response is dictated by the degree and chronicity of dentinal deformation.

Multiple factors influence the degree of tooth deformation during occlusal loading. Investigators have noted that preparation geometry has a direct impact on cuspal flexure. The width of the occlusal isthmus relative to the faciolingual dimension of the tooth as well as the ablation of marginal ridges directly impact on the degree of cuspal flexure.[199,219,270] MOD preparations have been shown to effect a 50% reduction in cuspal stiffness and resistance to fracture. Physical properties of the restorative material can also play a part in cuspal flexure. Studies have shown that polymerization shrinkage of certain resin composites can induce an inward deflection of cusps with resultant stresses on tooth structure.[272,273]

Symptomatology from cuspal flexure can result from two primary sources. It has been theorized that cuspal flexure results in dentin deformation, thus promoting the dentinal fluid flow that activates nerve endings in the odontoblast layer of the tooth. This is supported in part by an in vitro study that found that dentinal fluid flow could be induced by occlusal

loading of restored teeth.[103] A second source of pulpal pain is bacterial microleakage created by a gap at the restoration/dentin interface that is repeatedly opened during cycles of occlusal loading. If repeated cuspal flexure gives rise to a crack, dentinal exposure to bacteria and their by-products is even greater. It is likely that in vivo both dentinal fluid flow and bacterial access to dentinal surfaces work together to produce inflammation that is often manifested by thermal as well as biting sensitivity for the patient. In the instance of parafunctional habits, this is often combined with concussive periodontal forces to the periodontium that induce acute periradicular periodontitis, mobility, and radiographic changes.

On the cellular level, studies have shown increased levels of substance P after experimentally induced occlusal trauma.[45] Substance P is a modulator of both sensory and immune function in the dental pulp. Alterations in physiologic levels of this mediator could result in disruptions in the pain response as well as secondary stimulation of prostaglandin E2. Furthermore, the immunostimulatory ability of neuropeptides could initiate and maintain a chronic pulpal inflammation, possibly leading to necrosis. Although animal studies have suggested that pulp necrosis is a possible sequela to chronic occlusal trauma, there are no controlled clinical studies that confirm this.

Dentinal cracks expose tubules unoccluded by a smear layer and therefore offer a direct portal to the subjacent pulp. When dentinal tubules are freely exposed, there is an outward flow of dentinal fluid driven by relatively high pulpal tissue pressures. Dentinal fluid is composed of proteins such as fibrinogen and serum albumin, which can coagulate and effectively block the tubule lumen thereby limiting fluid egress and resultant dentin hypersensitivity. This phenomenon can occur within two days. As this serves as a short-term protective mechanism for the pulp, dentinal sclerosis and tertiary dentin formation ultimately can provide greater protection for the pulp and reduction of symptoms. Clinical interventions include the application of materials that occlude the tubules and extracoronal restorations to seal and prevent the propagation of cracks.

PULPAL REACTIONS TO IMPLANT PLACEMENT AND FUNCTION

Osseointegrated implants are now a common option for the replacement of missing teeth. The placement of implants requires multifaceted preoperative radiographic techniques, including intraoral, tomographic, cephalometric, and panoramic imaging.[264] This assures that implant placement fully rests in bone and does not compromise neighboring structures, including teeth. The lack of attention to the three-dimensional anatomy of the site of implant placement and the orientation of neighboring teeth may lead to the implant perforating the root and devitalizing the pulp.[162,249]

It is usually recommended that implants not be placed directly at a site where a periradicular lesion exists, particularly one with signs of purulence, as microbial irritants may interfere with osseointegration.[214] However, some data suggest that immediate implant placement in sites that have been adequately debrided is successful.[40] A systematic review generally corroborates this finding, provided that adequate preoperative, intraoperative, and postoperative antimicrobial measures are utilized.[50]

Case reports have also claimed that teeth with periradicular lesions may reduce the success of neighboring implants even if adequate endodontic treatment is performed.[248] To address this issue, a study was reported in which implants were placed to replace premolars in dogs; periradicular lesions were then induced, and some were treated nonsurgically or with surgical and nonsurgical treatments.[233] The results showed that the presence of treated or untreated periradicular lesions did not affect the long-term osseointegration of implants that were already osseointegrated. Clinical cases with complete resolution of periapical lesions that also involve neighboring implants, following adequate endodontic treatment, have been published.[155,244]

REFERENCES

1. About I, Murray PE, Franquin JC, et al: Pulpal inflammatory responses following non-carious class V restorations, *Oper Dent* 26:336, 2001.
2. Absi EG, Addy M, Adams D: Dentine hypersensitivity—the effect of toothbrushing and dietary compounds on dentine in vitro: an SEM study, *J Oral Rehabil* 19:101, 1992.
3. Addy M, Pearce N: Aetiological, predisposing and environmental factors in dentine hypersensitivity, *Arch Oral Biol* 39 (suppl):33S, 1994.
4. Ahlquist M, Franzen O, Coffey J, Pashley D: Dental pain evoked by hydrostatic pressures applied to exposed dentin in man: a test of the hydrodynamic theory of dentin sensitivity, *J Endod* 20:130, 1994.
5. Ahn J, Pogrel MA: The effect of 2% lidocaine with 1:100,000 epinephrine on pulpal and gingival blood flow, *Oral Surg Oral Med Oral Pathol Oral Radiol Endod* 85:197, 1998.
6. Al-Hiyasat AS, Barrieshi-Nusair KM, Al-Omari MA: The radiographic outcomes of direct pulp-capping procedures performed by dental students: a retrospective study, *J Am Dent Assoc* 137:1699, 2006.
7. Aljehani A, Yang L, Shi XQ: In vitro quantification of smooth surface caries with DIAGNOdent and the DIAGNOdent pen, *Acta Odontol Scand* 65:60, 2007.
8. Amano T, Muramatsu T, Amemiya K, et al: Responses of rat pulp cells to heat stress in vitro, *J Dent Res* 85:432, 2006.
9. Anderson DG, Chiego DJ Jr, Glickman GN, McCauley LK: A clinical assessment of the effects of 10% carbamide peroxide gel on human pulp tissue, *J Endod* 25:247, 1999.
10. Armstrong SR, Vargas MA, Fang Q, Laffoon JE: Microtensile bond strength of a total-etch 3-step, total-etch 2-step, self-etch 2-step, and a self-etch 1-step dentin bonding system through 15-month water storage, *J Adhes Dent* 5:47, 2003.
11. Asgary S, Eghbal MJ, Parirokh M, et al: A comparative study of histologic response to different pulp capping materials and a novel endodontic cement, *Oral Surg Oral Med Oral Pathol Oral Radiol Endod* 106:609, 2008.
12. Avellan NL, Sorsa T, Tervahartiala T, et al: Painful tooth stimulation elevates matrix metalloproteinase-8 levels locally in human gingival crevicular fluid, *J Dent Res* 84:335, 2005.
13. Awawdeh L, Lundy FT, Shaw C, et al: Quantitative analysis of substance P, neurokinin A and calcitonin gene-related peptide in pulp tissue from painful and healthy human teeth, *Int J* 35:30, 2002.
14. Baldissara P, Catapano S, Scotti R: Clinical and histological evaluation of thermal injury thresholds in human teeth: a preliminary study, *J Oral Rehabil* 24:791, 1997.
15. Banks P: Pulp changes after anterior mandibular subapical osteotomy in a primate model, *J Oral Maxillofac Surg* 5:39, 1977.
16. Barrieshi-Nusair KM, Qudeimat MA: A prospective clinical study of mineral trioxide aggregate for partial pulpotomy in cariously exposed permanent teeth, *J Endod* 32:731, 2006.
17. Barthel CR, Rosenkranz B, Leuenberg A, Roulet JF: Pulp capping of carious exposures: treatment outcome after 5 and 10 years: a retrospective study, *J Endod* 26:525, 2000.
18. Bauss O, Rohling J, Rahman A, Kiliaridis S: The effect of pulp obliteration on pulpal vitality of orthodontically intruded traumatized teeth, *J Endod* 34:417, 2008.
19. Bauss O, Rohling J, Sadat-Khonsari R, Kiliaridis S: Influence of orthodontic intrusion on pulpal vitality of previously traumatized maxillary permanent incisors, *Am J Orthod Dentofacial Orthop* 134:12, 2008.
20. Bergenholtz G, Ahlstedt S, Lindhe J: Experimental pulpitis in immunized monkeys, *Scand J Dent Res* 85:396, 1977.
21. Bergenholtz G, Cox CF, Loesche WJ, Syed SA: Bacterial leakage around dental restorations: its effect on the dental pulp, *J Oral Pathol* 11:439, 1982.
22. Bergenholtz G, Lindhe J: Effect of experimentally induced marginal periodontitis and periodontal scaling on the dental pulp, *J Clin Periodontol* 5:59, 1978.
23. Bergenholtz G, Nyman S: Endodontic complications following periodontal and prosthetic treatment of patients with advanced periodontal disease, *J Periodontol* 55:63, 1984.
24. Bergenholtz G, Warfvinge J: Migration of leukocytes in dental pulp in response to plaque bacteria, *Scand J Dent Res* 90:354, 1982.
24a. Bhingare AC, Ohno T, Tomura M, et al: Dental pulp dendritic cells migrate to regional lymph nodes, *J Dent Res* 93(3):288, 2014.
25. Bletsa A, Berggreen E, Brudvik P: Interleukin-1alpha and tumor necrosis factor-alpha expression during the early phases of orthodontic tooth movement in rats, *Eur J Oral Sci* 114:423, 2006.
26. Bogen G, Kim JS, Bakland LK: Direct pulp capping with mineral trioxide aggregate: an observational study, *J Am Dent Assoc* 139:305; quiz 305, 2008.
27. Botero TM, Shelburne CE, Holland GR, et al: TLR4 mediates LPS-induced VEGF expression in odontoblasts, *J Endod* 32:951, 2006.
28. Bouillaguet S: Biological risks of resin-based materials to the dentin-pulp complex, *Crit Rev Oral Biol Med* 15:47, 2004.
29. Bowles WR, Burke R, Sabino M, et al: Sex differences in neuropeptide content and release from rat dental pulp, *J Endod* 37:1098, 2011.
30. Bowles WR, Withrow JC, Lepinski AM, Hargreaves KM: Tissue levels of immunoreactive substance P are increased in patients with irreversible pulpitis, *J Endod* 29:265, 2003.
31. Brannstrom M: Dental and pulpal response. III. Application of an air stream to exposed dentin. Long observation periods, *Acta Odontol Scand* 18:234, 1960.
32. Brannstrom M: The effect of dentin desiccation and aspirated odontoblasts on the pulp, *J Prosthet Dent* 20:165, 1968.
33. Brannstrom M: Smear layer: pathological and treatment considerations, *Oper Dent Supplement* 3:35, 1984.
34. Brannstrom M, Lind PO: Pulpal response to early dental caries, *J Dent Res* 44:1045, 1965.
35. Butcher EO, Taylor AC: The effects of denervation and ischemia upon the teeth of the monkey, *J Dent Res* 30:265, 1951.
36. Byers MR, Narhi MV: Dental injury models: experimental tools for understanding neuroinflammatory interactions and polymodal nociceptor functions, *Crit Rev Oral Biol Med* 10:4, 1999.
37. Byers MR, Narhi MV, Mecifi KB: Acute and chronic reactions of dental sensory nerve fibers to cavities and desiccation in rat molars, *Anat Rec* 221:872, 1988.
38. Calland JW, Harris SE, Carnes DL Jr: Human pulp cells respond to calcitonin gene-related peptide in vitro, *J Endod* 23:485, 1997.
39. Camilleri J: Investigation of Biodentine as dentine replacement material, *J Dent* 41:600, 2013.
40. Casap N, Zeltser C, Wexler A, et al: Immediate placement of dental implants into debrided infected dentoalveolar sockets, *J Oral Maxillofac Surg* 65:384, 2007.
41. Cassidy N, Fahey M, Prime SS, Smith AJ: Comparative analysis of transforming growth factor-beta isoforms 1-3 in human and rabbit dentine matrices, *Arch Oral Biol* 42:219, 1997.
42. Caux C, Vanbervliet B, Massacrier C, et al: Regulation of dendritic cell recruitment by chemokines, *Transplantation* 73:S7, 2002.
43. Cavalcanti BN, Lage-Marques JL, Rode SM: Pulpal temperature increases with Er:YAG laser and high-speed handpieces, *J Prosthet Dent* 90:447, 2003.
44. Caviedes-Bucheli J, Ariza-Garcia G, Restrepo-Mendez S, et al: The effect of tooth bleaching on substance P expression in human dental pulp, *J Endod* 34:1462, 2008.
45. Caviedes-Bucheli J, Azuero-Holguin MM, Correa-Ortiz JA, et al: Effect of experimentally induced occlusal trauma on substance p expression in human dental pulp and periodontal ligament, *J Endod* 37:627, 2011.
46. Caviedes-Bucheli J, Moreno JO, Ardila-Pinto J, et al: The effect of orthodontic forces on calcitonin gene-related peptide expression in human dental pulp, *J Endod* 37:934, 2011.
47. Chabanski MB, Gillam DG: Aetiology, prevalence and clinical features of cervical dentine sensitivity, *J Oral Rehabil* 24:15, 1997.
48. Cheung GS, Lai SC, Ng RP: Fate of vital pulps beneath a metal-ceramic crown or a bridge retainer, *Int Endod J* 38:521, 2005.
49. Chng HS, Pitt Ford TR, McDonald F: Effects of prilocaine local anaesthetic solutions on pulpal blood flow in maxillary canines, *Endod Dent Traumatol* 12:89, 1996.
50. Chrcanovic BR, Martins MD, Wennerberg A: Immediate placement of implants into infected sites: a systematic review, *Clin Implant Dent Relat Res* 17(Suppl 1):e1, 2015.
51. Cohen JS, Reader A, Fertel R, et al: A radioimmunoassay determination of the concentrations of prostaglandins E2 and F2alpha in painful and asymptomatic human dental pulps, *J Endod* 11:330, 1985.
52. Coluzzi DJ: An overview of laser wavelengths used in dentistry, *Dent Clin North Am* 44:753, 2000.
53. Costa AM, Bezerra AC, Fuks AB: Assessment of the accuracy of visual examination, bite-wing radiographs and DIAGNOdent on the diagnosis of occlusal caries, *Eur Arch Paediatr Dent* 8:118, 2007.
54. Costa CA, Edwards CA, Hanks CT: Cytotoxic effects of cleansing solutions recommended for chemical lavage of pulp exposures, *Am J Dent* 14:25, 2001.
55. Costa CA, Giro EM, do Nascimento AB, et al: Short-term evaluation of the pulpo-dentin complex response to a resin-modified glass-ionomer cement and a bonding agent applied in deep cavities, *Dent Mater* 19:739, 2003.
56. Costa CA, Riehl H, Kina JF, et al: Human pulp responses to in-office tooth bleaching, *Oral Surg Oral Med Oral Pathol Oral Radiol Endod* 109:e59, 2010.

57. Cotton WR: Pulp response to an airstream directed into human cavity preparations, *Oral Surg Oral Med Oral Pathol* 24:78, 1967.

58. Cox CF, Bergenholtz G, Fitzgerald M, et al: Capping of the dental pulp mechanically exposed to the oral microflora: a 5 week observation of wound healing in the monkey, *J Oral Pathol* 11:327, 1982.

59. Cox CF, Hafez AA, Akimoto N, et al: Biocompatibility of primer, adhesive and resin composite systems on non-exposed and exposed pulps of non-human primate teeth, *Am J Dent* 11:S55, 1998.

60. Cvek M: A clinical report on partial pulpotomy and capping with calcium hydroxide in permanent incisors with complicated crown fracture, *J Endod* 4:232, 1978.

61. Cvek M, Granath L, Cleaton-Jones P, Austin J: Hard tissue barrier formation in pulpotomized monkey teeth capped with cyanoacrylate or calcium hydroxide for 10 and 60 minutes, *J Dent Res* 66:1166, 1987.

62. Czarnecki RT, Schilder H: A histological evaluation of the human pulp in teeth with varying degrees of periodontal disease, *J Endod* 5:242, 1979.

63. do Nascimento AB, Fontana UF, Teixeira HM, Costa CA: Biocompatibility of a resin-modified glass-ionomer cement applied as pulp capping in human teeth, *Am J Dent* 13:28, 2000.

64. Dummer PM, Hicks R, Huws D: Clinical signs and symptoms in pulp disease, *Int Endod J* 13:27, 1980.

65. Duran S, Guven O, Gunhan O: Pulpal and apical changes secondary to segmental osteotomy in the mandible: an experimental study, *J Craniomaxillofac Surg* 23:256, 1995.

66. Durand SH, Flacher V, Romeas A, et al: Lipoteichoic acid increases TLR and functional chemokine expression while reducing dentin formation in in vitro differentiated human odontoblasts, *J Immunol* 176:2880, 2006.

67. El Karim IA, Lamey PJ, Ardill J, et al: Vasoactive intestinal polypeptide (VIP) and VPAC1 receptor in adult human dental pulp in relation to caries, *Arch Oral Biol* 51:849, 2006.

68. El Karim IA, Lamey PJ, Linden GJ, et al: Caries-induced changes in the expression of pulpal neuropeptide Y, *Eur J Oral Sci* 114:133, 2006.

69. El Karim IA, Lamey PJ, Linden GJ, Lundy FT: Neuropeptide Y Y1 receptor in human dental pulp cells of noncarious and carious teeth, *Int Endod J* 41:850, 2008.

70. Elliott RD, Roberts MW, Burkes J, Phillips C: Evaluation of the carbon dioxide laser on vital human primary pulp tissue, *Pediatr Dent* 21:327, 1999.

71. Emshoff R, Kranewitter R, Brunold S, et al: Characteristics of pulpal blood flow levels associated with non-segmented and segmented Le Fort I osteotomy, *Oral Surg Oral Med Oral Pathol Oral Radiol Endod* 105:379, 2008.

72. Eversole LR, Rizoiu I, Kimmel AI: Pulpal response to cavity preparation by an erbium, chromium:YSGG laser-powered hydrokinetic system, *J Am Dent Assoc* 128:1099, 1997.

73. Faraco IM Jr, Holland R: Response of the pulp of dogs to capping with mineral trioxide aggregate or a calcium hydroxide cement, *Dent Traumatol* 17:163, 2001.

74. Farges JC, Keller JF, Carrouel F, et al: Odontoblasts in the dental pulp immune response, *J Exp Zoolog B Mol Dev Evol*, 312B:425, 2009.

75. Farges JC, Keller JF, Carrouel F, et al: Odontoblasts in the dental pulp immune response, *J Exp Zool B Mol Dev Evol* 312B:425, 2009.

76. Farges JC, Keller JF, Carrouel F, et al: O34-pathogen sensing by human odontoblasts, *Bull Group Int Rech Sci Stomatol Odontol* 49:90, 2010.

77. Farges JC, Romeas A, Melin M, et al: TGF-beta1 induces accumulation of dendritic cells in the odontoblast layer, *J Dent Res* 82:652, 2003.

78. Farik B, Munksgaard EC, Andreasen JO, Kreiborg S: Drying and rewetting anterior crown fragments prior to bonding, *Endod Dent Traumatol* 15:113, 1999.

79. Felton D: Long-term effects of crown preparation on pulp vitality, *J Dent Res* 68:1009 (abstract 139), 1989.

80. Ferracane JL, Condon JR: Rate of elution of leachable components from composite, *Dent Mater* 6:282, 1990.

81. Fitzgerald M, Hanks CT: In vivo study of resin diffusion through intact vital human dentin (abstract), *J Dent Res* 76:305, 1997.

82. Flecha OD, Azevedo CG, Matos FR, et al: Cyanoacrylate versus laser in the treatment of dentin hypersensitivity: a controlled, randomized, double-masked and non-inferiority clinical trial, *J Periodontol* 84:287, 2013.

83. Ford TR, Torabinejad M, Abedi HR, et al: Using mineral trioxide aggregate as a pulp-capping material, *J Am Dent Assoc* 127:1491, 1996.

84. Fosse G, Saele PK, Eide R: Numerical density and distributional pattern of dentin tubules, *Acta Odontol Scand* 50:201, 1992.

85. Fried K: Changes in pulpal nerves with aging, *Proc Finn Dent Soc* 88:517, 1992.

86. Fugaro JO, Nordahl I, Fugaro OJ, et al: Pulp reaction to vital bleaching, *Oper Dent* 29:363, 2004.

87. Fujitani M, Inokoshi S, Hosoda H: Effect of acid etching on the dental pulp in adhesive composite restorations, *Int Dent J* 42:3, 1992.

88. Garberoglio R, Brannstrom M: Scanning electron microscopic investigation of human dentinal tubules, *Arch Oral Biol* 21:355, 1976.

89. Gibson M, Sharif MO, Smith A, et al: A practice-based randomised controlled trial of the efficacy of three interventions to reduce dentinal hypersensitivity, *J Dent* 41:668, 2013.

90. Godoy BM, Arana-Chavez VE, Nunez SC, Ribeiro MS: Effects of low-power red laser on dentine-pulp interface after cavity preparation: an ultrastructural study, *Arch Oral Biol* 52:899, 2007.

91. Goodis HE, Schein B, Stauffer P: Temperature changes measured in vivo at the dentinoenamel junction and pulpodentin junction during cavity preparation in the Macaca fascicularis monkey, *J Endod* 14:336, 1988.

92. Graham L, Cooper PR, Cassidy N, et al: The effect of calcium hydroxide on solubilisation of bio-active dentine matrix components, *Biomaterials* 27:2865, 2006.

93. Gwinnett AJ, Tay F: Early and intermediate time response of the dental pulp to an acid etch technique in vivo, *Am J Dent* 11:S35, 1998.

94. Gwinnett AJ, Tay FR, Pang KM, Wei SH: Quantitative contribution of the collagen network in dentin hybridization, *Am J Dent* 9:140, 1996.

95. Hamersky PA, Weimer AD, Taintor JF: The effect of orthodontic force application on the pulpal tissue respiration rate in the human premolar, *Am J Orthod* 77:368, 1980.

96. Harada K, Sato M, Omura K: Blood-flow and neurosensory changes in the maxillary dental pulp after differing Le Fort I osteotomies, *Oral Surg Oral Med Oral Pathol Oral Radiol Endod* 97:12, 2004.

97. Harrington GW, Steiner DR, Ammons WF: The periodontal-endodontic controversy, *Periodontol 2000* 30:123, 2002.

98. Harris DM, White JM, Goodis H, et al: Selective ablation of surface enamel caries with a pulsed Nd:YAG dental laser, *Lasers Surg Med* 30:342, 2002.

99. Hartmann A, Azerad J, Boucher Y: Environmental effects on laser Doppler pulpal blood-flow measurements in man, *Arch Oral Biol* 41:333 1996.

100. Hasler JE, Mitchell DF: Painless pulpitis, *J Am Dent Assoc* 81:671, 1970.

101. Hayden MS, West AP, Ghosh S: NF-kappaB and the immune response, *Oncogene* 25:6758, 2006.

102. Heys DR, Cox CF, Heys RJ, Avery JK: Histological considerations of direct pulp capping agents, *J Dent Res* 60:1371, 1981.

103. Hirata K, Nakashima M, Sekine I, et al: Dentinal fluid movement associated with loading of restorations, *J Dent Res* 70:975, 1991.

104. Holland GR, Narhi MN, Addy M, et al: Guidelines for the design and conduct of clinical trials on dentine hypersensitivity, *J Clin Periodontol* 24:808, 1997.

105. Holland R, de Souza V, Nery MJ, et al: Reaction of dogs' teeth to root canal filling with mineral trioxide aggregate or a glass ionomer sealer, *J Endod* 25:728, 1999.

106. Horst OV, Horst JA, Samudrala R, Dale BA: Caries induced cytokine network in the odontoblast layer of human teeth, *BMC Immunol* 12:9, 2011.

107. Horst OV, Tompkins KA, Coats SR, et al: TGF-beta1 inhibits TLR-mediated odontoblast responses to oral bacteria, *J Dent Res* 88:333, 2009.

108. Horsted P, Sandergaard B, Thylstrup A, et al: A retrospective study of direct pulp capping with calcium hydroxide compounds, *Endod Dent Traumatol* 1:29, 1985.

109. Hume WR: An analysis of the release and the diffusion through dentin of eugenol from zinc oxide-eugenol mixtures, *J Dent Res* 63:881, 1984.

110. Hume WR, Gerzia TM: Bioavailability of components of resin-based materials which are applied to teeth, *Crit Rev Oral Biol Med* 7:172, 1996.

111. Hume WR, Kenney AE: Release of 3H-triamcinolone from Ledermix, *J Endod* 7:509, 1981.

112. Ikawa M, Komatsu H, Ikawa K, et al: Age-related changes in the human pulpal blood flow measured by laser Doppler flowmetry, *Dent Traumatol* 19:36, 2003.

113. Inoue H, Izumi T, Ishikawa H, Watanabe K: Short-term histomorphological effects of Er:YAG laser irradiation to rat coronal dentin-pulp complex, *Oral Surg Oral Med Oral Pathol Oral Radiol Endod* 97:246, 2004.

114. Inoue T, Miyakoshi S, Shimono M: Dentin/pulp adhesive resin interface: biological view from basic science to clinic. In Shimono M, Suda H, Takahashi K, editors: *Proceedings of the International Conference on Dentin/ Pulp Complex 1995*, Chiba, Japan, Chicago, 1996, Quintessence, pp 217-220.

115. Inoue T, Miyakoshi S, Shimono M: The in vitro and in vivo influence of 4-META/MMA-TBB resin components on dental pulp tissues, *Adv Dent Res* 15:101, 2001.

116. Isett J, Reader A, Gallatin E, et al: Effect of an intraosseous injection of depo-medrol on pulpal concentrations of PGE2 and IL-8 in untreated irreversible pulpitis, *J Endod* 29:268, 2003.

117. Izumi T, Inoue H, Matsuura H, et al: Changes in the pattern of horseradish peroxidase diffusion into predentin and dentin after cavity preparation in rat molars, *Oral Surg Oral Med Oral Pathol Oral Radiol Endod* 92:675, 2001.

118. Izumi T, Kobayashi I, Okamura K, Sakai H: Immunohistochemical study on the immunocompetent cells of the pulp in human non-carious and carious teeth, *Arch Oral Biol* 40:609, 1995.

119. Jaber L, Swaim WD, Dionne RA: Immunohistochemical localization of mu-opioid receptors in human dental pulp, *J Endod* 29:108, 2003.

120. Janeway CA Jr, Medzhitov R: Innate immune recognition, *Annu Rev Immunol* 20:197, 2002.

121. Jansson L, Ehnevid H, Lindskog S, Blomlof L: Relationship between periapical and periodontal status: a clinical retrospective study, *J Clin Periodontol* 20:117, 1993.

122. Jansson L, Sandstedt P, Laftman AC, Skoglund A: Relationship between apical and marginal healing in periradicular surgery, *Oral Surg Oral Med Oral Pathol Oral Radiol Endod* 83:596, 1997.

123. Jiang HW, Zhang W, Ren BP, et al: Expression of toll like receptor 4 in normal human odontoblasts and dental pulp tissue, *J Endod* 32:747, 2006.

124. Jontell M, Hanks CT, Bratel J, Bergenholtz G: Effects of unpolymerized resin components on the function of accessory cells derived from the rat incisor pulp, *J Dent Res* 74:1162, 1995.

125. Jukic S, Anic I, Koba K, et al: The effect of pulpotomy using CO2 and Nd:YAG lasers on dental pulp tissue, *Int Endod J* 30:175, 1997.

126. Kanjevac T, Milovanovic M, Volarevic V, et al: Cytotoxic effects of glass ionomer cements on human dental pulp stem cells correlate with fluoride release, *Med Chem* 8:40, 2012.

127. Katsuno K, Manabe A, Itoh K, et al: A delayed hypersensitivity reaction to dentine primer in the guinea-pig, *J Dent* 23:295, 1995.

128. Kawagishi E, Nakakura-Ohshima K, Nomura S, Ohshima H: Pulpal responses to cavity preparation in aged rat molars, *Cell Tissue Res* 326:111, 2006.

129. Keller JF, Carrouel F, Colomb E, et al: Toll-like receptor 2 activation by lipoteichoic acid induces differential production of pro-inflammatory cytokines in human odontoblasts, dental pulp fibroblasts and immature dendritic cells, *Immunobiology* 215:53, 2010.

130. Killough SA, Lundy FT, Irwin CR: Substance P expression by human dental pulp fibroblasts: a potential role in neurogenic inflammation, *J Endod* 35:73, 2009.

131. Kim S: Ligamental injection: a physiological explanation of its efficacy, *J Endod* 12:486, 1986.

132. Kim S, Edwall L, Trowbridge H, Chien S: Effects of local anesthetics on pulpal blood flow in dogs, *J Dent Res* 63:650, 1984.

133. Kim S, Trowbridge H, Suda H: Pulpal reaction to caries and dental procedures. In Cohen S, Burns RC, editors: *Pathways of the pulp*, ed 8, St. Louis, 2002, Mosby, pp 573-600.

134. Kimura Y, Wilder-Smith P, Yonaga K, Matsumoto K: Treatment of dentine hypersensitivity by lasers: a review, *J Clin Periodontol* 27:715, 2000.

135. Kimura Y, Yonaga K, Yokoyama K, et al: Histopathological changes in dental pulp irradiated by Er:YAG laser: a preliminary report on laser pulpotomy, *J Clin Laser Med Surg* 21:345, 2003.

136. Kina JF, Huck C, Riehl H, et al: Response of human pulps after professionally applied vital tooth bleaching, *Int Endod J* 43:572, 2010.

137. Koh ET, Ford TR, Kariyawasam SP, et al: Prophylactic treatment of dens evaginatus using mineral trioxide aggregate, *J Endod* 27:540, 2001.

138. Kohn MW, White RP Jr: Evaluation of sensation after segmental alveolar osteotomy in 22 patients, *J Am Dent Assoc* 89:154, 1974.

139. Kokkas AB, Goulas A, Varsamidis K, et al: Irreversible but not reversible pulpitis is associated with up-regulation of tumour necrosis factor-alpha gene expression in human pulp, *Int Endod J* 40:198, 2007.

140. Konno Y, Daimaruya T, Iikubo M, et al: Morphologic and hemodynamic analysis of dental pulp in dogs after molar intrusion with the skeletal anchorage system, *Am J Orthod Dentofacial Orthop* 132:199, 2007.

141. Koshiro K, Inoue S, Tanaka T, et al: In vivo degradation of resin-dentin bonds produced by a self-etch vs. a total-etch adhesive system, *Eur J Oral Sci* 112:368, 2004.

142. Koubi G, Colon P, Franquin JC, et al: Clinical evaluation of the performance and safety of a new dentine substitute, Biodentine, in the restoration of posterior teeth: a prospective study, *Clin Oral Investig* 17:243, 2013.

143. Koulaouzidou EA, Papazisis KT, Economides NA, et al: Antiproliferative effect of mineral trioxide aggregate, zinc oxide-eugenol cement, and glass-ionomer cement against three fibroblastic cell lines, *J Endod* 31:44, 2005.

144. Kuhnisch J, Bucher K, Henschel V, Hickel R: Reproducibility of DIAGNOdent 2095 and DIAGNOdent Pen measurements: results from an in vitro study on occlusal sites, *Eur J Oral Sci* 115:206, 2007.

145. Kvinnsland S, Heyeraas K, Ofjord ES: Effect of experimental tooth movement on periodontal and pulpal blood flow, *Eur J Orthod* 11:200, 1989.

146. Langeland K: Tissue response to dental caries, *Endod Dent Traumatol* 3:149, 1987.

147. Langeland K, Dowden WE, Tronstad L, Langeland LK: Human pulp changes of iatrogenic origin, *Oral Surg Oral Med Oral Pathol* 32:943, 1971.

148. Langeland K, Rodrigues H, Dowden W: Periodontal disease, bacteria, and pulpal histopathology, *Oral Surg Oral Med Oral Pathol* 37:257, 1974.

149. Lefebvre CA, Wataha JC, Bouillaguet S, Lockwood PE: Effects of long-term sub-lethal concentrations of dental monomers on THP-1 human monocytes, *J Biomater Sci Polym Ed* 10:1265, 1999.

150. Lepinski AM, Haegreaves KM, Goodis HE, Bowles WR: Bradykinin levels in dental pulp by microdialysis, *J Endod* 26:744, 2000.

151. Lesot H, Kubler MD: Experimental induction of odontoblast differentiation and stimulation during reparative processes, *Cells Materials* 3:201, 1993.

152. Levin LG, Rudd A, Bletsa A, Reisner H: Expression of IL-8 by cells of the odontoblast layer in vitro, *Eur J Oral Sci* 107:131, 1999.

153. Lier BB, Rosing CK, Aass AM, Gjermo P: Treatment of dentin hypersensitivity by Nd:YAG laser, *J Clin Periodontol* 29:501, 2002.

154. Lilja J, Nordenvall KJ, Branstrom M: Dentin sensitivity, odontoblasts and nerves under desiccated or infected experimental cavities. A clinical, light microscopic and ultrastructural investigation, *Swed Dent J* 6:93, 1982.

155. Lin S, Mayer Y: Treatment of a large periradicular lesion of endodontic origin around a dental implant with enamel matrix protein derivative, *J Periodontol* 78:2385, 2007.

156. Linde A: Dentin and entinogenesis. In Linde A, editor: *Noncollagenous proteins and proteoglycans in dentinogenesis*, Boca Raton, FL,1984, CRC Press, pp 55-92.

157. Litkowski LJ, Hack GD, Sheaffer HB, Greenspan DC: Occlusion of dentin tubules by 45s5 bioglass. Paper presented at Bioceramics, *Proceedings of the 10th international symposium on ceramics in medicine, October 1997*, Paris, France, 1997.

158. Liu HC, Lin CP, Lan WH: Sealing depth of Nd:YAG laser on human dentinal tubules, *J Endod* 23:691, 1997.

159. Loyd DR, Sun XX, Locke EE, et al: Sex differences in serotonin enhancement of capsaicin-evoked calcitonin gene-related peptide release from human dental pulp, *Pain* 153:2061, 2012.

160. Lupi-Pegurier L, Bertrand MF, Muller-Bolla M, et al: Comparative study of microleakage of a pit and fissure sealant placed after preparation by Er:YAG laser in permanent molars, *J Dent Child (Chic)* 70:134, 2003.

161. Lussi A, Hibst R, Paulus R: DIAGNOdent: an optical method for caries detection, *J Dent Res* 83 Spec No C:C80, 2004.

162. Margelos JT, Verdelis KG: Irreversible pulpal damage of teeth adjacent to recently placed osseointegrated implants, *J Endod* 21:479, 1995.

163. McCormack K, Davies R: The enigma of potassium ion in the management of dentine hypersensitivity: is nitric oxide the elusive second messenger? *Pain* 68:5, 1996.

164. McLachlan JL, Sloan AJ, Smith AJ, et al: S100 and cytokine expression in caries, *Infect Immun* 72:4102, 2004.

165. McLachlan JL, Smith AJ, Bujalska IJ, Cooper PR: Gene expression profiling of pulpal tissue reveals the molecular complexity of dental caries, *Biochim Biophys Acta* 1741:271, 2005.

166. Mente J, Geletneky B, Ohle M, et al: Mineral trioxide aggregate or calcium hydroxide direct pulp capping: an analysis of the clinical treatment outcome, *J Endod* 36:806, 2010.

167. Messer HM: Permanent restorations and the dental pulp. In Hargreaves KMG, Goodis HE, editors: *Seltzer and Bender's dental pulp*, Carol Stream, IL, 2002, Quintessence.

168. Michaelson PL, Holland GR: Is pulpitis painful? *Int Endod J* 35:829, 2002.

169. Mitchell DF, Tarplee RE: Painful pulpitis; a clinical and microscopic study, *Oral Surg Oral Med Oral Pathol* 13:1360, 1960.

170. Mjor IA: Bacteria in experimentally infected cavity preparations, *Scand J Dent Res* 85:599, 1977.

171. Mjor IA, Ferrari M: Pulp-dentin biology in restorative dentistry. Part 6: reactions to restorative materials, tooth-restoration interfaces, and adhesive techniques, *Quintessence Int* 33:35, 2002.

172. Mjor IA, Finn SB, Quigley MB: The effect of calcium hydroxide and amalgam on non-carious, vital dentine, *Arch Oral Biol* 3:283, 1961.

173. Murray PE, About I, Lumley PJ, et al: Postoperative pulpal and repair responses, *J Am Dent Assoc* 131:321, 2000.

174. Murray PE, Smith AJ, Garcia-Godoy F, Lumley PJ: Comparison of operative procedure variables on pulpal viability in an ex vivo model, *Int Endod J* 41:389, 2008.

175. Murray PE, Smith AJ, Windsor LJ, Mjor IA: Remaining dentine thickness and human pulp responses, *Int Endod J* 36:33, 2003.

176. Murray PE, Smyth TW, About I, et al: The effect of etching on bacterial microleakage of an adhesive composite restoration, *J Dent* 30:29, 2002.

177. Musselwhite JM, Klitzman B, Maixner W, Burkes EJ Jr: Laser Doppler flowmetry: a clinical test of pulpal vitality, *Oral Surg Oral Med Oral Pathol Oral Radiol Endod* 84:411, 1997.

178. Nakabayashi N, Kojima K, Masuhara E: The promotion of adhesion by the infiltration of monomers into tooth substrates, *J Biomed Mater Res* 16:265, 1982.

179. Nanda R, Legan HL, Langeland K: Pulpal and radicular response to maxillary osteotomy in monkeys, *Oral Surg Oral Med Oral Pathol* 53:624, 1982.

180. Nathanson D: Vital tooth bleaching: sensitivity and pulpal considerations, *J Am Dent Assoc* 128 (suppl):41S, 1997.

181. Nayyar S, Tewari S, Arora B: Comparison of human pulp response to total-etch and self-etch bonding agents, *Oral Surg Oral Med Oral Pathol Oral Radiol Endod* 104:e45, 2007.

182. Nixon CE, Saviano JA, King GJ, Keeling SD: Histomorphometric study of dental pulp during orthodontic tooth movement, *J Endod* 19:13, 1993.

183. Nomiyama K, Kitamura C, Tsujisawa T, et al: Effects of lipopolysaccharide on newly established rat dental pulp-derived cell line with odontoblastic properties, *J Endod* 33:1187, 2007.

184. Nowicka A, Lipski M, Parafiniuk M, et al: Response of human dental pulp capped with biodentine and mineral trioxide aggregate, *J Endod* 39:743, 2013.

185. Nup C, Rosenberg P, Linke H, Tordik P: Quantitation of catecholamines in inflamed human dental pulp by high-performance liquid chromatography, *J Endod* 27:73, 2001.

186. Nyborg H, Brannstrom M: Pulp reaction to heat, *J Prosthet Dent* 19:605, 1968.

187. Odor TM, Pitt Ford TR, McDonald F: Adrenaline in local anaesthesia: the effect of concentration on dental pulpal circulation and anaesthesia, *Endod Dent Traumatol* 10:167, 1994.

188. Okamura K: Histological study on the origin of dentinal immunoglobulins and the change in their localization during caries, *J Oral Pathol* 14:680, 1985.

189. Okamura K, Maeda M, Nishikawa T, Tsutsui M: Dentinal response against carious invasion: localization of antibodies in odontoblastic body and process, *J Dent Res* 59:1368, 1980.

190. Olgart L, Gazelius B, Sundstrom F: Intradental nerve activity and jaw-opening reflex in response to mechanical deformation of cat teeth, *Acta Physiol Scand* 133:399, 1988.

191. Orchardson R, Peacock JM, Whitters CJ: Effects of pulsed Nd:YAG laser radiation on action potential conduction in nerve fibres inside teeth in vitro, *J Dent* 26:421, 1998.

192. Orchardson R, Whitters CJ: Effect of HeNe and pulsed Nd:YAG laser irradiation on intradental nerve responses to mechanical stimulation of dentine, *Lasers Surg Med* 26:241, 2000.

193. Ozturk M, Doruk C, Ozec I, et al: Pulpal blood flow: effects of corticotomy and midline osteotomy in surgically assisted rapid palatal expansion, *J Craniomaxillofac Surg* 31:97, 2003.

194. Paakkonen V, Ohlmeier S, Bergmann U, et al: Analysis of gene and protein expression in healthy and carious tooth pulp with cDNA microarray and two-dimensional gel electrophoresis, *Eur J Oral Sci* 113:369, 2005.

195. Paakkonen V, Vuoristo JT, Salo T, Tjaderhane L: Comparative gene expression profile analysis between native human odontoblasts and pulp tissue, *Int Endod J* 41:117, 2008.

196. Palosaari H, Wahlgren J, Larmas M, et al: The expression of MMP-8 in human odontoblasts and dental pulp cells is down-regulated by TGF-beta1, *J Dent Res* 79, 2000.

197. Pameijer CH, Stanley HR: The disastrous effects of the "total etch" technique in vital pulp capping in primates [published erratum appears in *Am J Dent* 11:148, 1998], *Am J Dent* 11:S45, 1998.

198. Pamir T, Dalgar H, Onal B: Clinical evaluation of three desensitizing agents in relieving dentin hypersensitivity, *Oper Dent* 32:544, 2007.

199. Panitvisai P, Messer HH: Cuspal deflection in molars in relation to endodontic and restorative procedures, *J Endod* 21:57, 1995.

200. Pashley D: Pulpdentin complex. In Hargreaves KM, Goodis HE, editors: *Seltzer and Bender's The Dental Pulp*, Carol Stream, IL, 2002, Quintessence, p 66.

201. Pashley DH: The influence of dentin permeability and pulpal blood flow on pulpal solute concentrations, *J Endod* 5:355, 1979.

202. Pashley DH: In vitro simulations of in vivo bonding conditions, *Am J Dent* 4:237, 1991.

203. Pashley DH: Dynamics of the pulpo-dentin complex, *Crit Rev Oral Biol Med* 7:104, 1996.

204. Pashley DH, Kepler EE, Williams EC, Okabe A: Progressive decrease in dentine permeability following cavity preparation, *Arch Oral Biol* 28:853, 1983.

205. Pashley DH, Tay FR, Yiu C, et al: Collagen degradation by host-derived enzymes during aging, *J Dent Res* 83:216, 2004.

206. Pashley EL, Talman R, Horner JA, Pashley DH: Permeability of normal versus carious dentin, *Endod Dent Traumatol* 7:207, 1991.

207. Pepersack WJ: Tooth vitality after alveolar segmental osteotomy, *J Oral Maxillofac Surg* 1:85, 1973.

208. Perdigao J, Geraldeli S, Hodges JS: Total-etch versus self-etch adhesive: effect on postoperative sensitivity, *J Am Dent Assoc* 134:1621, 2003.

209. Perinetti G, Varvara G, Festa F, Esposito P: Aspartate aminotransferase activity in pulp of orthodontically treated teeth, *Am J Orthod Dentofacial Orthop* 125:88, 2004.

210. Peters DD, Baumgartner JC, Lorton L: Adult pulpal diagnosis. I. Evaluation of the positive and negative responses to cold and electrical pulp tests, *J Endod* 20:506, 1994.

211. Petersson K, Soderstrom C, Kiani-Anaraki M, Levy G: Evaluation of the ability of thermal and electrical tests to register pulp vitality, *Endod Dent Traumatol* 15:127, 1999.

212. Polat S, Er K, Akpinar KE, Polat NT: The sources of laser Doppler blood-flow signals recorded from vital and root canal treated teeth, *Arch Oral Biol* 49:53, 2004.

213. Premdas CE, Pitt Ford TR: Effect of palatal injections on pulpal blood flow in premolars, *Endod Dent Traumatol* 11:274, 1995.

214. Quirynen M, Gijbels F, Jacobs R: An infected jawbone site compromising successful osseointegration, *Periodontol 2000* 33:129, 2003.

215. Qvist V, Stoltze K, Qvist J: Human pulp reactions to resin restorations performed with different acid-etch restorative procedures, *Acta Odontol Scand* 47:253, 1989.

216. Rakich DR, Wataha JC, Lefebvre CA, Weller RN: Effects of dentin bonding agents on macrophage mitochondrial activity, *J Endod* 24:528, 1998.

217. Rakich DR, Wataha JC, Lefebvre CA, Weller RN: Effect of dentin bonding agents on the secretion of inflammatory mediators from macrophages, *J Endod* 25:114, 1999.

218. Ramsay DS, Artun J, Bloomquist D: Orthognathic surgery and pulpal blood flow: a pilot study using laser Doppler flowmetry, *J Oral Maxillofac Surg* 49:564, 1991.

219. Reeh ES, Messer HH, Douglas WH: Reduction in tooth stiffness as a result of endodontic and restorative procedures, *J Endod* 15:512, 1989.

220. Reeves R, Stanley HR: The relationship of bacterial penetration and pulpal pathosis in carious teeth, *Oral Surg Oral Med Oral Pathol* 22:59, 1966.

221. Reynolds RL: The determination of pulp vitality by means of thermal and electrical stimuli, *Oral Surg Oral Med Oral Pathol* 22:231, 1966.

222. Ritter AV, Leonard RH Jr, St Georges AJ, et al: Safety and stability of nightguard vital bleaching: 9 to 12 years post-treatment, *J Esthet Restor Dent* 14:275, 2002.

223. Rodd HD, Boissonade FM: Substance P expression in human tooth pulp in relation to caries and pain experience, *Eur J Oral Sci* 108:467, 2000.

224. Rodd HD, Boissonade FM: Innervation of human tooth pulp in relation to caries and dentition type, *J Dent Res* 80:389, 2001.

225. Rodd HD, Boissonade FM: Vascular status in human primary and permanent teeth in health and disease, *Eur J Oral Sci* 113:128, 2005.

226. Rotstein I, Simon JH: Diagnosis, prognosis and decision-making in the treatment of combined periodontal-endodontic lesions, *Periodontol 2000* 34:165, 2004.

227. Saito K, Nakatomi M, Ida-Yonemochi H, et al: The expression of GM-CSF and osteopontin in immunocompetent cells precedes the odontoblast differentiation following allogenic tooth transplantation in mice, *J Histochem Cytochem* 59:518, 2011.

228. Sato M, Harada K, Okada Y, Omura K: Blood-flow change and recovery of sensibility in the maxillary dental pulp after a single-segment Le Fort I osteotomy, *Oral Surg Oral Med Oral Pathol Oral Radiol Endod* 95:660, 2003.

229. Schmalz G, Krifka S, Schweikl H: Toll-like receptors, LPS, and dental monomers, *Adv Dent Res* 23:302, 2011.

230. Schroder U: Effects of calcium hydroxide-containing pulp-capping agents on pulp cell migration, proliferation, and differentiation, *J Dent Res* 64 Spec No:541, 1985.

231. Schuster GS, Caughman GB, Rueggeberg FA, et al: Alterations in cell lipid metabolism by glycol methacrylate (HEMA), *J Biomater Sci Polym Ed* 10:1121, 1999.

232. Seltzer S, Bender IB, Ziontz M: The dynamics of pulp inflammation: correlations between diagnostic data and actual histologic findings in the pulp, *Oral Surg Oral Med Oral Pathol* 16:846, 1963.

233. Shabahang S, Bohsali K, Boyne PJ, et al: Effect of teeth with periradicular lesions on adjacent dental implants, *Oral Surg Oral Med Oral Pathol Oral Radiol Endod* 96:321, 2003.

234. Silva AF, Tarquinio SB, Demarco FF, et al: The influence of haemostatic agents on healing of healthy human dental pulp tissue capped with calcium hydroxide, *Int Endod J* 39:309, 2006.

235. Simon JH, Lies J: Silent trauma, *Endod Dent Traumatol* 15:145, 1999.

236. Sloan AJ, Smith AJ: Stimulation of the dentine-pulp complex of rat incisor teeth by transforming growth factor-beta isoforms 1-3 in vitro, *Arch Oral Biol* 44:149, 1999.

237. Smith AJ: Pulpal responses to caries and dental repair, *Caries Res* 36:223, 2002.

238. Smith AJ, Lesot H: Induction and regulation of crown dentinogenesis: embryonic events as a template for dental tissue repair? *Crit Rev Oral Biol Med* 12:425, 2001.

239. Smith AJ, Tobias RS, Plant CG, et al: Preliminary studies on the in vivo morphogenetic properties of dentine matrix proteins, *Biomaterials* 11:22, 1990.

240. Smith JG, Smith AJ, Shelton RM, Cooper PR: Recruitment of dental pulp cells by dentine and pulp extracellular matrix components, *Exp Cell Res* 318:2397, 2012.

241. Soo-ampon S, Vongsavan N, Soo-ampon M, et al: The sources of laser Doppler blood-flow signals recorded from human teeth, *Arch Oral Biol* 48:353, 2003.

242. Stabholz A, Rotstein L, Neev J, Moshonov J: Efficacy of XeCl 308-nm excimer laser in reducing dye penetration through coronal dentinal tubules, *J Endod* 21:266, 1995.

243. Stanley HR: Pulp capping: conserving the dental pulp—can it be done? Is it worth it? *Oral Surg Oral Med Oral Pathol* 68:628, 1989.

244. Steiner DR: The resolution of a periradicular lesion involving an implant, *J Endod* 34:330, 2008.

245. Stenvik A: Pulp and dentine reactions to experimental tooth intrusion. (A histologic study—long-term effects), *Rep Congr Eur Orthod Soc* 449, 1969.

246. Stenvik A, Mjor IA: Pulp and dentine reactions to experimental tooth intrusion. A histologic study of the initial changes, *Am J Orthod* 57:370, 1970.

247. Stenvik A, Mjor IA: The effect of experimental tooth intrusion on pulp and dentine, *Oral Surg Oral Med Oral Pathol* 32:639, 1971.

248. Sussman HI: Endodontic pathology leading to implant failure—a case report, *J Oral Implantol* 23:112; discussion 15, 1997.

249. Sussman HI: Tooth devitalization via implant placement: a case report, *Periodontal Clin Investig* 20:22, 1998.

250. Swift EJ Jr, Trope M: Treatment options for the exposed vital pulp, *Pract Periodontics Aesthet Dent* 11:735; quiz 40, 1999.

251. Tagami J, Hosoda H, Burrow MF, Nakajima M: Effect of aging and caries on dentin permeability, *Proc Finn Dent Soc* 88 (suppl 1):149, 1992.

252. Takamori K: A histopathological and immunohistochemical study of dental pulp and pulpal nerve fibers in rats after the cavity preparation using Er:YAG laser, *J Endod* 26:95, 2000.

253. Tanabe K, Yoshiba K, Yoshiba N, et al: Immunohistochemical study on pulpal response in rat molars after cavity preparation by Er:YAG laser, *Eur J Oral Sci* 110:237, 2002.

254. Teixeira LS, Demarco FF, Coppola MC, Bonow ML: Clinical and radiographic evaluation of pulpotomies performed under intrapulpal injection of anaesthetic solution, *Int Endod J* 34:440, 2001.

255. Tjan AH, Grant BE, Godfrey MF 3rd: Temperature rise in the pulp chamber during fabrication of provisional crowns, *J Prosthet Dent* 62:622, 1989.

256. Tokita Y, Sunakawa M, Suda H: Pulsed Nd:YAG laser irradiation of the tooth pulp in the cat: I. Effect of spot lasing, *Lasers Surg Med* 26:398, 2000.

257. Tomson PL, Grover LM, Lumley PJ, et al: Dissolution of bio-active dentine matrix components by mineral trioxide aggregate, *J Dent* 35:636, 2007.

258. Torabinejad M, Kiger RD: A histologic evaluation of dental pulp tissue of a patient with periodontal disease, *Oral Surg Oral Med Oral Pathol* 59:198, 1985.

259. Tranasi M, Sberna MT, Zizzari V, et al: Microarray evaluation of age-related changes in human dental pulp, *J Endod* 35:1211, 2009.

260. Trantor IR, Messer HH, Birner R: The effects of neuropeptides (calcitonin gene-related peptide and substance P) on cultured human pulp cells, *J Dent Res* 74:1066, 1995.

261. Trowbridge H, Edwall L, Panopoulos P: Effect of zinc oxide-eugenol and calcium hydroxide on intradental nerve activity, *J Endod* 8:403, 1982.

262. Tsatsas BG, Frank RM: Ultrastructure of the dentinal tubular substances near the dentino-enamel junction, *Calcif Tissue Res* 9:238, 1972.

263. Turner DF, Marfurt CF, Sattelberg C: Demonstration of physiological barrier between pulpal odontoblasts and its perturbation following routine restorative procedures: a horseradish peroxidase tracing study in the rat, *J Dent Res* 68:1262, 1989.

264. Tyndall AA, Brooks SL: Selection criteria for dental implant site imaging: a position paper of the American Academy of Oral and Maxillofacial Radiology, *Oral Surg Oral Med Oral Pathol Oral Radiol Endod* 89:630, 2000.

265. Tziafas D: Basic mechanisms of cytodifferentiation and dentinogenesis during dental pulp repair, *Int J Dev Biol* 39:281, 1995.

266. Tziafas D, Kolokuris I: Inductive influences of demineralized dentin and bone matrix on pulp cells: an approach of secondary dentinogenesis, *J Dent Res* 69:75, 1990.

267. Umberto R, Claudia R, Gaspare P, et al: Treatment of dentine hypersensitivity by diode laser: a clinical study, *Int J Dent* 2012:858950, 2012.

268. Unemori M, Matsuya Y, Akashi A, et al: Composite resin restoration and postoperative sensitivity: clinical follow-up in an undergraduate program, *J Dent* 29:7, 2001.

269. Valderhaug J, Jokstad A, Ambjornsen E, Norheim PW: Assessment of the periapical and clinical status of crowned teeth over 25 years, *J Dent* 25:97, 1997.

270. Vale WA: Cavity preparation, *Ir Dent Rev* 2:33, 1956.

271. Vedtofte P: Pulp canal obliteration after Le Fort I osteotomy, *Endod Dent Traumatol* 5:274, 1989.

272. Versluis A, Douglas WH, Cross M, Sakaguchi RL: Does an incremental filling technique reduce polymerization shrinkage stresses? *J Dent Res* 75:871, 1996.

273. Versluis A, Tantbirojn D, Douglas WH: Distribution of transient properties during polymerization of a light-initiated restorative composite, *Dent Mater* 20:543, 2004.

274. von Troil B, Needleman I, Sanz M: A systematic review of the prevalence of root sensitivity following periodontal therapy, *J Clin Periodontol* 29 (suppl 3):173; discussion 95, 2002.

275. Vongsavan N, Matthews RW, Matthews B: The permeability of human dentine in vitro and in vivo, *Arch Oral Biol* 45:931, 2000.

276. Wakabayashi H, Hamba M, Matsumoto K, Tachibana H: Effect of irradiation by semiconductor laser on responses evoked in trigeminal caudal neurons by tooth pulp stimulation, *Lasers Surg Med* 13:605, 1993.

277. Wennberg A, Mjor IA, Heide S: Rate of formation of regular and irregular secondary dentin in monkey teeth, *Oral Surg Oral Med Oral Pathol* 54:232, 1982.

278. Wigdor H, Abt E, Ashrafi S, Walsh JT Jr: The effect of lasers on dental hard tissues, *J Am Dent Assoc* 124:65, 1993.

279. Yiu CK, King NM, Suh BI, et al: Incompatibility of oxalate desensitizers with acidic, fluoride-containing total-etch adhesives, *J Dent Res* 84:730, 2005.

280. Yoshiba K, Yoshiba N, Iwaku M: Class II antigen-presenting dendritic cell and nerve fiber responses to cavities, caries, or caries treatment in human teeth, *J Dent Res* 82:422, 2003.

281. Yoshiba N, Yoshiba K, Iwaku M, Ozawa H: Immunohistochemical localizations of class II antigens and nerve fibers in human carious teeth: HLA-DR immunoreactivity in Schwann cells, *Arch Histol Cytol* 61:343, 1998.

282. Yoshiba N, Yoshiba K, Nakamura H, et al: Immunohistochemical localization of HLA-DR-positive cells in unerupted and erupted normal and carious human teeth, *J Dent Res* 75:1585, 1996.

283. Yoshida S, Oshima K, Tanne K: Biologic responses of the pulp to single-tooth dento-osseous osteotomy, *Oral Surg Oral Med Oral Pathol Oral Radiol Endod* 82:152, 1996.

284. Yoshiyama M, Masada J, Uchida A, Ishida H: Scanning electron microscopic characterization of sensitive vs. insensitive human radicular dentin, *J Dent Res* 68:1498, 1989.

285. Zach L, Cohen G: Pulp response to externally applied heat, *Oral Surg Oral Med Oral Pathol* 19:515, 1965.

286. Zaia AA, Nakagawa R, De Quadros I, et al: An in vitro evaluation of four materials as barriers to coronal microleakage in root-filled teeth, *Int Endod J* 35:729, 2002.

287. Zhang J, Kawashima N, Suda H, et al: The existence of CD11c+ sentinel and F4/80+ interstitial dendritic cells in dental pulp and their dynamics and functional properties, *Int Immunol* 18:1375, 2006.

287a. Zhang J, Zhu LX, Cheng X, et al: Peng: Promotion of Dental Pulp Cell Migration and Pulp Repair by a Bioceramic Putty Involving FGFR-mediated Signaling Pathways, *B2 J Dent Res* 2015 Feb 27. pii: 0022034515572020.

288. Zhong S, Zhang S, Bair E, et al: Differential expression of microRNAs in normal and inflamed human pulps, *J Endod* 38:746, 2012.

CHAPTER 14

Microbiology of Endodontic Infections

JOSÉ F. SIQUEIRA, JR. | ISABELA N. RÔÇAS

CHAPTER OUTLINE

Apical periodontitis is essentially an inflammatory disease of microbial etiology primarily caused by infection of the root canal system.[196] Although chemical and physical factors can induce periradicular inflammation, a large body of scientific evidence indicates that endodontic infection is essential to the progression and perpetuation of the different forms of apical periodontitis.[16,86,120,250] Endodontic infection develops in root canals devoid of host defenses, as a consequence of either pulp necrosis (as a sequel to caries, trauma, periodontal disease, or invasive operative procedures) or pulp removal for treatment.

Although fungi and most recently archaea and viruses have been found in association with endodontic infections,[57,177,232,238,268] bacteria are the major microorganisms implicated in the pathogenesis of apical periodontitis. In advanced stages of the endodontic infectious process, bacterial organizations resembling biofilms can be observed adhered to the canal walls.[121,126,152,223] Consequently, apical periodontitis has been included in the roll of biofilm-related oral diseases.[92,228] Bacteria colonizing the root canal system enter in contact with the periradicular tissues via apical/lateral foramina or root perforations. As a consequence of the encounter between bacteria and host defenses, inflammatory changes take place in the periradicular tissues and give rise to the development of apical periodontitis. Depending on several bacterial and host-related factors, endodontic infections can lead to acute (symptomatic) or chronic (asymptomatic) apical periodontitis.

The ultimate goal of endodontic treatment is either to prevent the development of apical periodontitis or, in cases where the disease is already present, to create adequate conditions for periradicular tissue healing. The intent is to repair and preserve the tooth and associated periradicular bone. Because apical periodontitis is an infectious disease, the rationale for endodontic treatment is to eradicate the occurring infection or prevent microorganisms from infecting or reinfecting the root canal or the periradicular tissues. The cardinal principle of any health care profession is the thorough understanding of disease etiology and pathogenesis, which provides a framework for effective treatment. In this context, understanding the microbiologic aspects of apical periodontitis is the basis for endodontic practice and should be managed with an evidence-based approach. This chapter focuses on diverse aspects of endodontic microbiology, including pathogenetic, taxonomic, morphologic, and ecologic issues.

APICAL PERIODONTITIS AS AN INFECTIOUS DISEASE

The first recorded observation of bacteria in the root canal dates back to the 17th century and the Dutch amateur microscope builder Antony van Leeuwenhoek (1632-1723). He reported that the root canals of a decayed tooth "were stuffed with a soft matter" and that "the whole stuff" seemed to be

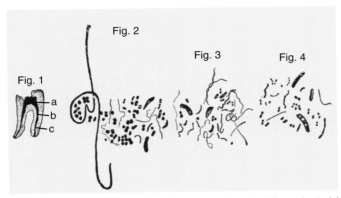

FIG. 14-1 Drawings from Miller's classic paper showing different bacterial forms in a root canal sample observed by microscopy.

alive.[46] At that time, the role of Leeuwenhoek's "animalcules" in disease causation was unsuspected. It took almost 200 years until his observation was confirmed and a cause-and-effect relationship between bacteria and apical periodontitis was suggested. This occurred specifically in 1894, when Willoughby Dayton Miller, an American dentist working at the laboratory of Robert Koch in Berlin, Germany, published a milestone study reporting the association between bacteria and apical periodontitis after an analysis of samples collected from root canals.[115] By means of bacterioscopy of the canal samples, he found bacterial cells in the three basic morphologies known at the time: cocci, bacilli, and spirilla (or spirochetes) (Fig. 14-1). Morphologically, the endodontic microbiota was clearly different in the coronal, middle, and apical parts of the root canal. Spirochetes were found in high frequencies in abscessed cases, and a pathogenic role was suspected for these bacteria. Most of the bacteria Miller observed under light microscopy could not be cultivated using the technology available at that time. Those bacteria were conceivably anaerobic bacteria, which were only successfully cultivated about 50 to 100 years later with the advent of anaerobic culture techniques. However, it is now widely recognized that a large number of bacterial species living in diverse environments still remain to be cultivated by current technology,[6,147] and the root canal is no exception (discussed later in this chapter). Based on his findings, Miller raised the hypothesis that bacteria were the causative agents of apical periodontitis.

Approximately 70 years after Miller's classic study, his assumptions were confirmed by an elegant study from Kakehashi and colleagues.[86] These authors investigated the response of exposed dental pulps to the oral cavity in conventional and germ-free rats. Histologic evaluation was performed and revealed that pulp necrosis and apical periodontitis lesions developed in all conventional rats; however, the exposed pulps of germ-free rats not only remained vital but also repaired themselves with hard-tissue formation. Dentin-like tissue sealed the exposure area and isolated the pulps again from the oral cavity.

The important role of bacteria in the etiology of apical periodontitis was further confirmed by Sundqvist's classic study.[250] This author applied advanced anaerobic culturing techniques to the evaluation of bacteria occurring in the root canals of teeth whose pulps became necrotic after trauma. Bacteria were found only in the root canals of teeth exhibiting radiographic evidence of apical periodontitis, confirming the

infectious cause of this disease. Anaerobic bacteria accounted for more than 90% of the isolates. Findings from Sundqvist's study also demonstrated that in the absence of infection, the necrotic pulp tissue itself and stagnant tissue fluid in the root canal cannot induce or perpetuate apical periodontitis lesions.

Möller and colleagues[120] also provided strong evidence about the microbial causation of apical periodontitis. Their study using monkeys' teeth demonstrated that only devitalized pulps that were infected induced apical periodontitis lesions, whereas devitalized and noninfected pulps showed an absence of significant pathologic changes in the periradicular tissues. In addition to corroborating the importance of microorganisms for the development of apical periodontitis, this study also confirmed that necrotic pulp tissue per se is unable to induce and maintain an apical periodontitis lesion.

Microorganisms causing apical periodontitis are primarily organized in biofilms colonizing the root canal system. Nair[126] was possibly the first to observe intracanal bacterial organizations adhered to the root canal walls, resembling biofilm structures. Several other morphologic studies found similar structures,[121,190,223] but it was not until the study of Ricucci and Siqueira[152] that the high prevalence of bacterial biofilms were consistently revealed in association with primary and post-treatment apical periodontitis (see the section Spatial Distribution of the Microbiota: Anatomy of Infection for a further discussion of biofilms in endodontic infections).

ROUTES OF ROOT CANAL INFECTION

Under normal conditions, the pulpodentin complex is sterile and isolated from oral microbiota by overlying enamel, dentin, and cementum. In the event that the integrity of these natural layers is breached (e.g., as a result of caries, trauma-induced fractures and cracks, restorative procedures, scaling and root planning, attrition, abrasion) or naturally absent (e.g., because of gaps in the cemental coating at the cervical root surface), the pulpodentin complex is exposed to the oral environment. The pulpodentin complex is then challenged by microorganisms present in caries lesions, saliva bathing the exposed area, or dental plaque formed on the exposed area. Microorganisms from subgingival biofilms associated with periodontal disease may also have access to the pulp via dentinal tubules at the cervical region of the tooth and lateral or apical foramina (see also Chapter 25). Microorganisms may also have access to the root canal any time during or after endodontic intervention, emphasizing the need for effective (fluid tight) use of the rubber dam.

Whenever dentin is exposed, the pulp is put at risk of infection as a consequence of the permeability of normal dentin dictated by its tubular structure[135] (Fig. 14-2). Dentinal tubules traverse the entire width of the dentin and have a conical conformation, with the largest diameter located near the pulp (mean, 2.5 μm) and the smallest diameter in the periphery, near the enamel or cementum (mean, 0.9 μm).[62] The smallest tubule diameter is entirely compatible with the cell diameter of most oral bacterial species, which usually ranges from 0.2 to 0.7 μm. One might assume that once exposed, dentin offers an unimpeded pathway for bacteria to reach the pulp via these tubules. However, it has been demonstrated that bacterial invasion of dentinal tubules occurs more rapidly with a nonvital pulp than with a vital pulp.[124] With a vital pulp, outward movement of dentinal fluid and the tubular contents (including

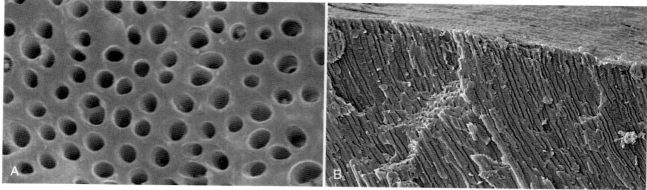

FIG. 14-2 **A,** Scanning electron micrographs of dentin showing tubules in cross-sectional view (magnification ×850). **B,** Longitudinal views (magnification ×130).

odontoblast processes, collagen fibrils, and the sheathlike lamina limitans that lines the tubules) influence dentinal permeability and can conceivably delay intratubular invasion by bacteria. Because of the presence of tubular contents, the functional or physiologic diameter of the tubules is only 5% to 10% of the anatomic diameter seen by microscopy.[113] Other factors such as dentinal sclerosis beneath a carious lesion, tertiary dentin, smear layer, and intratubular deposition of fibrinogen also reduce dentin permeability and thereby limit or even impede bacterial progression to the pulp via dentinal tubules.[137] Host defense molecules, such as antibodies and components of the complement system, may also be present in the dentinal fluid of vital teeth and can assist in the protection against deep bacterial invasion of dentin.[3,130,131] As long as the pulp is vital, dentinal exposure does not represent a significant route of pulpal infection, except when dentin thickness is considerably reduced or when the dentin permeability is significantly increased.

Most of the bacteria in the carious process are nonmotile; they invade dentin by repeated cell division, which pushes cells into tubules. Bacterial cells may also be forced into tubules by hydrostatic pressures developed on dentin during mastication.[114] Bacteria inside tubules under a deep carious lesion can reach the pulp even before frank pulpal exposure.[81] As mentioned, it has been assumed that the pulp will not be infected if it is still vital. The few bacteria that reach the pulp may not be significant, because the vital pulp can eliminate such a transient infection and rapidly clear or remove bacterial products. This efficient clearance mechanism tends to prevent injurious agents from reaching a high enough concentration to induce significant inflammatory reactions.[136] On the other hand, if the vitality of the pulp is compromised and the defense mechanisms are impaired, even a small amount of bacteria may initiate infection.

Direct exposure of the dental pulp to the oral cavity is the most obvious route of endodontic infection. Caries is the most common cause of pulp exposure, but bacteria may also reach the pulp via direct pulp exposure as a result of iatrogenic restorative procedures or trauma. The exposed pulp tissue comes in direct contact with oral bacteria from carious lesions, saliva, or plaque accumulated onto the exposed surface. Almost invariably, exposed pulps will undergo inflammation and necrosis and become infected. The time elapsed between pulp exposure and infection of the entire canal is unpredictable, but it is usually a slow process.[38]

The egress of microorganisms and their products from infected root canals through apical, lateral, or furcation foramina, dentinal tubules, and iatrogenic root perforations can directly affect the surrounding periodontal tissues and give rise to pathologic changes in these tissues. However, there is no consensus as to whether the opposite is true—that is, whether subgingival biofilms associated with periodontal disease can directly cause pulpal disease. Conceptually, microorganisms in subgingival plaque biofilms associated with periodontal disease could reach the pulp by the same pathways intracanal microorganisms reach the periodontium and could thereby exert harmful effects on the pulp. However, it has been demonstrated that although degenerative and inflammatory changes of different degrees may occur in the pulp of teeth with associated marginal periodontitis, pulpal necrosis as a consequence of periodontal disease only develops if the periodontal pocket reaches the apical foramen, leading to irreversible damage to the main blood vessels that penetrate through this foramen[98] (Fig. 14-3). After the pulp becomes necrotic, periodontal bacteria can reach the root canal system via exposed dentinal tubules at the cervical area of the root or via lateral and apical foramina to establish an endodontic infectious process.

It has been claimed that microorganisms can reach the pulp by *anachoresis*.[73] Theoretically, microorganisms can be transported in the blood or lymph to an area of tissue damage, where they leave the vessel, enter the damaged tissue, and establish an infection.[64,156] However, there is no clear evidence showing that this process can represent a route for root canal infection. It has been revealed that bacteria could not be recovered from unfilled root canals when the bloodstream was experimentally infected, unless the root canals were overinstrumented during the period of bacteremia, with resulting injury to periodontal blood vessels and blood seepage into the canal.[42] Another argument against anachoresis as a route for pulpal infection comes from the study by Möller and colleagues,[120] who induced pulpal necrosis in monkeys' teeth and reported that all cases of aseptic necrosis remained bacteria-free after 6 to 7 months of observation.

Bacteria have been isolated from traumatized teeth with necrotic pulps with apparently intact crowns.[250,278] Although anachoresis has been suggested to be the mechanism through which these traumatized teeth become infected,[73] current evidence indicates that the main pathway of pulpal infection in these cases is dentinal exposure due to enamel cracks.[106,107] Macro- and microcracks in enamel can be present in most teeth

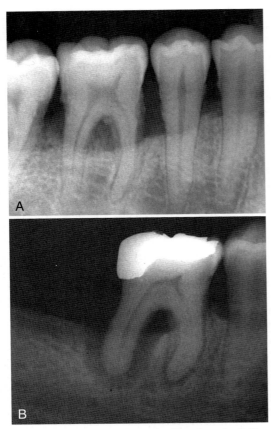

FIG. 14-3 Periodontal disease **(A)** mostly affects the pulp vitality when the subgingival biofilm reaches the apical foramen **(B)**.

(not only traumatized teeth) and do not necessarily end at the enamel-dentin junction; they can extend deep into the dentin.[107] A large number of dentinal tubules can be exposed to the oral environment by a single crack. These cracks can be clogged with dental plaque and provide portals of entry for bacteria. If the pulp remains vital after trauma, bacterial penetration into tubules is counteracted by the dentinal fluid and tubular contents, as discussed earlier, and pulpal health is not usually jeopardized. But if the pulp becomes necrotic as a consequence of trauma, it loses the ability to protect itself against bacterial invasion, and regardless of dentin thickness, dentinal tubules then will become true avenues through which bacteria can reach and colonize the necrotic pulp.

Whatever the route of bacterial access to the root canal, necrosis of pulp tissue is a prerequisite for the establishment of primary endodontic infections. To reiterate: if the pulp is vital, it can protect itself against bacterial invasion and colonization. If the pulp becomes necrotic due to caries, trauma, operative procedures, or periodontal disease, then it can be easily infected. This is because host defenses do not function in the necrotic pulp tissue, and those in the periradicular tissues do not reach deep into the root canal space.

Another situation in which the root canal system is devoid of host defenses relates to cases in which the pulp was removed for treatment. Microbial penetration in the canal can occur during treatment, between appointments, or even after root canal obturation. The main causes of microbial introduction into the canal *during treatment* include remnants of dental biofilm, calculus, or caries on the tooth crown; leaking rubber dam; contamination of endodontic instruments (e.g., after touching with the fingers); and contamination of irrigant solutions or other solutions of intracanal use (e.g., saline solution, distilled water, citric acid). Microorganisms can also enter the root canal system *between appointments* by leakage through the temporary restorative material; breakdown, fracture, or loss of the temporary restoration; fracture of the tooth structure; and in teeth left open for drainage. Microorganisms can penetrate the root canal system even *after completion of the root canal obturation* by leakage through the temporary or permanent restorative material; breakdown, fracture, or loss of the temporary/permanent restoration; fracture of the tooth structure; recurrent decay contaminating the root canal obturation; or delay in the placement of permanent restorations.[205]

MECHANISMS OF MICROBIAL PATHOGENICITY AND VIRULENCE FACTORS

The ability of a microorganism to cause disease is regarded as its *pathogenicity*. *Virulence* denotes the degree of pathogenicity of a microorganism, and *virulence factors* are the microbial products, structural cellular components, or strategies that contribute to pathogenicity. One example of bacterial strategy that contributes to pathogenicity includes the ability to coaggregate and form biofilms, which confers protection against microbial competitors, host defenses, and antimicrobial agents. Some microorganisms routinely cause disease in a given host and are called *primary pathogens*. Other microorganisms cause disease only when host defenses are impaired and are called *opportunistic pathogens*. Bacteria that make up the normal microbiota are usually present as harmless commensals and live in balance with the host. One of the greatest beneficial effects of human microbiota is probably the tendency to protect the host from exogenous infections by excluding other microorganisms. Nevertheless, in certain situations, the balance may be disturbed by a decrease in the normal level of resistance, and then the commensal bacteria are usually the first to take advantage. Most bacteria involved with endodontic infections are normal inhabitants of the oral microbiota that exploit changes in the balance of the host–bacteria relationship, becoming opportunistic pathogens.

Bacteria involved with the pathogenesis of primary apical periodontitis may have participated in the early stages of pulp inflammation and necrosis, or they may have gained entry into the root canal space any time after pulpal necrosis. In the former situation, involved bacteria are usually those present in the advanced front of caries lesions and from saliva bathing the affected area. Bacteria in caries lesions form authentic biofilms adhered to dentin (Fig. 14-4). Diffusion of bacterial products through dentinal tubules induces pulpal inflammation long before the tissue is exposed. After pulp exposure, the surface of the tissue can also be colonized and covered by bacteria present in the caries biofilm. The exposed pulp tissue is in direct contact with bacteria and their products and responds with severe inflammation. Some tissue invasion by bacteria may also occur. Bacteria in the battlefront have to survive the attack from the host defenses and at the same time acquire nutrients to keep themselves alive. In this bacteria–pulp clash, the latter invariably is "defeated" and becomes necrotic, so bacteria move forward and "occupy the territory"—that is, they colonize the necrotic tissue. These events advance through tissue compartments, coalesce, and move toward the apical part of the canal until virtually the entire root canal is necrotic and infected (Fig. 14-5). At this stage, involved bacteria can be regarded as the early root canal colonizers or pioneer species.

Early colonizers play an important role in the initiation of the apical periodontitis disease process. Moreover, they may significantly modify the environment, making it conducive to the establishment of other bacterial groups. These new species may have access to the canal via coronal exposure or exposed dentinal tubules, establish themselves, and contribute to a shift in the microbiota. Rearrangement in the proportions of the pioneer species and latecomers occurs, and as the environment changes, some early colonizers are expected to no longer participate in the consortium of advanced disease. With the passage of time, the endodontic microbiota becomes more and more structurally and spatially organized.

Some virulence attributes required for pathogens to thrive in other sites may be of no value for bacteria that reach the root canal after necrosis—for instance, the ability to evade host defenses. This is because latecomers face no significant opposition from host defenses, which are no longer active in the canal after necrosis. Although colonization may appear an easy task for late colonizers, other environmental factors (e.g., interaction with pioneer species, oxygen tension, nutrient availability) will determine whether new species entering the canal will succeed in establishing themselves and join the early colonizers to make up a dynamic mixed community in the root canal. Ultimately, the root canals of teeth with radiographically detectable apical periodontitis lesions harbor both early colonizers that managed to stay in the canals and late colonizers that managed to adapt to the new but propitious environmental conditions.[214]

Bacteria colonizing the necrotic root canal induce damage to the periradicular tissues and give rise to inflammatory changes. In fact, periradicular inflammation can be observed even before the frontline of infection reaches the apical foramen.[8,121,242,280] Bacteria exert their pathogenicity by wreaking havoc on the host tissues through direct or indirect mechanisms. Bacterial virulence factors that cause direct tissue harm include those that damage host cells or the intercellular matrix of the connective tissue. These factors usually involve secreted products, including enzymes, exotoxins, heat-shock proteins, and metabolic end products.[214] Furthermore, bacterial structural components, including lipopolysaccharide (LPS), peptidoglycan, lipoteichoic acid, fimbriae, flagella, outer membrane proteins and vesicles, lipoproteins, DNA, and exopolysaccharides, can act as modulins by stimulating the development of

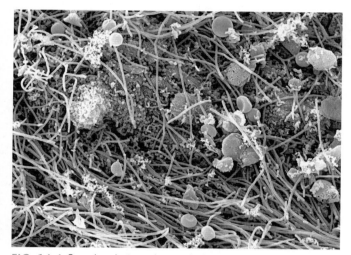

FIG. 14-4 Scanning electron micrograph showing a bacterial biofilm covering dentin in a deep carious lesion. Note the presence of different bacterial morphotypes (magnification ×3500). (From Torabinejad M, Walton RE: *Endodontics: principles and practice,* ed 4, St. Louis, 2009, Saunders/Elsevier.)

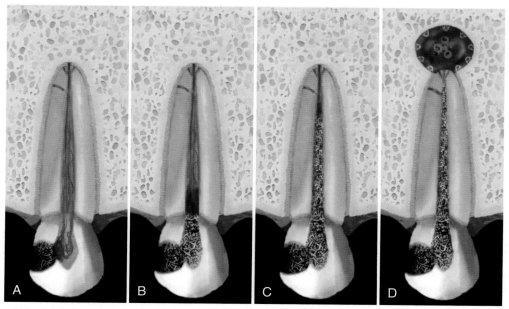

FIG. 14-5 Dynamics of pulp response from caries exposure **(A)** to pulp inflammation **(B)** to pulp necrosis **(C)** to apical periodontitis formation **(D)**.

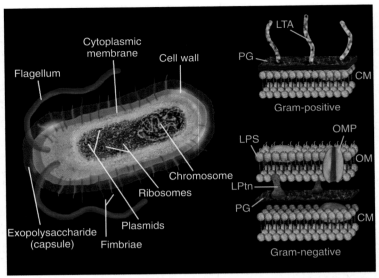

FIG. 14-6 Bacterial cell and its structural components that can act as virulence factors. *Right:* A detailed scheme of the bacterial cell walls from gram-positive and gram-negative bacteria. *CM,* cytoplasmic membrane; *LPS,* lipopolysaccharide (endotoxin); *LPtn,* lipoproteins; *LTA,* lipoteichoic acid; *OM,* outer membrane; *OMP,* outer membrane protein; *PG,* peptidoglycan.

host immune reactions capable not only of defending the host against infection but also of causing severe tissue destruction[80,214,265] (Fig. 14-6). For instance, inflammatory and noninflammatory host cells can be stimulated by bacterial components to release chemical mediators such as cytokines and prostaglandins, which are involved in the induction of bone resorption characteristically observed in asymptomatic (chronic) apical periodontitis lesions.[184] Another example of indirect damage caused by bacteria is the formation of purulent exudate in acute apical abscesses. Host defense mechanisms against bacteria emanating from the root canal appear to be the most important factor involved in the formation of purulent exudate associated with abscesses. Formation of oxygen-derived free radicals, such as superoxide and hydrogen peroxide, alongside the release of lysosomal enzymes by polymorphonuclear leukocytes, gives rise to destruction of the connective extracellular matrix, leading to pus formation.[264] Although direct damage caused by bacterial products may certainly be involved in the pathogenesis of apical periodontitis, bacterial indirect destructive effects seem to be more significant in this regard.[197]

Apical periodontitis is a multifactorial disease that is resultant of the interplay of many host and bacterial factors. Few if any of the putative endodontic pathogens are individually capable of inducing all of the events involved in the pathogenesis of the different forms of apical periodontitis. Probably, the process requires an integrated and orchestrated interaction of the selected members of the mixed endodontic microbiota and their respective virulence attributes. Although LPS is undoubtedly the most studied and quoted virulence factor, it sounds simplistic to ascribe to this molecule all responsibility for apical periodontitis causation. This statement is further reinforced by the fact that some cases of primary infections and many cases of secondary/persistent infections harbor exclusively gram-positive bacteria. Therefore, the involvement of other factors must not be overlooked. In fact, the pathogenesis of different forms of apical periodontitis and even the same

form in different individuals is unlikely to follow a stereotyped course with regard to the bacterial mediators involved.[197]

SPATIAL DISTRIBUTION OF THE MICROBIOTA: ANATOMY OF INFECTION

Mounting evidence indicates that apical periodontitis, like caries and periodontal diseases, is also a biofilm-related disease. Morphologic studies have shown that the root canal microbiota in primary infections is dominated by bacterial morphotypes that include cocci, rods, filaments, and spirilla (spirochetes) (Fig. 14-7). Fungal cells are sporadically found[190,223] (Fig. 14-8). Although planktonic bacterial cells suspended in a fluid phase and enmeshed in necrotic pulp tissue can be observed in the main root canal, most bacteria colonizing the root canal system usually grow in sessile multispecies biofilms adhered to the dentinal walls[121,126,223] (Fig. 14-9). Lateral canals, apical ramifications, and isthmuses connecting main canals may also be clogged with bacterial biofilms[125,151] (Figs. 14-10 and 14-11).

Bacterial cells from endodontic biofilms are often seen penetrating the dentinal tubules (Fig. 14-12). Dentinal tubule infection can occur in about 70% to 80% of the teeth evincing apical periodontitis lesions.[112,143] A shallow penetration is more common, but bacterial cells can be observed reaching approximately 300 μm in some teeth[223] (Fig. 14-13). Dividing cells are frequently observed within tubules during in situ investigations[223] (see Fig. 14-13), indicating that bacteria can derive nutrients within tubules, probably from degrading odontoblastic processes, denatured collagen, bacterial cells that die during the course of infection, and intracanal fluids that enter the tubules by capillarity.

Several putative endodontic pathogens have been shown to be capable of penetrating dentinal tubules in vitro, including *Porphyromonas endodontalis, Porphyromonas gingivalis, Fusobacterium nucleatum, Actinomyces israelii, Propionibacterium*

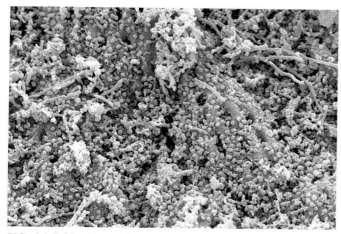

FIG. 14-7 Mixed bacterial population colonizing the root canal wall. Cocci are the predominant forms, but rods, filaments, and spirochetes are also observed. In some areas, coccoid cells are relatively apart from each other (magnification ×2200). (From Siqueira JF Jr, Rôças IN, Lopes HP: Patterns of microbial colonization in primary root canal infections, *Oral Surg Oral Med Oral Pathol Oral Radiol Endod* 93:174, 2002.)

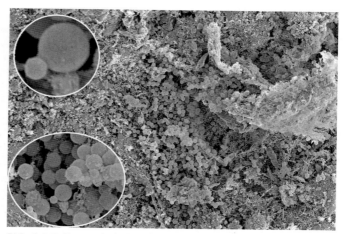

FIG. 14-8 Heavy colonization of yeast cells in the root canal of an extracted tooth with primary infection associated with apical periodontitis (magnification ×300). Note that some cells are in the stage of budding. A daughter cell is growing on the surface of the mother cell (insets: magnification ×2700 [*bottom*], magnification ×3500[*top*]). (From Siqueira JF Jr, Sen BH: Fungi in endodontic infections, *Oral Surg Oral Med Oral Pathol Oral Radiol Endod* 97:632, 2004.)

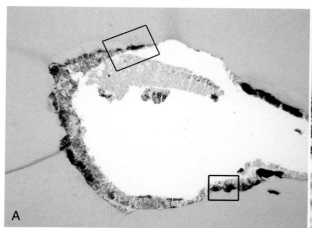

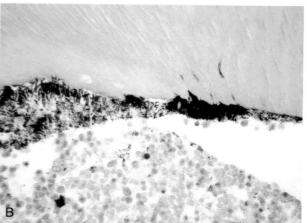

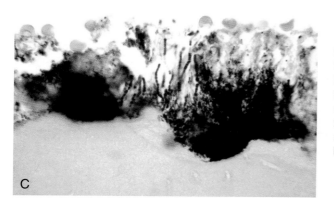

FIG. 14-9 A, Biofilm on the walls of a mesial root canal from a mandibular first molar (magnification ×100). The tooth was symptomatic, and an apical periodontitis lesion was present. Sections in B and C correspond to higher magnifications of the larger and smaller insets, respectively. Note the accumulation of polymorphonuclear neutrophils in the canal near the biofilm. (B, magnification ×400; C, magnification ×1000). Sections stained with a Taylor-modified Brown and Brenn technique. (Courtesy Dr. Domenico Ricucci.)

acnes, Enterococcus faecalis, Candida albicans, and streptococci.[107,141,201,224,273] In their clinical study, Peters and colleagues[143] isolated and identified bacteria present in root dentin at different depths, and the most common isolates belonged to the genera *Prevotella, Porphyromonas, Fusobacterium, Veillonella, Peptostreptococcus, Eubacterium, Actinomyces,* lactobacilli,

and streptococci. Using immunohistologic analysis, Matsuo and associates[112] observed the occurrence of *F. nucleatum, Pseudoramibacter alactolyticus, Eubacterium nodatum, Lactobacillus casei,* and *Parvimonas micra* inside dentinal tubules from the canal walls of extracted infected teeth with apical periodontitis.

Whereas bacteria present as planktonic cells in the main root canal may be easily accessed and eliminated by instruments and substances used during endodontic treatment, those organized in biofilms attached to the canal walls or located into isthmuses, lateral canals, and dentinal tubules are definitely more difficult to reach[125,267] and may require special therapeutic strategies to be eradicated.

BIOFILM AND COMMUNITY-BASED MICROBIAL PATHOGENESIS

Individual microorganisms proliferating in a habitat give rise to *populations*. Such populations often occur as microcolonies in the environment. Populations interact with one another to

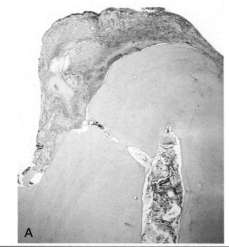

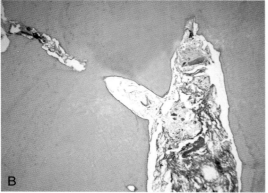

FIG. 14-10 **A,** Bacterial biofilm in the necrotic canal and in an apical ramification contiguous to inflamed periradicular tissues (magnification ×25). **B,** Higher magnification of **A** (magnification ×100). Sections stained with a Taylor-modified Brown and Brenn technique. (Courtesy Dr. Domenico Ricucci.)

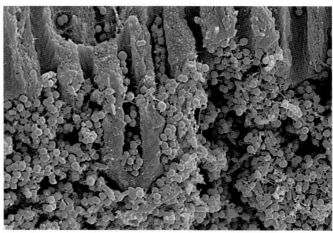

FIG. 14-12 Heavy infection of the root canal walls, mainly by cocci, but some small rods are also seen. Cocci are penetrating into dentinal tubules (magnification ×3500). (From Siqueira JF Jr, Rôças IN, Lopes HP: Patterns of microbial colonization in primary root canal infections, *Oral Surg Oral Med Oral Pathol Oral Radiol Endod* 93:174, 2002.)

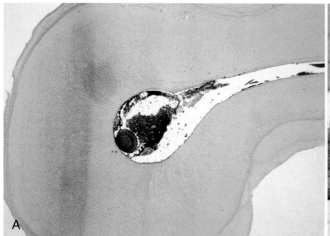

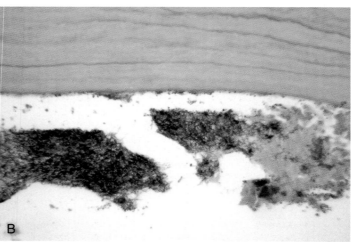

FIG. 14-11 Transverse sections of a maxillary second molar with fused mesial and palatal roots. **A,** Heavy bacterial infection of the canal, spreading to an isthmus (magnification ×25). **B,** Higher magnification of the isthmus clogged with bacteria (magnification ×400). Sections stained with a Taylor-modified Brown and Brenn technique. (Courtesy Dr. Domenico Ricucci.)

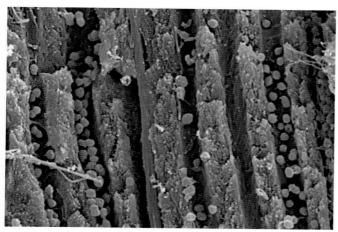

FIG. 14-13 Cocci in dentinal tubules approximately 300 μm from the main root canal (magnification ×5000). (From Siqueira JF Jr, Rôças IN, Lopes HP: Patterns of microbial colonization in primary root canal infections, *Oral Surg Oral Med Oral Pathol Oral Radiol Endod* 93:174, 2002.)

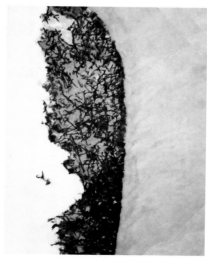

FIG. 14-14 Mixed bacterial biofilm adhered to the tooth surface (Brown and Brenn staining, magnification ×1000).

form a community. Thus, *community* refers to a unified assemblage of populations that coexist and interact at a given habitat. The community and habitat are part of a larger system called an *ecosystem,* which can be defined as a functional self-supporting system that includes the microbial community and its environment. In summary, the following hierarchy becomes apparent: ecosystem, community, population, and the single individual (cell).

Populations perform functions that contribute to the overall community and maintain the ecologic balance of the ecosystem. Each population occupies a functional role (*niche*) within the community. There are a limited number of niches within the community for which populations must compete. More competent populations occupy the niches and displace those less competent. As discussed later, highly structured and spatially organized microbial communities may exhibit properties that are greater than the sum of the component populations. In reality, complex microbial communities have been shown to be endowed with the ability to confront and withstand the challenges imposed by the environment by creating a mosaic of microenvironments that enable the survival and growth of the community members.

Historically, microbiologists dealing with infectious diseases have faced periods of "reductionism" and "holism."[95] *Reductionism* is based on the idea that the whole can be understood by examining smaller and smaller pieces of it, that is, all complex systems can be completely understood in terms of their individual components. Through reductionist approaches, individual species are isolated from complex mixed communities and metabolically and genetically studied so as to allow understanding of the community by examining every single constituent. However, it has become quite apparent for the microbiota associated with many human infectious diseases that the whole is very often greater than the simple sum of its parts. This concept has prompted microbiologists to adopt a holistic approach to understand the community behavior associated with pathogenesis of many infectious diseases known to have a polymicrobial etiology. *Holism* holds that any component cannot be thoroughly understood except in their relation to the whole. The holistic theory has been largely employed in

ecology: the interplay of the different parts composing the ecosystem will ultimately determine its properties.

It has been recognized that the biofilm (dental plaque) associated with caries and periodontal diseases represents a sophisticated community that exert functions essential for the biofilm architecture and physiology, with consequent pathogenetic implications. Recent evidence indicates that apical periodontitis can also develop as a result of collaborative activities of a biofilm community established in the root canal system.

Community profiling studies revealed that bacterial composition of the endodontic microbiota differs consistently between individuals suffering from the same disease.[32,108,168,229] This indicates that apical periodontitis has a heterogeneous etiology, where multiple bacterial combinations can play a role in disease causation. Interindividual variability is even more pronounced when different geographic locations are studied.[108,222] Moreover, community structure differs significantly between different disease forms (e.g., asymptomatic apical periodontitis versus acute apical abscess),[179,183,229] suggesting existence of a pattern associated with each form.

Biofilm and Bacterial Interactions

The community-forming ability can be regarded as essential for microbial survival in virtually all environments. Indeed, the majority of microorganisms in nature invariably grow and function as members of metabolically integrated communities, or biofilms.[35,110] *Biofilm* can be defined as a sessile multicellular microbial community characterized by cells that are firmly attached to a surface and enmeshed in a self-produced matrix of extracellular polymeric substance (EPS), usually a polysaccharide[35,47] (Fig. 14-14). The ability to form biofilms has been regarded as a virulence factor,[76] and biofilm infections account for an estimated 65% to 80% of bacterial infections that affect humans in the developed world.[34] Given its importance in varied aspects, there has been a high level of interest in the study of biofilm properties, not only in medical microbiology but also in different sectors of industrial and environmental microbiology.

Bacterial cells in biofilms form microcolonies (±15% by volume) that are embedded and nonrandomly distributed in the EPS matrix (±85% by volume) and separated by water channels.[37,47,240,244] Microcolonies are usually shaped as "towers" or "mushrooms." Dental biofilms can reach up to 300 or more cell layers in thickness.[240] Individual microcolonies may consist of a single bacterial species but more frequently are composed of several different species in a mixed community.

As the biofilm matures on the surface, extracellular polysaccharides are continually synthesized to form an extracellular matrix that eventually may constitute as much as 85% of the volume of the biofilm.[34] Although the matrix is primarily composed of polysaccharides, it can also contain proteins and nucleic acids.[76] The matrix is not only important physically as part of the scaffold that determines the biofilm structure, but it is also biologically active and can retain nutrients, water, and essential enzymes within the biofilm.[5] The matrix can also protect the biofilm community from exogenous threats and may participate in adherence to the surface.

Community members form distinct populations or microcolonies separated by open water channels that traverse the biofilm matrix and create primitive circulatory systems.[36] Fluid in these channels carries substrate, end products of bacterial metabolism, and signal molecules involved in bacterial interactions.[20] Thus, vital nutrients and communication molecules can diffuse, and wastes can be washed out through these channels.

Microcolonies that form in the biofilm arise from surface colonization by planktonic (unattached) bacterial cells. During the early stages of biofilm formation, bacteria bind to many host proteins and coaggregate with other bacteria. These interactions lead to changes in growth rate, gene expression, and protein production. It has been demonstrated by proteomic techniques or DNA arrays that genes expressed by cells in biofilms differed by 20% to 70% from those expressed by the same cells growing in planktonic culture.[15,132,185] Thus, bacteria in biofilms adopt a radically different phenotype compared with their planktonic counterparts. Within biofilms, some bacteria also use sophisticated systems of cell-cell communication (quorum sensing) to coordinate gene expression. Phenotypic heterogeneity in biofilms is also observed as a result of exposure of microcolonies to a variety of gradients (e.g., oxygen tension, pH, osmolarity, type and amounts of nutrients, cell density), which contribute to form diverse microenvironments throughout the biofilm structure.

Biofilm Community Lifestyle

Many naturally occurring biofilms have a highly diverse microbiota. These multispecies biofilms are not merely passive bacterial assemblages that are stuck to surfaces; they are complex biologic systems formed by populations (microcolonies) that are not randomly distributed but are spatially and functionally organized throughout the community. Indeed, populations are strategically positioned for optimal metabolic interaction, and the resultant architecture favors the ecologic role of the community in the ecosystem. The properties displayed by a multispecies biofilm community are mostly dictated by the interactions between populations, which create novel physiologic functions that cannot be usually observed with individual components. As a result, biofilm communities have a collective physiology, responding in concert to environmental challenges.

The biofilm community lifestyle affords a number of advantages to colonizing bacteria, including establishment of a broad habitat range for growth, increased metabolic diversity and efficiency, enhanced possibilities for genetic exchanges and bacterial intercommunications (quorum-sensing systems), and protection from external threats (competing microorganisms, host defenses, antimicrobial agents, and environmental stress).[111]

Biofilm organizations can also result in enhanced pathogenicity. To cause disease, bacteria must adhere to host surfaces, obtain nutrients from the host and multiply, invade tissues, overcome or evade the host defenses, and induce tissue damage. A diverse range of virulence traits are required for these particular stages of the disease process, and it is highly probable that each will require the concerted action of bacteria in a community. Similarly, it is possible that certain species can have more than one role in disease, and different species can perform similar functions. This helps explain why communities with different bacterial composition can be found in different individuals with similar disease. In multispecies communities, a broad spectrum of relationships may arise between the component species, ranging from no effect or reduced pathogenicity to additive or synergistic pathogenic effects. Endodontic abscesses are examples of polymicrobial infections whereby bacterial species that individually have low virulence and are unable to cause disease can do so when in association with others as part of a mixed consortium (pathogenic synergism).[21,39]

Resistance to Antimicrobial Agents

From a clinical standpoint, biofilm increased resistance to antimicrobial agents is of special concern. Bacteria arranged in biofilms are considered more resistant to antibiotics than the same cells grown in planktonic state. The antibiotic concentration required to kill bacteria in the biofilm is about 100 to 1000 times higher than that needed to kill the same species in planktonic state.[109] Several possible mechanisms are involved with biofilm resistance to antimicrobials.

Biofilm Structure May Restrict Penetration of Antimicrobial Agents

The agent may adsorb to and even inhibit the bacteria at the biofilm surface, but cells deeply located in the biofilm may remain relatively unaffected. The matrix in biofilms can also bind and retain neutralizing enzymes at concentrations that could inactivate the antimicrobial agent.[243]

Altered Growth Rate of Biofilm Bacteria

Many antibiotics can freely penetrate the biofilm matrix, but cells are often still protected. The occurrence of starved bacteria entering the stationary phase in biofilms seems to be a significant factor in the resistance of biofilm populations to antimicrobials. Bacteria grow slowly under conditions of low availability of nutrients in an established biofilm and as a consequence are much less susceptible than faster-dividing cells. Most antibiotics require at least some degree of cellular activity to be effective. Therefore, bacterial cells in stationary phase might represent a general mechanism of antibiotic resistance in the biofilm.[76]

Presence of "Persister" Bacteria

Increased tolerance of some biofilms to antibiotics may be largely due to the presence of a subpopulation of specialized survivor cells known as *persisters*.[89] It remains unclear whether these bacteria actually represent a distinct phenotype or are simply the most resistant cells within a population.[76]

APICAL PERIODONTITIS AS A BIOFILM-RELATED DISEASE

The evidence that apical periodontitis is a disease associated with polymicrobial biofilms comes mostly from in situ morphologic investigations.[25,121,125,126,152,153,154,186,223] These studies have observed that bacteria colonizing the root canal system of teeth with primary or posttreatment apical periodontitis usually formed sessile biofilm communities covering the walls of the main canal, apical ramifications, lateral canals, and isthmuses.

Although the concept of apical periodontitis as a biofilm-related disease has been built upon these observations, the prevalence of biofilms and their association with diverse presentations of apical periodontitis were only recently disclosed by Ricucci and Siqueira.[152] These authors evaluated the prevalence of biofilms in untreated teeth with primary apical periodontitis and treated teeth with posttreatment disease and looked for associations between biofilms and clinical/histopathologic conditions. Some of the most important findings of their study are as follows:

1. Intraradicular biofilms were generally observed in the apical segment of approximately 80% of the root canals of teeth with primary or posttreatment apical periodontitis.
2. Morphology of endodontic biofilms differed consistently from individual to individual (e.g., thickness, morphotypes, bacterial cells/extracellular matrix ratio).
3. Dentinal tubules underneath biofilms were often invaded by bacterial cells from the bottom of the biofilm community.
4. Biofilms were also commonly seen covering the walls of apical ramifications, lateral canals, and isthmuses.
5. Bacterial biofilms were more frequent in root canals of teeth with large apical periodontitis lesions. Because it takes time for apical periodontitis to develop and become radiographically visible, one can surmise that large lesions represent a longstanding pathologic process caused by an even "older" intraradicular infection. In longstanding infectious processes, involved bacteria may have had enough time and conditions to adapt themselves to the environment and set a mature and organized biofilm community. The fact that the apical root canal of teeth with large lesions harbors a large number of bacterial cells and species almost always organized in biofilms may help explain the long-held concept that treatment outcome is influenced by lesion size.[33,128]
6. The prevalences of intraradicular biofilms in teeth associated with apical cysts, abscesses, and granulomas were 95%, 83%, and 69.5%, respectively. Biofilms were significantly associated with epithelialized lesions. Because apical cysts develop as a result of epithelial proliferation in some granulomas,[102] it may be anticipated that the older the apical periodontitis lesion, the greater the probability of it becoming a cyst. Similar to teeth with large lesions, the age of the pathologic process may also help explain the high prevalence of biofilms in association with cysts.

7. Extraradicular biofilms were infrequent; they occurred in only 6% of the cases. Except for one case, they were always associated with intraradicular biofilms. All cases showing an extraradicular biofilm exhibited clinical symptoms. Thus, it seems that extraradicular infections in the form of biofilms or planktonic bacteria are not a common occurrence, are usually dependent on the intraradicular infection, and are more frequent in symptomatic teeth.
8. Bacteria were also seen in the lumen of the main canal, ramifications, and isthmuses as flocs and planktonic cells, either intermixed with necrotic pulp tissue or possibly suspended in a fluid phase. Bacterial flocs are sometimes regarded as "planktonic biofilms" and may originate from growth of cell aggregates/coaggregates in a fluid or they may have detached from biofilms.[77]

Some criteria have been proposed to establish a causal link between biofilms and a given infectious disease[77,134,152]:

1. Infecting bacteria are adhered to or associated with a surface.
2. Direct examination of the infected tissue shows bacteria forming clusters or microcolonies encased in an extracellular matrix.
3. The infection is generally confined to a particular site and although dissemination may occur, it is a secondary event.
4. The infection is difficult or impossible to eradicate with antibiotics in spite of the responsible microorganisms being susceptible to killing in the planktonic cell state.
5. Ineffective host clearance is evident, as suggested by the location of bacterial colonies in areas of the host tissue associated with host inflammatory cells. Accumulation of polymorphonuclear neutrophils and macrophages surrounding bacterial aggregates/coaggregates in situ considerably increases the suspicion of biofilm involvement with disease causation.
6. Elimination or significant disruption of the biofilm structure and ecology leads to remission of the disease process.

Based on findings from the Ricucci and Siqueira's study,[152] apical periodontitis can be considered to fulfill five of the six criteria. Bacterial aggregates/coaggregates are observed adhered to or at least associated with the dentinal root canal walls (criterion 1). Bacterial colonies are often seen encased in an amorphous extracellular matrix (criterion 2). Endodontic biofilms are frequently confined to the root canal system, in only a few cases extending to the external root surface, but dissemination through the lesion never occurred (criterion 3). In the great majority of cases, biofilms are directly faced by an accumulation of inflammatory cells, especially polymorphonuclear neutrophils (criterion 5).

As for criterion 4, it is widely known that intraradicular endodontic infections cannot be effectively treated by systemic antibiotic therapy, even though most endodontic bacteria in the planktonic cell state are susceptible to currently used antibiotics.[13,66,90] The lack of efficacy of systemic antibiotics against intraradicular infections is mainly because the drug does not reach endodontic bacteria that are located in an avascular necrotic space. The recognition of biofilms as the main mode of bacterial establishment in the root canal system further strengthens the explanations for the lack of antibiotic effectiveness against endodontic infections. Finally, there is a clear potential for fulfillment of criterion 6, because biofilms are frequently observed in canals of treated teeth with posttreatment apical periodontitis,[154] whereas teeth with a successful outcome show no biofilm infection of the root canal.[149]

METHODS FOR MICROBIAL IDENTIFICATION

The endodontic microbiota has been traditionally investigated by microbiologic culture methods. Culture is the process of propagating microorganisms in the laboratory by providing them with the required nutrients and proper physicochemical conditions, including temperature, moisture, atmosphere, salt concentration, and pH.[237] Essentially, culture analyses involve the following steps: sample collection and transport, dispersion, dilution, cultivation, isolation, and identification.[251] Endodontic samples are collected and transported to the laboratory in a viability-preserving, nonsupportive, anaerobic medium. They are then dispersed by sonication or vortex mixing, diluted, distributed onto various types of agar media, and cultivated under aerobic or anaerobic conditions. After a suitable period of incubation, individual colonies are subcultivated and identified on the basis of multiple phenotype-based aspects, including colony and cellular morphology, gram-staining pattern, oxygen tolerance, comprehensive biochemical characterization, and metabolic end-product analysis by gas-liquid chromatography. The outer cellular membrane protein profile as examined by gel electrophoresis, fluorescence under ultraviolet light, and susceptibility tests to selected antibiotics can be needed for identification of some species.[52] Marketed packaged kits that test for preformed enzymes have also been used for rapid identification of several species.

Culture analyses of endodontic infections have provided a substantial body of information about the etiology of apical periodontitis, composition of the endodontic microbiota in different clinical conditions, effects of treatment procedures in microbial elimination, susceptibilities of endodontic microorganisms to antibiotics, and so on. Advantages and limitations of culture methods are listed in Box 14-1; however, some important limitations of culture methods make a comprehensive analysis of the endodontic microbiota difficult to achieve.

The difficulties in culturing or identifying many microbial species are of special concern. Unfortunately, not all microorganisms can be cultivated under artificial conditions, and this is simply because the nutritional and physiologic needs of most microorganisms are still unknown. Investigations of many aquatic and terrestrial environments using culture-independent methods have revealed that the cultivable members of these systems represent less than 1% of the total extant population.[6,276] Furthermore, 50% to 80% of bacterial species composing the microbiota associated with diverse human sites, including the oral cavity, represent unknown and still uncultivated bacteria.[1,2,44,49,94,138,146,245]

That a given species has not been cultivated does not imply that this species will remain indefinitely impossible to cultivate. Myriad obligate anaerobic bacteria were uncultivable in the early 1900s, but further developments in anaerobic culturing techniques have to a large extent helped to solve this problem. It must be assumed that no single method or culture medium is suitable for isolating the vast diversity of microorganisms present in most environments.[70] Because we remain relatively unaware of the requirements for many bacteria to

grow, identification methods not based on cultivability are required.

In some situations, even the successful cultivation of a given microorganism does not necessarily mean that this microorganism can be successfully identified. Culture-dependent identification is based on phenotypic traits observed in reference strains, with predictable biochemical and physical properties under optimal growth conditions. However, many phenotype-related factors can lead to difficulties in identification and even to misidentification.[14,18,210,260] As a consequence of all these factors, phenotype-based identification does not always allow an unequivocal identification.

To sidestep the limitations of culturing, tools and procedures based on molecular biology have become available and have substantially improved the ability to achieve a more realistic description of the microbial world without the need for cultivation (Fig. 14-15). Molecular technology has also been applied to reliably identify cultivated bacteria, including strains with ambiguous or aberrant phenotypic behavior, rare isolates, poorly described or uncharacterized bacteria, and newly named species.[19,48,144,211,241,258]

Molecular approaches for microbial identification rely on certain genes that contain revealing information about the microbial identity. Of the several genes that have been chosen as targets for bacterial identification, the 16S rRNA gene (or 16S rDNA) has been the most widely used because it is universally distributed among bacteria, is long enough to be highly informative and short enough to be easily sequenced, possesses conserved and variable regions, and affords reliability for inferring phylogenetic relationships.[279] Similarly, the 18S rRNA gene of fungi and other eukaryotes has also been used extensively to identify these organisms.

BOX 14-1

Advantages and Limitations of Culture Methods

Advantages	Limitations
Broad-range nature, identification of unexpected species	Impossibility of culturing a large number of extant bacterial species
Allow quantification of all major viable cultivable microorganisms in samples	Not all viable bacteria can be recovered
Allow determination of antimicrobial susceptibilities of isolates	Once isolated, bacteria require identification using a number of techniques
Physiologic studies are possible	Misidentification of strains with ambiguous or aberrant phenotypic behavior
Pathogenicity studies are possible	Low sensitivity
Widely available	Strict dependence on the mode of sample transport
	Samples require immediate processing
	Costly, time consuming, and laborious, as for cultivation of anaerobes
	Specificity is dependent on experience of microbiologist
	Extensive expertise and specialized equipment needed to isolate anaerobes
	Takes several days to weeks to identify most anaerobes

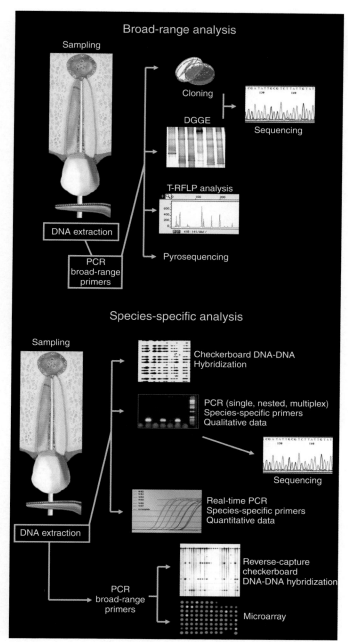

FIG. 14-15 Molecular biology methods used (or with potential to be used) in the study of endodontic infections. The choice for a particular technique will depend on the type of analysis to be performed. Some methods can be used for detection of target microbial species or groups and others for a broader analysis of the microbiota.

BOX 14-2

Advantages and Limitations of Molecular Biology Methods

Advantages

Detect both cultivable and as-yet-uncultivated species or strains

High specificity and accurate identification of strains with ambiguous or aberrant phenotypic behavior

Detect species directly in clinical samples

High sensitivity

Rapid; most assays take no more than minutes to a few hours to identify a microbial species

Do not require carefully controlled anaerobic conditions during sampling and transportation

Can be used during antimicrobial treatment

Anaerobic handling and expertise not required

Samples can be stored frozen for later analysis

DNA can be transported easily between laboratories

Detect dead microorganisms

Limitations

Most assays are qualitative or semiquantitative (exceptions: real-time PCR)

Most assays only detect one species or a few different species at a time (exceptions: broad-range PCR, checkerboard, microarray)

Most assays detect only the target species and fail to detect unexpected species (exception: broad-range PCR)

Some assays can be laborious and costly (e.g., broad-range PCR)

Biases in broad-range PCR introduced by homogenization procedures, preferential DNA amplification, and differential DNA extraction

Hybridization assays using whole genome probes detect only cultivable species

Can be very expensive

designed to detect specific target species directly in clinical samples.

Many molecular methods for the study of microorganisms exist; the choice of a particular approach depends on the questions being addressed.[218] Broad-range PCR followed by cloning and sequencing can be used to unravel the breadth of microbial diversity in a given environment. Bacterial community structures can be analyzed via pyrosequencing technology and by fingerprinting techniques such as denaturing gradient gel electrophoresis (DGGE) and terminal restriction fragment length polymorphism (T-RFLP). Fluorescence in situ hybridization (FISH) can measure the abundance of target species and provide information on their spatial distribution in tissues. Among other applications, DNA-DNA hybridization arrays (checkerboard techniques, DNA microarrays), species-specific single PCR, nested PCR, multiplex PCR, and quantitative real-time PCR can be used to survey large numbers of clinical samples for the presence of target species. Variations in PCR technology can also be used to type microbial strains. As with any other method, molecular methods have their own advantages and limitations (Box 14-2).

The Five Generations of Endodontic Microbiology Studies

Microbiologic studies for identification of the species participating in endodontic infections can be chronologically

Data from 16S rRNA gene sequences can be used for accurate and rapid identification of known and unknown bacterial species, using techniques that do not require cultivation. The 16S RNA gene of virtually all bacterial species in a given environment, including still uncultivated and uncharacterized bacteria, can be amplified by polymerase chain reaction (PCR) using broad-range (or universal) primers that are complementary to conserved regions of this gene. Sequencing of the variable regions flanked by the broad-range primers will provide information for accurate bacterial identification. Primers or probes that are complementary to variable regions can also be

TABLE 14-1

Generations of Studies for Microbiologic Identification in Endodontic Infections

Study Generation	Identification Method	Nature	Description and Findings
First	Culture	Open ended (broad range)	Revealed many cultivable species in association with apical periodontitis
Second	Molecular methods (e.g., PCR and its derivatives, original checkerboard assay)	Closed ended (species specific)	Target cultivable bacteria Confirmed and strengthened data from first generation Allowed inclusion of some culture-difficult species in the set of candidate endodontic pathogens
Third	Molecular methods (e.g., PCR-cloning-sequencing, T-RFLP)	Open ended (broad range)	Allowed a more comprehensive investigation of the bacterial diversity in endodontic infections Not only cultivable species but also as-yet-uncultivated and uncharacterized bacteria were identified
Fourth	Molecular methods (e.g., PCR, microarrays, reverse-capture checkerboard)	Closed ended (species specific)	Target cultivable and as-yet-uncultivated bacteria Large-scale clinical studies to investigate prevalence and association of species/phylotypes with endodontic infections
Fifth	Molecular methods (e.g., pyrosequencing)	Open ended (broad range)	Permit a deep-coverage and more comprehensive analysis of the diversity of endodontic infections

divided into five generations on the basis of the different strategic approaches used.[73] These generations are detailed in Table 14-1.

Impact of Molecular Methods in Endodontic Microbiology

Culture studies (first generation) identified a set of species thought to play an important role in the pathogenesis of apical periodontitis.[189,253] Further, not only have findings from culture-based methods been confirmed, but they have also been significantly supplemented with those from culture-independent molecular biology techniques, which constitute the other four generations of endodontic microbiology studies.[216] Molecular methods have confirmed and strengthened the association of many cultivable bacterial species with apical periodontitis and have also revealed new suspected endodontic pathogens.[212] The list of candidate pathogens has expanded to include culture-difficult species or as-yet-uncultivated bacteria that had never been found in endodontic infections by culturing approaches. The results from molecular studies impact remarkably on the knowledge of bacterial diversity in endodontic infections. More than 400 different bacterial species have already been detected in different types of endodontic infections.[216] Of these, about 45% were exclusively reported by molecular biology studies, compared with 32% detected by culture studies alone.[216] Twenty-three percent of the total bacterial species richness has been detected by application of both culture and molecular studies (Fig. 14-16). As a consequence, it becomes quite evident that the endodontic microbiota has been refined and redefined by molecular methods.[212]

TYPES OF ENDODONTIC INFECTIONS

Endodontic infections can be classified according to the anatomic location as intraradicular or extraradicular infection. *Intraradicular infection* is caused by microorganisms colonizing the root canal system and can be subdivided into three categories according to the time microorganisms entered the root canal system: *primary infection,* caused by microorganisms that initially invade and colonize the necrotic pulp tissue (initial or "virgin" infection); *secondary infection,* caused by microorganisms not present in the primary infection but introduced in the root canal at some time after professional intervention (i.e., *secondary* to intervention); and *persistent infection,* caused by microorganisms that were members of a primary or secondary infection and in some way resisted intracanal antimicrobial procedures and were able to endure periods of nutrient deprivation in treated canals. *Extraradicular infection* in turn is characterized by microbial invasion of the inflamed periradicular tissues and is a sequel to the intraradicular infection. Extraradicular infections can be dependent on or independent of the intraradicular infection.

DIVERSITY OF THE ENDODONTIC MICROBIOTA

Microbiota is a collective term for microorganisms and should replace terms such as *flora* and *microflora,* which perpetuate an outdated classification of microorganisms as plants.[43] *Diversity* refers to the number of different species present (richness) and their relative abundance (evenness) in a given ecosystem.[83]

The oral cavity harbors one of the highest accumulations of microorganisms in the body. Even though viruses, archaea, fungi, and protozoa can be found as constituents of the oral microbiota, bacteria are by far the most dominant inhabitants of the oral cavity. There are an estimated 10 billion bacterial cells in the oral cavity,[116] and culture-independent studies (microscopy and molecular biology technologies) have shown that over 50% to 60% of the oral microbiota still remains to be cultivated and fully characterized.[2,44,239] A high diversity of bacterial species has been revealed in the oral cavity by culturing approaches,[122] but application of molecular biology methods to the analysis of the bacterial diversity has revealed a still broader and more diverse spectrum of extant oral bacteria.[139] More than 1000 bacterial species/phylotypes have

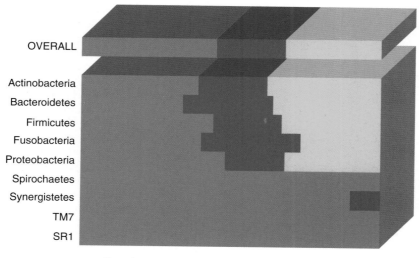

OVERALL

Actinobacteria
Bacteroidetes
Firmicutes
Fusobacteria
Proteobacteria
Spirochaetes
Synergistetes
TM7
SR1

■ Taxa detected in molecular studies
■ Taxa detected in both molecular and culture studies
□ Taxa detected in culture studies

FIG. 14-16 Percentage distribution of bacterial species/phylotypes found in endodontic infections according to the detection method. Data refer to the percentage of species or phylotypes overall or in each of the nine phyla that have endodontic representatives.

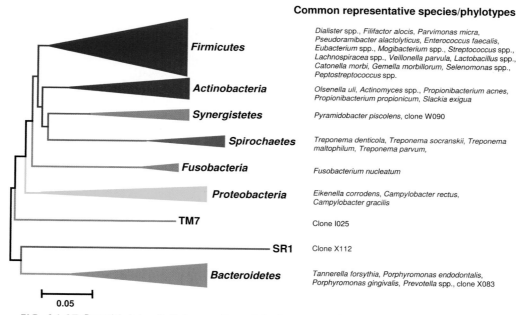

Common representative species/phylotypes

Firmicutes

Dialister spp., *Filifactor alocis, Parvimonas micra, Pseudoramibacter alactolyticus, Enterococcus faecalis, Eubacterium* spp., *Mogibacterium* spp., *Streptococcus* spp., *Lachnospiracea* spp., *Veillonella parvula, Lactobacillus* spp., *Catonella morbi, Gemella morbillorum, Selenomonas* spp., *Peptostreptococcus* spp.

Actinobacteria

Olsenella uli, Actinomyces spp., *Propionibacterium acnes, Propionibacterium propionicum, Slackia exigua*

Synergistetes

Pyramidobacter piscolens, clone W090

Spirochaetes

Treponema denticola, Treponema socranskii, Treponema maltophilum, Treponema parvum,

Fusobacteria

Fusobacterium nucleatum

Proteobacteria

Eikenella corrodens, Campylobacter rectus, Campylobacter gracilis

TM7

Clone I025

SR1

Clone X112

Bacteroidetes

Tannerella forsythia, Porphyromonas endodontalis, Porphyromonas gingivalis, Prevotella spp., clone X083

0.05

FIG. 14-17 Bacterial phyla with their respective endodontic representatives. *Right:* Example species or phylotypes for each phylum.

been found in the human oral cavity,[44] but advanced DNA pyrosequencing studies have indicated that this number may still have been largely underestimated.[4,72,88] Modern anaerobic culture and sophisticated molecular biology techniques have demonstrated that, at a broader taxonomic level, endodontic bacteria fall into nine phyla—namely, Firmicutes, Bacteroidetes, Spirochaetes, Fusobacteria, Actinobacteria, Proteobacteria, Synergistetes, TM7, and SR1[123,148,162,178-180,213,216] (Fig. 14-17). However, data from studies using pyrosequencing technology reveal that several other phyla may have been overlooked by previous identification techniques.[82,100,183,198,202] Fungi and

archaea are types of microorganisms that have been only occasionally found in endodontic infections.

Endodontic infections develop in a previously sterile place that does not contain a normal microbiota. Any species found has the potential to be an endodontic pathogen or at least play a role in the ecology of the endodontic microbial community. Culture and molecular studies reveal only prevalence of species; consequently, only association can be inferred. Causation is usually surmised on the basis of both frequency of detection and potential pathogenicity (in animal models or association with other human diseases), and several species

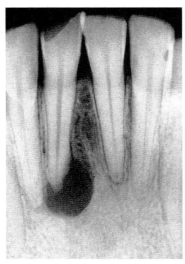

FIG. 14-18 Apical periodontitis due to primary intraradicular infection. Pulp is necrotic and lesion size is usually directly proportional to complexity of the microbiota involved.

have emerged as candidate endodontic pathogens. The following sections discuss specific aspects of each type of endodontic infection.

PRIMARY INTRARADICULAR INFECTION

Microbial Composition and Diversity

Primary intraradicular infection is infection of the necrotic pulp tissue (Fig. 14-18). It occurs in untreated teeth and is the cause of primary apical periodontitis. Participating microorganisms may be involved in earlier stages of pulp invasion (usually via caries) that culminated in inflammation and further necrosis, or they can be latecomers that took advantage of the environmental conditions in the root canal after pulp necrosis.

Primary infections are characterized by a mixed (multispecies) community conspicuously dominated by anaerobic bacteria. The number of bacterial cells may vary from 10^3 to 10^8 per root canal.[17,180,231,251,180,226,250,269] Molecular studies have disclosed a mean of 10 to 20 species/phylotypes per infected canal.[123,148,162,212,229] Canals of teeth with associated sinus tracts may exhibit a number of species close to the top of this range.[162] The size of apical periodontitis lesion has been shown to be proportional to the number of bacterial species and cells in the root canal.[162,227,250] A molecular study[162] demonstrated that the number of taxa per canal was clearly in direct proportion to the lesion size: small lesions (< 5 mm) harbored about 12 taxa, lesions from 5 to less than 10 mm harbored 16 taxa, and lesions over 10 mm harbored about 20 species. Some canals associated with large lesions may harbor even more than 40 taxa.[162] Therefore, the larger the lesion, the higher the bacterial diversity and density in the canal.

The most prevalent named bacterial species detected in primary infections, including abscessed cases, belong to diverse genera of gram-negative bacteria (i.e., *Fusobacterium, Dialister, Porphyromonas, Prevotella, Tannerella, Treponema, Pyramidobacter, Campylobacter,* and *Veillonella*) and gram-positive (*Parvimonas, Filifactor, Pseudoramibacter, Streptococcus, Propionibacterium,*

Olsenella, Actinomyces, Peptostreptococcus, and *Eubacterium*).[11,60,61,75,90,123,148,162,164,178,179,212,227,230,231,252,250,270] Bacterial prevalence in primary infections may vary from study to study as a function of several factors, such as sensitivity and specificity of the detection and identification methods, sampling technique, geographic location, and accuracy or divergence in clinical diagnosis and disease classification. Even so, the species most frequently detected are expected to be the same in most well-conducted studies. Figs. 14-19 to 14-21 display the most frequently detected species associated with asymptomatic apical periodontitis, symptomatic apical periodontitis, and acute apical abscesses, as revealed by studies from the authors' group using a highly sensitive molecular biology technique.

About 40% to 66% of the endodontic microbiota in primary infections is composed of species still uncultivated.[123,148,179] As for their abundance in these infections, as-yet-uncultivated phylotypes corresponded to about 40% of the clones sequenced.[179] Molecular studies investigating the breadth of bacterial diversity in infected root canals have disclosed the occurrence of uncultivated phylotypes belonging to several genera, including *Dialister, Prevotella, Solobacterium, Olsenella, Fusobacterium, Treponema, Eubacterium, Megasphaera, Veillonella,* and *Selenomonas,* as well as phylotypes related to the family *Lachnospiraceae* or the TM7 and Synergistetes phyla.[123,148,160,161,172,178,179,182,213,221] Some uncultivated phylotypes can even be among the most prevalent bacteria in primary intraradicular infections, and others may be associated with pain.[179] *Bacteroidetes* clone X083 is one of the most prevalent phylotypes found in endodontic infections.[162-164,219] Detection of as-yet-uncultivated phylotypes in samples from endodontic infections suggests that they can be previously unrecognized bacteria that play a role in the pathogenesis of different forms of apical periodontitis. The fact that they have not yet been cultivated and phenotypically characterized does not mean that they are not important.

Symptomatic Infections

Symptomatic apical periodontitis and acute apical abscesses are typical examples of endodontic infections causing severe symptoms. In these cases, the infection is located in the canal, but it has also reached the periradicular tissues and, in abscessed cases, can spread to other anatomic spaces. Acute apical abscesses are caused by bacteria that egress from the infected root canal and invade the periradicular tissues to establish an extraradicular infection and evoke purulent inflammation. Clinically, the disease leads to pain or swelling and has the potential to diffuse to sinuses and other fascial spaces of the head and neck to form a cellulitis or other complications (Fig. 14-22). The microbiota involved in endodontic abscesses is mixed and dominated by anaerobic bacteria[41,90,96,155,179,217,229] (see Fig. 14-19). Direct comparisons using molecular technology reveal an average of 12 to 18 taxa per abscess case, compared with 7 to 12 taxa present in root canals of teeth with asymptomatic lesions.[179,229] Uncultivated phylotypes constitute approximately 40% of the taxa found in abscesses and collectively represent more than 30% of the 16S rRNA gene sequences retrieved in clone libraries.[179]

Whereas microbial causation of apical periodontitis is well established, there is no strong evidence disclosing specific involvement of a single species with any particular sign or symptom of apical periodontitis. Some gram-negative anaerobic bacteria have been suggested to be involved with

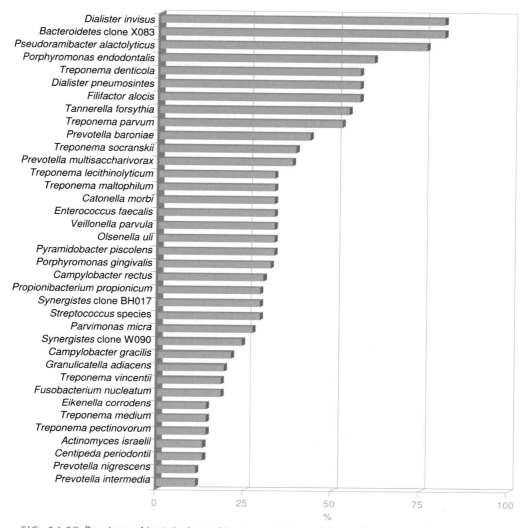

FIG. 14-19 Prevalence of bacteria detected in primary infections of teeth with asymptomatic (chronic) apical periodontitis. Data from the authors' studies using a taxon-specific nested-polymerase chain reaction protocol. (From references 159, 168, 211, and 210.)

symptomatic lesions,[67,71,169,179,250,266,281] but the same species may also be present in somewhat similar frequencies in asymptomatic cases,[11,61,75,85,230,231] so factors other than the mere presence of a given putative pathogenic species may play a role in the etiology of symptomatic endodontic infections.[193,199] These factors include differences in virulence ability among strains of the same species, bacterial interactions resulting in additive or synergistic effects among species in mixed infections, number of bacterial cells (infectious load), environmental cues regulating expression of virulence factors, host resistance; and concomitant herpesvirus infection. Association of some or all of these factors (instead of an isolated event) is likely to determine the occurrence and intensity of symptoms.[193,199]

Molecular studies using DGGE, T-RFLP, or pyrosequencing analysis have revealed that the structure of the endodontic bacterial communities in symptomatic teeth, including abscess cases, is significantly different from that of asymptomatic teeth.[179,183,229] Differences are represented by different dominant species in the communities and larger numbers of species in symptomatic cases. Differences in the type and load of dominant species and the resulting bacterial interactions may affect virulence of the whole bacterial community. Indeed, it has been shown that different species combinations may result in different outcomes because of the network of interactions.[170] The possibility exists that bacterial interactions result in communities that are more or less aggressive and consequently can cause host responses of corresponding intensity. This is consistent with the concept that the entire bacterial community is the unit of pathogenicity.

Geographic Influence

Findings from laboratories in different countries are often quite different regarding the prevalence of the species involved in endodontic infections. Although these differences may be attributed to variations in identification methodologies, a geographic influence in the composition of the root canal microbiota has been suspected. Studies using molecular biology techniques directly compared the endodontic microbiota of patients residing in distinct geographic locations and suggested that significant differences in the prevalence of some important species can actually exist.[10,157,204] In a more holistic approach, analysis of the bacterial community profiles of the microbiota

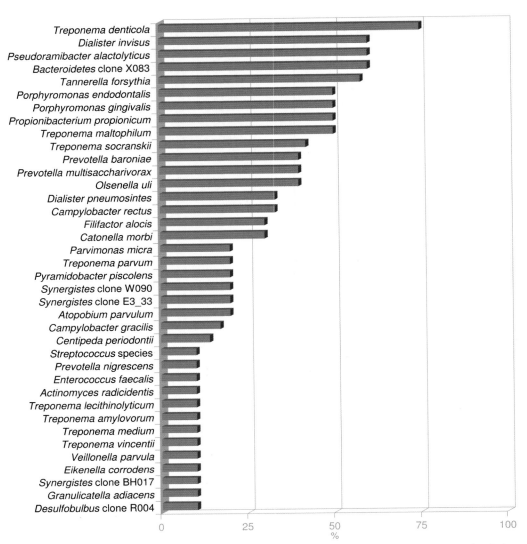

FIG. 14-20 Prevalence of bacteria detected in primary infections of teeth with symptomatic (acute) apical periodontitis. Data from the authors' studies using a taxon-specific nested-polymerase chain reaction protocol. (From references 159, 168, 211, and 210.)

associated with endodontic infections from different countries also revealed a geography-related pattern, with several species being exclusive for each location and others shared by the locations showing great differences in prevalence.[108,222] The factors that can lead to differences in the composition of the endodontic microbiota and the impact of these differences on therapy, particularly in abscessed cases requiring systemic antibiotic therapy, remain elusive.

Microbial Ecology and the Root Canal Ecosystem

A root canal with necrotic pulp provides a space for bacterial colonization and affords bacteria a moist, warm, nutritious, and anaerobic environment, which is by and large protected from the host defenses because of lack of active blood circulation in the necrotic pulp tissue. Also, the root canal walls are nonshedding surfaces conducive to persistent colonization and formation of complex communities. The necrotic root canal might be considered a fertile environment for bacterial growth,

with colonization not being a difficult task for virtually all oral bacterial species. Although a large number of bacterial species (about 100 to 200) can be found in the oral cavity of a particular individual,[139] only a limited assortment of these species (about 10 to 20) is consistently selected out for growth and survival within a root canal containing necrotic pulp tissue from the same individual. This indicates that ecologic determinants operate in the necrotic canal and dictate which species will succeed in colonizing this previously sterile environment. The major ecologic factors that determine the composition of the root canal microbiota include oxygen tension, type and amount of available nutrients, and bacterial interactions. Other factors such as temperature, pH, and receptors for adhesins may also be involved.

The root canal infection is a dynamic process, and different bacterial species apparently dominate at different stages.[259] Shifts in the composition of the microbiota are largely due to changes in environmental conditions, particularly in regard to oxygen tension and nutrient availability. In the initial phases of the pulpal infectious process, facultative bacteria

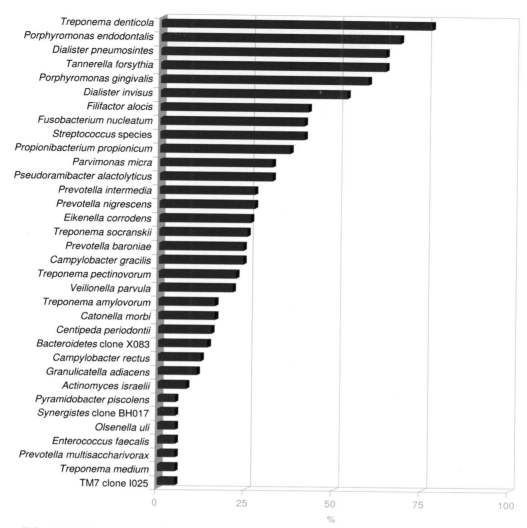

Treponema denticola
Porphyromonas endodontalis
Dialister pneumosintes
Tannerella forsythia
Porphyromonas gingivalis
Dialister invisus
Filifactor alocis
Fusobacterium nucleatum
Streptococcus species
Propionibacterium propionicum
Parvimonas micra
Pseudoramibacter alactolyticus
Prevotella intermedia
Prevotella nigrescens
Eikenella corrodens
Treponema socranskii
Prevotella baroniae
Campylobacter gracilis
Treponema pectinovorum
Veillonella parvula
Treponema amylovorum
Catonella morbi
Centipeda periodontii
Bacteroidetes clone X083
Campylobacter rectus
Granulicatella adiacens
Actinomyces israelii
Pyramidobacter piscolens
Synergistes clone BH017
Olsenella uli
Enterococcus faecalis
Prevotella multisaccharivorax
Treponema medium
TM7 clone I025

0   25   50   75   100
%

FIG. 14-21 Prevalence of bacteria detected in primary infections of teeth with acute apical abscesses. Data from the authors' studies using a taxon-specific nested-polymerase chain reaction protocol. (From references 159, 168, 211, and 210.)

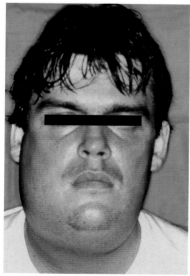

FIG. 14-22 Acute apical abscess. The infection has spread to other anatomic spaces to form cellulitis. (Courtesy Dr. Henrique Martins.)

predominate.[54] After a few days or weeks, oxygen is depleted within the root canal as a result of pulp necrosis and consumption by facultative bacteria. Further oxygen supply is interrupted with loss of blood circulation in the necrotic pulp. An anaerobic milieu develops and is highly conducive to the survival and growth of obligate anaerobic bacteria. With the passage of time, anaerobic conditions become even more pronounced, particularly in the apical third of the root canal; as a consequence, anaerobes will dominate the microbiota, outnumbering facultative bacteria (Fig. 14-23).

The main sources of nutrients for bacteria colonizing the root canal system include (1) the necrotic pulp tissue, (2) proteins and glycoproteins from tissue fluids and exudate that seep into the root canal system via apical and lateral foramina, (3) components of saliva that may coronally penetrate into the root canal, and (4) products of the metabolism of other bacteria. Because the largest amount of nutrients is available in the main canal, the most voluminous part of the root canal system, most of the infecting microbiota (particularly fastidious anaerobic species) is expected to be located in this region. Bacterial species that can best utilize and compete for nutrients in the root canal system will succeed in colonization.

In addition to being influenced by variations in oxygen levels, shifts in the composition of the microbiota colonizing the root canal system can also be dependent upon the dynamics of nutrient utilization. Saccharolytic species dominate the very early stages of the infectious process but are soon outnumbered by asaccharolytic species, which will dominate later stages.[254] Even though the necrotic pulp tissue can be regarded as a finite source of nutrients to bacteria (given the small volume of tissue that is progressively degraded), induction of periradicular inflammation guarantees a sustainable source of nutrients, particularly in the form of proteins and glycoproteins present in the exudate that seep into the canal. At this

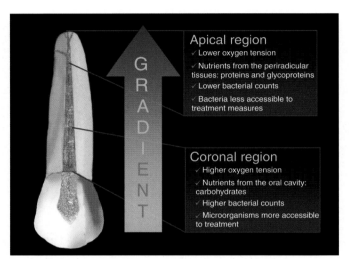

FIG. 14-23 Ecologic conditions in different areas of the root canal. A gradient of oxygen tension and nutrients (type and availability) is formed. Consequently, the microbiota residing in different parts can also differ in diversity, density, and accessibility to treatment procedures.

stage of the infectious process, bacteria that have a proteolytic capacity or establish a cooperative interaction with those that can utilize this substrate in the metabolism, start to dominate. Therefore, as the infectious process reaches the stage of induction of periradicular inflammation, proteins become the principal nutrient source, particularly in the apical part of the canal, favoring the establishment of anaerobic species that utilize peptides or amino acids in their metabolism (see Fig. 14-23).

Because primary endodontic infections are usually characterized by mixed communities, different bacterial species are in close proximity with one another, and interactions become inevitable. Thus, establishment of certain species in the root canal is also influenced by interactions with other species. In this regard, early colonizers play an important role in dictating which species will live along with them in the community. Bacterial interactions can be positive or negative. Positive interactions enhance the survival capacity of the interacting bacteria and enable different species to coexist in habitats where neither could exist alone. For instance, interbacterial nutritional interactions are important ecologic determinants that result in higher metabolic efficiency of the whole community. Nutritional interactions are mainly represented by food webs, including utilization of metabolic end products from one species by another and bacterial cooperation for the breakdown of complex host-derived substrates. Fig. 14-24 displays a complex array of interbacterial nutritional interactions that can take place in infected root canals, where the growth of some species can be dependent on products of the metabolism of other species. Moreover, one species can provide growth conditions favorable to another—for example, by reducing oxygen tension in the environment and favoring the establishment of anaerobes, or by releasing some proteinases that can provide protection from host defenses. Negative interactions in turn act as feedback mechanisms that limit population densities. Examples include competition (for nutrients and space) and amensalism (when one species produces a

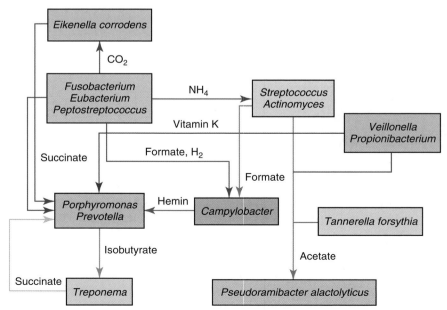

FIG. 14-24 Interbacterial nutritional interactions that can take place in infected root canals where growth of some species can be dependent on products of metabolism of other species.

substance that inhibits another species, including antibiotics such as penicillin).

Many species adhere directly to host surfaces, whereas other species adhere to bacteria already attached to the surface. The latter is called *coaggregation* and is a highly specific phenomenon with regard to the partners involved.[93] A given pair of species can attach to each other by means of specific receptor-adhesin interactions, which are usually lectin-like interactions (attachment of a specific protein on the surface of one species to a specific carbohydrate on the surface of the other). Coaggregation can favor colonization of host surfaces and also facilitate metabolic interactions between the partners. Coaggregation has been demonstrated for several pairs of bacterial taxa found in endodontic infections.[91]

Other Microorganisms in Endodontic Infections

Fungi

Fungi are eukaryotic microorganisms that may colonize the oral cavity, especially *Candida* species, but they have been only occasionally detected in primary intraradicular infections.[51,97,119,225] One molecular study[12] has, however, reported the occurrence of *C. albicans* in 21% of samples from primarily infected canals. Fungi are more frequently detected in canals of teeth with posttreatment disease (discussed later).

Archaea

Archaea consist of a highly diverse group of prokaryotes distinct from bacteria. Members of this domain have been traditionally recognized as extremophiles, but some of these microorganisms have also been found to flourish in nonextreme environments, including the human body.[50] To date, no member of the *Archaea* domain has been described as a human pathogen. Although studies have failed to detect archaea in samples from primary endodontic infections,[165,220] others detected a *Methanobrevibacter oralis*–like phylotype in some primarily infected canals.[268,270] Because these microorganisms have not been consistently detected in infected root canals, their role, if any, in the pathogenesis of apical periodontitis is questionable.

Viruses

Viruses are not cells but inanimate particles composed of a nucleic acid molecule (DNA or RNA) and a protein coat. On their own, they have no metabolism. In order to replicate the viral genome, they need to infect living cells and use the cell's machinery. Because viruses require viable host cells to infect and replicate themselves, they cannot thrive in the root canal with necrotic pulp. Viruses have been reported to occur in root canals only in teeth with vital pulps. For instance, the human immunodeficiency virus (HIV) has been detected in vital pulps of HIV-seropositive patients,[65] and some herpesviruses have been identified in both noninflamed and inflamed vital pulps.[99] Human cytomegalovirus (HCMV) and Epstein-Barr virus (EBV) have been detected in apical periodontitis lesions.[175] It has been hypothesized that HCMV and EBV may be implicated in the pathogenesis of apical periodontitis as a direct result of virus infection and replication or as a result of virally induced impairment of local host defenses, which might give rise to overgrowth of pathogenic bacteria in the very apical part of the root canal.[238] Bacterial challenge emanating from the canals

may cause an influx of virus-infected cells into the periradicular tissues. Reactivation of HCMV or EBV by tissue injury induced by bacteria may evoke impairment of host immune response in the periradicular microenvironment, changing the potential of local defense cells to mount an adequate response against infectious agents. In addition, herpesvirus may directly stimulate inflammatory cells to release proinflammatory cytokines.[117,275] Evidence of herpesvirus infection has been observed in symptomatic apical periodontitis lesions,[174,176] abscesses,[29,57] large lesions,[175-176] and lesions from HIV-positive patients.[177] However, the role of herpesviruses in the pathogenesis of apical periodontitis, if any, has still to be elucidated.

PERSISTENT/SECONDARY ENDODONTIC INFECTIONS

As defined earlier in this chapter, persistent intraradicular infections are caused by microorganisms that resisted intracanal antimicrobial procedures and survived in the treated canal. Involved microorganisms are remnants of a primary or secondary infection. The latter, in turn, is caused by microorganisms that at some time entered the root canal system secondary to clinical intervention. The moment can be during treatment, between appointments, or even after root canal filling. In any circumstance, if penetrating microorganisms manage to adapt themselves to the new environment, surviving and flourishing, a secondary infection is established. Species involved can be oral microorganisms or not, depending on the source of secondary infection.

Persistent and secondary infections are for the most part clinically indistinguishable. Exceptions include infectious complications (such as an apical abscess) arising after the treatment of noninfected vital pulps or cases in which apical periodontitis was absent at the time of treatment but present on the follow-up radiograph. Both situations are typical examples of secondary infections. Both persistent and secondary infections can be responsible for several clinical problems, including persistent exudation, persistent symptoms, interappointment flare-ups, and failure of the endodontic treatment, characterized by a posttreatment apical periodontitis lesion.

Persistent/Secondary Infections and Treatment Failure

Although there is some suggestion in the literature that extraradicular infection or nonmicrobial factors may be involved,[127,262] intraradicular infections, either persistent or secondary, can be regarded as the major causes of endodontic treatment failure (Fig. 14-25). This statement is supported by two strong evidence-based arguments. First, it has been demonstrated that there is an increased risk of adverse treatment outcome when bacteria are present in the canal at the time of obturation.[55,234,271] Second, most (if not all) root canal–treated teeth evincing persistent apical periodontitis lesions have been demonstrated to harbor an intraradicular infection.[101,103,145,154,159,181,210,255] Based on these arguments, studies investigating bacteria remaining in the root canals at the obturation stage disclose species that have the potential to influence the treatment outcome (*outcome into perspective*). On the other hand, studies dealing with the microbiota of root canal–treated teeth with apical periodontitis show the association of species with treatment failure, because the microorganisms detected

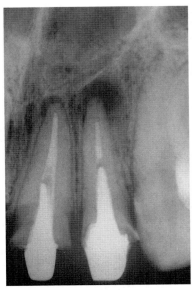

FIG. 14-25 Posttreatment apical periodontitis lesions in root canal–treated teeth. In poorly treated canals, the microbiota is similar to primary infections. In cases apparently well treated, fewer species are found. Regardless of treatment quality, persistent or secondary intraradicular infections are the main causative agents of endodontic treatment failure.

are likely to be participating in the etiology of posttreatment disease (*outcome already established*).

Bacteria at the Root Obturation Stage

Diligent antimicrobial treatment may still fail to completely eliminate bacteria from the infected root canal system. This is because persisting bacteria are either inaccessible or even resistant to treatment procedures. Whatever the cause of persistence, bacterial diversity and density in infected canals are substantially reduced after treatment. Root canal samples positive for bacterial growth after chemomechanical procedures, followed or not by intracanal medication, have been shown to harbor one to five bacterial species per case, and the number of persistent bacterial cells usually varies from 10^2 to 10^5 per sample.[24,180,207,208,234,269]

No single species has been significantly found to persist after treatment procedures. Gram-negative bacteria, which are common members of primary infections, are usually eliminated. Exceptions include some anaerobic rods, such as *F. nucleatum*, *Prevotella* species, and *Campylobacter rectus*, which are among the species found in postinstrumentation or postmedication samples.[24,68,142,180,226,234] Most studies on this subject have clearly revealed that when bacteria resist treatment procedures, gram-positive bacteria are more frequently present. Gram-positive facultatives or anaerobes often detected in these samples include streptococci, *P. micra*, *Propionibacterium* species, *P. alactolyticus*, *Actinomyces* species, lactobacilli, *E. faecalis*, and *Olsenella uli*.[24,26-28,31,68,140,142,164-166,180,203,207,208,234,257] This supports the notion that gram-positive bacteria can be more resistant to antimicrobial treatment measures and have the ability to adapt to the harsh environmental conditions in instrumented and medicated root canals. As-yet-uncultivated bacteria have also been detected in posttreatment samples,[133,180] indicating that they may also resist antimicrobial treatment.

Bacteria persisting in the root canal after chemomechanical procedures or intracanal medication will not always maintain an infectious process. This statement is supported by evidence that some apical periodontitis lesions healed even after bacteria were isolated from the canal at the obturation stage.[55,234] There are some possible explanations[215]:

- Residual bacteria may die after obturation because of toxic effects of the filling material or sealer, access denied to nutrients, or disruption of bacterial ecology.
- Residual bacteria may be present in quantities and virulence subcritical to sustaining periradicular inflammation.
- Residual bacteria remain in locations where access to periradicular tissues is denied.

Bacteria that resist intracanal procedures and are present in the canal at the time of obturation can influence the outcome of the endodontic treatment provided they do the following[215]:

- Have the ability to withstand periods of nutrient scarcity, scavenging for low traces of nutrients or assuming a dormant state or a state of low metabolic activity, to prosper again when the nutrient source is reestablished.
- Resist treatment-induced disturbances in the ecology of the bacterial community, including disruption of quorum-sensing systems, food webs, genetic exchanges, and disorganization of protective biofilm structures.
- Reach a critical population density (load) necessary to inflict damage to the host.
- Have unrestrained access to the periradicular tissues through apical/lateral foramina or iatrogenic root perforations.
- Possess virulence attributes that are expressed in the modified environment and reach concentrations adequate to directly or indirectly induce damage to the periradicular tissues.

In this context, it should not be forgotten that host resistance to infection is also an important and probably decisive counteracting factor.

Microbiota in Endodontically Treated Teeth

The microbiota in root canal–treated teeth with apical periodontitis also exhibits decreased diversity in comparison to primary infections. Canals apparently well treated harbor one to five species, but the number of species in canals with inadequate treatment can reach up to 10 to 20 species, which is similar to untreated canals (see Fig. 14-25).[145,168,181,210,255] The number of bacterial cells in treated teeth with posttreatment disease varies from 10^3 to 10^7 per canal.[17,140,167,187]

Several culture and molecular biology studies have revealed that *E. faecalis* is the most frequent species in root canal–treated teeth, with prevalence values reaching up to 90% of cases[118,145,159,171,167,187,210,255,283] (Fig. 14-26). Root canal–treated teeth are about nine times more likely to harbor *E. faecalis* than cases of primary infections.[171] This suggests that other members of a mixed bacterial consortium commonly present in primary infections can inhibit this species, and that the bleak environmental conditions within obturated root canals do not prevent its survival. The fact that *E. faecalis* has been commonly recovered from teeth treated at multiple visits or left open for drainage[233] suggests that this species is a secondary invader capable of colonizing the canal and resisting treatment. In other words, *E. faecalis* may cause secondary infections that later become

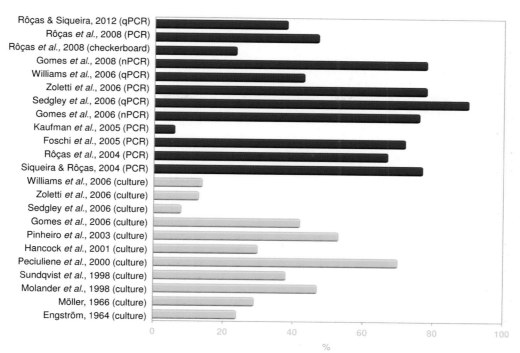

FIG. 14-26 Prevalence of *Enterococcus faecalis* in samples from root canal–treated teeth with apical periodontitis. Data from culture *(yellow bars)* and molecular *(blue bars)* studies follow.

Molecular Studies

1. Foschi F, Cavrini F, Montebugnoli L, et al: Detection of bacteria in endodontic samples by polymerase chain reaction assays and association with defined clinical signs in Italian patients, *Oral Microbiol Immunol* 20:289, 2005.
2. Gomes BP, Pinheiro ET, Jacinto RC, et al: Microbial analysis of canals of root-filled teeth with periapical lesions using polymerase chain reaction, *J Endod* 34:537, 2008.
3. Gomes BP, Pinheiro ET, Sousa EL, et al: *Enterococcus faecalis* in dental root canals detected by culture and by polymerase chain reaction analysis, *Oral Surg Oral Med Oral Pathol Oral Radiol Endod* 102:247, 2006.
4. Kaufman B, Spangberg L, Barry J, Fouad AF: *Enterococcus* spp. in endodontically treated teeth with and without periradicular lesions, *J Endod* 31:851, 2005.
5. Rôças IN, Hulsmann M, Siqueira JF Jr: Microorganisms in root canal-treated teeth from a German population, *J Endod* 34:926, 2008.
6. Rôças IN, Siqueira JF Jr: Characterization of microbiota of root canal-treated teeth with posttreatment disease, *J Clin Microbiol* 50:1721, 2012.
7. Rôças IN, Siqueira JF Jr, Santos KR: Association of *Enterococcus faecalis* with different forms of periradicular diseases, *J Endod* 30:315, 2004.
8. Sedgley C, Nagel A, Dahlen G, et al: Real-time quantitative polymerase chain reaction and culture analyses of *Enterococcus faecalis* in root canals, *J Endod* 32:173, 2006.
9. Siqueira JF Jr, Rôças IN: Polymerase chain reaction-based analysis of microorganisms associated with failed endodontic treatment, *Oral Surg Oral Med Oral Pathol Oral Radiol Endod* 97:85, 2004.
10. Williams JM, Trope M, Caplan DJ, Shugars DC: Detection and quantitation of *Enterococcus faecalis* by real-time PCR (qPCR), reverse transcription-PCR (RT-PCR), and cultivation during endodontic treatment, *J Endod* 32:715, 2006.
11. Zoletti GO, Siqueira JF Jr, Santos KR: Identification of *Enterococcus faecalis* in root-filled teeth with or without periradicular lesions by culture-dependent and -independent approaches, *J Endod* 32:722, 2006.

Culture Studies

1. Engström B: The significance of enterococci in root canal treatment, *Odontol Rev* 15:87, 1964.
2. Gomes BP, Pinheiro ET, Sousa EL, et al: *Enterococcus faecalis* in dental root canals detected by culture and by polymerase chain reaction analysis, *Oral Surgery Oral Medicine Oral Pathology Oral Radiology and Endodontology* 102:247, 2006.
3. Hancock HH 3rd, Sigurdsson A, Trope M, Moiseiwitsch J: Bacteria isolated after unsuccessful endodontic treatment in a North American population, *Oral Surg Oral Med Oral Pathol Oral Radiol Endod* 91:579, 2001.
4. Molander A, Reit C, Dahlen G, Kvist T: Microbiological status of root-filled teeth with apical periodontitis, *Int Endod J* 31:1, 1998.
5. Möller AJR: Microbial examination of root canals and periapical tissues of human teeth, *Odontol Tidskr* 74(suppl):1, 1966.
6. Peciuliene V, Balciuniene I, Eriksen HM, Haapasalo M: Isolation of *Enterococcus faecalis* in previously root-filled canals in a Lithuanian population, *J Endod* 26:593, 2000.
7. Pinheiro ET, Gomes BP, Ferraz CC, et al: Microorganisms from canals of root-filled teeth with periapical lesions, *Int Endod J* 36:1, 2003.
8. Sedgley C, Nagel A, Dahlen G, et al: Real-time quantitative polymerase chain reaction and culture analyses of *Enterococcus faecalis* in root canals, *J Endod* 32:173, 2006.
9. Sundqvist G, Figdor D, Persson S, Sjogren U: Microbiologic analysis of teeth with failed endodontic treatment and the outcome of conservative re-treatment, *Oral Surg Oral Med Oral Pathol Oral Radiol Endod* 85:86, 1998.
10. Williams JM, Trope M, Caplan DJ, Shugars DC: Detection and quantitation of *Enterococcus faecalis* by real-time PCR (qPCR), reverse transcription-PCR (RT-PCR), and cultivation during endodontic treatment, *J Endod* 32:715, 2006.
11. Zoletti GO, Siqueira JF Jr, Santos KR: Identification of *Enterococcus faecalis* in root-filled teeth with or without periradicular lesions by culture-dependent and -independent approaches, *J Endod* 32:722, 2006.

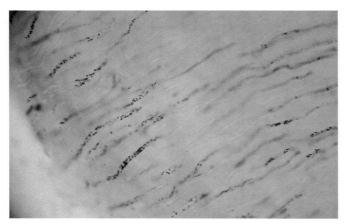

FIG. 14-27 Dentinal tubule infection by *Enterococcus faecalis* in dog's teeth after experimental infection. Notice that cells invaded the entire extent of some tubules up to the cementum (Brown and Brenn staining, ×1000).

persistent. *E. faecalis* is considered a transient species in the oral cavity; its source may be food.[282]

For a given microorganism to survive in endodontically treated teeth, it has to resist intracanal disinfection procedures and adapt to the harsh environmental conditions caused by treatment. The ability of *E. faecalis* to penetrate dentinal tubules, sometimes to a deep extent[74,201] (Fig. 14-27), can enable it to escape the action of endodontic instruments and irrigants used during chemomechanical preparation.[74,200] Moreover, its ability to form biofilms in root canals can be important for its resistance to and persistence after intracanal antimicrobial procedures.[45] *Enterococcus faecalis* is also resistant to calcium hydroxide[22]; such an ability to resist high pH values seems to be related to a functioning proton pump that drives protons into the cell to acidify the cytoplasm.[53] Unlike most putative endodontic pathogens frequently found in primary infections, *E. faecalis* may colonize root canals in single infections,[255] and such relative independence of living without deriving nutrients from other bacteria can be extremely important for its establishment in treated root canals. Finally, environmental cues can regulate gene expression in *E. faecalis*, affording this bacterium the ability to adapt to varying (and adverse) conditions.[84] Indeed, *E. faecalis* can enter a so-called viable but noncultivable (VBNC) state,[104] which is a survival mechanism adopted by several bacteria when exposed to unfavorable environmental conditions.[105] In the VBNC state, bacteria lose the ability to grow in culture media but maintain viability and pathogenicity and sometimes can resume division when optimal environmental conditions are restored. Studies have demonstrated that *E. faecalis* has the ability to survive in environments with scarcity of nutrients and then flourish when the nutrient source is reestablished.[59] It also has the capacity to recover from a prolonged starvation state in obturated canals,[188] suggesting that viable cells of this species, entombed at the time of canal obturation, may provide a long-term nidus for subsequent infection.

Taken together, all these properties help explain the significantly high prevalence of *E. faecalis* in root canal–treated teeth. Although association of this species with posttreatment disease is suggested by epidemiologic studies and supported by the species attributes that allow it to survive under unfavorable environmental conditions, causation is unproved. In fact, the

following findings from studies carried out in independent laboratories have questioned the status of *E. faecalis* as the main causative agent of endodontic failures:

- Despite being easily cultivated, *E. faecalis* is not detected in all studies evaluating the microbiota of root canal–treated teeth with posttreatment disease.[30,172]
- Even when present, *E. faecalis* is rarely one of the most dominant species in retreatment cases.[158,167,168,181]
- *E. faecalis* has been found not to be more prevalent in root canal–treated teeth with lesions when compared with treated teeth with no lesions.[87,283]

Other bacteria found in endodontically treated teeth with apical periodontitis include streptococci and some fastidious anaerobic species, such as *P. alactolyticus*, *Propionibacterium* species, *Filifactor alocis*, *Dialister pneumosintes*, *Dialister invisus*, *Tannerella forsythia*, *P. micra*, *Prevotella intermedia*, and *Treponema denticola*[7,69,118,145,158,167,168,181,210,213,255] (Fig. 14-28). Uncultivated phylotypes correspond to 55% of the taxa detected in treated canals, and collectively they can also be in high proportions, corresponding to about half of the 16S rRNA gene sequences retrieved in clone libraries.[181] Detection of uncultivated phylotypes helps explain why culture studies fail to detect bacteria in some treated root canals.

The bacterial community profiles in treated cases vary from individual to individual, indicating that distinct bacterial combinations can play a role in treatment failure.[168,181] All these findings strongly suggest that the microbiota of root canal–treated teeth with apical periodontitis is more complex than previously anticipated by culture studies.

Fungi are only occasionally found in primary infections, but *Candida* species have been detected in root canal–treated teeth in up to 18% of the cases.[30,51,118,119,140,145,210,255] Fungi gain access to root canals via contamination during endodontic therapy (secondary infection) or they overgrow after inefficient intracanal antimicrobial procedures that cause an imbalance in the primary endodontic microbiota.[232] *Candida albicans* is by far the most commonly detected fungal species in root canal–treated teeth. This species has several properties that can be involved in persistence following treatment, including its ability to colonize and invade dentin[191,192,224] and resistance to calcium hydroxide.[272,274]

EXTRARADICULAR INFECTIONS

Apical periodontitis lesions are formed in response to intraradicular infection and by and large constitute an effective barrier against spread of the infection to the alveolar bone and other body sites. In most situations, apical periodontitis inflammatory lesions succeed in preventing microorganisms from invading the periradicular tissues. Nevertheless, in some specific circumstances, microorganisms can overcome this defense barrier and establish an extraradicular infection. The most common form of extraradicular infection is the acute apical abscess, characterized by purulent inflammation in the periradicular tissues in response to a massive egress of virulent bacteria from the root canal. There are, however, other forms of extraradicular infection, which have been discussed as one of the possible etiologies of persistence of apical periodontitis lesions in spite of diligent root canal treatment.[194,263] These conditions entail the establishment of microorganisms in the periradicular tissues either by adherence to the apical external root surface in the form of extraradicular biofilm

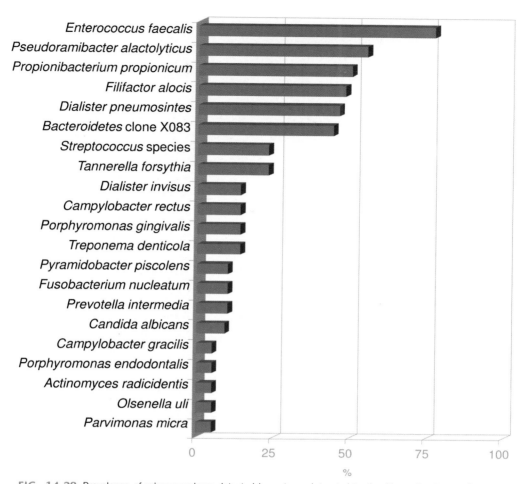

FIG. 14-28 Prevalence of microorganisms detected in root canal–treated teeth with posttreatment disease. Data from the authors' studies using a taxon-specific polymerase chain reaction assay. (From references 218 and 210.)

structures[129,261] or by formation of cohesive actinomycotic colonies within the body of the inflammatory lesion.[79]

Therefore, extraradicular infection can develop as follows[195]:

♦ It can be a result of direct advance of some bacterial species that overcome host defenses concentrated near or beyond the apical foramen, an extension of the intraradicular infectious process, or bacterial penetration into the lumen of pocket (bay) cysts, which are in direct communication with the apical foramen. The borderline between the infecting endodontic microbiota and the host defenses is often located intraradicularly, short of or at the apical foramen. In some cases, however, microorganisms may reach the periradicular tissues, and the borderline is then situated extraradicularly, beyond the boundaries of the apical foramen (Fig. 14-29). In the latter situation, the whole infectious process would be a continuum composed of an intraradicular and an extraradicular segment, in which the former fosters the latter (see Fig. 14-29). It has been suggested that in some cases, the extraradicular segment may become independent of the intraradicular component of the infectious process, but this has not been confirmed by scientific findings.

♦ It can result from bacterial persistence in the apical periodontitis lesion after remission of an acute apical abscess. The acute apical abscess is for the most part clearly dependent on the intraradicular infection; once the intraradicular infection is properly controlled by root canal treatment or tooth extraction and drainage of pus is achieved, the extraradicular infection is handled by the host defenses and usually subsides. Nonetheless, it should be appreciated that in some rare cases, bacteria that have participated in acute apical abscesses may persist in the periradicular tissues following resolution of the acute response and establish a persistent extraradicular infection associated with chronic periradicular inflammation, sometimes resulting in an actively draining sinus tract.

♦ It can be a sequel to apical extrusion of debris during root canal instrumentation (particularly after overinstrumentation). Bacteria embedded in dentinal chips can be physically protected from the host defense cells and therefore can persist in the periradicular tissues and sustain periradicular inflammation. The virulence and quantity of the involved bacteria, as well as the host's ability to deal with infection, will be decisive factors dictating whether an extraradicular infection will develop or not.

Conceivably, the extraradicular infection can be dependent on or independent of the intraradicular infection.[194] Independent extraradicular infections would be those that are no longer fostered by the intraradicular infection and can persist even after successful eradication of the latter. So far, it has been

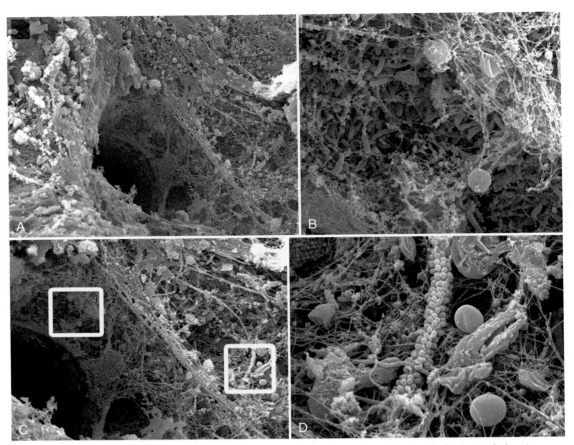

FIG. 14-29 Scanning electron micrograph showing extensive bacterial colonization in the very apical part of the canal, near and at the apical foramen (**A-B**, magnification ×550 and magnification ×850, respectively). **C,** Higher magnification of left inset in **B** showing a bacterial biofilm adhered to the very apical canal walls (magnification ×3700). **D,** Higher magnification of right inset in **B** showing a fully developed "corncob" in tissue meshwork adjacent to the apical foramen (magnification ×4000). (Modified from Siqueira JF Jr, Lopes HP: Bacteria on the apical root surfaces of untreated teeth with periradicular lesions: a scanning electron microscopy study, *Int Endod J* 34:216, 2001.)

suggested that the main bacterial species implicated in independent extraradicular infections are *Actinomyces* species and *Propionibacterium propionicum,* in a pathologic entity named *apical* (or periapical, periradicular) *actinomycosis*[23,79,236,256] (Fig. 14-30). These bacteria form cohesive colonies that may be collectively resistant to phagocytosis.[58] However, existence of apical actinomycosis as a self-sustained pathologic entity, no longer nurtured by the intraradicular infection, and its involvement as an exclusive cause of treatment failure is speculative and remains to be proved.[151,209]

It is still controversial whether chronic apical periodontitis lesions can harbor bacteria for very long beyond initial tissue invasion.[9] Studies using culture-dependent[247,262,277] or culture-independent molecular biology methods, such as checkerboard hybridization,[63,249] fluorescence in situ hybridization (FISH),[248] clone library analysis,[78] and pyrosequencing,[173] have reported the extraradicular occurrence of a complex microbiota associated with apical periodontitis lesions that did not respond favorably to the root canal treatment. Anaerobic bacteria have been reported as the dominant microorganisms in several of those lesions.[247,249] Apart from a discussion about whether contamination can be effectively prevented during surgical sampling of periradicular lesions, these studies did not

evaluate the bacteriologic conditions of the apical part of the root canal. This makes it difficult to ascertain whether those extraradicular infections were dependent on or independent of an intraradicular infection. Actually, findings from a study evaluating both the resected root ends and the apical periodontitis lesions from treated teeth suggested that the large majority of cases of extraradicular infections are maintained by a concomitant apical root canal infection.[246]

The incidence of extraradicular infections in untreated teeth is conceivably low.[126,206] Extraradicular biofilms are infrequent, and when present they are virtually always associated with intraradicular biofilms.[152] This is in consonance with the high success rate of nonsurgical root canal treatment.[40,150,235] Even in root canal–treated teeth with recalcitrant lesions in which a higher incidence of extraradicular bacteria has been reported, a high rate of healing following retreatment[56,235] indicates that the major cause of posttreatment disease is located within the root canal system, characterizing a persistent or secondary intraradicular infection. This has been confirmed by culture and by molecular and histobacteriologic studies investigating the microbiologic conditions of root canals associated with posttreatment apical periodontitis.[103,118,145,154,168,210,255]

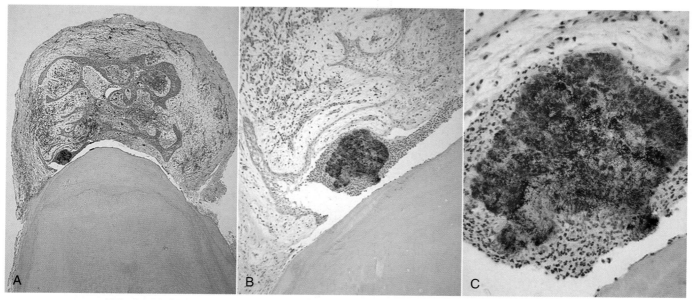

FIG. 14-30 Bacterial aggregate in an epithelialized apical periodontitis lesion, suggestive of actinomycosis. This case presented a severe flare-up in the past, but the tooth was asymptomatic at the time of extraction. **A,** Section not passing through the canal; note cyst cavity and bacterial aggregation on the left (magnification ×25). **B,** Detail of area with colony (magnification ×100). **C,** Higher magnification of colony, which is surrounded by neutrophils (magnification ×400). Sections stained with a Taylor-modified Brown and Brenn technique. (Courtesy Dr. Domenico Ricucci.)

REFERENCES

1. Aas JA, Griffen AL, Dardis SR, et al: Bacteria of dental caries in primary and permanent teeth in children and young adults, *J Clin Microbiol* 46:1407, 2008.
2. Aas JA, Paster BJ, Stokes LN, et al: Defining the normal bacterial flora of the oral cavity, *J Clin Microbiol* 43:5721, 2005.
3. Ackermans F, Klein JP, Frank RM: Ultrastructural localization of immunoglobulins in carious human dentine, *Arch Oral Biol* 26:879, 1981.
4. Ahn J, Yang L, Paster BJ, et al: Oral microbiome profiles: 16S rRNA pyrosequencing and microarray assay comparison, *PLoS ONE* 6:e22788, 2011.
5. Allison DG: The biofilm matrix, *Biofouling* 19:139, 2003.
6. Amann RI, Ludwig W, Schleifer KH: Phylogenetic identification and in situ detection of individual microbial cells without cultivation, *Microbiol Rev* 59:143, 1995.
7. Anderson AC, Hellwig E, Vespermann R, et al: Comprehensive analysis of secondary dental root canal infections: a combination of culture and culture-independent approaches reveals new insights, *PLoS One* 7:e49576, 2012.
8. Armada-Dias L, Breda J, Provenzano JC, et al: Development of periradicular lesions in normal and diabetic rats, *J Appl Oral Sci* 14:371, 2006.
9. Baumgartner JC: Microbiologic aspects of endodontic infections, *J Calif Dent Assoc* 32:459, 2004.
10. Baumgartner JC, Siqueira JF Jr, Xia T, Rôças IN: Geographical differences in bacteria detected in endodontic infections using polymerase chain reaction, *J Endod* 30:141, 2004.
11. Baumgartner JC, Watkins BJ, Bae KS, Xia T: Association of black-pigmented bacteria with endodontic infections, *J Endod* 25:413, 1999.
12. Baumgartner JC, Watts CM, Xia T: Occurrence of *Candida albicans* in infections of endodontic origin, *J Endod* 26:695, 2000.
13. Baumgartner JC, Xia T: Antibiotic susceptibility of bacteria associated with endodontic abscesses, *J Endod* 29:44, 2003.

14. Beighton D, Hardie JM, Whiley RA: A scheme for the identification of viridans streptococci, *J Med Microbiol* 35:367, 1991.
15. Beloin C, Valle J, Latour-Lambert P, et al: Global impact of mature biofilm lifestyle on Escherichia coli K-12 gene expression, *Mol Microbiol* 51:659, 2004.
16. Bergenholtz G: Micro-organisms from necrotic pulp of traumatized teeth, *Odontol Revy* 25:347, 1974.
17. Blome B, Braun A, Sobarzo V, Jepsen S: Molecular identification and quantification of bacteria from endodontic infections using real-time polymerase chain reaction, *Oral Microbiol Immunol* 23:384, 2008.
18. Bosshard PP, Abels S, Altwegg M, et al: Comparison of conventional and molecular methods for identification of aerobic catalase-negative gram-positive cocci in the clinical laboratory, *J Clin Microbiol* 42:2065, 2004.
19. Bosshard PP, Abels S, Zbinden R, et al: Ribosomal DNA sequencing for identification of aerobic gram-positive rods in the clinical laboratory (an 18-month evaluation), *J Clin Microbiol* 41:4134, 2003.
20. Bowden GH: The microbial ecology of dental caries, *Microb Ecol Health Dis* 12:138, 2000.
21. Brook I: Encapsulated anaerobic bacteria in synergistic infections, *Microbiol Rev Rev* 50:452, 1986.
22. Byström A, Claesson R, Sundqvist G: The antibacterial effect of camphorated paramonochlorophenol, camphorated phenol and calcium hydroxide in the treatment of infected root canals, *Endod Dent Traumatol* 1:170, 1985.
23. Byström A, Happonen RP, Sjogren U, Sundqvist G: Healing of periapical lesions of pulpless teeth after endodontic treatment with controlled asepsis, *Endod Dent Traumatol* 3:58, 1987.
24. Byström A, Sundqvist G: The antibacterial action of sodium hypochlorite and EDTA in 60 cases of endodontic therapy, *Int Endod J* 18:35, 1985.
25. Carr GB, Schwartz RS, Schaudinn C, et al: Ultrastructural examination of failed molar retreatment with secondary

apical periodontitis: an examination of endodontic biofilms in an endodontic retreatment failure, *J Endod* 35:1303, 2009.
26. Chavez de Paz L, Svensater G, Dahlen G, Bergenholtz G: Streptococci from root canals in teeth with apical periodontitis receiving endodontic treatment, *Oral Surg Oral Med Oral Pathol Oral Radiol Endod* 100:232, 2005.
27. Chavez de Paz LE, Dahlen G, Molander A, et al: Bacteria recovered from teeth with apical periodontitis after antimicrobial endodontic treatment, *Int Endod J* 36:500, 2003.
28. Chavez de Paz LE, Molander A, Dahlen G: Gram-positive rods prevailing in teeth with apical periodontitis undergoing root canal treatment, *Int Endod J* 37:579, 2004.
29. Chen V, Chen Y, Li H, et al: Herpesviruses in abscesses and cellulitis of endodontic origin, *J Endod* 35:182, 2009.
30. Cheung GS, Ho MW: Microbial flora of root canal-treated teeth associated with asymptomatic periapical radiolucent lesions, *Oral Microbiol Immunol* 16:332, 2001.
31. Chu FC, Leung WK, Tsang PC, et al: Identification of cultivable microorganisms from root canals with apical periodontitis following two-visit endodontic treatment with antibiotics/steroid or calcium hydroxide dressings, *J Endod* 32:17, 2006.
32. Chugal N, Wang JK, Wang R, et al: Molecular characterization of the microbial flora residing at the apical portion of infected root canals of human teeth, *J Endod* 37:1359, 2011.
33. Chugal NM, Clive JM, Spangberg LS: A prognostic model for assessment of the outcome of endodontic treatment: effect of biologic and diagnostic variables, *Oral Surg Oral Med Oral Pathol Oral Radiol Endod* 91:342, 2001.
34. Costerton B: Microbial ecology comes of age and joins the general ecology community, *Proc Natl Acad Sci U S A* 101:16983, 2004.
35. Costerton JW: *The biofilm primer*, Berlin, Heidelberg, 2007, Springer-Verlag.

36. Costerton JW, Lewandowski Z, Caldwell DE, et al: Microbial biofilms, *Annu Rev Microbiol* 49:711, 1995.

37. Costerton JW, Stewart PS, Greenberg EP: Bacterial biofilms: a common cause of persistent infections, *Science* 284:1318, 1999.

38. Cvek M, Cleaton-Jones PE, Austin JC, Andreasen JO: Pulp reactions to exposure after experimental crown fractures or grinding in adult monkeys, *J Endod* 8:391, 1982.

39. Dahlen G: Microbiology and treatment of dental abscesses and periodontal-endodontic lesions, *Periodontol 2000* 28:206, 2002.

40. de Chevigny C, Dao TT, Basrani BR, Marquis V, et al: Treatment outcome in endodontics: the Toronto study–phase 4: initial treatment, *J Endod* 34:258, 2008.

41. de Sousa EL, Ferraz CC, Gomes BP, et al: Bacteriological study of root canals associated with periapical abscesses, *Oral Surg Oral Med Oral Pathol Oral Radiol Endod* 96:332, 2003.

42. Delivanis PD, Fan VS: The localization of blood-borne bacteria in instrumented unfilled and overinstrumented canals, *J Endod* 10:521, 1984.

43. Dethlefsen L, Eckburg PB, Bik EM, Relman DA: Assembly of the human intestinal microbiota, *Trends Ecol Evol* 21:517, 2006.

44. Dewhirst FE, Chen T, Izard J, et al: The human oral microbiome, *J Bacteriol* 192:5002, 2010.

45. Distel JW, Hatton JF, Gillespie MJ: Biofilm formation in medicated root canals, *J Endod* 28:689, 2002.

46. Dobell C: *Antony van Leeuwenhoek and his "little animals,"* London, 1932, Staples Press.

47. Donlan RM, Costerton JW: Biofilms: survival mechanisms of clinically relevant microorganisms, *Clin Microbiol Rev* 15:167, 2002.

48. Drancourt M, Bollet C, Carlioz A, et al: 16S ribosomal DNA sequence analysis of a large collection of environmental and clinical unidentifiable bacterial isolates, *J Clin Microbiol* 38:3623, 2000.

49. Eckburg PB, Bik EM, Bernstein CN, et al: Diversity of the human intestinal microbial flora, *Science* 308:1635, 2005.

50. Eckburg PB, Lepp PW, Relman DA: Archaea and their potential role in human disease, *Infect Immun* 71:591, 2003.

51. Egan MW, Spratt DA, Ng YL, et al: Prevalence of yeasts in saliva and root canals of teeth associated with apical periodontitis, *Int Endod J* 35:321, 2002.

52. Engelkirk PG, Duben-Engelkirk J, Dowell VR Jr: *Principles and practice of clinical anaerobic bacteriology,* Belmont, CA, 1992, Star Publishing.

53. Evans M, Davies JK, Sundqvist G, Figdor D: Mechanisms involved in the resistance of *Enterococcus faecalis* to calcium hydroxide, *Int Endod J* 35:221, 2002.

54. Fabricius L, Dahlén G, Ohman AE, Möller AJR: Predominant indigenous oral bacteria isolated from infected root canals after varied times of closure, *Scand J Dent Res* 90:134, 1982.

55. Fabricius L, Dahlén G, Sundqvist G, et al: Influence of residual bacteria on periapical tissue healing after chemomechanical treatment and root filling of experimentally infected monkey teeth, *Eur J Oral Sci* 114:278, 2006.

56. Farzaneh M, Abitbol S, Friedman S: Treatment outcome in endodontics: the Toronto study. Phases I and II: orthograde retreatment, *J Endod* 30:627, 2004.

57. Ferreira DC, Paiva SS, Carmo FL, et al: Identification of herpesviruses types 1 to 8 and human papillomavirus in acute apical abscesses, *J Endod* 37:10, 2011.

58. Figdor D: *Microbial aetiology of endodontic treatment failure and pathogenic properties of selected species [odontological dissertation no.79],* Umea, Sweden, 2002, University of Umea.

59. Figdor D, Davies JK, Sundqvist G: Starvation survival, growth and recovery of *Enterococcus faecalis* in human serum, *Oral Microbiol Immunol* 18:234, 2003.

60. Foschi F, Cavrini F, Montebugnoli L, et al: Detection of bacteria in endodontic samples by polymerase chain reaction assays and association with defined clinical signs in Italian patients, *Oral Microbiol Immunol* 20:289, 2005.

61. Fouad AF, Barry J, Caimano M, et al: PCR-based identification of bacteria associated with endodontic infections, *J Clin Microbiol* 40:3223, 2002.

62. Garberoglio R, Brännström M: Scanning electron microscopic investigation of human dentinal tubules, *Arch Oral Biol* 21:355, 1976.

63. Gatti JJ, Dobeck JM, Smith C, et al: Bacteria of asymptomatic periradicular endodontic lesions identified by DNA-DNA hybridization, *Endod Dent Traumatol* 16:197, 2000.

64. Gier RE, Mitchell DF: Anachoretic effect of pulpitis, *J Dent Res* 47:564, 1968.

65. Glick M, Trope M, Bagasra O, Pliskin ME: Human immunodeficiency virus infection of fibroblasts of dental pulp in seropositive patients, *Oral Surg Oral Med Oral Pathol* 71:733, 1991.

66. Gomes BP, Jacinto RC, Montagner F, et al: Analysis of the antimicrobial susceptibility of anaerobic bacteria isolated from endodontic infections in Brazil during a period of nine years, *J Endod* 37:1058, 2011.

67. Gomes BP, Lilley JD, Drucker DB: Clinical significance of dental root canal microflora, *J Dent* 24:47, 1996.

68. Gomes BP, Lilley JD, Drucker DB: Variations in the susceptibilities of components of the endodontic microflora to biomechanical procedures, *Int Endod J* 29:235, 1996.

69. Gomes BP, Pinheiro ET, Jacinto RC, et al: Microbial analysis of canals of root-filled teeth with periapical lesions using polymerase chain reaction, *J Endod* 34:537, 2008.

70. Green BD, Keller M: Capturing the uncultivated majority, *Curr Opin Biotechnol* 17:236, 2006.

71. Griffee MB, Patterson SS, Miller CH, et al: The relationship of *Bacteroides melaninogenicus* to symptoms associated with pulpal necrosis, *Oral Surg Oral Med Oral Pathol* 50:457, 1980.

72. Griffen AL, Beall CJ, Campbell JH, et al: Distinct and complex bacterial profiles in human periodontitis and health revealed by 16S pyrosequencing, *ISME J* 6:1176, 2012.

73. Grossman LI: Origin of microorganisms in traumatized, pulpless, sound teeth, *J Dent Res* 46:551, 1967.

74. Haapasalo M, Ørstavik D: In vitro infection and disinfection of dentinal tubules, *J Dent Res* 66:1375, 1987.

75. Haapasalo M, Ranta H, Ranta K, Shah H: Black-pigmented *Bacteroides* spp. in human apical periodontitis, *Infect Immun* 53:149, 1986.

76. Hall-Stoodley L, Costerton JW, Stoodley P: Bacterial biofilms: from the natural environment to infectious diseases, *Nat Rev Microbiol* 2:95, 2004.

77. Hall-Stoodley L, Stoodley P: Evolving concepts in biofilm infections, *Cell Microbiol* 11:1034, 2009.

78. Handal T, Caugant DA, Olsen I, Sunde PT: Bacterial diversity in persistent periapical lesions on root-filled teeth, *J Oral Microbiol* 1:DOI:10.3402/jom.v1i0.1946, 2009.

79. Happonen RP: Periapical actinomycosis: a follow-up study of 16 surgically treated cases, *Endod Dent Traumatol* 2:205, 1986.

80. Henderson B, Poole S, Wilson M: Bacterial modulins: a novel class of virulence factors which cause host tissue pathology by inducing cytokine synthesis, *Microbiol Rev* 60:316, 1996.

81. Hoshino E, Ando N, Sato M, Kota K: Bacterial invasion of non-exposed dental pulp, *Int Endod J* 25:2, 1992.

82. Hsiao WW, Li KL, Liu Z, et al: Microbial transformation from normal oral microbiota to acute endodontic infections, *BMC Genomics* 13:345, 2012.

83. Huston MA: *Biological diversity*, Cambridge, UK, 1994, Cambridge University Press.

84. Jett BD, Huycke MM, Gilmore MS: Virulence of enterococci, *Clin Microbiol Rev* 7:462, 1994.

85. Jung IY, Choi BK, Kum KY, et al: Molecular epidemiology and association of putative pathogens in root canal infection, *J Endod* 26:599, 2000.

86. Kakehashi S, Stanley HR, Fitzgerald RJ: The effects of surgical exposures of dental pulps in germ-free and conventional laboratory rats, *Oral Surg Oral Med Oral Pathol* 20:340, 1965.

87. Kaufman B, Spangberg L, Barry J, Fouad AF: *Enterococcus* spp. in endodontically treated teeth with and without periradicular lesions, *J Endod* 31:851, 2005.

88. Keijser BJ, Zaura E, Huse SM, et al: Pyrosequencing analysis of the oral microflora of healthy adults, *J Dent Res* 87:1016, 2008.

89. Keren I, Kaldalu N, Spoering A, et al: Persister cells and tolerance to antimicrobials, *FEMS Microbiol Lett* 230:13, 2004.

90. Khemaleelakul S, Baumgartner JC, Pruksakorn S: Identification of bacteria in acute endodontic infections and their antimicrobial susceptibility, *Oral Surg Oral Med Oral Pathol Oral Radiol Endod* 94:746, 2002.

91. Khemaleelakul S, Baumgartner JC, Pruksakom S: Autoaggregation and coaggregation of bacteria associated with acute endodontic infections, *J Endod* 32:312, 2006.

92. Kishen A, Haapasalo M: Biofilm models and methods of biofilm assessment, *Endod Topics* 22:58, 2010.

93. Kolenbrander PE, Andersen RN, Blehert DS, et al: Communication among oral bacteria, *Microbiol Rev Mol Biol Rev* 66:486, 2002.

94. Kumar PS, Griffen AL, Moeschberger ML, Leys EJ: Identification of candidate periodontal pathogens and beneficial species by quantitative 16S clonal analysis, *J Clin Microbiol* 43:3944, 2005.

95. Kuramitsu HK, He X, Lux R, et al: Interspecies interactions within oral microbial communities, *Microbiol Rev Mol Biol Rev* 71:653, 2007.

96. Kuriyama T, Karasawa T, Nakagawa K, et al: Bacteriologic features and antimicrobial susceptibility in isolates from orofacial odontogenic infections, *Oral Surg Oral Med Oral Pathol Oral Radiol Endod* 90:600, 2000.

97. Lana MA, Ribeiro-Sobrinho AP, Stehling R, et al: Microorganisms isolated from root canals presenting necrotic pulp and their drug susceptibility in vitro, *Oral Microbiol Immunol* 16:100, 2001.

98. Langeland K, Rodrigues H, Dowden W: Periodontal disease, bacteria, and pulpal histopathology, *Oral Surg Oral Med Oral Pathol* 37:257, 1974.

99. Li H, Chen V, Chen Y, et al: Herpesviruses in endodontic pathoses: association of Epstein-Barr virus with irreversible pulpitis and apical periodontitis, *J Endod* 35:23, 2009.

100. Li L, Hsiao WW, Nandakumar R, et al: Analyzing endodontic infections by deep coverage pyrosequencing, *J Dent Res* 89:980, 2010.

101. Lin LM, Pascon EA, Skribner J, et al: Clinical, radiographic, and histologic study of endodontic treatment failures, *Oral Surg Oral Med Oral Pathol* 71:603, 1991.

102. Lin LM, Ricucci D, Lin J, Rosenberg PA: Nonsurgical root canal therapy of large cyst-like inflammatory periapical lesions and inflammatory apical cysts, *J Endod* 35:607, 2009.

103. Lin LM, Skribner JE, Gaengler P: Factors associated with endodontic treatment failures, *J Endod* 18:625, 1992.

104. Lleo MM, Bonato B, Tafi MC, et al: Resuscitation rate in different enterococcal species in the viable but nonculturable state, *J Appl Microbiol* 91:1095, 2001.

105. Lleo MM, Bonato B, Tafi MC, et al: Molecular vs culture methods for the detection of bacterial faecal indicators in groundwater for human use, *Lett Appl Microbiol* 40:289, 2005.

106. Love RM: Bacterial penetration of the root canal of intact incisor teeth after a simulated traumatic injury, *Endod Dent Traumatol* 12:289, 1996.

107. Love RM, Jenkinson HF: Invasion of dentinal tubules by oral bacteria, *Crit Rev Oral Biol Med* 13:171, 2002.

108. Machado de Oliveira JC, Siqueira JF Jr, Rôças IN, et al: Bacterial community profiles of endodontic abscesses from Brazilian and USA subjects as compared by denaturing gradient gel electrophoresis analysis, *Oral Microbiol Immunol* 22:14, 2007.

109. Mah TF, O'Toole GA: Mechanisms of biofilm resistance to antimicrobial agents, *Trends Microbiol* 9:34, 2001.

110. Marsh PD: Dental plaque as a microbial biofilm, *Caries Res* 38:204, 2004.

111. Marsh PD: Dental plaque: biological significance of a biofilm and community life-style, *J Clin Periodontol* 32(suppl 6):7, 2005.

112. Matsuo T, Shirakami T, Ozaki K, et al: An immunohistological study of the localization of bacteria invading root pulpal walls of teeth with periapical lesions, *J Endod* 29:194, 2003.

113. Michelich R, Pashley DH, Whitford GM: Dentin permeability: a comparison of functional versus anatomical tubular radii, *J Dent Res* 57:1019, 1978.

114. Michelich VJ, Schuster GS, Pashley DH: Bacterial penetration of human dentin in vitro, *J Dent Res* 59:1398, 1980.

115. Miller WD: An introduction to the study of the bacterio-pathology of the dental pulp, *Dent Cosmos* 36:505, 1894.

116. Mims C, Nash A, Stephen J: *Mims' pathogenesis of infectious diseases*, ed 5, San Diego, 2001, Academic Press.

117. Mogensen TH, Paludan SR: Molecular pathways in virus-induced cytokine production, *Microbiol Rev Mol Biol Rev* 65:131, 2001.

118. Molander A, Reit C, Dahlen G, Kvist T: Microbiological status of root-filled teeth with apical periodontitis, *Int Endod J* 31:1, 1998.

119. Möller AJR: Microbial examination of root canals and periapical tissues of human teeth. *Odontologisk Tidskrift* 74(suppl):1, 1966.

120. Möller AJR, Fabricius L, Dahlén G, et al: Influence on periapical tissues of indigenous oral bacteria and necrotic pulp tissue in monkeys, *Scand J Dent Res* 89:475, 1981.

121. Molven O, Olsen I, Kerekes K: Scanning electron microscopy of bacteria in the apical part of root canals in permanent teeth with periapical lesions, *Endod Dent Traumatol* 7:226, 1991.

122. Moore WEC, Moore LVH: The bacteria of periodontal diseases, *Periodontol 2000* 5:66, 1994.

123. Munson MA, Pitt-Ford T, Chong B, et al: Molecular and cultural analysis of the microflora associated with endodontic infections, *J Dent Res* 81:761, 2002.

124. Nagaoka S, Miyazaki Y, Liu HJ, et al: Bacterial invasion into dentinal tubules of human vital and nonvital teeth, *J Endod* 21:70, 1995.

125. Nair PN, Henry S, Cano V, Vera J: Microbial status of apical root canal system of human mandibular first molars with primary apical periodontitis after "one-visit" endodontic treatment, *Oral Surg Oral Med Oral Pathol Oral Radiol Endod* 99:231, 2005.

126. Nair PNR: Light and electron microscopic studies of root canal flora and periapical lesions, *J Endod* 13:29, 1987.

127. Nair PNR: On the causes of persistent apical periodontitis: a review, *Int Endod J* 39:249, 2006.

128. Ng YL, Mann V, Gulabivala K: A prospective study of the factors affecting outcomes of nonsurgical root canal treatment: part 1: periapical health, *Int Endod J* 44:583, 2011.

129. Noiri Y, Ehara A, Kawahara T, et al: Participation of bacterial biofilms in refractory and chronic periapical periodontitis, *J Endod* 28:679, 2002.

130. Okamura K, Maeda M, Nishikawa T, Tsutsui M: Dentinal response against carious invasion: localization of antibodies in odontoblastic body and process, *J Dent Res* 59:1368, 1980.

131. Okamura K, Tsubakimoto K, Uobe K, et al: Serum proteins and secretory component in human carious dentin, *J Dent Res* 58:1127, 1979.

132. Oosthuizen MC, Steyn B, Theron J, et al: Proteomic analysis reveals differential protein expression by Bacillus cereus during biofilm formation, *Appl Environ Microbiol* 68:2770, 2002.

133. Paiva SS, Siqueira JF Jr, Rôças IN, et al: Molecular microbiological evaluation of passive ultrasonic activation as a supplementary disinfecting step: a clinical study, *J Endod* 39:190, 2013.

134. Parsek MR, Singh PK: Bacterial biofilms: an emerging link to disease pathogenesis, *Annu Rev Microbiol* 57:677, 2003.

135. Pashley DH: Dentin-predentin complex and its permeability: physiologic overview, *J Dent Res* 64 Spec No:613, 1985.

136. Pashley DH: Clinical considerations of microleakage, *J Endod* 16:70, 1990.

137. Pashley DH: Dynamics of the pulpo-dentin complex, *Crit Rev Oral Biol Med* 7:104, 1996.

138. Paster BJ, Boches SK, Galvin JL, et al: Bacterial diversity in human subgingival plaque, *J Bacteriol* 183:3770, 2001.

139. Paster BJ, Olsen I, Aas JA, Dewhirst FE: The breadth of bacterial diversity in the human periodontal pocket and other oral sites, *Periodontol 2000* 42:80, 2006.

140. Peciuliene V, Reynaud AH, Balciuniene I, Haapasalo M: Isolation of yeasts and enteric bacteria in root-filled teeth with chronic apical periodontitis, *Int Endod J* 34:429, 2001.

141. Perez F, Calas P, de Falguerolles A, Maurette A: Migration of a Streptococcus sanguis strain through the root dentinal tubules, *J Endod* 19:297, 1993.

142. Peters LB, van Winkelhoff AJ, Buijs JF, Wesselink PR: Effects of instrumentation, irrigation and dressing with calcium hydroxide on infection in pulpless teeth with periapical bone lesions, *Int Endod J* 35:13, 2002.

143. Peters LB, Wesselink PR, Buijs JF, van Winkelhoff AJ: Viable bacteria in root dentinal tubules of teeth with apical periodontitis, *J Endod* 27:76, 2001.

144. Petti CA, Polage CR, Schreckenberger P: The role of 16S rRNA gene sequencing in identification of microorganisms misidentified by conventional methods, *J Clin Microbiol* 43:6123, 2005.

145. Pinheiro ET, Gomes BP, Ferraz CC, et al: Microorganisms from canals of root-filled teeth with periapical lesions, *Int Endod J* 36:1, 2003.

146. Preza D, Olsen I, Aas JA, et al: Bacterial profiles of root caries in elderly patients, *J Clin Microbiol* 46:2015, 2008.

147. Rappe MS, Giovannoni SJ: The uncultured microbial majority, *Annu Rev Microbiol* 57:369, 2003.

148. Ribeiro AC, Matarazzo F, Faveri M, et al: Exploring bacterial diversity of endodontic microbiota by cloning and sequencing 16S rRNA, *J Endod* 37:922, 2011.

149. Ricucci D, Lin LM, Spangberg LS: Wound healing of apical tissues after root canal therapy: a long-term clinical, radiographic, and histopathologic observation study, *Oral Surg Oral Med Oral Pathol Oral Radiol Endod* 108:609, 2009.

150. Ricucci D, Russo J, Rutberg M, et al: A prospective cohort study of endodontic treatments of 1,369 root canals: results after 5 years, *Oral Surg Oral Med Oral Pathol Oral Radiol Endod* 112:825, 2011.

151. Ricucci D, Siqueira JF Jr: Apical actinomycosis as a continuum of intraradicular and extraradicular infection: case report and critical review on its involvement with treatment failure, *J Endod* 34:1124, 2008.

152. Ricucci D, Siqueira JF Jr: Biofilms and apical periodontitis: study of prevalence and association with clinical and histopathologic findings, *J Endod* 36:1277, 2010.

153. Ricucci D, Siqueira J Jr: Fate of the tissue in lateral canals and apical ramifications in response to pathologic conditions and treatment procedures, *J Endod* 36:1, 2010.

154. Ricucci D, Siqueira JF Jr, Bate AL, Pitt Ford TR: Histologic investigation of root canal-treated teeth with apical periodontitis: a retrospective study from twenty-four patients, *J Endod* 35:493, 2009.

155. Robertson D, Smith AJ: The microbiology of the acute dental abscess, *J Med Microbiol* 58:155, 2009.

156. Robinson HBG, Boling LR: The anachoretic effect in pulpitis: bacteriologic studies, *J Am Dent Assoc* 28:268, 1941.

157. Rôças IN, Baumgartner JC, Xia T, Siqueira JF Jr: Prevalence of selected bacterial named species and uncultivated phylotypes in endodontic abscesses from two geographic locations, *J Endod* 32:1135, 2006.

158. Rôças IN, Hulsmann M, Siqueira JF Jr: Microorganisms in root canal-treated teeth from a German population, *J Endod* 34:926, 2008.

159. Rôças IN, Jung IY, Lee CY, Siqueira JF Jr: Polymerase chain reaction identification of microorganisms in previously root-filled teeth in a South Korean population, *J Endod* 30:504, 2004.

160. Rôças IN, Siqueira JF Jr: Detection of novel oral species and phylotypes in symptomatic endodontic infections including abscesses, *FEMS Microbiol Lett* 250:279, 2005.

161. Rôças IN, Siqueira JF Jr: Characterization of *Dialister* species in infected root canals, *J Endod* 32:1057, 2006.

162. Rôças IN, Siqueira JF Jr: Root canal microbiota of teeth with chronic apical periodontitis, *J Clin Microbiol* 46:3599, 2008.

163. Rôças IN, Siqueira JF Jr: Prevalence of new candidate pathogen: *Prevotella baroniae, Prevotella multisaccharivorax* and as-yet-uncultivated Bacteroidetes clone X083 in primary endodontic infections, *J Endod* 35:1359, 2009.

164. Rôças IN, Siqueira JF Jr: Identification of bacteria enduring endodontic treatment procedures by a combined reverse transcriptase-polymerase chain reaction and reverse-capture checkerboard approach, *J Endod* 36:45, 2010.

165. Rôças IN, Siqueira JF Jr: Comparison of the in vivo antimicrobial effectiveness of sodium hypochlorite and chlorhexidine used as root canal irrigants: a molecular microbiology study, *J Endod* 37:143, 2011.

166. Rôças IN, Siqueira JF Jr: In vivo antimicrobial effects of endodontic treatment procedures as assessed by molecular microbiologic techniques, *J Endod* 37:304, 2011.

167. Rôças IN, Siqueira JF Jr: Characterization of microbiota of root canal-treated teeth with posttreatment disease, *J Clin Microbiol* 50:1721, 2012.

168. Rôças IN, Siqueira JF Jr, Aboim MC, Rosado AS: Denaturing gradient gel electrophoresis analysis of bacterial communities associated with failed endodontic treatment, *Oral Surg Oral Med Oral Pathol Oral Radiol Endod* 98:741, 2004.

169. Rôças IN, Siqueira JF Jr, Andrade AFB, Uzeda M: Identification of selected putative oral pathogens in primary root canal infections associated with symptoms, *Anaerobe* 8:200, 2002.

170. Rôças IN, Siqueira JF Jr, Debelian GJ: Analysis of symptomatic and asymptomatic primary root canal infections in adult Norwegian patients, *J Endod* 37:1206, 2011.

171. Rôças IN, Siqueira JF Jr, Santos KR: Association of *Enterococcus faecalis* with different forms of periradicular diseases, *J Endod* 30:315, 2004.

172. Rolph HJ, Lennon A, Riggio MP, et al: Molecular identification of microorganisms from endodontic infections, *J Clin Microbiol* 39:3282, 2001.

173. Saber MH, Schwarzberg K, Alonaizan FA, et al: Bacterial flora of Dental periradicular lesions analyzed by the 454-pyrosequencing technology, *J Endod* 38:1484, 2012.

174. Sabeti M, Simon JH, Slots J: Cytomegalovirus and Epstein-Barr virus are associated with symptomatic periapical pathosis, *Oral Microbiol Immunol* 18:327, 2003.

175. Sabeti M, Slots J: Herpesviral-bacterial coinfection in periapical pathosis, *J Endod* 30:69, 2004.

176. Sabeti M, Valles Y, Nowzari H, et al: Cytomegalovirus and Epstein-Barr virus DNA transcription in endodontic symptomatic lesions, *Oral Microbiol Immunol* 18:104, 2003.

177. Saboia-Dantas CJ, Coutrin de Toledo LF, Sampaio-Filho HR, Siqueira JF Jr: Herpesviruses in asymptomatic apical periodontitis lesions: an immunohistochemical approach, *Oral Microbiol Immunol* 22:320, 2007.

178. Saito D, de Toledo Leonardo R, Rodrigues JLM, et al: Identification of bacteria in endodontic infections by sequence analysis of 16S rDNA clone libraries, *J Med Microbiol* 55:101, 2006.

179. Sakamoto M, Rôças IN, Siqueira JF Jr, Benno Y: Molecular analysis of bacteria in asymptomatic and symptomatic endodontic infections, *Oral Microbiol Immunol* 21:112, 2006.

180. Sakamoto M, Siqueira JF Jr, Rôças IN, Benno Y: Bacterial reduction and persistence after endodontic treatment procedures, *Oral Microbiol Immunol* 22:19, 2007.

181. Sakamoto M, Siqueira JF Jr, Rôças IN, Benno Y: Molecular analysis of the root canal microbiota associated with endodontic treatment failures, *Oral Microbiol Immunol* 23:275, 2008.

182. Sakamoto M, Siqueira JF Jr, Rôças IN, Benno Y: Diversity of spirochetes in endodontic infections, *J Clin Microbiol* 47:1352, 2009.

183. Santos AL, Siqueira JF Jr, Rôças IN, et al: Comparing the bacterial diversity of acute and chronic dental root canal infections, *PLoS One* 6:e28088, 2011.

184. Sasaki H, Stashenko P: Interrelationship of the pulp and apical periodontitis. In Hargreaves KM, Goodis HE, Tay FR, editors: *Seltzer and Bender's dental pulp*, ed 2, Chicago, 2012, Quintessence Publishing, p 277.

185. Sauer K, Camper AK, Ehrlich GD, et al: Pseudomonas aeruginosa displays multiple phenotypes during development as a biofilm, *J Bacteriol* 184:1140, 2002.

186. Schaudinn C, Carr G, Gorur A, et al: Imaging of endodontic biofilms by combined microscopy (FISH/cLSM—SEM), *J Microsc* 235:124, 2009.

187. Sedgley C, Nagel A, Dahlen G, et al: Real-time quantitative polymerase chain reaction and culture analyses of *Enterococcus faecalis* in root canals, *J Endod* 32:173, 2006.

188. Sedgley CM, Lennan SL, Appelbe OK: Survival of *Enterococcus faecalis* in root canals ex vivo, *Int Endod J* 38:735, 2005.

189. Seltzer S, Farber PA: Microbiologic factors in endodontology, *Oral Surg Oral Med Oral Pathol* 78:634, 1994.

190. Sen BH, Piskin B, Demirci T: Observation of bacteria and fungi in infected root canals and dentinal tubules by SEM, *Endod Dent Traumatol* 11:6, 1995.

191. Sen BH, Safavi KE, Spangberg LS: Colonization of *Candida albicans* on cleaned human dental hard tissues, *Arch Oral Biol* 42:513, 1997.

192. Sen BH, Safavi KE, Spangberg LS: Growth patterns of *Candida albicans* in relation to radicular dentin, *Oral Surg Oral Med Oral Pathol Oral Radiol Endod* 84:68, 1997.

193. Siqueira JF Jr: Microbial causes of endodontic flare-ups, *Int Endod J* 36:453, 2003.

194. Siqueira JF Jr: Periapical actinomycosis and infection with *Propionibacterium propionicum*, *Endod Topics* 6:78, 2003.

195. Siqueira JF Jr: Reaction of periradicular tissues to root canal treatment: benefits and drawbacks, *Endod Topics* 10:123, 2005.

196. Siqueira JF Jr: Microbiology of apical periodontitis. In Ørstavik D, Pitt Ford T, editors: *Essential endodontology*, ed 2, Oxford, UK, 2008, Blackwell Munksgaard, p 135.

197. Siqueira JF Jr: *Treatment of endodontic infections*, London, 2011, Quintessence Publishing.

198. Siqueira JF Jr, Alves FR, Rôças IN: Pyrosequencing analysis of the apical root canal microbiota, *J Endod* 37:1499, 2011.

199. Siqueira JF Jr, Barnett F: Interappointment pain: mechanisms, diagnosis, and treatment, *Endod Topics* 7:93, 2004.

200. Siqueira JF Jr, de Uzeda M: Disinfection by calcium hydroxide pastes of dentinal tubules infected with two obligate and one facultative anaerobic bacteria, *J Endod* 22:674, 1996.

201. Siqueira JF Jr, de Uzeda M, Fonseca ME: A scanning electron microscopic evaluation of in vitro dentinal tubules penetration by selected anaerobic bacteria, *J Endod* 22:308, 1996.

202. Siqueira JF Jr, Fouad AF, Rôças IN: Pyrosequencing as a tool for better understanding of human microbiomes, *J Oral Microbiol* 4:DOI:10.3402/jom.v4i0.10743, 2012.

203. Siqueira JF Jr, Guimarães-Pinto T, Rôças IN: Effects of chemomechanical preparation with 2.5% sodium hypochlorite and intracanal medication with calcium hydroxide on cultivable bacteria in infected root canals, *J Endod* 33:800, 2007.

204. Siqueira JF Jr, Jung IY, Rôças IN, Lee CY: Differences in prevalence of selected bacterial species in primary endodontic infections from two distinct geographic locations, *Oral Surg Oral Med Oral Pathol Oral Radiol Endod* 99:641, 2005.

205. Siqueira JF Jr, Lima KC: *Staphylococcus epidermidis* and *Staphylococcus xylosus* in a secondary root canal infection with persistent symptoms: a case report, *Aust Endod J* 28:61, 2002.

206. Siqueira JF Jr, Lopes HP: Bacteria on the apical root surfaces of untreated teeth with periradicular lesions: a scanning electron microscopy study, *Int Endod J* 34:216, 2001.

207. Siqueira JF Jr, Magalhães KM, Rôças IN: Bacterial reduction in infected root canals treated with 2.5% NaOCl as an irrigant and calcium hydroxide/camphorated paramonochlorophenol paste as an intracanal dressing, *J Endod* 33:667, 2007.

208. Siqueira JF Jr, Paiva SS, Rôças IN: Reduction in the cultivable bacterial populations in infected root canals by a chlorhexidine-based antimicrobial protocol, *J Endod* 33:541, 2007.

209. Siqueira JF Jr, Ricucci D: Periapikale aktinomykose. mikrobiologie, pathogenese und therapie, *Endodontie* 17:45, 2008.

210. Siqueira JF Jr, Rôças IN: Polymerase chain reaction-based analysis of microorganisms associated with failed endodontic treatment, *Oral Surg Oral Med Oral Pathol Oral Radiol Endod* 97:85, 2004.

211. Siqueira JF Jr, Rôças IN: Exploiting molecular methods to explore endodontic infections: Part 1-current molecular technologies for microbiological diagnosis, *J Endod* 31:411, 2005.

212. Siqueira JF Jr, Rôças IN: Exploiting molecular methods to explore endodontic infections: Part 2-redefining the endodontic microbiota, *J Endod* 31:488, 2005.

213. Siqueira JF Jr, Rôças IN: Uncultivated phylotypes and newly named species associated with primary and persistent endodontic infections, *J Clin Microbiol* 43:3314, 2005.

214. Siqueira JF Jr, Rôças IN: Bacterial pathogenesis and mediators in apical periodontitis, *Braz Dent J* 18:267, 2007.

215. Siqueira JF Jr, Rôças IN: Clinical implications and microbiology of bacterial persistence after treatment procedures, *J Endod* 34:1291, 2008.

216. Siqueira JF Jr, Rôças IN: Diversity of endodontic microbiota revisited, *J Dent Res* 88:969, 2009.

217. Siqueira JF Jr, Rôças IN: The microbiota of acute apical abscesses, *J Dent Res* 88:61, 2009.

218. Siqueira JF Jr, Rôças IN: Molecular analysis of endodontic infections. In Fouad AF, editors: *Endodontic microbiology*, Ames, Iowa, 2009, Wiley-Blackwell, p 68.

219. Siqueira JF Jr, Rôças IN, Alves FR, Silva MG: Bacteria in the apical root canal of teeth with primary apical periodontitis, *Oral Surg Oral Med Oral Pathol Oral Radiol Endod* 107:721, 2009.

220. Siqueira JF Jr, Rôças IN, Baumgartner JC, Xia T: Searching for Archaea in infections of endodontic origin, *J Endod* 31:719, 2005.

221. Siqueira JF Jr, Rôças IN, Cunha CD, Rosado AS: Novel bacterial phylotypes in endodontic infections, *J Dent Res* 84:565, 2005.

222. Siqueira JF Jr, Rôças IN, Debelian GJ, et al: Profiling of root canal bacterial communities associated with chronic apical periodontitis from Brazilian and Norwegian subjects, *J Endod* 34:1457, 2008.

223. Siqueira JF Jr, Rôças IN, Lopes HP: Patterns of microbial colonization in primary root canal infections, *Oral Surg Oral Med Oral Pathol Oral Radiol Endod* 93:174, 2002.

224. Siqueira JF Jr, Rôças IN, Lopes HP, et al: Fungal infection of the radicular dentin, *J Endod* 28:770, 2002.

225. Siqueira JF Jr, Rôças IN, Moraes SR, Santos KR: Direct amplification of rRNA gene sequences for identification of selected oral pathogens in root canal infections, *Int Endod J* 35:345, 2002.

226. Siqueira JF Jr, Rôças IN, Paiva SS, et al: Bacteriologic investigation of the effects of sodium hypochlorite and chlorhexidine during the endodontic treatment of teeth with apical periodontitis, *Oral Surg Oral Med Oral Pathol Oral Radiol Endod* 104:122, 2007.

227. Siqueira JF Jr, Rôças IN, Paiva SSM, et al: Cultivable bacteria in infected root canals as identified by 16S rRNA gene sequencing, *Oral Microbiol Immunol* 22:266, 2007.

228. Siqueira JF, Rôças IN, Ricucci D: Biofilms in endodontic infection, *Endod Topics* 22:33, 2010.

229. Siqueira JF Jr, Rôças IN, Rosado AS: Investigation of bacterial communities associated with asymptomatic and symptomatic endodontic infections by denaturing gradient gel electrophoresis fingerprinting approach, *Oral Microbiol Immunol* 19:363, 2004.

230. Siqueira JF Jr, Rôças IN, Souto R, et al: Checkerboard DNA-DNA hybridization analysis of endodontic infections, *Oral Surg Oral Med Oral Pathol Oral Radiol Endod* 89:744, 2000.

231. Siqueira JF Jr, Rôças IN, Souto R, et al: Microbiological evaluation of acute periradicular abscesses by DNA-DNA hybridization, *Oral Surg Oral Med Oral Pathol Oral Radiol Endod* 92:451, 2001.

232. Siqueira JF Jr, Sen BH: Fungi in endodontic infections, *Oral Surg Oral Med Oral Pathol Oral Radiol Endod* 97:632, 2004.

233. Siren EK, Haapasalo MP, Ranta K, et al: Microbiological findings and clinical treatment procedures in endodontic cases selected for microbiological investigation, *Int Endod J* 30:91, 1997.

234. Sjögren U, Figdor D, Persson S, Sundqvist G: Influence of infection at the time of root filling on the outcome of endodontic treatment of teeth with apical periodontitis, *Int Endod J* 30:297, 1997.

235. Sjögren U, Hagglund B, Sundqvist G, Wing K: Factors affecting the long-term results of endodontic treatment, *J Endod* 16:498, 1990.

236. Sjögren U, Happonen RP, Kahnberg KE, Sundqvist G: Survival of *Arachnia propionica* in periapical tissue, *Int Endod J* 21:277, 1988.

237. Slots J: Rapid identification of important periodontal microorganisms by cultivation, *Oral Microbiol Immunol* 1:48, 1986.

238. Slots J, Sabeti M, Simon JH: Herpesviruses in periapical pathosis: an etiopathogenic relationship? *Oral Surg Oral Med Oral Pathol Oral Radiol Endod* 96:327, 2003.

239. Socransky SS, Gibbons RJ, Dale AC, et al: The microbiota of the gingival crevice in man. 1. Total microscopic and viable counts and counts of specific organisms, *Arch Oral Biol* 8:275, 1963.

240. Socransky SS, Haffajee AD: Dental biofilms: difficult therapeutic targets, *Periodontol 2000* 28:12, 2002.

241. Song Y, Liu C, McTeague M, Finegold SM: 16S ribosomal DNA sequence-based analysis of clinically significant gram-positive anaerobic cocci, *J Clin Microbiol* 41:1363, 2003.

242. Stashenko P, Wang CY, Riley E, et al: Reduction of infection-stimulated periapical bone resorption by the biological response modifier PGG glucan, *J Dent Res* 74:323, 1995.

243. Stewart PS, Costerton JW: Antibiotic resistance of bacteria in biofilms, *Lancet* 358:135, 2001.

244. Stoodley P, Sauer K, Davies DG, Costerton JW: Biofilms as complex differentiated communities, *Annu Rev Microbiol* 56:187, 2002.

245. Suau A, Bonnet R, Sutren M, et al: Direct analysis of genes encoding 16S rRNA from complex communities reveals many novel molecular species within the human gut, *Appl Environ Microbiol* 65:4799, 1999.

246. Subramanian K, Mickel AK: Molecular analysis of persistent periradicular lesions and root ends reveals a diverse microbial profile, *J Endod* 35:950, 2009.

247. Sunde PT, Olsen I, Debelian GJ, Tronstad L: Microbiota of periapical lesions refractory to endodontic therapy, *J Endod* 28:304, 2002.

248. Sunde PT, Olsen I, Gobel UB, et al: Fluorescence in situ hybridization (FISH) for direct visualization of bacteria in periapical lesions of asymptomatic root-filled teeth, *Microbiology* 149:1095, 2003.

249. Sunde PT, Tronstad L, Eribe ER, et al: Assessment of periradicular microbiota by DNA-DNA hybridization, *Endod Dent Traumatol* 16:191, 2000.

250. Sundqvist G: *Bacteriological studies of necrotic dental pulps [odontologic dissertation no.7]*, Umea, Sweden, 1976, University of Umea.

251. Sundqvist G: Endodontic microbiology. In Spangberg LSW, editors: *Experimental endodontics*, Boca Raton, 1990, CRC Press, p 131.

252. Sundqvist G: Associations between microbial species in dental root canal infections, *Oral Microbiol Immunol* 7:257, 1992.

253. Sundqvist G: Taxonomy, ecology, and pathogenicity of the root canal flora, *Oral Surg Oral Med Oral Pathol* 78:522, 1994.

254. Sundqvist G, Figdor D: Life as an endodontic pathogen. Ecological differences between the untreated and root-filled root canals, *Endod Topics* 6:3, 2003.

255. Sundqvist G, Figdor D, Persson S, Sjogren U: Microbiologic analysis of teeth with failed endodontic treatment and the outcome of conservative re-treatment, *Oral Surg Oral Med Oral Pathol Oral Radiol Endod* 85:86, 1998.

256. Sundqvist G, Reuterving CO: Isolation of *Actinomyces israelii* from periapical lesion, *J Endod* 6:602, 1980.

257. Tang G, Samaranayake LP, Yip HK: Molecular evaluation of residual endodontic microorganisms after instrumentation, irrigation and medication with either calcium hydroxide or Septomixine, *Oral Dis* 10:389, 2004.

258. Tang YW, Ellis NM, Hopkins MK, et al: Comparison of phenotypic and genotypic techniques for identification of unusual aerobic pathogenic gram-negative bacilli, *J Clin Microbiol* 36:3674, 1998.

259. Tani-Ishii N, Wang CY, Tanner A, Stashenko P: Changes in root canal microbiota during the development of rat periapical lesions, *Oral Microbiol Immunol* 9:129, 1994.

260. Tanner A, Lai C-H, Maiden M: Characteristics of oral gram-negative species. In Slots J, Taubman MA, editors: *Contemporary oral microbiology and immunology*, St Louis, 1992, Mosby, p 299.

261. Tronstad L, Barnett F, Cervone F: Periapical bacterial plaque in teeth refractory to endodontic treatment, *Endod Dent Traumatol* 6:73, 1990.

262. Tronstad L, Barnett F, Riso K, Slots J: Extraradicular endodontic infections, *Endod Dent Traumatol* 3:86, 1987.

263. Tronstad L, Sunde PT: The evolving new understanding of endodontic infections, *Endod Topics* 6:57, 2003.

264. Trowbridge HO, Emling RC: *Inflammation. A review of the process*, ed 5, Chicago, 1997, Quintessence.

265. van Amersfoort ES, van Berkel TJC, Kuiper J: Receptors, mediators, and mechanisms involved in bacterial sepsis and septic shock, *Clin Microbiol Rev* 16:379, 2003.

266. van Winkelhoff AJ, Carlee AW, de Graaff J: *Bacteroides endodontalis* and others black-pigmented *Bacteroides* species in odontogenic abscesses, *Infect Immun* 49:494, 1985.

267. Vera J, Siqueira JF Jr, Ricucci D, et al: One- versus two-visit endodontic treatment of teeth with apical periodontitis: a histobacteriologic study, *J Endod* 38:1040, 2012.

268. Vianna ME, Conrads G, Gomes BPFA, Horz HP: Identification and quantification of archaea involved in primary endodontic infections, *J Clin Microbiol* 44:1274, 2006.

269. Vianna ME, Horz HP, Gomes BP, Conrads G: *In vivo* evaluation of microbial reduction after chemo-mechanical preparation of human root canals containing necrotic pulp tissue, *Int Endod J* 39:484, 2006.

270. Vickerman MM, Brossard KA, Funk DB, et al: Phylogenetic analysis of bacterial and archaeal species in symptomatic and asymptomatic endodontic infections, *J Med Microbiol* 56:110, 2007.

271. Waltimo T, Trope M, Haapasalo M, Ørstavik D: Clinical efficacy of treatment procedures in endodontic infection control and one year follow-up of periapical healing, *J Endod* 31:863, 2005.

272. Waltimo TM, Orstavik D, Siren EK, Haapasalo MP: *In vitro* susceptibility of *Candida albicans* to four disinfectants and their combinations, *Int Endod J* 32:421, 1999.

273. Waltimo TM, Orstavik D, Siren EK, Haapasalo MP: *In vitro* yeast infection of human dentin, *J Endod* 26:207, 2000.

274. Waltimo TM, Siren EK, Orstavik D, Haapasalo MP: Susceptibility of oral *Candida* species to calcium hydroxide in vitro, *Int Endod J* 32:94, 1999.

275. Wara-Aswapati N, Boch JA, Auron PE: Activation of interleukin 1beta gene transcription by human cytomegalovirus: molecular mechanisms and relevance to periodontitis, *Oral Microbiol Immunol* 18:67, 2003.

276. Ward DM, Weller R, Bateson MM: 16S rRNA sequences reveal numerous uncultured microorganisms in a natural community, *Nature* 345:63, 1990.

277. Wayman BE, Murata SM, Almeida RJ, Fowler CB: A bacteriological and histological evaluation of 58 periapical lesions, *J Endod* 18:152, 1992.

278. Wittgow WC Jr, Sabiston CB Jr: Microorganisms from pulpal chambers of intact teeth with necrotic pulps, *J Endod* 1:168, 1975.

279. Woese CR: Bacterial evolution, *Microbiol Rev Rev* 51:221, 1987.

280. Yamasaki M, Kumazawa M, Kohsaka T, et al: Pulpal and periapical tissue reactions after experimental pulpal exposure in rats, *J Endod* 20:13, 1994.

281. Yoshida M, Fukushima H, Yamamoto K, et al: Correlation between clinical symptoms and microorganisms isolated from root canals of teeth with periapical pathosis, *J Endod* 13:24, 1987.

282. Zehnder M, Guggenheim B: The mysterious appearance of enterococci in filled root canals, *Int Endod J* 42:277, 2009.

283. Zoletti GO, Siqueira JF Jr, Santos KR: Identification of *Enterococcus faecalis* in root-filled teeth with or without periradicular lesions by culture-dependent and -independent approaches, *J Endod* 32:722, 2006.

CHAPTER 15

Pathobiology of Apical Periodontitis

LOUIS M. LIN | GEORGE T.-J. HUANG

CHAPTER OUTLINE

Periradicular tissues consist of cementum, periodontal ligament, and alveolar bone. *Cementum* is a mineralized, avascular connective tissue and consists of three different types. Acellular afibrillar cementum covers the teeth at and along the cementoenamel junction. Acellular extrinsic fiber cementum is confined to the coronal half of the root. Cellular intrinsic fiber cementum is present on the apical half of the root where no acellular extrinsic fiber cementum has been laid down.[192] Many growth factors, such as insulin-like growth factor-1 (IGF-1), fibroblast growth factors (FGFs), epidermal growth factor (EGF), bone morphogenetic proteins (BMPs), transforming growth factor-β (TGF-β), and platelet-derived growth factor (PDGF), are contained in the cementum matrix.[47,88,164] These growth factors may be released under certain conditions,

as they have been shown to be associated with cementoblast proliferation, migration, and differentiation during cementum wound healing.[88]

The *periodontal ligament* is a soft, specialized connective tissue that connects the cementum to the alveolar bone. Periodontal ligament contains heterogeneous cell populations and extracellular matrix (ECM).[144,192] The cells of the periodontal ligament include osteoblasts, osteoclasts, fibroblasts, epithelial cell rests of Malassez, macrophages, cementoblasts, and undifferentiated mesenchymal cells (stem cells).[192] Fibroblasts, osteoblasts, and epithelial cells are differentiated cells that have retained the ability to undergo limited cell divisions and proliferation upon stimulation by appropriate signals. Multipotent mesenchymal stem cells of the periodontal ligament are capable of differentiating into cementoblast-like cells and periodontal ligament cells as well as osteoblasts.[112,182,233] The ECM of the periodontal ligament consists of collagen fibers, fibronectin, elastin, other noncollagenous proteins, and proteoglycans. The ECM serves as stratum for cell adhesion and promotes cell spreading and cytoskeletal organization. The collagen fibers (Sharpey fiber) of the periodontal ligament connect the tooth with the alveolar bone. The periodontal ligament is highly vascularized and innervated. The tissue apical to the dentino-cemental junction should be considered as part of the periodontal ligament because cementum is not a normal component of the pulp tissue.

Epithelial cell rests of Malassez (ERM), the remnants of the Hertwig epithelial root sheath that disintegrates after tooth development, are present in the periodontal ligament near the root surface in all teeth after root formation.[209] They are nests of epithelial cells connected as a network and surrounded by a basal lamina.[192,230] ERM are quiescent in normal periodontal ligament[192] but can be stimulated to proliferate in apical periodontitis.[158] They are believed to be the cellular source that when properly stimulated can form radicular cysts in certain apical periodontitis lesions.[158,184,200]

Alveolar bone or *alveolar process* is that part of bone of the jaws housing the sockets for the teeth. It consists of outer cortical plate, a central spongy or cancellous bone, and bone lining the sockets.[192] Bone matrix contains IGFs, TGF-β, BMPs, FGF, and PDGF.[40,250] These growth factors are essential for osteoblast progenitor cell proliferation, migration, and differentiation during bone wound healing.[161]

The response of the periradicular tissues to various injuries is similar to that of other connective tissues elsewhere in the body. The response is manifested as an inflammatory reaction regulated by both innate and adaptive immune mechanisms. Although microbial infection of the pulp in the root canals is the primary cause of apical periodontitis,[119,178,184] the pathologic changes of the periapical tissues in apical periodontitis are usually not directly caused by microbes themselves, but rather by their toxins, noxious metabolic by-products, and disintegrated pulp tissue in the root canal system. These irritants are capable of inducing both innate and adaptive immune responses; they can either activate nonantigenic pathways or serve as antigens to activate adaptive responses. The subsequent inflammatory responses are diverse and can involve changes in microvasculature, transmigration of blood-borne cells and plasma proteins out of the blood circulation into the tissue space, and activation of sensory nerves. In addition, endothelial cells, mast cells, platelets, fibroblasts, neutrophils, macrophages, dendritic cells, innate and adaptive immune cells, immunoglobulins, inflammatory mediators, proinflammatory cytokines, chemokines, and neuropeptides are also involved in the inflammatory response. Apical periodontitis can be protective or destructive, depending on the dynamic interaction between microbial insult and the host's defenses in the periapical tissues. Unfortunately, the bacterial biofilm formed in the root canal system with necrotic pulp is protected from host's defenses and antibiotic therapy because of a lack of blood circulation in the root canal system. Consequently, any attempt of wounded periradicular tissues to repair/ regenerate is futile, because bacterial toxins and noxious metabolic by-products in the root canal system continuously egress into the periapical area and irritate the periapical tissues. Emerging lines of evidence suggest that under most conditions,

bacterial biofilms in the complex root canal system can be greatly reduced, but not eliminated, by conventional endodontic procedures such as mechanical instrumentation, antiseptic irrigation, and intracanal medication. If microbes in the root canal system are effectively eliminated or entombed within the root canal by filling material, and the root canal system is adequately sealed and protected from coronal microleakage, then periradicular tissues have the ability to restore their original structures by means of a repair/regeneration process. Nevertheless, the presence of posttreatment apical periodontitis may be due to persistent microbial biofilms,[76] and this recognition has spurred considerable research into treating biofilms (see Chapters 13 and 14).

APICAL PERIODONTITIS

Prevalence

Epidemiologic study of apical periodontitis documents that the prevalence of apical periodontitis varies among patients aged 20 to 30 (33% prevalence of apical periodontitis), 30 to 40 (40%), 40 to 50 (48%), 50 to 60 (57%), and older than 60 years of age (62%).[203] Most studies on the prevalence of apical periodontitis are from European and Scandinavian countries.[70,117,237] According to a survey by the American Dental Association in 1990, an estimated 14 million root canal treatments were performed in the United States alone.[9] Apical periodontitis is a prevalent health problem.[71]

ETIOLOGY

The etiology, pathogenesis, and histopathology of apical periodontitis are similar to that of marginal periodontitis (see also Chapter 25). Both diseases are caused by bacterial infection and involve pathologic changes of alveolar bone, periodontal ligament, and cementum. Marginal periodontitis affects coronal periodontal tissues, whereas apical periodontitis affects apical periodontal tissues. Bone loss is one of characteristic features in both diseases: crestal bone is lost in marginal periodontitis, and apical bone undergoes resorption in apical periodontitis.

Apical periodontitis can be caused by both exogenous and endogenous factors. Exogenous factors include microbes and their toxins and noxious metabolic by-products, chemical agents, mechanical irritation, foreign bodies, and trauma. Endogenous factors include the host's metabolic products, such as urate and cholesterol crystals,[188] as well as cytokines or other inflammatory mediators that activate osteoclasts.[252] These irritants can activate nonantigenic pathways or antigenic pathways to induce innate and adaptive immunoinflammatory responses, respectively.

In the root canal system, infection of the pulp tissue caused by caries or other pathways is the primary cause of apical periodontitis.[119,178,184,261] The classic study by Kakehashi and colleagues[119] demonstrated that pulp necrosis and periradicular inflammation developed in conventional rats when the pulps of teeth were exposed to oral microorganisms. However, in germ-free laboratory rats, no pulp necrosis and periradicular inflammation occurred even when the pulps of teeth were exposed to the oral environment and packed with sterile food debris. A similar response occurs in humans. Using bacterial culturing, it has been demonstrated that traumatized human teeth with intact crowns and necrotic pulps *without bacterial contamination* did not show radiographic evidence of periapical bone destruction. In contrast, if bacteria were isolated from traumatized teeth with intact crowns and necrotic pulps, then radiographic evidence of periradicular bone destruction was observed.[261] These important findings have been replicated in nonhuman primate experiments. When the pulps of intact vital teeth were intentionally devitalized under aseptic conditions and left in the root canals with bacteria-tight, sealed coronal restoration for 6 months to 1 year, no periradicular inflammatory reaction was observed.[156,178] Taken together, there is considerable evidence that bacteria constitute a major etiologic factor in the development of apical periodontitis.

Bacterial toxins (e.g., lipopolysaccharide [LPS], lipoteichoic acid [LTA]) and noxious metabolic by-products that egress from the root canal system into the periapical tissues are capable of inducing a periapical inflammatory reaction.[53,64,226,311] These substances can activate the innate immune system via receptors that recognize the stereotypic pathogen-associated molecular patterns (PAMPs) that are found in the structure of these toxins. Different classes of microbes express different molecular patterns that are recognized by different pattern recognition receptors (PRRs) or Toll-like receptors (TLRs) on host cells, such as phagocytes, dendritic cells, and B lymphocytes.[1,171,172] PRRs or TLRs are encoded in the germline. In mammalian species, there are at least 10 TLRs, and each appears to have a distinct function in innate immune recognition.[171] For example, LPS can stimulate sensory nerve fibers to release calcitonin gene–related peptide (CGRP) and substance P (SP)[61,107] to cause vasodilation and increased vascular permeability. LPS and lipoproteins can also activate TLRs on dendritic cells to stimulate T lymphocyte differentiation.[4] Certain subtypes of TLRs recognize the common shared structural features of various toxins (i.e., PAMPS). Because the TLRs are synthesized before an infection, they are classified as part of the innate immune system.

Apical periodontitis can be caused either by entry into the periapical tissues of bacterial toxins, enzymes, and noxious metabolic by-products or by direct invasion of the periapical tissues by microbes originating from the root canal system. It is important to differentiate between apical inflammation and apical infection. *Apical inflammation* is the periapical tissue reaction to irritants emerging from the root canal system that manifests as vasodilation, increased vascular permeability, and exudation. In contrast, *apical infection* is due to the physical presence of pathogenic microorganisms in the periapical tissues that subsequently produce tissue damage. There can be infection without inflammation, for instance, in a severely immunocompromised patient. There can also be inflammation without infection, such as in a myocardial infarct, cerebral infarct, and physical or chemical injury.[165] In diseases caused by infection, bacteria are usually present in the involved tissues or organs,[294] such as acute necrotizing gingivitis, marginal periodontitis, actinomycosis, tuberculosis, and bacterial bronchitis. Although apical periodontitis is primarily an infectious disease, bacteria are usually not present in the periapical tissues but in the root canal system,[139,184,296] except in certain cases of apical periodontitis associated with abscess formation,[201,291,303] or with a draining sinus tract,[90,203,301] or extraradicular endodontic infection.[260,284] One major current hypothesis is that apical periodontitis is triggered by entry into the periapical tissues of bacterial toxins, enzymes, and noxious metabolic by-products.[269] The mere presence of bacteria (colonization) in some apical periodontitis lesions does not necessarily denote

a periradicular infection. Periapical infection is related to both virulence and the number and specific combinations of microorganisms in the periapical tissues.[264] Bacteria may be temporarily present in the inflamed periradicular tissues only to be killed by the host's defense mechanisms when the focus of infection in the root canal system is effectively eliminated by mechanical instrumentation, antiseptic irrigation, and intracanal medication. For instance, the majority of apical periodontitis lesions with abscess formation or draining sinus tracts heal satisfactorily after nonsurgical root canal treatment without the need for systemic antimicrobial therapy.[203]

Primary root canal infection in untreated root canals is a polymicrobial mix with approximately equal proportions of gram-positive and gram-negative species, dominated by obligate anaerobes (see Chapter 14).[262,264] In root-filled teeth with apical periodontitis, gram-positive microorganisms, with a relatively equal distribution of facultative and anaerobic species, appear to dominate other microorganisms.[176,265] A high prevalence of *E. faecalis* is frequently observed in filled root canals associated with persistent apical periodontitis.[94,124,176,206,244,264] These issues are described in greater detail in Chapter 14.

Physical (overinstrumentation, overfilling) and chemical (irrigants, intracanal medication, root canal filling materials) insults,[230] as well as traumatic injury[10,11] to the periapical tissues, can also cause apical periodontitis, depending on the severity of injury and cytotoxicity of the chemicals. Foreign bodies, such as root canal filling materials, have been shown to cause persistent periapical inflammation.[133,187,205,313] However, the possibility of bacterial contamination in foreign body–induced apical periodontitis lesions was not carefully ruled out in many studies, so it is possible that the foreign bodies served as carriers for the microorganisms. In addition, foreign bodies have the odd property of favoring infection,[315] as they can lower the infectious dose of bacteria (LL) and cause granulocytes to develop phagocytic defect or loss of ammunition (LL, OK).[314] Although most root canal filling materials are not inert and are capable of inducing certain degrees of inflammation, in general they are biocompatible and well tolerated by periapical tissues.[99]

It has been demonstrated histologically that periodontal disease could cause inflammatory pulpal and periapical disease.[140]

INFECTION: A CONFLICT BETWEEN HOST AND PARASITES

Every infection is a race between the capabilities of the microorganism to multiply, spread, and cause disease and the ability of the host to control and finally eliminate the microorganisms.[294] The host has physical barriers—surface epithelium, enamel, and dentin—as well as innate and adaptive immune defenses to prevent pulpal and periapical infection. Nevertheless, parasites also possess weapons, leading to inhibition of phagocytosis, inhibited lysosomal function, reduced killing by phagocytes, inactivation of complement system and immunoglobulins, and specific mechanisms that permit invasion of the host's physical barriers.[294] Infection of a tissue can manifest different histopathologic features as a result of specific host-parasite interactions that occur. Many infections are asymptomatic in more than 90% of individuals.[294] For instance, pulp necrosis and chronic apical periodontitis caused by root canal infection are usually asymptomatic, and patients are often surprised to find out that this infection has been present for a sufficient time to lead to destruction of periapical bone. Therefore, there is no simple correlation between infection and clinical symptoms of apical periodontitis, except in cases of symptomatic apical periodontitis and acute apical abscess.

PATHOGENESIS

When pulps are infected/inflamed, many innate and adaptive immune cells release elevated amounts of various inflammatory mediators, including cytokines, chemokines, and neuropeptides. As the pulpal inflammation spreads, the inflammatory mediators begin to alter the physiology of the periapical tissues. Clinically, the observable changes on radiographic examination are widening of the periodontal ligament space or development of apical osteolytic lesions due to bone resorption. The loss of bone is mainly caused by activated osteoclasts. Many cytokines, such as interleukin (IL)-1, IL-11, IL-17, and tumor necrosis factor α (TNF-α), are found to have the ability to induce osteoclast progenitor cell differentiation and activation.[24,252] The inflammation-induced bone resorption in the periapical tissues is accompanied by recruitment of immune cells that essentially build a defensive line against the spread of microbial invasion from the root canal.[170] The pathogenesis of apical periodontitis involves innate and adaptive immune responses as well as sensory nerve response in the periapical tissues. Immune cells present in human periradicular lesions consist of lymphocytes, macrophages, plasma cells, neutrophils, dendritic cells, and natural killer (NK) cells with the former two types as the majority.[151,169] The characteristic features of innate and adaptive immunity are summarized in Table 15-1.

Innate Immune Response

Specificity of Innate Immune Response

In recent years, the concept of the nonspecific nature of innate immunity has changed since identification of a network of germline-encoded receptors, the pattern-recognition receptors (PRRs) mentioned earlier, that recognize specific molecular motifs of microorganisms.[5,171] PRRs can be expressed on the cell surface (macrophages, dendritic cells, neutrophils, NK cells, B cells), in intracellular compartments, or secreted into the blood and tissue fluids.[115] There are numerous microbial constitutive and conserved products such as the pathogen-associated molecular patterns (PAMPs), also noted earlier. Importantly, the PRRs of the innate immune system recognize PAMPs.[5,171]

The specificity of innate immunity is due to the recognition of PAMPs of microorganisms by PRRs, such as *Toll-like receptors* (TLRs), of the host's cells. Activation of PRRs triggers numerous host responses, including opsonization, activation of complement and coagulation cascades, phagocytosis, activation of proinflammatory signaling pathways, and induction of apoptosis.[115] For example, TLR4/CD14 is the receptor for the gram-negative bacterial LPS. TLR4-mutated C3H/HeJ mice (LPS hyporesponsive) have reduced response to gram-negative bacteria and are highly susceptible to infection by *Salmonella typhimurium* or *Neisseria meningitidis*.[48] Importantly, there is a reduced expression of IL-1 and IL-12 and decreased periradicular bone destruction in TLR-4 deficient mice when teeth are subjected to pulpal exposures and infection with a mixture

TABLE 15-1		
Features of Innate and Adaptive Immunity		
Property	**Innate**	**Adaptive**
Recognition	Structures shared by groups of related microbes (conserved molecular patterns)	Antigens of microbes and of nonmicrobial antigens (details of molecular structure)
Diversity	Limited	Very large
Memory	None	Yes
Receptors	Encoded in the genome	Encoded in gene segments (somatic recombination)
Blood proteins	Complement	Antibodies
Cells	Macrophages Neutrophis	Lymphocytes Antigen-presenting cells NK cells
Action time	Immediate activation of effectors	Delayed activation of effectors
Response	Costimulatory molecules, cytokines	
(IL-1, IL-6)		
IL-2	Clonal expansion	
Chemokines (IL-8)	Effector cytokines (IL-4, IFN*r*)	

IFN, interferon; *IL*, interleukin; *NK*, natural killer.
Data from Janeway CA, Medzhitov R: Innate immune recognition, *Annu Rev Immunol* 20:197, 2002; Abbas AK, Lichtman AH, Pober JS: *Cellular and molecular immunology*, ed 5, Philadelphia, 2003, Saunders.

of four anaerobic pathogens: *Prevotella intermedia*, *Fusobacterium nucleatum*, *Streptococcus intermedius* (G+), and *Peptostreptococcus micros* (G+).[106] In addition, LPS is shown to be capable of inducing pain via direct activation of TLR4/CD14 expressed on nociceptive sensory neurons.[293] Thus, the TLR4 PRR receptor is importantly involved in odontogenic infections.

Components such as lipoteichoic acid (LTA) of gram-positive bacterial cell walls can also stimulate innate immunity in a way similar to LPS. TLR2 plays a major role in detecting gram-positive bacteria and is involved in the recognition of a variety of microbial components, including LTA, lipoproteins, and peptidoglycan. The importance of TLR2 in the host defense against gram-positive bacteria has been demonstrated using TLR2-deficient (TLR2−/−) mice, which were found to be highly susceptible to challenge with *Staphylococcus aureus* or *Streptococcus pneumoniae*.[66,270] LTA also stimulates leukocytes to release inflammatory mediators, including TNF-α, IL-1β, IL-6, IL-8, and prostaglandin (PG) E2, which are known to play a role in various phases of the inflammatory response. All of these inflammatory mediators have been detected in periapical samples, and each has a well-known tissue-damaging effect by activating various host responses.

The innate immune response to bacterial infection induces expression of proinflammatory cytokines, chemokines, and costimulators, which are essential for activation and influence of the nature of adaptive immune response.[4,172] The innate immune system is capable of recognizing nonself and self-antigens, whereas the adaptive immune system does not; thus, many autoimmune diseases are disorders of adaptive immunity.[172]

Nonspecific Innate Immune Response

The primary nonspecific innate immune defense mechanism in apical periodontitis is phagocytosis of microbes by specialized phagocytes such as polymorphonuclear leukocytes (PMNs) and macrophages. Tissue inflammation leads to the recruitment of PMNs from the blood circulation into the periradicular tissue. Activated PMNs exhibit an abrupt increase in oxygen consumption, the well-known respiratory burst, resulting in the release of oxygen radicals, a family of extremely destructive, short-lived substances that destroy nearby microorganisms and host cells.[15] Phagocytosed microbes or foreign particles are exposed to a toxic environment containing specific and azurophil granules and oxygen-derived free radicals and are eventually degraded.[194] PMNs also possess an extracellular killing mechanism via neutrophil extracellular traps (NETs), which are extracellular structures composed of chromatin with specific proteins from the neutrophilic granules. Upon activation (e.g., by IL-8, LPS, bacteria, fungi, activated platelets), neutrophils start a cellular program called *apoptosis* that leads to their death and the formation of NETs, which have antimicrobial activities.[30,77] Besides their role in the innate immunity as professional phagocytes, macrophages also serve as antigen-presenting cells by expressing MHC (major histocompatibility complex) class II molecules that interact with antigen-specific clones of T-helper lymphocytes. Circulating monocytes are the precursors of both tissue macrophages and many dendritic cell subsets.[1,126,234] The details of the immunologic activities of neutrophils and macrophages in periapical pathosis are described in Chapters 12 and 13.

Adaptive/Specific Immune Response

The specificity of adaptive immunity is regulated at genetic levels in B and T lymphocytes through a complex process leading to the generation of molecules that recognize and bind to foreign or self-antigens. These molecules are specific receptors on T cells (T-cell antigen receptors or TCRs) and on B cells (B-cell antigen receptors or BCRs; also termed *immunoglobulins*). TCRs on T cells interact with antigens that are presented by antigen presenting cells expressing MHC molecules along with other accessory molecules, whereas BCRs on B cells interact with antigens directly. BCRs may be secreted in the blood circulation or in the tissues as antibodies. The variable region of both TCR and BCR proteins are rearranged at the genomic level via genetic recombination of the V(D)J segments. The estimated total diversity after this recombination for TCR is approximately 10^{21} and for BCR is approximately 10^{16} that generates the repertoire of different individual T and B cell clones.[1,116] Each T or B cell clone generated in the bone marrow carries a specific TCR and BCR. They undergo a positive and negative selection process through which most clones are deleted via apoptosis because they bind to self-antigens. This initial "negative screening" process reduces the potential for autoimmune disorders. Only those that do not interact with self-antigens are released into the lymphatic system and blood circulation. The naive T cells circulate back and forth between the lymphatic system and blood circulation until they encounter foreign antigens presented by antigen-presenting cells. About 97% of T cells undergo apoptosis, and only a small percentage of these cells are exported to the periphery as mature T cells.[1]

The interaction between TCR and the antigen peptide/MHC complex and costimulators activates T cells, leading to the synthesis of T-cell growth factor, IL-2, and its receptor that causes T-cell clonal expansion/proliferation. Some of these T cells differentiate into armed, effector T cells, and others become memory cells. There are a number of T-cell subpopulations, categorized by their functions: (1) T helper cells (T_H), (2) T regulatory cells (T_{reg}), (3) T suppressor cells (T_S), and (4) T cytotoxic (cytolytic) (T_C) cells.[1,56,290] Some of them can be distinguished by their cell surface markers, cytokine profiles, or transcriptional factors. See also Chapter 13 for additional details.

Upon antigen stimulation, naive CD4 T cells proliferate and differentiate into T_H0, which are subsequently committed to develop into T_H1 or T_H2 cells. Monocytoid DC (dendritic cell) (DC1) induces T_H1-type responses; plasmacytoid DC (DC2) selectively induces T_H2 responses. Each subset of T_H cells has distinct functions and cytokine profiles. T_H1 cells mainly produce IL-2 and interferon (IFN)-γ, which activate macrophages and induce B cells to produce opsonizing antibody. T_H2 cells produce IL-4, -5, -10, and -13, which activate B cells to make neutralizing antibody. T_H0 can also develop into T_H17 under the activation of IL-6 and TGF-β and produce IL-17, a powerful pro-inflammatory cytokine. Overall, T_H1 and T_H2 have mutually inhibitory effects.[1] The development of CD4 T_H cells involves the encounter of antigen presented by antigen-presenting cells (APCs) in association with class II MHC. All cells express MHC class I, but only certain cells express class II MHC. These class II MHC–expressing cells constitute the body's population of APCs and consist of (1) dendritic cells, (2) macrophages, (3) B cells, (4) vascular endothelial cells, and (5) epithelial cells. The former three are considered "professional" APCs, because they are dedicated to this function. The latter two APCs are quiescent under normal conditions but can be induced to express class II MHC when exposed to elevated concentrations of IFN-γ.[1,116]

Dendritic cells and macrophages phagocytose foreign antigens, whereas B cells utilize the membrane-bound immunoglobulin to bind and internalize antigens. Other APCs endocytose foreign antigens into the cytoplasm for antigen processing. The processed antigens are partially degraded into small peptides. Many of them are 10 to 30 amino acids long and capable of binding onto the newly synthesized class II MHC molecules before the antigen/class II MHC complex is transported to the surface of cells and presented to TCRs of CD4$^+$ T cells.

Although controversial, evidence has suggested that CD8$^+$ T_S and CD8$^+$ CTLs represent distinct subpopulations of CD8$^+$ T cells. T_S are MHC class I–restricted CD8$^+$/CD28$^-$ T_S cells, which act on antigen-presenting cells (APC) by a contact-dependent manner, rendering them tolerogenic to T_H cells. They inhibit the proliferation of T_H cells.[50,316] T cytotoxic cells (CD8^+T_C), also known as *cytolytic T lymphocytes* (CTLs), are a subset of T cells that kill target cells expressing MHC-associated peptide antigens. The majority of T_C express CD8 and recognize antigens degraded in the cytosol and expressed on the cell surface in association with class I MHC molecules of the target cells. Functional T_C acquire specific membrane-bound cytoplasmic granules, including a membrane pore-forming protein called *perforin* or *cytolysin* and enzymes called *granzymes*.[1]

The role of B cells in adaptive immunity is mainly the production of antibodies that constitute the host humoral immune response. The V(D)J gene recombination occurs in both heavy and light (κ and λ) chains. A recombinase system, which is an enzymatic complex consisting of several enzymes—including recombination activating gene 1 and 2 (RAG-1, RAG-2), terminal deoxynucleotidyl transferase (TdT), DNA ligase IV, Ku proteins, and XRCC4—is essential for successful recombination. This recombinase system is also used for TCR recombination. Mature IgM/IgD coexpressing B cells undergo isotype switching via a process called *switch recombination* after encountering antigen. The rearranged V(D)J gene segment recombines with a downstream C region gene (γ, ε, or α), and the intervening DNA sequence is deleted. This gives rise to other classes of immunoglobulins (IgG, IgE, IgA) besides IgM. In addition to isotype switching, activated B cells also undergo somatic mutation in the V region gene, leading to affinity maturation of antibodies and alternative splicing of VDJ RNA to membrane or secreted immunoglobulin mRNA. A large quantity of antibody is secreted when B cells terminally differentiate into plasma cells.[1,116] The ability of antigens to selectively stimulate the differentiation of plasma cells supports the clinical finding that plasma cells isolated from periapical lesions secrete antibodies specific for the particular bacteria found in the adjacent root canal system.

The immune response and the role of lymphocyte subpopulations in apical periodontitis lesions were investigated by employing lymphocyte-deficient rodents as study models. T-cell deficiency appears to accelerate bone loss at the early phase of apical periodontitis lesions (2 weeks) but does not affect the overall course of lesion development.[271,295] Using RAG (recombination activating)-2 SCID mice (both T- and B-cell-deficient), it was found that approximately a third of the RAG-2 mice developed endodontic abscesses, whereas no immunocompetent controls had abscesses.[273] In another study, specific RAG 2 knockout (k/o) mice were used to determine which immune element was important for the defense mechanism in endodontic infection. The results demonstrated that B cells, but not T cells, played a pivotal role in preventing dissemination of endodontic infection.[105] Therefore, both T and B cells mediate the observed immune responses in apical periodontitis lesions.[170]

Neurogenic Inflammation

Certain primary afferent nerve fibers, upon stimulation by various irritants, release neuropeptides, which cause vasodilation, protein extravasation, and recruitment/regulation of immune cells such as macrophages, neutrophils, mast cells, and lymphocytes. This phenomenon is termed *neurogenic inflammation*.[26,29] Pivotal neuropeptides in the induction of neurogenic inflammation are CGRP, for vasodilation, and SP, for the induction of protein extravasation. Neuropeptides and their receptors are widely distributed throughout the body. During inflammation, there is a sprouting of afferent fibers[38,39,96] and local increases in inflammatory mediators that trigger neuropeptide release, leading to neurogenic inflammation.[26,43] Besides the cardinal functions of the key neuropeptides that cause the first sign of inflammation—vasodilation and increased vascular permeability—the role of these

neuropeptides in the process of inflammation is now known to be far more complex. In the development of chronic apical periodontitis lesions, neuropeptides are also involved in immune regulation, bone resorption, and wound healing. At sufficient concentrations, SP increases the secretion of IL-1, TNF-α, and IL-6 from macrophages and stimulates T-lymphocyte proliferation and enhances antigen-induced IFN-γ production by T cells.[253] Certain neuropeptides, such as SP, upregulate immune and inflammatory responses, whereas other neuropeptides, such as vasoactive intestinal peptide (VIP) and neuropeptide Y (NPY), inhibit inflammatory responses. Synergistic interactions among neuropeptides, such as CGRP and other inflammatory mediators, eicosanoids, and bradykinin, suggest a complex interplay between these molecules in the immune response.[83,211,253]

In chronic apical periodontitis lesions, specific receptors for SP and CGRP are expressed in certain immune cells, including macrophages and lymphocytes. Both CGRP and VIP may play a role in inhibiting bone resorption by suppressing osteoclastic functions. The level of VIP in apical periodontitis lesions is inversely related to lesion size. Osteoclast cell culture studies have demonstrated that the presence of greater concentrations of VIP leads to a decrease in their ability to form lacunae of osseous resorption, causing rapid cytoplasmatic contraction and reduced cell mobility. VIP exerts an effect on macrophages to block the production of TNF-α, IL-6, and IL-12, suggesting that VIP could have a role in controlling growth of apical periodontitis lesions.[43]

The major innate and adaptive immune responses and neurogenic inflammation in the pathogenesis of apical periodontitis caused by root canal infection are illustrated in Fig. 15-1.

DIAGNOSIS

Correlation Between Clinical and Histologic Findings

Clinical diagnosis of inflammatory periapical disease is mainly based on clinical signs or symptoms, duration of disease, pulp tests, percussion, palpation, and radiographic findings (see also Chapter 1). In contrast, a histologic diagnosis is a morphologic and biologic description of cells and extracellular matrix of diseased tissues. The clinical diagnosis represents a provisional diagnosis based on signs, symptoms, and testing results, whereas the histologic diagnosis is a definitive diagnosis of tissue disease.

Similar to pulpitis,[231,238] apical periodontitis is not always symptomatic or painful. Although many inflammatory mediators (histamine, bradykinin, prostaglandins) and proinflammatory cytokines (IL-1, IL-6, TNF, nerve growth factor [NGF]), as well as neuropeptides (SP, CGRP), are capable of sensitizing and activating nociceptive sensory nerve fibers,[96,97] other mediators such as endogenous opioids and somatostatin released by inflammatory cells during inflammation are able to inhibit firing of sensory nerve fibers.[102,236] Activation of nociceptive sensory nerve fibers may also be related to concentrations of inflammatory mediators. The complexity of these findings supports the clinical observation that there is no good correlation between clinical symptoms and histopathologic findings of apical periodontitis.[27,159] For example, many teeth with apical periodontitis are free of symptoms.

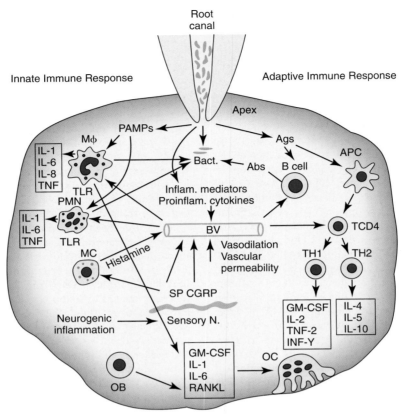

FIG. 15-1 Major innate and adaptive immune responses and neurogenic inflammation in the pathogenesis of apical periodontitis. *APC,* antigen presenting cell; *GM-CSF,* granulocyte/monocyte colony-stimulating factor; *MC,* mast cell; *Mφ,* macrophage; *OB,* osteoblast; *OC,* osteoclast; *PAMPs,* pathogen-associated molecular patterns; *PMN,* polymorphonuclear leukocyte; *RANKL,* receptor activator of nuclear factor κB ligand; *TLR,* Toll-like receptor. (Courtesy Dr. Lin.)

Correlation Between Radiographic and Histologic Findings

Radiography is designed to detect pathologic changes at tissue not cellular levels. Even using sensitive imaging systems such as ultrasound, cone-beam computed tomography, and other technologies, it is impossible to detect the presence of inflammatory cells or other subtle changes in the periapical tissues. Using conventional radiographic and histologic methods in the same cadavers, evidence of inflammation was often observed in the periapical tissues of endodontically treated teeth with normal radiographic features.[17,36,85] This finding is supported by the fact that lesions localized in the cancellous bone may not be visible radiographically unless they involve cortical bone (see also Chapter 2).[20,22,109] In addition, radiographic findings are unable to predict asymptomatic apical periodontitis (granuloma) from asymptomatic apical periodontitis with cyst formation (radicular cyst).[141,267] Accordingly, radiographic findings and histopathologic features of apical periodontitis have a poor correlation based on available case series studies.

The absence of clinical symptoms and negative periapical radiographic findings of endodontically involved teeth does not necessarily indicate absence of apical periodontitis.[17] By the same token, clinical success of endodontically involved teeth (i.e., absence of signs and symptoms and negative periapical radiographic findings) after nonsurgical root canal therapy does not necessarily imply complete histologic healing

of periapical lesions. Thus, currently available diagnostic methods used in endodontics, such as percussion, palpation, and pulp tests (cold, heat, electric), are not sensitive enough to provide histologic diagnosis of an inflammatory periapical disease. In fact, all endodontic tests are basically used to examine the functions of nociceptive sensory nerves and not the pathologic changes of the pulp or periapical tissues. Until we have more advanced and sophisticated clinical diagnostic technologies, we will continue to face the problem of clinical diagnosis of inflammatory periapical disease. Nevertheless, the treatment of various types of apical periodontitis lesions is basically the same: nonsurgical root canal therapy. Interestingly, this treatment does provide a consistently good clinical outcome, as measured by either clinical signs of success or survival of the treated tooth. Future research should focus on developing testing methods that provide greater insight into the status of the periapical tissue.

HISTOPATHOLOGY

The study of the histopathology of diseased tissues and organs has gone through an interesting evolution. It began at macroscopic, light microscopic, and then electron microscopic observations of diseased tissues and organs. Nowadays, histopathology focuses on cellular and molecular biology of diseased tissues and organs. Biochemical disorders occur inside the cells before light and electron microscopic observable morphologic changes of cell injury. Cell death (protein denaturation) occurs before observable morphologic changes of cell necrosis. Gene transformation or mutation occurs before observable morphologic changes of neoplastic cells.[165]

Based on etiology, clinical signs and symptoms, and duration of the disease process, the World Health Organization (WHO) classifies disease of periapical tissues into many categories.[307] There are also many classifications of inflammatory periradicular disease in several endodontic textbooks[110,203,282] and by the American Board of Endodontists, depending on clinical manifestations and histologic appearances. In addition, the American Association of Endodontists held a consensus conference on diagnostic terms in the fall of 2008. Traditionally, there has been a lack of consensus on clinical diagnostic terminology of pulpal and periapical disease in the endodontic community because of the paucity of studies with high levels of evidence. Because this chapter focuses on pathobiology of apical periodontitis, inflammatory periapical disease will be classified based on histologic appearances and cell biology of the injured periapical tissues. To avoid confusion between histologic and clinical diagnosis, readers are encouraged to read the chapters related to clinical examination, radiographic interpretation, and clinical diagnosis of inflammatory periapical disease (see Chapters 1, 2, and 3).

The histopathologic analysis of a diseased tissue or organ only shows structural changes of cells and extracellular matrix at the time the tissue or organ is removed. Therefore, it does not represent the complete kinetics or spectrum of disease development. Histologic classification of apical periodontitis is based on types of cells participating in inflammatory responses in the periapical tissues. In general, inflammation can be divided into acute and chronic responses, depending on types of cells present at the site of injured tissue.[137,165,248,299] Acute inflammatory response is characterized by participation of neutrophilic leukocytes and chronic inflammatory response by participation of macrophages and lymphocytes. However, many factors, such as severity of tissue injury, specific etiology, host's resistance, and particular tissue involved, can modify the course and morphologic variations as well as cell biology of both acute and chronic inflammatory responses.[137,165] Acute and chronic inflammatory responses are in fact not rigid phases of a single programmed event but two overlapping responses with partially different triggering mechanisms and programs.[165]

SYMPTOMATIC APICAL PERIODONTITIS

It is a general belief that the development of apical periodontitis follows total pulp necrosis. This belief is based on (1) the pulpal strangulation theory due to a generalized increase in pulpal interstitial pressure inside the uncompromised pulp space during pulpal inflammation that causes collapse of venules and cessation of blood flow[96] and (2) animal and human studies that concluded that uncontaminated necrotic pulps that are intentionally devitalized or accidentally traumatized are generally incapable of inducing periapical inflammation unless they are infected.[156,178,261] However, if the vital pulps become infected due to caries or other pathways, periapical inflammation can develop even when inflamed, but vital tissue is still present in the apical portion of the root canal. Most of our information related to the histopathology of apical periodontitis comes from analysis of longstanding, chronic human lesions caused by caries or from time-course studies of development of apical periodontitis induced by artificial root canal infection in animals. In these instances, the moment of transition from pulpitis to apical periodontitis was not captured. In fact, apical periodontitis has been demonstrated to be a direct extension of apical pulpitis into the periapical tissues before total pulp necrosis caused by root canal infection (Fig. 15-2).[135,154,155,214,215,268] For example, Kovacevic and colleagues[135] studied the transition from pulpitis to apical periodontitis in dogs' teeth by artificial exposure of pulps to the

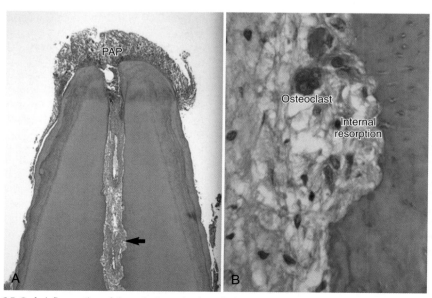

FIG. 15-2 A, Inflammation of the pulp tissue in the apical root canal extends into the periapical tissues in a mature tooth (H&E, magnification: ×100). **B,** Arrow in (**A**). High magnification of the pulp tissue in the apical root canal in **A**. The pulp tissue is vital and infiltrated with chronic inflammatory cells. Note resorption of canal wall and multinucleated clast cells (H&E magnification: ×200). (Courtesy Dr. Domenico Ricucci, Rome, Italy.)

oral cavity and observed that pulpitis was coupled with an acute apical periodontitis. Similarly, Kimberly and Byers[128] demonstrated that periapical changes, including sprouting of nerve fibers, appeared 3 to 5 weeks following establishment of irreversible pulpitis subsequent to pulp exposure lesions in animals. Yamasaki and coworkers[310] and Stashenko and colleagues[255] also showed that periapical inflammatory infiltrates, increased osteoclast numbers, and bone destruction were apparent well in advance of total pulpal necrosis, with vital pulp tissue still present in the apical portion of the root canal. The biologic basis for these observations appears to hinge on the apical development of pulpal infection/inflammation leading to the diffusion of many inflammatory mediators, pro-inflammatory cytokines, chemokines, and bacterial toxins into the periapical area[154] prior to total pulpal necrosis.

The development of acute apical periodontitis largely reflects the innate immune system and is the first line of active defense against irritants from the root canal. Acute apical periodontitis is an immediate defense reaction to irritants and does not require exquisite specificity and memory. Characteristic features of acute apical periodontitis are similar to the typical acute inflammatory reaction and consist of vasodilation, increased vascular permeability, and transmigration of leukocytes from the blood vessels into perivascular tissue space. The beneficial actions of acute inflammation are (1) infiltration of leukocytes to the injured tissue to phagocytose and kill microbial agents; (2) accumulation and activation of humoral factors such as immunoglobulins, complement factors, and plasma proteins in the injured tissue to recruit more neutrophils and macrophages; and (3) neutralization or degradation of bacterial toxins and their harmful metabolic by-products.[137,165]

Cell Biology

The inflammatory response is a dynamic interaction between host defense mechanisms and microbial insults. The interlacing activation and control pathways of cellular and humoral components involved in the inflammatory response are complex. The cells involved—neutrophils, monocytes/macrophages, platelets, mast cells, T lymphocytes, B lymphocytes, NK cells, dendritic cells, endothelial cells, fibroblasts, eosinophils, and basophils—each have numerous functions that are activated and modulated by a multiplicity of biochemical messengers.[1,137,165] *Cell activation* means that the cell acquires the ability to perform one or more new functions or to perform normal functions at a higher rate[1]; it often results in transcription of new genes and synthesis of new proteins.[1]

Mast Cells

Histamine stored in the cytoplasmic granules of mast cells is the mediator that first appears in acute inflammation to induce vasodilation and increased vascular permeability; mast cells are the designated triggers of acute inflammation. They are widely distributed in perivascular tissue spaces and originate in the bone marrow from precursor cells. Mature mast cells contain numerous cytoplasmic granules, which are the source of vasoactive mediators. The preformed histamine is released by mast cell degranulation and can be triggered by (1) physical stimuli such as cold, heat, and mechanical trauma; (2) binding of IgE-specific antigen to mast cells and membrane-bound IgE antibodies; (3) binding of complement components (C3a and C5a) to their complementary receptors on mast cells; and (4) stimulation by neuropeptide (SP) and cytokines (IL-1, IL-8).[1,29,137,165]

In addition, activated mast cells secret cytokines (TNF-α, IL-1, IL-3, IL-4, IL-5, IL-6, IL-13), prostaglandins, and leukotrienes to enhance inflammatory defense mechanisms.[1,37,126]

Endothelial Cells

Endothelial cells are important players in the inflammatory response. Without the participation of endothelial cells, the host is unable to deliver its cellular and humoral defense components from the circulating blood to the site of tissue injury. Inflammatory mediators, complement components, proinflammatory cytokines, nitric oxide, neuropeptides, and bacterial toxins can all affect endothelial cells, resulting in vasodilation and increased vascular permeability.[1,137,165] IL-1 and TNF released by activated macrophages and NK cells can stimulate endothelial cells to express intercellular adhesion molecules (ICAMs), such as ICAM-1, ICAM-2, ICAM-3, vascular cell adhesion molecule (VCAM), and platelet endothelial cell adhesion molecule (PECAM), which enhance leukocyte adhesion to endothelial cells and transmigration through the blood vessels.[1,137,148,165] IL-1, TNF, and LPS also can activate endothelial cells to synthesize chemokine (IL-8), a potent chemotactic mediator for neutrophils.[1]

Polymorphonuclear Neutrophilic Leukocytes

Polymorphonuclear neutrophilic leukocytes (PMNs) are the principal effector cells in acute apical periodontitis. They are derived from bone marrow stem cells. Neutrophils have a lobulated nucleus and contain primary or azurophil (elastase and myeloperoxidase) and secondary or specific (lysozyme and other protease) granules in their cytoplasm.[126,137,165] Neutrophils are only present in the blood circulation. They are the first leukocytes to transmigrate through the blood vessels into perivascular tissue space and then are directed toward the wound or irritants, peaking at 24 to 48 hours. The transmigration of neutrophilic leukocytes from the blood vessels into perivascular space involves complex cellular and molecular biology. Following vasodilation and increased vascular permeability, leukocyte margination, rolling, capture, and activation in the blood vessel and then transmigration through the blood vessel are mediated by an intricate interaction of cell adhesion molecules expressed on leukocytes (L-selectin, integrins) and on endothelial cells (P- and E-selectins, ICAM, VCAM, PECAM-1). Neutrophil rolling is mediated by interaction between leukocyte selectin ligands and P-selectins on endothelial cells. Leukocyte sticking is mediated by interaction between leukocyte integrins and ICAMs and VCAMs on endothelial cells. Leukocyte transmigration is mediated by interaction between PECAM-1 on both leukocytes and endothelial cells.[165] Chemokines (IL-8) increase the affinity of leukocyte integrins for their ligands on endothelial cells.[1] Once transmigrating through the junction between endothelial cells and basement membrane into the perivascular tissue space, neutrophilic leukocytes are directed toward stimuli by chemotactic factors or chemotaxins, such as bacterial products (fLMP), C3a, C5a, leukotriene B4 (LTB4), platelet-activating factor (PAF), fibrinopeptides, dead cells, and chemokines (IL-8) by receptor-mediated mechanisms.[1,137,165,248]

Neutrophils can be activated by bacteria and pathogen-associated molecular patterns (also known as the TLRs, described earlier). They can also be stimulated by IL-1, TNF, and chemokines produced by activated macrophages and NK cells to enhance the phagocytic activity of infectious agents and synthesis of defensins, which are broad-spectrum antibiotics.[1] Neutrophilic leukocytes are terminally differentiated cells and short lived—within hours to a few days. Most neutrophilic leukocytes in acute inflammatory response die as a result of apoptosis or programmed cell death. The apoptotic neutrophils are phagocytosed by macrophages.[89,137,165] However, some neutrophilic leukocytes die after a furious battle against microbial infection and release intracellular proteolytic lysosomal enzymes, oxygen-derived active metabolites, nitric oxide, proinflammatory cytokines, eicosanoids, and matrix metalloproteinases into tissue to intensify inflammation and tissue damage.[137,165] The release of lysosomal enzymes by neutrophils and macrophages can also occur by lysosomal suicide due to rupture of phagolysosome in the cytosol, regurgitation during phagocytosis of irritants, or frustrated phagocytosis of indigestible foreign bodies.[137,165] The main effector functions of neutrophilic leukocytes are phagocytosis, killing of microbes, and release of inflammatory mediators (including proinflammatory cytokines) to recruit more leukocytes to prevent spread of infection.

Macrophages

Macrophages make their appearance as a second wave in acute apical periodontitis within 48 to 96 hours. Macrophages are blood-borne but have a counterpart in the connective tissue.[165] Blood monocytes transmigrate through the blood vessel into the tissues and become macrophages. Mature macrophages have an irregular-shaped nucleus and contain abundant lysosomes and many phagocytic vesicles (phagosomes). Monocytes use mechanisms similar to neutrophils to adhere to endothelial cells in high endothelial venule–expressing adhesion molecules for mononuclear leukocytes (ICAM for macrophages and VCAM for lymphocytes); they then transmigrate through the blood vessel and are directed toward the site of tissue injury by chemotactic factors.[165]

Macrophages can be activated by bacteria, PAMPs, and interferon-r (INF-r) and produce numerous products: lysosomal enzymes, coagulation factors, bioactive lipids, reactive oxygen species, chemokines, cytokines/growth factors, and angiogenesis factors.[137,165,248] Macrophages are the most dynamic and versatile leukocytes. The main functions of macrophages are numerous. They include phagocytosis of microbes and foreign bodies, production of inflammatory mediators, initiation of the immune response, cleanup operation of necrotic cells and tissue, induction of systemic effects (fever, acute phase reaction, cachexia), synthesis of molecules or cytokines affecting cell and vascular growth in wound healing, as well as antibacterial and antiviral defenses.[165] Tissue macrophages are not terminally differentiated cells and are able to undergo mitosis. Their life span is from several weeks to months.

Activated neutrophilic leukocytes and macrophages are capable of phagocytosing and killing pathogens. They recognize microbes through TLRs and receptors for the Fc fragment of immunoglobulin IgG as well as complement component C3b on their cell surface. C3b opsonization and antibody coating of microbes enhance recognition and phagocytosis of pathogens by activated neutrophilic leukocytes and macrophages.[1,137,165] Activated neutrophilic leukocytes are effective in phagocytosing and killing extracellular microbes, whereas macrophages activated by IFN-r produced by NK cells and T_H1 cells are more effective in phagocytosing and killing

intracellular microbes.[1] Killing of phagocytosed microbes by neutrophilic leukocytes and macrophages is mediated through oxygen-dependent and oxygen-independent mechanisms. Oxygen-dependent mechanisms are more effective in killing all kinds of bacteria than oxygen-independent mechanisms.[1,137,248] The effector molecules of an oxygen-dependent system are hydrogen peroxide, superoxide anion, hydroxyl radical, singlet oxygen, and hypochlorite. An oxygen-independent system is also important in killing microbes and is dependent on lysozymes, defensins, and lactoferrin contained in phagocyte granules.[1,137,165,248] Some antimicrobial peptides and other oxygen-independent mechanisms possessed by phagocytes are specialized for killing of certain groups of microbes.[1,248]

Microbes phagocytosed by phagocytes are enclosed in membrane-bound phagosomes in the cytosol. The phagosomes fuse with lysosomes to form phagolysosomes. Irritants such as microbes, foreign protein antigens, and dead cells inside the phagolysosome are destroyed or degraded by proteolytic enzymes stored in lysosomes.[1] There are also granules that are fused with the nascent phagosome and release their contents into the phagosome. Some of these granules have direct antimicrobial action, such as defensins and the bactericidal permeability-increasing protein azurocidin. Others are proteases, such as elastase and cathepsins, lactoferrin, and peroxidase myeloperoxidase. Lysosomal enzymes, reactive oxygen intermediates, and nitric oxide released by neutrophils and macrophages indiscriminately kill not only bacteria but also tissue cells. Much of periapical tissue damage that occurs during acute inflammation can be attributed to release of proteolytic lysosomal enzymes and matrix metalloproteinases from disintegrated neutrophilic leukocytes and macrophages rather than to bacteria and their toxins.[1,165]

Platelets

Platelets normally circulate in the blood but also play an important role in inflammation. They are small cytoplasmic fragments derived from the megakaryocyte.[126] Platelets are essential for blood clotting, hemostasis, and fibrinolysis. Platelets produce vasoactive amines (PAF, serotonin), chemokines, and growth factors (PGDF, FGF, TGF) during inflammation.[165]

Natural Killer Cells

NK cells may also be players in acute apical periodontitis. They are a subset of lymphocytes found in blood and lymphoid tissues. NK cells are derived from the bone marrow stem cells but lack the specific T-cell receptor for antigen recognition.[1] NK cells also possess TLRs for microbial constitutive and conserved products. The effector functions of NK cells are to lyse virus-infected cells without expressing class 1 MHC molecules and to secret IFN-r to activate macrophages. Antibody-coated cells, cells infected by viruses, some intracellular bacteria, and IL-2 released by activated macrophages can activate NK cells. Viruses have been isolated in apical periodontitis lesions.[218,249] NK cells kill target cells by antibody-dependent cell-mediated cytotoxicity because NK cells express receptor for the Fc fragment of IgG.[1] NK cells provide a link between the innate and adaptive immune systems.[115]

Inflammatory Mediators

Numerous biochemical mediators are involved in the acute innate inflammatory response. They are mainly derived from

TABLE 15-2

Major Mediators in Inflammation

Mediator	Source	Effector Cells and Tissues	Mediator	Source	Effector Cells and Tissues
Vasodilator			Chemokines	Macrophages Neutrophils Endothelial cells Fibroblasts	Endothelial cells
Histamine	Mast cells Platelets	Endothelial cells	**Leukocyte Activation and Chemotaxis**		
Prostaglandins	Leukocytes Mast cells	Endothelial cells	C3a, C5a	Plasma	Leukocytes
Nitric oxide	Endothelial cells Macrophages	Vascular smooth muscle	Leukotriene B4	Mast cells Leukocytes	Leukocytes
CGRP	Sensory nerve	Endothelial cells	Chemokines (IL-8)	Macrophages Neutrophils Endothelial cells Fibroblasts	Leukocytes
Fibrin degradation products	Plasma	Endothelial cells			
Increased Vascular Permeability			Fibrinopeptides	Plasma	Leukocytes
Bradykinin	Plasma	Endothelial cells	Bacterial products (fMLP)	Bacteria	Leukocytes
Leukotrienes C4, D4, E4	Leukocytes Mast cells	Endothelial cells	TNF	Activated macrophages Dead cells	Leukocytes
PAF	Leukocytes Mast cells Endothelial cells	Endothelial cells	**Opsonins**		
C3a, C5a	Plasma	Endothelial cells	C3b, C5b, immunoglobulins	Plasma	Microbes
Fibrinopeptides	Plasma	Endothelial cells	**Tissue Damage**		
Substance P	Sensory nerve	Endothelial cells	Lysosomal enzymes	Neutrophils Macrophages	Cells and tissues
Increased Expression of Endothelial Adhesion Molecules (Selectin, ICAM, VCAM, PEAM)			Free oxygen radicals	Activated leukocytes	Cells and tissues
TNF	Activated macrophages NK cells	Endothelial cells	Nitric oxide	Macrophages	Cells and tissues
IL-1	Activated macrophages NK cells	Endothelial cells	Bacterial products (LPS)	Bacteria	Cells and tissues

CGRP, calcitonin gene–related peptide; *fMLP,* formyl-methionyl-leucyl-phenylalanine; *IL-1,* interleukin-1; *PAF,* platelet activation factor; *NK cell,* natural killer cell; *TNF,* tumor necrosis factor.
Data from Kumar V, Abbas AK, Fausto N, et al: *Robbins and Cotran pathologic basis of disease,* ed 8, Philadelphia, 2010, Saunders; Slauson DO, Cooper BJ: *Mechanisms of disease,* ed 3, St Louis, 2002, Mosby; Majno G, Joris I: *Cell, tissues, and disease,* ed 2, Oxford, 2004, Oxford University Press; Abbas AK, Lichtman, Pober JS: *Cellular and molecular immunology,* ed 5, Philadelphia, 2003, Saunders.

plasma and cells. The main biologic functions of inflammatory mediators are to cause vasodilation and increased vascular permeability and recruit inflammatory cells, mainly neutrophilic leukocytes and macrophages from blood circulation to the site of tissue injury. Some mediators can also cause tissue damage. The major mediators involved in vascular changes, cell recruitment, and tissue damage in the acute inflammatory response are listed in Table 15-2.

All listed inflammatory mediators have been shown to be present in apical periodontitis.[278,279] Bradykinin is the product of kinin-system activation; fibrinopeptides, the products of blood-clotting system activation; and fibrin degradation products, the products of fibrinolytic-system activation. Kinin, fibrinolytic, and clotting systems are initiated by activated Hageman factor. Prostaglandins and leukotrienes are the products of arachidonic acid metabolism. Activated phospholipase A2 splits cell membrane phospholipid molecules into arachidonic

acid and platelet activating factor. Arachidonic acid molecules can be processed along two pathways: the cyclooxygenase pathway, which leads to production of prostaglandins and thromboxanes, and the lipoxygenase pathway, which produces leukotrienes.[137,165]

Complement components, such as C3a, C3b, C5a, C5b, and C5-C9, are products of the complement cascade, which can be activated by two pathways. The classic pathway is initiated by activation of C1 by multimolecular aggregates of IgG or IgM antibody complexed with specific antigen. The alternate pathway is activated by microbial cell components (lipopolysaccharide, teichoic acid) and plasmin. C3a and C5a are anaphylatoxins that stimulate mast cells and basophils to release histamine. They also cause phagocytes to release lysosomal enzymes. C3b is an opsonin and can coat bacteria to enhance phagocytosis by phagocytes. In addition, C3b can also bind to antibody bound to antigen or microbes. C5a is a strong chemotaxin for neutrophils. C5b-C9 is a membrane attack complex and able to cause cell lysis if activated on the host cell and bacterial cell membrane.[137,165]

Besides inflammatory mediators, the inflammatory response is also dependent upon the timing and extent of various cytokine and chemokine secretions. IL-1, TNF, IL-6, IL-12, and IFN-γ are present in the acute inflammatory response.[1,91] IL-6 is produced by activated mononuclear phagocytes, endothelial cells, and fibroblasts in response to microbial infection and other cytokines, such as IL-1 and TNF. IL-6 stimulates the synthesis of acute-phase proteins by hepatocytes.[1] The major source of IL-12 is activated mononuclear phagocytes and dendritic cells. IL-12 provides a link between innate and adaptive immune responses.[1] IFN-r is produced by activated NK cells, T_H1 cells, and cytotoxic T cells and can activate macrophages and enhance their microbial killing ability. IL-1β and TNF are associated with apical bone resorption during chronic apical periodontitis.[252]

Chemokines are a large family of structurally homologous cytokines that stimulate leukocyte movement and regulate the transmigration of leukocytes from the blood vessel to tissue space.[1] They are produced by leukocytes, endothelial cells, and fibroblasts. The secretion of chemokines is induced by microbial infection, TNF, and IL-1.[1,91,240] Different types of leukocytes express different chemokine receptors.[1]

Neuropeptides are released via axon reflexes of afferent sensory neurons in response to various stimuli. Neuropeptides, as mediators of the inflammatory process, are described in detail in the Neurogenic Inflammation section of this chapter. Inflammatory mediators such as histamine, kinins, prostaglandins, and proinflammatory cytokines are capable of sensitizing and activating sensory nerves to release neuropeptides.[29,96,97,213,225]

Histopathology

The acute inflammatory response is practically immutable in all vascularized living tissues, largely due to the programmed actions of the innate immune system. Initially, blood vessels are engorged by a local infiltration of inflammatory cells, mainly activated neutrophilic leukocytes and some macrophages in the apical periodontal ligament of the infected/inflamed root canal. In addition, sprouting of sensory nerve fibers has been shown early in the inflamed periapical tissues.[39,128] Several studies have also demonstrated the presence of inflamed vital pulp tissue with intact nerve fibers in the apical portion of the root canal in association with apical periodontitis.[154,214,215,255,310] This explains the clinical observation that a patient may experience some pain if an instrument is introduced into the canal short of the apex in some teeth with apical periodontitis lesions.

In primary acute apical periodontitis, apical bone destruction is usually not observed radiographically because the duration of acute response is short, and activated neutrophilic leukocytes and macrophages are not able to resorb bone. Only osteoclasts are capable of resorbing bone, and they have to differentiate from the monocyte/macrophage cell lineage in the blood circulation. However, in a rat model experiment, Stashenko and colleagues[255] showed histologically that periapical inflammatory cell infiltration increases osteoclast numbers, and that bone destruction was apparent well in advance of total pulpal necrosis.

Bacteria are usually not present in acute apical periodontitis lesions.

Clinical Features

As discussed earlier, there is no correlation between clinical and radiographic findings and histologic appearance of inflammatory periapical disease. Teeth with acute apical periodontitis are usually symptomatic and painful to bite and percussion, which results from mechanical allodynia and hyperalgesia.[125] Pain is induced by sensitization and activation of nociceptive sensory nerve fibers by inflammatory mediators, proinflammatory cytokines, nerve growth factor, and pressure.[125] Sprouting of sensory nerve fibers in inflamed periapical tissues could also increase receptive field size in teeth with apical periodontitis.[38,39] Radiographic examination usually does not show periapical bone destruction of the involved tooth in acute apical periodontitis, although occasional slight widening of the apical periodontal ligament space and loss of the apical lamina dura of the involved tooth may be present.

Outcomes

The fundamental purpose of the acute inflammatory response is to restore the structural and functional integrity of damaged tissue by eliminating irritants as soon as possible.[137,165,299] Tissue damage can also occur in acute inflammation by release of lysosomal enzymes, toxic oxygen radicals, and nitric acid from disintegrated neutrophilic leukocytes and macrophages into tissue.[165] Depending on the dynamic interaction between host defenses and microbial insults, acute apical periodontitis can result in (1) restitution of normal periapical tissues if irritants are immediately eliminated by root canal therapy, (2) abscess formation if massive invasion of periapical tissues by highly pyogenic bacteria occurs, (3) organization by scarring if extensive destruction of periapical tissues results, or (4) progression to chronic apical inflammation if irritants continue to persist.

Abscess is a focal localized collection of purulent exudate in a tissue or an organ.[137] It is a morphologic variation of acute and chronic inflammation.[137,165,299] The development of an abscess in apical periodontitis lesions is probably caused by invasion of a combination of specific pyogenic bacteria in the inflamed periapical tissues.[32,201,263,291] Neutrophilic leukocytes are the predominant cells in acute apical periodontitis with abscess formation. Abscess begins as a furious battle between highly virulent pathogens and an army of neutrophilic leukocytes. The pathogens produce massive toxins to kill neutrophils. As neutrophils attack the pathogens, they secrete lysosomal enzymes that digest not only the dead cells but also some live ones. Many neutrophils die fighting against pathogens. The resulting purulent fluid is poorly oxygenated and has a low pH. The bactericidal ability of leukocytes appears to be impaired because of the deprivation of oxygen and interference of respiratory burst. The purpose of respiratory burst is to generate bactericidal agents.[15,165] However, the phagocytic activity of leukocytes is not impaired in anaerobic conditions.[165]

Histologically, apical abscess formation is characterized by local collection of suppurative or purulent exudate composed of dead and live neutrophilic leukocytes, disintegrated tissue cells, degraded extracellular matrix, and lysosomal enzymes released by dead neutrophilic leukocytes. It also contains dead and live bacteria and bacterial toxins released by dead bacteria in the inflamed periapical tissues. Abscess formation also involves destruction of periodontal ligament and sometimes periapical bone—especially in chronic apical periodontitis

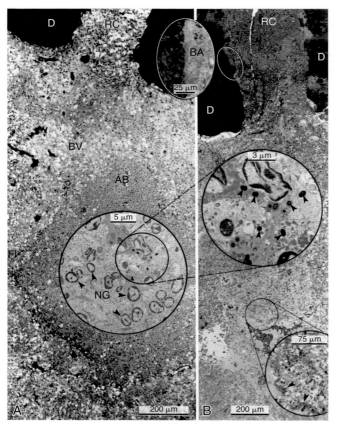

FIG. 15-3 Structure of a secondary periapical abscess. **A,** Axial section of an abscessed apical periodontitis. The microabscess (AB) contains a focus of neutrophils (NG inset in **A**). Note the phagocytosed bacteria in one of the neutrophils (further magnified in large inset in **B**). A secondary abscess forms when bacteria (BA in oval inset) from the apical root canal (RC) advance into the chronic apical periodontitis lesion (**B**). Note the tissue necrosis immediately in front of the apical foramen and the bacterial front in the body of the lesion *(arrowheads in lower inset). BV,* blood vessels; *D,* dentin. (*A,* magnification: ×130; *B,* magnification: ×100; oval inset, magnification: ×400; inset in *A,* magnification: ×2680; upper inset in *B,* magnification: ×4900; lower inset in **B,** magnification: ×250.) (From Nair PNR: Apical periodontitis: a dynamic encounter between root canal infection and host response, *Periodontol 2000* 13:121, 1997.)

with abscess formation—and a surrounding layer of viable neutrophilic leukocytes and a band of fibrovascular granulation tissue. Both layers are thought to serve as protective barriers to prevent the spread of infection. Epithelial cell proliferation is scanty in acute apical periodontitis with abscess formation (Fig. 15-3).[44,215,230]

Clinically, teeth with acute apical abscess formation usually have symptoms such as pain to biting and percussion. The periapical area of the involved tooth may be tender to palpation. Intraoral or extraoral swelling is often present. Because of a sudden outpouring of suppurative exudate in the periapical area, tissue pressure increases such that mechanical stimuli are capable of activating terminals of nociceptive neurons in the inflamed periapical tissues. The severe pain of an acute apical abscess can be due to activation of nociceptors by inflammatory mediators and sensitization to mechanical stimuli due to increased interstitial pressures.[232] If the periapical purulent exudate can be evacuated through the root canal

(or through incision and drainage when indicated) during root canal therapy, the patient usually experiences an immediate relief of acute pain. Radiographically, the involved teeth may show slight widening of the apical periodontal ligament space to loss of apical lamina dura. In chronic apical abscess, the involved teeth may be symptomatic or asymptomatic. If an intraoral or extraoral draining sinus tract is present, swelling is usually absent. Radiographic bone destruction is obvious in teeth with chronic apical abscess formation.

In most cases, if the source of infection in the root canal is eliminated by root canal therapy, the abscess will heal by reabsorption of the pus in teeth with an acute apical abscess. Phagocytes will kill all bacteria in the abscess. The continued influx of leukocytes stops because the chemotactic stimuli have been removed, and the existing neutrophilic leukocytes die of apoptosis. Finally, macrophages move in to clean up necrotic neutrophilic leukocytes and disintegrated tissue cells. In chronic apical abscess formations, wound healing will take place mainly by means of regeneration and to some degree by tissue repair. However, if bacterial virulence and numbers of pathogens overwhelm the host's defenses, the abscess may break through the cortical bone, periosteum, and oral mucosa or facial skin to develop an intraoral or extraoral draining sinus tract. Sometimes, the uncontrolled abscess may spread along the fascial planes of the head and neck to develop serious cellulitis (see also Chapter 18).[142,230]

ASYMPTOMATIC APICAL PERIODONTITIS: APICAL GRANULOMA, CHRONIC APICAL PERIODONTITIS

If pathogens in the root canal are not eliminated, the symptomatic apical periodontitis may progress to become an asymptomatic apical periodontitis. Asymptomatic apical periodontitis is characterized by the persistence of inflammatory stimuli, adaptation of the host's response to stimuli, presence of adaptive immune responses, and initiation of the repair process.[137,165,248,299] Chronic inflammation is good news and bad news. The good news is that the host's defenses are able to maintain an active defense against the invading microorganisms and toxins; the bad news is that the host response is inadequate to eliminate these factors.[165]

Asymptomatic apical periodontitis is a form of adaptive immune response that requires exquisite specificity and memory. The adaptive immune response enhances bacterial killing compared with the innate immune response. Traditionally, the terms *asymptomatic chronic apical periodontitis* and *periapical granuloma* are used interchangeably. A granuloma is a focal area of *granulomatous inflammation,* which is a histologic term for a chronic inflammatory reaction.[137,165,294] Granulomatous inflammation is characterized by the presence of activated macrophages with modified epithelioid cells in diseases such as tuberculosis, leprosy, syphilis, cryptococcosis, sarcoidosis, rheumatic fever, and foreign body granuloma.[101,137,165,304] The presence of poorly digestible irritants (nonantigenic or antigenic), T cell–mediated immunity to irritants, or both appears to be necessary for granuloma formation.[1,137,165] A granuloma is relatively avascular,[137,165] whereas a chronic apical periodontitis is very vascular. Histologically, some but not all chronic apical periodontitis lesions may show some features of granulomatous inflammation,[137,165] so the terms *apical granuloma* and *asymptomatic chronic apical periodontitis* should not be used interchangeably. A *granuloma* is best considered a histologic term used to describe a specific form of chronic inflammation such as foreign body granuloma or immune granuloma.[137,165]

The foreign body reaction is a specific subtype of chronic inflammation.[137,165,299] Foreign materials such as root canal filling materials, paper points, cotton fibers, and surgical sutures can trigger a foreign body giant cell granuloma.[133,187,313] If activated macrophages are unable to engulf large indigestible foreign particles, they can fuse to form giant cells on the surface of the particles and continuously release lysosomal enzymes, inflammatory mediators, and proinflammatory cytokines as a result of frustrated phagocytosis. Giant cells appear to be at least as active metabolically as a regular macrophage.[165] In addition, foreign bodies can favor infection in several ways, as they can be a source of bacterial biofilm[51,197] and they lower the infectious dose of bacteria to induce infection. For example, if a small, sterile plastic cage is implanted under the skin of a guinea pig, as few as 100 *Staphylococcus aureus* are sufficient to infect the tissue, whereas even 10^9 bacteria (i.e., a million-fold increase in dose) fails to produce an abscess in normal guinea pig skin.[315] Finally, foreign bodies can make the infection hard to treat because bacteria in biofilms can switch on appropriate genes and cover themselves with a thick layer of biopolymer that is resistant to both host defense mechanisms and antimicrobial agents.[118,165]

Cell Biology

Macrophages and Lymphocytes

Macrophages and lymphocytes are the primary players in asymptomatic apical periodontitis.[3,52,79,122,132,258,259,280,312] Lymphocytes are blood-borne and have counterparts in the connective tissue.[165] Macrophages play a dual role in host defenses. In the innate immune response, activated macrophages phagocytose microbes, dead cells, and foreign bodies and produce inflammatory mediators and proinflammatory cytokines to enhance the host defense against stimuli. In the adaptive immune response, activated macrophages function as APCs. They phagocytose and present the processed foreign antigens in association with MHC to T cells. Thus, activated macrophages are effector cells of adaptive immune response.

Lymphocytes are the only cells in the body capable of specifically recognizing and distinguishing different antigenic determinants; they are responsible for the two defining characteristics of the adaptive immune response: specificity and memory. The functions of lymphocytes were described earlier in the section on the adaptive immune response.

Dendritic Cells

Dendritic cells play a vital role in asymptomatic apical periodontitis. They have been shown to be present in apical periodontitis lesions in rats.[120,202] Dendritic cells are accessory immune cells derived from bone marrow stem cells and may be related to the mononuclear phagocyte lineage.[1] They function as antigen-presenting cells for naive T lymphocytes and are important for the initiation of adaptive immune responses to protein antigen.[1] Activated dendritic cells produce IL-12, which is a key inducer of cell-mediated immunity.

Osteoclasts

Periapical bone destruction is a hallmark of asymptomatic apical periodontitis. During the chronic stage of apical periodontitis, both osteoclast and osteoblast activity decrease,[297] so the periapical osteolytic lesion remains stationary. Based on magnified radiographic and automated image analysis, periapical bone destruction was observed at 7 days after the pulps of experimental teeth were exposed to oral microorganisms in animal studies. A period of rapid bone destruction took place between 10 and 20 days, with slower bone resorption thereafter.[297] The stationary phase of bone resorbing activity was correlated to asymptomatic apical periodontitis.[297] Increased expression of bone resorptive cytokines such as IL-1, IL-6, and TNF was related to the period of active bone resorption.[298] T_H cells appear to outnumber T_S cells during the active stage of periapical bone destruction in induced rat periapical lesions, but T_S cells dominate T_H cells during the stationary stage of bone destruction.[256]

Bone resorption is caused by osteoclasts. The formation of osteoclasts involves differentiation of the osteoclast precursor from the monocyte-macrophage cell lineage in bone marrow. Several cytokines and growth factors, such as granulocyte/macrophage colony-stimulating factor (GM-CSF), RANKL (receptor activator of nuclear factor κB ligand), osteoprotegerin (OPG), IL-1, IL-6, TNF, as well as prostaglandins, bradykinin, kallidin, and thrombin, have been shown to mediate osteoclast progenitor cell differentiation.[24,40,65,147,180,208,272] Parathyroid hormone is capable of stimulating osteoblasts to synthesize GM-CSF and RANKL. Bone stromal cells and T cells also produce RANKL. Osteoclast progenitor cells express receptor activator of nuclear factor κB (RANK). OPG, a decoy receptor for RANKL secreted by osteoblasts, negatively regulates the differentiation of osteoclasts by absorbing RANKL and reducing its ability to activate the RANK pathway.[126]

RANKL activates the RANK pathway on osteoclast progenitor cells, resulting in differentiation of these cells along the osteoclast lineage. Proinflammatory cytokines, IL-1, TNF, and IL-6 also mediate the differentiation of osteoclast progenitor cells to osteoclasts. The differentiation of the mononuclear osteoclast progenitor cells terminates with fusion to latent multinucleated osteoclasts, which are finally activated to become bone-resorbing osteoclasts. The mature osteoclasts then attach to mineralized bone surface after osteoblasts have primed the unmineralized bone surface and released chemotactic factor to attract osteoclasts.[190] Osteoclasts attach to bone by the vitronectin receptor (integrin superfamily), expressed preferentially in the sealing zone. Vitronectin has binding sites for the arginine-glycine-aspartic amino acid (RDG) sequences present in many extracellular matrix proteins, including osteopontin, bone sialoprotein, and fibronectin, on the surface of the exposed mineralized bone.[81] When bound to bone extracellular matrix, osteoclasts develop a ruffled border. Inside the ruffled border, osteoclasts use ATP to drive H^+ pumps, leading to the acidification of the extracellular compartment. They subsequently secrete proteolytic lysosomal enzymes and carbonic anhydrase to degrade both the mineralized and unmineralized components of bone.[16,18,28,272] (See Fig. 15-5 for the mechanism of bone resorption by osteoclasts in apical periodontitis.)

The resorption of root cementum or dentin in apical periodontitis lesions is less well understood than resorption of bone. Bone is constantly remolding (resorption and deposition) through physiologic and functional processes and thus is much easier to study. In contrast, cementum and dentin are more stable. The cells responsible for dental hard-tissue resorption are called *odontoclasts*.[219] It has been shown in

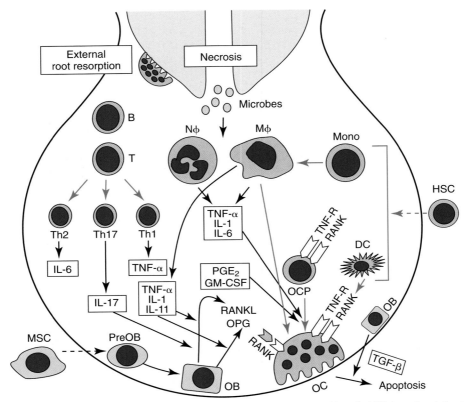

FIG. 15-4 Bone resorption by osteoclasts in apical periodontitis. *DC*, dendritic cell; *HSC*, hematopoietic stem cell; *Mφ*, macrophage; *MSC*, mesenchymal stromal cell; *Nφ*, neutrophil; *OB*, osteoblast; *OC*, osteoclast; *OCP*, osteoclast precursor; *OPG*, osteoprotegerin; *RANK*, receptor activator of nuclear factor κB; *RANKL*, receptor activator of nuclear factor κB ligand. (Courtesy Dr. Huang.)

ultrastructure and gene expression studies that odontoclasts and osteoclasts are similar.[220,221] Therefore, it is believed that the cellular mechanisms of bone, cementum, and dentin resorption are similar.[221] Nevertheless, little is known about how the precursors of the odontoclasts appear and what causes odontoclast differentiation and activation to resorb dentin and cementum. Bone resorption by osteoclasts in apical periodontitis is illustrated in Fig. 15-4.

Epithelial Cell Rests of Malassez

Proliferation of epithelial cell rests of Malassez (ERM) is evident in approximately 52% of inflammatory periapical lesions collected from extracted teeth.[186] It is a form of pathologic (inflammatory) hyperplasia. This type of hyperplasia is caused by stimulation of growth factors and cytokines produced during the inflammatory response. Hyperplasia is a self-limiting process and is reversible when the causative stimulus is eliminated.[137,165,248] During periapical inflammation, innate and adaptive immune cells and stromal cells (e.g., activated macrophages, neutrophilic leukocytes, NK cells, T cells, fibroblasts) in the periapical tissues produce many inflammatory mediators (e.g., prostaglandin, histamine), proinflammatory cytokines (e.g., IL-1, IL-6, TNF), and growth factors (e.g., PDGF, epidermal growth factor [EGF], keratinocyte growth factor [KGF], FGF). These inflammatory mediators, proinflammatory cytokines,[35,46,87,173,223] and growth factors[78,111,160,177,198,276] are capable of stimulating epithelial cell rests to proliferate (Fig. 15-5). The

extent of cellular proliferation appears to be related to the degree of inflammatory cell infiltration.[214,215]

Fibroblasts

Fibroblasts are important cells in chronic inflammation and wound healing. They are derived from undifferentiated mesenchymal cells and exist in all connective tissues. They synthesize and secret proteoglycans, glycoproteins, and precursor molecules of various types of collagens and elastin.[126] In chronic inflammation, fibroblast migration and proliferation are triggered by multiple growth factors (TGF-β, PDGF, EGF, FGF) and the fibrogenic cytokines, IL-1 and TGF-α, produced by activated platelets, macrophages, endothelial cells, and inflammatory cells.[137,165] In turn, activated fibroblasts produce an array of cytokines such as IL-1, IL-6, and granulocyte/macrophage colony-stimulating factor, which influence leukocyte development. Fibroblasts stimulated by inflammation also produce matrix metalloproteinase to degrade the proteins that comprise the extracellular matrix.[165,287]

Fibrovascular granulation tissue is also a prominent feature of chronic apical periodontitis as a repair process. Migration and proliferation of endothelial cells from preexisting capillaries and venules into the site of chronic inflammation is called *neovascularization*. It is mediated by angiogenesis factors, such as vascular endothelial growth factor (VEGF) and TGF-β, produced by activated macrophages, platelets, and endothelium.[165,248] Neovascularization supplies oxygen and nutrients

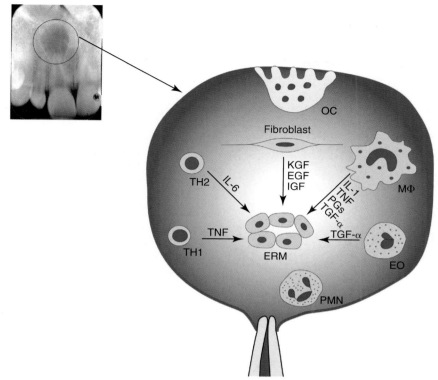

FIG. 15-5 Schematic illustration of the major mechanisms that activate proliferation of epithelial cell rests in apical periodontitis. (From Lin LM, Huang GT-J, Rosenberg P: Proliferation of epithelial cell rests, formation of apical cysts, and regression of apical cysts after periapical wound healing, *J Endod* 33:908, 2007.)

for the support of metabolically active macrophages and fibroblasts during wound healing.

Inflammatory Mediators

Many inflammatory mediators present in symptomatic apical periodontitis are also expressed in asymptomatic apical periodontitis. In addition, several different cytokines and growth factors are secreted by cells such as activated macrophages, lymphocytes, dendritic cells, and fibroblasts, in the chronic/adaptive inflammatory response described earlier.

Histopathology

Macrophages and lymphocytes are predominant cells in asymptomatic apical periodontitis lesions (Fig. 15-6). Occasionally, foamy macrophages and giant cells are seen, especially associated with cholesterol crystal deposits, which are products of disintegrated cell membranes. Cholesterol crystals are present in approximately 18% to 44% of all apical periodontitis lesions.[33,286] Bone resorption is a hallmark of asymptomatic apical periodontitis. Multinucleated osteoclasts may sometimes be seen in resorptive Howship lacunae. Proliferation of epithelial cell rests is often present in asymptomatic apical periodontitis lesions. ERM proliferate in three dimensions and form irregular strands or islands of epithelium, which are often infiltrated by varying degrees of inflammatory cells (see Fig. 15-6, *B*). A key feature of asymptomatic apical periodontitis is a proliferation of fibrovascular granulation tissue that is an attempt to prevent further spread of infection/inflammation and to repair wounded periapical tissues.

Little information is available concerning cemental changes in apical periodontitis. Using a scanning electron microscope,

Simon and associates[242] observed that projections, depressions, and fibers of cementum were haphazardly arranged in root canal infection under scanning electron microscopy. There was an increase of mineralized projections, cementum lacunae, and surface resorptions and a decrease in fibers. All these changes may provide a more favorable condition for attachment of bacterial biofilm on the apical external root surface in extraradicular infection.

It is a general belief that asymptomatic apical periodontitis lesions are usually devoid of innervation, so local anesthesia may not be necessary if teeth with asymptomatic apical periodontitis require root canal therapy. However, light and transmission electron microscopic studies have demonstrated that teeth with chronic apical periodontitis were well innervated (Fig. 15-7).[153,168] This explains why instruments accidentally introduced into inflamed periapical tissues without local anesthesia can cause the patient pain.

External root resorption that involves cementum or both cementum and dentin usually occurs in asymptomatic apical periodontitis lesions.[143,292] Fortunately, cementum and dentin appear to be less readily resorbed than bone by inflammatory processes.[92] However, the radiographic presence of root "blunting" should be interpreted by the astute clinician as evidence for resorption of dentin and cementum, and the working length of the instrumentation and obturation phases of nonsurgical endodontic treatment should be adjusted by a corresponding amount.

Using light and transmission electron microscopy and microbiologic culturing, bacteria have been shown to be present in many asymptomatic apical periodontitis lesions.[2,114,284,300] Inadvertent contamination is a major concern

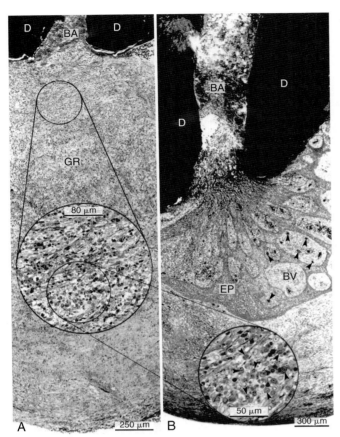

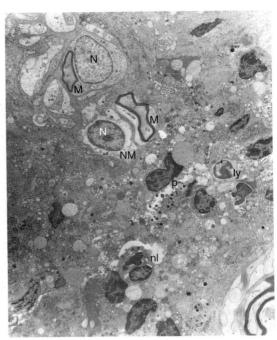

FIG. 15-7 Presence of intact myelinated and nonmyelinated nerve fibers in chronic apical periodontitis lesion. *ly,* Lymphocyte; *M,* myelinated nerve fiber; *N,* nucleus of Schwann cell; *nl,* neutrophilic leukocyte; *NM,* nonmyelinated nerve fiber; *p,* plasma cell (EM, magnification: ×1600). (From Lin L, Langeland K: Innervation of inflammatory periapical lesions, *Oral Surg Oral Med Oral Pathol Oral Radiol Endod* 51:535, 1981.)

FIG. 15-6 Chronic asymptomatic apical periodontitis without (**A**) and with (**B**) epithelium (EP). The root canal contains bacteria (BA) in **A** and **B**. The lesion in **A** has no acute inflammatory cells, even at the mouth of the root canal with visible bacteria at the apical foramen (BA). Note the collagen-rich maturing granulation tissue (GR) infiltrated with plasma cells and lymphocytes (inset in **A** and **B**). *BV,* blood vessels; *D,* dentin. (**A**, magnification: ×80; **B**, magnification: ×60; inset in **A**, magnification: ×250; inset in **B**, magnification: ×400.) (From Nair PNR: Apical periodontitis: a dynamic encounter between root canal infection and host response, *Periodontol 2000* 13:121, 1997.)

when culturing bacteria from these lesions. Under meticulous transmission electron microscopic examination, Nair[183] was unable to observe bacteria in most asymptomatic apical periodontitis lesions. If bacteria are present in the inflamed periapical tissues, they are usually found inside the phagocytes (Fig. 15-8).[154] Importantly, the mere presence of bacteria in the inflamed periapical tissues (colonization) does not necessarily imply periapical infection. Bacteria have to be able to establish an infectious process, such as survival and tissue destruction, in the inflamed periapical tissues to be considered etiologic factors for the resulting infection. Most apical periodontitis lesions are not infected; nonsurgical root canal therapy of teeth with apical periodontitis can achieve a high success rate, provided root canal infection is controlled.

Clinical Features

Involved teeth are usually asymptomatic and show an ill-defined or well-defined periapical radiolucent lesion. The chronic apical abscess and associated sinus tract are usually asymptomatic. Occasionally, the sinus tract from an apical abscess may drain along the root surface and opens into the

gingival sulcus. This leads to the development of a deep, narrow pseudopocket that often mimics a periodontal pocket or a vertical root fracture (see Chapter 25 for details).

Outcomes

Asymptomatic apical periodontitis may result in (1) regeneration or repair of the periapical tissues after root canal therapy, (2) severe periapical tissue destruction, (3) acute exacerbation, (4) development of an abscess with an intraoral or extraoral draining sinus tract, or (5) development of a serious cellulitis.

ASYMPTOMATIC APICAL PERIODONTITIS WITH CYST FORMATION: RADICULAR CYST, CHRONIC APICAL PERIODONTITIS WITH CYST FORMATION

The radicular cyst is unique because no cysts in the body have similar pathogenesis. It is believed that the radicular cyst is likely formed by inflammatory proliferation of epithelial cell rests in the inflamed periodontal ligament.[158,189,200,274] The radicular cyst is a pathologic cavity completely lined by nonkeratinized stratified squamous epithelium of variable thickness in a three-dimensional structure in an apical periodontitis lesion. A radicular cyst can be a "pocket cyst" (i.e., attached to the apical foramen) or a "true cyst" (no attachment to the root structure), but it cannot form by itself. Therefore, a radicular cyst should not be considered a separate disease entity from asymptomatic apical periodontitis. A radicular cyst (pocket or true) is classified as an inflammatory and not a

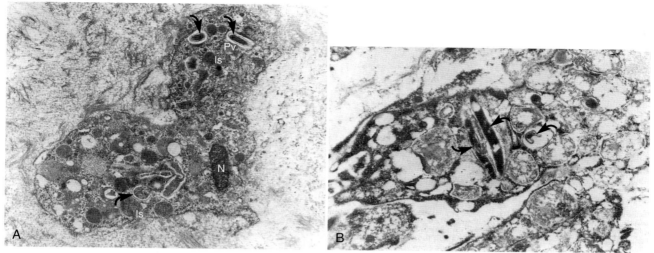

FIG. 15-8 Bacteria phagocytosed by phagocytes in chronic apical periodontitis lesion. **A,** Bacteria *(arrows)* in phagosome of a neutrophil. *Is,* Lysosome; *N,* part of nucleus; *Pv,* phagocytic vacuole (EM, magnification: ×6300). **B,** Part of the cell structure of a macrophage. Note longitudinally and cross-cut bacteria cells with unit membrane *(arrows)* in phagocytic vacuoles (EM, magnification: ×10,000). (From Lin L, Langeland K: Light and electron microscopic study of teeth with carious pulp exposures, *Oral Surg Oral Med Oral Pathol* 51:292, 1981.)

neoplastic lesion in the WHO Histological Typing of Odontogenic Tumors, Jaw Cysts and Allied Lesions.[136] The prevalence of radicular cysts in apical periodontitis lesions from extracted teeth ranges from 15% to 20%.[186]

Cell Biology

In addition to the presence of all chronic inflammatory cells, the epithelial cells are the most prominent cell type found in asymptomatic apical periodontitis with cyst formation. ERM can be considered unipotent or restricted-potential stem cells. They can be stimulated to divide symmetrically and asymmetrically into basal cells (stem cells) and suprabasal squamous cells of lining epithelium of radicular cysts.[158] Many theories about apical cyst formation have been proposed. The nutritional deficiency theory assumes that when islands of epithelium keep growing, the central cells of the epithelial island will move farther away from their source of nutritional supply and undergo necrosis and liquefaction degeneration. The products accumulated attract neutrophils and granulocytes into the necrotic area. Microcavities then coalesce to form a cyst cavity lined by stratified squamous epithelium.[274] The abscess theory postulates that when an abscess is formed in connective tissue, epithelial cells proliferate and line the abscess cavity because of their inherent tendency to cover exposed connective-tissue surface.[189,200] The theory of merging of epithelial strands proposes that proliferating epithelial strands merge in all directions to form a three-dimensional spherelike structure composed of fibrovascular connective tissue, with varying degrees of inflammatory cells trapped, that gradually degenerates due to lack of blood supply. This leads to formation of a cyst cavity.[158] Regardless of how a radicular cyst (pocket or true) is formed, it is likely caused by inflammatory proliferation (hyperplasia) of epithelial cell rests in these lesions.

It has been speculated that radicular cyst expansion is caused by increased osmotic pressure in the cyst cavity,[277] but this hypothesis overlooks the cellular aspects of cyst growth and the biochemistry of bone destruction.[72,173] Radicular cyst expansion is likely caused by degradation of fibrous connective tissue capsule by matrix metalloproteinases, which are produced by activated neutrophils, fibroblasts, and macrophages[275] and bone resorption. The ERM have also been shown to be capable of secreting a bone resorbing factor.[25] Most inflammatory mediators and proinflammatory cytokines that stimulate proliferation of epithelial cell rests also mediate bone resorption in apical periodontitis lesions.

Inflammatory Mediators

Mediators are basically similar to those present in chronic apical periodontitis.

Histopathology

Two types of cysts have been described in chronic apical periodontitis lesions. The pocket cyst's lumen opens into the root canal of the involved tooth (Fig. 15-9).[185,186,241] The true cyst is completely enclosed by a lining epithelium, and its lumen has no communication with the root canal of the involved tooth (Fig. 15-10).[185,186,241] Apical cysts are lined by hyperplastic, nonkeratinized stratified squamous epithelium of variable thickness, which is separated from the fibrovascular connective tissue capsule by a basement membrane. Both the lining epithelium and the connective tissue capsule are usually infiltrated with inflammatory cells,[235] indicating that inflammatory cells are attracted to these tissues by chemotactic irritants, either in the root canal system or in the periapical tissues. In nonproliferating epithelium, there is less inflammatory cell infiltration.[44,230] Occasionally, mucous cell metaplasia or ciliated respiratory-type cells are present in cystic epithelial lining.[195] The epithelial cells of lining epithelium do not show any characteristic features of neoplastic changes, such as pleomorphism, lack of polarity, nuclear enlargement, large nucleoli, abnormal nuclear/cytoplasmic ratio, hyperchromatism, or abnormal mitosis. Unlike odontogenic keratocysts and calcifying odontogenic cysts, the basal cells of radicular cystic lining epithelium are incapable of proliferation by themselves without stimulation of growth factors or cytokines released by innate

FIG. 15-9 A, A well-developed pocket cyst in apical periodontitis lesion. **B,** Note the saclike epithelial lumen. **C-D,** Sequential axial serial section passing through the apical foramen in the root canal plane (RC) shows the continuity of the lumen with the root canal. *D,* dentin (**A, C,** magnification: ×16; **B, D,** magnification: ×40). (From Nair PNR: Non-microbial etiology: foreign body reaction maintaining post-treatment apical periodontitis, *Endod Topics* 6:96, 2003.)

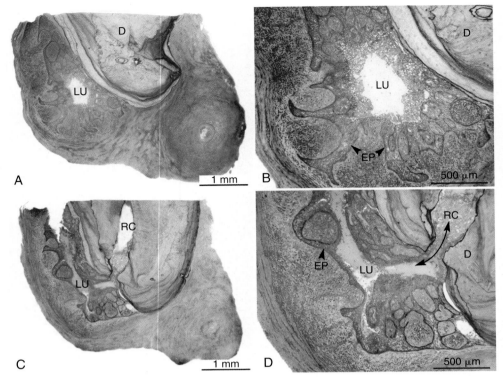

FIG. 15-10 A, Two distinct cysts lined by epithelium in apical periodontitis lesion. There is no evidence of communication with the foramen in serial sections (H&E, magnification: ×25). **B,** Cyst cavity on the left side in **A.** Accumulation of foamy macrophages (H&E, magnification: ×50; inset magnification: ×1000). **C,** Lower part of cavity in **B.** Dense infiltration of neutrophilic leukocytes (H&E, magnification: ×1000). **D,** Cyst cavity on the right side in **A.** Necrotic tissue debris in the lumen; infiltration of inflammatory cells in the epithelium (H&E, magnification: ×50). **E,** Cystic wall in **D.** Cyst's lining epithelium is infiltrated with acute and chronic inflammatory cells. *LU,* Lumen (H&E, magnification: ×1000). **F,** Foamy macrophages, neutrophilic leukocytes, and necrotic tissue inside the cyst *(inset),* but no bacteria (Brown & Brenn, magnification: ×25, inset magnification: ×1000). **G,** Area indicated by an *open arrow* in **F.** Bacterial colonies in the apical foramen (Brown & Brenn, magnification: ×1000). (From Ricucci D, Pascon EA, Pitt Ford TR, Langeland K: Epithelium and bacteria in periapical lesions, *Oral Surg Oral Med Oral Pathol Oral Radiol Endod* 101:241, 2006.)

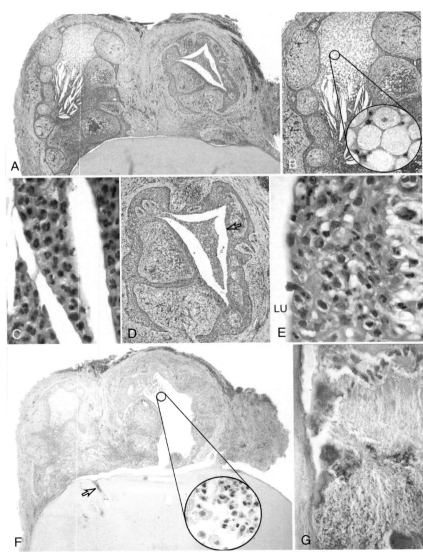

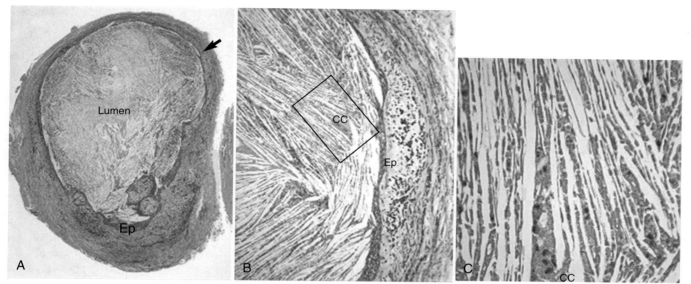

FIG. 15-11 A, A radicular cyst in which the lumen is completely filled with cholesterol crystals (H&E, magnification: ×25). **B,** High magnification of cholesterol crystals in **A** (H&E, magnification: ×100). **C,** High magnification of rectangular area in **B.** Multinucleated giant cells associated with cholesterol crystals (H&E, magnification: ×400). (Courtesy Dr. Ricucci, Rome, Italy.)

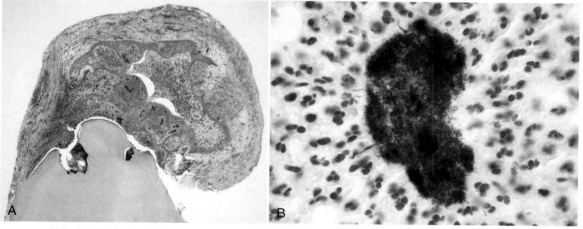

FIG. 15-12 A, An apical true cyst in apical periodontitis lesion. Bacterial colonies are seen in the foraminal areas (Brown & Brenn, magnification: ×25). **B,** Bacterial colonies in the cyst lumen, surrounded by inflammatory cells (Brown & Brenn, magnification: ×400). (From Ricucci D, Bergenholtz G: Histologic features of apical periodontitis in human biopsies, *Endod Topics* 8:68, 2004, Fig. 6.)

and adaptive immune cells during periapical inflammation. The lumen of cysts may contain inflammatory exudates, cholesterol crystals, clear fluid, or bacterial colonies (Figs. 15-11 and 15-12).[186,215]

Clinical Features

The involved tooth is usually asymptomatic. Periapical osteolytic lesions of endodontically involved teeth may sometimes show a well-demarcated radiolucency surrounded by a rim of radiopaque border.

Outcomes

There is no direct evidence demonstrating whether asymptomatic apical periodontitis with cyst formation (pocket and true) can or cannot regress after nonsurgical root canal therapy.

Unfortunately, apical cysts cannot be diagnosed clinically and can only be diagnosed after surgical biopsy or extraction of teeth with apical periodontitis. Clinical outcome studies have shown that after proper nonsurgical root canal therapy, teeth with apical periodontitis heal in 78% of cases.[247] Therefore, it is speculated that some cysts, especially pocket cysts, may heal after nonsurgical root canal therapy.[185] Apical true cysts are less likely to heal after nonsurgical root canal therapy because of their self-sustaining nature; surgical intervention is necessary.[185] Nonetheless, similar to the periapical pocket cyst, a periapical true cyst is also formed within an apical periodontitis lesion and is not a neoplastic lesion. Any disease caused by inflammation/infection should be able to heal if the causative irritant/irritants are removed, unless the irritant/irritants are neoplasm-inducing agents or a carcinogen.

ASYMPTOMATIC APICAL PERIODONTITIS WITH REACTIVE BONE FORMATION: CONDENSING OSTEITIS OR CHRONIC FOCAL SCLEROSING OSTEOMYELITIS

Asymptomatic apical periodontitis with reactive bone formation is analogous to chronic osteomyelitis with proliferative periostitis. The etiology and pathogenesis of these two diseases are not well understood. It is generally believed that both lesions are caused by a long-term, low-grade inflammation/infection or a high resistance of local tissue to inflammation/infection.[195,210] Instead of bone resorption, the inflammation induces reactive bone formation of alveolar trabecular or spongy bone around the periapex of endodontically involved teeth.

Cell Biology

As described previously, during the chronic stage of apical periodontitis, both osteoclast and osteoblast activity decreases.[297] However, in asymptomatic apical periodontitis with reactive bone formation, osteoblasts appear to be stimulated to produce more bone. It is not clear what factor/factors stimulate osteoblasts to produce more bone mass. It could be due to increased expression of growth factors/cytokines, such as TGF-β, BMP, PDGF, and transcription factor Cbfa1 (core-binding factor family).[126]

Histopathology

There is an excessive apposition of bone mass without bone resorption in the apical area. As the bone marrow spaces become smaller and obliterated, the bone resembles compact bone that is infiltrated by a small number of lymphocytes. The compact bone has few lacunae, and many of them are empty of osteocytes. It has many prominent resting and reversal lines, similar to an idiopathic osteosclerosis or a Pagetoid appearance.[44,195,210]

Clinical Features

The lesion is usually observed in young patients, and the mandibular first molar is most commonly involved. The teeth often have gross carious lesions and can be vital or nonvital. They are usually asymptomatic. Radiographically, the lesion may have a well-defined or ill-defined radiopaque mass associated with the apex of an endodontically involved tooth. The lamina dura around the root apex is usually intact.

Outcomes

Most apical periodontitis lesions with reactive bone formation demonstrate healing after nonsurgical root canal therapy. The excessive compact bone in most cases will be remodeled to normal appearance.[69]

PERIAPICAL LESIONS OF NONENDODONTIC ORIGIN

Many periapical lesions are not of endodontic origin and should be considered in the differential diagnosis of apical periodontitis. These lesions include (but are not limited to) trauma,[10,11] foreign bodies,[133,187,313] host metabolic by-products,[188] advanced periodontal disease,[140] fibro-osseous lesions, and benign and malignant tumors.[195] A complete description of these lesions is beyond the scope of this chapter; the interested reader is encouraged to seek the cited references.

EXTRARADICULAR ENDODONTIC INFECTION

Extraradicular endodontic infection implies that bacteria have established an infectious process outside the root canal system in the periapical area.[243,260,284] Extraradicular endodontic infection can only be diagnosed after surgical biopsy or microbiologic sampling or molecular detection of therapy-resistant periapical lesions during apical surgery. The method of sample collection should be carefully reviewed, because contamination is a problem in bacteriologic study of apical periodontitis lesions during apical surgery.

Extraradicular endodontic infection can be a part of intraradicular infection or an independent entity without an intraradicular component. To be considered an independent extraradicular infection, the presence of pathogens in the root canal system must be completely ruled out, because intraradicular bacteria pose more potential problems than extraradicular bacteria in periapical inflammation. Bacteria in the complex root canal system are well protected from root canal procedures (i.e., mechanical instrumentation, antiseptic irrigation, intracanal medication), host defenses, and antimicrobial therapy because of a lack of blood circulation and areas resistant to access (e.g., isthmi; see Chapter 6). In our opinion, the independent extraradicular infection probably does not occur often and is usually associated with apical actinomycosis.[95,266] Bacteria have been observed as biofilm on the apical external root surface.[243,283] In addition, viruses have also been isolated from apical periodontitis lesions.[149,218,249] If microbiologic root canal cultures are not completely reliable (because bacteria may remain in the complex root canal system),[222] then interpretation of independent extraradicular infections as endodontic treatment failures should be carefully evaluated.

Although virulence and number of pathogens, as well as the host's defenses, determine whether extraradicular infection will develop or not, the development of extraradicular infection is still not fully understood. What are the predisposing factors to extraradicular infection? How are bacteria able to evade the host's powerful defenses in order to colonize and establish an infectious process in the periapical tissues? Are all extraradicular infections resistant to nonsurgical root canal therapy? For instance, are bacteria present in apical periodontitis with abscess formation?[32,90,263,291] Importantly, most periapical abscesses heal after proper nonsurgical root canal therapy. Similarly, most apical periodontitis lesions with draining sinus tracts also heal after proper nonsurgical root canal therapy, because the primary source of infection in the root canal system is removed. The preponderance of evidence does not support the consistent presence of an independent periapical infection in endodontic infections.

APICAL PERIODONTITIS AND SYSTEMIC DISEASES

Information concerning apical periodontitis and systemic diseases is limited. Clinical and radiographic studies have shown that there is a greater prevalence of periapical lesions in diabetics than in nondiabetics.[21] Type 2 diabetes mellitus is significantly associated with an increased prevalence of apical periodontitis.[229] Other findings demonstrated that type 2 diabetes is associated with increased risk of a poor response by the periradicular tissues to odontogenic pathogens.[31] In rodent models, diabetic conditions enhance the development of periradicular lesions and increase mortality.[73,113,131] Mice deficient in P/E-selectin are shown to be more prone to infection-mediated early-onset periodontal disease.[196]

Genetic polymorphisms may also play a role in the individual's response to various diseases. Haplotype analyses have indicated that a variant of the IL-1β gene was likely to be most important for early-onset periodontitis risk.[62] In a Chinese male population, it was reported that the polymorphisms of IL1A+4845 and IL1B-511 might play an important role in determining generalized aggressive periodontitis susceptibility. A possible combined effect of the polymorphism of IL1B-511 and smoking on this type of periodontitis susceptibility was suggested.[150] In a study on patients from Chile, the heterozygous inheritance of the IL1B+3954 gene was found significantly higher in periodontitis cases than in control patients. The prevalence of a positive genotype (at least one allele of the two variants present at each locus) is significantly higher in cases (26%) than in controls (10%) and significantly associated with periodontitis, irrespective of smoking status and periodontitis severity.[162] Those displaying high-producer IL6 genotype, intermediate and high-producer IL1B genotypes, and low-producer TNFA genotype tend to exhibit symptomatic dental abscesses.[57]

Apical periodontitis was once considered a focus of infection, and the microorganisms from the focus could disseminate through blood circulation to remote parts of the body, where secondary disease occurred.[108] Even though bacteremias do occur during root canal treatment of teeth with apical periodontitis when instrumentation is carried through the apical foramen into the periapical tissues, the incidence and magnitude of bacteremias is not clinically significant for a healthy person and in fact appears to be lower than that observed by flossing.[19,58,59] Microorganisms in the blood circulation are rapidly eliminated by the host's humoral and cellular defense components within minutes.[19,59] However, bacteremia may pose a potential danger to immunocompromised patients or patients with congenital heart valve disease.[58] No correlation between apical periodontitis and coronal heart disease and rheumatoid arthritis has been observed.[41,181] There is insufficient evidence to support that apical periodontitis could serve as a focus of infection and cause significant systemic diseases.[68,204]

GENETIC AND SYSTEMIC DISEASE RISK FACTORS OF PERSISTENT APICAL PERIODONTITIS

Genetic Risk Factors

Genetic polymorphism in the population plays an important role in the variation of the susceptibility and development of diseases among individuals. Knowledge on the polymorphism of key genes that are involved in disease development will help us to understand and establish prevention or treatment strategies for the diseases. Because of the completion of the Human Genome Project, many advanced molecular technologies have been developed including high-throughput screening and sequencing which further help gather the information on polymorphism in human populations. There are different types and causes of genetic polymorphisms. Single nucleotide polymorphisms (SNPs) that have a single base variation resulting from insertion or deletion of a base are considered the most common type of genetic polymorphism.[42]

Occurrence of SNP within the coding region of a gene may produce an altered protein, which may lead to altered function (termed functional SNPs). Occurrence of SNP within the promoter region of a gene may alter gene regulation, which may cause reduction/inhibition or overexpression of gene expression. Functional SNPs alter amino acid sequence or interfere with the transcriptional factor binding, whereas nonfunctional SNPs do not affect the regulation of protein expression. Many SNPs have no effect on cell function, but some could predispose people to disease or influence their response to drugs. Besides SNPs, there are single amino-acid polymorphisms (SAAPs or SAPs) of proteins, which may result from RNA editing independent of SNPs.[308]

A genetic polymorphism is defined as alleles or variants that appear in at least 1% of the population. The 1% cutoff excludes mutations that may have occurred in a single family. In most polymorphisms, one allele dominates and appears with < 99% frequency (for example, 65%) in the population. In a biallelic situation, some authors term the dominant allele as normal (N-allele or allele 1) and it occurs in < 99%, whereas the rarer allele (R-allele or allele 2) is present in >1% in the population.[227,245] It has been long known that genetic polymorphisms are associated with increased severity of inflammatory diseases.[98] Both endodontic and periodontic diseases are mainly an infectious disease caused by microbial infection. They share common features in terms of inflammation and bone resorption. Studies have implicated association of periodontitis or apical periodontitis with several gene polymorphisms such as IL-1, IL-6, IL-8, FcγR, tumor necrosis factor receptor superfamily member 1B (TNFRSF1B), (selenoprotein S) SEPS1, and matrix metalloproteinases (MMPs).[7,45,129,134,174,175,309]

It has long been observed that the proinflammatory cytokine interleukin-1 (IL-1) genotype is a severity factor in adult periodontal disease.[134] The specific periodontitis-associated IL-1 genotype has a variant in the IL-1B gene that is associated with high levels of IL-1 production. Gene polymorphism studies suggest that the frequency of IL-1β genotypes (IL-1β+3953 restriction fragment length biallelic polymorphism) is increased in patients with advanced adult periodontitis compared to early and moderate combined, and to healthy controls.[84] A more recent study showed that IL-1β levels in gingival crevicular fluid is increased with severity of disease and correlates well with clinical signs of incipient disease.[254] This suggests that some individuals, when challenged by bacterial accumulations, may respond with a higher level of inflammatory activities, therefore leading to more severe periodontitis. Both FcγRIIa (CD32) and FcγRIIIb (CD16) influence polymorphonuclear leukocyte phagocytic function and therefore their polymorphisms may also influence inflammatory disease development. It was reported that the FcγR IIIb-NA2 allotype represents a risk factor for recurrence of adult periodontitis,[129] and the FcγRIIIa-158V allele and possibly FcγRIIIb-NA2 may be associated with severity of chronic periodontitis in a Japanese population[130]; whereas the FcγRIIa-H/H131 genotype may be associated with chronic periodontitis risk (and disease severity) in Caucasian smokers.[309] FcγRIIIa and FcγRIIIb genotypes may impose an additional risk of periodontal bone loss in a German population.[174]

The polymorphisms of two other genes involved in inflammation, *SEPS1* and *TNFRSF1B*, have been found to be involved in determining host individual susceptibility to aggressive periodontitis, and there is the potential association between *IL-6* and *FcγR* polymorphisms and the aggressive periodontitis in a Caucasian-Italian population.[224]

The genetic polymorphisms have been involved in the development of apical periodontitis reports. Two genetic conditions—carriage of allele H131 of the *FcγRIIa* gene and a combination of this allele with allele NA2 of the *FcγRIIIb* gene—have been reported to be associated with posttreatment apical periodontitis,[245] whereas polymorphism in the *FcγRIIIa* does not influence the patient's response to endodontic treatment of teeth with apical periodontitis in a Brazilian population.[246] So far there has been only one report on *IL-1* polymorphism association with apical periodontitis in an American population.[179] In this study, patients with persistent apical periodontitis showed an increased prevalence in the genotype composed of allele 2 of *IL-1β* polymorphism when compared with those who experienced complete healing after acceptable root canal therapy (70.6% versus 24.6%). This outcome suggests that specific genetic markers associated with IL-1β production may predict increased susceptibility to persistent apical periodontitis. An earlier paper that studied a Brazilian population did not find an association between IL1 polymorphism and persistent apical periodontitis; however, allele 1 (for *IL-1A* and *IL-1B*) was always detected higher in diseased than in healthy/healing individuals, although not statistically significant.[245] This lack of statistical difference could be due to small sample size or different population pools.

The polymorphism of the IL-8 gene, a potent chemokine that attracts neutrophils to the site of infection, has also been shown to influence the development of different forms of apical periodontitis.[7] *IL8/CXCL8-251 T* allele, which is associated with higher production of IL8/CXCL8, is also associated with a higher risk of developing acute suppurative form of apical periodontitis. *IL8/CXCL8 -251 A* allele, which is associated with lower production of IL8/CXCL8, is associated with chronic nonsuppurative form of apical periodontitis. SNP of other inflammation-associated genes, matrix metalloproteinases (MMPs) 2 and MMP3, also show influence on periapical lesion formation.[175] Thus, markers in MMP3 and MMP2 genes could also help predict host susceptibility to developing periapical lesions and the healing response.

Systemic Disease Risk Factors

Many systemic diseases have been linked to periodontal disease[127,199] because they contribute to either a decreased host's resistance to infection or dysfunction in the connective tissue of periodontium, increasing patient susceptibility to immuno-inflammation-induced destruction.[14] However, the similar systemic diseases do not appear to link to apical periodontitis, possibly because periodontitis is an open lesion and apical periodontitis is a closed lesion.

Diabetes mellitus (DM), a systemic disease, has been well documented to be associated with a high prevalence of apical periodontitis.[21,74,113,163,167,228] DM is a chronic disorder of carbohydrate, fat and protein metabolism, and a defective or deficient insulin secretory response.[137] Hyperglycemia is characteristic of DM and has profound effects on cell metabolisms, especially endothelial cells such as increased polyol pathway flux, increased formation of advanced glycation end products, hyperglycemia-induced activation of protein kinase C, and

increased hexosamine pathway flux.[34] The tissue most frequently affected by hyperglycemia is microvasculature, whereby endothelial cells are not able to transport intracellular glucose effectively.[34] Because of damage to vasculature (atherosclerosis), blood circulation, innate and adaptive immuno-inflammatory mechanism, and phagocyte function are impaired,[34,137] thus leading to pulp necrosis and predisposition to pulpal infection and subsequent apical periodontitis.[21]

Sickle cell anemia is the prototype of hereditary globinopathies, characterized by the production of structurally abnormal hemoglobulin.[137] The red blood cells are sickle shaped. Accumulation of distorted red cells could cause vasoocclusion, which could lead to anoxia, infarcts, and necrosis of tissue.[100] The occurrence of asymptomatic pulp necrosis in clinically intact permanent teeth has been reported.[13,123,239] Pulp necrosis could predispose to pulpal infection and apical periodontitis because of a lack of defense mechanism.

Sjögren syndrome is a chronic, systemic autoimmune disorder.[195] It involves salivary glands resulting in xerostomia. The lack of salivary cleansing action predisposes the patient to dental caries. If the caries is not prevented or treated early, it would impose risk of pulpal infection and apical periodontitis.

Radiation therapy of head and neck malignant lesions is associated with a high occurrence of caries.[104] If untreated, the radiation caries could lead to pulpal infection and subsequent apical periodontitis. It has been shown that a radiation dose 66 to 72.2 Gy (gray) in the head and neck region was associated with a high prevalence of caries and apical periodontitis because of a change in microflora favorable for carious development.[103]

However, there is no clear-cut direct causation or mechanism between systemic disease risk factors and the incidence or persistence of apical periodontitis without prior caries and pulp infection.

WOUND HEALING OF APICAL PERIODONTITIS

Periapical Wound Healing After Nonsurgical Root Canal Therapy

Understanding wound healing is as important as knowing the pathogenesis of disease, because satisfactory wound healing is the ultimate goal of treatment. If we are able to understand the mechanisms of periapical wound healing, we can design treatment approaches that maximize favorable conditions for wound healing to occur, such as effective disinfection of the root canal system in nonsurgical root canal therapy, control of periapical inflammation by medication, or incorporation of growth factors in bone grafts in surgical endodontic therapy (see also Chapters 12 and 21).

Interestingly, healing begins as soon as inflammation starts. When irritants (microbial and nonmicrobial) in the canal systems or in the periapical tissues are eliminated by nonsurgical or surgical endodontic therapy, inflammatory mediators are no longer produced in the periapical tissues because of the reduction of inflammatory cells. Inflammatory mediators already present are inactivated by the body's control mechanisms to prevent an inflammatory reaction from going unchecked. This process precedes wound healing. Although a great deal of information is known about what turns on the inflammation, relatively little is known about what turns off the inflammatory system after elimination of irritants. Examples of host antiinflammatory control mechanisms are (1) enzyme destruction of inflammatory activators; (2) natural inhibitors of inflammatory mediators (opioids, somatostatin, glucocorticoids); (3) relative balance between intracellular levels of cyclic AMP (adenosine monophosphate) and cyclic GMP (guanosine monophosphate); (4) the antiphlogistic role of histamine; (5) inhibitors of the complement system[287]; and (6) antiinflammatory cytokines, such as IL-4, IL-10, IL-13, and TGF-β.[93,193] In addition, the major cellular inducer of inflammation, neutrophilic leukocytes, undergo apoptosis,[89] and the major cellular player of wound healing, macrophages, secrete antiinflammatory molecules such as lipoxins, resolvins, and protectins.[137,165,193]

The process of wound healing is tightly regulated by cell-to-cell cross-talk, cell-to–extracellular matrix interactions, and cell surface receptors, as well as the temporal and spatial expression of a variety of cytokines, growth factors, and neuropeptides and apoptosis (Table 15-3).[29,86,89,257,302] All these cellular and humoral factors operate together in either an antagonistic or synergistic manner and are precisely orchestrated during wound healing. This results in a highly organized response permitting regeneration of the original tissue architecture. Wound healing appears to be a programmed event. Much information concerning the pathogenesis of apical periodontitis has been gained from animal studies.[75,119,281] Although studies of wound healing of teeth with apical periodontitis after nonsurgical root canal therapy and endodontic surgery are available in a few animal experiments and a human

TABLE 15-3
Important Growth Factors/Cytokines in Wound Healing

Cytokines	Major Source	Target Cells and Major Effects
EGF	Macrophages, platelets, fibroblasts	Epithelial cells, fibroblasts, endothelial cells
FGF	Macrophages, endothelial cells	Endothelial cells (angiogenesis), mesenchymal cells
TGF-α	Macrophages, platelets, keratinocytes	Angiogenesis, fibroblasts
TGF-β	Macrophages, platelets	Similar to EGF
PDGF	Macrophages, platelets, endothelial cells	Chemoattractant for macrophages, fibroblasts
VEGF	Macrophages, epithelial cells	Angiogenesis
IGF	Fibroblasts, epithelial cells	Granulation tissue formation, reepithelialization
CSF	Multiple cells	Macrophages, granulation tissue formation
SP, CGRP	Sensory nerve	Endothelial cells, fibroblasts, keratinocytes

CGRP, calcitonin gene–related peptide; *CSF*, colony-stimulating factor; *EGF*, epidermal growth factor; *FGF*, fibroblast growth factor; *IGF*, insulin-like growth factor; *PDGF*, platelet-derived growth factor; *TGF*, transforming growth factor; *VEGF*, vascular endothelial growth factor.
Modified from Majno G, Joris I: *Cell, tissues, and disease*, ed 2, Oxford, 2004, Oxford University Press; Slauson DO, Cooper BJ: *Mechanisms of disease*, ed 3, St Louis, 2002, Mosby; Werner S, Grose R: Regulation of wound healing by growth factors and cytokines, *Physiol Rev* 83:835, 2003.

study,[12,145,146] no studies of wound healing of apical periodontitis lesions with cyst formation after nonsurgical root canal therapy exist in the literature.

Wound healing of apical periodontitis lesions after proper nonsurgical root canal therapy follows the general principle of wound healing of connective tissues elsewhere in the body, with the formation of fibrovascular granulation tissue, removal of necrotic tissue and dead bacteria by activated macrophages, and finally repair or regeneration of the wounded tissue. Healing of apical periodontitis lesions is largely accomplished by regeneration and to some degree by fibrosis. Local tissue resident cells involved in periapical wound healing are osteoblasts and bone marrow mesenchymal stem cells in alveolar bone and multipotent stem cells in the periodontal ligament.[233] During periapical wound healing, many unwanted hyperplastic cells (e.g., endothelial cells, fibroblasts, epithelial cells) are deleted by apoptosis,[60,86,89] and the extracellular matrix is remodeled by metalloproteinases. Pathologic processes such as extensive fibrosis do not occur often, and the damaged periapical tissues can be restored mostly to their original structure by the process of regeneration.

The temporal and spatial relationship between alveolar bone, cementum, and periodontal ligament during periapical wound healing after nonsurgical root canal therapy cannot be clearly delineated. Nevertheless, wound healing appears to recapitulate the embryonic morphogenesis of damaged tissues or organs in many instances. The process of periapical wound healing after nonsurgical root canal therapy may be similar to wound healing following guided tissue regeneration in periodontal therapy: regeneration of new cementum, new alveolar bone, and new periodontal ligament.[67,285] Both nonsurgical root canal therapy and guided tissue regeneration therapy in periodontal disease are intended to remove irritants and provide a favorable microenvironment conducive to regeneration of periodontal tissues damaged by apical periodontitis and marginal periodontitis, respectively.

During periapical wound healing, the cells of viable periodontal ligament from adjacent root surfaces proliferate to cover the root surfaces in which the periodontal ligament was damaged by apical periodontitis and removed by macrophages. Proteins derived from the Hertwig epithelial root sheath (i.e., enamel matrix proteins) are required for cementoblast differentiation from ectomesenchymal stem cells in the dental follicle during tooth development.[251] The cells of the Hertwig epithelial root sheath are absent in mature teeth.[192,230]

Nevertheless, the extracellular matrix and growth factors of cementum (i.e., IGF-1, FGFs, EGF, BMP, TGF-β, PDGF) sequestered after cemental resorption in mature teeth are capable of inducing proliferation, migration, attachment, and differentiation of multipotent stem cells in the periodontal ligament into cementoblast-like cells and produce cementoid tissue on the root surface denuded of periodontal ligament.[88,233] This is similar to reparative dentin formation by pulp stem cells in direct pulp capping procedures where growth factors such as TGF-β are released from dentin matrix binding sites.[191,217,289] Root resorption that involves cementum or both cementum and dentin can only be repaired by cementoid tissue, because multipotent stem cells of the periodontal ligament are incapable of differentiating into odontoblasts that produce dentin.[233]

Bone has a remarkable capacity for regeneration in response to injury. During periapical wound healing, the osteoprogenitor cells or mesenchymal cells lining the surfaces of endosteum—stimulated by TGF-β, BMPs, IGFs, PDGF, VEGF, and cytokines released by stromal cells, osteoblasts, platelets, and bone matrix after bone resorption—can undergo proliferation and differentiation into osteoblasts and produce bone matrix.[6,161] When one of the cortical bone plates (buccal or lingual/palatal) is destroyed, osteoprogenitor cells in the inner layer of periosteum beneath the oral mucosa—stimulated by TGF-β, BMPs, IGFs, PDGF, and VEGF—are also capable of proliferation and differentiation into osteoblasts and can produce bone matrix.[126,161] If both buccal and lingual/palatal cortical bone plates are destroyed by large apical periodontitis lesions, it is possible that the lesion may be repaired with fibrous scar tissue because of extensive destruction of the periosteum beneath the oral mucosa.[12] Accordingly, a guided tissue regeneration procedure using membrane barriers and bone grafts is recommended to prevent ingrowth of fibroblasts from periosteum or submucosa into the bony defect and to enhance periapical wound healing if periapical surgery is necessary.[54,55] The cellular and molecular mechanisms of excess scar tissue formation in periapical wound healing are not completely understood. Growth factors/cytokines may play an important role in regulating fibroblast gene expression and excess scar tissue formation.[288]

The newly regenerated periodontal ligament will finally undergo remodeling into a mature periodontal ligament, with one group of collagen fibers (Sharpey fibers) inserted into the newly formed cementum and another group of collagen fibers inserted into the newly formed alveolar bone. Thereby, regeneration of damaged periapical tissues, cementum, periodontal ligament, and alveolar bone is completed.

Periapical Wound Healing After Surgical Endodontic Therapy

The mechanism of periapical wound healing after nonsurgical and surgical endodontic therapy is similar, but the kinetics of healing of the periapical wound after endodontic surgery is faster than nonsurgical endodontic therapy.[138] In surgical endodontic therapy, a clinician removes irritants, such as necrotic cells, tissue debris, and bacteria in the periapical lesions, which is called *surgical debridement*.[157,165] In contrast, in nonsurgical endodontic therapy, activated macrophages perform bacterial killing and cleanup of periapical lesions, which is called *biologic debridement*.[165] Surgical debridement is very effective and of course quite rapid, whereas biologic debridement takes time. However, endodontic surgery is more invasive. In addition, proper case selection is more important in endodontic surgery than in nonsurgical endodontic therapy. The distinctive difference between nonsurgical and surgical endodontic therapy is that the goal of nonsurgical endodontic therapy is to remove primary microbial etiology from the root canal system, and the goal of surgical endodontic therapy is often to seal microbial etiology within the root canal system by root-end filling in most cases (see also Chapter 21).

Can Radicular Cysts in Apical Periodontitis Lesions Regress After Nonsurgical Endodontic Therapy?

Based on histology and cell biology, no studies have ever shown that apical true cysts are different from apical pocket cysts. It was suggested that pocket cysts in apical periodontitis

lesions might regress after nonsurgical root canal therapy by the mechanism of apoptosis or programmed cell death, based on molecular cell biology.[158] In contrast, apical true cysts may be less likely to heal after nonsurgical root canal therapy because of their self-sustaining nature.[185] Histologically, inflammatory cell infiltration is always present in the lining epithelium or fibrous connective tissue capsule of apical true cysts.[185,214,215] This indicates there is continued presentation of irritants (such as bacteria)—present in the root canal system, the periapical tissues, or the lumen of cysts—to attract inflammatory cells to the cystic lining epithelium or fibrous connective tissue capsule.[186,214,215] It is not known if epithelial cells of apical true cysts alone are capable of acting as autocrine cells and secreting growth factors to sustain their own survival. It is important to realize that the apical true cyst is completely different from the odontogenic keratocyst, which is self-sustaining because it is a neoplastic lesion. Biologically, it is unlikely that the hyperplastic epithelial cells of inflammatory apical true cysts would suddenly transform into cells that behave like self-sustaining neoplasms. Any disease caused by infection should be able to regress after removal of its causative irritant(s), unless the irritants themselves are neoplasm-inducing agents or carcinogens, such as some viruses and human malignant tumors.[165,294] From pathogenesis, histology, and molecular cell biology, apical true cysts are similar to pocket cysts. Accordingly, apical true cysts, similar to pocket cysts, may be able to regress after nonsurgical root canal therapy by the mechanism of apoptosis if root canal infection is effectively under control.[158] This prediction is consistent with the high level of healing observed after nonsurgical root canal treatment.

In apical periodontitis lesions with cyst formation, the cysts have to regress before the periapical tissues can be restored to their original architecture. It is not known what matrix serves as a scaffold for endothelial cells, fibroblasts, and osteoblasts to migrate into the lumen of regressing cysts after nonsurgical root canal therapy. Complete regression of radicular cysts after nonsurgical root canal therapy could be due to any of several possible scenarios. Regression of radicular cysts and regeneration of bone may occur concurrently; or during regression of radicular cysts, part of the cystic lining epithelium could disintegrate due to apoptosis of local epithelial cells. Together with degradation of the basal lamina by matrix metalloproteinases, this could allow a fibrous connective tissue capsule to grow into the lumen of radicular cysts. Eventually, the cystic lining epithelium will completely regress or become remnants of epithelial cell rests remaining in the periodontal ligament.

Taken together, our knowledge of cyst mechanisms and healing offers tantalizing clinical implications and clearly supports the conclusion that more studies are required to understand the complex mechanisms of regression of inflammatory apical cysts, both pocket and true.

FACTORS INFLUENCING PERIAPICAL WOUND HEALING AFTER ENDODONTIC THERAPY

Local and systemic factors may affect periapical wound healing. Infection will complicate and prevent wound healing, foreign bodies can impair wound healing,[187,313] and nutrition can also affect wound healing.[305] Diabetes was reported to reduce the likelihood of healing of apical periodontitis lesions after nonsurgical root canal therapy.[74] Impaired nonspecific immune response and disorders of the vascular system appeared to have a significant influence on the success rate of nonsurgical root canal therapy on teeth with apical periodontitis.[166] However, immunocompromised patients, such as HIV patients, responded as well as counterpart patients after nonsurgical endodontic therapy.[49,82,207] Although smoking has not been shown to be associated with increased incidence of apical periodontitis and prognosis of nonsurgical root canal therapy,[23,63] smoking may increase complications of periapical surgery, such as pain and swelling.[80]

Patients receiving radiotherapy of jaws and bisphosphonate therapy have a risk of developing osteonecrosis of jawbones,[212,216,306] so nonsurgical root canal therapy is recommended for these patients.[121,152] However, for endodontic surgery, the guidelines of the American Association of Oral and Maxillofacial Surgeons position paper on bisphosphonate-related osteonecrosis of the jaws are highly recommended.[8] For asymptomatic patients who have taken an oral bisphosphonate for less than 3 years and have no clinical risk factors, endodontic surgery is not contraindicated.[8] Nevertheless, the patient's physician should be consulted. Any kind of surgical procedure should be avoided for patients receiving intravenous bisphosphonate.[8] To prevent the complication of osteonecrosis, if patients are going to receive radiation of jaws or bisphosphonate therapy, nonsurgical or surgical endodontic therapy should be completed before the initiation of radiation or bisphosphonate therapy.[8]

REFERENCES

1. Abbas AK, Lichtman AH, Pober JS: *Cellular and molecular immunology*, Philadelphia, 2007, Saunders.
2. Abous-Rass M, Bogen G: Microorganisms in closed periapical lesions, *Int Endod J* 31:39, 1998.
3. Akamine A, Hashiguchi I, Toriya Y, Maeda K: Immunohistochemical examination of the localization of macrophages and plasma cells in induced rat's periapical lesions, *Endod Dent Traumatol* 10:121, 1994.
4. Akira S, Takeda K, Kaisho T: Toll-like receptors: critical proteins linking innate and acquired immunity, *Nature Immunol* 2:675, 2001.
5. Akira S, Uematsu S, Takeuchi O: Pathogen recognition and innate immunity, *Cell* 124:783, 2006.
6. Al-Aql ZS, Alagl AS, Graves DT, et al: Molecular mechanisms controlling bone formation during fracture healing and distraction osteogenesis, *J Dent Res* 87:107, 2008.
7. Amaya MP, Criado L, Blanco B, et al: Polymorphisms of pro-inflammatory cytokine genes and the risk for acute suppurative or chronic nonsuppurative apical periodontitis in a Colombian population, *Int Endod J* 46:71, 2013.
8. American Association of Oral and Maxillofacial Surgeons: *Position paper on bisphosphonate-related osteonecrosis of the jaws*. Rosemont, IL, 2006, AAOMS Board of Trustees, September.
9. American Dental Association: *1990 survey of dental services rendered*. Chicago, 1994, American Dental Association.
10. Andreasen FM: Transient apical breakdown and its relation to color and sensitivity changes after luxation injuries to teeth, *Endod Dent Traumatol* 2:9, 1986.
11. Andreasen JO, Andreasen FM: *Textbook and color atlas of traumatic injuries to the teeth*, ed 3, Copenhagen, 1994, Munksgaard.
12. Andreasen JO, Rud J: Modes of healing histologically after endodontic surgery in 70 cases, *Int Oral Surg* 1:148, 1972.
13. Andrews CH, England MC, Kemp WB: Sickle cell anemia: an etiological factor in pulp necrosis, *J Endod* 9:249, 1986.
14. Armitage GC: Periodontal diagnoses and classification of periodontal disease, *Periodontology 2000* 34:9, 2004.
15. Babior BM: The respiratory burst of phagocytes, *J Clin Invest* 73:599, 1984.
16. Baron R: Molecular mechanisms of bone resorption by the osteoclasts, *Anat Rec* 224:317, 1989.
17. Barthel CR, Zimmer S, Trope M: Relationship of radiologic and histologic signs of inflammation in human root-filled teeth, *J Endod* 30:75, 2004.
18. Bartkiewicz M, Hernando N, Reddy SV, et al: Characterization of the osteoclast vacuolar H+-ATPase B-subunit. *Gene* 160:157, 1995.

19. Baumgartner JC, Heggers JP, Harrison JW: The incidence of bacteremias related to endodontic procedures. I. Non-surgical endodontics, *J Endod* 2:135, 1976.
20. Bender IB: Factors influencing the radiographic appearance of bone lesions, *J Endod* 8:161, 1982.
21. Bender IB, Bender AB: Diabetes mellitus and the dental pulp, *J Endod* 29:383, 2003.
22. Bender IB, Seltzer S: Roentgenographic and direct observation of experimental lesions in bone: 1, *J Am Dent Assoc* 62:152, 1961.
23. Bergstrom J, Babcan J, Eliasson S: Tobacco smoking and dental periapical condition, *Eur J Oral Sci* 112:115, 2004.
24. Bezerra MC, Carvalho JF, Prokopowitsch AS, Pereira RM: RANK, RANKL and osteoprotegerin in arthritic bone loss, *Braz J Med Biol Res* 38:161, 2005.
25. Birek C, Heersche JN, Jez D, Brunette DM: Secretion of a bone resorbing factor by epithelial cells cultured from porcine rests of Malassez, *J Periodontal Res* 18:75, 1983.
26. Birklein F, Schmelz M: Neuropeptides, neurogenic inflammation and complex regional pain syndrome (CRPS), *Neurosci Lett* 437:199, 2008.
27. Block RM, Bushell A, Rodrigues H, Langeland K: A histopathologic, histobacteriologic, and radiographic study of periapical endodontic surgical specimens, *Oral Surg Oral Med Oral Pathol* 42:656, 1976.
28. Boyle WJ, Simonet WS, Lacey DL: Osteoclast differentiation and activation, *Nature* 423:337, 2003.
29. Brian SD: Sensory peptides: their role in inflammation and wound healing, *Immunopharmacology* 37:133, 1997.
30. Brinkmann V, Zychlinsky A: Beneficial suicide: why neutrophils die to make NETs, *Nat Rev Microbiol* 5:577, 2007.
31. Britto LR, Katz J, Guelmann M, Heft M: Periradicular radiographic assessment in diabetic and control individuals, *Oral Surg Oral Med Oral Pathol Oral Radiol Endod* 96:449, 2003.
32. Brook I, Fraizier EH, Gher ME: Aerobic and anaerobic microbiology of periapical abscess, *Oral Microbiol Immunol* 6:123, 1991.
33. Browne RM: The origin of cholesterol in odontogenic cysts in man, *Arch Oral Biol* 16:107, 1971.
34. Brownless M: The pathobiology of diabetes complications: a unifying mechanism, *Diabetes* 54:1615, 2005.
35. Brunette DM: Cholera toxin and dibutyl cyclic-AMP stimulate the growth of epithelial cells derived from epithelial cell rests from porcine periodontal ligament, *Arch Oral Biol* 29:303, 1984.
36. Brynolf I: A histological and roentgenological study of the periapical region of human upper incisors, *Odontol Rev* 18(suppl 11):1, 1967.

37. Burd PR, Rogers HW, Gordon JR, et al: Interleukin 3-dependent and -independent mast cells stimulated with IgE and antigen express multiple cytokines, *J Exp Med* 170:245, 1989.
38. Byers MR, Narhi MVO: Dental injury models: experimental tools for understanding neuroinflammatory nociceptor functions, *Crit Rev Oral Biol* 10:4, 1999.
39. Byers MR, Taylor PE, Khayat BG, Kimberly CL: Effects of injury and inflammation on the pulp and periapical nerves, *J Endod* 16:78, 1990.
40. Canalis E, McCarthy TL, Centrella M: Growth factors and cytokines in bone cell metabolism, *Annu Rev Med* 42:17, 1991.
41. Caplan DJ, Chasen JB, Krall EA, et al: Lesions of endodontic origin and risk of coronary heart disease, *J Dent Res* 85:996, 2006.
42. Cargill M, Altshuler D, Ireland J, et al: Characterization of single-nucleotide polymorphisms in coding regions of human genes, *Nat Genet* 22:231, 1999.
43. Caviedes-Bucheli J, Muñoz HR, Azuero-Holguín MM, Ulate E: Neuropeptides in dental pulp: the silent protagonists, *J Endodon* 34:773, 2008.
44. Cawson RA, Everson JW: *Oral pathology and diagnosis*, Philadelphia, 1987, Saunders.
45. Chai L, Song YQ, Zee KY, Leung WK: SNPs of Fc-gamma receptor genes and chronic periodontitis, *J Dent Res* 89:705, 2010.
46. Chedid M, Rubin JS, Csaky KG, Aaronson SA: Regulation of keratinocyte growth factor gene expression by interleukin 1, *J Biol Chem* 269:10753, 1994.
47. Cochran DL, Wozney JM: Biological mediators for periodontal regeneration, *Periodontol 2000* 19:40, 1999.
48. Cook DN, Pisetsky DS, Schwartz DA: Toll-like receptors in the pathogenesis of human disease, *Nat Immunol* 5:975, 2004.
49. Cooper H: Root canal treatment in patients with HIV infection, *Int Endod J* 26:369, 1993.
50. Cortesini R, LeMaoult J, Ciubotariu R, Cortesini NS: CD8+CD28- T suppressor cells and the induction of antigen-specific, antigen-presenting cell-mediated suppression of T_H reactivity, *Immunol Rev* 182:201, 2001.
51. Costerton JW, Geesey GG, Chen KJ: How bacteria stick, *Sci Am* 238:86, 1978.
52. Cymerman JJ, Cymerman DH, Walters I, Nevins AJ: Human T lymphocyte subpopulations in chronic periapical lesions, *J Endod* 10:9, 1984.
53. Dahlen G, Magnusson BC, Moller A: Histological and histochemical study of the influence of lipopolysaccharide extracted from *Fusobacterium nucleatum* on the periapical tissues in the monkey Macaca fascicularis, *Arch Oral Biol* 26:591, 1981.
54. Dahlin C, Gottlow J, Linde A, Nyman S: Healing of maxillary and mandibular bone defects using a membrane

technique: an experimental study in monkeys, *Scand J Plast Reconstr Hand Surg* 24:13, 1990.

55. Dahlin C, Linde A, Gottlow J, Nyman S: Healing of bone defects by guided tissue regeneration, *Plast Reconstr Surg* 81:672, 1988.

56. Damoiseaux J: Regulatory T cells: back to the future, *Neth J Med* 64:4, 2006.

57. de Sa AR, Moreira PR, Xavier GM, et al: Association of CD14, IL1B, IL6, IL10 and TNFA functional gene polymorphisms with symptomatic dental abscesses, *Int Endod J* 40:563, 2007.

58. Debelian GJ, Olsen I, Transtad L: Systemic diseases caused by oral microorganisms, *Endod Dent Traumatol* 10:5, 1994.

59. Debelian GJ, Olsen I, Transtad L: Bacteremia in conjunction with endodontic therapy, *Endod Dent Traumatol* 11:142, 1995.

60. Desmouliere A, Redard M, Darby I, Gabbiani G: Apoptosis mediates the decrease in cellularity during the transition between granulation tissue and scar, *Am J Pathol* 146:56, 1995.

61. Dickerson C, Undem B, Bullock B, Winchurch RA: Neuropeptides regulation of proinflammatory cytokine responses, *J Leukocyte Biol* 63:602, 1998.

62. Diehl SR, Wang Y, Brooks CN, et al: Linkage disequilibrium of interleukin-1 genetic polymorphisms with early-onset periodontitis, *J Periodontol* 70:418, 1999.

63. Duncan HF, Pitt Ford TR: The potential association between smoking and endodontic disease, *Int Endo J* 39:843, 2006.

64. Dwyer TG, Torabinejad M: Radiographic and histologic evaluation of the effect of endotoxin on the periapical tissues of the cat, *J Endod* 7:31, 1980.

65. Dziak R: Biochemical and molecular mediators of bone metabolism, *J Periodontol* 64:407, 1993.

66. Echchannaoui H, Frei K, Schnell C, et al: Toll-like receptor 2-deficient mice are highly susceptible to *Streptococcus pneumoniae* meningitis because of reduced bacterial clearing and enhanced inflammation, *J Infect Dis* 186:798, 2002.

67. Egelberg J: Regeneration and repair of periodontal tissues, *J Periodontal Res* 22:233, 1987.

68. Ehrmann EH: Focal infection: the endodontic point of view, *Oral Surg Oral Med Oral Pathol* 44:628, 1977.

69. Eliasson S, Halvarson C, Ljunheimer C: Periapical condensing osteitis and endodontic treatment, *Oral Surg Oral Med Oral Pathol* 57:195, 1984.

70. Eriksen HM, Bjertness E: Prevalence of apical periodontitis and results of endodontic treatment in middle-aged adults in Norway, *Dent Traumatol* 7:1, 1991.

71. Figdor D: Apical periodontitis: a very prevalent problem, *Oral Surg Oral Med Oral Pathol Oral Radiol Endod* 94:65, 2002.

72. Formigli L, Orlandini SZ, Tonelli P, et al: Osteolytic processes in human radicular cysts: morphological and biochemical results, *J Oral Pathol Med* 24:216, 1995.

73. Fouad AF, Barry J, Russo J, et al: Periapical lesion progression with controlled microbial inoculation in a type I diabetic mouse model, *J Endod* 28:8, 2002.

74. Fouad AF, Burleson J: The effect of diabetes mellitus on endodontic treatment outcome: data from an electronic patient record, *J Am Dent Assoc* 134:43, 2003.

75. Fouad AF, Walton RE, Rittman BR: Induced periapical lesions in ferret canines: histological and radiographic evaluation, *Dent Traumatol* 8:56, 1992.

76. Friedman S: Considerations and concepts of case selection in the management of post-treatment endodontic disease (treatment failure), *Endod Topics* 1:54, 2002.

77. Fuchs TA, Abed U, Goosmann C, et al: Novel cell death program leads to neutrophil extracellular traps, *J Cell Biol* 176:231, 2007.

78. Gao Z, Falitz CM, Mackenzie IC: Expression of keratinocyte growth factor in periapical lesions, *J Dent Res* 75:1658, 1996.

79. Gao Z, Mackenzie IC, Rittman BR, et al: Immunocytochemical examination of immune cells in periapical granulomas and odontogenic cysts, *J Oral Pathol* 17:84, 1988.

80. Garcia B, Penerrocha M, Marti E, et al: Pain and swelling after periapical surgery related to oral hygiene and smoking, *Oral Surg Oral Med Oral Pathol Oral Radiol Endod* 104:271, 2007.

81. Giachelli CM, Steitz S: Osteopontin: a versatile regulator of inflammation and biomineralization, *Matrix Biol* 19:615, 2000.

82. Glick M, Abel SN, Muzyka BC, DeLorenzo M: Dental complications after treating patients with AIDS, *J Am Dent Assoc* 125:296, 1994.

83. Gonzalez-Rey E, Chorny A, Delgado M: Regulation of immune tolerance by anti-inflammatory neuropeptides, *Nat Rev Immunol* 7:52, 2007.

84. Gore EA, Sanders JJ, Pandey JP, et al: Interleukin-1beta+3953 allele 2: association with disease status in adult periodontitis, *J Clin Periodontol* 25:781, 1998.

85. Green TL, Walton RE, Taylor JK, Merrell P: Radiographic and histologic findings of root canal treated teeth in cadaver, *Oral Surg Oral Med Oral Pathol Oral Radiol Endod* 83:707, 1997.

86. Greenhalgh DG: The role of apoptosis in wound healing, *Int J Biochem Cell Biol* 30:1019, 1998.

87. Grossman RM, Kreuger J, Yourish D, et al: Interleukin-6 is expressed in high levels in psoriatic skin and stimulates proliferation of cultured human keratinocyte, *Proc Nat Acad Sci U S A* 86:6367, 1989.

88. Grzesik WJ, Narayanan AS: Cementum and periodontal wound healing and regeneration, *Crit Rev Oral Biol Med* 13:474, 2002.

89. Haanen C, Vermes IV: Apoptosis and inflammation, *Mediators Inflamm* 4:5, 1995.

90. Haapasalo M, Ranta K, Ranta H: Mixed anaerobic periapical infection with sinus tract, *Endod Dent Traumatol* 3:83, 1987.

91. Hahn C-L, Liewehr FR: Innate immune responses of the dental pulp to caries, *J Endod* 33:643, 2007.

92. Hammarstrom L, Lindskog S: General morphological aspects of resorption of teeth and alveolar bone, *Int Endod J* 18:93, 1985.

93. Hanada T, Yoshimura A: Regulation of cytokine signaling and inflammation, *Cytokine Growth Factor Rev* 13:413, 2002.

94. Hancock HH III, Sigurdsson A, Trope M, Moiseiwitsch J: Bacteria isolated after unsuccessful endodontic treatment in a North American population, *Oral Surg Oral Med Oral Pathol Oral Radiol Endod* 91:579, 2001.

95. Happonen RP: Periapical actinomycosis: a follow-up study of 16 surgically treated cases, *Endod Dent Traumatol* 2:205, 1986.

96. Hargreaves KM, Goodis HE: *Dental pulp*, Chicago, 2002, Quintessence.

97. Hargreaves KM, Swift JQ, Roszkowski MT, et al: Pharmacology of peripheral neuropeptide and inflammatory mediator release, *Oral Surg Oral Med Oral Pathol* 78:503, 1994.

98. Hart TC, Kornman KS: Genetic factors in the pathogenesis of periodontitis, *Periodontol 2000* 14:202, 1997.

99. Hauman CHJ, Love RM: Biocompatibility of dental materials used in contemporary endodontic therapy: a review. Part 2. Root-canal filling materials, *Int Endod J* 36:147, 2003.

100. Hebble PR, Vercellotti GM, Nath KA: A systems biology consideration of the vasculopathy of the sickle cell anemia: the need for multi-modality chemo-prophylaxis, *Cardiovasc Hematol Disord Drug Targets* 9:271, 2009.

101. Hirsh BC, Johnson WC: Concepts of granulomatous inflammation, *Int J Dermatol* 23:90, 1984.

102. Hirvonen T, Hippi P, Narhi M: The effect of an opioid antagonist and somatostatin antagonist on the nerve function in normal and inflamed dental pulps, *J Dent Res* 77:1329, 1998.

103. Hommez GG, De Meerkeer GO, De Neve WJ, De Meer RJG: Effect of radiation dose on the prevalence of apical periodontitis: a dosimetric analysis, *Clin Oral Invest* 16:1543, 2012.

104. Hong CHL, Napenas JJ, Hodgson BD, et al, editors: A systematic review of dental disease in patients undergoing cancer therapy, *Support Care Cancer* 18:1007, 2010.

105. Hou L, Sasakj H, Stashenko P: B-Cell deficiency predisposes mice to disseminating anaerobic infections: protection by passive antibody transfer, *Infect Immun* 68:5645, 2000.

106. Hou L, Sasaki H, Stashenko P: Toll-like receptor 4-deficient mice have reduced bone destruction following mixed anaerobic infection, *Infect Immun* 68:4681, 2000.

107. Hou L, Wang X: PKC and PKA, but not PKG mediate LPS-induced CGRP release and $(Ca^{2+})_i$ elevation in DRG neurons of neonatal rats, *J Neurosci Res* 66:592, 2001.

108. Hunter W: Oral sepsis as a cause of disease, *Br Med J* 2:215, 1900.

109. Huumonen S, Orstavik D: Radiological aspects of apical periodontitis, *Endod Topics* 1:3, 2002.

110. Ingle J, Bakland L, Baugartner C: *Ingle's endodontics*, ed 6, Hamilton, 2008, BC Decker.

111. Irwin CR, Schor SL, Ferguson NW: Expression of EGF-receptor on epithelial and stromal cells of normal and inflamed gingiva, *J Periodont Res* 26:388, 1991.

112. Isaka J, Ohazama A, Kobayashi M, et al: Participation of periodontal ligament cells with regeneration of alveolar bone, *J Periodontol* 72:314, 2001.

113. Iwama A, Nishigaki N, Nakamura K, et al: The effect of high sugar intake on the development of periradicular lesions in rats with type 2 diabetes, *J Dent Res* 82:322, 2003.

114. Iwu C, MacFarlane TW, MacKenzie D, Stenhouse D: The microbiology of periapical granulomas, *Oral Surg Oral Med Oral Pathol* 69:502, 1990.

115. Janeway CA, Medzhitov R: Innate immune recognition, *Annu Rev Immunol* 20:197, 2002.

116. Janeway CA, Travers P, Walport M, Shlomchik MJ: *Immunobiology: the immune system in health and disease*, ed 6, New York, 2005, Garland Science.

117. Jimenez-Pinzon A, Segura-Egea JJ, Poyato-Ferrera M, et al: Prevalence of apical periodontitis and frequency of root-filled teeth in an adult Spanish population, *Int Endod J* 37:167, 2004.

118. Johnson GM, Lee DA, Regelmann WE, et al: Interference with granulocyte function by Staphylococcus epidermidis slime, *Infect Immun* 54:13, 1986.

119. Kakehashi S, Stanley H, Fitzgerald R: The effect of surgical exposures of dental pulps in germ-free and conventional laboratory rats, *Oral Surg Oral Med Oral Pathol* 20:340, 1965.

120. Kaneko T, Okiji T, Kan L, et al: Ultrastructural analysis of MHC class II molecule-expressing cells in experimentally induced periapical lesions in the rat, *J Endod* 27:337, 2001.

121. Katz H: Endodontic implications of bisphosphonate-associated osteonecrosis of the jaws: a report of three cases, *J Endod* 31:831, 2005.

122. Kawashima N, Okiji T, Kosaka T, Suda H: Kinetics of macrophages and lymphoid cells during the development of experimentally induced periapical lesions in rat molars, *J Endod* 22:311, 1996.

123. Kaya AD, Aktener BO, Unsal P: Pulp necrosis with sickle cell anemia, *Int Endod J* 37:602, 2004.

124. Kayaoglu G, Orstavik D: Virulence factors of *Enterococcus faecalis*: relationship to endodontic disease, *Crit Rev Oral Biol Med* 15:308, 2004.

125. Khan AA, Hargreaves KM: Dental pain. In Trup JC, Sommer C, Hugger A, editors: *The puzzle of orofacial pain*, Basel, 2007, Karger.

126. Kierszenbaum AL: *Histology and cell biology*, St. Louis, 2002, Mosby.

127. Kim J, Amar S: Periodontal disease and systematic conditions: a bidirectional relationship, *Odontology* 94:10, 2006.

128. Kimberly CL, Byers MR: Inflammation of rat molar pulp and periodontium causes increased calcitonin gene-related peptide and axonal sprouting, *Ant Rec* 222:289, 1988.

129. Kobayashi T, Westerdaal NA, Miyazaki A, et al: Relevance of immunoglobulin G Fc receptor polymorphism to recurrence of adult periodontitis in Japanese patients, *Infect Immun* 65:3556, 1997.

130. Kobayashi T, Yamamoto K, Sugita N, et al: The Fc gamma receptor genotype as a severity factor for chronic periodontitis in Japanese patients, *J Periodontol* 72:1324, 2001.

131. Kohsaka T, Kumazawa M, Yamasaki M, Nakamura H: Periapical lesions in rats with streptozotocin-induced diabetes, *J Endod* 22:418, 1996.

132. Kopp W, Schwarting R: Differentiation of T lymphocyte subpopulations, macrophages, and HLA-DR-restricted cells of apical granulation tissue, *J Endod* 15:72, 1989.

133. Koppang HS, Koppang R, Solheim T, et al: Cellulose fibers from endodontic paper points as an etiological factor in postendodontic periapical granulomas and cysts, *J Endod* 15:369, 1989.

134. Kornman KS, Crane A, Wang HY, et al: The interleukin-1 genotype as a severity factor in adult periodontal disease, *J Clin Periodontol* 24:72, 1997.

135. Kovacevic M, Tamarut T, Jonjic N, et al: The transition from pulpitis to periapical periodontitis in dog's teeth, *Aust Endod J* 34:12, 2008.

136. Kramer IR, Pindberg JJ, Shear M: *WHO histological typing of odontogenic tumors*, ed 2, Geneva, 1992, Springer Verlag.

137. Kumar V, Abbas AK, Fausto N, et al, editors: *Robbins and Cotran pathologic basis of disease*, ed 8, Philadelphia, 2010, Saunders.

138. Kvist T, Reit C: Results of endodontic retreatment: a randomized clinical study comparing surgical and nonsurgical procedures, *J Endod* 25:814, 1999.

139. Langeland K, Block RM, Grossman LI: A histopathological and histobacteriologic study of 35 periapical endodontic surgical specimens, *J Endod* 3:8, 1977.

140. Langeland K, Rodrigues H, Dowden W: Periodontal disease, bacteria and pulpal histopathology, *Oral Surg Oral Med Oral Pathol* 37:257, 1974.

141. Lalonde ER: A new rationale for the management of periapical granulomas and cysts: an evaluation of histopathological and radiographic findings, *J Am Dent Assoc* 80:1056, 1970.

142. Laskin DM: Anatomic considerations in diagnosis and treatment of odontogenic infections, *J Am Dent Assoc* 69:308, 1964.

143. Laux M, Abbott PV, Pajarola G, Nair PNR: Apical inflammatory root resorption: a correlative radiographic and histological assessment, *Int Endod J* 33:483, 2000.

144. Lekic P, Rojas J, Birek C, et al: Phenotypic comparison of periodontal ligament cells in vivo and in vitro, *J Periodontal Res* 36:71, 2001.

145. Leonardo MR, Hemandez MEFT, Silva LAB, Tanomaru-Filho M: Effect of a calcium hydroxide-based root canal dressing on periapical repair in dogs: a histological study, *Oral Surg Oral Med Oral Pathol Oral Radiol Endod* 102:680, 2006.

146. Leonardo MR, Silva LAB, Utrilla LS, et al: Calcium hydroxide root canal sealers—histologic evaluation of apical and periapical repair after endodontic treatment, *J Endod* 23:232, 1997.

147. Lerner UH: Inflammation-induced bone remodeling in periodontal disease and the influence of post-menopausal osteoporosis, *J Dent Res* 85:596, 2006.

148. Ley K: Molecular mechanisms of leukocyte recruitment in the inflammatory process, *Cardiovasc Res* 32:733, 1996.

149. Li H, Chen V, Chen Y, et al: Herpesviruses in endodontic pathosis: association of Epstein-Barr virus with irreversible pulpitis and apical periodontitis, *J Endod* 35:23, 2009.

150. Li QY, Zhao HS, Meng HX, et al: Association analysis between interleukin-1 family polymorphisms and generalized aggressive periodontitis in a Chinese population, *J Periodontol* 75:1627, 2004.

151. Liapatas S, Nakou M, Rontogianni D: Inflammatory infiltrate of chronic periradicular lesions: an immunohistochemical study, *Int Endod J* 36:464, 2003.

152. Lilly JP, Cox D, Arcuri M, Krell KV: An evaluation of root canal treatment in patients who have received irradiation to the mandible and maxilla, *Oral Surg Oral Med Oral Pathol Oral Radiol Endod* 86:224, 1998.

153. Lin L, Langeland K: Innervation of inflammatory periapical lesions, *Oral Surg Oral Med Oral Pathol* 51:535, 1981.

154. Lin L, Langeland K: Light and electron microscopic study of teeth with carious pulp exposures, *Oral Surg Oral Med Oral Pathol* 51:292, 1981.

155. Lin L, Shovlin F, Skribner J, Langeland K: Pulp biopsies from the teeth associated with periapical radiolucency, *J Endod* 10:436, 1984.

156. Lin LM, Di Fiore PM, Lin JL, Rosenberg PA: Histological study of periradicular tissue responses to uninfected and infected devitalized pulps in dogs, *J Endod* 32:34, 2006.

157. Lin LM, Gaengler P, Langeland K: Periapical curettage, *Int Endod J* 29:220, 1996.

158. Lin LM, Huang G T-J, Rosenberg P: Proliferation of epithelial cell rests, formation of apical cysts, and regression of apical cysts after periapical wound healing, *J Endod* 33:908, 2007.

159. Lin LM, Pascon EA, Skribner J, et al: Clinical, radiographic, and histological study of endodontic treatment failures, *Oral Surg Oral Med Oral Pathol* 11:603, 1991.

160. Lin LM, Wang SL, Wu-Wang C, et al: Detection of epidermal growth factor receptor in inflammatory periapical lesions, *Int Endod J* 29:179, 1996.

161. Linkhart TA, Mohan S, Baylink DJ: Growth factors for bone growth and repair, *Bone* 19:1S, 1996.

162. Lopez NJ, Jara L, Valenzuela CY: Association of interleukin-1 polymorphisms with periodontal disease, *J Periodontol* 76:234, 2005.

163. Lopez-Lopez J, Jane-Salas E, Estrugo-Devesa A, et al editors: Periapical and endodontic status of type 2 diabetic patients in Catalonia, Spain: a cross-sectional study, *J Endod* 37:598, 2011.

164. MacNeil RL, Somerman MJ: Development and regeneration of the periodontium: parallels and contrasts, *Periodontol* 19:8, 1999.

165. Majno G, Joris I: *Cells, tissues, and disease*, ed 2, Oxford, 2004, Oxford University Press.

166. Marending M, Peters OA, Zehnder M: Factors affecting the outcome of orthograde root canal therapy in a general dentistry hospital practice, *Oral Surg Oral Med Oral Pathol Oral Radiol Endod* 99:119, 2005.

167. Marotta PS, Fontes TV, Armada L, et al, editors: Type 2 diabetes mellitus and the prevalence of apical periodontitis and endodontic treatment in an adult Brazilian population, *J Endod* 38:297, 2012.

168. Martinelli C, Rulli MA: The innervation of chronic inflammatory human periapical lesions, *Arch Oral Biol* 12:593, 1967.

169. Marton IJ, Kiss C: Characterization of inflammatory cell infiltrate in dental periapical lesions, *Int Endod J* 26:131, 1993.

170. Marton IJ, Kiss C: Protective and destructive immune reactions in apical periodontitis, *Oral Microbiol Immunol* 15:139, 2000.

171. Medzhitove R: Toll-like receptors and innate immunity, *Nat Rev Immunol* 1:135, 2001.

172. Medzhitov R, Janeway C Jr: Innate immunity, *New Engl J Med* 343:338, 2000.

173. Meghji S, Qureshi W, Henderson B, Harris M: The role of endotoxin and cytokines in the pathogenesis of odontogenic cysts, *Arch Oral Biol* 41:523, 1996.

174. Meisel P, Carlsson LE, Sawaf H, et al: Polymorphisms of Fc gamma-receptors RIIa, RIIIa, and RIIIb in patients with adult periodontal diseases, *Genes Immun* 2:258, 2001.

175. Menezes-Silva R, Khaliq S, Deeley K, et al: Genetic susceptibility to periapical disease: conditional contribution of MMP2 and MMP3 genes to the development of periapical lesions and healing response, *J Endod* 38:604, 2012.

176. Molander A, Reit C, Dahlen G, Kvist T: Microbiological status of root-filled teeth with apical periodontitis, *Int Endod J* 31:1, 1998.

177. Moldauer I, Velez I, Kuttler S: Upregulation of basic fibroblast growth factor in human periapical lesions, *J Endod* 32:408, 2006.

178. Moller AJR, Fabricius L, Dahlen G, et al: Influence on periapical tissues of indigenous oral bacteria and necrotic pulp tissue in monkeys, *Scand J Dent Res* 89:29, 1981.

179. Morsani JM, Aminoshariae A, Han YW, et al: Genetic predisposition to persistent apical periodontitis, *J Endod* 37:455, 2011.

180. Mundy GR: Inflammatory mediators and the destruction of bone, *J Periodont Res* 26:213, 1991.

181. Murray CA, Saunders WP: Root canal treatment and general health: a review of the literature, *Int Endod J* 33:1, 2000.

182. Nagatomo K, Komaki M, Sekiya Y, et al: Stem cell properties of human periodontal ligament cells, *J Periodontal Res* 41:303, 2006.

183. Nair PNR: Light and electron microscopic studies on root canal flora and periapical lesions, *J Endod* 13:29, 1987.

184. Nair PNR: Apical periodontitis: a dynamic encounter between root canal infection and host response, *Periodontol 2000* 13:121, 1997.

185. Nair PNR: New perspectives on radicular cysts: do they heal?, *Int Endod J* 31:155, 1998.

186. Nair PNR, Pajarola G, Schroeder HE: Types and incidence of human periapical lesions obtained with extracted teeth, *Oral Surg Oral Med Oral Pathol* 81:93, 1996.

187. Nair PNR, Sjogren U, Krey G, Sundqvist G: Therapy-resistant foreign body giant cell granuloma at the periapex of a root-filled human tooth, *J Endod* 26:225, 1990.

188. Nair PNR, Sjogren U, Sundqvist G: Cholesterol crystals as an etiological factor in non-resolving chronic inflammation: an experimental study in guinea pigs, *Eur J Oral Sci* 106:644, 1998.

189. Nair PNR, Sundqvist G, Sjogren U: Experimental evidence supports the abscess theory of development of radicular cysts, *Oral Surg Oral Med Oral Pathol Oral Radiol Endod* 106:294, 2008.

190. Nakamura I, Takahashi N, Sasaki T, et al: Chemical and physical properties of extracellular matrix are required for the actin ring formation in osteoclasts, *J Bone Miner Res* 11:1873, 1996.

191. Nakashima M: Induction of dentin formation on canine amputated pulp by recombinant human bone morphogenic proteins (BMP)-2 and -4, *J Dent Res* 73:1515, 1994.

192. Nanci A: *Ten Cate's oral histology: development, structure, and function*, ed 7, St. Louis, 2008, Mosby.

193. Nathan C: Points of control in inflammation, *Nature* 420:846, 2002.

194. Nauseef WM: How human neutrophils kill and degrade microbes: an integrated view. *Immunol Rev* 219:88, 2007.

195. Neville BW, Damm DD, Allen CM, Bouquot JE: *Oral and maxillofacial pathology*, ed 3, St. Louis, 2009, Saunders.

196. Niederman R, Westernoff T, Lee C, et al: Infection-mediated early-onset periodontal disease in P/E-selectin-deficient mice, *J Clin Periodontol* 28:569, 2001.

197. Noirti Y, Ehara A, Kawahara T, et al: Participation of bacterial biofilms in refractory and chronic periapical periodontitis, *J Endod* 28:679, 2002.

198. Nordlund L, Hormia M, Saxen L, Thesleff I: Immunohistochemical localization of epidermal growth factor receptors in human gingival epithelia, *J Periodont Res* 26:333, 1991.

199. Nualart Groslimus ZC, Morales Chavez MC, Slvestre Donat FJ: Periodontal disease associated to systemic genetic disorders, *Med Oral Pathol Oral Cir Bucal* 12:E211, 2007.

200. Oehlers FAC: Periapical lesions and residual dental cysts, *Br J Oral Surg* 8:103, 1970.

201. Oguntebi B, Slee AM, Tanzer JM, Langeland K: Predominant microflora associated with human dental periradicular abscesses, *J Clin Microbiol* 15:964, 1982.

202. Okiji T, Kawashima N, Kosaka T, et al: Distribution of Ia antigen-expressing nonlymphoid cells in various stages of induced periapical lesions in rat molars, *J Endod* 20:27, 1994.

203. Orstavik D, Pitt Ford TR: *Essential endodontology: prevention and treatment of apical periodontitis*, ed 2, Philadelphia, 2008, Wiley-Blackwell.

204. Pallasch TJ, Wahl MJ: Focal infection: new age or ancient history? *Endod Topics* 4:32, 2003.

205. Pascon EA, Leonardo MR, Safavi K, Langeland K: Tissue reaction to endodontic materials: methods, criteria, assessment, and observations, *Oral Surg Oral Med Oral Pathol* 2:222, 1991.

206. Peciuliene V, Reynaud AH, Balciuniene I, Haapasalo M: Isolation of yeasts and enteric bacteria in root-filled teeth with chronic apical periodontitis, *Int Endod* 34:429, 2001.

207. Quesnell BT, Alves M, Hawkinson RW, et al: The effect of human immunodeficiency virus on endodontic treatment outcome, *J Endod* 31:633, 2005.

208. Reddy SV, Roodman GD: Control of osteoclast differentiation, *Crit Rev Eukaryotic Gene Expression* 8:1, 1998.

209. Reeve CM, Wentz FM: The prevalence, morphology, and distribution of epithelial cell rests in the human periodontal ligament, *Oral Surg* 15:785, 1962.

210. Regezi JA, Scubba JJ, Jordan RCK: *Oral pathology: clinical pathologic correlations*, ed 5, St. Louis, 2008, Saunders.

211. Reinke E, Fabry Z: Breaking or making immunological privilege in the central nervous system: the regulation of immunity by neuropeptides, *Immunol Lett* 104:102, 2006.

212. Reuther T, Schuster T, Mende U, Kubler A: Osteoradionecrosis of the jaws as a side effect of radiotherapy of head and neck tumor patients—a report of a thirty year retrospective review, *Int J Oral Maxillofacial Surg* 32:289, 2003.

213. Richardson JD, Vasko MR: Cellular mechanisms of neurogenic inflammation, *J Pharmacol Exp Ther* 302:839, 2002.

214. Ricucci D, Bergenholtz G: Histologic features of apical periodontitis in human biopsies, *Endod Topics* 8:68, 2004.

215. Ricucci D, Pascon EA, Pitt Ford TR, Langeland K: Epithelium and bacteria in periapical lesions, *Oral Surg Oral Med Oral Pathol Oral Radiol Endod* 101:241, 2006.

216. Ruggiero SL, Drew SJ: Osteonecrosis of the jaws and bisphosphonate therapy, *J Dent Res* 86:1013, 2007.

217. Rutherford RB, Spangberg L, Tucker M, et al: The time-course of the induction of reparative dentin formation in monkeys by recombinant human osteogenic protein-1, *Arch Oral Biol* 39:833, 1994.

218. Sabeti M, Simon JH, Howzari H, Slot J: Cytomegalovirus and Epstein-Barr virus active infection in periapical lesions of teeth with intact crowns, *J Endod* 29:321, 2003.

219. Sahara N, Toyoki A, Ashizawa Y, et al: Cytodifferentiation of the odontoclast prior to the shedding of human deciduous teeth: an ultrastructural and cytochemical study, *Anat Rec* 244:33, 1996.

220. Sasaki T: Differentiation and functions of osteoclasts and odontoclasts in mineralized tissue resorption, *Microscopy Res Tech* 61:483, 2003.

221. Sasaki T, Sasaki T, Motegi N, et al: Dentin resorption mediated by odontoclasts in physiological root resorption of human deciduous teeth, *Am J Anat* 183:303, 1988.

222. Sathorn C, Parashos P, Messer HH: How useful is root canal culturing in predicting treatment outcome? *J Endod* 33:220, 2007.

223. Saunder DN: Interleukin-1 in dermatological disease. In Bomford R, Henderson B, editors: *Interleukin-1, inflammation and disease*, North Holland, 1989, Elsevier.

224. Scapoli C, Mamolini E, Carrieri A, et al: Gene-gene interaction among cytokine polymorphisms influence susceptibility to aggressive periodontitis, *Genes Immun* 12:473, 2011.

225. Schaffer M, Beiter T, Becker HD, Hunt TK: Neuropeptides: mediators of inflammation and tissue repair?, *Arch Surg* 133:1107, 1998.

226. Schoenfeld SE, Greening AB, Glick DH, et al: Endotoxic activity in periapical lesions, *Oral Surg Oral Med Oral Pathol Oral Radiol Endod* 53:82, 1982.

227. Schork NJ, Fallin D, Lanchbury JS: Single nucleotide polymorphisms and the future of genetic epidemiology, *Clin Genet* 58:250, 2000.

228. Segura-Egea JJ, Castellanos-Cosano L, Machuca G, et al, editors: Diabetes mellitus, periapical inflammation and endodontic treatment outcome, *Med Oral Patol Cir Bucal* 17:e356, 2012.

229. Segura-Egea JJ, Jimenez A, Rios-Santos JV, et al: High prevalence of apical periodontitis amongst type 2 diabetic patients, *Int Endod J* 38:564, 2005.

230. Seltzer S: *Endodontology*, ed 2, Philadelphia, 1988, Lea & Febiger.

231. Seltzer S, Bender IB, Zionitz M: The dynamics of pulp inflammation: correlation between diagnostic data and actual histological finding in the pulp. Part 1 and Part 2, *Oral Surg Oral Med Oral Pathol* 16:846, 1963.

232. Seltzer S, Naidorf IJ: Flare-ups in endodontics: 1. Etiological factors, *J Endod* 11:472, 1985.

233. Seo B-M, Miura M, Gronthos S, et al: Investigation of multipotent postnatal stem cells from human periodontal ligament, *Lancet* 364:149, 2004.

234. Serbina NV, Jia T, Hohl TM, Pamer EG: Monocyte-mediated defense against microbial pathogens, *Ann Rev Immunol* 26:421, 2008.

235. Shear M: The histogenesis of dental cysts, *Dent Pract* 13:238, 1963.

236. Shimono M, Suda H, Maeda T, editors: *Dentin/pulp complex*, New York, 1996, Quintessence.

237. Sidaravicius B, Aleksejuniene J, Eriksen HM: Endodontic treatment and prevalence of apical periodontitis in an adult population of Vilnius, Lithuania, *Dent Traumatol* 15:210, 2000.

238. Sigurdsson A: Pulpal diagnosis, *Endod Topics* 5:12, 2003.

239. Silva Costa CP, Abreu Fonseca EB, Carvalho Souza S de F: Association between sickle cell anemia and pulp necrosis, *J Endod* 39:177, 2013.

240. Silva TA, Garlet GP, Fukada SY, et al: Chemokines in oral inflammatory diseases: apical periodontitis and periodontal disease, *J Dent Res* 86:306, 2007.

241. Simon JHS: Incidence of periapical cysts in relation to root canal, *J Endod* 6:116, 1980.

242. Simon JHS, Yonemoto GS, Bakland LK: Comparison of cellular cementum in normal and diseased teeth—a scanning electron microscope study, *J Endod* 7:370, 1981.

243. Siqueira JF, Lopes HP: Bacteria on the apical root surfaces of untreated teeth with periradicular lesions: a scanning electron microscopy study, *Int Endod J* 34:216, 2001.

244. Siqueira JF Jr, Rocas IN: Polymerase chain reaction-based analysis of microorganisms associated with failed endodontic treatment, *Oral Surg Oral Med Oral Pathol Oral Radiol Endod* 97:85, 2004.

245. Siqueira JF Jr, Rocas IN, Provenzano JC, et al: Relationship between Fcgamma receptor and interleukin-1 gene polymorphisms and post-treatment apical periodontitis, *J Endod* 35:1186, 2009.

246. Siqueira JF Jr, Rocas IN, Provenzano JC, Guilherme BP: Polymorphism of the FcgammaRIIIa gene and post-treatment apical periodontitis, *J Endod* 37:1345, 2011.

247. Sjogren U, Hagglund B, Sundqvist G, Wing K: Factors affecting the long-term results of endodontic treatment, *J Endod* 16:498, 1990.

248. Slauson DO, Cooper BJ: *Mechanisms of disease*, ed 3, St. Louis, 2002, Mosby.

249. Slots J, Nowzari H, Sabeti M: Cytomegalovirus infection in symptomatic periapical pathosis, *Int Endod J* 37:519, 2004.

250. Solheim E: Growth factors in bone, *Int Orthop* 22:410, 1998.

251. Sonoyama W, Seo B-M, Yamaza T, Shi S: Human Hertwig's epithelial root sheath cells play crucial roles in cementum formation, *J Dent Res* 86:594, 2007.

252. Stashenko F: The role of immune cytokines in the pathogenesis of periapical lesions, *Endod Dent Traumatol* 6:89, 1990.

253. Stashenko P, Teles R, D'Souza R: Periapical inflammatory responses and their modulation, *Crit Rev Oral Biol Med* 9:498, 1998.

254. Stashenko P, Van Dyke T, Tully P, et al: Inflammation and genetic risk indicators for early periodontitis in adults, *J Periodontol* 82:588, 2011.

255. Stashenko P, Wang CY, Riley E, et al: Reduction of infection-stimulated bone periapical bone resorption by the biological response modifier PGG glucan, *J Dent Res* 74:323, 1995.

256. Stashenko P, Yu SM: T helper and T suppressor cell reversal during the development of induced rat periapical lesions, *J Dent Res* 68:830, 1989.

257. Steed DL: The role of growth factors in wound healing, *Surg Clin North Am* 77:575, 1997.

258. Stern MH, Dreizen S, Mackler BF, et al: Quantitative analysis of cellular composition of human periapical granulomas, *J Endod* 7:117, 1981.

259. Stern MH, Dreizen S, Mackler BF, et al: Isolation and characterization of inflammatory cells from the human periapical granuloma, *J Dent Res* 61:1408, 1982.

260. Sunde P, Olsen I, Debelian G, Transtad L: Microbiota of periapical lesions refractory to endodontic therapy, *J Endod* 28:304, 2002.

261. Sundqvist G: *Bacteriological studies of necrotic dental pulps*, Sweden, 1976, Dissertation, Umea.

262. Sundqvist G: Taxonomy, ecology, and pathogenicity of the root canal flora, *Oral Surg Oral Med Oral Pathol* 78:522, 1994.

263. Sundqvist G, Eckerbom MI, Larsson AP, Sjogren UT: Capacity of anaerobic bacteria from necrotic pulp to induce purulent infection, *Infect Immun* 25:685, 1979.

264. Sundqvist G, Figdor D: Life as an endodontic pathogen, *Endod Topics* 6:3, 2003.

265. Sundqvist G, Figdor D, Persson S, Sjogren U: Microbiological analysis of teeth with failed endodontic treatment and the outcome of conservative re-treatment, *Oral Surg Oral Med Oral Pathol Oral Radiol Endod* 85:86, 1998.

266. Sundqvist G, Reuterving CO: Isolation of *Actinomyces israelii* from periapical lesion, *J Endod* 6:60, 1980.

267. Syrjanen S, Tammisalo E, Lilja R, Syrjanen K: Radiographical interpretation of the periapical cysts and granulomas, *Dentomaxillofac Radiol* 11:89, 1982.

268. Tagger M, Massler M: Periapical tissue reactions after pulp exposure in rat molars, *Oral Surg Oral Med Oral Pathol* 39:304, 1975.

269. Takahashi K: Microbiological, pathological, inflammatory, immunological and molecular biological aspects of periradicular disease, *Int Endod J* 31:311, 1998.

270. Takeuchi O, Hoshino K, Akira S: Cutting edge: TLR2-deficient and MyD88-deficient mice are highly susceptible to *Staphylococcus aureus* infection, *J Immunol* 165:5392, 2000.

271. Tani N, Kuchiba K, Osada T, et al: Effect of T-cell deficiency on the formation of periapical lesions in mice: histological comparison between periapical lesion formation in BALB/c and BALB/c nu/nu mice, *J Endod* 21:195, 1995.

272. Teitelbaum SL, Tondravi MM, Ross FP: Osteoclasts, macrophages, and the molecular mechanisms of bone resorption, *J Leukocyte Biol* 61:381, 1997.

273. Teles R, Wang CY, Stashenko P: Increased susceptibility of RAG-2 SCID mice to dissemination of endodontic infections, *Infect Immun* 65:3781, 1997.

274. Ten Cate AR: The epithelial cell rests of Malassez and the genesis of the dental cyst, *Oral Surg Oral Med Oral Pathol* 34:56, 1972.

275. Teronen O, Salo T, Laitinen J, et al: Characterization of interstitial collagenases in jaw cyst wall, *Eur J Oral Sci* 103:141, 1995.

276. Thesleff I: Epithelial cell rests of Malassez bind epidermal growth factor intensely, *J Periodont Res* 22:419, 1987.

277. Toller PA: The osmolality of fluids from cysts of the jaws, *Br Dent J* 129:275, 1970.

278. Torabinejad M: Mediators of acute and chronic periradicular lesions, *Oral Surg Oral Med Oral Pathol* 78:511, 1994.

279. Torabinejad M, Eby WC, Naidorf IJ: Inflammatory and immunological aspects of the pathogenesis of human periapical lesions, *J Endod* 11:479, 1985.

280. Torabinejad M, Kiger RD: Identification and relative concentration of B and T lymphocytes in human chronic periapical lesions, *J Endod* 11:122, 1985.

281. Torabinejad M, Kiger RD: Experimentally induced alterations in periapical tissues of the cat, *J Dent Res* 59:87, 1980.

282. Torabinejad M, Walton RE: *Endodontics: principles and practice*, ed 4, St. Louis, 2009, Saunders.

283. Tronstad L, Barnett F, Cervone F: Periapical bacterial plaque in teeth refractory to endodontic treatment, *Dent Traumatol* 6:73, 1990.

284. Tronstad L, Barnett F, Riso K, Slots J: Extraradicular endodontic infection, *Dent Traumatol* 3:86, 1987.

285. Trombelli L, Lee MB, Promsudthi A, et al: Periodontal repair in dogs: histologic observations of guided tissue regeneration with a prostaglandin E1 analog/methacrylate composite, *Clin Periodontol* 26:381, 1999.

286. Trott JR, Chebeb F, Galindo Y: Factors related to cholesterol formation in cysts and granulomas, *J Cand Dent Assoc* 38:76, 1973.

287. Trowbridge H, Emling RC: *Inflammation: a review of the process*, ed 5, Chicago, 1997, Quintessence Publishing.

288. Tuan T-L, Nichter LS: The molecular basis of keloid and hypertrophic scar formation, *Mol Med Today* 4:19, 1998.

289. Tzaifas D, Alvanou A, Papadimitrious S, et al: Effects of recombinant basic fibroblast growth factor, insulin-like growth factor-II and transforming growth factor-β 1 on dog dental pulp cells in vivo, *Arch Oral Biol* 43:431, 1998.

290. van Oosterhout AJ, Bloksma N: Regulatory T-lymphocytes in asthma, *Eur Respir J* 26:918, 2005.

291. van Winkelhoff AJ, Carless AW, de Graaff J: Bacteroides endodontalis and other black-pigmented Bacteroides species in odontogenic abscesses, *Infect Immun* 49:494, 1985.

292. Vier FV, Figueiredo JA: Prevalence of different periapical lesions associated with human teeth and their correlation with the presence and extension of apical external root resorption, *Int Endod J* 35:710, 2002.

293. Wadachi R, Hargreaves KW: Trigeminal nociceptors express TLR-4 and CD14: a mechanism for pain due to infection, *J Dent Res* 85:49, 2006.

294. Wakelin D, Roitt I, Mims C, et al, editors: *Mims' medical microbiology*, ed 4, Philadelphia, 2008, Mosby.

295. Wallstrom JB, Torabinejad M, Kettering J, McMillan P: Role of T cells in the pathogenesis of periapical lesions: a preliminary report, *Oral Surg Oral Med Oral Pathol* 76:213, 1993.

296. Walton RE, Ardjmand K: Histological evaluation of the presence of bacteria in induced periapical lesions in monkeys, *J Endod* 18:216, 1992.

297. Wang CY, Stashenko P: Kinetics of bone-resorbing activity in developing periapical lesions, *J Dent Res* 70:1362, 1991.

298. Wang CY, Tani-Ishii N, Stashenko P: Bone resorptive cytokine gene expression in developing rat periapical lesions, *Oral Microbiol Immunol* 12:65, 1997.

299. Warren JR, Scarpelli DG, Reddy JK, Kanwar YS: *Essentials of general pathology*, New York, 1987, Macmillan Publishing.

300. Wayman BE, Murata SM, Almeida RJ, Fowler CB: A bacteriological and histological evaluation of 58 periradicular lesions, *J Endod* 18:152, 1992.

301. Weiger R, Manncke B, Werner H, Lost C: Microbial flora of sinus tracts and root canals of non-vital teeth, *Endod Dent Traumatol* 11:15, 1995.

302. Werner S, Grose R: Regulation of wound healing by growth factors and cytokines, *Physiol Rev* 83:835, 2003.

303. Williams BL, McCann GF, Schoenknecht FD: Bacteriology of dental abscesses of endodontic origin, *J Clin Microbiol* 18:770, 1983.

304. Williams GT, Williams WJ: Granulomatous inflammation—a review, *J Clin Pathol* 36:723, 1983.

305. Williams JZ, Barbul A: Nutrition and wound healing, *Surg Clin North Am* 83:571, 2003.

306. Woo S-B, Hellstein JW, Kalmar JR: Systematic review: bisphosphonates and osteonecrosis of the jaws, *Ann Int Med* 144:753, 2006.

307. World Health Organization: *Application of the international classification of disease to dentistry and stomatology*, ed 3, Geneva, 1995, WHO.

308. Wu JR, Zeng R: Molecular basis for population variation: from SNPs to SAPs, *FEBS Lett* 586:2841, 2012.

309. Yamamoto K, Kobayashi T, Grossi S, et al: Association of Fcgamma receptor IIa genotype with chronic periodontitis in Caucasians, *J Periodontol* 75:517, 2004.

310. Yamasaki M, Kumazawa M, Kohsaka T, et al: Pulp and periapical tissue reactions after experimental pulpal exposure in rats, *J Endod* 20:13, 1994.

311. Yamasaki M, Nakane A, Kumazawa M, et al: Endotoxin and gram-negative bacteria in the rat periapical lesion, *J Endod* 18:501, 1992.

312. Yu SM, Stashenko P: Phenotypic characterization of inflammatory cells in induced rat periapical lesions, *J Endod* 13:535, 1987.

313. Yusulf H: The significance of the presence of foreign material periapically as a cause of failure of root treatment, *Oral Surg Oral Med Oral Pathol* 54:566, 1982.

314. Zimmerli W, Lew PD, Walvogel FA: Pathogenesis of foreign body infection: evidence for a local granulocyte defect, *J Clin Invest* 73:1191, 1984.

315. Zimmerli W, Waldvogel FA, Vaudaux P, Nydegger UE: Pathogenesis of foreign body infection: description and characteristics of an animal model, *J Infect Dis* 146:487, 1982.

316. Zimring JC, Kapp JA: Identification and characterization of CD8+ suppressor T cells, *Immunol Res* 29:303, 2004.

CHAPTER 16

Root Resorption

SHANON PATEL | CONOR DURACK | DOMENICO RICUCCI

CHAPTER OUTLINE

Dental resorption is the loss of dental hard tissues as a result of clastic activities.[90] It may occur as a physiologic or pathologic phenomenon. Root resorption in the primary dentition is a normal physiologic process except when the resorption occurs prematurely.[22,23] The initiating factors involved in physiologic root resorption in the primary dentition are not completely understood, although the process appears to be regulated by cytokines and transcription factors that are similar to those involved in bone remodeling.[60,123] Unlike bone, which undergoes continuous physiologic remodeling throughout life, root resorption of permanent teeth does not occur naturally and is invariably inflammatory in nature. Thus, root resorption in the permanent dentition is a pathologic event; if left untreated, it may result in premature loss of the affected teeth.

Root resorption may be broadly classified into two types, external and internal, based on the location of the resorption in relation to the root surface.[8,105] Internal root resorption was reported as early as 1830.[19] Compared with external root resorption, internal root resorption is a relatively rare occurrence, and its etiology and pathogenesis have not been completely elucidated.[72,91] Nevertheless, internal root resorption (IRR) poses diagnostic concerns to the clinician because it is often confused with external cervical resorption (ECR). An incorrect diagnosis may result in inappropriate treatment in certain cases.[57,58,88,89,91]

GENERAL HISTOLOGIC FEATURES

Osteoclasts are motile, multinucleated giant cells that are responsible for bone resorption. They are formed by the fusion of mononuclear precursor cells of the monocyte-macrophage lineage derived from the spleen or bone marrow; osteoblasts and osteocytes, on the other hand, are derived from skeletal precursor cells.[77,101] Osteoclasts are recruited to the site of injury or irritation by the release of many proinflammatory cytokines. To perform their function, osteoclasts must attach themselves to the bone surface. On contact with mineralized extracellular matrices, the actin cytoskeleton of an actively resorbing osteoclast is reorganized to produce an organelle-free zone of sealing cytoplasm (clear zone) associated with the osteoclast's cell membrane; this enables the osteoclast to achieve intimate contact with the hard tissue surface.[92] The clear zone surrounds a series of fingerlike projections (podosomes) of cell membrane, known as the *ruffled border,* beneath which bone resorption occurs. The resorptive area within the clear zone, therefore, is isolated from the extracellular environment, creating an acidic microenvironment for the resorption of hard tissues.

Odontoclasts, which are the cells that resorb dental hard tissues (Fig. 16-1), are morphologically similar to osteoclasts.[49] Odontoclasts differ from osteoclasts in that they are smaller, have fewer nuclei, and have smaller sealing zones, possibly as a result of differences in their respective resorption substrata.[74] Osteoclasts and odontoclasts resorb their target tissues in a similar manner.[92] The two cells have similar enzymatic properties,[84] show similar cytologic features, and create resorption depressions, termed *Howship lacunae,* on the surface of the mineralized tissues (see Fig. 16-1).[92] Odontoclasts are polarized in relation to dental tissue and have a ruffled border, located inside a clear zone, that is in intimate contact with their

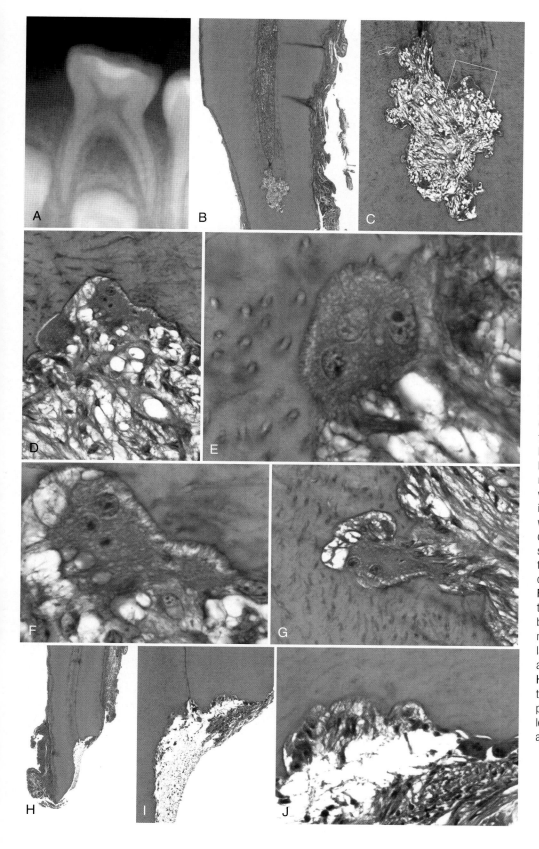

FIG. 16-1 Light microscopy images of a deciduous tooth showing both physiologic and pathologic (inflammatory) resorption. **A,** Tooth 7.5 in a 9-year-old boy. Extensive exposure of a mesial pulp horn occurred during caries excavation, and pulp capping was performed. The patient was brought to the dental office 4 months after the treatment because of severe spontaneous pain. The radiograph shows radiolucencies on both apices and interradicularly. The parents did not accept any treatment and requested extraction. **B,** Longitudinal section taken on a mesiodistal plane, passing approximately at the center of the mesial root. (Hematoxylin-eosin (H&E) stain; original magnification ×25.) **C,** Detail of the resorption area apically in **B** (original magnification ×100). **D,** Magnification of the area demarcated by the rectangle in **C.** Two odontoclasts are present in an area of dentin being resorbed, surrounded by fibroblasts and inflammatory cells (original magnification ×400). **E,** High-power view of the area indicated by the arrow in **C.** An odontoclast is in close contact with the dentin in a Howship lacuna. Its cytoplasm appears vacuolated and shows a more intense staining reaction than the cytoplasm of the adjacent cells (original magnification ×1000). **F,** High-power view of the upper odontoclast in **D.** The characteristic ruffled border can be distinguished (original magnification ×1000). **G,** Howship lacuna with an odontoclast in another area (original magnification ×400). **H** to **J,** Progressive magnification of the mesial root apex. The resorption process may be physiologic at this level (original magnification ×16, ×100, and ×400).

dental substratum.[67,92] Wesselink et al.[119] demonstrated that odontoclasts can simultaneously have two areas of ruffled border, which can resorb bone and hard dental tissue concurrently. Based on this evidence, Jones and Boyd[67] and Pierce[92] have stated that odontoclasts and osteoclasts are effectively the same cell type, differing only in their respective substrata. Wedenberg and Yumita[117] demonstrated that rat osteoclasts resorbed fully mineralized human dentin ex vivo, but did not attach to demineralized dentin or predentin. These researchers concluded that osteoclasts and odontoclasts are probably the same cell.

At high-power magnification, the cytoplasm of the odontoclasts appears vacuolated and shows a more intense staining reaction than the cytoplasm of the adjacent cells. Where odontoclasts are in contact with the tooth surface, the characteristic brush border can be seen, but the hematoxyphilic zone lining the lacunae is absent.[49] When odontoclasts are observed with an electron microscope, the most striking features are the large number of mitochondria and vacuoles in the cytoplasm and the scarcity of endoplasmic reticulum. An abundance of cytoplasmic ribosomes can be seen. The nucleoli are fairly large and centrally located in the nucleus. Close to the nucleus, the Golgi apparatus appears as a narrow zone of fine canals. Where the odontoclasts are in contact with the tooth surface, the ruffled border (corresponding to the brush border) may be observed with the light microscope. The ruffled border consists of cytoplasmic folds that create a system of canals extending 2 to 3 μm into the cytoplasm. In undecalcified sections, mineral crystals could be observed in these canals.[49]

Although mononuclear dendritic cells share a common hematopoietic lineage with the multinucleated osteoclasts, they have previously been regarded solely as immunologic defense cells. Recent studies have indicated that immature dendritic cells function also as osteoclast precursors and have the potential to transdifferentiate into osteoclasts.[102] Because dendritic cells are present in the dental pulp, it is possible they also may function as precursors of odontoclasts.

From a molecular signaling perspective, the OPG/RANKL/RANK transcription factor system[25] that controls clastic functions during bone remodeling has also been identified in root resorption.[109] The system is responsible for the differentiation of clastic cells from their precursors by means of complex cell-cell interactions with osteoblastic stromal cells. Similar to periodontal ligament cells that are responsible for external root resorption,[111] the human dental pulp has recently been shown to express osteoprotegerin (OPG) and receptor activator of NF-κb ligand (RANKL) messenger ribonucleic acids (mRNAs).[110] Osteoprotegerin, a member of the tumor necrosis factor superfamily, has the ability to inhibit clastic functions by acting as a decoy receptor that binds to RANKL and reduces its affinity for RANK receptors on the surface of clastic precursors. This results in inhibition of the regulation of clastic cell differentiation. Thus, it is possible that the OPG/RANKL/RANK system may be actively involved in the differentiation of odontoclasts during root resorption.

We know that osteoclasts do not adhere to nonmineralized collagen matrices.[106] It has been suggested that the presence of a noncollagenous, organic component in dentin (odontoblast layer and predentin) prevents (internal) resorption of the root canal wall, and precementum prevents (external) resorption of the external root surface.[114,116] Similar to osteoclasts, odontoclasts may bind to extracellular proteins containing the

arginine-glycine–aspartic acid (RGD) sequence of amino acids by means of integrins.[98] The latter are specific surface adhesion glycoprotein membrane receptors containing different α and β subunits. In particular, $\alpha_v\beta_3$ integrin plays a key role in the adhesion of clastic cells.[81] Extracellular matrix proteins containing the RGD peptide sequence, particularly osteopontin, present on the surface of mineralized tissues and serve as binding sites of clastic cells.[65] The osteopontin molecule contains different domains, with one domain binding to apatites in the denuded dentin and another domain binding to integrin receptors in the plasma membranes of clastic cells. Thus, osteopontin serves as a linker molecule that optimizes the attachment of a clastic cell to mineralized tissues, mediating the rearrangement of its actin cytoskeleton.[33] It has been speculated that the lack of RGD peptides in predentin reduces the binding of odontoclasts, thereby conferring resistance of the canal walls to IRR.

Once the clastic cells have established contact with the cementum, any subsequent resorption is self-limiting unless the bound cells are subject to continued stimulation.[8] Therefore, in addition to the precipitating events discussed previously, progressive root resorption requires a source of stimulation for the resorbing cells. Stimulating factors vary and are related to the site and type of resorption, in addition to the cause of the predisposing damage to the predentin or precementum. Examples include persistent pressure and forces associated with continued orthodontic treatment; persistent impacted teeth; untreated cysts, granulomas, and tumors; endodontic inflammation and/or infection; and periodontal inflammation and/or infection.[50]

EXTERNAL INFLAMMATORY RESORPTION

Introduction

External inflammatory resorption (EIR) affects the surface of the root and is a relatively frequent sequel to dental luxation[4] and avulsion[14] injuries. It is a progressive condition with a potentially precipitous onset, and it is capable of advancing rapidly, such that an entire root surface may be resorbed within a few months if the tooth is left untreated.[10,14] It also affects teeth diagnosed with chronic periapical periodontitis (Figs. 16-2 through 16-5).[70]

The prevalence of EIR after luxation injuries ranges from almost 5%[4] to 18%.[35] It affects 30% of replanted avulsed teeth.[11,12] EIR is the most common form of external resorption root resorption after luxation and avulsion injuries.[35]

Clinical treatment of EIR is based on effective removal of the causal agent; namely, infected necrotic pulpal tissue in the root canal space.[41] Treatment should be carried out as soon as the resorptive process has been diagnosed. The earlier EIR is diagnosed and treated, the better the prognosis is for the affected tooth.[38]

The diagnosis of EIR in clinical situations is based solely on the radiographic demonstration of the process.[3] In some cases, the initial radiographic signs of EIR can be visualized as early as 2 weeks after replantation of avulsed teeth.[14] However, the limitations of conventional radiographic imaging in dentistry have been well reported. The diagnostic yield of radiographs is reduced by adjacent anatomic noise,[20,56,69,95] geometric distortion,[56] and compression of three-dimensional (3D) structures onto a two-dimensional (2D) shadowgraph.[34,87,113] These limitations may result in late diagnosis of EIR after dental trauma.

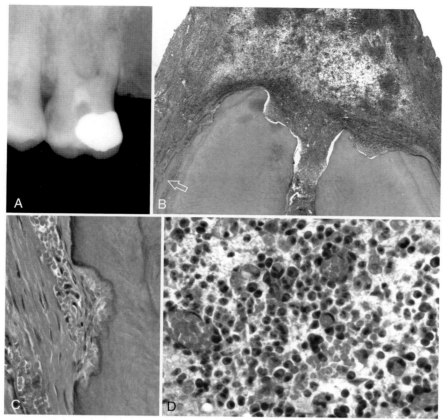

FIG. 16-2 External apical inflammatory resorption. **A,** Maxillary first molar in a 46-year-old female patient that was causing severe pain. The radiographs revealed material in the pulp chamber, a large distal caries, and apical radiolucencies. The tooth was extracted. **B,** Palatal root apex extracted with the pathologic tissue attached. Note the ingrowth of granulation tissue into the foramen and the massive resorption of the apical profile. Also note the resorption of lacunae on the left radicular profile. (H&E stain; original magnification ×25.) **C,** High magnification of the area of the external radicular profile indicated by the arrow in **B.** A resorption lacuna can be seen in the cementum. (H&E stain; original magnification ×400.) **D,** View from the center of the apical periodontitis lesion showing severe concentration of chronic inflammatory cells (mostly plasma cells) (original magnification ×400).

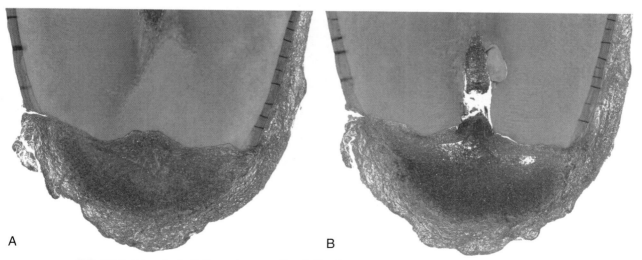

FIG. 16-3 External apical inflammatory resorption. **A,** Mandibular second premolar extracted with the periapical lesion attached. This histologic section, which did not pass through the canal, shows extensive apical resorption. (H&E stain; original magnification ×25.) **B,** Section taken approximately 120 sections away encompasses the apical foramen. In addition to resorption, the opposite phenomenon can be observed; that is, a large calcification partly embedded in the right apical dentin wall (original magnification ×25).

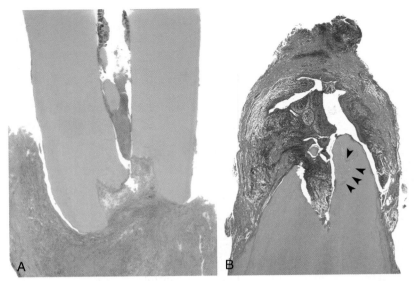

FIG. 16-4 External apical inflammatory resorption. **A,** Mesial root of a mandibular first molar extracted with a periapical lesion attached. This section passes through the canal and the foramen. Extensive resorption of the foramen has occurred, and a calcification can be seen more coronally. Note that the tissue in the apical canal and in the resorptive defect appears structured and continuous with the apical periodontitis lesion. A thick biofilm can be discerned layering the root canal walls more coronally. (Taylor's modified Brown & Brenn stain; original magnification ×25). **B,** Palatal root of a maxillary first molar extracted with the periapical lesion attached. A cyst cavity is present in the body of the lesion. Resorption of the foramen is present, and a portion of the right dentin wall has been replaced by bone *(arrowheads)*. (H&E stain; original magnification ×25.)

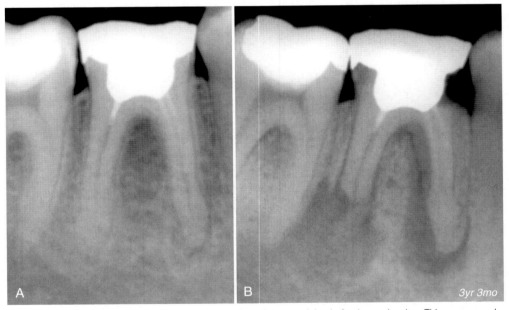

FIG. 16-5 Apical resorption. **A,** A 22-year-old male patient complained of pain on chewing. This was caused by a molar that had been treated endodontically 1 year earlier. A radiograph showed obturation material only at the root canal orifices and a periapical radiolucency on the mesial root. Endodontic retreatment was recommended, but the patient declined this treatment. **B,** The patient returned 3 years and 3 months later because of an abscess that was causing severe pain. A radiograph disclosed destructive mesial caries and large periapical radiolucencies on both roots, along with resorption of the whole apical third of the distal root.

When the occurrence of EIR is correlated with the specific types of luxation injury, it is clear that this type of resorption is often associated with the severity of the luxation injury. Andreasen and Vestergaard Pedersen[4] prospectively followed up 637 permanent luxated teeth in 400 patients for up to 10 years. In that cohort, there were no reported cases of EIR after concussion injuries and only one case after subluxation injuries, which represented only 0.5% of the total number of subluxated teeth. Six percent of extrusively luxated teeth and 3% of laterally luxated teeth developed EIR. However, EIR was a healing complication in 38% of intrusive luxation injuries.[4] Crona-Larsson et al.[35] also reported a higher prevalence of EIR after more severe luxation injuries, with 60% of extrusively luxated teeth and 22% of intruded teeth affected by the complication. They reported EIR to be a much more frequent occurrence after lateral luxation (16.7%) and subluxation injuries (3.8%) relative to the findings of Andreasen and Vestergaard Pedersen.

Etiology and Pathogenesis of External Inflammatory Resorption

A specific set of conditions is required for the initiation and progression of EIR. Under normal conditions, permanent teeth are resistant to resorption.[115-117] Although the mechanisms that protect teeth against root resorption have not been fully elucidated, it is generally accepted that odontoclasts do not adhere to the nonmineralized layers covering the external root surface and the root canal wall (i.e., the precementum and predentin, respectively).[8,59,115-117] Similarly, it has been shown that, between episodes of physiologic resorption, the surface of bone is impervious to osteoclastic activity because it is covered by a layer of nonmineralized collagen fibrils, to which the osteoclast is incapable of binding.[32]

Traumatic dental injuries (e.g., intrusion, lateral luxation, and avulsion) and subsequent replantation often result in contusion injuries to the periodontal ligament (PDL).[8] Damage to the precementum, with a resultant breach in its integrity, is the precipitating factor in all types of external resorption.[8,9] In the subsequent wound healing process, necrotic PDL tissue remnants are excavated and removed by macrophages and osteoclasts.[44] A critical factor is that the precementum may be stripped from the root surface during the injury and the damaged cementum and bone may also be phagocytosed, resulting in exposure of the underlying dentin to osteoclastic and odontoclastic activity.[44] External root resorption may ensue, but the precise type depends on the severity of the initial injury, the stage of root development, and the pulp status of the affected tooth.[8,9] Once the clastic cells have established contact with the cementum or dentin, any subsequent resorption is self-limiting unless the cells are subject to continued stimulation.[7] As already mentioned, odontoclasts do not adhere to the nonmineralized layers covering the external root surface.[8,59,115-117] Therefore, damage to the precementum, with a resultant breach in the integrity of these layers, is the precipitating factor in all types of ERR.[8,9] Damage to the precementum and underlying tooth structure allow circulating odontoclasts to bind to the underlying mineralized dentin and cementum.[115]

The pathogenesis of EIR can be explained as follows. Contusion injuries to the PDL, after a traumatic dental injury (TDI) involving the periodontal structures, initiate wound healing, during which osteoclasts and macrophages are attracted to the site of the injury to remove the damaged tissue. The initial injury causes a breach in the integrity of the protective precementum. This permits odontoclasts to bind to and resorb the underlying mineralized cementum and dentin in a manner similar to the development of surface resorption.[9] However, EIR differs from surface resorption in that it is a progressive event that relies on microbial stimulation from the infected necrotic pulp of the affected tooth for its progression.[7] Therefore, it is more commonly associated with tooth avulsions[11,12]

and moderate to severe luxation injuries, which have the potential to compromise pulp vitality.[4] If the strength of the initial osteoclast attack is sufficient to expose patent dentinal tubules beneath the cementum, a communication is created between the pulp space and the external root surface and adjacent periodontal tissues.[7,15] Microbes and/or their toxins (e.g., lipopolysaccharide, muramyl dipeptide, and lipoteichoic acid),[16] located in the root canal and the dentinal tubules, diffuse through the tubules and directly stimulate the resorbing osteoclasts. The resorption process intensifies and accelerates.[7] The resorbed mineralized tissue is replaced by granulation tissue, which ultimately invades the pulp space if the process continues.[16]

Pressure on the root surface during orthodontic treatment[71] and from impacted teeth,[122] cysts,[104] and tumors[73] may also denude the protective precementum from the root surface and therefore initiate ERR.

Histologic Appearance

The histologic appearance of EIR is characterized by saucer- or bowl-shaped areas of resorption in both the cementum and dentin, with concomitant inflammation in the adjacent periodontal membrane. Howship lacunae are a common feature of the resorption cavities, and histologic sections show that the lacunae sometimes are occupied by odontoclasts. The inflammatory reaction in the periodontal membrane appears intense and consists of a mixed-cell infiltrate that includes plasma cells, lymphocytes, and polymorphonuclear leukocytes in a granulation tissue matrix. Proliferation of capillaries in the areas of inflammation is also a feature.[15] EIR can be identified histologically 1 week after experimental replantation of teeth.[6]

Clinical Features

The tooth in question may look normal, but it will not respond positively to vitality testing. In advanced cases, signs of pulpal and/or periapical periodontitis may be present (e.g., discolored tooth, sinus present, and/or tenderness to percussion and/or palpation).

Radiographic Features

As mentioned, diagnosis of EIR is based solely on radiographic demonstration of the process.[3,14] EIR is characterized radiographically by radiolucent, concave, and sometimes ragged bowl-shaped excavations along the root surface, with corresponding and associated radiolucencies in the adjacent alveolar bone. Complete loss of the lamina dura is seen in the area of the resorption.[15] The initial radiographic signs of EIR can often be seen as early as 3 to 4 weeks after a TDI involving the periodontal tissues[15] and, if it will develop, EIR is always seen within 1 year after the injury.[5]

EIR can have a rapid onset and aggressive progression, such that complete resorption of an entire root can occur within 3 months. The diagnostic potential of a number of radiographic imaging systems has been investigated, with varying degrees of success.

Conventional intraoral radiographic imaging (digital or film based) is currently the clinical reference standard for the detection of ERR after luxation and avulsion injuries.[46,47] However, it has been well documented that this form of imaging is an inadequate method of detecting simulated ERR, especially when the cavity sizes are small.[3] Clinical studies have also demonstrated that conventional radiography grossly underestimates the extent of inflammatory root resorption.[45]

Andreasen et al.[3] performed ex vivo experiments investigating the diagnostic accuracy of conventional radiographic imaging in the detection of simulated EIR and surface resorption. The simulated resorption cavities were located on the mesial, distal, or lingual surfaces and in the cervical, middle, or apical thirds. Nine preoperative radiographs and nine postoperative radiographs of each specimen were taken, for a total of 90 radiographs for the five specimens. The radiographs differed in the angulation between the specimen and the x-ray beam and also in the exposure time.

More than 50% of the medium and large cavities were identified, but none of the small cavities could be visualized on the radiographs, regardless of the horizontal x-ray beam angle or film density. The trabecular arrangement (noise) of the alveolar bone concealed the small cavities. Simulated resorption cavities on the proximal surfaces of the teeth were significantly easier to identify than lesions on the lingual aspect of the root. However, the position of the cavities along the root length (coronal, middle, or apical third) had no bearing on the examiners' ability to identify them. Cavities were more readily identified on high-contrast films; the availability of preoperative radiographs and multiple angled views of the specimens increased the chances of identifying the cavities.[3]

Chapnick[31] used an experimental design similar to that of Andreasen et al.[3] to further examine the efficacy of conventional radiography in the detection of simulated ERR. Multiple angled radiographs and alterations in exposure parameters were also used in this study in an attempt to maximize the diagnostic yield of the radiographs. Although the examiners were able to identify some small simulated resorption cavities, these defects were significantly more difficult to detect than medium or large ones. In agreement with Andreasen et al.,[3] Chapnick concluded that conventional radiography is an inadequate method of detecting early ERR.

Goldberg et al.[54] concluded that *"radiology is not a very accurate procedure for achieving an early and precise diagnosis of resorption defects."*

The studies discussed to this point all used film-based conventional, intraoral radiography. Borg et al[24] concluded that charged coupled device (CCD) and photostimulable phosphor plate (PSP) digital systems are as sensitive as film-based radiography in the detection of simulated ERR. In a similar investigation, Kamburoğlu et al.[68] found that, although the CCD system used in their study performed as well as their conventional film radiographs, the PSP system was significantly less accurate at identifying the artificial cavities. In agreement with Andreasen et al.[3] and Goldberg et al.,[54] this study further reported that lesions created on the proximal root surfaces were easier to detect than those on the buccal/lingual surfaces and that the best results were achieved when multiple angled views and preoperative radiographs were available to the examiners at the same time.[68]

Clinical studies directly comparing the ability of intraoral radiographs and cone beam computed tomography (CBCT) to detect and diagnose EIR are limited. One clinical study reported that CBCT is superior to conventional radiography in diagnosing and determining the extent of nonspecific inflammatory resorption on root surfaces.[45] D'Addazio et al.[40] compared the ability of CBCT and periapical radiography to detect simulated external resorption cavities of about 2 mm in diameter in a human ex vivo model. Although both imaging modalities were 100% sensitive in the detection of the lesions, only CBCT could accurately assess the position of the defects on the root surface and their relationship to the root canal, even though multiple angled periapical radiographs of the test teeth were available to the examiners.

Alqerban et al.[1] compared the ability of two CBCT systems and conventional panoramic radiography to detect simulated external surface resorption lesions of varying sizes associated with canine impaction. The authors reported that with small and medium field of view (FOV), CBCT systems were superior to conventional panoramic radiography in the detection of simulated external resorption cavities regardless of the cavity size. There was no statistical difference between the diagnostic ability of the CBCT systems. However, conventional panoramic radiography is rarely used in endodontic-specific investigations. Intraoral radiography is currently the imaging technique of choice for assessing traumatically injured permanent teeth, which may develop EIR.[46,47]

A more recent study by the King's College London (KCL) group concluded that CBCT was a reliable and valid method of detecting simulated EIR, and performed significantly better than intraoral periapical radiography. Durack et al.[43] found that changing the exposure parameters so as to halve the radiation dose did not have a negative effect on the diagnostic yield of the reconstructed images.

Management

Clinical treatment of EIR is based on effective removal of the causal agent, the infected necrotic pulpal tissue in the root canal space. This arrests the resorption process and creates an environment conducive to hard tissue repair of the damaged root surface.[36,37,41] Therefore, it is essential to initiate root canal treatment as soon as radiographic signs of EIR are identified.[38] An exception to this is replanted teeth with closed apices; in these cases, root canal treatment should be carried out 7 to 10 days after replantation, even if there are no radiographic signs of EIR.[47] The earlier the resorption is diagnosed and treated, the better the prognosis is for the affected tooth. Failure to diagnose and treat the condition may result in tooth loss.

Effective chemomechanical debridement of the root canal space is fundamental to the success of the root canal treatment and the inhibition and cessation of EIR.[37,41] In principle, the specific root canal protocol used is irrelevant, as long as the biologic objectives are met. Long-term dressing of the root canal with calcium hydroxide may be beneficial in the treatment of established EIR; however, this protocol should be used judiciously because of the associated risk of root fracture.[13]

In many cases the EIR is extensive, rendering the tooth unsalvageable and requiring extraction.

Follow-up and Prognosis of External Inflammatory Resorption

Healing of EIR is characterized radiographically by cessation of the resorption process, resolution of the radiolucency in the adjacent bone, and reestablishment of the PDL space.[14] As mentioned previously, in untreated cases, EIR can progress so rapidly that an entire root can be resorbed within 3 months.[14,37] The prognosis is especially poor for untreated immature teeth.[14]

EXTERNAL CERVICAL RESORPTION

Introduction

External cervical resorption (ECR) is a form of root resorption that originates on the external root surface but may invade root dentin in any direction and to varying degrees. ECR generally develops immediately apical to the epithelial attachment of the tooth. In healthy teeth with a normal periodontal attachment, this is in the tooth's cervical region, a feature that gave rise to the name. However, in teeth that have developed gingival recession and lost periodontal support and/or have developed a long junctional epithelium, the resorptive defect may arise at a more apical location.

ECR has also been referred to as *invasive cervical resorption*,[62] *supraosseous extracanal invasive resorption*,[48] *peripheral inflammatory root resorption*,[53] and *subepithelial external root resorption*.[107] The authors of this chapter prefer the term *external cervical resorption* because it describes the nature and location of the lesions.

Etiology and Pathogenesis

The exact etiology and pathogenesis of ECR have not been fully elucidated. It is accepted that the resorptive process is the same for ECR as it is for any other type of resorption: a breach in the protective non-mineralized layers must exist to allow the clastic cells to bind to the underlying dentin, and the same cells must be stimulated to perpetuate the process. However, in ECR only some of the factors that predispose the root surface to clastic activity have been identified.

The anatomic profile of the cementoenamel junction (CEJ) is variable, and the junction between the enamel and the cementum in this region is not contiguous in all teeth. This may lead to exposed areas of unprotected dentin, which are vulnerable to osteoclastic activity, in the cervical region of some teeth.[83]

Heithersay[61] investigated the potential predisposing factors in 257 cases of ECR in 222 patients. Orthodontic treatment, dental trauma, oral surgery, periodontal therapy, bruxism, intracoronal restorations, delayed eruption, enamel stripping, and dental developmental defects were all identified as potential predisposing factors, either alone or in combination. Orthodontic treatment was the most common, sole predisposing factor identified, with a history of treatment in 21% of the patients and 24% of the teeth assessed. Dental trauma was the only identifiable predisposing factor for ECR in 14% of the examined teeth. Oral surgical procedures (particularly those in which the cervical region of the affected tooth was involved) were identified as the sole etiologic factor in 6% of the cases. Specific surgical procedures included extraction of partially and fully erupted third molar teeth adjacent to the affected tooth, exposure of unerupted canines or supernumerary teeth, transplantation of canine teeth, and surgical amputation of periodontally compromised teeth. Intracoronal bleaching was highlighted as the only evident predisposing factor in 5% of patients affected. A combination of predisposing factors was identified in a number of cases. For example, 4.3% of the affected teeth had a combined history of orthodontic treatment and another potential predisposing factor, primarily dental trauma and/or intracoronal bleaching. In addition, of the patients assessed, 7.7% had a history of bleaching and dental trauma; 1.8% had a history of dental trauma, bleaching, and orthodontic treatment;

and 0.9% had a history of bleaching and orthodontic treatment only.

Although the data provided in this study are valuable and arguably the most comprehensive information available on the potential causes of ECR, no definitive cause-and-effect relationship has been established. In the cases affected by a combination of predisposing factors, it was impossible to determine definitively whether the development of ECR was the result of one specific event or a combination of factors, or if any of the potential causes identified were in fact contributory. In 15% of the patients examined in Heithersay's study, no potential predisposing factor was identified. Furthermore, intracoronal restorations were attributed as possible predisposing factors only when no other potential cause could be identified.[61]

There are conflicting views on the manner in which the resorptive process is sustained once the clastic cells have bound to the root dentin in ECR. One view is that microorganisms originating from the gingival sulcus provide the stimulus for continued resorption.[50,105] The opposing hypothesis, by Heithersay,[62] suggests that ECR is a type of "benign proliferative fibrovascular or fibro-osseous disorder" in which microorganisms play no active role and are either absent from the site of resorption or invade it only secondarily.

Histologic Appearance

The histologic profile of ECR is similar to that of other forms of resorption, with certain unique features reflecting the invasive nature of the process. In the early stages, granulation (fibrovascular) tissue occupies the resorptive cavity, and odontoclasts may be evident in lacunae on the resorbing front of the defect.[61] Acute inflammatory cells are often absent from the site of resorption in the early stages of ECR, but secondary bacterial colonization of the site of resorption may occur at a later stage.[39,62]

The resorptive cavity advances toward the subjacent root canal system and typically extends either circumferentially around, or in an apicocoronal direction through, the radicular dentin without communicating with the root canal. Narrow "channels" of resorption extend through the dentin and may communicate with the periodontal ligament.[61] However, perforation of the root canal wall usually occurs only at a late stage because the predentin affords protection against the resorbing cells.[61,64] Consequently, the pulpal tissue adjacent to the site of resorption has a normal histologic appearance until the root canal has been invaded.[61]

As the lesion progresses, bonelike tissue is deposited in the resorptive cavity in direct contact with the adjacent dentin; this is an attempt to repair the previous tissue destruction.[61]

Clinical Features

The clinical features of ECR are variable (Figs. 16-6 and 16-7). The process is very often quiescent and asymptomatic, especially in the earlier stages, and absence of clinical signs and symptoms is very common; the diagnosis is commonly made as a result of a chance radiographic finding. A pink or red discoloration may develop at the cervical region of the tooth; when present, this often is the feature that alerts the patient or clinician to the possible existence of a problem. The discoloration is due to the fibrovascular granulation tissue occupying the resorptive defect, which has a reduced thickness of enamel and dentin at its peripheries because of the loss of hard tissue. The granulation tissue imparts a pink hue to the tooth, through the

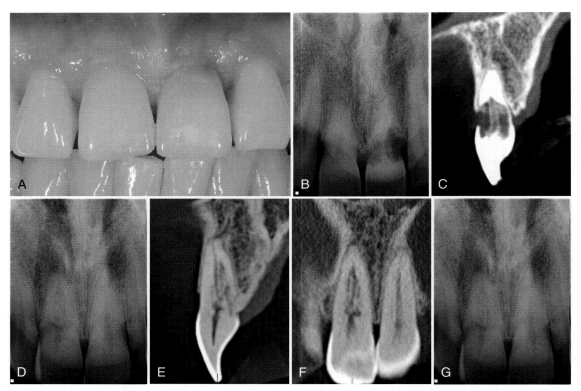

FIG. 16-6 External cervical resorption (ECR). **A,** A 55-year-old female patient presented with an asymptomatic "pink spot." She had no history of any predisposing factors. **B,** A periapical radiograph revealed radiolucent defects on the proximal aspects of the upper left central incisor; note the ragged borders. **C,** A reconstructed coronal cone beam computed tomography (CBCT) slice reveals the true extent of the ECR lesion. Note that the root canal wall appears to be intact. Inhibitory factors in the root canal wall/odontoblastic layer prevented the ECR lesion from penetrating the root canal. **D,** A 41-year-old male patient presented as a new patient. Routine radiographic examination revealed a poorly defined periapical radiolucency in the root of the upper right central incisor. The appearance is suggestive of ECR; the patient had orthodontic treatment in his early teens and remembered "knocking the tooth" at least twice when he was very young. Reconstructed sagittal **(E)** and coronal **(F)** CBCT slices revealed the true nature of the ECR lesion and showed that the lesion was not amenable to treatment. The treatment options were discussed with the patient, and it was decided to review the tooth periodically. **G,** The 4-year radiograph shows no change in size of this asymptomatic lesion.

thinned enamel and dentin, in the region of the resorption.[90] The granulation tissue may perforate the enamel or dentin at the gingival margin, giving the appearance of mild gingival hyperplasia. The discoloration, sometimes referred to as a "pink spot," can be quite subtle and is often a chance finding by the patient, the dentist or, increasingly, the dental hygienist. However, it is a relatively rare feature of ECR. Furthermore, it must occur at a site where it is readily identifiable (e.g., labial surface of an anterior tooth) to be noticed. Loss of periodontal attachment may occur in the region of the resorption, and probing of the resorptive defect or the associated periodontal pocket causes the granulation tissue to bleed profusely.[89]

As the process progresses, perforation of the root canal wall and bacterial contamination of the pulp may occur. The affected tooth may develop pulpitis and the associated clinical symptoms. Pulp necrosis and chronic periapical periodontitis may eventually develop. Clinical signs and symptoms may be the first indication of a problem with the affected tooth; they may include tooth discoloration, spontaneous localized pain, tenderness on mastication, tenderness to percussion, tenderness to palpation over the apical region of the tooth, a draining sinus, and/or buccal sulcus swelling.

Radiographic Features

The radiographic appearance of ECR depends on the location, the extent of invasion, and the relative proportions of fibro-osseous and fibrovascular tissue occupying the resorptive cavity. All ECR defects present as a radiolucency of varying radiodensity, often in but not confined to the cervical region of the affected tooth or teeth (see Figs. 16-6 and 16-7; also Figs. 16-8 and 16-9).

The lesion tends to be radiolucent when the defect is predominantly fibrovascular, granulomatous tissue. However, in cases with some fibro-osseous inclusions (i.e., more longstanding lesions), the radiolucency may adapt a more cloudy appearance. In advanced cases with extensive repair of the tissue destruction, significant deposition of fibro-osseous tissue gives the defect a mottled radiographic appearance (Fig. 16-10).

The margins of the lesion may vary from poorly to well defined, depending on the depth of the defect and the proportion and distribution of osseous inclusions in the lesion. Although lesions with irregular margins are more common, some ECR defects may have smooth and/or well-defined margins.

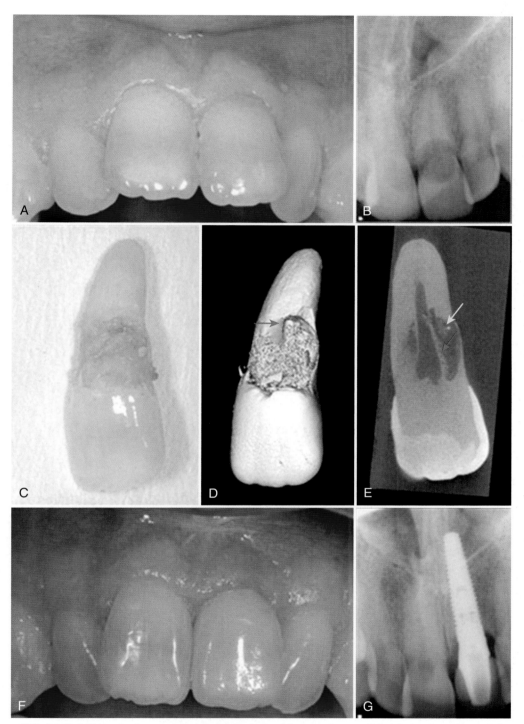

FIG. 16-7 A, This patient's upper left central incisor had a pink spot and was cavitated. **B,** A radiograph revealed an unusual presentation of ECR; the lesion is circular and has well-defined margins. Note that the outline of the root canal is visible and intact through the radiolucent lesion. **C,** The tooth was unrestorable and was extracted; note the large amount of granulation tissue. **D,** Three-dimensional reconstruction of the extracted tooth from microtomography data revealed bonelike tissue below the overlying granulation tissue. Note the intact root canal wall *(red arrow)*. **E,** Coronal reconstruction from a microtomography scan reveals how the predentin *(red arrow)* prevented the ECR defect from invading the root canal. In addition, bonelike tissue can be seen *(yellow arrow)*. Posttreatment view **(F)** and radiograph **(G)** after replacement of the upper left central incisor with an implant-retained crown. (From Patel S, Kanagasingam S, Pitt Ford T: External cervical resorption: a review, *J Endod* 35:616, 2009.)

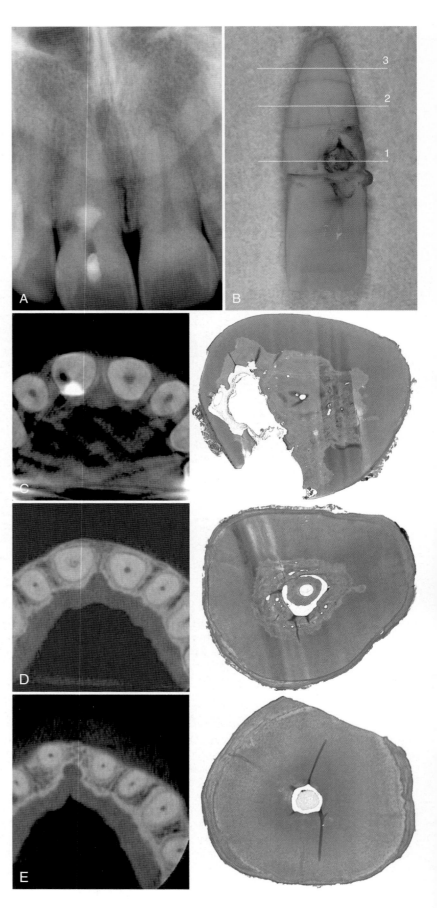

FIG. 16-8 External cervical resorption (ECR) with replacement. **A,** Radiograph of a maxillary central incisor of a 34-year-old female patient who recalled being struck in the face with a cricket ball when she was 11 years old. The dentist mistakenly diagnosed the resorptive defect as caries and attempted to manage it accordingly. The tooth was asymptomatic; however, a 4-mm periodontal probing depth was identified on the palatal aspect of the tooth. A cone beam computed tomography (CBCT) scan confirmed an ECR defect. The tooth was deemed unrestorable and was extracted with the patient's consent. **B,** Palatal view of the tooth at the end of the demineralization process, while immersed in the clearing agent. The tooth was separated into four portions, which were embedded separately in paraffin blocks. **C,** CBCT axial section passing through the coronal third at the level of line 1 in **B.** The corresponding histologic section shows that most of the dentin has been replaced by a bonelike tissue. The root canal is no longer present. (H&E stain; original magnification ×8.) **D,** CBCT axial section passing through the middle third at the level of line 2 in **B.** The root canal can be appreciated at this level, although reduced in size, but it appears to be encircled by bonelike tissue (original magnification ×8). **E,** CBCT axial section taken from the apical third at the level of line 3 in **B.** At this level the canal is the same size as that of the contralateral tooth. The histologic section confirmed the absence of bonelike tissue (original magnification ×8).

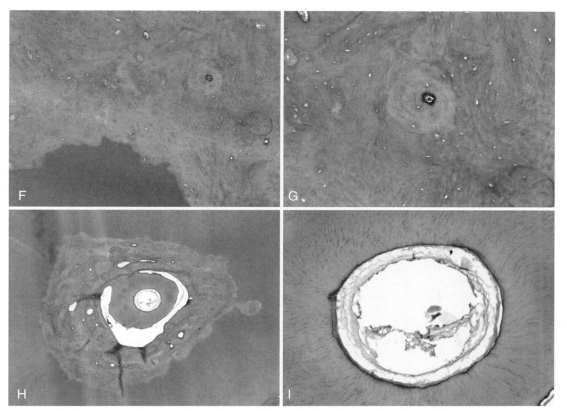

FIG. 16-8, cont'd **F,** Detail from **C** showing the transition from dentin to bonelike tissue (original magnification ×100). **G,** Higher magnification of **F.** The metaplastic tissue does not show the lamellar structure typical of bone (original magnification ×400). **H,** Detail of the canal in **D.** The metaplastic bonelike tissue has concentrically replaced a consistent portion of dentin, leaving in place a reduced layer of the original dentin (original magnification ×25). **I,** High-power view confirms that the tissue surrounding the canal is dentin (original magnification ×400). *Considerations:* The resorption process, followed by replacement with a bonelike tissue, started in the cervical area and extended in an apical direction, tunneling dentin circumferentially up to the transition between the middle and apical thirds of the tooth.

Despite its often cervical location, ECR may commence apical to this region, reflecting the position of the epithelial attachment of the affected tooth. In teeth with a normal periodontal attachment, the invasive nature of the process may result in the lesion extending some distance apical and/or coronal to the cervical location where it started. Furthermore, the tissue destruction at the site of onset may sometimes be minimal and/or not evident on conventional radiographs due to its location on the root surface. In these instances the lesion may appear to have originated at a location where significant tissue destruction, evident radiographically, has occurred. This may be some distance from the actual point of origin. This feature has come to light only since the advent of assessment of ECR with CBCT.

The radiographic features of ECR are very similar to those of Internal Root Resorption (IRR) (discussed later), and differentiating between them, especially in the absence of clinical signs, may be challenging. It is useful to trace the outline of the root canal walls as they approach and pass through the resorption defect on the radiograph. In cases of ECR, the outline of the canal wall should be visible and intact and should maintain its course as it passes through the defect. This is due to the fact that the resorptive lesion lies on the external surface of the root and is not in communication with

the root canal; it is merely superimposed on the defect radiographically. In cases of IRR, it should be possible to trace the outline of the root canal through the resorptive defect because the defect is an extension of the root canal wall and is continuous with it.[51] Although this is a useful diagnostic feature, it does have some shortcomings. First, the outline of the root canal wall may be obscured by calcified tissue in the resorptive defect (ECR or IRR). Second, when ECR has resulted in extensive tissue destruction, perforation of the root canal wall may have allowed communication between the canal wall and the external defect.

Parallax radiographs should always be used to obtain further information about the nature of the resorptive process. In addition to a paralleled periapical radiograph, another radiograph should be taken with a shift (parallax) in the horizontal angulation of the x-ray tube in relation to the image receptor. In cases of ECR, the position of the resorptive defect moves relative to the root canal. If the lesion is located palatally/lingually, the defect moves in the same direction as the x-ray tube shift. If the lesion is located buccally, it moves in the opposite direction. This is sometimes referred to as the "same lingual, opposite buccal" (SLOB) rule. In contrast, internal resorptive defects maintain their position relative to the root canal because the defects are an extension of the root canal system.

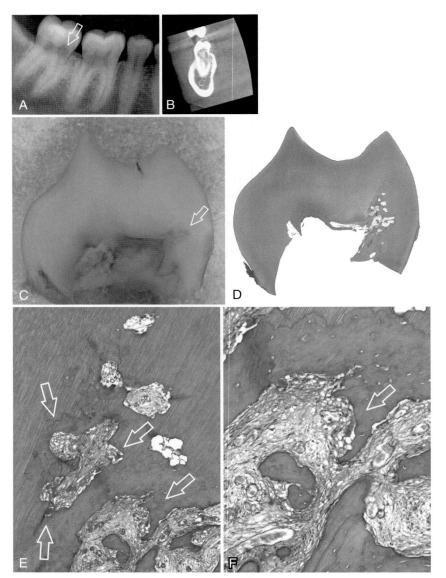

FIG. 16-9 External cervical resorption with replacement. **A,** Mandibular first and second molars in a 27-year-old female patient. The patient had symptoms of irreversible pulpitis associated with the lower right second molar; the lower right first molar was asymptomatic. **B,** CBCT scan taken through the second molar at the level of the area indicated by the arrow in **A.** Note massive resorption involving the crown and root. **C,** Mesial portion of the crown of the second molar after clearing. **D,** Section taken on a buccolingual plane. Overview shows resorption and replacement on the lingual side, corresponding to the area indicated by the arrow in **C.** (H&E stain; original magnification ×6.) **E,** Detail of the area indicated by the arrow in **C.** Several areas of resorption, with replacement by metaplastic tissue, can be seen (original magnification ×100). **F,** Magnification of the area indicated by the right lower arrow in **E.** The metaplastic tissue closely resembles bone (original magnification ×400).

CBCT has allowed 3D assessment of the nature, position, and extent of the resorptive defect, eliminating diagnostic confusion and providing essential information about the restorability and subsequent management of the tooth. CBCT is particularly useful if the clinician is not sure whether the ECR cavity has perforated the root canal wall (and thus for determining the need for root canal treatment). A CBCT scan eliminates the need for exploratory treatment. A clinical study by Patel et al.[88] comparing the ability of conventional radiographs and CBCT to diagnose and to differentiate accurately between IRR and ECR showed that CBCT was significantly more accurate (100%) than periapical radiographs at

diagnosing the presence and nature of the root resorption. These researchers also concluded that the correct treatment plan should incorporate the additional information provided by CBCT.[88]

Management

The fundamental treatment objectives in ECR are to excavate the resorptive defect, halt the resorptive process, restore the hard tissue defect with an aesthetic filling material, and prevent and monitor the tooth for recurrence. Endodontic treatment of the affected tooth is necessary when the resorptive process has perforated the root canal wall. Surgical access

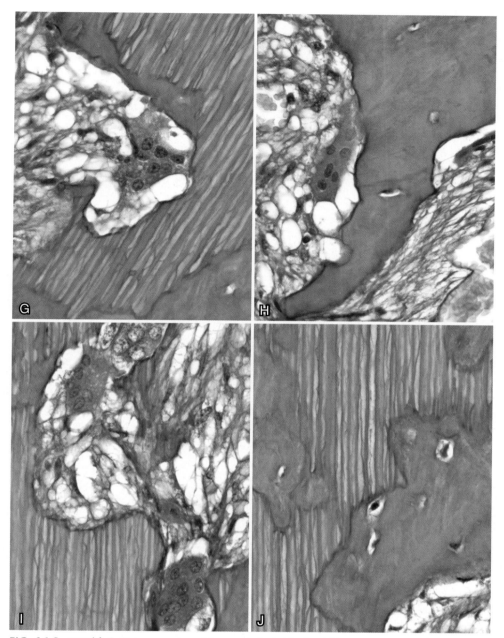

FIG. 16-9, cont'd G, High-power view of the area indicated by the right upper arrow in E. Note the lacuna in dentin occupied by a multinucleated clastic cell (original magnification ×1000). H, High-power view of the metaplastic bone tissue in the area indicated by the arrow in F. A bone trabecula is being resorbed by a typical osteoclast (original magnification ×1000). I, High-power view of the area indicated by the left lower arrow in E. A Howship lacuna with odontoclasts can be seen (original magnification ×1000). J, High-power view of the area indicated by the left upper arrow in E. Note the islands of bone tissue, with typical osteocytes, surrounded by dentin (original magnification ×1000). *Considerations:* In this case the metaplastic tissue was similar to normal lamellar bone. It is interesting that the bone tissue was undergoing remodeling, as evidenced by the presence of osteoclasts. Osteoclasts and odontoclasts can be observed in the same area and show morphologic similarity.

to the site of resorption is gained by raising a mucoperiosteal flap, the dimensions of which should allow visualization of the full extent of the defect (see Fig. 16-10). Once access has been achieved, the resorptive cavity is excavated. Fibrovascular granulomatous tissue is readily removed with a hand excavator. However, defects containing significant amounts of fibro-osseous tissue (especially when the latter is contiguous with the adjacent dentin) require discriminate

removal of the tissue with ultrasonic instruments. It may be extremely difficult to differentiate between sound dentin and fibro-osseous deposits; therefore, use of the surgical operating microscope is essential. Frequent intraoperative radiographs may be necessary to ensure accurate removal of unwanted, hard resorptive tissue and to prevent unnecessary removal of sound dental tissue. The value of a preoperative CBCT scan in these cases cannot be overemphasized. The scan allows

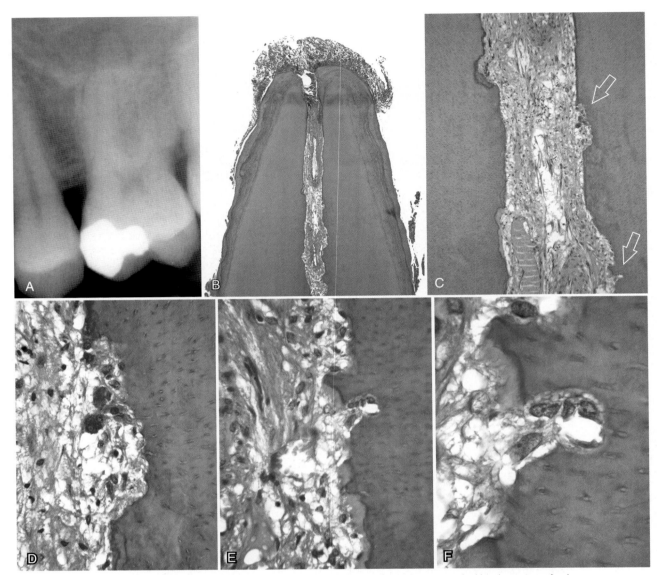

FIG. 16-10 Early internal root resorption. **A,** A 54-year-old male patient presented with a long story of pain on chewing and with cold stimuli. Recently the pain had become continuous and severe. The maxillary first molar, which had a mesial amalgam restoration, did not respond to sensitivity tests. A radiograph showed a periapical radiolucency on the palatal root. After removal of the restorative materials, a crack line involving the pulp chamber floor was diagnosed, and the tooth was extracted. **B,** Some pathologic tissue remained attached to the palatal root apex at extraction. A longitudinal section passing at the center of the canal demonstrated vital connective tissue in the apical third. (H&E stain; original magnification ×16.) **C,** Detail of the canal in B. Note the connective tissue with vessels and relatively few inflammatory cells, in addition to the resorption lacunae on the root canal walls (original magnification ×1000). **D,** High-power view of the area of the canal wall indicated by the upper arrow in C. Note the resorption lacuna with odontoclasts (original magnification ×1000). **E** and **F,** Progressive magnification of the area of the canal wall indicated by the lower arrow in C. Note the Howship lacuna housing clastic cells. Predentin is present in some areas of the wall, but it is absent in the areas with active resorption (original magnification ×400 and ×1000).

accurate interpretation of the full extent of the defect in all planes. True measurements can be made from the scan and related to clinical reference points, reducing greatly the need for subjective tissue removal.

Once the resorptive tissue has been removed, the cavity may be treated with a 90% aqueous solution of trichloracetic acid; this causes coagulation necrosis of the resorptive tissue without damaging the periodontal tissue.[61] The acid also penetrates and treats small channels of resorption that are not accessible to mechanical instrumentation.[89] Once the defect has been excavated and treated with trichloroacetic acid, any undermined dentin or enamel at the peripheries of the cavity are removed with a bur in a high-speed handpiece, and the cavity is restored with an aesthetically acceptable restorative material, such as composite resin or glass ionomer cement. Biodentine may prove to be a particularly suitable material for restoring these defects[30,85] because it may combine acceptable aesthetics with the ability to support PDL attachment.

Once the cavity has been restored, the mucoperiosteal flap is replaced and secured in position. If perforation of the root canal wall has occurred, root canal treatment should be carried out. Access to the root canal system should be gained under a rubber dam before the resorptive defect is assessed. The root canal should be prepared in the area of the defect as normal, using saline as an irrigant. A tapered gutta-percha (GP) point then should be placed in the canal to maintain its patency during the excavation and restoration of the resorptive defect and to provide a barrier against which the final restoration can be condensed. The rubber dam is removed, and surgical treatment of the resorptive defect can be carried out as described, without any risk of the resorptive debris entering the root canal system. After repositioning of the mucoperiosteal flap, root canal treatment can be completed in the normal manner, without fear of extrusion of infected tissue, irrigants, or medicaments into the periodontal tissues.

Heithersay[62] advocated a nonsurgical approach to the treatment of ECR. In this technique, a 90% aqueous solution of trichloroacetic acid is applied to the resorptive tissue in the defect until coagulation necrosis occurs. The necrosed tissue is then excavated, and the defect is restored with glass ionomer cement.

The treatment of ECR depends on the severity, extent, and location of the resorptive defect and the restorability of the tooth. Heithersay[61] developed a four-stage classification system for ECR based on the depth of penetration of the resorption in a buccolingual and apicocoronal direction. He examined the prognosis of treatment in 101 cases of ECR in 94 patients using the nonsurgical protocol referred to previously, and related the success rates for treatment to the classification of the lesion.[61] He reported a 100% success rate for class I and class II lesions, a 77.8% success rate for class III lesions, and a 12.5% success rate for class IV lesions. This emphasizes the poorer outcome that can be expected for more advanced cases. A major limitation of the Heithersay classification is that it is valid only if the ECR lesion is confined to the proximal aspect of the tooth, because lesions are assessed on 2D radiographs. If the ECR lesion is located on and/or extends to the labial and/or buccal (proximal) aspects of the tooth, the true nature of the lesion cannot be accurately assessed with radiographs.[86,89]

INTERNAL ROOT RESORPTION

Introduction

Internal root resorption (IRR) is a form of root resorption that originates in and affects the root canal wall.[9] It is further classified as either inflammatory or replacement. The replacement type is associated with the deposition of mineralized tissue in the root canal space after the initial loss of dentin (initial dentin loss is a feature of both types).[9] Because their characteristics are largely similar, the two types of IRR are discussed together.

Etiology and Pathogenesis of Internal Root Resorption

For IRR to occur, the outermost protective odontoblast layer and the predentin of the canal wall must be damaged, resulting

in exposure of the underlying mineralized dentin to odontoclasts (Fig. 16-11).[106,115]

The precise injurious events necessary to bring about such damage have not been completely elucidated. Various etiologic factors have been proposed for the loss of predentin, including trauma, caries and periodontal infections, excessive heat generated during restorative procedures on vital teeth, calcium hydroxide procedures, vital root resections, anachoresis, orthodontic treatment, cracked teeth, or simply idiopathic dystrophic changes in normal pulps.[5,18,28,93,112] In a study of 25 teeth with internal resorption, trauma was found to be the most common predisposing factor, responsible for 45% of the cases examined.[29] The suggested etiologies in the other cases were inflammation as a result of carious lesions (25%) and carious/periodontal lesions (14%). The cause of the internal resorption in the remaining teeth was unknown. Other reports in the literature support the view that trauma[5,116,118] and pulpal inflammation/infection[58,118] are the major contributory factors in the initiation of internal resorption.

Wedenberg and Lindskog[115] reported that IRR could be a transient or progressive event. In an in vivo primate study, the root canals were accessed in 32 incisors with the predentin intentionally damaged. The access cavities in half of the teeth were sealed; those in the other half were left open to the oral cavity. The teeth were extracted at intervals of 1, 2, 6, and 10 weeks. The authors noted only a transient colonization of the damaged dentin by multinucleated clastic cells in the teeth that had been sealed (i.e., transient internal root resorption). Those teeth were free of bacterial contamination, and no signs of active hard tissue resorption occurred. The teeth that were left unsealed during the experimental period showed signs of extensive bacterial contamination of pulpal tissue and dentinal tubules. Those teeth demonstrated extensive and prolonged colonization of the damaged dentin surface by clastic cells and signs of mineralized tissue resorption (progressive internal root resorption). As previously mentioned, damage to the odontoblast layer and predentin of the canal wall is a prerequisite for initiation of internal root resorption.[116] However, progression of internal root resorption depends on bacterial stimulation of the clastic cells involved in hard tissue resorption. Without this stimulation, the resorption is self-limiting.[116]

For IRR to continue, the pulp tissue apical to the resorptive lesion must have a viable blood supply; this provides clastic cells and their nutrients, and the infected necrotic coronal pulp tissue provides stimulation for those clastic cells (see Fig. 16-11).[105] Bacteria may enter the pulp canal through dentinal tubules, carious cavities, cracks, fractures, and lateral canals. In the absence of a bacterial stimulus, the resorption is transient and may not advance to the stage that can be diagnosed clinically and radiographically. Therefore, the pulp apical to the site of resorption must be vital for the resorptive lesion to progress (see Fig. 16-11). If left untreated, internal resorption may continue until the inflamed connective tissue filling the resorptive defect degenerates, advancing the lesion in an apical direction. Ultimately, if left untreated, the pulp tissue apical to the resorptive lesion undergoes necrosis and the bacteria infect the entire root canal system, resulting in apical periodontitis.[96]

Histologic Appearance

Wedenberg and Zetterqvist[118] reported on the histologic nature of IRR. The authors specifically examined the histologic,

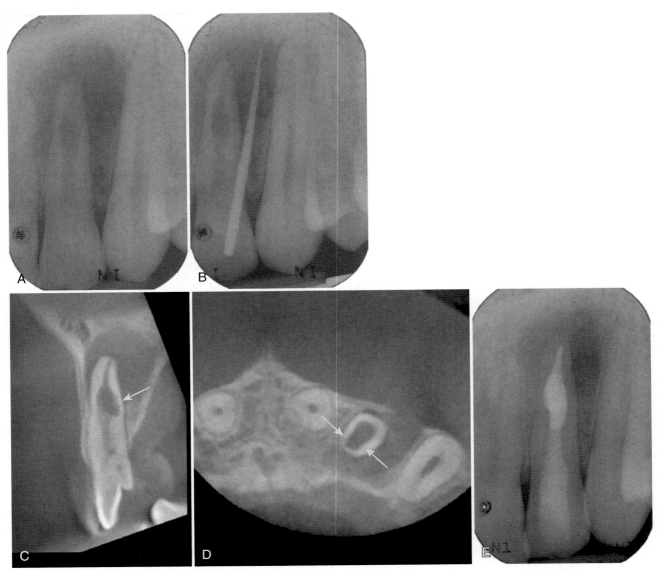

FIG. 16-11 **A** and **B,** Parallax views of the maxillary left lateral incisor showing internal root resorption with necrosis. A gutta-percha point has been used to track the sinus. The reconstructed sagittal **(C)** and axial **(D)** slices from a CBCT scan reveal that the lesion has resorbed the palatal aspect of the root *(arrows)* and has nearly perforated the root wall. **E,** The tooth has been obturated with gutta-percha using a thermoplasticized technique. (From Patel S, Ricucci D, Durack C, Tay F: Internal root resorption: a review, *J Endod* 36:1107, 2010.)

enzyme histochemical, and scanning electron micrographic (SEM) features of the resorptive process in a small sample of primary and secondary teeth extracted due to progressive IRR. The histologic and enzyme histochemical profiles were identical for the two groups, but the resorptive process appeared to occur more rapidly in the primary teeth. The pulpal tissue was populated to varying degrees in all teeth with an inflammatory infiltrate composed predominantly of lymphocytes and macrophages, with some neutrophils. The connective tissue in the pulp spaces was less vascular than healthy pulpal tissue and resembled periodontal membrane connective tissue with relatively more cells and fibers. The odontoblast layer and predentin were absent from the affected dentinal walls, which were populated by large, multinucleated odontoclasts occupying

resorption lacunae. The odontoclasts showed evidence of active resorption (see Fig. 16-11). They were accompanied by mononuclear cells, believed to be odontoclast precursors, which populated the connective tissue adjacent to the site of resorption. Both types of cell displayed tartarate-resistant acid phosphatase (TRAP) activity.

Interestingly, the root canal wall was incompletely lined with a mineralized tissue resembling bone or cementum in all of the examined teeth.[118] Furthermore, islands of calcified tissue of a similar nature occupied the pulpal space in three of the cases. Islands of mineralized tissue occupying the root canal space are the defining feature of internal replacement resorption.[9] The authors suggested that deposition of this mineralized tissue is likely to be part of a coupling process, at the end of a period of resorption, in which osteoblasts are attracted to the affected site and participate in bone formation.[118]

Clinical Features

The clinical features of IRR largely depend on the histologic status of the affected pulp, the extent of the hard tissue destruction caused by the resorptive process, and the position of the resorptive cavity in the root canal space. In the active stages of resorption, bacterial contamination of vital pulpal tissue may cause an acute inflammatory response, leading to clinical symptoms of pulpitis. With the onset of pulpal necrosis and an established bacterial colonization of the root canal space, clinical signs and symptoms associated with acute or chronic apical periodontitis may develop. Sinus tract(s) may occur and may be associated with suppuration in the periapical tissues or possibly at the site of a perforation of the root canal wall caused by the hard tissue destruction. Extensive resorption of the coronal pulp may result in a pink or red discoloration visible through the crown of the affected tooth; this is caused by granulomatous tissue extending into and occupying the resorptive defect.[75] Although often reported as a common clinical indicator of the process, these pink spots actually are rare in cases of IRR. They may occur relatively more frequently in cases of ECR, but they are not very common with that resorption type, either. Often the affected tooth is asymptomatic, and clinical signs are absent.

Radiographic Features and Diagnosis

The diagnosis of any type of root resorption depends on radiographic demonstration of its presence. The two-dimensional nature of conventional radiographic imaging makes the detection and differentiation of the various types of resorption challenging. This is especially true when attempts are made to differentiate between IRR and ECR, which may have similar radiographic features.[57,90,91,105] Much has been reported in the literature about the "typical" radiographic features of IRR. Gartner et al.[51] reported that lesions of IRR present radiographically as radiolucencies of uniform density that have a smooth outline and are symmetrically distributed over the root of the affected tooth (Fig. 16-12). The authors further reported that the outline of the root canal wall should not be traceable through the resorption defect because the root canal wall balloons out. Other authors have described IRR lesions as oval, circumscribed radiolucencies in continuity with the root canal wall.[82] Although certain cases of IRR may have some or all of these radiographic features, many do not; each case should be assessed individually before a diagnosis is made.

IRR can occur at any location in the root canal system and may manifest radiographically as a radiolucency with variable shape, radiodensity, outline, and symmetry in relation to the root canal. Internal inflammatory root resorption lesions are more likely be uniformly radiolucent, whereas in internal replacement (metaplastic) root resorption, the defect has a somewhat mottled or clouded appearance as a result of the radiopaque nature of the calcified material occupying the lesion (Fig. 16-13).[91] ECR lesions may contain predominantly granulomatous tissue, predominantly calcified tissue, or a mixture of the two; therefore, they may have a radiodensity similar to either type of internal resorption, which complicates the clinical differentiation of the disease process. As noted by Gartner et al.,[51] the best practice is to trace the outline of the root canal wall as it approaches and leaves

the resorption defect. An IRR cavity is continuous with the normal root canal walls because it is essentially an extension of them. As such, in teeth with single canals affected by IRR, the canal walls should not be traceable through the defect. This is in contrast to ECR, in which the lesion lies buccal or palatal/lingual to the defect and is consequently superimposed on the canal system when viewed on conventional radiographs. In this situation the canal walls should maintain their normal course as they pass through the resorption defect, allowing them to be traced through it. However, it should be noted that in teeth with multiple canals, a canal that has been unaffected by IRR may be superimposed onto the IRR resorption defect on conventional radiographs. When the guidelines outlined by Gartner et al.[51] are used, this may lead to misdiagnosis.

Parallax radiographs must always be used to obtain further information about the resorptive process. In addition to a paralleled periapical radiograph, a radiograph should be taken with a shift in the horizontal angulation of the x-ray tube in relation to the image receptor. IRR lesions maintain their position relative to the root canal system on the angled view. ECR lesions move in the same direction as the x-ray tube shift if they are lingually/palatally positioned and move in the opposite direction if they are buccally located.[51] This diagnostic technique, coupled with tracing of the root canal/pulp chamber outline through the lesion, has been the most reliable aid in the differential diagnosis of IRR when conventional radiography is used. However, as discussed previously, the amount of information available from conventional radiographic imaging is limited. This can lead to misdiagnoses and incorrect treatment in the management of IRR and invasive cervical resorption.

The use of CBCT as a diagnostic and treatment planning tool in the management of IRR has been reported in the literature.[21] Information such as the position, extent, and dimensions of an IRR lesion, in addition to the presence of any associated perforation, can be obtained from a CBCT scan. The same scan can differentiate between ECR and IRR, removing any doubt about the diagnosis that may have arisen with the conventional radiographic examination.

Management

Once a diagnosis of IRR has been made, the extent of the hard tissue destruction must be assessed and a clinical decision must be made about the prognosis of the affected tooth. If the affected tooth is salvageable and has a reasonable prognosis, root canal treatment is necessary. As with any infected tooth, the main purpose of the root canal treatment is to remove the intraradicular bacteria and disinfect the root canal space. If the resorptive process is still active, the treatment serves an adjunctive purpose, which is to eliminate the vital apical tissue that is sustaining and stimulating the resorbing cells.

The nature of the resorptive process in cases of IRR presents the endodontist with unique operative challenges. In teeth with active resorption, profuse bleeding from the granulomatous and inflamed pulpal tissues may impair visibility in the initial stages of treatment and may provide a stubborn source of mild hemorrhage when attempts are made to dry the canal after chemomechanical preparation. Furthermore, the irregularly concave nature of resorption defects makes them inaccessible to direct mechanical debridement.

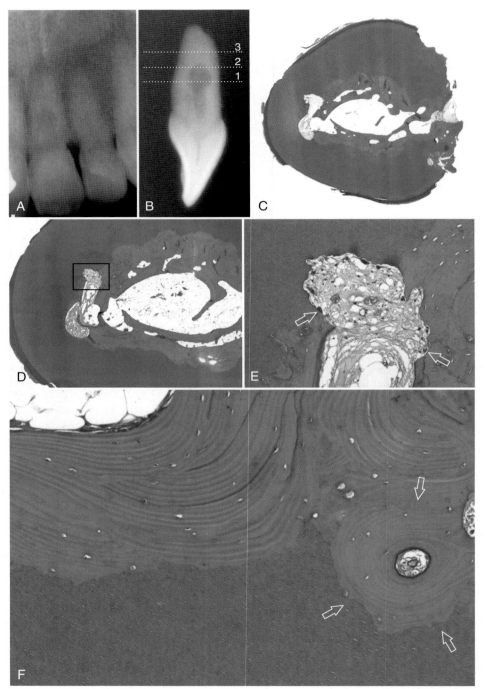

FIG. 16-12 Light microscopy images of a tooth with internal (root canal) replacement resorption. The tooth belonged to a 44-year-old male patient who was referred to the first author for management of a perforated root. The tooth was asymptomatic on examination, but there was a history of previous trauma. **A,** Radiograph of a maxillary central incisor with a radiolucent lesion in the middle third of the root canal. The radiolucent lesion appears to be mottled, which suggests internal root resorption with metaplasia. **B,** Clinical radiograph of the tooth after extraction, taken at a 90-degree angle, showing the continuity of the resorptive lesion with the canal space. **C,** Cross section taken approximately at the level of line 1 in Fig. 16-12, *B*. The low-magnification overview shows that the dentin around the root canal had been replaced by an ingrowth of bone tissue, and the root appears to have been perforated on the distopalatal aspect. (H&E stain; ×8.) **D,** Higher magnification of Fig. 16-12, *C*. (H&E stain; ×16.) **E,** High magnification of the area demarcated by the rectangle in Fig. 16-12, *D*. The intraradicular dentin has been resorbed. (H&E stain; ×100.) **F,** High-magnification view taken from the right part of Fig. 16-12, *C,* showing that the resorbed dentin has been replaced by lamellar bone. Osteocytes are present in lacunae between the lamellae. A characteristic cross section of an osteon can be seen on the right *(open arrows),* with concentric lamellae surrounding a vascular structure. (H&E stain; ×100.)

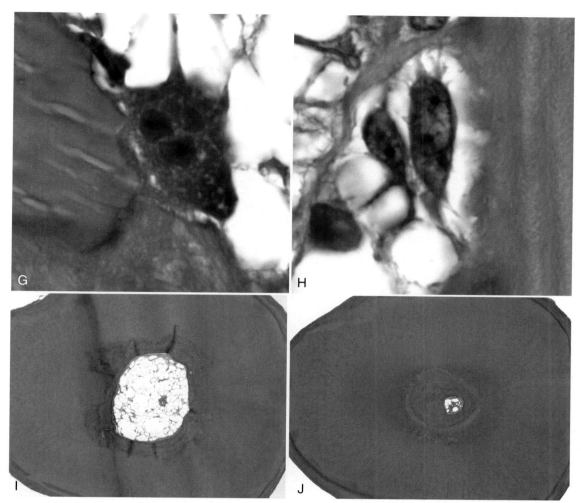

FIG. 16-12, cont'd **G,** High-magnification view of the area indicated by the left open arrow in Fig. 16-12, *E*. A multinucleated resorbing cell (odontoclast) can be seen in a dentinal lacuna, indicating active resorption of the dentinal wall. (H&E stain; ×1000.) **H,** High-magnification view of the bone surface indicated by the right arrow in Fig. 16-12, *E*. The large cells are osteoblast-like cells. Once they produced mineralized tissue, they were embedded in the bone lacunae, assuming the characteristics of osteocytes. (H&E stain; ×1000.) **I,** Cross section taken approximately at the level of line 2 in Fig. 16-12, *B*. The root canal is still large at this level and is surrounded by a relatively thin layer of newly formed bone. (H&E stain; ×16.) **J,** Cross section taken approximately at the level of line 3 in Fig. 16-12, *B*. At this level the root canal appears consistently narrowed by a dense layer of newly formed bone. (H&E stain; ×16.) (From Patel S, Ricucci D, Durack C, Tay F: Internal root resorption: a review, *J Endod* 36:1107, 2010.)

Chemomechanical Debridement of the Root Canal

The complex anatomic and morphologic features of root canal systems provide unique recesses that may harbor microorganisms in infected teeth. Endodontic instruments and passively delivered irrigants fail to penetrate into these secluded spaces and niches.[80,97,99] The use of ultrasonic instruments to aid the penetration of endodontic irrigants has been shown to improve the removal of organic debris and biofilms from the root canal space.[26] Given the inaccessibility of IRR defects to normal instrumentation and passive irrigation, ultrasonic activation of irrigants should be considered an essential step in the treatment of these cases (see Fig. 16-11). However, even when this adjunctive measure is used, microbes may persist in confined areas after chemomechanical debridement.[26] As such, an intracanal antibacterial medicament should be used to further reduce the microbial load and improve the disinfection of the root canal space.[99] Calcium hydroxide is an antibacterial, interappointment, endodontic medicament that has been shown to eradicate bacteria persisting in the root canal space after root canal treatment.[27,100] Also, when used in conjunction with sodium hypochlorite, it potentiates the effect of that irrigant in the removal of organic debris from the root canal system.[2,108] Based on this evidence the authors advocate the use of calcium hydroxide as an intracanal, antibacterial medicament to supplement the conventional chemomechanical debridement of the root canal system.[91]

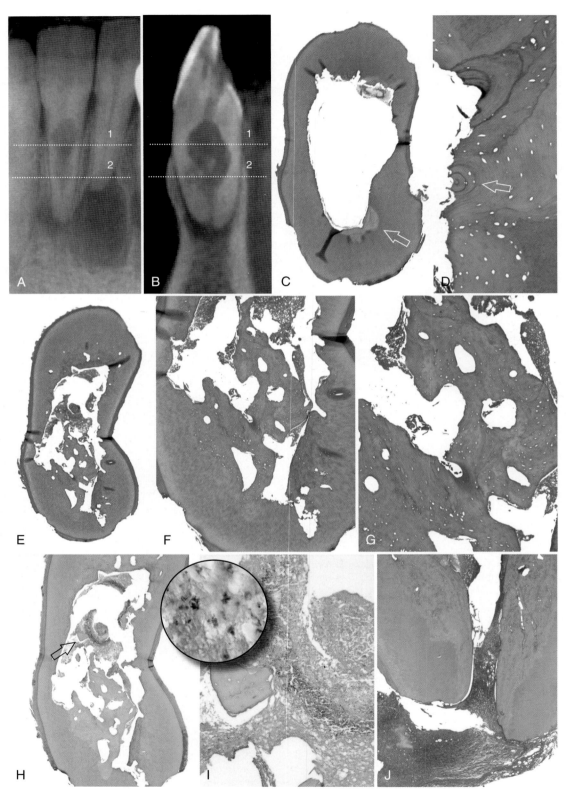

FIG. 16-13 Light microscopy images of a variant of internal (root canal) replacement resorption with tunneling resorption. The lower right lateral incisor belonged to a 39-year-old former boxer who had suffered a jaw fracture in a boxing match in his early twenties and was placed in intermaxillary fixation. The patient developed symptoms 20 years later and complained of pain associated with his lower incisors. **A,** Radiograph of the mandibular right incisors. The lower right central incisor had asymptomatic apical periodontitis associated with a necrotic and infected pulp. The lower right lateral incisor showed a large area of internal root resorption. The tooth did not respond to sensitivity tests. **B,** Sagittal CBCT slice shows some calcified tissue in the resorptive defect. **C,** Cross section taken at the level of line 1 in Fig. 16-13, *A* and *B.* The overview shows that the canal was apparently empty at this level. (H&E stain; ×6.) **D,** High magnification of the area indicated by the arrow in Fig. 16-13, *C.* Lamellar bone filling an area of previous resorption. Note the osteon structure *(arrow).* (H&E stain; ×100.) **E,** Cross section taken at the level of line 2 in Fig. 16-13, *A* and *B.* Overview shows that the canal lumen was partly occupied by necrotic remnants, partly by bonelike tissue. (H&E stain; ×8.) **F,** High magnification of the lower part in Fig. 16-13, *E.* (H&E stain; ×50.) **G,** Higher magnification of Fig. 16-13, *F.* Bone trabeculae are surrounded by necrotic debris. (H&E stain; ×100.) **H,** Cross section taken from the same area as that in Fig. 16-13, *E.* (Taylor's modified Brown & Brenn [TBB] stain; ×16.) **I,** High magnification of the area indicated by the arrow in Fig. 16-13, *H.* A fragment of bonelike tissue can be seen surrounded by bacteria-colonized necrotic tissues. (TBB stain; ×100; inset ×1000.) **J,** Longitudinal section passing approximately through the center of the root apex. Dentin walls have been resorbed and replaced by a bonelike tissue. (H&E stain; ×16.) (From Patel S, Ricucci D, Durack C, Tay F: Internal root resorption: a review, *J Endod* 36:1107, 2010.)

Obturation

One of the fundamental objectives of endodontic treatment is to fill the disinfected root canal space completely with an appropriate material. In IRR, the hard tissue defects caused by the resorptive process are challenging to fill adequately. To obturate the resorptive defect, the root-filling material must be able to flow. Gutta-percha is widely regarded as the gold standard filling material in endodontics. It can plasticize when pressure is applied, and it becomes flowable with the application of heat. Gencoglu et al.[52] examined the ability of different obturation systems and techniques to fill the defects in artificially created internal resorptive cavities ex vivo. They found that Obtura II (ObII) and Microseal (MS) thermoplastic gutta-percha systems produced significantly better fills in simulated resorptive cavities than did Thermafill, soft core systems (SCS), and cold lateral condensation (CLC). In a similar study Goldberg et al.[55] demonstrated that the Obtura II system filled simulated resorptive defects statistically better than CLC, Thermafill, and a hybrid technique. Gencoglu et al.[52] reported that the Obtura II and Microseal systems produced fills with greater gutta-percha–to-sealer (GP/sealer) ratios than did the other techniques examined. These findings were corroborated in the study by Goldberg et al.[55]

Because root canal sealers shrink on setting[120] and dissolve and degrade to varying degrees in the presence of moisture,[78] fillings with higher GP/sealer ratios reduce the risk of void formation and leakage of contaminants into the root canal system, with potentially positive benefits for the treatment outcome.

Stamos and Stamos[103] and Wilson and Barnes[121] reported on cases of internal resorption in which the Obtura system was successfully used to obturate the canal. In light of the evidence presented, the Obtura and Microseal systems apparently can be expected to produce the best technical results for obturating canals with IRR.

When choosing the appropriate materials and methods for filling resorptive defects of IRR, the clinician first must establish the presence and extent of any perforations in the wall of the affected root. This information can be readily obtained from an appropriate CBCT scan. If perforation has occurred, mineral trioxide aggregate (MTA) should be considered the material of choice to repair the root wall. MTA is biocompatible,[79] has superior sealing properties when used as a retrograde filling material,[17] and has proved effective in the repair of lateral and furcal root perforations in animal studies.[76] Furthermore, the material is well tolerated in the periapical tissues, and when used as a root-end filling material in the absence of infection, it supports almost complete regeneration of the adjacent periodontium.[94] These are desirable properties in the context of perforation repair because of the very real possibility of unintentional extrusion of the material when a perforating internal resorptive defect is repaired in an orthograde manner. However, the flow properties of MTA are significantly poorer than those of heated GP. Its use as an effective filling material in IRR depends on adequate ultrasonic activation of the material to disperse it into the recesses of the defect.[21] Use of a dental operating microscope and the correct equipment to deliver the material are essential.

A hybrid technique to obturate canals affected by perforating internal resorption also may be used. In these cases the canal apical to the resorption defect is filled with GP. The GP can then be used as a barrier against which the MTA can be packed. Hsiang-Chi Hsien et al.[63] successfully used this technique to treat a perforating IRR defect in a maxillary incisor. Jacobowitz and de Lima[66] described a case in which a maxillary central incisor with a large, perforating internal resorption defect had a poor prognosis and initially was designated for extraction. The tooth subsequently was successfully treated in an orthograde manner with white MTA and gutta-percha.[66]

Clinical situations arise in which a perforating resorptive defect causes extensive dental hard tissue destruction that fails to respond to or is not amenable to repair with an orthograde approach. Surgical treatment may be needed in these cases. For the reasons discussed already, MTA would be the material of choice to repair these perforations. In cases that have not already been treated in a nonsurgical manner, the operator first must access the root canal as for orthograde treatment. A well-fitting, tapered GP point or an appropriately sized finger spreader is then positioned in the canal to occlude it and to provide a barrier against which the MTA can be packed once surgical access to the defect has been gained. The barrier also prevents inadvertent deposition of the MTA into the apical third of the canal. The perforation is then exposed surgically and repaired with the MTA. The canal can be shaped, disinfected, and obturated with thermoplasticized GP once the MTA has set.

If the resorptive process has caused sufficient tissue destruction to render the tooth unrestorable, extraction is the most appropriate treatment option. If the tooth has been weakened by the disease process to the extent that fracture of the tooth root is likely, the patient may elect to have the tooth extracted. The presence of a perforating resorptive defect is certainly not a contraindication to treatment, but a perforation of significant size will have a bearing on the decision to surgically treat or extract the tooth. CBCT is an invaluable component of the clinician's armamentarium in the treatment of IRR.[42] A CBCT scan gives the clinician a 3D view of the tooth, the resorptive defect, and the adjacent anatomy. The clinician thus has the information necessary to determine a prognosis for the tooth and/or its amenability to surgical repair. If extraction of the affected tooth is indicated, the scan may be used as a diagnostic and treatment planning tool for provision of a dental implant–retained prosthesis. Bhuva et al.[21] described a case in which CBCT was used as a treatment planning tool in the successful treatment of a case of IRR. As mentioned previously, CBCT has been found to be highly accurate in revealing the nature of the resorptive lesion, and this leads to the selection of the most suitable treatment plan.

SUMMARY

- The prevalence, etiology, and pathogenesis of various types of root resorption are not fully understood, and more research is required in these areas.
- More clinical data are required on the presenting features of ECR because this particular type of resorption may vary significantly in its presentation.
- Early detection of root resorption is essential for successful management and favorable outcomes.
- CBCT is an excellent diagnostic tool for confirming the presence of ECR and IRR and also for appreciating the true nature of these conditions and managing them.

REFERENCES

1. Alqerban A, Jacobs R, Souza PC, Willems G: In-vitro comparison of 2 cone beam computed tomography systems and panoramic imaging for detecting simulated canine impaction-induced external root resorption in maxillary lateral incisors, *Am J Orthod Dentofacial Orthop* 136:764e1, 2009.
2. Andersen M, Lund A, Andreasen JO, Andreasen FM: In vitro solubility of human pulp tissue in calcium hydroxide and sodium hypochlorite, *Endod Dent Traumatol* 1:170, 1992.
3. Andreasen FM, Sewerin I, Mandel U, Andreasen JO: Radiographic assessment of simulated root resorption cavities, *Endod Dent Traumatol* 3:21, 1987.
4. Andreasen FM, Vestergaard Pedersen B: Prognosis of luxated permanent teeth: the development of pulp necrosis, *Endod Dent Traumatol* 1:207, 1985.
5. Andreason JO: Luxation of permanent teeth due to trauma: a clinical and radiographic follow up study of 189 injured teeth, *Scand J Dent Res* 19:273, 1970.
6. Andreasen JO: A time-related study of periodontal healing and root resorption activity after replantation of mature permanent incisors in monkeys, *Swed Dent J* 4:101, 1980.
7. Andreasen JO: Relationship between surface and inflammatory root resorption and changes in the pulp after replantation of permanent incisors in monkeys, *J Endod* 7:294, 1981.
8. Andreasen JO: Review of the root resorption systems and models: etiology of root resorption and the homeostatic mechanisms of the periodontal ligament. In Davidotch D, editor: *The biological mechanisms of tooth eruption and root resorption*, Birmingham, Ala, 1988, EBSCO Media.
9. Andreasen JO, Andreasen FM: Root resorption following traumatic dental injuries, *Proceedings of the Finnish Dental Society* 88:95, 1991.
10. Andreasen JO, Andreasen FM: Avulsions. In Andreasen JO, Andreasen FM, Andersson L, editors: *Textbook and colour atlas of traumatic injuries to the teeth*, ed 4, Oxford, 2007, Blackwell Munksgaard.
11. Andreasen JO, Borum MK, Andreasen FM: Replantation of 400 avulsed permanent incisors. Part 3. Factors related to root growth, *Endod Dent Traumatol* 11:69, 1995.
12. Andreasen JO, Borum MK, Jacobsen HL, Andreasen FM: Replantation of 400 avulsed permanent incisors. Part 2. Factors related to pulpal healing, *Endod Dent Traumatol* 11:59, 1995.
13. Andreasen JO, Farik B, Munksgaard EC: Long-term calcium hydroxide as a root canal dressing may increase risk of root fracture, *Dent Traumatol* 18:134, 2002.
14. Andreasen JO, Hjørting-Hansen E: Replantation of teeth. I. Radiographic and clinical study of 110 human teeth replanted after accidental loss, *Acta Odontol Scand* 24:263, 1966.
15. Andreasen JO, Hjørting-Hansen E: Replantation of teeth. II. Histological study of 22 replanted anterior teeth in humans, *Acta Odontol Scand* 24:287, 1966.
16. Andreasen JO, Løvschall H: Response of oral tissues to trauma. In Andreasen JO, Andreasen FM, Andersson L, editors: *Textbook and colour atlas of traumatic injuries to the teeth*, ed 4, Oxford, 2007, Blackwell Munksgaard.
17. Aqrabawi J: Sealing ability of amalgam, super EBA cement and MTA when used as retrograde filling materials, *Br Dent J* 188:266, 2000.
18. Ashrafi MH, Sadeghi EM: Idiopathic multiple internal resorption: report of case, *J Dent Child* 47:196, 1980.
19. Bell T: *The anatomy, physiology, and disease of the teeth*, Philadelphia, 1830, Carey & Lee.
20. Bender IB, Seltzer S: Roentgenographic and direct observation of experimental lesions in bone. I, *J Am Dent Assoc* 62:152, 1961.
21. Bhuva B, Barnes JJ, Patel S: The use of limited cone beam computed tomography in the diagnosis and management of a case of perforating internal root resorption, *Int Endod J* 44:777, 2011.

22. Bille ML, Kvetny MJ, Kjaer I: A possible association between early apical resorption of primary teeth and ectodermal characteristics of the permanent dentition, *Eur J Orthod* 30:346, 2008.
23. Bille ML, Nolting D, Kvetny MJ, Kjaer I: Unexpected early apical resorption of primary molars and canines, *Eur Arch Paediatr Dent* 8:144, 2007.
24. Borg E, Källqvist A, Gröndahl K, Gröndahl H-G: Film and digital radiography for detection of simulated root resorption cavities, *Oral Surg Oral Med Oral Pathol Oral Radiol Endod* 86:110, 1998.
25. Boyce BF, Xing L: Functions of RANKL/RANK/OPG in bone modeling and remodeling, *Arch Biochem Biophys* 473:139, 2008.
26. Burleson A, Nusstein J, Reader A, Beck M: The in vivo evaluation of hand/rotary/ultrasound instrumentation in necrotic human mandibular molars, *J Endod* 33:782, 2007.
27. Byström A, Claesson R, Sundqvist G: The antibacterial effect of camphorated paramonochlorophenol, camphorated phenol and calcium hydroxide in the treatment of infected root canals, *Endod Dent Traumatol* 1:170, 1985.
28. Cabrini R, Maisto O, Manfredi E: Internal resorption of dentine: histopathologic control of eight cases after pulp amputation and capping with calcium hydroxide, *Oral Surg Oral Med Oral Pathol* 10:90, 1957.
29. Çalişkan M, Türkün M: Prognosis of permanent teeth with internal resorption: a clinical review, *Endod Dent Traumatol* 13:75, 1997.
30. Camilleri J: Investigation of Biodentine as dentine replacement material, *J Dent* 41:600, 2013.
31. Chapnick L: External root resorption: an experimental radiographic evaluation, *Oral Surg Oral Med Oral Pathol* 67:578, 1989.
32. Chow J, Chambers TJ: An assessment of the prevalence of organic matter on bone surfaces, *Calcif Tissue Int* 50:118, 1992.
33. Chung CJ, Soma K, Rittling SR, et al: OPN deficiency suppresses appearance of odontoclastic cells and resorption of the tooth root induced by experimental force application, *J Cell Physiol* 214:614, 2008.
34. Cohenca N, Simon JH, Mathur A, Malfaz JM: Clinical indications for digital imaging in dentoalveolar trauma. Part 2. Root resorption, *Dent Traumatol* 23:105, 2007.
35. Crona-Larsson G, Bjarnasan S, Norén JG: Effect of luxation injuries on permanent teeth, *Endod Dental Traumatol* 7:199, 1991.
36. Cvek M: Treatment of non-vital permanent incisors with calcium hydroxide. II. Effect on external root resorption in luxated teeth compared with effect of root filling with gutta percha, *Odontol Revy* 24:343, 1973.
37. Cvek M: Prognosis of luxated non-vital maxillary incisors treated with calcium hydroxide and filled with gutta-percha: a retrospective clinical study, *Endod Dent Traumatol* 8:45, 1992.
38. Cvek M: Endodontic management and the use of calcium hydroxide in traumatized permanent teeth. In Andreasen JO, Andreasen FM, Andersson L, editors: *Textbook and colour atlas of traumatic injuries to the teeth*, ed 4, Oxford, 2007, Blackwell Munksgaard.
39. Cvek M, Lindvall AM: External root resorption following bleaching of pulpless teeth with oxygen peroxide, *Endod Dent Traumatol* 1:56, 1985.
40. D'Addazio PS, Campos CN, Özcan M, et al: A comparative study between cone-beam computed tomography and periapical radiographs in the diagnosis of simulated endodontic complications, *Int Endod J* 44:218, 2011.
41. Dumsha T, Hovland EJ: Evaluation of long-term calcium hydroxide treatment in avulsed teeth: an in vivo study, *Int Endod J* 28:7, 1995.
42. Durack C, Patel S: Cone beam computed tomography in endodontics, *Braz Dent J* 23:179, 2012.

43. Durack C, Patel S, Davies J, et al: Diagnostic accuracy of small volume cone beam computed tomography and intraoral periapical radiography for the detection of simulated external inflammatory root resorption, *Int Endod J* 44:136, 2011.
44. Ehnevid H, Lindskog S, Jansson L, Blomlöf L: Tissue formation on cementum surfaces in vivo, *Swed Dent J* 17:1, 1993.
45. Estrela C, Reis Bueno M, Alencar AHG, et al: Method to evaluate inflammatory root resorption by using cone beam computed tomography, *J Endod* 35:1491, 2009.
46. Flores MT, Andersson L, Andreasen JO, et al: Guidelines for the management of traumatic dental injuries. I. Fractures and luxations of permanent teeth, *Dent Traumatol* 23:66, 2007.
47. Flores MT, Andersson L, Andreasen JO, et al: Guidelines for the management of traumatic dental injuries. II. Avulsion of permanent teeth, *Dent Traumatol* 23:130, 2007.
48. Frank AL, Blakland LK: Nonendodontic therapy for supraosseous extracanal invasive resorption, *J Endod* 13:348, 1987.
49. Furseth R: The resorption process of human teeth studied by light microscopy, microradiography and electron microscopy, *Arch Oral Biol* 12:417, 1968.
50. Fuss Z, Tsesis I, Lin S: Root resorption: diagnosis, classification and treatment choices based on stimulation factors, *Ental Traumatol* 19:175, 2003.
51. Gartner AH, Mark T, Somerlott RG, Walsh LC: Differential diagnosis of internal and external cervical resorption, *J Endod* 2:329, 1976.
52. Gencoglu N, Yildrim T, Garip Y, et al: Effectiveness of different gutta percha techniques when filling experimental internal resorptive cavities, *Int Endod J* 41:836, 2008.
53. Gold SI, Hasselgren G: Peripheral inflammatory root resorption: a review of the literature with case reports, *J Clin Periodontol* 19:523, 1992.
54. Goldberg F, De Silvio A, Dreyer C: Radiographic assessment of simulated external root resorption cavities in maxillary incisors, *Endod Dent Traumatol* 14:133, 1998.
55. Goldberg F, Massone EJ, Esmoris M, Alfie D: Comparison of different techniques for obturating experimental internal resorptive cavities, *Endod Dent Traumatol* 16:116, 2000.
56. Gröndahl H-G, Huumonen S: Radiographic manifestations of periapical inflammatory lesions, *Endod Topics* 8:55, 2004.
57. Gulabivala K, Searson LJ: Clinical diagnosis of internal resorption: an exception to the rule, *Int Endod J* 28:255, 1995.
58. Haapasalo M, Endal U: Internal inflammatory root resorption: the unknown resorption of the tooth, *Endod Topics* 14:60, 2006.
59. Hammarström L, Lindskog S: General morphological aspects of resorption of teeth and alveolar bone, *Int Endod J* 18:93, 1985.
60. Harokopakis-Hajishengallis E: Physiologic root resorption in primary teeth: molecular and histological events, *J Oral Sci* 49:1, 2007.
61. Heithersay GS: Invasive cervical resorption: an analysis of potential predisposing factors, *Quintessence Int* 30:83, 1999.
62. Heithersay GS: Invasive cervical resorption, *Endod Topics* 7:73, 2004.
63. Hsien HC, Cheng YA, Lee Y, et al: Repair of perforating internal resorption with mineral trioxide aggregate: a case report, *J Endod* 29:538, 2003.
64. Iqbal MK: Clinical and scanning electron microscopic features of invasive cervical resorption in a maxillary molar, *Oral Med Oral Pathol Oral Radiol Endod* 103:e49, 2007.
65. Ishijima M, Rittling SR, Yamashita T, et al: Enhancement of osteoclastic bone resorption and suppression of

osteoblastic bone formation in response to reduced mechanical stress do not occur in the absence of osteopontin, *J Exp Med* 193:399, 2001.

66. Jacobowitz M, de Lima RKP: Treatment of inflammatory internal root resorption with mineral trioxide aggregate: a case report, *Int Endod J* 41:1, 2008.

67. Jones SJ, Boyd A: A resorption of dentine and cementum in vivo and in vitro. In Davidotch Z, editor: *The biological mechanisms of tooth eruption and root resorption*, Birmingham, Ala, 1988, EBSCO Media.

68. Kamburoğlu K, Tsesis I, Kfir A, Kaffe I: Diagnosis of artificially induced external root resorption using conventional intraoral film radiography, CCD, and PSP: an ex vivo study, *Oral Surg Oral Med Oral Pathol Oral Radiol Endod* 106:885, 2008.

69. Kundel HL, Revesz G: Lesion conspicuity, structured noise, and film reader error, *Am J Roentgenol* 126:1233, 1976.

70. Laux M, Abbott PV, Pajarola G, Nair PN: Apical inflammatory root resorption: a correlative radiographic and histological assessment, *Int Endod J* 33:483, 2000.

71. Levander E, Malmgren O: Evaluation of the risk of root resorption during orthodontic treatment: a study of upper incisors, *Eur J Orthod* 10:30, 1988.

72. Levin L, Trope M: Root resorption. In Hargreaves KM, Goodis HE, editors: *Seltzer and Bender's dental pulp*, Chicago, 2002, Quintessence.

73. Li BL, Long X, Wang S, et al: Clinical and radiologic features of desmoplastic ameloblastoma, *J Oral Maxillofac Surg* 69:2173, 2011.

74. Lindskog S, Blomlöf L, Hammarström L: Repair of periodontal tissues in vivo and in vitro, *J Clin Periodontol* 10:188, 1983.

75. Lyroudia KM, Dourou VL, Pantelidou OC, et al: Internal root resorption studied by radiography, stereomicroscope and computerized 3D reconstructive method, *Endod Dent Traumatol* 18:148, 2002.

76. Main C, Mirzayan N, Shabahang S, Torabinejad M: Repair of root perforations using mineral trioxide aggregate: a long term study, *J Endod* 30:80, 2004.

77. McHugh KP, Shen Z, Crotti TN, et al: Role of cell matrix interactions in osteoclast differentiation, *Adv Exp Med Biol* 602:107, 2007.

78. McMichen FR, Pearson G, Rahbaran S, Gulabivala K: A comparative study of selected physical properties of five root-canal sealers, *Int Endod J* 36:629, 2003.

79. Mitchell PJ, Pitt Ford TR, Torabinejad M, McDonald F: Osteoblast biocompatibility of mineral trioxide aggregate, *Biomaterials* 20:167, 1999.

80. Nair PNR, Henry S, Cano V, Vera J: Microbial status of apical root canal system of human mandibular first molars with primary apical periodontitis after "one-visit" endodontic treatment, *Oral Surg Oral Med Oral Pathol Oral Radiol Endod* 99:231, 2005.

81. Nakamura I, Duong LE, Rodan SB, Rodan GA: Involvement of alpha(v)beta3 integrinsin osteoclast function, *J Bone Miner Metab* 25:337, 2007.

82. Ne RF, Witherspoon DE, Gutmann JL: Tooth resorption, *Quintessence Int* 30:9, 1999.

83. Neuvald L, Consolaro A: Cementoenamel junction: microscopic analysis and external cervical resorption, *J Endod* 26:503, 2000.

84. Nilsen R, Magnusson BC: Enzyme histochemistry of induced heterotopic bone formation in guinea pigs, *Arch Oral Biol* 24:833, 1979.

85. Nowicka A, Lipski M, Parafiniuk M, et al: Response of human dental pulp capped with Biodentine and mineral trioxide aggregate, *J Endod* 39:743, 2013.

86. Patel S, Dawood A: The use of cone beam computed tomography in the management of external cervical resorption lesions, *Int Endod J* 40:730, 2007.

87. Patel S, Dawood A, Whaites E, Pitt Ford T: New dimensions in endodontic imaging. Part 1. Conventional and alternative radiographic systems, *Int Endod J* 42:447, 2009.

88. Patel S, Dawood A, Wilson R, et al: The detection and management of root resorption lesions using intraoral radiography and cone beam computed tomography: an in vivo investigation, *Int Endod J* 42:831, 2009.

89. Patel S, Kanagasingham S, Pitt Ford T: External cervical resorption: a review, *J Endod* 35:616, 2009.

90. Patel S, Pitt Ford T: Is the resorption external or internal?, *Dent Update* 34:218, 2007.

91. Patel S, Ricucci D, Durak C, Tay F: Internal root resorption: a review, *J Endod* 36:1107, 2010.

92. Pierce AM: Experimental basis for the management of dental resorption, *Endod Dent Traumatol* 5:255, 1989.

93. Rabinowitch BZ: Internal resorption, *Oral Surg Oral Med Oral Pathol* 33:263, 1972.

94. Regan JD, Gutmann JL, Witherspoon DE: Comparison of Diaket and MTA when used as root-end filling materials to support regeneration of the periradicular tissues, *Int Endod J* 35:840, 2002.

95. Revesz G, Kundel HL, Graber MA: The influence of structured noise on the detection of radiologic abnormalities, *Invest Radiol* 6:479, 1974.

96. Ricucci D: Apical limit of root canal instrumentation and obturation. Part 1. Literature review, *Int Endod J* 31:384, 1998.

97. Ricucci D, Langeland K: Apical limit of root canal instrumentation and obturation. Part 2. A histological study, *Int Endod J* 31:394, 1998.

98. Schaffner P, Dard MM: Structure and function of RGD peptides involved in bone biology, *Cell Mol Life Sci* 60:119, 2003.

99. Siqueira JF, Rôças IN, Santos SRLD, et al: Efficacy of instrumentation techniques and irrigation regimens in reducing the bacterial population within root canals, *J Endod* 3:181, 2002.

100. Sjogren U, Figdor D, Spångberg L, Sundqvist G: The antimicrobial effect of calcium hydroxide as a short-term intracanal dressing, *Int Endod J* 24:119, 1991.

101. Soltanoff CS, Yang S, Chen W, Li YP: Signaling networks that control the lineage commitment and differentiation of bone cells, *Crit Rev Eukaryot Gene Expr* 19:1, 2009.

102. Speziani C, Rivollier A, Gallois A, et al: Murine dendritic cell transdifferentiation into osteoclasts is differentially regulated by innate and adaptive cytokines, *Eur J Immunol* 37:747, 2007.

103. Stamos DE, Stamos DG: A new treatment modality for internal resorption, *J Endod* 12:315, 1986.

104. Suei Y, Taguchi A, Nagasaki T, Tanimoto K: Radiographic findings and prognosis of simple bone cysts of the jaws, *Dentomaxillofac Radiol* 39:65, 2010.

105. Tronstad L: Root resorption: etiology, terminology and clinical manifestations, *Endod Dent Traumatol* 4:241, 1988.

106. Trope M: Root resorption of dental and traumatic origin: classification based on etiology, *Pract Periodontics Aesthet Dent* 10:515, 1998.

107. Trope M: Root resorption due to dental trauma, *Endod Topics* 1:79, 2002.

108. Türkün M, Cengiz T: The effects of sodium hypochlorite and calcium hydroxide on tissue dissolution and root canal cleanliness, *Int Endod J* 30:335, 1997.

109. Tyrovola JB, Spyropoulos MN, Makou M, Perrea D: Root resorption and the OPG/RANKL/RANK system: a mini review, *J Oral Sci* 50:367, 2008.

110. Uchiyama M, Nakamichi Y, Nakamura M, et al: Dental pulp and periodontal ligament cells support osteoclastic differentiation, *J Dent Res* 88:609, 2009.

111. Wada N, Maeda H, Tanabe K, et al: Periodontal ligament cells secrete the factor that inhibits osteoclastic differentiation and function: the factor is osteoprotegerin/osteoclastogenesis inhibitory factor, *J Periodont Res* 36:56, 2001.

112. Walton RE, Leonard LA: Cracked tooth: an etiology for "idiopathic" internal resorption?, *J Endod* 12:167, 1986.

113. Webber RL, Messura JK: An in vivo comparison of diagnostic information obtained from tuned-aperture computed tomography and conventional dental radiographic imaging modalities, *Oral Surg Oral Med Oral Pathol Oral Radiol Endod* 88:239, 1999.

114. Wedenberg C: Evidence for a dentin-derived inhibitor of macrophage spreading, *Scand J Dent Res* 95:381, 1987.

115. Wedenberg C, Linskog S: Experimental internal resorption in monkey teeth, *Endod Dent Traumatol* 6:221, 1985.

116. Wedenberg C, Lindskog S: Evidence for a resorption inhibitor in dentine, *Eur J Oral Sci* 95:205, 1987.

117. Wedenberg C, Yumita S: Evidence for an inhibitor of osteoclast attachment in dentinal matrix, *Endod Dent Traumatol* 6:255, 1990.

118. Wedenberg C, Zetterqvist L: Internal resorption in human teeth: a histological, scanning electron microscopic and enzyme histochemical study, *J Endod* 6:255, 1987.

119. Wesselink PR, Beertsen W, Everts V: Resorption of the mouse incisor after the application of cold to the periodontal attachment apparatus, *Calcif Tissue Int* 39:11, 1986.

120. Wiener BH, Schilder H: A comparative study of important physical properties of various root canal sealers. II. Evaluation of dimensional changes, *Oral Surg Oral Med Oral Pathol* 32:928, 1971.

121. Wilson PR, Barnes IE: Treatment of internal root resorption with thermoplasticized gutta-percha: a case report, *Int Endod J* 20:94, 1987.

122. Yamaoka M, Furusawa K, Ikeda M, Hasegawa T: Root resorption of mandibular second molar teeth associated with the presence of the third molars, *Aust Dent J* 44:112, 1999.

123. Yildirim S, Yapar M, Sermet U, et al: The role of dental pulp cells in resorption of deciduous teeth, *Oral Surg Oral Med Oral Pathol Oral Radiol Endod* 105:113, 2008.

CHAPTER 17

Diagnosis of Nonodontogenic Toothache

DONNA MATTSCHECK | ALAN S. LAW | DONALD R. NIXDORF

CHAPTER OUTLINE

An unthinking dentist is a bad dentist. Perfect technique misapplied is at least as unconscionable as sloppy work.

—*Marjorie Jeffcoat*

A nonodontogenic toothache is, of course, an oxymoron. How can one have a toothache that is not odontogenic in etiology? The answer lies in the differentiation of people's perceptions of where they sense their pain, termed the *site of the pain,* from the location of a pathophysiologic process giving rise to the pain that may or may not be in the same region, termed the *source of the pain.* This concept of the attribution of pain to an anatomic region that is different from the location of the etiologic process is generically known as the *referred pain phenomenon* and can occur in multiple areas of the body. Thus, a nonodontogenic toothache has a source of pain that is not the tooth the patient has indicated, clearly demonstrating the diagnostic challenge (Fig. 17-1).

Pain is common. It causes human suffering and has significant socioeconomic effects. Pain is a motivator that provokes individuals to seek care. But protracted chronic pain debilitates and can significantly impair the quality and productivity of a person's life. One survey revealed that 66% of respondents reported experiencing pain or discomfort over a 6-month period. Significantly, 40% of respondents reported that this pain affected them to a "high degree."[19] A study published in 2003 estimated the lost productive work time attributed to common pain conditions among active workers to cost $61.2 billion per year.[127] One investigator reported that over a 6-month period, 22% of Americans experienced at least one of five types of facial pain. Of these pains, the most common type (12.2%) was toothache.[81]

Although toothache is the most common pain entity occurring in the facial region,[81] many other types of pain can occur in the same general area. A primary responsibility of a dental practitioner is to diagnose pathologic entities associated with the oral cavity and masticatory apparatus. Many of these pathologic entities have pain as a primary component of their presentation. Because dental practitioners are sought out daily for the alleviation of odontogenic pain, it is imperative for them to have a basic working knowledge of other types of facial pain in order to make an accurate diagnosis and properly select care for patients. It is paramount to realize that not all pain entities presenting as toothache are of odontogenic origin. The presenting toothache may be a heterotopic symptom of another disorder. A heterotopic symptom is perceived to originate from a site that is different from the tissue that is actually the source of the pain. This is in contrast to primary pain, in which the perceived site of pain is the actual tissue from which the pain originates. Before discussing pain entities that mimic toothache, it is helpful to understand the neurobiologic mechanisms of orofacial pain.

REVIEW OF NEUROANATOMY

Somatic Structures

To understand the pathways by which orofacial pain occurs, one must first gain a basic understanding of the structures involved in its transmission to higher brain centers (see also Chapter 4). Structures of the orofacial region can be divided

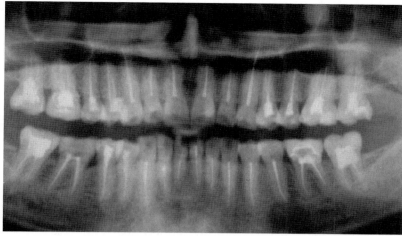

FIG. 17-1 Pantomogram of a patient who has undergone several endodontic procedures without resolution of her chief complaint. (Courtesy Dr. Jeffrey Okeson, Lexington, Kentucky.)

into two broad categories: somatic and neural structures. Somatic structures are those that make up the different non-neural tissues and organs. The somatic structures can be further anatomically divided into superficial and deep structures. Superficial structures include the skin, mucosa, and gingiva; pain that arises from these superficial structures is usually well localized (e.g., a sharp explorer penetrating the gingiva results in well-localized pain). Deep structures include musculoskeletal and visceral tissues. Pains from these deep structures are typically poorly localized and diffuse in nature.

Neural Structures

Neural structures involved in the perception of pain include the afferent (toward the brain) and efferent (away from the brain) regulation of somatic structures. Nerve impulses are transmitted from orofacial structures to the brain via the peripheral nervous system, whereas modulation and interpretation of these impulses into what we feel as pain occurs in the central nervous system. Pain can arise solely from either central or peripheral nervous tissue but heterotopic pain, which is often involved with nonodontogenic toothache, likely requires central modulation to occur.

Peripheral Nervous System

Pain arises as a result of tissue damage, or the potential for tissue damage, and is transmitted via terminal nerve fibers known as primary afferent nerve fibers. Two major classes of nociceptive (or pain-sensing) primary afferent nerve fibers can detect potentially damaging noxious stimuli: the A-delta and C fibers. Both fiber types have a wide distribution throughout the skin, oral mucosa, and tooth pulp. In addition, separate classes of nerve fibers exist that are involved in detecting non-noxious stimuli such as vibration and in proprioception. These fibers can be found in the periodontal ligament, skin, and oral mucosa and include the A-beta fibers.

Primary Afferent Neurons

Primarily the trigeminal, or fifth cranial, nerve detects and encodes noxious stimuli for the orofacial region. The majority of cell bodies of the trigeminal sensory fibers are in the trigeminal ganglion located on the floor of the middle cranial fossa.

The peripheral axons of the trigeminal ganglion run in three divisions—the ophthalmic (V1), maxillary (V2), and mandibular (V3)—which innervate most of the oral mucosa, the temporomandibular joint, the anterior two thirds of the tongue, the dura of the anterior and middle cranial fossae, the tooth pulp, the gingiva, and the periodontal membrane.

In the peripheral nervous system, these neurons or nerves are referred to as primary afferent (i.e., sensory) fibers. The primary afferent fibers can broadly be divided into A-beta fibers, which transmit light touch or proprioceptive information, and A-delta and C fibers, which encode pain. The tooth is densely innervated by afferent nerve fibers, which are believed to transmit mainly pain in response to thermal, mechanical, or chemical stimuli. The majority of dental nerves are C fibers that innervate the central pulp, most of which terminate beneath the odontoblasts.[23]

A-beta Fibers

The rapidly conducting myelinated neurons that respond to light touch are called A-beta fibers. Under normal conditions, activation of the A-beta fibers by high-intensity stimulation results in low-frequency output in the central nervous system. Activation of A-beta fibers normally is interpreted as nonpainful mechanical stimulation[133] or, under certain conditions, can be perceived as a "prepain" sensation.[23] A-beta fibers also have been shown to undergo phenotypic changes that allow them to encode painful stimuli under certain inflammatory conditions.[98]

A-delta Fibers

The A-delta fibers are lightly myelinated, have a faster conduction velocity than C fibers, and are believed to transmit a sharp or pricking sensation. A-delta fibers respond primarily to noxious mechanical stimuli rather than to chemical or thermal stimuli. Other A-delta fibers may be polymodal (responding to mechanical, chemical, and thermal stimuli)[13] or respond only to cold/mechanical[78] or hot/mechanical noxious stimuli.[39]

In the tooth pulp, A-delta fibers traverse the odontoblastic layer and terminate in the dentinal tubules.[25] Because of their location and their sensitivity to mechanical stimulation, A-delta fibers are believed to respond to stimuli that result in

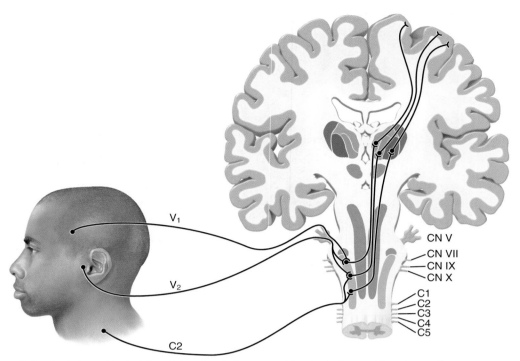

FIG. 17-2 A graphic depiction of the trigeminal nerve entering the brainstem. The primary afferent neuron synapses with a second-order neuron in the trigeminal nucleus. The second-order neuron carries pain information to the thalamus, from which it is sent to the cerebral cortex for interpretation. (Redrawn from Okeson JP: *Bell's orofacial pains,* ed 5, Chicago, 1995, Quintessence Publishing.)

movement of fluid within the dentinal tubules (e.g., osmotic, mechanical probing, or thermal stimuli applied to the external surface of the tooth).[18] Consistent with the hypothesized mechanism of dentinal pain is the fact that the stimuli that cause dentinal fluid movement result in a sharp pain associated with A-delta fiber activation.[95] When intense noxious stimuli activate the A-delta fibers, the input to the central nervous system consists of high-frequency action potentials.

C Fibers

The C fibers are unmyelinated, have slower conduction velocity, and are associated with a dull, aching, or burning sensation. Most C fibers are polymodal, responding to mechanical, thermal, and chemical stimuli. Because of the difference in conduction velocities, A-delta fibers are believed to transmit early, shooting pain, whereas C fibers would transmit late, dull pain. Noxious stimuli that exceed the receptor threshold of these nociceptive primary afferent terminals result in action potentials that travel centrally, signaling tissue damage. In the pulp tissue, the more centrally located C fibers respond to thermal, mechanical, and chemical stimuli and are believed to be sensitized by inflammation.[39] All visceral structures are innervated primarily by afferent fibers conducting nociceptive information such as that carried by A-delta and C fibers.

Central Nervous System

The primary afferent fibers are responsible for the transduction and transmission of sensory information to higher brain centers, and they do so by synapsing on neurons located within the trigeminal nucleus, which spans the midbrain and cervical spinal cord. This point marks the beginning of the central

nervous system and is the point at which processing of pain information begins (Fig. 17-2).

Just as there are different types of sensory neurons in the periphery, in the trigeminal nucleus there are also different types of neurons that receive nociceptive input from the periphery. The ascending neurons located in the trigeminal nucleus are known collectively as *second-order* or *projection neurons* and can be subdivided into three distinct groups of neurons based on the type of information they receive: (1) low-threshold mechanoreceptors, (2) nociceptive-specific, and (3) wide dynamic range neurons.

The primary central site of termination for nociceptive fibers is the subnucleus caudalis, located in the most caudal region of the trigeminal nucleus,[39,57,144] which anatomically and functionally resembles the dorsal horn of the spinal cord and has been referred to as the medullary dorsal horn.[57] Four major components of nociceptive processing are located in the dorsal horn of the subnucleus caudalis: central terminals of afferents, local circuit neurons (interneurons), projection neurons, and descending neurons.[71] Within the subnucleus caudalis, the A-delta and C fibers terminate primarily in the outer laminae (I and IIa) and lamina V. Local circuit neurons are composed of islet cells (which are thought to be inhibitory) and stalked cells (which are believed to be excitatory).[38] Combined, the local circuit neurons may modulate nociceptive transmission from the primary afferents to the projection neurons.

The fourth component of the dorsal horn are the terminal endings of descending neurons. The descending neurons originate in the nucleus raphe magnus (NRM), the medullary reticular nuclei, and the locus ceruleus (LC). Descending brainstem neurons release serotonin (from the NRM) or norepinephrine (from the LC), which may inhibit the activity of projection neurons directly or by activating local opioid interneurons. These neurons are responsible for the endogenous abatement of pain; blockade of their activity increases pain transmission and reduces pain thresholds.

Second-Order Neurons

Projection neurons have axons that cross to the contralateral medulla to ascend in the trigeminothalamic tract and project to the ventral posterior medial and intralaminar nuclei of the thalamus, where additional neurons project to the cortex. Projection neurons involved in the transmission of painful stimuli can be divided into two classes: wide dynamic range and nociceptive-specific neurons. Wide dynamic range neurons receive input from mechanoreceptors, thermoreceptors, and nociceptors, whereas nociceptive-specific neurons are excited solely by nociceptors. These two types of projection neurons may be responsible for signaling the severity and location of pain, respectively.[79]

Multiple primary afferent neurons may synapse on a single projection (i.e., convergence). This occurs to a much greater degree in deep tissues as opposed to cutaneous tissues. Primary afferent fibers of nontrigeminal origin such as those derived from vagus, glossopharyngeal, facial, and cervical spinal ganglia have been shown to converge and synapse onto trigeminal projection neurons located as far caudal as spinal level C4.[74] This phenomenon of convergence may result in the clinical finding of pain that radiates beyond an area of tissue injury. Convergence may also explain why pain appears to be associated with a site other than the injured area. Interestingly, when projection neurons receive input from superficial and deep structures, the more superficial inputs usually predominate.[121] Thus, pain originating from deep structures would typically be referred to superficial areas (e.g., pain originating from the jaw muscles would typically be referred to the face rather than deeper structures).

Autonomic Nervous System

The stellate ganglia supply the entire sympathetic innervation of the orofacial region, which is located bilaterally at the level of the seventh cervical vertebra. Under normal conditions, sympathetic stimulation has no influence on sensory function. However, afferent sympathetic fibers in an area of trauma may become involved in the response to pain and may also play a role in chronic pain states. Specifically, C fibers in the area of partial nerve injury may become responsive to sympathetic nerve stimulation. The modulation of nociception by the sympathetic nervous system has been shown such that release of pain neurotransmitters may be altered in the presence of sympathetic agonists and by blockade of the sympathetic nervous system, using antagonists.[70] Whether the effects of sympathetic nerve fibers on pain transmission are direct (via homeostatic regulation) or indirect remains unclear. The parasympathetic division of the autonomic nervous system has not been shown to be involved in the development or modulation of pain.

REVIEW OF NEUROPHYSIOLOGY

Peripheral Sensitization

After tissue insult there is an inflammatory reaction that often produces pain. The severity of pain that follows is related to several aspects of the injury, such as the type, extent, and location; the innervation of the tissue; and the phase of the inflammation. In the nociceptive system, tissue injury can manifest itself as increased responsiveness or reduced thresholds to a noxious stimulus, referred to as hyperalgesia. Hyperalgesia can be partially accounted for by sensitization of nociceptors (primary hyperalgesia) and by central nervous system mechanisms (secondary hyperalgesia).

In the absence of tissue damage, activation of C or A-delta fibers produces a transient pain. This pain is believed to serve as a physiologic warning. When there is tissue injury, afferent fibers may be activated by lower intensity stimuli than usual, and the quality of pain may be more persistent and intense. This phenomenon is due, in part, to the sensitization of nociceptors, including an increase in spontaneous activity.

At the site of tissue injury, there are a number of inflammatory mediators that can directly or indirectly sensitize primary afferent nociceptors (see Chapter 12 for more details). These inflammatory mediators may be released from the local tissue cells, circulating and resident immune cells, vasculature and endothelial smooth muscle cells, and peripheral nervous system cells.

Central Sensitization

After peripheral tissue injury there is an afferent barrage from C fibers resulting from peripheral tissue inflammation, decreased afferent thresholds, and spontaneous firing of afferent fibers. When a second-order neuron receives a prolonged barrage of nociceptive input, the second-order neuron may also become sensitized. This results in a phenomenon referred to as central sensitization.[17] The result of central sensitization is enhanced processing (i.e., amplification) of neural impulses that are being transmitted to higher brain centers. Two effects of central sensitization are secondary hyperalgesia and referred pain.

Secondary hyperalgesia is an increased response to painful stimulation at the site of pain resulting from central nervous system changes. This is in contrast to primary hyperalgesia, which is a lowered pain threshold resulting from sensitization of peripheral neurons. Secondary hyperalgesia might be felt in superficial (e.g., gingiva or skin) or deep structures (e.g., muscles or teeth).

Terminology

In general, as research progresses and uncovers new ways for us to look at pain, the terminology changes. This can introduce some confusion, especially when older terms are used. Therefore, it may be helpful to present contemporary definitions of some of the basic terms and review some of the previously mentioned terms (Box 17-1).

CLINICAL ENTITIES THAT CAN PRESENT AS TOOTHACHE

Sources of Odontogenic Toothache

Before considering heterotopic pains that may present as toothache, it is important to fully understand odontogenic pain as a primary source for toothache. Only two structures serve as sources for primary odontogenic pain: the pulp–dentin complex and the periradicular tissues. The innervation of the pulp is similar to that of other deep visceral tissues, and in various states of pathosis will have pain characteristics similar to deep

BOX 17-1
Types of Pain

Pain
An unpleasant sensory and emotional experience associated with actual or potential tissue damage or described in terms of such damage.[86]

Nociceptive Pain
Pain arising from activation of nociceptors.[86]

Neuropathic Pain
Pain arising as a direct consequence of a lesion or disease affecting the somatosensory system.[86,135]

Peripheral Sensitization
Increased responsiveness and reduced thresholds of nociceptors to stimulation of their receptive fields.[86]

Central Sensitization
Increased responsiveness of nociceptive neurons in the central nervous system to their normal or subthreshold afferent input.[86]

Heterotopic Pain
Any pain that is felt in an area other than its true source is heterotopic pain. There are three types of heterotopic pain: referred, central, and projected.[105,106] Referred pain is pain felt in an area innervated by a nerve different from the one that mediates the primary pain. Referred pain cannot be provoked by stimulation of the area where the pain is felt; rather, it is brought on by manipulation of the primary source of pain (Fig. 17-3). In addition, referred pain cannot be arrested unless the primary source of pain is anesthetized. The referral of pain tends to occur in a laminated fashion (Fig. 17-4). This is because peripheral nociceptors enter the spinal trigeminal tract in a laminated fashion. As a result there are general referral patterns in the face. In addition, the referral of pain is usually in a cephalad or upward direction. This is evidenced clinically in that pain from mandibular molars typically is referred to maxillary molars, as opposed to premolars or incisors.

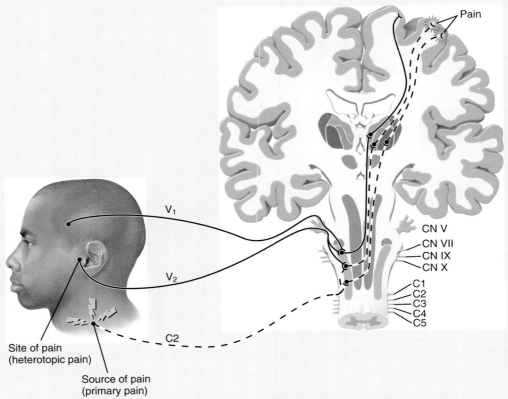

FIG. 17-3 Illustration of pain that is referred from an area innervated by one nerve *(C2)* to an area innervated by a different nerve *(V₂)*. Note that this phenomenon occurs secondary to the convergence of different neurons onto the same second-order neuron in the trigeminal nucleus. The sensory cortex perceives two locations of pain. One area is the trapezius region that represents the source of pain. The second area of perceived pain is felt in the temporomandibular joint area, which is only a site of pain, not a source of pain. This pain is heterotopic (referred). (Redrawn from Okeson JP: *Bell's orofacial pains,* ed 5, Chicago, 1995, Quintessence Publishing.)

BOX 17-1
Types of Pain—cont'd

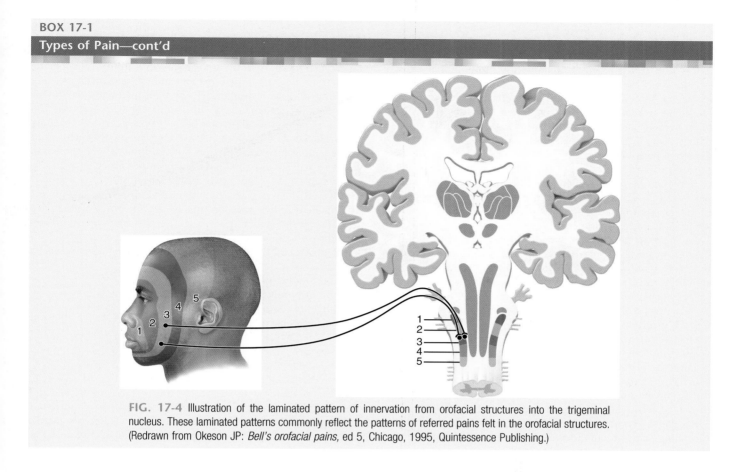

FIG. 17-4 Illustration of the laminated pattern of innervation from orofacial structures into the trigeminal nucleus. These laminated patterns commonly reflect the patterns of referred pains felt in the orofacial structures. (Redrawn from Okeson JP: *Bell's orofacial pains,* ed 5, Chicago, 1995, Quintessence Publishing.)

visceral tissues. The primary nociceptors of the pulp that respond to inflammation are the slow-conducting, high-threshold C fibers. Because their threshold is high and they rarely terminate in dentinal tubules, C fibers do not respond to normal or nonpathologic dentinal stimulation. C fibers typically conduct pain that is associated with tissue damage. In addition, C fibers respond in a threshold manner that can be termed "all or nothing." For example, a slightly cold stimulus that is below the C fiber threshold will fail to produce any sensation. Only when a stimulus is intense enough to reach the threshold will the C fiber fire, resulting in the sensation of pain.

Pulpal pain is mediated by C fibers and is dull, aching, or throbbing in nature. This is in contrast to the quick, short, sharp sensation produced by A-delta fibers that mediate dentinal pain. Therefore, when pulp testing, it is meaningful to note not only whether the patient perceived the stimulus but also the nature of the stimulus perceived. A simple notation would be to use an "s" (short) to indicate a response more typical of an A-delta fiber (dentinal pain) or a "p" (prolonged) to indicate the response was more indicative of a C fiber response (pulpal pain).

Tissue inflammation can result in sensitization of nerve fibers. When peripheral nociceptors (e.g., pulpal C fibers) are sensitized, the threshold of firing in response to a given stimulus (e.g., temperature and pressure) is lowered. In states of sensitization these nociceptors can be provoked with a less intense stimulus. The threshold for excitation is still "all or nothing" but the required level of stimulation has decreased. These fibers can become so sensitized that they may fire at as

low a temperature threshold as body temperature,[95] normally not sufficient to stimulate a C fiber. In fact, they can become so sensitized that they will fire in response to the normal pulse pressure of cardiac contraction, eliciting a complaint of "I can feel my heartbeat in my tooth" or "my tooth is throbbing." Sensitized C fibers can even fire without provocation, resulting in spontaneous pain.

Similar to deep visceral tissues, the pulpal nociceptors demonstrate a high degree of convergence in the central nervous system. In a study of cat brain, 74% of the neurons tested in the subnucleus caudalis showed convergence from multiple tooth pulps.[22] In addition, the dental pulp has little to no proprioceptive neurons. The high degree of convergence from pulp tissue and the lack of proprioceptive information provided are the key factors in why purely pulpal pain can be so difficult for patients to localize. In addition to reducing localization of pain, convergence increases the referral of pain to tissues not actually affected by the inflammation. The fact that neurons from the pulps of mandibular teeth converge with those of maxillary teeth can result in pain from a mandibular pulpitis being referred to the maxillary arch. Because the patient may poorly localize pulpal pain, it is important for the clinician to localize the source of the pain. This is often accomplished through the use of tests that are employed in an attempt either to reproduce the eliciting stimulus of a patient's pain or to eliminate the pain. For example, pulpal pain should be aggravated with hot or cold stimulation and should be eliminated or significantly reduced with local anesthetic.

Unlike pulpal pain, pain of periradicular origin is easier to localize. Mechanoreceptors are numerous in the periodontal ligament (PDL) and are most densely concentrated in the apical one third.[87] Once inflammation from pulpal disease extends into the periodontal ligament, patients are able to locate the source of the pain much more readily. As a musculoskeletal structure, the PDL responds to noxious stimulation in a graded fashion—that is, the degree of discomfort a patient feels in relation to periradicular pain depends on the degree of peripheral sensitization and the amount of provocation to this structure. A sensitized PDL will be uncomfortable to a patient if percussed lightly but more uncomfortable if percussed heavily. This is known as a graded response. It is, therefore, appropriate to record periradicular testing such as percussion and palpation in terms of degrees of tenderness (versus "all or nothing"). As with pulpal pain, pain of periradicular origin should also have an identifiable etiology. Periradicular pain tends to be dull, aching, or throbbing and should resolve completely with local anesthesia. If pain of suspected periradicular origin is nonresponsive to local anesthetic, it is a strong indication that the pain may be nonodontogenic in origin.

The tooth is unique in the human body in that it has a visceral-like component, the pulp, and a musculoskeletal component, the periodontal ligament. Therefore, odontogenic pain can have a wide variety of presentations. Tooth pain can be diffuse or well localized, mild or intense, or spontaneous or provoked with various stimuli applied at various intensities. The quality can vary between sharp and dull and aching or throbbing. This potential for extreme variability makes it possible for toothaches to mimic or be mimicked by many other types of pain that occur in the head and neck. In addition, because both the pulp tissue and periodontal ligament can be categorized as deep somatic tissue, continued nociceptive input from odontogenic pain has a great propensity to produce central excitatory effects such as secondary hyperalgesia, referred pain, secondary co-contraction of muscles, myofascial trigger points, and autonomic changes. These effects add to the complexity of diagnosing odontogenic pain and differentiating tooth pain from other sources in the region.

Sources of Nonodontogenic Toothache

This chapter provides information that will help the dental clinician to identify toothaches with a nonodontogenic etiology. The clinician must have a thorough knowledge of all possible causes of orofacial pain, which includes both odontogenic and nonodontogenic conditions. This knowledge prevents misdiagnosis and allows for proper treatment selection and referral if necessary. For information about treatment of these disorders, other references should be used.

Consensus on the exact taxonomy with diagnostic criteria and their interrelationships among various orofacial pain disorders has not been established. Various health care professions involved in the diagnosis and treatment of such pains have used different terms in the literature. This, of course, can and has led to confusion, especially within what we refer to as neuropathic pain. The terms used in the literature are diverse, and they overlap in meaning to an unknown degree; for example, *phantom tooth pain* and *atypical odontalgia* are used interchangeably. At other times the literature uses the same terms to describe seemingly different disorders; for example, trigeminal neuralgia has the connotation of an idiopathic pain

disorder characterized either as intense, intermittent lightning bolt–type pain within one or more distributions of the trigeminal nerve, or as continuous pain that is often mild to moderate in intensity that arises in association with injury to a specific branch of the trigeminal nerve. Efforts have resulted in a working diagnostic framework for neuropathic pains.[135] Our classification scheme uses this framework to enhance the clarity of communication and follows the American Academy of Orofacial Pain's guidelines for assessment, diagnosis, and management for orofacial pain,[30] even though the application of these criteria to pains that present in the orofacial region is known to be associated with misclassification.[35]

Overall, one can classify the nonodontogenic reasons for toothache into five broad groups of pain disorders:

1. Musculoskeletal and other nonprogressive pains arising from somatic structures
2. Neurovascular pain, otherwise known as headache disorders
3. Neuropathic pains
4. Pain of purely psychologic origin, otherwise known as psychogenic toothache
5. Pain associated with a pathologic process

Musculoskeletal and Somatic Pain
Myofascial Pain

Although any deep somatic tissue type in the head and neck has the propensity to induce central excitatory effects and therefore cause referral of pains to teeth, pains of muscular origin appear to be the most common.[46] Myofascial pain (MFP) emanates from small foci of hyperexcitable muscle tissue. Clinically these areas feel like taut bands or knots and are termed *trigger points*.[134] Typically the pain is described as a diffuse, constant, dull, aching sensation; this may lead the clinician to a misdiagnosis of pulpal pain. Another potentially misleading characteristic of masticatory muscle pain is that patients may report pain when chewing. This feature is similar to pain that is periradicular, not pulpal, in origin. On further investigation, it should become clear that the pain is triggered by contraction of masticatory muscles rather than loading of periodontal ligaments. Palpation of the muscles of mastication should reproduce the pain, whereas percussion of the teeth should not. The intensity of the pain will increase and can be perceived in a distant site. Myofascial pain that is perceived to emanate from a tooth is a referred type of heterotopic pain—that is, the pain is felt in an area other than the nerve branch that innervates the trigger point. Typically muscles that refer pain to teeth are the masseter, temporalis, and lateral pterygoid; muscles of the neck and nonmuscular deep structures of the face can also be a source for this type of pain.[134,142]

Although the definitive pathogenesis of MFP is unknown, authors have theorized that muscles may become disturbed through injury or sustained contraction such as clenching.[45,105] Clinically this muscular contraction might occur as a parafunctional habit or as a protective response by localized muscle to an ongoing deep noxious input such as dental pain. Considering this theory and what is witnessed clinically, trigger points appear to be induced or aggravated by toothache. It also appears that trigger points can persist after the toothache has been resolved. This can be confusing for the clinician and frustrating for the patient. It is important to realize the relationship of these two entities. MFP can mimic toothache, and toothaches may induce the development of MFP.

Toothaches of myofascial origin may arise with or without evidence of pulpal or periapical pathosis. Definitive diagnosis is based on lack of symptoms after pulp testing and percussion or palpation sensitivity, or failure to resolve symptoms with local anesthetic blockade. In contrast, jaw function and palpation of the masticatory muscle(s) elicit toothaches of myofascial origin. Typically, local anesthetic infiltration into the trigger point(s) will resolve symptoms.

Common therapeutic modalities used to treat myofascial pain include deep massage, relaxation techniques, "spray and stretch," muscle relaxants, and trigger point injections. Deep massage and relaxation techniques have the advantage of being noninvasive and easily administered. Spray and stretch involves an application of a vapor coolant spray to the skin overlying the trigger point, followed by a gentle stretching of the muscle. Trigger point injections are used for both the diagnosis and treatment of myofascial pain. Specifically, if the pain complaint is diminished on injection of the trigger point(s), then the source of the pain has been confirmed. The therapeutic efficacy of a trigger point injection varies. Some patients might experience lasting relief with one injection or several, whereas others may not. See the Additional Tests section for further information about trigger point injections.

Pain of Sinus or Nasal Mucosal Origin

Sinus/nasal mucosal pain is another source of pain that can mimic toothache.[1,2,28,138] Sinus pain can exhibit symptoms of fullness or pressure below the eyes but is generally not particularly painful unless the nasal mucosa is also affected.[37] Pain from the nasal mucosa tends to be dull and aching and can also have a burning quality typical of visceral mucosal pain. In general, these pains are of viral, bacterial, or allergic etiology. Other symptoms consistent with these types of disease (e.g., congestion or nasal drainage) should be noted in the patient history.

Typical of deep visceral-like tissues, sinus/nasal mucosal pain can induce central excitatory effects such as secondary hyperalgesia, referral of pain, and autonomic changes. It is this tendency that gives sinus/nasal pain the ability to masquerade as toothache. Secondary hyperalgesia, seen clinically as a concentric spread of pain beyond the area of tissue injury, results in tenderness of the mucosa in the area of the maxillary sinuses as well as tenderness to percussion of several maxillary teeth. Teeth tender to percussion and palpation suggest periradicular inflammation. Autonomic sequelae might present as edema or erythema in the area, which could suggest a dental abscess. However, when an etiology for pulpal and therefore periradicular pathosis is absent, sinus/nasal mucosal disease should be suspected. The three cardinal symptoms of acute rhinosinusitis are (1) purulent nasal discharge, (2) nasal obstruction, and (3) facial pain-pressure-fullness.[118] Other symptoms of sinus disease include sensitivity to palpation of structures overlying sinuses (i.e., paranasal tenderness) and a throbbing or increased pain sensation when the head is placed lower than the heart. Dental local anesthetic blockade will not abate sinus/nasal mucosal pain, although topical nasal anesthetic will.

Patients with suspected sinus/nasal mucosal disease should be referred to an otolaryngologist for further diagnosis and treatment. Physical examination as well as adjunctive tests may be necessary for a definitive diagnosis. Tests may include nasal cytologic and ultrasound studies and the use of nasal endoscopes, in addition to imaging tests such as radiology and computed tomographic imaging.[36,125] Treatment of sinus/nasal mucosal pain is dependent on the etiology (e.g., bacterial, viral, allergic, or obstructive).

Salivary Gland Pain

Pain referred from one or more of the salivary glands may be perceived as tooth pain; the authors have not encountered this response in clinical practice, but it has been reported to present as a nonodontogenic toothache.[80,115] Because the primary somatosensory innervation of the major salivary glands comes from the mandibular branch, it is conceivable that such a presentation will occur most often in mandibular teeth.

Neurovascular Pain

Neurovascular pains, otherwise and interchangeably referred to as headache disorders, have qualities similar to pulpal pain. These types of pain can be intense, often pulsatile, and are known to occur only in the head. The International Headache Society (Oxford, UK) has developed a classification system that is widely accepted even though validation studies of these criteria have yet to be published. The interested reader should consult the classification system for more details on this topic.[56] Primary neurovascular pain disorders are thought to be a referred pain phenomenon, meaning that intracranial branches of the trigeminal nerve become sensitized via incompletely understood mechanisms and the associated pain and symptoms are perceived in the somatic structures of the head. Most commonly people report pain presenting in the forehead, back of the head, and temples but also in the sinuses, jaws, and teeth.

The current understanding of the pathophysiology of headaches implies that dental disease and treatments are not likely to be a cause of a person developing a headache disorder, but rather, because the same neuroanatomic circuitry is involved, these aspects of dentistry can be thought of as an inciting event, similar to the analogy that exercise producing increased demands on the cardiovascular system can be an inciting event for an acute myocardial infarction. For this reason, dental clinicians should be aware of the diagnostic status of their patients, because patients with headache disorders are likely to experience more peritreatment pain complications that are related to the innate hyperexcitability of the trigeminal nervous system in these people.

Of most interest to the dental clinician are the primary headache disorders, which make up the bulk of the headache disorders that occur within the population and have been reported to present as nonodontogenic toothache. To simplify thinking, these primary headache disorders can be grouped into three major subdivisions: (1) migraine, (2) tension-type headache, and (3) cluster headache and other trigeminal autonomic cephalalgias (TACs).

Migraine is a common headache experienced by about 18% of females and 6% of males.[82,128] It is associated with significant amounts of disability, which is the motivating factor that brings the patient to seek care and the reason why this type of headache is the one most often seen in medical clinics.[131] Migraine has been reported to present as toothache[4,26,34,52,96,103] and is likely the most common neurovascular disorder to do so. In addition, people with migraine headaches are thought of as having increased regional pain sensitivity that has diagnostic and treatment implications for the clinician.[102]

Migraine headaches typically last between 4 and 72 hours. They tend to be unilateral in presentation and pulsatile in quality, with a moderate to severe intensity to the pain. Patients may also experience nausea or vomiting, as well as photophobia or phonophobia, which are different from toothache. The headache is usually aggravated with routine physical activity, such as walking up stairs. Caffeine/ergotamine compounds have been used widely in the past as abortive agents for migraine headaches, but in contemporary times they have been replaced with triptans, such as sumatriptan and rizatriptan.[93] Of note, migraine headaches may partially or fully abate with the use of nonsteroidal anti-inflammatory medications in a similar fashion as toothaches.

Tension-type headache is the most frequent headache disorder experienced, with a wide range of reported prevalence (41% to 96%).[117,123] The concept of tension-type headache pain presenting as toothache has not been reported in the literature to our knowledge, likely because the construct of what a tension-type headache is has not been clearly defined. Some research supports the notion that a tension-type headache has a significant musculoskeletal component to the pain,[129] whereas other research suggests otherwise. Tension-type headaches are likely a heterogeneous group of similarly presenting head pains that have overlapping pathophysiologic mechanisms, which has led some researchers to consider aspects of tension-type headache to be the same as musculoskeletal orofacial pain, otherwise known as temporomandibular disorders (TMDs).[55] This has further been supported by data from a TMD validation study to derive criteria for such headaches that are of TMD origin.[6,122]

Cluster headaches and other TACs are rare neurovascular disorders that are strictly unilateral pains defined by the concurrent presentation of at least one ipsilateral autonomic symptom—such as nasal congestion, rhinorrhea, lacrimation, eyelid edema, periorbital swelling, facial erythema, ptosis, or miosis—that occurs with the pain. The major distinguishing features between these headache disorders are the duration and frequency of the pain episodes, as well as the gender most often afflicted. Cluster headache is the most common of the group, occurring in men three to four times more often than in women, with pain episodes lasting between 15 minutes and 2 hours that occur at a frequency of eight episodes per day to one every other day. These headaches come in clusters, with active periods of 2 weeks to 3 months,[56] thus the name. Elimination of pain after 10 minutes with inhalation of 100% oxygen is diagnostic for cluster headache,[49] whereas sublingual ergotamine and sumatriptan are also effective acute treatments for cluster headache.[42] Paroxysmal hemicrania, which has a 3 : 1 female predilection, presents with characteristics similar to those of cluster headache but with a frequency of more than five per day and a duration lasting 2 to 30 minutes.[56] This headache disorder has a 100% response to indomethacin but is refractory to other treatments,[65] thus underscoring the need for obtaining an accurate diagnosis from an experienced clinician.

From a nonodontogenic perspective, cluster headache[4,14,21,51] and almost all the other TACs have been reported in the literature to present as nonodontogenic toothache.[4,11,12,31,92,110,120] The concurrent autonomic features, such as discoloration or swelling in the anterior maxilla, might compound the diagnostic problem by suggesting tooth abscess. It is important to note that neurovascular headaches tend to be episodic with complete remission between episodes, whereas toothache pain usually has at least some background pain that stays between any exacerbations. Provocation of the tooth should not result in a clear increase in pain but cause a slight alteration because this tissue has become hypersensitized. Local anesthetic is unpredictable in these cases and can mislead the clinician. Management by the typical clinician is to determine that the pain is not of odontogenic origin and then to refer the patient to an appropriate care provider. Other neurovascular disorders not classified as primary headaches have been reported to present as nonodontogenic toothache, such as cough headache.[91] One would not expect a dental clinician who does not have a specific focus on orofacial pain to arrive at such a specific diagnosis but rather to be aware of and sensitive to the fact that more obscure headache disorders exist and should be considered in the differential diagnosis of a nonodontogenic toothache that is not easily classified.

Neuropathic Pain

All previously described pain entities can be classified as somatic pain. That is, they are a result of noxious stimulation of somatic structures. These impulses are transmitted by normal neural structures, and their clinical characteristics are related to stimulation of normal neural structures. Neuropathic pain actually arises from abnormalities in the neural structures themselves, specifically the somatosensory system. The clinical examination generally reveals no somatic tissue damage, and the response to stimulation of the tissue is disproportionate to the stimulus. For this reason, neuropathic pains can be misdiagnosed as psychogenic pain simply because a local cause cannot be readily identified. There are many ways to categorize neuropathic pain in the orofacial region. For the purposes of this chapter and ease of discussion, neuropathic pain is divided into four subcategories: neuralgia, neuroma, neuritis, and neuropathy. It should be acknowledged that these subcategories are arbitrary and are not mutually exclusive.

Neuralgia

As alluded to previously, not all uses of the term *neuralgia* refer to what is often thought of as the classic trigeminal neuralgia or tic douloureux. Sometimes the term *neuralgia* is used to describe pain felt along a specific peripheral nerve distribution, such as with postherpetic neuralgia and occipital neuralgia, as opposed to a focus of pain disorders that have similar characteristics and are thought to have common underlying pathophysiologic mechanisms. When used in the generic sense to describe pains that present intraorally, the term can lead to a great deal of confusion.

Although deviations are not uncommon, trigeminal neuralgia is characteristically an intense, sharp shooting pain that is most often unilateral. Ipsilateral to the perceived location of the symptoms is an area that, on stimulation such as light touch, elicits sharp shooting pain. The area that elicits the pain is referred to as a trigger zone, and it can be in the distribution of the resultant pain or in a different distribution—but is always ipsilateral. Although most patients present with a characteristic trigger zone, not all patients will present with this finding. An important characteristic of trigger zones is that the response to the stimulus is not proportional to the intensity of the stimulus—that is, slight pressure on a trigger zone results in severe pain. In addition, once triggered, pain typically subsides within a few minutes until triggered again. This is in contrast to odontogenic pain, which may come and go but does not do so in such a predictable and repeatable manner. Finally, the trigger for odontogenic pain is an area that has no sensory abnormalities (e.g., dysesthesia or paresthesia).

Trigger zones for trigeminal neuralgia tend to be related to areas of dense somatosensory innervation, such as the lips and teeth. For this reason, triggers that elicit this type of pain may include chewing and may lead both the patient and clinician to think of a diagnosis of odontogenic pain. In addition, because the trigger involves peripheral input, anesthetizing the trigger zone may diminish symptoms. This can be very misleading to the clinician if the assumption is that local anesthetic blocks only odontogenic pain.

Because symptoms can be quite severe, patients may consent to or even insist on treatment even though the clinical findings do not definitively support an odontogenic etiology. The possibly misleading symptoms, along with the willingness of the patient to consent to what may seem to be desperate measures, emphasize the importance of a thorough history and clinical evaluation. The absence of a dental etiology for the symptoms (e.g., large restorations, dental trauma, or recent dental treatment) in the presence of the characteristic sharp shooting pain should alert the clinician to consider trigeminal neuralgia in the differential diagnosis. In general, these individuals should be referred to a neurologist or orofacial pain/oral medicine clinician for a complete diagnostic workup and treatment, because case series have suggested 15% to 30% of patients have secondary reasons for their pain,[58,143] such as brain tumors and multiple sclerosis.

Trigeminal neuralgia typically presents in individuals older than 50 years of age. The etiology is thought to be irritation/compression of the root of the trigeminal nerve, prior to the gasserian ganglion, possibly as a result of carotid artery pressure. Individuals with multiple sclerosis develop trigeminal neuralgia more frequently than the general population. For this reason, a person younger than 40 years of age who develops trigeminal neuralgia should also be screened for multiple sclerosis[147] or other intracranial pathosis.[58]

The two general treatment options for trigeminal neuralgia are pharmacologic and surgical procedures. Because of the possible complications associated with surgery, this form of treatment is usually considered only after attempting pharmacologic therapies. Several medications, including carbamazepine, baclofen, gabapentin, and more recently pregabalin and oxcarbazepine, have been used to treat trigeminal neuralgia. Drugs aimed at relieving nociception, such as nonsteroidal antiinflammatory agents, have no significant benefit in these patients, nor do opioid-based analgesics. Clinical trials support carbamazepine as a first-line drug for treating trigeminal neuralgia.[8] In patients who experience pain relief from carbamazepine, the effect is usually rapid; most will report a decrease in severity of symptoms within the first couple of days.

What is thought to be a variation of trigeminal neuralgia, and may also mimic toothache, is pretrigeminal neuralgia. Pretrigeminal neuralgia, as the name suggests, has been described as symptoms that are different from those of classic trigeminal neuralgia but that respond to pharmacotherapy like classic trigeminal neuralgia and, over time (usually weeks to 3 years), take on the classic characteristics of trigeminal neuralgia. The definitive features include the presence of a dull aching or burning pain that is less paroxysmal in nature but still triggered by a light touch within the orofacial region, with variable periods of remission.[48] The subsequent onset of true neuralgic pain may be sudden or may appear several years later,[105] which emphasizes the need for long-term follow-up of these patients to obtain an accurate final diagnosis.

Neuroma

The term *neuroma* has been around for many years and is often overused in an attempt to describe other types of neuropathic pain. A traumatic neuroma, also known as an amputation neuroma, is a proliferative mass of disorganized neural tissue at the site of a traumatically or surgically transected nerve. A part of the diagnosis, therefore, is confirmation of a significant event that would account for the damage to the nerve. Symptoms will not develop until the neural tissue on the proximal stump has had time to proliferate, typically about 10 days after the event. Tapping over the area of a neuroma elicits volleys of sharp electrical pain (i.e., Tinel sign) similar to trigeminal neuralgia. In contrast to trigeminal neuralgia, there should be a zone of anesthesia peripheral to the area of the neuroma[111] that can be identified by checking for loss of pinprick sensibility, such as with the use of an explorer.

Treatment of a neuroma involves pharmacologic management, often via local measures, and may involve surgical coaptation of the nerve with prognosis being variable and dependent on adequate distal nerve tissue and the time interval between injury and reconstruction.[148] Therefore, early recognition and referral are of key importance to prevent significant distal nerve degeneration.[76] Although neuromas most commonly develop in the area of the mental foramen, lower lip, and tongue, there is some evidence that they can also form in extraction sites and after pulpal extirpation. Neuromas were found to form in extraction sites between 4 and 6 months after removal of the tooth in an experimental animal model.[69] Although not all neuromas that form are painful, this could be a potential explanation for ongoing pain in extraction sites after healing has appeared to occur.[111] It is interesting to ponder the possibility of neuroma formation in deafferentation injuries such as pulpectomy and the implications this might have on continued PDL sensitivity after adequate root canal treatment. For treatment of neuromas that are not amenable to surgical correction, see the Neuropathy section of this chapter.

Neuritis

Neuritis is a condition caused by inflammation of a nerve or nerves secondary to injury or infection of viral or bacterial etiology. In general, pain from a virally induced neuritis, such as recurrent herpes simplex or herpes zoster, is associated with skin or mucosal lesions (Fig. 17-5). This presentation does not result in much of a diagnostic challenge, but pain can precede the vesicular outbreak by many days or even weeks.[47] Because neuritic disorders are caused by reactivation of a virus that has been dormant in the trigeminal ganglion, they are considered projected pain with distribution within the dermatomes innervated by the affected peripheral nerves. The nerves affected by the virus may solely supply deeper tissues and therefore may not produce any cutaneous lesions. In the absence of skin or mucosal lesions, a viral neuritis can be difficult to diagnose[47,60,67] and should be considered in the differential diagnosis of a patient with a history of primary herpes zoster infection. Bacterial infection of the sinuses or dental abscess can also cause neural inflammation that may result in pain. This pain occurs simultaneously with pain of the infected tissues and usually

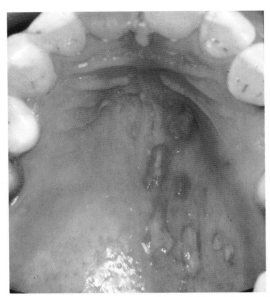

FIG. 17-5 Herpes zoster involving the maxillary division of the left trigeminal nerve of the palate of a 45-year-old male. He complained of a deep, diffuse dull ache of his maxillary left quadrant for 1 week before this vesicular outbreak.

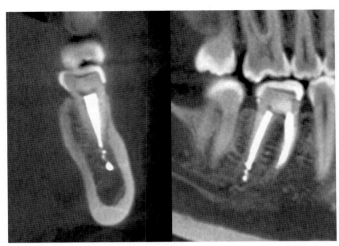

FIG. 17-6 Extrusion of the filling material from the distal canal of tooth #30 of a 36-year-old female. Her complaint was of extreme pain after completion of the root canal treatment followed by sharp, burning continuous pain that could be made worse by a light touch of the tooth.

dissipates once the etiology is addressed. In susceptible individuals, virally or bacterially induced neuritis may produce a postinfection neuropathy of the infected nerve. The pain is fairly constant and can be dull, aching, and burning. Also, the pain may be accompanied by allodynia, a painful response to normally non-noxious stimulation such as light brushing of the skin. Oral acyclovir has become the most common treatment for acute herpetic outbreaks and has been shown to be efficacious in decreasing the duration and severity of pain after herpes zoster infection. Efficacy is based only on administration in the prevesicular, not the vesicular, stage. The addition of prednisolone to acyclovir produces only slight benefits over acyclovir alone. Neither acyclovir alone nor its combination with prednisolone appears to reduce the frequency of postherpetic neuralgia.[140]

Localized traumatic injury can also induce neuritis. This injury can be chemical, thermal, or mechanical in nature. A classic endodontic example of a chemical injury to a nerve is the overextension of a highly neurotoxic paraformaldehyde-containing paste (e.g., Sargenti paste) onto the inferior alveolar nerve canal. Chemical trauma can be due to certain toxic components of the endodontic filling materials (such as eugenol), irrigating solutions (such as sodium hypochlorite), or intracanal medicaments (such as formocresol) (Fig. 17-6).[94] Mechanical compression, in addition to thermal trauma, may be a factor when thermoplasticized material is overextended, using an injectable[50] or carrier-based technique. Mechanical nerve trauma is more commonly associated with oral surgical procedures, such as orthognathic surgery, and third molar extraction.

Neuritic complications have also been documented after mandibular implant surgery at a rate of 5% to 15%, with permanent neuropathies, which are discussed later, resulting in approximately 8% of these cases.[66] It is unfortunate that traumatic neuritis is often misdiagnosed as a posttreatment chronic infection and that the area is reentered and debrided.

Additional surgical insult further traumatizes the nerve, prolonging the already present nociceptive barrage, which puts the patient at an increased risk of developing central hyperalgesia. Undiagnosed and mistreated cases of acute neuritis not only lead to unnecessary dental procedures but may also aggravate the neuritis and, therefore, the neuritic pain has a greater chance of becoming chronic, something that is often referred to as neuropathic pain.

Neuritic pain typically is a persistent, nonpulsatile burning often associated with sensory aberrations such as paresthesia, dysesthesia, or anesthesia. The pain can vary in intensity, but when stimulated, the pain provoked is disproportionate to the stimulus.

Treatment of acute neuritis is based on its etiology. In instances of chemical trauma (e.g., Sargenti paste) where an obvious irritant is present, surgical debridement of the nerve to remove any substance that can continue to irritate the nerve is an important aspect of treatment. With neuritis secondary to mechanical compression (e.g., implant placement) of a nerve, nerve decompression by removal of the implant fixture is indicated. Such localized, acute, traumatically induced neuritis is inflammatory in nature and, therefore, can also benefit from supportive pharmacotherapies such as steroids. For management of neuritis that is not responsive to the previously cited treatments, medications used to treat neuropathic pain may be used (see Neuropathy). For neuritis occurring secondary to an infection, such as one of odontogenic or viral etiology, treatment is directed at eliminating the offending pathogen and minimizing injury to the afferent nerves.

Neuropathy

In this chapter we use the word *neuropathy* as the preferred term for localized, sustained nonepisodic pain secondary to an injury or change in a neural structure. Historically, other terms have been used including *atypical facial pain*. This term suggests pain that is felt in a branch of the trigeminal nerve and that does not fit any other pain category. Pain of an unknown source that is perceived in a tooth may be labeled *atypical odontalgia*. Pain that persists after the tooth has been extracted

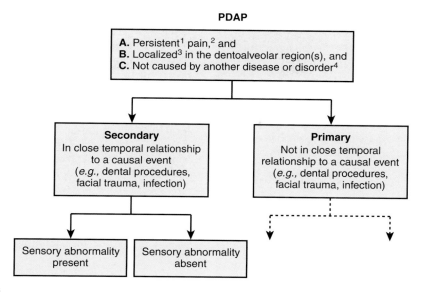

FIG. 17-7 Diagnostic criteria for persistent dentoalveolar pain disorder (PDAP).

is referred to as *phantom tooth pain*. The major limitation in the use of all these terms is that they merely suggest an area where a pain of unknown etiology exists and completely lack any information regarding the pathophysiology. Although each of these terms has been extensively described in the literature,[88,89] probably none actually represents one discrete condition but rather a collection of various conditions. Based on these thoughts, a consensus process resulted in proposing new terminology, persistent dentoalveolar pain disorder (PDAP), and diagnostic criteria (Fig. 17-7).[99]

Once a nerve has been sensitized via injury or disease it may remain so and present as a peripherally sensitized nerve. This peripheral sensitization and the ongoing pain (nociceptive barrage) that accompanies it can induce changes in the central nervous system. *Peripheral* sensitization and *central* sensitization can potentially impact the clinical presentation of a neuropathy. A typical clinical course of someone with an undiagnosed neuropathy might consist of treatment for a toothache. When the pain does not resolve with nonsurgical root canal treatment, it might then be followed by apical surgery and then perhaps an extraction. The extraction site might then be explored and debrided in a misguided attempt to remove any potential source of the patient's ongoing pain. After each treatment, there tends to be a reduction of the pain for a short time and then a return to its original, or even increased, level of pain intensity. It is likely that this is a result of a new neural injury consisting of reorganization and resprouting that increases the inhibition of nerve firing for a time. Surgical approaches to neuropathies are not effective because they do not desensitize the nerve. On the contrary, surgical intervention may aggravate the situation by inflicting an additional neural injury in the periphery and contributing to the already present nociceptive input. This intervention therefore puts the patient at increased risk of developing

persistent pain, which is supported by a couple of long-term observational studies[3,113] and further supported by the observation that patients with pain following root canal therapy did not uniformly experience elimination of this pain with apicoectomy surgery.[108]

A diagnosis of neuropathy is based primarily on history and examination with the use of selected diagnostic tests to rule out other potential etiologies. The history should reveal some inflammation-inducing event (see the earlier sections Neuritis and Neuroma), although the nature of the initial insult is not always identified, as seemingly spontaneous development of such pains has been reported.[99] Typically, the examination is grossly unremarkable with no evidence of local tissue damage, leaving the clinician to rely mainly on the patient's report of symptoms. Although quality of pain is no longer thought to be capable of distinguishing neuropathic pains from others, patients repeatedly reported several features that may be key for identification purposes (Box 17-2).[40] Regarding examination features, the area where the pain is perceived may be hyperalgesic or allodynic—that is, noxious stimulation to the area will be perceived as more painful or non-noxious stimulation will now be perceived as painful. This phenomenon is documented by reports where standardized applications of stimuli to the affected tissue are performed and demonstrate exaggerated responses.[85,90,146] Besides gain in sensory function, loss of function has also been observed,[85] which is more in line with a general definition for neuropathic pain.[135] Furthermore, maintenance of pain following local anesthesia to the affected region[83] and a lack of pain reduction with fentanyl and ketamine[7] all suggest the role of a central pain-related mechanism.

Research related to the diagnostic imaging of cases that may be PDAP suggests two roles: first, to identify pathosis contributing to the pain presentation and, second, as a means of

---

BOX 17-2

Recurrent Patient-Reported Themes Regarding Their Persistent Dentoalveolar Pain Disorder (PDAP)

◆ Difficult for patients to respond to history taking because their words do not adequately describe what they feel; therefore time may be needed to obtain the necessary information

◆ Well localized to a region within the dentoalveolar structures

◆ Pain is perceived to be deep in the tissues, rather than on the surface

◆ Continuous pain, one that never stops and seems to always be there

◆ Pain has the sensation of feeling pressure with a dull ache quality

◆ Complex and confounding descriptors, such as itching, tingling, or pricking, are sometimes present

---

obtaining a positive finding for this enigmatic chronic pain disorder. As for the first role, diagnostic imaging is recommended to assess for odontogenic-related pathosis and other regionally presenting disease, as most pain in the dentoalveolar region is tooth-related. For patients suspected of having PDAP, the diagnostic yield of cone-beam computed tomography (CT) was reported to be superior to PA radiograph, but the findings were of questionable significance.[112] For patients without local pathosis and PDAP, magnetic resonance imaging (MRI) of the brain revealed several cases of intracranial findings thought to be related to the pain presentation (e.g., cysts, tumors, infarcts).[104] This is consistent with the clinical experience of one of the authors, which has led to brain imaging being routine prior to a diagnosis of PDAP being rendered. As for the second role of diagnostic imaging, conventional dental radiographic techniques have consistently been found not to be able to identify patients with PDAP, thus prompting pilot investigation into other imaging techniques. Results suggest high levels of sensitivity and specificity can be reached using thermography[64] revealing a "cold" image profile.[63] On the contrary, results suggest that a technetium-99 bone scan had low sensitivity and specificity for detecting dentoalveolar regions with chronic pain,[32] and MRI techniques do not seem to have been studied.

Neuropathic disorders have a predilection for women but can affect both genders. These patients are usually older than 30 years of age and may have a history of migraine.[126] In the orofacial region, neuropathies are most commonly seen in the maxillary premolar area and molar region.[61,108]

Neuropathies can be classified on the basis of their clinical presentation and response to therapies. *Peripheral neuropathy* may develop after sensitization of a peripheral nerve and presents clinically as described previously. Diagnosis of peripheral neuropathy is based on its favorable response to peripheral neural blockade. Treatment is directed at decreasing the sensitization of peripheral nerves and reducing ectopic neuronal firing. Topical as well as systemic medications can be used to treat cutaneous peripheral neuropathies. Topical medications include topical anesthetics, capsaicin-containing compounds, and anticonvulsants, as well as nonsteroidal anti-inflammatory drugs (NSAIDs), sympathomimetic agents, and N-methyl-D-aspartate (NMDA) receptor-blocking agents[109] with encouraging results.[72]

The clinical presentation of a *central neuropathy* is similar to that of a peripheral neuropathy. After sensitization of peripheral nerves and the accompanying nociceptive barrage, the pain is nonremitting and lacks evidence of tissue insult. Unlike its peripheral counterpart, allodynia and secondary hyperalgesia are clearly present—that is, the area of pain is significantly larger than the initial site of injury. The most telling sign that a neuropathy has taken on a more central component is that local anesthetics are no longer effective. Therefore, the treatment must be directed toward the central processing of pain. This is done with medications such as NMDA receptor agonists (ketamine), gabapentin, tricyclic antidepressants, and opioids. The prognosis for a central neuropathy is not as good as for a peripheral neuropathy, as central neuropathic pain tends to become more refractory with time. Treatment is often based on the management of pain, rather than its cure, and sometimes is best performed in a multidisciplinary chronic pain clinic facility.

The last variation of neuropathic pain is sympathetically enhanced or maintained pain. In cases of sympathetically maintained pain (SMP), peripheral nerve fibers upregulate the expression of adrenergic receptors, making them responsive and sensitive to sympathetic input. SMP may also have a central component, whereby the constant sympathetic drive alters neuronal excitability. Neuronal injury may induce sprouting of sympathetic axons into the trigeminal spinal nucleus because basket-like formations of sympathetic fibers have been reported around the cell bodies of sensory neurons in the dorsal root ganglia.[141] Increases in sympathetic drive, such as with stress and fever, may aggravate SMP. Diagnosis of sympathetically maintained pain is based on blocking sympathetic outflow to the affected region via sympathetic nerve blocks. In the orofacial region this would require a stellate ganglion block. The block is considered diagnostic for SMP if it effectively decreases the patient's pain. Multiple blocks can also be used as a form of therapy. Other therapies include drugs that target peripheral α_2-adrenoceptors (agonists) or α_1-adrenoceptors (antagonists), such as guanethidine, phentolamine, and clonidine. SMP presenting in the orofacial region is extremely rare[54] and therefore makes clinicians prone to deriving a falsely positive diagnosis of this condition.[101] Furthermore, researchers have failed to produce SMP-type pain in animals,[10] something that is presumed to be due to the fact that the efferent nerve fibers in the head and neck region run with the blood vessels as opposed to the afferent nerves, as they do elsewhere in the human body. For these reasons, the likelihood of this type of pain presenting as "toothache" is extremely low and thus does not require much discussion here.

Psychogenic Toothache

Psychogenic toothache falls within a group of mental disorders known as somatoform disorders. The name is derived from the fact that the patient has somatic complaints yet lacks a physical cause. Because these patients lack a physical cause for pain, they also present without local tissue changes. Patients with somatoform disorders are not fabricating the symptoms, nor are they consciously seeking benefit. It is important to make a distinction between somatoform disorders and factitious pain or malingering behavior.[5] In factitious pain there are physical or psychological symptoms that are produced by the individual and are under voluntary control. Malingering is similar to factitious pain with the added characteristic that the symptoms are presented for obvious and recognizable benefit. This category poses a significant diagnostic challenge. Lacking evidence of local tissue damage is typical of heterotopic pain entities previously discussed in this chapter. It is important to emphasize that psychogenic pain is rare. When arriving at this diagnosis it is critical that all other potential diagnoses have been ruled out.

The diagnosis of psychogenic toothache is one of exclusion and is based on the clinician's awareness of other heterotopic pain characteristics and behavior. Of particular note are centrally emanating pains, cardiac pain, neurovascular pain, and neuropathic pain. Adding to the diagnostic difficulty is that comorbid psychological disorders are commonly present with chronic intraoral pain disorders, including those erroneously presenting as toothache.[84,130] This has led to the current thinking that psychological disorders (i.e., depression, anxiety, somatization) may not be related to the initiation or perpetuation of chronic pain disorders but rather are a consequence of living with chronic pain.

Psychogenic pain is known to be precipitated by severe psychologic stress. These pains present a general departure from the characteristics of any other pain condition—that is, they may not fit normal anatomic distributions or physiologically plausible patterns. The pain may be felt in multiple teeth and may jump around from one tooth to another. The intensity of pain reported tends to be more severe than is reflected by the patient's level of concern about the condition. Patients' responses to therapy are variable and include a lack of response or an unusual or unexpected response. Early identification of psychogenic pain and referral to a psychologist or psychiatrist is necessary to avoid irreversible and unnecessary dental treatment.

Toothache Referred from a Distant Organic Source

A variety of pathologies that seem to be unrelated have been reported to present as nonodontogenic toothache.[107,115] The only common link that can be identified is that branches of cranial nerves innervate the involved tissues, and hence the trigeminal nucleus processes nociceptive input. Therefore, conceivably, any somatic structure with cranial nerve innervation has the potential to cause pain that the patient perceives as a toothache. For this reason, once dentoalveolar etiologies for such pain have been ruled out, all possible sources of nonodontogenic pain including distant pathology should be considered in the differential diagnosis. Several of these types of organic pathologies that have been reported to present as toothache are described in the following sections.

Cardiac and Thoracic Structures

Cardiac pain has been cited as the cause of nonodontogenic toothache in a number of case reports.[9,41,62,77,97,136] Classically, cardiac pain presents as a crushing substernal pain that most commonly radiates to the left arm, shoulder, neck, and face. Although not as common, anginal pain may present solely as dental pain, generally felt in the lower left jaw.[16] Similar to pain of pulpal origin, cardiac pain can be spontaneous and diffuse, with a cyclic pattern that fluctuates in intensity from mild to severe. The pain can also be intermittent and the patient may be completely asymptomatic at times. The quality of cardiac pain when referred to the mandible is chiefly aching and sometimes pulsatile. Cardiac pain may be spontaneous or increased with physical exertion, emotional upset, or even the ingestion

of food.[9] Cardiac pain cannot be aggravated by local provocation of teeth. Anesthetizing the lower jaw or providing dental treatment will not reduce the pain. It can be decreased with rest or a dose of sublingual nitroglycerin. Diagnosis of cardiac pain, along with immediate referral, is mandatory to avoid impending myocardial infarction.

Besides pain of cardiac origin, other chest structures have been reported to produce nonodontogenic toothache pain. Various cancerous lesions of the lungs have been described to present a mandibular pain, with the pain being both ipsilateral and contralateral to the side where the tumor is present.[24,59] Furthermore, diaphragmatic pain is mediated via the phrenic nerve and may present as nonodontogenic tooth pain.[15]

Intracranial Structures

Space-occupying lesions within and around the brain are known to impinge on structures innervated with somatosensory fibers, such as the dural and perivascular tissues, causing pain. These pains are highly variable, with a common complaint being headache or head pain. Just as intracranially derived pain may be referred to the face and jaws in neurovascular disorders, it may also present as a toothache.[137] To outline the vast differences in clinical features of such pain, intracranial lesions have also been reported to cause trigeminal neuralgic pain in response to treatment of what was first thought to be toothache.[29] This extreme variability has been observed by one of the authors, which leads to the recommendation that if local etiologic factors are not readily identified in a patient with toothache symptoms, magnetic resonance brain imaging should be considered.

Throat and Neck Structures

Nonodontogenic toothache has been reported to arise from various structures of the neck, but these reports are sparse and hence it is not possible to draw conclusions regarding how patients with these pain-provoking disorders may present. Squamous cell carcinoma of the lateral pharyngeal surface presenting as ipsilateral mandibular molar pain has been observed by one of the authors. This finding is consistent with previous reports of nonodontogenic pain being associated with smooth muscle tumors of a similar location.[139] Vascular structures of the neck have also been implicated in the production of toothache symptoms, with a report of a patient initially presenting for dental care when pain was from the result of a life-threatening carotid artery dissection.[119]

Craniofacial Structures

Clinically, pain from other craniofacial structures has been observed as being the most common reason for organic pathologies presenting as nonodontogenic toothache, likely because these structures are innervated by branches of the trigeminal nerve. Tumors in the maxillary sinus[27,43,145] and jaw,[132] as well as metastatic disease, particularly within the mandible,[33,53,114,124] have been reported. The clinical presentation of symptoms is highly variable, but a common feature is sensory loss along the distribution of the nerve, the result of pain arising from nerve impingement. This underscores the need for regional imaging techniques, such as pantomography or computed tomography (CT) (as opposed to just periapical radiographs). This is especially true in patients who have a history of cancer. One must also not forget that nerve impingement anywhere along the distribution of the trigeminal nerve, even within the cranial vault itself,[20] can elicit nonodontogenic tooth pain.

Vascular structures within the craniofacial region have also been reported to present as nonodontogenic toothache, with arteritis being the pain-provoking pathology.[68,73] These pains have been described as a continuous dull pain that can sometimes be made worse with jaw function. The stereotypical presentation includes a history of eyesight changes, such as blurred vision, and the examination feature of pulseless, indurated temporal arteries that are painful to palpation. A laboratory finding of an elevated erythrocyte sedimentation rate (ESR) is suggestive of the disorder, and diagnosis is confirmed by temporal artery biopsy. Treatment includes administration of corticosteroids; therefore, because permanent blindness is a possible sequela if cranial arteries are left unmanaged, immediate referral to the appropriate medical colleague is indicated.

Frequency of Nonodontogenic Toothache

The prevalence of nonodontogenic toothache in the population is unknown, as is the prevalence of such a presentation for dental care. Specific to endodontics, pain is thought to be present in 5.3% of patients 6 or more months following treatment,[100] with about half of those individuals being estimated to have nonodontogenic etiologies accounting for their complaint of that pain.[100] At present, the proportion of such patients having the aforementioned nonodontogenic pain diagnosis is unknown. It remains unclear how this nonodontogenic pain is related to the endodontic diagnosis and subsequent treatment.

TAKING A PATIENT'S HISTORY

Pain diagnosis is largely based on the patient's subjective history; however, patients rarely give all pertinent diagnostic information about their pain of their own accord. Often it is necessary to carefully extract the details of the patient's pain complaint through systematic and thorough questioning. This is known as "taking a history," and it involves both careful listening and astute questioning. Fig. 17-8 is an example of a basic diagnostic workup for odontogenic pain. It can be easily used to obtain histories of typical odontogenic pain by circling

all descriptors that apply and then filling in the remaining blanks. As the details of a patient's pain complaint are gathered, the clinician should be mentally progressing through an algorithm of possible diagnoses, as each detail should lend itself to one type of pain over another. After completing a thorough and accurate history of the complaint(s) (Fig. 17-9), often the diagnosis has already been narrowed down to one particular pain entity. This is particularly true with odontogenic pain. The only question that will remain is "which tooth is it?" It is critical to keep in mind that whereas patients will provide information about the perceived site of pain, it is the clinician's examination that will reveal the true source of their pain. With more complicated pain complaints, the clinician may have a list of possible diagnoses. This is known as a differential diagnosis. This differential will guide the examination and testing in an effort to confirm one diagnosis while ruling out all others. If after completing the subjective examination all items on the differential are outside the clinician's scope of practice, then the clinician should continue the examination until he or she has a firm idea of the possible diagnosis so that a proper referral can be made. In addition, it is paramount that all odontogenic sources have been ruled out and that this information is communicated to the health care provider to which the patient is referred. If no differential can be formulated after the history has been

---

Sufficient for pain of odontogenic origin.

Subjective

Pain: (Circle all appropriate)   Level (0-10) _____

Well-localized	Diffuse	Intermittent
Spontaneous	Elicited (cold, hot, chewing)	Throbbing
Constant	Fluctuant	
Dull ache	Sharp shooting	

Onset _____

Progression (F/I/D) _____

Aggravating factors _____

Relieving factors _____

FIG. 17-8 Example of a form to evaluate odontogenic pain.

Chief complaint
Prioritize complaints _____
Specify location _____
VAS 0-10 _____
Initial onset
When did you first notice this? _____
Progression
Frequency _____
Intensity _____
Duration _____
Previous similar complaints
Have you ever had this type of pain before? _____
Characterize complaint
Daily, not daily _____
Constant, fluctuant, intermittent _____
Duration _____
Temporal pattern _____
Quality _____
Aggravating factors
What makes this pain worse? Be specific! _____
Alleviating factors
What makes this pain better? _____
How much better? _____
Associated factors
Swelling _____
Discoloration _____
Numbness _____
Relationship to other complaints
Would your jaw hurt if your tooth didn't hurt? _____
Prior consults/treatment
Who? _____
When? _____
What was the diagnosis? _____
What was done? _____
How did it affect the pain? _____

FIG. 17-9 Example of a form to evaluate pain history.

taken, then the history should be redirected to the patient to confirm that the information is complete and accurate. If the patient is unable to provide sufficient information regarding the pain complaint, then it may be helpful to have the patient keep a pain history, detailing the aspects of the pain on a daily basis. Of utmost importance is to avoid treatment when the diagnosis is uncertain. Diagnostic therapy (i.e., "let's do a root canal treatment and see if it helps") may result in costly treatment that does not improve the patient's condition and could be a factor in aggravating and perpetuating a patient's pain. Treatment should always specifically address a diagnosis.

A complete medical history along with current medications and drug allergies should always be ascertained. It is also important to make note of demographic information, as patients of certain genders and ages are more at risk for some disorders compared with others.

Recording a patient's *chief complaint* in the patient's own words is a medical legal necessity but falls short of constituting a thorough pain history. A complete history begins with a patient's general pain complaint—for example, "My tooth hurts." Patients may have more than one pain complaint—for example, "My tooth hurts and it is starting to make my jaw hurt." All pain complaints should be noted and investigated separately. Understanding the specific components of the complaints makes it possible to discern the relationship between them—that is, either the complaints are wholly separate and two types of pathosis are present, or one source of pain is merely creating a heterotopic pain that is wholly secondary to the first.

Begin with determining the *location* at which the patient perceives the pain. Aspects of the location involve localization and migration. Pain should be definable as either well localized or diffuse and either superficial or deep. Easily localized superficial pain tends to be cutaneous or neurogenic. Musculoskeletal pain is felt deeply and is more localizable once it is provoked. Deep, diffuse pain is suggestive of deep somatic pain, be it visceral or musculoskeletal. Both tissue types are involved in a high degree of nociceptor convergence in the trigeminal nucleus and, therefore, much more likely to be involved in creating heterotopic pain. Typical referral patterns of deep somatic pain tend to follow peripheral dermatomes that reflect the laminations in the trigeminal nucleus. Referred pain also tends to occur in a cephalad direction. Therefore, referred pain from a deep somatic tissue such as tooth pulp, cardiac tissue, or skeletal muscle will respect this pattern. Pain that spreads distally along a nerve branch is much more indicative of a projected type of heterotopic pain. Projected pains imply a neurogenic source and possibly one that is secondary to impingement from intracranial pathosis. Recall that superficial sources of pain are not likely to be involved in referral, so if a patient is indicating that the pain is superficial and spreading, this is highly suggestive of a neurogenic rather than a cutaneous source.

Assessment of the *intensity* of pain is easily accomplished using a verbal analog scale. This question is best phrased, "On a scale of one to ten, zero being no pain and ten being the worst pain you can imagine, how bad is your pain?" Not only can intensity provide insight about pain type; it can also help guide posttreatment pain management as well as provide a baseline for response to therapies.

Identifying the *onset* of pain may provide information regarding etiology. Question if the onset followed a particular event such as a dental appointment or a traumatic injury. Beware of these relationships, as they can be misleading. Having a temporal correlation does not necessarily ensure a cause-and-effect relationship. The onset of pain may be either gradual or sudden. Severe pain of sudden onset can signal a more serious problem. Pain that has been present over a protracted period of time, particularly if the pain has been unchanging, is highly suggestive of a nonodontogenic pain source.

Other *temporal* aspects of pain include frequency and duration. The clinician should ask the patient, "How often does the pain occur and how long does it last?" These temporal aspects may establish patterns that point more clearly to one condition over another.

Progression of the patient's pain over time should be noted. Whether pain is better, worse, or unchanging since its onset should be broken down into three factors: frequency, intensity, and duration. Static pain that does not change over time is typically not odontogenic in origin.

The *quality* of pain—that is, "what it feels like"—is a critical aspect of a pain history. Knowledge of pain characteristics as they relate to tissue types is essential. Pain quality can be difficult for patients to describe, and it is often necessary to provide them with a list of descriptors from which to choose. In instances of odontogenic pain, the list is fairly short. The deep visceral and musculoskeletal components of a tooth limit true odontogenic pain to having qualities that are dull, aching, or throbbing. If there is an aspect of sharpness to the pain, it is helpful to understand whether the sharpness is stabbing in nature, which would indicate A-delta fiber–mediated dentinal pain, or whether it is electrical in nature, which would indicate neuralgia. Common examples of pain descriptors and their respective pain types are listed in Table 17-1.

Factors that precipitate or aggravate the patient's pain complaint are of key importance in diagnosis. Not only do aggravating factors suggest the tissue types that may be involved, but they also aid in directing the objective tests. When gathering information, it is important to be specific. If a patient reports pain while eating, keep in mind that many structures are stimulated during mastication, such as muscles, temporomandibular joints (TMJs), mucosa, PDLs, and, potentially, pulps. Be specific as to the aggravating factor. The lack of any aggravating factors indicates that the pain is not of odontogenic origin.

Alleviating factors can provide insight as to the nature of the pain. If a medication relieves the pain, it is critical to know the specific medication, its dosage, and the degree to which the pain was attenuated. It is equally important to know what has no effect on the intensity of the pain. For example, if a pain of midlevel intensity is completely unresponsive to anti-inflammatory drugs, then it is probably not inflammatory in origin.

TABLE 17-1

Examples of Pain Descriptors

Origin	Quality of Pain
Muscular	Dull, aching
Neurogenic	Shocking, burning
Vascular	Throbbing, pulsatile

Associated factors such as swelling, discoloration, and numbness must be ascertained, as well as their correlation with symptoms. Swelling of acute onset suggests an infection, and its concurrent pain would be of inflammatory origin. Swelling that comes and goes with the intensity of pain suggests an autonomic component. The same can be said for discoloration, such as redness. Numbness or any other type of sensory aberrations should be recorded. If the altered sensation is a major component of the pain complaint, then it should be investigated separately and its relationship to the pain determined. Pains that occur with sensory aberrations tend to have a strong neurogenic component.

If the patient complains of more than one pain, an effort should be made during the subjective history to determine the *relationship of the complaints*. One pain might serve as an aggravating factor to the other. There may be a correlation as to the onset, intensity, or progression of the complaints. Also, keep in mind that patients may actually have more than one type of pathosis occurring concurrently and there may be no relationship whatsoever. Ask whether there have been any *previous similar complaints* and, if so, what happened. Recurrence of similar pains might reveal a pattern that lends itself to a particular pain diagnosis.

It is critical to gain knowledge of any prior consultations that have occurred. Details regarding the type of clinician, actual workup performed, and diagnosis rendered will help to narrow down a differential. Any treatment that was performed should be ascertained along with its effect on the chief complaint.

PATIENT EXAMINATION

As stated previously, the purpose of the history is to gather information about a patient's pain complaint in order to formulate a list of possible diagnoses based on specific pain characteristics. Poor or improper symptom analysis will lead to a false differential, and any testing will therefore have limited meaning. Performing a general examination including an extraoral, intraoral, and hard and soft tissue assessment is requisite to confirm the health of various structures and to identify possible pain-producing etiologies. When a patient presents with a toothache, the pain is usually of odontogenic origin. Diagnostic procedures are often limited to confirming a suspect tooth rather than identifying a nonodontogenic source of pain. Standard pulpal and periradicular tests serve to aid in both ruling in odontogenic pain and therefore ruling out nonodontogenic pain as a diagnosis. Remember that the site of pain is determined by patient history, but the true source of the pain should be revealed with testing. If the chief complaint cannot be reproduced with standard tests then additional tests may be necessary to narrow down a differential diagnosis. For details on general examinations and standard tests, please refer to Chapter 1.

Additional Tests

Further tests should be chosen with forethought in an effort to develop a workable differential that can guide the clinician toward a meaningful consultation or an appropriate referral for the patient. These tests may consist of palpation or provocation of various structures, sensory testing, or diagnostic blocks. The application of these tests is not covered in detail in this chapter. For more information about the application and interpretation of these tests, please consult other sources.

Palpation and percussion are common tests to differentiate odontogenic pain from pain of sinus origin. Palpation of the sinuses consists of firm pressure placed over the involved sinus (usually maxillary). In addition, pain of sinus origin may be provoked with a lowering of the patient's head.

If pain of muscular origin is suspected, then an attempt to reproduce this pain can be done by palpation of the muscles of mastication or provocation via functional manipulation. The temporalis, deep and superficial masseter, medial pterygoid, and digastric muscles should be palpated in an effort to discover tenderness or trigger points that reproduce the pain complaint. The medial pterygoid is only partially accessible to palpation and may need to be functionally tested by stretching the muscle (opening wide) or contracting the muscle (biting firmly). The lateral pterygoid may be difficult if not impossible to palpate intraorally and therefore is more appropriately assessed by functional manipulation. Pain emanating from this muscle may be increased by protruding the jaw against resistance. Exacerbating the chief complaint by muscular function provides a strong indication of a myofascial source of pain.

Because of the complexity of innervation and the occurrence of heterotopic pain in the orofacial region, it may be difficult to definitively determine the origin of pain by testing alone. It cannot be stressed enough that primary pain should not only be provoked by local manipulation but also be relieved by anesthetic blocking. In diagnostic anesthesia the relief of pain has a typical onset and duration, depending on the particular anesthetic used. In addition, the pain should be completely diminished or else suspicion of a central component or a coexisting disorder should arise. The use of diagnostic anesthesia may be necessary and useful in augmenting the diagnostic workup (Fig. 17-10). Topical anesthetic can be helpful in the investigation of cutaneous pain and peripheral neuropathies. Anesthetic injection including peripheral nerve blocks can be used to determine whether the etiology of the pathosis is peripheral to the area of the block. Pain that persists after the onset of usual signs of anesthesia suggests a central component. The patient's history and general examination are of key importance in differentiating between the pain of a central neuropathy and the central pain emanating from an intracranial mass.

Pain that is primarily muscular, as suggested by trigger points discovered on examination, can be further investigated by local anesthetic injection into the trigger point. Trigger point injections are typically performed with either a 27- or a 25-gauge needle and a minimally myotoxic anesthetic such as 2% lidocaine or 3% mepivacaine without a vasoconstrictor. Myofascial trigger point injections may temporarily relieve pain at the trigger point as well as at the site of referral.

Sympathetic efferent activity can play a role in the enhancement or maintenance of chronic pain. In the head and neck, sympathetic activity flows through the stellate ganglion located bilaterally near the first rib. When there is suspicion of a sympathetic component to a patient's pain, a stellate ganglion block can be used to provide diagnostic insight. A trained anesthesiologist usually performs this procedure. An effective block delivered to the stellate ganglion will interrupt sympathetic outflow to the ipsilateral side of the face, resulting in a partial Horner syndrome. This is evidenced by flushing, congestion, lacrimation, miosis of the pupil, ptosis, and anhidrosis.[75] A sympathetic blockade that diminishes or eliminates a pain state may guide future treatment such as repeated blocks or systemic

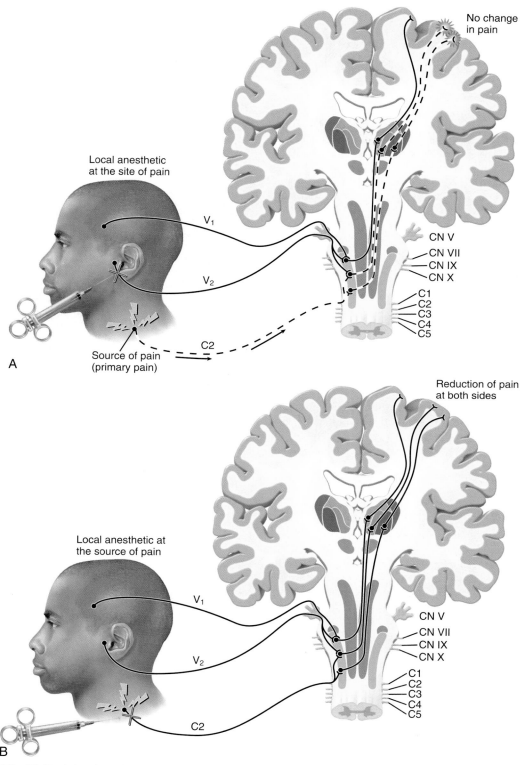

FIG. 17-10 **A,** Local anesthetic at the site of pain fails to reduce the pain. **B,** Local anesthetic at the source of pain reduces the pain at the source as well as at the site. (Redrawn from Okeson JP: *Bell's orofacial pains,* ed 5, Chicago, 1995, Quintessence Publishing.)

treatment with sympathetically active drugs (e.g., clonidine and prazosin).[116]

Neurologic conditions, both peripheral and central, can present as pain in the orofacial region. A role of the clinician is to help rule out gross neurologic conditions secondary to intracranial pathosis. Systemic complaints such as nausea, dizziness, or changes in one of the special senses should raise suspicion of intracranial pathosis. A neurologic screening examination including a gross sensory and motor evaluation of cranial nerves II through XII should be performed. For details on cranial nerve examination, please refer to other sources.[44] Investigation of sharp/dull differentiation as well as light touch discrimination between the different branches of the trigeminal nerve can provide insight as to the location and etiology of the pathosis.

Case Studies

Case 1

A 56-year-old male presents with a chief complaint of "This tooth still hurts and it's getting worse. It even hurts when I smile." He has a history of angina secondary to a 70% occlusion of his right coronary artery. He also reports a history of hypercholesterolemia. He has no history of myocardial infarction and denies any other significant medical history. The patient is taking lovastatin (Mevacor, 400 mg/day), nifedipine (Procardia, 60 mg once per day), and atenolol (50 mg once per day). He has no known drug allergy.

The patient was referred by a periodontist for evaluation of continued pain associated with tooth #3. He had been receiving periodontal maintenance therapy for generalized moderate adult periodontitis for more than 5 years. He had root canal treatment and a mesial buccal root amputation of tooth #3 as treatment for a localized area of advanced periodontitis 6 months ago.

Subjective History

After careful questioning, it becomes apparent that the patient is experiencing pain of two different qualities: an intermittent ache associated with tooth #3 and an intermittent sharp shooting pain also associated with tooth #3. The intermittent dull ache was of gradual onset 9 months ago. This pain was unaffected by the nonsurgical root canal treatment and root amputation. This pain has increased in frequency, intensity, and duration over the past 3 months. There is no temporal component. The dull ache is aggravated by biting and by the occurrence of the sharp shooting pain. The sharp shooting pain had a sudden onset 6 months ago. It has also increased in frequency, intensity, and duration without a temporal component. It can occur spontaneously or when the patient is "smiling big." The patient reports that the sharp shooting pain can also be aggravated by pressing lightly on his face in the area overlying #3, but not by pressing intraorally on #3.

Examination

The coronal portion of the amputated mesiobuccal root had been restored with IRM (Intermediate Restorative Material; DENTSPLY Caulk, Milford, DE). No cracks, fractures, sinus tracts, or swelling is detected. There are generalized probing depths of 4 mm throughout the upper right sextant. Tooth #3 has an 8-mm-broad probing defect mesially with bleeding on probing. For the results of clinical testing, see Table 17-2.

TABLE 17-2

Case 1: Clinical Results of Testing

Test	Tooth #2	Tooth #3	Tooth #4
Endo Ice*	+ (s)†	−	+ (s)
Percussion	−	+	−
Palpation	−	−	−

*Endo Ice (Coltène/Whaledent, Cuyahoga Falls, Ohio) is used to detect pulp vitality.
†s, pain of short duration.

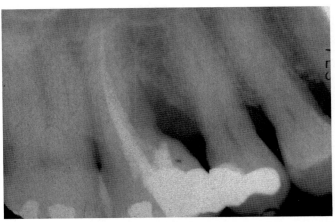

FIG. 17-11 Periapical radiograph showing prior nonsurgical root canal treatment and mesiobuccal root amputation of tooth #3.

A periapical radiograph (Fig. 17-11) shows evidence of prior nonsurgical root canal treatment and mesiobuccal root amputation of tooth #3. Mild to moderate horizontal bone loss is evident in the quadrant. No radiographic evidence of caries or apical radiolucencies is noted.

Additional Tests

In the absence of a clear etiology, a more extensive extraoral examination is performed. Cranial nerves II through XII are intact. The sharp shooting pain is predictably produced with light brushing of the skin over the area of tooth #3. This examination increases the patient's subjective complaint of a dull ache associated with tooth #3. With the likelihood of two possible sources of pain existing, a diagnostic anesthetic block of tooth #3 is performed: buccal infiltration of tooth #3 with 27 mg of 3% mepivacaine without epinephrine. After 3 minutes the patient no longer reports a dull ache at tooth #3 and he is nontender to percussion. His sharp shooting pain can still be initiated with light brushing of the skin over the area of tooth #3 and continues to cause a dull ache in the area of tooth #3. Diagnoses of trigeminal neuralgia and advanced localized adult periodontitis of tooth #3 are made. The patient is referred to a neurologist for evaluation and treatment. The diagnosis of trigeminal neuralgia is confirmed and he is placed on carbamazepine at 100 mg/day.

Case 2

A 28-year-old male presents with a chief complaint of "My teeth on the right side hurt." His medical history is not significant. He denies any systemic disease and has no known drug allergies. He is currently taking 600 mg of ibuprofen as needed for pain. He is taking no other medications. The patient was referred by his general clinician for evaluation of pain associated with his teeth on the right side.

Subjective History

After careful questioning, it is determined that the patient is experiencing pain of two different types. The most distressing pain to the patient is a diffuse, right-sided, constant low-grade dull ache (3/10 on a verbal analog scale [VAS]). The onset was gradual, beginning 2 years ago. The pain has recently increased in intensity and duration. This pain is aggravated by opening wide and increases in intensity after the occurrence of a sharp pain that is induced by biting down. There is no notable temporal component, and the patient has made no attempts to obtund the pain.

His other pain type had a sudden onset approximately 4 months ago. This pain is localized to the area of the right first molars. It is an intermittent sharp shooting pain (8/10 on VAS) that occurs when biting.

Examination

Tooth #3 has an occlusal amalgam with cracks evident on the mesial marginal ridge and the buccal groove. Tooth #30 has an occlusal amalgam, and cracks are noted on the mesial and distal marginal ridges of the tooth. There are no swellings or sinus tracts and no probing greater than 4 mm on the right side. A periapical radiograph demonstrates no evidence of caries or apical radiolucencies. The patient's sharp pain is reproduced with a bite test applied to the mesial lingual cusp of tooth #30. After the bite test, the patient reports that his dull ache has intensified. For the results of clinical testing see Table 17-3. Thirty seconds after pulp testing has been completed, the patient again reports that his dull ache has intensified.

Additional Tests

In consideration of an uncertain diagnosis, a more extensive examination is performed. Palpation and provocation tests of

the muscles of mastication reveal a trigger point in the patient's right deep masseter. Palpation of this trigger point immediately intensifies his "toothache." A trigger point injection of 3% mepivacaine without epinephrine is done in an effort to clarify a diagnosis. After a trigger point injection, all tests are repeated. Palpation of the trigger point no longer produces pain. The bite test and cold test still produce a short sharp pain but are no longer followed by a dull ache.

Diagnoses of reversible pulpitis secondary to a cracked tooth #31 and myofascial pain of the right masseter are made. The patient is given home care instructions for treatment of his myofascial pain, and he is referred to his general clinician for cuspal coverage of both teeth #3 and #30.

SUMMARY

As clinicians who are frequently called on to diagnose and treat complaints of orofacial pain, it is important to have a thorough knowledge of the odontogenic and nonodontogenic causes. The basis for this knowledge begins with an understanding of the anatomy and physiology of the pain system, and how alterations in this system can result in pain that is poorly localized and therefore misdiagnosed. A realization that pain does not always originate in the structures in which they are felt, along with an understanding of the neurobiologic basis of heterotopic pain, is necessary to ensure accurate diagnosis of orofacial pain.

There are several indicators that a toothache may be nonodontogenic in origin. Red flags for nonodontogenic pain include toothaches that have no apparent etiology for pulpal or periradicular pathosis; pain that is spontaneous, poorly localized, or migratory; and pain that is constant and nonvariable. In addition, pain that is described as burning, pricking, or "shocklike" is less likely to be pulpal or periradicular in origin.

A thorough pain history and an examination of dental and nondental structures are essential to differentiate between odontogenic and nonodontogenic sources of pain. Examples of key components of the pain history and examination are included in this chapter for reference. In addition, the chapter has focused on the more common nonodontogenic sources of orofacial pain. As stated previously, the role of the dental clinician is to diagnose and treat disorders of the oral cavity and masticatory structures. In the event that a nondental pathosis is suspected, a differential diagnosis of probable disorders is essential as part of a referral to a more appropriate health care provider. In addition, an understanding of any potential role or interaction of dental structures in the patient's pain complaint should be communicated as part of the referral.

TABLE 17-3

Case 2: Clinical Results of Testing

Test	Tooth					
	#2	#3	#4	#31	#30	#29
Endo Ice	+ (s)	+ (s)	+ (s)	+ (s)	+ (s)	+ (s)
Percussion	−	−	−	−	−	−
Palpation	−	−	−	−	−	−

REFERENCES

1. Abu-Bakra M, Jones NS: Prevalence of nasal mucosal contact points in patients with facial pain compared with patients without facial pain, *J Laryngol Otol* 115:629, 2001.
2. Albin R, Wiener J, Gordon R, Willoughby JH: Diagnosis and treatment of pansinusitis: report of case, *J Oral Surg* 37:604, 1979.
3. Allerbring M, Haegerstam G: Chronic idiopathic orofacial pain: a long-term follow-up study, *Acta Odontol Scand* 62:66, 2004.
4. Alonso AA, Nixdorf DR: Case series of four different headache types presenting as tooth pain, *J Endod* 32:1110, 2006.
5. American Psychiatric Association: *Diagnostic and statistical manual of mental disorders (DSM-IV)*, Washington, DC, 1994, American Psychiatric Association, p 447.
6. Anderson GC, John MT, Ohrbach R, et al: Influence of headache frequency on clinical signs and symptoms of TMD in subjects with temple headache and TMD pain, *Pain* 152:765, 2011.
7. Baad-Hansen L, Juhl GI, Jensen TS, et al: Differential effect of intravenous S-ketamine and fentanyl on atypical odontalgia and capsaicin-evoked pain, *Pain* 129:46, 2007.
8. Backonja M: Use of anticonvulsants for treatment of neuropathic pain, *Neurology* 59(5 suppl 2):S14, 2002.
9. Batchelder B, Krutchkoff DJ, Amara J: Mandibular pain as the initial and sole clinical manifestation of coronary insufficiency, *J Am Dent Assoc* 115:710, 1987.

10. Benoliel R, Eliav E, Tal M: No sympathetic nerve sprouting in rat trigeminal ganglion following painful and non-painful infraorbital nerve neuropathy, *Neurosci Lett* 297:151, 2001.

11. Benoliel R, Sharav Y: Paroxysmal hemicrania: case studies and review of the literature, *Oral Surg Oral Med Oral Pathol Oral Radiol Endod* 85:285, 1998.

12. Benoliel R, Sharav Y: SUNCT syndrome: case report and literature review, *Oral Surg Oral Med Oral Pathol Oral Radiol Endod* 85:158, 1998.

13. Besson J, Chaouch A: Peripheral and spinal mechanisms of nociception, *Physiol Rev* 67:67, 1987.

14. Bittar G, Graff-Radford SB: A retrospective study of patients with cluster headaches, *Oral Surg Oral Med Oral Pathol* 73:519, 1992.

15. Blows WT: Diaphragmatic cramp as a possible cause of noncardiac chest pain and referred mandibular pain, *J Neurosci Nurs* 31:187, 1999.

16. Bonica J: *The management of pain with special emphasis on the use of analgesic block in diagnosis, prognosis and therapy*, Philadelphia, 1953, Lea & Febiger.

17. Bonica J: *The management of pain*, Philadelphia, 1990, Lea & Febiger, 1990.

18. Brannstrom M, Johnson G, Nordenvall KJ: Transmission and control of dentinal pain: resin impregnation for the desensitization of pain, *J Am Dent Assoc* 99:612, 1979.

19. Brattberg J, Thorslund M, Wickman A: The prevalence of pain in a general population. The results of a postal study in a county in Sweden, *Pain* 37:215, 1989.

20. Brazis PW, Wharen RE, Czervionke LF, et al: Hemangioma of the mandibular branch of the trigeminal nerve in the Meckel cave presenting with facial pain and sixth nerve palsy, *J Neuroophthalmol* 20:14, 2000.

21. Brooke RI: Periodic migrainous neuralgia: a cause of dental pain, *Oral Surg Oral Med Oral Pathol* 46:511, 1978.

22. Broton J, Hu JW, Sessle BJ: Effects of temporomandibular joint stimulation on nociceptive and nonnociceptive neurons of the cat's trigeminal subnucleus caudalis (medulla dorsal horn), *J Neurophysiol* 59:1575, 1988.

23. Brown A, Beeler WJ, Kloka AC, Fields RW: Spatial summation of pre-pain and pain in human teeth, *Pain* 21:1, 1985.

24. Buddery DJ: Mandible pain, *Br Dent J* 194:121, 2003.

25. Byers M: Dental sensory receptors, *Int Rev Neurobiol* 25:39, 1984.

26. Campbell JK: Facial pain due to migraine and cluster headache, *Semin Neurol* 8:324, 1988.

27. Chan YW, Guo YC, Tsai TL, et al: Malignant fibrous histiocytoma of the maxillary sinus presenting as toothache, *J Chin Med Assoc* 67:104, 2004.

28. Chen YH, Tseng CC, Chao WY, et al: Toothache with a multifactorial etiology: a case report, *Endod Dent Traumatol* 13:245, 1997.

29. Cirak B, Kiymaz N, Arslanoglu A: Trigeminal neuralgia caused by intracranial epidermoid tumor: report of a case and review of the different therapeutic modalities, *Pain Physician* 7:129, 2004.

30. de Leeuw R: Differential diagnosis of orofacial pain. In de Leeuw R, editor: *Orofacial pain: guidelines for assessment, diagnosis, and management*, Hanover Park, IL, 2008, Quintessence Publishing, p 49.

31. Delcanho RE, Graff-Radford SB: Chronic paroxysmal hemicrania presenting as toothache, *J Orofac Pain* 7:300, 1993.

32. DeNucci DJ, Chen CC, Sobiski C, Meehan S: The use of SPECT bone scans to evaluate patients with idiopathic jaw pain, *Oral Surg Oral Med Oral Pathol Oral Radiol Endod* 90:750, 2000.

33. Dewan K, Owens J, Silvester K: Maintaining a high level of suspicion for recurrent malignant disease: report of a case with periapical involvement, *Int Endod J* 40:900, 2007.

34. Dodick DW: Migraine with isolated face pain: a diagnostic challenge, *Cephalalgia* 27:1199, 2007.

35. Drangsholt MT, Svennson P, Nguyen KL: Which orofacial pain conditions are neuropathic? A systematic review using NEUPSIG '08 criteria, World Congress on Pain, International Association for the Study of Pain, August 2008.

36. Druce H: Diagnosis of sinusitis in adults: History, physical examination, nasal cytology, echo, and rhinoscope, *J Allergy Clin Immunol* 90:436, 1992.

37. Druce H, Slavin RG: Sinusitis: critical need for further study, *J Allergy Clin Immunol* 88:675, 1991.

38. Dubner R, Bennet G: Spinal and trigeminal mechanisms of nociception, *Ann Rev Neurosci* 6:381, 1983.

39. Dubner R, Hayes RL, Hoffman DS: Neural and behavioral correlates of pain in the trigeminal system, *Res Publ Assoc Res Nerv Ment Dis* 58:63, 1980.

40. Durham J, Exley C, John MT, Nixdorf DR: Persistent dentoalveolar pain: the patient's experience, *J Orofac Pain* 27:6, 2013.

41. Durso BC, Israel MS, Janini ME, Cardoso AS: Orofacial pain of cardiac origin: a case report, *Cranio* 21:152, 2003.

42. Ekborn K: Treatment of cluster headache: clinical trials, design and results, *Cephalalgia* 15:33, 1995.

43. Ellinger RF, Kelly WH: Maxillary sinus lymphoma: a consideration in the diagnosis of odontogenic pain, *J Endod* 15:90, 1989.

44. Evans RW: *Saunders manual of neurologic practice*, Philadelphia, 2003, Elsevier Science.

45. Fricton J: Masticatory myofascial pain: an explanatory model integrating clinical, epidemiological and basic science research, *Bull Group Int Research Sci Stomatol Odontol* 41:14, 1999.

46. Fricton JR: Critical commentary: A unified concept of idiopathic orofacial pain: clinical features, *J Orofac Pain* 13:185, 1999.

47. Fristad I, Bardsen A, Knudsen GC, Molven O: Prodromal herpes zoster: a diagnostic challenge in endodontics, *Int Endod J* 35:1012, 2002.

48. Fromm GH, Graff-Radford SB, Terrence CF, Sweet WH: Pre-trigeminal neuralgia, *Neurology* 40:1493, 1990.

49. Gallagher R, Mueller L, Ciervo CA: Increased prevalence of sensing types in men with cluster headaches, *Psychol Rev* 87:555, 2000.

50. Gatot A, Peist M, Mozes M: Endodontic overextension produced by injected thermopolasticized gutta-percha, *J Endod* 15:273, 1989.

51. Gaul C, Gantenbein AR, Buettner UW, et al: Orofacial cluster headache, *Cephalalgia* 28:903, 2008.

52. Gaul C, Sandor PS, Galli U, et al: Orofacial migraine, *Cephalalgia* 27:950, 2007.

53. Gaver A, Polliack G, Pilo R, et al: Orofacial pain and numb chin syndrome as the presenting symptoms of a metastatic prostate cancer, *J Postgrad Med* 48:283, 2002.

54. Giri S, Nixdorf D: Sympathetically maintained pain presenting first as temporomandibular disorder, then as parotid dysfunction, *Tex Dent J* 124:748, 2007.

55. Glaros A, Urban D, Locke J: Headache and temporomandibular disorders: evidence for diagnostic and behavioural overlap, *Cephalalgia* 27:542, 2007.

56. Goadsby PJ: The international classification of headache disorders, ed 2, *Cephalgia* 24 (suppl 1):1-160, 2004.

57. Gobel S, Falls W, Hockfield S: The division of the dorsal and ventral horns of the mammalian caudal medulla into eight layers using anatomic criteria. In Anderson D, Matthews B, editors: *Pain in the trigeminal region*, proceedings of a symposium held in the Department of Physiology, University of Bristol, England, on July 25-27, 1977, Amsterdam, 1977, Elsevier Press, p 443.

58. Goh B, Poon CY, Peck RH: The importance of routine magnetic resonance imaging in trigeminal neuralgia diagnosis, *Oral Surg Oral Med Oral Pathol Oral Radiol Endod* 92:424, 2001.

59. Goldberg HL: Chest cancer refers pain to face and jaw: a case review, *Cranio* 15:167, 1997.

60. Goon WW, Jacobsen PL: Prodromal odontalgia and multiple devitalized teeth caused by a herpes zoster infection of the trigeminal nerve: report of case, *J Am Dent Assoc* 116:500, 1988.

61. Graff-Radford SB, Solberg WK: Atypical odontalgia, *J Craniomandib Disord* 6:260, 1992.

62. Graham LL, Schinbeckler GA: Orofacial pain of cardiac origin, *J Am Dent Assoc* 104:47, 1982.

63. Gratt BM, Graff-Radford SB, Shetty V, et al: A 6-year clinical assessment of electronic facial thermography, *Dentomaxillofac Radiol* 25:247, 1996.

64. Gratt BM, Pullinger A, Sickles EA, Lee JJ: Electronic thermography of normal facial structures: a pilot study, *Oral Surg Oral Med Oral Pathol* 68:346, 1989.

65. Greenberg DA, Aminoff MJ, Simon RP: *Clinical neurology*, New York, 2002, McGraw-Hill, p 390.

66. Gregg J: Neuropathic complications of mandibular implant surgery: review and case presentations, *Ann R Australas Coll Dent Surg* 15:176, 2000.

67. Gregory WB Jr, Brooks LE, Penick EC: Herpes zoster associated with pulpless teeth, *J Endod* 1:32, 1975.

68. Guttenberg SA, Emery RW, Milobsky SA, Geballa M: Cranial arteritis mimicking odontogenic pain: report of case, *J Am Dent Assoc* 119:621, 1989.

69. Hansen H: Neuro-histological reactions following tooth extractions, *Int J Oral Surg* 9:411, 1980.

70. Hargreaves K, Bowles WR, Jackson DL: Intrinsic regulation of CGRP release by dental pulp sympathetic fibers, *J Dent Res* 82:398, 2003.

71. Hargreaves K, Dubner R: *Mechanisms of pain and analgesia*, Amsterdam, 1991, Elsevier Press.

72. Heir G, Karolchek S, Kalladka M, et al: Use of topical medication in orofacial neuropathic pain: a retrospective study, *Oral Surg Oral Med Oral Path Oral Radiol Endod* 105:466, 2008.

73. Hellmann DB: Temporal arteritis: a cough, toothache and tongue infarction, *JAMA* 287:2996, 2002.

74. Jacquin MF, Renehan WE, Mooney RD, Rhoades RW: Structure-function relationships in rat medullary and cervical dorsal horns. I. Trigeminal primary afferents, *J Neurophysiol* 55:1153, 1986.

75. Kisch B: Horner's syndrome, an American discovery, *Bull Hist Med* 25:284, 1951.

76. Kraut R, Chahal O: Management of patients with trigeminal nerve injuries after mandibular implant placement, *J Am Dent Assoc* 133:1351, 2002.

77. Kreiner M, Okeson JP, Michelis V, et al: Craniofacial pain as the sole symptom of cardiac ischemia: a prospective multicenter study, *J Am Dent Assoc* 138:74, 2007.

78. Lamotte R, Campbell JN: Comparison of responses of warm and nociceptive C-fiber afferents in monkey with human judgements of thermal pain, *J Neurophysiol* 41:509, 1978.

79. LeBars D, Dickenson AH, Besson JM, Villanueva L: Aspects of sensory processing through convergent neurons. In Yaksh TL, editor: *Spinal afferent processing*, New York, 1986, Plenum Press.

80. Li Y, Li HJ, Huang J, et al: Central malignant salivary gland tumors of the jaw: retrospective clinical analysis of 22 cases, *J Oral Maxillofac Surg* 66:2247, 2008.

81. Lipton J, Ship JA, Larach-Robinson D: Estimated prevalence and distribution of reported orofacial pain in the United States, *J Am Dent Assoc* 124:115, 1993.

82. Lipton RB, Stewart WF, Diamond S, et al: Prevalence and burden of migraine in the United States: data from the American Migraine Study II, *Headache* 41:646, 2001.

83. List T, Leijon G, Helkimo M, et al: Effect of local anesthesia on atypical odontalgia—A randomized controlled trial, *Pain* 122:306, 2006.

84. List T, Leijon G, Helkimo M, et al: Clinical findings and psychosocial factors in patients with atypical odontalgia: a case-control study, *J Orofac Pain* 21:89, 2007.

85. List T, Leijon G, Svensson P: Somatosensory abnormalities in atypical odontalgia: a case-control study, *Pain* 139:333, 2008.

86. Loeser JD, Treede RD: The Kyoto protocol of IASP basic pain terminology, *Pain* 137:473, 2008.

87. Long A, Loeschr AR, Robinson PP: A quantitative study on the myelinated fiber innervation of the periodontal ligament of cat canine teeth, *J Dent Res* 74:1310, 1995.
88. Marbach J, Raphael KG: Phantom tooth pain: a new look at an old dilemma, *Pain Med* 1:68, 2000.
89. Melis M, Lobo SL, Ceneviz C, et al: Atypical odontalgia: a review of the literature, *Headache* 43:1060, 2003.
90. Moana-Filho EJ, Nixdorf DR, Bereiter DA, et al: Evaluation of a magnetic resonance-compatible dentoalveolar tactile stimulus device, *BMC Neurosci* 11:142, 2010.
91. Moncada E, Graff-Radford SB: Cough headache presenting as a toothache: a case report, *Headache* 33:240, 1993.
92. Moncada E, Graff-Radford SB: Benign indomethacin-responsive headaches presenting in the orofacial region: eight case reports, *J Orofac Pain* 9:276, 1995.
93. Mondell B: A review of the effects of almotriptan and other triptans on clinical trial outcomes that are meaningful to patients with migraine, *Clin Ther* 25:331, 2003.
94. Morse D: Infection-related mental and inferior alveolar nerve paresthesia: literature review and presentation of two cases, *J Endod* 23:457, 1997.
95. Nahri M: The neurophysiology of the teeth, *Dent Clin North Am* 34:439, 1990.
96. Namazi MR: Presentation of migraine as odontalgia, *Headache* 41:420, 2001.
97. Natkin E, Harrington GW, Mandel MA: Anginal pain referred to the teeth: report of a case, *Oral Surg Oral Med Oral Pathol* 40:678, 1975.
98. Neumann S, Doubell TP, Leslie T, Woolf CJ: Inflammatory pain hypersensitivity mediated by phenotypic switch in myelinated primary sensory neurons, *Nature* 384:360, 1996.
99. Nixdorf DR, Drangsholt MT, Ettlin DA, et al: International RDC-TMD Consortium: Classifying orofacial pains: a new proposal of taxonomy based on ontology, *J Oral Rehabil* 39:161, 2012.
100. Nixdorf DR, Moana-Filho EJ, Law AS, et al: Frequency of persistent tooth pain after root canal therapy: a systematic review and meta-analysis, *J Endod* 36:224, 2010.
101. Nixdorf DR, Sobieh R, Gierthmuhlen J: Using an n-of-1 trial to assist in clinical decision making for patients with orofacial pain, *J Am Dent Assoc* 143:259, 2012.
102. Nixdorf DR, Velly AM, Alonso AA: Neurovascular pains: implications of migraine for the oral and maxillofacial surgeon, *Oral Maxillofac Surg Clin North Am* 20:221, vi, 2008.
103. Obermann M, Mueller D, Yoon MS, et al: Migraine with isolated facial pain: a diagnostic challenge, *Cephalalgia* 27:1278, 2007.
104. Ogutcen-Toller M, Uzun E, Incesu L: Clinical and magnetic resonance imaging evaluation of facial pain, *Oral Surg Oral Med Oral Path Oral Radiol Endod* 97:652, 2004.
105. Okeson J: *Orofacial pain: guidelines for assessment, diagnosis and management*, Chicago, 1996, Quintessence Publishing.
106. Okeson JP: *Bell's orofacial pains: the clinical management of orofacial pain*, ed 6, Chicago, 2005, Quintessence Publishing.
107. Okeson JP, Falace DA: Nonodontogenic toothache, *Dent Clin North Am* 41:367, 1997.
108. Oshima K, Ishii T, Ogura Y, et al: Clinical investigation of patients who develop neuropathic tooth pain after endodontic procedures, *J Endod* 35:958, 2009.

109. Padilla M, Clark GT, Merrill RL: Topical medications for orofacial neuropathic pain: a review, *J Am Dent Assoc* 131:184, 2000.
110. Pareja JA, Antonaci F, Vincent M: The hemicrania continua diagnosis, *Cephalalgia* 21:940, 2001.
111. Peszkowski M, Larsson AJ: Extraosseous and intraosseous oral traumatic neuromas and their association with tooth extraction, *J Oral Maxillofac Surg* 48:963, 1990.
112. Pigg M, List T, Petersson K, et al: Diagnostic yield of conventional radiographic and cone-beam computed tomographic images in patients with atypical odontalgia, *Int Endod J* 44:1092, 2011.
113. Pigg M, Svensson P, Drangsholt M, List T: 7-year follow-up of patients diagnosed with atypical odontalgia: a prospective study, *J Orofac Pain* 27:151, 2013.
114. Pruckmayer M, Glaser C, Marosi C, Leitha T: Mandibular pain as the leading clinical symptom for metastatic disease: nine cases and review of the literature, *Ann Oncol* 9:559, 1998.
115. Quail G: Atypical facial pain: a diagnostic challenge, *Aust Fam Physician* 34:641, 2005.
116. Raja S, Davis KD, Campbell JN: The adrenergic pharmacology of sympathetically-maintained pain, *J Reconstr Microsurg* 8:63, 1992.
117. Rasmussen BK, Jensen R, Schroll M, Olesen J: Epidemiology of headache in a general population—a prevalence study, *J Clin Epidemiol* 44:1147, 1991.
118. Rosenfeld RM, Andes D, Bhattacharyya N, et al: Clinical practice guideline: adult sinusitis, *Otolaryngol Head Neck Surg* 137(suppl):S1, 2007.
119. Roz TM, Schiffman LE, Schlossberg S: Spontaneous dissection of the internal carotid artery manifesting as pain in an endodontically treated molar, *J Am Dent Assoc* 136:1556, 2005.
120. Sarlani E, Schwartz AH, Greenspan JD, Grace EG: Chronic paroxysmal hemicrania: a case report and review of the literature, *J Orofac Pain* 17:74, 2003.
121. Schaible HG: Basic mechanisms of deep somatic tissue. In McMahon SB, Koltzenburg M, editors: *Textbook of pain*, Philadelphia, 2006, Elsevier, p 621.
122. Schiffman E, Ohrbach R, List T, et al: Diagnostic criteria for headache attributed to temporomandibular disorders, *Cephalalgia* 32(9):683, 2012.
123. Schwartz BS, Stewart WF, Simon D, Lipton RB: Epidemiology of tension-type headache, *JAMA* 279:381, 1998.
124. Selden HS, Manhoff DT, Hatges NA, Michel RC: Metastatic carcinoma to the mandible that mimicked pulpal/periodontal disease, *J Endod* 24:267, 1998.
125. Setzen G, Ferguson BJ, Han JK, et al: Clinical consensus statement: appropriate use of computed tomography for paranasal sinus disease, *Otolaryngol Head Neck Surg* 147(5):808, 2012.
126. Sicuteri F, Nicolodi M, Fusco BM, Orlando S: Idiopathic pain as a possible risk factor for phantom tooth pain, *Headache* 31:577, 1991.
127. Stewart W, Ricci JA, Chee E, et al: Lost productive time and cost due to common pain conditions in the US workforce, *JAMA* 290:2443, 2003.
128. Stewart WF, Lipton RB, Celentano DD, Reed ML: Prevalence of migraine headache in the United States: relation to age, income, race, and other sociodemographic factors, *JAMA* 267:64, 1992.

129. Svennson P: Muscle pain in the head: overlap between temporomandibular disorders and tension-type headaches, *Curr Opin Neurol* 20:320, 2007.
130. Takenoshita M, Sato T, Kato Y, et al: Psychiatric diagnoses in patients with burning mouth syndrome and atypical odontalgia referred from psychiatric to dental facilities, *Neuropsychiatr Dis Treat* 6:699, 2010.
131. Tepper SJ, Dahlof CG, Dowson A, et al: Prevalence and diagnosis of migraine in patients consulting their physician with a complaint of headache: data from the Landmark Study, *Headache* 44:856, 2004.
132. Thomas G, Pandey M, Mathew A, et al: Primary intraosseous carcinoma of the jaw: pooled analysis of world literature and report of two new cases, *Int J Oral Maxillofac Surg* 30:349, 2001.
133. Torebjork H, Lundberg LE, LaMotte RH: Pain, hyperalgesia and activity in nociceptive C units in humans after intradermal injection of capsaicin, *J Physiol* 448:749, 1992.
134. Travell JG, Simons DG: *Myofascial pain and dysfunction: the trigger point manual*, Baltimore, 1983, Williams & Wilkins, p 1.
135. Treede RD, Jensen TS, Campbell JN, et al: Neuropathic pain: redefinition and a grading system for clinical and research purposes, *Neurology* 70:1630, 2008.
136. Tzukert A, Hasin Y, Sharav Y: Orofacial pain of cardiac origin, *Oral Surg Oral Med Oral Pathol* 51:484, 1981.
137. Uehara M, Tobita T, Inokuchi T: A case report: toothache caused by epidermoid cyst manifested in cerebellopontine angle, *J Oral Maxillofac Surg* 65:560, 2007.
138. Webb DJ, Colman MF, Thompson K, Wescott WB: Acute, life-threatening disease first appearing as odontogenic pain, *J Am Dent Assoc* 109:936, 1984.
139. Wertheimer-Hatch L, Hatch GF 3rd, Hatch KF, et al: Tumors of the oral cavity and pharynx, *World J Surg* 24:395, 2000.
140. Wood M, Johnson RW, McKendrick MW, et al: A randomized trial of acyclovir for 7 days or 21 days with and without prednisolone for treatment of acute herpes, *N Engl J Med* 330:896, 1994.
141. Woolf C: Phenotype modification of primary sensory neurons: the role of nerve growth factor in the production of persistent pain, *Philos Trans R Soc Lond B Biol Sci* 351:441, 1996.
142. Wright EF: Referred craniofacial pain patterns in patients with temporomandibular disorder, *J Am Dent Assoc* 131:1307, 2000.
143. Yang J, Simonson TM, Ruprecht A, et al: Magnetic resonance imaging used to assess patients with trigeminal neuralgia, *Oral Surg Oral Med Oral Pathol Oral Radiol Endod* 81:343, 1996.
144. Yokota T: Neural mechanisms of trigeminal pain, *Pain*, New York, 1985, McGraw-Hill.
145. Yoon JH, Chun YC, Park SY, et al: Malignant lymphoma of the maxillary sinus manifesting as a persistent toothache, *J Endod* 27:800, 2001.
146. Zagury JG, Eliav E, Heir GM, et al: Prolonged gingival cold allodynia: a novel finding in patients with atypical odontalgia, *Oral Surg Oral Med Oral Pathol Oral Radiol Endod* 111:312, 2011.
147. Zakrzewska JM: Diagnosis and differential diagnosis of trigeminal neuralgia, *Clin J Pain* 18:14, 2002.
148. Zuniga J: Surgical management of trigeminal neuropathic pain, *Atlas Oral Maxillofac Surg Clin North Am* 9:59, 2001.

CHAPTER 18

Management of Endodontic Emergencies

SAMUEL O. DORN | GARY SHUN-PAN CHEUNG

EMERGENCY CLASSIFICATIONS

The proper diagnosis and effective management of acute dental pain are possibly the most rewarding and satisfying aspects of providing dental care. An endodontic emergency is defined as pain or swelling caused by various stages of inflammation or infection of the pulpal or periapical tissues. The cause of dental pain is typically from caries, deep or defective restorations, or trauma. Sometimes occlusion-related pain can also mimic acute dental pain (Fig. 18-1). Bender[8] stated that patients who manifest severe or referred pain almost always had a previous history of pain with the offending tooth. Approximately 85% of all dental emergencies arise as a result of pulpal or periapical disease, which would necessitate either extraction or endodontic treatment to relieve the symptoms.[38,68] It has also been estimated that about 12% of the U.S. population experienced a toothache in the preceding 6 months.[65]

Determining a definitive diagnosis can sometimes be challenging and even frustrating for the clinician; but a methodical, objective, and subjective evaluation, as described in Chapter 1, is imperative before developing a proper treatment plan. Unfortunately, on the basis of the diagnosis, there are conflicting opinions on how to best clinically manage various endodontic emergencies. According to surveys of board certified endodontists by Dorn and associates in 1977[22,23] and 1990[31] and by Lee in 2009,[63] there are seven clinical presentations that are considered endodontic emergencies:

1. Irreversible pulpitis with normal periapex
2. Irreversible pulpitis with symptomatic apical periodontitis
3. Necrotic pulp with symptomatic apical periodontitis, with no swelling

4. Necrotic pulp, fluctuant swelling, with drainage through the canal
5. Necrotic pulp, fluctuant swelling, with no drainage through the canal
6. Necrotic pulp, diffuse facial swelling, with drainage through the canal
7. Necrotic pulp, diffuse facial swelling, with no drainage through the canal

There are other endodontic emergencies that were not discussed in these surveys. These emergencies pertain to traumatic dental injuries, as discussed in Chapter 20, to teeth that have had previous endodontic treatment, as discussed in Chapters 8 and 19, and endodontic flare-ups that may occur between treatment sessions. Of course, there are also many types of facial pain that have a nonodontogenic origin; these are described in detail in Chapter 17.

In the decades between the previously cited surveys, there have been several changes pertaining to the preferred clinical management of endodontic emergencies. Many of these treatment modifications have occurred because of the more contemporary armamentarium and materials as well as new evidence-based research and the presumption of empirical clinical success.

EMERGENCY ENDODONTIC MANAGEMENT

Because pain is both a psychological and biologic entity, as discussed in Chapters 4 and online Chapter 28, the management of acute dental pain must take into consideration both the physical symptoms and the emotional status of the

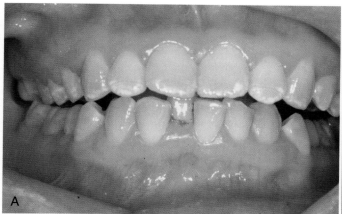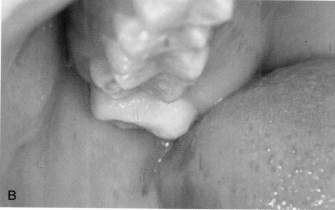

FIG. 18-1 **A,** Patient complained of acute pain on biting at the lower right molar. **B,** The pain was resolved after removal of an overerupted upper right wisdom tooth. Notice the presence of wear facet on the mesial marginal ridge and surface of this tooth before extraction.

patient. The patient's needs, fears, and coping mechanisms must be compassionately understood. This assessment and the clinician's ability to build rapport with the patient are key factors in the comprehensive success of the patient's management.[8,30,48,91]

The methodical steps for determining an accurate diagnosis, based on evaluation of the patient's chief complaint, review of the medical history, and the protocols used for an objective and subjective diagnosis, are described in detail in Chapter 1. Once it has been determined that endodontic treatment is necessary, it is incumbent on the clinician to take the proper steps necessary to manage the acute dental emergency.

As described in Chapters 3 and 29, the clinician has a responsibility to inform the patient of the recommended treatment plan and to advise the patient of the treatment alternatives, the risks and benefits that pertain, and the expected prognosis under the present circumstances. Given this information, the patient may elect extraction over endodontics, or possibly request a second opinion. The treatment plan should never be forced on a patient. The informed course of treatment is made jointly between the patient and the clinician.

In the event of an endodontic emergency, the clinician must determine the optimal mode of endodontic treatment pursuant to the diagnosis. Treatment may vary depending on the pulpal or periapical status, the intensity and duration of pain, and whether there is diffuse or fluctuant swelling. Paradoxically, as discussed later, the mode of therapy that we tend to choose has been directed more from surveys of practicing endodontists rather than from controlled clinical studies or research investigations.

Teeth with Vital Pulps

As described in Chapter 1, teeth with vital pulps can have one of the following presentations:

- *Normal.* The teeth are asymptomatic with no objective pathoses.
- *Reversible pulpitis.* There is a reversible sensitivity to cold or osmotic changes (i.e., sweet, salty, and sour).
- *Irreversible pulpitis.* The sensitivity to temperature changes is more intense and with a longer duration.

Reversible Pulpitis

Reversible pulpitis can be induced by caries, exposed dentin, recent dental treatment, and defective restorations. Conservative removal of caries, protection of dentin, and a proper restoration will typically resolve the symptoms. However, the symptoms from exposed dentin, specifically from gingival recession and cervically exposed roots, can often be difficult to alleviate. Topical applications of desensitizing agents and the use of certain dentifrices have been helpful in the management of dentin hypersensitivity; the etiology, physiology, and management of this are discussed in Chapter 12.

Irreversible Pulpitis

The diagnosis of irreversible pulpitis can be subcategorized as asymptomatic or symptomatic. *Asymptomatic* irreversible pulpitis pertains to a tooth that has no symptoms, but has deep caries or tooth structure loss that, if left untreated, will cause the tooth to become symptomatic or nonvital. On the other hand, the pain from *symptomatic* irreversible pulpitis is often an emergency condition that requires immediate treatment. These teeth exhibit intermittent or spontaneous pain, whereby exposure to extreme temperatures, especially cold, will elicit intense and prolonged episodes of pain, even after the source of the stimulus is removed.

In 1977,[22,23] 187 board-certified endodontists responded to a survey to determine how they would manage various endodontic emergencies. Ten years later, 314 board-certified endodontists responded to the same questionnaire in order to determine whether there had been any changes in how these emergencies were managed.[31] The clinical management of emergency treatment of a tooth with irreversible pulpitis with or without a normal periapex seemed to be fairly similar by removing the inflamed pulp tissue either by pulpotomy or complete instrumentation.[75] In a similar survey conducted in 2009,[63] most respondents stated that they cleaned to the level of the "apex," as confirmed with an electronic apex locator; this suggests a change in the management of endodontic cases based on the advent of a more contemporary armamentarium. In general, the most current survey indicates that there is a trend toward more cleaning and shaping of the canal when irreversible pulpitis presents with a normal periapex, compared with performing just pulpectomies as described in the 1977 survey. None of the individuals surveyed in the 1990 or 2009 poll stated that they would manage these emergencies by establishing any type of drainage by trephinating the apex, making an incision, or leaving the tooth open for an extended period of time.

In addition, for vital teeth, the 1977 survey did not even broach the concept of completing the endodontics in one visit, whereas in the 1988 study about one third of the respondents indicated that they would complete these vital cases in a single visit and the response rose to 79% in the most recent survey. Since the early 1980s, there seems to have been an increase in the acceptability of providing endodontic therapy in one visit, especially in cases of vital pulps, with most studies revealing an equal number, or fewer, flare-ups after single-visit endodontic treatment.[24,78,83,88,90,98] However, this has not come without controversy, with some studies showing otherwise,[111] contending that there is more posttreatment pain after single-visit endodontics, and possibly a lower long-term success rate. Unfortunately, time constraints at the emergency visit often make the single-visit treatment option not practical.[4]

If root canal therapy is completed at a later date, medicating the canal with calcium hydroxide has been suggested to reduce the chances of bacterial growth in the canal between appointments in most studies,[17] but not all.[13,17] One randomized clinical study showed that a dry cotton pellet was as effective in relieving pain as a pellet moistened with camphorated monochlorophenol (CMCP), metacresylacetate (Cresatin), eugenol, or saline.[40] Sources of infection, such as caries and defective restorations, should be completely removed to prevent recontamination of the root canal system between appointments.[40] The concept of single- versus multiple-visit endodontics is described in greater detail in Chapter 11.

For emergency management of vital teeth that are not initially sensitive to percussion, occlusal reduction has not been shown to be beneficial.[19,31] However, the clinician should be cognizant of the possibility of occlusal interferences and prematurities that might cause tooth fracture under heavy mastication. In vital teeth in which the inflammation has extended periapically, which will present with pretreatment pain to percussion, occlusal reduction has been reported to reduce posttreatment pain.[31,74,89]

Antibiotics are not recommended for the emergency management of irreversible pulpitis[53,99] (see Chapters 11 and 14), as placebo-controlled clinical trials have demonstrated that antibiotics have no effect on pain levels in patients with irreversible pulpitis.[72]

Most endodontists and endodontic textbooks recommend the emergency management of *symptomatic* irreversible pulpitis to involve the initiation of root canal treatment,[17,31,39,63,103] with complete pulp removal and total cleaning of the root canal system. Unfortunately, in an emergency situation, the allotted time necessary for this treatment is often an issue. Given the potential time constraints and inevitable differences in skill level between clinicians, it may not be feasible to complete the total canal cleaning at the initial emergency visit. Subsequently, especially with multirooted teeth, a pulpotomy (removal of the coronal pulp or tissue from the widest canal) has been advocated for emergency treatment of irreversible pulpitis.[15,39,103] In a clinical study of various emergency procedures, it has been demonstrated that this treatment is highly effective for alleviating acute dental pain due to irreversible pulpitis.[15]

To assist the clinician in assessing the level of difficulty of a given endodontic case, the American Association of Endodontists (Chicago, IL) has developed the "AAE Endodontic Case Difficulty Assessment Form and Guidelines" (Fig. 18-2). This form is intended to make case selection more efficient, more consistent, and easier to document, as well as to provide a more objective ability to determine when it may be necessary to refer the patient to another clinician who may be better able to manage the complexities of the case.

Pulpal Necrosis with Acute Apical Abscess
No Swelling

Over the years, the proper methodology for the emergency endodontic management of necrotic teeth has been controversial. In a 1977 survey of board-certified endodontists,[22,23] it was reported that, in the absence of swelling, most respondents would completely instrument the canals, keeping the file short of the radiographic apex. However, when swelling was present, the majority of those polled in 1977 preferred to leave the tooth open, with instrumentation extending beyond the apex to help facilitate drainage through the canals. Years later and again validated in a 2009 study, most respondents favored complete instrumentation regardless of the presence of swelling. Also, it was the decision of 25.2% to 38.5% of the clinicians to leave these teeth open in the event of diffuse swelling; 17.5% to 31.5% left the teeth open in the presence of a fluctuant swelling. However, as discussed later, there is currently a trend toward not leaving teeth open for drainage. There is also another trend: when treatment is done in more than one visit, most endodontists will use calcium hydroxide as an intracanal medicament.[63]

Care should be taken not to push necrotic debris beyond the apex during root canal instrumentation, as this has been shown to promote more posttreatment discomfort.[13,31,87,96] Crown-down instrumentation techniques have been shown to remove most of the debris coronally rather than pushing it out the apex. The use of positive-pressure irrigation methods, such as needle-and-syringe irrigation, also poses a risk of expressing debris or solution out of the apex.[10,20] Improvements in technology, such as electronic apex locators, have facilitated increased accuracy in determining working length measurements, which in turn may allow for a more thorough canal debridement and less apical extrusion. These devices are now used by an increased number of clinicians.[56,63]

Trephination

In the absence of swelling, trephination is the surgical perforation of the alveolar cortical plate to release, from between the cortical plates, the accumulated inflammatory and infective tissue exudate that causes pain. Its use has been historically advocated to provide pain relief in patients with severe and recalcitrant periradicular pain.[22,23] The technique involves an engine-driven perforator entering through the cortical bone and into the cancellous bone, often without the need for an incision,[16] in order to provide a pathway for drainage from the periradicular tissues. Although more recent studies have failed to show the benefit of trephination in patients with irreversible pulpitis with symptomatic apical periodontitis[69] or necrotic teeth with symptomatic apical periodontitis,[74] there remain some advocates who recommend trephination for managing acute and intractable periapical pain.[45] The clinician should understand that local anesthesia may be difficult for cases with acute inflammation or infection.[49] Extreme care must be taken when carrying out a trephination procedure to guard against inadvertent and possibly irreversible injury to the tooth root or surrounding structures, such as the mental foramen, intra-alveolar nerve, or maxillary sinus.

Necrosis and Single-Visit Endodontics

Although single-visit endodontic treatment for teeth diagnosed with irreversible pulpitis is not contraindicated,[2,83,85,90,112] performing single-visit endodontics on necrotic and previously treated teeth is not without controversy. In cases of necrotic teeth, although research[24] has indicated that there may be no difference in posttreatment pain if the canals are filled at the time of the emergency versus a later date, some studies[97,104] have questioned the long-term prognosis of such treatment, especially in cases of symptomatic apical periodontitis. Several studies,[25,60] including a CONSORT (Consolidated Standards of Reporting Trials) meta-analysis,[84] have shown no difference in outcome between single-visit and two-visit treatments. The concept of single- versus multivisit endodontics is further discussed in Chapters 3 and 11.

AAE Endodontic Case Difficulty Assessment Form and Guidelines

PATIENT INFORMATION

Name________________

Address________________

City/State/Zip________________

Phone________________

DISPOSITION

Treat in Office: Yes ☐ No ☐

Refer Patient to:

____

Date:________________

Guidelines for Using the AAE Endodontic Case Difficulty Assessment Form

The AAE designed the Endodontic Case Difficulty Assessment Form for use in endodontic curricula. The Assessment Form makes case selection more efficient, more consistent and easier to document. Dentists may also choose to use the Assessment Form to help with referral decision making and record keeping.

Conditions listed in this form should be considered potential risk factors that may complicate treatment and adversely affect the outcome. Levels of difficulty are sets of conditions that may not be controllable by the dentist. Risk factors can influence the ability to provide care at a consistently predictable level and impact the appropriate provision of care and quality assurance.

The Assessment Form enables a practitioner to assign a level of difficulty to a particular case.

LEVELS OF DIFFICULTY

MINIMAL DIFFICULTY	Preoperative condition indicates routine complexity (uncomplicated). These types of cases would exhibit only those factors listed in the MINIMAL DIFFICULTY category. Achieving a predictable treatment outcome should be attainable by a competent practitioner with limited experience.
MODERATE DIFFICULTY	Preoperative condition is complicated, exhibiting one or more patient or treatment factors listed in the MODERATE DIFFICULTY category. Achieving a predictable treatment outcome will be challenging for a competent, experienced practitioner.
HIGH DIFFICULTY	Preoperative condition is exceptionally complicated, exhibiting several factors listed in the MODERATE DIFFICULTY category or at least one in the HIGH DIFFICULTY category. Achieving a predictable treatment outcome will be challenging for even the most experienced practitioner with an extensive history of favorable outcomes.

Review your assessment of each case to determine the level of difficulty. If the level of difficulty exceeds your experience and comfort, you might consider referral to an endodontist.

The AAE Endodontic Case Difficulty Assessment Form is designed to aid the practitioner in determining appropriate case disposition. The American Association of Endodontists neither expressly nor implicitly warrants any positive results associated with the use of this form. This form may be reproduced but may not be amended or altered in any way.

FIG. 18-2 The American Association of Endodontists (AAE) Endodontic Case Difficulty Assessment Form and Guidelines, developed to assist the clinician in assessing the level of difficulty of a given endodontic case and to help determine when referral may be necessary.

Continued

AAE Endodontic Case Difficulty Assessment Form

CRITERIA AND SUBCRITERIA	MINIMAL DIFFICULTY	MODERATE DIFFICULTY	HIGH DIFFICULTY
A. PATIENT CONSIDERATIONS			
MEDICAL HISTORY	☐ No medical problem (ASA Class 1*)	☐ One or more medical problems (ASA Class 2*)	☐ Complex medical history/serious illness/disability (ASA Classes 3-5*)
ANESTHESIA	☐ No history of anesthesia problems	☐ Vasoconstrictor intolerance	☐ Difficulty achieving anesthesia
PATIENT DISPOSITION	☐ Cooperative and compliant	☐ Anxious but cooperative	☐ Uncooperative
ABILITY TO OPEN MOUTH	☐ No limitation	☐ Slight limitation in opening	☐ Significant limitation in opening
GAG REFLEX	☐ None	☐ Gags occasionally with radiographs/treatment	☐ Extreme gag reflex which has compromised past dental care
EMERGENCY CONDITION	☐ Minimum pain or swelling	☐ Moderate pain or swelling	☐ Severe pain or swelling
B. DIAGNOSTIC AND TREATMENT CONSIDERATIONS			
DIAGNOSIS	☐ Signs and symptoms consistent with recognized pulpal and periapical conditions	☐ Extensive differential diagnosis of usual signs and symptoms required	☐ Confusing and complex signs and symptoms: difficult diagnosis ☐ History of chronic oral/facial pain
RADIOGRAPHIC DIFFICULTIES	☐ Minimal difficulty obtaining/interpreting radiographs	☐ Moderate difficulty obtaining/interpreting radiographs (e.g., high floor of mouth, narrow or low palatal vault, presence of tori)	☐ Extreme difficulty obtaining/interpreting radiographs (e.g., superimposed anatomical structures)
POSITION IN THE ARCH	☐ Anterior/premolar ☐ Slight inclination (<10°) ☐ Slight rotation (<10°)	☐ 1st molar ☐ Moderate inclination (10-30°) ☐ Moderate rotation (10-30°)	☐ 2nd or 3rd molar ☐ Extreme inclination (>30°) ☐ Extreme rotation (>30°)
TOOTH ISOLATION	☐ Routine rubber dam placement	☐ Simple pretreatment modification required for rubber dam isolation	☐ Extensive pretreatment modification required for rubber dam isolation
MORPHOLOGIC ABERRATIONS OF CROWN	☐ Normal original crown morphology	☐ Full coverage restoration ☐ Porcelain restoration ☐ Bridge abutment ☐ Moderate deviation from normal tooth/root form (e.g., taurodontism, microdens) ☐ Teeth with extensive coronal destruction	☐ Restoration does not reflect original anatomy/alignment ☐ Significant deviation from normal tooth/root form (e.g., fusion, dens in dente)
CANAL AND ROOT MORPHOLOGY	☐ Slight or no curvature (<10°) ☐ Closed apex <1 mm diameter	☐ Moderate curvature (10-30°) ☐ Crown axis differs moderately from root axis. Apical opening 1-1.5 mm in diameter	☐ Extreme curvature (>30°) or S-shaped curve ☐ Mandibular premolar or anterior with 2 roots ☐ Maxillary premolar with 3 roots ☐ Canal divides in the middle or apical third ☐ Very long tooth (>25 mm) ☐ Open apex (>1.5 mm in diameter)
RADIOGRAPHIC APPEARANCE OF CANAL(S)	☐ Canal(s) visible and not reduced in size	☐ Canal(s) and chamber visible but reduced in size ☐ Pulp stones	☐ Indistinct canal path ☐ Canal(s) not visible
RESORPTION	☐ No resorption evident	☐ Minimal apical resorption	☐ Extensive apical resorption ☐ Internal resorption ☐ External resorption
C. ADDITIONAL CONSIDERATIONS			
TRAUMA HISTORY	☐ Uncomplicated crown fracture of mature or immature teeth	☐ Complicated crown fracture of mature teeth ☐ Subluxation	☐ Complicated crown fracture of immature teeth ☐ Horizontal root fracture ☐ Alveolar fracture ☐ Intrusive, extrusive or lateral luxation ☐ Avulsion
ENDODONTIC TREATMENT HISTORY	☐ No previous treatment	☐ Previous access without complications	☐ Previous access with complications (e.g., perforation, non-negotiated canal, ledge, separated instrument) ☐ Previous surgical or nonsurgical endodontic treatment completed
PERIODONTAL-ENDODONTIC CONDITION	☐ None or mild periodontal disease	☐ Concurrent moderate periodontal disease	☐ Concurrent severe periodontal disease ☐ Cracked teeth with periodontal complications ☐ Combined endodontic/periodontal lesion ☐ Root amputation prior to endodontic treatment

*American Society of Anesthesiologists (ASA) Classification System

Class 1: No systemic illness. Patient healthy.
Class 2: Patient with mild degree of systemic illness, but without functional restrictions, e.g., well-controlled hypertension.
Class 3: Patient with severe degree of systemic illness which limits activities, but does not immobilize the patient.

Class 4: Patient with severe systemic illness that immobilizes and is sometimes life threatening.
Class 5: Patient will not survive more than 24 hours whether or not surgical intervention takes place.

www.asahq.org/clinical/physicalstatus.htm

FIG. 18-2, cont'd

Swelling

Tissue swelling may be associated with an acute periradicular abscess at the time of the initial emergency visit, or it may occur as an inter-appointment flare-up or as a postendodontic complication. Swellings may be localized or diffuse, fluctuant or firm. Localized swellings are confined within the oral cavity, whereas a diffuse swelling, or cellulitis, is more extensive, spreading through adjacent soft tissues and dissecting tissue spaces along fascial planes.[92]

Swelling may be controlled by establishing drainage through the root canal or by incising the fluctuant swelling. As discussed later and in Chapter 14, antibiotics may be recruited

as part of the management of swelling, especially when there are systemic manifestations of the infection, such as fever and malaise. The principal modality for managing swelling secondary to endodontic infections is to achieve drainage and remove the source of the infection.[36,92] When the swelling is localized, the preferred avenue is drainage through the root canal (Fig. 18-3). However, it is also possible to achieve drainage with an incision and iodoform gauze drain before entering the canal. In this manner, the canal can be dried and the endodontic treatment completed in one visit. The dentist should see the patient the following day to remove the drain. Complete canal debridement and disinfection[37,106] are paramount

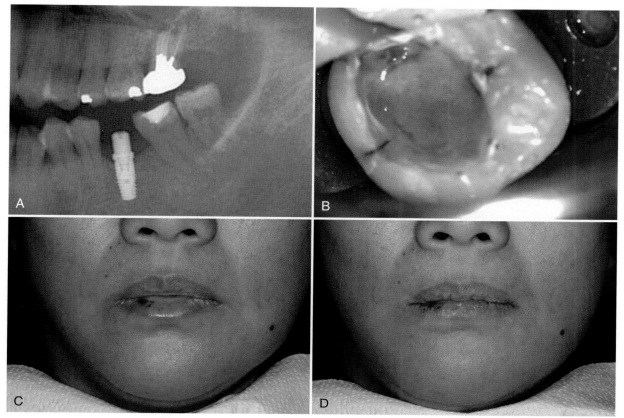

FIG. 18-3 Drainage of pus through the root canal. **A,** Acute apical abscess arising from the lower left first molar with little radiographic radiolucency. **B,** Drainage through the canals. **C,** Extracoronal swelling bear angle of left mandible before drainage. **D,** Reduction in the extent of swelling after drainage.

for success regardless of observable drainage, because the presence of any bacteria remaining within the root canal system will compromise the resolution of the acute infection.[67] In the presence of persistent swelling, gentle finger pressure to the mucosa overlying the swelling may help facilitate drainage through the canal. Once the canals have been cleaned and allowed to dry, the access should be closed.[17,31,39] In these cases, when not completing the treatment in a single visit, there has been a trend to use calcium hydroxide as the intracanal medicament.[63]

FASCIAL SPACE INFECTIONS

If bacteria from the infected root canal gain entry into the periradicular tissues and the immune system is unable to suppress the invasion, an otherwise healthy patient eventually shows signs and symptoms of an acute apical abscess, which can in turn evolve to cellulitis. Clinically, the patient experiences swelling and mild to severe pain. Depending on the relationship of the apices of the involved tooth to the muscular attachments, the swelling may be localized to the vestibule or extend into a fascial space. The patient may also have systemic manifestations, such as fever, chills, lymphadenopathy, headache, and nausea. Because the reaction to the infection may occur quickly, the involved tooth may or may not show radiographic evidence of a widened periodontal ligament space. In most cases, the tooth elicits a positive response to percussion, and the periradicular area is tender to palpation. The tooth

now becomes a *focus of infection* because it leads to periradicular infection and secondary spread to the fascial spaces of the head and neck, resulting in cellulitis and systemic signs and symptoms of infection.

In such cases, treatment may involve incision for drainage, root canal treatment, or extraction in order to remove the source of the infection. Antibiotic therapy may be indicated in patients with a compromised host resistance, the presence of systemic symptoms, or fascial space involvement. Fascial space infections of odontogenic origin are infections that have spread into the fascial spaces from the periradicular area of a tooth, the focus of infection. They are *not* examples of the theory of focal infection, which describes the dissemination of bacteria or their products from a distant focus of infection. Rather, this is an example of the local spread of infection from an odontogenic source.

Fascial spaces are potential anatomic areas that exist between the fascia and underlying organs and other tissues. During infection, these spaces are formed as a result of the spread of purulent exudate. The spread of infections of odontogenic origin into the fascial spaces of the head and neck is determined by the location of the root end of the involved tooth in relation to its overlying buccal or lingual cortical plate and the relationship of the apex to the attachment of a muscle (Fig. 18-4, *A*). For example, if the source of the infection is a mandibular molar whose apices lie closer to the lingual cortical plate and *above* the attachment of the mylohyoid muscle of the floor of the mouth, the purulent exudate may break through

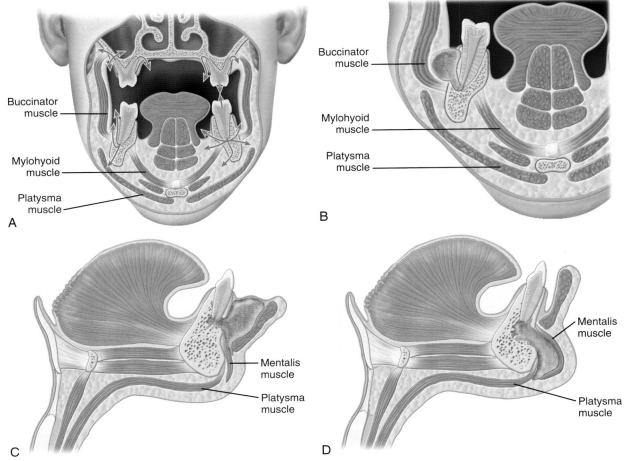

FIG. 18-4 **A,** Spread of odontogenic infections. **B,** Mandibular buccal vestibule (posterior tooth). **C,** Mandibular buccal vestibule (anterior tooth). **D,** Mental space. *Continued*

the lingual cortical plate and into the *sublingual* space. However, if the apices lie *below* the attachment of the mylohyoid muscle, the infection may spread into the *submandibular* space.

As described by Hohl and colleagues,[47] the fascial spaces of the head and neck can be categorized into four anatomic groups:

- The mandible and below
- The cheek and lateral face
- The pharyngeal and cervical areas
- The midface

Swellings of and below the mandible include six anatomic areas or fascial spaces:

- The buccal vestibule
- The body of the mandible
- The mental space
- The submental space
- The sublingual space
- The submandibular space

The *mandibular buccal vestibule* is the anatomic area amid the buccal cortical plate, the overlying alveolar mucosa, and the buccinator muscle (posterior) or the mentalis muscle (anterior) (Figs. 18-4, *B* and *C*). In this case, the source of the infection is a mandibular posterior or anterior tooth in which the purulent exudate breaks through the buccal cortical plate, and the apex or apices of the involved tooth lie

above the attachment of the buccinator or mentalis muscle, respectively.

The *space of the body of the mandible* is the potential anatomic area between the buccal or lingual cortical plate and its overlying periosteum. The source of infection is a mandibular tooth in which the purulent exudate has broken through the overlying cortical plate but not yet perforated the overlying periosteum. Involvement of this space can also occur as a result of a postsurgical infection.

The *mental space* (Fig. 18-4, *D*) is the potential bilateral anatomic area of the chin that lies between the mentalis muscle superiorly and the platysma muscle inferiorly. The source of the infection is an anterior tooth in which the purulent exudate breaks through the buccal cortical plate, and the apex of the tooth lies below the attachment of the mentalis muscle.

The *submental space* (Fig. 18-4, *E*) is the potential anatomic area between the mylohyoid muscle superiorly and the platysma muscle inferiorly. The source of the infection is an anterior tooth in which the purulent exudate breaks through the lingual cortical plate, and the apex of the tooth lies below the attachment of the mylohyoid muscle.

The *sublingual space* (Fig. 18-4, *F*) is the potential anatomic area between the oral mucosa of the floor of the mouth superiorly and the mylohyoid muscle inferiorly. The lateral boundaries of the space are the lingual surfaces of the mandible. The

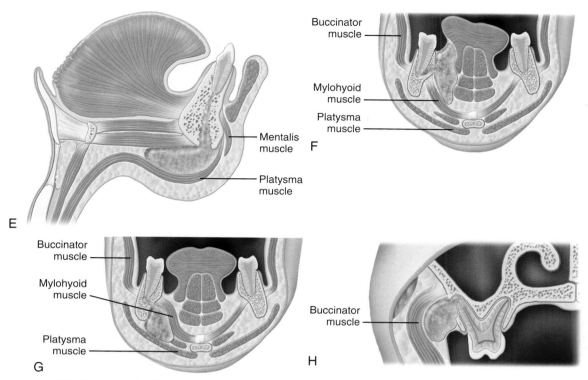

FIG. 18-4, cont'd   E, Submental space. F, Sublingual space. G, Submandibular space. H, Maxillary buccal vestibule.

source of infection is any mandibular tooth in which the purulent exudate breaks through the lingual cortical plate, and the apex or apices of the tooth lie above the attachment of the mylohyoid muscle.

The *submandibular space* (Fig. 18-4, *G*) is the potential space between the mylohyoid muscle superiorly and the platysma muscle inferiorly. The source of infection is a posterior tooth, usually a molar, in which the purulent exudate breaks through the lingual cortical plate and the apices of the tooth lie below the attachment of the mylohyoid muscle. If the submental, sublingual, and submandibular spaces are involved at the same time, a diagnosis of Ludwig angina is made. This life-threatening cellulitis can advance into the pharyngeal and cervical spaces, resulting in airway obstruction.

Swellings of the lateral face and cheek include four anatomic areas or fascial spaces:

◆ The buccal vestibule of the maxilla
◆ The buccal space
◆ The submasseteric space
◆ The temporal space

Anatomically, the *buccal vestibular space* (Fig. 18-4, *H*) is the area between the buccal cortical plate, the overlying mucosa, and the buccinator muscle. The superior extent of the space is the attachment of the buccinator muscle to the zygomatic process. The source of infection is a maxillary posterior tooth in which the purulent exudate breaks through the buccal cortical plate, and the apex of the tooth lies below the attachment of the buccinator muscle.

The *buccal space* (Fig. 18-4, *I*) is the potential space between the lateral surface of the buccinator muscle and the medial surface of the skin of the cheek. The superior extent of the space is the attachment of the buccinator muscle to the

zygomatic arch, whereas the inferior and posterior boundaries are the attachment of the buccinator to the inferior border of the mandible and the anterior margin of the masseter muscle, respectively. The source of the infection can be either a posterior mandibular or maxillary tooth in which the purulent exudate breaks through the buccal cortical plate, and the apex or apices of the tooth lie above the attachment of the buccinator muscle (i.e., maxilla) or below the attachment of the buccinator muscle (i.e., mandible).

As the name implies, the *submasseteric space* (Fig. 18-4, *J*) is the potential space between the lateral surface of the ramus of the mandible and the medial surface of the masseter muscle. The source of the infection is usually an impacted third molar in which the purulent exudate breaks through the lingual cortical plate, and the apices of the tooth lie very close to or within the space.

The *temporal space* (Fig. 18-4, *K*) is divided into two compartments by the temporalis muscle. The *deep temporal space* is the potential space between the lateral surface of the skull and the medial surface of the temporalis muscle; the *superficial temporal space* lies between the temporalis muscle and its overlying fascia. The deep or superficial temporal spaces are involved indirectly if an infection spreads superiorly from the inferior pterygomandibular or submasseteric spaces, respectively.

Swellings of the pharyngeal and cervical areas include the following fascial spaces:

◆ The pterygomandibular space
◆ The parapharyngeal spaces
◆ The cervical spaces

The *pterygomandibular space* (Fig. 18-4, *L*) is the potential space between the lateral surface of the medial pterygoid muscle and the medial surface of the ramus of the mandible.

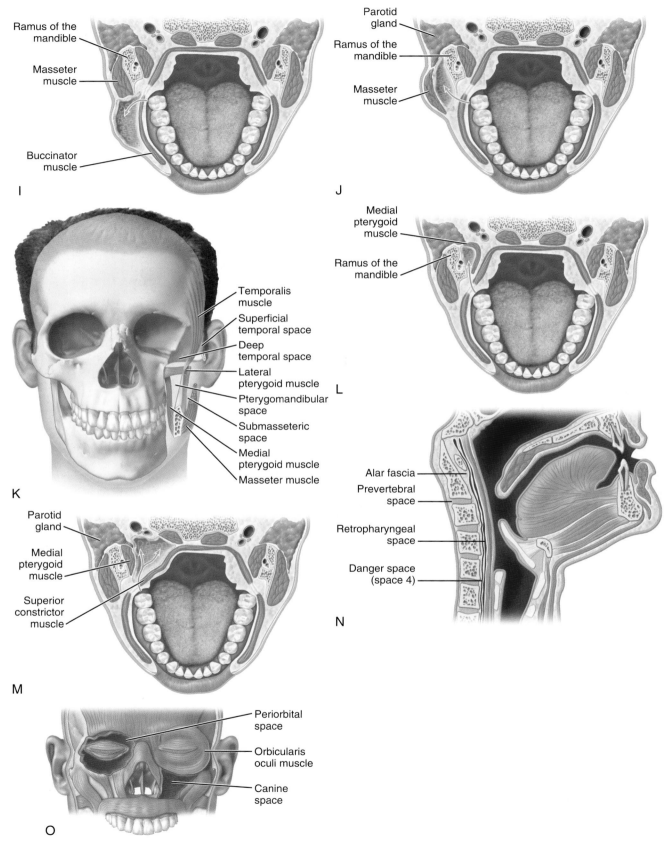

FIG. 18-4, cont'd **I,** Buccal space. **J,** Submasseteric space. **K,** Temporal space. **L,** Pterygomandibular space. **M,** Parapharyngeal spaces. **N,** Cervical spaces. **O,** Canine (infraorbital) and periorbital space.

The superior extent of the space is the lateral pterygoid muscle. The source of the infection is mandibular second or third molars in which the purulent exudate drains directly into the space. In addition, contaminated inferior alveolar nerve injections can lead to infection of the space.

The *parapharyngeal spaces* comprise the lateral pharyngeal and retropharyngeal spaces (Fig. 18-4, *M*). The *lateral pharyngeal space* is bilateral and lies between the lateral surface of the medial pterygoid muscle and the posterior surface of the superior constrictor muscle. The superior and inferior margins of the space are the base of the skull and the hyoid bone, respectively, and the posterior margin is the *carotid space,* or sheath, which contains the common carotid artery, internal jugular vein, and the vagus nerve. Anatomically, the *retropharyngeal space* lies between the anterior surface of the prevertebral fascia and the posterior surface of the superior constrictor muscle and extends inferiorly into the retroesophageal space, which extends into the posterior compartment of the mediastinum. The pharyngeal spaces usually become involved as a result of the secondary spread of infection from other fascial spaces or directly from a peritonsillar abscess.

The cervical spaces comprise the pretracheal, retrovisceral, danger, and prevertebral spaces (Fig. 18-4, *N*). The *pretracheal space* is the potential space surrounding the trachea. It extends from the thyroid cartilage inferiorly into the superior portion of the anterior compartment of the mediastinum to the level of the aortic arch. Because of its anatomic location, odontogenic infections do not spread to the pretracheal space. The *retrovisceral space* comprises the retropharyngeal space superiorly and the retroesophageal space inferiorly. The space extends from the base of the skull into the posterior compartment of the mediastinum to a level between vertebrae C6 and T4. The *danger space* (i.e., space 4)[26,33] is the potential space between the alar and prevertebral fascia. Because this space is composed of loose connective tissue, it is considered an actual anatomic space extending from the base of the skull into the posterior compartment of the mediastinum to a level corresponding to the diaphragm. It is not unknown for odontogenic infection to spread into this space, if left untreated and undiagnosed.[32] The consequence can be fatal. The *prevertebral space* is the potential space surrounding the vertebral column. As such, it extends from vertebra C1 to the coccyx. A retrospective study showed that 71% of cases in which the mediastinum was involved arose from the spread of infection from the retrovisceral space (21% from the carotid space and 8% from the pretracheal space).[64]

Swellings of the midface consist of four anatomic areas and spaces:
- The palate
- The base of the upper lip
- The canine spaces
- The periorbital spaces

Odontogenic infections can spread into the areas between the palate and its overlying periosteum and mucosa and the base of the upper lip, which lies superior to the orbicularis oris muscle, even though these areas are not considered actual fascial spaces. The source of infection of the palate is any of the maxillary teeth in which the apex of the involved tooth lies close to the palate. The source of infection of the base of the upper lip is a maxillary central incisor in which the apex lies close to the buccal cortical plate and above the attachment of the orbicularis oris muscle.

The *canine,* or *infraorbital, space* (Fig. 18-4, *O*) is the potential space between the levator anguli oris muscle inferiorly and the levator labii superioris muscle superiorly. The source of infection is the maxillary canine or first premolar in which the purulent exudate breaks through the buccal cortical plate, and the apex of the tooth lies above the attachment of the levator anguli oris muscle. There is a chance for the infection to spread from the infraorbital space into the cavernous sinus in the cranium via the valveless veins of the face and anterior skull base.[26]

The *periorbital space* (see Fig. 18-4, *O*) is the potential space that lies deep to the orbicularis oculi muscle. This space becomes involved through the spread of infection from the canine or buccal spaces. Infections of the midface can be very dangerous because they can result in *cavernous sinus thrombosis,* a life-threatening infection in which a thrombus formed in the cavernous sinus breaks free, resulting in blockage of an artery or the spread of infection. Under normal conditions, the angular and ophthalmic veins and the pterygoid plexus of veins flow into the facial and external jugular veins. If an infection has spread into the midfacial area, however, edema and the resultant increased pressure from the inflammatory response cause the blood to back up into the cavernous sinus. Once in the sinus, the blood stagnates and clots. The resultant infected thrombi remain in the cavernous sinus or escape into the circulation.[77,115]

MANAGEMENT OF ABSCESSES AND CELLULITIS

The two most important elements of effective patient management for the resolution of an odontogenic infection are correct diagnosis and removal of the cause. When endodontic treatment is possible and preferred, in an otherwise healthy patient, chemomechanical preparation of the infected root canals and incision for drainage of any fluctuant periradicular swelling usually provide prompt improvement of the clinical signs and symptoms. The majority of cases of endodontic infections can be treated effectively without the use of systemic antibiotics. The appropriate treatment is removal of the cause of the inflammatory condition.

Antibiotics are *not* recommended for irreversible pulpitis, symptomatic apical periodontitis, draining sinus tracts, after endodontic surgery, to prevent flare-ups, or after incision for drainage of a localized swelling (without cellulitis, fever, or lymphadenopathy).[28,46,72,86,110] When the ratio of risk to benefit is considered in these situations, antibiotic use may put the patient at risk for side effects of the antimicrobial agent and select for resistant microorganisms. Analgesics (not antibiotics) are indicated for controlling the pain.

Antibiotics in conjunction with appropriate endodontic treatment are recommended for progressive or persistent infections with systemic signs and symptoms such as fever (over 100°F or 37°C), malaise, cellulitis, unexplained trismus, and progressive or persistent swelling (or both). In such cases, antibiotic therapy is indicated as an adjunct to debridement of the root canal system, which is a reservoir of microorganisms. In addition, aggressive incision for drainage is indicated for any infection marked by cellulitis. Incision for drainage is indicated whether the cellulitis is indurated or fluctuant. It is important to provide a pathway of drainage to prevent further spread of the abscess or cellulitis. An incision for drainage allows decompression of the increased tissue pressure associated with edema and provides significant pain relief. Furthermore, the incision provides a draining pathway not only for bacteria and their products but also for the inflammatory mediators associated with the spread of cellulitis.

A minimum inhibitory concentration of antibiotic may not reach the source of the infection because of decreased blood flow and because the antibiotic must diffuse through the edematous fluid and pus. Drainage of edematous fluid and purulent exudate improves circulation to the tissues associated with an abscess or cellulitis, providing better delivery of the antibiotic to the area. Placement of a drain may not be indicated for localized fluctuant swellings if complete evacuation of the purulent exudate is believed to have occurred.

For effective drainage, a vertically oriented stab incision is made through the mucoperiosteum in the most dependent site of the swelling. The incision must be long enough to allow blunt dissection using a curved hemostat or periosteal elevator under the periosteum for drainage of pockets of inflammatory exudate. A rubber dam drain or a Penrose drain is indicated for any patient with a progressive abscess or cellulitis to maintain an open pathway for drainage. A more detailed description is given later.

Patients with cellulitis should be followed on a daily basis to ensure that the infection is resolving. The best practical guide for determining the duration of antibiotic therapy is clinical improvement of the patient. When clinical evidence indicates that the infection is certain to resolve or is resolved, antibiotics should be administered for no longer than 1 or 2 days more.

Endodontic treatment should be completed as soon as possible after the incision for drainage. The drain can usually be removed 1 or 2 days after improvement. If no significant clinical improvement occurs, the diagnosis and treatment must be reviewed carefully. Consultation with a specialist and referral may be indicated for severe or persistent infections. Likewise, patients requiring extraoral drainage should be referred to a clinician trained in the technique.

INCISION FOR DRAINAGE

Establishing drainage from a localized soft tissue swelling is sometimes necessary. This can be accomplished through the *incision for drainage* of the area.[73] Incision for drainage is indicated whether the cellulitis is indurated or fluctuant,[92] and it is used when a pathway for drainage is needed to prevent further spread of infection. Incision for drainage allows decompression from the increased tissue pressure associated with edema and can provide significant pain relief for the patient; noteworthy is that often pain decreases when the soft tissues swell due to the relief of pressure within the bone. The incision also provides a pathway not only for bacteria and bacterial by-products but also for the inflammatory mediators that are associated with the spread of cellulitis.

The basic principles of incision for drainage are as follows:
- Anesthetize the area.
- Make a vertically oriented incision at the site of greatest fluctuant swelling.
- Dissect gently, through the deeper tissues, and thoroughly explore all parts of the abscess cavity, eventually extending to the offending roots that are responsible for the pathosis.

This will allow compartmentalized areas of inflammatory exudates and infection to be disrupted and evacuated.
- To promote drainage, the wound should be kept clean with warm saltwater mouth rinses. Intraoral heat application to infected tissues results in a dilation of small vessels, which subsequently intensifies host defenses through increased vascular flow.[36,92]
- A drain should be placed to prevent the incision from closing too early. The preferable type of drain is ½-inch iodoform gauze, which is more comfortable and less traumatic to the patient.(Fig. 18-5). The patient should be seen the following day to remove the drain.
- In many cases, the endodontic treatment can be completed in one visit after the drain is placed. The drainage allows for the ability to dry the instrumented canal, and completing the endodontic treatment eliminates the source of the infection, enabling the periapical lesion to heal quicker.

A diffuse swelling may develop into a life-threatening medical emergency. Because the spread of infection can traverse between the fascial planes and muscle attachments, vital structures can be compromised and breathing may be impeded. Two examples are Ludwig's angina and cervical fasciitis.[32] It is imperative that the clinician be in constant communication with the patient to ensure that the infection does not worsen and that medical attention is provided as necessary. Antibiotics and analgesics should be prescribed, and the patient should be monitored closely for the next several days or until there is improvement. Individuals who show signs of toxicity, elevated body temperature, lethargy, central nervous system (CNS) changes, or airway compromise should be referred to an oral surgeon or medical facility for immediate care and intervention.

SYMPTOMATIC TEETH WITH PREVIOUS ENDODONTIC TREATMENT

The emergency management of teeth with previous endodontic treatment may be technically challenging and time consuming. This is especially true in the presence of extensive restorations, including posts and cores, crowns, and bridgework. However, the goal remains the same as for the management of necrotic teeth: remove contaminants from the root canal system and establish patency to achieve drainage.[85] Gaining access to the periapical tissues through the root canals may require removal of posts and obturation materials, as well as negotiating blocked or ledged canals. Failure to complete root canal debridement and achieve periapical drainage may result in continued painful symptoms, in which case a trephination procedure or apicoectomy may be indicated. The ability, practicality, and feasibility to adequately retreat the root canal system must be carefully assessed before the initiation of treatment, as conventional retreatment might not be the optimal treatment plan. This is further discussed in Chapter 8.

LEAVING TEETH OPEN

On rare occasions, canal drainage may continue from the periapical spaces (Fig. 18-6). In these cases, the clinician may opt to step away from the patient for some time to allow the drainage to continue and hopefully resolve on the same treatment visit.[103]

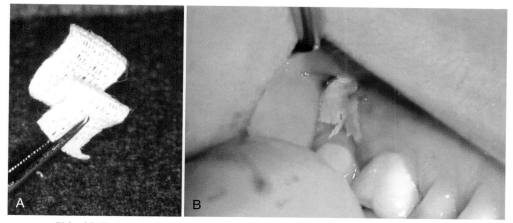

FIG. 18-5 **A,** Iodoform gauze cut to proper length. **B,** Iodoform gauze drain after 24 hours.

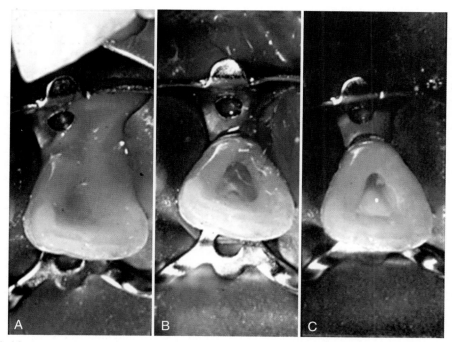

FIG 18-6 Nonvital infected tooth with active drainage from the periapical area through the canal. **A,** Access opened and draining for 1 minute. **B,** Drainage after 2 minutes. **C,** Canal space dried after 3 minutes.

Historically, in the presence of acutely painful necrotic teeth with no swelling or diffuse swelling, 19.4% to 71.2% of surveyed endodontists would leave the tooth open between visits.[22,23] However, the more current literature makes it clear that this form of treatment would impair uneventful resolution and create more complicated treatment.[5,7,113] For this reason, *leaving teeth open between appointments is not recommended.* Foreign objects have been found in teeth left open for drainage (Fig. 18-7). There has even been a documented case report of a foreign object being found to enter the periapical tissues through a tooth that had been left open for drainage.[95] In addition, leaving a tooth open provides an opportunity for oral microorganisms to invade and colonize the root canal system if the tooth is left open for an extended period.

SYSTEMIC ANTIBIOTICS FOR ENDODONTIC INFECTIONS

A hundred years ago, infectious diseases were the major recognized causes of death in the world. The advent of antibiotics resulted in a significant decline in the incidence of life-threatening infections and heralded a new era in the therapy of infectious diseases; but the enthusiasm generated turned out to be premature. Over the years, microbial evolutionary responses to the selective pressure exerted by antibiotics have resulted in microbial species resistant to virtually every known antibiotic agent.[41] The rapid emergence of resistant microbial strains comes as a consequence of the astonishing power of natural selection among microorganisms. If a given member of

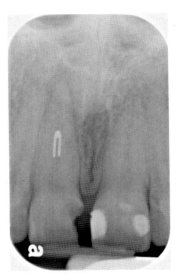

FIG. 18-7 Foreign object in tooth left open to drain. Patient used a sewing needle to clear out food particles that were blocking the canal and broke the needle in the tooth.

a microbial community possesses genes of resistance against a certain antibiotic and the community is persistently exposed to the drug, the resistant microorganism is selected to emerge and multiply to the detriment of the susceptible portion of the community. Passing on the genes responsible for resistance via plasmids and quorum sensing[41] has also been shown to encourage the survival of the microbial community. The emergence of multidrug-resistant strains of several bacterial species capable of causing life-threatening infections has been reported.[41,66,82,100,114] Antibiotic resistance among obligately anaerobic bacteria is increasing, with resistance to penicillins, clindamycin, and cephalosporins noted at community hospitals and major medical centers.[42,43]

Among oral bacteria, there have been reports on emerging resistance to commonly used antibiotics. Resistance has been found in *F. nucleatum* strains for penicillin, amoxicillin, and metronidazole, in *P. intermedia* for tetracycline and amoxicillin, and in *A. actinomycetemcomitans* for amoxicillin and azithromycin.[59,107] Macrolides (erythromycin and azithromycin) have presented decreased activity against *Fusobacterium* and nonpigmented *Prevotella* species.[44,58,59] Production of beta-lactamase by oral bacteria has also been reported, with the most prominent beta-lactamase-producing bacteria belonging to the anaerobic genus *Prevotella*.[9,12,27,34,108] Kuriyama and colleagues[58] revealed that beta-lactamase production was detected in 36% of the black-pigmented *Prevotella* and 32% of the nonpigmented *Prevotella* species isolated from pus samples of oral abscesses. Susceptibility of *Prevotella* strains to several cephalosporins, erythromycin, and azithromycin has been found to correlate with amoxicillin susceptibility; amoxicillin-resistant strains can be similarly resistant to these other antibiotics.[59] This finding suggests that there is little value in the use of oral cephalosporins and macrolides in managing endodontic abscesses, particularly when penicillin-resistant strains are evident. Other enzyme-producing oral anaerobic species include strains of *F. nucleatum*, *P. acnes*, *Actinomyces* species, and *Peptostreptococcus* species.[12,27,34,108] Facultative bacteria such as *Capnocytophaga* and *Neisseria* species have also been detected

among the beta-lactamase producers.[34] Bacteria that produce beta-lactamases protect not only themselves but also other penicillin-susceptible bacteria present in a mixed community by releasing free beta-lactamase into the environment.[11]

Overuse and misuse of antibiotics has been considered the major cause for the emergence of multidrug-resistant strains. Improper use of antibiotics includes use in cases with no infection, erroneous choice of the agent, dosage or duration of therapy, and excessive use in prophylaxis.[80,81] Antibiotics are used in clinical practice far more often than necessary. Antibiotic therapy is actually warranted in about 20% of the individuals who are seen for clinical infectious disease, but they are prescribed up to 80% of the time. To complicate matters further, in up to 50% of cases, recommended agents, doses, or duration of therapy are incorrect.[66]

The appalling rise in the frequency of multidrug resistance among leading pathogens should cause great concern and incite a commitment to act carefully and responsibly. A single erroneous use of antibiotics can be a significant contribution to the current scenario of increasing microbial resistance. Diseases that were effectively treated in the past with a given antibiotic may now require the use of another drug, usually more expensive and potentially more toxic, to achieve effective antimicrobial treatment. Unfortunately, even the new drug may not be effective.

Antibiotics are defined as naturally occurring substances of microbial origin or similar synthetic (or semisynthetic) substances that have antimicrobial activity in low concentrations and inhibit the growth of or kill selective microorganisms. The purpose of antibiotic therapy is to aid the host defenses in controlling and eliminating microorganisms that temporarily have overwhelmed the host defense mechanisms.[80] Based on the earlier discussion, it becomes clear that the most important decision in antibiotic therapy is not so much *which* antibiotic should be employed but *whether* antibiotics should be used at all.[79] One should bear in mind that antibiotics are very useful drugs classically employed to treat or help treat infectious disease and provide prophylaxis in carefully selected cases.

The majority of infections of endodontic origin are treated without the need for antibiotics. As mentioned, the absence of blood circulation in a necrotic pulp prevents antibiotics from reaching and eliminating microorganisms present in the root canal system; therefore, the source of infection is often unaffected by systemic antibiotic therapy. Antibiotics can, however, help impede the spread of the infection and development of focal infections in medically compromised patients and provide a valuable adjunct for managing selected cases of endodontic infection. In addition to the indications for systemic antibiotics discussed earlier for acute abscesses and cellulitis, antibiotics are also prescribed for prophylaxis in medically compromised patients during routine endodontic therapy, in some cases of persistent exudation not resolved after revision of intracanal procedures, and after the replantation of avulsed teeth.

Selection of antibiotics in clinical practice is either empirical or based on the results of microbial sensitivity tests. For diseases with known microbial causes, empirical therapy may be used. This is especially applicable to infections of endodontic origin, because culture-dependent antimicrobial tests of anaerobic bacteria can take too long to provide results about their susceptibility to antibiotics (7 to 14 days).

Therefore, it is preferable to opt for an antimicrobial agent whose spectrum of action includes the most commonly detected bacteria. Most of the bacterial species involved with endodontic infections, including abscesses, are susceptible to penicillins,[6,51,55,59] which make them first-line drugs of choice. Because the use of antibiotics is restricted to severe infections or prophylaxis, it seems prudent to use amoxicillin, a semisynthetic penicillin with a broad spectrum of antimicrobial activity and one that is well absorbed in the alimentary canal. In more serious cases, including life-threatening conditions, combining amoxicillin with clavulanic acid or metronidazole may be required to achieve optimum antimicrobial effects as a result of the extended spectrum of action to include penicillin-resistant strains.[59] In patients allergic to penicillins or in cases refractory to amoxicillin therapy, clindamycin is indicated. Clindamycin has strong antimicrobial activity against oral anaerobes.[55,57,59,61]

The risk/benefit ratio should always be evaluated prior to prescribing antibiotics. Appropriately selected patients will benefit from systemically administered antibiotics. A restrictive and conservative use of antibiotics is highly recommended in endodontic practice. Indiscriminate use (including cases of a reversible or irreversible pulpitis) is contrary to sound clinical practice, as it may cause a selective overgrowth of intrinsically resistant bacteria, predisposing patients to secondary and super-infections, rendering drugs ineffective against potentially fatal medical infectious diseases.

ANALGESICS

As a more thorough description of pain medications can be found in Chapter 4, the following information is merely a summary of pain control using analgesics. Because pulpal and periapical pain involves inflammatory processes, the first choice of analgesics is nonsteroidal anti-inflammatory drugs (NSAIDs).[63] However, no pain medication can replace the efficacy of thoroughly cleaning the root canal system to rid the tooth of the source of infection.[35]

Aspirin has been used as an analgesic for more than 100 years. In some cases, it may be more effective than 60 mg of codeine[18]; its analgesic and antipyretic effects are equal to those of acetaminophen, and its anti-inflammatory effect is more potent.[21] However, aspirin's side effects include gastric distress, nausea, and gastrointestinal ulceration. In addition, its analgesic effect is inferior to that of ibuprofen, 400 mg. When NSAIDs and aspirin are contraindicated, such as in patients for whom gastrointestinal problems are a concern, acetaminophen is the preferred nonprescription analgesic. A recommended maximum daily dose of 4 g of acetaminophen is currently in force, and a further reduction of this dosage has been proposed to reduce the chance of acetaminophen-related liver toxicity.[62,93]

For moderate to severe pain relief, ibuprofen, an NSAID, has been found to be superior to aspirin (650 mg) and acetaminophen (600 mg) with or without codeine (60 mg). Also, ibuprofen has fewer side effects than the combinations with opioid.[18,52] The maximal dose of 3.2 g in a 24-hour period should not be exceeded. Patients who take daily doses of aspirin for its cardioprotective benefit can take occasional doses of ibuprofen; however, it would be prudent to advise such patients to avoid regular doses of ibruprofen.[1] These patients would gain more relief by taking a selective cyclooxygenase (COX)-2 inhibitor, such as diclofenac or celecoxib.

Because of their anti-inflammatory effect, NSAIDs can suppress swelling to a certain degree after surgical procedures. The good analgesic effect combined with the additional anti-inflammatory benefit make NSAIDs, especially ibuprofen, the drug of choice for acute dental pain in the absence of any contraindication to their use. Ibuprofen has been used for more than 30 years and has been thoroughly evaluated.[21] If the NSAID alone does not have a satisfactory effect in controlling pain, then the addition of an opioid may provide additional analgesia. However, in addition to other possible side effects, opioids may cause nausea, constipation, lethargy, dizziness, and disorientation.

LABORATORY DIAGNOSTIC ADJUNCTS

Chapter 14 discusses culturing techniques and indications. Because the results of culturing for anaerobic bacteria usually require at least 1 to 2 weeks, it is not considered routine in the management of an acute endodontic emergency. Thus, in an endodontic emergency, antibiotic treatment, *when indicated* (see Chapter 18), should begin immediately, because oral infections can progress rapidly.

FLARE-UPS

An endodontic flare-up is defined as an acute exacerbation of a periradicular pathosis after the initiation or continuation of nonsurgical root canal treatment.[3] The incidence may be from 2% to 20% of cases.[50,70,76,109] A meta-analysis of the literature, using strict criteria, showed the flare-up frequency to be about 8.4%.[105] Endodontic flare-ups are more prevalent among females under the age of 20 years and may occur more in maxillary lateral incisors; in mandibular first molars, when there are large periapical lesions; and in the retreatment of previous root canals.[102] The presence of pretreatment pain may also be a predictor of potential posttreatment flare-ups.[50,102,109] Fortunately, there is no decrease in the endodontic success for cases that had a treatment flare-up.[54]

Endodontic flare-ups may occur for a variety of reasons, including preparation beyond the apical terminus, over-instrumentation, pushing dentinal and pulpal debris into the periapical area,[36] incomplete removal of pulp tissue, overextension of root canal filling material, chemical irritants (such as irrigants, intracanal medicaments, and sealers), hyperocclusion, root fractures, and microbiologic factors.[94] Although many of these cases can be pharmacologically managed (see Chapter 18), recalcitrant cases may require periapical surgery, reentry into the tooth, the establishment of drainage either through the tooth or via trephination, or, at a minimum, adjustment of the occlusion.[19,89,94] The prophylactic use of antibiotics to decrease the incidence of flare-ups has been met with some controversy. Whereas earlier investigators[71] found that antibiotic administration before treatment of necrotic teeth decreased the incidence of flare-ups, more recent studies found antibiotic use either less effective than analgesics or to have no effect in reducing interappointment emergencies or posttreatment symptoms.[86,110,101]

CRACKED AND FRACTURED TEETH

Described in detail in Chapter 1 and Chapter 21, cracks and incomplete fractures can be difficult to locate and diagnose, but their detection can be an important component in the management of an acute dental emergency. In the early stages, cracks are small and difficult to discern. Removal of filling materials, applications of dye solutions, selective loading of cusps, transillumination, and magnification are helpful in their detection. As the crack or fracture becomes more extensive, it can become easier to visualize. Because cracks are difficult to find and their symptoms can be so variable, the name *cracked tooth syndrome* has been suggested,[14] even though it is not truly a syndrome. Cracks in vital teeth often exhibit a sudden and sharp pain, especially during mastication. Cracks in nonvital or obturated teeth tend to have more of a "dull ache" but can still be sensitive to mastication.

The determination of the presence of a crack or fracture is paramount because the prognosis for the tooth may be directly dependent on the extent of the crack or fracture. Management of cracks in vital teeth may be as simple as a bonded restoration or a full coverage crown. However, even the best efforts to manage a crack may be unsuccessful, often requiring endodontic treatment or extraction. Fractures in nonvital or obturated teeth may be more challenging. In addition, it must be determined whether the crack or fracture was the cause of pulpal necrosis and whether there has been extensive periodontal breakdown. If so, the prognosis for the tooth is generally poor; thus extraction is recommended.

SUMMARY

The management of endodontic emergencies is an important part of a dental practice. It can often be a disruptive part of the day for the clinician and staff, but it is an invaluable solution for the distressed patient. Methodical diagnosis and prognostic assessment are imperative, with the patient being informed of the various treatment alternatives.

ACKNOWLEDGMENTS

The authors acknowledge the outstanding work of Drs. J. Craig Baumgartner, Jeffrey W. Hutter, and Louis Berman in previous editions of this text.

REFERENCES

1. Abramowicz M, editor: Do NSAIDs interfere with the cardioprotective effects of aspirin? *Med Lett Drugs Ther* 46:61, 2004.
2. Albahaireh ZS, Alnegrish AS: Postobturation pain after single and multiple-visit endodontic therapy: a prospective study, *J Dent* 26:227, 1998.
3. American Association of Endodontics: *Glossary of endodontic terms*, ed 7, Chicago, 2003, American Association of Endodontists.
4. Ashkenaz PJ: One-visit endodontics, *Dent Clin North Am* 28:853, 1984.
5. Auslander WP: The acute apical abscess, *N Y State Dent J* 36:623, 1970.
6. Baumgartner JC, Xia T: Antibiotic susceptibility of bacteria associated with endodontic abscesses, *J Endod* 29:44, 2003.
7. Bence R, Meyers RD, Knoff RV: Evaluation of 5,000 endodontic treatment incidents of the open tooth, *Oral Surg Oral Med Oral Pathol* 49:82, 1980.
8. Bender IB: Pulpal pain diagnosis: a review, *J Endod* 26:175, 2000.
9. Bernal LA, Guillot E, Paquet C, Mouton C: Beta-lactamase producing strains in the species *Prevotella intermedia* and *Prevotella nigrescens*, *Oral Microbiol Immunol* 13:36, 1998.
10. Boutsioukis C, Psimma Z, Kastrinakis E: The effect of flow rate and agitation technique on irrigant extrusion *ex vivo*, *Int Endod J* 47:487, 2014.
11. Brook I: beta-Lactamase-producing bacteria in mixed infections, *Clin Microbiol Infect* 10:777, 2004.
12. Brook I, Frazier EH, Gher ME Jr: Microbiology of periapical abscesses and associated maxillary sinusitis, *J Periodontol* 67:608, 1996.
13. Bystrom A, Claesson R, Sundqvist G: The antibacterial effect of camphorated paramonochlorophenol, camphorated phenol and calcium hydroxide in the treatment of infected root canals, *Endod Dent Traumatol* 1:170, 1985.
14. Cameron CE: The cracked tooth syndrome, *J Am Dent Assoc* 93:971, 1976.
15. Carrotte P. Endodontics: part 3. Treatment of endodontic emergencies, *Br Dent J* 197:299, 2004.
16. Chestner SB, Selman AJ, Friedman J, Heyman RA: Apical fenestration: solution to recalcitrant pain in root canal therapy, *J Am Dent Assoc* 77:846, 1986.

17. Chong BS, Pitt Ford TR: The role of intracanal medication in root canal treatment, *Int Endod J* 25:97, 1992.
18. Cooper SA, Beaver WT: A model to evaluate mild analgesics in oral surgery outpatients, *Clin Pharmacol Ther* 20:241, 1976.
19. Creech JH, Walton RE, Kaltenbach R: Effect of occlusal relief on endodontic pain, *J Am Dent Assoc* 109:64, 1984.
20. Desi P, Himel V: Comparative safety of various intracanal irrigation systems, *J Endod* 35:545,2009.
21. Dionne RA, Phero JC, Becker DE: *Management of pain and anxiety in the dental office*, Philadelphia, 2002, Saunders.
22. Dorn SO, Moodnik RM, Feldman MJ, Borden BG: Treatment of the endodontic emergency: a report based on a questionnaire—part I, *J Endod* 3:94, 1977.
23. Dorn SO, Moodnik RM, Feldman MJ, Borden BG: Treatment of the endodontic emergency: a report based on a questionnaire—part II, *J Endod* 3:153, 1977.
24. Eleazer PD, Eleazer KR: Flare-up rate in pulpally necrotic molars in one-visit versus two-visit endodontic treatment, *J Endod* 24:614, 1998.
25. Field JW, Gutmann JL, Solomon ES, Rakuskin H: A clinical radiographic retrospective assessment of the success rate of single-visit root canal treatment, *Int Endod J* 37:70, 2004.
26. Flynn TR: Anatomy of oral and maxillofacial infections. In Topazian RG, Goldberg MH, Hupp JR, editors: *Oral and maxillofacial infections*, ed 4, Philadelphia, 2002, WB Saunders, pp 188-213.
27. Fosse T, Madinier I, Hitzig C, Charbit Y: Prevalence of betalactamase-producing strains among 149 anaerobic gram negative rods isolated from periodontal pockets, *Oral Microbiol Immunol* 14:352, 1999.
28. Fouad AF, Rivera EM, Walton RE: Penicillin as a supplement in resolving the localized acute apical abscess, *Oral Surg Oral Med Oral Pathol Oral Radiol Endod* 81:590, 1996.
29. Reference deleted in proofs.
30. Gatchel RJ: Managing anxiety and pain during dental treatment, *J Am Dent Assoc* 123:37, 1992.
31. Gatewood RS, Himel VT, Dorn S: Treatment of the endodontic emergency: a decade later, *J Endod* 16:284, 1990.

32. Goldberg MH, Topazian RG: Odontogenic infections and deep fascial space infections of dental origin. In Topazian RG, Goldberg MH, Hupp JR, editors: *Oral and maxillofacial infections*, ed 4, Philadelphia, 2002, WB Saunders, pp 158-187.
33. Grodinsky M, Holyoke EA: The fasciae and fascial spaces of the head, neck, and adjacent regions, *Am J Anat* 63:367, 1938.
34. Handal T, Olsen I, Walker CB, Caugant DA: Beta-lactamase production and antimicrobial susceptibility of subgingival bacteria from refractory periodontitis, *Oral Microbiol Immunol* 19:303, 2004.
35. Hargreaves KM, Keiser K: New advances in the management of endodontic pain emergencies, *J Calif Dent Assoc* 32:469, 2004.
36. Harrington GW, Natkin E: Midtreatment flare-ups, *Dent Clin North Am* 36:409, 1992.
37. Harrison JW: Irrigation of the root canal system, *Dent Clin North Am* 28:797, 1984.
38. Hasler JF, Mitchel DF: Analysis of 1628 cases of odontalgia: a corroborative study, *J Indianap Dist Dent Soc* 17:23 1963.
39. Hasselgren G: Pains of dental origin, *Dent Clin North Am* 12:263, 2000.
40. Hasselgren G, Reit C: Emergency pulpotomy: pain relieving effect with and without the use of sedative dressings, *J Endod* 15:254, 1989.
41. Hayward CMM, Griffin GE: Antibiotic resistance: the current position and the molecular mechanisms involved, *Br J Hosp Med* 52:473, 1994.
42. Hecht DW: Prevalence of antibiotic resistance in anaerobic bacteria: worrisome developments, *Clin Infect Dis* 39:92, 2004.
43. Hecht DW, Vedantam G, Osmolski JR: Antibiotic resistance among anaerobes: what does it mean? *Anaerobe* 5:421, 1999.
44. Heimdahl A, von Konow L, Satoh T, Nord CE: Clinical appearance of orofacial infections of odontogenic origin in relation to microbiological findings, *J Clin Microbiol* 22:299, 1985.
45. Henry BM, Fraser JG: Trephination for acute pain management, *J Endod* 29:144, 2003.
46. Henry M, Reader A, Beck M: Effect of penicillin on postoperative endodontic pain and swelling in symptomatic necrotic teeth, *J Endod* 27:117, 2001.

47. Hohl TH, Whitacre RJ, Hooley JR, Williams B: *A self instructional guide: diagnosis and treatment of odontogenic infections,* Seattle, 1983, Stoma Press.

48. Holmes-Johnson E, Geboy M, Getka EJ: Behavior considerations, *Dent Clin North Am* 30:391, 1986.

49. Horrobin DF, Durnad LG, Manku MS: Prostaglandin E 1 modifies nerve conduction and interferes with local anesthetic action, *Prostaglandins* 14:103, 1997.

50. Imura N, Zuolo ML: Factors associated with endodontic flareups: a prospective study, *Int Endod J* 28:261, 1995.

51. Jacinto RC, Gomes BP, Ferraz CC, et al: Microbiological analysis of infected root canals from symptomatic and asymptomatic teeth with periapical periodontitis and the antimicrobial susceptibility of some isolated anaerobic bacteria, *Oral Microbiol Immunol* 18:285, 2003.

52. Jain AK, Ryan JR, McMahon G: Analgesic efficacy of low-dose ibuprofen in dental extraction, *Pharmacotherapy* 6:318, 1986.

53. Keenan JV, Farman AG, Fedorowica Z, Newton JT: A Cochrane Systematic Review finds no evidence to support the use of antibiotics for pain relief in irreversible pulpitis, *J Endod* 32:87, 2006.

54. Kerekes K, Tronstad L: Long-term results of endodontic treatment performed with a standardized technique, *J Endod* 5:83, 1979.

55. Khemaleelakul S, Baumgartner JC, Pruksakorn S: Identification of bacteria in acute endodontic infections and their antimicrobial susceptibility, *Oral Surg Oral Med Oral Pathol Oral Radiol Endod* 94:746, 2002.

56. Kim E, Lee SJ: Electronic apex locator [Review], *Dent Clin North Am* 48:35, 2004.

57. Kuriyama T, Karasawa T, Nakagawa K, et al: Bacteriologic features and antimicrobial susceptibility in isolates from orofacial odontogenic infections, *Oral Surg Oral Med Oral Pathol Oral Radiol Endod* 90:600, 2000.

58. Kuriyama T, Karasawa T, Nakagawa K, et al: Incidence of beta-lactamase production and antimicrobial susceptibility of anaerobic gram-negative rods isolated from pus specimens of orofacial odontogenic infections, *Oral Microbiol Immunol* 16:10, 2001.

59. Kuriyama T, Williams DW, Yanagisawa M, et al: Antimicrobial susceptibility of 800 anaerobic isolates from patients with dentoalveolar infection to 13 oral antibiotics, *Oral Microbiol Immunol* 22:285, 2007.

60. Kvist T, Molander A, Dahlen G, Reit C: Microbiological evaluation of one- and two-visit endodontic treatment of teeth with apical periodontitis: a randomized, clinical trial, *J Endod* 30:572, 2004.

61. Lakhassassi N, Elhajoui N, Lodter JP, et al: Antimicrobial susceptibility variation of 50 anaerobic periopathogens in aggressive periodontitis: an interindividual variability study, *Oral Microbiol Immunol* 20:244, 2005.

62. Larson AM, Polson J, Fontana RJ, et al: Acetaminophen-induced acute liver failure: results of a United States multicenter, prospective study, *Hepatology* 42:1364, 2005.

63. Lee M, Winkler J, Hartwell G, et al: Current trends in endodontic practice: emergency treatments and technological armamentarium, *J Endod* 35:35, 2009.

64. Levitt GW: The surgical treatment of deep neck infections, *Laryngoscope* 81:403, 1970.

65. Lipton JA, Ship JA, Larach-Robinson D: Estimated prevalence and distribution of reported orofacial pain in the United States, *J Am Dent Assoc* 124:115, 1993.

66. Madigan MT, Martinko JM, Parker J: *Brock biology of microorganisms,* ed 9, Upper Saddle River, NJ, 2000, Prentice-Hall.

67. Matusow RJ, Goodall LB: Anaerobic isolates in primary pulpal–alveolar cellulitis cases: endodontic resolutions and drug therapy considerations, *J Endod* 9:535, 1983.

68. Mitchell DF, Tarplee RE: Painful pulpitis: a clinical and microscopic study, *Oral Surg* 13:1360, 1960.

69. Moos HL, Bramwell JD, Roahen JO: A comparison of pulpectomy alone versus pulpectomy with trephination for the relief of pain, *J Endod* 22:422, 1996.

70. Morse DR, Koren LZ, Esposito JV, et al: Asymptomatic teeth with necrotic pulps and associated periapical radiolucencies: relationship of flare-ups to endodontic instrumentation, antibiotic usage and stress in three separate practices at three different time periods, *Int J Psychosom* 33:5, 1986.

71. Morse DR, Furst ML, Belott RM, et al: Infectious flare-ups and serious sequelae following endodontic treatment: a prospective randomized trial on efficacy of antibiotic prophylaxis in cases of asymptomatic pulpal–periapical lesion, *Oral Surg* 64:96, 1987.

72. Nagle D, Reader A, Beck M, Weaver J: Effect of systemic penicillin on pain in untreated irreversible pulpitis, *Oral Surg Oral Med Oral Pathol* 90:636, 2000.

73. Natkin E: Treatment of endodontic emergencies, *Dent Clin North Am* 18:243, 1974.

74. Nusstein J, Reader A, Nist R, et al: Anesthetic efficacy of the supplemental intraosseous injection, *J Endod* 24:487, 1998.

75. Nyerere JW, Matee MI, Simon EN: Emergency pulpotomy in relieving acute dental pain among Tanzanian patients, *BMC Oral Health* 6:1, 2006.

76. Oginni AO, Udoye CI: Endodontic flare-ups: comparison of incidence between single and multiple visit procedures in patients attending a Nigerian teaching hospital, *BMC Oral Health* 4:4, 2004.

77. Ogundiya DA, Keith DA, Mirowski J: Cavernous sinus thrombosis and blindness as complications of an odontogenic infection, *Oral Maxillofac Surg* 47:1317, 1989.

78. Oliet S: Single-visit endodontics: a clinical study, *J Endod* 24:614, 1998.

79. Pallasch TJ: Antibiotics in endodontics, *Dent Clin North Am* 23:737, 1979.

80. Pallasch TJ: Pharmacokinetic principles of antimicrobial therapy, *Periodontol 2000* 10:5, 1996.

81. Pallasch TJ, Slots J: Antibiotic prophylaxis and the medically compromised patient, *Periodontol 2000* 10:107, 1996.

82. Patel R: Clinical impact of vancomycin-resistant enterococci, *J Antimicrob Chemother* 51(suppl 3):iii13, 2003.

83. Pekruhn RB: The incidence of failure following single-visit endodontic therapy, *J Endod* 12:68, 1986.

84. Penesis VA, Fitzgerald PI, Fayad MI, et al: Outcome of one-visit and two-visit endodontic treatment of necrotic teeth with apical periodontitis: a randomized controlled trial with one-year evaluation, *J Endod* 34:251, 2008.

85. Peters LB, Wesselink PR: Periapical healing of endodontically treated teeth in one and two visits obturated in the presence or absence of detectable microorganisms, *Int Endod J* 35:660, 2002.

86. Pickenpaugh L, Reader A, Beck M, et al: Effect of prophylactic amoxicillin on endodontic flare-up in asymptomatic, necrotic teeth, *J Endod* 27:53, 2001.

87. Reddy SA, Hicks ML: Apical extrusion of debris using two hand and two rotary instrumentation techniques, *J Endod* 24:180, 1998.

88. Roane JB, Dryden JA, Grimes EW: Incidence of postoperative pain after single- and multiple-visit endodontic procedures, *Oral Surg Oral Med Oral Pathol* 55:68, 1983.

89. Rosenberg PA, Babick PJ, Schertzer L, Leung A: The effect of occlusal reduction on pain after endodontic instrumentation, *J Endod* 24:492, 1998.

90. Rudner WL, Oliet S: Single-visit endodontics: a concept and a clinical study, *Compend Contin Educ Dent* 2:63, 1981.

91. Rugh JD: Psychological components of pain, *Dent Clin North Am* 31:579, 1987.

92. Sandor GK, Low DE, Judd PL, Davidson RJ: Antimicrobial treatment options in the management of odontogenic infections, *J Can Dent Assoc* 64:508, 1998. Comment in *J Can Dent Assoc* 65:602, 1999.

93. Schilling A, Corey R, Leonard M, Eghtesad B: Acetaminophen: old drug, new warnings, *Cleve Clin J Med* 77:19, 2010, doi: 10.3949/ccjm.77a.09084.

94. Seltzer S, Naidorf IJ: Flare-ups in endodontics. 1. Etiological factors, *J Endod* 11:472, 1985.

95. Simon JH, Chimenti RA, Mintz GA: Clinical significance of the pulse granuloma, *J Endod* 8:116, 1982.

96. Siqueira JF, Rocas IN: Microbial causes of endodontic flareups, *Int Endod J* 36:433, 2003.

97. Sjogren U, Figdor D, Persson S, Sundqvist G: Influence of infection at the time of root filling on the outcome of endodontic treatment of teeth with apical periodontitis, *Int Endod J* 30:297, 1997.

98. Southard DW, Rooney TP: Effective one-visit therapy for the acute periapical abscess, *J Endod* 10:580, 1984.

99. Sutherland S, Matthews DC. Emergency management of acute apical periodontitis in the permanent dentition: a systematic review of the literature, *J Can Dent Assoc* 69:160, 2003.

100. Tendolkar PM, Baghdayan AS, Shankar N: Pathogenic enterococci: new developments in the 21st century, *Cell Mol Life Sci* 60:2622, 2003.

101. Torabinejad M, Dorn SO, Eleazer PD, et al: The effectiveness of various medications on postoperative pain following root canal obturation, *J Endod* 20:427, 1994.

102. Torabinejad M, Kettering JD, McGraw JC, et al: Factors associated with endodontic interappointment emergencies of teeth with necrotic pulps, *J Endod* 14:261, 1988.

103. Torabinejad M, Walton R: *Endodontics: principles and practice,* ed 4, St. Louis, 2009, Saunders.

104. Trope ME, Delano EO, Orstavik D: Endodontic treatment of teeth with apical periodontitis: single vs. multivisit treatment, *J Endod* 25:345, 1999.

105. Tsesis I, Faivishevsky V, Fuss Z, Zukerman O: Flare-ups after endodontic treatment: a meta-analysis of literature, *J Endod* 34:1177, 2008.

106. Turkun M, Cengiz T: The effects of sodium hypochlorite and calcium hydroxide in tissue dissolution and root canal cleanliness, *Int Endod J* 30:335, 1997.

107. van Winkelhoff AJ, Herrera D, Oteo A, Sanz M: Antimicrobial profiles of periodontal pathogens isolated from periodontitis patients in The Netherlands and Spain, *J Clin Periodontol* 32:893, 2005.

108. van Winkelhoff AJ, Winkel EG, Barendregt D, et al: beta-Lactamase producing bacteria in adult periodontitis, *J Clin Periodontol* 24:538, 1997.

109. Walton R, Fouad A: Endodontic interappointment flare-ups: a prospective study of incidence and related factors, *J Endod* 18:172, 1992.

110. Walton RE, Chiappinelli J: Prophylactic penicillin: effect on posttreatment symptoms following root canal treatment of asymptomatic periapical pathosis, *J Endod* 19:466, 1993.

111. Weiger R, Axmann-Krcmar D, Löst C: Prognosis of conventional root canal treatment reconsidered, *Endod Dent Traumatol* 14:1, 1998.

112. Weiger R, Rosendahl R, Lost C: Influence of calcium hydroxide intracanal dressings on the prognosis of teeth with endodontically induced periapical lesions, *Int Endod J* 33:219, 2000.

113. Weine FS, Healey HJ, Theiss EP: Endodontic emergency dilemma: leave tooth open or keep it closed? *Oral Surg Oral Med Oral Pathol* 40:531, 1975.

114. Whitney CG, Farley MM, Hadler J, et al: Increasing prevalence of multidrug-resistant Streptococcus pneumoniae in the United States, *N Engl J Med* 343:1917, 2000.

115. Yun MW, Hwang CF, Lui CC: Cavernous sinus thrombus following odontogenic and cervicofacial infection, *Eur Arch Otorhinolaryngol* 248:422, 1991.

CHAPTER 19

Managing Iatrogenic Endodontic Events

YOSHITSUGU TERAUCHI

An iatrogenic event is defined as a procedure "induced inadvertently by a physician or surgeon" (Merriam-Webster dictionary). This is true for dentistry as well, with cases of endodontic malpractice being among the most prevalent in dentistry.[57,111,252] These occurrences are not limited to the United States, with other countries reporting similar percentages of endodontic malpractice claims.[225]

Although iatrogenic accidents cannot be prevented with absolute certainty, their occurrences can be greatly reduced with the aid of the "Three Ts": training, technique, and technology. Incumbent with the first (training) is expertise with the other two factors, especially regarding technology and, more specifically, the dental operating microscope. It has proved itself indispensable in locating canals,[155,157,250,277] removing separated instruments,[279] repairing perforations,[234] and enhancing the delivery of quality care.[150] The superior visualization permits more accurate clinical evaluations, allowing for a precise assessment of the challenge and the appropriate treatment plan for its resolution. This instrument is indispensable for all of the treatment scenarios that follow, which are therefore assumed to be performed with the aid of magnification.

SODIUM HYPOCHLORITE (NaOCl)

Often happening without warning, the progression of events following sodium hypochlorite extrusion into periradicular tissues is both rapid and startling to witness. In addition to the physical outcomes, the experience is likely to leave the patient wary of both the procedure and practitioner.

Although the properties and methods of delivering sodium hypochlorite are covered in Chapter 6, the gravity of the consequences of its misuse merits a brief highlight. Sodium hypochlorite is an effective irrigating solution in concentrations ranging from 0.5% to 6%[127,317] and is able to disrupt the biofilm,[45] dissolve necrotic tissues,[184] and remove organic components of the smear layer.[17] However, it is extremely cytotoxic, irrespective of the tissue it contacts,[202] with concentrations as low as 0.01% lethal to fibroblasts in vitro.[116] NaOCl injection into vital tissue initiates hemolysis and ulceration, damages endothelial and fibroblast cells, and inhibits neutrophil migration.[89,91] A study investigating the physical effects of NaOCl on bone ex vivo found degradation of the organic matrix collagen and no sign of living cellular contents (Fig. 19-1).[140]

The majority of reported NaOCl complications appear to be due to an inaccurate working length, iatrogenic widening of the radicular foramen, lateral perforation of the root, or wedging of the irrigation needle.[147,271] The pattern of facial distention is comparable to that encountered with a cervicofacial emphysema (discussed later), dissecting fascial spaces in a similar fashion, with the concomitant tissue destruction magnifying the effect and impeding recovery. This swelling is further exacerbated by the presence of effervescing agents such

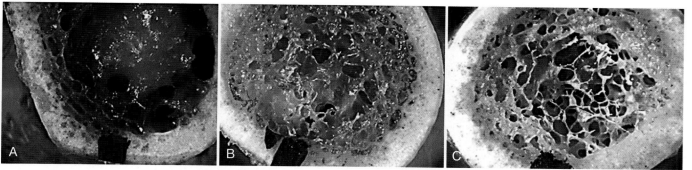

FIG. 19-1 Femur shaft cross sections (**A**) untreated bone section; (**B**) saline-treated bone; (**C**) NaOCl-treated bone section. Grossly, NaOCl caused significant changes in cancellous structure, leaving large structural craters of apparent demineralization. (From Kerbl FM, DeVilliers P, Litaker M, Eleazer PD: Physical effects of sodium hypochlorite on bone: an ex vivo study, *J Endod* 38:357, 2012.)

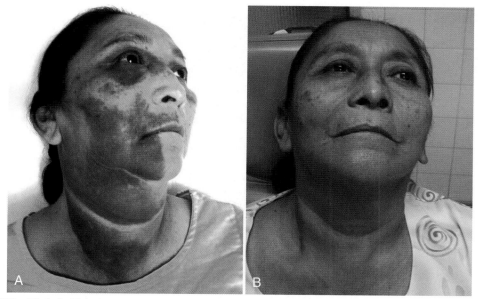

FIG. 19-2 A, Clinical presentation 3 days following the extrusion of NaOCl during treatment of the maxillary right canine. The patient had difficulty opening her right eye, and the swelling had extended to the submandibular/sublingual regions on the affected side; she also experienced limited mouth opening. There was altered sensation infraorbitally and in the region of the upper right lip, but no reported paresthesia of the alveolar or facial nerves. **B,** One month post extrusion, the ecchymosis had resolved, with a return of sensation and full function. Therapy was completed without incident. (From de Sermeño RF, da Silva LA, Herrera H: Tissue damage after sodium hypochlorite extrusion during root canal treatment, *Oral Surg Oral Med Oral Pathol Oral Radiol Endod* 108:e46, 2009.)

as hydrogen peroxide, potentiating the effect of the hypochlorite and amplifying soft tissue involvement.[20,161] The initial patient reaction to the fluid insult is severe and immediate pain, with marked edema or bruising that may continue to extend over the injured side of the face, cheek, or lips (Fig. 19-2). There may be spontaneous and profuse hemorrhaging from the canal space, and, in the case of maxillary posterior teeth, the patient may report periorbital pain,[21,89] chlorine taste, or irritation of the throat.[63] The amount that has been expressed into the periradicular area, the spatial location of the fluid introduction, and the proximity to sensitive anatomic structures will dictate the severity and duration of the reaction. Paresthesia, either transient[21] or permanent,[223] can occur, especially if interventional treatment is not rendered immediately.

In addition to sensory deprivation, motor nerve dysfunction secondary to irreversible chemical damage has been reported (Fig. 19-3).[206] In this case, there was distinct loss of upper lip and cheek function, with problems in the musculature. In mandibular teeth, extension into the submandibular, submental or sublingual regions can compromise the airway, compelling immediate hospitalization and surgical intervention to avert a life-threatening episode.[30]

Upon realizing that an extrusion event has occurred, it is imperative that the clinician cease further treatment and immediately engage in measures targeted at diminishing the effect of the chemical; ignoring the event reduces outcomes.[162,223] Treatment protocols are empirical and are predicated on cause and severity. With the emphasis on pain control, local

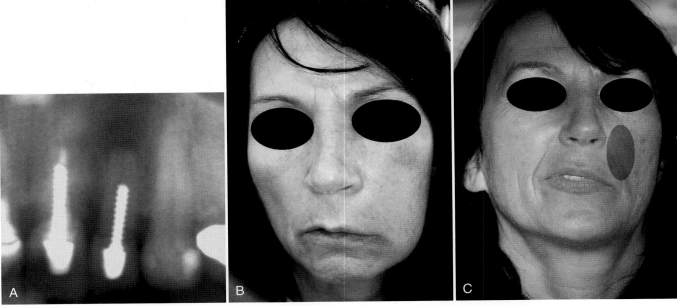

FIG. 19-3 A, Radiograph of the maxillary left lateral incisor (#10, #22) before post removal. Radicular root resection had been completed, and the canal space is empty. Prior to re-cementation, the canal was irrigated with 3% NaOCl, precipitating the extrusion event. **B,** Twenty-four hours post extrusion, there was altered sensation infraorbitally and from the upper left lip to the left lip corner. In addition, the buccal branch of the facial nerve was affected, as evidenced by a distinct loss of upper lip and cheek function (the corner of the mouth could not be pulled up by the mimic musculature). The mouth opening was limited to 20 mm **(C)**, 3 years post incident. The weakness of the mimic musculature of the left face side is clearly visible. Attempts to laugh resulted in a hanging left lip corner secondary to the weakness of the motor innervation by the facial nerve. In the gray-marked area there is a permanent hypoesthesia. (From Pelka M, Petschelt A: Permanent mimic musculature and nerve damage caused by sodium hypochlorite: a case report, *Oral Surg Oral Med Oral Pathol Oral Radiol Endod* 106:e80, 2008.)

anesthetics and analgesics can be administered, along with cold compresses, in an effort to moderate swelling and edema. Directed at diluting the effect of the extrusion, it has been suggested that the clinician immediately irrigate the canal with normal saline to encourage bleeding, both diluting the irritant and removing it from the site of the injury.[63,179] In addition, clinicians may immediately irrigate the canal and periradicular areas of the extrusion with saline, using a negative pressure irrigation device with the cannula placed at the radicular foramen. In one report, the subsequent reaction was short lived with this approach.[235]

After one day, warm compresses are substituted for the cold, and warm oral rinses are prescribed to stimulate the local microcirculation. Antibiotics are usually prescribed, and their administration commensurate with the severity of hard and soft tissue destruction and necrosis; milder cases can be treated with oral medications, whereas severe presentations are better controlled and modulated in a hospital setting with intravenous routes of delivery. The use of corticosteroids is equivocal; the control of the spreading edema must be balanced with the increased risk of infection. The patient should be monitored closely; a marked increase in the size or extent of the swelling or signs of impending airway obstruction mandate immediate referral to the hospital or a maxillofacial surgeon for more aggressive treatment and management. Lastly, reassuring patients that recovery, in spite of their current appearance, is usually complete and uneventful, will ease their anxiety. They should be informed as to why it occurred and what to expect during their recovery. Recovery should be monitored and documented daily until the resolution is imminent.

Prevention involves attention to detail and an appreciation for fluid dynamics. In summary, the clinician should do the following:

◆ Establish an accurate working length and avoid overinstrumentation/enlargement of the radicular foramen.
◆ If irrigating using positive pressure, employ a small side-vented needle placed no closer than 2 mm from the working length. Express the fluid slowly and observe that it is venting through the access cavity.[29]
◆ Carefully assess the canal integrity for signs of perforation or other large portals of fluid egress.
◆ Avoid wedging the needle tip in the canal space or inserting it beyond the working length.
◆ Confirm the identity of the solution prior to injection or irrigation.[104]

INSTRUMENT SEPARATION

The introduction of NiTi rotary instruments into endodontics revolutionized the way the root canal system is instrumented. However, with the advent of rotary NiTi files, there has also been a perceived increase in the occurrence of separated instruments,[84,242] with some reports indicating that separation of NiTi rotary instruments occurs more frequently than hand instruments.[294] On radiographic examination, separated instruments can usually be discerned by the distinct radiopacity within the canal. However, if the canal with a separated instrument is subsequently obturated with radiopaque materials, it may not be visualized in the radiograph. Upon removal of filling materials from the canal, a separated instrument may be visualized under the dental operating microscope (DOM) or become apparent on radiographs for the first time (Fig. 19-4).

Causes of Instrument Separation

A common cause for instrument separation is improper use.[84,245] Typical examples of improper use include inadequate access, overuse of the instrument, too much radicular pressure during instrumentation,[247,291] and the continuous use of a large

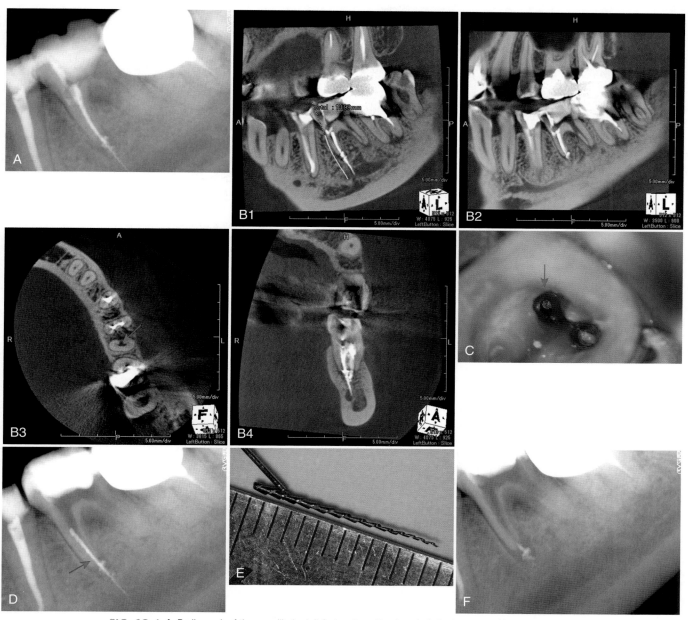

FIG. 19-4 **A,** Radiograph of the mandibular left first molar with a long indistinct separated instrument obviously longer than 4.5 mm in the mesial root that is extruded beyond the radicular foramen. **B1,** Sagittal view of CBCT showing the radicular end of the separated instrument is extended into the IAN and it measures 14 mm on it. **B2,** Sagittal view of CBCT showing root perforation in the distal canal (*yellow arrow*). **B3,** Axial view of CBCT showing the perforation in the distal canal (*yellow arrow*). **B4,** Coronal view of CBCT showing the radicular end of the separated instrument is in the IAN. **C,** Separated instrument in the mesiobuccal canal upon removal of root filling materials (*red arrow*) **D,** Radiograph showing removal of the root fillings in the mesiobuccal canal revealed the overall length of the separated instrument (*red arrow*). **E,** Retrieved separated instruments measuring 14 mm on the ruler. **F,** Radiograph showing completion of separated instrument removal.   *Continued*

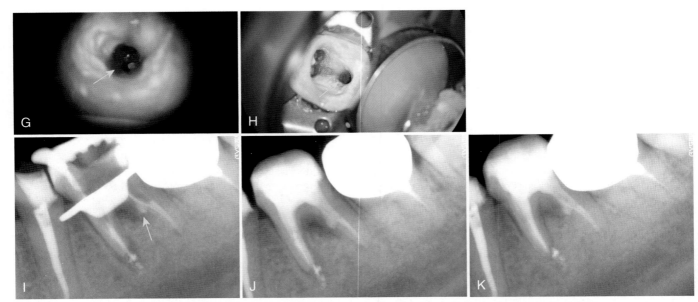

FIG. 19-4, cont'd **G**, Perforation site in the distal canal (*yellow arrow*). **H**, Perforation repaired with MTA (*yellow arrow*). **I**, Postoperative radiograph showing root canal fillings in all the canals and perforation repair (*yellow arrow*). **J**, One-month postoperative radiograph revealing the periradicular lesions still present. **K**, Three-month postoperative radiograph showing periradicular healing.

instrument in a curved canal.[107,219] Additional contributing factors are operator experience,[200,285] rotational speed,[53,169] canal curvature (radius),[170,219] instrument design and technique,[33,152] torque setting,[83] manufacturing process,[5] the type of NiTi alloys used,[88] the type of rotational motion (continuous rotations versus reciprocating motions),[205] the type of tooth,[51,191,258] and absence of a glide path.[204] Based on these factors, it is not surprising that the reported incidence of separated NiTi files ranges from 0.4% to 23%.[5,7,210,221,248,272]

Separated instruments seem to occur more frequently in molars than anterior teeth, especially in mandibular molars. This high incidence of instrument fracture in molars may be related to accessibility to the canal, diameter of the root canal, and root canal curvature.[51,191,258] Endodontists have reported the incidence of instrument separation to be about 5%.[5,200] The clinician must inform the patient of the instrument separation and treatment options as well as potential complications of both the separated instrument retention and its attempted removal.

Endodontic instruments fracture as a result of cyclic fatigue or torsional fatigue[47] or a combination of both types of fatigue.[245,257,296] Cyclic fatigue is caused by repetitive compressive and tensile stresses acting on the outer portion of a file rotating in a curved canal, leading to cyclic failure without previous signs of plastic deformation.[200] Torsional failure occurs when the tip of the instrument binds but the shank of the file (driven by the handpiece) continues to rotate.[245] Shear fracture of the material then occurs when the maximum strength of the material is exceeded.[154] Clinically, cyclic fatigue seems to be more prevalent in curved root canals, whereas torsional failure might happen even in a straight canal.[43,316] Cyclic-fatigued instruments are reported to become less resistant to torsional fatigue failure,[145] whereas the use of rotary instruments at a high torque setting is reported to increase the risk of cyclic fatigue failure.[84] Interestingly, the use of reciprocal motions (as opposed to rotational motions) is reported to

extend the life span of an instrument[56,315] and increase cyclic fatigue resistance.[205] It is recommended that instruments designed for reciprocating motion be used for shaping a severely curved canal and that the instruments used to prepare such curved root canals be discarded after use to prevent instrument fracture.

Management of Separated Instruments

Management of separated instruments includes nonsurgical orthograde (mechanical or chemical) or surgical approaches. The mechanical removal involves the use of tools dedicated to separated instrument removal such as extractors, wire loops, post removal systems, ultrasonics, and laser irradiation (see also Chapter 8). The chemical removal involves the use of chemical solvents for instrument corrosion and electrochemical process for instrument dissolution. Surgical approaches include radicular surgery, intentional replantation, root amputation, or hemisection.

For a nonsurgical approach in removing a separated file, various methods and devices have been developed (see also Chapter 8). When a separated instrument extends above the root canal orifice, it can often be easily removed with a hemostat, Steiglitz forceps, a modified Castroviejo needle holder,[78] or a Perry plier.[304] A spoon excavator or a Caulfield retriever can also be used to engage and remove the separated instrument with coronally directed pressure. In the event that a hand file can bypass the separated instrument, a "braiding technique" can be used whereby several Hedstrom files are inserted along the bypassed instrument, the files are twisted to grasp the separated instrument, and it is then extracted as one unit. When a fractured instrument is below the canal orifice and cannot be bypassed, one basic method for removing the separated instrument requires the exposure of approximately 2 mm of the coronal portion of the separated file. This allows the use of an extracting device for engaging the file, securing it, and removing it. The Masserann kit (Micro-Mega, Besancon, France) is a popular system for the removal of separated instruments located within the straight part of the canal. This kit involves the use of trephine burs to expose the coronal portion of the separated instrument and for creating a space for an extractor. An extractor is then used to grasp and remove the separated instrument. The limitation of this system is that it cannot be used for cases involving separated instruments located beyond the midroot or in a curved canal, as this technique involves a considerable amount of dentin sacrifice that can weaken the root structure and increase the risk of perforation.[313] An alternative to the Masserann kit is the Endo Safety System.[306] This system differs from the Masserann kit in that it uses smaller diameter trephine burs and the extractor has its own unique mechanism for grasping instruments. The Endo Extractor (Brasseler Inc., Savannah, GA) can also be used in these types of cases. This system consists of a trephine bur to expose the coronal portion of the separated instrument and a hollow tube extractor that is threaded over the exposed portion of the separated instrument and bonded to it with cyanoacrylate adhesive.[92] The Canal Finder System (FaSociété Endo Technique, Marseilles, France) or the EndoPuls System (EndoTechnic, San Diego, CA) provides a different approach to a separated instrument. The system is composed of a handpiece and files that are designed exclusively for the system.[164] The system produces a vertical movement with a maximum amplitude of 1 to 2 mm, which decreases when the speed increases.[126] This vertical movement of the file will also help bypass an instrument fragment. The flutes of the file can mechanically engage with the separated instrument, and with the vertical vibration, the instrument fragment can be loosened or even retrieved.[125] The mechanical movement of the file can get aggressive, so the clinician must use caution to avoid root perforation, especially in a curved canal. These systems are technique sensitive and therefore results can vary between cases.

Ultrasonic instruments are very effective for the removal of separated instruments.[42,185,241] However, it is important to realize that separated NiTi files tend to fracture repeatedly when ultrasonics are applied to them for broken file removal, whereas stainless steel instruments are more resistant and more easily removed with ultrasonics than NiTi instruments.[241,279,301] Small ultrasonic instruments allow continuous and improved vision of the field of operation. The use of ultrasonics, especially when performed under the microscope, enhances the removal process and can provide relatively safe removal of separated instruments.[191,279,300] The ultrasonic tip is placed on the staging platform between the exposed portion of the separated file and the canal wall, and it is vibrated around it in a counterclockwise direction, applying an unscrewing force to the separated file. This technique will help with removing most rotary instruments that have a clockwise cutting action. If it is known that the separated file has a counterclockwise cutting action, then a clockwise rotation will be needed. The energy applied will aid in loosening the file, and occasionally the file will suddenly exit out of the canal.

However, the use of ultrasonics does have some drawbacks. Upon ultrasonic activation, a separated file can be accidentally extruded into the bone, either radicularly or through a perforation. In addition, the ultrasonic activation of a separated instrument has been reported to separate small fragments from the original fragment,[41] further complicating the management of the case. Smaller fragments of a file are considered more difficult to remove than longer fragments.[170,219,241] These smaller fragments of a separated file can often be pushed back into a more radicular and narrow level of the canal, which would eventually increase the risk of perforation and extra dentin sacrifice upon attempted fragment removal.

The success rate for removing separated files varies from 33% to 95%[7,51,221,240,301] with the time required for using ultrasonic techniques varying between 3 to over 60 minutes.[9,185,285] The variations in success rates are due to the location of fractured instruments, the diameter of the root canal,[258] the degree of canal curvature,[9,220,268] the radius of curvature,[9,219] operator experience,[9,285] operator fatigue, and the length of the separated instrument.[284] Visualization and accessibility to the separated instrument play a major role in file retrieval.[51] In general, the success rate for removal is high for separated files located before the canal curvature, moderate for those located at the curvature, and low for those located beyond the curvature.[170,305] The success rate is also more favorable when the canal curvature is less and the radius of curvature is longer.[9] The combination of ultrasonic techniques and microscopes typically improves success rates in file removal.[51,82,191,301]

It has been recommended that removal attempts of separated instruments from root canals should not exceed 45 to 60 minutes because the success rates may drop with increased treatment time.[279] The reduced success rate could be related to operator fatigue or overenlargement of the canal, which compromises the integrity of the tooth and increases the risk of perforation. Any case where the separated instrument can be visualized under the DOM may be considered less challenging to manage. If the separated instrument is considered irretrievable after a sufficient attempt, the case should be completed by having the separated file incorporated as part of the obturation and kept under observation.[74,79,221,269]

Conditions for Separated Instrument Removal Attempts

File removal can be attempted in either a dry or a wet environment. Dry conditions provide better visibility when using the dental operating microscope, preventing fewer additional procedural accidents.[242,268,279,300] However, heat generation by ultrasonics is inevitable,[96,113,156,173,258,268,279,300] and a temperature rise above 10° C on the external root surface can damage the periodontal tissues.[66,280] In addition, the separated instrument will be susceptible to secondary heat when ultrasonic tips are in contact with the file.[286,300] Therefore, it is recommended that water or some other irrigant be used while the ultrasonic tip is activated at the lowest possible power setting.[37,70,175,300] In addition, the irrigating solution used in the canal should be EDTA solution; the use of an ultrasonic tip as an adjunct with EDTA solution enhances the canal wall cleanliness.[256]

Separated Instrument Removal Technique

The majority of separated instruments are NiTi,[272] with the mean length of separated instruments being 2.5 to 3.5 mm.[135] Many NiTi rotary instruments used have a .04 to .08 taper range with a tip size of #20 to #30, resulting in a coronal diameter of about 0.30 mm to 0.58 mm. If the coronal diameter of the separated instrument is smaller than 0.45 mm, then a #3 modified Gates Gliden bur (#3 MGG bur from the FRK, DentalCadre, Seattle, WA) should be used to enlarge the canal to the separated instrument, followed by the micro-trephine bur (DentalCadre) for exposing the coronal portion of the

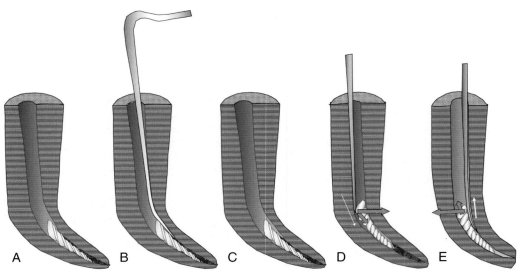

FIG. 19-5 **A,** Separated file around the curve after the canal enlargement with a NiTi rotary file. **B,** Space needs to be created on the inside curve with the spoon ultrasonic tip, followed by the straight tip. **C,** Thin space created on the inner curve. **D,** Ultrasonic forces applied to the separated instrument from the outside curvature will reorient it in a radicular direction. **E,** Ultrasonic forces applied to the separated instrument from the inside curvature will reorient it in a coronal direction rather than a radicular direction.

separated instrument, with less risk than ultrasonics for secondary fracture of the separated instrument.[285,286] The inner diameter of the micro-trephine bur is 0.45 mm and it is then used, in a counter clockwise rotation, with the intent of unscrewing the separated instrument. This bur should be used at 600 rpm in wet conditions; if the rotational speed exceeds 600 rpm, unintentional ledge formation may occur, especially in a curved canal.

If the coronal diameter of the separated instrument is larger than 0.45 mm or the canal curvature is greater than 15 degrees, a larger NiTi rotary instrument, with tip size 0.1 mm (two sizes) larger than the coronal diameter of the separated instrument, should be used to enlarge the canal coronal to the separated instrument, followed by ultrasonic instruments to expose the coronal portion.

Firstly, the spoon tip with the concave portion facing the separated instrument (DentalCadre) will be introduced into the thin gap between the separated instrument and the inside curve of the canal to create one quarter space of the circle around the separated instrument. Secondly, the straight tip (DentalCadre) is introduced to expand the space to complete the semicircular space on the inside curve. The ultrasonic tip should always be applied to the area on the inner canal curve being extended in the radicular direction (Fig. 19-5). If the ultrasonic tip is placed in the space outside the curve and ultrasonic energy is given to the separated instrument from the outside of the curve, the force applied will redirect the separated instrument in an apical direction, eventually pushing it more apically and making the instrument retrieval more difficult, whereas the force applied from the inside of the curve to the separated instrument will consequently reorient the separated instrument in a coronal direction. In most cases, the coronal one third of the separated file is the main portion engaged in the canal wall. This portion is typically resistant to mechanical force for disengagement due to the highly stressed concentration on the coronal one third of the

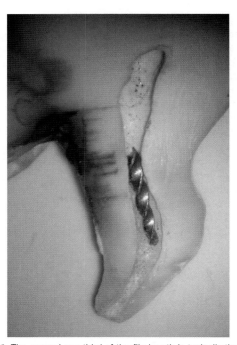

FIG. 19-6 The coronal one third of the file length is typically the part to be stuck in the canal wall, whereas the radicular portion of the file is typically not in contact with the canal wall. Stress is concentrated mostly on the coronal one third of the file length.

separated file. Therefore, the dentin wall contacting the coronal third of the separated file has to be eliminated to free it and facilitate its removal (Fig. 19-6). It is recommended that the ultrasonic tip be used in a counter clockwise direction to trough around the coronal aspect of a separated instrument.[240] However, a fatigued separated instrument is already extremely susceptible to secondary fracture by ultrasonic activation.[286,300]

For this reason it is safer to cut only a semicircular trough on one side of the separated instrument behind which there is dentin wall support,[286] and a pulsing motion should be applied to it while ultrasonics is activated to prevent instrument fracture and temperature rise, especially in dry conditions.[66,280,286,300] Just a thin space created on one side of the coronal third of the separated instrument is enough to free the separated instrument from being engaged in the canal wall. Especially in a curved canal, ultrasonic activation should always apply to the thin space created between the separated fragment and the inside curve, and the dentin wall supporting the separated file fragment must always be present behind the ultrasonic activation site to prevent secondary fracture. The radicular extent to be created along the separated instrument should be approximately as long as one third of the fragment length. For example, if the separated file fragment is 3 mm long, the semicircular space needs to be extended radicularly about 1 mm on the inside curve to help the ultrasonic tip loosen it. This process of extending the space in an apical direction must continue until it is confirmed that the separated file is seen dancing with ultrasonics under the DOM. The root canal preparation for instrument retrieval is done when the movement of the separated instrument is confirmed. The ultrasonic tip used for this purpose should be as thin as possible, allowing the clinician to both visualize the operative field and prevent overenlargement of the canal wall. During this ultrasonic preparation phase, the separated file may come out by ultrasonic activation at any moment (Fig. 19-7).

When the separated instrument is not visible upon the straight line access to it, instrument retrieval is considered challenging and it requires expertise and a little bit of guesswork to remove it. First, the microexplorer (DentalCadre) is precurved to meet the separated instrument, and then radiographs are taken with the microexplorer in the canal to confirm that it is in the space between the separated instrument and the inside curve. Next, the straight tip is precurved the same way as the microexplorer was precurved to get into the inner thin space, and the ultrasonic tip is activated to extend the space apically until the separated instrument gets loosened (Fig. 19-8).

Once the root canal preparation for instrument retrieval is completed, it is important to confirm that the canal wall is smooth from the separated file to the coronal extent, with no protrusions on the outside canal wall. Following the ultrasonic loosening of the coronal portion of the separated instrument, the canal is filled with EDTA solution to enhance the ultrasonic effect (see Fig. 19-7, B). A retrospective study and the author's empirical findings show that when the separated instrument is shorter than 4.5 mm, the clinician will most likely be able to retrieve it with ultrasonics alone (Fig. 19-9).[284] Ultrasonic activation should be applied in push-pull motions in the space created between the separated file and the inside curvature of the canal until the separated file is removed (see Fig. 19-7, C and D).

If the separated instrument is longer than 4.5 mm, or if it is seen moving with ultrasonic activation, but the instrument retrieval with ultrasonics was not successful, then the loop device (DentalCadre, Seattle, WA) should be applied to it to capture the coronal portion of the separated file and pull the file fragment out of the canal.[284] The probability is that an instrument fragment longer than 4.5 mm is touching all over the canal walls, which creates more friction as it is reoriented in a coronal direction and makes it more resistant to instrument retrieval with ultrasonics alone, requiring more mechanical force to pull it out of the canal. The coronal portion of the separated instrument needs to be peripherally exposed by at least 0.7 mm (see Fig. 19-10, A), and a semicircular space needs to be created and extended apically on the inside curvature of the canal the same way as in the root canal preparation for ultrasonic instrument retrieval until the separated instrument is seen dancing with ultrasonics. The loop size must be adjusted to fit the coronal diameter of the separated file using

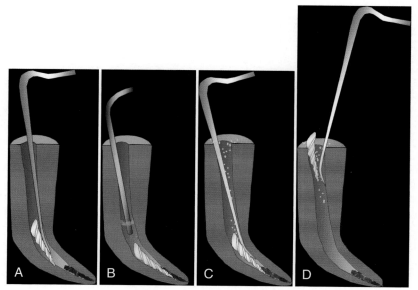

FIG. 19-7   **A,** Separated file may accidentally come out with ultrasonic activation during a preparation phase. **B,** EDTA solution is put into the canal to take advantage of cavitation and acoustic streaming effects for instrument retrieval. **C,** Ultrasonics must be activated within the space created. **D,** Separated file is removed from the canal with ultrasonics in the presence of EDTA solution.

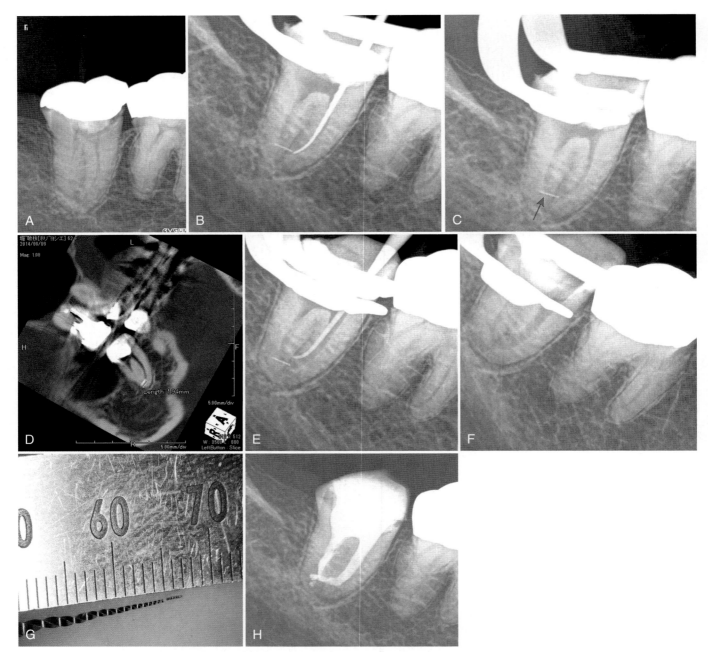

FIG. 19-8 A, Preoperative radiograph showing deep caries lesions underneath the crown with meager looking pulp-capping materials on the pulp chamber. The tooth was diagnosed with irreversible pulpitis. **B,** NiTi rotary instrument (ProTaper NEXT X1) was separated in the mesial canal during root canal instrumentation. **C,** Interoperative radiograph showing an instrument fractured beyond the severe curve (*red arrow*). **D,** Separated instrument measured 1.94 mm on the axial view of CBCT. **E,** Interoperative radiograph showing the location of the curved microexplorer in relation to the separated instrument in the mesial canal. **F,** Interoperative radiograph showing the separated instrument was removed with the curved straight ultrasonic tip activated inside the curve. **G,** Retrieved separated instrument measured actually 2 mm on a ruler in contrast with the coronal portion of the fractured instrument. **H,** Postoperative radiograph showing the final root fillings, which reveals dentin sacrifice for removal of the separated instrument was minimum.

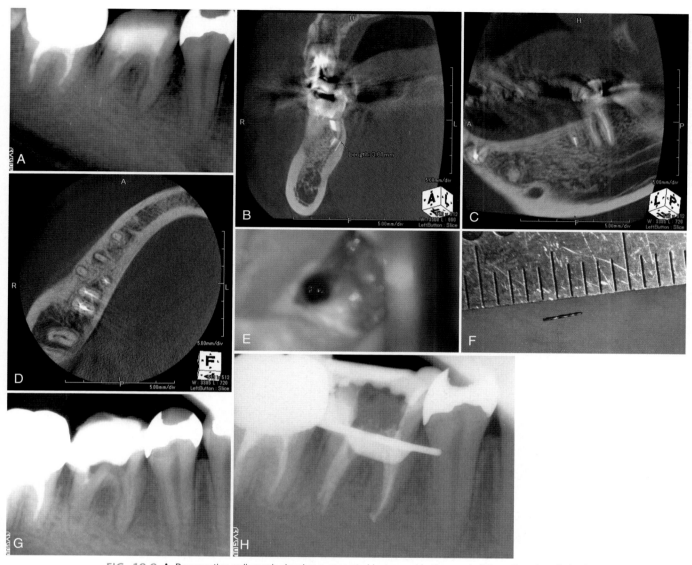

FIG. 19-9 A, Preoperative radiograph showing a separated instrument in the canal of the radix entomolaris of the mandibular right first molar. **B,** Coronal view of CBCT showing the separated instrument measuring 3.01 mm beyond the curve of the radix entomolaris, which suggests the separated instrument can be removed with ultrasonics alone. **C,** Sagittal view of CBCT showing the radicular end of the separated instrument is beyond the radicular foramen (*white arrow*). **D,** Axial view of CBCT showing the separated instrument in the canal of the radix entomolaris (*white arrow*). **E,** Magnification of the coronal portion of the separated instrument in the canal (*white arrow*). Removal of this instrument was considered easy as it was visible under the DOM. A small space was created on the inside curve of the canal with the FRK-12 ultrasonic tip. **F,** Retrieved instrument measuring 3 mm on a ruler. **G,** Interoperative radiograph taken after the separated instrument was removed (*white arrow*). **H,** Postoperative radiograph showing root fillings in all the canals revealing the dentin sacrifice for removal of the separated instrument from the radix entomolaris was not significant, compared to the root canal space on the preoperative radiograph.

an endodontic explorer such as a DG16 Endo Explorer (Hu-Friedy, Chicago, IL) (Fig. 19-11). The tip of a DG16 is placed in the loop and the loop is contracted around it. The apical portion of the DG16 is used to make the loop size smaller and the coronal portion is used to make it larger when the loop is tightened around it. The loop is then pre-bent at 45 degrees (Fig. 19-10, *B* and *C*) to facilitate the placement of the loop over the separated instrument. The loop is then brought into the canal and placed over the exposed portion of the separated file as the loop is pushed back at 90 degrees upon

it. Subsequently, the loop is tightened over the separated instrument by sliding down the handle (Fig. 19-10, *C*). The separated instrument will be retrieved by pulling the loop out of the canal in various directions in swaying motions to dislodge it from the canal walls (Fig. 19-10, *D*). A couple of pull motions in several directions will usually dislodge the file fragment and complete the case for separated file removal.

Surgical approaches for the management of separated instruments represent a second category of procedures for dealing with this iatrogenic event (see also Chapter 9).

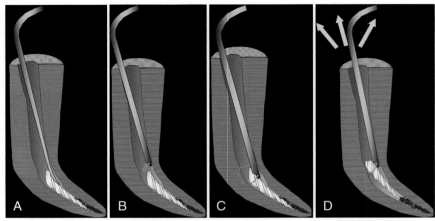

FIG. 19-10 **A,** Coronal portion of the separated file should be exposed at least 0.7 mm above the bottom of the space created around it. **B,** Approaching the separated file with the loop bent at 45 degrees against it. **C,** Loop is pushed back at 90 degrees as it is placed over the separated file. Removal with the loop requires the diameters of the loop device (0.16 mm ~ 0.45 mm) and the separated instrument and a depth of at least 0.7 mm. **D,** Separated file is pulled out with the loop device in various directions.

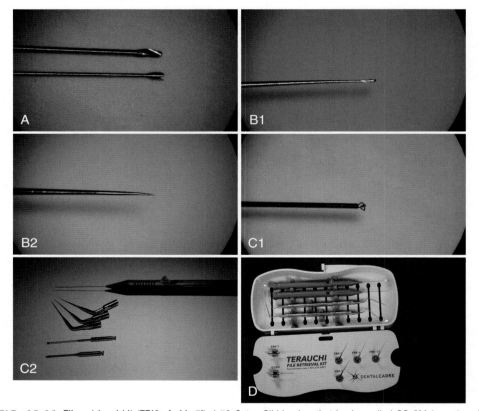

FIG. 19-11 **File retrieval kit (FRK). A,** Modified #3 Gates Glidden bur that is also called GG-3M (upper) and microtrephine bur that is also called FRK-T (lower). **B1,** FRK-6 ultrasonic tip (the tip portion looks like a spoon and is also called a spoon tip. It has a micro-concave on the spoon, which turns toward the handpiece at the 6 o'clock position. **B2,** FRK-S ultrasonic tip (the tip portion looks like a sharp spear and is also called a straight tip). **C1,** Yoshi loop, which captures a separated instrument. This micro-lasso is comprised of a tiny wire loop at the end of a stainless steel cannula, with a sliding handle that tightens the loop when pulled. **C2,** Yoshi loop holding a separated file from an actual case. Note that the loop holding the files requires 0.7 mm in length and width. **D,** File retrieval kit (FRK) in an autoclavable cassette case. The kit includes a GG-3M, FRK-T, FRK-6 ultrasonic tip, FRK-12 ultrasonic tip, FRK-S ultrasonic tip, Yoshi loop, gutta-percha removal (GPR) instrument, and a microexplorer instrument.

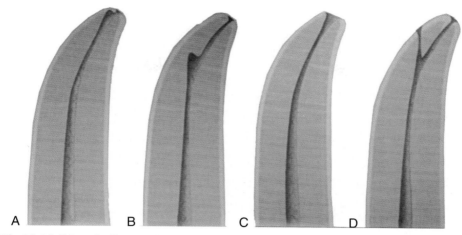

FIG. 19-12 Schematic diagrams showing the most common preparation errors. **A,** Radicular zip. **B,** Ledge. **C,** Radicular zip with perforation. **D,** Ledge with perforation.

Surgical approaches should be considered in the following situations[174]:

◆ As a last resort if other nonsurgical approaches fail, post-treatment disease develops, and the tooth is strategically important to retain

◆ As a first approach when periradicular pathosis is present at the time of instrument separation, especially if the separated instrument is found in the apical third of the canal coexistent presumably with persistent extraradicular infection

◆ As a first approach when the radicular portion of the separated instrument is already outside the root, when an orthograde approach is unsuccessful, or when a significant amount of dentin must be sacrificed for instrument removal

Prognosis

When an endodontic instrument separates in a canal during cleaning and shaping procedures and if it hinders adequate cleaning of the canal, then the prognosis may be affected. Moreover, attempts to remove a separated instrument from a curved canal may cause additional complications such as excessive removal of dentin structure, secondary instrument fracture, root perforation, or even root fracture.[113,246,268,272] However, there are cases in which the prognosis is not compromised, depending on what stage of instrumentation the file fracture occurred, the preoperative diagnosis of the pulp and periradicular tissues, and whether or not the separated file can be removed or bypassed.[272] The presence of a separated instrument per se in a canal or outside the root does not necessarily condemn the case to postoperative disease. Rather, it is the residual presence of any infected tissue that determines the prognosis. The closer the root canal preparation is to the terminus at the time of instrument separation, the better the outcome will be.[291] It has been suggested that instrument separation occurring in a later stage of canal instrumentation, especially if it is at the apex, has the best prognosis because the canal is probably well debrided and may be relatively free from microorganisms.[290] If the preoperative canal is not infected, and no radicular periodontitis is associated with the root, then the presence of the separated instrument should not affect the prognosis[50] and the separated instrument can be incorporated into root canal filling materials. If the separated file can be removed predictably without sacrificing a significant amount

of dentin, the prognosis will not be reduced. In other words, the treatment prognosis depends more on the removal of microbial infection than on instrument removal.

LEDGE FORMATION

Ledges may be created as a result of instrumentation causing radicular transportation, which also causes zipping of the canal and possible canal perforation (Fig. 19-12). The Glossary of Endodontic Terms of the American Association of Endodontists[10] defines a ledge as "an artificial irregularity created on the surface of the root canal wall that impedes the placement of an instrument to the apex of an otherwise patent canal." Canal transportation[10] is defined as "the removal of canal wall structure on the outside curve in the radicular half of the canal due to the tendency of files to restore themselves to their original linear shape during canal preparation." The presence of a ledge hinders adequate shaping and cleaning of the canal in the areas radicular to the ledge. Consequently, there is a possible causal relationship between ledge formation and an unfavorable endodontic treatment outcome.[48,49,99,105,112,137,188,319]

Causes of Ledge Formation

Ledge formation can occur during biomechanical preparation of the canal system, especially when the canals are more curved. There are a number of factors associated with ledge formation such as the instrumentation technique, instrument type, root canal curvature, tooth type, working length, master radicular file size, clinician's level of expertise, and canal location. Failure to precurve the instruments, the inability to achieve a proper glide path to the apex, and forcing large files into curved canals are perhaps the most common reasons for ledge formation.[131] The incidence of ledge formation was reported to increase significantly when the curvature of the canal was greater than 20 degrees; more than 50% of the canals in the study were ledged when the canal curvature was greater than 30 degrees.[99] Jafarzadeh[134] described 14 possible causes of ledge formation (Box 19-1).

Management of Ledge Formation

Once a canal is ledged, the endodontic treatment becomes difficult and the prognosis may be compromised. When a ledge is formed, early recognition of its location, using radiographs including CBCT and magnification, will facilitate its management.[105] The canal is usually "straightened" at the point where the file stops negotiating the curve, and there is suddenly a looser feeling of the file within the canal, with no more tactile sensation of the tip of the instrument binding in the canal. If the radiograph reveals that the tip of the instrument deviates away from the canal curvature, then it is highly likely that a ledge formation has occurred on the canal wall.

When a ledge formation is identified, the shortest file possible that can reach the working length should be selected to bypass the ledge. Shorter instruments have more stiffness and allow the clinician's fingers to be placed closer to the tip of the instrument, which consequently provides greater tactile sensation and more control over the instrument.[134] It usually requires determination, perseverance, and patience to bypass a ledge once it is formed.[48] The successful management of a ledge depends on whether both the ledge and the orifice of the original pathway can be visualized, reached, or felt with instruments.[166] Any case where the ledge can be visualized under the DOM may be considered less complex to treat. Cases whereby the ledge is not directly visible are more difficult to treat, as tactile sensation and negotiation require patience and experience.[48] However, 3D radiographic images obtained from CBCT reveal the locations and the directions of both the ledge and the original pathway to the canal terminus, which provides additional information for diagnosis and therefore helps the clinician manage the ledge formation with a more predictable outcome and negotiate the original canal.[203]

Bypassing a Ledge

Using Hand Instruments

Precurving of a #8 or #10 hand file is a critical step in bypassing a ledge. The small file should have a distinct curve at the tip (that is, in the radicular 2 to 3 mm) (Fig. 19-13). This file should be used initially to negotiate past the ledge and explore the original pathway of the canal to the radicular foramen.[48,131,299]

A rubber stopper with a directional indicator is valuable in this situation because the indicator can be pointed in the same direction as the bend placed in the instrument.[131] A slight rotation of the file combined with a "pecking" motion can often help advance the instrument to the full working length of the canal.[131,299] Whenever resistance to negotiation is met, the file should be retracted slightly, rotated, and then advanced again with the precurved tip facing in a different direction. This action should be repeated until the file consistently bypasses the ledge.[131] If this technique is unsuccessful, the clinician should flare the canal coronal to the ledge in an anticurvature direction to obtain wider straight-line access to the original pathway of the canal beyond the ledge, followed by a #10 K-file with the tip precurved to bypass the ledge (see Fig. 19-13). Small hand files dedicated to the microscopic use (such as the micro-opener with #10/.06 taper) may help flare the orifice of the original pathway beyond the ledge. The use of such small micro–hand files under the DOM with magnification and illumination helps the clinician locate the original pathway and facilitate bypassing the ledge. The micro-opener is available only in 16 mm and it is short enough to provide tactile sensation and better control. However, in some cases a longer instrument is required to reach the ledge present in the radicular third of a long canal. In these instances, a hand instrument holder such as an EndoHandle (Venta, Logan, UT) may help the clinician easily negotiate the canal radicular to the ledge. Any hand files can be attached to the handle for microscopic use. Other hand instruments are available specifically for this purpose (microexplorer instrument, DentalCadre and ELES instrument, DenMat Lompoc, CA) that are long enough to reach the ledge formed in the radicular third. Both of the instruments are made of stainless steel. The microexplorer is used to explore the original canal and penetrate a narrow canal beyond the ledge, while the ELES is used to reduce the ledge as the tip portion is coated with fine diamond particles. They can be used in sequence to reduce or remove the ledge. The microexplorer instrument can be precurved as it has a smooth surfaced tip to get into the original pathway beyond the ledge (Fig. 19-14), whereas the ELES instrument has diamond coating on the tip to enlarge the original pathway (Fig. 19-15). The microexplorer instrument has a 0.1 mm biconical tip with a .08 taper for the first 1-mm portion from the radicular end and a .06 taper for the next 10-mm portion, which gives the instrument more stability in push-pull motions than a .02 tapered K-file, while the tip diameter of the ELES instrument is 0.2 mm with a .06 taper. The maximum diameter of the microexplorer instruments is 0.78 mm, which provides stability and maintains a high visibility under the DOM when it is precurved. On the other hand, the maximum diameter of the ELES instrument is 0.68 mm, which provides flexibility and visibility even around a curve. Once the first microexplorer instrument has successfully bypassed the ledge, subsequently the ELES instrument can be used to enlarge and reestablish the original pathway (Fig. 19-16), followed by hand instruments (such as ProTaper S1 and S2 hand instruments, DENTSPLY Tulsa Dental Specialties, Tulsa, OK) to both reduce the ledge and complete the shape. #15/.04 and #15/.06 Vortex Blue rotary files (DENTSPLY Tulsa Dental Specialties) can also be precurved with ease and used as hand files in short pumping motions to reduce the ledge after the preliminary enlargement of the original pathway with the micro-hand instruments.

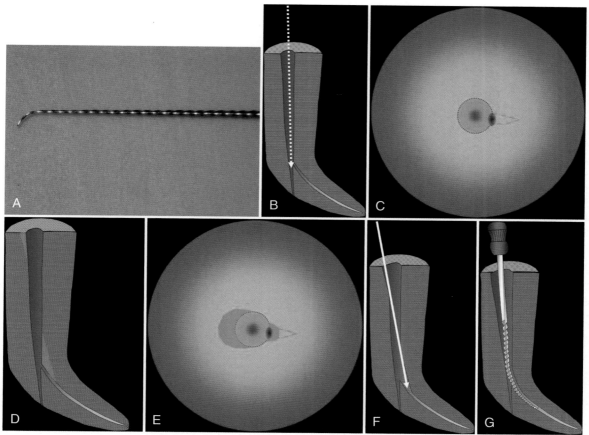

FIG. 19-13 A, Ledge removal instrument (microexplorer) to explore a canal for impediments and to penetrate a narrow canal beyond a ledge. B, Ledge is formed with perforation in a radicular straight direction. C, Microscopic view showing the ledged canal in the center and a narrow access to the original pathway on the right side. D, The canal orifice as well as the access to the original pathway needs to be flared in an anticurvature direction *(red portions)*. E, Microscopic view showing red portions to be removed for easy access to the original pathway. F, Access to the original pathway was flared to facilitate file insertion. G, Bypassing file used in short push-pull strokes to create a distinct pathway to the original canal as the final glide path.

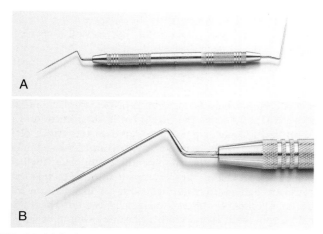

FIG. 19-14 Ledge removal instrument (Microexplorer) to explore and penetrate a canal.

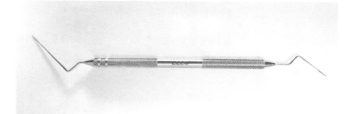

FIG. 19-15 Ledge removal instrument with diamond coating (ELES) to bypass/eliminate/reduce a ledge and enlarge the orifice of the original pathway.

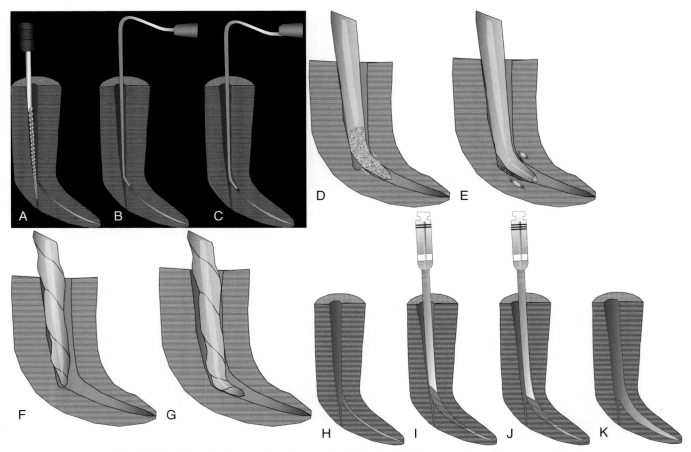

FIG. 19-16 Schematic diagrams showing bypassing the ledge with ledge removal hand instruments. **A**, Ledge is created in a radicular straight direction around a curve. **B**, Original pathway is explored and opened up with the microexplorer instrument in short push-pull strokes. **C**, Original pathway is widened with the ELES instrument. **D**, ELES instrument used in push-pull motions to reduce the ledge. **E**, Precurved straight ultrasonic tip can also be used here to reduce the ledge instead of the ELES instrument. **F**, File with a biconical tip is brought into the canal to eliminate/reduce the ledge and negotiate the original canal. The primary cone of the biconical tip has no cutting tip. As it hits the curve or irregularities on the canal wall, it will slip alongside the curve and scoot over the irregularities. **G**, Secondary cone of the biconical tip removes the points at the transition angles and provides a smooth surface that guides the tip portion into the original pathway. **H**, Orifice of the original canal beyond the ledge needs to be enlarged for easy file insertion after the ledge has been bypassed successfully. **I**, Orifice of the original canal can be efficiently widened with a precurved instrument such as a ProTaper S1 hand file and a #15/.04 Vortex Blue rotary file used as a hand file, and the apical patency established. **J**, Original canal can be sequentially prepared with more tapered NiTi files. **K**, Postoperative canal showing the ledge is significantly eliminated.

Using Ultrasonic Tips

Small diameter ultrasonic tips improve visibility with the added benefit of reducing the need for sacrificing sound dentin in bypassing or removing the ledge.[167] The only drawback to the thinner tips could be that they are more prone to fracture during ultrasonic activation.[298] Therefore, thinner ultrasonic tips should be activated in a pulsing fashion at the lowest possible power setting to prevent fracture and heat generation.

The use of longer ultrasonic tips may also facilitate bypassing or reducing the ledge in the radicular third as long as it is performed under the DOM. The orifice of the original canal just coronal to the ledge should be enlarged. If the ledged portion of the canal can be visualized under the DOM, then ultrasonic instruments should be used over hand instruments (Fig. 19-17). First, an appropriate size of a small diameter

ultrasonic tip (such as the straight ultrasonic tip, DentalCadre, Seattle, WA) is selected and precurved in the direction of the original canal. Then it is simply placed in the orifice of the original pathway to the radicular foramen and activated, which will automatically enlarge the opening of the true canal in a few seconds. Ultrasonic tips can cut dentin faster than hand instruments and widen the orifice of the original pathway more easily so that files can consecutively be placed into the original canal for root canal preparation. Ultrasonics should be used on the lowest power setting to avoid overextending the ledge, as ultrasonics may get very aggressive in cutting.[243] Once the orifice of the original pathway gets wide enough for file insertion, negotiation files need to be placed into the canal to establish patency and to smooth out the irregularities on the canal wall that may have been created with ultrasonics,

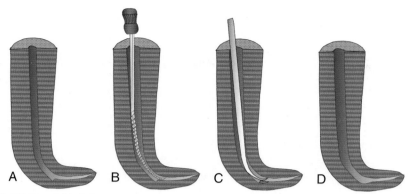

FIG. 19-17 Non-visible ledge removal with ultrasonics. **A,** Ledge formed beyond the curve. CBCT is taken to locate both the ledge and the original pathway. **B,** Canal coronal to the ledge is flared in an anticurvature direction with NiTi rotary files in brushing motions. Original pathway to the canal terminus is explored with a #10 precurved K-file or the precurved microexplorer instrument and radiographs are taken with it inserted in the canal to see if it is in the original canal beyond the ledge. **C,** Straight ultrasonic tip is precurved the same way as the hand instrument used and placed in the canal to eliminate/reduce the ledge. The red portion needs to be smoothed out to facilitate the insertion of an instrument into the original pathway. **D,** Postoperative canal showing the ledge is significantly reduced.

followed by root canal preparation with NiTi rotary or hand files (Figs. 19-18, 19-19).

Using Rotary Instruments

Pre-curved rotary PathFiles are also beneficial for negotiating past a ledge. First the radicular 2 to 3 mm of the #13 PathFile is precurved at 30 to 45 degrees and is rotated at 100 rpm or slower as it is brought slowly into the canal and moved radicularly. If a ledge or sharp radicular curvature is encountered, the instrument is withdrawn about 1 mm and immediately reinserted. This allows the precurved tip to move to a different orientation within the canal as it is reinserted. This may require one or two withdrawals and re-insertions to negotiating the original canal. This procedure is followed in sequence by the #16 and #19 PathFiles to preliminarily enlarge the original pathway and reduce the ledge prior to the conventional root canal preparation with NiTi rotary instruments.

Potential Complications of Removal or Bypassing a Ledge

During ledge removal or bypassing a ledge, complications can occur, including root fracture, root perforation, worsening the ledge, and instrument separation. Since a ledge is likely to form around a curve, attempts to bypass or eliminate it may often involve dentin sacrifice, which may eventually compromise the integrity of the tooth and increase the risk of perforation or root fracture. Care should be taken not to remove excessive root structure or overstress the instruments during the ledge removal process. If a ledge cannot be bypassed with any of the techniques described earlier, and if signs or symptoms of the periradicular lesion persist, then the treatment options are limited to surgical intervention such as periradicular surgery or intentional replantation.[131]

Prevention of Ledge Formation

Passive step-back and balanced force techniques are two beneficial methods of canal preparation that reduce the chances of ledge formation.[131,299] Moreover, it has been proposed that an advantage of the step-back technique is that this method tends to minimize procedural errors such as transportation and ledge formation.[298] Each file is used in sequence with circumferential filing to remove any irregularities before a larger diameter file is placed. The effective use of circumferential filing, especially with Hedström files, will ensure smoothness of the canal walls and flaring toward the coronal end of the canal, which will help to prevent the formation of ledges.[105,299] Precurving the instruments and not forcing them into the canal is one of the most important considerations in the prevention of ledge formation.[131]

The use of NiTi files and instruments with noncutting tips helps to maintain original root canal curvatures.[131] The concept of use of these instruments is that the rounded tip does not cut into the wall but will slip alongside it.[130,131] In addition to the tip design, flexibility of an instrument also plays an important role for keeping the instrument centered in the canal, with NiTi instruments favored over stainless steel instruments.[121,128,196] Compared to stainless steel instruments, NiTi instruments offered less canal transportation, more dentin conservation, and reduced risk of zipping or stripping curved canals.[69,95,201]

Prognosis

A ledge in a canal is analogous to any intracanal obstruction that hinders the cleaning and shaping of the root canal to the radicular terminus. The presence of a non-negotiated ledge may have a similar prognosis as a canal with a retained separated instrument. If the ledge can be bypassed or eliminated, and if the canal beyond the ledge can be cleaned without excessive enlargement or perforation, then the prognosis should not be that greatly reduced.[290,291] The amount of debris and bacteria left in the canal apical to the ledge greatly influences the prognosis.

PERFORATIONS (NONSURGICAL)

The topic of nonsurgical perforations, whether by caries, access bur, or post drill, and whether occurring in the furcation or

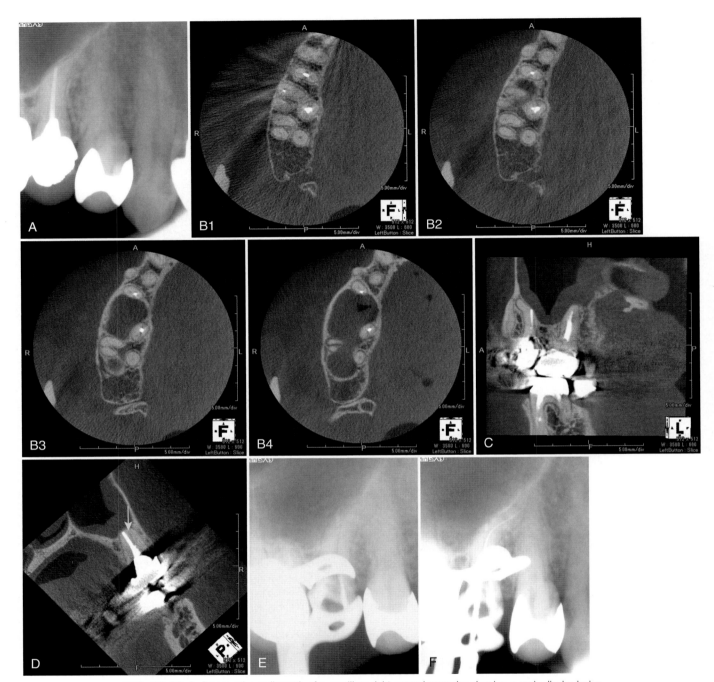

FIG. 19-18 **A,** Preoperative radiograph of a maxillary right second premolar showing a periradicular lesion. Note the root filling in a radicular straight direction deviates away from the radicular foramen. **B,** A series of CBCT images in axial view from the coronal third to the middle third (**B1** to **B4**) reveals the original pathway (*red arrows*) curves in a mesiobuccal direction with the root filling turning away from the original canal. **C,** CBCT image in sagittal view clearly shows the original pathway in relation to the root filling. **D,** CBCT image in coronal view also shows the root filling alongside the original pathway (*red arrow*). **E,** Radiograph showing the root filling coronal to the ledge was removed. Original pathway to the radicular foramen was enlarged with an ultrasonic tip. **F,** Radiograph showing the original canal beyond the ledge was renegotiated with a #10 K-file.

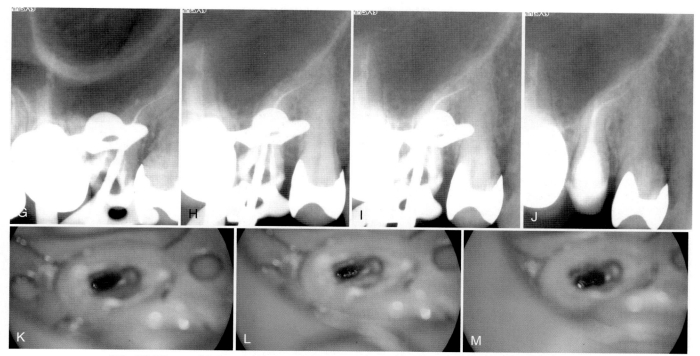

FIG. 19-18, cont'd **G,** Radiograph showing the original canal was flared with a TF adaptive SM1 rotary file used as a hand file in push-pull motions. **H,** Radiograph showing the original canal was sequentially more tapered with a TF Adaptive SM2 rotary file used as a hand file. **I,** Radiograph showing the final root canal preparation of the original canal with a #20/.06 Vortex Blue rotary file used as a hand file. **J,** Postoperative radiograph showing the obturation of the original canal. **K,** Magnification of the original canal orifice side by side with the root filling in the ledged canal. Note the locations of the original canal and the ledge are exactly the same as shown on the axial view of CBCT **B3. L,** Magnification of the original canal showing it was flared with the precurved straight ultrasonic tip. **M,** Magnification of the original canal showing the original canal was completely shaped to the canal terminus with NiTi instruments.

canal space, has been extensively discussed in other chapters of this text. For ease of reference, the various locations and topics are as follows:

- Chapter 8: Nonsurgical Retreatment. Clinical examples of nonsurgical repair of furcation and midlevel perforations, with descriptions of the latest techniques and materials, illustrated with clinical photographs and radiographs. Listed also are the appropriate literature references, indications and contraindications for the repairs presented, and protocols for treatment management.
- Chapter 5: Tooth Morphology and Access Cavity Preparation. Diagrams of perforations and repairs.
- Chapter 29: Endodontic Records and Legal Responsibilities. Legal implications and clinician responsibilities.
- Chapter 26: Effects of Age and Systemic Health on Endodontics. Radiographs of perforations secondary to endodontic attempts in calcified canals.

RADICULAR EXTRUSION OF ROOT CANAL FILLING MATERIALS

The extrusion of root filling materials beyond the radicular foramen may occur either when the canal is obturated or during the removal of obturation materials. Radicularly extruded materials such as obturating materials, necrotic pulp tissue, bacteria, medicaments, and irrigants have been associated with posttreatment inflammation and flare-up or the lack of radicular healing.[186,254,261,289] In vivo histologic studies show the most favorable histologic outcome when the root filling material remains within the radicular constriction. When gutta-percha is extruded into the periradicular tissue, there can be a severe inflammatory reaction.[232] However, other materials such as ProRoot MTA (DENTSPLY Tulsa Dental Specialties) are more biocompatible[1,98,144] and do not seem to produce much periradicular inflammation if extruded beyond the root of the tooth.[75,267]

Studies show that almost all instrumentation techniques promote the radicular extrusion of debris including root filling materials.[8,122,283] Furthermore, gutta-percha and Resilon filling materials obtained from teeth associated with refractory radicular periodontitis have indicated the presence of bacterial biofilm and *E. faecalis*.[102,187,196,255] Another study stressed the possibility of gutta-percha–centered *E. faecalis* biofilm as well as the role of tissue fluids such as saliva and serum in the biofilm formation.[90] *E. faecalis* adheres well to gutta-percha with and without canal sealers, with the biofilm formation more effective when it is in contact with serum in periradicular tissues. Because bacterial biofilm is considered the primary cause of chronic and recurrent endodontic infections,[292] it is crucial to keep gutta-percha filling materials within the canal system as much as possible to prevent potential periradicular periodontitis.

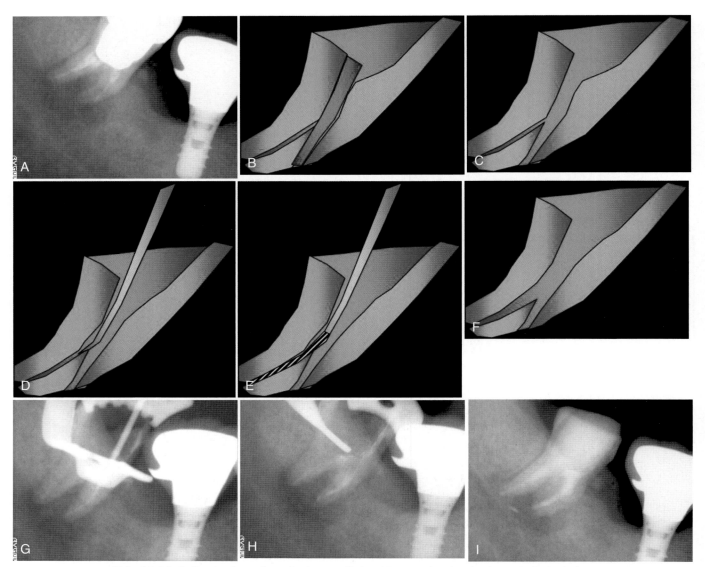

FIG. 19-19 **A,** Preoperative radiograph of a mandibular right second molar showing periradicular lesions associated with the mesial and distal roots. Note the root filling in the mesial root deviates away from the center of the root. **B,** Schematic diagram showing gutta-percha root filling materials in the ledged canal of the mesial root. **C,** Root filling materials were removed chemomechanically from the mesial root. **D,** Original pathway to the radicular foramen was explored and enlarged with the microexplorer and a pre-curved FRK-S ultrasonic tip. **E,** Original canal beyond the ledge was renegotiated with a #10 K-file, followed by a #15 K file. **F,** Schematic diagram showing the original canal shaped to the canal terminus. **G,** Interoperative radiograph showing root canal preparation of the original canal with a ProTaper S1 file. **H,** Postoperative radiograph showing root canals filled with MTA both in mesial and distal roots. **I,** Three-month postoperative radiograph showing periradicular healing.

Uncontrolled obturation can cause the extrusion of root canal filling materials into the maxillary sinus[67] or into the territory of the inferior alveolar nerve (IAN).[214] Serious complications such as maxillary sinusitis, aspergillosis infection, paresthesia, dysesthesia, and similar neural complications may occur after extruding the root filling materials into such sensitive areas.[176]

Endodontic-related paresthesia can be caused mechanically or chemically via the passage of endodontic materials into the vicinity of the major nerves such as the IAN or its branches.[3] These materials include root canal irrigants, sealers, and paraformaldehyde-containing pastes.[297] Because of the potential

for chemical degeneration of the nerve axons, the use of paraformaldehyde-containing pastes is not recommended for endodontic obturation.[183,217] The optimum pH of an endodontic medicament should be as close as possible to that of body fluids, which is around 7.35. Significantly higher or lower pHs are likely to cause cellular necrosis of tissues when they are in direct contact with these materials. The clinician must also consider the pH of some of the routinely used endodontic and related dental materials. It has been reported that an alkaline pH of root canal sealers could neutralize the lactic acid from osteoclasts and prevent dissolution of mineralized components of teeth; therefore, root canal sealers, especially calcium silicate–based cements or sealers, can contribute to hard tissue formation by activating alkaline phosphatase.[276] Commonly used endodontic medicaments are as follows[39,87,226,260]:

- Formocresol: pH 12.45 +/− 0.02
- Sodium hypochlorite: pH 11 to 12
- Calcium hydroxide (Calyxl): pH 10 to 14
- ProRoot MTA: pH 11.7 to 7.12 at 3 hours to 28 days
- Endosequence BC Sealer: pH 10.31 to 11.16 at 3 hours to 240 hours
- MTA Fillapex: pH 9.68 to 7.76 at 3 hours to 168 hours
- AH plus: pH 7.81 to 7.17 at 3 hours to 240 hours
- Antibiotic-corticosteroid paste (Ledermix): pH 8.13 +/− 0.01
- Eugenol: pH 4.34 +/−0.05
- Iodoform paste: pH 2.90 +/−0.02

Neural damage from these materials may be permanent and can cause neuropathic pain (i.e., dysesthesia) or anesthesia.

Orbital pain and headache may occur secondary to the local compression of overextended material into the maxillary sinus.[311] Sinus infection caused by zinc-oxide-eugenol–based filling materials extruded into the maxillary sinus is often associated with aspergillus growth[18,19,93,151,236] (Fig. 19-20). Although aspergillosis of the paranasal sinuses is a relatively rare finding in non-immunocompromised patients, it is known as an opportunistic infection.[143] Many studies have demonstrated that maxillary sinus aspergillosis is generally caused by extruded root canal filling material containing zinc oxide and formaldehyde.[18,19,151,163,274] Besides maxillary sinus infections, the overextension of root filling materials such as gutta-percha into the maxillary sinus may also cause mechanical irritation.[149] When paresthesia is involved, it is thought to occur more from mechanical or thermal insult to the affected neurons.[217] In addition, although such substances are not considered toxic,[270] they may cause an additional foreign body reaction. Inflammation caused by mechanical irritation is likely to persist until the extruded materials are removed, and it may become permanent secondary to the mechanical, thermal, or chemical insult.[114] The incidence of IAN damage has been reported to be up to 1% of cases when performing a root canal filling of a lower premolar.[148] This overextension may cause an unnecessary mechanical or chemical irritation, which hinders repair of the periradicular tissue and thus diminishes the probability of a successful prognosis. The patient may also experience sharp, localized posttreatment pain, which may or may not resolve. When the inferior alveolar nerve is injured, the pain is not only located in the immediate periradicular area but may radiate and refer to the surrounding or distant structures.[195]

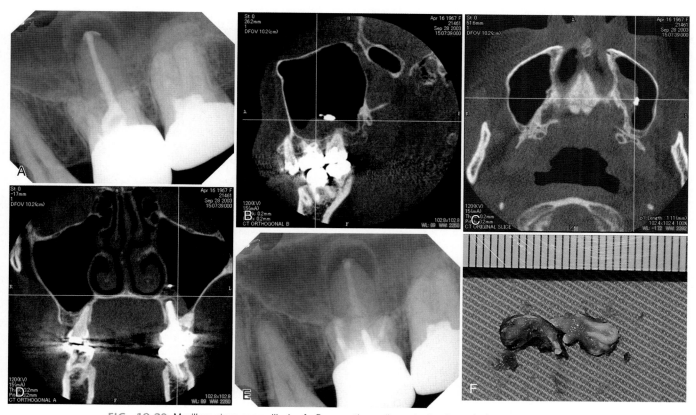

FIG. 19-20 Maxillary sinus aspergillosis. **A,** Preoperative radiograph showing a lesion associated with the palatal root, from which the extrusion of the root filling materials occurred in the maxillary sinus. **B,** CBCT image in sagittal view showing the relation between mucositis on the maxillary sinus floor and the gutta-percha filling material. **C,** CBCT image in axial view showing the relation between mucositis on the mesial wall of the maxillary sinus and the extruded root filling materials. **D,** CBCT image in coronal view showing the relation between the palatal root and the extruded root filling materials. **E,** Postoperative radiograph of orthograde root canal retreatment on the maxillary left first molar showing the mesiobuccal, distobuccal, and palatal root canals were adequately filled without overextension of the filling materials. **F,** Aspergillus was found on the filling materials retrieved from the maxillary sinus.

One study with a 10-year follow-up reported that the overall success rate of endodontic treatment was 91%, with the best prognosis achieved when the obturation was under 0 to 2 mm from the apex.[262] Consequently, radicular extrusion of root canal filling materials must be avoided as much as possible to obtain optimal results.

Causes of Extrusion of Obturation Materials Beyond the Radicular Foramen

The extrusion of obturation material that was thought to be the cause of endodontic failure is reported to be as low as 3%,[266] with the majority of causes thought to be more from coronal leakage. However, several researchers have seen a higher frequency of failure and unhealed periradicular lesions in cases where the root filling material had extruded beyond the radicular foramen.[23,34,209] Overextension of the root canal filling materials occurs mainly for lack of material control.[36,106] The degree of extrusion of obturation materials into periradicular tissues depends on the techniques used for root canal preparation and obturation,[233] which include accidental overinstrumentation and incorrect canal working length measurement. Caution should also be taken when obturating a canal with open apices and larger minor foramen diameters, which are often found in cases with radicular inflammatory resorption. Warm vertical compaction techniques produce a homogeneous obturation that adapts well to the canal walls[249,309] but may result in the extrusion of gutta-percha filling into the periradicular tissues.[36] Carrier-based obturation was also found to have more radicular extrusion of gutta-percha when compared with warm vertical compaction.[158] The type of canal shaping may also be a contributing factor. The canal shape created with the Profile GT system is more prone to extrusion of gutta-percha when obturated with the carrier-based technique than the canal shape created using Profile 0.06 instruments. The Profile GT system created a more parallel preparation coronally and a tapered preparation radicularly, whereas the Profile 0.06 system created a preparation with uniform taper from the apex to its most coronal extent.[233] Therefore, possibly the more continuously tapered the canal shape is, the less obturation material is extruded beyond the radicular foramen.

When endodontic retreatment is performed, irritants in the form of root filling materials can be extruded into the periradicular tissues.[8,122,283] Techniques involving push-pull filing strokes usually create a greater mass of debris than those involving some sort of rotational motions.[6,32,76,142,178,222]

Management of Obturation Materials Extruded Beyond the Radicular Foramen

Nonsurgical Management of Extrusion of Obturation Materials

Methods to remove the gutta-percha filling material from the root canal include the use of heat-carrying instruments, ultrasonics, solvents, and rotary or hand files. Mechanized methods to remove filling materials are faster but possibly not more effective than manual methods.[141,282] Heat-carrying instrument may damage the periradicular tissues if the removal attempts extend beyond the radicular foramen. The complete removal of gutta-percha from the root canal system has proven difficult.[108,282] Poorly compacted gutta-percha obturation can easily be removed with Hedstrom files and solvents such as

chloroform,[46,132] although the extruded portion of root canal fillings will often remain in the periradicular tissue[46] (Fig. 19-21). The relative ease of gutta-percha removal suggests a failure of previous endodontic treatment, possibly related to poor obturation compaction or canal shaping, which resulted in both radicular extrusion and failure of the radicular seal. Comparatively, well-filled canals with radicular extrusion do not appear to have a significant failure rate.[13,132] On the other hand, the extrusion of the MTA root filling material into the periradicular tissues does not appear to negatively affect the periradicular healing due to the high biocompatibility and antibacterial properties that the calcium silicate–based cement possesses,[171,281] compared to gutta-percha filling materials (Fig. 19-22).

When gutta-percha is overextended into the periradicular space, removal can be attempted by inserting a new Hedstrom file, usually a #15 or #20, into the radicular obturation, using a gentle clockwise rotation to a depth of 0.5 to 1 mm beyond the radicular constriction. The file is then slowly and firmly withdrawn with no rotation, thereby engaging and removing the overextended material.[180] This technique works frequently, but care must be taken not to force the instrument, or further extrusion of the gutta-percha or separation of the file may result. The overextended radicular portion of the gutta-percha should not be softened with heat or solvent, because this application can decrease the likelihood of the Hedstrom file engaging the obturation, hindering its retrieval.[273] In addition, care should be taken not to overextend the file into the area of the inferior alveolar nerve canal, which could cause irreversible damage to the associated nerves.

The use of rotary NiTi files that are specifically designed for gutta-percha removal appears to be effective[124,265] include Pro-Taper Universal Retreatment files (DENTSPLY Tulsa Dental Specialties), Mtwo R rotary files (VDW, Munich, Germany), R-Endo retreatment files (Micromega, Besancon, France), and hand instruments such Micro-debriders (DENTSPLY Maillefer, Ballaigues, Switzerland), EGPR-L/R/U/D (G. Hartzell & Son, Concord, CA), and the gutta-percha removal instrument (DentalCadre). The self-adjusting file (SAF) (ReDent-Nova, Ra'anana, Israel) is also effective in removing obturation material, especially the remaining gutta-percha after conventional retreatment. Its variable shape and scraping motion allow it to touch a higher percentage of root canal walls than rotary instruments, facilitating effective cleaning.[181] Literature has shown that significantly less debris was extruded with the rotary retreatment files during endodontic retreatment compared with other traditional techniques using Hedström files with chloroform,[124] although all techniques resulted in some radicular extrusion.[124,265] ProTaper Universal Retreatment files have been reported to remove gutta-percha from the canals in large pieces around the spirals of instruments, whereas Hedström files generally remove gutta-percha in small increments.[124] Furthermore, a combination of both rotary instruments for initial quick removal of gutta-percha and hand instruments to refine and complete the cleaning of the canal, especially in the radicular third of the root, shows the better protocol for obtaining clean canal walls during endodontic retreatment.[24,129]

In difficult retreatment cases where root canal fillings persistently remain in the periradicular tissues, the use of a solvent, such as chloroform, may help to dissolve the remaining gutta-percha. In addition, chloroform has been reported to be capable of reducing the intracanal levels of *Enterococcus*

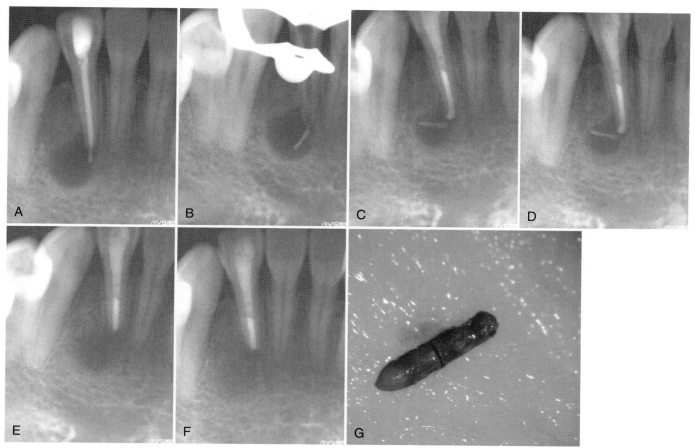

FIG. 19-21 Root filling materials extruded beyond the radicular foramen. **A,** Preoperative radiograph showing overextension of the root filling material with a large lesion associated with the root. **B,** Root filling in the canal was mechanically removed, but the extruded portion of it remained in the periradicular tissues. **C,** MTA was filled in the canal with the extruded portion remaining in the lesion. **D,** Six-month postoperative radiograph showing the reduced size of the lesion, but the lesion surrounding the extruded portion stayed the same in size for the next 6 months, indicating infection of the extruded gutta-percha point. The extruded portion was surgically removed from the lesion at this point. **E,** 3-month follow-up radiograph after the surgery showing the healing lesion. **F,** 12-month follow-up radiograph after the surgery showing a more periradicular healing. **G,** Gutta-percha point retrieved from the lesion.

faecalis.[62,182] When chloroform is used during the early stages of gutta-percha removal, more filling material will remain in the canal and some of it may be extruded beyond the radicular foramen.[124,172] Although the carcinogenicity of chloroform in humans is suspect, chloroform is regarded as a safe and effective endodontic solvent, when used carefully.[44,177]

Unlike rotary instruments, the EGPR-L/R/U/D hand instruments and the gutta-percha removal instrument are 30 mm in length, allowing them to remove obturation material not only from the radicular third of the canal but also from the periradicular tissues through the radicular foramen. The microdebriders are designed to be used in conjunction with a dental operating microscope. They have a Hedström cutting configuration with a standard .02 taper in sizes 20 and 30 with 16 mm of cutting flutes, which may not be long enough to reach the gutta-percha filling material beyond the radicular foramen. The EGPR instrument has a tiny projection on one side of the tip for scratching and engaging the gutta-percha filling left on the canal wall. The overall diameter of the tip is 0.3 mm and the length of the projection is 0.1 mm. This hand instrument

works like a scraper on the canal wall. First, a small hole is created with a small diameter ultrasonic tip between the canal wall and the root filling material, and the instrument is brought into the canal with the projection facing away from the gutta-percha filling. When the radicular portion comes down to the bottom of the hole created, the projection is turned back on the gutta-percha filling so that it can be hooked on the projection pressed against it. Then the gutta-percha filling should be scraped and come apart in large pieces from the canal wall (Fig. 19-23, *A* to *C*).

The gutta-percha removal instrument has a tiny conical harpoon-shaped tip that is sharp and small enough to penetrate into a mass of gutta-percha filling and hook it on the rim on the return stroke. The tip portion of this instrument has a .40 taper with the minimum tip diameter of 0.1 mm and the maximum diameter of 0.3 mm with a 0.2-mm diameter shank supporting the tip portion. The 0.1-mm gap between the 0.3-mm and the 0.2-mm diameters works practically as a tiny circular projection over the shank portion that can hook a mass of gutta-percha fillings. Gutta-percha fillings can be separated

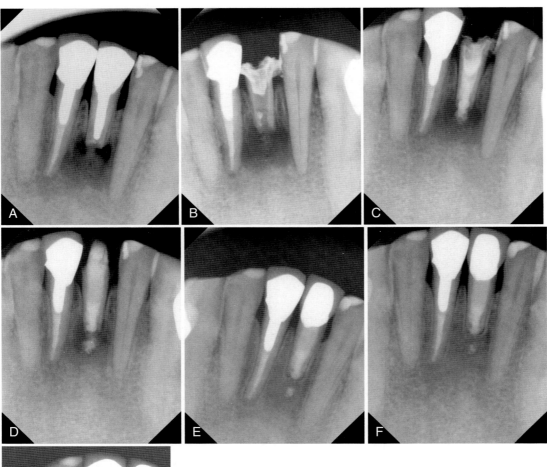

FIG. 19-22 **A,** Preoperative radiograph showing a large periradicular lesion associated with the root of the mandibular left incisor. **B,** Interoperative radiograph showing the cast post and the root filling in the canal was mechanically removed. Calcium hydroxide was placed as an intracanal dressing on the first appointment. **C,** Postoperative radiograph on the second appointment showing the canal was obturated with MTA, which resulted in overextension of the material into the periradicular tissues. **D,** Six-month postoperative radiograph showing the significantly reduced size of the lesion. **E,** One-year postoperative radiograph showing a nice periradicular healing with a residual of the MTA root filling extruded into the periradicular tissues. **F,** Three-year postoperative radiograph showing the tooth has maintained healthy periradicular tissues with the extruded MTA filling reduced in size. **G,** Twelve-year postoperative radiograph showing the tooth has maintained healthy periradicular tissues with the extruded MTA filling completely absorbed in the bone.

from the canal wall by wedging the tip between the gutta-percha and the canal wall. The gutta-percha filling can also be hooked by pressing the projecting rim against it, and then the gutta-percha filling should be removed in large pieces from the canal wall.

It is recommended that a small hole be created in the center of the gutta-percha filling with a small diameter ultrasonic tip to facilitate the root filling removal with the hand gutta-percha removal instrument placed into the hole. If the gutta-percha filling is poorly adapted to the canal wall with a large radicular diameter, the insertion space for the hand instrument should be created between the canal wall and the gutta-percha filling to avoid radicular extrusion of the root filling materials with the hand instrument or an ultrasonic tip. When a small amount

of gutta-percha filling remains on the inside curve or in the radicular third of the canal after the mechanical removal attempts, chloroform should be filled in the canal and the gutta-percha removal instrument can be used to agitate it in short push-and-pull motions in the canal, or even outside the canal if root filling is extruded beyond the radicular foramen, to actively dissolve the residual root filling.

Management of Tissue Damage Caused by Extrusion of Root Canal Filling Materials

When root canal filling material extends into the periradicular spaces, tissue damage may occur. The majority of these cases are managed by nonsurgical methods such as analgesics, cold

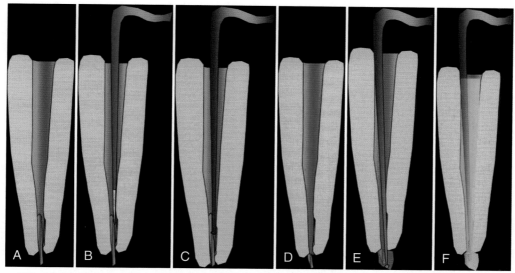

FIG. 19-23 Diagrams showing removal of gutta-percha filling materials extruded beyond the radicular foramen. **A,** Solid gutta-percha filling extruded beyond the radicular foramen. **B,** Small space is created between the canal wall and the gutta-percha filling with a thin ultrasonic tip (such as a FRK-S ultrasonic tip). **C,** Gutta-percha removal hand instrument, such as the GPR instrument and the EGPR instrument, is brought into the canal with the tiny projection pressed against the gutta-percha filling to pull it out. **D,** Extruded gutta-percha root filling portion separated from the coronal portion within the canal. **E,** Chloroform is filled in the canal using a gutta-percha removal hand instrument and agitating it to dissolve the extruded portion. **F,** Gutta-percha filling material is diluted and dissolved with the hand instrument in push-and-pull motions.

packs, corticosteroids, and antibiotics.[72] Dexamethasone is a corticosteroid that has been widely used in dentistry, and it seems to decrease periradicular inflammation caused by a foreign body[183] with minimal side effects.[52] If the tissue damage is extended to the IAN or maxillary sinus, a different approach may be necessary.

SINUS PERFORATION

There is a close proximity of maxillary premolars and molars to the sinus, and the apices of these teeth can be less than 2 mm from the floor of the sinus.[61] Pathologic destruction of the sinus floor may predispose a maxillary sinus communication,[253] producing an oroantral communication,[80,165,239,302] also known as an OAC. In general, exposure of the sinus lumen is well tolerated,[133,208] with no overt repercussions on healing. One investigator[302] found no significant difference in the healing of the mucosa in patients with and without intraoperative perforations and regeneration of the membrane, complete with cilia, in approximately 5 months following complete removal.[22] However, introduction of foreign materials during the access or apical resection/manipulation can initiate thickening of the sinus mucosa with symptoms of maxillary sinusitis.[65]

Conventional radiographs appear to be of limited value in predicting the potential for OAC, with the position of the root tip, periapical lesion, or outline of the lesion not statistically significant in that respect.[197] In contrast, a CBCT survey of the intended surgical field is much more informative, providing accurate measurements of the osseous thickness, distance to the sinus floor, and presence of pathosis.[28]

Maxillary sinus complications secondary to the extrusion of root canal filling material need to be managed differently. Approximately 10% of all patients with chronic sinusitis are found to have an aspergilloma.[101,168] It has been suggested that

root canal treated teeth with overextension of the root canal sealer into the maxillary sinus might be the main cause for aspergillosis in healthy patients.[18,19] Surgical intervention is usually the most predictable method for removing extruded root canal filling material and allowing for adequate healing secondary to IAN or sinus complications.[287]

INFERIOR ALVEOLAR NERVE (IAN) INJURY

Prior to considering any treatment to resolve IAN damage, the etiology must be first determined. Common causes of injury to the IAN are listed in Box 19-2.[226] The IAN may be damaged when an increase in temperature proximal to the IAN is greater than 10° C.[68] IAN damage has been suggested to occur in up to 1% of mandibular premolars that receive root canal treatment.[68] The type of sealer cement used may influence the symptoms of IAN damage.[189] If the patient exhibits neuropathic signs after the local anesthesia has worn off, posttreatment radiographs should be exposed to observe the possibility of any obturation material extending into the IAN canal.

Management should be performed by immediate removal of endodontic materials within 24 to 48 hours via periapical surgery, tooth extraction, or surgical debridement, whichever will be the most effective option with the least potential damage to the IAN.[59,153,214,226]

Nonsurgical Causes of IAN Injury

Trigeminal nerve injury is the most challenging consequence of contemporary dental surgical procedures with significant medical-legal repercussions (see also Chapter 29).[38] An approximate estimation places the incidence if IAN injury at 5%, with approximately one third of these patients afflicted with neuropathies, including neuropathic pain.[228] Neuropathic pain is characterized by symptoms that differ significantly from other chronic pain states, including paresthesia, either as a tingling or formication (ants crawling on the skin), burning or shooting pain, electric shock and evoked pain in the form of hyperalgesia, and mechanical allodynia. There is almost always an area of abnormal sensation, and the patient's maximum pain is often coexistent with the site of sensory deficit.[227] This is an important diagnostic feature, as the sensory deficit is usually to noxious and thermal stimuli, indicating damage to small diameter afferent fibers of the spinothalamic tract.[224]

The highest incidence of reported damage to the inferior alveolar and lingual nerves is associated with third molar extractions.[15,118,119] Local anesthesia was the second most common cause of nerve injury, and its exact mechanism can be confusing. It may be physical (needle damage, epineural/perineural hemorrhage) or chemical (local anesthetic contents). Reports have implicated certain local anesthetics of high concentrations (prilocaine 4% and articaine 4%) with IAN neuropathies (see also Chapter 4).[14,110,120,216]

A relatively small percentage of IAN injury cases (8%) are associated with an endodontic procedure.[229] Mandibular second molars are most commonly associated with this population, but cases involving treatment of mandibular first molars and premolars have also been reported.[148] The three primary factors responsible for instigating IAN damage during endodontic treatment are as follows:

1. Chemical factors: cytotoxic materials employed either in the preparation (e.g., irrigation liquids, intracanal medicaments)[2,91] or the obturation of the canal space[238]
2. Mechanical factors: repeated insertions of endodontic instruments through the apex into the IAN and surrounding tissues[57]
3. Thermal factors: inappropriate/prolonged heat application[71]

The presence of bone between the apices and the IAN canal does not necessarily protect against injury to the nerve. Research has provided an enlightening explanation to this puzzle (Figs. 19-24, 19-25, and 19-26).[288] Using fresh cadaver specimens (mandibles), researchers examined the true anatomic relationship among the root apices, inferior alveolar nerve, and the artery. They drew the following conclusions:

◆ There was never any compact layer of cortical bone surrounding the mandibular nerve sheath. In some cases a slightly denser cancellous bone was found, but it was replete with multiple perforations that would not afford significant resistance to penetration.[115]

◆ The proximity of the IAN canal to the apices of the second molars was < 1 mm, and it was more variable (1 to 4 mm) with first molars. This could explain the higher percentages of paresthesias reported with these teeth.

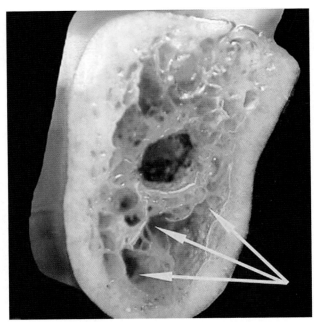

FIG. 19-24 Cross section of mandible in the molar region showing the presence of bone vacuoles *(yellow arrows)*. (From Tilotta-Yasukawa F, Millot S, El Haddioui A, et al: Labiomandibular paresthesia caused by endodontic treatment: an anatomic and clinical study, *Oral Surg Oral Med Oral Pathol Oral Radiol Endod* 102:e47, 2006.)

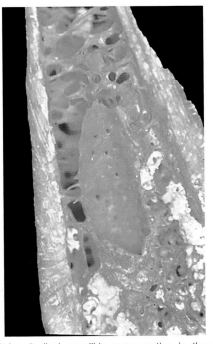

FIG. 19-25 Longitudinal mandible cross section in the molar region showing the spongy bone cover of the neurovascular bundle. Note the multiple fenestrations and honeycombed trabeculations. (From Tilotta-Yasukawa F, Millot S, El Haddioui A, et al: Labiomandibular paresthesia caused by endodontic treatment: an anatomic and clinical study, *Oral Surg Oral Med Oral Pathol Oral Radiol Endod* 102:e47, 2006.)

◆ The mandibular artery ran along the superomedial side of the IAN up to the first molar, and then crossed on the upper side until the mental foramen. Perforation of this vessel, with the concomitant hemorrhage exerting pressure on the pedicle, could feasibly produce a paresthetic event via the resulting ischemia.[58]

◆ Only with root apices in direct contact with the IAN canal were extrusions able to penetrate the nerve. If cancellous bone was interspersed between the apices and pedicle, the spread of the extrusion through the trabeculations remained at the periphery of the sheath.

◆ The low density of trabeculations and presence of numerous vacuoles provided an avenue for the diffusion of extruded irrigation fluids and obturation materials toward the IAN bundle. In a tooth with apical resorption, the foramen is frequently enlarged[310]; these two factors in concert could explain the occurrence of sensory symptoms in the absence of clinical or radiographic signs of overexpression or close proximity to the mandibular nerve.

Prevention is the key to successful treatment. Damage, either directly to the IAN or to the vessel(s) that nourish it, will result in sensory events that may be transient or permanent. Pretreatment radiographic assessment using periapical images is mandatory; in critical cases, CBCT may be more appropriate and precise in establishing proximity (Fig. 19-27). Every attempt should be undertaken to confine the instrumentation and irrigation processes to within the canal space; damage from extrusions can be chemical or mechanical in origin,[251] and toxic products can easily diffuse through the trabecular spaces and vacuoles surrounding the nerve bundle. This latency in diffusion, and the potential onset of paresthetic symptoms, dictates close monitoring for 72 hours postoperatively in cases where extrusion is apparent.[214] Imprudent heat application during thermoplastic compaction of gutta-percha may also lead to IAN injury.[26]

There is a strong correlation between duration, origin, significance of the injury, and the prognosis for resolution of the paresthesia. The longer the irritation persists, either chemical of mechanical, the more fibers are involved in a degenerative process and the more likely the paresthesia will become permanent.[244] If injury to the nerve is demonstrated by postoperative neuropathy and radiographs confirm the presence of a significant extrusion into the IAN canal, management entails the surgical removal of the offending material.[214,226,228] However, in spite of the best efforts to eliminate the causative agent, the symptoms may persist because of the associated chemical damage to the nerve. If sensory improvement has not been evident after 2 months, with or without repair during interventional surgery, then the prognosis for recovery is poor, and steps should be taken to alleviate the patient's concerns through counseling and systemic medications for chronic pain.[229]

Surgical Causes of IAN Injury

Surgical endodontic procedures need to be designed to minimize trauma to nerves including the IAN, mental nerve, and mental foramen. Although the mental foramen is most often

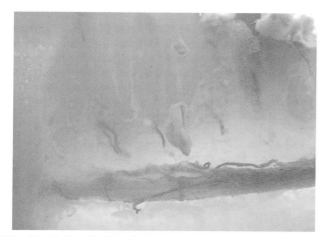

FIG. 19-26 Overfill of the distal root under direct observation. Note the proximity of the extruded material to the artery and nerve bundle (pedicle). (From Tilotta-Yasukawa F, Millot S, El Haddioui A, et al: Labiomandibular paresthesia caused by endodontic treatment: an anatomic and clinical study, *Oral Surg Oral Med Oral Pathol Oral Radiol Endod* 102:e47, 2006.)

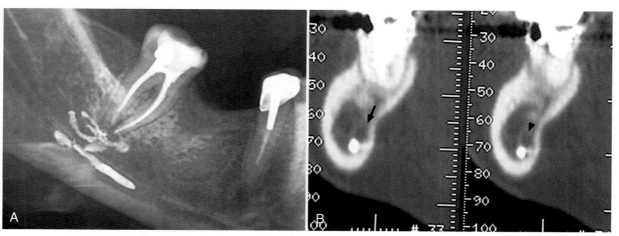

FIG. 19-27 **A,** Panoramic radiograph demonstrating significant overfilling and extension in the radicular vacuoles and overlying the mandibular canal. **B,** A coronal CT section demonstrating that the extruded material is lateral and below the mandibular bundle *(arrows)*. The patient's sensory complications were temporary. (From Tilotta-Yasukawa F, Millot S, El Haddioui A, et al: Labiomandibular paresthesia caused by endodontic treatment: an anatomic and clinical study, *Oral Surg Oral Med Oral Pathol Oral Radiol Endod* 102:e47, 2006.)

located apically to the second premolar,[190,211–213] it can vary in anterior-posterior locations,[139,193] coronal-apical locations,[77] and number. Pogrel[215] concluded that the severity of the injury was proportional to the process by which the injury was created, and these processes included scalpel blade wounding/transection, crushing, and stretching damages. These would be analogous to the dissection and reflection of the flap, improper retraction location/application, and postoperative edema.

If the transected ends are closely approximated following the injury, either naturally or surgically, proliferating axons will attempt to bridge the gap and, if they find a perineural tube to populate, gradually restore function. However, in cases where the gap is beyond a critical length, a neuroma may develop at the proximal end. Neuromas consist of dense fibrous tissue intermingled with nerve fascicles, with a disproportionate proliferation of unmyelinated fibers. Treatment, if initiated within 3 months of the initial event, often entails resection of the neuroma and repair by tension-free anastomosis or nerve grafting.

Careful presurgical assessment via radiographs and CBCT provides critical information on the size, location, and spatial relation of the planned surgery to nearby trigeminal nerves.[27] Before exiting the mandibular canal, the nerve often loops anteriorly, then superior and posteriorly in the apical portion of the premolar region.[100] If an apical procedure is planned in an area commensurate with this anatomic variant, then CBCT is warranted and strongly advised. Controlled reflection of the tissue overlying the suspected location of the foramen will diminish the incidence of transection. Cautious reflection of the flap will reveal evidence of tissue "funneling" at its base (Fig. 19-28); this is the telltale sign of the exiting nerve bundle.[194] This exiting tissue, upon discovery, can be marked with a dot of gentian violet or methylene blue dye. By highlighting it in this fashion, the surgeon can avoid unintentional impingement with a retractor. The tissues should be minimally distended and the underside of the flap kept well hydrated.

Transient paresthesia may occur in cases where a protracted surgical procedure, inadvertent stretching, or excessive post-operative edema has occurred. Appropriate reevaluation appointments include neurosensory testing and mapping the outline of the sensory deficit. Return of sensation within the first 4 weeks indicates a neuropraxia and implies an excellent prognosis.

Prognosis

Although the prognosis in the case of the IAN damage caused by resorbable or inert material is favorable, as it is dissolved over time, the toxicity of the material, whether chemical or pH, may cause permanent damage if left in place.[195] In addition, pressure from the material on the IAN may be caused by a hematoma or inflammatory, which can also contribute to temporary or permanent IAN damage.[72,195]

The prognosis of the IAN damage depends on the severity of the direct injury to the nerve, toxicity of the irritant, the amount and speed of its resorption, and how rapidly the causative agent is removed.[195,198,214] Because the paresthesia can be of both a mechanical and a chemical nature, removal of the excess material might not be sufficient if the nerve fibers have already undergone degeneration from a chemical irritant. Nevertheless, paresthesia caused by an instant irritation of the nerve, like a minor overinstrumentation or swelling from infection or minor inflammation, usually subsides within days. If no signs of healing are observed within 6 months, the chances of healing are considered much lower, although normal sensory function might still return after this time.[94,288] Counseling and therapeutic management are indicated within 48 hours for injuries caused by endodontic treatment or local anesthetic injections.[81]

Radiographs, especially CBCT, are often useful in revealing the extent of tissue damage in relation to hard tissues (e.g., the size and location of the lesion or the location of extruded materials in relation to the mandibular canal or the maxillary sinus).[26,85,94]

Prevention of Complications Due to Nerve Injury

Prevention of complications during root canal treatment should be the main focus, as once permanent nerve injury has occurred the patient may not regain normal sensation.[307] Careful consideration should also focus on the distance between the root apices and the mandibular canal. For mandibular first molars, this distance varies between 1 and 4 mm, and for mandibular second and third molars, the distance can be less than 1 mm.[288] With mandibular premolars, the proximity of a mental foramen should always be considered.[192] In addition, a study using CBCT has shown that the mesiobuccal root apex of maxillary second molars is frequently in very close proximity with the sinus floor[199] (Fig. 19-29).

CERVICOFACIAL SUBCUTANEOUS EMPHYSEMA

Subcutaneous emphysema is defined as the penetration of air or other gases beneath the skin and submucosa, resulting in soft tissue distention. A specific type, termed *cervicofacial subcutaneous emphysema* (CFSE), is a relatively rare occurrence and may be limited to traumatic, iatrogenic, or spontaneous events.

The first recorded instance was reported by Turnbull in 1900.[293] It details the account of a musician inducing CFSE by

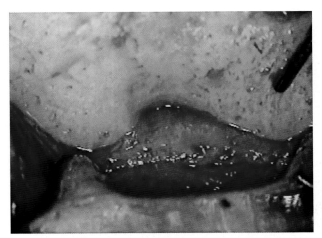

FIG. 19-28 Full-thickness reflection of the flap in the region of the premolar root apices reveals the mental nerve exiting the foramen; note how the tissue "funnels" from the reflected flap to the foramen. (From Tilotta-Yasukawa F, Millot S, El Haddioui A, et al: Labiomandibular paresthesia caused by endodontic treatment: an anatomic and clinical study, *Oral Surg Oral Med Oral Pathol Oral Radiol Endod* 102:e47, 2006.)

playing his bugle immediately after the extraction of a mandibular tooth; the subsequent swelling resolved a few days after he ceased playing the instrument. Indeed, most early reports of CFSE usually follow tooth extractions and were the result of activities the patient engaged in that raised intraoral pressures.[259] With the introduction of air-driven handpieces, there was an increased risk of CFSE.[11,54,314] Although tooth extraction, especially of mandibular third molars, remains the most commonly reported reason for CFSE,[41,54,123,237,312,314] it can also result from restorative treatment,[40,86,136,275,295] periodontal surgery,[81,264] crown and bridge treatments,[97,318] and root canal therapy.[25,127,138,207,278,295,308]

Compressed air, delivered through an air syringe, a high-speed handpiece, or a combination of the two during the operative procedure is associated with 71% of the cases.[117] A more recent study[12] reviewing 47 computed tomography (CT)–documented cases of CFSE found the exclusive cause was the high-speed handpiece in 66% of these patients. Other means of introducing air into the facial spaces include the following:

◆ Use of the dental laser (Er:YAG) in the gingival pocket: compressed air is used to cool the tip but is of sufficient pressure to dissect the sulcular wound.[4]
◆ Hydrogen peroxide beyond the canal space: most often reported when the fluid is introduced through a perforation in the canal[25] or over instrumented apex.[138]
◆ Lack of rubber dam isolation: a compressed air syringe was implemented to increase visibility in these molar retreatments, with air infiltration through the gingival sulcus.[60,146]
◆ Barotrauma secondary to Boerhaave syndrome: spontaneous rupture of the distal esophagus as a result of intractable vomiting, causing an increase in intraluminal esophageal pressure.[103]

The deposition of air beyond the canal space is a function of both the diameter of the canal at the apex[64] and the position of the syringe tip.[263] An air emphysema has the potential to spread along the facial planes in a similar manner (Fig. 19-30 and Fig. 19-31). Air entering the parapharyngeal and retropharyngeal spaces can lead to soft tissue infections,[73] airway compromise,[230] optic nerve damage,[35] and even death.[55,231] The majority of the cases, however, present as a soft, skin-colored swelling without redness that occurs during or shortly after the dental appointment. The cervicofacial swelling is always associated with crepitus (a crunchy feeling to the tissues upon

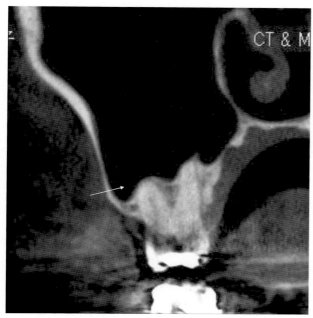

FIG. 19-29 CBCT image in coronal view showing that the mesiobuccal root apex of a maxillary second molar is in close proximity with the sinus floor.

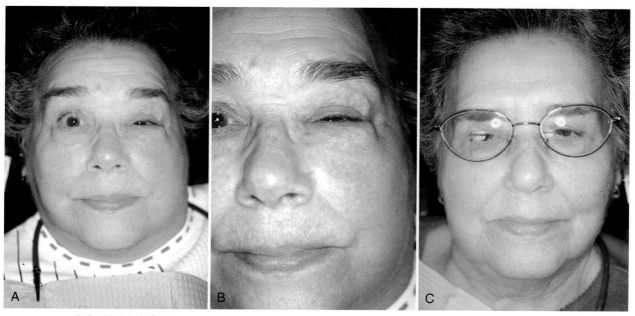

FIG. 19-30 **A,** Facial presentation after the rubber dam was removed. **B,** Close-up view reveals marked distention of the left suborbital region, with ptosis of the eye and loss of the nasolabial fold. There was marked crepitus upon palpation, but the patient was pain-free. **C,** She was placed on an antibiotic regime, as per the protocol, 2 days after the incident, the emphysema has resolved and the tissues are normal in color and texture.

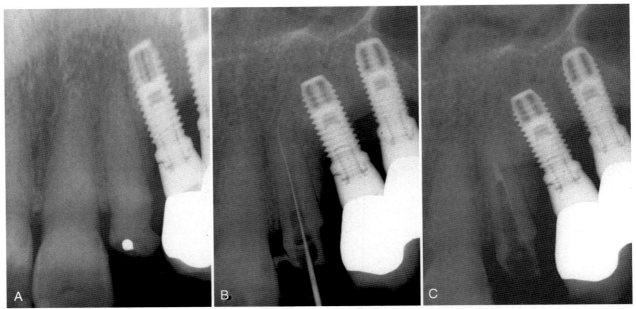

FIG. 19-31 A, Preoperative radiograph tooth #10[136]; dystrophic calcification has obliterated the pulp chamber and the coronal half of the canal space. **B,** A #10 file inserted to estimated working length; the file is actually through a facial perforation of the root at the radicular extent of the ultrasonic excavation. Repeated drying of the canal space using an air syringe forced air through the perforation site and precipitated the emphysema seen in Fig. 19-26 (*A* and *B*). **C,** The radicular perforation site was sealed with mineral trioxide aggregate (MTA) before the canal space was obturated. The tooth has remained asymptomatic since the incident.

palpation), which may not be palpable before a latency period of several hours. The more serious presentation of pneumomediastinum is characterized by dyspnea with a brassy voice, chest or back pain, and Hamman sign (a bubbling or crunching sound caused by air or movement accompanied by cardiac pulsation).[109] Secondary complications such as pyogenic mediastinitis or necrotizing fasciitis must be considered, and appropriate means taken to evaluate and manage them (blood cultures, broad-spectrum intravenous antibiotics).[60] Differential diagnosis should include an allergic reaction (more pronounced dermal signs prior to cardiac/respiratory symptoms), hematoma (a rapid accumulation of fluid without initial discoloration and without crepitation), and angioneurotic edema (a defined, circumscribed area of edema, often preceded by a burning sensation in the mucous membranes or skin).[81]

Treatment is largely empirical and dependent on the extent of the CFSE. Antibiotics are usually prescribed due to the nonsterility of the air supply and the possibility of necrotic debris or microorganisms forced into surrounding tissues.[230] Administration of 100% oxygen via a non-rebreather mask is reported to hasten the resolution of the emphysema because the oxygen,

which replaces the trapped air, is more readily absorbed at the site.[146] More severe presentations warrant hospitalization with intravenous antibiotics, where the extent and regression of the CFSE can be closely monitored using CT scans and complications can be managed more effectively.[31] Resolution, barring any severe complications, is characteristically rapid and uneventful, with the patients returning to their normal appearance within 4 to 7 days. A reevaluation of the cause of the emphysema should be examined and corrected before treatment resumes, especially in instances of a perforation.

From an endodontic perspective, minimizing compressed air at the site, from either a high-speed handpiece or an air syringe, is key to preventing this consequence. Isolation with a rubber dam, the use of paper points or high-volume aspiration for drying canal spaces, and avoiding the use of hydrogen peroxide during the procedure will also reduce the risk of introducing or entrapping air beneath the overlying tissues. For endodontic microsurgery, the use of a rear-exhausting high-speed handpiece for root resection as well as ultrasonics for root end preparation would decrease the likelihood of precipitating a CFSE during root end procedures.[16]

REFERENCES

1. Abbasipour F, Rastgar A, Bakhtiar H, et al: The nociceptive and anti-nociceptive effects of white mineral trioxide aggregate, *Int Endod J* 42:794, 2009.
2. Ahlgren FK, Johannessen AC, Hellem S: Displaced calcium hydroxide paste causing inferior alveolar nerve paraesthesia: report of a case, *Oral Surg Oral Med Oral Pathol Oral Radiol Endod* 96:734, 2003.
3. Ahonen M, Tjaderhane L: Endodontic-related paresthesia: a case report and literature review, *J Endod* 37:1460, 2011.
4. Mitsunaga S, Iwai T, Aoki N, et al: Cervicofacial subcutaneous and mediastinal emphysema caused by air

cooling spray of dental laser, *Oral Surg Oral Med Oral Pathol Oral Radiol* 115:e13, 2013.
5. Alapati SB, Brantley WA, Svec TA, et al: SEM observations of nickel-titanium rotary endodontic instruments that fractured during clinical use, *J Endod* 31:40, 2005.
6. Albrecht LJ, Baumgartner JC, Marshall JG: Evaluation of apical radicular debris removal using various sizes and tapers of ProFile GT files, *J Endod* 30:425, 2004.
7. Al-Fouzan KS: Incidence of rotary ProFile instrument fracture and the potential for bypassing in vivo, *Int Endod J* 36:864, 2003.

8. Al-Omari MA, Dummer PM: Canal blockage and debris extrusion with eight preparation techniques, *J Endod* 21:154, 1995.
9. Alomairy KH: Evaluating two techniques on removal of fractured rotary nickel-titanium endodontic instruments from root canals: an in vitro study, *J Endod* 35:559, 2009.
10. American Association of Endodontists: *Glossary of endodontic terms*, ed 7, Chicago, 2003, American Association of Endodontists.
11. American Association of Oral and Maxillofacial Surgeons, Council on Dental Materials, Instruments and Equipment:

Air-driven handpieces and air emphysema, *J Am Dent Assoc* 123:108, 1992.

12. Arai I, Aoki T, Yamazaki H, et al: Pneumomediastinum and subcutaneous emphysema after dental extraction detected incidentally by regular medical checkup: a case report, *Oral Surg Oral Med Oral Pathol Oral Radiol Endod* 107:e33, 2009.

13. Augsburge RA, Peters DD: Radiographic evaluation of extruded obturation materials, *J Endod* 16:492, 1990.

14. Bartling R, Freeman K, Kraut RA: The incidence of altered sensation of the mental nerve after mandibular implant placement, *J Oral Maxillofac Surg* 57:1408, 1999.

15. Bataineh AB: Sensory nerve impairment following mandibular third molar surgery, *J Oral Maxillofac Surg* 59:1012; discussion 7, 2001.

16. Battrum DE, Gutmann JL: Implications, prevention and management of subcutaneous emphysema during endodontic treatment, *Endod Dent Traumatol* 11:109, 1995.

17. Baumgartner JC, Mader CL: A scanning electron microscopic evaluation of four root canal irrigation regimens, *J Endod* 13:147, 1987.

18. Beck-Mannagetta J, Necek D, Grasserbauer M: Solitary aspergillosis of maxillary sinus, a complication of dental treatment, *Lancet* 2:1260, 1983.

19. Beck-Mannagetta J, Necek D, Grasserbauer M: Zahnaerztliche Aspekte der solitaeren Kieferhoehlen-Aspergillose, *Z Stomatol* 83:283, 1986.

20. Becker GL, Cohen S, Borer R: The sequelae of accidentally injecting sodium hypochlorite beyond the root apex: report of a case, *Oral Surg Oral Med Oral Pathol* 38:633, 1974.

21. Becking AG: Complications in the use of sodium hypochlorite during endodontic treatment: report of three cases, *Oral Surg Oral Med Oral Pathol* 71:346, 1991.

22. Benninger MS, Sebek BA, Levine HL: Mucosal regeneration of the maxillary sinus after surgery, *Otolaryngol Head Neck Surg* 101:33, 1989.

23. Bergenholtz G, Lekholm U, Milthon R, Engstrom B: Influence of apical overinstrumentation and overfilling on re-treated root canals, *J Endod* 5:310, 1979.

24. Betti LV, Bramante CM: Quantec SC rotary instruments versus hand files for gutta-percha removal in root canal retreatment, *Int Endod J* 34:514, 2001.

25. Bhat KS: Tissue emphysema caused by hydrogen peroxide, *Oral Surg Oral Med Oral Pathol* 38:304, 1974.

26. Blanas N, Kienle F, Sandor GK: Inferior alveolar nerve injury caused by thermoplastic gutta-percha overextension, *J Can Dent Assoc* 70:384, 2004.

27. Bornstein MM, Lauber R, Sendi P, von Arx T: Comparison of periapical radiography and limited cone-beam computed tomography in mandibular molars for analysis of anatomical landmarks before apical surgery, *J Endod* 37:151, 2011.

28. Bornstein MM, Wasmer J, Sendi P, et al: Characteristics and dimensions of the Schneiderian membrane and apical bone in maxillary molars referred for apical surgery: a comparative radiographic analysis using limited cone beam computed tomography, *J Endod* 38:51, 2012.

29. Boutsioukis C, Verhaagen B, Versluis M, et al: Evaluation of irrigant flow in the root canal using different needle types by an unsteady computational fluid dynamics model, *J Endod* 36:875, 2010.

30. Bowden JR, Ethunandan M, Brennan PA: Life-threatening airway obstruction secondary to hypochlorite extrusion during root canal treatment, *Oral Surg Oral Med Oral Pathol Oral Radiol Endod* 101:402, 2006.

31. Breznick DA, Saporito JL: Iatrogenic retropharyngeal emphysema with impending airway obstruction, *Arch Otolaryngol Head Neck Surg* 115:1367, 1989.

32. Brown DC, Moore BK, Brown CE, Newton CW: An in vitro study of apical extrusion of sodium hypochlorite during endodontic canal preparation, *J Endod* 12:587, 1995.

33. Bryant ST, Thompson SA, al-Omari MA, Dummer PM: Shaping ability of ProFile rotary nickel-titanium instruments with ISO sized tips in simulated root canals: part 1, *Int Endod J* 31:275, 1998.

34. Buckley M, Sprangberg LSW: The prevalence and technical quality of endodontic treatment in an American subpopulation, *Oral Pathol Oral Radiol Endod* 79:92, 1995.

35. Buckley MJ, Turvey TA, Schumann SP, Grimson BS: Orbital emphysema causing vision loss after a dental extraction, *J Am Dent Assoc* 120:421; discussion 423, 1990.

36. Budd CS, Weller RN, Kulild JC: A comparison of thermoplasticized injectable gutta-percha obturation techniques, *J Endod* 17:260, 1991.

37. Budd JC, Gekelman D, White JM: Temperature rise of the post and on the root surface during ultrasonic post removal, *Int Endod J* 38:705, 2005.

38. Caissie R, Goulet J, Fortin M, Morielli D: Iatrogenic paresthesia in the third division of the trigeminal nerve: 12 years of clinical experience, *J Can Dent Assoc* 71:185, 2005.

39. Candeiro GTM, Correia FC, Duarte MAH, et al: Evaluation of radiopacity, ph, release of calcium ions, and flow of a bioceramic root canal Sealer, *J Endod* 38:842, 2012.

40. Chan DC, Myers T, Sharaway M: A case for rubber dam application—subcutaneous emphysema after Class V procedure, *Oper Dent* 32:193, 2007.

41. Chen SC, Lin FY, Chang KJ: Subcutaneous emphysema and pneumomediastinum after dental extraction, *Am J Emerg Med* 17:678, 1999.

42. Chenail BL, Teplitsky PE: Orthograde ultrasonic retrieval of root canal obstructions, *J Endod* 13:186, 1987.

43. Cheung GS, Peng B, Bian Z, et al: Defects in ProTaper S1 instruments after clinical use: fractographic examination, *Int Endod J* 38:802, 2005.

44. Chutich MJ, Kaminski EJ, Miller DA, Lautenschlager EP: Risk assessment of the toxicity of solvents of gutta-percha used in endodontic retreatment, *J Endod* 24:213, 1998.

45. Clegg MS, Vertucci FJ, Walker C, et al: The effect of exposure to irrigant solutions on apical dentin biofilms in vitro, *J Endod* 32:434, 2006.

46. Cohen S, Burns RC: *Pathways of the pulp*, ed 3, St. Louis, 1984, CV Mosby, pp 291-292.

47. Cohen S, Burns RC: *Pathways of the pulp*, ed 5, St. Louis, 1991, Mosby.

48. Cohen S, Burns RC: *Pathways of the pulp*, ed 8, St Louis, 2002, Mosby, pp 94, 242-252, 530, 870, 910.

49. Cohen S, Hargreaves KM: *Pathways of the pulp*, ed 9, St Louis, 2006, Mosby, pp 992-994.

50. Crump MC, Natkin E: Relationship of broken root canal instruments to endodontic case prognosis: a clinical investigation, *J Am Dent Assoc* 80:1341, 1970.

51. Cuje J, Bargholz C, Hulsmann M: The outcome of retained instrument removal in a specialist practice, *Int Endod J* 43:545, 2010.

52. Dan AE, Thygesen TH, Pinholt EM: Corticosteroid administration in oral and orthognathic surgery: a systematic review of the literature and meta-analysis, *J Oral Maxillofac Surg* 68:2207, 2010.

53. Daugherty DW, Gound TG, Comer TL: Comparison of fracture rate, deformation rate, and efficiency between rotary endodontic instruments driven at 150 rpm and 350 rpm, *J Endod* 27:93, 2001.

54. Davies DE: Pneumomediastinum after dental surgery, *Anaesth Intensive Care* 29:638, 2001.

55. Davies JM, Campbell LA: Fatal air embolism during dental implant surgery: a report of three cases, *Can J Anaesth* 37:112, 1990.

56. De-Deus G, Moreira EJ, Lopes HP, Elias CN: Extended cyclic fatigue life of F2 Pro-Taper instruments used in reciprocating movement, *Int Endod J* 43:1063, 2010.

57. Dempf R, Hausamen JE: Lesions of the inferior alveolar nerve arising from endodontic treatment, *Aust Endod J* 26:67, 2000.

58. Denio D, Torabinejad M, Bakland LK: Anatomical relationship of the mandibular canal to its surrounding structures in mature mandibles, *J Endod* 18:161, 1992.

59. Dorn S, Garther A: Case selection and treatment planning. In Cohen S, Burns RC, editors: *Pathways of the pulp*, ed 7, St Louis, 1998, Mosby, p 60.

60. Durukan P, Salt O, Ozkan S, et al: Cervicofacial emphysema and pneumomediastinum after a high-speed air drill endodontic treatment procedure, *Am J Emerg Med* 30:2095.e3, 2012.

61. Eberhardt JA, Torabinejad M, Christiansen EL: A computed tomographic study of the distances between the maxillary sinus floor and the apices of the maxillary posterior teeth, *Oral Surg Oral Med Oral Pathol* 73:345, 1992.

62. Edgar SW, Marshall JG, Baumgartner JC: The antimicrobial effect of chloroform on Enterococcus faecalis after gutta-percha removal, *J Endod* 32:1185, 2006.

63. Ehrich DG, Brian JD Jr, Walker WA: Sodium hypochlorite accident: inadvertent injection into the maxillary sinus, *J Endod* 19:180, 1993.

64. Eleazer PD, Eleazer KR: Air pressures developed beyond the apex from drying root canals with pressurized air, *J Endod* 24:833, 1998.

65. Ericson S, Finne K, Persson G: Results of apicoectomy of maxillary canines, premolars and molars with special reference to oroantral communication as a prognostic factor, *Int J Oral Surg* 3:386, 1974.

66. Eriksson AR, Albrektsson T: Temperature threshold levels for heat-induced bone tissue injury: a vital-microscopic study in the rabbit, *J Prosthet Dent* 50:101, 1983.

67. Erisen R, Yucel T, Kucukay S: Endomethasone root canal filling material in the mandibular canal: a case report, *Oral Surg Oral Med Oral Pathol* 68:343, 1989.

68. Escoda-Francoli J, Canalda-Sahli C, Soler A, et al: Inferior alveolar nerve damage because of overextended endodontic material: a problem of sealer cement biocompatibility? *J Endod* 33:1484, 2007.

69. Esposito P, Cunnington C: A comparison of canal preparation with nickel-titanium and stainless steel instruments, *J Endod* 21:173, 1995.

70. Ettrich CA, Labossiere PE, Pitts DL, et al: An investigation of the heat induced during ultrasonic post removal, *J Endod* 33:1222, 2007.

71. Fanibunda K, Whitworth J, Steele J: The management of thermomechanically compacted gutta percha extrusion in the inferior dental canal, *Br Dent J* 184:330, 1998.

72. Farren ST, Sadoff RS, Penna KJ: Sodium hypochlorite chemical burn: case report, *N Y State Dent J* 74:61, 2008.

73. Feinstone T: Infected subcutaneous emphysema: report of case, *J Am Dent Assoc* 83:1309, 1971.

74. Feldman G, Solomon C, Notaro P, Moskowitz E: Retrieving broken endodontic instruments, *J Am Dent Assoc* 88:588, 1974.

75. Felippe MC, Felippe WT, Marques MM, Antoniazzi JH: The effect of the renewal of calcium hydroxide paste on the apexification and periapical healing of teeth with incomplete root formation, *Int Endod J* 38:436, 2005.

76. Ferraz CC, Gomes NV, Gomes BP, et al: Apical extrusion of debris and irrigants using two hand and three engine-driven instrumentation techniques, *Int Endod J* 34:354, 2001.

77. Fishel D, Buchner A, Hershkowith A, Kaffe I: Roentgenologic study of the mental foramen, *Oral Surg Oral Med Oral Pathol* 41:682, 1976.

78. Fors UGH, Berg JO: A method for the removal of separated endodontic instruments from root canals, *J Endod* 9:156, 1983.

79. Fox J, Moodnik RM, Greenfield E, Atkinson JS: Filling root canals with files: radiographic evaluation of 304 cases, *N Y State Dent J* 38:154, 1972.

80. Freedman A, Horowitz I: Complications after apicoectomy in maxillary premolar and molar teeth, *Int J Oral Maxillofac Surg* 28:192, 1989.

81. Fruhauf J, Weinke R, Pilger U, et al: Soft tissue cervicofacial emphysema after dental treatment: report of 2 cases with emphasis on the differential diagnosis of angioedema, *Arch Dermatol* 141:1437, 2005.

82. Fu M, Zhang Z, Hou B: Removal of broken files from root canals by using ultrasonic techniques combined with dental microscope: a retrospective analysis of treatment outcome, *J Endod* 37:619, 2011.

83. Gambarini G: Rational for the use of low-torque endodontic motors in root canal instrumentation, *Endod Dent Traumal* 16:95, 2000.

84. Gambarini G: Cyclic fatigue of nickel-titanium rotary instruments after clinical use with low-and high-torque endodontic motors, *J Endod* 27:772, 2001.

85. Gambarini G, Plotino G, Grande NM, et al: Differential diagnosis of endodonticrelated inferior alveolar nerve paraesthesia with cone beam computed tomography: a case report, *Int Endod J* 44:176, 2011.

86. Gamboa Vidal CA, Vega Pizarro CA, Almeida Arriagada A: Subcutaneous emphysema secondary to dental treatment: case report, *Medicina Oral, Patologia Oral y Cirugia Bucal* 12:E76, 2007.

87. Gandolfi MG, Siboni F, Primus CM, Prati C: Ion release, porosity, solubility, and bioactivity of MTA plus tricalcium silicate, *J Endod* 40:1632, 2014.

88. Gao Y, Shotton V, Wilkinson K, et al: Effects of raw material and rotational speed on the cyclic fatigue of ProFile Vortex rotary instruments, *J Endod* 36:1205, 2010.

89. Gatot A, Arbelle J, Leiberman A, Yanai-Inbar I: Effects of sodium hypochlorite on soft tissues after its inadvertent injection beyond the root apex, *J Endod* 17:573, 1991.

90. George S, Basrani B, Kishen A: Possibilities of gutta-percha-centered infection in endodontically treated teeth: an in vitro study, *J Endod* 36:1241, 2010.

91. Gernhardt CR, Eppendorf K, Kozlowski A, Brandt M: Toxicity of concentrated sodium hypochlorite used as an endodontic irrigant, *Int Endod J* 37:272, 2004.

92. Gettleman BH, Spriggs KA, ElDeeb ME, Messer HH: Removal of canal obstructions with the endo extractor, *J Endod* 17:608, 1991.

93. Giardino L, Pontieri F, Savoldi E, Tallarigo F: Aspergillus mycetoma of the maxillary sinus secondary to overfilling of a root canal, *J Endod* 32:692, 2006.

94. Giuliani V, Lajolo C, Deli G, et al: Inferior alveolar nerve paresthesia caused by endodontic pathosis: a case report and review of the literature, *Oral Surg Oral Med Oral Pathol Oral Radiol Endod* 92:670, 2001.

95. Glickman GN, Koch KA: 21st century endodontics, *J Am Dent Assoc* 131:39, 2000.

96. Gluskin AH, Ruddle CJ, Zinman EJ: Thermal injury through intraradicular heat transfer using ultrasonic devices: precautions and practical preventive strategies, *J Am Dent Assoc* 136:1286, 2005.

97. Goorhuis H, Rothrock SG: Cervicofacial and thoracic barotrauma following a minor dental procedure, *Pediatr Emerg Care* 9:29, 1993.

98. Gorduysus M, Avcu N, Gorduysus O, et al: Cytotoxic effects of four different endodontic materials in human periodontal ligament fibroblasts, *J Endod* 33:1450, 2007.

99. Greene KJ, Krell KV: Clinical factors associated with ledged canals in maxillary and mandibular molars, *Oral Surg Oral Med Oral Pathol* 70:490, 1990.

100. Greenstein G, Tarnow D: The mental foramen and nerve: clinical and anatomical factors related to dental implant placement: a literature review, *J Periodontol* 77:1933, 2006.

101. Grigorin D, Brambule J, Delacretaz J: La sinusite maxillaire fungique, *Dermatologica* 159:180, 1979.

102. Guerreiro-Tanomaru JM, De Faria-Jnior NB, Duarte MAH, et al: Comparative analysis of Enterococcus faecalis biofilm formation on different substrates, *J Endod* 39:346, 2013.

103. Gulati A, Baldwin A, Intosh IM, Krishnan A: Pneumomediastinum, bilateral pneumothorax, pleural effusion, and surgical emphysema after routine apicectomy caused by vomiting, *Br J Oral Maxillofac Surg* 46:136, 2008.

104. Gursoy UK, Bostanci V, Kosger HH: Palatal mucosa necrosis because of accidental sodium hypochlorite injection instead of anaesthetic solution, *International Endod J* 39:157, 2006.

105. Gutmann JL, Dumsha TC, Lovdahl PE, Hovland EJ: *Problem solving in endodontics*, ed 3, St Louis, 1997, Mosby, pp 96-100, 117.

106. Gutmann JL, Rakusin H: Perspectives on root canal obturation with thermoplasticized injectable gutta-percha, *Int Endod J* 20:261, 1987.

107. Haikel Y, Serfaty R, Bateman G, et al: Dynamic and cyclic fatigue of engine-driven rotary nickel-titanium endodontic instruments, *J Endod* 25:434, 1999.

108. Hammad M, Qualtrough A, Silikas N: Three-dimensional evaluation of effectiveness of hand and rotary instrumentation for retreatment of canals filled with different materials, *J Endod* 34:1370, 2008.

109. Hamman L: Spontaneous mediastinal emphysema, *Bull Johns Hopkins Hosp* 54:46, 1961.

110. Handschel J, Figgener L, Joos U: [Forensic evaluation of injuries to nerves and jaw bone after wisdom tooth extraction from the viewpoint of current jurisprudence], *Mund Kiefer Gesichtschir* 5:44, 2001.

111. Hapcook CP Sr: Dental malpractice claims: percentages and procedures, *J Am Dent Assoc* 137:1444, 2006.

112. Harty FJ, Parkins BJ, Wengraf AM: Success rate in root canal therapy: a retrospective study of conventional cases, *Br Dent J* 128:65, 1970.

113. Hashem AA: Ultrasonic vibration: temperature rise on external root surface during broken instrument removal, *J Endod* 33:1070, 2007.

114. Hauman CH, Chandler NP, Tong DC: Endodontic implications of the maxillary sinus: a review, *Int Endod J* 35:127, 2002.

115. Heasman PA: Variation in the position of the inferior dental canal and its significance to restorative dentistry, *J Dent* 16:36, 1988.

116. Heling I, Rotstein I, Dinur T, et al: Bactericidal and cytotoxic effects of sodium hypochlorite and sodium dichloroisocyanurate solutions in vitro, *J Endod* 27:278, 2001.

117. Heyman SN, Babayof I: Emphysematous complications in dentistry, 1960-1993: an illustrative case and review of the literature, *Quintessence Int* 26:535, 1995.

118. Hillerup S: Iatrogenic injury to oral branches of the trigeminal nerve: records of 449 cases, *Clin Oral Investig* 11:133, 2007.

119. Hillerup S: Iatrogenic injury to the inferior alveolar nerve: etiology, signs and symptoms, and observations on recovery, *Int J Oral Maxillofac Surg* 37:704, 2008.

120. Hillerup S, Jensen R: Nerve injury caused by mandibular block analgesia, *Int J Oral Maxillofac Surg* 35:437, 2006.

121. Himel V, Ahmed K, Wood D, et al: An evaluation of nitinol and stainless steel files used by students during a laboratory proficiency exam, *Oral Surg* 79:232, 1995.

122. Hinrichs RE, Walker WA, Schindler WG: A comparison of amounts of apically extruded debris using handpiece-driven nickel-titanium instrument systems, *J Endod* 24:102, 1998.

123. Horowitz I, Hirshberg A, Freedman A: Pneumomediastinum and subcutaneous emphysema following surgical extraction of mandibular third molars: three case reports, *Oral Surg Oral Med Oral Pathol* 63:25, 1987.

124. Huang X, Ling J, Gu L: Quantitative evaluation of debris extruded apically by using ProTaper Universal Tulsa Rotare System in endodontic retreatment, *J Endod* 33:1102, 2007.

125. Hulsmann M: Removal of fractured root canal instruments using the Canal Finder System, *Dtsch Zahnarztl Z* 45:229, 1990.

126. Hulsmann M: Methods for removing metal obstructions from the root canal, *Endod Dent Traumatol* 9:223, 1993.

127. Hulsmann M, Hahn W: Complications during root canal irrigation: literature review and case reports, *Int Endod J* 33:186, 2000.

128. Hulsmann M, Peters OA, Dummer PMH: Mechanical preparation of root canals: shaping goals, techniques and means, *Endod Topics* 10:30, 2005.

129. Hülsmann M, Stotz S: Efficacy, cleaning ability and safety of different devices for gutta-percha removal in root canal retreatment, *Int Endod J* 30:227, 1997.

130. Ingle JI: *PDQ endodontics*, London, 2005, BC Decker, p 220.

131. Ingle JI, Bakland LK: *Endodontics*, ed 5, London, 2002, BC Decker, pp 412, 482-489, 525-538, 695, 729, 769, 776.

132. Ingle JI, Luebke RG, Zidell JD, et al: Obturation of the radicular space. In Ingle JI, Taintor JF, editors: *Endodontics*, ed 3, Philadelphia, 1985, Lea & Febiger, pp 223-307.

133. Ioannides C, Borstlap WA: Apicoectomy on molars: a clinical and radiographical study, *Int J Oral Surg* 12:73, 1983.

134. Jafarzadeh H, Abbott PV: Ledge formation: review of a great challenge in endodontics, *J Endod* 33:1155, 2007.

135. Jiang LM, Verhaagen B, Versluis M, van der Sluis LWM: The influence of the orientation of an ultrasonic file on the cleaning efficacy of ultrasonic activated irrigation, *J Endod* 36:1372, 2010.

136. Josephson GD, Wambach BA, Noordzji JP: Subcutaneous cervicofacial and mediastinal emphysema after dental instrumentation, *Otolaryngol Head Neck Surg* 124:170, 2001.

137. Kapalas A, Lambrianidis T: Factors associated with root canal ledging during instrumentation, *Endod Dent Traumatol* 16:229, 2000.

138. Kaufman AY: Facial emphysema caused by hydrogen peroxide irrigation: report of a case, *J Endod* 7:470, 1981.

139. Kekere-Ekun TA: Antero-posterior location of the mental foramen in Nigerians, *Afr Dent J* 3:2, 1989.

140. Kerbl FM, DeVilliers P, Litaker M, Eleazer PD: Physical effects of sodium hypochlorite on bone: an ex vivo study, *J Endod* 38:357, 2012.

141. Kfir A, Tsesis I, Yakirevich E, et al: The efficacy of five techniques for removing root filling material: microscopic versus radiographic evaluation, *Int Endod J* 45:35, 2012.

142. Khademi A, Yazdizadeh M, Feizianfard M: Determination of the minimum instrumentation size for penetration of irrigants to the apical third of root canal systems, *J Endod* 32:417, 2006.

143. Khongkhunthian P, Reichart PA: Aspergillosis of the maxillary sinus as a complication of overfilling root canal material into the sinus: report of two cases, *J Endod* 27:476, 2001.

144. Kim EC, Lee BC, Chang HS, et al: Evaluation of the radiopacity and cytotoxicity of Portland cements containing bismuth oxide, *Oral Surg Oral Med Oral Pathol Oral Radiol Endod* 105:e54, 2008.

145. Kim JY, Cheung GS, Park SH, et al: Effect from cyclic fatigue of nickel-titanium rotary files on torsional resistance, *J Endod* 38:527, 2012.

146. Kim Y, Kim MR, Kim SJ: Iatrogenic pneumomediastinum with extensive subcutaneous emphysema after endodontic treatment: report of 2 cases, *Oral Surg Oral Med Oral Pathol Oral Radiol Endod* 109:e114, 2010.

147. Kleier DJ, Averbach RE, Mehdipour O: The sodium hypochlorite accident: experience of diplomates of the American Board of Endodontics, *J Endod* 34:1346, 2008.

148. Knowles KI, Jergenson MA, Howard JH: Paresthesia associated with endodontic treatment of mandibular premolars, *J Endod* 29:768, 2003.

149. Kobayashi A: Asymptomatic aspergillosis of the maxillary sinus associated with foreign body of endodontic origin: report of a case, *Int J Oral Maxillofac Surg* 24:243, 1995.

150. Koch K: The microscope: its effect on your practice, *Dent Clin North Am* 41:619, 1997.

151. Kopp W, Fotter R, Steiner H, et al: Aspergillosis of the paranasal sinuses, *Radiology* 156:715, 1985.

152. Kosti E, Zinelis S, Lambrianidis T, Margelos J: A comparative study of crack development in stainless-steel Hedström files used with step-back or crown-down techniques, *J Endod* 30:38, 2004.

153. Kothari P, Hanson N, Cannell H: Bilateral mandibular nerve damage following root canal therapy, *Br Dent J* 180:189, 1996.

154. Kramkowski TR, Bahcall J: An in vitro comparison of torsional stress and cyclic fatigue resistance of ProFile GT and ProFile GT Series X rotary nickel-titanium files, *J Endod* 35:404, 2009.

155. Krasner P, Rankow HJ: Anatomy of the pulp-chamber floor, *J Endod* 30:5, 2004.

156. Kremeier K, Pontius O, Klaiber B, Hulsmann M: Nonsurgical endodontic management of a double tooth: a case report, *Int Endod J* 40:908, 2007.

157. Kulild JC, Peters DD: Incidence and configuration of canal systems in the mesiobuccal root of maxillary first and second molars, *J Endod* 16:311, 1990.

158. Kytridou V, Gutmann JL, Nunn MH: Adaptation and sealability of two contemporary obturation techniques in the absence of the dentinal smear layer, *Int Endod J* 32:464, 1999.

159. Lambrianidis T: Ledge formation. In *Iatrogenic complications during endodontic treatment.* Thessaloniki, Greece, 1996, Univ Studio Press.

160. Reference deleted in proofs.

161. Lee J, Lorenzo D, Rawlins T, Cardo VA Jr: Sodium hypochlorite extrusion: an atypical case of massive soft tissue necrosis, *J Oral Maxillofac Surg* 69:1776, 2011.

162. Lee JS, Lee JH, Lee JH, et al: Efficacy of early treatment with infliximab in pediatric Crohn's disease, *World J Gastroenterol* 16:1776, 2010.

163. Legent F, Billet J, Beauvillain C, et al: The role of dental canal fillings in the development of aspergillus sinusitis: a report of 85 cases, *Arch Otorhinolaryngol* 246:318, 1989.

164. Levy G: [Canal Finder System 89: improvements and indications after 4 years of experimentation and use], *Rev Odontostomatol (Paris)* 19:327, 1990.

165. Lin L, Chance K, Shovlin F, et al: Oroantral communication in periapical surgery of maxillary posterior teeth, *J Endod* 11:40, 1985.

166. Ling JQ, Wei X, Gao Y: Evaluation of the use of dental operating microscope and ultrasonic instruments in the management of blocked canals, *Zhonghua Kou Qiang Yi Xue Za Zhi* 38:324, 2003; review article 1162.

167. Liu R, Kaiwar A, Shemesh H, et al: Incidence of apical root cracks and apical dentinal detachments after canal preparation with hand and rotary files at different instrumentation lengths, *J Endod* 39:129, 2013.

168. Loidolt D, Mangge H, Wilders-Trushing M, et al: In vivo and in vitro suppression of lymphocyte function in aspergillus sinusitis, *Arch Otorhinolaryngol* 246:321, 1989.

169. Lopes HP, Ferreira AA, Elias CN, et al: Influence of rotational speed on the cyclic fatigue of rotary nickel-titanium endodontic instruments, *J Endod* 35:1013, 2009.

170. Lopes HP, Moreira EJ, Elias CN, et al: Cyclic fatigue of ProTaper instruments, *J Endod* 33:55, 2007.

171. Lovato KF, Sedgley CM: Antibacterial activity of EndoSequence Root Repair Material and ProRoot MTA against clinical isolates of Enterococcus faecalis, *J Endod* 37:1542, 2011.

172. Ma J, Al-Ashaw AJ, Shen Y, et al: Efficacy of ProTaper Universal Rotary Retreatment System for gutta-percha removal from oval root canals: a micro-computed tomography study, *J Endod* 38:1516, 2012.

173. Madarati A, Watts DC, Qualtrough AE: Opinions and attitudes of endodontists and general dental practitioners in the UK towards the intracanal fracture of endodontic instruments: part 2, *Int Endod J* 41:1079, 2008.

174. Madarati AA, Hunter MJ, Dummer PMH: Management of intracanal separated instruments, *J Endod* 39:569, 2013.

175. Madarati AA, Qualtrough AJ, Watts DC: Efficiency of a newly designed ultrasonic unit and tips in reducing temperature rise on root surface during the removal of fractured files, *J Endod* 35:896, 2009.

176. Manisal Y, Yücel T, Erişen R: Overfilling of the root, *Oral Surg Oral Med Oral Pathol* 68:773, 1989.

177. McDonald MN, Vire DE: Chloroform in the endodontic operatory, *J Endod* 18:301, 1992.

178. McKendry DJ: Comparison of balanced forces, endosonic and step-back filing instrumentation techniques: quantification of extruded apical debris, *J Endod* 16:24, 1990.

179. Mehdipour O, Kleier DJ, Averbach RE: Anatomy of sodium hypochlorite accidents, *Compend Contin Educ Dent* 28:544, 548, 550, 2007.

180. Metzger Z, Ben-Amar A: Removal of overextended gutta-percha root canal fillings in endodontic failure cases, *J Endod* 21:287, 1995.

181. Metzger Z, Teperovich E, Zary R, et al: The self-adjusting file (SAF). Part 1: respecting the root canal anatomy—a new concept of endodontic files and its implementation, *J Endod* 36:679, 2010.

182. Molander A, Reit C, Dahen G, Kvist T: Microbiological status of root-filled teeth with apical periodontitis, *Int Endod J* 31:1, 1998.

183. Morse DR: Endodontic-related inferior alveolar nerve and mental foramen paresthesia, *Compend Contin Educ Dent* 18:963, 1997.

184. Naenni N, Thoma K, Zehnder M: Soft tissue dissolution capacity of currently used and potential endodontic irrigants, *J Endod* 30:785, 2004.

185. Nagai O, Tani N, Kayaba Y, et al: Ultrasonic removal of separated instruments in root canals, *Int Endod J* 19:298, 1986.

186. Nair PN: On the causes of persistent apical periodontitis: a review, *Int Endod J* 39:249, 2006.

187. Nair PNR, Henry S, Cano V, Vera J: Microbial status of apical root canal system of human mandibular first molars with primary apicalr periodontitis after "one-visit" endodontic treatment, *Oral Surg Oral Med Oral Pathol Oral Radiol Endod* 99:231, 2005.

188. Namazikhah MS, Mokhlis HR, Alasmakh K: Comparison between a hand stainless steel K file and a rotary NiTi 0.04 taper, *J Calif Dent Assoc* 28:421, 2000.

189. Neaverth E: Disabling complications following inadvertent overextension of a root canal filling material, *J Endod* 15:135, 1989.

190. Neiva RF, Gapski R, Wang HL: Morphometric analysis of implant-related anatomy in Caucasian skulls, *J Periodontol* 75:1061, 2004.

191. Nevares G, Cunha RS, Zuolo ML, et al: Success rates for removing or bypassing fractured instruments: a prospective clinical study, *J Endod* 38:442, 2012.

192. Ngeow WC: Is there a "safety zone" in the mandibular premolar region where damage to the mental nerve can be avoided if periapical extrusion occurs? *J Can Dent Assoc* 76:a61, 2010.

193. Ngeow WC, Yuzawati Y: The location of the mental foramen in a selected Malay population, *J Oral Sci* 45:171, 2003.

194. Niemczyk SP: Essentials of endodontic microsurgery, *Dent Clin North Am* 54:375, 2010.

195. Nitzan DW, Stabholz A, Azaz B: Concepts of accidental overfilling and overinstrumentation in the mandibular canal during root canal treatment, *J Endod* 9:81, 1983.

196. Noiri Y, Ehara A, Kawahara T, et al: Participation of bacterial biofilms in refractory and chronic periapical periodontitis, *J Endod* 28:679, 2002.

197. Oberli K, Bornstein MM, von Arx T: Periapical surgery and the maxillary sinus: radiographic parameters for clinical outcome, *Oral Surg Oral Med Oral Pathol Oral Radiol Endod* 103:848, 2007.

198. Ozkan BT, Celik S, Durmus E: Paresthesia of the mental nerve stem from periapical infection of mandibular canine tooth: a case report, *Oral Surg Oral Med Oral Pathol Oral Radiol Endod* 105:e28, 2008.

199. Pagin O, Centurion BS, Rubira-Bullen LRF, Capelozza ALA: Maxillary sinus and posterior teeth: accessing close relationship by cone-beam computed tomographic scanning in a Brazilian population, *J Endod* 39:748, 2013.

200. Parashos P, Gordon I, Messer HH: Factors influencing defects of rotary nickel titanium endodontic instruments after clinical use, *J Endod* 30:722, 2004.

201. Park H: A comparison of greater taper files, profiles, and stainless steel files to shape curved root canals, *Oral Surg Oral Med Oral Pathol Oral Radiol* 9:715, 2001.

202. Pashley EL, Birdsong NL, Bowman K, Pashley DH: Cytotoxic effects of NaOCl on vital tissue, *J Endod* 11:525, 1985.

203. Patel S, Dawood A, Ford TP, Whaites E: The potential applications of cone beam computed tomography in the management of endodontic problems, *Int Endod J* 40:818, 2007.

204. Patino PV, Biedma BM, Liebana CR, et al: The influence of a manual glide path on the separation rate of NiTi rotary instruments, *J Endod* 31:114, 2005.

205. Pedull E, Grande NM, Plotino G, et al: Influence of continuous or reciprocating motion on cyclic fatigue resistance of 4 different nickel-titanium rotary instruments, *J Endod* 39:258, 2013.

206. Pelka M, Petschelt A: Permanent mimic musculature and nerve damage caused by sodium hypochlorite: a case report, *Oral Surg Oral Med Oral Pathol Oral Radiol Endod* 106:e80, 2008.

207. Penna KJ, Neshat K: Cervicofacial subcutaneous emphysema after lower root canal therapy, *N Y State Dent J* 67:28, 2001.

208. Persson G: Periapical surgery of molars, *Int J Oral Surg* 11:96, 1982.

209. Petersson K, Petersson A, Olsson B, et al: Technical quality of root fillings in an adult Swedish population, *Endod Dent Traumatol* 2:99, 1986.

210. Pettiette MT, Conner D, Trope M: Procedural errors with the use of nickel-titanium rotary instruments in undergraduate endodontics, *J Endod* 28:259, 2002.

211. Phillips JL, Weller RN, Kulild JC: The mental foramen: 1. Size, orientation, and positional relationship to the mandibular second premolar, *J Endod* 16:221, 1990.

212. Phillips JL, Weller RN, Kulild JC: The mental foramen: 2. Radiographic position in relation to the mandibular second premolar, *J Endod* 18:271, 1992.

213. Phillips JL, Weller RN, Kulild JC: The mental foramen: 3. Size and position on panoramic radiographs, *J Endod* 18:383, 1992.

214. Pogrel MA: Damage to the inferior alveolar nerve as the result of root canal therapy, *J Am Dent Assoc* 138:65, 2007.

215. Pogrel MA, Le H: Etiology of lingual nerve injuries in the third molar region: a cadaver and histologic study, *J Oral Maxillofac Surg* 64:1790, 2006.

216. Pogrel MA, Thamby S: Permanent nerve involvement resulting from inferior alveolar nerve blocks, *J Am Dent Assoc* 131:901, 2000.

217. Poveda R, Bagan JV, Diaz Fernandez JM, et al: Mental nerve paresthesia associated with endodontic paste within the mandibular canal: report of a case, *Oral Surg Oral Med Oral Pathol Oral Radiol Endod* 102:e46, 2006.

218. Powell SE, Wong PD, Simon JH: A comparison of the effect of modified and nonmodified instrument tips on apical canal configuration: part II, *J Endod* 14:224, 1988.

219. Pruett JP, Clement DJ, Carnes DL Jr: Cyclic fatigue testing of nickel-titanium endodontic instruments, *J Endod* 23:77, 1997.

220. Rahimi M, Parashos P: A novel technique for the removal of fractured instruments in the apical third of curved root canals, *Int Endod J* 42:264, 2009.

221. Ramirez-Salomon M, Soler-Bientz R, de la Garza-Gonzalez R, et al: Incidence of Lightspeed separation and the potential for bypassing, *J Endod* 23:586, 1997.

222. Reddy SA, Hicks ML: Apical extrusion of debris using two hand and two rotary instrumentation techniques, *J Endod* 24:180, 1998.

223. Reeh ES, Messer HH: Long-term paresthesia following inadvertent forcing of sodium hypochlorite through perforation in maxillary incisor, *Endod Dent Traumatol* 5:200, 1989.

224. Rehm S, Koroschetz J, Baron R: An update on neuropathic pain, *Eur Neur Rev* 3:125, 2008.

225. Rene N, Owall B: Dental malpractice in Sweden, *J Law Ethics Dent* 4:16, 1991.

226. Renton T: Prevention of iatrogenic inferior alveolar nerve injuries in relation to dental procedures, *Dent Update* 37:350, 354, 358, passim, 2010.

227. Renton T, Dawood A, Shah A, et al: Post-implant neuropathy of the trigeminal nerve: a case series, *Br Dent J* 212:E17, 2012.

228. Renton T, Yilmaz Z: Profiling of patients presenting with posttraumatic neuropathy of the trigeminal nerve, *J Orofac Pain* 25:333, 2011.

229. Renton T, Yilmaz Z: Managing iatrogenic trigeminal nerve injury: a case series and review of the literature, *Int J Oral Maxillofac Surg* 41:629, 2012.

230. Reznick JB, Ardary WC: Cervicofacial subcutaneous air emphysema after dental extraction, *J Am Dent Assoc* 120:417, 1990.

231. Rickles NH, Joshi BA: A possible case in a human and an investigation in dogs of death from air embolism during root canal therapy, *J Am Dent Assoc* 67:397, 1963.

232. Ricucci D, Langeland K: Apical limit of root-canal instrumentation and obturation, *Int Endod J* 31:394, 1998.

233. Robinson MJ, McDonald NJ, Mullally PJ: Apical extrusion of thermoplasticized obturating material in canals instrumented with Profile 0.06 or Profile GT, *J Endod* 30:418, 2004.

234. Roda RS: Root perforation repair: surgical and nonsurgical management, *Pract Proced Aesthet Dent* 13:467; quiz 474, 2001.

235. Roda RS: Personal communication, 2013.

236. Ross IS: Some effects of heavy metals on fungal cells, *Transactions of the British Mycology Society* 64:175, 1975.

237. Rossiter JL, Hendrix RA: Iatrogenic subcutaneous cervicofacial and mediastinal emphysema, *J Otolaryngol* 20, 1981.

238. Rowe AH: Damage to the inferior dental nerve during or following endodontic treatment, *Br Dent J* 155:306, 1983.

239. Rud J, Rud V: Surgical endodontics of upper molars: relation to the maxillary sinus and operation in acute state of infection, *J Endod* 24:260, 1998.

240. Ruddle CJ: Micro-endodontic non-surgical retreatment, *Dent Clin North Am* 41:429, 1997.

241. Ruddle CJ: Nonsurgical retreatment. In Cohen S, Burns RC, editors: *Pathways of the pulp*, ed 8, St. Louis, 2002, CV Mosby, p 875.

242. Ruddle CJ: Nonsurgical retreatment, *J Endod* 30:827, 2004.

243. Sabala CL, Roane JB, Southard LZ: Instrumentation of curved canals using a modified tipped instrument: a comparison study, *J Endod* 14:59, 1988.

244. Sakkal S, Gagnon A, Lemian L: [Paresthesia of the mandibular nerve caused by endodontic treatment: a case report], *J Can Dent Assoc* 60:556, 1994.

245. Sattapan B, Nervo GJ, Palamara JE, Messer HH: Defects in rotary nickel-titanium files after clinical use, *J Endod* 26:161, 2000.

246. Saunders JL, Eleazer PD, Zhang P, Michalek S: Effect of a separated instrument on bacterial penetration of obturated root canals, *J Endod* 30:177, 2004.

247. Schafer E, Dzepina A, Danesh G: Bending properties of rotary nickel-titanium instruments, *Oral Surg Oral Med Oral Pathol Oral Radiol Endod* 96:757, 2003.

248. Schafer E, Schulz-Bongert U, Tulus G: Comparison of hand stainless steel and nickel titanium rotary instrumentation: a clinical study, *J Endod* 30:432, 2004.

249. Schilder H: Filling root canals in three dimensions, *Dent Clin North Am* 11:723, 1967.

250. Schwarze T, Baethge C, Stecher T, Geurtsen W: Identification of second canals in the mesiobuccal root of maxillary first and second molars using magnifying loupes or an operating microscope, *Aust Endod J* 28:57, 2002.

251. Scolozzi P, Lombardi T, Jaques B: Successful inferior alveolar nerve decompression for dysesthesia following endodontic treatment: report of 4 cases treated by mandibular sagittal osteotomy, *Oral Surg Oral Med Oral Pathol Oral Radiol Endod* 97:625, 2004.

252. Selbst AG: Understanding informed consent and its relationship to the incidence of adverse treatment events in conventional endodontic therapy, *J Endod* 16:387, 1990.

253. Selden HS: The endo-antral syndrome: an endodontic complication, *J Am Dent Assoc* 119:397, 401, 1989.

254. Seltzer S, Naidorf IJ: Flare-ups in endodontics. I. Etiological factors, *J Endod* 11:472, 1985.

255. Senges C, Wrbas KT, Altenburger M, et al: Bacterial and Candida albicans adhesion on different root canal filling materials and sealers, *J Endod* 37:1247, 2011.

256. Serafino C, Gallina G, Cumbo E, et al: Ultrasound effects after post space preparation: an SEM study, *J Endod* 32:549, 2006.

257. Setzer FC, Bohme CP: Influence of combined cyclic fatigue and torsional stress on the fracture point of nickel-titanium rotary instruments, *J Endod* 39:133, 2013.

258. Shen Y, Peng B, Cheung GS: Factors associated with the removal of fractured NiTi instruments from root canal systems, *Oral Surg Oral Med Oral Pathol Oral Radiol Endod* 98:605, 2004.

259. Shovelton DS: Surgical emphysema as a complication of dental operations, *Br Dent J* 102:125, 1957.

260. Silva EJ, Rosa TP, Herrera DR, et al: Evaluation of cytotoxicity and physicochemical properties of calcium silicate-based endodontic sealer MTA Fillapex, *J Endod* 39:274, 2013.

261. Siqueira JF: Microbial causes of endodontic flare-ups, *Int Endod J* 36:453, 2003.

262. Sjögren U: Success and failure in endodontics, Umeå University Dissertation N. 60 33, 1996.

263. Smatt Y, Browaeys H, Genay A, et al: Iatrogenic pneumomediastinum and facial emphysema after endodontic treatment, *Br J Oral Maxillofac Surg* 42:160, 2004.

264. Snyder MB, Rosenberg ES: Subcutaneous emphysema during periodontal surgery: report of a case, *J Periodontol* 48:790, 1997.

265. Somma F, Cammarota G, Plotino G: The effectiveness of manual and mechanical instrumentation for the retreatment of three different root canal filling materials, *J Endod* 34:466, 2008.

266. Song M, Kim HC, Lee W, Kim E: Analysis of the cause of failure in nonsurgical endodontic treatment by microscopic inspection during endodontic microsurgery, *J Endod* 37:1516, 2011.

267. Sousa CJ, Loyola AM, Versiani MA, et al: A comparative histological evaluation of the biocompatibility of materials used in apical surgery, *Int Endod J* 37:738, 2004.

268. Souter NJ, Messer HH: Complications associated with fractured file removal using an ultrasonic technique, *J Endod* 31:450, 2005.

269. Souyave LC, Inglis AT, Alcalay M: Removal of fractured endodontic instruments using ultrasonics, *Br Dent J* 159:251, 1985.

270. Spangberg L, Langeland K: Biologic effects of dental materials. 1. Toxicity of root canal filling materials on HeLa cells in vitro, *Oral Surg* 35:402,1973.

271. Spencer HR, Ike V, Brennan PA: Review: the use of sodium hypochlorite in endodontics—potential complications and their management, *Br Dent J* 202:555, 2007.

272. Spili P, Parashos P, Messer HH: The impact of instrument fracture on outcome of endodontic treatment, *J Endod* 31:845, 2005.

273. Stabholz A, Friedman S: Endodontic retreatment—case selection and technique. Part 2: treatment planning for retreatment, *J Endod* 14:607, 1988.

274. Stammberger H, Jakse R, Beaufort F: Aspergillosis of the paranasal sinuses: x-ray diagnosis, histopathology and clinical aspects, *Ann Otol Rhinol Laryngol* 93:251, 1984.

275. Steelman RJ, Johannes PW: Subcutaneous emphysema during restorative dentistry, *International Journal of Paediatric Dentistry/the British Paedodontic Society [and] the International Association of Dentistry for Children* 17:228, 2007.

276. Stock CJ: Calcium hydroxide: root resorption and perio-endo lesions, *Br Dent J* 158:325–34, 1985.

277. Stropko JJ: Canal morphology of maxillary molars: clinical observations of canal configurations, *J Endod* 25:446, 1999.

278. Sujeet K, Shankar S: Images in clinical medicine. Prevertebral emphysema after a dental procedure, *New Engl J Med* 356:173, 2007.

279. Suter B, Lussi A, Sequeira P: Probability of removing fractured instruments from root canals, *Int Endod J* 38:112, 2005.

280. Sweatman TL, Baumgartner JC, Sakaguchi RL: Radicular temperatures associated with thermoplastic gutta percha, *J Endod* 27:512, 2001.

281. Tahan E, Çelik D, Er K, Taşdemir T: Effect of unintentionally extruded mineral trioxide aggregate in treatment of tooth with periradicular lesion: a case report, *J Endod* 36:760, 2010.

282. Takahashi CM, Cunha RS, De Martin AS, et al: In vitro evaluation of the effectiveness of ProTaper Universal rotary retreatment system for gutta-percha removal with or without a solvent, *J Endod* 35:1580, 2009.

283. Tanalp J, Kaptan F, Sert S, et al: Quantitative evaluation of the amount of apically extruded debris using 3 different rotary instrumentation systems, *Oral Surg Oral Med Oral Pathol Oral Radiol Endod* 101:252, 2006.

284. Terauchi Y: Separated file removal, *Dentistry Today* 31:110, 2012.

285. Terauchi Y, O'Leary L, Kikuchi I, et al: Evaluation of the efficiency of a new file removal system in comparison with two conventional systems, *J Endod* 33:585, 2007.

286. Terauchi Y, O'Leary L, Yoshioka T, Suda H: Comparison of the time required to create secondary fracture of separated file fragments using ultrasonic vibration under various canal conditions, *J Endod* 39:1300, 2013.

287. Thompson SA, Dummer PMH: Shaping ability of Quantec Series 2000 rotary nickel-titanium instruments in simulated root canals: part 2, *Int Endod J* 31:268, 1998.

288. Tilotta-Yasukawa F, Millot S, El Haddioui A, et al: Labiomandibular paresthesia caused by endodontic treatment: an anatomic and clinical study, *Oral Surg Oral Med Oral Pathol Oral Radiol Endod* 102:e47, 2006.

289. Tinaz AC, Alacam T, Uzun O, et al: The effect of disruption of apical constriction on periapical extrusion, *J Endod* 31:533, 2005.

290. Torabinejad M, Lemon RR: Procedural accidents. In Walton RE, Torabinejad M, editors: *Principles and practice of endodontics*, ed 3, Philadelphia, 2002, WB Saunders, p 310.

291. Torabinejad M, Walton RE, editors: *Principles and practice of endodontics*, ed 4, St. Louis, 2009, Saunders.

292. Tronstad L, Sunde PT: The evolving new understanding of endodontic infections, *Endod Topics* 6:57, 2003.

293. Turnbull A: Remarkable coincidence in dental surgery [letter], *Br Med J* 1:1131, 1900.

294. Tzanetakis GN, Kontakiotis EG, Maurikou DV, et al: Prevalence and management of instrument fracture in the postgraduate endodontic program at the Dental School of Athens: a five-year retrospective clinical study, *J Endod* 34:675, 2008.

295. Uehara M, Okumura T, Asahina I: Subcutaneous cervical emphysema induced by a dental air syringe: a case report, *Int Dent J* 57:286, 2007.

296. Ullmann CJ, Peters OA: Effect of cyclic fatigue on static fracture loads in ProTaper nickel-titanium rotary instruments, *J Endod* 31:183, 2005.

297. Vasilakis GJ, Vasilakis CM: Mandibular endodontic-related paresthesia, *General Dent* 52:334, 2004.
298. Walton RE: Current concepts of canal preparation, *Dent Clin North Am* 36:309, 1992.
299. Walton RE, Torabinejad M: *Principles and practice of endodontics*, ed 3, Philadelphia, 2002, WB Saunders, pp 184, 222-223, 319.
300. Ward JR, Parashos P, Messer HH: Evaluation of an ultrasonic technique to remove fractured rotary nickel-titanium endodontic instruments from root canals: an experimental study, *J Endod* 29:756, 2003.
301. Ward JR, Parashos P, Messer HH: Evaluation of an ultrasonic technique to remove fractured rotary nickel-titanium endodontic instruments from root canals: clinical cases, *J Endod* 29:764, 2003.
302. Watzek G, Bernhart T, Ulm C: Complications of sinus perforations and their management in endodontics, *Dent Clin North Am* 41:563, 1997.
303. Weine F: *Endodontic therapy*, ed 5, St Louis, 1996, Mosby, pp 324-330, 545.
304. Weisman MI: The removal of difficult silver cones, *J Endod* 9:210, 1983.
305. Wilcox LR, Roskelley C, Sutton T: The relationship of root canal enlargement to finger-spreader induced vertical root fracture, *J Endod* 23:533, 1997.
306. Wong R, Cho F: Microscopic management of procedural errors, *Dent Clin North Am* 41:455, 1997.
307. Worthington P: Injury to the inferior alveolar nerve during implant placement: a formula for protection of the patient and clinician, *Int J Oral Maxillofac Implants* 19:731, 2004.
308. Wright KJ, Derkson GD, Riding KH: Tissue-space emphysema, tissue necrosis, and infection following use of compressed air during pulp therapy: case report, *Pediatr Dentistry* 13:110, 1991.
309. Wu MK, Kast'akova A, Wesselink PRL: Quality of cold and warm gutta-percha in oval canals in mandibular premolars, *J Endod* 24:223, 1998.
310. Wu MK, Wesselink PR, Walton RE: Apical terminus location of root canal treatment procedures, *Oral Surg Oral Med Oral Pathol Oral Radiol Endod* 89:99, 2000.
311. Yaltirik M, Berberoglu HK, Koray M, et al: Orbital pain and headache secondary to overfilling of a root canal, *J Endod* 29:771, 2003.
312. Yang SC, Chiu TH, Lin TJ, Chan HM: Subcutaneous emphysema and pneumomediastinum secondary to dental extraction: a case report and literature review, *Kaohsiung J Med Sci* 22:641, 2006.
313. Yoldas O, Oztunc H, Tinaz C, Alparslan N: Perforation risks associated with the use of Masserann endodontic kit drills in mandibular molars, *Oral Surg Oral Med Oral Pathol Oral Radiol Endod* 97:513, 2004.
314. Yoshimoto A, Mitamura Y, Nakamura H, Fujimura M: Acute dyspnea during dental extraction, *Respiration* 69:369, 2002.
315. You SY, Bae KS, Baek SH, et al: Lifespan of one nickel-titanium rotary file with reciprocating motion in curved root canals, *J Endod* 36:1991, 2010.
316. Yum J, Cheung GS, Park JK, et al: Torsional strength and toughness of nickel-titanium rotary files, *J Endod* 37:382, 2011.
317. Zehnder M: Root canal irrigants, *J Endod* 32:389, 2006.
318. Zemann W, Feichtinger M, Karcher H: Cervicofacial and mediastinal emphysema after crown preparation: a rare complication, *Int J Prosthodont* 20:143, 2007.
319. Zuolo ML, Walton RE, Imura N: Histologic evaluation of three endodontic instrument/preparation techniques, *Endod Dent Traumatol* 8:125, 1992.

Expanded Clinical Topics

CHAPTER 20

The Role of Endodontics After Dental Traumatic Injuries

MARTIN TROPE | FREDERIC BARNETT | ASGEIR SIGURDSSON | NOAH CHIVIAN

CHAPTER OUTLINE

A traumatic injury to the tooth results in damage to many dental and periradicular structures, making the management and consequences of these injuries multifactorial. Knowledge of the interrelating healing patterns of these tissues is essential. This chapter concentrates on the role of the dentinopulpal complex in the pathogenesis of disease subsequent to dentinal trauma and how treatment of this complex can contribute to favorable healing after an injury.

UNIQUE ASPECTS OF DENTAL TRAUMA

Most dental trauma occurs in the 7- to 12-year-old age group and is mainly due to falls and accidents near home or school.[23,143] It occurs primarily in the anterior region of the mouth, affecting the maxillary more than the mandibular jaw.[28] Serious accidents, such as automobile crashes, can affect any tooth and can occur in all age ranges. In many cases, after a traumatic dental injury, endodontic treatment is provided to caries-free, single-rooted, young permanent teeth. If quick and correct treatment for these teeth is provided after injury, the potential for a successful endodontic outcome is very good.

MOST COMMON TYPES OF DENTAL TRAUMA

Crown Fractures

Most crown fractures occur in young, caries-free anterior teeth.[95,107] This makes maintaining or regaining pulp vitality essential. Luckily, vital pulp therapy supports a good prognosis in these situations if correct treatment and follow-up procedures are carefully followed.

Crown-Root Fractures

Crown-root fractures are first treated periodontally to ensure that there is a sufficient and good margin to allow restoration. If the tooth can be maintained from a periodontal point of view, then the pulp is treated as for a crown fracture.

Root Fractures

A surprisingly large number of pulps in root-fractured teeth will survive this rather dramatic injury. In almost every case, the apical segment stays vital, and in many cases, the coronal segment stays vital or regains vitality subsequent to the injury. If the coronal segment permanently loses vitality, it should be treated as an immature permanent tooth with nonvital pulp. *The apical segment rarely needs treatment.*

Luxation Injuries and Avulsion

Luxation injuries and avulsion often result in pulp necrosis and damage to the cemental protective layer of the root. The potential complication of pulp infection in a root that has lost its cemental protective layer makes these injuries potentially catastrophic. Correct emergency and follow-up evaluation, which may include timely endodontic treatment, is critical.

FOLLOW-UP AFTER DENTAL TRAUMA

The reader is referred to Chapter 1 for specific descriptions of pulp tests, but a few general statements about pulp tests on traumatized teeth may be helpful in trying to interpret the results.

For decades, controversy has surrounded the validity of thermal and electric tests on traumatized teeth. Only generalized impressions may be gained from these tests following a traumatic injury. They are in reality sensitivity tests for nerve function and do not indicate the presence or absence of blood circulation within the pulpal space. It is assumed that subsequent to traumatic injury, the conduction capability of the nerve endings and/or sensory receptors is sufficiently deranged to inhibit the nerve impulse from an electrical or thermal stimulus. This makes the traumatized tooth vulnerable to false-negative readings from such tests.[123]

Teeth that give a response at the initial examination cannot be assumed to be healthy and to continue to give a response over time. Teeth that yield no response cannot be assumed to have necrotic pulps because they may give a response at later follow-up visits. It has been demonstrated that it may take as long as 9 months for normal blood flow to return to the coronal

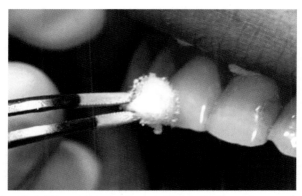

FIG. 20-1 Difluorodichloromethane (-40° F [-40° C]) gas is sprayed on a cotton pellet and then placed on the incisal edge of the maxillary incisor.

pulp of a traumatized fully formed tooth. As circulation is restored, the responsiveness to pulp tests returns.[73]

The transition from a negative response to a positive response at a subsequent test may be considered a sign of a healing pulp. The repetitious finding of responses may be taken as a sign of a healthy pulp. The transition from a response to no response may be taken as an indication that the pulp is probably undergoing degeneration and therefore an intervention in the form of endodontic treatment might be indicated. The persistence of no response would suggest that the pulp has been irreversibly damaged, but even this is not absolute.[32]

Thermal and electrical pulp tests of all anterior teeth (canine to canine) of the maxillary and mandibular jaws should be performed at the time of the initial examination and carefully recorded to establish a baseline for comparison with subsequent repeated tests in later months. These tests should be repeated at 3 weeks; at 3, 6, and 12 months; and at yearly intervals after the trauma. The purpose of the tests is to establish a trend as to the physiologic status of the pulps of these teeth. Particularly in traumatized teeth, carbon dioxide snow (CO_2, -78° C) or dichlorodifluoromethane (-40° C) placed on the incisal third of the facial surface gives more accurate responses than a water-ice pencil (Fig. 20-1).[71,72] The intense cold seems to penetrate the tooth and covering splints or restorations and reach the deeper areas of the tooth. Neither the dry ice nor the dichlorodifluoromethane spray forms ice water, which could disperse over adjacent teeth or gingiva to give a false-positive response. In trauma evaluation, there is no question that using water-ice pencils should be avoided because of this. Dichlorodifluoromethane spray is a very inexpensive alternative to CO_2 snow; its coldness elicits much more reliable responses than water-ice. The electrical pulp test relies on electrical impulses directly stimulating the nerves of the pulp. These tests have limited value in young teeth but are useful when the dentinal tubules are closed and do not allow dentinal fluid to flow in them. This situation is typical of teeth in elderly patients or in traumatized teeth that are undergoing premature sclerosis. In these situations, the thermal tests that rely on fluid flow in the tubules cannot be used, and the electrical pulp test becomes important.

Laser Doppler flowmetry (LDF) was introduced in the early 1970s for measurement of blood flow in the retina.[88] The technique has also been used to assess blood flow in other tissue systems, such as the skin and renal cortex. It uses a beam of

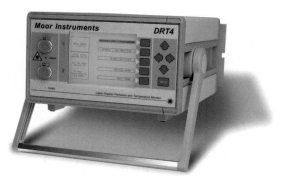

FIG. 20-2 Laser Doppler machine. (Courtesy Moor Instruments, Devon, United Kingdom.)

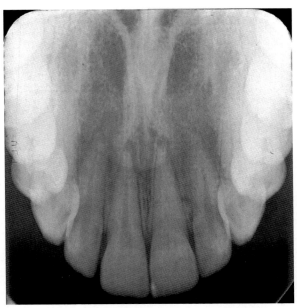

FIG. 20-3 An occlusal film of a luxation injury of central incisors. Both were diagnosed to be laterally luxated with apical translocation. Note that the left central is completely obliterated and has a history of being luxated some years prior.

infrared (780 to 820 nm) or near-infrared (632.8 nm) light that is directed into the tissue by optical fibers. As light enters the tissue, it is scattered by moving red blood cells and stationary tissue cells. Photons that interact with moving red blood cells are scattered, and the frequency shifts according to the Doppler principle. Photons that interact with stationary tissue cells are scattered but not Doppler shifted. A portion of the light is returned to a photodetector, and a signal is produced (Fig. 20-2).

Attempts have been made to use LDF technology for pulp vitality diagnosis in traumatized teeth because this would provide a more accurate reading of the vitality status of the pulp.[113,175,176] Studies have shown promising results, indicating that laser Doppler can detect blood flow more consistently and earlier than the standard vitality tests would be expected to render a response. In a study on young dogs, laser Doppler was able to correctly detect blood flow as early as 2 to 3 weeks after avulsion of an immature tooth and at the same time indicate no flow in those that would remain necrotic.[176]

Presently the cost of a laser Doppler flowmetry machine limits its use in private dental offices; these are used primarily in hospitals and teaching institutions.

RADIOGRAPHIC EXAMINATIONS

Radiographic imaging is essential for thorough examination, diagnosis, and management of dentoalveolar trauma. Imaging may reveal root fractures, subgingival crown fractures, tooth displacements, bone fractures, root resorptions, and embedded foreign objects. A single radiograph, even a panoramic image, is insufficient to properly diagnose just about any dental trauma case. In its 2012 guidelines for the management of traumatic dental injuries, and in the current recommendations on its interactive website (*www.dentaltraumaguide.org*), the International Association of Dental Traumatology (IADT) has recommended taking at least four different radiographs for almost every injury[65-67]: a direct 90-degree on the axis of the tooth, two with different vertical angulations, and one occlusal film (Fig. 20-3).

Multiple radiographs increase the likelihood of diagnosing root fractures, tooth displacement, and other possible injuries. However, two-dimensional (2D) imaging methods have well-known inherent limitations, and their lack of three-dimensional (3D) information may prevent proper diagnosis and adversely affect long-term treatment outcomes. The interpretation of an image can be confounded by a number of factors, including the regional anatomy and superimposition of both the teeth and surrounding dentoalveolar structures. As a result of superimposition, periapical radiographs reveal only limited aspects (i.e., a 2D view) of the true 3D anatomy.[44,119] Additionally, there is often geometric distortion of the anatomic structures imaged with conventional radiographic methods.[3] These problems can be overcome by using cone beam computed tomography (CBCT) imaging techniques, which produce accurate 3D images of the teeth and surrounding dentoalveolar structures and have shown promise in improving the clinician's ability to properly diagnose luxation injuries, alveolar fractures, root fractures, and root resorption (Fig. 20-4).[42,43]

In instances of soft tissue laceration, it is advisable to radiograph the injured area before suturing to be sure that no foreign objects have been embedded. A soft tissue radiograph with a normal-sized film briefly exposed at reduced kilovoltage should reveal the presence of many foreign substances, including tooth fragments (Fig. 20-5).

Cone Beam Computed Tomography and Dentoalveolar Trauma

CBCT is accomplished by using a rotating gantry to which an x-ray source and detector are fixed (see Chapter 2). A divergent pyramidal or cone-shaped source of ionizing radiation is directed through the middle of the area of interest onto an area x-ray detector on the opposite side of the patient. The x-ray source and detector rotate around a fixed fulcrum within the region of interest. During the exposure sequence, hundreds of planar projection images are acquired of the field of view (FOV) in an arc of at least 180°. In this single rotation, CBCT provides precise, essentially immediate, and accurate 3D radiographic images. Because CBCT exposure incorporates the

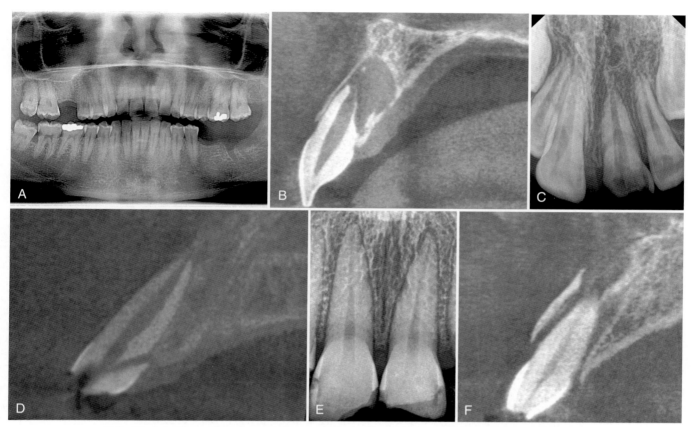

FIG. 20-4 **A,** Panoramic radiograph taken on a patient with past history of dentoalveolar trauma. Tooth #9 appeared to have arrested root development with a periapical radiolucency. **B,** Sagittal view of tooth #9 of same patient from CBCT imaging. This revealed that tooth #9 had arrested root development, a large PA radiolucency, and extensive root resorption along the palatal surface that was *not* evident on the panoramic image. **C,** Periapical radiograph of tooth #9 with extensive complicated crown fracture. The clinical examination revealed the crown fracture extended subgingivally on the palatal aspect. **D,** Sagittal view of tooth #9 of same patient from CBCT imaging. This revealed that the apical extent of the fractured palatal portion extended just apical to the crest of bone. The correct diagnosis of this injury was complicated crown-root fracture. **E,** Periapical radiograph of teeth #8, #9 revealed crown fractures. **F,** Sagittal view of tooth #9 of same patient from CBCT imaging. This revealed that tooth #9 suffered a lateral luxation displacement injury with extensive concomitant alveolar fracture. The necessary treatment of repositioning and splinting was apparent.   *Continued*

entire FOV, only one rotational sequence of the gantry is necessary to acquire enough data for image reconstruction.

CBCT has been suggested as an adjunct imaging tool when the true nature of the dentoalveolar root fracture and dental injuries cannot be confidently diagnosed from a conventional examination and radiographs.[43,111,120] However, it has been repeatedly demonstrated that the use of CBCT provides improved diagnostic images in cases of dentoalveolar injury.* Perhaps the use of CBCT imaging for dentoalveolar injuries will be considered "best practice" sometime in the near future.

Root Resorption

Because the development and progression of root resorption occur without clinical signs or symptoms, their early detection is challenging. The definitive diagnosis of root resorption,

therefore, depends on its radiographic demonstration, which in turn is limited by the diagnostic accuracy of the imaging device used to determine its presence (see Chapter 16).[120] The radiodensity of the root requires that a significant amount of root substance be removed to cause enough contrast on the radiograph to allow it to be detected. Thus, only resorptive defects on the mesial or distal aspects of the root can be predictably detected after some time; the facial and palatal or lingual aspects are much harder to see. To overcome these difficulties, it is essential to take as many different horizontal-angled radiographs as feasible in cases of suspected root resorption. Early detection of small resorption defects has been shown to be poor with conventional dental radiographs, and the extent of the resorptive defect is grossly underestimated compared to CBCT.[31,57,61]

The available literature supports the use of CBCT as a diagnostic tool to assess the true nature of teeth diagnosed with root resorption to improve diagnosis and aid management. This should ultimately improve the prognosis of teeth with

---

*References 30, 31, 42-44, 57, 61, 103, 111, 119, and 120.

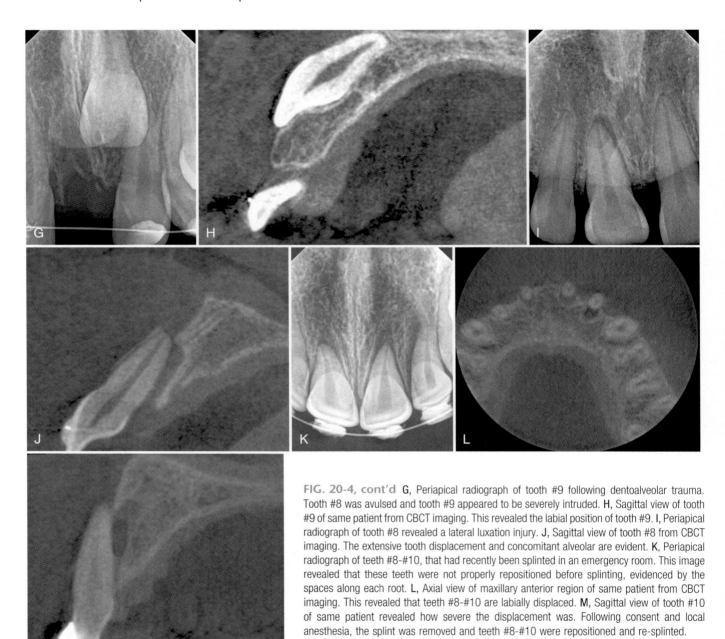

FIG. 20-4, cont'd **G,** Periapical radiograph of tooth #9 following dentoalveolar trauma. Tooth #8 was avulsed and tooth #9 appeared to be severely intruded. **H,** Sagittal view of tooth #9 of same patient from CBCT imaging. This revealed the labial position of tooth #9. **I,** Periapical radiograph of tooth #8 revealed a lateral luxation injury. **J,** Sagittal view of tooth #8 from CBCT imaging. The extensive tooth displacement and concomitant alveolar are evident. **K,** Periapical radiograph of teeth #8-#10, that had recently been splinted in an emergency room. This image revealed that these teeth were not properly repositioned before splinting, evidenced by the spaces along each root. **L,** Axial view of maxillary anterior region of same patient from CBCT imaging. This revealed that teeth #8-#10 are labially displaced. **M,** Sagittal view of tooth #10 of same patient revealed how severe the displacement was. Following consent and local anesthesia, the splint was removed and teeth #8-#10 were repositioned and re-splinted.

root resorption that require endodontic management (see Fig. 20-4, *A, B*).[120]

Horizontal (Transverse) Root Fractures

There is a significant risk of misdiagnosing the true location of a root fracture in anterior teeth when intraoral radiography is used because of the possibility of the oblique course of the fracture line in the sagittal plane. It has been shown that horizontal root fracture can be detected sooner using CBCT than with periapical views, and the fracture can be assessed in coronal, axial and cross-sectional views (see Fig. 20-4, *C, D*).[98] Compared to conventional radiographs, CBCT increased the

accuracy of diagnosing the actual nature of horizontal root fractures.[30,111]

Luxation Injuries

As previously mentioned, conventional intraoral radiography provides poor sensitivity in the detection of minimal tooth displacements and root and alveolar fractures.[103] CBCT has significantly improved the ability to accurately diagnose traumatic injuries and has the potential to overcome most of the technical limitations of the plain-film projection (see Fig. 20-4, *E-M*).*

---

*References 30, 31, 42, 43, 57, 61, 98, 103, 111, and 120.

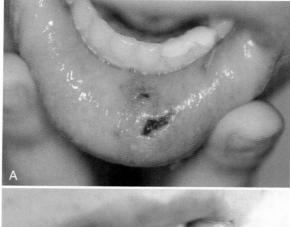
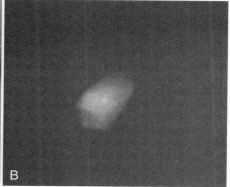
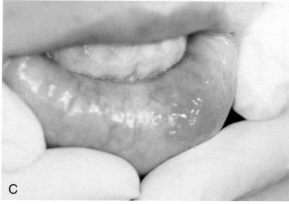

FIG. 20-5 Patient sustained complicated crown fractures on the left lower incisors and later on the canine tooth. **A,** An emergency pulp capping; Band-Aid composite was placed on the teeth. Six days later the patient was referred to the clinic because of a poorly healed laceration on the lip. **B,** Radiograph of the lip revealed a portion of the lateral crown still in the lip. The patient was anesthetized and the crown removed. **C,** Healing was quick and uneventful.

CROWN FRACTURES

As already mentioned, the primary aim from an endodontic point of view is to maintain pulp vitality after crown fractures.

Crown Infraction

Crown infraction can be defined as an incomplete fracture of or a crack in the enamel, without loss of tooth structure.[16]

Biologic Consequences

Crown infractions are injuries that carry little danger of resulting in pulp necrosis. Meticulous follow-up over a 5-year period is the most important endodontic preventive measure in these cases. If, at any follow-up examination, the reaction to sensitivity tests changes, or if, on radiographic assessment, signs of apical or periradicular periodontitis develop or the root appears to have stopped development or is obliterating, endodontic intervention should be considered.

Uncomplicated Crown Fracture

Uncomplicated crown fracture can be defined as fracture of the enamel only or the enamel and dentin without pulp exposure.[16]

Incidence

Uncomplicated crown fracture is likely to be the most commonly reported dental injury. It is estimated to account for at least one third to one half of all reported dental trauma.

Biologic Consequences

Uncomplicated crown fractures are also injuries that have little danger of resulting in pulp necrosis. In fact, the biggest danger to the health of the pulp is through iatrogenic causes during the aesthetic restoration of these teeth.

Treatment

There are two key issues in the treatment of crown fractures. First, all exposed dental tubules need to be closed as soon as reasonably possible. If the broken-off piece is not available or if it is not possible to reattach it and there is no time to do a full composite restoration at the time of the emergency appointment, a composite Band-Aid or temporary coverage should be placed on all exposed dentin. This prevents any ingress of bacteria into the tubules and reduces the patient's discomfort. The second issue is the remaining dentin thickness. Several studies have confirmed that if the remaining dentin is more than 0.5 mm thick, the tooth can be restored with the restoration of choice, including etching and bonding, and no special attention needs to be given to the pulp.[3,46,60,115,151] However, if the remaining dentin is less than this thickness, a protective layer of hard-setting calcium hydroxide in the deepest part of the dentin exposure does reduce, if not completely prevent, reactive inflammation of the underlying pulp, which is a significantly different reaction compared to the negative reaction to composite bonding systems.[3,46,60,115,151]

Complicated Crown Fracture

A *complicated crown fracture* involves enamel, dentin, and pulp (Fig. 20-6).[1]

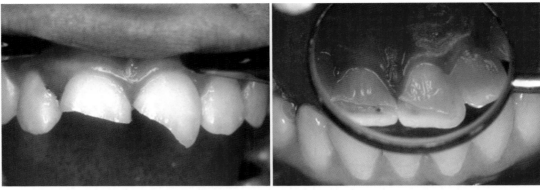

FIG. 20-6 Complicated crown fracture involving enamel, dentin, and pulp.

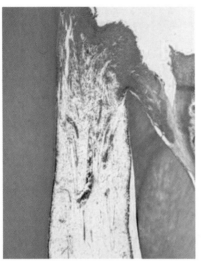

FIG. 20-7 Histologic appearance of the pulp within 24 hours of a traumatic exposure. The pulp proliferated over the exposed dentinal tubules. There is approximately 1.5 mm of inflamed pulp below the surface of the fracture.

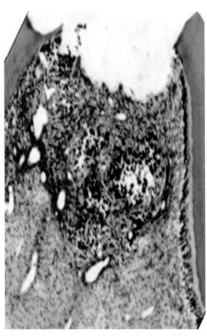

FIG. 20-8 Histologic appearance of the pulp days after a traumatic exposure. Superficial necrosis above a zone of inflamed pulp is seen.

Incidence

Complicated crown fractures occur in 0.9% to 13% of all dental injuries.[40,130,153]

Biologic Consequences

A crown fracture involving the pulp, if left untreated, always results in pulp necrosis.[97] However, the manner and time sequence in which the pulp becomes necrotic allow a great deal of potential for successful intervention to maintain pulp vitality. The first reaction after the injury is hemorrhage and local inflammation (Fig. 20-7).

Subsequent inflammatory changes are usually proliferative but can be destructive over time. A proliferative reaction is favored in traumatic injuries because the fractured surface is usually flat, allowing salivary rinsing with little chance of impaction of contaminated debris. Unless impaction of contaminated debris is obvious, it is expected that in the first 24 hours after the injury, a proliferative response with inflammation extending not more than 2 mm into the pulp will be present (see Fig. 20-7).[49,52,82] In time, the bacterial challenge results in local pulpal necrosis and a slow apical progression of the pulpal inflammation (Fig. 20-8).

Treatment

Treatment options for complicated crown fracture are (1) vital pulp therapy, comprising pulp capping, partial pulpotomy, or full pulpotomy; and (2) pulpectomy. The choice of treatment depends on the stage of development of the tooth, the time between trauma and treatment, concomitant periodontal injury, and the restorative treatment plan.

Stage of Development of the Tooth

Loss of vitality in an immature tooth can have catastrophic consequences. Root canal treatment on a tooth with a blunderbuss canal is time consuming and difficult. It is probably more important that necrosis of an immature tooth leaves it with thin dentinal walls that are susceptible to fracture both during and after the apexification procedure.[99] Every effort must be made to keep the tooth vital, at least until the apex and cervical root have completed their development.

Removal of the pulp in a mature tooth is not as significant as in an immature tooth because a pulpectomy in a mature tooth has an extremely high success rate.[142] However, it has been shown that under optimal conditions, vital pulp therapy (rather than removal) can be carried out successfully on a mature tooth.[110,172] Therefore, this form of therapy can be an option under certain circumstances, even though a pulpectomy is the treatment that affords the most predictable success.

In an immature tooth, vital pulp therapy should always be attempted if at all feasible because of the tremendous advantages of maintaining the vital pulp.

Time Between Trauma and Treatment

For 48 hours after a traumatic injury, the initial reaction of the pulp is proliferative, with no more than a 2-mm depth of pulpal inflammation (see Fig. 20-8). After 48 hours, chances of direct bacterial contamination of the pulp increase, with the zone of inflammation progressing apically[52]; as time passes, the likelihood of successfully maintaining a healthy pulp decreases.

Concomitant Attachment Damage

A periodontal injury compromises the nutritional supply of the pulp. This fact is particularly important in mature teeth, in which the chance of pulp survival is not as good as for immature teeth.[13,59]

Restorative Treatment Plan

Unlike in an immature tooth, in which the benefits of maintaining vitality of the pulp are so great, pulpectomy is a viable treatment option in a mature tooth. As pointed out, if performed under optimal conditions, vital pulp therapy after traumatic exposures can be successful. If the restorative treatment plan is simple and a composite resin restoration will suffice as the permanent restoration, this treatment option should be given serious consideration. If a more complex restoration is to be placed (e.g., a crown or bridge abutment), pulpectomy may be the more predictable treatment method.

Vital Pulp Therapy: Requirements for Success

Vital pulp therapy has an extremely high success rate if the following requirements can be met (also see Chapter 23).

- *Treatment of a noninflamed pulp.* Treatment of a healthy pulp has been shown to be an important requirement for successful therapy.[152,162] Vital pulp therapy of the inflamed pulp yields an inferior success rate,[152,162] so the optimal time for treatment is in the first 24 hours when pulp inflammation is superficial. As time between the injury and therapy increases, pulp removal must be extended apically to ensure that noninflamed pulp has been reached.
- *Bacteria-tight seal.* In our opinion, this requirement is the most critical factor for successful treatment.[152] Challenge by bacteria during the healing phase causes failure (see also Chapter 14).[45] If the exposed pulp is effectively sealed from bacterial leakage, successful healing of the pulp with a hard tissue barrier will occur independent of the dressing placed on the pulp and after more extended time periods between accident and treatment.[46,80]
- *Pulp dressing.* Calcium hydroxide has traditionally been used for vital pulp therapy. Its main advantage is that it is antibacterial[39,141] and disinfects the superficial pulp. Pure calcium hydroxide causes necrosis of about 1.5 mm of pulp tissue, which removes superficial layers of inflamed pulp if present (Fig. 20-9).[112] The high pH (12.5) of calcium hydroxide causes a liquefaction necrosis in the most superficial layers.[134] The toxicity of calcium hydroxide appears to be neutralized as the deeper layers of pulp are affected, causing a coagulative necrosis at the junction of the necrotic and vital pulp, resulting in only mild irritation. This mild irritation initiates an inflammatory response, and in the absence of

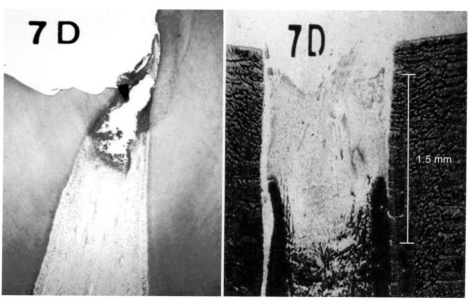

FIG. 20-9 Pulp necrosis of 1.5 mm as a result of the high pH of calcium hydroxide.

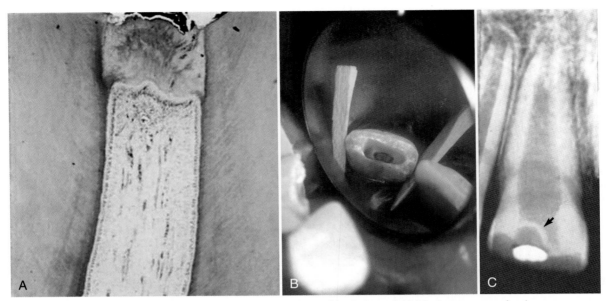

FIG. 20-10 Hard tissue barrier after calcium hydroxide partial pulpotomy. **A,** Histologic appearance of replacement odontoblasts and a hard tissue barrier. **B,** Clinical appearance of the barrier on removal of the coronal restoration 3 months after placement of the calcium hydroxide. **C,** Radiographic appearance of the hard tissue barrier.

bacteria,[134] the pulp will heal with a hard tissue barrier (Fig. 20-10).[133,134] Hard-setting calcium hydroxide does not cause necrosis of the superficial layers of pulp; it has also been shown to initiate healing with a hard tissue barrier.[150,159]

The major disadvantage of calcium hydroxide is that it does not seal the fractured surface. Therefore, an additional material must be used to ensure that bacteria do not challenge the pulp, particularly during the critical healing phase.

Many materials, such as zinc oxide eugenol,[25,162] tricalcium phosphate,[84] and composite resin,[24] have been proposed as medicaments for vital pulp therapy. None to this date have afforded the predictability of calcium hydroxide used in conjunction with a well-sealed coronal restoration.[60,102,139,151] In a dog study, for example, pulps capped directly with various adhesive agents showed moderate to severe inflammatory reactions, with progressive extension of tissue necrosis with time and total absence of continuous hard tissue bridge formation.[102] Application of a calcium hydroxide–based material was characterized by inflammatory cell infiltration, limited tissue necrosis, and partial to complete hard tissue bridging.[102] In a similar study on human teeth in vivo, it was found that Scotchbond Multi-Purpose Plus (3M, St. Paul, MN) caused inflammatory changes when applied directly to exposed pulp tissue; however, direct capping with Dycal followed by sealing with Scotchbond Multi-Purpose Plus showed favorable results in pulp tissue.[151]

Currently, bioceramic materials are considered the pulp capping agents of choice.[4] Mineral trioxide aggregate (MTA), a first-generation bioceramic material, has been shown to be a good pulp capping agent.[62,116,118,174] It has a high pH, similar to that of calcium hydroxide, when unset[156] and after setting creates an excellent bacteria-tight seal.[157] It is also hard enough to act as a base for a final restoration.[156] Yet MTA does not enjoy the same popularity as calcium hydroxide as a pulp capping agent in the treatment of traumatic exposures. There are

probably three main reasons. The first is likely to be that because MTA needs a moist environment for at least 6 hours to set properly, the treatment becomes a two-step procedure, compared with a one-step procedure for other medicaments. Using MTA as a pulp capping agent thus necessitates that a wet cotton pellet be placed over it until it is set, and then the permanent restoration can be fabricated at a later time. The second likely reason is that originally, MTA was gray in color and reported to cause discoloration in the tooth crown when used as a capping agent in anterior teeth.[37] To counter this discoloration problem, a new white version of MTA was marketed a few years ago. Initially there were some concerns that the pulp did not respond to the white version as favorably as it had to the gray one.[121] Relatively few studies have been done comparing the white MTA to the gray one, but most have indicated that the pulp seems to react as well to one as the other.[91,116,131] Unfortunately, the white MTA has been found to discolor in a similar fashion to the gray, presumably because of the bismuth oxide filler in the material.

The third likely reason is that recently, newer generation bioceramic materials have come to the market that have the same positive properties as MTA but not the disadvantages described previously. They set quickly enough for a one-visit procedure and do not discolor the tooth. These materials are now considered superior to calcium hydroxide as the capping agent for traumatic pulp exposures.

Treatment Methods
Pulp Capping
Pulp capping implies placing the dressing directly on the pulp exposure without any removal of the soft tissue.[24]

Indications
There are few indications for pulp capping when traumatic pulp exposures are treated. The success rate of this procedure

(80%),[69,125] compared to partial pulpotomy (95%),[49] indicates that a superficial pulp cap should not be considered after traumatic pulp exposures. The lower success rate is not difficult to understand because superficial inflammation develops soon after the traumatic exposure. If the treatment is at the superficial level, a number of inflamed (rather than healthy) pulps will be treated, lowering the potential for success. In addition, a bacteria-tight coronal seal is much more difficult to attain in superficial pulp capping because there is no depth to the cavity to aid in creating the seal, as there is with a partial pulpotomy.

It must be acknowledged that the studies suggesting that an inflamed pulp is contraindicated for an attempt at pulp capping were performed in the 1970s with amalgam as the standard coronal restoration. If we consider that amalgam leaks and calcium hydroxide washes out in the presence of moisture as the reasons for the poor results, then it may be poor coronal seal, rather than the inflamed pulp, that leads to the failure in these cases. More recent studies suggest that with the bioceramic as the pulp cap, the inflamed pulp is not the impediment as previously thought, but rather that the seal seems to be the major factor for success. Thus this material used as a base in these situations may give us more leeway for capping the inflamed pulp.

However in a situation of a traumatic pulp exposure of a tooth (injuries in which most patients are young [large pulps]), the patient typically presents for treatment within 48 hours because of sensitivity and aesthetic concerns. Therefore, the pulpal inflammation is usually only superficial. In these cases, we still feel it is prudent to remove the superficial layer of inflammation and place a bioceramic agent for pulp capping.

Partial Pulpotomy

Partial pulpotomy implies the removal of coronal pulp tissue to the level of healthy pulp. Knowledge of the reaction of the pulp after a traumatic injury makes it possible to accurately determine this level. This procedure is commonly called the *Cvek pulpotomy.*

Indications

As for pulp capping.

Technique

Administration of an anesthetic (possibly without a vasoconstrictor), rubber dam placement, and superficial disinfection are performed. A 1- to 2-mm deep cavity is prepared into the pulp, using a high-speed handpiece with a sterile diamond bur of appropriate size and copious water coolant (Fig. 20-11).[77] A slow-speed bur or spoon excavator should be avoided. If bleeding is excessive, the pulp is amputated deeper until only moderate hemorrhage is seen. Excess blood is carefully removed by rinsing with sterile saline, and the area is dried with a sterile cotton pellet. Use of 5% sodium hypochlorite (NaOCl; bleach) has been recommended to rinse the pulpal wound.[46] The bleach causes chemical amputation of the blood coagulum; removes damaged pulp cells, dentin chips, and other debris; and provides hemorrhage control with minimal damage to the "normal" pulp tissue underneath.

Care must be taken not to allow a blood clot to develop because this would compromise the prognosis.[49,133] A thin layer of pure calcium hydroxide is mixed with sterile saline or anesthetic solution to a thick mix and carefully placed on the pulp stump. If the pulp size does not permit additional loss of pulp tissue, a commercial hard-setting calcium hydroxide can be used.[150] The prepared cavity is filled with a material with the best chance of a bacteria-tight seal (zinc oxide eugenol or glass ionomer cement) to a level flush with the fractured surface. The material in the pulpal cavity and all exposed dentinal tubules are etched and restored with bonded composite resin. Alternatively, after hemostasis has been obtained, the pulp can be capped with MTA, a wet cotton pellet can be placed on top of it, and the access can be temporized for the appropriate time. The cotton pellet needs to be removed as early as possible and the tooth then restored with composite restoration.

Follow-Up

The follow-up is the same as for pulp capping. Emphasis is placed on evidence of maintenance of responses to sensitivity tests and radiographic evidence of continued root development (Fig. 20-12).

Prognosis

This method affords many advantages over pulp capping. Superficial inflamed pulp is removed during preparation of the pulpal cavity. Calcium hydroxide disinfects dentin and pulp and removes additional pulpal inflammation. Most important, space is provided for a material that can achieve a bacteria-tight seal to allow pulpal healing with hard tissue under optimal conditions. Additionally, coronal pulp remains, which allows sensitivity testing to be carried out at the follow-up visits. The prognosis is extremely good (94% to 96%).[49,70]

Full Pulpotomy

Full pulpotomy involves removal of the entire coronal pulp to a level of the root orifices. This level of pulp amputation is chosen arbitrarily because of its anatomic convenience. Because inflamed pulp sometimes extends past the canal orifices into the root pulp, many mistakes are made that result in treatment of an inflamed rather than a noninflamed pulp.

Indications

Full pulpotomy is indicated when it is anticipated that the pulp is inflamed to the deeper levels of the coronal pulp. Traumatic exposures after more than 72 hours and carious exposure of a young tooth with a partially developed apex are two examples of cases in which this treatment may be indicated. Because of the likelihood that the dressing will be placed on an inflamed pulp, full pulpotomy is contraindicated in mature teeth. In the immature tooth, benefits outweigh risks for this treatment form only with incompletely formed apices and thin dentinal walls.

Technique

The procedure begins with administration of an anesthetic, rubber dam placement, and superficial disinfection, as for pulp capping and partial pulpotomy. The coronal pulp is removed as in partial pulpotomy, but to the level of the root orifices. A calcium hydroxide dressing, a bacteria-tight seal, and a coronal restoration are carried out as for partial pulpotomy.

Follow-Up

Follow-up is the same as for pulp capping and partial pulpotomy. A major disadvantage of this treatment method is that

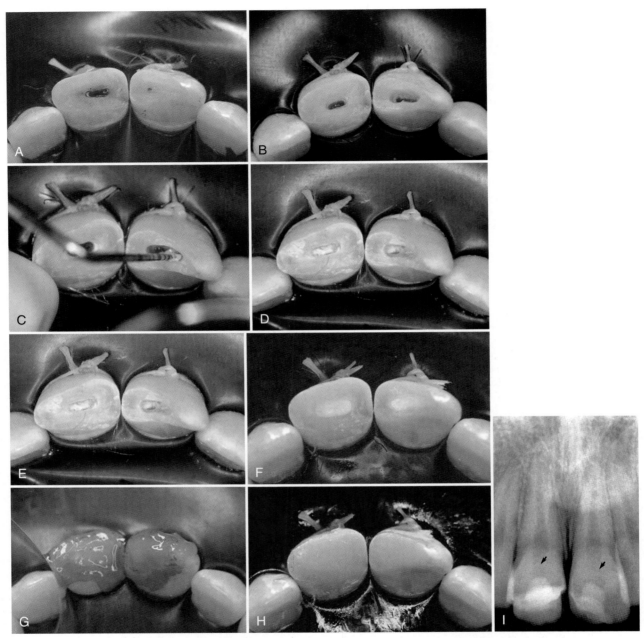

FIG. 20-11 Cvek partial pulpotomy. **A**, The fractured teeth are cleaned and disinfected; a rubber dam is placed. **B**, Cavities are prepared at high speed with a round diamond bur 1 to 2 mm into the pulpal tissue. **C**, Calcium hydroxide on a plugger (**D**) is placed on the soft tissue of the pulp. **E**, Care is taken to avoid smearing the walls of the preparation with the calcium hydroxide. **F**, Cavity preparations are filled with glass ionomer cement. The exposed dentin is etched (**G**) and then covered with composite resin (**H**). **I**, Radiograph 6 months later shows formation of hard tissue barriers in both teeth. (Courtesy Dr. Alessandra Ritter, Chapel Hill, NC.)

sensitivity testing is not possible, owing to the loss of coronal pulp, so radiographic follow-up is extremely important to assess for signs of apical periodontitis and to ensure the continuation of root formation.

Prognosis

Because cervical pulpotomy is performed on pulps that are expected to have deep inflammation and the site of pulp amputation is arbitrary, many more mistakes are made that lead to treatment of the inflamed pulp. Consequently the prognosis, which is in the range of 75%, is poorer than for partial pulpotomy.[74] Because of the inability to evaluate pulp status after full pulpotomy, some authors have recommended pulpectomy routinely after the roots have fully formed (Fig. 20-13). This philosophy is based on the pulpectomy procedure having a success rate in the range of 95%, whereas if apical periodontitis develops, the prognosis of root canal treatment drops significantly to about 80%.[136,142]

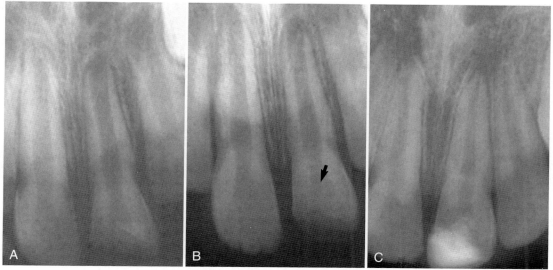

FIG. 20-12 Continued root development after partial pulpotomy. **A,** Radiograph of immature tooth with a complicated crown fracture. **B,** At the time of placement of calcium hydroxide after partial pulpotomy. **C,** Follow-up radiograph confirming that the pulp maintained vitality and the root continued to develop.

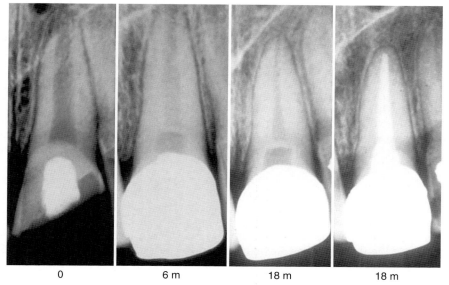

| 0 | 6 m | 18 m | 18 m |

FIG. 20-13 Successful pulpotomy followed by a pulpectomy at 18 months. (Courtesy Dr. Leif Tronstad, Oslo, Norway.)

Pulpectomy

Pulpectomy implies removal of the entire pulp to the level of the apical foramen.

Indications

Pulpectomy is indicated in a complicated crown fracture of mature teeth if conditions are not ideal for vital pulp therapy or if it is foreseeable that restoring the tooth would require placement of a post. This procedure is no different from root canal treatment of a vital nontraumatized tooth.

Treatment of the Nonvital Pulp

Immature Tooth: Apexification

Indications

Apexification should be performed in teeth with open apices and thin dentinal walls in which standard instrumentation techniques cannot create an apical stop to facilitate effective root canal filling.

Biologic Consequences

A nonvital immature tooth presents a number of difficulties for adequate endodontic treatment. The canal is often wider apically than coronally, necessitating the use of a filling technique with softened filling material to mold it to the shape of the apical part of the canal. Because the apex is extremely wide, no barrier exists to stop this softened material from moving into and traumatizing the apical periodontal tissues. Also, the lack of apical stop and extrusion of material through the canal might result in a canal that is underfilled and susceptible to leakage. An additional problem in immature teeth with thin dentinal walls is their susceptibility to fracture, both during and after treatment.[50]

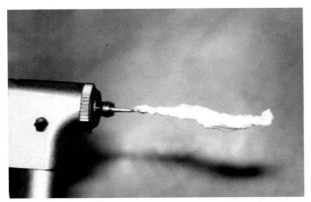

FIG. 20-14 Creamy mix of calcium hydroxide on a Lentulo spiral instrument ready for placement into the canal.

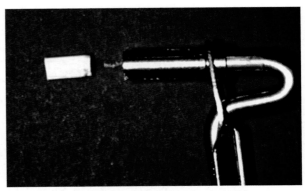

FIG. 20-15 Thick mix of calcium hydroxide.

These problems are overcome by stimulating the formation of a hard tissue barrier to allow for optimal filling of the canal and by reinforcing the weakened root against fracture, both during and after apexification.[101,154]

Technique

Disinfection of the Canal

In most cases nonvital teeth are infected,[29,138] so the first phase of treatment is to disinfect the root canal system to ensure periapical healing.[39,53] The canal length is estimated with a parallel preoperative radiograph, and after access to the canals has been prepared, a file is placed to this estimated length. When the length has been confirmed radiographically, very light filing (because of the thin dentinal walls) is performed with copious irrigation with 0.5% NaOCl.[54,147] A lower strength of NaOCl is used because of the increased danger of placing the agent through the apex in immature teeth. The increased volume of irrigant used compensates for this lower concentration of NaOCl. An irrigation needle that can passively reach close to the apical length is useful in disinfecting the canals of these immature teeth. The canal is dried with paper points and a creamy mix of calcium hydroxide (toothpaste thickness) spun into the canal with a Lentulo spiral instrument (Fig. 20-14). Additional disinfecting action of calcium hydroxide is effective after its application for at least 1 week,[141] so continuation of treatment can take place any time after 1 week. Further treatment should not be delayed more than 1 month because the calcium hydroxide could be washed out by tissue fluids through the open apex, leaving the canal susceptible to reinfection.

Hard Tissue Apical Barrier

Traditional Method

Formation of the hard tissue barrier at the apex requires a similar environment to that required for hard tissue formation in vital pulp therapy: a mild inflammatory stimulus to initiate healing and a bacteria-free environment to ensure that inflammation is not progressive.

As with vital pulp therapy, calcium hydroxide is used for this procedure.[50,83,85] Pure calcium hydroxide powder is mixed with sterile saline (or anesthetic solution) to a thick (powdery) consistency (Fig. 20-15). The calcium hydroxide is packed against the apical soft tissue with a plugger or thick point to initiate hard tissue formation. This step is followed by backfilling with calcium hydroxide to completely fill the canal. The calcium hydroxide is meticulously removed from the access cavity to the level of the root orifices, and a well-sealing, temporary filling is placed in the access cavity. A radiograph is taken; the canal should appear to have become calcified, indicating that the entire canal has been filled with the calcium hydroxide (Fig. 20-16). Because calcium hydroxide washout is evaluated by its relative radiodensity in the canal, it is prudent to use a calcium hydroxide mixture without the addition of a radiopaquer, such as barium sulfate. These additives do not wash out as readily as calcium hydroxide, so if they are present in the canal, evaluation of washout is impossible.

At 3-month intervals, a radiograph is exposed to evaluate whether a hard tissue barrier has formed and if the calcium hydroxide has washed out of the canal. This is assessed to have occurred if the canal can be seen again radiographically. If no washout is evident, the calcium hydroxide can be left intact for another 3 months. Excessive calcium hydroxide dressing changes should be avoided if at all possible because the initial toxicity of the material is thought to delay healing.[104]

When completion of a hard tissue barrier is suspected, the calcium hydroxide should be washed out of the canal with NaOCl. A file of a size that can easily reach the apex can be used to gently probe for a stop at the apex. When a hard tissue barrier is indicated radiographically and can be probed with an instrument, the canal is ready for filling.

Bioceramic Barrier

The creation of a physiologic hard tissue barrier, although quite predictable, takes anywhere from 3 to 18 months with calcium hydroxide. The disadvantages of this long time period are that the patient is required to present for treatment multiple times and the tooth may fracture during treatment before the thin, weak roots can be strengthened. In addition, one study has indicated that long-term treatment with calcium hydroxide may weaken the roots and make them even more susceptible to fracture.[19]

Bioceramic material has been used to create a hard tissue barrier quickly after disinfection of the canal (see earlier in the section Traditional Method) (Fig. 20-17). Calcium sulfate is pushed through the apex to provide a resorbable extraradicular barrier against which to pack the bioceramic material. The material is mixed and placed into the apical 3 to 4 mm of the canal in a manner similar to the placement of calcium hydroxide. A wet cotton pellet should be placed against the bioceramic material and left for at least 6 hours. After the material

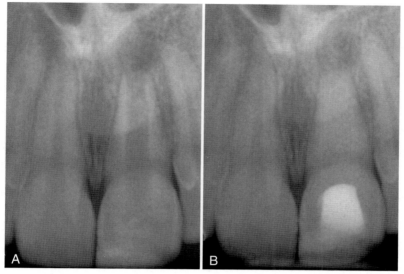

FIG. 20-16 **A** and **B**, Root canal that "disappears" after placement of a thick mix of pure calcium hydroxide and then over time washes out again. (Courtesy Dr. Cecilia Bourguignon, Paris, France.)

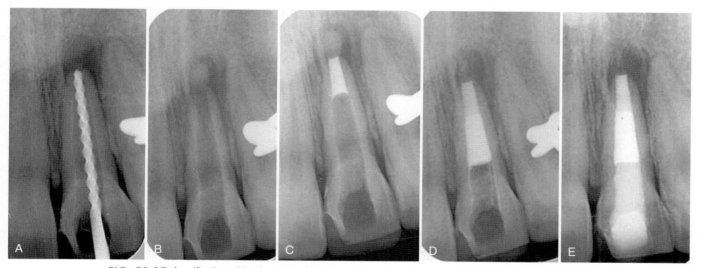

FIG. 20-17 Apexification with mineral trioxide aggregate (MTA). **A**, The canal is disinfected with light instrumentation, copious irrigation, and a creamy mix of calcium hydroxide for 1 month. **B**, Calcium sulfate is placed through the apex as a barrier against which the MTA is placed. **C**, A 4-mm MTA plug is placed at the apex. **D**, The body of the canal is filled with the Resilon obturation system. **E**, A bonded resin is placed below the cementoenamel junction (CEJ) to strengthen the root. (Courtesy Dr. Marga Ree. Purmerend, Netherlands)

has fully set, the entire canal is filled with a root-filling material. The cervical canal is then reinforced with composite resin to below the marginal bone level (described later) (see Fig. 20-17).

A number of case reports have been published using this apical barrier technique,[75,87,109] and it has steadily gained popularity with clinicians. Presently, no prospective long-term outcome study is available comparing its success rate with that of the traditional calcium hydroxide technique.

Filling the Root Canal
Because the apical diameter is larger than the coronal diameter of most of these canals, a softened filling technique is indicated in these teeth (see Chapter 7). Care must be taken to avoid excessive lateral force during filling, owing to the thin walls of

the root. If the hard tissue barrier was produced by long-term calcium hydroxide therapy, it consists of irregularly arranged layers of coagulated soft tissue, calcified tissue, and cementum-like tissue (Fig. 20-18). Included also are islands of soft connective tissue, giving the barrier a "Swiss cheese" consistency.[33,48] Because of the irregular nature of the barrier, it is not unusual for cement or softened filling material to be pushed through it into the apical tissues during filling (Fig. 20-19). Formation of the hard tissue barrier might be some distance short of the radiographic apex because the barrier forms wherever the calcium hydroxide contacts vital tissue. In teeth with wide, open apices, vital tissue can survive and proliferate from the periodontal ligament a few millimeters into the root canal. Filling should be completed to the level of the hard tissue barrier and not forced toward the radiographic apex.

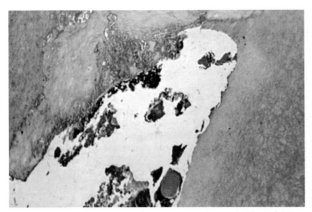

FIG. 20-18 Histologic appearance of hard tissue barrier after calcium hydroxide apexification. The barrier is composed of cementum and bone with soft tissue inclusions.

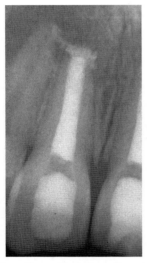

FIG. 20-19 Root filing with a soft technique after calcium hydroxide apexification. Sealer and softened filling material is expressed through the "Swiss cheese" holes in the barrier.

Reinforcement of Thin Dentinal Walls

The apexification procedure has become a predictably successful procedure (see the section Prognosis),[68] but thin dentinal walls still present a clinical problem. Should secondary injuries occur, teeth with thin dentinal walls are more susceptible to fractures that render them unrestorable.[56,158] It has been reported that approximately 30% of these teeth will fracture during or after endodontic treatment.[101] Consequently, some clinicians have questioned the advisability of the apexification procedure and have opted for more radical treatment procedures, including extraction followed by extensive restorative procedures, such as dental implants. Studies have shown that intracoronal bonded restorations can internally strengthen endodontically treated teeth and increase their resistance to fracture.[76,99] Thus, after root filling, the material should be removed to below the marginal bone level and a bonded resin filling placed (see Fig. 20-17).

Follow-Up

Routine recall evaluation should be performed to determine success in the prevention or treatment of apical periodontitis.

Restorative procedures should be assessed to ensure that they in no way promote root fractures.

Prognosis

Periapical healing and the formation of a hard tissue barrier occur predictably with long-term calcium hydroxide treatment (79% to 96%).[50,101] However, long-term survival is jeopardized by the fracture potential of the thin dentinal walls of these teeth. It is expected that the newer techniques of internally strengthening the teeth described earlier will increase their long-term survivability.

Pulp Revitalization

Revitalization of a necrotic pulp has been considered possible only after avulsion of an immature permanent tooth that was reimplanted within 40 minutes (discussed later). The advantages of pulp revascularization lie in the possibility of further root development and reinforcement of dentinal walls by deposition of hard tissue, thus strengthening the root against fracture (see also Chapter 10). After reimplantation of an avulsed immature tooth, a unique set of circumstances exists that allows regeneration to take place. The young tooth has an open apex and is short, which allows new tissue to grow into the pulp space relatively quickly. The pulp is necrotic but usually neither degenerated nor infected, so it acts as a matrix into which the new tissue can grow. It has been experimentally shown that the apical part of a pulp may remain vital and after reimplantation proliferate coronally, replacing the necrotized portion of the pulp.[26,117,145] Because in most cases the crown of the tooth is intact and caries free, bacterial penetration into the pulp space through cracks[106] and defects will be a slow process. The race between new tissue growth and infection of the pulp space favors the new tissue.

Regeneration of pulp tissue in a necrotic infected tooth with apical periodontitis was thought to be impossible until about a decade ago.[114] However, if it is possible to create an environment similar to that described for the avulsed tooth, regeneration will probably occur. If the canal is effectively disinfected, a matrix into which new tissue can grow is provided, and coronal access is effectively sealed. Regeneration should occur as in an avulsed immature tooth.

Banchs and Trope[25] wrote one of the first case reports that suggest it may be possible to replicate the unique circumstances of an avulsed tooth. The case (Fig. 20-20) described the treatment of an immature second mandibular premolar that had radiographic and clinical signs of apical periodontitis, along with a sinus tract. The canal was disinfected without mechanical instrumentation but with copious irrigation with 5.25% NaOCl, followed by placement of an intracanal mixture of antibiotics consisting of equal amounts of ciprofloxacin, metronidazole, and minocycline for 3 weeks.[89]

The antibiotic mixture was rinsed out after 3 weeks, and a blood clot was produced to the level of the cementoenamel junction to provide a matrix for ingrowth of new tissue; this was followed by a deep coronal restoration to provide a bacteria-tight seal. Clinical and radiographic evidence of healing appeared as early as 22 days; the large radiolucency had disappeared within 2 months; and at the 24-month recall, it was obvious that the root walls were thick and development of the root below the restoration was similar to that of the adjacent and contralateral teeth. More recently, published cases and case series reports have further supported that it is possible

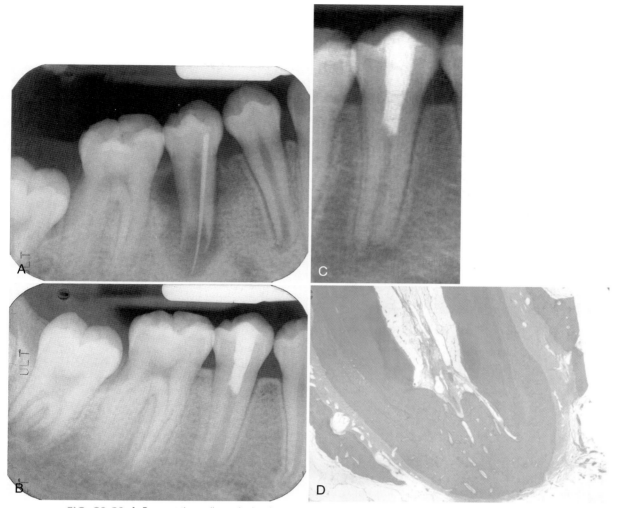

FIG. 20-20 **A,** Preoperative radiograph showing an immature root with periradicular periodontitis and a traced sinus tract to the apex of the root. **B,** Radiographic checkup 7 months after treatment that included application of a mixture of ciprofloxacin, metronidazole, and minocycline. **C,** At 24-month checkup, showing continued root development both in length and width of the root. **D,** Histologic slide from Thibodeau et al.[155] showing thickened root walls, apical development, and healing of apical periodontitis in a dog tooth where a periapical lesion had been created in an immature tooth.

to have ingrowths of tissue followed by new apposition of dentin and continuation of root formation.[96,155] Studies have also confirmed the potent antibacterial properties of the triantibiotic paste used in these cases.

There has been an explosion of studies in the last few years aimed at making the procedure more predictable both in healing of apical periodontitis and in promoting pulp and not nonspecific connective tissue (see Chapter 10).

The minocycline in the triantibiotic paste causes unacceptable discoloration of the teeth; this has led to many studies on eliminating or replacing this antibiotic in the paste, or eliminating the tripaste. Studies are underway to find a synthetic matrix that can act as a more predictable scaffold for new ingrowth of tissue than the blood clot that was used in these examples.[155,173]

Studies are also underway on stem cells and growth factors aimed at a more predictable production of odontoblasts and thus pulp cells.

The procedure described here can be attempted in most cases, and if after 3 months there are no signs of regeneration, the more traditional treatment methods can be initiated.

Mature Tooth
Conventional endodontic therapy is recommended for mature teeth with closed apex.

CROWN-ROOT FRACTURE

Crown-root fracture is a periodontal rather than an endodontic challenge. The tooth must be treated periodontally to enable a well-sealed coronal restoration. This could be accomplished by simple gingivectomy if the extent of the root component of the fracture is large. Alternatively, the tooth could be orthodontically or surgically extruded such that the exposed surface of the root fracture is treatable. Once the feasibility of the coronal restoration is assured, the particular crown fracture is treated as previously described.

ROOT FRACTURE

Root fracture implies fracture of the cementum, dentin, and pulp. These injuries are relatively infrequent, occurring in less than 3% of all dental injuries.[177] Immature teeth with vital pulps rarely sustain horizontal root fractures.[7] When a root fractures horizontally, the coronal segment is displaced to a varying degree, but generally the apical segment is not displaced. Because the apical pulpal circulation is not disrupted, pulp necrosis in the apical segment is extremely rare. Permanent pulpal necrosis of the coronal segment, requiring endodontic treatment, occurs in about 25% of cases.[8,9,93]

Diagnosis and Clinical Presentation

The clinical presentation of a root fracture is similar to that of luxation injuries. The extent of displacement of the coronal segment is usually indicative of the location of the fracture and can vary from none, simulating a concussion injury (apical fracture), to severe, simulating an extrusive luxation (cervical fracture).

Radiographic examination for root fractures is extremely important. Because root fractures are usually oblique (facial to palatal) (Fig. 20-21), one periapical radiograph may easily miss it. It is imperative to take at least three angled radiographs (45°, 90°, and 110°) so that at least at one angulation, the x-ray beam passes directly through the fracture line to make it visible on the radiograph (Fig. 20-22).

Treatment

Emergency treatment involves repositioning the segments into close proximity as much as possible. In the case of severe displacement of the coronal segment, its apical extension is frequently lodged in (if not perforating through) the cortical bone facial to the tooth. Forcing the crown facially is not possible, and the two segments will not be properly aligned. The only way to accomplish reapproximation of the two segments is to release the coronal segment from the bone by gently pulling it slightly downward with finger pressure or extraction forceps and, once it is loose, rotating it back to its original position (Fig. 20-23). The traditionally recommended[124] splinting protocol has been changed from 2 to 4 months with rigid splinting to a semirigid splint to adjacent teeth for 2 to 4 weeks.[18] If a long time has elapsed between the injury and treatment, repositioning of the segments close to their original position probably will not be possible; this compromises the long-term prognosis for the tooth.

Healing Patterns

Investigators[21] have described four types of responses to root fractures.

1. *Healing with calcified tissue.* Radiographically, the fracture line is discernible, but the fragments are in close contact (Fig. 20-24, *A*).
2. *Healing with interproximal connective tissue.* Radiographically, the fragments appear separated by a narrow radiolucent line, and the fractured edges appear rounded (Fig. 20-24, *B*).
3. *Healing with interproximal bone and connective tissue.* Radiographically, the fragments are separated by a distinct bony ridge (Fig. 20-24, *C*).
4. *Interproximal inflammatory tissue without healing.* Radiographically, a widening of the fracture line and/or a developing radiolucency corresponding to the fracture line becomes apparent (Fig. 20-24, *D*).

The first three healing patterns are considered successful. The teeth are usually asymptomatic and respond positively to sensitivity testing. Coronal yellowing is possible because calcific metamorphosis of the coronal segment is not unusual (see Fig. 20-29).[94,177]

The fourth type of root fracture response is typical when the coronal segment loses its vitality. The infective products in the coronal pulp cause an inflammatory response and typical radiolucencies at the fracture line (see Fig. 20-24, *D*).[21]

Treatment of Complications

Coronal Root Fractures

Historically it had been thought that fractures in the cervical segment had a poor prognosis, and extraction of the coronal segment was recommended. Research does not support this treatment; in fact, if these coronal segments are adequately splinted, chances of healing do not differ from those for midroot or apical fractures (Fig. 20-25).[177] However, if the fracture occurs at the level of or coronal to the crest of the alveolar bone, the prognosis is extremely poor.

If reapproximation of the fractured segments is not possible, extraction of the coronal segment is indicated. The level of fracture and length of the remaining root are evaluated for restorability. If the apical root segment is long enough, gentle orthodontic eruption of this segment can be carried out to enable fabrication of a restoration.

Midroot and Apical Root Fractures

Permanent pulpal necrosis occurs in 25% of root fractures.[48,93] Initially it is likely that in many cases the pulp in the coronal segment will become necrotic after the injury; however, because of a very large apical opening in the coronal segment, revascularization is possible if the segments are well reapproximated.

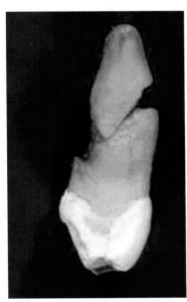

FIG. 20-21 Extracted root after a root fracture. Note the oblique angle of the fracture.

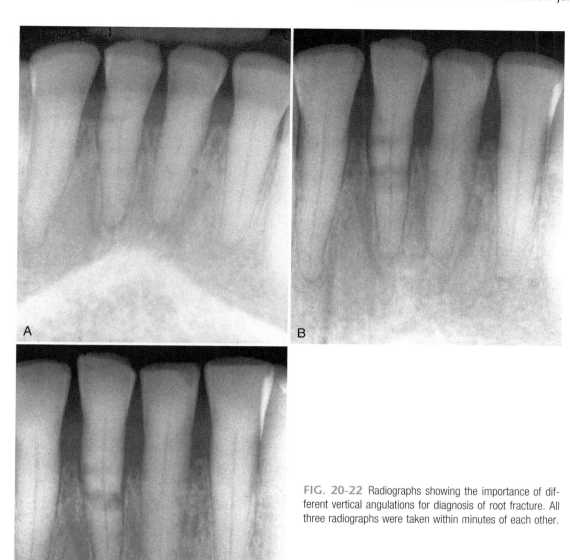

FIG. 20-22 Radiographs showing the importance of different vertical angulations for diagnosis of root fracture. All three radiographs were taken within minutes of each other.

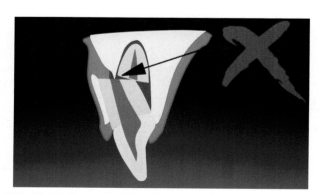

FIG. 20-23 Figure of facial root fracture manipulated back into place.

In most cases, permanent necrosis occurs in the coronal segment, with only the apical segment remaining vital. Therefore, endodontic treatment is indicated in the coronal root segment unless periapical pathology is seen in the apical segment. In most cases the pulpal lumen is wide at the apical extent of the coronal segment, and long-term calcium hydroxide treatment or an MTA apical plug is indicated (see the section Apexification). The coronal segment is filled after a hard tissue barrier has formed apically in the coronal segment and periradicular healing has taken place.

In rare cases in which both the coronal and apical pulp are necrotic, treatment is more complicated. Endodontic treatment through the fracture is extremely difficult. Endodontic manipulations, medicaments, and filling materials all have a

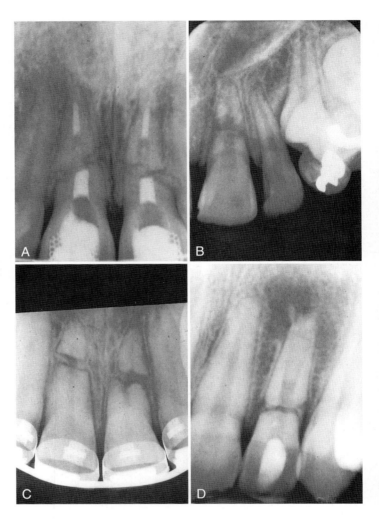

FIG. 20-24 Healing patterns after horizontal root fractures. **A,** Healing with calcified tissue. **B,** Healing with interproximal connective tissue. **C,** Healing with bone and connective tissue. **D,** Interproximal connective tissue without healing.

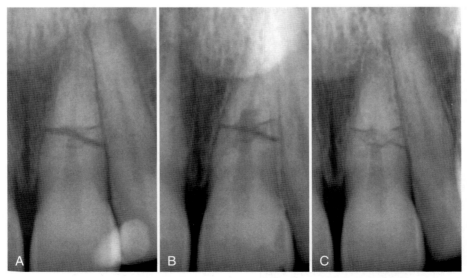

FIG. 20-25 Internal root resorption in the root fracture area; tooth was diagnosed with compound midroot fracture. **A,** Coronal portion was repositioned and then splinted to the lateral incisor with a composite splint. **B,** At 6-month recall, the pulp responded normally to cold, but an internal root-resorptive defect was noted on radiograph. No treatment was indicated, because the pulp did respond normally to vitality tests. **C,** At 42-month recall, the tooth was still asymptomatic, and the pulp still responded to vitality tests. The resorptive defect had healed, and signs of dystrophic calcifications were evident in the apical and coronal segments.

detrimental effect on healing of the fracture site. If healing of the fracture has been completed and is followed by necrosis of the apical segment, the prognosis is much improved.

In more apical root fractures, necrotic apical segments can be surgically removed. This is a viable treatment if the remaining coronal root segment is long enough to provide adequate periodontal support. Removal of the apical segment in midroot fractures leaves the coronal segment with a compromised attachment; endodontic implants have been used to provide additional support to the tooth.

Follow-Up

After the splinting period is completed, follow-up is as for all dental traumatic injuries: at 3, 6, and 12 months and yearly thereafter.

Prognosis

The following factors influence repair:

1. The degree of dislocation and mobility of the coronal fragment are extremely important in determining outcome.[7,17,94,148,177] Increased dislocation and coronal fragment mobility result in a poorer prognosis.
2. Immature teeth are seldom involved in root fractures, but in the unlikely event they are, the prognosis is good.[17,92]
3. The quality of treatment is vital to successful repair. The prognosis improves with quick treatment, close reduction of the root segments, and semirigid splinting for 2 to 4 weeks.[18]

Complications include pulp necrosis and root canal obliteration. Pulp necrosis can be treated successfully[48,93] by treating the coronal segment with calcium hydroxide to stimulate hard tissue barrier formation. Root canal obliteration is common if the root segment (coronal or apical) remains vital.

LUXATION INJURIES

Definitions

The types of luxation injury can be defined as follows:

1. *Concussion* implies no displacement, normal mobility, and sensitivity to percussion.
2. *Subluxation* implies sensitivity to percussion, increased mobility, and no displacement.
3. *Lateral luxation* implies displacement labially, lingually, distally, or incisally.
4. *Extrusive luxation* implies displacement in a coronal direction.
5. *Intrusive luxation* implies displacement in an apical direction into the alveolus.

Definitions 1 through 5 describe injuries of increasing magnitude in terms of intensity of the injury and subsequent sequelae.

Incidence

Luxation injuries as a group are the most common of all dental injuries, with a reported incidence ranging from 30% to 44%.[55]

Treatment

Teeth that are concussed or subluxated do not need any immediate treatment. Responses to vitality tests should be investigated and noted. Even after mild injury, such as subluxation,

the pulp might be unresponsive to vitality tests for several weeks if not months.[144] When the pulp is unresponsive initially after the trauma, patients should be recalled on a regular basis and monitored for any additional signs of infection of the root canal (discussed later).

Teeth with lateral and extrusive luxation should be repositioned as soon as possible. In lateral luxation, the apex might be perforating the facial bone plate, and the tooth must be slightly and gently pulled down to loosen the hold before it is repositioned in its original position. Current IADT guidelines call for 2 weeks of physiologic splinting in cases of extrusion luxation and 4 weeks for lateral luxation. A decision on root canal therapy follows the guidelines for avulsion (discussed later). If the tooth has a fully formed apex and was diagnosed to have moved into (if not through) the cortical plate (apical translocation), there is a good likelihood of the pulp being devitalized; therefore, endodontic treatment should be initiated as early as 2 weeks after the injury. If the apex is still not fully formed, waiting for signs of revascularization is strongly recommended.

Permanent teeth that are intruded are not likely to spontaneously re-erupt, especially if the apex is fully formed.[100] Alternative treatment, such as orthodontic extrusion or immediate surgical repositioning, should be considered. If orthodontic extrusion is planned for an intruded tooth, it should be initiated as soon as possible and should not be delayed longer than 2 to 3 weeks after the trauma. Only a few studies have evaluated the true efficacy of this approach. One study[168] using a dog model indicated that severely intruded teeth showed signs of ankylosis as early as 11 to 13 days after the trauma, despite initiation of orthodontic movement 5 to 7 days after the injury.

For the surgical approach, one study[47] (using a dog model) concluded that "a careful immediate surgical repositioning of a severely intruded permanent tooth with complete root formation has many advantages with few disadvantages." Another investigation,[58] a retrospective study of 58 intruded human teeth, indicated that surgical repositioning resulted in a predictable outcome, with only five of the teeth lost over the observation period. However, it was also observed that less surgical manipulation positively influenced the healing. If an intruded tooth is immediately reimplanted, it should be splinted for at least 4 weeks, but in most cases the splint needs to be left on the tooth longer.

Biologic Consequences

Luxation injuries result in damage to the attachment apparatus (periodontal ligament and cemental layer), the severity of which depends on the type of injury sustained (concussion least, intrusion most). The apical neurovascular supply to the pulp is also affected to varying degrees, resulting in an altered or nonvital tooth.

Healing can be favorable or unfavorable. Favorable healing after a luxation injury occurs if the initial physical damage to the root surface and the resultant inflammatory response to the damaged external root surface are again covered with cementum. An unfavorable response occurs when there is direct attachment of bone to the root, with the root ultimately being replaced by bone.

There are two resorption responses in which the pulp plays an essential role:

1. In *external* inflammatory root resorption, the *necrotic infected pulp* provides the stimulus for periodontal

inflammation in the ligament space. If the cementum has been damaged, the inflammatory stimulators in the pulp space are able to diffuse through the dentinal tubules and stimulate an inflammatory response over large areas of the periodontal ligament. Because of the lack of cemental protection, the periodontal inflammation includes root resorption in addition to the expected bone resorption.

2. With *internal* inflammatory root resorption, the inflamed pulp is the tissue involved in resorbing the root structure. The pathogenesis of internal root resorption is not completely understood. Here it is thought that coronal necrotic infected pulp provides a stimulus for a pulpal inflammation in the more apical parts of the remaining vital pulp.[7] If the internal root surface has lost its precemental protection during an injury, internal root resorption occurs in the area adjacent to the inflamed pulp. Thus, both the necrotic infected pulp and the inflamed pulp contribute to this type of root resorption.

External Root Resorption
Caused by an Injury (Alone) to the External Root Surface

If an injury harms the attachment, the by-products of this mechanical damage stimulate an inflammatory response. The healing response depends on the extent of the initial damage.

Localized Injury: Healing with Cementum

When the injury is localized (e.g., after concussion or subluxation injury), mechanical damage to the cementum occurs, resulting in a local inflammatory response and a localized area of root resorption. If no further inflammatory stimulus is present, periodontal healing and root surface repair occur within 14 days (Fig. 20-26).[78] The resorption is localized to the area of mechanical damage, and treatment is not required because it is free of symptoms and not even visualized radiographically in most cases. In a minority of cases, however, small radiolucencies can be seen on the root surface if the radiograph is taken at a specific angle. It is important to avoid misinterpreting these cases as progressive. The pulp is not involved. If the pulp responds to sensitivity tests, this is a clue that no treatment should be performed. A wait-and-see attitude can allow spontaneous healing to take place. It is important to realize that in the initial stages, radiolucency could be followed by spontaneous repair, and endodontic treatment should *not* be initiated.

Diffuse Injury: Healing by Osseous Replacement

When the traumatic injury is severe (e.g., intrusive luxation or avulsion with extended dry time), involving diffuse damage on more than 20% of the root surface, an abnormal attachment can occur after healing takes place.[105] The initial reaction, as always, is inflammation in response to the severe mechanical damage to the root surface. After the initial inflammatory response, a diffuse area of root surface devoid of cementum results. Cells in the vicinity of the denuded root now compete to repopulate it. Often cells that are precursors of bone, rather than the slower-moving periodontal ligament cells, move across from the socket wall and populate the damaged root. Bone comes into contact with the root without an intermediate attachment apparatus. This phenomenon is termed *dentoalveolar ankylosis.*[105] However, the ankylosis and osseous replacement that follows cannot be reversed and can be considered a physiologic process because bone resorbs and reforms throughout life. Thus root is resorbed by osteoclasts, but in the reforming stage, bone is laid down instead of dentin, slowly replacing the root with bone. This process is termed *osseous replacement* (Fig. 20-27).[164] The initial inflammation to remove the mechanical debris of the traumatic injury is a pathologic response that in the authors' opinion may be reversed. In these traumatic cases, however, the resorptive phase includes the root (Fig. 20-28).

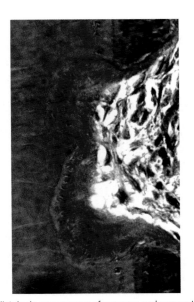

FIG. 20-27 Histologic appearance of osseous replacement. There is direct contact between bone and root structure. Resorptive defects are seen in the bone and root tissue, which is the normal physiologic process of bone turnover. The resorptive defects are filled by new bone and additional areas resorbed. In this way the entire root is replaced by bone at a rate dependent on the metabolic rate of the patient.

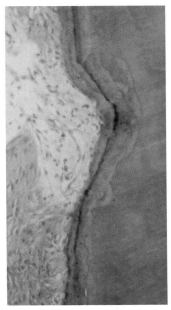

FIG. 20-26 Histologic section showing previous root resorptive defect healed with new cementum and periodontal ligament.

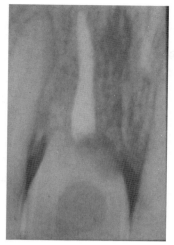

FIG. 20-28 Radiographic appearance of osseous replacement. The root acquires the radiographic appearance of the surrounding bone (without a lamina dura). Note that radiolucencies typical of active inflammation are not present.

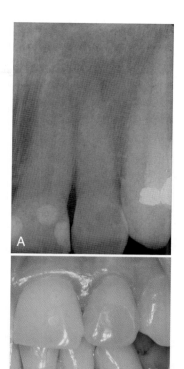

FIG. 20-29 A, Pulp canal calcification after a luxation injury. Radiographic appearance of a calcified maxillary lateral incisor; note that despite calcification, it has now become necrotic and infected, evident by the periapical lesion. B, The typical yellow appearance of the tooth caused by thickened dentin in the pulp chamber.

Treatment

Treatment strategies for limiting the effect of the traumatic injury to the periodontal structures are outside the scope of this chapter. However, in general they involve minimizing the initial inflammatory response to the injury. The initial inflammation is destructive in nature and increases the surface area of root to be covered in the healing phase.[20] The smaller the surface area to be covered by new cementum, the higher the chances of favorable repair.

A study has indicated that if Ledermix, a drug combining corticosteroid and tetracycline, is placed in the root canal immediately after a severe trauma in which osseous replacement is expected, favorable healing occurs at a very high rate.[38] In a more recent study, it was shown that triamcinolone (the corticosteroid portion of the Ledermix paste) was as effective as Ledermix at inhibiting external root resorption.[41] Both of these studies were done on young dogs and need to be replicated in human studies.

Caused by an Injury to the External Root Surface and Inflammatory Stimulus in the Root Canal

Recognized inflammatory stimuli that cause root resorption are pressure, pulp space infection, and sulcular infection. This chapter focuses on pulp space infection.

Consequences of Apical Neurovascular Supply Damage

Pulp Canal Obliteration (Calcification)

Pulp canal obliteration is common after luxation injuries (Fig. 20-29). The frequency of pulp canal obliteration appears inversely proportional to pulp necrosis. The exact mechanism of pulp canal obliteration is unknown. It has been theorized that the sympathetic/parasympathetic control of blood flow to the odontoblasts is altered, resulting in uncontrolled reparative dentin.[7,15] Another theory is that hemorrhage and blood clot formation in the pulp after injury form a nidus for subsequent calcification if the pulp remains vital.[7,15] One study[11] found that pulp canal obliteration could usually be diagnosed within the first year after injury and was more frequent in teeth with open

apices (>0.7 mm radiographically), those with extrusive and lateral luxation injuries, and those that had been rigidly splinted.[11]

Pulp Necrosis

The factors most important for the development of pulp necrosis are the type of injury (concussion least, intrusion most) and the stage of root development (mature apex more than an immature apex).[10] Pulp necrosis is most likely to lead to infection of the root canal system, with problematic consequences.

Pulp Space Infection

Pulp space infection in conjunction with damage to the external root surface results in periradicular root and bone resorption and continues in its active state as long as the pulpal stimulus (infection) remains. When the root loses its cemental protection, lateral periodontitis with root resorption can result (Fig. 20-30).

To have pulp space infection, the pulp must first become necrotic. Necrosis occurs after a fairly serious injury in which displacement of the tooth results in severing of the apical blood vessels. In mature teeth, pulp regeneration cannot occur, and usually by 3 weeks, the necrotic pulp becomes infected. (For details of the typical bacterial contents of a traumatized necrotic pulp, the reader is referred to Chapter 14 or to Bergenholtz.[29]) Because a serious injury is required for pulp necrosis, areas of cemental covering of the root usually are also affected, resulting in loss of its protective (insulating) quality. Now bacterial toxins can pass through the dentinal tubules and

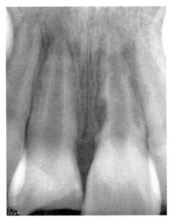

FIG. 20-30 Inflammatory root resorption caused by a pulp space infection. Note the radiolucencies in the root and surrounding bone. (Courtesy Dr. Fred Barnett.)

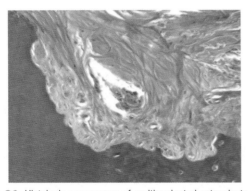

FIG. 20-31 Histologic appearance of multinucleated osteoclasts (dentino-clasts) resorbing the dentin of the root.

stimulate an inflammatory response in the periodontal ligament. The result is resorption of the root and bone. The periodontal infiltrate consists of granulation tissue with lymphocytes, plasma cells, and polymorphonuclear leukocytes. Multinucleated giant cells resorb the denuded root surface, and this continues until the stimulus (pulp space bacteria) is removed (Fig. 20-31).[160] Radiographically the resorption is observed as progressive radiolucent areas of the root and adjacent bone (see Fig. 20-30).

Treatment
Assessing attachment damage caused by the traumatic injury and minimizing the subsequent inflammation should be the focus of the emergency visit. The clinician's attention to pulp space infection should ideally be 7 to 10 days after the injury.[166,167] Root canal disinfection removes the stimulus to the periradicular inflammation, thus the resorption will stop.[78,166,167] In most cases a new attachment will form, but if a large area of root is affected, osseous replacement can result by the mechanism already described. Again, treatment principles include prevention of pulp space infection or elimination of the bacteria if they are present in the pulp space.
1. Prevention of pulp space infection
   a. *Reestablish the vitality of the pulp.* If the pulp stays vital, the canal will be free of bacteria, and external inflammatory root resorption will not occur. In severe injuries

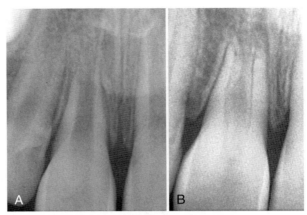

FIG. 20-32 Revascularization of immature root. A tooth with an open apex was replanted soon after the avulsion. The checkup radiograph 12 years later confirms that regrowth has taken place into the pulp chamber. It appears that a bone plug has grown in, and new periodontal ligament has formed, with a lamina dura within the pulp canal. (Courtesy Dr. Cecilia Bourguignon, Paris, France.)

in which vitality has been lost, it is possible under some circumstances to promote revascularization of the pulp. Revascularization is possible in young teeth with incompletely formed apices if the teeth are replaced in their original position within 60 minutes of the injury (Fig. 20-32).[51] If the tooth has been avulsed, soaking it in doxycycline for 5 minutes or covering the root with minocycline powder before replantation has been shown to double or triple the revascularization rate.[51,127] Even under the best conditions, however, revascularization fails to occur on many occasions, and a diagnostic dilemma results. If the pulp revascularizes, external root resorption will not occur, and the root will continue to develop and strengthen. If the pulp becomes necrotic and infected, the subsequent external inflammatory root resorption that develops could result in loss of the tooth in a very short time. At present, the diagnostic tools available cannot detect a vital pulp in this situation before approximately 6 months after successful revascularization. This period of time is obviously unacceptable because by that time the teeth that have not revascularized could be lost to the resorption process. Recently the laser Doppler flowmeter or the pulse oximeter have been shown to have diagnostic potential for the detection of revascularization in immature teeth (Fig. 20-33). These devices appear to detect the presence of vital tissue in the pulp space by 4 weeks after the traumatic injury.[176]
   b. *Prevent root canal infection by initiating root canal treatment at 7 to 10 days.* In teeth with closed apices, revascularization cannot occur. These teeth should be endodontically treated within 7 to 10 days of the injury, before the ischemically necrosed pulp becomes infected.[166,167] Theoretically, treating teeth within this time period can be considered equivalent to treating a tooth with a vital pulp, and the endodontic treatment could be completed in one visit if possible. However, efficient treatment is extremely difficult so soon after a serious traumatic injury, and in the authors' opinion, it is beneficial to start the endodontic treatment with chemomechanical preparation, after which an intracanal

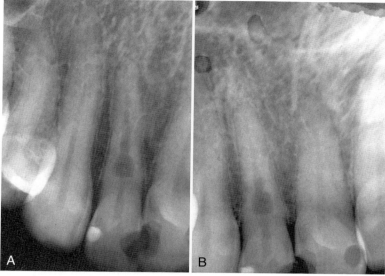

FIG. 20-33 Angled radiographs to show internal resorption. Radiographs from two different horizontal projections depict **(A)** the lesion within the confines of the root canal on both views and **(B)** the adjacent bone intact on both views.

dressing with a creamy mix of calcium hydroxide is placed (see Fig. 20-14).[166] Then, the clinician can fill the canal at his or her convenience after periodontal healing of the injury is complete, approximately 1 month after the instrumentation visit. There appears to be no necessity for long-term calcium hydroxide treatment in cases in which the endodontic treatment is started within 10 days of the injury.[166]

2. *Eliminate pulp space infection.* When root canal treatment is initiated later than 10 days after the accident or if active external inflammatory resorption is observed, the preferred antibacterial protocol consists of microbial control followed by long-term dressing with densely packed calcium hydroxide.[167] Calcium hydroxide can effect an alkaline pH in the surrounding dentinal tubules (Fig. 20-34), kill bacteria, and neutralize endotoxin, a potent inflammatory stimulator.

The first visit consists of the microbial control phase, with cleaning and shaping of the canal and the placement of a creamy mix of calcium hydroxide using a Lentulo spiral. The patient is seen in approximately 1 month, at which time the canal is filled with a dense mix of calcium hydroxide. Once filled, the canal should appear radiographically to be calcified because the radiodensity of calcium hydroxide in the canal is usually similar to that of the surrounding dentin (see Fig. 20-16). A radiograph is then exposed at 3-month intervals. At each visit the tooth is tested for symptoms of periodontitis. In addition to stopping the resorptive process, calcium hydroxide washout is assessed. Because the root surface is so radiodense as to make assessment of healing difficult, the adjacent bone healing is assessed. If adjacent bone has healed, it is assumed that the resorptive process has stopped in the root as well; then the canal can be obturated with the permanent root filling material (Fig. 20-35).

Internal Root Resorption

Internal root resorption is rare in permanent teeth. Internal resorption is characterized by an oval-shaped enlargement of

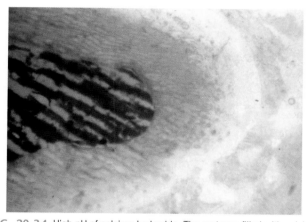

FIG. 20-34 High pH of calcium hydroxide. The root was filled with calcium hydroxide and then cut in cross section. A pH indication shows the high pH in the canal and surrounding root, whereas the surrounding tissue is a neutral pH.

the root canal space.[16] External resorption, which is much more common, is often misdiagnosed as internal resorption.

Etiology

Internal root resorption is characterized by resorption of the internal aspect of the root by multinucleated giant cells adjacent to the granulation tissue in the pulp (Fig. 20-36). Chronic inflammatory tissue is common in the pulp, but only rarely does it result in resorption. There are different theories on the origin of the pulpal granulation tissue involved in internal resorption. The most logical explanation is that it is inflamed pulp tissue caused by an infected coronal pulp space. Communication between the coronal necrotic tissue and the vital pulp is through appropriately oriented dentinal tubules (see Fig. 20-36).[170] One investigator[170] reports that resorption of the

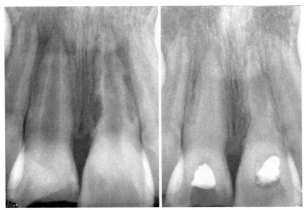

FIG. 20-35 Healing of external inflammatory root resorption after calcium hydroxide treatment. The radiolucencies seen before treatment have disappeared with the reestablishment of the lamina dura. (Courtesy Dr. Fred Barnett.)

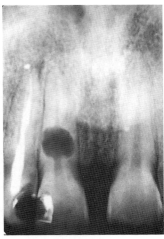

FIG. 20-37 A maxillary incisor with internal root resorption. Uniform enlargement of the pulp space is apparent. Outline of the canal cannot be seen in the resorptive defect.

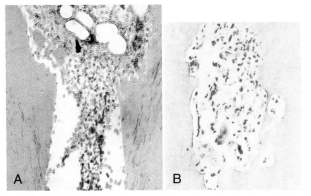

FIG. 20-36 Histologic appearance of internal root resorption. **A,** Section stained with Brown and Brenn. Bacteria are seen (in the dentinal tubules) communicating between the necrotic coronal segment and the apical granulomatous tissue and resorbing cells. **B,** An area of active internal root resorption. (Courtesy Dr. Leif Tronstad, Oslo, Norway.)

dentin is frequently associated with deposition of hard tissue resembling bone or cementum and not dentin. He postulates that the resorbing tissue is not of pulpal origin but is "metaplastic" tissue derived from the pulpal invasion of macrophage-like cells. Others[149] concluded that the pulp tissue was replaced by periodontium-like connective tissue when internal resorption was present. In addition to the requirement of the presence of granulation tissue, root resorption takes place only if the odontoblastic layer and predentin are lost or altered.[160]

Reasons for the loss of predentin adjacent to the granulation tissue are not obvious. Trauma frequently has been suggested as a cause.[135,171] Another reason for the loss of predentin might be extreme heat produced when cutting on dentin without an adequate water spray. The heat presumably would destroy the predentin layer, and if later the coronal aspect of the pulp becomes infected, the bacterial products could initiate the typical inflammation in conjunction with resorbing giant cells in the vital pulp adjacent to the denuded root surface. Internal root resorption has been produced experimentally by the application of diathermy.[170]

Clinical Manifestations

Internal root resorption is usually asymptomatic and is first recognized clinically through routine radiographs. For internal resorption to be active, at least part of the pulp must be vital. The coronal portion of the pulp is often necrotic, whereas the apical pulp that includes the internal resorptive defect can remain vital. Therefore, a negative sensitivity test result does not rule out active internal resorption. It is also possible that the pulp becomes nonvital after a period of active resorption, giving a negative sensitivity test, radiographic signs of internal resorption, and radiographic signs of apical inflammation. Traditionally, the pink tooth has been thought pathognomonic of internal root resorption. The pink color is due to the granulation tissue in the coronal dentin undermining the crown enamel. The pink tooth can also be a feature of subepithelial external inflammatory root resorption, which must be ruled out before a diagnosis of internal root resorption is made.

Radiographic Appearance

The usual radiographic presentation of internal root resorption is a fairly uniform radiolucent enlargement of the pulp canal (Fig. 20-37). Because the resorption is initiated in the root canal, the resorptive defect includes some part of the root canal space, so the original outline of the root canal is distorted.

Histologic Appearance

Like that of other inflammatory resorptive defects, the histologic picture of internal resorption is granulation tissue with multinucleated giant cells (see Fig. 20-35). An area of necrotic pulp is found coronal to the granulation tissue. Dentinal tubules containing microorganisms and communicating between the necrotic zone and the granulation tissue can sometimes be seen (see Fig. 20-36).[140,160,167,170] Unlike external root resorption, the adjacent bone is not affected with internal root resorption.

Treatment

Treatment of internal root resorption is conceptually very easy. Because the resorptive defect is the result of the inflamed pulp and the blood supply to the tissue is through the apical

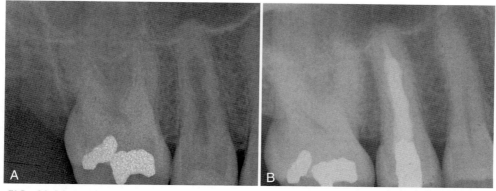

FIG. 20-38 **A,** Internal root resorption in a maxillary premolar with a history of trauma 7 years before the diagnosis (patient's head slammed against side window during an automobile accident). **B,** Three-year follow-up radiograph after endodontic treatment.

foramina, endodontic treatment that effectively removes the blood supply to the resorbing cells is the treatment approach. After adequate anesthesia has been obtained, the canal apical to the internal defect is explored, and a working length short of the radiographic apex is used. The apical canal is thoroughly cleaned and shaped to ensure that the blood supply to the tissue resorbing the root is cut off.

By completion of the root canal instrumentation, it should be possible to obtain a blood-free and dry canal with paper points. Calcium hydroxide is spun into the canal to facilitate the removal of the tissue in the irregular defect at the next visit. At the second visit, the tooth and defect are filled with a warm gutta-percha technique (Fig. 20-38).

Diagnostic Features of External Versus Internal Root Resorption

It is often very difficult to distinguish external from internal root resorption, so misdiagnosis and incorrect treatment may result. The following sections present a list of typical diagnostic features of each resorptive type.

Radiographic Features

A change of angulation of x-rays should give a fairly good indication of whether a resorptive defect is internal or external. A lesion of internal origin appears close to the canal, whatever the angle of the x-ray (see Fig. 20-37). A defect on the external aspect of the root moves away from the canal as the angulation changes (Fig. 20-39). By using the buccal object rule, it is usually possible to distinguish whether the external root defect is buccal or lingual-palatal.

With internal resorption, the outline of the root canal is usually distorted, and the root canal and radiolucent resorptive defect appear contiguous (see Fig. 20-37). When the defect is external, the root canal outline appears normal and can usually be seen "running through" the radiolucent defect (Fig. 20-40).

External inflammatory root resorption is always accompanied by resorption of the bone in addition to the root (Fig. 20-41); radiolucencies will be apparent in the root and the adjacent bone. Internal root resorption does not involve the bone, and as a rule the radiolucency is confined to the root (see Fig. 20-37). On rare occasions, if the internal defect perforates the root, the bone adjacent to it is resorbed and appears radiolucent on the radiograph.

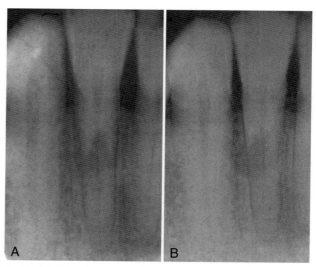

FIG. 20-39 External root resorption. Radiographs from two different horizontal projections depict movement of the lesion to outside the confines of the root canal.

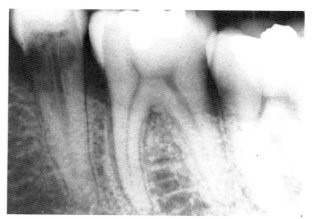

FIG. 20-40 External root resorption on a mandibular premolar 6 years after completing orthodontic treatment. Note the mottled appearance of the resorptive defect and the outline of the root canal within the defect.

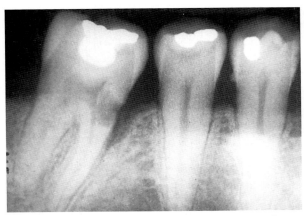

FIG. 20-41 Mandibular molar with subepithelial external inflammatory resorption on its mesial aspect. Note the small opening into the root and the extensive resorption in the dentin; however, the pulp is not exposed. Also note that a resorptive defect is present in the adjacent bone, appearing on the radiograph as similar to an infrabony pocket.

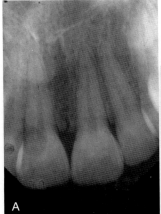
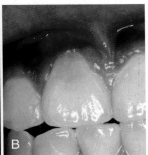

FIG. 20-42 Pink spot of subepithelial external inflammatory root resorption. A, Radiographic appearance. B, Clinical appearance.

Vitality Testing

External inflammatory resorption in the apical and lateral aspects of the root involves an infected pulp space, so no response to sensitivity tests supports the diagnosis. However, because subepithelial external root resorption does not involve the pulp (the bacteria are thought to originate in the sulcus of the tooth), a normal response to sensitivity testing is usually associated with this type of resorption. Internal root resorption usually occurs in teeth with vital pulps and responses to sensitivity testing. In teeth that exhibit internal root resorption, it is common to register a no-response to sensitivity testing because often the coronal pulp has been removed or is necrotic, and the active resorbing cells are more apical in the canal. Also, the pulp might have become necrotic after active resorption took place.

Pink Spot

With apical and lateral external root resorption, the pulp is nonvital, so the granulation tissue that produces the pink spot is not present in these cases. For subepithelial external (Fig. 20-42) and internal root resorption, the pink spot due to the granulation tissue undermining the enamel is a possible sign.

Summary of Possible Diagnostic Features

- ◆ External inflammatory root resorption due to pulp infection.
  - • *Apical:* No response of the pulp to thermal or electric stimuli, with or without a history of trauma.
  - • *Lateral:* History of trauma, no response of the pulp to thermal or electric stimuli, lesion moves on angled x-rays, root canal visualized radiographically overlying the defect, bony radiolucency also apparent.
- ◆ Subepithelial external inflammatory root resorption due to sulcular infection. History of trauma (often forgotten, or its long-term risks not appreciated by the patient); positive pulp sensitivity test; lesion located at the attachment level of the tooth; lesion moves on angled x-rays; root canal outline is undistorted and can be visualized radiographically; crestal bony defect associated with the lesion; pink spot possible.
- ◆ Internal root resorption. History of trauma, crown preparation, or pulpotomy; responsive pulp to thermal or electric stimuli likely, may occur at any location along the root canal (not only attachment level); lesion stays associated with the root canal on angled x-rays, radiolucency contained in the root without an adjacent bony defect; pink spot possible.

Most misdiagnoses of resorptive defects are made between subepithelial external and internal root resorptions. The diagnosis should always be confirmed as treatment proceeds. If root canal therapy is the treatment of choice for an apparent internal root resorption, the bleeding within the canal should cease quickly after pulp extirpation because the blood supply of the granulation tissue is the apical blood vessels. If bleeding continues during treatment, and particularly if it is still present at the second visit, the source of the blood supply is external, and treatment for perforating external resorption should be carried out. On obturation, it should be possible to fill the entire canal from within in internal resorption. Failure to achieve this should make the clinician suspicious of an external lesion that perforates the root. Finally, if the blood supply of an internal resorption defect is removed on pulp extirpation, any continuation of the resorptive process on recall radiographs should alert the clinician to the possibility that an external resorptive defect was misdiagnosed.

CLINICAL MANAGEMENT OF THE AVULSED TOOTH

Favorable healing after an avulsion injury requires quick emergency intervention followed by evaluation and possible treatment at decisive times during the healing phase. The urgency of the emergency visit and the multidisciplinary nature of follow-up evaluations require that both the public and clinicians from many dental disciplines be knowledgeable about the treatment strategies involved.

Consequences of Tooth Avulsion

Tooth avulsion results in attachment damage and pulp necrosis. The tooth is "separated" from the socket due mainly to tearing of the periodontal ligament that leaves viable periodontal ligament cells on most of the root surface. In addition, small and localized cemental damage occurs from the crushing of the tooth against the socket.

If the periodontal ligament left attached to the root surface does not dry out, the consequences of tooth avulsion are usually minimal.[14,146] The hydrated periodontal ligament cells will maintain their viability and repair after replantation, with minimal destructive inflammation as a by-product. Because the areas of the crushing injury are localized, inflammation stimulated by the damaged tissues will be correspondingly limited, and favorable healing with new replacement cementum is likely to occur after the initial inflammation subsides (see Fig. 20-26).

If excessive drying occurs before replantation, the damaged periodontal ligament cells elicit a severe inflammatory response over a diffuse area on the root surface. Unlike the situation described earlier, in which the area to be repaired after the initial inflammatory response is small, here a large area of root surface is affected that must be repaired by new tissue. The slower moving cementoblasts cannot cover the entire root surface in time, and it is likely that in certain areas, bone will attach directly onto the root surface. In time, through physiologic bone recontouring, the entire root will be replaced by bone. As earlier noted, this has been termed *osseous replacement* or *replacement resorption* (see Figs. 20-27 and 20-28).[20,163]

Pulpal necrosis always occurs after an avulsion injury. Although a necrotic pulp itself is not of consequence, the necrotic tissue is extremely susceptible to bacterial contamination. If revascularization does not occur or effective endodontic therapy is not carried out, the pulp space inevitably becomes infected. The combination of bacteria in the root canal and cemental damage on the external surface of the root results in an external inflammatory resorption that can be very serious and can lead to rapid loss of the tooth (see Fig. 20-30).[160]

The consequences after tooth avulsion appear to be directly related to the severity and surface area of the inflammation on the root surface and resultant damaged root surface that must be repaired. Treatment strategies should always be considered in the context of limiting the extent of the periradicular inflammation, thus tipping the balance toward favorable responses (cemental) rather than unfavorable ones (osseous replacement or inflammatory resorption).

Treatment Objectives

Treatment is directed at avoiding or minimizing resultant inflammation due to the two main consequences of the avulsed tooth: attachment damage and pulpal infection.

Attachment damage as a direct result of the avulsion injury cannot be avoided. However, considerable additional damage can occur to the periodontal ligament in the time that the tooth is out of the mouth (primarily because of drying). Treatment is directed at minimizing this damage (and the resultant inflammation) so that the fewest possible complications result. When severe additional damage cannot be avoided and osseous replacement of the root is considered certain, steps are taken to slow the replacement of the root by bone to maintain the tooth in the mouth for as long as possible.

In the open apex tooth, all efforts are made to promote revascularization of the pulp, thus avoiding pulp space infection. When revascularization fails (in the open apex tooth) or is not possible (in the closed apex tooth), all treatment efforts are made to prevent or eliminate toxins from the root canal space.

Clinical Management

Emergency Treatment at the Accident Site

Replant if possible or place in an appropriate storage medium. As mentioned, damage to the attachment apparatus that occurred

during the initial injury is unavoidable but usually minimal. However, all efforts must be made to minimize necrosis of the remaining periodontal ligament while the tooth is out of the mouth. Pulpal sequelae are not a concern initially and are dealt with at a later stage of treatment.

The single most important factor to assure a favorable outcome after replantation is the speed with which the tooth is replanted.[16,22] Of utmost importance is the prevention of drying, which causes loss of normal physiologic metabolism and morphology of the periodontal ligament cells.[22,146] Every effort should be made to replant the tooth within the first 15 to 20 minutes.[27] This usually requires emergency personnel at the site of the injury with some knowledge of treatment protocol. The clinician should communicate clearly with the person at the site of the accident. Ideally this information should have been given at an earlier time; for example, as an educational offering to school nurses or athletic trainers. Failing this, the information can be given over the phone. The aim is to replant a clean tooth with an undamaged root surface as gently as possible, after which the patient should be brought to the office immediately. If doubt exists that the tooth can be replanted adequately, the tooth should quickly be stored in an appropriate medium until the patient can get to the dental office for replantation. Suggested storage media, in order of preference, are milk, saliva (either in the vestibule of the mouth or in a container into which the patient expectorates), physiologic saline, and water.[86] Water is the least desirable storage medium because the hypotonic environment causes rapid cell lysis and increased inflammation on replantation.[35,36]

Cell culture media in specialized transport containers, such as Hank's Balanced Salt Solution (HBSS), have shown superior ability to maintain the viability of the periodontal ligament fibers for extended periods.[165] Presently they are considered impractical because they need to be present at the accident site before the injury occurs. However, if we consider that more than 60% of avulsion injuries occur close to home or school,[81] it seems reasonable to assume that it would be beneficial to have these media available in emergency kits at these sites. It would also be advantageous to have them in ambulances and in the kits of emergency response personnel who are likely to treat the more serious injuries in which teeth might otherwise be sacrificed to a more serious life-threatening situation.

Management in the Dental Office
Emergency Visit
Prepare socket, prepare root, replant, construct a functional splint, and administer local and systemic antibiotics.

Recognizing that a dental injury might be secondary to a more serious injury is essential. The attending dental clinician is likely to be the first health care provider the patient sees after a head injury, so ruling out any injuries to the brain (e.g., concussion) and/or central nervous system (CNS) in general is paramount. If on examination a CNS injury is suspected, immediate referral to the appropriate expert is the first priority, above and beyond the dental injury. Once a CNS injury has been ruled out, the focus of the emergency visit is the attachment apparatus. The aim is to replant the tooth with a minimum of irreversibly damaged cells (that will cause inflammation) and the maximal number of periodontal ligament cells that have the potential to regenerate and repair the damaged root surface.

Diagnosis and Treatment Planning

If the tooth was replanted at the site of injury, a complete history is taken to assess the likelihood of a favorable outcome. The position of the replanted tooth is assessed and adjusted if necessary. On rare occasions, the tooth may be gently removed to prepare the root to increase the chances of a favorable outcome (discussed later).

If the patient presents with the tooth out of the mouth, the storage medium should be evaluated and the tooth placed in a more appropriate medium if required. HBSS is presently considered the best medium for this purpose. Milk or physiologic saline is also appropriate for storage purposes.

The medical and accident histories are taken, and a clinical exam is carried out, with emphasis on questions about when, how, and where the injury occurred.

The clinical examination should include an examination of the socket to ascertain whether it is intact and suitable for replantation. The socket is gently rinsed with saline, and when it has been cleared of the clot and debris, its walls are examined directly for the presence, absence, or collapse of the socket wall. The socket and surrounding areas, including the soft tissues, should be radiographed. Three vertical angulations are required for diagnosis of the presence of a horizontal root fracture in adjacent teeth.[16] The remaining teeth in both the upper and lower jaws should be examined for injuries, such as crown fractures. Any soft tissue lacerations should be noted and, if tooth fragments are missing, explored.

PREPARATION OF THE ROOT

Preparation of the root depends on the maturity of the tooth (open versus closed apex) and on the dry time of the tooth before it was placed in a storage medium. A dry time of 60 minutes is considered the point where survival of root periodontal ligament cells is unlikely.

Extraoral Dry Time Less Than 60 Minutes

Closed Apex
The root should be rinsed of debris with water or saline and replanted in as gentle a fashion as possible.

If the tooth has a closed apex, revascularization is not possible,[51] but because the tooth was dry for less than 60 minutes (replanted or placed in appropriate medium), the chance for periodontal healing exists. Most important, the chance of a severe inflammatory response at the time of replantation is lessened. A dry time of less than 15 to 20 minutes is considered optimal, and periodontal healing would be expected.[14,27,146]

A continuing challenge is the treatment of the tooth that has been dry for more than 20 minutes (periodontal cell survival is assured) but less than 60 minutes (periodontal cell survival unlikely). In these cases, logic suggests that the root surface consists of some cells with the potential to regenerate and some that will act as inflammatory stimulators.

Open Apex
Gently rinse off debris, soak in doxycycline for 5 minutes or cover with minocycline, replant.

In an open apex tooth, revascularization of the pulp and continued root development are possible (see Fig. 20-32). Investigators[51] found in monkeys that soaking the tooth in doxycycline (1 mg in approximately 20 mL of physiologic saline) for 5 minutes before replantation significantly enhanced complete revascularization. This result was confirmed later in dogs by other investigators.[127,176] A study found that covering the root with minocycline (Arestin, OraPharma, Warminster, Pennsylvania), which attaches to the root for approximately 15 days, further increased the revascularization rate in dogs.[127] Although animal studies do not provide us with a prediction of the rate of revascularization in humans, it is reasonable to expect that the same enhancement of revascularization that occurred in two animal species also will occur in humans. As for a closed apex tooth, the open apex tooth is gently rinsed and replanted.

Extraoral Dry Time More Than 60 Minutes

Closed Apex
Remove the periodontal ligament by placing in acid for 5 minutes, soak in fluoride, replant.

When the root has been dry for 60 minutes or more, survival of the periodontal ligament cells is not expected.[22,146] In such cases the root should be prepared to be as resistant to resorption as possible (attempting to slow the osseous replacement process). These teeth should be soaked in acid for 5 minutes to remove all remaining periodontal ligament and thus remove the tissue that would initiate the inflammatory response on replantation. The tooth should then be soaked in 2% stannous fluoride for 5 minutes and replanted.[34,137] A few years ago, studies were published that indicated that an enamel matrix protein, Emdogain (Straumann USA, Andover, Massachusetts), could be beneficial in teeth with extended extraoral dry times, not only to make the root more resistant to resorption, but also, possibly, to stimulate the formation of new periodontal ligament from the socket (see Fig. 20-8).[64,90] Unfortunately, more recent studies have shown that the positive effect of Emdogain is only temporary, and most of these teeth start to resorb after a few years.[132]

If the tooth has been dry for more than 60 minutes and no consideration is given to preserving the periodontal ligament, the endodontics may be performed extraorally. In the case of a tooth with a closed apex, no advantage exists to this additional step at the emergency visit. However, in a tooth with an open apex, endodontic treatment performed after replantation involves a long-term apexification procedure. In these cases, completing the root canal treatment extraorally, in which a seal in the blunderbuss apex is easier to achieve, may be advantageous. When endodontic treatment is performed extraorally, it must be performed aseptically with the utmost care to achieve a root canal system that is thoroughly disinfected.

Open Apex
Replant? If yes, treat as with closed apex tooth. Endodontic treatment may be performed out of the mouth.

Because these teeth are in young patients in whom facial development is usually incomplete, many pediatric clinicians consider the prognosis to be so poor and the potential complications of an ankylosed tooth so severe, they recommend that these teeth not be replanted. Considerable debate exists as to whether it would be beneficial to replant the root even though it will inevitably be lost due to osseous replacement. If the patients are followed carefully and the root submerged by decoronation procedure at the appropriate time,[6,63,67] the height, and more important, the width of the alveolar bone will be maintained, allowing for easier permanent restoration at the appropriate time when the child's facial development is complete.

PREPARATION OF THE SOCKET

The socket should be left undisturbed before replantation.[16] Emphasis is placed on removal of obstacles in the socket to facilitate replacement of the tooth into the socket.[78] It should be lightly aspirated if a blood clot is present. If the alveolar bone has collapsed or may interfere with replantation, a blunt instrument should be inserted carefully into the socket in an attempt to reposition the wall.

SPLINTING

A splint that allows for physiologic movement of the tooth during healing and that is in place for a minimal period results in a decreased incidence of ankylosis.[3,12,78] Semirigid (physiologic) fixation for 1 to 2 weeks is recommended.[3,5,67] The splint should allow movement of the tooth, should have no memory (so the tooth is not moved during healing), and should not impinge on the gingiva and/or prevent maintenance of oral hygiene in the area. Many splints satisfy the requirements of an acceptable device. A new titanium trauma splint (TTS) has recently been shown to be particularly effective and easy to use (Fig. 20-43).[169] After the splint is in place, a radiograph should be exposed to verify the positioning of the tooth and as a preoperative reference for further treatment and follow-up. When the tooth is in the best possible position, adjusting the bite to ensure that it has not been splinted in a position causing traumatic occlusion is important. One week is sufficient to create periodontal support to maintain the avulsed tooth in position.[164] Therefore, the splint should be removed after 1 to 2 weeks. The only exception is with avulsion in conjunction with alveolar fractures, for which 4 to 8 weeks is the suggested time of splinting.[164]

MANAGEMENT OF THE SOFT TISSUES

Soft tissue lacerations of the socket gingiva should be tightly sutured. Lacerations of the lip are fairly common with these types of injuries. The clinician should approach lip lacerations with some caution; a plastic surgery consult might be prudent.

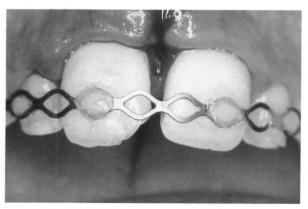

FIG. 20-43   Titanium trauma splint (TTS) in place.

If these lacerations are sutured, care must be taken to clean the wound thoroughly beforehand because dirt or even minute tooth fragments left in the wound affect healing and the aesthetic result.

ADJUNCTIVE THERAPY

Systemic antibiotics given at the time of replantation and before endodontic treatment are effective in preventing bacterial invasion of the necrotic pulp and therefore subsequent inflammatory resorption.[79] Tetracycline has the additional benefit of decreasing root resorption by affecting the motility of the osteoclasts and reducing the effectiveness of collagenase.[128] The administration of systemic antibiotics is recommended, beginning at the emergency visit and continuing until the splint is removed.[79] For patients not susceptible to tetracycline staining, the antibiotic of choice is doxycycline twice daily for 7 days at the appropriate dosage for patient age and weight.[128,129] Penicillin V 1000 mg as a loading dose, followed by 500 mg 4 times daily for 7 days, has also been shown to be beneficial. The bacterial content of the sulcus also should be controlled during the healing phase. In addition to stressing to the patient the need for adequate oral hygiene, the use of chlorhexidine rinses for 7 to 10 days is helpful.

As stated previously, a recent series of studies by our research group found great benefit in removal of the pulp contents at the emergency visit and placing Ledermix or corticosteroid into the root canal.[38,41] Apparently the use of the medicament was able to shut down the inflammatory response after replantation to allow for more favorable healing compared to those teeth that did not have the medicament.

The need for analgesics should be assessed on an individual case basis. The use of pain medication stronger than nonprescription nonsteroidal antiinflammatory drugs (NSAIDs) is unusual. The patient should be sent to a physician for consultation regarding a tetanus booster within 48 hours of the initial visit.

Second Visit

The second visit should take place 1 to 2 weeks after the trauma. At the emergency visit, emphasis was placed on the preservation and healing of the attachment apparatus. The focus of the second visit is the prevention or elimination of potential irritants from the root canal space. These irritants, if present, provide the stimulus for the progression of the inflammatory response, bone and root resorption. Also at this visit, the course of systemic antibiotics is completed; the chlorhexidine rinses can be stopped. At this appointment the splint is removed; the tooth might still have class I or class II mobility after splint removal, but all indications are that it will continue to heal better without the splint.[3]

ENDODONTIC TREATMENT

Extraoral Time Less Than 60 Minutes

Closed Apex
Initiate endodontic treatment after 1 to 2 weeks. When endodontic treatment is delayed or signs of resorption are present, provide long-term calcium hydroxide treatment before obturation.

No chance exists for revascularization of teeth with closed apices; therefore, endodontic treatment should be initiated at the second visit 7 to 10 days later.[13,51] If therapy is initiated at this optimum time, the pulp should be necrotic without (or with minimal) infection.[108,166] Endodontic therapy with an effective interappointment antibacterial agent[166] over a relatively short period (1 to 2 weeks) is sufficient to ensure effective disinfection of the canal.[141] Long-term calcium hydroxide treatment should always be considered if the injury occurred more than 2 weeks before initiation of the endodontic treatment or especially if radiographic evidence of resorption is present.[166]

The root canal is thoroughly cleaned and shaped, irrigated, and then filled with a thick (powdery) mix of calcium hydroxide and sterile saline (anesthetic solution is also an acceptable vehicle) (see Fig. 20-15). The canal is obturated when a radiographically intact periodontal membrane can be demonstrated around the root (see Fig. 20-35). Calcium hydroxide is an effective antibacterial agent[39,141] and favorably influences the local environment at the resorption site, theoretically promoting healing.[161] It also changes the environment in the dentin to a more alkaline pH, which may slow the action of the resorptive cells and promote hard tissue formation.[161] However, changing of the calcium hydroxide should be kept to a minimum (not more than every 3 months) because it has a necrotizing effect on the cells attempting to repopulate the damaged root surface.[104]

Calcium hydroxide is considered the drug of choice in the prevention and treatment of inflammatory root resorption, but it is not the only medicament recommended in these cases. Some attempts have been made not only to remove the stimulus for the resorbing cells, but also to affect them directly. The antibiotic-corticosteroid paste Ledermix is effective in treating inflammatory root resorption by inhibiting the spread of dentinoclasts[122] without damaging the periodontal ligament; however, its ability to diffuse through the human tooth root has been demonstrated,[1] and its release and diffusion are enhanced when it is used in combination with calcium hydroxide paste.[2]

Open Apex

Avoid endodontic treatment and look for signs of revascularization. At the first sign of an infected pulp, initiate apexification procedure.

Teeth with open apices have the potential to revascularize and continue root development; initial treatment is directed toward reestablishing the blood supply (Fig. 20-44).[51,127,175] The initiation of endodontic treatment is avoided if at all possible, unless definite signs of pulp necrosis are present (e.g., periradicular inflammation). An accurate diagnosis of pulp vitality is extremely challenging in these cases. After trauma, a diagnosis of necrotic pulp is particularly undesirable because infection in these teeth is potentially more harmful due to cemental damage accompanying the traumatic injury. External inflammatory root resorption can be extremely rapid in these young teeth because the tubules are wide and allow irritants to move freely to the external surface of the root.[51,175]

Patients are recalled every 3 to 4 weeks for pulp vitality testing. Studies indicate that thermal tests with carbon dioxide snow (−78° C) or dichlorodifluoromethane (−40° C) placed at the incisal edge or pulp horn are the best methods of sensitivity testing, particularly in young permanent teeth.[71,72,117] One of these two tests must be included in the pulp vitality testing. Recent reports confirm the superiority of the laser Doppler

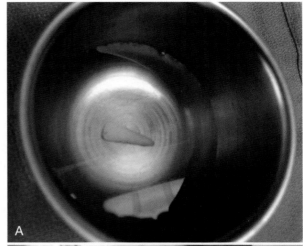
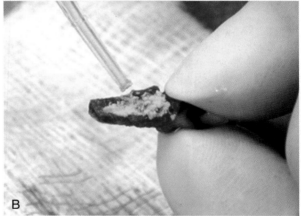

FIG. 20-44 **A,** Avulsed tooth soaking in doxycycline. **B,** Minocycline powder placed on the root surface before replantation.

flowmeter in the diagnosis of revascularization of traumatized immature teeth[176]; however, the cost of such an instrument precludes its use in the average dental office. Radiographic signs (apical breakdown and/or signs of lateral root resorption) and clinical signs (pain on percussion and palpation) of pulp pathosis are carefully assessed. At the first sign of pathosis, endodontic treatment should be initiated, and after disinfection of the root canal space, an apexification procedure should be carried out.

Extraoral Time More Than 60 Minutes

Closed Apex

Teeth with closed apices are treated endodontically in the same way as teeth that had an extraoral time of less than 60 minutes.

Open Apex (if Replanted)

If endodontic treatment was not performed out of the mouth, initiate apexification procedure.

The chance of revascularization in these teeth is extremely poor,[163,167] so no attempt is made to revitalize them. An apexification procedure is initiated at the second visit if root canal treatment was not performed at the emergency visit. If endodontic treatment was performed at the emergency visit, the second visit is a recall visit to assess initial healing only.

TEMPORARY RESTORATION

Effectively sealing the coronal access is essential to prevent infection of the canal between visits. Recommended temporary restorations are reinforced zinc oxide eugenol cement, acid etch composite resin, or glass ionomer cement. The depth of the temporary restoration is critical to its sealability. A depth of at least 4 mm is recommended, so a cotton pellet should not be placed; the temporary restoration is placed directly onto the calcium hydroxide in the access cavity. Calcium hydroxide should be removed from the walls of the access cavity before the temporary restoration is placed because calcium hydroxide is soluble and washes out when it comes into contact with saliva, leaving a defective temporary restoration.

After initiation of the root canal treatment, the splint is removed. If time does not permit complete removal of the splint at this visit, the resin tacks are smoothed so as not to irritate the soft tissues; the remaining resin is removed at a later appointment.

At this appointment, healing is usually sufficient to allow a detailed clinical examination of the teeth surrounding the avulsed tooth. Pulp vitality tests, reaction to percussion and palpation, and periodontal probing measurements should be carefully recorded for reference at follow-up visits.

Root Filling Visit

This visit should take place at the clinician's convenience or after long-term calcium hydroxide therapy, when an intact lamina dura is traced.

If the endodontic treatment was initiated 1 to 2 weeks after the avulsion and a thorough examination confirms normality, filling of the root canal at this visit is acceptable. Long-term use of calcium hydroxide is also a proven option for these cases. If endodontic treatment was initiated more than 2 weeks after the avulsion or active resorption is visible, the pulp space

must first be disinfected before root filling. Traditionally, the reestablishment of a lamina dura (see Fig. 20-35) is a radiographic sign that the canal bacteria have been controlled. When an intact lamina dura can be traced throughout, root filling can take place.

The canal is cleaned, shaped, and irrigated under strict asepsis (i.e., a rubber dam). After completion of cleaning and shaping, the canal can be filled.

PERMANENT RESTORATION

Much evidence exists that coronal leakage caused by defective temporary and permanent restorations results in a clinically relevant amount of bacterial contamination of the root canal after root filling.[126] Therefore, the tooth should receive a permanent restoration as soon as possible. The depth of restoration is important for a tight seal, so the deepest restoration possible should be made. A post should be avoided if possible. Because most avulsions occur in the anterior region of the mouth where aesthetics is important, composite resins combined with dentin bonding agents are recommended in these cases.

Follow-Up Care

Follow-up evaluations should take place at 3 months, 6 months, and yearly for at least 5 years. If osseous replacement is identified (see Fig. 20-28), a more closely monitored follow-up schedule is indicated. In the case of inflammatory root resorption (see Fig. 20-30), a new attempt at disinfection of the root canal space by standard retreatment might reverse the process. Teeth adjacent to and surrounding the avulsed tooth or teeth may show pathologic changes long after the initial accident, so these teeth, too, should be tested at follow-up visits and the results compared to those collected soon after the accident.

REFERENCES

1. Abbott PV, Heithersay GS, Hume WR: Release and diffusion through human tooth roots in vitro of corticosteroid and tetracycline trace molecules from Ledermix paste, *Endod Dent Traumatol* 4:55, 1988.
2. Abbott PV, Hume WR, Heithersay GS: Effects of combining Ledermix and calcium hydroxide pastes on the diffusion of corticosteroid and tetracycline through human tooth roots in vitro, *Endod Dent Traumatol* 5:188, 1989.
3. About I, Murray PE, Franquin JC, et al: The effect of cavity restoration variables on odontoblast cell numbers and dental repair, *J Dent* 29:109, 2001.
4. Accorinte L, Holland R, Reis A, et al: Evaluation of mineral trioxide aggregate and calcium hydroxide cement as pulp-capping agents in human teeth, *J Endod* 34:1, 2008.
5. Andersson L, Friskopp J, Blomlof L: Fiber-glass splinting of traumatized teeth, *ASDC J Dent Child* 50:21, 1983.
6. Andersson L, Malmgren B: The problem of dentoalveolar ankylosis and subsequent replacement resorption in the growing patient, *Aust Endod J* 25:57, 1999.
7. Andreasen FM: Pulpal healing after luxation injuries and root fracture in the permanent dentition, *Endod Dent Traumatol* 5:111, 1989.
8. Andreasen FM, Andreasen JO: Resorption and mineralization processes following root fracture of permanent incisors. *Endod Dent Traumatol* 4:202, 1988.
9. Andreasen FM, Andreasen JO, Bayer T: Prognosis of root-fractured permanent incisors: prediction of healing modalities, *Endod Dent Traumatol* 5:11, 1989.
10. Andreasen FM, Pedersen BV: Prognosis of luxated permanent teeth: the development of pulp necrosis, *Endod Dent Traumatol* 1:207, 1985.
11. Andreasen FM, Zhijie Y, Thomsen BL, Andersen PK: Occurrence of pulp canal obliteration after luxation injuries in the permanent dentition, *Endod Dent Traumatol* 3:103, 1987.
12. Andreasen JO: Etiology and pathogenesis of traumatic dental injuries: a clinical study of 1,298 cases, *Scand J Dent Res* 78:329, 1970.
13. Andreasen JO: Luxation of permanent teeth due to trauma: a clinical and radiographic follow-up study of 189 injured teeth,. *Scand J Dent Res* 78:273, 1970.
14. Andreasen JO: Effect of extra-alveolar period and storage media upon periodontal and pulpal healing after replantation of mature permanent incisors in monkeys, *Int J Oral Surg* 10:43, 1981.
15. Andreasen JO: Review of root resorption systems and models: etiology of root resorption and the homeostatic mechanisms of the periodontal ligament. In Davidovitch Z, editor: *The biological mechanisms of tooth eruption and resorption*, Birmingham, Ala, 1989, EB-SCOP Media.
16. Andreasen JO, Andreasen FM, Andersson L: *Textbook and color atlas of traumatic injuries to the teeth*, ed 4, Hoboken, NJ, 2007, Wiley-Blackwell.
17. Andreasen JO, Andreasen FM, Mejare I, Cvek M: Healing of 400 intra-alveolar root fractures. Part 1. Effect of pre-injury and injury factors such as sex, age, stage of root development, fracture type, location of fracture and severity of dislocation, *Dent Traumatol* 20:192, 2004.
18. Andreasen JO, Andreasen FM, Mejare I, Cvek M: Healing of 400 intra-alveolar root fractures. Part 2. Effect of treatment factors such as treatment delay, repositioning, splinting type and period and antibiotics, *Dent Traumatol* 20:203, 2004.
19. Andreasen JO, Farik B, Munksgaard EC: Long-term calcium hydroxide as a root canal dressing may increase risk of root fracture, *Dent Traumatol* 18:134, 2002.
20. Andreasen JO, Hjorting-Hansen E: Replantation of teeth. I. Radiographic and clinical study of 110 human teeth replanted after accidental loss, *Acta Odontol Scand* 24:263, 1966.
21. Andreasen JO, Hjorting-Hansen E: Intraalveolar root fractures: radiographic and histologic study of 50 cases, *J Oral Surg* 25:414, 1967.
22. Andreasen JO, Kristerson L: The effect of limited drying or removal of the periodontal ligament: periodontal healing after replantation of mature permanent incisors in monkeys, *Acta Odontol Scand* 39:1, 1981.
23. Andreasen JO, Ravn JJ: Epidemiology of traumatic dental injuries to primary and permanent teeth in a Danish population sample, *Int J Oral Surg* 1:235, 1972.
24. Arakawa M, Kitasako Y, Otsuki M, Tagami J: Direct pulp capping with an auto-cured sealant resin and a self-etching primer, *Am J Dent* 16:61, 2003.

25. Banchs F, Trope M: Revascularization of immature permanent teeth with apical periodontitis: new treatment protocol? *J Endod* 30:196, 2004.

26. Barrett AP, Reade PC: Revascularization of mouse tooth isografts and allografts using autoradiography and carbon-perfusion, *Arch Oral Biol* 26:541, 1981.

27. Barrett EJ, Kenny DJ: Avulsed permanent teeth: a review of the literature and treatment guidelines, *Endod Dent Traumatol* 13:153, 1997.

28. Bastone EB, Freer TJ, McNamara JR: Epidemiology of dental trauma: a review of the literature, *Aust Dent J* 45:2, 2000.

29. Bergenholtz G: Micro-organisms from necrotic pulp of traumatized teeth, *Odontol Revy* 25:347, 1974.

30. Bernardes RA, de Moraes IG, Duarte MAH, Azevedo BC: Use of cone-beam volumetric tomography in the diagnosis of root fractures, *Oral Surg Oral Med Oral Pathol Oral Radiol Endod* 108:270, 2009.

31. Bernardes RA, de Paulo RS, Pereira LO, et al: Comparative study of cone beam computed tomography and intraoral periapical radiographs in diagnosis of lingual-simulated external root resorptions, *Dent Traumatol* 28:268, 2012.

32. Bhaskar SN, Rappaport HM: Dental vitality tests and pulp status, *J Am Dent Assoc* 86:409, 1973.

33. Binnie WH, Rowe AH: A histological study of the periapical tissues of incompletely formed pulpless teeth filled with calcium hydroxide, *J Dent Res* 52:1110, 1973.

34. Bjorvatn K, Selvig KA, Klinge B: Effect of tetracycline and SnF2 on root resorption in replanted incisors in dogs, *Scand J Dent Res* 97:477, 1989.

35. Blomlof L: Milk and saliva as possible storage media for traumatically exarticulated teeth prior to replantation, *Swed Dent J Suppl* 8:1, 1981.

36. Blomlof L, Lindskog S, Andersson L, et al: Storage of experimentally avulsed teeth in milk prior to replantation, *J Dent Res* 62:912, 1983.

37. Bortoluzzi EA, Broon NJ, Bramante CM, et al: Mineral trioxide aggregate with or without calcium chloride in pulpotomy, *J Endod* 34:172, 2008.

38. Bryson EC, Levin L, Banchs F, et al: Effect of immediate intracanal placement of Ledermix Paste on healing of replanted dog teeth after extended dry times, *Dent Traumatol* 18:316, 2002.

39. Bystrom A, Claesson R, Sundqvist G: The antibacterial effect of camphorated paramonochlorophenol, camphorated phenol and calcium hydroxide in the treatment of infected root canals, *Endod Dent Traumatol* 1:170, 1985.

40. Canakci V, Akgul HM, Akgul N, Canakci CF: Prevalence and handedness correlates of traumatic injuries to the permanent incisors in 13 17-year-old adolescents in Erzurum, Turkey, *Dent Traumatol* 19:248, 2003.

41. Chen H, Teixeira FB, Ritter AL, et al: The effect of intracanal anti-inflammatory medicaments on external root resorption of replanted dog teeth after extended extra-oral dry time, *Dental Traumatol* 24:74, 2008.

42. Cohenca N, Simon JH, Roges R, et al: Clinical indications for digital imaging in dento-alveolar trauma. Part 1. Traumatic injuries, *Dent Traumatol* 23:95, 2007.

43. Cohenca N, Simon JH, Marhtur A, Malfaz JM: Clinical indications for digital imaging in dento-alveolar trauma. Part 2. Root resorption, *Dent Traumatol* 23:105, 2007.

44. Cotton TP, Geisler TM, Holden DT, et al: Endodontic applications of cone beam volumetric tomography, *J Endod* 33:1121, 2007.

45. Cox CF, Keall CL, Keall HJ, et al: Biocompatibility of surface-sealed dental materials against exposed pulps. *J Prosthet Dent* 57:1, 1987.

46. Cox CF, Tarim B, Kopel H, et al: Technique sensitivity: biological factors contributing to clinical success with various restorative materials, *Adv Dent Res* 15:85, 2001.

47. Cunha RF, Pavarini A, Percinoto C, et al: Influence of surgical repositioning of mature permanent dog teeth following experimental intrusion: a histologic assessment, *Dent Traumatol* 18:304, 2002.

48. Cvek M: Treatment of non-vital permanent incisors with calcium hydroxide. IV. Periodontal healing and closure of the root canal in the coronal fragment of teeth with intra-alveolar fracture and vital apical fragment: a follow-up, *Odontol Revy* 25:239, 1974.

49. Cvek M: A clinical report on partial pulpotomy and capping with calcium hydroxide in permanent incisors with complicated crown fracture, *J Endod* 4:232, 1978.

50. Cvek M: Prognosis of luxated non-vital maxillary incisors treated with calcium hydroxide and filled with gutta-percha: a retrospective clinical study, *Endod Dent Traumatol* 8:45, 1992.

51. Cvek M, Cleaton-Jones P, Austin J, et al: Effect of topical application of doxycycline on pulp revascularization and periodontal healing in reimplanted monkey incisors, *Endod Dent Traumatol* 6:170, 1990.

52. Cvek M, Cleaton-Jones PE, Austin JC, Andreasen JO: Pulp reactions to exposure after experimental crown fractures or grinding in adult monkeys, *J Endod* 8:391, 1982.

53. Cvek M, Hollender L, Nord CE: Treatment of non-vital permanent incisors with calcium hydroxide. VI. A clinical, microbiological and radiological evaluation of treatment in one sitting of teeth with mature or immature root, *Odontol Revy* 27:93, 1976.

54. Cvek M, Nord CE, Hollender L: Antimicrobial effect of root canal debridement in teeth with immature root: a clinical and microbiologic study, *Odontol Revy* 27:1, 1976.

55. Da Silva AC, Passeri LA, Mazzonetto R, et al: Incidence of dental trauma associated with facial trauma in Brazil: a 1-year evaluation, *Dent Traumatol* 20:6, 2004.

56. Deutsch AS, Musikant BL, Cavallari J, et al: Root fracture during insertion of prefabricated posts related to root size, *J Prosthet Dent* 53:786, 1985.

57. Durack C, Patel S, Davies J, et al: Diagnostic accuracy of small volume cone beam computed tomography and intraoral periapical radiography for the detection of simulated external inflammatory root resorption, *Int Endod J* 44:136, 2011.

58. Ebeleseder KA, Santler G, Glockner K, et al: An analysis of 58 traumatically intruded and surgically extruded permanent teeth, *Endod Dent Traumatol* 16:34, 2000.

59. Eklund G, Stalhane I, Hedegard B: A study of traumatized permanent teeth in children aged 7-15 years. III. A multivariate analysis of post-traumatic complications of subluxated and luxated teeth, *Sven Tandlak Tidskr* 69:179, 1976.

60. Ersin NK, Eronat N: The comparison of a dentin adhesive with calcium hydroxide as a pulp-capping agent on the exposed pulps of human and sheep teeth, *Quintessence Int* 36:271, 2005.

61. Estrela C, Reis Bueno M, Alencar AHG: Method to evaluate inflammatory root resorption by using cone beam computed tomography, *J Endod* 35:1491, 2009.

62. Faraco IM Jr, Holland R: Response of the pulp of dogs to capping with mineral trioxide aggregate or a calcium hydroxide cement, *Dent Traumatol* 17:163, 2001.

63. Filippi A, Pohl Y, von Arx T: Decoronation of an ankylosed tooth for preservation of alveolar bone prior to implant placement, *Dent Traumatol* 17:93, 2001.

64. Filippi A, Pohl Y, von Arx T: Treatment of replacement resorption with Emdogain: preliminary results after 10 months, *Dent Traumatol* 17:134, 2001.

65. Flores MT, Malmgren B, Andersson L, et al: Guidelines for the management of traumatic dental injuries. I. Fractures and luxations of permanent teeth, *Dent Traumatol* 23:66, 2007.

66. Flores MT, Malmgren B, Andersson L, et al: Guidelines for the management of traumatic dental injuries. II. Avulsion of permanent teeth, *Dent Traumatol* 23:130, 2007.

67. Flores MT, Malmgren B, Andersson L, et al: Guidelines for the management of traumatic dental injuries. III. Primary teeth, *Dent Traumatol* 23:196, 2007.

68. Frank AL: Therapy for the divergent pulpless tooth by continued apical formation, *J Am Dent Assoc* 72:87, 1966.

69. Fuks AB, Bielak S, Chosak A: Clinical and radiographic assessment of direct pulp capping and pulpotomy in young permanent teeth, *Pediatr Dent* 4:240, 1982.

70. Fuks AB, Cosack A, Klein H, Eidelman E: Partial pulpotomy as a treatment alternative for exposed pulps in crown-fractured permanent incisors, *Endod Dent Traumatol* 3:100, 1987.

71. Fulling HJ, Andreasen JO: Influence of maturation status and tooth type of permanent teeth upon electrometric and thermal pulp testing, *Scand J Dent Res* 84:286, 1976.

72. Fuss Z, Trowbridge H, Bender IB, et al: Assessment of reliability of electrical and thermal pulp testing agents, *J Endod* 12:301, 1986.

73. Gazelius B, Olgart L, Edwall B: Restored vitality in luxated teeth assessed by laser Doppler flowmeter, *Endod Dent Traumatol* 4:265, 1988.

74. Gelbier MJ, Winter GB: Traumatised incisors treated by vital pulpotomy: a retrospective study, *Br Dent J* 164:319, 1988.

75. Giuliani V, Baccetti T, Pace R, Pagavino G: The use of MTA in teeth with necrotic pulps and open apices, *Dent Traumatol* 18:217, 2002.

76. Goldberg F, Kaplan A, Roitman M, et al: Reinforcing effect of a resin glass ionomer in the restoration of immature roots in vitro, *Dent Traumatol* 18:70, 2002.

77. Granath LE, Hagman G: Experimental pulpotomy in human bicuspids with reference cutting technique, *Acta Odontol Scand* 29:155, 1971.

78. Hammarstrom L, Lindskog S: General morphological aspects of resorption of teeth and alveolar bone, *Int Endod J* 18:93, 1985.

79. Hammarstrom L, Pierce A, Blomlof L, et al: Tooth avulsion and replantation: a review, *Endod Dent Traumatol* 2:1, 1986.

80. Hebling J, Giro EM, Costa CA: Biocompatibility of an adhesive system applied to exposed human dental pulp, *J Endodontol* 25:676, 1999.

81. Hedegard B, Stalhane I: A study of traumatized permanent teeth in children 7-15 years. I, *Sven Tandlak Tidskr* 66:431, 1973.

82. Heide S, Mjor IA: Pulp reactions to experimental exposures in young permanent monkey teeth, *Int Endod J* 16:11, 1983.

83. Heithersay GS: Calcium hydroxide in the treatment of pulpless teeth with associated pathology, *J Br Endod Soc* 8:74, 1962.

84. Heller AL, Koenigs JF, Brilliant JD, et al: Direct pulp capping of permanent teeth in primates using a resorbable form of tricalcium phosphate ceramic, *J Endod* 1:95, 1975.

85. Herforth A, Strassburg M: Therapy of chronic apical periodontitis in traumatically injuring front teeth with ongoing root growth. *Dtsch Zahnarztl Z* 32:453, 1977.

86. Hiltz J, Trope M: Vitality of human lip fibroblasts in milk, Hanks Balanced Salt Solution and Viaspan storage media, *Endod Dent Traumatol* 7:69, 1991.

87. Holland R, Bisco Ferreira L, de Souza V, et al: Reaction of the lateral periodontium of dogs' teeth to contaminated and noncontaminated perforations filled with mineral trioxide aggregate, *J Endod* 33:1192, 2007.

88. Holloway GA Jr, Watkins DW: Laser Doppler measurement of cutaneous blood flow. *J Invest Dermatol* 69:306, 1977.

89. Hoshino E, Kurihara-Ando N, Sato I, et al: In-vitro antibacterial susceptibility of bacteria taken from infected root dentine to a mixture of ciprofloxacin, metronidazole and minocycline, *Int Endod J* 29:125, 1996.

90. Iqbal MK, Bamaas N: Effect of enamel matrix derivative (Emdogain) upon periodontal healing after replantation of permanent incisors in beagle dogs, *Dent Traumatol* 17:36, 2001.

91. Iwamoto CE, Erika A, Pameijer CH, et al: Clinical and histological evaluation of white ProRoot MTA in direct pulp capping, *Am J Dent* 19:85, 2006.

92. Jacobsen I: Root fractures in permanent anterior teeth with incomplete root formation, *Scand J Dent Res* 84:210, 1976.

93. Jacobsen I, Kerekes K: Diagnosis and treatment of pulp necrosis in permanent anterior teeth with root fracture, *Scand J Dent Res* 88:370, 1980.

94. Jacobsen I, Zachrisson BU: Repair characteristics of root fractures in permanent anterior teeth, *Scand J Dent Res* 83:355, 1975.

95. Jarvinen S: Fractured and avulsed permanent incisors in Finnish children: a retrospective study, *Acta Odontol Scand* 37:47, 1979.

96. Jung IY, Lee SJ, Hargreaves KM: Biologically based treatment of immature permanent teeth with pulpal necrosis: a case series, *J Endod* 34:876, 2008.

97. Kakehashi S, Stanley HR, Fitzgerald RJ: The effect of surgical exposures on dental pulps in germ-free and conventional laboratory rats, *Oral Surg* 20:340, 1965.

98. Kamburoglu K, Ilker Cebeci AR, Grondahl HG: Effectiveness of limited cone-beam computed tomography in the detection of horizontal root fracture, *Dent Traumatol* 25:256, 2009.

99. Katebzadeh N, Dalton BC, Trope M: Strengthening immature teeth during and after apexification, *J Endod* 24:256, 1998.

100. Kenny DJ, Barrett EJ, Casas MJ: Avulsions and intrusions: the controversial displacement injuries. *J Can Dent Assoc* 69:308, 2003.

101. Kerekes K, Heide S, Jacobsen I: Follow-up examination of endodontic treatment in traumatized juvenile incisors, *J Endod* 6:744, 1980.

102. Koliniotou-Koumpia E, Tziafas D: Pulpal responses following direct pulp capping of healthy dog teeth with dentine adhesive systems, *J Dent* 33:639, 2005.

103. Kositbowornchai S, Nuansakul R, Sikram S, et al: Root fracture detection: a comparison of direct digital radiography with conventional radiography, *Dentomaxillofac Radiol* 30:106, 2001.

104. Lengheden A, Blomlof L, Lindskog S: Effect of delayed calcium hydroxide treatment on periodontal healing in contaminated replanted teeth, *Scand J Dent Res* 99:147, 1991.

105. Lindskog S, Pierce AM, Blomlof L, Hammarstrom L: The role of the necrotic periodontal membrane in cementum resorption and ankylosis, *Endod Dent Traumatol* 1:96, 1985.

106. Love RM: Bacterial penetration of the root canal of intact incisor teeth after a simulated traumatic injury, *Endod Dent Traumatol* 12:289, 1996.

107. Love RM, Ponnambalam Y: Dental and maxillofacial skeletal injuries seen at the University of Otago School of Clinicianry, New Zealand, 2000-2004, *Dent Traumatol* 24:170, 2008.

108. Lundin SA, Noren JG, Warfvinge J: Marginal bacterial leakage and pulp reactions in Class II composite resin restorations in vivo, *Swed Dent J* 14:185, 1990.

109. Maroto M, Barberia E, Planells P, Vera V: Treatment of a non-vital immature incisor with mineral trioxide aggregate (MTA), *Dent Traumatol* 19:165, 2003.

110. Masterton JB: The healing of wounds of the dental pulp: an investigation of the nature of the scar tissue and of the phenomena leading to its formation, *Dent Pract Dent Rec* 16:325, 1966.

111. May JJ, Cohenca N, Peters OA: Contemporary management of horizontal root fractures to the permanent dentition: diagnosis, radiologic assessment to include cone-beam computed tomography, *Pediatr Dent* 35:120, 2013.

112. Mejare I, Hasselgren G, Hammarstrom LE: Effect of formaldehyde-containing drugs on human dental pulp evaluated by enzyme histochemical technique, *Scand J Dent Res* 84:29, 1976.

113. Mesaros S, Trope M, Maixner W, Burkes EJ: Comparison of two laser Doppler systems on the measurement of blood flow of premolar teeth under different pulpal conditions, *Int Endod J* 30:167, 1997.

114. Myers WC, Fountain SB: Dental pulp regeneration aided by blood and blood substitutes after experimentally

115. induced periapical infection, *Oral Surg Oral Med Oral Pathol* 37:441, 1974.

115. Murray PE, Smith AJ, Windsor LJ, Mjor IA: Remaining dentine thickness and human pulp responses, *Int Endod J* 33:36, 2003.

116. Nair PN, Duncan HF, Pitt Ford TR, Luder HU: Histological, ultrastructural and quantitative investigations on the response of healthy human pulps to experimental capping with mineral trioxide aggregate: a randomized controlled trial, *Int Endod J* 41:128, 2008.

117. Ohman A: Healing and sensitivity to pain in young replanted human teeth: an experimental, clinical and histological study, *Odontol Tidskr* 73:166, 1965.

118. Parirokh M, Kakoei S: Vital pulp therapy of mandibular incisors: a case report with 11-year follow up, *Aust Endod J* 32:75, 2006.

119. Patel S, Dawood A, Pitt Ford T, Whaites E: The potential applications of cone beam computed tomography in the management of endodontic problems, *Int Endod J* 40:818, 2007.

120. Patel S, Durack C, Abella F, et al: Cone beam computed tomography in endodontics: a review, *Int Endod J* 48:3, 2015.

121. Perez AL, Spears R, Gutmann JL, Opperman LA: Osteoblasts and MG-63 osteosarcoma cells behave differently when in contact with ProRoot MTA and White MTA, *Int Endod J* 36:564, 2003.

122. Pierce A, Lindskog S: The effect of an antibiotic/corticosteroid paste on inflammatory root resorption in vivo, *Oral Surg Oral Med Oral Pathol* 64:216, 1987.

123. Pileggi R, Dumsha TC, Myslinksi NR: The reliability of electric pulp test after concussion injury, *Endod Dent Traumatol* 12:16, 1996.

124. Rabie G, Barnett F, Tronstad L: Long-term splinting of maxillary incisor with intra alveolar root fracture, *Endod Dent Traumatol* 4:99, 1988.

125. Ravn JJ: Follow-up study of permanent incisors with complicated crown fractures after acute trauma, *Scand J Dent Res* 90:363, 1982.

126. Ray HA, Trope M: Periapical status of endodontically treated teeth in relation to the technical quality of the root filling and the coronal restoration, *Int Endod J* 28:12, 1995.

127. Ritter AL, Ritter AV, Murrah V, et al: Pulp revascularization of replanted immature dog teeth after treatment with minocycline and doxycycline assessed by laser Doppler flowmetry, radiography, and histology, *Dent Traumatol* 20:75, 2004.

128. Sae-Lim V, Wang CY, Choi GW, Trope M: The effect of systemic tetracycline on resorption of dried replanted dogs' teethl, *Endod Dent Traumatol* 14:127, 1998.

129. Sae-Lim V, Wang CY, Trope M: Effect of systemic tetracycline and amoxicillin on inflammatory root resorption of replanted dogs' teeth, *Endod Dent Traumatol* 14:216, 1998.

130. Saroglu I, Sonmez H: The prevalence of traumatic injuries treated in the pedodontic clinic of Ankara University, Turkey, during 18 months, *Dent Traumatol* 18:299, 2002.

131. Sawicki L, Pameijer CH, Emerich K, Adamowicz-Klepalska B: Histological evaluation of mineral trioxide aggregate and calcium hydroxide in direct pulp capping of human immature permanent teeth, *Am J Dent* 21:262, 2008.

132. Schjott M, Andreasen JO: Emdogain does not prevent progressive root resorption after replantation of avulsed teeth: a clinical study, *Dental Traumatol* 21:46, 2005.

133. Schroder U: Reaction of human dental pulp to experimental pulpotomy and capping with calcium hydroxide (thesis), *Odont Revy* 24(Suppl 25):97, 1973.

134. Schroder U, Granath LE: Early reaction of intact human teeth to calcium hydroxide following experimental pulpotomy and its significance to the development of hard tissue barrier, *Odontol Revy* 22:379, 1971.

135. Seltzer S: *Endodontology*, Philadelphia, 1988, Lea & Febiger.

136. Seltzer S, Bender IB, Turkenkopf S: Factors affecting successful repair after root canal therapy, *J Am Dent Assoc* 52:651, 1963.

137. Selvig KA, Zander HA: Chemical analysis and microradiography of cementum and dentin from periodontically diseased human teeth, *J Periodontol* 33:103, 1962.

138. Shuping GB, Orstavik D, Sigurdsson A, Trope M: Reduction of intracanal bacteria using nickel-titanium rotary instrumentation and various medications, *J Endod* 26:751, 2000.

139. Silva GA, Lanza LD, Lopes-Junior N, et al: Direct pulp capping with a dentin bonding system in human teeth: a clinical and histological evaluation, *Oper Dent* 31:297, 2006.

140. Silverman S: The dental structures in primary hyperparathyroidism, *Oral Surg* 15:426, 1962.

141. Sjogren U, Figdor D, Spangberg L, Sundqvist G: The antimicrobial effect of calcium hydroxide as a short-term intracanal dressing, *Int Endod J* 24:119, 1991.

142. Sjogren U, Hagglund B, Sundqvist G, Wing K: Factors affecting the long-term results of endodontic treatment, *J Endod* 16:498, 1990.

143. Skaare AB, Jacobsen I: Dental injuries in Norwegians aged 7-18 years, *Dent Traumatol* 19:67, 2003.

144. Skieller V: The prognosis for young teeth loosened after mechanical injuries, *Acta Odontol Scand* 18:171, 1960.

145. Skoglund A, Tronstad L: Pulpal changes in replanted and autotransplanted immature teeth of dogs, *J Endod* 7:309, 1981.

146. Soder PO, Otteskog P, Andreasen JO, Modeer T: Effect of drying on viability of periodontal membrane, *Scand J Dent Res* 85:164, 1977.

147. Spangberg L, Rutberg M, Rydinge E: Biologic effects of endodontic antimicrobial agents, *J Endod* 5:166, 1979.

148. Stalhane I, Hedegard B: Traumatized permanent teeth in children aged 7-15 years, *Sven Tandlak Tidskr* 68:157, 1975.

149. Stanley HR: Diseases of the dental pulp. In Tieck RW, editors: *Oral pathology*, New York, 1965, McGraw-Hill.

150. Stanley HR, Lundy T: Dycal therapy for pulp exposures, *Oral Surg Oral Med Oral Pathol* 34:818, 1972.

151. Subay RK, Demirci M: Pulp tissue reactions to a dentin bonding agent as a direct capping agent, *J Endod* 31:201, 2005.

152. Swift EJ Jr, Trope M: Treatment options for the exposed vital pulp, *Pract Periodontics Aesthet Dent* 11:735, 1999.

153. Tapias MA, Jimenez-Garcia R, Lamas F, Gil AA: Prevalence of traumatic crown fractures to permanent incisors in a childhood population: Mostoles, Spain, *Dent Traumatol* 19:119, 2003.

154. Teixeira FB, Teixeira EC, Thompson JY, Trope M: Fracture resistance of roots endodontically treated with a new resin filling material, *J Am Dent Assoc* 135:646, 2004.

155. Thibodeau B, Teixeira F, Yamauchi M, et al: Pulp revascularization of immature dog teeth with apical periodontitis, *J Endod* 33:680, 2007.

156. Torabinejad M, Hong CU, McDonald F, Pitt Ford TR: Physical and chemical properties of a new root-end filling material, *J Endod* 21:349, 1995.

157. Torabinejad M, Rastegar AF, Kettering JD, Pitt Ford TR: Bacterial leakage of mineral trioxide aggregate as a root-end filling material, *J Endod* 21:109, 1995.

158. Trabert KC, Caput AA, Abou-Rass M: Tooth fracture: a comparison of endodontic and restorative treatments, *J Endod* 4:341, 1978.

159. Tronstad L: Reaction of the exposed pulp to Dycal treatment, *Oral Surg Oral Med Oral Pathol* 38:945, 1974.

160. Tronstad L: Root resorption: etiology, terminology and clinical manifestations, *Endod Dent Traumatol* 4:241, 1988.

161. Tronstad L, Andreasen JO, Hasselgren G, et al: pH changes in dental tissues after root canal filling with calcium hydroxide, *J Endod* 7:17, 1980.

162. Tronstad L, Mjor IA: Capping of the inflamed pulp, *Oral Surg Oral Med Oral Pathol* 34:477, 1972.

163. Trope M: Root resorption of dental and traumatic origin: classification based on etiology, *Pract Periodontics Aesthet Dent* 10:515, 1998.

164. Trope M: Clinical management of the avulsed tooth: present strategies and future directions, *Dent Traumatol* 18:1, 2002.

165. Trope M, Friedman S: Periodontal healing of replanted dog teeth stored in Viaspan, milk and Hank's Balanced Salt Solution, *Endod Dent Traumatol* 8:183, 1992.

166. Trope M, Moshonov J, Nissan R, et al: Short vs long-term calcium hydroxide treatment of established inflammatory root resorption in replanted dog teeth, *Endod Dent Traumatol* 11:124, 1995.

167. Trope M, Yesilsoy C, Koren L, et al: Effect of different endodontic treatment protocols on periodontal repair and root resorption of replanted dog teeth, *J Endod* 18:492, 1992.

168. Turley PK, Joiner MW, Hellstrom S: The effect of orthodontic extrusion on traumatically intruded teeth, *Am J Orthod* 85:47, 1984.

169. von Arx T, Filippi A, Buser D: Splinting of traumatized teeth with a new device: TTS (titanium trauma splint), *Dent Traumatol* 17:180, 2001.

170. Wedenberg C, Lindskog S: Experimental internal resorption in monkey teeth, *Endod Dent Traumatol* 1:221, 1985.

171. Wedenberg C, Zetterqvist L: Internal resorption in human teeth: a histological, scanning electron microscopic, and enzyme histochemical study, *J Endod* 13:255, 1987.

172. Weiss M: Pulp capping in older patients, *N Y State Dent J* 32:451, 1966.

173. Windley W, Teixeira F, Levin L, et al: Disinfection of immature teeth with a triple antibiotic paste, *J Endod* 31:439, 2005.

174. Witherspoon DE, Small JC, Harris GZ: Mineral trioxide aggregate pulpotomies: a case series outcomes assessment, *J Am Dent Assoc* 137:610, 2006.

175. Yanpiset K, Trope M: Pulp revascularization of replanted immature dog teeth after different treatment methods, *Endod Dent Traumatol* 16:211, 2000.

176. Yanpiset K, Vongsavan N, Sigurdsson A, Trope M: Efficacy of laser Doppler flowmetry for the diagnosis of revascularization of reimplanted immature dog teeth, *Dent Traumatol* 17:63, 2001.

177. Zachrisson BU, Jacobsen I: Long-term prognosis of 66 permanent anterior teeth with root fracture, *Scand J Dent Res* 83:345, 1975.

CHAPTER 21

Cracks and Fractures

ZVI METZGER | LOUIS H. BERMAN | AVIAD TAMSE

CHAPTER OUTLINE

Root cracks and fractures can be two of the most frustrating aspects of endodontic and restorative dentistry. The diagnosis can be difficult; the symptoms can be either vague or specific, yet they are often insufficient for a definitive diagnosis; the radiographic evaluation can be evasive. Clinical management of the crack or fracture depends on its extent. Prevention of a potential crack or fracture is a fundamental principle, and early detection is imperative.

UNOBSERVED TRAUMA

Tooth fracture is commonly associated with impact trauma. A car accident, a fall from a bicycle, and an accidental blow to the face are among the common causes. These types of traumatic fractures mainly occur in the anterior segment of the mouth and are covered elsewhere in this book (see Chapter 20). In contrast, the cracks and fractures described in this chapter are often not associated with a traumatic event that the patient can remember. These cracks and fractures are frequently the result of an accumulating, unobserved trauma resulting from either normal or excessive occlusal forces that are repetitively applied[22,34,45,47,70,71,90] without the patient's awareness.

DIAGNOSTIC CHALLENGE

Three categories of cracks and fractures are discussed in this chapter: cracked and fractured cusps, cracked and split teeth, and vertical root fractures. Each is often undiagnosed or misdiagnosed for a relatively long time.[16,19,80] The astute clinician can usually diagnose a pulpitis, apical periodontitis, or an abscess after appropriate diagnostic tests and clinical assessments are performed. However, because of the wide variety of clinical presentations from cracks and fractures, the diagnosis is less straightforward.[16,18,78] To complicate the diagnosis, not one of the three entities necessarily exhibits a radiographic manifestation in the early stages, depriving the dentist of one of the most objective diagnostic tools.

Symptoms from one of these conditions may be present for *several months* before an accurate diagnosis is made,[5,16,19] which may be frustrating for both the patient and the dentist, and often causes the patient to develop a subsequent loss of trust and confidence in the dentist.

The final diagnosis is typically reached at a relatively late stage of these conditions, often after complications have already occurred. Complications may include a catastrophic fracture of the tooth or cusp or significant periradicular bone loss associated with a vertical root fracture as seen by radiographic examination (see also Chapter 2). For this reason, this chapter emphasizes the *early diagnosis* of these conditions. The collection of signs and symptoms associated with each of the three categories of cracks and fractures may be confusing unless the clinician considers these indicators as representing a continuous process examined at a given time point.

FRACTURE MECHANICS

Fracture mechanics is the field of biomechanics concerned with the propagation of *cracks* in a given material until the formation of the final catastrophic *fracture*.[7,52] Many terms have been loosely used in the dental literature to describe the clinical entities that are the subject of this chapter.[5,9,18,35] Here, the term

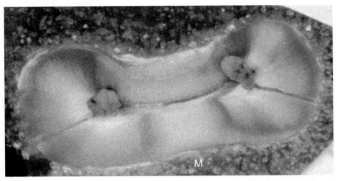

FIG. 21-1 Complete vertical root fracture. A cross section of a mesial root of a mandibular molar with a complete vertical root fracture. The fracture is in the buccolingual plane and extends from the buccal convexity of the root to its lingual convexity.

crack will be used in the biomechanical sense: a *partial discontinuity* in a material that may propagate and eventually lead to a complete discontinuity, also known as a *fracture*.[7,52] In this context, a cusp may be described as *cracked*, a condition leading with time to a *fractured cusp*. A *cracked tooth* may be so called until a final fracture occurs that separates the tooth into two parts, a condition termed a *split tooth*. Similarly, microcracks may appear in the radicular dentin of an endodontically treated tooth, and these cracks may propagate with time until a *vertical root fracture* occurs, at which point the full thickness of the dentinal wall shows discontinuity: a through-and-through fracture. Such a fracture may be *incomplete*, involving one wall of the root, or *complete*, separating the root into two parts[80] (Fig. 21-1).

CRACKED AND FRACTURED CUSPS

Definition

A *cracked cusp* is characterized by a crack between a cusp and the rest of the tooth structure, to the extent of allowing microscopic flexure upon mastication. This crack typically does not involve the pulp. With time, the crack may propagate, eventually resulting in a *fractured cusp*.[5]

Diagnosis

Patient History

In the case of a cracked cusp, the patient history is the most important tool for making a diagnosis. The patient will likely complain about pain when chewing, to the extent of not being able to chew on the side on which the crack occurred.[18,35,69] The patient will also often state that the condition existed for a relatively long time and that his or her dentist could not find the source or glean any information from radiography.[3,16,47] When asked whether the pain is sharp or dull, patients will typically report a sharp pain that makes them immediately stop chewing on that side. The diagnostic challenge is attempting to determine which cusp of which tooth is involved, as patients often have difficulties determining the specific location of the discomfort.[16,18,35,69] Because the pain has a pulpal origin, the patient's proprioception may not be accurate, as no periodontal ligament is involved. Occasionally, the pain upon chewing may radiate to nondental locations on the same side of the face,[16,47,71] as also described in Chapters 4 and 17.

Clinical Manifestation
Early Manifestation

The typical characteristic of cracked cusps is a sharp pain upon chewing, although the affected tooth may not be sensitive, or only selectively sensitive, to percussion.[70] The tooth is vital, and its response to a cold stimulus may be normal; but with time, this response may resemble a pulpitis, which may be either localized or referred to other odontogenic or nonodontogenic locations.[16,47,71]

Cracked cusps are often associated with extensive occlusal restorations,[3,29,71,78] which may undermine and weaken the cusp and predispose it to initiating or perpetuating a crack from occlusal forces. Nevertheless, cracked cusps may also be present in intact teeth or teeth with smaller restorations.[13,70]

Late Manifestation

With time, a crack may propagate and result in a fractured cusp. If the fracture line occurs coronally to the periodontal ligament the fractured portion will simply separate from the tooth. However, if the fracture line extends subgingivally, gingival fibers or the periodontal ligament will often retain the fractured cusp. Initially, it may be possible to move the cusp by wedging a sharp explorer into the fracture line, making the fractured cusp more visible. Often, from continued mastication, a localized and more acute type of pain may emerge secondary to the movement of the fractured fragment in the coronal PDL. The pulpal pain that is typical at an earlier stage (the cracked cusp) will typically resolve once a complete fracture occurs.

Diagnosis

A cracked cusp may be diagnosed, to a large extent, on the basis of the patient history. To locate the affected tooth, a *biting test* should be performed using a Tooth Slooth (Professional Results, Laguna Niguel, CA) or a similar device[9,12] (Fig. 21-2). The device is composed of a small pyramid with a flattened top that is placed on a selective cusp, while the wider part of the device is applied to several opposing teeth while the patient occludes (see Fig. 21-2). The application of these forces to a cracked cusp will generate a sharp pain, which may occur upon pressure or released.[3,34,43] The patient will typically state that this sensation has reproduced the sensation of the chief complaint.

Magnification with such devices as loupes or an operating microscope can be helpful when looking for a crack. If the tooth does not have an extensive intracoronal restoration, *transillumination* may also assist in revealing the crack line. If the tooth has a large restoration, the removal of the restoration may facilitate the effective use of this diagnostic tool (Fig. 21-3). The light source should be intense but with small dimensions (Fig. 21-4); it is applied to the tooth at the area of the suspected cusp fracture, with the lights of the dental unit, microscope, and room extinguished. The light penetrates the tooth structure up to the crack, leaving the part beyond the crack relatively dark (see Fig. 21-3). However, when large intracoronal restorations are present, this type of examination may be less effective.

Once the crack propagates, resulting in a fractured cusp, the diagnosis becomes more straightforward: the fractured cusp will either be missing or moved by wedging an explorer into the fracture line (Fig. 21-5).

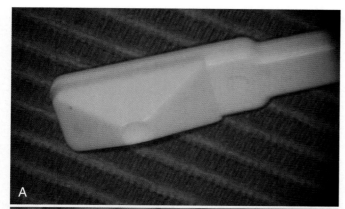

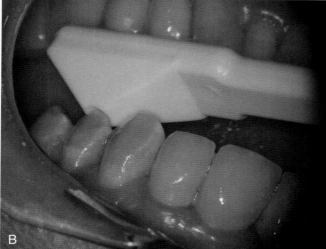

FIG. 21-2 A Tooth Slooth device. A, The Tooth Slooth device. **B,** Application for a bite test: the tip of the pyramid is touching the tested cusp while the wide base is supported by multiple contacts.

Etiology

Extensive intracoronal restorations may be a predisposing factor for cracked and fractured cusps.[3,29,71,78] Otherwise, the etiology of these conditions is similar to that of cracked teeth (see Cracked and Split Teeth, Etiology).

Treatment Planning

Cracked Cusp

Treatment should consist of protecting the affected cusp from occlusal forces, both to prevent pain while chewing and to prevent the propagation of the crack into a full fracture. A full-coverage crown or onlay is recommended,[5,16,39] although bonded composite restorations have also been proposed.[28,64] One should keep in mind that if the cracked cusp is not protected, the tooth may eventually fracture. If the fracture plane extends apically into the root, the tooth will be potentially nonrestorable.[5,9,12] Endodontic treatment is indicated only if signs and symptoms of pulpal pathosis are observed. In addition, if the removal of the cracked cusp and associated restoration will result in little or no remaining coronal tooth structure, then elective root canal treatment may be necessary for prosthetic reasons. When such a treatment plan is selected, one should also perform an occlusal reduction of the tooth as soon as possible to remove the tooth from active occlusion. The

patient should be instructed to be careful when chewing until the tooth is restored with a crown.

Fractured Cusp

The treatment of a fractured cusp depends on the amount of tooth structure remaining. If the missing part is limited in size, then the conservative restoration of a bonded composite resin may be indicated to cover the exposed dentin. In contrast, when a larger fragment has fractured and is either removed or missing, a full crown or an onlay may be necessary.

In certain cases, when cracked cusps are found in intact teeth or in teeth with no extensive restoration, it is difficult to predict the direction in which the crack is propagating. Therefore, in these cases, when considering endodontic and restorative treatment, the patient should be advised as to the potential decrease in prognosis, as described later.

CRACKED AND SPLIT TEETH

Definition

A *cracked tooth* exhibits a crack that incompletely separates the tooth crown into two parts. If the crack is allowed to propagate longitudinally, the tooth will eventually fracture into two fragments, resulting in a *split tooth*.

Diagnosis

Patient History

In cases of a cracked tooth, the patient history may be similar to that for a cracked cusp—namely, sharp pain upon mastication and prolonged failure of the dentist to diagnose the source of the pain.[16,19] Similar to a cracked cusp, the diagnosis of a cracked tooth is often made on the basis of the patient history alone. Often it is challenging for the practitioner to determine the location of the offending tooth. With time, the patient may report that he or she *used to have* a sharp pain and now experiences great sensitivity to cold stimuli; the patient may even report, at a later stage, that the pain has subsided. These observations are consistent with pulpitis or pulp necrosis, which may develop in the affected tooth with time.[13]

Clinical Manifestation
Early Manifestation

Cracked teeth may have extensive restorations with a weakened crown, or they may have minimal or no restorations. A cracked tooth begins with a crack in the clinical crown, which may gradually propagate in an apical direction.[3,5,28,47] Such cracks typically run in the mesiodistal direction, often splitting the crown into the buccal and lingual fragments. In the early stages, the tooth may be vital and painful to mastication. The pain may be sharp, to the extent that the patient is unable to chew on the affected side. This condition may persist for an extended period of time.[16,18,19] The pain may be localized or referred to any tooth, maxillary or mandibular, on the same side of the mouth.[16,47,71] No radiographic manifestations are present at these early stages, as the crack is microscopic and runs perpendicular to the x-ray beam. The affected tooth may or may not be sensitive to percussion at this point, and pulp testing may be normal or indicative of increased sensitivity to cold stimuli.

Late Manifestation

The late manifestation of a cracked tooth may include *pulp involvement* and eventually the *loss of pulp vitality*[13] or apical

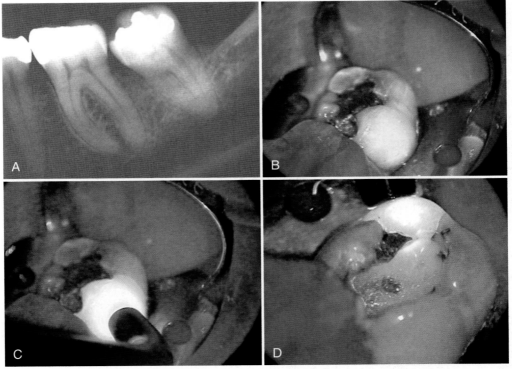

FIG. 21-3 Transillumination for the detection of a cracked cusp/tooth. An intense but small light source is applied to the suspect tooth, preferably in relative darkness. The light is transmitted through the tooth structure but is reflected from the crack plane, leaving the area behind the crack in darkness.

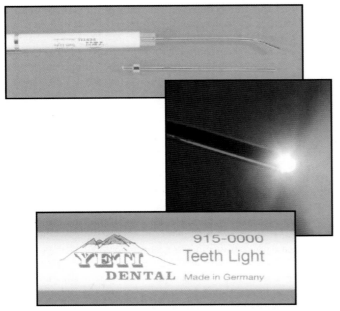

FIG. 21-4 Light source for transillumination. The light source should be intense yet with small dimensions, such as the simple battery-operated device manufactured by Yeti Dental (Engen, Germany).

propagation of the fracture, resulting in a *split tooth*. In one investigation,[13] 27 nonvital molar and premolar teeth that had minimal or no restorations or caries were studied. Upon extraction, these teeth were examined under a surgical operating microscope or using micro–computed tomography (CT)

analysis. In each of these teeth, a longitudinal crack was observed, which extended to the pulp. Although the study had a limited sample size, the clinician should understand the potentially poor prognosis from cracked teeth, especially when the crack is suspected to be the cause of pulp necrosis.[13]

Pulp involvement occurs more often in cases of centrally located cracks (i.e., extending from marginal ridge to marginal ridge through the central fossa) than in cracks with a more buccal or lingual location.[18,90] These centrally located cracks commonly affect the roof of the pulp chamber at a later stage. Consequently, pulp vitality may be compromised and later lost due to bacterial penetration through the crack. The pulp may first become reversibly or irreversibly inflamed and later necrotic and infected. The sharp pain upon mastication that is typical of the early stage may disappear once pulp vitality is lost. Moreover, apical periodontitis in an apparently intact molar may be a late manifestation of an untreated case of a cracked tooth.[13] When pulp necrosis occurs, the radiographic manifestation may be an apical radiolucency, which is undistinguishable from that of apical periodontitis (Fig. 21-6).

A crack may propagate with time through the pulp chamber and into the root, resulting in a complete fracture that separates the tooth into two parts, a condition termed *split tooth*. When this split occurs, the resulting parts of the tooth may be movable by wedging a sharp explorer into the fissure.[5,9] Later, more evident movement of the parts may be observed. The radiographic presentation at such a late stage may eventually develop into a diffuse radiolucency surrounding the root. At this late stage, narrow isolated deep periodontal pockets may be present.[9] However, such pockets are typically located

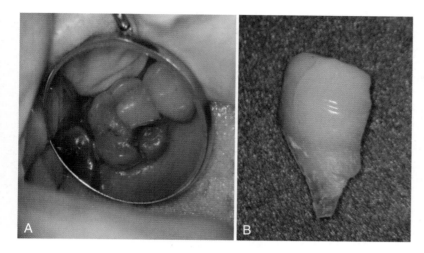

FIG. 21-5 A fractured cusp. A, The mesiopalatal cusp of a maxillary first right molar was fractured. The fractured cusp was movable and was retained by the periodontal ligament. **B,** The cusp was removed, and the tooth was considered restorable. It was treated with root canal treatment and a crown.

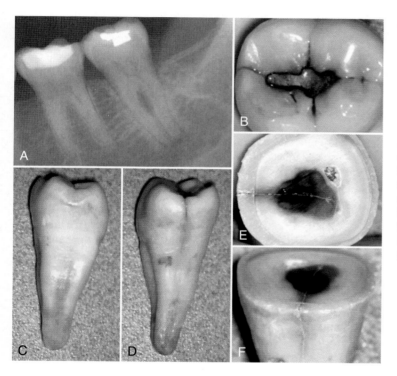

FIG. 21-6 A case of fracture-induced necrosis. A tooth with minimal or no restoration or caries is unlikely to become nonvital. **A,** This radiograph of a mandibular second molar shows a restoration that is distant from the pulp chamber, yet the tooth is nonvital and symptomatic. **B,** On occlusal examination, a slight crack is observed on the distal marginal ridge. **C,** After extraction, the mesial aspect of the crown and root shows no indication of a fracture. **D,** However, the distal aspect of the crown and coronal root shows the fracture. **E, F,** When the crown is sectioned, the crack can be observed to extend well into the pulp chamber.

mesially or distally and, if adjacent teeth are present, they will be difficult, if not impossible, to detect.

Cracked and split teeth may present with a large and variable collection of signs and symptoms that are potentially confusing.[16,18,78] Only by being aware of the *process* leading from early to late manifestations can clinicians interpret these signs and symptoms and identify the specific point they are encountering on the potential timeline of this process.

A definitive combination of factors, signs, and symptoms that, when collectively observed, allows the clinician to conclude the existence of a specific disease state is termed a *syndrome*. However, given the multitude of signs and symptoms that cracked roots can present with, it is often difficult to achieve an objective definitive diagnosis. For this reason, the terminology of *cracked tooth syndrome*[18] should be avoided.

Diagnosis

As in the case of a cracked cusp, early detection is imperative in order to resolve the patient's symptoms as well as increasing the prognosis. However, the use of the Tooth Slooth device (see Fig. 21-2) may or may not provide as clear a result for a symmetrically cracked tooth, as each of the parts of the tooth may be rather stable. Asking the patient to chew on a cotton roll[9] or on the tip of a cotton-tip applicator placed at a particular site may reproduce the pain. Nevertheless this method may not indicate whether the source is a maxillary or mandibular tooth and need further measures to pinpoint the involved tooth. *Magnification* using either loupes or an operating microscope can be helpful for detecting a fracture line. In addition, dyes, such as methylene blue or tincture of iodine, which are applied either to the outer surface of the crown or to the dentin after the removal of an existing intracoronal restoration, can be helpful for visualizing the crack (see Fig. 21-3). Transillumination can also be applied to the suspected tooth and, if the tooth has no restorations, this method may yield an impressively straightforward diagnosis (see Fig. 21-3). Anesthetizing the suspected tooth, followed by asking the patient to chew again on the cotton roll, may further confirm the diagnosis and finally differentiate the origin as a mandibular or maxillary tooth. At a later stage, when splitting of the tooth has occurred, wedging of a sharp explorer into the fracture line will provide a clear diagnosis of a split tooth.

Generally speaking, the diagnosis of a crack in a tooth can be difficult. When there are signs and symptoms of a pulpitis or necrosis, it is incumbent upon the clinician to determine the source that initiated the signs and symptoms. In the case of a problematic tooth with no apparent reason for the pulpitis or necrosis, like a tooth with minimal or no caries, restoration, or trauma, a crack or fracture must be considered.[13] In some cases, an objective diagnosis may not be possible; however, with the possibility of a crack or fracture, the patient should be advised of a potential decrease in the endodontic or restorative prognosis.[5,12]

Etiology

Masticatory forces are the cause of cracked teeth.[22,34,45,47,70,71,90] Thus, the dietary habit of chewing on coarse food has been proposed as a contributing factor.[22,90] Bruxism or clenching of the teeth as well as occlusal prematurities are also frequent causes of cracked teeth.[18,22,34,45,47,70,71,90] For this reason, certain teeth may be more prone to developing cracks, such as mandibular second molars and maxillary premolars.[18] Masticatory habits such as chewing ice may also predispose teeth to cracks. The term *fatigue root fracture,* proposed by Yeh,[90] encompasses all of these causes.

In certain cases, traumatic injuries, such as a severe upward blow to the mandible (e.g., during a car or sports accident) can also cause a tooth crack or fracture. Another potential cause is the unexpected chewing of a hard object (e.g., a cherry pit or an unpopped corn kernel in popcorn). The occlusal forces applied by the first molars are as high as 90 kg,[45] which, when fully applied unexpectedly, may damage the tooth structure. However, in most cases, a tooth crack can be attributed to no specific cause other than normal or excessive masticatory forces.[22,34,45,47,70,71,90]

Treatment Planning

Cracked Tooth

When a cracked tooth is either suspected or determined, the patient should be informed that the prognosis is reduced and sometimes questionable.[5,9,12] Protecting a tooth from the propagation of a crack and improving comfort while chewing are the principal goals in the treatment of cracked teeth. Both goals can often be immediately achieved by placing an orthodontic band around the tooth[3,9,16] or by placing a provisional crown. These procedures allow the clinician to evaluate the extent of pulp involvement by checking whether the pulpal symptoms subside in response to the intervention.[3,9,16]

Protecting the tooth from further splitting forces by the placement of a permanent crown is essential in these cases.[3,5,9,16,39] Unfortunately, a crown alone is often not sufficient to resolve symptoms, and endodontic treatment may be considered prior to the placement of the permanent crown, depending on the pulpal symptoms.[9]

A root canal treatment followed by a permanent crown has the benefit of immediately eliminating the long-lasting, painful symptoms as well as early protection from occlusal forces that may cause propagation of a cracked tooth to become a split tooth. Nevertheless, when 127 cracked teeth with reversible pulpitis were treated with a crown alone, 20% of these teeth converted to irreversible pulpitis within 6 months and required root canal treatment.[51] In contrast, none of the other teeth needed a root canal over a 6-year evaluation period.[51] However, it should also be understood that varying percentages of crowned teeth, cracked or noncracked, may also require endodontic treatment, merely from the trauma of the crown preparation. By comparison, it has been shown that when suspected cracked teeth were restored with resin bonded restorations, only 7% required subsequent endodontic treatment or extraction.[64]

After removal of an intracoronal restoration or when penetrating the dentin to prepare for endodontic access, one may observe discoloration along the crack in the dentin. Once the access cavity has been completed, the floor and the distal and mesial walls of the pulp chamber should be carefully inspected to check for the presence and extent of any cracks. Upon evaluating 245 restored teeth, cracks were observed preoperatively in 23.3% of the teeth; however, when the restorations were removed, 60% of these teeth were found to have cracks.[1] Methylene blue dye may be helpful in this type of examination. If a crack is found that reaches from the mesial wall, through the floor of the pulp chamber and into the distal wall, then the prognosis for the tooth is poor, and extraction should be considered (see Fig. 21-6).[5,9,12] If the crack does not reach the pulp chamber or is limited to the coronal parts of the mesial or distal wall, the subsequent protection of the tooth with a crown may save the tooth. Nevertheless, as mentioned previously, the patient should be advised that the treatment success may be compromised and that long-term follow-up will be required.[5,9,12]

Given that such cracks occasionally occur in teeth with minimal or no restorations and that all of the pain may cease once the pulp is removed, it may be tempting to limit the final restoration to an intracoronal amalgam or composite restoration. This temptation should be resisted by all means, as the forces that caused the crack are still present, and the apical propagation of the crack and loss of the tooth is still likely.

Split Tooth

When the tooth is split either through its whole length or diagonally (Fig. 21-7), extraction is typically the only treatment option.[5,9] However, if the fracture line is such that the split results in large and small segments, and if the removal of the small fragment preserves enough tooth structure that is restorable, then retention and restoration of the tooth may be considered.[5]

VERTICAL ROOT FRACTURE (VRF)

Definition

A *vertical root fracture* (VRF) is a longitudinally oriented complete or incomplete fracture initiated in the root at any level and is usually directed buccolingually[5] (Figs. 21-1 and 21-8 through 21-11). By definition, these types of fractures do not arise from the propagation of a fracture that originated in the crown. This definition separates a VRF from a split tooth,

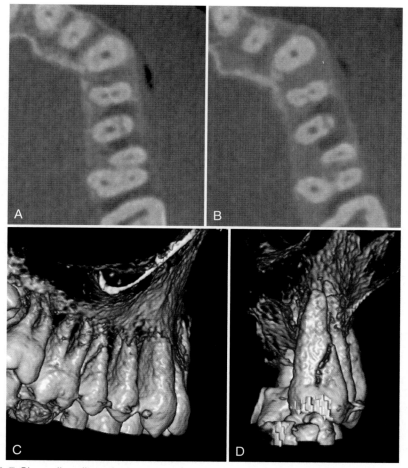

FIG. 21-7 Diagonally split tooth. A maxillary right second premolar presented with a mesiodistal coronal fracture. **A, B,** CBCT axial views revealing a mesiodistal fracture at two different levels, with associated mesial and distal bone loss. The more coronal view has mesial and buccal bone loss **(A)**. A more apical view reveals mesial, distal, and buccal bone loss **(B)**. **C, D,** the three-dimensional reconstruction clearly reveals the nature and direction of the fracture and defined the tooth as unrestorable. Both bone loss and the thick dimensions of the fracture line indicate a longstanding case in which bone resorption allowed opening of the fracture to dimensions that could be detected by CBCT. It is unlikely that such clear demonstration of the fracture line could appear at earlier stages of its formation. (Courtesy Dr. Anda Kfir, Tel Aviv, Israel.)

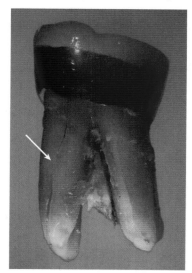

FIG. 21-8 Diagonal VRF in a molar. A lingual view of a right first mandibular molar revealing a diagonal VRF in the mesial root.

which begins with a crack of the crown that propagates apically into the root as a longitudinal fracture. Although both are catastrophic longitudinal factures, a vertical root fracture should be clearly differentiated from a split tooth in that the causes, origins, and typical planes of fracture are substantially different.

Diagnosis

Patient History

In the case of a VRF, a patient may complain of pain or sensitivity related or adjacent to a given tooth. Sensitivity and discomfort while chewing are also common complaints.[80] Swelling may occasionally occur in the area. There is often a long history of failing to diagnose the cause of the pain and discomfort. A history of repeated clinical and radiographic examinations that revealed no cause for the pain is also common in VRF cases. After recent endodontic retreatment, if the symptoms remain and the dentist is unable to determine the cause of the symptoms, the patient may lose confidence in the dentist. Often retreatment or surgical retreatment may have

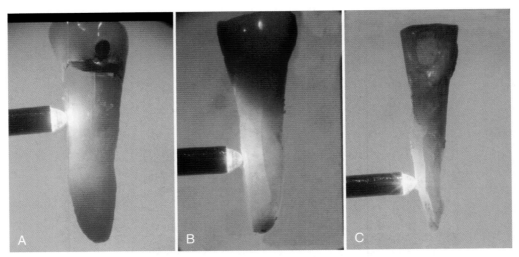

FIG. 21-9 **Three types of VRFs. A,** A coronally located VRF extending apically as far as one third of the root. **B,** A midroot VRF extending along the middle third of the root. **C,** An apically located VRF extending coronally as far as the apical two thirds of the root.

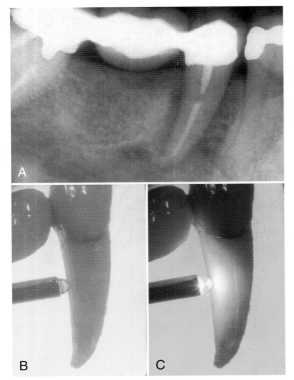

FIG. 21-10 **Radiographic presentation of VRF-associated bone loss.** A second right mandibular bicuspid was endodontically treated and restored using a short post. Two years later the patient started experiencing discomfort and sensitivity upon chewing. Initially no radiographic signs were present. This lasted for 9 months until a radiograph **(A)** revealed an extensive bone resorption and the tooth extracted. **A,** A large radiolucent lesion was present along the root on the distal side. **B,** The tooth was extracted, but the buccal VRF was not readily evident. **C,** Transillumination with an intense but small light source was used after extraction to clearly demonstrate the VRF. (Courtesy Dr. Ramy Levi, Israel.)

been attempted to reveal the accurate diagnosis.[1] Unfortunately, such ineffective treatment attempts may only worsen the dentist-patient relationship.

Clinical Manifestations
Susceptible Teeth and VRF Location
Vertical root fractures are commonly associated with endodontically treated teeth with or without a post.[5] Nevertheless, VRFs can also occur in teeth with no previous root canal treatment.[22] The most susceptible sites and tooth groups are the maxillary and mandibular premolars, the mesial roots of the mandibular molars, the mesiobuccal roots of the maxillary molars, and the mandibular incisors.[81] However, VRFs may occasionally occur in other teeth and roots as well.

Vertical root fractures may progress in the buccolingual direction in these teeth and roots, which are typically narrow mesiodistally and wide buccolingually.[40] However, VRFs may also propagate diagonally, thus affecting the mesial or distal aspect of the root (see Fig. 21-8). VRFs may be initiated at any root level.[5] They may be initiated at the apical part of the root and propagate coronally (see Fig. 21-9, C). Nevertheless, certain VRFs originate at the coronal, cervical part of the root and extend apically (see Fig. 21-9, A), and in other cases, a VRF may be initiated as a midroot fracture (see Figs. 21-9, B; 21-10, C; and 21-11, D).

It is commonly believed that VRFs begin as microcracks at the root canal surface of the radicular dentin and gradually propagate outward until the full thickness of the radicular dentin is fractured.[5,10,21,56,87] Studies[14,17,50,76,91] indicate that microcracks can also be initiated at the outer surface of the root and propagate inward. Therefore, the correlation between microcracks in the radicular dentin and the formation of VRFs should be further investigated.

Early Manifestation
In the early stages of a VRF, there may be pain or discomfort on the affected side of the tooth. In particular, the tooth may feel uncomfortable and sensitive upon chewing, although this pain is often of a dull nature, as opposed to the sharp pain typical of

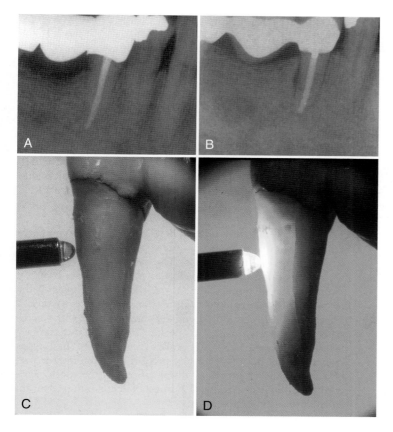

FIG. 21-11 Small isolated radiographic presentation of VRF-associated bone loss. A second right mandibular bicuspid was endodontically treated and restored with no dowel. A year later the patient started complaining about sensitivity on the lingual side. Three months later the radiograph (**A**) was taken and the tooth extracted. A small radiolucent lesion was present along the root on the distal side. The tooth was extracted, but the lingual VRF was not readily evident (**B**). Transillumination with an intense but small light source was used after extraction to clearly demonstrate the VRF (**C, D**). (Courtesy Dr. Ramy Levi, Israel.)

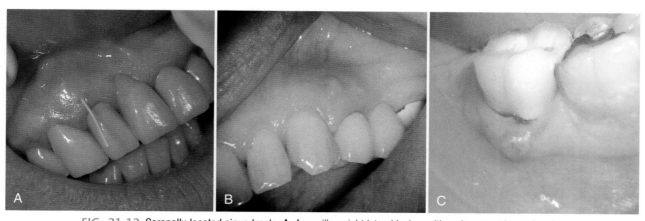

FIG. 21-12 Coronally located sinus tracts. A, A maxillary right lateral incisor with a sinus tract located at the attached gingiva, an uncommon location for sinus tract drainage from a chronic periapical abscess. Maxillary lateral incisors are *not* among the teeth with high prevalence of VRFs. **B,** A draining sinus tract at a coronal location originating from a buccal VRF in the first left maxillary premolar. **C,** A draining sinus tract at the gingival margin of a right first mandibular molar with a buccal VRF in the mesial root. (*A and B,* Courtesy Dr. Russ Paul, Zichron Yaakov, Israel.)

a cracked cusp or tooth with a vital pulp. As the fracture and subsequent infection progresses, swelling often occurs, and a sinus tract may be present at a location more coronal than a sinus tract associated with a case of chronic apical abscess[79,81] (Fig. 21-12). These signs and symptoms are frequently similar to those encountered from nonhealing root canal treatment.[57,86] In the early stages, radiographic findings are unlikely because (1) the root canal filling may obstruct the detection of the fracture (Fig. 21-13, *A*), and (2) the bone destruction (which still

has limited mesiodistal dimensions) may be obstructed by the superimposed root structure (Fig. 21-14).

A deep, narrow, and isolated periodontal pocket may be associated with the root, which often cannot be explained by, as it is inconsistent with, the surrounding periodontal examination.[79,81,85] This specific type of periodontal defect occurs secondary to the bony dehiscence caused by the vertical root fracture. It is substantially different from the pockets caused by advanced periodontitis (discussed later).

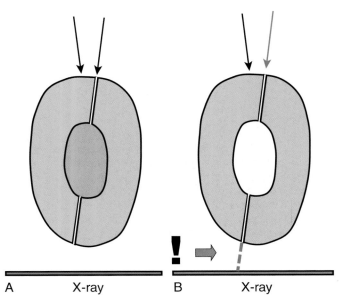

FIG. 21-13 Radiographic examination of filled versus empty canals. **A,** The buccolingual projection of a filled root will fail to detect a VRF at an early stage. **B,** The removal of the root filling and use of radiography at different mesiodistal angulations may reveal the VRF.

Late Manifestation

A longstanding vertical root fracture is easier to detect. The major destruction of the alveolar bone adjacent to the root has already occurred, allowing the VRF to be more likely revealed in a periapical radiograph (see Fig. 21-7). One of the most typical signs is the *J-shaped* or *halo radiolucency*, which is a combination of periapical and periradicular radiolucency (i.e., bone loss apically and along the side of the root, extending coronally)[82,83] (Fig. 21-15). In addition, the pocket along the fracture, which was initially tight and narrow, may become wider and easier to detect. In longstanding cases in which the bone destruction is extensive, the segments of the root may also separate, resulting in a radiograph that clearly reveals an objective root fracture (Fig. 21-16).

Diagnosis
Importance of Early Diagnosis

Accurate and timely diagnosis is crucial in VRF cases, allowing the extraction of the tooth or root before extensive damage to the alveolar bone can occur. Early diagnosis is particularly important when implants are a potential part of the future restorative procedure; when an extraction is performed at an early stage, the uncomplicated placement of an implant is likely. When the tooth is extracted after extensive damage has already occurred (see Fig. 21-14), bone regeneration procedures may be required,[42] adding cost and time to the restoration procedure.

The American Association of Endodontists stated in 2008[5] that a sinus tract and a narrow, isolated periodontal probing defect associated with a tooth that has undergone a root canal treatment, with or without post placement, can be considered pathognomonic for the presence of a VRF.

However, the combination of the following two factors makes the early diagnosis difficult: (1) many of the clinical symptoms associated with VRFs mimic apical periodontitis or periodontal disease, and (2) the narrow and tight pocket associated with

early stages of VRF is difficult to detect using rigid probes (see the VRF Pocket section). Consequently, a delay in the accurate diagnosis or a misdiagnosis of a VRF may often occur.

Misdiagnosis of VRFs

Certain cases of longstanding VRFs are so discernible that no dentist can miss the diagnosis (see Fig. 21-16). Nevertheless, two retrospective case series, one by Fuss and colleagues[32] and the other by Chan and associates,[22] reported that general practitioners often misdiagnose VRFs. The teeth that were extracted in these studies had often been diagnosed as endodontic failures or refractive periodontal pockets, only to realize after extraction that in some of them the actual cause was a VRF.

VRF Pockets

The pockets that are typical of the early stages of VRFs differ substantially from the deep pockets associated with advanced periodontal disease. The deep pockets associated with periodontal disease develop as a result of the bacterial biofilm that initially accumulates at the cervical areas of the tooth and the destructive host response to these bacteria.[38] Therefore, deep periodontal pockets are typically wider coronally and relatively loose. This pocket structure allows the easy insertion of rigid periodontal probes (Fig. 21-17). These types of periodontal pockets typically present with the deeper part of a pocket at the mesial or distal aspects of the tooth. Periodontal disease often affects groups of teeth rather than an isolated location of a single tooth.

The pockets associated with VRFs develop due to bacterial penetration into the fracture, triggering a destructive host response that occurs in the periodontal ligament along the entire length of the fracture. These bacteria may leak from an infected root canal[87]; however, when the VRF extends to the cervically exposed root, the microbes in the fracture may also originate from the oral cavity. In the early stages, the periodontal ligament is affected and destroyed along the longitudinal opening of the fracture, initially with a limited resorption to the adjacent bone. This permits the penetration of a periodontal probe. The pocket associated with a VRF is typically isolated and present only in a limited area adjacent to the affected tooth. This pocket is often located at the buccal or lingual convexity of the tooth. In the early stages, the pocket is deep but has a narrow coronal opening (see Fig. 21-17). The insertion of a probe first requires the detection of the coronal opening; often, light pressure is necessary for the insertion of the probe. Because the pocket is narrow, probe insertion may result in the blanching of the surrounding tissue (Fig. 21-18). This is specially the case when a plastic probe is used, as its coronal part is thicker than an equivalent metal probe (Figs. 21-18 and 21-19).

The pocket associated with the early stages of a VRF is quite different from a common periodontal pocket. This difference has been widely recognized, and terms such as *osseous defect*[28] and *probing defect*[5] have been used to emphasize the point. Nevertheless, these pockets do possess enough unique features to justify them being specifically termed a *VRF pocket*.

Rigid metal periodontal probes may be ineffective in probing VRF pockets in the early stages of a VRF. Given that the pocket is deep, narrow, and tight, the bulge of the tooth's crown may prevent the insertion of a metal probe into the pocket (see Fig. 21-19). A flexible probe should be used instead, such as a probe available from Premier Dental Products (Plymouth

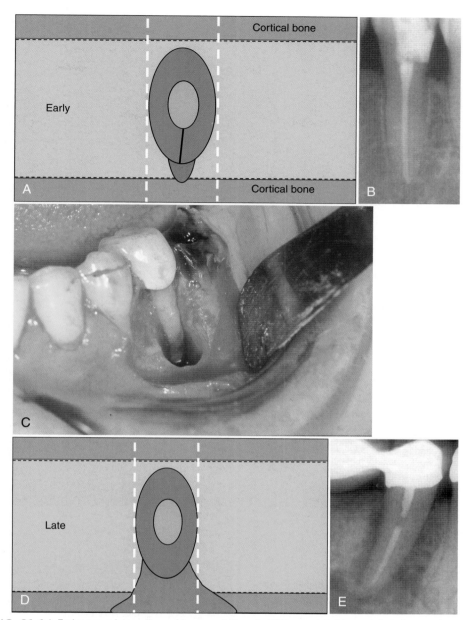

FIG. 21-14 Early versus late radiographic presentation of a VRF-associated bone defect. At an early stage, a bone defect *(red)* is not likely to be detected in a periapical radiograph, as the root will overlap with the defect **(A, B)**. At later stages, when major damage has occurred to the cortical plate **(C)**, the bone defect may be large enough to extend beyond the silhouette of the root **(C, D)** and appear as a radiolucent defect along the root **(E)**. (Surgical image courtesy Dr. Devora Schwartz-Arad, Ramat-Hasharon, Israel.)

Meeting, Pennsylvania) (see Fig. 21-19) or a similar device. This type of flexible probe should be included on every endodontic examination tray and is an essential tool when checking for potential VRF pockets.

A typical VRF pocket was observed in 67% of the VRF cases reported by Tamse and colleagues.[81] However, because the early detection of such pockets is technique sensitive and because traditional metal probes were used in the aforementioned study, the incidence of these pockets may in fact be higher than reported. When a typical VRF pocket is located on the convex flank of the root on the buccal or lingual side, it is likely that the root has a VRF. In contrast, when such a pocket

is located at the furcation of a molar, the pocket may indicate either a VRF or a sinus tract from an apical abscess that found a point of least resistance at the furcation area. In cases with a furcation pocket, when a VRF diagnosis cannot be conclusively determined, a positive healing response to the elimination of infection by initiating root canal retreatment may differentiate between these two types of pathoses.

Coronally Located Sinus Tract

Sinus tracts that originate from a chronic apical abscess are typically detected at the site of least bone resistance, against the apical part of the root or in the area of the junction of the

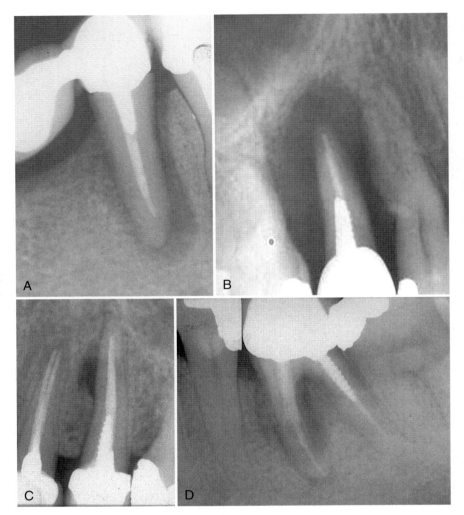

FIG. 21-15 Radiographic presentations of long-standing VRFs. **A,** J-shaped "halo" associated with a VRF in a second right mandibular premolar. **B,** Extensive bone damage associated with a complete VRF in a second right maxillary premolar. **C,** Limited bone damage associated with a midroot VRF in a second left maxillary premolar. **D,** Bone damage associated with a VRF in the mesial root of a first left mandibular molar. All such presentations are typical of longstanding VRFs.

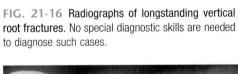

FIG. 21-16 Radiographs of longstanding vertical root fractures. No special diagnostic skills are needed to diagnose such cases.

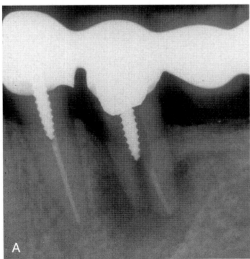

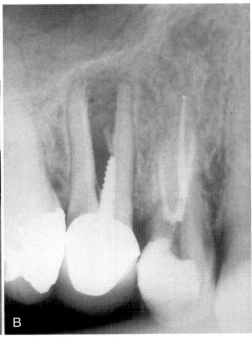

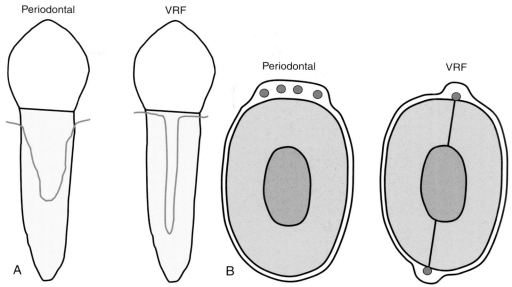

FIG. 21-17 **VRF pocket. A,** Periodontal pockets *(left)* are wide coronally, whereas VRF pockets *(right)* are narrow and deep. **B,** Periodontal pockets *(left)* are loose and allow probing at various sites, whereas VRF pockets *(right)* are narrow and tight. If not checked carefully at every millimeter of the sulcus, an early VRF pocket can easily be missed. Please note that periodontal pockets appear more commonly in the proximal sides of the root, whereas VRF pockets are more common on the buccal or lingual sides.

attached gingiva and the oral mucosa. Sinus tracts that are associated with a VRF pocket are often found in a more coronal position, as the source is not from a periapical lesion[80] (see Fig. 21-12).

In four clinical retrospective case series, coronally located sinus tracts were found in 13% to 35% of these cases.[58,79,81,85] As in the case of a VRF pocket, if the sinus tract is located at the furcation of a molar, this observation does not necessarily indicate a VRF, as periapical abscesses from a failing root canal treatment can also drain in this coronal location.

Radiographic Features

A definitive VRF diagnosis can sometimes be made based on the radiographic appearance of a thin radiolucent line extending longitudinally down the root.[72] Such lines, however, are difficult to detect and are commonly not seen in routine orthoradial, periapical radiographs because either the root canal filling has "masked" the fracture line or the angulation of the radiograph is not optimal for discerning the fracture (see Fig. 21-13) (Figs. 21-20 and 21-21). Rud and Omnell[72] claimed that it was possible to observe fracture lines in 35.7% of cases, but many of these cases were not true VRF instances. In clinical practice, it is still rare to observe a VRF on a radiograph, especially when only a single periapical radiograph is taken. Such an observation requires the x-ray beam to align with the plane of the fracture as well as the fracture line not being superimposed over the radiopaque root filling (Fig. 21-20, *A*). Therefore, two or three periapical radiographs should be exposed from different horizontal angulations when a fracture is suspected[80] (see Figs. 21-21 and 21-22).

In most VRF cases, the clinician must make *interpretations* or *predictions* based on the various patterns of periradicular bone destruction, which, unfortunately, are also shared by other periodontal and endodontic-like lesions.[58,75,88]

In the early stages of a VRF, no radiolucent bone lesions may be observed[20] (see Fig. 21-14), which may be the reason why VRFs often remain undetected, delaying diagnosis and treatment. Rud and Omnell[72] correlated the direction of the fracture, the degree of bone destruction, and the radiographic appearance, and emphasized that the extent of bone destruction around a fractured root depends on the location of the root fracture and the time elapsed since the inception of the fracture. The significance of time was confirmed by Meister and colleagues,[58] who demonstrated that immediate radiographic detection is difficult due to the time required for bone resorption to occur or for the fractured segments to separate and be radiographically visible. In a study of the patterns of bone resorption in 110 VRF cases, Lustig and associates[57] found that in 72% of patients with either chronic signs and symptoms (i.e., pertaining to a sinus tract, osseous defect, or mobility) or acute exacerbations, there was greater bone loss recorded compared to patients for whom a VRF diagnosis was made at an early stage.[57]

Despite the difficulty of diagnosing *early stage* VRFs in endodontically treated teeth, there are often several radiographic signs associated with *later stages* that are strong indicators of VRF.

The J-shaped or halo appearance, a combination of periapical and periradicular radiolucencies, was associated with a high probability of a VRF in a double-blind radiographic study involving 102 endodontically treated maxillary premolars[82] (see Fig. 21-15). An angular resorption of the crestal bone along the root on one or both sides, without the involvement of the periapical area, mimicking a "periodontal radiolucency" (see Fig. 21-15), was found in 14% of the cases. Tamse and coworkers[83] also reported the radiographic appearance of "halo" (see Fig. 21-10) and "periodontal" radiolucencies (see Fig. 21-10) in vertically fractured mesial roots of

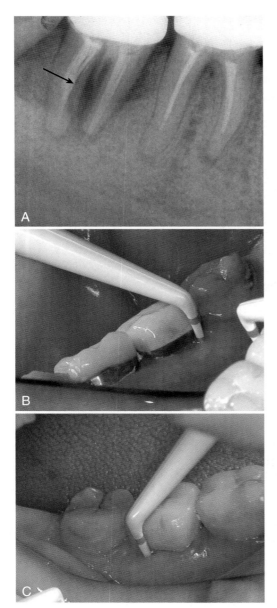

FIG. 21-18 Tight VRF pockets. A, The distal root of a second right mandibular molar with a VRF. VRF pockets were found on both the lingual (**B**) and the buccal (**C**) sides. VRF pockets are tight, so inserting a probe into these pockets causes pressure blanching of the surrounding tissues.

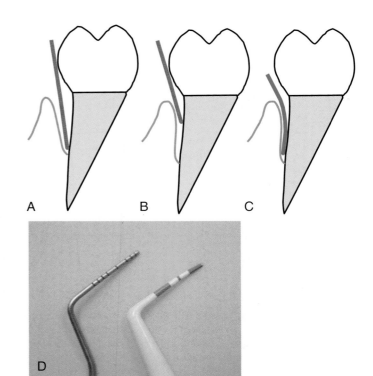

FIG. 21-19 Rigid versus flexible probes. A, In a loose periodontal pocket, a rigid metal probe can easily reach the depth of the pocket. **B,** In a tight, early-stage VRF pocket, a rigid probe may be of limited value, as the bulge of the crown often prevents the insertion of the probe into the tight, deep pocket. **C,** A flexible probe (**D**) is more likely to detect VRF pockets at an early stage.

mandibular molars (37% and 29%, respectively). In that study, the use of these two variables, combined with bifurcation involvement (63%) and the presence of an amalgam dowel (67%), predicted fracture in 78% of the cases. Others have reported similar findings.[24,62] Despite the different sample sizes, study designs, and objectives, the most common radiographic feature in these studies was a lateral radiolucency appearing longitudinally along the root and a halo appearance.

Radiolucency in the Bone Along Root

The type of periradicular radiolucency associated with a vertical root fracture is not and should not be interpreted as a thickening of the PDL. Instead, it represents a substantial destruction of the cortical plate of the alveolar bone[57] (see Fig. 21-14). In the case of a VRF in the buccolingual plane, often the bone resorption is limited at early stages, and any associated radiolucency may be obscured by the superimposition of the root (see Fig. 21-14). As the bone loss increases, the radiolucency becomes greater than the dimensions of the root, allowing it to be detected more clearly in the above-mentioned manner (see Fig. 21-14). As the VRF progresses to an intermediate stage, radiographs taken at different horizontal angulations may detect bone resorption (see Fig. 21-22), whereas a conventional orthoradial radiograph may not (see Figs. 21-14 and 21-22). This radiographic feature should be differentiated from a split tooth, in which the fracture plane is typically mesiodistal, with the bone resorption occurring in the earlier stages on the mesial or distal aspects of the root.

Radiograph of Empty Canal

As mentioned previously, the direct clinical detection of an early stage VRF from a periapical radiograph is unlikely, especially when there has been endodontic treatment. Because most VRFs are in the buccolingual plane, the radiopaque obturation often obstructs the view of the hairline radiolucency of the fracture (see Figs. 21-13 and 21-20). When a VRF is suspected, one may initiate root canal retreatment, removing the root obturation, and taking radiographs at two or three different horizontal angulations. The detection of a hairline radiolucency may provide a more definitive diagnosis of a VRF[80] (see Figs. 21-20 and 21-21).

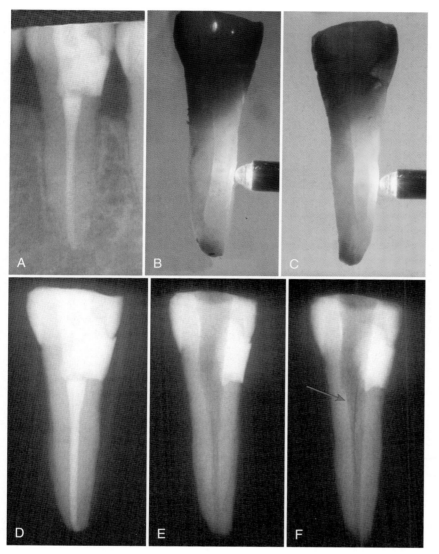

FIG. 21-20 **Radiography of an ex vivo empty canal.** The second left mandibular bicuspid underwent a root canal treatment, with no post required. Thirteen months later, the patient complained about pain and sensitivity to palpation on the lingual side. A radiograph provided no further information (**A**). An isolated, 7-mm pocket was detected on the lingual side, and the tooth was extracted. Midroot VRFs were visible on the buccal (**B**) and lingual sides (**C**). An ex vivo radiograph of the same tooth with no findings (**D**). The root filling was removed, and radiographs were taken from different mesiodistal angulations (**E, F**). One of the radiographs clearly revealed the VRF (**F**).

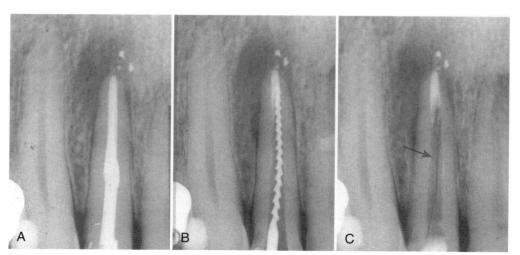

FIG. 21-21 **Radiography of an empty canal: a clinical case.** The right maxillary lateral incisor underwent a root canal treatment a few years ago. The patient complained about occasional pain on the palatal side. The tooth was sensitive to percussion and palpation on the palatal side. Radiography revealed a periapical radiolucency (**A**). An isolated, deep, and narrow pocket was found on the palatal side of the root. Both the patient and the referring dentist were reluctant to extract the tooth, assuming that the pocket could potentially be a sinus tract, and decided on retreatment. A radiograph taken with a file during the process (**B**) could have missed essential information that was obscured by the file, which was an evident VRF (**C**).

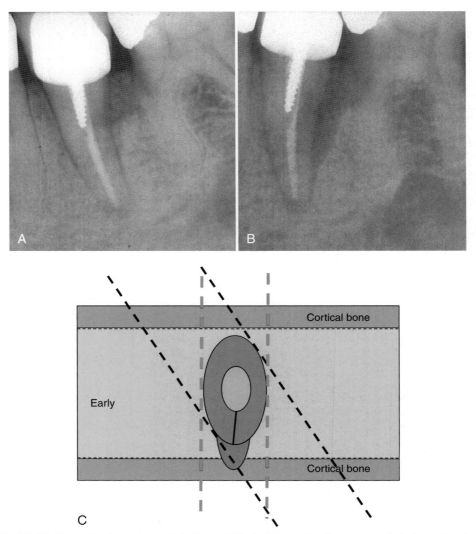

FIG. 21-22 Diagonal radiographs for detection of VRF. **A,** Orthoradial radiograph: very limited bone loss is seen. **B,** A different horizontal angulation reveals a radiolucent lesion along the root. **C,** Schematic presentation. Although a radiograph in an orthoradial direction *(blue lines)* cannot pick up the radiolucency along the root, diagonal angulation *(black lines)* may do so, as in **B.**

Cone-Beam Computed Tomography in VRF Diagnosis

Modern cone-beam computed tomography (CBCT) has a much smaller radiation dose compared to traditional medical spiral CT imaging, thus rendering CBCT a reasonable diagnostic tool for the use in selected endodontic cases.[6,31,31a,65]

One of the unique features of CBCT is its ability to study the suspected tooth and associated bone in an axial plane. Axial views may provide detailed information regarding the cross-sectional appearance of the tooth and its surrounding bone (Fig. 21-23). With the CBCT devices currently available, the width of an unseparated fracture may be too small and undetectable (see Fig. 21-23) (SEDENTEXCT guidelines[31]). Traditional planar, periapical radiographs are also of limited value for the *early* detection of VRFs. More specifically, bone damage or separation of the fragments is only radiographically evident at a relatively late stage. Several studies suggested that the detection of early-stage VRFs by a CBCT scan set to an axial view may be possible.[41,42,59] Yet such detection may greatly depend on the resolution of the machine (i.e., the voxel size). At a voxel size of 0.3 mm, the detection of early, unseparated VRFs is not reliable; however, when smaller voxel sizes were used in these in vitro studies, the reliability greatly increased.[41,42,59] Although the detection level of a fracture is thought to be twice the voxel size of CBCT imaging, there is presently no literature available to support this theory. Therefore, given that the smallest voxel size currently available for a CBCT device is about 0.075 mm, CBCT imaging would not be able to visualize a root fracture unless the fracture width was greater than 0.15 mm. It should also be noted that the intracanal presence of gutta-percha or a metal post often causes artifacts that make it extremely difficult to differentiate a VRF from such artificial lines.[59]

Although early VRFs may still be below the detection level of many CBCT machines, the *early destruction of the bone* along the suspected fracture may be visible in the cancellous bone (i.e., with an axial view) at relatively early stages, whereas this early bone destruction would not be detectable in traditional planar, periapical radiographs; such bone resorption may help to establish a VRF diagnosis (see Fig. 21-23).

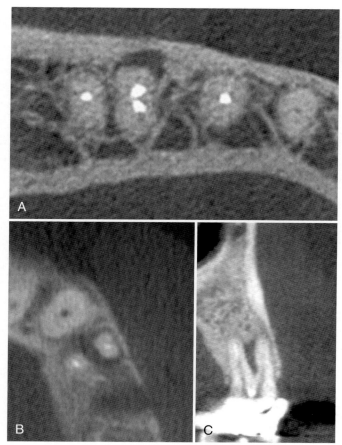

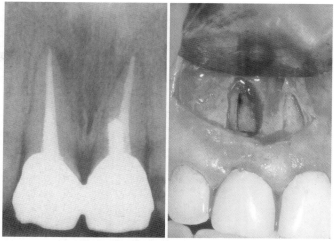

FIG. 21-24 **An apical VRF with no pockets.** The right maxillary central incisor was symptomatic despite an apparently adequate obturation. A radiolucent area was present around the apex, but no pockets were detected. Apical surgery was attempted, only to reveal a VRF at the apical part of the root that did not (yet) extend into the gingival margin and thus did not present with a typical VRF pocket. A semilunar flap design was used in this case, which was intended for apicoectomy. If surgical exploration for suspected VRF was initially intended, a conventional full flap would have been used. (Courtesy Dr. Ram Zeev, Rehovot, Israel.)

FIG. 21-23 **"Invisible" bone destruction associated with early VRFs.** **A,** Buccal VRF was present in the mesial root of a first left mandibular molar. At this early stage a typical VRF pocket was evident, yet no associated bone destruction was observed in a periapical radiograph. The VRF-associated bone destruction was evident in an axial plane of a CBCT. **B,** A VRF was present in the palatal side of the buccal root of the first maxillary premolar. A draining sinus tract was present with no radiographic signs to explain it. **C,** CBCT revealed a radiolucent lesion on the palatal side of the buccal root, which was verified, after extraction, as caused by VRF. Please note that in neither of these cases could the actual VRF fracture line be seen in the CBCT scan. (*B,* Courtesy Dr. Anda Kfir, Tel Aviv.)

With likely increased resolution in the near future, CBCT may become an important diagnostic tool for the detection of VRFs. For the present, neither the most updated Joint Position Statement of the American Association of Endodontists and American Academy of Oral and Maxillofacial Radiology (2010), nor the European Society of Endodontology position statement on the use of CBCT in endodontics (2014) recommend the use of CBCT for diagnosis of VRF.[6,31a]

Improvements of CBCT imaging—such as achieving a better signal-to-noise ratio, obtaining a smaller voxel size, and by applying advanced algorithms to segment fracture lines—may promise the potential to enhance the ability to detect early-stage VRFs in the future.

Exploratory Surgery

When clinical and radiographic evaluations are equivocal in detecting a suspected vertical root fracture, exploratory surgery may be indicated. When a full-thickness flap is raised and the

granulation tissue is removed, a VRF may often be directly visualized[80] (see Figs. 21-14 and 21-24). The bone resorption pattern associated with a VRF is mostly seen as a bony dehiscence, with the greater bone destruction being present on the buccal cortical plate located over the offending root. In a small percentage of the cases, fenestration can also be seen.[57] Furthermore, it has been shown that the longer a VRF-related infection persists, the greater the resulting periradicular bone destruction.[57]

Etiology

Vertical root fractures may arise from a series of factors, some of which are natural whereas others are iatrogenic, arising from dental procedures such as endodontic treatment and the restorative procedures that follow it. The most common dental procedure contributing to vertical root fractures is endodontic treatment.[11]

Most vertical root fractures occur in endodontically treated teeth.[11,24] VRFs usually do not occur during the actual obturation of the root canal, but rather they occur long after the procedure has been completed.[81]

The etiology of VRFs is multifactorial.[33,79] It is likely that in the presence of one or an accumulation of more predisposing factors, the repeated functional or parafunctional occlusal loads may eventually lead, over months or even years, to the development of a VRF. Predisposing factors may include natural ones, such as the anatomy of the root, or iatrogenic ones, such as the excessive forces during root canal instrumentation, excessive tooth structure removal, or excessive obturation pressure.

Natural Predisposing Factors
Shape of Root Cross Section

One of the common anatomic features shared by teeth that typically develop VRFs is an oval cross section of the root, with

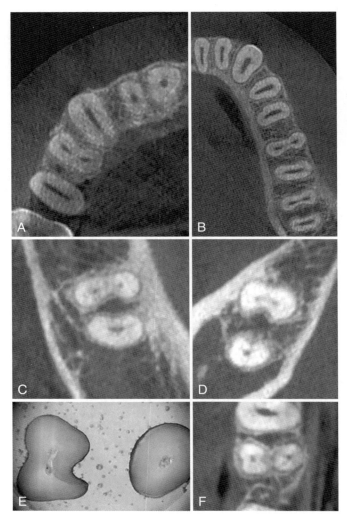

FIG. 21-25 Anatomic predisposing factors. A, An axial view of CBCT scan of a maxilla, revealing oval canals in the maxillary canine and second premolar. B, An axial view of a mandible, revealing oval canals in incisors, canine, premolars, and distal roots of the mandibular molars. Oval anatomy combined with endodontic treatment has been associated with a higher incidence of VRFs. C, D, Concavities on the distal aspect of the mesial roots of mandibular molar may establish a "danger zone" in which excessive instrumentation, combined with straightening of the canal, may result in a thinner dentin wall that may allow strain concentration. E, F, Concavities in the palatal side of the buccal root of maxillary first premolar (E, sections; F, axial view from a CBCT). These depressions may also represent a potential danger zone. Neither the concavity in C and D nor the concavity in E and F would be evident in a planar periapical radiograph. It should be noted that CBCT scans should not be used for routine screening but should be limited to the indications delineated in the joint statement of the American Association of Endodontists (AAE) and the American Academy of Oral and Maxillofacial Radiology (AAOMR).[5,6]

a buccolingual diameter being larger than the mesiodistal diameter.[36,40] These teeth include the maxillary and mandibular premolars, the mesial roots of the mandibular molars, and the mandibular incisors (Fig. 21-25, A and B). Such anatomy is easily observed in the axial plane of a CBCT scan (see Fig. 21-25, A and B). The fracture in these teeth typically starts in the buccolingual plane, specifically at the highest convexity of the oval root[21,80] (see Fig 21-25, A and B). This conclusion,

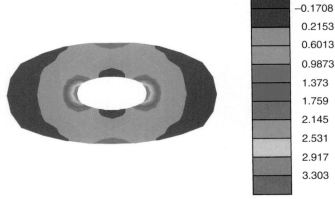

	−0.1708
	0.2153
	0.6013
	0.9873
	1.373
	1.759
	2.145
	2.531
	2.917
	3.303

FIG. 21-26 Finite element analysis of the strain distribution in an oval root. Note the strain concentration on the inner side of the highest convexity of the remaining dentin wall. Red and orange represent areas of higher strains than blue areas. (From Lertchirakarn V, Palamara J, Messer HH: Patterns of vertical fractures: factors affecting stress distribution in the root canal, *J Endod* 29:523, 2003.)

derived from large case series, is also supported by finite element analysis.[64] Such analysis clearly demonstrated strain concentration on the inner side of the remaining dentin wall at the highest convexity point (i.e., the buccal and lingual sides of the oval roots)[54,55] (Fig. 21-26).

Occlusal Factors

Excessive occlusal loads or concentration of such loads may be another natural predisposing factor. Load concentrations, such as those caused by occlusal prematurities in maxillary premolars, and excessive occlusal forces, specifically in the case of mandibular second molars, are examples.[18] In combination with other natural and iatrogenic predisposing factors, excessive occlusal loads may, over time, lead to VRFs.

Preexisting Microcracks

Preexisting microcracks may be present in the radicular dentin, likely resulting from repeated forces of mastication or occlusal parafunction.[15,63] Such fractures were also recently reported by Barreto and colleagues,[10] who have found these microcracks in 40% of intact maxillary incisors and canines.

Iatrogenic Predisposing Factors

Root Canal Treatment

VRFs mostly appear in endodontically treated teeth[5,80]; therefore, endodontic treatment per se may be considered an iatrogenic predisposing factor. Teeth were once thought to be more susceptible to fracturing after endodontic treatment because of a decrease in hydration.[43] However, later studies found no difference in the properties of dentin, as a material, after endodontic procedures.[46,75]

Although the physical characteristics of the dentin, as a material, may not be compromised by endodontic treatment, the radicular dentin, as a structure, may be compromised by the accumulative or combined effect of several natural or iatrogenic factors associated with the endodontic treatment and the restoration of endodontically treated teeth. This may be the reason for the often-reported association of VRF with endodontically treated teeth.

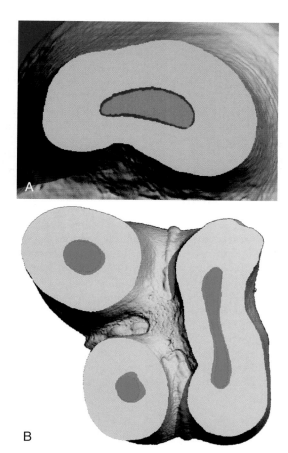

B

FIG. 21-27 Minimally invasive endodontic preparation. In this preparation, a uniform layer of dentin was removed from all around the root canal wall using a self-adjusting file, as opposed to shaping the canal into a circular cross section using rotary endodontic files. (*A,* From Metzger Z, Teperovich E, Zary R, et al: The self-adjusting file (SAF). Part 1: respecting the root canal anatomy—a new concept of endodontic files and its implementation, *J Endod* 36:679, 2010. *B,* From Solomonov M: Eight months of clinical experience with the self-adjusting file system, *J Endod* 37:881, 2011. Image from ongoing study by Solomonov and Paque F.)

It is incumbent for the clinician to recognize this effect and take efforts to minimize any steps that may contribute to the development of a root fracture during endodontic treatment.

Excessive Root Canal Preparation

Excessive root canal preparation may be a predisposing factor for VRF development.[89] In one study, cracks detected by transillumination were more frequent when the same teeth were subjected to a gradually increasing endodontic canal preparation.[89] To reduce the risk of VRFs, less invasive methods may be considered, such as minimally invasive endodontic instrumentation[60,66] (Fig. 21-27; see also Chapter 6).

Microcracks Caused by Rotary Instrumentation

Shemesh and colleagues[76] and others[2,10,14,17,44,77,91] observed that root canal preparation using nickel-titanium rotary and reciprocating files often results in microcracks in the remaining radicular dentin (Fig. 21-28). This finding, which was originally noted for single-root teeth, has been further supported by Yoldas and coworkers,[91] who studied microcrack formation from rotary files in the mesial roots of mandibular molars. Each

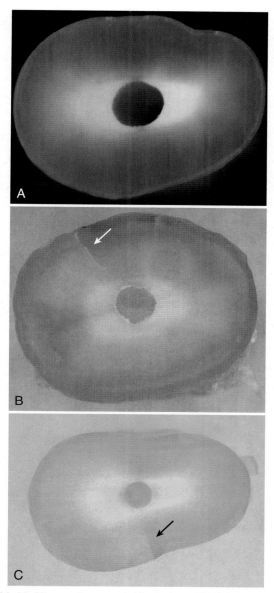

FIG. 21-28 Microcracks generated in single-root teeth by rotary nickel-titanium files. A, Control: hand instrumentation, generating no microcracks. **B, C,** Rotary instrumentation: microcracks generated in the remaining radicular dentin *(arrows).* (Courtesy Dr. H. Shemesh, Amsterdam, Holland.)

of the rotary file systems examined in this study caused frequent microcracks in the dentin, whereas both hand instrumentation with files and the self-adjusting file (see Chapter 6) did not cause such cracks (Fig. 21-29).

A finite element analysis by Kim and colleagues[50] supports and may explain these findings. These researchers reported that rotary files induce strain on the dentin, as measured in the surface layers of the root dentin, which likely exceeds the elasticity of the dentin, causing subsequent microcracks, as also reported by Shemesh, Bier, Adorno, Yoldas, and Bürklein, along with their research associates as well as by others.[2,10,14,17,44,76,77,91] Additional stress, by either root obturation with lateral compaction[10,76] or by retreatment[77] that was applied to roots that were previously instrumented with rotary files, caused some of the microcracks to propagate and become

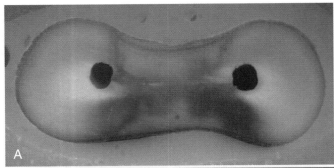

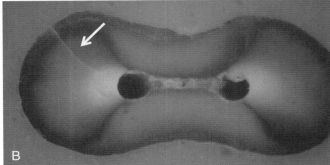

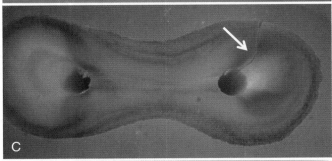

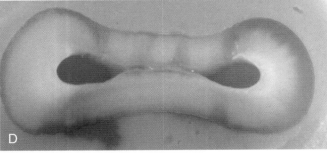

FIG. 21-29 Microcracks generated in mesial roots of mandibular molars by rotary nickel-titanium files. **A,** Control: hand instrumentation, generating no microcracks. Rotary instrumentation: microcracks generated in the remaining radicular dentin *(arrows).* **B,** A partial-thickness crack. **C,** A full-thickness fracture. **D,** Self-adjusting file instrumentation: no microcracks generated. (From Yoldas O, Yilmaz S, Atakan G, et al: Dentinal microcrack formation during root canal preparation by different NiTi rotary instruments and the self-adjusting file, *J Endod* 38:232, 2012.)

through-and-through fractures that were indistinguishable from VRFs.[10,76,77]

The relationship of these various findings to the subsequent clinical creation of a VRF has yet to be confirmed. In any event, considering the basic principles of fracture mechanics, the creation of microcracks should at least be considered as a potential predisposing factor.

Uneven Thickness of Remaining Dentin

The instrumentation of root canals often results in uneven thickness of the remaining dentin, particularly when curved canals are straightened by instrumentation.[67] Uneven dentin thickness can also occur upon excessive instrumentation of the mesial roots of the mandibular molars or first maxillary premolars, which may exhibit a distal or mesial concavity, respectively, that is not detectable in a common planar, periapical radiograph (Fig. 21-25, *C* and *D*). These areas, which have been referred to as "danger zones,"[30] may be characterized by a decrease in the remaining dentin thickness in which the application of internal strain may potentially lead to a fracture. The anatomic groove that is often found on the palatal side of the buccal root of maxillary bifurcated premolars is another example of such a hidden danger zone[48] (Fig. 21-25, *E* and *F*).

Lingual access, which is commonly used in incisors, may also result in a thinner buccal wall in the apical area as compared with the lingual wall. This phenomenon may be especially pronounced when thick, and thus rigid, instruments are used excessively. When lateral compaction was applied ex vivo in a similar case, the strain concentration was recorded on the thinner buccal side of the apical part of the tooth (Figs. 21-30 and 21-31).

The use of flexible nickel-titanium files and minimally invasive instrumentation with instruments such as the self-adjusting file may reduce such risks (see also Fig. 21-27 and Chapter 6).

Methods of Obturation

Certain obturation techniques, such as lateral compaction, involve the application of internal pressure with a spreader, which may cause strains[27,73] and subsequent propagation of microcracks into fractures across the full dentin thickness.[10,76] Other obturation methods may create less pressure, such as thermoplasticized gutta-percha, and may reduce the risk of VRFs (see Chapter 7).

Type of Spreader Used

The use of a more rigid and thick stainless-steel hand spreader may lead to increased strain in the radicular dentin and can result in an increased incidence of root fracture.[27,73] The introduction of more flexible finger spreaders, which have smaller diameter, may greatly reduce such risks.[27] Among the finger spreaders, devices composed of nickel-titanium allow insertion with less force than stainless-steel finger spreaders.[74] The nickel-titanium spreaders also allow a further reduction in the strain induced in the radicular dentin during obturation compared to traditional stainless-steel finger spreaders[68] (Fig. 21-32).

Post Design

Post selection, design, and seating have a significant effect on the strain distribution in the root. Excessively long or thick posts are considered a predisposing factor for VRFs.[23,25,61] The use of posts carries an inherent risk of root fracture, particularly if excessive sound dentin is removed during preparation. Posts should only be used when essential for core retention and should be avoided whenever a sufficient coronal tooth structure is available for the secure retention of the crown.[4,37]

Crown Design

When considering endodontically treated teeth, crowns with a ferrule margin (i.e., supported by a sound tooth structure all

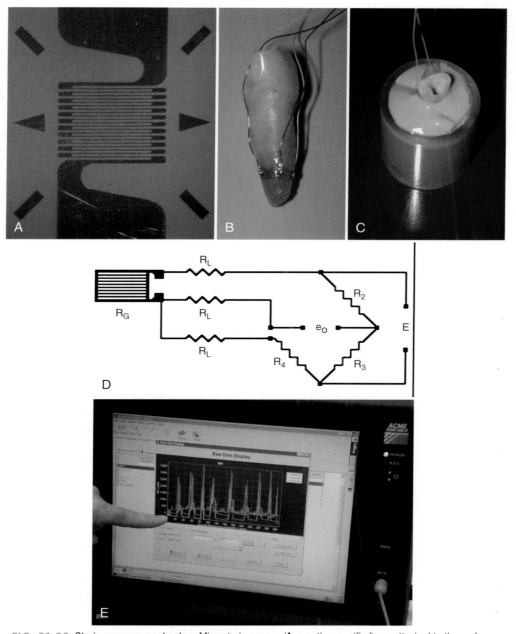

FIG. 21-30 **Strain measurement setup.** Microstrain gauges (**A,** greatly magnified) are attached to the surface of the root in the area(s) of interest (**B**). The tooth is embedded in a cylinder composed of flexible dental-impression material (**C**), and the strain gauge or gauges are wired with a 3/4 Wheatstone bridge circuit (**D**) and connected to a data collection system (**E**). The continuous registration of the force applied to the spreader and the strain that develops in a given area of the root allows for the analysis presented in Figs. 21-31 and 21-32. (From Pilo R: Development of strains and mechanical failure in dental roots undergoing root canal obturation and prosthetic rehabilitation. PhD thesis, Tel Aviv University, 2007, supervised by Zvi Metzger and T. Brosh.)

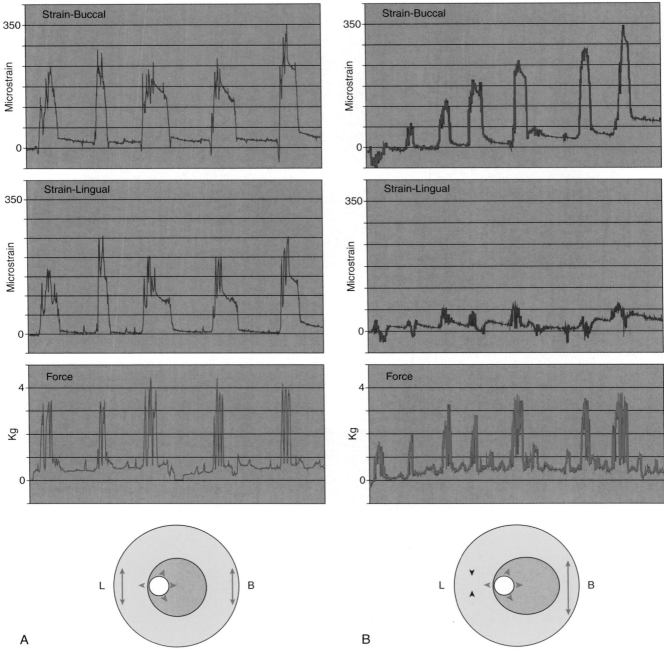

FIG. 21-31 Strain during lateral compaction: even versus uneven wall thickness. A pattern of the strain that develops in the buccal and lingual dentin of the apical area of a maxillary central incisor during lateral compaction. **A,** The thicknesses of the remaining buccal and lingual dentin were similar (even). Each manual insertion of the spreader was registered as a force peak. The tension strain was recorded for each insertion and was *similar* on the buccal and lingual sides. **B,** The thickness of the remaining dentin was lower on the buccal side than on the lingual side (uneven) due to the lingual access and rigidity of the instruments used. Each manual insertion of the spreader was registered as a force peak. The tension strain was recorded for each insertion on the buccal side, whereas compression was recorded on the lingual side. (From Pilo R: Development of strains and mechanical failure in dental roots undergoing root canal obturation and prosthetic rehabilitation. PhD thesis, Tel Aviv University, 2007, supervised by Zvi Metzger and T. Brosh.)

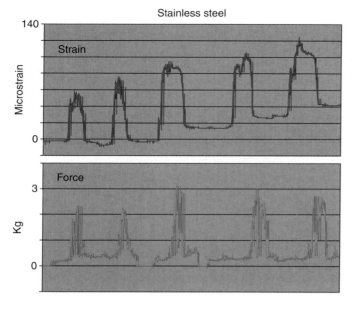

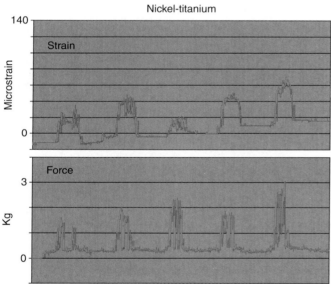

FIG. 21-32 **Strain caused by stainless-steel versus nickel-titanium finger spreaders.** The force applied to the finger spreader during lateral compaction caused strain on the buccal side of the apical part of the maxillary central incisors. Upper panels: the force and strain registered with a stainless-steel finger spreader. Lower panels: the root filling was removed, and another cycle of lateral compaction was completed for the same tooth using a nickel-titanium finger spreader. The spreader dimensions and depth of insertion were similar in both cycles. The nickel-titanium finger spreader required less force and generated lower strains than the stainless-steel finger spreader. (From Pilo R: Development of strains and mechanical failure in dental roots undergoing root canal obturation and prosthetic rehabilitation. PhD thesis, Tel Aviv University, 2007, supervised by Zvi Metzger and T. Brosh.)

around and beyond the gingival margins of the core) provide better strain distribution than similar restorations that are supported by the post and core alone.[4] This design may help to avoid yet another potential predisposing factor for VRFs.[26]

Conclusions

In conclusion, even though endodontic treatment may be necessary in many occasions, the impact of each of the iatrogenic predisposing factors should be minimized as much as possible, as they are likely to have a cumulative deleterious effect.

TREATMENT PLANNING

Prevention is the key to managing vertical root fractures. There are many predisposing factors and iatrogenic causes of these fractures, all of which should be minimized as much as clinically possible. VRFs may be present in teeth subjected to retreatment but are rarely present also in teeth that have never undergone endodontic treatment.[22] Therefore, comprehensive clinical, radiographic, and *periodontal examination* is imperative when evaluating any tooth that is planned for endodontic treatment or retreatment. A flexible periodontal probe is mandatory in such examinations.

When a VRF is determined to be present, extraction of the affected tooth or root is recommended as soon as possible. Any delay may increase the potential for additional periradicular bone loss and possibly compromise the placement of an endosseous implant. Thus the measures and means that may allow the dentist to make the diagnosis at early stages are important. Attempts to "repair" a fracture by filling the crevice with a variety of restorative materials have been reported; however, none of these repairs is considered a reliable long-term solution.[8,49,53,84]

SUMMARY

Because of the wide variety of different types of cracks and fractures in teeth, there may be a myriad of symptoms and presentations that may appear at different stages of the crack or fracture development, making their diagnosis often difficult. The awareness that many of these symptoms represent *stages in an evolving process* may make their interpretation easier for the operator.

The extensiveness of a crack may directly alter the prognosis assessment and treatment plan for a given tooth; the presence of a fracture may lead to the demise of a tooth and may compromise the periradicular bone. Therefore, developing a diagnosis, prognosis assessment, and treatment plan for teeth with suspected cracks and fractures is essential, with an emphasis on early detection. In addition, endodontic and restorative procedures should focus on minimizing any offending and predisposing factors that may perpetuate cracks and fractures.

REFERENCES

1. Abbott PV: Assessing restored teeth with pulp and periapical diseases for the presence of cracks, caries and marginal breakdown, *Aust Dent J* 49:33, 2004.
2. Adorno CG, Yoshioka T, Suda H: Crack initiation on the apical root surface caused by three different nickel-titanium rotary files at different working lengths, *J Endod* 37:522, 2011.
3. Alior JE: Managing incomplete tooth fractures, *J Am Dent Assoc* 131:1186, 2000.
4. American Association of Endodontists: *Restoration of endodontically treated teeth. Endodontics; colleagues for excellence*, Chicago, spring/summer 2004, American Association of Endodontists.
5. American Association of Endodontists: *Cracking the cracked tooth code: detecting and treatment of various longitudinal tooth fractures. Endodontics; colleagues for excellence*, Chicago, summer 2008, American Association of Endodontists.
6. American Association of Endodontists and American Academy of Oral and Maxillofacial Radiology: AAE and AAOMR joint position statement: use of cone-beam computed tomography in endodontics, *J Endod* 37:274, 2011.
7. Anderson TL: *Fracture mechanics: fundamentals and applications*, ed 3, Oxford, 2005, Taylor & Francis.
8. Arakawa S: Treatment of root fractures by CO_2 and Nd:YAG lasers, *J Endod* 22:662, 1996.
9. Bakland LK: Tooth infractions. In Ingle JI, Bakland LK, Baumgartner JC, editors: *Ingle's endodontics*, ed 6, Hamilton, ON, 2008, BC Decker.
10. Barreto MS, Moraes RA, da Rosa RA, et al: Vertical root fractures and dentin defects: effects of root canal preparation, filling and mechanical cycling, *J Endod* 38:1135, 2012.
11. Bender IB: Adult root fracture, *J Am Dent Assoc* 107:413, 1983.
12. Berman LH, Hartwell GR: Diagnosis. In Hargreaves KM, Cohen S, editors, *Cohen's pathways of the pulp*, ed 10, New York, 2011, Elsevier, p 2.
13. Berman LH, Kuttler S: Fracture necrosis: diagnosis, prognosis assessment, and treatment recommendations, *J Endod* 36:442, 2010.
14. Bier CA, Shemesh H, Tanomaru-Filho M, et al: The ability of different nickel-titanium rotary instruments to induce dentinal damage during canal preparation, *J Endod* 35:236, 2009.
15. Boyarsky H, Davis R: Root fracture with dentin retained post, *Am J Dent* 5:11, 1992.
16. Brynjulfsen A, Fristad I, Grevstad T, Hals-Kvinsland I: Incompletely fractured teeth associated with diffuse longstanding orofacial pain: diagnosis and treatment outcome, *Int Endod J* 35:461, 2002.
17. Bürklein S, Tsotsis P, Schäfer E: Incidence of dentinal defects after root canal preparation: reciprocating versus rotary instrumentation, *J Endod* 39:501, 2013.
18. Cameron CE: Cracked tooth syndrome, *J Am Dent Assoc* 68:405, 1964.
19. Cameron CE: The cracked tooth syndrome: additional findings, *J Am Dent Assoc* 93:971, 1976.
20. Caplan DJ, Weintraub JA: Factors related to loss of root canal filled teeth, *J Publ Health Dent* 57:31, 1997.
21. Chai H, Tamse A: Fracture mechanisms analysis of vertical root fracture from condensation of gutta-percha, *J Biomech* 45:1673, 2012.
22. Chan CP, Lin CP, Tseng SC, Jeng JH: Vertical root fracture in endodontically versus non-endodontically treated teeth, *Oral Surg Oral Med Oral Pathol Oral Radiol Endod* 87:504, 1999.
23. Cheung W: A review of the management of endodontically treated teeth, *J Am Dent Assoc* 136:611, 2005.
24. Cohen S, Blanco L, Berman L: Vertical root fractures—clinical and radiographic diagnosis, *J Am Dent Assoc* 134:434, 2003.

25. Cooney JP, Caputo AA, Trabert KC: Retention and stress distribution of tapered-end endodontic posts, *J Prosthet Dent* 55:540, 1986.
26. da Silva NR, Raposo LH, Versluis A, et al: The effect of post, core, crown type, and ferrule presence on the biomechanical behavior of endodontically treated bovine anterior teeth, *J Prosth Dent* 104:306, 2010.
27. Dang DA, Walton RE: Vertical root fracture and root distortion effect of spreader design, *J Endod* 15:294, 1989.
28. Davis R, Overton JD: Efficacy of bonded and nonbonded amalgam in treatment of teeth with incomplete fractures, *J Am Dent Assoc* 131:469, 2000.
29. Eakle WS, Maxwell EH, Braly BV: Fractures of posterior teeth in adults, *J Am Dent Assoc* 112:215, 1986.
30. El Ayouti A, Chu A-L, Kimionis I, et al: Efficacy of rotary instruments with greater taper in preparing oval root canals, *Int Endod J* 41:1088, 2008.
31. European Commission for Radiation Protection: Radiation protection No 172, Cone Beam CT for dental and maxillofacial radiology: evidence-based guidelines, SEDENTEXCT project, www.sedentexct.eu, 2012.
31a. European Society of Endodontology position statement: The use of CBCT in endodontics, *Int Endod J* 47:502, 2014.
32. Fuss Z, Lustig J, Katz A, Tamse A: An evaluation of endodontically treated vertically fractured roots: impact of operative procedures, *J Endod* 1:46, 2001.
33. Fuss Z, Lustig J, Tamse A: Prevalence of vertical root fractures in extracted endodontically treated teeth, *Int Endod J* 32:283, 1999.
34. Geurdsen W, Schwarze T, Günay H: Diagnosis, therapy and prevention of the cracked tooth syndrome, *Quintessence Int* 34:409, 2003.
35. Gibbs JW: Cuspal fracture odontalgia, *Dent Dig* 60:158, 1954.
36. Gluskin AH, Radke RA, Frost SL, Watanbe LG: The mandibular incisor: rethinking guidelines for post and core design, *J Endod* 21:33, 1995.
37. Goodcare CJ, Baba NZ: Restoration of endodontically treated teeth. In Ingle JI, Bakland LK, Baumgartner JC, editors: *Ingle's endodontics*, ed 6, Hamilton, ON, 2008, BC Decker, p 1431.
38. Graves DT, Oates T, Garlet GP: Review of osteoimmunology and the host response in endodontic and periodontal lesions, *J Oral Microbiol* 3:5304—DOI: 10.3402/jom.v3i0.5304, 2011.
39. Guthrie RC, DiFiore PM: Treating the cracked tooth with full crown, *J Am Dent Assoc* 122:71, 1991.
40. Gutmann JL: The dentin-root complex: anatomic and biologic considerations in restoring endodontically treated teeth, *J Prosth Dent* 67:458, 1992.
41. Hassan B, Metska ME, Ozok AR, et al: Detection of vertical root fractures in endodontically treated teeth by a cone beam computed tomography scan, *J Endod* 35:719, 2009.
42. Hassan B, Metska ME, Ozok AR, et al: Comparison of five cone beam computed tomography systems for the detection of vertical root fractures, *J Endod* 36:126, 2010.
43. Helfer AR: Determination of the moisture content of vital and pulpless teeth, *Oral Surg* 34:661, 1972.
44. Hin ES, Wu M-K, Wesselink PR, Shemesh H: Effects of self-adjusting file, Mtwo, and ProTaper on the root canal wall, *J Endod* 39:262, 2013.
45. Homewood CI: Cracked tooth syndrome: incidence, clinical findings and treatment, *Aust Dent J* 43:217, 1998.
46. Huang TJ, Schilder H, Nathanson D: Effects of moisture content and endodontic treatment on some mechanical properties of human dentin, *J Endod* 18:209, 1991.
47. Kahler B, Moule A, Stenzel D: Bacterial contamination of cracks in symptomatic vital teeth, *Aust Endod J* 26:115, 2000.
48. Katz A, Wasenstein-Kohn S, Tamse A, Zukerman O: Residual dentin thickness in bifurcated maxillary premolars after root canal and dowel space preparation, *J Endod* 32:202, 2006.

49. Kawai K, Masaka N: Vertical root fracture treated by bonding fragments and rotational replantation, *Dent Traumatol* 18:42, 2002.
50. Kim HC, Lee MH, Yum J, et al: Potential relationship between design of nickel-titanium rotary instruments and vertical root fracture, *J Endod* 36:1195, 2010.
51. Krell KV, Rivera EM: A six year evaluation of cracked teeth diagnosed with reversible pulpitis: treatment and prognosis, *J Endod* 33:1405, 2007.
52. Kruzic JJ, Nalla RK, Kinney JH, Ritchie RO: Mechanistic aspects of in vitro fatigue-crack growth in dentin, *Biomaterials* 26:1195, 2005.
53. Kudou Y, Kubota M: Replantation with intentional rotation of complete vertically fractured root using adhesive resin, *Dent Traumatol* 18:115, 2003.
54. Lertchirakarn V, Palamara J, Messer HH: Patterns of vertical fractures: Factors affecting stress distribution in the root canal, *J Endod* 29:523, 2003.
55. Lertchirakarn V, Palamara JEA, Messer HH: Finite element analysis and strain-gauge studies of vertical root fracture, *J Endod* 29:529, 2003.
56. Liu R, Kaiwar A, Shemesh H, et al: Incidence of apical root cracks and apical dentinal detachments after canal preparation with hand and rotary files at different instrumentation lengths, *J Endod* 39:129, 2013.
57. Lustig JP, Tamse A, Fuss Z: Pattern of bone resorption in vertically fractured endodontically treated teeth, *Oral Surg Oral Med Oral Pathol Oral Radiol Endod* 90:224, 2000.
58. Meister F, Lommel TJ, Gerstein H: Diagnosis and possible causes of vertical root fractures, *Oral Surg Oral Med Oral Pathol Oral Radiol Endod* 49:243, 1980.
59. Melo SLS, Bortoluzzi EA, Abreu M Jr, et al: Diagnostic ability of a cone-beam computed tomography scan to assess longitudinal root fractures in prosthetically treated teeth, *J Endod* 36:1879, 2010.
60. Metzger Z, Teperovich E, Zary R, et al: The self-adjusting file (SAF). Part 1: respecting the root canal anatomy—a new concept of endodontic files and its implementation, *J Endod* 36:679, 2010.
61. Morando G, Leupold RJ, Reiers JC: Measurements of hydrostatic pressure during simulated post cementation, *J Prosthet Dent* 74:586, 1995.
62. Nikopoulou-Karayanni K, Bragger U, Lang NP: Patterns of periodontal destruction associated with incomplete root fractures, *Dentomaxillofac Radiol* 26:321, 1997.
63. Onnink PA, Davis RD, Wayman BE: An in vitro comparison of incomplete root fractures associated with obturation technique, *J Endod* 20:32, 1994.
64. Opdam NJ, Roeters JJ, Loomans BA, Bronkhorst EM: Seven-year clinical evaluation of painful cracked teeth restored with a direct composite restoration, *J Endod* 34:808, 2008.
65. Patel S, Dawood A, Ford TP, Whaites E: The potential applications of cone beam computed tomography in the management of endodontic problems, *Int Endod J* 40:818, 2007.
66. Peters OA, Paqué F: Root canal preparation of maxillary molars with the self-adjusting file: A micro-computed tomographic study, *J Endod* 37:53, 2011.
67. Peters OA, Peters CL, Schönenberg K, Barbakow F: ProTaper rotary root canal preparation assessment of torque and force in relation to canal anatomy, *Int Endod J* 36:93, 2003.
68. Pilo R: *Development of strains and mechanical failure in dental roots undergoing root canal obturation and prosthetic rehabilitation*. PhD thesis, Tel Aviv University, 2007.
69. Ritchey B, Mendenhall R, Orban B: Pulpitis resulting from incomplete tooth fracture, *Oral Surg Oral Med Oral Pathol Oral Radiol Endod* 10:665, 1957.
70. Roh BD, Lee YE: Analysis of 154 cases of teeth with cracks, *Dent Traumatol* 22:118, 2006.
71. Rosen H: Cracked tooth syndrome, *J Prosthet Dent* 47:36, 1982.

72. Rud J, Omnell KA: Root fracture due to corrosion, *Scand J Dent Res* 78:397, 1970.

73. Saw L-H, Messer HH: Root strains associated with different obturation techniques, *J Endod* 21:314, 1995.

74. Schmidt KJ, Walker TL, Johnson JD, Nicoll BK: Comparison of nickel-titanium and stainless steel spreader penetration and accessory cone fit in curved canals, *J Endod* 26:42, 2000.

75. Sedgley CM, Messer HH: Are endodontically treated teeth more brittle? *J Endod* 18:332, 1992.

76. Shemesh H, Bier CA, Wu MK, et al: The effects of canal preparation and filling on the incidence of dentinal defects, *Int Endod J* 42:208, 2009.

77. Shemesh H, Roeleveld AC, Wesselink PR, Wu MK: Damage to root dentin during retreatment procedures, *J Endod* 37:63, 2011.

78. Snyder DE: The cracked tooth syndrome and fractured posterior cusp, *Oral Surg Oral Med Oral Pathol Oral Radiol Endod* 41:698, 1976.

79. Tamse A: Iatrogenic vertical root fractures in endodontically treated teeth, *Endod Dent Traumatol* 4:190, 1988.

80. Tamse A: Vertical root fractures of endodontically treated teeth. In Ingle JI, Bakland LK, Baumgartner JC, editors: *Ingle's endodontics*, ed 6, Hamilton, ON, 2008, BC Decker, p 676.

81. Tamse A, Fuss Z, Lustig J, Kaplavi J: An evaluation of endodontically treated vertically fractured teeth, *J Endod* 25:506, 1999.

82. Tamse A, Fuss Z, Lustig JP, et al: Radiographic features of vertically fractured endodontically treated maxillary premolars, *Oral Surg Oral Med Oral Pathol Oral Radiol Endod* 88:348, 1999.

83. Tamse A, Kaffe I, Lustig J, et al: Radiographic features of vertically fractured endodontically treated mesial roots of mandibular molars, *Oral Surg Oral Med Oral Pathol Oral Radiol Endod* 101:797, 2006.

84. Taschieri S, Tamse A, del Fabbro M, et al: A new surgical technique for preservation of endodontically treated teeth with coronally located vertical root fractures: a prospective study, *Oral Surg Oral Med Oral Pathol Oral Radiol Endod* 110:45, 2010.

85. Testori T, Badino M, Castagnola M: Vertical root fractures in endodontically treated teeth: a clinical survey of 36 cases, *J Endod* 19:87, 1993.

86. Tsesis A, Rosen E, Tamse A, et al: A diagnosis of vertical root fractures in endodontically treated teeth based on clinical and radiographic indices: a systematic review, *J Endod* 36:1455, 2010.

87. Walton RE, Michelich RJ, Smith GN: The histopathogenesis of vertical root fractures, *J Endod* 10:48, 1984.

88. Walton RE, Torabinejad M: *Principles and practice of endodontics*, ed 3, Philadelphia, 2002, WB Saunders, p 516.

89. Wilcox LR, Roskelley C, Sutton T: The relationship of root canal enlargement to finger-spreader induced vertical root fracture, *J Endod* 23:533, 1997.

90. Yeh CJ: Fatigue root fracture: a spontaneous root fracture in non-endodontically treated teeth, *British Dent J* 182:261, 1997.

91. Yoldas O, Yilmaz S, Atakan G, et al: Dentinal microcrack formation during root canal preparations by different Ni-Ti rotary instruments and the self-adjusting file, *J Endod* 38:235, 2012.

CHAPTER 22

Restoration of the Endodontically Treated Tooth

DIDIER DIETSCHI | SERGE BOUILLAGUET | AVISHAI SADAN

CHAPTER OUTLINE

SPECIAL FEATURES OF ENDODONTICALLY TREATED TEETH

Once endodontic therapy is completed, the tooth must be adequately restored. Indeed, given the large impact that poor or missing restorations have on the survival of endodontically treated teeth, one could make the argument that the restoration is actually the last step of endodontic therapy. However, it is important to realize that endodontically treated teeth are structurally different from nontreated vital teeth. Major changes following treatment include altered tissue physical characteristics, loss of tooth structure, and possibly discoloration. Research has analyzed these tissue modifications at different levels, including tooth composition, dentin microstructure, and tooth macrostructure. These studies indicate that it is critical to understand the implication of such features on tooth biomechanics, as they will largely influence the restorative approach and means (Table 22-1). Additional in vitro studies dealing with the complexity of the nonvital tooth substrate are reported in the literature; ultimately, clinical studies have documented the global effect of these changes on the long-term survival of endodontically treated teeth.

Compositional Changes in Nonvital Teeth and the Influence of Endodontic Therapy

The loss of pulpal vitality is accompanied by a slight change in tooth moisture content. This loss of moisture (9%) is attributed to a change in free water but not in water bonded to the organic and inorganic components.[65,69] This alteration was associated with a slight change in values for the Young modulus and proportional limit.[75] However, no decrease in compressive and tensile strength values was associated with this change in water content.[75] Only one study showed no difference in moisture content between vital and nonvital teeth.[123] No difference in collagen cross-linkage was found between vital and nonvital dentin.[140] Thus, nonvital teeth undergo rather minor changes in physical characteristics.

Sodium hypochlorite and chelators such as ethylenediamine tetra-acetic acid (EDTA), cyclohexane-1,2-diaminetetraacetic acid (CDTA), ethylene glycol-bis-(β-amino-ethyl ether) N,N,N′,N′-tetra-acetic acid (EGTA), and calcium hydroxide $(Ca[OH]_2)$ commonly used for canal irrigation and disinfection interact with root dentin, with either mineral content

TABLE 22-1

Specific Tissue Modifications and Possible Clinical Implications Following Loss of Vitality or Endodontic Treatment

Alteration Level	Specific Changes	Possible Clinical Implication
Composition	Collagen structure Tooth moisture Mineral composition and content	Increased tooth fragility Reduced adhesion to substrate
Dentin structure	Elasticity modulus and behavior Tensile and shear strength Microhardness	Increased tooth fragility
Tooth macrostructure	Resistance to deformation Resistance to fracture Resistance to fatigue	Increased tooth fragility Reduced retention/stability of the prosthesis

(chelators) or organic substrate (sodium hypochlorite).[78,116,119] Chelators mainly deplete calcium by complex formation and also affect noncollagenous proteins (NCPs), leading to dentin erosion and surface softening.[78,82,144] Depending on concentration, duration of exposure, and other factors (see Chapter 6), sodium hypochlorite can demonstrate a proteolytic action by hydrolysis of long peptide chains such as collagen.[68] These alterations are likely to impact dentin and root structure and alter bonding properties of this substrate.

Dentin Structure and Properties in Nonvital and Endodontically Treated Teeth

It is important to know that dentin displays a range of normal variations in its physical properties which must be distinguished from alterations related to loss of vitality or endodontic treatment. For instance, dentin microhardness and elasticity actually vary between peritubular and intertubular dentin and depend on tooth location. Peritubular dentin presents an elasticity modulus of 29.8 GPa, whereas intertubular dentin ranges from 17.7 GPa (close to pulp) to 21.1 GPa (close to the root surface).[70,85,101] Most if not all the decreases in hardness on approaching the pulp can be attributed to changes in hardness of the intertubular dentin.[84,85] Overall dentin elasticity modulus is considered to be in the range of 16.5 to 18.5 Gpa.[15,32,50,86,121,138]

The changes in mineral density due to the variation in the number and diameter of tubules within the tooth may also contribute to variations in the properties of dentin. Not surprisingly, dentin hardness values are inversely related to dentin tubule density.[124] Ultra microindentation measurements also demonstrated significantly higher values for hardness and elasticity modulus when forces were parallel to the tubules rather than perpendicular.[133] Differences in maximum strength and compressive strength were also found to vary according to tubule orientation.[121] The ultimate tensile strength (UTS) of human dentin is lowest when the tensile force is parallel to tubule orientation, showing the influence of dentin

microstructure and anisotropy of the tissue.[93] No difference was found in the Young modulus of aged, transparent dentin (also called *sclerotic*) and normal dentin,[19,87,167] but the mineral concentration significantly increases and crystallite size is slightly smaller in transparent dentin, in relation with closure of the tubule lumens. Transparent dentin, unlike normal dentin, exhibits almost no yielding before failure. Its fracture toughness is also lowered by about 20%, whereas the fatigue lifetime is deleteriously affected.[87]

Interestingly, comparisons between vital and nonvital dentin of contralateral teeth demonstrate no or only minor differences in microhardness values after periods ranging up to 10 years after treatment.[94,154] Thus, the literature does not support a widely held belief that attributes particular weakness or brittleness to nonvital dentin. Others have suggested that nonvital teeth in older patients may have greater risk for fracture because the age-related generation of secondary or tertiary dentin would be lost. However, this is not the case because the only impact of age-related tissue changes is the aforementioned reduction in fracture toughness and fatigue lifetime attributed to dentin sclerosis.[87]

The chemicals used for canal irrigation and disinfection, as already mentioned, interact with mineral and organic contents and then reduce dentin elasticity and flexural strength to a significant extent,[64,157] as well as microhardness.[33,77,146] On the contrary, disinfectants like eugenol and formocresol increase dentin tensile strength by way of protein coagulation and chelation with hydroxyapatite (eugenol). Dentin hardness, however, did not prove to be influenced by the latter products.[112]

In conclusion, a possible decrease in tooth strength can be attributed to dentin aging and to a smaller extent to dentin alteration by endodontic irrigants.

Fracture Resistance and Tooth Stiffness of Nonvital and Endodontically Treated Teeth

In contrast to the aforementioned factors, the major changes in tooth biomechanics appear to be due to the loss of hard tissue following decay, fracture, or cavity preparation (including the access cavity prior to endodontic therapy).

The loss of hard tooth structure following a conservative access cavity preparation affects tooth stiffness by only 5%.[91,169] The influence of subsequent canal instrumentation and obturation lead only to a slight reduction in the resistance to fracture[91,169] and ultimately have little effect on tooth biomechanics.[91,137,169] From a clinical perspective, one can expect alteration of tooth biomechanics only in cases of nonconservative canal preparation or through the chemical or structural alteration triggered by endodontic irrigants, as previously mentioned.

In fact, the largest reduction in tooth stiffness results from excessive access preparation, especially the loss of marginal ridges. The literature reports a 20% to 63% and a 14% to 44% reduction in tooth stiffness following occlusal and MOD cavity preparations, respectively.[44,92,137] It was shown that an endodontic access cavity combined with an MOD preparation results in maximum tooth fragilization. The cavity depth, isthmus width, and configuration are therefore highly critical to the reduction in tooth stiffness and risk of fracture (Fig. 22-1).[74,83,96,122] This important point has profound clinical implications.

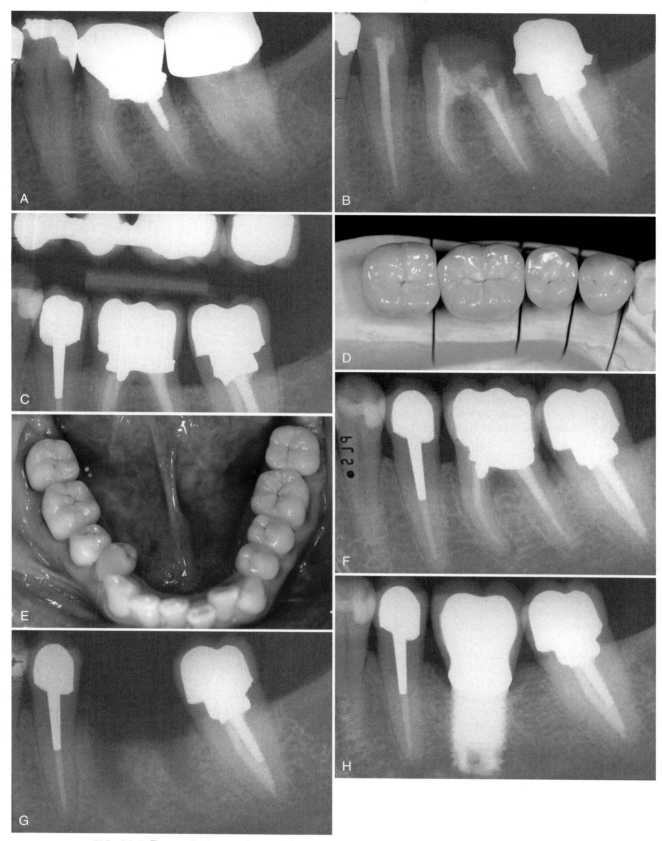

FIG. 22-1 The negative impact of poor initial biomechanical status on restoration success. **A, B,** Preoperative radiographic views following the removal of the old metallic foundation. **C,** A new amalgam core, using post and self-anchorage into mesial root structure, was performed. **D,** Prosthetic restorations on working model. **E,** Full arch view after 3 years. **F,** The tooth is symptomatic due to furcation involvement and periapical lesion. **G,** This untreatable tooth was finally extracted and replaced by an implant. **H,** Eight-year postoperative radiograph showing a stable situation. Other teeth with less extensive biomechanical damage overcame functional stresses.

The presence of residual hard tissue in the cervical area (which constitutes the *ferrule* for restorations) and a larger amount of residual mineralized tissue in general increase tooth resistance to fracture. It actually allows the axial walls of the crown to encircle the tooth, providing restoration retention and stabilization and reducing cervical tensile stresses.[6,23,161] Crown preparations with as little as 1 mm coronal extension of dentin above the margin double the fracture resistance of preparations, compared to those where the core terminates on a flat surface immediately above the margin[103,161]; therefore, a minimal 1-mm ferrule (and ideally 2 to 3 mm) is considered necessary to stabilize the restoration.[161] However, the widths of preparation shoulder and crown margin do not appear to influence fracture strength.[2] Taken together, the height of the ferrule is one of the most important elements in the long-term survival of restorations. These considerations have led to the conclusion that the most important part of the restored tooth is the tooth itself, and no contemporary restorative material or combination of materials will perfectly substitute for lost tooth structure.

Aesthetic Changes in Nonvital and Endodontically Treated Teeth

Several aesthetic changes may also occur in nonvital or endodontically treated teeth. For example, color change or darkening of nonvital teeth is a common clinical observation (Fig. 22-2). In addition, incomplete endodontic treatment can contribute to discoloration. For instance, inadequate cleaning and shaping can leave necrotic tissue in coronal pulp horns, resulting in tooth darkening. In addition, root canal filling materials (gutta-percha and root canal sealer cements, MTA-like materials) retained in the coronal aspect of anterior teeth can detract from the aesthetic appearance. Opaque substances also adversely affect the color and translucency of most uncrowned teeth. Biochemically altered dentin modifies tooth color and appearance. It is generally accepted that organic substances present in dentin (e.g., hemoglobin) might play an important role in this color change and also food and drink pigment penetration triggered by the absence of pulpal pressure. However, the respective contribution of these two phenomena and precise

physicochemical mechanisms leading to discoloration are poorly understood or described in the literature.[34,67,131]

Thin gingival tissue or, in general, thin biotype is considered a negative factor for aesthetic outcome of restorative and prosthetic treatment of discolored teeth.[110,111,118]

Endodontic treatment and subsequent restoration of teeth in the aesthetic zone require careful control of procedures and materials to retain a translucent, natural appearance. It is therefore strongly recommended that one avoid the use of potentially staining endodontic cements and clean all material residues left in the pulpal chamber and access cavity.

RESTORATIVE MATERIALS AND OPTIONS

As described previously, endodontic treatment, particularly excessive access preparations, can result in significant loss and weakening of tooth structure. Tooth structure lost during endodontic treatment increases the risk of crown fracture, with fatigue mechanisms mediating the fracture of roots over time. Restorations of endodontically treated teeth are designed to (1) protect the remaining tooth from fracture, (2) prevent reinfection of the root canal system, and (3) replace the missing tooth structure.

According to the amount of tissue to be replaced, restorations of endodontically treated teeth rely on different materials and clinical procedures. As a general rule, most structurally damaged teeth should be restored with an artificial crown.

Although the use of a crown built on post and core is a traditional approach, others have advocated the use of direct composite resins for restoring small defects in endodontically treated teeth. More recently, indirect restorations such as overlays or endocrowns made of composite resins or ceramics have also been used. The selection of appropriate restorative materials and techniques is dictated by the amount of remaining tooth structure. This is far more relevant to the long-term prognosis of endodontically treated teeth than any properties of post, core, or crown materials.

Direct Composite Restorations

When a minimal amount of coronal tooth structure has been lost after endodontic therapy, a direct resin composite restoration may be indicated. Composite resins are a mixture of a polymerized resin network reinforced by inorganic fillers. Contemporary composites have compressive strengths of about 280 MPa, and the Young modulus of composite resins is generally about 10 to 16 GPa, which is close to that of dentin.[134]

When properly cured, resin composites are highly aesthetic, exhibit high mechanical properties, and can reinforce the remaining tooth structure through bonding mechanisms. Typically, 500 to 800 mW/cm² of blue light for 30 to 40 seconds is necessary to polymerize an increment of composite that must be 1- to 3-mm thick. Unfortunately, the shrinkage that accompanies polymerization of contemporary composite resins remains a significant problem to the long-term success of these restorations. The use of an incremental filling technique, which helps to reduce shrinkage stresses during polymerization, is highly recommended. The amount of shrinkage will also depend on the shape of the cavity preparation and the ratio of bonded to unbonded (or free) surfaces.[36] This so-called C-factor is a clinically relevant predictor of the risk of debonding and leakage; restorations with high C-factors (> 3.0) are at greatest risk for debonding.[175] In other words, a direct composite

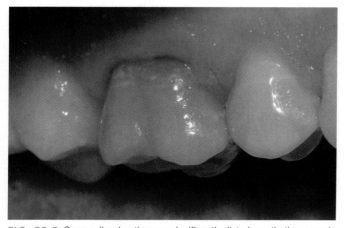

FIG. 22-2 Severe discoloration can significantly disturb aesthetics, even in the lateral area of the smile. When not treatable with bleaching agents or veneers, this condition might justify tooth preparation for a full crown.

restoration may be indicated when only one proximal surface of the tooth has been lost; using an incremental filling technique is mandatory.

Classically, direct composite restorations have been placed in anterior teeth that have not lost tooth structure beyond the endodontic access preparation. In such cases, the placement of a direct composite restoration offers an immediate sealing of the tooth, which prevents coronal leakage and recontamination of the root canal system with bacteria. In vitro studies have demonstrated that the fracture resistance of small bonded restorations is nearly as great as that of intact teeth.[57,136]

Although direct composite resins may also be used for small restorations in posterior teeth, they are contraindicated when more than a third of coronal tissue has been lost. In one study,[136] it was reported that the resistance to fracture of endodontically treated teeth is reduced by 69% in cases where MOD cavities are present.[137] Under such conditions, a direct composite restoration may not be appropriate to prevent the tooth structure from fracture and reinfection. Furthermore, resin composite materials may require the use of reinforcing in vitro fibers to increase their mechanical resistance. Although most studies on the clinical performance of direct composite restorations were conducted on vital teeth, one clinical report indicates that direct in vitro fiber-reinforced composite restorations may represent a valuable alternative to conventional restorations of endodontically treated teeth.[37] On the contrary, inserting an in vitro fiber post in the root canal of an endodontically treated tooth before bonding a direct MOD restoration significantly reduces its fracture resistance compared to the same composite restoration without a post.[160]

Indirect Restorations: Composite or Ceramic Onlays and Overlays

Ceramic or resin composite onlays and endocrowns can also be used to restore endodontically treated teeth. Whereas overlays incorporate a cusp or cusps by covering the missing tissue, endocrowns combine the post in the canal, the core, and the crown in one component.[88,142] Both onlays and endocrowns allow for conservation of remaining tooth structure, whereas the alternative would be to completely eliminate cusps and perimeter walls for restoration with a full crown.[58] Onlays and overlays are generally constructed in the laboratory from either hybrid resin composite or ceramics.

Ceramics are a material of choice for long-term aesthetic indirect restorations because their translucency and light transmission mimic enamel. Whereas traditional feldspathic porcelains were sintered from a slurry, new ceramic materials may be cast, machined, pressed, or slip-cast, in addition to being sintered. New materials either are variations of feldspathic porcelains (e.g., In-Ceram, Cerec, IPS Empress) or may be fabricated from other ceramic systems, including alumina, zirconia, or silica.[3,38] Among these newer compositions is lithium disilicate, which offers high strength, high fracture toughness, and a high degree of translucency. Physical properties of these materials have improved to the point where they can survive high stress-bearing situations such as posterior restorations in endodontically treated teeth.[46,73] Researchers have examined 140 partial Cerec restorations (Vita MKII, feldspathic porcelain) adhesively cemented to endodontically treated teeth and found this treatment approach satisfactory after an observation period of 55 months.[9] Their results indicate that survival rates are higher for molars than for premolars.

Onlays, overlays, and endocrowns can also be fabricated from resin composites processed in the laboratory. Using various combinations of light, pressure, and vacuum, these fabrication techniques are claimed to increase the conversion rate of the polymer and consequently the mechanical properties of the restorative material. Other investigations have described the application of glass fiber–reinforced composite endocrowns on premolars and molars as single restorations or as abutment for fixed partial dentures.[58,59] One in vitro study by another research team indicates that composite inlays can partially restore the resistance to fracture of endodontically treated molars and prevent catastrophic fractures after loading.[28] Other investigators reported that composite resin MZ100 increased the fatigue resistance of overlay-type restorations in endodontically treated molars when compared to porcelain MKII.[97] Another study used three-dimensional finite element analysis to estimate bone resorption around endocrowns made up of high-(alumina) or low-elastic modulus materials (resin composites). They concluded that the higher resilience of resin composite restorations acts positively against the risk of periodontal bone resorption by reducing the amount of force transferred to root dentin.[4]

Full Crowns

When a significant amount of coronal tooth structure has been lost by caries, restorative procedures, and endodontics, a full crown may be the restoration of choice. In a few cases, the crown can be directly built on the remaining coronal structure, which has been prepared accordingly (see the Core Materials section). More frequently, the cementation of a post inside the root canal is necessary to retain the core material and the crown.[164] The core is anchored to the tooth by extension into the root canal through the post and replaces missing coronal structure. The crown covers the core and restores the aesthetics and function of the tooth.

An additional role of the post and core is to protect the crown margins from deformation under function and thereby to prevent coronal leakage. Because most endodontic sealers do not completely seal the root canal space, the coronal seal provided by the placement of a post and core will positively influence the outcome of the endodontic treatment.[148] The post's ability to anchor the core is also an important factor for successful reconstruction, because the core and the post are usually fabricated of different materials. Finally, the luting material used to cement the post, the core, and the crown to the tooth will also influence the longevity of the restoration. The post, the core, and their luting or bonding agents together form a *foundation restoration* to support the future crown.[106]

The Foundation Restoration: General Considerations

Although many materials and techniques can be used to fabricate a foundation restoration, no combination of materials can substitute for tooth structure. As a general rule, the more tooth structure that remains, the better the long-term prognosis of the restoration. The coronal tooth structure located above the gingival level will help to create a ferrule.[6,100,128] The *ferrule* is formed by the walls and margins of the crown, encasing at least 2 to 3 mm of sound tooth structure. A properly executed ferrule significantly reduces the incidence of fracture in endodontically treated teeth by reinforcing the tooth at its external surface and dissipating forces that concentrate at the narrowest circumference of the tooth.[95,173] A longer ferrule increases fracture resistance significantly. The ferrule also resists lateral forces from posts and leverage from the crown in function and increases the retention and resistance of the restoration. To be successful, the crown and crown preparation together must meet five requirements:

1. The ferrule (dentin axial wall height) must be at least 2 to 3 mm.
2. The axial walls must be parallel.
3. The restoration must completely encircle the tooth.
4. The margin must be on solid tooth structure.
5. The crown and crown preparation must not invade the attachment apparatus.

Root anatomy can also have significant influence over post placement and selection. Root curvature, furcations, developmental depressions, and root concavities observed at the external surface of the root are all likely to be reproduced inside the root canal (see also Chapter 5). Within the same root, the shape of the canal will vary between the cervical level and the apical foramen.[62] As a result, severe alteration of the natural shape of the canal is often necessary to adapt a circular post inside the root. This increases the risk of root perforation, especially in mesial roots of maxillary and mandibular molars that exhibit deep concavities on the furcal surface of their mesial root.[16,89] The tooth is also weakened if root dentin is sacrificed to place a larger-diameter post. A study using three-dimensional electronic speckle-pattern interferometry (ESPI) evaluated the effects of root canal preparation and post placement on the rigidity of human roots.[93] ESPI has the major advantage of being able to assess tooth deformation in real time and can be used repeatedly on the same root because of the nondestructive nature of the test. Study results indicate that root deformability increases significantly after the preparation of a post space. Thus, preservation of root structure is also a guiding principle in the decision to use a post, the selection of the post, and the preparation of the post space. This is a reason why not every endodontically treated tooth needs a post and why more conservative approaches that do not rely on the use of a post are currently being developed. However, a post may be used in the root of a structurally damaged tooth in which additional retention is needed for the core and coronal restoration. Posts should provide as many of the following clinical features as possible:

- Maximal protection of the root from fracture
- Maximal retention within the root and retrievability
- Maximal retention of the core and crown
- Maximal protection of the crown margin seal from coronal leakage
- Pleasing aesthetics, when indicated
- High radiographic visibility
- Biocompatibility

From a mechanical point of view, an endodontic post should not break, should not break the root, and should not distort or allow movement of the core and crown. An ideal post would have an optimal combination of resilience, stiffness, flexibility, and strength. *Resilience* is the ability to deflect elastically under force without permanent damage. It is a valuable quality in endodontic posts, but too much flexibility in a narrow post compromises its ability to retain the core and crown under functional forces. *Stiffness* describes a material's ability to resist deformation when stressed. The stiffness of a material is an inherent physical property of that material, regardless of size. However, the actual flexibility of a post depends both on the diameter of a specific post and on the modulus of elasticity of the post's material. Posts with a lower modulus of elasticity are more flexible than posts of the same diameter with a higher modulus of elasticity. Posts made of nonstiff materials (low modulus of elasticity) are more resilient, absorb more impact force, and transmit less force to the root than stiff posts, but low-modulus posts fail at lower levels of force than do high-modulus posts.[99,120,143]

Excessive flexing of the post and micromovement of the core are particular risks in teeth with minimal remaining tooth structure, because these teeth lack their own cervical stiffness as a result of the missing dentin. Post flexion can also distort and open crown margins. Open margins can result in potentially devastating caries or endodontic leakage and apical reinfection. Extensive caries extending into the root can be as irreparable as root fracture. Because rigid posts flex and bend less than nonrigid posts, they can limit movement of the core and possible disruption of the crown margins and cement seal. However, the force must go somewhere. Force from a stiff post is transmitted to the root, next to the apex of the post. An attempt to strengthen a weak root by adding a stiff post can instead make the root weaker as a result of the force concentration of a stiff rod in a more flexible material. Stress concentration in the post/root complex can lead to the self-destructive process of cracking and fracturing. Root fracture is particularly a risk in teeth with minimal remaining tooth structure to support a ferrule.

Roots also flex under force, which is a function of both the modulus of elasticity of dentin and the diameter of the root. Dentin is relatively flexible, and posts can be flexible or stiff. Although no material can behave exactly like dentin, a post with functional behavior similar to that of dentin is beneficial when the post must be placed next to dentin. Posts have been developed with a modulus of elasticity closer to dentin than that offered by traditional metal posts. But posts are significantly narrower than roots, and the actual deflection of a post within dentin is a function of both the modulus of elasticity and the diameter. The modulus of elasticity of various posts, compared with that of dentin, represents only one aspect of flexion.

In summary, an ideal post would be resilient enough to cushion an impact by stretching elastically, thereby reducing the resulting stress to the root. It would then return to normal without permanent distortion. At the same time, this ideal post would be stiff enough not to distort, permanently bend, or structurally fail under mastication forces. Finally, the perfect post would combine the ideal level of flexibility and strength in a narrow-diameter structure, which is dictated by root canal morphology. Current post systems are designed to provide the best compromise between the desired properties and inherent limitations of available materials.

Why Roots Fracture

Structures subjected to low but repeated forces can appear to fracture suddenly for no apparent reason. This phenomenon, also known as *fatigue failure,* occurs when a material or a tissue is subjected to cyclic loading. Fatigue may be characterized as a progressive failure phenomenon that proceeds by the initiation and propagation of cracks; many failures of teeth or materials observed in the mouth are fatigue-related. Because teeth are subjected to fluctuating cycles of loading and unloading during mastication, fatigue failure of dentin, posts, cores, crown margins, or adhesive components is likely to occur.[153] Mechanical loading will favor the propagation of microcracks that will progress from the coronal to the apical region of the tooth.

Initial failure of crown margins from fatigue loading is clinically undetectable. However, when measured in vitro, early failure resulted in significant leakage of crown margins, extending between the tooth, restoration, and post space. Particularly in teeth with minimal remaining tooth structure, fatigue can cause endodontic posts to bend permanently or break, or it can cause a fiber-matrix complex to disintegrate.

Fatigue failure of nonvital teeth restored with a post is more catastrophic because it may result in a complete fracture of the root. A post placed into a dentin root will function physically like any structural rod anchored in another material. This means that the forces applied on the post are transmitted to the root dentin with characteristic patterns depending on the modulus of elasticity of both the post and the dentin. If the post has a higher modulus than the dentin, the stress concentration is adjacent to the bottom of the post (Fig. 22-3). This is evident in clinical cases of root fracture originating at the apex of a rigid post.

When the stiffness of the endodontic post is similar to that of dentin, stresses are not concentrated in the dentin adjacent to the apex of the post but rather are dissipated by both the coronal and the root dentin (see Fig. 22-3). A resilient post can also prevent a sudden blow by stretching elastically, which reduces the transient forces against the tooth, but a post that is too elastic becomes too flexible for retaining a core and a crown when the tooth cannot do so on its own. A resilient post that is overloaded fails with less force than a stiffer post. This limits the amount of resilience that can be designed into a post.

Direct Foundation Restorations

In general, the evolution of foundation restorations has been to diminish invasiveness and eliminate some components in selected cases. When a sufficient amount of tissue is present at the periphery of the prepared tooth, a direct foundation restoration is indicated. In the direct technique, a prefabricated post is cemented inside the root canal, and the core is built directly on the prepared tooth. For other clinical situations, an indirect custom-cast post and core may be indicated.

Various materials can be used to fabricate a direct foundation restoration. Although there is growing interest in using resin-based materials such as resin composites or fiber-reinforced resin posts, more traditional materials such as amalgam are still used for that purpose.[27] For clarity, the components used for fabricating a direct foundation restoration (e.g., the endodontic post and core material) are described individually.

Posts

The large number of post designs and materials available on the market reflects the absence of consensus in that field. Based on what manufacturers or clinicians consider the most important properties, posts can be fabricated from metal (gold, titanium, stainless steel), ceramic, or fiber-reinforced resins. As a general rule, a post needs retention and resistance. Whereas *post retention* refers to the ability of a post to resist vertical

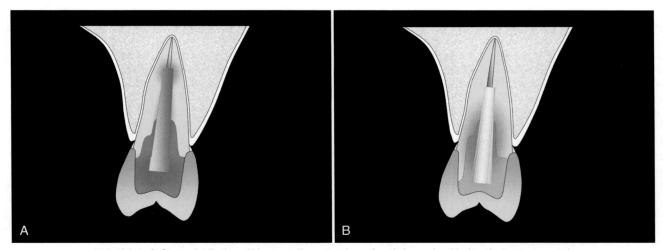

FIG. 22-3 **A,** Stress distribution within a metallic post and core foundation and residual tooth structure, according to photoelastic and FEM studies. The post is cemented and usually penetrates the apical portion of the root. Functional stresses accumulate inside the foundation, slightly around the post and further inside the canal, around the apex of the post; there is less stress buildup in the cervical area compared to that with a fiber post (as shown in Fig. 22-3, *B*). This configuration more ideally protects the coronocervical structures, but when failing, it results in severe untreatable root fractures. **B,** Stress distribution within a fiber post/composite foundation and residual tooth structure, according to photoelastic and FEM studies. The post is bonded to the canal walls and penetrates the canal less apically. Functional stresses mainly accumulate around the post in the cervical area. This configuration protects the cervical area less efficiently but tends to prevent untreatable root fractures. The presence of a ferrule is mandatory. (Adapted from Dietschi D, Duc O, Krejci I, Sadan A: Biomechanical considerations for the restoration of endodontically treated teeth: a systematic review of the literature—Part 1. Composition and micro- and macrostructure alterations, *Quintessence Int* 38:733, 2007.)

forces, *resistance* refers to the ability of the tooth/post combination to withstand lateral and rotational forces. Resistance is influenced by the presence of a ferrule, the post's length and rigidity, and the presence of antirotational features. A restoration lacking resistance form is not likely to be a long-term success, regardless of the retentiveness of the post.

Prefabricated Metallic Posts

Prefabricated metallic posts are frequently used for the fabrication of a direct foundation restoration. These posts are classified several ways, including by alloy composition, retention mode, and shape. Materials used to fabricate metallic posts include gold alloys, stainless steel, or titanium alloys. Metallic posts are very strong and, with the exception of the titanium alloys, very rigid.[90] One study indicates that the flexural strength of stainless steel posts is about 1430 MPa and that flexural modulus approximates 110 GPa.[130] On the other hand, titanium posts are less rigid (66 GPa) but exhibit a flexural strength (1280 MPa) similar to stainless steel.

The retention of prefabricated posts inside the root canal is also essential for successful restorations. Two basic concepts have been used to promote the retention of endodontic posts: active posts and passive posts. Active posts derive their primary retention directly from the root dentin by the use of threads. Most active posts are threaded and are intended to be screwed into the walls of the root canal. A major concern about threaded posts has been the potential for vertical root fracture during placement. As the post is screwed into place, it introduces great stresses within the root, causing a wedging effect.[163] Therefore, it is generally accepted that *the use of threaded posts should be avoided.* Furthermore, the improved retention once offered by threaded posts can now be achieved with adhesive luting cements (discussed later).[117] Passive posts are passively placed in close contact to the dentin walls, and their retention primarily relies on the luting cement used for cementation. The shape of a passive post may be either tapered or parallel.[139] A parallel post is more retentive than a tapered post but also requires removal of more root dentin during the preparation of the post space. Parallel posts are reported to be less likely to cause root fractures than tapered posts, although they are less conforming to the original shape of the root.[79,152,161] Unfortunately, modern techniques for root canal preparation use tapered nickel-titanium (NiTi) rotary shaping files, which result in a very wide tapered and unretentive canal exhibiting a significant divergence from apical to coronal.[145] Longer posts are often necessary to accommodate this problem and offer adequate retention; adequate length in the root canal is considered to be greater than 6 mm. When teeth are protected by crowns with an adequate ferrule, longer posts do not further increase fracture resistance.[80] Posts designed with mechanical locking features in the heads and roughened surface texture can show better retention of the core.[29]

Fiber Posts

A fiber post consists of reinforcing fibers embedded in a resin-polymerized matrix. Monomers used to form the resin matrix are typically bifunctional methacrylates (Bis-GMA, UDMA, TEGDMA), but epoxies have also been used. Common fibers in today's fiber posts are made of carbon, glass, silica, or quartz but the type, volume content, and uniformity of the fibers and the matrix are proprietary and vary among fiber post systems. These differences in the manufacturing process may reflect the large variations observed among different types of fiber posts subjected to a fatigue-resistance test.[63] Fibers are commonly 7 to 20 μm in diameter and are used in a number of configurations, including braided, woven, and longitudinal. The original fiber posts consisted of carbon fibers embedded in epoxy resin, but quartz-fiber posts are currently preferred for their favorable mechanical properties, aesthetic qualities, and ability to chemically bond to the polymer matrix.[49] One study indicates that the flexural strength of glass-, silica-, or quartz-fiber posts approximates 1000 MPa and that flexural modulus is about 23 GPa.[35] Current fiber posts are radiopaque and may also conduct the light for polymerization of resin-based luting cements. A light-transmitting post results in better polymerization of resin composites in the apical area of simulated root canals, as measured by hardness values.[141,174] To enhance bonding at the post/core/cement interfaces, several physicochemical pretreatments such as silanization or sand blasting of the post surface have been described. Research indicates that silanization, hydrofluoric etching, and sandblasting (with 30 to 50 μm Al_2O_3) do not modify the mechanical properties of different glass-, silica-, or quartz-fiber posts.[5]

It is generally accepted that bonding fiber posts to root canal dentin can improve the distribution of forces applied along the root, thereby decreasing the risk of root fracture and contributing to the reinforcement of the remaining tooth structure.[12,18] A well-adapted adhesively cemented fiber post is considered the most retentive with the least stress generated on the canal walls. In a retrospective study that evaluated three types of bonded fiber posts, investigators reported a 3.2% failure of 1306 fiber posts in recalls of 1 to 6 years.[54] More recently, another study reported survival rates of 98.6% and 96.8% for parallel-sided and tapered fiber posts, respectively, placed in anterior teeth covered with full-ceramic crowns after a mean observation period of 5.3 years.[156]

Zirconia posts are composed of zirconium dioxide (ZrO_2) partially stabilized with yttrium oxide and exhibit a high flexural strength. Zirconia posts are aesthetic, partially adhesive, rigid, but also brittle. Zirconia posts cannot be etched, and available literature suggests that bonding resins to these materials is less predictable and requires substantially different bonding methods than conventional ceramics.[11] When a composite core is built on a zirconia post, core retention may also be a problem. Controversies exist about the efficiency of airborne particle abrasion at establishing a durable resin bond to zirconia posts treated or not treated with a coupling agent.[1,127] Overall, there are concerns about the rigidity of zirconia posts, which tends to make those posts too brittle. Other reports indicate that the rigidity of zirconia posts negatively affects the quality of the interface between the resin core material and dentin when subjected to fatigue testing.[40,43]

Core Materials

The core replaces carious, fractured, or missing coronal structure and helps to retain the final restoration. Desirable physical characteristics of a core include (1) high compressive and flexural strength, (2) dimensional stability, (3) ease of manipulation, (4) short setting time, and (5) the ability to bond to both tooth and post. Core materials include composite resin, cast metal or ceramic, amalgam, and sometimes glass-ionomer materials. The core is anchored to the tooth by extension into the coronal aspect of the canal or through the endodontic post. The importance of retention between the post, the core, and the tooth increases as remaining tooth structure decreases.

Composite Resin Core

Composite core materials take a number of strategies to enhance their strength and resistance; metal may be added, filler levels may be greater, or faster-setting ionomers may be used.[134] Composite core materials have been shown to exhibit slightly better mechanical values than conventional materials, but improvements are negligible.[176] However, they appear to be superior to silver-glass-ionomer cement and amalgam.[30] The advantages of composite core resins are adhesive bonding to tooth structure and many posts, ease of manipulation, rapid setting, and translucent or highly opaque formulations. Composite cores have been shown to protect the strength of all-ceramic crowns equally to amalgam cores. Bond strength of composite cores to dentin depends on a complete curing of the resin materials, so dentin bonding agents must be chemically compatible with composite core materials. Self-cure composite resins require self-cure adhesives and are mostly incompatible with light-cure adhesives.[26] However, no adhesive has been shown to completely eliminate microleakage at the margins of the restoration.[17] A degradation of the resin core or the marginal integrity of the crown can result in invasion of oral fluids. Therefore, as with all buildup materials for decimated teeth, more than 2 mm of sound tooth structure should remain at the margin for optimal composite resin core function.

Composite core materials can be used in association with metallic, fiber, or zirconia posts. This is frequently observed in the presence of structurally compromised teeth. They may provide some protection from root fracture in teeth restored with metal posts compared with amalgam or gold cores. Loosening of the post, core, and crown with composite core can occur, but composite cores have been shown to fail more favorably than amalgam or gold.[129] A retrospective study of the clinical performance of fiber posts indicates that fiber posts and cores have a failure rate ranging between 7% and 11% after a service period of 7 to 11 years and that post loosening may also occur.[53] Composite core materials are typically two-paste, self-cured composites, but light-curing materials are also available. The use of light-curing composite core materials generally eliminates the risk of chemical incompatibility between adhesives and self-curing resin core materials. Bonding light-cured resin composites to the irregular structure of the pulp chamber and canal orifices might eliminate the need for a post when sufficient tooth structure remains. Research indicates that bonding to the dentin walls of the pulp chamber is easier and superior to resin dentin bonds made on dentin canal walls.[7]

Amalgam Core

Dental amalgam is a traditional core buildup material with a long history of clinical success. Although there are many variations in the alloy's composition, more recent formulations have high compressive strength (400 MPa after 24 hours), high tensile strength, and a high modulus of elasticity. High-copper alloys tend to be stiffer (60 GPa) than low-copper alloys.

Amalgam can be used with or without a post. In the 1980s, investigators described the amalcore.[113] With the amalcore technique, amalgam is compacted into the pulp chamber and 2 to 3 mm coronally of each canal. The following criteria were considered for the application of this technique: the remaining pulp chamber should be of sufficient width and depth to provide adequate bulk and retention of the amalgam restoration, and an adequate dentin thickness around the pulp chamber was required for the tooth-restoration continuum rigidity and strength. The fracture resistance of the amalgam coronal-radicular restoration with four or more millimeters of chamber wall was shown to be adequate, although the extension into the root canal space had little influence.[81]

Amalgam can also be used in combination with a prefabricated metallic post when the retention offered by the remaining coronal tissue needs to be increased. Amalgam cores are highly retentive when used with a preformed metal post in posterior teeth; they require more force to dislodge than cast posts and cores.[102] Others have suggested the use of adhesive resins to bond amalgam to coronal tissue.[155]

Significant disadvantages of amalgam cores are the "nonadhesive nature" of the material, the potential for corrosion, and subsequent discoloration of the gingiva or dentin. Amalgam use is declining worldwide because of legislative, safety, and environmental issues.

Glass Ionomer Core and Modified Glass Ionomer Core

Glass ionomer and resin-modified glass ionomer cements are adhesive materials useful for small buildups or to fill undercuts in prepared teeth. The rationale for using glass ionomer materials is based on their cariostatic effect resulting from fluoride release. However, their low strength and fracture toughness result in brittleness, which contraindicates the use of glass-ionomer buildups in thin anterior teeth or to replace unsupported cusps. They may be indicated in posterior teeth in which (1) a bulk of core material is possible, (2) significant sound dentin remains, and (3) caries control is indicated.[172]

Resin-modified glass ionomer materials are a combination of glass ionomer and composite resin technologies and have properties of both materials. Resin-modified glass ionomers have moderate strength, greater than glass ionomers but less than composite resins. As a core material, they are adequate for moderate-sized buildups, but hygroscopic expansion can cause fracture of ceramic crowns and fragilized roots.[158] The bond to dentin is close to that of dentin-bonded composite resin and significantly higher than traditional glass ionomers. Today, resin composites have replaced glass ionomer materials for core fabrication.

Indirect Foundation Restorations: Cast Post and Core

For many years, use of the cast metal post and core has been the traditional method for fabricating the foundation restoration of a prosthetic crown. Classically, smooth-sided, tapered posts conforming to the taper of the root canal are fabricated from high noble alloys, although noble and base-metal classes of dental alloys have also been used. Noble alloys used for post and core fabrication have high stiffness (approximately 80 to 100 GPa), strength (1500 MPa), hardness, and excellent resistance to corrosion.[31]

One advantage of the cast post/core system is that the core is an integral extension of the post and that the core does not depend on mechanical means for retention on the post. This construction prevents dislodgment of the core from the post and root when minimal tooth structure remains. However, the cast post/core system also has several disadvantages. Valuable tooth structure must be removed to create a path of insertion or withdrawal. Second, the procedure is expensive because two appointments are needed, and laboratory costs may be significant. The laboratory phase is technique sensitive. Metal casting of a pattern with a large core and a small-diameter post can result in porosity in the gold at the post/core interface. Fracture of the metal at this interface under function results in failure of the restoration. Most important, the cast post/core system has a higher clinical rate of root fracture than preformed posts.[47,159]

Studies on cast post retention have shown that the post must fit the prepared root canal as closely as possible to be perfectly retained. When a ferrule is present, custom cast posts and cores exhibit a higher fracture resistance compared to composite cores built on prefabricated metallic posts or carbon posts.[98] Cast posts are also known to exhibit the least amount of retention and are associated with a higher failure rate compared to prefabricated parallel-sided posts. In a classic retrospective study (1 to 20 years) of 1273 endodontically treated teeth in general practice, 245 (19.2%) were restored with tapered cast posts and cores. Among these, 12.7% were deemed failures. This failure rate was higher than that for the other passive post systems used. Of particular concern was the fact that 39% of the failures led to unrestorable teeth requiring extraction. Thirty-six percent of the failures were due to loss of retention, and 58% were due to the fracture of the root. It has been suggested that tapered smooth-sided posts have a "wedging" effect under functional loading, and it is this that leads to increased risk of root fracture.[162]

One 6-year retrospective study reported a success rate higher than 90% using a cast post and core as a foundation restoration.[8] The lower failure rate and fewer root fractures were attributed to the presence of an adequate ferrule and careful tooth preparation. Attention has also been drawn to the fact that the higher failure rate may be due to the fact that nearly half of the posts were shorter than recommended from the literature. A venting groove for the cement along the axis of the post results in less stress on residual tissues.

Luting Cements

A variety of cements have been used to cement endodontic posts and include traditional cements, glass ionomer cements, and resin-based luting cements.

Traditional Cements

Zinc phosphate cements or polycarboxylate cements are still used for cementation of posts and crowns. They are generally supplied as a powder and a liquid, and their physical properties are highly influenced by the mixing ratio of the components. Their compressive strength is about 100 MPa, and elastic moduli are lower than that of dentin (5 to 12 GPa). Zinc phosphate cement is mostly used for cementing metal restorations and posts; film thickness of the zinc phosphate cement is less than 25 μm. These cements provide retention through mechanical means and have no chemical bond to the post or to dentin but provide clinically sufficient retention for posts in teeth with adequate tooth structure.

Glass Ionomer Luting Cements

Glass ionomer cements are a mixture of glass particles and polyacids, but resin monomers may also be added. Depending on the resin content, glass ionomer cements can be classified as either conventional or resin-modified glass ionomer cements. Conventional glass ionomer cements have compressive strengths ranging between 100 and 200 MPa; the Young modulus is generally about 5 GPa. They are mechanically more resistant than zinc phosphate cements, and they can bond to dentin with values ranging between 3 and 5 MPa. Some authors still recommend the use of glass ionomer cements for the cementation of metallic posts. Major advantages of conventional glass ionomer cements are their ease of manipulation, chemical setting, and ability to bond to both tooth and post. On the contrary, resin-modified glass ionomer cements are not indicated for post cementation, because these cements exhibit hygroscopic expansion that can promote fracture of the root.

Resin-Based Luting Cements

Today there is a trend toward the use of adhesive cements for bonding endodontic posts during the restoration of nonvital teeth. The rationale for using adhesive cements is based on the premise that bonding posts to root canal dentin will reinforce the tooth and help retain the post and the restoration.[48] Contemporary resin-based luting cements have been shown to exhibit compressive strengths around 200 MPa and elastic moduli between 4 and 10 GPa.[24] These materials may be polymerized through a chemical reaction, a photopolymerization process, or a combination of both mechanisms. Photopolymerization of these resin-based materials is often necessary to maximize strength and rigidity.

Most luting cements require a pretreatment of the root canal dentin with either etch-and-rinse or self-etching adhesives. Both types of adhesives have been shown to form hybrid layers along the walls of the post spaces.[10] However, bonding to root canal dentin may be compromised by the use of endodontic irrigants such as sodium hypochlorite, hydrogen peroxide, or their combination.[115] Because these chemicals are strong oxidizing agents, they leave behind an oxygen-rich layer on the dentin surface that inhibits the polymerization of the resin.[151] Previous research has shown that the bond strength of C&B Metabond to root canal dentin was reduced by half when the dentin was previously treated with 5% sodium hypochlorite (NaOCl) or 15% EDTA/10% urea peroxide (RC Prep, Premier Dental, Plymouth Meeting, PA).[107] Other reports indicate that the contamination of the dentin walls by eugenol diffusing from endodontic sealers may also affect the retention of bonded posts.[66,168] Further, it is difficult to control the amount of moisture left in a root canal after acid etching, making impregnation of collagen fibers with etch-and-rinse adhesives problematic. The use of self-etching adhesives has been proposed as an alternative for the cementation of endodontic posts, because self-etching adhesives are generally used on dry dentin and do not require rinsing of the etchant. However, their efficiency at infiltrating thick smear layers like those produced during post space preparation remains controversial.[104,171] More recently, dual-curing adhesives have been developed to ensure a better polymerization of the resin deep inside the root canal. Dual-cured adhesives contain ternary catalysts to offset the acid-base reaction between the acidic monomers and the basic amines along the composite/adhesive interface.[105]

Although both self-curing and light-curing luting cements can be used for cementation of prefabricated endodontic posts, most resin cements have a dual-curing process that requires light exposure to initiate the polymerization reaction. Dual-curing cements are preferred because there are concerns as to whether light-curing materials are properly cured, especially in areas of difficult light access such as the apical portion of the root canal. However, it has been reported that photocured composites generate more shrinkage stress and exhibit less flow than chemically cured composites.[52] Contraction stresses induced by polymerization also depend on the geometry of the post space and the thickness of the resin film. Previous research indicates that the restriction of flow of resin cements by the configuration of the root canal can significantly increase the contraction stress at the adhesive interface.[51,166]

In recent years, a number of techniques have been used to measure the adhesion of resin-based luting cements to root canal dentin. These methods include the pull-out tests, the microtensile bond strength tests, and the push-out tests.[45,61] Although laboratory tests confirmed that bond strengths ranging between 10 and 15 MPa can be obtained with modern resin-based luting cement, there is also evidence that frictional retention is a factor contributing to post retention.[14] It is generally accepted that bonding to dentin of the pulp chamber is more reliable than bonding to root canal dentin, especially at the apical level.[126] The lowered bond strength values recorded at the apical third of the root canal are likely to be related to the reduced number of dentinal tubules available for dentin hybridization. Shorter posts may be used when successful bonding occurs between fiber-reinforced posts and root dentin, because current adhesive luting cements can assist in the retention of posts in the root canal space.[132]

Another factor that may influence the performance of resin-based luting cements is the thickness of the cement layer. The cementation of endodontic fiber posts with thicker cement layers might be required when posts do not perfectly fit inside the root canal. Although a slight increase in cement thickness (up to 150 microns) does not significantly affect the performance of adhesive luting cements applied to root canal dentin, thicker layers may be detrimental to bond quality.[76,150]

One study indicates that bond strength to radicular dentin might be maximized by adopting procedures that compensate for polymerization stresses.[13] The bonding procedures are realized in two separate steps. The initial step allows optimal resin film formation and polymerization along the root canal walls, leading to more ideal resin-dentin hybridization without stresses imposed by the placement of the post. A second step bonds the post to the cured resin film. The polymerization shrinkage that occurs during the initial adhesive coating step reduces the effects of stress imposed when the resin-coated post polymerizes, thereby preserving the bond integrity.

Although the bonding performance of resin-based luting cements is well documented, other reports indicate that resin-dentin bonds degrade over time.[22,56] The loss of bond strength and seal are attributed to the degradation of the hybrid layer created at the dentin-adhesive interface. This is particularly true for etch-and-rinse adhesives, because the gelatinization of collagen fibers caused by phosphoric acids may restrict the diffusion of the resin within the interfibrillar spaces and may leave unprotected fibers available for degradation. Removing organic components from the demineralized dentin prior to bonding procedures has been suggested. The use of dilute NaOCl (0.5%) after acid etching or the conditioning of dentin smear layers with EDTA (0.1 M, pH 7.4) has been shown to produce more durable resin-dentin bonds made with single-step etch-and-rinse adhesives.[149]

Other research indicates that the degradation of denuded collagen fibrils exposed in incompletely infiltrated hybrid layers is driven by an endogenous proteolytic mechanism involving the activity of matrix metalloproteinases (MMPs).[21,125] The release of MMPs such as collagenases has been evidenced in both coronal and root dentin of fully developed teeth of young patients.[147] Researchers suggest that conditioning root canal dentin with a broad-spectrum protease inhibitor such as chlorhexidine (2 wt% chlorhexidine digluconate solution) might be useful for the preservation of dentin bond strength over time.[20]

Interestingly, these dentin-conditioning procedures, which may improve the resistance of the resin-dentin bond to chemical degradation, also act as antibacterial agents; this might be of interest in the endodontic context.

Self-Adhesive Cements

More recently, self-adhesive resin cements have been introduced as an alternative to conventional resin-based luting cements. Self-adhesive luting cements contain multifunctional phosphoric acid methacrylates that react with hydroxyapatite and simultaneously demineralize and infiltrate dental hard tissue.[108] They do not require any pretreatment of the tooth substrates, and their clinical application is accomplished in a single step. Therefore, the self-etching capability of these new cements reduces the risk for incomplete impregnation of the conditioned tissue by the resins and reduces technique sensitivity. The elastic moduli of chemically cured self-adhesive resin cements are relatively low (4 to 8 GPa) but generally increase when a dual-curing process is used. It is therefore recommended that all dual-cured resin cements receive maximal light to achieve superior material properties wherever clinically possible.[135] Adhesion performance to dentin was found comparable to multistep luting cements, but bonding to enamel without prior phosphoric acid etching is not recommended.[72] However, their long-term clinical performances need to be assessed before making a general recommendation for their use.

PRETREATMENT EVALUATION AND TREATMENT STRATEGY

Before any therapy is initiated, the tooth must be thoroughly evaluated to ensure treatment success. Each tooth must be examined individually and in the context of its contribution to the overall treatment plan and rehabilitation. This assessment includes endodontic, periodontal, biomechanical, and aesthetic evaluations. Planning of the restoration for endodontically treated teeth brings together all aforementioned biomechanical and clinical factors, as well as the various materials and procedures designed to address them.

Pretreatment Evaluation

Endodontic Evaluation

The prerestorative examination should include an inspection of the quality of existing endodontic treatment. New restorations, particularly complex restorations, should not be placed on abutment teeth with a questionable endodontic prognosis. Endodontic retreatment is indicated for teeth showing radiographic signs of apical periodontitis or clinical symptoms of inflammation. Restorations that require a post need a post space, which is prepared by removal of gutta-percha from the canal. Canals obturated with a silver cone or other inappropriate filling material should be endodontically retreated before starting any restorative therapy. Because the probability for periapical tissue to heal after endodontic retreatment is reasonably high, the chances to retain a well-restored tooth in asymptomatic function over time are excellent.[119]

Periodontal Evaluation

Maintenance of periodontal health is also critical to the long-term success of endodontically treated teeth. The periodontal condition of the tooth must therefore be determined before the start of endodontic therapy and restorative phase. The following conditions are to be considered as critical for treatment success:

- Healthy gingival tissue
- Normal bone architecture and attachment levels to favor periodontal health
- Maintenance of biologic width and ferrule effect before and after endodontic and restorative phases

If one or more of the aforementioned conditions are not met owing to preexisting pathology or structural defects, treatment success or even feasibility can be compromised, sometimes suggesting extraction of weak teeth and replacement with dental implants rather than conventional therapy.

Biomechanical Evaluation

All previous events, from initial decay or trauma to final root canal therapy, influence the biomechanical status of the tooth and the selection of restorative materials and procedures. The biomechanical status can even justify the decision to extract extremely mutilated teeth that do not deserve extensive treatments that carry a limited probability of success. Important clinical factors include the following:

- The amount and quality of remaining tooth structure
- The anatomic position of the tooth
- The occlusal forces on the tooth
- The restorative requirements of the tooth

Teeth with minimal remaining tooth structure are at increased risk for the following clinical complications[114,165,170] (see Fig. 22-1 and Fig. 22-4):

- Root fracture
- Coronal-apical leakage

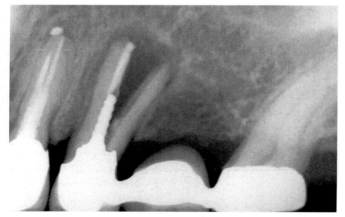

FIG. 22-4 Failure of prosthetic foundations can have dramatic consequences on both overlying restorations and surrounding tissues. A better understanding of compositional and structural changes that affect tooth resistance to repeated functional forces is mandatory to improve treatment success in endodontically treated teeth.

- Recurrent caries
- Dislodgment or loss of the core/prosthesis
- Periodontal injury from biologic width invasion

The amount and quality of remaining tooth substrate are far more important to the long-term prognosis of the restored tooth than any restorative material properties. One must consider that no restorative material can truly substitute for dentin or enamel and that a minimal amount of intact structure is mandatory to justify tooth maintenance and its strategic importance to the overall treatment plan. The presence of healthy adjacent teeth available as abutments or the option of dental implants are additional factors to be analyzed when justifying the restoration of endodontically treated teeth.

Tooth Position, Occlusal Forces, and Parafunctions

Teeth are subjected to cyclic axial and nonaxial forces. The teeth and associated restorations must resist these forces to limit potential damages such as wear or fracture. The degree and direction of forces depend on the location of the tooth in the arch, the occlusal scheme, and the patient's functional status.

In most occlusal schemes, anterior teeth protect posterior teeth from lateral forces through anterolateral guidance. In the context of very steep anterior guidance and deep vertical overbite, maxillary anterior teeth are sustaining higher protrusive and lateral forces from the mandibular anterior teeth. Restorations of damaged anterior teeth with heavy function should therefore be designed to resist flexion. Restorative components should be stronger than would be required for teeth with an edge-to-edge relationship and therefore vertical forces.

Posterior teeth normally carry more vertical forces, especially when maintaining canine and anterior guidance; they also sustain greater occlusal loads than anterior teeth, and restorations must be planned to protect posterior teeth against fracture. In the case of parafunctions, protection by anterior contacts is likely to be reduced or lost and posterior teeth then submitted to more lateral stresses, generating a higher demand for restorative materials.

The literature reports that average biting forces vary between 25 and 75 N in the anterior region and between 40 and 125 N for the posterior region of the mouth, depending on food type, dental status (dentate or edentulous), and patient anatomy and functional habits.[55,71] Those forces can easily reach 1000 N or above in case of parafunctions, showing how potentially destructive they can be for intact teeth and even more so for nonvital, fragilized teeth. Parafunctional habits (clenching and bruxism) are major causes of fatigue or traumatic injury to teeth, including wear, cracks, and fractures. Teeth that show extensive wear or sequelae from parafunctions, especially heavy lateral function, require components with the highest physical properties to protect restored teeth against fracture.

In general, modern strategy focuses on tissue preservation and also on the use of adhesion to stabilize the restoration for improved short- and long-term service. However, in certain conditions like reduced tooth support, conventional materials are not obsolete.

Aesthetic Evaluation and Requirements

Anterior teeth, premolars, and often the maxillary first molar, along with the surrounding gingiva, compose the aesthetic zone of the mouth. Changes in the color or translucency of the visible tooth structure, along with thin soft tissues or

TABLE 22-2

Clinical Protocols for Restoring Nonvital Teeth with Partial Restorations (Most Likely Procedures)

Treatment Approach	Indications	Tooth Preparation (Critical Guidelines)	Interface Treatment		Restoration Fabrication
			Tooth	Restoration	
Composite restoration	Minimal tissue loss	None	DBA	—	Direct multilayer
Veneer	Limited tissue loss	≥ 1 mm Buccal reduction, lingual enamel present, minimal to moderate discoloration only	DBA	1. Sandblasting or etching 2. Silane 3. Bonding resin	CP direct multilayer *or* *In laboratory:* Etchable CER: fired, pressed, or CAD-CAM
Overlay (composite/ ceramics)	Thin remaining walls	Minimum 2 mm occlusal reduction	DBA + composite lining	1. Sandblasting or etching 2. Silane 3. Bonding resin	*In laboratory:* CP: hand-shaped, light or heat cured, CAD-CAM Etchable CER: fired, pressed, or CAD-CAM
Endocrown (composite/ ceramics)	Loss of occlusal anatomy	Minimum 2 mm occlusal reduction, extension into pulpal chamber	DBA + composite lining	1. Sandblasting or etching 2. Silane 3. Bonding resin	*In laboratory:* CP: hand-shaped, light or heat cured, CAD-CAM Etchable CER: fired, pressed, or CAD-CAM

CAD-CAM, computer-aided design/computer-aided machined; *CER,* ceramic; *CP,* composite; *DBA,* dentin bonding agent.

biotype, diminish the chance for a successful aesthetic treatment outcome.

Potential aesthetic complications should be investigated before endodontic therapy is initiated. For instance, metal or dark carbon fiber posts or amalgam placed in the pulpal chamber can result in unacceptable aesthetic results, such as a grayish appearance of the overlying prosthetic restoration (especially with modern, more translucent full-ceramic crowns) or gingival discoloration from the underlying cervical area or root (see Fig. 22-1). All teeth located in the aesthetic zone also require critical control of endodontic filling materials in the coronal third of the canal and the pulp chamber to avoid or reduce the risk of discoloration. Careful selection of restorative materials, careful handling of tissues, and timely endodontic intervention are important for preserving the natural appearance of nonvital teeth and gingiva.

Treatment Strategy

General Principles and Guidelines

The post, the core, and their luting or bonding agents together form the *foundation restoration* to support the coronal restoration of endodontically treated teeth. The evolution of foundation restorations has been to diminish invasiveness, to use adhesion rather than macromechanical anchorage, and to eliminate intraradicular components in selected cases. These changing clinical concepts derive from both an improved understanding of tooth biomechanics and advances in restorative materials.

The foundation and its different constituents are then aimed at providing the best protection against leakage-related caries, fracture, or restoration dislodgment. Therefore, all aforementioned local and general parameters are to be systematically analyzed in order to select the best treatment approach and restorative materials. Prosthetic requirements are also to be taken into consideration to complete each case analysis. In general, abutments for fixed or removable partial dentures

clearly dictate more extensive protective and retentive features than do single crowns, owing to greater transverse and torquing forces. This modern biomechanical treatment strategy is summarized in Figure 22-5.

Structurally Sound Anterior Teeth

Anterior teeth can lose vitality as a result of a trauma with no or minimal structural damage. They generally do not require a crown, core, or post; restorative treatment is limited to sealing the access cavity and direct composite fillings. Discoloration, whenever present, is addressed by nonvital bleaching, or, for untreatable or relapsing ones, with conservative restorative approaches such as direct or indirect veneers (Table 22-2).

Nonvital Posterior Teeth with Minimal/ Reduced Tissue Loss

The loss of vitality in posterior teeth resulting from trauma, decay, or a restorative procedure does not necessarily lead to extreme biomechanical involvement and therefore allows, in certain conditions, for conservative restorations.

Occlusal cavities or mesio/disto-occlusal cavities can be restored with either direct- or indirect-adhesive intracoronal restorations, providing residual walls are thick enough (proximal ridges and buccolingual walls more than 1.5-mm thickness). The three additional clinical factors that must be analyzed to ensure optimal treatment success are the configuration factor (C-factor), cavity volume, and dentin quality. For instance, a large class I cavity with contaminated and sclerotic dentin would clearly be a contraindication to the direct approach, despite the fact that it apparently falls within the indications of direct techniques. Conservative options must, however, always be analyzed under the light of functional and occlusal environment. They can only be considered in the absence of parafunctions and with anterior guidance, which limits overall functional loading and lateral or flexural forces.

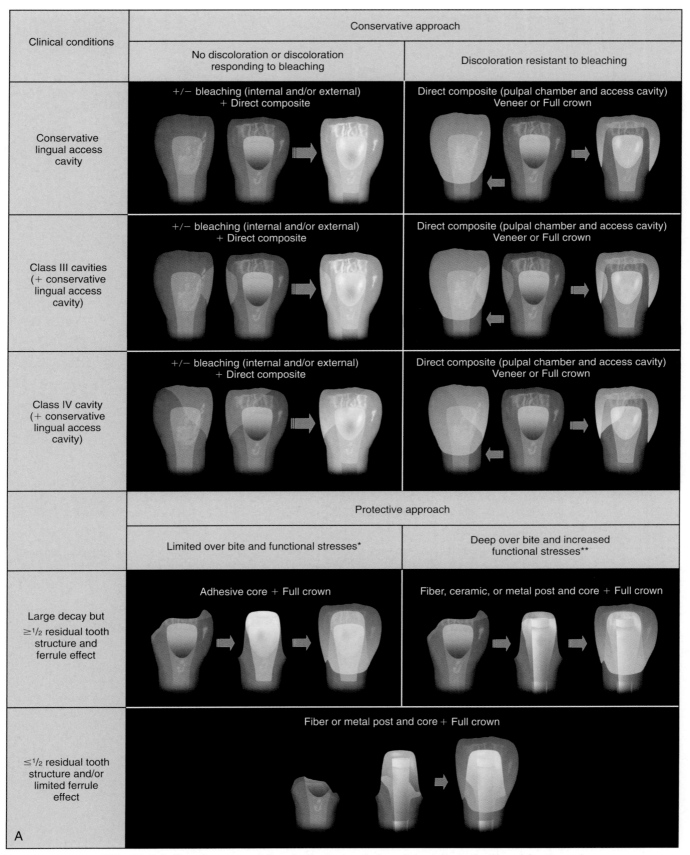

FIG. 22-5 A, Current recommendations for the treatment of nonvital anterior teeth. *Normal function and anterior guidance; **moderate to severe parafunctions and abnormal occlusion/anterior guidance.

Continued

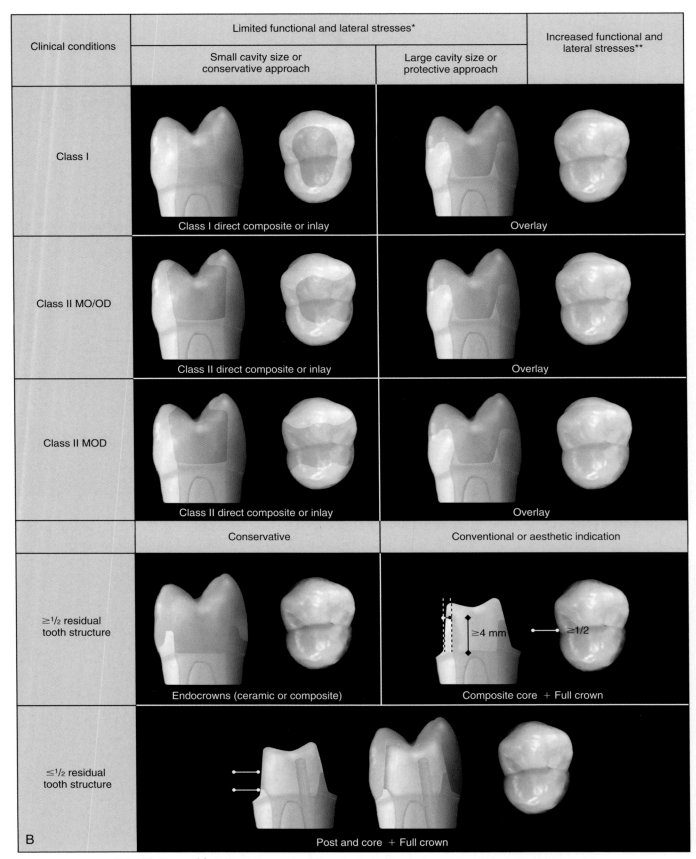

Clinical conditions	Limited functional and lateral stresses*		Increased functional and lateral stresses**
	Small cavity size or conservative approach	Large cavity size or protective approach	
Class I	Class I direct composite or inlay	Overlay	
Class II MO/OD	Class II direct composite or inlay	Overlay	
Class II MOD	Class II direct composite or inlay	Overlay	
	Conservative	Conventional or aesthetic indication	
≥¹/₂ residual tooth structure	Endocrowns (ceramic or composite)	≥4 mm ≥1/2 Composite core + Full crown	
≤¹/₂ residual tooth structure	Post and core + Full crown		

FIG. 22-5, cont'd B, Current recommendations for the treatment of nonvital posterior teeth. *Relatively flat anatomy and canine guidance, normal function; **group guidance, steep occlusal anatomy, parafunctions.

In less favorable biomechanical conditions (e.g.,) group guidance, steep occlusal anatomy, bruxism, clenching a protective approach with full occlusal coverage (onlay or overlay) is mandated to minimize the risk of fatigue failures (see Table 22-2).

Structurally Compromised Teeth

The decision for placing a post as well as the selection of a post system (rigid or nonrigid) depends once again on the amount and quality of remaining tooth structure and the anticipated forces sustained by this tooth (Table 22-3).

In general, rigid posts made of stiff materials (metal and ceramics) are indicated for teeth with minimal tooth structure

that rely on the post to hold the core and crown. Because rigid posts flex and bend less than other types of posts, they are supposed to limit movement of the core and possible disruption of the crown margins and cement seal. But one must remember that stiff posts transmit more stresses to the root, next to the post apex, when conventionally cemented. An attempt to strengthen a weak root by adding a stiff post can instead make the root weaker as a result of the force concentration behavior of a stiff rod in a more flexible material. Adhesion therefore plays a crucial role, because a well-bonded post can help absorb stresses more evenly throughout the remaining tooth structure. Benefit and increased risk of fissure and

TABLE 22-3

Clinical Protocols for Restoring Nonvital Teeth with Full Prosthetic Restorations (Most Likely Procedures)

Treatment Approach	Indications	Tooth Preparation (Critical Guidelines)	Foundation		Restoration	
			Post	Core	Fabrication	Luting
Composite core	Reduced walls but > ½ crown height	Maintain all residual structures > 1 mm thickness (after core prep.)	—	DBA + composite Dual or LC, incremental	*In laboratory:* PFM or full ceramic restoration: slip-casting, pressed, or CAD-CAM	Coating, sandblasting, or etching + silane and Dual or SA cement
Composite core + ceramic post	More than ½ coronal structure lost, reduced wall height	Maintain all residual structures > 1 mm thickness (after core prep.)	Sandblasting or coating/silane + DBA + Dual cement or SA cement	DBA + composite Dual or LC, incremental	*In laboratory:* PFM or full ceramic restoration: slip-casting, pressed, or CAD-CAM	Coating, sandblasting, or etching + silane and Dual or SA cement
Composite core + in vitro fiber post	More than ½ coronal structure lost, reduced wall height	Maintain all residual structures > 1 mm thickness (after core prep.)	Sandblasting or coating/silane + DBA + Dual cement or SA cement	DBA + composite Dual or LC, incremental	*In laboratory:* PFM or full ceramic restoration: slip-casting, pressed, or CAD-CAM	Coating, sandblasting, or etching + silane and Dual or SA cement
Composite core + metal post	More than ⅔ coronal structure lost, reduced wall height	Maintain all residual structures > 1 mm thickness (after core prep.)	Sandblasting or coating/silane + DBA + Dual cement or SA cement	DBA + composite Dual or LC, incremental	*In laboratory:* PFM or full ceramic restoration: slip-casting, pressed, or CAD-CAM	Coating, sandblasting, or etching + silane and Dual or SA cement
Amalgam core (+/− metal post)	Alternative to composite core with metal post	Maintain all residual structures > 1 mm thickness (after core prep.)	No tt + nonadhesive cement or sandblasting/ coating/silane + DBA + Dual cement or SA cement	Amalgam placement in retentive cavity/ preparation	*In laboratory:* PFM restoration	Coating, sandblasting, or etching + silane and Dual or SA cement
Cast gold post and core (+/− porcelain)	More than ¾ coronal structure lost	Maintain all residual structures > 1 mm thickness (after core prep.) Internal walls are divergent	No tt/sandblasting + nonadhesive cement or sandblasting/ coating/silane + DBA + Dual cement or SA cement	No tt + nonadhesive cement or DBA + Dual cement or SA cement	*In laboratory:* PFM or full ceramic restoration: Zirconia/ CAD-CAM	Coating, sandblasting, or etching + silane and Dual or SA cement

CAD-CAM, computer-aided design/computer-aided machined; *CER*, ceramic; *DBA*, dentin bonding agent; *Dual*, dual curing; *LC*, light curing; *PFM*, porcelain fused to metal; *SA*, self-adhesive.

fracture must then be appropriately weighed against adhesion potential inside the root and post type, composition, and surface treatment.

In structurally sound teeth, nonrigid posts flex with the tooth under functional forces, reducing the transfer of force to the root and reducing the risk of root fracture. Flexion is of course related to post diameter. In structurally compromised teeth, which lack cervical stiffness from dentin and ferrule effect, excessive post flexion can be detrimental to the marginal seal and prosthesis longevity, so fiber posts are generally contraindicated.

White or translucent fiber posts are generally preferred underneath full-ceramic restorations, whereas stronger black carbon fiber posts, which can reflect through gingiva, tooth structure, or ceramic restorations, are usually used in teeth to be restored with gold or porcelain fused to metal crowns, as well as in zirconia-based restorations. The literature has largely overemphasized the impact of post color on restoration aesthetics. Metal or carbon post color can be masked with resin opaquer and gold post and core ceramized to enhance aesthetic integration. Such procedures can help to approach a more ideal restoration biomechanical behavior through the fabrication of rigid but more aesthetic foundations. Upper lateral and lower incisors, together with extremely thin biotype, are probably the only real aesthetic contraindication for metal or carbon fiber posts.

In cases of extreme tooth fragility secondary to caries, fracture, previous overenlargement of the root canal system, or immaturity, residual root structure can be unified and reinforced with adhesive bonding and composite before placing a normal-diameter post, forming an altogether cohesive unit, as previously described.

In conclusion, in a damaged tooth that is to be restored with a nonrigid post, 2 to 3 mm of cervical tooth structure must ideally remain to allow creation of a restoration as a whole that is resistant to flexion. Teeth with minimal tooth structure and limited ferrule effect need additional cervical stiffness from a more rigid post to resist distortion. In this situation, adhesive cementation is preferred to conventional cementation.

Structurally Compromised Anterior Teeth

Restoration of endodontically treated teeth becomes more complex as teeth or supporting structures become increasingly affected. A nonvital anterior tooth that has lost significant tooth structure requires restoration with a crown, supported and retained by a core and possibly a post as well.

When less than half the core height is present, or when remaining walls are extremely thin (less than 1 mm on more than three fourths of the tooth circumference), a post is needed to increase retention and stabilize and reinforce the foundation. Many post options are available nowadays, including titanium, fiber-reinforced resin, and ceramics. Adhesion is now the preferred mode of post cementation unless a long-term contamination of root dentin is obvious (e.g., with eugenol), making adhesion highly questionable.

In the latter situation or in the presence of flared canals (possibly as well when a limited ferrule effect is present), cast gold post and core are still considered a feasible option. Actually, in this extremely unfavorable biomechanical environment, this traditional treatment approach provides a higher rigidity in the cervical area, which is mandatory for restoration stability. Here, a fiber-reinforced composite foundation having

higher flexibility might present less favorable biomechanical behavior, such as suggested by FEM studies[42] (see Fig. 22-3 and Table 22-2). Tooth extraction and implant placement or bonded bridge (particularly for lateral incisors) are also to be considered in this situation.

In the aesthetic zone, the post should not detract from the aesthetics of the coronal tooth structure, ceramic crown, or gingiva. Current restorative procedures allow fabrication of highly aesthetic ceramic coronal restorations that have no metal substructure. When such restorations with remarkably lifelike color and vitality are selected, it usually implies the use of nonmetal aesthetic posts, either ceramic or resin fiber-reinforced ones.

Structurally Compromised Posterior Teeth

Slightly decayed posterior teeth in the context of parafunctions or significantly fragilized premolars and molars require cuspal protection afforded by onlay restoration, endocrown, or a full crown. The need for a post and core depends on the amount of remaining tooth structure. When remaining walls (buccal and lingual) provide more than 3 to 4 mm height (from the pulpal chamber floor) and 1.5 to 2 mm thickness, core and restoration stability are granted through macromechanical retention or adhesion; then, posts are not needed (see Fig. 22-5). With current treatment strategy, *the post has become the exception rather than the rule for the restoration of nonvital posterior teeth*.

Additional Procedures

Periodontal crown lengthening surgery or orthodontic extrusion can expose additional root structure to allow restoration of a severely damaged tooth. In the smile frame, crown lengthening might, however, be limited by aesthetically adverse consequences (proximal attachment reduction); basically, buccal crown lengthening only can be considered as a potential indication for this procedure. In the posterior region, crown lengthening is limited by tooth and furcation anatomy or by loss of bone structure, which complicates future implant placement. As regards to orthodontic extrusion, root length and anatomy are the limiting factors of this procedure; short roots or conical anatomy are contraindications to orthodontic extrusion. Once again, when a long-lasting, functional restoration cannot be predictably created, it might be better to extract the tooth than to pursue heroic efforts to restore an extremely weak tooth, using complex, expensive, and unpredictable procedures.

CLINICAL PROCEDURES

The restoration of a nonvital tooth may include several restorative components such as the post, the core, and the overlying restoration. Within the same tooth, several interfaces such as post to radicular dentin, core to coronal dentin, core to post, and core to overlying restoration will be created. According to the biomechanical status, some or all restorative components and interfaces will be present and need to be addressed.

General clinical guidelines for restoring endodontically treated teeth with either partial or full crown restorations are presented in Table 22-2, with specific procedures for tooth preparation and treatment of the different interfaces involved. Clinical steps for all recommended treatment options are presented in Figures 22-6 through 22-14.

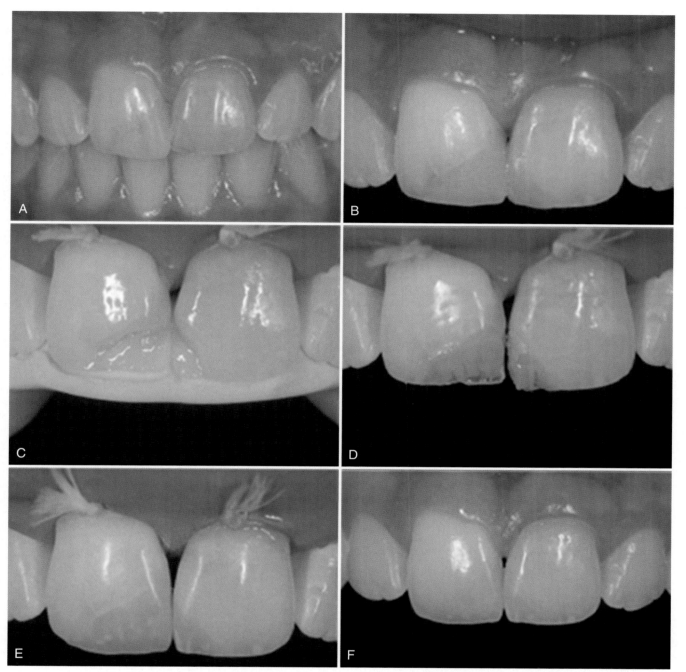

FIG. 22-6 Direct composite restorations on front teeth (following bleaching). Nonvital anterior tooth with sufficient amount of residual tissue and intact, healthy neighboring teeth, usually in rather young patients. **A,** Preparation. Existing restorative material and all remnants of endodontic sealer and gutta-percha were removed from the cavity to expose a clean dentin substrate. Opaque cement can be used to mark the entrance of the roots to facilitate eventual retreatment or for the later placement of a post. **B,** Bleaching procedures. Two sessions of internal bleaching were needed to adapt the color of both traumatized anterior teeth (tooth #11), using a mixture of 3% hydrogen peroxide and sodium perborate powder. Each bleaching session extended over a 10-day period. Between sessions and until the given delay to proceed with final restoration (1 to 2 weeks up to 6 to 8 weeks), access cavity is closed with either a temporary filling material or flowable resin composite. **C, D,** Restorative procedures. A layer of adhesive is applied over all cavity surfaces. An etch-and-rinse system is frequently preferred when the dentinal tissue is highly sclerotic or was contaminated (e.g., by eugenol). A hard cement such as glass ionomer (not a resin-modified glass ionomer because of water uptake and further expansion) was used for dentin replacement, before adding enamel composite to close the lingual cavity. A full resin composite restoration can also be considered to fill in the lingual cavity (dentin + enamel masses) in consideration of the material's hydrophobic nature, which could presumably prevent or limit penetration of water-soluble pigments from the oral cavity. Two or three layers are usually used to replace the missing tissue, preferably following the "natural layering concept," which aims to build up the restoration with two basic masses, namely dentin and enamel, with the help of a silicone index. **E, F,** Postoperative views. The two conservative restorations are shown after finishing and polishing, with the rubber dam still in place (**E**) and after several weeks (**F**). Note that aesthetic integration cannot be evaluated before full rehydration has occurred (4 to 6 hours at least).

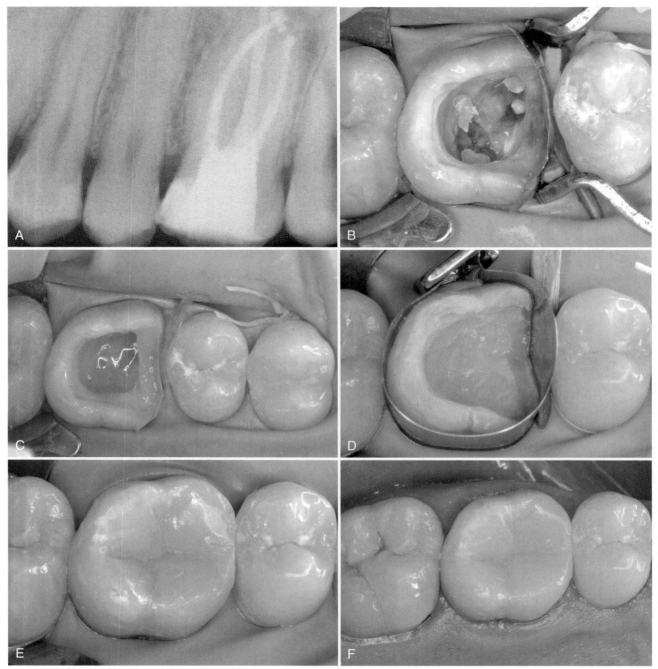

FIG. 22-7 Direct composite restoration on posterior tooth. Nonvital posterior tooth with sufficient amount of residual tissue and mostly intact, rather healthy, neighboring teeth. No significant discoloration of buccal tooth substrate and absence of severe parafunctions or group guidance or other unfavorable occluso-functional condition. **A,** Preparation. Existing restorative material and all remnants of endodontic sealer and gutta-percha are removed from the cavity to expose a clean dentin substrate. Opaque cement can be used to mark the entrance of the roots to facilitate eventual retreatment or for a later placement of a post. **B,** Adhesive procedure. An etch-and-rinse adhesive system was used here owing to the presence of sclerotic and contaminated dentin. **C-E,** Restoration base and layering technique. Resins or glass ionomer cements can be used for dentin replacement, before adding enamel composite to close the lingual cavity. A full resin composite restoration can also be considered to fill in the lingual cavity (dentin + enamel masses) in consideration of the material's hydrophobic nature, which could presumably prevent or limit penetration of water-soluble pigments from the oral cavity. A dentin composite mass is used to replace missing dentinal tissue, and enamel composite is used to build up proximal walls and the occlusal anatomy. **F,** The postoperative view demonstrates the advantage of this conservative approach in the context of teeth with appropriate biomechanical status.

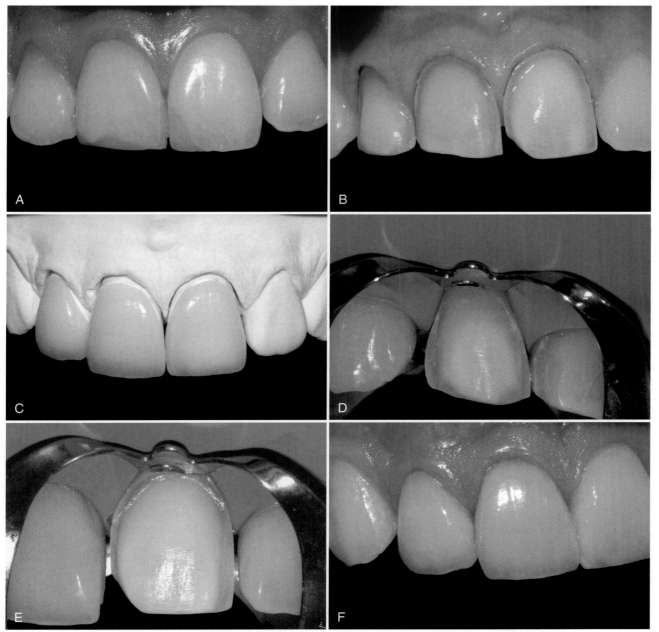

FIG. 22-8 Veneer. Nonvital anterior tooth with sufficient amount of residual tissue and rather healthy neighboring teeth. Discoloration resisted bleaching or relapsed, despite several retreatments. Preferably thick biotype to limit the risk of gingival recession and loss of aesthetic integration. **A,** Closing the lingual cavity. A hard cement such as glass ionomer (not resin-modified glass ionomer because of water uptake and possible expansion) can be used for dentin replacement, before adding enamel composite to close the lingual cavity. A full resin composite restoration can also be considered to fill in the lingual cavity (dentin + enamel masses) in consideration of the material's hydrophobic nature, which could presumably prevent or limit penetration of water-soluble pigments from the oral cavity. **B,** Preparation. A sufficient amount of buccal tooth structure must be removed to allow for a good aesthetic result (preparation depth is dictated by the discoloration severity). Cervical margins closely follow gingival contours, preventing soft-tissue impingement, but they assume complete coverage of discolored tooth structure. **C, D,** Adhesive procedure. Hydrophobic bonding systems are preferred to wet-etched enamel when no dentin is exposed. An etch-and-rinse adhesive system is preferred when dentin is exposed (here, in the presence of significant areas of sclerotic dentin). Restoration. Ceramic is etched and silanated. Just before cementation, a last layer of bonding resin is applied but not light-cured until placement. **E,** Luting technique. A light-curing, highly filled, translucent and fluorescent restorative material is preferably used for cementation. This allows better control of restoration placement and minimal wear and fatigue of the cement layer. **F,** Postoperative view. The postoperative view demonstrates satisfactory aesthetics. This approach is sometimes suitable to meet a patient's high aesthetic demands.

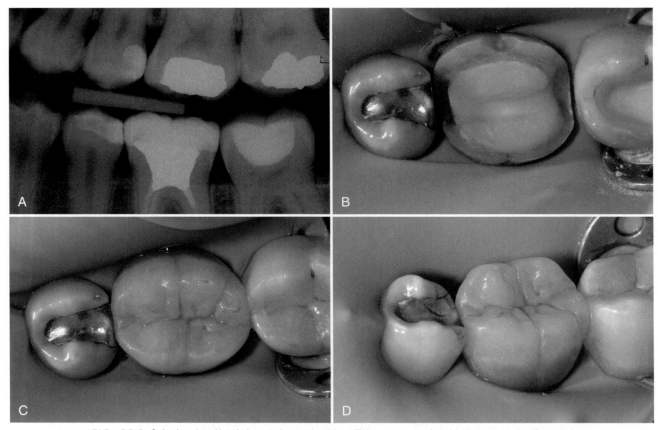

FIG. 22-9 Onlay/overlay. Nonvital posterior tooth with sufficient amount of residual tissue to justify partial restoration. Preparation involves both proximal surfaces or only two surfaces, but in a less favorable occluso-functional environment (thin walls). No significant discoloration of visible buccal tooth substrate. Option is favorable for short clinical crowns. **A, B,** Preparation. Existing restorative material and all remnants of endodontic sealer and gutta-percha are removed from the cavity to expose a clean dentin substrate. Opaque cement can be used to mark the entrance of the roots to facilitate eventual retreatment or for the later placement of a post. Thin and weak occlusal walls are removed until reaching sufficient thickness for the restoration (1.5 to 2 mm in occlusal-free and occlusal areas, respectively). Adhesive procedure: an etch-and-rinse adhesive system is preferably used here owing to the presence of sclerotic and contaminated dentin (a self-etch adhesive system can also be used). A resin composite base is made with a restorative composite or preferably with flowable composite (for limited volume and thickness) to smooth internal angles, fill undercuts, and, when needed, relocate cervical margins occlusally. **C, D,** After impression and model fabrication, the restoration is generated in the laboratory to optimize restoration anatomy, function, and aesthetics. The restoration can be made of different tooth-colored materials: ceramics (fired, pressed, or CAD-CAM generated) or resin composite. This treatment option provides optimal tissue conservation, function, and aesthetics and is a good alternative to full crowns.

Tooth Preparation

The most important part of the restored tooth is the tooth itself. As described earlier, thickness and height of remaining dentin walls or cusps along with functional occlusal conditions are the determining factors in choosing the most appropriate restorative solution.

For partial intracoronal restorations, maximal tissue conservation is the only consideration for the clinician. In other situations, the selected restorative approach will usually necessitate some tooth preparation to comply with restoration design and thickness. Onlays, overlays, and endocrowns require about 1.5 to 2 mm occlusal space to guarantee restoration resistance to functional loads. For full crowns, a ferrule is needed to encircle the vertical walls of sound tooth structure above the restoration

margin (1.5 to 3 mm), thus preventing a coincidence between core and restoration limits. Other preparation requirements presented in this chapter are to be respected to ensure treatment success. This means that a 4- to 5-mm height and 1-mm thickness of sound, suprabony tooth structure should be available to accommodate both the periodontal biologic width and the restorative ferrule.

Post Placement

The post is an extension of the foundation into the root of structurally damaged teeth, needed for core and coronal restoration stability and retention. The post is cemented or bonded into the root, according to tissue quality and post and core choice. The post performs both a mechanical and

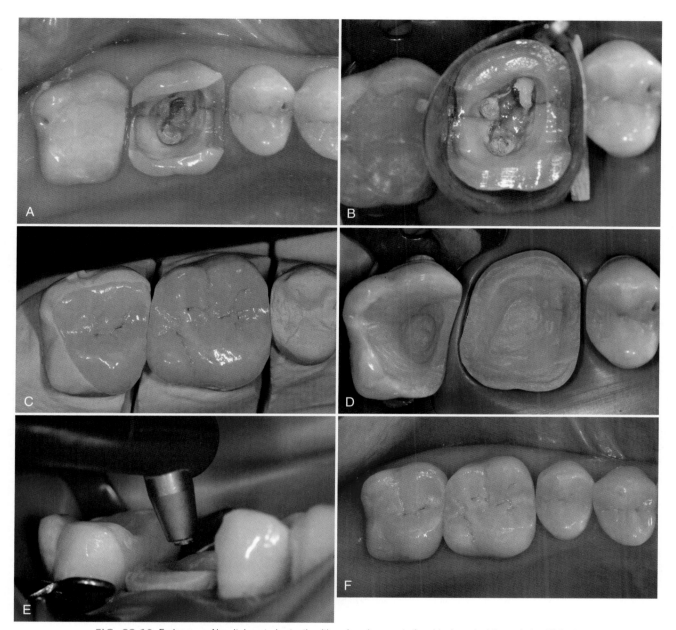

FIG. 22-10 Endocrown. Nonvital posterior tooth with reduced amount of residual cervical tissue but sufficient tissue to provide supragingival restoration margins and good stabilization within former pulpal chamber. No or limited discoloration in visible buccal tooth substrate. Favorable option for short clinical crowns. **A, B,** Preparation. Existing restorative material and all remnants of endodontic sealer and gutta-percha are removed from the cavity to expose a clean dentin substrate. Opaque cement can be used to mark the entrance of the roots to facilitate eventual retreatment or for the later placement of a post. Thin and weak walls are removed until reaching sufficient thickness (1.5 mm minimum); as much residual cervical structure as possible is then maintained to avoid restoration interference with periodontal tissues. **C,** Prosthetic restoration on working model. **D,** Restoration base. Adhesive procedures: An etch-and-rinse adhesive system is preferably used here owing to the presence of sclerotic and contaminated dentin (a self-etch adhesive system can also be used). Restoration base: A resin composite base is made with a restorative composite or preferably with flowable composite (for limited volume and thickness) to smooth internal angles, fill undercuts, and, when needed, relocate cervical margins occlusally. **E,** Impression and restoration fabrication. After impression and model fabrication, the restoration is generated in the laboratory to optimize restoration anatomy, function, and aesthetics. The restoration can be made of different tooth-colored materials: ceramics (fired, pressed, or CAD-CAM generated) or resin composite. **F,** Postoperative result. Despite their relatively rare application, endocrowns combine biomechanical advantages with facilitation of clinical procedures and minimal if any involvement of biologic width. It is an interesting alternative to full crowns. (From Rocca GT, Bouillaguet S: Alternative treatments for the restoration of nonvital teeth, *Rev Odont Stomat* 37:259, 2008.)

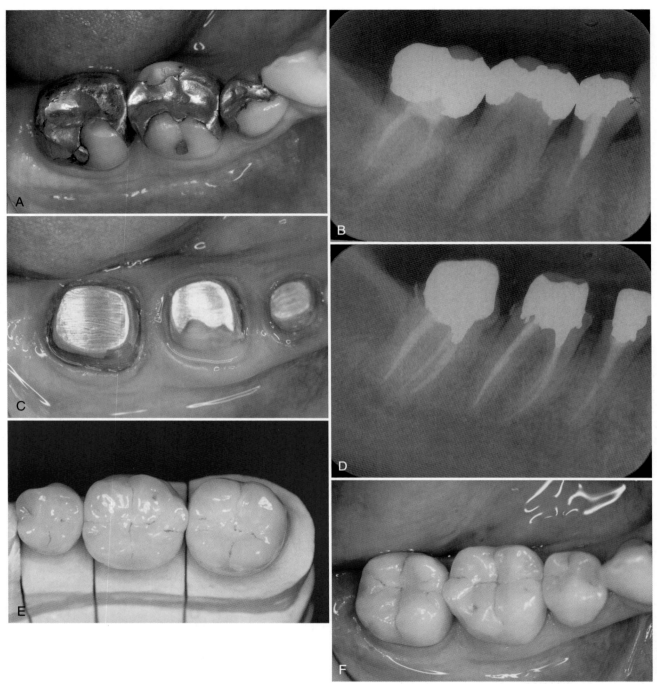

FIG. 22-11 Amalgam core. Nonvital posterior teeth with reduced tooth structure and wall height. Amalgam core stability is granted by extension of the restoration into the coronal portion of the canal (curved roots) and post (only if straight root anatomy) and remaining pulpal chamber undercuts. Today, this option is considered obsolete or historical because of the intrinsic staining of amalgam, the nonadhesive technique, and the less-than-ideal biomechanical behavior of amalgam. **A, B,** Preparation. Existing restorative material and all remnants of endodontic sealer and gutta-percha are removed from the cavity to expose a clean dentin substrate. Thin and weak walls are removed until reaching sufficient thickness (1.5 to 2 mm); existing retentions are used to stabilize the amalgam core, together with a post. The metal post (with passive and anatomic design, preferably made of titanium) extends into the root for about the same length as its coronal extension. **C-E,** Restoration fabrication. After placing a matrix or cupper ring to envelop the preparation, amalgam is compacted into the cavity, superior root canal portion, and around the post until the appropriate coronal volume is restored. Preparation of cores is made to manage optimal space for porcelain fused to metal (PFM) crowns. **F,** Posttreatment result. This treatment approach is feasible for teeth already restored with amalgam cores and when PFM restorations are mandated. Satisfactory aesthetics can be attained with intrasulcular restoration margins.

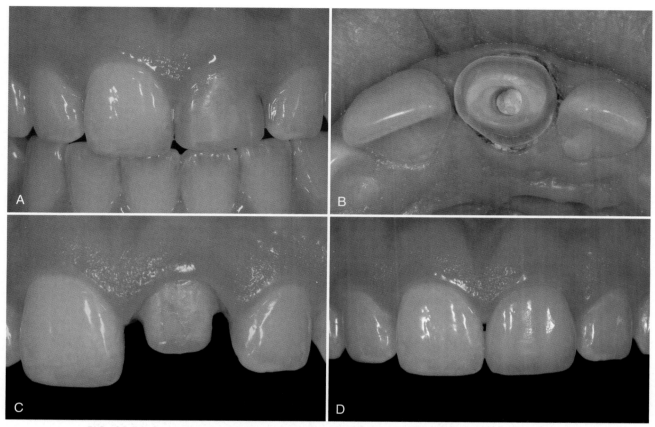

FIG. 22-12 Composite core (without post). Nonvital tooth with more than half the coronal structure left and sufficient wall thickness. Core stability is granted by adhesion, remaining pulpal chamber, and residual wall height. **A, B,** Preparation. Existing restorative material and all remnants of endodontic sealer and gutta-percha are removed from the cavity to expose a clean dentin substrate. The tooth is prepared to evaluate precisely the height and thickness of residual tooth structure. Half of the abutment height and more than 1.5 mm wall thickness must be present to restore the tooth without a post. If aforementioned conditions are met, a thin layer of hard cement (calcium hydroxide, zinc phosphate, or glass ionomer; not resin-modified glass ionomer) is applied at the entrance of the root canal to enable possible retreatment in the future. **C,** Adhesive procedures and core fabrication. All walls are covered with the adhesive system (etch-and-rinse or self-etch) before applying in layers a direct light-curing restorative composite or a self-curing material, in case of limited restoration volume. **D,** Postoperative view. The advantage of this approach is the ease of application and excellent aesthetics. It is considered a good restorative solution for highly aesthetic ceramic crowns placed on teeth with limited tissue loss and discoloration.

biologic function by protecting the apical seal from bacterial contamination in case of coronal leakage. These functions should not be attained at the expense of tooth strength; post space preparation should be as conservative as possible to avoid an increased risk of root fracture. It is important to point out again that a post does not strengthen or reinforce a tooth. This elusive goal would only be achieved in a case of perfect cohesion between post and tooth substrate, nowadays only partially achievable. Therefore, the clinician must keep in mind that inherent strength of the tooth and its resistance to root fracture comes mostly from the remaining tooth structure and the surrounding alveolar bone. The tooth is weakened if dentin is sacrificed to place a larger-diameter post.

The post should be long enough to meet aforementioned biomechanical demands without jeopardizing root integrity.

The standard parameters for post placement in a tooth with normal periodontal support are as follows:
1. In case of nonadhesive cementation (metal posts only)[60]:
   - Two thirds the length of the canal
   - A radicular extension at least equal to the coronal length of the core
   - One half the bone-supported length of the root
2. In case of adhesive cementation (fiber posts)[41,136]:
   - One third to one half the length of the canal, maximum
   - A radicular extension about the coronal length of the core

The first step for all types of post and core restorations is removal of gutta-percha and endodontic cement from the future post space. This procedure generally is best accomplished by the clinician providing the endodontic service, because that person has a clear knowledge of the size and form

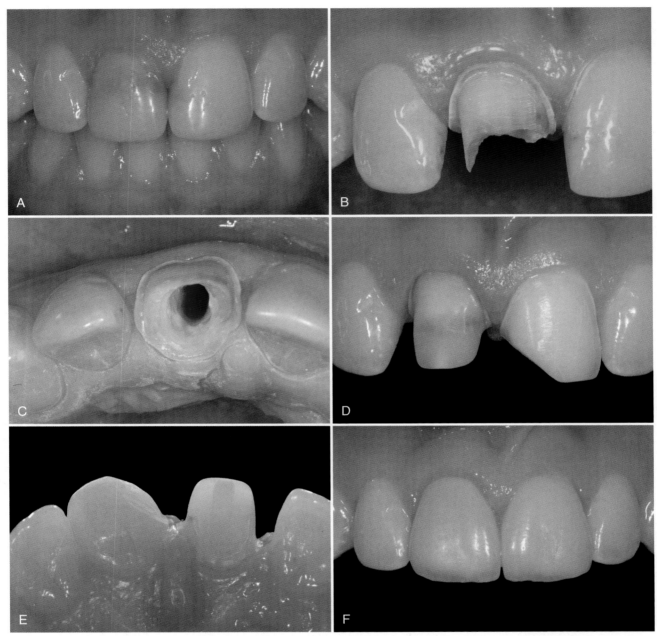

FIG. 22-13 Composite core with white post (resin-reinforced fiber or zirconia post). Nonvital tooth with less than half the coronal structure left or insufficient wall thickness. Core stability is improved through adhesion and a tooth-colored post (resin-reinforced fiber or ceramic posts). **A,** Preoperative view. **B, C,** Preparation. Existing restorative material and all remnants of endodontic sealer and gutta-percha are removed from the cavity to expose a clean dentin substrate. The tooth is prepared to evaluate precisely the height and thickness of residual tooth structure. If less than half of the abutment height or 1.5-mm wall thickness remain, the abutment requires a post to increase core retention and foundation stability. **D, E,** Post-and-core fabrication. Post placement: The post space is prepared with ad hoc instruments until reaching a length equivalent to core height or slightly less depending on remaining wall height. Increased length is not needed, because retention is predominantly achieved through adhesion. Any tooth-colored post can be used, but fiber posts are usually preferred to limit stress buildup into the root structure, even though they provide less rigidity to the foundation. Post cementation: A self-curing adhesive system is applied on all cavity walls and into post preparation before luting the post with a dual-cured composite cement or, as a simple alternative, a self-adhesive cement (then, no adhesive is used). Core fabrication: The remaining core volume is built up in layers, using a direct light-curing restorative composite or with a single increment of a self-curing material when only limited volume is to be completed. **F,** Postoperative view. The primary advantage of this approach is the excellent aesthetic outcome. It is considered a good restorative solution for highly aesthetic ceramic crowns placed on teeth with more tissue loss but moderate discoloration.

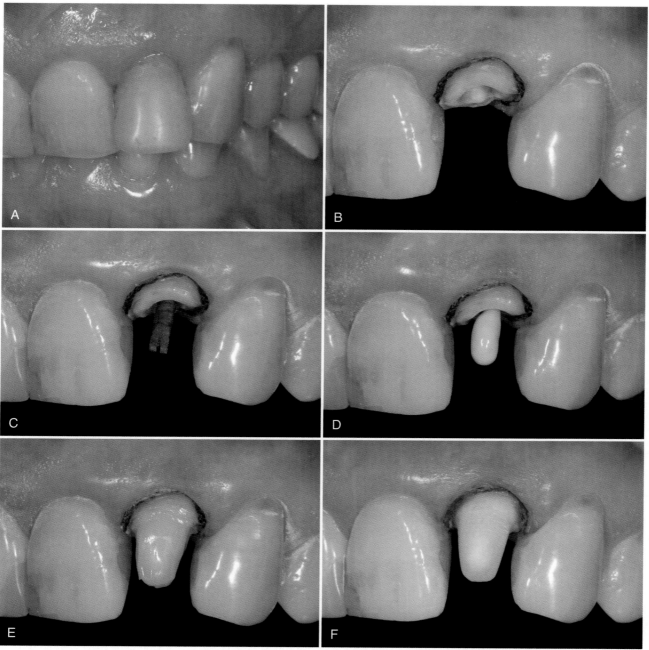

FIG. 22-14 Composite core with prefabricated metal post. Nonvital tooth with reduced coronal structure and ferrule effect or insufficient wall thickness. Core stability is improved through adhesion and a metal (opacified) post (titanium posts are usually preferred). **A,** Preoperative view. **B,** Preparation. Existing restorative material and all remnants of endodontic sealer and gutta-percha are removed from the cavity to expose the remaining tooth structure and a clean dentin substrate. The absence of coronal tissue and ferrule effect mandates the use of a more rigid post (ceramic posts are considered too rigid and contraindicated in this situation). **C-F,** Post and core fabrication. Post space preparation: The post space is prepared with ad hoc instruments until reaching a length equivalent to about core height. More length is not needed, because retention is predominantly achieved through adhesion. Post preparation: The metal post (titanium here) is sandblasted (silicoating can be used to increase adhesion; i.e., Rocatec or CoJet systems, 3M), followed by silane application. An opaque resin or flowable composite can be used to mask metal dark color and improve aesthetics. Post cementation: A self-curing adhesive system is applied on all cavity walls and into post preparation before luting the post with a dual-cured composite cement or, as a simple alternative, a self-adhesive cement (then, no adhesive is used). Core fabrication: The remaining core volume is built up in layers, using a direct light-curing restorative composite or a single increment of a self-curing material when only limited volume is to be completed.

of the canal system. The initial post space preparation procedure is similar for most standardized post and core systems. The space, cleared of gutta-percha, has the form of the canal after cleaning and shaping. Proprietary systems are supplied with a series of drills to prepare the internal surface of the canal. The goal of post space formation is to remove little or no dentin from the root canal.

Adhesive Procedures

In general, both self-etch and etch-and-rinse adhesive systems can be used successfully on root dentin, both systems having a well-documented proof of efficacy. However, the use of etch-and-rinse adhesive systems may be advantageous in the presence of highly sclerotic or contaminated dentin, because phosphoric acids will etch dentin more deeply than self-etching primers. When treating the canal in the perspective of post cementation, a dual-curing adhesive system is preferably used to optimize polymerization. Self-adhesive cements have also demonstrated satisfactory performance for post cementation.

Partial Restorations

In the case of limited to moderate coronal substance loss, the restorative strategy for endodontically treated front teeth varies, from direct composite restoration using the same layering or application techniques as for vital teeth (possibly with the contribution of intracoronal or extracoronal bleaching) to full veneers, when discoloration is not fully treatable or tends to relapse. From a restorative standpoint, it is only necessary to mention that a 1- to 2-week delay is mandatory prior to adhesively restoring a bleached tooth. For more extensive restoration, it is even advised to wait up to 6 weeks or more (depending on the extent and duration of bleaching treatment) to allow for tooth final color stabilization and to proceed with shade selection.[39] Figures 22-6 and 22-7 describe the clinical steps involved in the restoration of moderately decayed front teeth using direct composite and bleaching or veneers.

In posterior teeth exhibiting limited to moderate tissue loss, direct to indirect partial or full occlusal restorations are proposed. Their benefit is to take advantage of residual tooth structure to stabilize the restoration and minimize the potential impact of a prosthetic rehabilitation on periodontal tissues. For instance, second molars definitely profit from a conservative approach using adhesively luted intracoronal and full occlusal coverage restorations. An endocrown is a modification of the aforementioned concept, with extension of the restoration into the pulpal chamber as an additional retentive and stabilization structure. Figures 22-8, 22-9, and 22-10 describe the clinical steps involved in the restoration of moderately decayed posterior teeth using onlays, overlays, and endocrowns.

Foundation Restoration Underneath Full Crowns

If significant coronal substance loss justifies a full-tooth coverage, the strategy for foundation fabrication varies as follows:
- Amalgam core with/without metal post
- Composite core without post
- Composite post with fiber or ceramic post
- Composite with prefabricated metal post
- Cast gold post and core

Amalgam Core

A coronal-radicular amalgam foundation may be realized with or without a post (Figs. 22-11 through 22-14). The amalgam coronal-radicular core without a post is indicated for posterior teeth that have a large pulp chamber and lateral walls at least 4 mm high. This restoration extends slightly into the coronal portion of the canals (1 to 1.5 mm). The core is then retained by a combination of the divergence of the canals and natural undercuts in the pulp chamber. A single, homogeneous material is used for the entire restoration, rather than the dual phases of a conventional preformed post and core.

When shorter lateral walls are present, a post is mandatory to improve core stability and retention. The preferred roots for post placement for molars are the palatal root in the upper jaw and the distal root in the lower jaw. Other roots, thinner and presenting more pronounced curvatures, are normally not indicated for post placement. Coronal-radicular amalgam foundations are not indicated for premolars owing to their smaller dimensions; adhesive foundations or cast gold post and core are preferred.

Cast Gold Post and Core

Cast gold post and core restorations can be fabricated with either direct or indirect techniques.

Direct Technique

In the direct technique, a castable post and core pattern is fabricated in the mouth on the prepared tooth. A preformed plastic post pattern is seated in the post space. To gain a path of withdrawal, undercuts are blocked out with resin composite rather than by removing healthy dentin structure. Acrylic resin is added to create a core directly attached to the post pattern. The finished pattern is removed from the tooth and cast in the laboratory.

Indirect Technique

With the indirect technique, a final impression of the prepared tooth and post space is made (Fig. 22-15). As with the direct technique, the path of withdrawal is made by undercut blockout, not by dentin removal. The castable final post and core pattern are fabricated on a die from this impression. The crown margins need not be accurately reproduced at this stage. Proprietary systems provide matched drills, impression posts, and laboratory casting patterns of various diameters. An impression post (preferably a repositionable one) is fitted to the post space, and a final impression is made that captures the form of the remaining coronal tooth structure and picks up the impression post. In the laboratory, a die reproduces the post space and the residual coronal tooth structure for fabrication of the post and core pattern.

With both techniques, the fabrication of a temporary crown with intraradicular retention is needed. This provisional restoration must stay in the mouth only for a limited time to prevent decementation or canal reinfection. This is why this approach is less popular today and replaced by direct techniques in most cases.

The cast post and core is cemented at the second appointment. The cementation process must be passive in nature and an evacuation groove made on post side to facilitate cement expulsion and limit seating pressure. Rapid seating, excessive cement, and heavy seating pressure (e.g., occlusal force) can

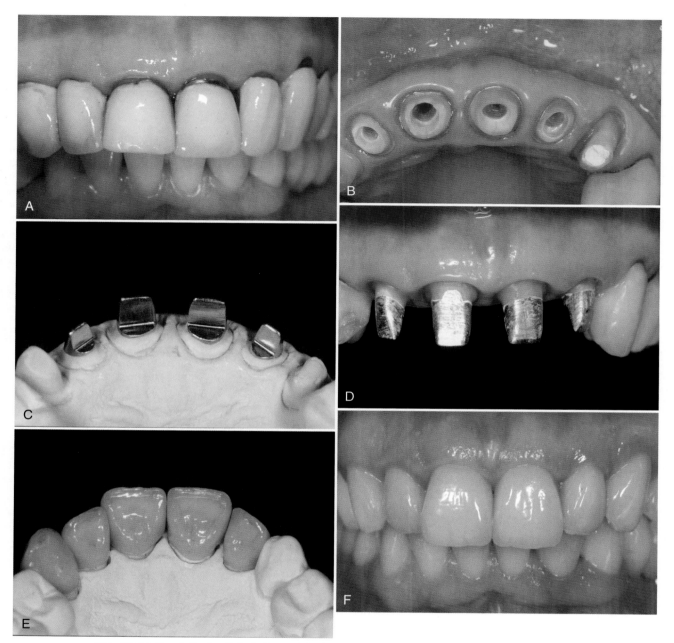

FIG. 22-15 Nonvital teeth with limited coronal structure or numerous abutments. Indirect post and core fabrication helps to achieve proper parallelism and core anatomy. Core retention is assumed by a conventional or adhesive cement. Today, this solution is considered mostly for extended metal-ceramic restorations or sometimes for multiple full-ceramic restorations. **A,** Preoperative view. **B,** Preparation. Existing restorative material and all remnants of endodontic sealer and gutta-percha are removed from the cavity to expose the remaining tooth structure and a clean dentin substrate. Despite the indirect approach, all healthy coronal structures must be maintained to improve foundation stability. Access cavity and coronal walls are prepared with minimal convergence (6 to 10 degrees) to allow for easy insertion. **C, D,** Cast gold post and core fabrication and luting. Post space preparation: The post space is prepared with ad hoc instruments until reaching a length equivalent to about core height or more. More length is needed here, as retention cannot always be achieved through adhesion (endodontic retreatment or highly sclerotic contaminated dentin). Then a conventional glass ionomer or zinc phosphate cement is used. Post and core preparation: The gold post is sandblasted (or eventually sandblasted and coated if adhesive procedures are possible) using Rocatec or CoJet systems, 3M + silane. Post cementation: The post and core is luted with the aforementioned conventional cements or adhesive technique. Next, a self-curing adhesive system is applied on all cavity walls and into post preparation (before the insertion of the post and core) and covered with a dual-cured composite cement or, as a simple alternative, a self-adhesive cement (then, no adhesive is used). **E, F,** Restoration fabrication and placement. A second impression is needed for the final prosthetic work to optimize restoration precision and quality. Lab-made PFM or full ceramic crowns are made with optimal foundation design and alignment.

produce high hydraulic pressures inside the root that may be great enough to crack the root.

Crown Preparation and Temporary Restoration

When a coronal restoration is indicated, the amount of tooth structure remaining after final preparation is the most important determinant of the design of the post and core. In addition, the underlying sound tooth structure provides greater resistance to fracture than any post and core type, design, or material. Natural tooth structure should always be carefully preserved during all phases of post space and crown preparation. Otherwise, preparation of endodontically treated teeth is not different from that for vital teeth, with the exception of severely discolored teeth, which require a slightly deeper chamfer to hide discoloration with the prosthetic structure and intrasulcular margins to reduce the visibility of a dark cervical tooth structure.

Provisional crowns for endodontically treated teeth must be used only for short periods of time because the loss of cement seal—which is, of course, symptom free—can lead to leakage, canal reinfection, and even serious carious invasion, thereby jeopardizing the success of endodontic treatment and even resulting in tooth loss.

SUMMARY

Endodontically treated teeth represent a singular situation because of the attendant qualitative and quantitative alterations of the dental substrate. Current literature indicates that treatment success relies on an effective coronal seal that will prevent canal reinfection and an adequate restoration that will resist functional stresses applied to the remaining tooth structure. The purpose of this chapter is to help the clinician make treatment planning decisions concerning the restorative options available for endodontically treated teeth.

REFERENCES

1. Akgungor G, Sen D, Aydin M: Influence of different surface treatments on the short-term bond strength and durability between a zirconia post and a composite resin core material, *J Prosthet Dent* 99:388, 2008.
2. Al-Wahdani A, Gutteridge DL: An in vitro investigation into the effects of retained coronal dentine on the strength of a tooth restored with a cemented post and partial core restoration, *Int Endod J* 35:913, 2002.
3. Anusavice KJ, editor: *Phillips' science of dental materials,* ed 11, St. Louis, 2003, Saunders.
4. Aversa R, Apicella D, Perillo L, et al: Non-linear elastic three-dimensional finite element analysis on the effect of endocrown material rigidity on alveolar bone remodeling process, *Dent Mater* 25:678, 2009.
5. Balbosh A, Kern M: Effect of surface treatment on retention of glass-fiber endodontic posts, *J Prosthet Dent* 95:218, 2006.
6. Barkhodar RA, Radke R, Abbasi J: Effect of metal collars on resistance of endodontically treated teeth to root fracture, *J Prosthet Dent* 61:676, 1989.
7. Belli S, Zhang Y, Pereira PN, et al: Regional bond strengths of adhesive resins to pulp chamber dentin, *J Endod* 27:527, 2001.
8. Bergman B, Lundquist P, Sjögren U, Sundquist G: Restorative and endodontic results after treatment with cast posts and cores, *J Prosthet Dent* 61:10, 1989.
9. Bindl A, Richter B, Mormann WH: Survival of ceramic computer-aided design/manufacturing crowns bonded to preparations with reduced macroretention geometry, *Int J Prosthodont* 18:219, 2005.
10. Bitter K, Paris S, Mueller J, et al: Correlation of scanning electron and confocal laser scanning microscopic analyses for visualization of dentin/adhesive interfaces in the root canal, *J Adhes Dent* 11:7, 2009.
11. Blatz MB, Sadan A, Kern M: Resin-ceramic bonding: a review of the literature, *J Prosthet Dent* 89:268, 2003.
12. Boschian Pest L, Cavalli G, et al: Adhesive post-endodontic restorations with fiber posts: push-out tests and SEM observations, *Dent Mater* 18:596, 2002.
13. Bouillaguet S, Bertossa B, Krejci I, et al: Alternative adhesive strategies to optimize bonding to radicular dentin, *J Endod* 33:1227, 2007.
14. Bouillaguet S, Troesch S, Wataha JC, et al: Microtensile bond strength between adhesive cements and root canal dentin, *Dent Mater* 19:199, 2003.
15. Bowen RL, Rodriguez MS: Tensile strength and modulus of elasticity of tooth structure and several restorative materials, *J Am Dent Assoc* 64:378, 1962.

16. Bower RC: Furcation morphology relative to periodontal treatment, *J Periodontol* 50:366, 1979.
17. Breschi L, Mazzoni A, Ruggeri A, et al: Dental adhesion review: aging and stability of the bonded interface, *Dent Mater* 24:90, 2008.
18. Butz F, Lennon AM, Heydecke G, Strub JR: Survival rate and fracture strength of endodontically treated maxillary incisors with moderate defects restored with different post-and-core systems: an in vitro study, *Int J Prosthodont* 14:58, 2001.
19. Carrigan PG, Morse DR, Furst L, Sinai JH: A scanning electron microscopic evaluation of human dentinal tubules according to age and location, *J Endod* 10:359, 1984.
20. Carrilho MR, Carvalho RM, de Goes MF, et al: Chlorhexidine preserves dentin bond in vitro, *J Dent Res* 86:90, 2007.
21. Carrilho MR, Tay FR, Donnelly AM, et al: Host-derived loss of dentin matrix stiffness associated with solubilization of collagen, *J Biomed Mater Res B Appl Biomater* 90:373, 2009.
22. Carrilho MR, Tay FR, Pashley DH, et al: Mechanical stability of resin-dentin bond components, *Dent Mater* 21:232, 2005.
23. Cathro PR, Chandler NP, Hood JA: Impact resistance of crowned endodontically treated central incisors with internal composite cores, *Endod Dent Traumatol* 12:124, 1996.
24. Ceballos L, Garrido MA, Fuentes V, Rodríguez J: Mechanical characterization of resin cements used for luting fiber posts by nanoindentation, *Dent Mater* 23:100, 2007.
25. Reference deleted in proofs.
26. Christensen G: Core buildup and adhesive incompatibility, *Clin Res Assoc Newsl* 24:6, 2000.
27. Christensen G: Posts: a shift away from metal? *Clin Res Assoc Newsl* 28:1, 2004.
28. Cobankara FK, Unlu N, Cetin AR, Ozkan HB: The effect of different restoration techniques on the fracture resistance of endodontically-treated molars, *Oper Dent* 33:526, 2008.
29. Cohen BI, Pagnillo MK, Newman I, et al: Retention of a core material supported by three post head designs, *J Prosthet Dent* 83:624, 2000.
30. Combe EC, Shaglouf AM, Watts DC, Wilson NH: Mechanical properties of direct core build-up materials, *Dent Mater* 15:158, 1999.

31. Council on Dental Materials, Instruments, and Equipment, American Dental Association: Classification system for cast alloys, *J Am Dent Assoc* 109:766, 1984.
32. Craig RG, Peyton FA: Elastic and mechanical properties of human dentin, *J Dent Res* 52:710, 1958.
33. Cruz-Filho AM, Souza-Neto MD, Saquy PC, Pecora JD: Evaluation of the effect of EDTAC, CDTA and EGTA on radicular dentin microhardness, *J Endod* 27:183, 2001.
34. Dahl JE, Pallesen U: Tooth bleaching—a critical review of the biological aspects, *Crit Rev Oral Biol Med* 14:292, 2003.
35. D'Arcangelo C, D'Amario M, Vadini M, et al: Influence of surface treatments on the flexural properties of fiber posts, *J Endod* 33:864, 2007.
36. Davidson CL, Feilzer AJ: Polymerization shrinkage and polymerization shrinkage stress in polymer-based restoratives, *J Dent* 25:435, 1997.
37. Deliperi S, Bardwell DN: Reconstruction of nonvital teeth using direct fiber-reinforced composite resins: a pilot clinical study, *J Adhes Dent* 11:71, 2009.
38. Denry IL: Recent advances in ceramics for dentistry, *Crit Rev Oral Biol Med* 7:134, 1996.
39. Dietschi D, Ardu S, Krejci I: A new shading concept based on natural tooth color applied to direct composite restorations, *Quintessence Int* 37:91, 2006.
40. Dietschi D, Ardu S, Rossier-Gerber A, Krejci I: Adaptation of adhesive post and cores to dentin after in vitro occlusal loading: evaluation of post material influence, *J Adhes Dent* 8:409, 2006.
41. Dietschi D, Duc O, Krejci I, Sadan A: Biomechanical considerations for the restoration of endodontically treated teeth: a systematic review of the literature–Part 1—Composition and micro- and macrostructure alterations, *Quintessence Int* 38:733, 2007.
42. Dietschi D, Duc O, Krejci I, Sadan A: Biomechanical considerations for the restoration of endodontically treated teeth: a systematic review of the literature, Part II—Evaluation of fatigue behavior, interfaces, and in vivo studies, *Quintessence Int* 39:117, 2008.
43. Dietschi D, Romelli M, Goretti A: Adaptation of adhesive posts and cores to dentin after fatigue testing, *Int J Prosthodont* 10:498, 1997.
44. Douglas WH: Methods to improve fracture resistance of teeth. In Vanherle G, Smith DC, editors: *Proceedings of the international symposium on posterior composite resin dental restorative materials,* Utrecht, Netherlands, 1985, Peter Szulc, p 433.

45. Drummond JL: In vitro evaluation of endodontic posts, *Am J Dent* 13:5B, 2000.

46. Drummond JL, King TJ, Bapna MS, Koperski RD: Mechanical property evaluation of pressable restorative ceramics, *Dent Mater* 16:226, 2000.

47. Drummond JL, Toepke TR, King TJ: Thermal and cyclic loading of endodontic posts, *Eur J Oral Sci* 107:220, 1999.

48. Duncan JP, Pameijer CH: Retention of parallel-sided titanium posts cemented with six luting agents: an in vitro study, *J Prosthet Dent* 80:423, 1998.

49. Duret B, Reynaud M, Duret F: New concept of coronoradicular reconstruction: the Composipost (1), *Chir Dent Fr* 542:69, 1990.

50. Duret B, Reynaud M, Duret F: Un nouveau concept de reconstitution corono-radiculaire: le composipost (1), *Chir Dent Fr* 540:131, 1990.

51. Feilzer A, De Gee AJ, Davidson CL: Setting stress in composite resin in relation to configuration of the restoration, *J Dent Res* 66:1636, 1987.

52. Feilzer A, De Gee AJ, Davidson CL: Setting stresses in composite for two different curing modes, *Dent Mater* 9:2, 1993.

53. Ferrari M, Cagidiaco MC, Goracci C, et al: Long-term retrospective study of the clinical performance of fiber posts, *Am J Dent* 20:287, 2007.

54. Ferrari M, Vichi A, Mannocci F, Mason PN: Retrospective study of the clinical performance of fiber posts, *Am J Dent* 13(Spec No):9BB, 2000.

55. Fontijn-Tekamp FA, Slagter AP, Van Der Bilt A, et al: Biting and chewing in overdentures, full dentures, and natural dentitions, *J Dent Res* 79:1519, 2000.

56. García-Godoy F, Tay FR, Pashley DH, et al: Degradation of resin-bonded human dentin after 3 years of storage, *Am J Dent* 20:109, 2007.

57. Gelb MN, Barouch E, Simonsen RJ: Resistance to cusp fracture in class II prepared and restored premolars, *J Prosthet Dent* 55:184, 1986.

58. Göhring TN, Peters OA: Restoration of endodontically treated teeth without posts, *Am J Dent* 16:313, 2003.

59. Gohring TN, Roos M: Inlay-fixed partial dentures adhesively retained and reinforced by glass fibers: clinical and scanning electron microscopy analysis after five years, *Eur J Oral Sci* 113:60, 2005.

60. Goodacre CJ, Spolnik KJ: The prosthodontic management of endodontically treated teeth: a literature review, II, Maintaining the apical seal, *J Prosthodont* 4:51, 1995.

61. Goracci C, Tavares AU, Fabianelli A, et al: The adhesion between fiber posts and root canal walls: comparison between microtensile and push-out bond strength measurements, *Eur J Oral Sci* 112:353, 2004.

62. Grandini S, Goracci C, Monticelli F, et al: SEM evaluation of the cement layer thickness after luting two different posts, *J Adhes Dent* 7:235, 2005.

63. Grandini S, Goracci C, Monticelli F, et al: Fatigue resistance and structural characteristics of fiber posts: three-point bending test and SEM evaluation, *Dent Mater* 21:75, 2005.

64. Grigoratos D, Knowles J, Ng YL, Gulabivala K: Effect of exposing dentin to sodium hypochlorite on its flexural strength and elasticity modulus, *Int J Endod J* 34:113, 2001.

65. Gutmann JL: The dentin root complex: anatomic and biologic considerations in restoring endodontically treated teeth, *J Prosthet Dent* 67:458, 1992.

66. Hagge MS, Wong RD, Lindemuth JS: Retention strengths of five luting cements on prefabricated dowels after root canal obturation with a zinc oxide/eugenol sealer: 1, Dowel space preparation/cementation at one week after obturation, *Prosthodont* 11:168, 2002.

67. Hattab FN, Qudeimat MA, al-Rimawi HS: Dental discoloration: an overview, *J Esthet Dent* 11:291, 1999.

68. Hawkins CL, Davies MJ: Hypochlorite-induced damage to proteins: formation of nitrogen-centered radicals from lysine residues and their role in protein fragmentation, *Biochem J* 332:617, 1998.

69. Helfer AR, Melnick S, Shilder H: Determination of the moisture content of vital and pulpless teeth, *Oral Surg Oral Med Oral Pathol* 34:661, 1972.

70. Herr P, Ciucchi B, Holz J: Méthode de positionnement de répliques destinée au contrôle clinique des matériaux d'obturation, *J Biol Buccale* 9:17, 1981.

71. Hidaka O, Iwasaki M, Saito M, Morimoto T: Influence of clenching intensity on bite force balance, occlusal contact area, and average bite pressure, *J Dent Res* 78:1336, 1999.

72. Hikita K, Van Meerbeek B, De Munck J, et al: Bonding effectiveness of adhesive luting agents to enamel and dentin, *Dent Mater* 23:71, 2007.

73. Holand W, Rheinberger V, Apel E, et al: Clinical applications of glass-ceramics in dentistry, *J Mater Sci Mater Med* 17:1037, 2006.

74. Hood JAA: Methods to improve fracture resistance of teeth. In Vanherle G, Smith DC, editors: *Proceedings of the international symposium on posterior composite resin dental restorative materials*, Utrecht, Netherlands, 1985, Peter Szulc, p 443.

75. Huang TJ, Shilder H, Nathanson D: Effect of moisture content and endodontic treatment on some mechanical properties of human dentin, *J Endod* 18:209, 1992.

76. Huber L, Cattani-Lorente M, Shaw L, et al: Push-out bond strengths of endodontic posts bonded with different resin-based luting cements, *Am J Dent* 20:167, 2007.

77. Hulsmann M, Heckendorf M, Shafers F: Comparative in-vitro evaluation of three chelators pastes, *Int Endod J* 35:668, 2002.

78. Hulsmann M, Heckendorff M, Lennon A: Chelating agents in root canal treatment: mode of action and indications for their use, *Int Endod J* 36:810, 2003.

79. Isidor F, Brondum K: Intermittent loading of teeth with tapered, individually cast or prefabricated, parallel-sided posts, *Int J Prosthodont* 5:257, 1992.

80. Isidor F, Brøndum K, Ravnholt G: The influence of post length and crown ferrule length on the resistance to cyclic loading of bovine teeth with prefabricated titanium posts, *Int J Prosthodont* 12:78, 1999.

81. Kane JJ, Burgess JO, Summitt JB: Fracture resistance of amalgam coronal-radicular restorations, *J Prosthet Dent* 63:607, 1990.

82. Kawasaki K, Ruben J, Stokroos I, et al: The remineralization of EDTA-treated human dentine, *Caries Res* 33:275, 1999.

83. Khera SC, Goel VK, Chen RCS, Gurusami SA: Parameters of MOD cavity preparations: a 3D FEM study, *Oper Dent* 16:42, 1991.

84. Kinney JH, Balooch M, Marshall SJ, et al: Atomic force microscope measurements of the hardness and elasticity of peritubular and intertubular human dentin, *J Biomech Eng* 118:133, 1996.

85. Kinney JH, Balooch M, Marshall SJ, et al: Hardness and Young's modulus of human peritubular and intertubular dentine, *Arch Oral Biol* 41:9, 1996.

86. Kinney JH, Marshall SJ, Marshall GW: The mechanical properties: a critical review and re-evaluation of the dental literature, *Crit Rev Oral Biol Med* 14:13, 2003.

87. Kinney JH, Nallab RK, Poplec JA, et al: Age-related transparent root dentin: mineral concentration, crystallite size, and mechanical properties, *Biomaterials* 26:3363, 2005.

88. Krejci I, Lutz F, Füllemann J: Tooth-colored inlays/overlays, Tooth-colored adhesive inlays and overlays: materials, principles and classification, *Schweiz Monatsschr Zahnmed* 102:72, 1992.

89. Kuttler S, McLean A, Dorn S, Fischzang A: The impact of post space preparation with Gates-Glidden drills on residual dentin thickness in distal roots of mandibular molars, *J Am Dent Assoc* 135:903, 2004.

90. Lambjerg-Hansen H, Asmussen E: Mechanical properties of endodontic posts, *J Oral Rehabil* 24:882, 1997.

91. Lang H, Korkmaz Y, Schneider K, Raab WH: Impact of endodontic treatments on the rigidity of the root, *J Dent Res* 85:364, 2006.

92. Larsen TD, Douglas WH, Geistfeld RE: Effect of prepared cavities on the strength of teeth, *Oper Dent* 6:2.5, 1981.

93. Lertchirakarn V, Palamara JE, Messer HH: Anisotropy of tensile strength of root dentin, *J Dent Res* 80:453, 2001.

94. Lewinstein I, Grajower R: Root dentin hardness of endodontically treated teeth, *J Endod* 7:421, 1981.

95. Libman WJ, Nicholls JI: Load fatigue of teeth restored with cast posts and cores and complete crowns, *Int J Prosthodont* 8:155, 1995.

96. Linn J, Messer HH: Effect of restorative procedures on the strength of endodontically treated molars, *J Endod* 20:479, 1994.

97. Magne P, Knezevic A: Simulated fatigue resistance of composite resin versus porcelain CAD/CAM overlay restorations on endodontically treated molars, *Quintessence Int* 40:125, 2009.

98. Marchi GM, Mitsui FH, Cavalcanti AN: Effect of remaining dentine structure and thermal-mechanical aging on the fracture resistance of bovine roots with different post and core systems, *Int Endod J* 41:969, 2008.

99. Martinez-Insua A, da Silva L, Rilo B, Santana U: Comparison of the fracture resistances of pulpless teeth restored with a cast post and core or carbon fiber post with a composite core, *J Prosthet Dent* 80:527, 1998.

100. McLean A: Criteria for the predictably restorable endodontically treated tooth, *J Can Dent Assoc* 64:652, 1998.

101. Meredith N, Sheriff M, Stechell DJ, Swanson SA: Measurements of the microhardness and Young's modulus of human enamel and dentine using an indentation technique, *Arch Oral Biol* 41:539, 1996.

102. Millstein PL, Ho J, Nathanson D: Retention between a serrated steel dowel and different core materials, *J Prosthet Dent* 65:480, 1991.

103. Milot P, Stein RS: Root fracture in endodontically treated teeth related to post selection and crown design, *J Prosthet Dent* 68:428, 1992.

104. Miyasaka K, Nakabayashi N: Combination of EDTA conditioner and Phenyl-P/HEMA self-etching primer for bonding to dentin, *Dent Mater* 15:153, 1999.

105. Monticelli F, Ferrari M, Toledano M: Cement system and surface treatment selection for fiber post luting, *Med Oral Patol Oral Cir Bucal* 13:E214, 2008.

106. Morgano SM, Brackett SE: Foundation restorations in fixed prosthodontics: current knowledge and future needs, *J Prosthet Dent* 82:643, 1999.

107. Morris MD, Lee KW, Agee KA, et al: Effect of sodium hypochlorite and RC-Prep on bond strengths of resin cement to endodontic surfaces, *J Endod* 27:753, 2001.

108. Moszner N, Salz U, Zimmermann J: Chemical aspects of self-etching enamel-dentin adhesives: a systematic review, *Dent Mater* 21:895, 2005.

109. Reference deleted in proofs.

110. Muller HP, Eger T: Gingival phenotypes in young male adults, *J Clin Periodontol* 24:65, 1997.

111. Muller HP, Eger T: Masticatory mucosa and periodontal phenotype: a review, *Int J Periodontics Restorative Dent* 22:172, 2002.

112. Nakano F, Takahashi H, Nishimura F: Reinforcement mechanism of dentin mechanical properties by intracanal medicaments, *Dent Mater J* 18:304, 1999.

113. Nayyar A, Zalton RE, Leonard LA: An amalgam coronal-radicular dowel and core technique for endodontically treated posterior teeth, *J Prosthet Dent* 43:511, 1980.

114. Nicopoulou-Karayianni K, Bragger U, Lang NP: Patterns of periodontal destruction associated with incomplete root fractures, *Dentomaxillofac Radiol* 26:321, 1997.

115. Nikaido T, Takano Y, Sasafuchi Y, et al: Bond strengths to endodontically-treated teeth, *Am J Dent* 12:177, 1999.

116. Nikiforuk G, Sreebny L: Demineralization of hard tissues by organic chelating agents at neutral pH, *J Dent Res* 32:859, 1953.

117. Nissan J, Dmitry Y, Assif D: The use of reinforced composite resin cement as compensation for reduced post length, *J Prosthet Dent* 86:304, 2001.

118. Olsson M, Lindhe J: Periodontal characteristics in individuals with varying form of the upper central incisors, *J Clin Periodontol* 18:78, 1991.

119. Orstavik D, Pitt Ford T, editors: *Essential endodontology: prevention and treatment of apical periodontitis*, ed 2, 2008, Munksgaard Blackwell.

120. Ottl P, Hahn L, Lauer HCH, Lau YH: Fracture characteristics of carbon fibre, ceramic and non-palladium endodontic post systems at monotonously increasing loads, *J Oral Rehabil* 29:175, 2002.

121. Palamara JE, Wilson PR, Thomas CD, Messer HH: A new imaging technique for measuring the surface strains applied to dentine, *J Dent* 28:141, 2000.

122. Panitvisai P, Messer HH: Cuspidal deflection in molars in relation to endodontic and restorative procedures, *J Endod* 21:57, 1995.

123. Papa J, Cain C, Messer HH: Moisture content of vital vs endodontically treated teeth, *Endod Dent Traumatol* 10:91, 1994.

124. Pashley D, Okabe A, Parham P: The relationship between dentin microhardness and tubule density, *Endod Dent Traumatol* 1:176, 1985.

125. Pashley DH, Tay FR, Yiu C, et al: Collagen degradation by host-derived enzymes during aging, *J Dent Res* 83:216, 2004.

126. Perdigão J, Lopes MM, Gomes G: Interfacial adaptation of adhesive materials to root canal dentin, *J Endod* 33:259, 2007.

127. Phark JH, Duarte S Jr, Blatz M, Sadan A: An in vitro evaluation of the long-term resin bond to a new densely sintered high-purity zirconium-oxide ceramic surface, *J Prosthet Dent* 101:29, 2009.

128. Pierrisnard L, Hohin F, Renault P, Barquins M: Coronoradicular reconstruction of pulpless teeth: a mechanical study using finite element analysis, *J Prosthet Dent* 88:442, 2002.

129. Pilo R, Cardash HS, Levin E, Assif D: Effect of core stiffness on the in vitro fracture of crowned, endodontically treated teeth, *J Prosthet Dent* 88:302, 2002.

130. Plotino G, Grande NM, Bedini R, et al: Flexural properties of endodontic posts and human root dentin, *Dent Mater* 23:1129, 2007.

131. Plotino G, Grande NM, Pameijer CH, Somma F: Nonvital tooth bleaching: a review of the literature and clinical procedures, *J Endod* 34:394, 2008.

132. Pontius O, Hutter JW: Survival rate and fracture strength of incisors restored with different post and core systems and endodontically treated incisors without coronoradicular reinforcement, *J Endod* 28:710, 2002.

133. Poolthong S, Mori T, Swain MV: Determination of elastic modulus of dentin by small spherical diamond indenters, *Dent Mater* 20:227, 2001.

134. Powers JM, Sakaguchi RL: *Craig's restorative dental materials*, ed 12, St. Louis, 2006, Mosby.

135. Radovic I, Monticelli F, Goracci C, et al: Self-adhesive resin cements: a literature review, *J Adhes Dent* 10:251, 2008.

136. Reeh ES, Douglas WH, Messer HH: Stiffness of endodontically treated teeth related to restoration technique, *J Dent Res* 68:540, 1989.

137. Reeh ES, Messer HH, Douglas WH: Reduction in tooth stiffness as a result of endodontic and restorative procedures, *J Endod* 15:512, 1989.

138. Rees JS, Jacobsen PH, Hickman J: The elastic modulus of dentine determined by static and dynamic methods, *Clin Mater* 17:11, 1994.

139. Ricketts DN, Tait CM, Higgins AJ: Post and core systems, refinements to tooth preparation and cementation, *Br Dent J* 198:533, 2005; review.

140. Rivera EM, Yamauchi M: Site comparisons of dentine collagen cross-links from extracted human teeth, *Arch Oral Biol* 38:541, 1993.

141. Roberts HW, Leonard DL, Vandewalle KS, et al: The effect of a translucent post on resin composite depth of cure, *Dent Mater* 20:617, 2004.

142. Rocca GT, Bouillaguet S: Alternative treatments for the restoration of non-vital teeth, *Rev Odont Stomat* 37:259, 2008.

143. Rosentritt M, Furer C, Behr M, et al: Comparison of in vitro fracture strength of metallic and tooth-coloured posts and cores, *J Oral Rehabil* 27:595, 2000.

144. Rosentritt M, Plein T, Kolbeck C, et al: In vitro fracture force and marginal adaptation of ceramic crowns fixed on natural and artificial teeth, *Int J Prosthodont* 13:387, 2000.

145. Ruddle CJ: Nickel-titanium rotary instruments: current concepts for preparing the root canal system, *Aust Endod J* 29:87, 2003.

146. Saleh AA, Ettman WM: Effect of endodontic irrigation solutions on microhardness of root canal dentin, *J Dent* 27:43, 1999.

147. Santos J, Carrilho M, Tervahartiala T, et al: Determination of matrix metalloproteinases in human radicular dentin, *J Endod* 35:686, 2009.

148. Saunders WP, Saunders EM: Coronal leakage as a cause of failure in root-canal therapy: a review, *Endod Dent Traumatol* 10:105, 1994.

149. Sauro S, Mannocci F, Toledano M, et al: EDTA or H3PO4/NaOCl dentine treatments may increase hybrid layers' resistance to degradation: a microtensile bond strength and confocal-micropermeability study, *J Dent* 37:279, 2009.

150. Schmage P, Pfeiffer P, Pinto E, et al: Influence of oversized dowel space preparation on the bond strengths of FRC posts, *Oper Dent* 34:93, 2009.

151. Schwartz RS: Adhesive dentistry and endodontics, Part 2: bonding in the root canal system—the promise and the problems: a review, *J Endod* 32:1125, 2006.

152. Schwartz RS, Robbins JW: Post placement and restoration of endodontically treated teeth: a literature review, *J Endod* 30:289, 2004.

153. Scotti R, Malferrari S, Monaco C: Clarification on fiber posts: prosthetic core restoration, pre-restorative endodontics, *Proceedings from the 6th International Symposium on Adhesive and Restorative Dentistry*, p 7, 2002.

154. Sedgley CM, Messer HH: Are endodontically treated teeth more brittle? *J Endod* 18:332, 1992.

155. Setcos JC, Staninec M, Wilson NH: Bonding of amalgam restorations: existing knowledge and future prospects, *Oper Dent* 25:121, 2000; review.

156. Signore A, Benedicenti S, Kaitsas V, et al: Long-term survival of endodontically treated, maxillary anterior teeth restored with either tapered or parallel-sided glass-fiber posts and full-ceramic crown coverage, *J Dent* 37:115, 2009.

157. Sim TP, Knowles JC, Ng YL, et al: Effect of sodium hypochlorite on mechanical properties of dentine and tooth surface strain, *Int Endod J* 33:120, 2001.

158. Sindel J, Frandenberger R, Kramer N, Petschelt A: Crack formation in all-ceramic crowns dependent on different core build-up and luting materials, *J Dent* 27:175, 1999.

159. Sirimai S, Riis DN, Morgano SM: An in vitro study of the fracture resistance and the incidence of vertical root fracture of pulpless teeth restored with six post-and-core systems, *J Prosthet Dent* 81:262, 1999.

160. Soares CJ, Soares PV, de Freitas Santos-Filho PC, et al: The influence of cavity design and glass fiber posts on biomechanical behavior of endodontically treated premolars, *J Endod* 34:1015, 2008.

161. Sorensen JA, Engelman MJ: Ferrule design and fracture resistance of endodontically treated teeth, *J Prosthet Dent* 63:529, 1990.

162. Sorensen JA, Martinoff MD: Intracoronal reinforcement and coronal coverage: a study of endodontically treated teeth, *J Prosthet Dent* 51:780, 1984.

163. Standlee JP, Caputto AA, Holcomb JP: The Dentatus screw: comparative stress analysis with other endodontic dowel designs, *J Oral Rehabil* 9:23, 1982.

164. Summit JB, Robbins JW, Schwart RS: *Fundamentals of operative dentistry—a contemporary approach*, ed 3, Hanover Park, Illinois, 2006, Quintessence.

165. Tamse A, Fuss Z, Lustig J: An evaluation of endodontically treated vertically fractured teeth, *J Endod* 25:506, 1999.

166. Tay FR, Loushine RJ, Lambrechts P, et al: Geometric factors affecting dentin bonding in root canals: a theoretical modeling approach, *J Endod* 31:584, 2005.

167. Tidmarsch BG, Arrowsmith MG: Dentinal tubules at the root ends of apisected teeth: a scanning electron microscopy study, *Int Endod J* 22:184, 1989.

168. Tjan AH, Nemetz H: Effect of eugenol-containing endodontic sealer on retention of prefabricated posts luted with adhesive composite resin cement, *Quintessence Int* 23:839, 1992.

169. Trope M, Ray HL: Resistance to fracture of endodontically treated roots, *Oral Surg Oral Med Oral Pathol* 73:99, 1992.

170. Vire DE: Failure of endodontically treated teeth: classification and evaluation, *J Endod* 17:338, 1991.

171. Watanabe I, Saimi Y, Nakabayashi N: Effect of smear layer on bonding to ground dentin—relationship between grinding conditions and tensile bond strength, *Shika Zairyo Kikai* 13:101, 1994.

172. Wiegand A, Buchalla W, Attin T: Review on fluoride-releasing restorative materials—fluoride release and uptake characteristics, antibacterial activity and influence on caries formation, *Dent Mater* 23:343, 2007.

173. Wu MK, Pehlivan Y, Kontakiotis EG, Wesselink PR: Microleakage along apical root fillings and cemented posts, *J Prosthet Dent* 79:264, 1998.

174. Yoldas O, Alaçam T: Microhardness of composites in simulated root canals cured with light transmitting posts and glass-fiber reinforced composite posts, *J Endod* 31:104, 2005.

175. Yoshikawa T, Sano H, Burrow MF, et al: Effects of dentin depth and cavity configuration on bond strength, *J Dent Res* 78:898, 1999.

176. Yüzügüllü B, Ciftçi Y, Saygili G, Canay S: Diametral tensile and compressive strengths of several types of core materials, *J Prosthodont* 17:102, 2008.

CHAPTER 23

Vital Pulp Therapy

GEORGE BOGEN | SERGIO KUTTLER | NICHOLAS CHANDLER

CHAPTER OUTLINE

"There is nothing permanent except change."

—Heraclitus

Vital pulp therapy is designed to preserve and maintain pulpal health in teeth that have been exposed to trauma, caries, restorative procedures, and anatomic anomalies. The treatment can be completed for permanent teeth that show reversible pulpal injuries, and the outcomes depend on a variety of factors.[63,162,215] The prime objective in vital pulp therapy is to initiate the formation of tertiary reparative dentin or calcific bridge formation. This procedure is essential for the preservation of involved immature permanent teeth where root development may be incomplete and preservation of arch integrity is critical during maxillofacial development.[288]

Recent advances in pulp biology and dental materials have provided alternative treatment strategies for healthy and partially inflamed pulps. Vital pulps can be successfully treated if the clinician has an improved understanding of diagnosis and case selection, hemostasis, caries removal, magnification systems, bioactive capping materials, bonded composites, and other restorative materials. The treatment is particularly valuable in young permanent teeth that have not attained their complete adult length and exhibit thin-walled roots and wide-open apices.[52,219,350]

Immature teeth may require up to 5 years or more to gain apical closure after emergence into the oral cavity. They are characterized by large dentinal tubules that allow increased permeability for microbial penetration.[53] The vulnerability and perceived poor prognosis of vital pulp treatment for immature permanent teeth have prompted aggressive treatment recommendations that include extraction.[350] Alternately, with an accurate diagnosis and early intervention, new strategies for pulp preservation promote a domain for continued hard tissue formation that encourages apexogenesis. Maintaining pulp vitality in these teeth reduces the probability of fracture, through continued growth and natural strengthening of the tooth structures.[78,94]

The introduction of mineral trioxide aggregate (MTA) and other bioceramic or calcium silicate-based cements (CSCs), along with advanced treatment strategies, has markedly changed the long-held concept that pulp capping after carious pulp exposure should be avoided. According to Seltzer and Bender,[289,290] "Pulp capping is a questionable procedure even under ideal circumstances." They further stated that "pulp capping should be discouraged for carious pulp exposures, since microorganisms and inflammation are invariably associated." The perception that outcomes for direct pulp capping in a carious field are inconsistent and problematic is based on traditional protocols and materials that did not generate a favorable milieu for hard tissue formation.[139,197,235,334] This perspective has encouraged clinicians to deliver alternative treatments, such as pulpotomy or pulpectomy, particularly in immature permanent teeth.[53,350] This rigid approach is further complicated by the difficulty in

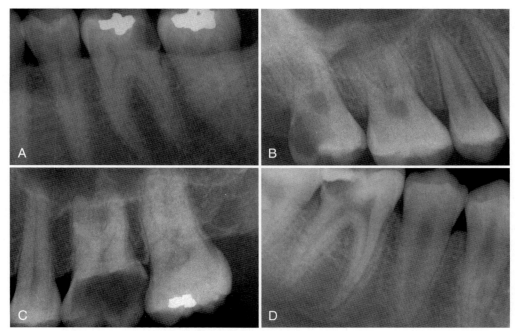

FIG. 23-1 Radiographs of carious molars in patients aged 12 to 38 years. **A**, Mandibular left first molar in a 23-year-old with minor symptoms. **B**, Asymptomatic maxillary right molar in a 16-year-old. **C**, Asymptomatic maxillary left first molar in a 38-year-old. **D**, Deep caries in the mandibular right first molar of a 12-year-old. All patients were referred to the endodontist for root canal treatment based on radiographic observation. They exhibited normal vitality with cold testing, and all were treated successfully with vital pulp therapy. (© Dr. George Bogen.)

establishing the appropriate diagnosis because clinical signs, symptoms, and radiographic evidence may not accurately reflect the histologic condition of the involved pulp tissue (Fig. 23-1).[165] However, based on a better understanding of pulp physiology, caries microbiology, and the inflammatory mechanisms responsible for irreversible changes in pulp tissue, teeth with the potential for repair and continued vitality can now be more readily identified and predictably treated.[335]

Advances in our knowledge of pulpal physiology and immunology, together with recently introduced dental materials, have markedly changed the treatment approaches for teeth with involved pulps. Bioactive CSCs, such as MTA, have changed the perception that treating direct carious pulp exposures is unpredictable and therefore contraindicated. From the introduction of indirect pulp capping by Pierre Fauchard in the eighteenth century, dentistry has recognized the innate reparability of the dental pulp when exposed to injury.[99] Subsequent advances have been complemented by newly developed dental materials that provide superior sealing properties and protect the pulp from microorganisms and their toxic by-products.

A goal in vital pulp therapy has been to identify bioactive pulp capping and pulpotomy agents and implement a consistent treatment regimen that favors pulp preservation. It is recognized that outcomes for vital pulp therapy can vary, depending on the age of the patient, extent of bacterial contamination, and degree of pulp inflammation. Perhaps of greater importance may be the choice of pulp capping material and the quality of the permanent restoration.[63] Appropriate case selection, through a detailed differential diagnosis using multiple tests paired with a careful radiographic interpretation,

is paramount for establishing the best treatment for the problem tooth. In its guidelines, the American Academy of Pediatric Dentistry (AAPD) states, "Teeth exhibiting provoked pain of short duration relieved with over-the-counter analgesics, by brushing, or upon the removal of the stimulus without signs and symptoms of irreversible pulpitis, have a clinical diagnosis of reversible pulpitis and are candidates for vital pulp therapy."[13]

In young patients, assessment of pulpal status before treatment is often difficult, but the probability of favorable outcomes increases with a diagnosis of reversible pulpitis or normal pulp (AAPD). Furthermore, subjective and sometimes negative patient reports or pain associated with cold testing does not absolutely signify that the pulp capping or pulpotomy procedure will be unsuccessful. Because pulpal disease is microbial in nature,[179] this chapter describes the microbiology of caries and the associated physiologic reactivity of pulp tissue. Based on the understanding that pulp tissue has an innate potential for repair in the absence of bacterial contamination, the chapter reviews new treatment concepts in vital pulp therapy intended for the ultimate preservation of the pulpally involved permanent tooth.[72,172]

THE LIVING PULP

As reviewed in Chapter 12, the dental pulp is a highly vascular and innervated loose connective tissue that has the unusual distinction of being enclosed within a rigid envelope composed of enamel, dentin, and cementum.[321,362] These hard tissues impart mechanical support and offer protection from the oral microbiota.[200] When these tissues are examined together embryologically and histologically, they may be referred to as the *dentin-pulp complex.*[68,339] The pulp tissue accomplishes several important functions, including immune cell defense and surveillance, nutrition, dentinogenesis, and proprioceptor recognition.[309] Healthy pulp tissue can generate reparative hard tissue, secondary, and peritubular dentin in response to assorted biologic and pathologic stimuli.[309] The maintenance of dental pulp vitality, therefore, is essential to the long-term retention and normal functioning of the tooth.

The dental pulp encompasses four distinct structural zones: a cell-rich zone, and core, composed of major vessels and nerves; a cell-free zone; and the odontoblastic layer that lines the entire pulp periphery.[321] The cell-rich zone demonstrates a greater density of undifferentiated mesenchymal cells and fibroblasts than is present in the pulp proper. The central pulp core consists of nerve fibers, blood vessels, fibroblasts, undifferentiated mesenchymal stem cells, immunocompetent cells, ground substance, and collagen fibers. The cell-free zone of Weil is subjacent to the odontoblast layer and is linked by capillaries, fibroblastic processes, and an extensive network of unmyelinated nerve fibers. The odontoblastic zone lines the pulp circumference as an epithelioid layer and includes the large, columnar-shaped odontoblasts, nerve fibers, capillaries, and dendritic cells.[186]

Vital pulp tissue comprises various cell populations that include fibroblasts or pulpoblasts, undifferentiated mesenchymal cells, odontoblasts, macrophages, dendritic cells, and other immunocompetent cells. The cells of the subodontoblastic layer and odontoblasts form a thin border between the inside margin of the dentin and the periphery of the pulp; this border is known as the *Höehl cell layer.*[130] The odontoblasts are tall, columnar-shaped cells separated from the mineralized dentin by predentin and characterized by processes that extend into the dentin and possibly to the dentinoenamel junction.[137,298,321,354] Odontoblasts are credited with formation of the mineralized predentin-dentin matrix, which is composed of an assortment of molecules, including phosphoproteins, glycoproteins, proteoglycans, and sialoproteins.[186] Repair mechanisms in the dental pulp are similar to those observed in normal connective tissue injured by trauma. When the enamel and dentin are challenged and the pulp exposed to advancing microorganisms, inflammatory changes can induce pulp necrosis, which precedes progressive pathologic changes that can include infection and its complications.[35,44]

Pressoreceptors and proprioreceptors protect the dentin-pulp complex against excessive occlusal loading while circulating immune competent cells confront bacterial challenges. Pulpless teeth with minimal remaining tooth structure that undergo root-filling procedures and are restored with post and core systems combined with cuspal coverage restorations are more vulnerable to irreparable fracture because of the loss of any protective proprioceptive mechanisms.[225,273,307] Investigations have shown that moisture depletion from dentin and the relative reduction of tooth stiffness are minimal after root canal treatment.[154,175,206] Although root canal treatment can prolong tooth survival, the cumulative loss of tooth structure from it and restorative care may precipitate tooth loss.[54,89,346] Root-filled teeth also demonstrate an increased susceptibility to recurrent caries, either because of poor marginal integrity of the permanent restoration or as a result of the modification of the biologic environment in these teeth.[226]

The pulp undergoes physiologic, pathologic, and defensive changes during its life.[240,333] These age-related transitions

include continued dentin apposition, causing gradual narrowing of pulp volume and circumference.[96,241] The atrophy results in fibrosis, dystrophic calcification, degeneration of odontoblasts, and increased cellular apoptosis.[33,96] The aging of human dental pulp cells is primarily characterized by the formation of reactive oxygen species and senescence-related beta-galactosidase activity.[199] In addition, sensitivity to dental pain is reduced due to a decrease in fast-conducting A-delta fibers and diminished pulp repair, partly attributed to decreases in the levels of substances such as alkaline phosphatase.[217,295] An array of extracellular matrix macromolecules regulated by pulp cell activity contributes to tissue differentiation and growth, defense mechanisms, reactions to inflammatory stimuli, and the formation of calcified tissues.[333]

A comparison analysis of gene expression levels that reflect the activity of biologic cell function, proliferation, differentiation, and development found them markedly higher in young pulps compared to older dental pulps.[333] Analyses of young dental pulps indicated a greater expression level in cell and tissue differentiation, proliferation, and development of the lymphatic, hematologic, and immune systems compared to older dental pulps where the apoptosis pathway is highly expressed.[333] Although A-beta fiber function remains constant with aging, a decrease in A-delta fibers with age may reduce the perception of dental pain transmitted by these faster-conducting fibers.[217] Pulp volume and root canal lumen dimensions also diminish with advancing age as a result of continual deposition of dentin.[96,241] These age-related changes in tissue differentiation and organization, growth regulation, defense mechanisms, responses to inflammatory stimuli, and the deposition of calcified tissue are regulated by pulp cell activity and an assortment of extracellular matrix molecules.[333]

PULPAL RESPONSE TO CARIES*

The advance of invading microorganisms in carious lesions is the essential cause of pulpal inflammation and potential tissue necrosis. Acidogenic gram-positive bacteria, predominantly oral streptococci and lactobacilli, produce metabolic by-products during active caries that demineralize enamel and dentin.[147] Immune responses and pulpal inflammation occur when the caries front advances to within 1.5 mm of the pulp and bacterial antigens and metabolites diffuse through the dentinal tubules.[32,174,255] The main by-product in active carious lesions is lactic acid, which contributes to the demineralization of tooth structure. If the bacterial challenge continues, immune cell responses lead to increased inflammation and edema, initially characterized clinically by pulpal pain. Inflammation is a complex protective biologic response designed to remove injurious stimuli produced by pathogens and reestablish pulpal equilibrium. Prolonged inflammation in the low-compliance environment of the pulp space eventually leads to pulp disintegration and apical pathosis.[147,328]

The caries invasion is initially blocked by protective innate immune responses; it progresses to an adaptive immune response when bacteria directly approach the pulp.[146] The pioneer microbes during caries progression first encounter a positive outward flow of dentinal fluid, characterized by the deposition of immunoglobulins and serum proteins that slow

---

*Adapted from Hahn and Liewehr.[146-148]

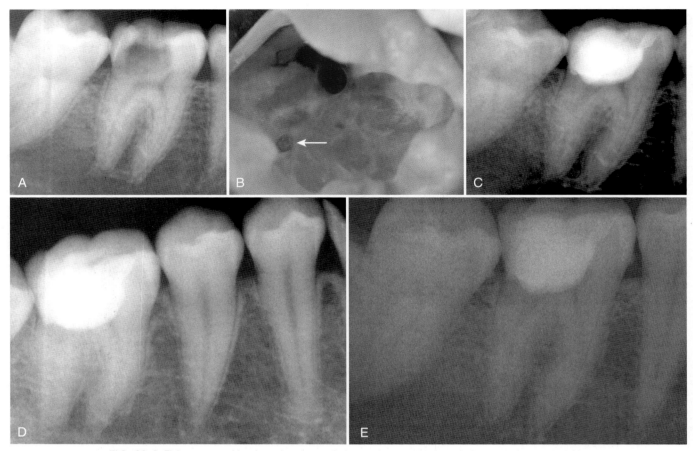

FIG. 23-2 Eighteen-year-old patient who presented with a carious mandibular right first molar that was sensitive to chewing. Cold testing elicited a short, nonlingering but painful response. **A,** Preoperative radiograph showing deep caries near the pulpal roof. **B,** Photograph after caries excavation using caries detector dye and 5-minute sodium hypochlorite hemostasis. Note the distobuccal pulp horn exposure and reactionary (reparative) dentin over the distolingual horn *(arrow).* **C,** Radiograph after bonded composite placement at the second visit, after confirmation of mineral trioxide aggregate (MTA) curing and continued pulp vitality. **D,** Three-year radiographic recall. Patient was asymptomatic and had normal responses on cold testing. **E,** Thirteen-year, 6 month radiographic review. Patient was asymptomatic and responded to vitality testing. The bonded composite restoration was intact and had no marginal degradation. (© Dr. George Bogen.)

the diffusion of bacterial antigens.[147] Potent microbial metabolites, such as lipoteichoic acid and lipopolysaccharide, also activate the innate immune system. The bacterial by-products stimulate signaling by Toll-like receptors in odontoblasts when the odontoblasts first encounter the carious front. They also stimulate proinflammatory cytokines, including interleukin-1, interleukin-8, interleukin-12, tumor necrosis factor alpha, vascular endothelial growth factor, and transforming growth factor beta (TGF-β).[108,156,361] Vascular endothelial growth factor promotes vascular permeability and angiogenesis. Dentin mineralization and matrix metalloproteinase secretion are also induced by the increased expression of TGF-β. Caries bacteria also activate complement pathways and induce the proinflammatory cytokine interferon gamma, which is responsible for killing phagocytosed bacteria by activated macrophages.[160] Odontoblasts also participate in the adaptive response to microbial invasion of dentin by the synthesis of a modified mineralized matrix known as *reactionary dentin,* a structurally altered hard tissue characterized by diminished tubularity.[62] As

microorganisms advance toward the pulp, the modified helical structure in reparative dentin effectively constricts tubular lumen diameter and forms an active barrier against advancing pathogens (Fig. 23-2).[61]

As pulpitis progresses, vasoactive neuropeptides contribute to increased vascular permeability and intrapulpal blood flow. Increases in neuropeptide concentration and nerve sprouting characterize neurogenic inflammation, which can cause a transient increase in interstitial tissue pressure and contribute to painful pulpitis.[47,277] Immune cells attempt to control neurogenic inflammation with the secretion of peptides such as somatostatin and β-endorphin.[243] The primary effector cells in innate responses include natural killer cells, neutrophils, monocytes, and macrophages. Immature dendritic cells and T cells contribute to immunosurveillance during the progression of caries. Macrophages participate in the innate and adaptive immune responses by eliminating both pathogens and senescent cells while contributing to tissue homeostasis by repairing and remodeling tissue after inflammation.[146]

Cytokines are small, cell-signaling proteins secreted by innate immune cells that induce phagocyte extravasation during inflammation. Chemokines secreted by odontoblasts, fibroblasts, immature dendritic cells, and macrophages stimulate leukocyte recruitment by directing monocyte and neutrophil migration extravascularly to sites of infection.[146] Persistent infection engages the adaptive immune system, which can lead to edema and increased intrapulpal pressure, causing tissue destruction, acute phase protein production, and cell death, leading to tissue necrosis.[148] As the caries front progresses to the pulp, prompt clinical intervention, through removal of decay and bacterial antigens before irreversible pulpitis commences, can resolve pulpal inflammation and promote recovery.

REPARATIVE BRIDGE FORMATION

The foremost objective in vital pulp therapy is to encourage protective hard tissue barrier formation after injury. The process is initiated when regenerated odontoblast-like cells recruited from the cell-rich zone and subodontoblastic layer advance the repair of pulpodental defects after migration of highly vascularized tissue to the site. The repair process after pulp capping is characterized by four steps: (1) moderate inflammation, (2) recruitment and advance of dedicated adult reserve stem (progenitor) cells, (3) proliferation of the progenitor cells, and (4) terminal differentiation.[132] Strong evidence supports the role of inflammation as a prerequisite for tissue repair to proceed.[104]

The osteoblast/odontoblast-like progenitors responsible for reparative calcific bridge formation are either fibroblasts, inflammatory cells that undergo phenotypic conversion, or potentially resident stem cells activated by cytokines released during the inflammatory process.[130] Progenitor cell differentiation may also be modulated during inflammation by activation of antigen-presenting dendritic cells or triggered by specific odontoblast and fibroblast membrane receptors.[130] Currently, the origin of the differentiated odontoblast-like cells remains controversial. Fibroblasts, perivascular cells, bone marrow stem cells, and undifferentiated mesenchymal stem cells have all been proposed as potential progenitors.[338] A recent histologic study, however, suggests that the amorphous, atubular calcified repair tissue formed subjacent to the calcium hydroxide (CH) placed on the pulp wound in the absence of odontoblasts is produced by pulpal fibroblasts.[276a] Therefore, such mineralized hard tissue is not genuine dentin, but repair tissue that has been called "reparative dentin," for lack of a better term.

Odontoblast replacement in nonhuman primates directly after pulp exposures capped with CH has been examined during the cell migration and replication stages.[111] Newly differentiating odontoblast-type cells showing initial matrix formation were demonstrated as early as day 8 at the CH-pulp interface. The continual influx of labeled differentiating cells indicated that the original derivation was from the deeper, central pulp tissue that required two DNA replications before terminal differentiation.[111] Investigations have also indicated that reparative bridge mineralization may be more dependent on the extracellular matrix than on the capping material selected.[171,189,259]

During healing, initial calcification immediately after pulp amputation is characterized by a proliferation of extracellular matrix vesicles situated between the forming cells and the injured pulp surface.[152,264] The formation of needle-like crystals and osmophilic material within vesicles proceeds with an accumulation of crystals and aggregate at the calcified fronts, along with the disappearance of the vesicular membrane. The crystals produced during the calcification process are associated with phosphate and calcium ions, similar to fundamental calcification processes shown by other normal and pathologic calcified tissues.[152] Defects in pulpal healing and dentinal bridge formation are associated with different pulp capping materials and include pulpal inflammation, bacterial microleakage, operative debris, and tunnel defects.[188]

PROCEDURES FOR GENERATING HARD TISSUE BARRIERS

Direct Pulp Capping

The treatment options for permanent teeth that encourage pulp preservation include direct and indirect pulp capping and partial or complete pulpotomy. *Direct pulp capping* is defined as "placing a dental material directly on a mechanical or traumatic vital pulp exposure" and "sealing the pulpal wound to facilitate the formation of reparative dentin and maintenance of the vital pulp."[12] The procedure is indicated for pulp exposures incurred as a result of caries removal, trauma, or tooth preparation. When mechanical exposures occur during tooth preparation, the exposed tissue is generally not inflamed. However, in cases of trauma or carious exposure, the degree of inflammation is the key predetermining prognostic factor. According to the American Association of Endodontists, "In a carious pulp exposure, underlying pulp is inflamed to a varying or unknown extent."[12] The major challenge in direct pulp capping is the proper identification and removal of the acutely inflamed or necrotic tissue compromised by longstanding exposure to oral microorganisms.[210]

Pulpotomy

Pulpotomy, or *pulp amputation,* is a more intrusive procedure defined as "the removal of the coronal portion of the vital pulp as a means of preserving the vitality of the remaining radicular portion: may be performed as emergency procedure for temporary relief of symptoms or therapeutic measure, as in the instance of a Cvek pulpotomy."[12] After complete amputation of the coronal pulp, a capping material is placed over the pulp floor and the remaining exposed tissue in the canal orifices. Dressing materials of varying toxicity have been used for this purpose, including ferric sulfate, creosote, phenol, zinc oxide eugenol, polycarboxylate cement, glutaraldehyde, CH, and formaldehyde; some of these dressing materials embalm any remaining tissue.[265]

The procedure is recommended for primary teeth for which short-term outcomes are generally favorable. Formocresol has been the accepted "standard" universal pulpotomy agent in primary teeth and is recommended for young adult teeth; however, it has considerable drawbacks that put into question its continued use in humans.[195,196,281,318] It has been identified as carcinogenic and genotoxic, and experiments have shown a high incidence of internal resorption in nonhuman primate models.[120,203,207] Changes in the root canal system apical to formocresol placement can also create challenges when orthograde root canal treatment is attempted.[278] Comparative studies have demonstrated MTA to be an appropriate replacement for formocresol for primary molar pulpotomy.[48,164,306] Recent investigations also support the use of MTA and other CSCs for application in pulpotomy procedures in permanent teeth.[17,300]

Partial Pulpotomy

Partial pulpotomy (shallow pulpotomy, or Cvek pulpotomy) is defined as the removal of a small portion of the vital coronal pulp as a means of preserving the remaining coronal and radicular pulp tissues.[12] After the pulp has been exposed and is visualized after hemostasis, inflamed or necrotic tissue is removed to uncover deeper, healthy pulp tissue in the pulp chamber.[77,257] Partial pulpotomy and direct pulp capping can be viewed as similar procedures, but they differ in the amount of vital pulp tissue remaining after treatment. Partial pulpotomy is the preferred option in elective treatment procedures for teeth diagnosed with anatomic anomalies, such as dens invaginatus.

Indirect Pulp Capping

Indirect pulp capping is defined by the AAPD as "a procedure performed in a tooth with a deep carious lesion approximating the pulp but without signs or symptoms of pulp degeneration. Indirect pulp treatment is indicated in a permanent tooth diagnosed with a normal pulp with no signs or symptoms of pulpitis or with a diagnosis of reversible pulpitis."[13] The treatment can be completed as a one-step or two-step procedure (stepwise technique) with the objective of arresting the active carious lesion.[37] Indirect pulp capping has been shown to be an effective technique for caries and patient management in the primary dentition, but it remains controversial in permanent teeth.[46,107,116,210,212] The technique is similar for both primary and permanent teeth, except that permanent teeth require reentry for the removal of residual carious tissue; reentry also is considered necessary to confirm reactionary dentin formation.[53,178] However, data from a recent investigation have questioned the need to reopen cavities to remove residual infected dentin in a subsequent visit.[209]

The treatment requires prudent case selection, including identification of asymptomatic patients with no suspicion of irreversible pulpitis. Pulp exposures are avoided during caries excavation by removal of the superficial demineralized necrotic dentin and then the removal of the peripheral dentin.[119] After excavation, the remaining carious dentin is lined with CH and sealed with a provisional material, such as intermediate restorative material (IRM) or a resin-modified glass ionomer (RMGI). The patient returns in 8 to 12 weeks for placement of a permanent coronal restoration. Advocates of indirect pulp capping argue that pulp healing can be compromised if the carious dentin barrier is removed during excavation and that the prognosis of vital pulp therapy (direct exposure) is unfavorable.[36] A challenging aspect of indirect pulp capping is determining the exact boundary point where caries excavation is terminated. Therefore, the technique is based primarily on subjective criteria and the operator's skill.[201] Further complicating the process is the presence of potential voids under the provisional restoration; during the mineralization process, these can permit dentin to lose volume during desiccation. Another drawback is the rapid reactivation of dormant lesions after restoration failure.[36] However, in younger patients with management issues, indirect pulp capping has shown promising results for immature permanent teeth in which the apical foramina are large, the canal walls are thin, and pulp vascularization is pronounced.[88,138,201,323]

INDICATIONS FOR VITAL PULP THERAPY

Vital pulp therapy is recommended for all teeth diagnosed with reversible pulpitis or partially inflamed pulps in which the remaining healthy tissue can be conserved to generate a hard tissue barrier that seals and protects the pulp from future microbial insult. The introduction of new bioactive materials, along with modified protocols, make more teeth with deep caries, traumatic injuries, and mechanical exposures viable candidates for innovative pulp therapies designed to potentiate and maintain pulpal survival. Treatment outcomes for direct pulp capping and pulpotomy procedures depend on multiple factors, beginning with a differential diagnosis that takes into account pulp testing, radiographic evaluation, clinical evaluation, and the patient history to determine a rational prognosis. Outcomes also depend on case selection, hemostatic agents, choice of pulp capping material, and the integrity of the sealed permanent restoration. The underlying purpose in vital pulp therapy is to avoid or delay root canal therapy and advanced restorative care because these, together, may reduce long-term tooth survival compared to teeth with vital pulps.*

MATERIALS FOR VITAL PULP THERAPY

A variety of pulp dressing materials have been investigated and used over the past century to encourage bridge formation and pulp preservation. A short list of compounds includes CH products, calcium phosphate, zinc oxide, calcium-tetracycline chelate, zinc phosphate and polycarboxylate cements, Bioglass, Emdogain, antibiotic and growth factor combinations, Ledermix, calcium phosphate ceramics, cyanoacrylate, hydrophilic resins, RMGI cements, hydroxyapatite compounds and, recently, MTA and other CSCs.† Other strategies designed to arrest invasive caries and promote repair of underlying tissues include the use of lasers, ozone technology, silver diamine fluoride, and bioactive agents that stimulate pulpal defense mechanisms.‡ Retrospective investigations have shown varying success rates of 30% to 85% for direct pulp capping in humans, depending on the method, hemostatic agent, and dressing material used.§ The search to identify and produce the ideal pulp capping material continues, and remarkable progress has been made in pulp preservation research in the past decade.

Calcium Hydroxide

Calcium hydroxide has long been considered the universal standard for vital pulp therapy materials. The introduction of CH into dentistry is credited to Hermann in the 1920s.[158] Although the material demonstrates many advantageous properties, long-term study outcomes in vital pulp therapy have been inconsistent.[21,28,30,165] Desirable characteristics of CH include an initial high alkaline pH, which is responsible for stimulating fibroblasts and enzyme systems. It neutralizes the low pH of acids, shows antibacterial properties, and promotes pulp tissue defense mechanisms and repair. The drawbacks of CH include weak marginal adaptation to dentin, degradation and dissolution over time, and primary tooth resorption.

---

*References 54, 55, 89, 234, 251, 282, 314, 331, and 346.
†References 31, 34, 113, 155, 161, 182, 262, 265, 308, 311, 360, and 368.
‡References 45, 67, 79, 132, 239, 261, 279, 367, and 369.
§References 21, 26, 30, 81, 151, 222, and 349.

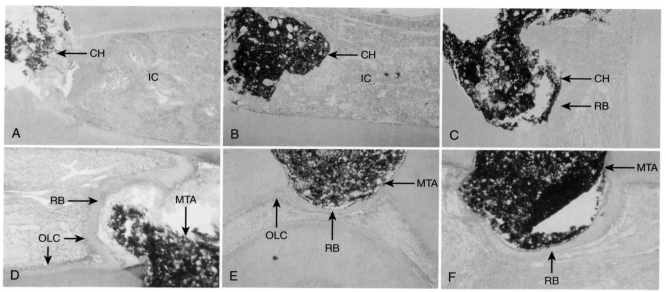

FIG. 23-3 Reparative bridge formation compared in dog pulps using mineral trioxide aggregate *(MTA)* and calcium hydroxide *(CH)*. A, Two-week pulp response to CH showing inflammatory cells *(IC)*. B, Tissue specimen showing lack of bridge formation and disorganized tissue proximal to CH. C, An 8-week specimen with partial reparative bridge (RB) formation subjacent to CH. D, Two-week pulpal response to MTA showing notable barrier formation and layer of organized odontoblast-like cells *(OLC)*. E, Pulp tissue section demonstrating complete calcificbridge formation proximal to MTA at 4 weeks. F, Sample section pulp capped with MTA at the 8-week period showing organized hard tissue formation with no inflammatory cell infiltrate. (Loma Linda University, Loma Linda, California.)

Reparative bridge formation subjacent to CH can also be characterized by tunnel defects.* Histologically, CH demonstrates cytotoxicity in cell cultures and has been shown to induce pulp cell apoptosis.[14,131,287]

Tunnel defects have been demonstrated in reparative hard tissue bridges associated with both CH and CSCs.[10] However, the primary difference between the two pulp therapy agents is that CH products are absorbable over time and dimensionally unstable. The slow disintegration of the CH after hard tissue barrier formation can allow microleakage, thus permitting a slow ingress of microorganisms through calcific bridge defects. This can induce subsequent pulpal degeneration, further leading to potential dystrophic calcification and pulpal necrosis. Over extended periods, this problematic outcome of CH pulp capping can complicate nonsurgical root canal treatment if required.[237]

Clinical retrospective investigations have shown variable success rates over 2- to 10-year recall periods for direct CH pulp capping in humans.[21,28,30,165] Two current studies have examined the efficacy of CH as a direct pulp capping agent. One study examined the survival rate of 248 pulp-capped teeth that were diagnosed either as having normal pulps or as exhibiting spontaneous pain; the researchers found an overall survival rate of 76.3% with an average recall period of 6.1 years.[81] Treatment outcomes were less favorable for teeth showing spontaneous pain, in older compared to younger patients, and in teeth restored with glass ionomer cements. The probability of pulps becoming nonvital after CH pulp capping was greater within the first 5 years of treatment.

The second study observed 1,075 teeth directly pulp capped with a CH-based agent; these teeth had either healthy pulps or showed signs of reversible pulpitis.[349] Inclusion criteria limited pulp chamber roof exposures to no larger than 2 mm in diameter. Successful outcomes were 80.1% after 1 year and 68% after 5 years; this diminished to 58.7% after a 9-year observation period.

The results of the two studies indicate increasing failure rates over time, attributable to absorption of the material under permanent restorations proximal to mineralized bridges with tunnel defects. Another investigation has confirmed decreasing success rates with CH pulp capping with extended recall periods.[222] Calcium hydroxide clearly has many favorable characteristics as a vital pulp therapy agent. However, the material also demonstrates inherent physical weaknesses and can no longer be considered the preferred universal agent in vital pulp therapy (Fig. 23-3).[105,162a,222,224a,247]

Resin-Modified Glass Ionomer Cements and Hydrophilic Resins

Adhesive systems were introduced in the early 1980s as potential agents for direct pulp capping of cariously and mechanically exposed pulps.[170,216,355] These materials include RMGI cements, composite resins, and hydrophilic resins. Hydrophilic resins and RMGI cements initially showed favorable outcomes in preliminary pulp capping investigations with nonhuman primates based on standards set by the International Organization for Standardization (ISO).[71,315-317] However, the transitional use of these materials in human subjects did not demonstrate the corresponding biocompatibility or consistent reparative bridge formation.[2,90,131,153,166,235] Investigations that

---

*References 14, 25, 73, 74, 131, 134, 238, and 286.

have examined responses of resin-based materials in human teeth have demonstrated unfavorable histologic reactions when the material is placed directly or in close proximity to pulp tissue.[2,95,143,236,274] Histologic sections from these studies typically demonstrate the presence of inflammatory cell infiltrates consistent with pulp cell cytotoxicity, subclinical adhesive failures at the pulp interface, and a profound absence of biocompatibility.*

Research data have shown that increasing concentrations of triethylene glycol dimethacrylate (TEGDMA), a common dentin bonding compound, differentially increase the levels of apoptotic and necrotic cell populations after direct exposure.[305] Moreover, even low levels of TEGDMA diminish alkaline phosphatase activity and calcium deposition, thus inhibiting pulp cell mineralization and potential reparative bridge formation.[127] Alternatively, adhesive resins have shown some promise when combined with additives or growth factors, such as hydroxyapatite powder, dental matrix protein-derived synthetic peptides, calcium chloride (CaCl$_2$), calcium phosphate, and antibacterial agents, including 12-methacryloyloxydodecylpyridinium bromide (MDPB).[76,183,312] It is evident that bonding agents used for direct pulp capping do not predictably generate a favorable environment for pulp healing and hard tissue formation.[299] However, hydrophilic resins and RMGI cements provide excellent seals when they are combined with light-cured composites in permanent restorations and then placed directly over pulp capping materials such as MTA.[20,101,249]

Mineral Trioxide Aggregate (MTA)

Mineral trioxide aggregate was introduced as a pulp capping material by Torabinejad and associates in the mid-1990s.[113] Most preliminary experimental and current clinical data in vital pulp therapy are based on the proprietary material ProRoot MTA (Tulsa/Dentsply, Tulsa, Oklahoma). The cement consists of hydraulic calcium silicate powder containing various oxide compounds, including calcium oxide, ferric oxide, silicon oxide, sodium and potassium oxides, magnesium oxide, and aluminum oxide.[51] The material exhibits favorable physiochemical characteristics that stimulate reparative dentinogenesis by recruitment and activation of hard tissue–forming cells, contributing to matrix formation and mineralization.[260] Soluble cytokines and growth factors that mediate wound repair of the dentin-pulp complex are nested in the extracellular matrix, and MTA stimulates reparative hard tissue formation by sequestering these growth factors and cytokines embedded in the surrounding dentin matrix.[190,191,327,340] Calcium hydroxide and calcium silicate hydrate, the principal by-products formed during hydration of mixed MTA, contribute to a sustained alkaline pH.[50,117] The setting properties of the hydroscopic silicate cements are not affected by the presence of tissue fluids or blood.[329]

During the setting process, the gradual release of calcium ions encourages reparative barrier formation by promoting signaling molecules, such as vascular endothelial growth factor (VEGF), macrophage colony-stimulating factor (MCSF), TGF-β, and interleukins IL-1β and IL-1α.[214,267] MTA demonstrates superior marginal adaptation to dentin compared to CH-based agents; MTA forms an adherent interfacial layer during mineral nucleation at the dentin surface that appears similar in composition to hydroxyapatite when examined with X-ray diffraction, energy-dispersive X-ray analysis, and scanning electron microscopy (SEM).[260,283,330]

If the pulp is injured, wound healing and the repair process can advance only after the initiation of the inflammatory reaction.[130,205] Similar to CH, MTA induces an inflammatory cascade that results from calcium ion release and the creation of an alkaline environment, producing tissue necrosis. Both MTA and CH have been shown to stimulate and increase the Höehl cell mitosis index in rodent models.[82,83] MTA activates the migration of progenitor cells from the central pulp to the injury site and promotes their proliferation and differentiation into odontoblast-like cells without inducing pulp cell apoptosis.[260] MTA also stimulates in vitro the production of messenger ribonucleic acid (mRNA) and increases protein expression of the mineralized matrix genes and cellular markers crucial for mineralization after matrix formation.[260]

Gray MTA has been shown to enhance cell proliferation and survival of cultured human dental pulp stromal cells.[267] The biocompatibility of set MTA up-regulates the expression of transcription factors, angiogenic factors, and gene products, such as dentin sialoprotein, osteocalcin, and alkaline phosphatase.[266] Odontoblast signaling proteins are essential in the differentiation of progenitor cells into the odontoblast-like cells responsible for repair and hard tissue deposition.[266,267] After MTA pulp capping, both sialoprotein and osteopontin have been observed in the fibrodentin matrix at the exposure site during the process of reparative hard tissue formation.[194]

Dental pulp cells differentiate into the odontoblastic cell line in the presence of the signaling molecules, such as TGF-β, heme oxygenase-1 enzyme, and bone morphogenetic proteins BMP-2, BMP-4, and BMP-7.[141] MTA most likely up-regulates fibroblast secretion of BMP-2 and TGF-β1 and therefore stimulates and promotes mineralization and hard tissue regeneration.* MTA induces a time-dependent environment that is proinflammatory and promotes wound regeneration through up-regulation of cytokines.[275] Immunohistochemical analyses show that cytokines, including myeloperoxidase, inducible nitric oxide synthase, VEGF, nuclear factor-kappa B (NF-κB), activating protein-1, and cyclooxygenase-2, show increased expression in the presence of MTA. Cytokine up-regulation is responsible for inducing biomineralization by producing apatite-like clusters on collagen fibrils at the MTA-dentin interface. MTA does not affect the generation of reactive oxygen species, thereby positively influencing cell survival. MTA also has been shown to improve the secretion of IL-1β, Il-6, and IL-8.[49,57,66] However, an inhibitory effect on dental pulp cells has been demonstrated in the presence of MTA, which may be attributed to the release of aluminum ions.[231] The data indicate that MTA promotes a biocompatible, noncytotoxic, antibacterial environment and surface morphology that are favorable for reparative calcific bridge formation. MTA stimulates the release of the dentin matrix components necessary for hard tissue repair and regeneration in mechanically exposed healthy and partially inflamed pulps (Figs. 23-4 to 23-6).†

Calcium Silicate–Based Cements (CSCs)

A variety of new bioactive CSCs or bioceramic materials have been developed since the introduction of MTA.[85,128,198]

---

*References 2, 90, 236, 258, 274, and 299.

*References 84, 141, 142, 149, 291, 313, and 357.
†References 6, 113, 142, 230, 247, 276, and 326.

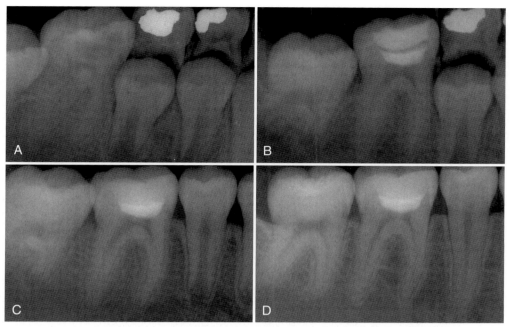

FIG. 23-4 Symptomatic mandibular right first molar in a 9-year-old patient. **A,** Preoperative film; cold testing evoked a short period of discomfort. **B,** Postoperative radiograph after sodium hypochlorite hemostasis, direct mineral trioxide aggregate (MTA) pulp caps on 0.5- and 1-mm exposures, and wet cotton pellet with Photocore® provisionalization. **C,** One-year radiographic review; tooth responds normally to cold vitality test. **D,** Control radiograph at 8 years. Patient was asymptomatic and exhibited normal pulp testing response. (© Dr. George Bogen.)

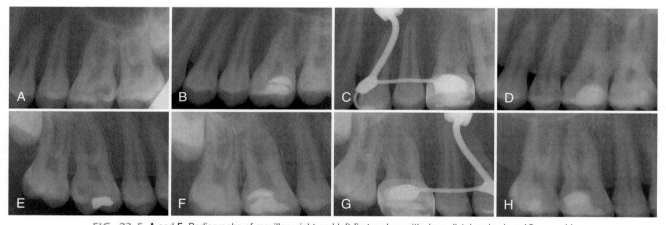

FIG. 23-5 **A** and **E,** Radiographs of maxillary right and left first molars with deep distal caries in a 12-year-old patient. **B** and **F,** Posttreatment radiographs after direct mineral trioxide aggregate (MTA) pulp caps, wet cotton pellets, and Photocore provisionalization. **C** and **G,** One-year radiographic recall; the patient was in active orthodontic treatment. **D** and **H,** Radiographic controls taken 7.5 years after MTA direct pulp caps. Note caries in maxillary left second premolar in **D** (patient was advised). The patient was asymptomatic and tested normal on cold tests at the 1- and 7.5-year recall periods for both molars. (© Dr. George Bogen.)

Preliminary investigations with CSCs have demonstrated physiochemical and bioinductive properties comparable to those of MTA, indicating the potential future application of these materials in vital pulp therapy.[42,98] Some of these tricalcium-based materials include BioAggregate (Innovative Bioceramix, Vancouver, British Columbia), Biodentine (Septodont, Cambridge, Ontario, Canada), MTA-Angelus, MTA Bio, and MTA Branco (MTA-Angelus, Londrina PR, Brazil).[133,202] Other formulations include EndocemMTA (Maruchi, Wonju-si, Gangwon-do, South Korea) and Endosequence root repair material (Brasseler USA, Savannah, Georgia). Additional compounds are currently undergoing clinical investigations to establish their safety and efficacy.[16,242]

The main components of MTA and the new CSCs are tricalcium silicate and dicalcium silicate, major components of Portland cement. Hydraulic tricalcium silicates promote reparative barrier formation by up-regulation of transcription factors after gaining immediate strength on hydration. However, research data are limited on direct pulp capping and pulpotomy treatments in humans using these new bioceramic products.

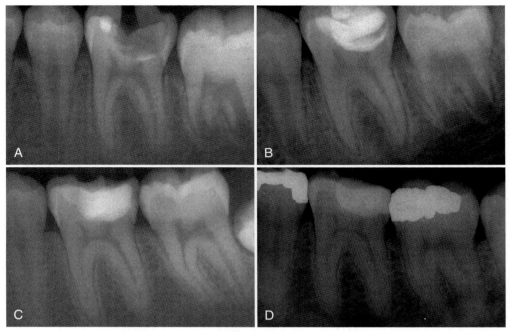

FIG. 23-6 Direct pulp capping of a mandibular left molar in an 11-year-old patient. **A,** Pretreatment radiograph showing large carious lesion after loss of a temporary restoration. **B,** Radiograph after mineral trioxide aggregate (MTA) placement with moist cotton pellet, and an unbonded Photocore® interim restoration was placed over a 2-mm pulp exposure. **C,** Four-year radiographic recall. The molar responded normally to carbon dioxide (CO_2) ice testing. **D,** Thirteen-year recall radiograph showing typical periapical structures and completed root formation. Cold testing responses were normal, and the patient was asymptomatic. (© Dr. George Bogen.)

BioAggregate is a bioinductive tricalcium cement that can induce mineralization in osteoblast cells by increasing levels of osteocalcin, collagen type 1, and osteopontin gene expression.[363] Hydration of the cement results in the formation of calcium silicate hydrate and CH, showing high concentrations of silica and calcium phosphate.[136] This characteristic is consistent with materials used in vital pulp therapy to promote hard tissue formation. Investigations using X-ray diffraction show the material to have a composition similar to that of MTA, but BioAggregate contains tantalum rather than bismuth oxide to provide radiopacity.[268] BioAggregate demonstrates remarkable biocompatibility compared to MTA, inducing cell differentiation in both human periodontal ligament and gingival fibroblasts.[356] Both fresh and set mixtures of MTA and BioAggregate have shown antimicrobial properties effective against *Enterococcus faecalis* in vitro when combined with equal amounts of human dentin powder.[366] The material also shows a greater resistance to dislodgement in an acidic environment compared to MTA, in addition to higher fracture resistance when used as a filling material.[150,336]

Biodentine is a tricalcium silicate–based cement that also demonstrates exceptional bioactive properties with potential for both direct and indirect pulp capping procedures. The cement has a short setting time of 10 minutes and does not induce genotoxic or cytotoxic effects when measured with the Ames mutagenicity test. It is considered a biocompatible dentin replacement material for use under various restorative materials as a base or liner, and it does not alter human pulp fibroblast cytodifferentiation.[198] SEM analysis demonstrates the sealing ability of Biodentine to be similar to that of MTA;

Biodentine forms needle-like crystals resembling apatite at the dentin interface.[91] The material induces odontoblast-like cell differentiation, stimulates biomineralization, and promotes hard tissue formation when used as a pulp capping material.[293,365]

Another promising material for vital pulp therapy is MTA-Angelus, which has a basic formulation of 25% bismuth oxide and 75% Portland cement. The composition eliminates calcium sulfate, providing a short setting time of 10 minutes, which is preferable for one-visit pulp capping or pulpotomy procedures (Fig. 23-7).[42] Variations in bismuth oxide and the presence of iron characterize the chemical composition of MTA-Angelus, and the crystalline structures formed on hydration are similar to gray and white ProRoot MTA.[302] MTA-Angelus and ProRoot MTA have been compared experimentally as pulp capping agents in intact, caries-free human teeth.[5] Histomorphologic examination of extracted teeth revealed that the two materials produced similar responses with regard to inflammation and hard tissue formation.[5,193] MTA-Angelus also demonstrates antifungal properties and a lower compressive strength than ProRoot MTA.[29,180]

Endosequence root repair material shows low cytotoxicity, antibacterial activity against *E. faecalis,* and strong potential as a pulp capping material.[80,370] Another material, calcium-enriched mixture (CEM) cement, has also demonstrated excellent physical and biologic properties in vital pulp therapy investigations.[17-19,256]

This new generation of CSCs appears promising when used as vital pulp therapeutic agents and current investigations appear to support these materials' future potential.

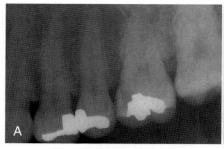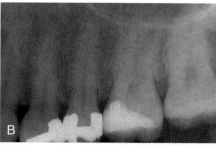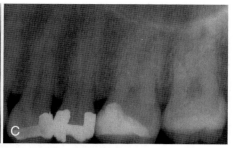

FIG. 23-7 Thirty-four-year old patient who presented with sensitivity to hot, cold, and sweet foods. **A,** Preoperative radiograph of maxillary left first molar showing mesial caries and an occlusal amalgam restoration. **B,** Posttreatment radiograph after 1.5-mm wide pulp exposure, direct "fast set" mineral trioxide aggregate (MTA-Angelus) pulp cap, and bonded composite restoration. The tooth was symptomatic for 1 hour after the local anesthetic had dissipated. **C,** Two-year radiographic review; the tooth has a normal response to cold testing. (© Dr. George Bogen.)

MTA APPLICATIONS IN VITAL PULP THERAPY

Direct Pulp Capping with MTA

Controlled prospective investigations on direct pulp capping in humans using MTA against cariously exposed pulps are limited. Collectively, most studies are inconsistent with regard to case selection, treatment strategies, and clinical protocols.[232] The subsequent spectrum of outcomes is reflected by the absence of standardized guidelines for caries removal, hemostatic agents, single- versus two-visit delivery sequences, and the choice and placement of a capping material.

Unsatisfactory outcomes for direct capping due to variations in treatment delivery and protocols were clearly demonstrated in a cohort investigation completed by predoctoral dental students.[229] Fifty-one direct MTA pulp caps completed in a carious field were radiographically and clinically evaluated for a 12- to 27-month period. The overall success rates using Kaplan-Meier analysis were 67.7% at 1 year and 56.2% at 2 years. The poor outcome can be attributed to an absence of strict control protocols with regard to caries removal, selection of hemostatic agents, and appropriate magnification, illumination, and thickness combined with area coverage of MTA. As a result, the investigation concluded that the amount of hemorrhaging after pulp exposure was not a determining factor in the clinical outcome, contrary to other findings.[63,215]

More impressive results for pulp maintenance and continued vitality after direct pulp capping procedures have been demonstrated in several other contemporary studies.[4,6,204,222] An investigation examined 30 immature permanent teeth exhibiting wide-open apices directly pulp capped with MTA and restored temporarily with IRM.[109] Definitive permanent composite restorations were placed 2 weeks later, after confirmation of pulp vitality. In these cariously exposed immature permanent teeth, the success rate at a 2-year review was 93%.

Another observational investigation examined direct pulp capping after carious exposures of mature and immature permanent teeth completed using MTA in a two-visit sequence.[40] Forty-nine teeth were examined in patients aged 7 to 45 years over a 1- to 9-year period, with an average 3.94-year observation time. The study incorporated a strict protocol that included detector dye–aided caries excavation using the dental operating microscope, 5.25% to 6% sodium hypochlorite (NaOCl)

hemostasis, thick MTA placement on pulp exposures and surrounding dentin, coupled with adhesion-based permanent restorations placed at a subsequent visit to compensate for the delayed setting properties of ProRoot MTA. Based on subjective symptomatology, cold testing, and radiographic evaluation, 97.96% of teeth showed a favorable outcome. All 15 patients with immature apices showed continued root formation, with apical closure over a 6- to 10-year period; five patients with large or multiple exposures exhibited pulpal calcification (Fig. 23-8).

The improved survival outcomes seen in this MTA pulp capping study can be credited to changes in established treatment protocols and the incorporation of improved pulp capping materials. Progress in the caries removal process, magnification systems, NaOCl hemostasis, MTA selection, and adhesion technology take advantage of advances in vital pulp therapy to surpass the outcomes seen with accepted traditional methods (Figs. 23-9 and 23-10).

The unique physiochemical properties of MTA also promote a superior environment for pulpal repair and bridge formation, compared to CH products.[162a,204,222,224a,247] MTA is a hygroscopic cement that sets in the presence of blood and serum, produces a gap-free interface with dentin, and generates a sustained alkaline pH; in addition, the surface morphology of the hardened cement allows for predictable bonding with current adhesion systems. Growth factors necessary for hard tissue formation are activated by MTA through the gradual release of calcium ions during cement curing.[190] The small particle size and alkaline pH contribute to the entombment of remaining cariogenic bacteria at the dentin-MTA interface, impeding bacterial ingression and caries progression and discouraging continued pulpal injury.[250,359a]

Pulpotomy with MTA

The decision to remove a small or large portion of the coronal pulp is based on visual inspection of the pulp tissue and the ability to achieve hemostasis after pulp exposure during either caries excavation or exposure as a result of trauma (partial or shallow pulpotomy). The coronal pulp tissue can also be removed completely to the pulp floor or cervical area (pulpotomy) in the case of molars and some premolars.[118,122] The AAPD guidelines state, "A pulpotomy is performed in a tooth with extensive caries but without evidence of radicular pathology when caries removal results in a carious or mechanical

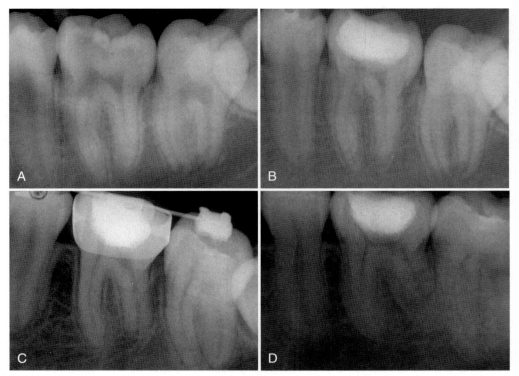

FIG. 23-8 An 11-year-old who presented with deep occlusal caries in a mandibular left first molar. Responses to cold testing were normal, although the patient complained of a sleepless night. **A,** Preoperative radiograph. **B,** Radiograph after direct mineral trioxide aggregate (MTA) pulp caps were applied, followed by composite restoration placement on the second visit. The tooth had two large exposures, 1.5 and 2 mm in diameter. **C,** Three-year radiographic review with molar in full banding during orthodontic treatment. **D,** Radiographic review at 9.5 years showing no evidence of periapical pathosis or notable pulp calcification. Carbon dioxide cold testing indicated normal vitality. (© Dr. George Bogen.)

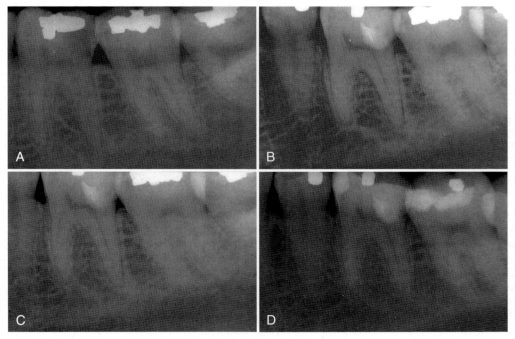

FIG. 23-9 **A,** Deep caries in a partially symptomatic mandibular left first molar in a 29-year-old patient. **B,** Direct pulp cap with mineral trioxide aggregate (MTA); the final restoration was placed during the second visit after MTA curing. **C,** Radiographic recall at 1 year. **D,** Seven-year recall radiograph showing regular periapical appearance. The molar responded normally to cold testing at both follow-up visits. (© Dr. George Bogen.)

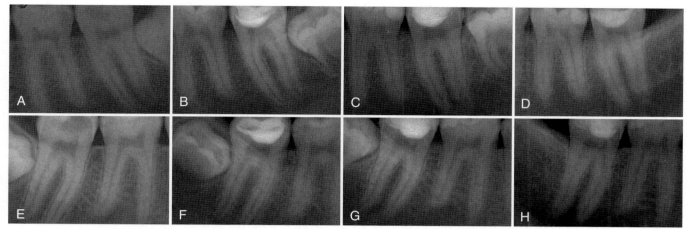

FIG. 23-10 **A** and **E**, Radiographs of mandibular left and right second molars with deep distal caries in a 22-year-old patient. **B** and **F**, Posttreatment radiographs after direct gray mineral trioxide aggregate (MTA) pulp caps, wet cotton pellets, and Photocore® provisionalization. **C** and **G**, Two-year radiographic recalls. **D** and **H**, Radiographic controls taken 10 years after pulp capping. Both teeth responded positive to cold tests at the 2- and 10-year recall periods. The third molars had been extracted. (© Dr. George Bogen.)

pulp exposure."[13] If bleeding cannot be controlled after 10 minutes of direct exposure to NaOCl after removal of unhealthy tissue, complete removal of the coronal pulp to the pulp floor is the preferred option.

Sodium hypochlorite serves as an excellent diagnostic tool to differentiate irreversible from reversible pulpitis and to help determine whether to proceed with partial pulpotomy, complete pulpotomy, or pulpectomy. This decision can be of paramount importance in young permanent teeth with open apices, in which removal of tissue contaminated by microorganisms can reverse symptoms and stabilize inflamed tissue.[64,100] Investigations have shown that the proliferative response of pulp tissue after exposure progresses several millimeters into the pulp from the injury site.[77] The removal of 1 to 3 mm of peripheral tissue to access the deeper, healthy tissue, in cases of trauma or when carious exposures reveal inflamed tissue, ensures pulp survival (Fig. 23-11).

Partial pulpotomy for treating direct pulp exposures in immature permanent teeth using CH products has been shown to be a reliable treatment option with proper case selection.* However, improved success rates ranging from 93% to 100% have been demonstrated using MTA for pulpotomies in permanent teeth.[28,272,352] Moreover, pulpotomies completed with MTA in primary molar teeth do not show pathologic complications such as internal resorption, which typically are seen with CH, formocresol, and ferric sulfate.[97]

It has been recommended that pulpectomy be avoided in immature permanent teeth with vital canal tissue so as to protect the remaining radicular pulp tissue and thus encourage continued root development and apexogenesis.[112,287,303] However, with the introduction of MTA, predictable root-end closure and maturogenesis can be achieved with new approaches using regenerative, revascularization, and apexogenesis procedures (Fig. 23-12).† Although controversy remains regarding the type and quality of tissue produced in regenerative procedures for nonvital teeth, current treatment options for

immature teeth strengthen roots by increasing wall thickness and root length.[177,211]

Complete pulpotomy for mature irreversibly inflamed permanent molars represents a novel approach in treating symptomatic teeth while preserving pulp canal tissue.[17] A current randomized clinical trial compared full pulpotomies completed with MTA and CEM; the study examined postoperative pain, along with radiographic and clinical outcomes in patients diagnosed with irreversible pulpitis.[18] At a 1-year follow-up for 413 pulpotomized teeth, the clinical success rates were 98% for MTA and 97% for CEM. Similarly, the radiographic success rates were 95% for MTA and 92% for CEM. Most patients experienced a significant reduction in pain intensity postoperatively over a 7-day period. This conservative strategy for irreversibly inflamed teeth may be beneficial for patients in underserved areas globally.

VITAL PULP THERAPY TECHNIQUES

Diagnosis

A differential diagnosis based on symptoms and clinical findings is the goal in the assessment of pulp vitality. However, an accurate determination of the pulpal condition before treatment initiation can be more challenging in younger patients.[304] Establishing a diagnosis of reversible versus irreversible pulpitis in immature teeth can be complicated by subjective symptoms and testing responses that may not accurately reflect the histopathologic condition of the involved pulp.[52] However, efforts should be directed toward the ultimate goal of pulpal preservation and continued apexogenesis in immature permanent teeth.[38,39] A diagnosis of irreversible pulpitis, based on signs and symptoms, along with clinical testing procedures, does not preclude vital pulp therapy options. Regardless of the treatment choice of pulp capping or partial or complete pulpotomy, preservation of the radicular pulp and apical papilla allows for root maturation in cases of trauma or deep caries.[121,122,140,292]

Acceptable diagnostic quality intraoral radiographs of the involved tooth must be taken to evaluate accurately the extent

---

*References 27, 121, 213, 220, 256, 272, and 332.
†References 39, 41, 110, 129, 169, 244, 322, and 353.

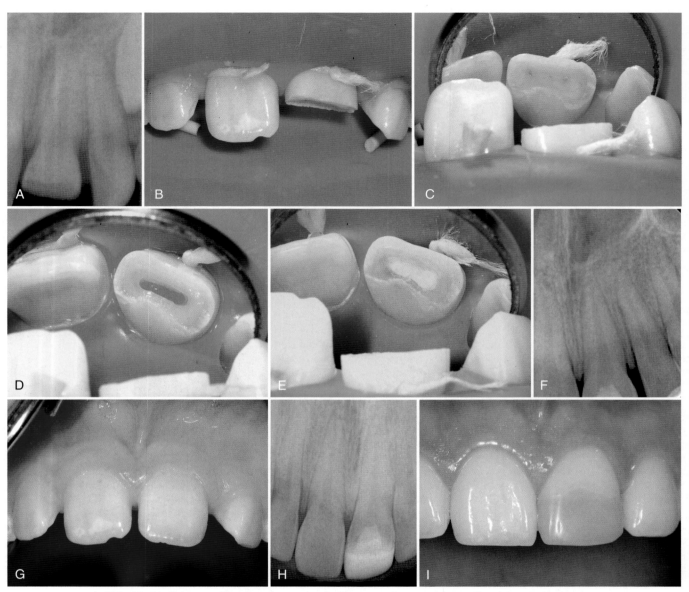

FIG. 23-11 Eight-year-old patient who presented with a crown fracture of the maxillary left central incisor 2 hours after trauma. **A,** Periapical radiograph of the traumatized tooth revealed immature root formation with a horizontal crown fracture. **B** and **C,** Dental dam isolation showing a complicated crown fracture with three pulp exposures. **D,** Incisal view after partial pulpotomy. **E,** Incisal view after hemostasis and mineral trioxide aggregate (MTA) placement. **F,** Control radiograph after 5 years showing apexogenesis with absence of apical pathosis. **G,** Clinical photograph of reattached tooth fragment after adhesive bonding. **H,** Radiographic recall at 7 years with recently placed composite after loss of coronal fragment. Pulp testing showed normal vitality with no evidence of pathosis. **I,** Clinical photograph showing slight discoloration of the composite 1 year after placement. (Courtesy Dr. Katharina Bücher and Dr. Jan Kühnisch, Munich, Germany.)

of root formation and periradicular or furcation changes associated with the periodontal ligament and supporting bone.[219] In young permanent teeth, the stage of root development directly influences the diagnosis and treatment options.[53] Because the faciolingual dimension of most immature roots is greater than the mesiodistal dimension, apical closure may be difficult to determine radiographically.[53,187] Teeth that demonstrate radiographic evidence of deep caries should not be planned for aggressive procedures, such as pulpectomy, without the benefit of thermal (cold) testing (see Fig. 23-1).

Before arriving at treatment decisions, the clinician should carefully assess all available information; the medical history, patient report, radiographic evidence, clinical evaluation, and vitality (cold) testing are recommended. Periodontal probing, mobility assessment, and the presence of any localized swelling or sinus tracts should be recorded during the evaluation. Radiographs, including bite wings and periapical views, should be evaluated for periapical and furcation pathosis, resorptive defects, and pulpal calcification resulting from trauma or previous restorations.

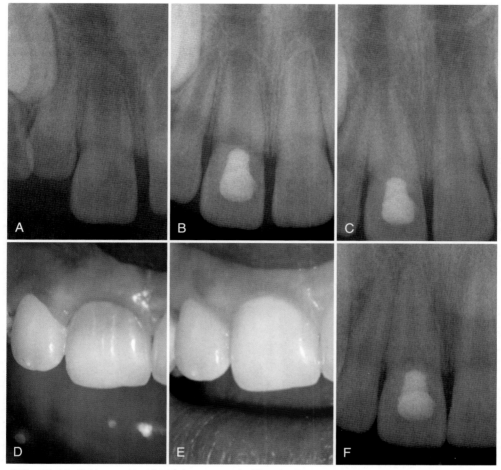

FIG. 23-12 Eight-year-old patient who presented with pulp exposure after traumatic injury. **A,** Periapical radiograph of maxillary right central incisor showing wide-open, immature apex. **B,** Radiograph 6 months after pulp amputation with a high speed diamond bur, saline irrigation, white mineral trioxide aggregate (MTA) partial pulpotomy, and placement of adhesive composite restoration. **C,** Two-year radiographic review; note apical maturation. **D,** Photograph showing coronal staining at 4-year recall. **E,** Photograph after MTA removal, reparative bridge confirmation, and internal bleaching with sodium perborate for 6 days. The hard tissue bridge was covered with a thin layer of phosphate cement before bleaching. **F,** Four-year radiographic review after MTA removal and bonded composite placement. Note presence of thick reparative calcific bridge and complete apical closure. The incisor remained asymptomatic and responded normally to cold testing at all time periods. (Courtesy Dr. Michael Hülsmann, Göttingen, Germany.)

Subjective symptomatology can be reviewed after clinical and radiographic assessments preclude the presence of unconditional irreversible pulpal disease. Patients with deep carious lesions often experience sensitivity to cold, heat, or sweet or acidic foods, and cold tests may evoke a short lingering response of 1 to 2 seconds. This may not be a definitive indicator that the pulp is irreversibly damaged. Determination of the pulpal condition with the aid of contemporary testing methods can be challenging, even for veteran clinicians, because of possible excessive responses to pulp percussion and palpation testing in children.[123,181,350] Clinical evidence indicates that cold testing with carbon dioxide ice is a more reliable prognosticator of pulp status in immature permanent teeth than electronic testing devices.[53] However, a diagnosis of irreversible pulpitis or pulp necrosis should be considered for teeth that generate pain on percussion.

Recent clinical investigations have demonstrated that a diagnosis of symptomatic irreversible pulpitis and acute apical periodontitis may not proscribe pulp capping and pulpotomy procedures when MTA or other CSCs that have been shown to reverse the inflammatory process are used.[64,100] Clinically, the difference between reversible and irreversible pulpitis is often determined on the basis of the duration and intensity of pain.[122] Unprovoked spontaneous pain of long duration or unrelenting symptoms forcing sleep deprivation are consistent with irreversible pulp inflammation or an acute periapical abscess.[350]

Another important consideration in the differential diagnosis is a patient with displacement trauma, which can display a transient apical breakdown radiographically that mimics periapical radiolucencies.[15] Teeth that experience luxation-type injuries can discolor and may not respond to cold testing for up to 4 months before they recover normal color and vitality. Also, biologically or pharmacokinetically immunosuppressed patients may not respond to conventional treatments because of abnormal function of related repair mechanisms.[208,343] Most clinical investigations clearly indicate that successful outcomes for vital pulp therapy decrease as the patient's age increases. Although aging of the pulp diminishes pulpal volume, vascularity, and host immune responses, functional repair mechanisms can still provide favorable treatment outcomes in older patients (Fig. 23-13).[1,234]

The initial pulpal diagnosis can be confirmed after visualization of the exposed pulp and during hemostasis assessment. If no hemorrhaging is seen, this area of the tissue is most likely necrotic, and the tissue must be removed with a high-speed round diamond bur until bleeding is evident (Fig. 23-14). After hemostasis with NaOCl, a large bulk of MTA can be placed directly against the remaining tissue. Alternatively, if hemorrhage control cannot be achieved after 10 minutes of direct contact with 3% to 6% NaOCl, the pulp is likely to be irreversibly involved, and a full pulpotomy or pulpectomy is recommended.

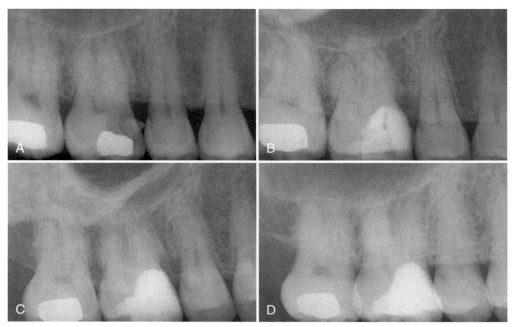

FIG. 23-13 Fifty-one-year-old patient who presented with a deeply carious but asymptomatic maxillary right first molar. **A,** Preoperative radiograph reveals extensive mesial caries and an occlusal amalgam. **B,** Postoperative radiograph after 1.5-mm pulpal exposure, sodium hypochlorite hemostasis, mineral trioxide aggregate (MTA) direct pulp cap, wet cotton pellet placement, and Photocore® provisionalization. **C,** Radiograph 1 week after pulp capping and placement of a permanent bonded composite restoration. The patient was asymptomatic and showed a positive response to cold testing. **D,** One-year radiographic recall; cold testing revealed normal vitality. (© Dr. George Bogen.)

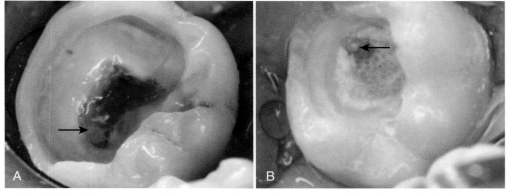

FIG. 23-14 Clinical examples of diseased pulp tissues after sodium hypochlorite hemostasis. **A,** Photograph of exposed pulp tissue of a mandibular right first molar in a 13-year-old patient. Note necrotic pulp tissue *(arrow)* that was subsequently removed with the remaining coronal pulp during a complete pulpotomy procedure. **B,** Clinical presentation of mandibular right molar in a 7-year-old patient after pulp exposure during caries excavation using a caries detector dye. Note the extruded seminecrotic, nonhemorrhagic tissue *(arrow)*. The tooth later underwent mineral trioxide aggregate (MTA) partial pulpotomy and permanent restoration. (© Dr. George Bogen.)

Although the size of the pulp exposure has no significant bearing on the final outcome, some clinicians falsely assume that larger exposures have an unfavorable prognosis.[215] Pulp sizes are underestimated on radiographs.[58-60] The size of the pulp exposures may also be overestimated, which could affect the decision-making process, leading clinicians to abandon more conservative vital pulp options.[135] Pulp dimensions may also vary with various racial groups and between genders.[59,296,345]

Teeth that have a history of trauma or previous restorations or that display pulpal calcification have a poorer prognosis than teeth showing only initial caries. In the selection of a specific vital pulp treatment, it is important to consider the remaining tooth structure and future restorative plan. In patients with uncontrolled caries or extensive loss of coronal structure, in which full coverage is indicated, pulpotomy rather than pulp capping is recommended.[43,52,324]

Caries Removal

The main objective in caries removal is the identification and complete removal of the infected tissue while preserving sound tooth structure; this contributes to pulpal protection and continued vitality. Caries removal is enhanced with the aid of a caries detector dye and optical magnification; however, some studies have indicated that dyes can cause excessive and unnecessary removal of healthy tooth structure.[24,218,359]

Caries removal has traditionally been completed somewhat subjectively using hand instruments and slow-speed burs. The procedure is performed using an explorer and tactile sense to differentiate soft from hard dentin to determine infected from noninfected dental tissue. However, this method can have shortcomings because clinicians may leave decay at the dentinoenamel junction and unnecessarily remove dentin that still has the potential to remineralize under a sealed restoration.[124] Furthermore, it has been found that the ability to remove caries varies among operators and during different time periods for the same operator.[124,125]

Investigators in the early 1970s used SEM to identify two different layers of carious dentin.[125] Teeth show two distinct layers of carious dentin as the result of gram-positive bacteria releasing lactic acid as their main by-product. The outside carious layer subjacent to the dentinoenamel junction exhibited demineralized hydroxyapatite crystals that were dissolved by acidic bacterial byproducts; this layer also featured unbound and altered collagen denatured by microbial proteolytic enzymes.[271] A fuchsin dye suspended in propylene glycol was used to reveal that this necrotic and infected layer could be selectively stained, identified, and removed objectively, thus preserving the inner carious layer that remained capable of remineralization. A highly significant difference in the total colony-forming units in stained and unstained dentin has been demonstrated.[364]

The second demineralized carious layer proximal to the pulp featured degraded hydroxyapatite crystals but contained collagen with intact intermolecular cross-links unaffected by cariogenic acids and not stainable with caries detector dyes.[125,126,285] If the second inner layer can be identified and preserved during caries excavation, the remaining pulp tissue and odontoblasts subjacent to the carious zone will be subjected to less trauma, which contributes to pulpal protection and survival.[245,280] The second layer proximal to the pulp has a stronger capacity to remineralize when paired with bonded composite restorations to prevent bacterial microleakage.[233,245]

The two carious layers have been further classified into four zones (pink, light pink, transparent, and apparently normal) when analyzed by atomic force microscopy and transverse digital microradiography.[271] Consistent with previous investigations, the four zones reinforce the concept that increasing levels of demineralization decrease the peritubular dentin rating and mechanical properties of dentin.[271]

Caries detector dyes can be considered a valuable tool in caries excavation when attempts are made to preserve remineralizable dentin and to minimize trauma to the pulp.[87,168,173] Investigations in human, dog, and nonhuman primate models have demonstrated this regenerative characteristic in caries-affected dentin.[178,184,233,319,320] Several studies have questioned the efficacy of caries removal using a caries detector dye. Not all stainable dentin can be classified as infected, and the absence of staining does not eliminate the potential for residual cariogenic bacteria.[185,271] However, dyes allow the operator to visually inspect, under magnification, infected dentin that may have been overlooked, particularly at the dentinoenamel junction, a situation that may compromise the outcome for vital pulp therapy.[185,358] Although a compromise, it may be preferable clinically to inadvertently remove a small excess amount of dentin than to leave infected tissue with active caries.

Hemostatic Agents

A wide range of hemostatic solutions and methods have been recommended to control a bleeding pulp exposure. These include various concentrations of NaOCl; 2% chlorhexidine; MTAD (DENTSPLY Tulsa Dental Specialties, Tulsa, Oklahoma); 30% hydrogen peroxide (Superoxol); ferric sulfate; disinfectants, such as Tubulicid (Global Dental Products, North Bellmore, New York); epinephrine; direct pressure with cotton pellets soaked in sterile water or saline; and the use of lasers.[8] Sodium hypochlorite in concentrations of 1.5% to 6% is currently regarded as the most effective, safe, and inexpensive hemostatic solution for pulp capping and partial and complete pulpotomy procedures.[145,351] First used as a wound antiseptic during World War I and referred to as Dakin's solution, NaOCl became a valuable hemostatic agent in dentistry for direct pulp exposures in the late 1950s.[144,163,310] The antimicrobial solution provides hemostasis and disinfection of the dentin-pulp interface, chemical amputation of the blood clot and fibrin, biofilm removal, clearance of dentinal chips, and removal of damaged cells at the mechanical exposure site.[27,97,144,212] Concentrations of 1.5% to 6% in direct contact with pulp tissue do not appear to adversely alter pulp cell recruitment, cytodifferentiation, and hard tissue deposition.[92] Sodium hypochlorite also shows excellent efficacy as a hemostatic agent at lower dilutions (0.5%).[337]

When direct pulp exposures occur in a carious field, the ability to attain hemostasis remains the most crucial factor in the success of vital pulp therapy. This was demonstrated in an innovative study that examined outcomes of teeth directly pulp capped with a hard-setting CH after pulp exposures were generated during caries excavation.[215] Caries removal during the investigation was aided by a caries detector dye, and 10% NaOCl was used for hemostasis. The 2-year success rate was 81.8%. A statistical analysis of key factors revealed that preoperative thermal responses, percussion sensitivity, the diameter of the exposure, the age of the patient, and the tooth type and location had no significant influence on the outcome. The degree of bleeding and its control at the time of exposure constituted the most critical predictor for outcome assessment.

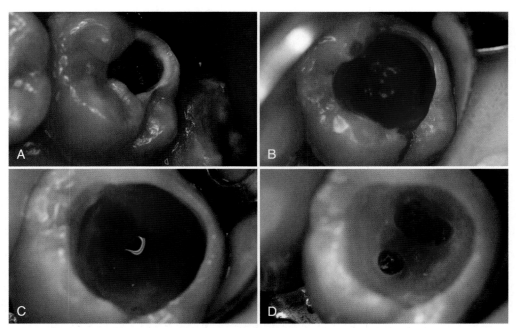

FIG. 23-15 Clinical sequence showing a cariously involved maxillary right first molar in an asymptomatic 20-year-old patient. **A,** Large occlusal-buccal carious lesion. **B,** Caries detector dye staining after initial removal of debris and infected dentin. **C,** Occlusal view of pulp roof exposure with 6% sodium hypochlorite hemostatic solution. **D,** Two large pulp exposures (2 mm and 2 · 4 mm) after caries removal and sodium hypochlorite hemostasis. Note that bleeding is absent and there is no evidence of necrotic tissue. (© Dr. George Bogen.)

When hemostasis can be attained, pulpal repair and reparative dentin formation can proceed normally, in the absence of microbial challenges, when MTA is used as the pulp dressing.[63,179]

Sodium hypochlorite is not only an effective hemostatic agent, it can also be considered an invaluable diagnostic tool for assessing the difference between irreversibly and reversibly inflamed pulps (Fig. 23-15). During the inflammatory process, as cariogenic bacteria approach the pulp, higher levels of immunoglobulins (e.g., IgA, IgG, IgM) and inflammatory markers have been detected, including elastase and prostaglandin E_2.[248] The presence of these mediators can contribute to increased intrapulpal pressure and may play a critical role in the pathogenesis of the irreversibly inflamed pulp.[248,325]

The coronal pulp must be considered irreversibly inflamed when hemorrhage cannot be arrested after 5 to 10 minutes of direct exposure to NaOCl. If bleeding continues, partial or complete removal of the coronal pulp is indicated, with the goal of gaining hemostasis before MTA placement (Figs. 23-16 and 23-17). Sodium hypochlorite has demonstrated effective hemostatic and antiseptic properties in humans without adversely affecting pulp repair, healing, and tertiary dentinogenesis.[92] An investigation into pulp-capped human third molars treated with either CH or a self-etching adhesive system histologically examined pulps at 30 and 60 days after the use of 2.5% NaOCl for hemostasis.[102] Histologic evidence demonstrated no impairment of the repair process after the use of NaOCl, although CH appeared to outperform the resin-based pulp capping agent. Current data clearly support the use of 1.25% to 6% NaOCl solutions in humans as a safe and appropriate hemostatic agent for direct pulp capping and pulpotomies.*

---

*References 3, 22, 92, 102, 144, 162, 215, 337, 342, and 351.

Treatment Considerations

An important and often unrecognized aspect of direct pulp capping in a carious field is the potential survival of undetected cariogenic bacteria, in dentinal tubules of the dentin adjacent to the exposure site, after caries removal. These microorganisms can compromise treatment even after meticulous caries excavation and NaOCl disinfection. Unfortunately, traditional pulp capping protocols have directed clinicians to place pulp dressings only at the exposure site, without considering the adjacent dentin. Therefore, it is recommended that MTA or CSC be placed over the exposure sites and most of the surrounding dentin with the goal of entombing residual microorganisms.[359a] This notable change in pulp capping strategy can improve treatment outcomes in symptomatic and asymptomatic teeth featuring extensive caries and multiple exposures after caries excavation.[39] Together with an extensive application of MTA or CSC, a cement thickness of 1.5 mm or greater increases the likelihood of bacterial neutralization and minimizes further microbial challenges.

This concept in pulp capping with MTA becomes more critical in one-step pulp capping protocols that use slow-set CSCs covered with RMGI cements. These cements are water-based bonding agents and are not affected by small amounts of water on the dentin or MTA/CSC surface.[86] Unset RMGI cement has an initial pH of about 1.5 and demonstrates no polymerization shrinkage stress, and the material acts as a self-etching primer. Although the bond strength reaches only 25% of comparable resin bonding systems (approximately 10 MPa), the bond is reliable and resistant to disintegration.[86] Although the active chemical constituents are inflammatory and toxic when used for pulp capping and placed directly on exposed pulp tissue, RMGI cements produce only mild inflammatory

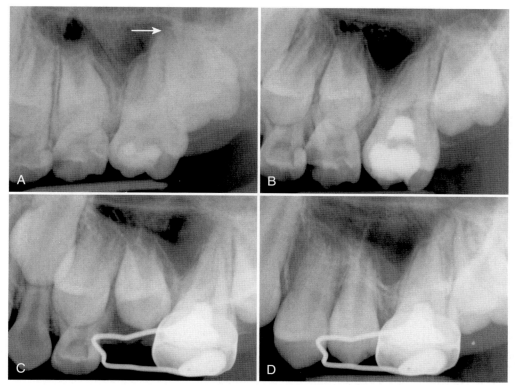

FIG. 23-16 Seven-year-old patient who presented with a symptomatic maxillary left first molar. **A,** Periapical radiograph showing open palatal apex and a coronal provisional restoration. **B,** Radiograph taken after sodium hypochlorite hemostasis and mineral trioxide aggregate (MTA) pulpotomy. **C,** One-year radiographic recall showing advancing apical maturation and a banded space maintainer. The patient was asymptomatic. **D,** Two-year radiographic recall; the tooth showed no pathosis, and the molar was firm and in full function. (© Dr. George Bogen.)

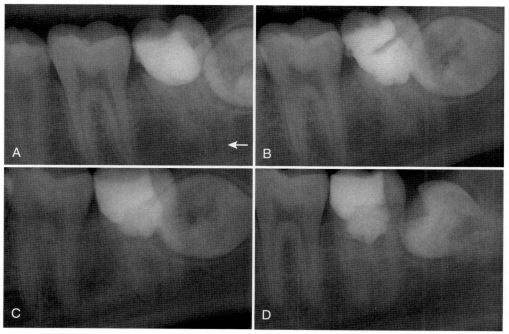

FIG. 23-17 Twelve-year-old patient who received an unsatisfactory previous pulpotomy treatment. **A,** Recently completed pulpotomy in tooth #18 using zinc oxide eugenol (ZOE). Note the carious lesion in the distal aspect of the second premolar and the open apex in the distal root of the second molar *(arrow).* **B,** Radiograph after removal of ZOE and placement of mineral trioxide aggregate (MTA) with a Cavit® provisional. **C,** Radiograph of bonded adhesive composite restoration over cured MTA pulpotomy. **D,** Four-year radiographic control demonstrating maturation and closure of the distal root apex. (© Dr. George Bogen.)

changes to vital pulp tissue when indirectly placed on the remaining dentin.[70,95,159,192]

Resin Modified Glass Ionomer cements have substantial antimicrobial properties, and there are no known physiochemical properties of unset MTA that would adversely affect the set of RMGI materials. However, the challenge during one-step pulp capping procedures with RMGI cements in conjunction with a larger volume of unset MTA is adequate adhesion of the RMGI to the remaining dentin and wet MTA during composite placement.[26] This situation creates great difficulty when contemporary bonding protocols require air blasting during primer and resin placement because the RMGI can be easily dislodged from the unset MTA. In this instance, it may be advisable to place an unbonded amalgam restoration over the RMGI/MTA/dentin interface, if feasible.[250] A reduction in MTA coverage and probable thickness to accommodate RMGI adhesion can compromise favorable outcomes in vital pulp therapy, and either a two-step treatment sequence or fast-set CSCs should be considered.

TREATMENT RECOMMENDATIONS*

Two-Visit MTA Pulp Capping

1. After differential diagnosis, it is determined that the tooth demonstrates either a normal pulp or reversible pulpitis. The tooth should have a normal radiographic appearance and be restorable without crown lengthening procedures. After profound local anesthesia has been obtained, the tooth is isolated with a dental dam and additionally sealed with an agent, such as Oraseal (Ultradent Products, South Jordan, Utah) or a similar product, if saliva leakage is present. The clinical crown is then disinfected with NaOCl or chlorhexidine. Optical magnification and illumination are highly recommended. A high-speed diamond or carbide bur is used to remove undermined enamel, and soft debris is removed with a spoon excavator.

2. After the carious dentin has been exposed and air-dried, a caries detector dye is applied for 10 seconds, and the tooth is washed and dried with a two-way syringe. Caries removal is completed with spoon excavators and/or slow-speed #6-2 carbide round burs until minimal (light pink) or no deeply stained dentin is evident. The dentin is washed and dried again, and the caries detector is reapplied on the dentin for 10 seconds. The process is repeated meticulously until no or only light pink staining is evident (usually 5 to 7 applications).

3. Bleeding can be controlled by the placement of a cotton pellet moistened with 3% to 6% NaOCl for 20 to 60 seconds if pulp exposure occurs during the caries removal process. The staining and caries removal are continued carefully around the exposure site(s) until minimal or no staining is visible. Areas of reparative dentin should be left intact.

4. Direct pulp exposures that occur during caries removal should be hemorrhaging to some degree. A 3% to 6% NaOCl solution, with or without a cotton pellet, is placed directly against the exposure or exposures for a contact time of 1 to 10 minutes. If the tissue appears normal while

hemorrhaging, no tissue amputation is indicated. The diagnosis is changed to irreversible pulpitis when hemostasis cannot be obtained within 10 minutes; more aggressive treatment should then be initiated. If bleeding is not evident after pulpal exposure, a high-speed round diamond bur is used to remove tissue until bleeding and healthy tissue are evident. A second application of NaOCl after tissue removal should stop any hemorrhaging. A pulpotomy or pulpectomy must also be considered if the entire axial wall or pulpal roof is removed during caries excavation (Fig. 23-18).

5. The dentin should be gently washed with water and dried to remove excess NaOCl before MTA is applied. The material is mixed according to the manufacturer's instructions (3:1, MTA:H_2O) to a consistency similar to wet sand. An MTA carrier gun or a hand instrument (spoon excavator or Glick) is used to bring the cement to the site in bulk. The MTA should be placed directly over the exposed pulp tissue, including all surrounding dentin. The material is gently patted down with a small moist cotton pellet or a dry pellet if the mixture is too wet. The cement placed should have a minimum thickness of 1.5 mm. MTA inadvertently forced into the pulp chamber will not affect the outcome adversely. For the final bonded restoration to provide an effective seal, a region of dentin and enamel measuring approximately 1.5 to 2 mm should be cleared circumferentially around the MTA with a small (2 mm) moist cotton pellet or sponge brush.

6. A custom-fabricated, flat (1 to 2 mm), moist cotton pellet or gauze is placed over the entire mass of the MTA. The moist pellet or gauze may require placement in two sections if the cavity involves a proximal preparation with an exposure on the axial wall. If the decision is made to complete the restorative treatment on the same day, a large moist cotton pellet can be placed; the patient is instructed not to eat or chew because this may disrupt the unset MTA. A bonded restoration can be placed after a 4-hour waiting period.

7. After placement of MTA and coverage with a wet, flat cotton pellet or gauze, a durable and removable provisional material is used. Unbonded Photocore® (Kuraray America, Inc., New York, New York) is recommended as a reliable option because of its ease of handling and unique polymerization characteristics. Teeth should be conservatively removed from occlusion if thin cusps are present as a result of extensive caries removal. Unless amalgam is the designated restorative material, restorations such as IRM or zinc oxide eugenol (ZOE) (eugenol based) may reduce the bond strengths of adhesive resins and their use with bonding materials remains controversial.[56a,269a]

8. The return appointment can be scheduled 1 to 10 days after MTA placement. The patient is asked about sensitivity, mastication comfort, and pain before the local anesthetic is given. To confirm continued normal vitality before anesthesia, the tooth is cold tested with carbon dioxide (CO_2) ice or Hygienic Endo-Ice (Coltène/Whaledent, Cuyahoga Falls, Ohio). After profound anesthesia is obtained, the tooth is isolated with a dental dam. The provisional material is removed with a high-speed diamond or carbide bur using water coolant. The cotton pellet or gauze is removed, and the embedded cotton fibers are removed with a spoon excavator or similar hand instrument. Magnification and

---

*Adapted from Bogen and Chandler.[38]

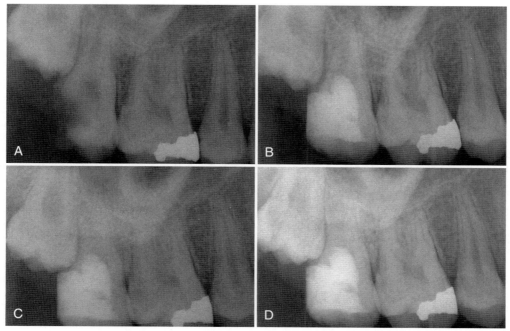

FIG. 23-18 Radiographic sequence of treatment of a maxillary right second molar in a 14-year-old patient, previously recommended for extraction because of advanced caries. **A,** Preoperative radiograph showing extensive caries at the occlusal level of the erupting third molar. The patient was asymptomatic but had pain on cold testing. **B,** Postoperative radiograph after complete exposure of axial wall during caries excavation, mineral trioxide aggregate (MTA) pulpotomy, and placement of flowable resin-modified glass ionomer cement over wet MTA with bonded composite placement. **C,** One-year radiographic recall. **D,** Two-year radiographic control showing absence of apical disease. The molar was functioning normally and without symptoms. (© Dr. George Bogen.)

illumination are strongly recommended to guide the operator. A bonded composite restoration is placed, following the manufacturer's recommendations, after the MTA has been checked to ensure proper curing.

9. After completion of the permanent bonded restoration, the occlusion is checked and adjusted as required. Subjective symptomatology and cold testing should be evaluated at 6 weeks. Radiographic follow-up, cold testing, and subjective symptomatology can be reevaluated at 6 and 12 months if the initial follow-up appears favorable. Yearly or biannual recalls are recommended.

One-Step Pulp Capping

The manufacturer of MTA (ProRoot MTA, DENTSPLY Tulsa Dental Specialties) recommends that pulp capping be completed in one visit. In some instances, treatment of the immature permanent tooth can be difficult, particularly in young patients with challenging medical or behavioral problems that require treatment under sedation. The manufacturer of MTA recommends the following protocol when one-step treatment is indicated.

1. With dental dam isolation, complete a cavity preparation outline using high-speed burs under constant water cooling.
2. If caries is present, excavate using a round bur in a handpiece at low speed or use hand instruments.
3. Rinse the cavity and exposure site (or sites) with 2.6% to 5% NaOCl. Heavy bleeding may be controlled with a cotton pellet moistened with NaOCl.
4. Prepare ProRoot MTA according to mixing instructions.

5. Using a small ball applicator or similar device, apply a small amount of ProRoot MTA over the exposure.
6. Remove excess moisture at the site with a dry cotton pellet.
7. Apply a small amount of Dyract flow flowable compomer (Dentsply International, York, Pennsylvania) (or an equivalent light-cured resin–glass ionomer liner) to cover the ProRoot MTA and light cure according to the material's instructions.
8. Etch the remaining cavity walls with 34% to 37% phosphoric acid gel for 15 seconds. Rinse thoroughly.
9. Dry the cavity gently, leaving the dentin moist but not wet. Apply Prime and Bond NT material or an equivalent bonding material. Cure according to its instructions.
10. Place TPH Spectrum (Dentsply Caulk, Milford, Delaware) composite material or an equivalent composite resin to complete the restoration. Cure according to its instructions.
11. At the next appointment, assess the pulp vitality. Pulp vitality and status should be assessed radiographically every 3 to 6 months or as needed.

The authors recommend the following modifications: Caries removal can be completed under magnification and illumination with the aid of a caries detector dye (step 2). During MTA placement against the exposure site (step 5), a larger bulk of MTA be placed that includes most of the surrounding dentin at a thickness of at least 1.5 mm. One-step pulp capping and pulpotomy procedures can also be completed with the faster-setting hydraulic tricalcium silicate materials.

THE PERMANENT RESTORATION

The placement and quality of the permanent restoration can be crucial to the long-term maintenance of pulp vitality and may be more significant than the actual pulp treatment.[11,114,157,221,227] The aim of the final restoration is to complement the sealing ability of the pulp capping/pulpotomy material and effectively defend the pulp from further microbial challenges. The selection of the restorative material, procedure execution, and adherence to proper restorative protocols can all contribute to minimizing potential restorative microleakage. It has been proposed that microleakage around restorations may be more detrimental to vital pulp tissue than unfilled cavity preparations directly exposed to the oral environment.[284] An important consideration in both mature and immature permanent teeth is the conservation of the remaining tooth structure, which ultimately contributes to favorable long-term retention and function.[69,93,167,301] The incorporation of adhesive restorative materials as definitive final restorations minimizes tooth reduction, encourages anatomic preservation, and thus provides better pulpal protection and repair potential.[124,143]

Technologic advances in dental materials have increased treatment options in the restoration of teeth that have undergone vital pulp procedures. Permanent restorations for pulp capped or pulpotomized permanent teeth can include composite resins, bonded or unbonded amalgam restorations, and cuspal coverage restorations. However, the more conservative the restorative treatment, the greater the probability of pulp survival.[124] Vital pulp therapy must be considered an injury to an already challenged connective tissue, and every effort should be directed toward minimizing further injurious procedures.[1] Factors that affect the repair mechanisms in pulp tissue can include the age of the patient, the depth and size of the cavity preparation, and the choice of restorative material.[246]

Amalgam remains the most widely used restorative material because of its ease of placement, proven durability, and low cost. However, drawbacks include potential health risks to dental personnel, esthetic limitations, and a high modulus of elasticity that can increase the incidence of cuspal fracture or coronal infractions.[9,114] This is a major concern in immature permanent teeth, in which cusps are unprotected, requiring further tooth reduction by placement of stainless steel crowns.[75,106,297,348,350] The implementation of bonding resins or RMGI liners in conjunction with amalgam placement can improve sealing ability and reduce potential microleakage. Even though amalgam restorations remain a safe and predictable long-term restorative option, the technology driving adhesion dentistry continues to improve as new composites and bonding resins evolve.[115,263]

Total-etch and self-etching systems produce excellent bond strength to enamel, dentin, and cured tricalcium silicate cements.[20,249] The most durable bond strengths generated with contemporary materials are achieved using selective etching of the enamel with 40% phosphoric acid, followed by two-step self-etching adhesive systems.[56,253,341] Current advances in adhesive technology have also shown that beneath the resin-interfused hybrid layer, an acid-base–resistant zone is formed that enhances the resistance of normal dentin to recurrent caries. This reinforced layer (termed "super dentin") forms when monomer penetration and polymerization occur, and it demonstrates an ability to restrict (inhibit) primary and secondary caries.[252] As a result of their simplifications and improved bonding strengths, modern adhesives have proved to be a predictable partner that complements vital pulp therapy. It is imperative that all bonding procedures strictly follow the manufacturer's recommendations and include dental dam placement.[56]

POSTOPERATIVE FOLLOW-UP AND RECALL

After treatment completion, the pulp status must be assessed periodically to ensure continued pulp vitality, normal function, and apical closure in immature teeth. Radiographic evaluation and cold testing most accurately assess continued pulp health and are excellent predicators for measuring survival rates. Recalls can address postoperative sensitivity, pulpal degeneration or necrosis, and indications for more extensive endodontic care, such as pulpectomy and root canal treatment Radiographic and clinical review also allows detection of emerging complications, including recurrent caries, poor hygiene, restoration failures, cuspal fractures, and other potentially adverse conditions.

Patient compliance for recall in asymptomatic cases can be challenging compared to patients who had unsuccessful pulp treatments that became irreversibly inflamed or advanced to symptomatic apical periodontitis. Because some parents do not practice regular preventive care and may not have a strong background in basic oral health care, recall compliance rates for children can be unpredictable.[176,270] Although recall intervals have traditionally been based on the conventional 6-month checkup and oral prophylaxis period, this generally accepted practice has come into question for accurate follow-up assessment.[228] It may be preferable to establish recall rates individually, based on patient need, symptomatology, the caries index, periodontal status, and craniofacial development assessment in younger patients.[254,344]

A tentative diagnosis of tooth survivability can be made at the 3-month recall.[215] One study demonstrated that the prognosis for long-term pulp survival can be established at an observation period of 21 to 24 months.[215] A 5- to 10-day review period can be beneficial diagnostically when the patient returns for the final restoration in the two-visit MTA pulp capping protocol. Thereafter, if cold testing reveals normal vitality, recall reviews can be scheduled, if possible, at 6 weeks and at 6 and 12 months depending on patient compliance.[40]

The paramount objective in vital pulp therapy is to promote the physiologic formation and maturation of the root end (apexogenesis). Radiographic evidence of root-end closure in immature adult teeth is a reliable prognostic marker of continued pulp vitality (Fig. 23-19).[23] Apexogenesis after direct pulp capping or pulpotomy procedures using MTA should proceed normally in healthy patients at a progressive rate.[27,269,347,353] The observed root maturation should also follow a predictable pattern of tooth development that coincides with the contralateral teeth in the same patient when the teeth are compared radiographically and viewed chronologically.[23]

Observation of contralateral tooth development can be an invaluable method of measuring the success of vital pulp therapy when using MTA. Alternatively, in traumatized teeth that exhibit necrotic pulps and periradicular pathosis, MTA and CH can be used as an apical plug to stimulate the apical papilla to promote barrier formation, which may otherwise require 5 to 20 months for completion (apexification).[7,65,294]

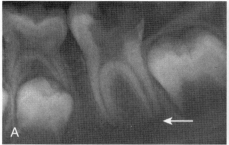
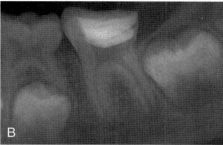
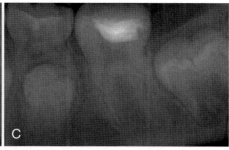

FIG. 23-19 **A,** Radiograph of a symptomatic mandibular first molar with deep caries in a 7-year-old patient who presented with an open distal root apex *(arrow).* **B,** The patient received a mineral trioxide aggregate (MTA) direct pulp cap and bonded restoration in a two-visit sequence. **C,** Radiographic recall after 14 months showing maturation and apical closure. The tooth showed a positive response to carbon dioxide (CO_2) ice testing. (© Dr. George Bogen.)

If MTA is substituted for CH in vital pulp therapy procedures, similar time periods for apical maturation can be anticipated.[103,223,224]

In the absence of microbial challenges, the human dental pulp demonstrates an exceptional regenerative capacity when treated with MTA and similar bioactive substances. Together with our advances in pulp biology and dental materials, changes in treatment protocols and delivery that encourage dental pulp preservation and survival will ultimately contribute to improved dental health for all patients needing vital pulp therapy.

ACKNOWLEDGEMENT

We wish to thank Dr. Leif K. Bakland for his contributions to this chapter.

REFERENCES

1. Abou-Rass M: The stressed pulp condition: an endodontic-restorative diagnostic concept, *J Prosthet Dent* 48:264, 1982.
2. Accorinte Mde L, Loguercio AD, Reis A, et al: Adverse effects of human pulps after direct pulp capping with different components from a total-etch, three-step adhesive system, *Dent Mater* 21:599, 2005.
3. Accorinte Mde L, Loguercio AD, Reis A, et al: Response of human pulp capped with a bonding agent after bleeding control with hemostatic agents, *Oper Dent* 30:147, 2005.
4. Accorinte ML, Loguercio AD, Reis A, et al: Response of human dental pulp capped with MTA and calcium hydroxide powder, *Oper Dent* 33:488, 2008.
5. Accorinte MLR, Loguercio AD, Reis A, et al: Evaluation of two mineral trioxide aggregate compounds as pulp-capping agents in human teeth, *Int Endod J* 42:122, 2009.
6. Aeinehchi M, Eslami B, Ghanberiha M, et al: Mineral trioxide aggregate (MTA) and calcium hydroxide as pulp-capping agents in human teeth: a preliminary report, *Int Endod J* 36:225, 2003.
7. Aggarwal V, Miglani S, Singla M: Conventional apexification and revascularization induced maturogenesis of two non-vital, immature teeth in same patient: 24 months follow up of a case, *J Conserv Dent* Jan-Mar; 15(1):68-72, 2012.
8. Akashi G, Kato J, Hirai Y: Pathological study of pulp treated with chemicals after Er:YAG laser preparation, *Photomed Laser Surg* 24:698, 2006.
9. Akerboom HB, Advokatt JB, Van Amerongen WE, et al: Long-term evaluation of rerestoration of amalgam restorations. *Community Dent Oral Epidemiol* 21:45, 1993.
10. Al-Hezaimi K, Salameh Z, Al-Fouzan K, et al: Histomorphometric and micro-computed tomography analysis of pulpal response to three different pulp capping materials, *J Endod* 37:507, 2011.
11. Alptekin T, Ozer F, Unlu N, et al: In vivo and in vitro evaluations of microleakage around Class I amalgam and composite restorations, *Oper Dent* 35:641, 2010.

12. American Association of Endodontists: *Glossary of endodontic terms,* ed 8, Chicago, 2012.
13. American Academy of Pediatric Dentistry, Clinical Affairs Committee, Pulp Therapy Subcommittee: Guideline on pulp therapy for primary and immature permanent teeth: reference manual 2012-13, *Pediatr Dent* 34:222, 2012.
14. Andelin WE, Shabahang S, Wright K, et al: Identification of hard tissue after experimental pulp capping using dentin sialoprotein (DSP) as a marker, *J Endod* 29:646, 2003.
15. Andreasen F: Transient apical breakdown and its relation to color and sensibility changes, *Endod Dent Traumatol* 2:9, 1986.
16. Arruda RA, Cunha RS, Miguita KB, et al: Sealing ability of mineral trioxide aggregate (MTA) combined with distilled water, chlorhexidine, and doxycycline, *J Oral Sci* 54:233, 2012.
17. Asgary S, Eghbal MJ: Treatment outcomes of pulpotomy in permanent molars with irreversible pulpitis using biomaterials: a multi-center randomized controlled trial, *Acta Odontol Scand* 71:130, 2013.
18. Asgary S, Eghbal MJ, Ghoddusi J, et al: One-year results of vital pulp therapy in permanent molars with irreversible pulpitis: an ongoing multicenter, randomized, non-inferiority clinical trial, *Clin Oral Investig* 17:431, 2013.
19. Asgary S, Moosavi SH, Yadegari Z, Shahriari S: Cytotoxic effect of MTA and CEM cement in human gingival fibroblast cells: scanning electronic microscope evaluation, *N Y State Dent J* 78:51, 2012.
20. Atabek D, Sillelioğlu H, Olmez A: Bond strength of adhesive systems to mineral trioxide aggregate with different time intervals, *J Endod* 38:1288, 2012.
21. Auschill TM, Arweiler NB, Hellwig E, et al: Success rate of direct pulp capping with calcium hydroxide, *Schweiz Monatsschr Zahnmed* 113:946, 2003.
22. Bal C, Alacam A, Tuzuner T, et al: Effects of antiseptics on pulpal healing under calcium hydroxide pulp capping: a pilot study, *Eur J Dent* 5:265, 2011.

23. Ballesio I, Marchetti E, Mummolo S, et al: Radiographic appearance of apical closure in apexification: follow-up after 7-13 years, *Eur J Paediatr Dent* 7:29, 2006.
24. Banerjee A, Kidd EA, Watson TF: In vitro validation of carious dentin removed using different excavation criteria, *Am J Dent* 16:228, 2003.
25. Barnes IM, Kidd EA: Disappearing Dycal, *Br Dent J* 147:111, 1979.
26. Barrieshi-Nusair KM, Hammad HM: Intracoronal sealing comparison of mineral trioxide aggregate and glass ionomer, *Quintessence Int* 36:539, 2005.
27. Barrieshi-Nusair KM, Qudeimat MA: A prospective clinical study of mineral trioxide aggregate for partial pulpotomy in cariously exposed permanent teeth, *J Endod* 32:731, 2006.
28. Barthel CR, Rosenkranz B, Leuenberg A, et al: Pulp capping of carious exposures treatment outcome after 5 and 10 years: a retrospective study, *J Endod* 26:525, 2000.
29. Basturk FB, Nekoofar MH, Günday M, et al: The effect of various mixing and placement techniques on the compressive strength of mineral trioxide aggregate, *J Endod* 39:111, 2013.
30. Baume LJ, Holz J: Long term clinical assessment of direct pulp capping, *Int Endod J* 31:251, 1981.
31. Beagrie GS, Main JH, Smith DC, et al: Polycarboxylate cement as a pulp capping agent, *Dent J* 40:378, 1974.
32. Bergenholtz G: Effect of bacterial products on inflammatory reactions in the dental pulp, *Scand J Dent Res* 85:122, 1977.
33. Bernick S, Nedelman C: Effect of aging on the human pulp, *J Endod* 1:88, 1975.
34. Bhaskar SN, Beasley JD, Ward JP, et al: Human pulp capping with isosbutyl cyanoacrylate, *J Dent Res* 51:58, 1972.
35. Bjørndal L, Darvann T, Thylstrup A: A quantitative light microscopic study of the odontoblast and subodontoblastic reactions to active and arrested enamel caries without cavitation, *Caries Res* 32:59, 1998.

36. Bjørndal L, Larsen T, Thylstrup A: A clinical and microbiological study of deep carious lesions during stepwise excavation using long treatment intervals, *Caries Res* 31:411, 1997.

37. Bjørndal L, Reit C, Bruun G, et al: Treatment of deep caries lesions in adults: randomized clinical trials comparing stepwise vs direct complete excavation, and direct pulp capping vs partial pulpotomy, *Eur J Oral Sci* 118:290, 2010.

38. Bogen G, Chandler NP: Vital pulp therapy. In Ingle JI, Bakand LK, Baumgartner JC, editors: *Ingle's endodontics*, ed 6, Hamilton, Ontario, 2008, Decker.

39. Bogen G, Chandler NP: Pulp preservation in immature permanent teeth, *Endod Topics* 23:131, 2012.

40. Bogen G, Kim JS, Bakland LK: Direct pulp capping with mineral trioxide aggregate: an observational study, *J Am Dent Assoc* 139:305, 2008.

41. Bogen G, Kuttler S: Mineral trioxide aggregate obturation: a review and case series, *J Endod* 35:777, 2009.

42. Bortoluzzi EA, Broon NJ, Bramante CM, et al: Sealing ability of MTA and radiopaque Portland cement with or without calcium chloride for root-end filling, *J Endod* 32:897, 2006.

43. Brambilla E, García-Godoy F, Strohmenger L: Principles of diagnosis and treatment of high-caries-risk subjects, *Dent Clin North Am* 44:507, 2000.

44. Brännström M, Lind PO: Pulpal response to early dental caries, *J Dent Res* 44:1045, 1965.

45. Burke FJ: Ozone and caries: a review of the literature, *Dent Update* 39:271, 2012.

46. Büyükgüral B, Cehreli ZC: Effect of different adhesive protocols vs calcium hydroxide on primary tooth pulp with different remaining dentin thicknesses: 24-month results, *Clin Oral Investig* 12:91, 2008.

47. Byers MR, Taylor PE, Khayat BG, et al: Effects of injury and inflammation on pulpal and periapical nerves, *J Endod* 16:78, 1990.

48. Caicedo R, Abbott PV, Alongi DJ, et al: Clinical, radiographic and histological analysis of the effects of mineral trioxide aggregate used in direct pulp capping and pulpotomies of primary teeth, *Aust Dent J* 51:297, 2006.

49. Camargo SE, Camargo CH, Hiller KA, et al: Cytotoxicity and genotoxicity of pulp capping materials in two cell lines, *Int Endod J* 42:227, 2009.

50. Camilleri J: Characterization of hydration products of mineral trioxide aggregate, *Int Endod J* 41:408, 2008.

51. Camilleri J, Montesin FE, Brady K, et al: The constitution of mineral trioxide aggregate, *Dent Mater* 21:297, 2005.

52. Camp J: Pediatric endodontic treatment. In Cohen S, Burns RC, editors: *Pathways of the pulp*, ed 7, St Louis, 1998, Mosby.

53. Camp JH, Fuks AB: Pediatric endodontics: endodontic treatment for the primary and young permanent dentition. In Cohen S, Hargreaves K, editors: *Pathways of the pulp*, ed 9, St Louis, 2006, Mosby/Elsevier.

54. Caplan DJ, Cai J, Yin G, et al: Root canal filled versus non-root canal filled teeth: a retrospective comparison of survival times, *J Public Health Dent* 65:90, 2005.

55. Caplan DJ, Kolker J, Rivera EM, et al: Relationship between number of proximal contacts and survival of root treated teeth, *Int Endod J* 35:193, 2002.

56. Cardoso MV, de Almeida Neves A, Mine A, et al: Current aspects on bonding effectiveness and stability in adhesive dentistry, *Aust Dent J* 56(Suppl 1):31, 2011.

56a. Carvalho CN, de Oliveira Bauer JR, Loguercio AD, et al: Effect of ZOE temporary restoration on the resin-dentin bond strength using different adhesive strategies. *J Esthet Restor Dent* 19:144, 2007.

57. Cavalcanti BN, Rode Sde M, Franca CM, et al: Pulp capping materials exert an effect of the secretion of IL-1β and IL-8 by migrating human neutrophils, *Braz Oral Res* 25:13, 2011.

58. Chandler NP, Ng BP, Monteith BD: Radiographic recognition and distribution of approximal carious lesions

59. Chandler NP, Pitt Ford TR, Monteith BD: Coronal pulp size in molars: a study of bitewing radiographs, *Int Endod J* 36:757, 2003.

60. Chandler NP, Pitt Ford TR, Monteith BD: Pulp size in molars: underestimation on radiographs, *J Oral Rehabil* 31:764, 2004.

61. Charadram N, Austin C, Trimby P, et al: Structural analysis of reactionary dentin formed in response to polymicrobial invasion, *J Struct Biol* S1047-8477(12)00339-5:1310, 2012.

62. Charadram N, Farahani RM, Harty D, et al: Regulation of reactionary dentin formation by odontoblasts in response to polymicrobial invasion of dentin matrix, *Bone* 50:265, 2012.

63. Cho SY, Seo DG, Lee SJ, et al: Prognostic factors for clinical outcomes according to time after direct pulp capping, *J Endod* 39:327, 2013.

64. Chueh LH, Chiang CP: Histology of irreversible pulpitis premolars treated with mineral trioxide aggregate pulpotomy, *Oper Dent* 35:370, 2010.

65. Chueh LH, Huang GT: Immature teeth with periradicular periodontitis or abscess undergoing apexogenesis: a paradigm shift, *J Endod* 32:1205, 2006.

66. Ciasca M, Aminoshariae A, Jin G, et al: A comparison of the cytotoxicity and proinflammatory cytokine production of EndoSequence root repair material and ProRoot mineral trioxide aggregate in human osteoblast cell culture using reverse-transcriptase polymerase chain reaction, *J Endod* 38:486, 2012.

67. Cohen BD, Combe EC: Development of new adhesive pulp capping materials, *Dent Update* 21:57, 1994.

68. Cohenca N, Paranjpe A, Berg J: Vital pulp therapy, *Dent Clin North Am* 57:59, 2013.

69. Convery LP: Conserving the immature first permanent molar, *J Ir Dent Assoc* 14:76, 1968.

70. Costa CAS, Ribeiro AP, Giro EM, et al: Pulp response after application of two resin modified glass ionomer cements (RMGICs) in deep cavities of prepared human teeth, *Dent Mater* 27:158, 2011.

71. Cox CF, Hafez AA, Akimoto N, et al: Biocompatibility of primer, adhesive and resin composite systems on non-exposed and exposed pulps of non-human primate teeth, *Am J Dent* 11:S55, 1998.

72. Cox CF, Keall CL, Keall HJ, et al: Biocompatibility of surface-sealed dental materials against exposed pulps, *J Prosthet Dent* 57:1, 1987.

73. Cox CF, Sübay RK, Ostro E, et al: Tunnel defects in dentinal bridges: their formation following direct pulp capping, *Oper Dent* 21:4, 1996.

74. Cox CF, Suzuki S: Re-evaluating pulp protection: calcium hydroxide liners vs cohesive hybridization, *J Am Dent Assoc* 125:823, 1994.

75. Croll TP, McKay MS, Castaldi CR: Impaction of permanent posterior teeth by overextended stainless steel margins, *J Pedod* 5:240, 1981.

76. Cui C, Zhou XN, Chen WM: Self-etching adhesives: possible new pulp capping agents to vital pulp therapy, *Front Med* 5:77, 2011.

77. Cvek M: A clinical report on partial pulpotomy and capping with calcium hydroxide in permanent incisors with complicated root fractures, *J Endod* 4:232, 1978.

78. Cvek M: Prognosis of luxated non-vital maxillary incisors treated with calcium hydroxide and filled with gutta-percha: a retrospective clinical study, *Endod Dent Traumatol* 8:45, 1992.

79. Dähnhardt JE, Jaeqqi T, Lussi A: Treating open carious lesions in anxious children with ozone: a prospective controlled clinical study, *Am J Dent* 19:267, 2006.

80. Damas BA, Wheater MA, Bringas JS, et al: Cytotoxicity comparison of mineral trioxide aggregates and EndoSequence bioceramic root repair materials, *J Endod* 37:372, 2011.

81. Dammaschke T, Leidinger J, Schäfer E: Long-term evaluation of direct pulp capping: treatment outcomes

in New Zealand undergraduate dental students, *N Z Dent J* 101:106, 2005.

over an average period of 6.1 years, *Clin Oral Investig* 14:559, 2010.

82. Dammaschke T, Stratmann U, Wolff P, et al: Direct pulp capping with mineral trioxide aggregate: an immunohistologic comparison with calcium hydroxide in rodents, *J Endod* 36:814, 2010.

83. Dammaschke T, Wolff P, Saqheri D, et al: Mineral trioxide aggregate for direct pulp capping: an histologic comparison with calcium hydroxide in rat molars, *Quintessence Int* 41:20, 2010.

84. D'Antò V, Di Caprio MP, Ametrano G, et al: Effect of mineral trioxide aggregate on mesenchymal stem cells, *J Endod* 36:1839, 2010.

85. Darvell BW, Wu RC: "MTA"—an hydraulic silicate cement: review update and setting reaction, *Dent Mater* 27:407, 2011.

86. Davidson CL: Advances in glass ionomer cements, *J Appl Oral Sci* 14:3, 2006.

87. De Almeida Neves A, Coutinho E, Cardoso MV, et al: Current concepts and techniques for caries excavation and adhesion to residual dentin, *J Adhes Dent* 13:7, 2011.

88. De Assunção Pinheiro IV, Borges BC, De Lima KC: In vivo assessment of secondary caries and dentin characteristics after traditional amalgam restorations, *Eur J Dent* 6:263, 2012.

89. De Backer H, Van Maele G, Decock V, et al: Long-term survival of complete crowns, fixed dental prostheses, and cantilever prostheses with post and cores on root-canal treated teeth, *Int J Prosthodont* 20:229, 2007.

90. De Mendonça AA, De Oliveira CF, Hebling J, et al: Influence of thicknesses of smear layer on the transdentinal cytotoxicity and bond strength of a resin-modified glass-ionomer cement, *Braz Dent J* 23:379, 2012.

91. Déjou J, Raskin A, Colombani J, et al: Physical, chemical and mechanical behavior of a new material for direct posterior fillings, *Eur Cell Mater* 10(Suppl 4):22, 2005.

92. Demir T, Cehreli ZC: Clinical and radiographic evaluation of adhesive pulp capping in primary molars following hemostasis with 1.25% sodium hypochlorite: 2-year results, *Am J Dent* 20:182, 2007.

93. Dennison JB, Hamilton JC: Treatment decisions and conservation of tooth structure, *Dent Clin North Am* 49:825, 2005.

94. Desai S, Chandler N: The restoration of permanent immature anterior teeth, root filled using MTA: a review, *J Dent* 37:652, 2009.

95. Do Nascimento ABL, Fontana UF, Teixeira HM, et al: Biocompatibility of a resin-modified glass-ionomer cement applied as pulp capping in human teeth, *Am J Dent* 13:28, 2000.

96. Domine L, Holz J: The aging of the human pulp-dentin organ, *Schweiz Monatsschr Zahnmed* 101:725, 1991.

97. Doyle TL, Casas MJ, Kenny DJ, et al: Mineral trioxide aggregate produces superior outcomes in vital primary molar pulpotomy, *Pediatr Dent* 32:41, 2010.

98. Dreger LA, Felippe WT, Reyes-Carmona JF, et al: Mineral trioxide aggregate and Portland cement promote biomineralization in vivo, *J Endod* 38:324, 2012.

99. Dummet CO, Kopel M: Pediatric endodontics. In Ingle JI, Bakland LK, editors: *Endodontics*, ed 5, Hamilton, Ontario, 2002, Decker.

100. Eghbal MJ, Asgary S, Baglue RA, et al: MTA pulpotomy of human permanent molars with irreversible pulpitis, *Aust Endod J* 35:4, 2009.

101. Eid AA, Komabayashi T, Watanabe E, et al: Characterization of the mineral trioxide aggregate-resin modified glass ionomer cement interface in different setting conditions, *J Endod* 38:1126, 2012.

102. Elias RV, Demarco FF, Tarquinio SB, et al: Pulp responses to the application of a self-etching adhesive in human pulps after controlling bleeding with sodium hypochlorite, *Quintessence Int* 38:67, 2007.

103. El-Meligy OA, Avery DR: Comparison of mineral trioxide aggregate and calcium hydroxide as pulpotomy agents in

young permanent teeth (apexogenesis), *Pediatr Dent* 28:399, 2006.

104. Eming SA, Krieg T, Davidson JM: Inflammation in wound repair: molecular and cellular mechanisms, *J Invest Dermatol* 127:514, 2007.

105. Eskandarizadeh A, Shahpasandzadeh MH, Shahpasandzadeh M, et al: A comparative study on dental pulp response to calcium hydroxide, white and grey mineral trioxide aggregate as pulp capping agents, *J Conserv Dent* 14:351, 2011.

106. Ettinger RL, Kambhu PP, Asmussen CM, et al: An in vitro evaluation of the integrity of stainless steel crown margins cemented with different luting agents, *Spec Care Dent* 18:78, 1998.

107. Falster CA, Araujo FB, Straffon LH, et al: Indirect pulp treatment: in vivo outcomes of an adhesive resin system vs calcium hydroxide for protection of the dentin-pulp complex, *Pediatr Dent* 24:241, 2002.

108. Farges JC, Carrouel F, Keller JF, et al: Cytokine production by human odontoblast-like cells upon Toll-like receptor-2 engagement, *Immunobiology* 216:513, 2011.

109. Farsi N, Alamoudi N, Balto K, et al: Clinical assessment of mineral trioxide aggregate (MTA) as direct pulp capping in young permanent teeth, *Pediatr Dent* 31:72, 2006.

110. Felippe WT, Felippe MC, Rocha MJ: The effect of mineral trioxide aggregate on the apexification and periapical healing of teeth with incomplete root formation, *Int Endod J* 39:2, 2006.

111. Fitzgerald M, Chiego DJJ, Heys DR: Autoradiographic analysis of odontoblast replacement following pulp exposure in primate teeth, *Arch Oral Biol* 35:707, 1990.

112. Fong CD, Davis MJ: Partial pulpotomy for immature permanent teeth: its present and future, *Pediatr Dent* 24:29, 2002.

113. Ford TR, Torabinejad M, Abedi HR, et al: Using mineral trioxide aggregate as a pulp-capping material, *J Am Dent Assoc* 127:1491, 1996.

114. Forss H, Widström E: The post-amalgam era: a selection of materials and their longevity in primary and young permanent dentitions, *Int J Paediatr Dent* 13:158, 2003.

115. Forss H, Widström E: Reasons for restorative therapy and longevity of restorations in adults, *Acta Odontol Scand* 62:82, 2004.

116. Franzon R, Casagrande L, Pinto AS, et al: Clinical and radiographic evaluation of indirect pulp treatment in primary molars: 36 months follow-up, *Am J Dent* 20:189, 2007.

117. Fridland M, Rosado R: MTA solubility: a long term study, *J Endod* 31:376, 2005.

118. Fuks AB: Pulp therapy for the primary and young permanent dentitions, *Dent Clin North Am* 44:571, 2000.

119. Fuks AB: Vital pulp therapy with new materials for primary teeth: new directions and treatment perspectives, *J Endod* 34:S18, 2008.

120. Fuks AB, Bimstein E, Bruchim A: Radiographic and histologic evaluation of the effect of two concentrations of formocresol on pulpotomized primary and young permanent teeth in monkeys, *Pediatr Dent* 5:9, 1983.

121. Fuks AB, Gavra S, Chosack A: Long-term follow up of traumatized incisors treated by partial pulpotomy, *Pediatr Dent* 15:334, 1993.

122. Fuks AB, Heling I: Pulp therapy for the young permanent dentition. In Pinkham JR, Casamassimo PS, Fields HW, et al, editors: *Pediatric dentistry: infancy through adolescence*, ed 24, St Louis, 2005, Saunders/Elsevier.

123. Fulling HJ, Andreasen JO: Influence of maturation status and tooth type of permanent teeth upon electrometric and thermal pulp testing procedures, *Scand J Dent Res* 84:286, 1976.

124. Fusayama T: *A simple pain-free adhesive restorative system by minimal reduction and total etching*, St Louis, 1993, Ishiyaku Euro America Publishing.

125. Fusayama T, Kurosaki N: Structure and removal of carious dentin, *Int Dent J* 22:401, 1972.

126. Fusayama T, Okuse K, Hosoda H: Relationship between hardness, discoloration, and microbial invasion in carious dentin, *J Dent Res* 45:1033, 1966.

127. Galler KM, Schwiki H, Hiller KA, et al: TEGDMA reduces mineralization in dental pulp cells, *J Dent Res* 90:257, 2011.

128. Gandolfi MG, Ciapetti G, Taddei P, et al: Apatite formation on bioactive calcium-silicate cements for dentistry affects surface topography and human marrow stromal cells proliferation, *Dent Mater* 26:974, 2010.

129. Garcia-Godoy F, Murray PE: Recommendations for using regenerative endodontic procedures in permanent immature traumatized teeth, *Dent Traumatol* 28:33, 2012.

130. Goldberg M, Farges JC, Lacerda-Pinheiro S, et al: Inflammatory and immunological aspects of dental pulp repair, *Pharmacol Res* 58:137, 2008.

131. Goldberg M, Lasfargues JJ, Legrand JM: Clinical testing of dental materials–histological considerations, *Dent J* 22:S25, 1994.

132. Goldberg M, Six N, Decup F, et al: Bioactive molecules and the future of pulp therapy, *Am J Dent* 16:66, 2003.

133. Gonçalves JL, Viapiana R, Miranda CE, et al: Evaluation of physico-chemical properties of Portland cements and MTA, *Braz Oral Res* 24:277, 2010.

134. Goracci G, Mori G: Scanning electron microscopic evaluation of resin-dentin and calcium hydroxide dentin-interface with resin composite restorations, *Quintessence Int* 27:129, 1996.

135. Gracia TB: *Accuracy of size estimations by dentists of simulated pulp exposures and cavity preparations. MDS (endodontics) research report*, Dunedin, New Zealand, 2006, University of Otago.

136. Grech L, Mallia B, Camilleri J: Characterization of set intermediate restorative material, Biodentine, Bioaggregate and a prototype calcium silicate cement for use as root-end filling materials, *Int Endod J* 46:632, 2012.

137. Grötz KA, Duschner H, Reichert TE, et al: Histotomography of the odontoblast processes at the dentine-enamel junction of permanent healthy human teeth in the confocal laser scanning microscope, *Clin Oral Investig* 2:21, 1998.

138. Gruythuysen RJ, Van Strijp AJ, Wu MK: Long-term survival of indirect pulp treatment performed in primary and permanent teeth with clinically diagnosed deep carious lesions, *J Endod* 36:1490, 2010.

139. Gudkina J, Mindere A, Locane G, et al: Review of the success of pulp exposure treatment of cariously and traumatically exposed pulps in immature permanent incisors and molars, *Stomatologija* 14:71, 2012.

140. Gutmann JL, Heaton JF: Management of the open (immature) apex. Part 1. Vital teeth, *Int Endod J* 14:166, 1981.

141. Guven G, Cehreli ZC, Ural A, et al: Effect of mineral trioxide aggregate cements on transforming growth factor beta-1 and bone morphogenetic protein production by human fibroblasts in vitro, *J Endod* 33:447, 2007.

142. Guven EP, Yalvac ME, Sahin F, et al: Effect of calcium hydroxide–containing cement, mineral trioxide aggregate, and enamel matrix derivative on proliferation and differentiation of human tooth germ stem cells, *J Endod* 37:650, 2011.

143. Gwinnett J, Tay FR, Pang KM, et al: Quantitative contribution of collagen network in dentin hybridization, *Am J Dent* 9:140,1996.

144. Hafez AA, Cox CF, Tarim B, et al: An in vivo evaluation of hemorrhage control using sodium hypochlorite and direct capping with a one- or two-component adhesive system in exposed nonhuman primate pulps, *Quintessence Int* 33:261, 2002.

145. Haghgoo R, Abbasi F: A histopathological comparison of pulpotomy with sodium hypochlorite and formocresol, *Iran Endod J* 7:60, 2012.

146. Hahn CL, Liewehr FR: Innate immune responses of the dental pulp to caries, *J Endod* 33:643, 2007.

147. Hahn CL, Liewehr FR: Relationships between caries bacteria, host responses, and clinical signs and symptoms of pulpitis, *J Endod* 33:213, 2007.

148. Hahn CL, Liewehr FR: Update on the adaptive immune responses of the dental pulp, *J Endod* 33:773, 2007.

149. Ham KA, Witherspoon DE, Gutmann JL, et al: Preliminary evaluation of BMP-2 expression and histological characteristics during apexification with calcium hydroxide and mineral trioxide aggregate, *J Endod* 31:275, 2005.

150. Hashem AA, Wanees Amin SA: The effect of acidity on dislodgment resistance of mineral trioxide aggregate and bioaggregate in furcation perforations: an in vitro comparative study, *J Endod* 38:245, 2012.

151. Haskell EW, Stanley HR, Chellemi J, et al: Direct pulp capping treatment: a long-term follow-up, *J Am Dent Assoc* 97:607, 1978.

152. Hayashi Y: Ultrastructure of initial calcification in wound healing following pulpotomy, *J Oral Pathol* 11:174, 1982.

153. Hebling J, Giro EMA, DeSouza Costa CA: Biocompatibility of an adhesive system applied to exposed human dental pulp, *J Endod* 25:676, 1999.

154. Helfer AR, Melnick S, Schilder H: Determination of the moisture content of vital and pulpless teeth, *Oral Surg Oral Med Oral Pathol* 34:661, 1972.

155. Heller AL, Koenigs JF, Brilliant JD, et al: Direct pulp capping of permanent teeth in primates using a resorbable form of tricalcium phosphate ceramic, *J Endod* 1:95, 1975.

156. Henderson B, Wilson M: Cytokine induction by bacteria: beyond lipopolysaccharide, *Cytokine* 8:269, 1996.

157. Henderson HZ, Setcos JC: The sealed composite resin restoration, *ASDC J Dent Child* 52:300, 1985.

158. Hermann BW: Dentinobliteration der Wurzelkanale nach Behandlung mit Calcium, *Zahnärztl Rdsch* 39:887, 1930.

159. Herrera M, Castillo A, Bravo M, et al: Antibacterial activity of resin adhesives, glass ionomer and resin-modified glass ionomer cements and a compomer in contact with dentin caries samples, *Oper Dent* 25:265, 2000.

160. Hessle CC, Andersson B, Wold AE: Gram-positive and Gram-negative bacteria elicit different patterns of pro-inflammatory cytokines in human monocytes, *Cytokine* 30:311, 2005.

161. Higashi T, Okamoto H: Influence of particle size of hydroxyapatite as a capping agent on cell proliferation of cultured fibroblasts, *J Endod* 22:236, 1996.

162. Hilton TJ: Keys to clinical success with pulp capping: a review of the literature, *Oper Dent* 34:615, 2008.

162a. Hilton TJ, Ferracane JL, Mancl L: Northwest Practice-based Research Collaborative in Evidence-based Dentistry (NWP). Comparison of CaOH with MTA for direct pulp capping: a PBRN randomized clinical trial. *J Dent Res* 92:16S, 2013.

163. Hirota K: A study on the partial pulp removal (pulpotomy) using four different tissue solvents, *J Jpn Stomatol Soc* 26:1588, 1959.

164. Holan G, Eidelman E, Fuks A: Long-term evaluation of pulpotomy in primary molars using mineral trioxide aggregate or formocresol, *Pediatr Dent* 27:129, 2005.

165. Hørsted P, Søndergaard B, Thylstrup A, et al: A retrospective study of direct pulp capping with calcium hydroxide compounds, *Endod Dent Traumatol* 1:29, 1985.

166. Hörsted-Bindslev P, Vilkinis V, Sidlauskas A: Direct capping of human pulps with a dentin bonding system or with calcium hydroxide cement, *Oral Surg Oral Med Oral Pathol Oral Radiol Endod* 96:591, 2003.

167. Hosoda H, Fusayama T: A tooth substance saving restorative technique, *Int Dent J* 34:1, 1984.

168. Hosoya Y, Taguchi T, Arita S, et al: Clinical evaluation of polypropylene glycol–based caries detecting dyes for primary and permanent carious dentin, *J Dent* 36:1041, 2008.

169. Huang GT: A paradigm shift in endodontic management of immature teeth: conservation of stem cells for regeneration, *J Dent* 36:379, 2008.

170. Inokoshi S, Iwaku M, Fusayama T: Pulpal response to a new adhesive resin material, *J Dent Res* 61:1014, 1982.

171. Inoue H, Muneyuki H, Izumi T, et al: Electron microscopic study on nerve terminals during dentin bridge formation after pulpotomy in dog teeth, *J Endod* 23:569, 1997.

172. Ishizaka R, Hayashi Y, Iohara K, et al: Stimulation of angiogenesis, neurogenesis and regeneration by side population cells from dental pulp, *Biomaterials* 34:1888, 2013.

173. Itoh K, Kusunoki M, Oikawa M, et al: In vitro comparison of three caries dyes, *Am J Dent* 22:195, 2009.

174. Izumi T, Kobayashi I, Okamura K, et al: Immunohistochemical study on the immunocompetent cells of the pulp in human non-carious and carious teeth, *Arch Oral Biol* 40:609, 1995.

175. Jameson MW, Hood JAA, Tidmarsh BG: The effects of dehydration and rehydration on some mechanical properties of human dentine, *J Biomech* 26:1055, 1993.

176. Jamieson WJ, Vargas K: Recall rates and caries experience of patients undergoing general anesthesia for dental treatment, *Pediatr Dent* 29:253, 2007.

177. Jeeruphan T, Jantarat J, Yanpiset K, et al: Mahidol study 1: comparison of radiographic and survival outcomes of immature teeth treated with either regenerative endodontic or apexification methods—a retrospective study, *J Endod* 38:1330, 2012.

178. Jordan RE, Suzuki M: Conservative treatment of deep carious lesions, *J Can Dent Assoc* 37:337, 1971.

179. Kakehashi S, Stanley HR, Fitzgerald RT: The effects of surgical exposures of dental pulps in germ-free and conventional laboratory rats, *Oral Surg Oral Med Oral Pathol* 20:340, 1965.

180. Kangarlou A, Sofiabadi S, Asgary S, et al: Assessment of antifungal activity of ProRoot mineral trioxide aggregate and mineral trioxide aggregate–Angelus, *Dent Res J (Isfahan)* 9:256, 2012.

181. Karibe H, Ohide Y, Kohno H, et al: Study on thermal pulp testing of immature permanent teeth, *Shigaku* 77:1006, 1989.

182. Kashiwada T, Takagi M: New restoration and direct pulp capping systems using adhesive composite resin, *Bull Tokyo Med Dent Univ* 38:45, 1991.

183. Kato C, Suzuki M, Shinkai K, et al: Histopathological and immunohistochemical study on the effects of a direct pulp capping experimentally developed adhesive resin system containing reparative dentin-promoting agents, *Dent Mater J* 30:583, 2011.

184. Kato S, Fusayama T: Recalcification of artificially decalcified dentin in vivo, *J Dent Res* 49:1060, 1970.

185. Kidd EA, Ricketts DN, Beighton D: Criteria for caries removal at the enamel-dentine junction: a clinical and microbiological study, *Br Dent J* 180:287, 1996.

186. Kim S, Heyeraas KJ, Haug SR: Structure and function of the dentin-pulp complex In Ingle JI, Bakand LK, Baumgartner JC, editors: *Ingle's endodontics*, ed 6, Hamilton, Ontario, 2008, Decker.

187. Kim YJ, Chandler NP: Determination of working length for teeth with wide or immature apices: a review, *Int Endod J* 46:483, 2013.

188. Kitasako Y, Murray PE, Tagami J, et al: Histomorphometric analysis of dentinal bridge formation and pulpal inflammation, *Quintessence Int* 33:600, 2002.

189. Kitasako Y, Shibata S, Arakawa M, et al: A light and transmission microscopic study of mechanically exposed monkey pulps: dynamics of fiber elements during early dentin bridge formation, *Oral Surg Oral Med Oral Pathol Oral Radiol Endod* 89:224, 2000.

190. Koh ET, Pitt Ford TR, Torabinejad M, et al: Mineral trioxide aggregate stimulates cytokine production in human osteoblasts, *J Bone Min Res* 10S:S406, 1995.

191. Koh ET, Torabinejad M, Pitt Ford TR, et al: Mineral trioxide aggregate stimulates a biological response in human osteoblasts, *J Biomed Mater Res* 37:432, 1997.

192. Kotsanos N, Arizos S: Evaluation of a resin modified glass ionomer serving both as indirect pulp therapy and as restorative material for primary molars, *Eur Arch Paediatr Dent* 12:170, 2011.

193. Koulaouzidou EA, Economides N, Beltes P, et al: In vitro evaluation of the cytotoxicity of ProRoot MTA and MTA Angelus, *J Oral Sci* 50:397, 2008.

194. Kuratate M, Yoshiba K, Shigetani Y, et al: Immunohistochemical analysis of nestin, osteopontin, and proliferating cells in the reparative process of exposed dental pulp capped with mineral trioxide aggregate, *J Endod* 34:970, 2008.

195. Kurji ZA, Sigal MJ, Andrews P, et al: A retrospective study of a modified 1-minute formocresol pulpotomy technique. Part 1. Clinical and radiographic findings, *Pediatr Dent* 33:131, 2011.

196. Kurji ZA, Sigal MJ, Andrews P, et al: A retrospective study of a modified 1-minute formocresol pulpotomy technique. Part 2. Effect on exfoliation times and successors, *Pediatr Dent* 33:139, 2011.

197. Langeland K: Management of the inflamed pulp associated with deep carious lesion, *J Endod* 7:169, 1981.

198. Laurent P, Camps J, De Méo M, et al: Induction of specific cell responses to a Ca(3)SiO(5)–based posterior restorative material, *Dent Mater J* 24:1486, 2008.

199. Lee YH, Kim GE, Cho HJ, et al: Aging of in vitro pulp illustrates change of inflammation and dentinogenesis, *J Endod* 39:340, 2013.

200. Leeson TS, Leeson CR, Paparo AA: *Atlas of histology: the digestive system*, Philadelphia, 1988, Saunders.

201. Leksell E, Ridell K, Cvek M, et al: Pulp exposure after stepwise versus direct complete excavation of deep carious lesions in young posterior permanent teeth, *Endod Dent Traumatol* 12:192, 1996.

202. Lessa FC, Aranha AM, Hebling J, et al: Cytotoxic effects of White MTA and MTA-Bio cements on odontoblast-like cells (MDPC-23), *Braz J* 21:24, 2010.

203. Lewis B: The obsolescence of formocresol, *J Calif Dent Assoc* 38:102, 2010.

204. Leye Benoist F, Gaye Ndiaye F, Kane AW, et al: Evaluation of mineral trioxide aggregate (MTA) versus calcium hydroxide cement (Dycal) in the formation of a dentine bridge: a randomised controlled trial, *Int Dent J* 62:33, 2012.

205. Lin LM, Rosenberg PA: Repair and regeneration in endodontics, *Int Endod J* 44:889, 2011.

206. Linn J, Messer HH: Effect of restorative procedures on the strength of endodontically treated molars, *J Endod* 20:479, 1994.

207. Lucas Leite AC, Rosenblatt A, Da Silva Calixto M, et al: Genotoxic effect of formocresol pulp therapy of deciduous teeth, *Mutat Res* 747:93, 2012.

208. Mahmoud SH, Grawish Mel-A, Zaher AR, et al: Influence of selective immunosuppressive drugs on the healing of exposed dogs' dental pulp capped with mineral trioxide aggregate, *J Endod* 36:95, 2010.

209. Maltz M, Garcia R, Jardim JJ, et al: Randomized trial of partial vs stepwise caries removal: 3-year follow-up, *J Dent Res* 91:1026, 2012.

210. Marchi JJ, De Araujo FB, Fröner AM, et al: Indirect pulp capping in the primary dentition: a 4 year follow-up study, *J Clin Pediatr Dent* 31:68, 2006.

211. Martin G, Ricucci D, Gibbs JL, et al: Histological findings of revascularized/revitalized immature permanent molar with apical periodontitis using platelet-rich plasma, *J Endod* 39:138, 2013.

212. Mass E, Zilberman U: Long-term radiologic pulp evaluation after partial pulpotomy in young permanent molars, *Quintessence Int* 42:547, 2011.

213. Mass E, Zilberman U, Fuks AB: Partial pulpotomy: another treatment option for cariously exposed permanent molars, *J Dent Child* 62:342, 1995.

214. Matsumoto S, Hayashi M, Suzuki Y, et al: Calcium ions released from mineral trioxide aggregate convert the differentiation pathway of C2C12 cells into osteoblast lineage, *J Endod* 39:68, 2013.

215. Matsuo T, Nakanishi T, Shimizu H, et al: A clinical study of direct pulp capping applied to carious-exposed pulps, *J Endod* 22:551, 1996.

216. Matsuura T, Katsumata T, Matsuura T, et al: Histopathological study of pulpal irritation of dental adhesive resin. Part 1. Panavia EX, *Nihon Hotetsu Shika Gakkai Zasshi* 31:104, 1987.

217. Matysiak M, Dubois JP, Ducastelle T, et al: Morphometric analysis of human pulp myelinated fibers during aging, *J Biol Buccale* 14:69, 1986.

218. McComb D: Caries-detector dyes: how accurate and useful are they? *J Can Dent Assoc* 66:195, 2000.

219. McDonald RE, Avery DR, Dean JA: Treatment of deep caries, vital pulp exposure, and pulpless teeth. In Dean JA, Avery DR, McDonald RE, editors: *McDonald and Avery's dentistry of the child and adolescent*, ed 9, St Louis, 2011, Mosby/Elsevier.

220. Mejàre I, Cvek M: Partial pulpotomy in young permanent teeth with deep carious lesions, *Endod Dent Traumatol* 9:238, 1993.

221. Memarpour M, Mesbahi M, Shafiei F: Three-and-a-half-year clinical evaluation of posterior composite resin in children, *J Dent Child* 77:92, 2010.

222. Mente J, Geletneky B, Ohle M, et al: Mineral trioxide aggregate or calcium hydroxide direct pulp capping: an analysis of the clinical treatment outcome, *J Endod* 36:806, 2010.

223. Mente J, Hage N, Pfefferie T, et al: Mineral trioxide aggregate apical plugs in teeth with open apical foramina: a retrospective analysis of treatment outcome, *J Endod* 35:1354, 2009.

224. Mente J, Leo M, Panagidis D, et al: Treatment outcome of mineral trioxide aggregate in open apex teeth, *J Endod* 39:20, 2013.

224a. Mente J, Hufnagel S, Leo M, et al: Treatment of mineral trioxide aggregate or calcium hydroxide direct pulp capping: long-term results. *J Endod* 40:1746, 2014.

225. Mentink AG, Meeuwissen R, Käyser AF, et al: Survival rate and failure characteristics of the all metal post and core restoration, *J Oral Rehabil* 20:455, 1993.

226. Merdad K, Sonbul H, Bukhary S, et al: Caries susceptibility of endodontically versus nonendodontically treated teeth, *J Endod* 37:139, 2011.

227. Mertz-Fairhurst EJ, Call-Smith KM, Shuster GS, et al: Clinical performance of sealed composite restorations placed over caries compared with sealed and unsealed amalgam restorations, *J Am Dent Assoc* 115:689, 1987.

228. Mettes D: Insufficient evidence to support or refute the need for 6-monthly dental check-ups: What is the optimal recall frequency between dental checks? *Evid Based Dent* 6:62, 2005.

229. Miles JP, Gluskin AH, Chambers D, et al: Pulp capping with mineral trioxide aggregate (MTA): a retrospective analysis of carious pulp exposures treated by undergraduate dental students, *Oper Dent* 35:20, 2010.

230. Min KS, Park HJ, Lee SK, et al: Effect of mineral trioxide aggregate on dentin bridge formation and expression of dentin sialoprotein and heme oxygenase-1 in human pulp, *J Endod* 34:666, 2008.

231. Minamikawa H, Yamada M, Deyama Y, et al: Effect of N-acetylcysteine on rat dental pulp cells cultured on mineral trioxide aggregate, *J Endod* 37:637, 2011.

232. Miyashita H, Worthington HV, Qualtrough A, et al: Pulp management for caries in adults: maintaining pulp vitality, *Cochrane Database Syst Rev* 18:CD004484, 2007.

233. Miyauchi H, Iwaku M, Fusayama T: Physiological recalcification of carious dentin, *Bull Tokyo Med Dent Univ* 25:169, 1978.

234. Mjör IA: Pulp-dentin biology in restorative dentistry. Part 5. Clinical management and tissue changes associated with wear and trauma, *Quintessence Int* 32:771, 2001.

235. Mjör IA: Pulp-dentin biology in restorative dentistry. Part 7. The exposed pulp, *Quintessence Int* 33:113, 2002.

236. Modena KC, Casas-Apayco LC, Atta MT: Cytotoxicity and biocompatibility of direct and indirect pulp capping materials, *J Appl Oral Sci* 17:544, 2009.

237. Mohammadi Z, Dummer PMH: Properties and applications of calcium hydroxide in endodontics and dental traumatology, *Int Endod J* 44:697, 2011.

238. Moretti AB, Sakai VT, Oliveira TM, et al: The effectiveness of mineral trioxide aggregate, calcium hydroxide and formocresol for pulpotomies in primary teeth, *Int Endod J* 41:547, 2008.

239. Moritz A, Schoop U, Goharkhay K, et al: The CO_2 laser as an aid in direct pulp capping, *J Endod* 24:248, 1998.

240. Morse DR: Age-related changes of the dental pulp complex and their relationship to systemic aging, *Oral Surg Oral Med Oral Pathol* 72:721, 1991.

241. Morse DR, Esposito JV, Schoor RS: A radiographic study of aging changes of the dental pulp and dentin in normal teeth, *Quintessence Int* 24:329, 1993.

242. Mozayeni MA, Milani AS, Marvasti LA, et al: Cytotoxicity of calcium enriched mixture cement compared with mineral trioxide aggregate and intermediate restorative material, *Aust Dent J* 38:70, 2012.

243. Mudie AS, Holland GR: Local opioids in the inflamed dental pulp, *J Endod* 32:319, 2006.

244. Murray PE, Garcia-Godoy F, Hargreaves KM: Regenerative endodontics: a review of current status and a call for action, *J Endod* 33:377, 2007.

245. Murray PE, Hafez AA, Smith AJ, et al: Histomorphometric analysis of odontoblast-like cell numbers and dentine bridge secretory activity following pulp exposure, *Int Endod J* 36:106, 2003.

246. Murray PE, Smith AJ: Saving pulps: a biological basis—an overview, *Prim Dent Care* 9:21, 2002.

247. Nair PNR, Duncan HF, Pitt Ford TR, et al: Histological, ultrastructural and quantitative investigations on the response of healthy human pulps to experimental pulp capping with mineral trioxide aggregate: a randomized controlled trial, *Int Endod J* 41:128, 2008.

248. Nakanishi T, Matsuo T, Ebisu S: Quantitative analysis of immunoglobulins and inflammatory factors in human pulpal blood from exposed pulps, *J Endod* 21:131, 1995.

249. Neelakantan P, Grotra D, Subbarao CV, et al: The shear bond strength of resin-based composite to white mineral trioxide aggregate, *J Am Dent Assoc* 143:e40, 2012.

250. Neelakantan P, Rao CV, Indramohan J: Bacteriology of deep carious lesions underneath amalgam restorations with different pulp-capping materials: an in vivo analysis, *J Appl Oral Sci* 20:139, 2012.

251. Ng YL, Mann V, Gulabivala K: A prospective study of the factors affecting outcomes of non-surgical root canal treatment. Part 2. Tooth survival, *Int Endod J* 44:610, 2011.

252. Nikaido T, Inoue G, Takagaki T, et al: New strategy to create "Super Dentin" using adhesive technology: reinforcement of adhesive-dentin interface and protection of tooth structures, *Jpn Dent Sci Rev* 47:31, 2011.

253. Nikaido T, Weerasinghe DD, Waidyasekera K, et al: Assessment of the nanostructure of acid-base resistant zone by the application of all-in-one adhesive systems: super dentin formation, *Biomed Mater Eng* 19:163, 2009.

254. Nikiforuk G: Optimal recall intervals in child dental care, *J Can Dent Assoc* 63:618, 1997.

255. Nissan R, Segal H, Pashley D, et al: Ability of bacterial endotoxin to diffuse through human dentin, *J Endod* 21:62, 1995.

256. Nosrat A, Seifi A, Asgary S: Pulpotomy in caries-exposed immature permanent molars using calcium-enriched mixture cement or mineral trioxide aggregate: a randomized clinical trial, *Int J Paediatr Dent* 23:56, 2013.

257. Nosrat IV, Nosrat CA: Reparative hard tissue formation following calcium hydroxide application after partial pulpotomy in cariously exposed pulps of permanent teeth, *Int Endod J* 31:221, 1998.

258. Nowicka A, Parafiniuk M, Lipski M, et al: Pulpo-dentin complex response after direct capping with self-etch adhesive systems, *Folia Histochem Cytobiol* 50:565, 2012.

259. Oguntebi BR, Heaven T, Clark AE, et al: Quantitative assessment of dentin bridge formation following pulp-capping in miniature swine, *J Endod* 21:79, 1995.

260. Okiji T, Yoshiba K: Reparative dentinogenesis induced by mineral trioxide aggregate: a review from the biological and physicochemical points of view, *Int J Dent* 464:280, 2009.

261. Olivi G, Genovese MD, Maturo P, et al: Pulp capping: advantages of using laser technology, *Eur J Paediatr Dent* 8:89, 2007.

262. Olsson H, Davies JR, Holst KE, et al: Dental pulp capping: effect of Emdogain Gel on experimentally exposed human pulps, *Int Endod J* 38:186, 2005.

263. Opdam NJ, Bronkhorst EM, Loomans BA, et al: 12-year survival of composite vs amalgam restorations, *J Dent Res* 89:1063, 2010.

264. Orhan EO, Maden M, Sengüüven B: Odontoblast-like cell numbers and reparative dentine thickness after direct pulp capping with platelet-rich plasma and enamel matrix derivative: a histomorphometric evaluation, *Int Endod J* 45:317, 2012.

265. Ørstavik D, Pitt Ford TR: *Essential endodontology: prevention and treatment of apical periodontitis*, Oxford, England, 1998, Blackwell Science,.

266. Paranjpe A, Smoot T, Zhang H, et al: Direct contact with mineral trioxide aggregate activates and differentiates human dental pulp cells, *J Endod* 37:1691, 2011.

267. Paranjpe A, Zhang H, Johnson JD: Effects of mineral trioxide aggregate on human pulp cells after pulp-capping procedures, *J Endod* 36:1042, 2010.

268. Park JW, Hong SH, Kim JH, et al: X-ray diffraction analysis of white ProRoot MTA and Diadent BioAggregate, *Oral Surg Oral Med Oral Pathol Oral Radiol Endod* 109:155, 2010.

269. Patel R, Cohenca N: Maturogenesis of a cariously exposed immature permanent tooth using MTA for direct pulp capping: a case report, *Dent Traumatol* 22:328, 2006.

269a. Peutzfeldt A, Asmussen E: Influence of eugenol-containing temporary cement on self-etching adhesives to dentin. *J Adhes Dent* 8:31, 2006.

270. Primosch RE, Balsewich CM, Thomas CW: Outcomes assessment an intervention strategy to improve parental compliance to follow-up evaluations after treatment of early childhood caries using general anesthesia in a Medicaid population, *ASDC J Dent Child* 68:102, 2001.

271. Pugach MK, Strother J, Darling CL, et al: Dentin caries zones: mineral, structure, and properties, *J Dent Res* 88:71, 2009.

272. Qudeimat MA, Barrieshi-Nusair KM, Owais AI: Calcium hydroxide vs mineral trioxide aggregates for partial pulpotomy of permanent molars with deep caries, *Eur Arch Paediatr Dent* 8:99, 2007.

273. Randow K, Glantz PO: On cantilever loading of vital and non-vital teeth: an experimental clinical study, *Acta Odontol Scand* 44:271, 1986.

274. Ranly DM, Garcia-Godoy F: Current and potential pulp therapies for primary and young permanent teeth, *J Dent* 28:153, 2000.

275. Reyes-Carmona JF, Santos AS, Figueiredo CP, et al: Host-mineral trioxide aggregate inflammatory molecular signaling and biomineralization ability, *J Endod* 36:1347, 2010.

276. Reyes-Carmona JF, Santos AR, Figueiredo CP, et al: In vivo host interactions with mineral trioxide aggregate and calcium hydroxide: inflammatory molecular signaling assessment, *J Endod* 37:1225, 2011.

276a. Ricucci D, Loghin S, Lin LM, et al: Is hard tissue formation in the dental pulp after the death of the primary odontoblasts a regenerative or a reparative process? *J Dent* 42:1156, 2014.

277. Rodd HD, Boissonade FM: Comparative immunohistochemical analysis of the peptidergic innervation of human primary and permanent tooth pulp, *Arch Oral Biol* 47:375, 2002.

278. Rölling I, Hasselgren G, Tronstad L: Morphologic and enzyme histochemical observations on the pulp of human primary molars 3 to 5 years after formocresol treatment, *Oral Surg Oral Med Oral Pathol* 42:518, 1976.

279. Rosenblatt A, Stamford TC, Niederman R: Silver diamine fluoride: a caries "silver fluoride bullet", *J Dent Res* 88:116, 2009.

280. Roth KK, Müller M, Ahrens G: Staining of carious dentin with Kariesdetektor, *Dtsch Zahnärztl Z* 44:460, 1989.

281. Rothman MS: Formocresol pulpotomy: a practical procedure for permanent teeth, *Gen Dent* 25:39, 1977.

282. Salvi GE, Siegrist Guldener BE, Amstad T, et al: Clinical evaluation of root filled teeth restored with or without post-and-core systems in a specialist practice setting, *Int Endod J* 40:209, 2007.

283. Sarkar NK, Caicedo R, Ritwik P, et al: Physiochemical basis of the biologic properties of mineral trioxide aggregate, *J Endod* 31:97, 2005.

284. Sasafuchi Y, Otsuki M, Inokoshi S, et al: The effects on pulp tissue of microleakage in resin composite restorations, *J Med Dent Sci* 46:155, 1999.

285. Sato Y, Fusayama T: Removal of dentin guided by Fuchsin staining, *J Dent Res* 55:678, 1976.

286. Schröder U: Effect of calcium hydroxide–containing pulp capping agents on pulp cell migration, proliferation, and differentiation, *J Dent Res* 66:1166, 1985.

287. Schröder U: Pedodontic endodontics. In Koch G, Poulsen S, editors: *Pediatric dentistry: a clinical approach*, Copenhagen, 2001, Munksgaard.

288. Seale NS, Coll JA: Vital pulp therapy for the primary dentition, *Gen Dent* 58:194, 2010.

289. Seltzer S, Bender IB: Some influences affecting repair of the exposed pulps of dogs' teeth, *J Dent Res* 37:678, 1958.

290. Seltzer S, Bender IB: *The dental pulp*, ed 3, Philadelphia, 1984, Lippincott.

291. Seo MS, Hwang KG, Lee J, et al: The effect of mineral trioxide aggregate on odontogenic differentiation in dental pulp stem cells, *J Endod* 39:242, 2013.

292. Shabahang S, Torabinejad M: Treatment of teeth with open apices using mineral trioxide aggregate, *Pract Periodontics Aesthet Dent* 12:315, 2000.

293. Shayegan A, Jurysta C, Atash R, et al: Biodentine used as a pulp-capping agent in primary pig teeth, *Pediatr Dent* 34:202, 2012.

294. Sheehy EC, Roberts GJ: Use of calcium hydroxide for apical barrier formation and healing in non-vital immature permanent teeth: a review, *Br Dent J* 183:241, 1997.

295. Shiba H, Nakanishi K, Rashid F, et al: Proliferative ability and alkaline phosphatase activity with in vivo cellular aging in human pulp cells, *J Endod* 29:9, 2003.

296. Shields ED, Altschuller B, Choi EY, et al: Odontometric variation among American black, European, and Mongoloid populations, *J Craniofac Genet Dev Biol* 10:7, 1990.

297. Shiflett K, White SN: Microleakage of cements for stainless steel crowns, *Pediatr Dent* 19:103, 1997.

298. Sigal MJ, Pitaru S, Aubin JE, et al: A combined scanning electron microscopy and immunofluorescence study demonstrating that the odontoblast process extends to the dentinoenamel junction in human teeth, *Anat Rec* 210:453, 1984.

299. Silva GA, Gava E, Lanza LD, et al: Subclinical failures of direct pulp capping of human teeth by using a dentin bonding system, *J Endod* 39:182, 2013.

300. Simon S, Perard M, Zanini M, et al: Should pulp chamber pulpotomy be seen as a permanent treatment? Some preliminary thoughts, *Int Endod J* 46:79, 2013.

301. Simonsen RJ: Conservation of tooth structure in restorative dentistry, *Quintessence Int* 16:15, 1985.

302. Song JS, Mante FK, Romanow WJ, et al: Chemical analysis of powder and set forms of Portland cement, gray ProRoot MTA, white ProRoot MTA, and gray MTA-Angelus, *Oral Surg Oral Med Oral Pathol Oral Radiol Endod* 102:809, 2006.

303. Sonoyama W, Liu Y, Yamaza T, et al: Characterization of the apical papilla and its residing stem cells from human immature teeth: a pilot study, *J Endod* 34:166, 2008.

304. Souza RA, Gomes SC, Dantas Jda C, et al: Importance of the diagnosis in the pulpotomy of immature permanent teeth, *Braz Dent J* 18:244, 2007.

305. Spagnuolo G, Galler K, Schmalz G, et al: Inhibition of phosphatidylinositol 3-kinase amplifies TEGDMA-induced

apoptosis in primary human pulp cells, *J Dent Res* 83:703, 2004.

306. Srinivasan D, Jayanthi M: Comparative evaluation of formocresol and mineral trioxide aggregate as pulpotomy agents in deciduous teeth, *Ind J Dent Res* 22:385, 2011.

307. Stanley HR: Pulp capping—conserving the dental pulp: Can it be done? Is it worth it? *Oral Surg Oral Med Oral Pathol* 68:628, 1989.

308. Stanley HR, Clark AE, Pameijer CH, et al: Pulp capping with a modified bioglass formula (#A68 modified), *Am J Dent* 14:227, 2001.

309. Stockton LW: Vital pulp capping: a worthwhile procedure, *J Can Dent Assoc* 65:328, 1999.

310. Sudo C: A study on partial pulp removal (pulpotomy) using NaOCl (sodium hypochlorite), *J Jpn Stomatol Soc* 26:1012, 1959.

311. Sveen OB: Pulp capping of primary teeth with zinc oxide eugenol, *Odontol Tidskr* 77:427, 1969.

312. Taira Y, Shinkai K, Suzuki M, et al: Direct pulp capping effect with experimentally developed adhesive resin systems containing reparative dentin-promoting agents on rat pulp: mixed amounts of additives and their effect on wound healing, *Odontology* 99:135, 2011.

313. Takita T, Hayashi M, Takeichi O, et al: Effect of mineral trioxide aggregate on proliferation of cultured human dental pulp cells, *Int Endod J* 39:415, 2006.

314. Tang W, Wu Y, Smales RJ: Identifying and reducing risks for potential fractures in endodontically treated teeth, *J Endod* 36:609, 2010.

315. Tarim B, Hafez AA, Cox CF: Pulpal response to a resin-modified glass-ionomer material on nonexposed and exposed monkey pulps, *Quintessence Int* 29:535, 1998.

316. Tarim B, Hafez AA, Suzuki SH, et al: Biocompatibility of compomer restorative systems on nonexposed dental pulps of primate teeth, *Oper Dent* 22:149, 1997.

317. Tarim B, Hafez AA, Suzuki SH, et al: Biocompatibility of Optibond and XR-Bond adhesive systems in nonhuman primate teeth, *Int J Periodontics Restorative Dent* 18:86, 1998.

318. Tate AR: Formocresol performs better than calcium hydroxide as a pulpotomy technique over 2-year period, *J Evid Based Dent Pract* 11:65, 2011.

319. Tatsumi T: Physiological remineralization of artificially decalcified monkey dentin under adhesive composite resin restoration, *Kokubyo Gakkai Zasshi* 56:47, 1989.

320. Tatsumi T, Inokoshi S, Yamada T, et al: Remineralization of etched dentin, *J Prosthet Dent* 67:617, 1992.

321. Ten Cate AR: Dentin-pulp complex. In *Oral histology*, ed 4, St Louis, 1994, Mosby.

322. Thibodeau B, Trope M: Pulp revascularization of a necrotic infected immature permanent tooth: case report and review of the literature, *Pediatr Dent* 29:47, 2007.

323. Thompson V, Craig RG, Curro FA, et al: Treatment of deep carious lesions by complete excavation or partial removal: a critical review, *J Am Dent Assoc* 139:705, 2008.

324. Tinanoff N, Douglass JM: Clinical decision making for caries management in children, *Pediatr Dent* 24:386, 2002.

325. Tjäderhane L: The mechanism of pulpal wound healing, *Aust Endod J* 28:68, 2002.

326. Tomson PL, Grover LM, Lumley PJ, et al: Dissolution of bio-active dentine matrix components by mineral trioxide aggregate, *J Dent* 35:636, 2007.

327. Tomson PL, Lumley PJ, Alexander MY, et al: Hepatocyte growth factor is sequestered in dentine matrix and promotes regeneration-associated events in dental pulp cells, *Cytokine* 61:622, 2013.

328. Tønder KJ: Vascular reactions in the dental pulp during inflammation, *Acta Odontol Scand* 41:247, 1983.

329. Torabinejad M, Higa RK, McKendry DJ, et al: Dye leakage of four root end filling materials: effects of blood contamination, *J Endod* 20:159, 1994.

330. Torabinejad M, Smith PW, Kettering JD, et al: Comparative investigation of marginal adaptation of mineral trioxide aggregate and other commonly used root-end filling materials, *J Endod* 21:295, 1995.

331. Torbjörner A, Karlsson S, Odman PA: Survival rate and failure characteristics for two post designs, *J Prosthet Dent* 73:439, 1995.

332. Trairatvorakul C, Koothiratrakarn A: Calcium hydroxide partial pulpotomy is an alternative to formocresol pulpotomy based on a 3-year randomized trial, *Int J Paediatr Dent* 22:382, 2012.

333. Tranasi M, Sberna MT, Zizzari V, et al: Microarray evaluation of age-related changes in human dental pulp, *J Endod* 35:1211, 2009.

334. Tronstad L, Mjör IA: Capping of the inflamed pulp, *Oral Surg Oral Med Oral Pathol* 34:477, 1972.

335. Trope M, McDougal R, Levin L, et al: Capping the inflamed pulp under different clinical conditions, *J Esthet Restor Dent* 14:349, 2002.

336. Tuna EB, Dinçol ME, Gençay K, et al: Fracture resistance of immature teeth filled with Bioaggregate, mineral trioxide aggregate and calcium hydroxide, *Dent Traumatol* 27:174, 2011.

337. Tüzüner T, Alacam A, Altunbas DA, et al: Clinical and radiographic outcomes of direct pulp capping therapy in primary molar teeth following haemostasis with various antiseptics: a randomised controlled trial, *Eur J Paediatr Dent* 13:289, 2012.

338. Tziafas D: Basic mechanisms of cytodifferentiation and dentinogenesis during dental pulp repair, *Int J Dev Biol* 39:281, 1995.

339. Tziafas D: Dentinogenic potential of the dental pulp: facts and hypothesis, *Endod Topics* 17:42, 2007.

340. Tziafas D, Pantelidou O, Alvanou A, et al: The dentinogenic effect of mineral trioxide aggregate (MTA) in short-term capping experiments, *Int Endod J* 35:245, 2002.

341. Van Meerbeek B, Peumans M, Poitevin A, et al: Relationship between bond-strength tests and clinical outcomes, *Dent Mater* 26:e100, 2010.

342. Vargas KG, Packham B, Lowman D: Preliminary evaluation of sodium hypochlorite for pulpotomies in primary molars, *Pediatr Dent* 28:511, 2006.

343. Wang CH, Chueh LH, Chen SC, et al: Impact of diabetes mellitus, hypertension, and coronary artery disease on tooth extraction after nonsurgical endodontic treatment, *J Endod* 37:1, 2011.

344. Wang NJ, Aspelund GØ: Preventive care and recall intervals: targeting of services in child dental care in Norway, *Community Dent Health* 27:5, 2010.

345. Wang Y, Zheng QH, Zhou XD, et al: Evaluation of the root and canal morphology of mandibular first permanent molars in a western Chinese population by cone-beam computed tomography, *J Endod* 36:1786, 2010.

346. Wegner PK, Freitag S, Kern M: Survival rate of endodontically treated teeth with posts after prosthetic restoration, *J Endod* 32:928, 2006.

347. Weisleder R, Benitez CR: Maturogenesis: Is it a new concept? *J Endod* 29:776, 2003.

348. White SN, Ingles S, Kipnis K: Influence of marginal opening on microleakage of cemented artificial crowns, *J Prosthet Dent* 71:257, 1994.

349. Willershausen B, Willershausen I, Ross A, et al: Retrospective study on direct pulp capping with calcium hydroxide, *Quintessence Int* 42:165, 2011.

350. Winters J, Cameron AC, Widmer RP: Pulp therapy for primary and immature permanent teeth. In Cameron AC, Widmer RP, editors: *Handbook of pediatric dentistry*, ed 3, Philadelphia, 2008, Mosby/Elsevier.

351. Witherspoon DE: Vital pulp therapy with new materials: new directions and treatment perspectives—permanent teeth, *J Endod* 34:S25, 2008.

352. Witherspoon DE, Small JC, Harris GZ: Mineral trioxide aggregate pulpotomies: a case series outcomes assessment, *J Am Dent Assoc* 137:610, 2006.

353. Witherspoon DE, Small JC, Regan JD, et al: Retrospective analysis of open apex teeth obturated with mineral trioxide aggregate, *J Endod* 34:1171, 2008.

354. Yamada T, Nakamura K, Iwaku M, et al: The extent of the odontoblast process in normal and carious human dentin, *J Dent Res* 62:798, 1983.

355. Yamani T, Yamashita A, Takeshita N, et al: Histopathological evaluation of the effects of a new dental adhesive resin on dog dental pulps, *J Jpn Prosthet Soc* 30:671, 1986.

356. Yan P, Yuan Z, Jiang H, et al: Effect of Bioaggregate on differentiation of human periodontal ligament fibroblasts, *Int Endod J* 43:1116, 2010.

357. Yasuda Y, Ogawa M, Arakawa T, et al: The effect of mineral trioxide aggregate on the mineralization ability of rat dental pulp cells: an in vitro study, *J Endod* 34:1057, 2008.

358. Yazici AR, Baseren M, Gokalp S: The in vitro performance of laser fluorescence and caries-detector dye for detecting residual carious dentin during tooth preparation, *Quintessence Int* 36:417, 2005.

359. Yip HK, Stevenson AG, Beeley JA: The specificity of caries detector dyes in cavity preparation, *Br Dent J* 176:417, 1994.

359a. Yoo JS, Chang SW, Oh SR, et al: Bacterial entombment by intratubular mineralization following orthograde mineral trioxide aggregate obturation: a scanning electron microscopy study. *Int J Oral Sci* 6:227, 2014.

360. Yoshimine Y, Maeda K: Histologic evaluation of tetracalcium phosphate-based cement as a direct pulp-capping agent, *Oral Surg Oral Med Oral Pathol* 79:351, 1995.

361. Yoshimura A, Lien E, Ingalls RR, et al: Cutting edge: recognition of Gram-positive bacterial cell wall components by the innate immune system occurs via Toll-like receptor 2, *J Immunol* 163:1, 1999.

362. Yu C, Abbott PV: An overview of the dental pulp: its functions and responses to injury, *Aust Dent J Supplement* 52:S4, 2007.

363. Yuan Z, Peng B, Jiang H, et al: Effect of bioaggregate on mineral-associated gene expression in osteoblast cells, *J Endod* 36:1145, 2010.

364. Zacharia MA, Munshi AK: Microbiological assessment of dentin stained with a caries detector dye, *J Clin Pediatr Dent* 19:111, 1995.

365. Zanini M, Sautier JM, Berdal A, et al: Biodentine induces immortalized murine pulp cell differentiation into odontoblast-like cells and stimulates biomineralization, *J Endod* 38:1220, 2012.

366. Zhang H, Pappen FG, Haapasalo M: Dentin enhances the antibacterial affect of mineral trioxide aggregate, *J Endod* 35:221, 2009.

367. Zhang W, McGrath C, Lo EC, et al: Silver diamine fluoride and education to prevent and arrest root caries among community-dwelling elders, *Caries Res* 47:284, 2013.

368. Zhang W, Walboomers XF, Jansen JA: The formation of tertiary dentin after pulp capping with a calcium phosphate cement, loaded with PLGA microparticles containing TGF-beta-1, *J Biomed Mater Res A* 85:439, 2008.

369. Zhi QH, Lo EC, Lin HC: Randomized clinical trial on effectiveness of silver diamine fluoride and glass ionomer in arresting dentine caries in preschool children, *J Dent* 40:962, 2012.

370. Zoufan K, Jiang J, Komabayashi T, et al: Cytotoxicity evaluation of Gutta Flow and Endo Sequence BC sealers, *Oral Surg Oral Med Oral Pathol Oral Radiol Endod* 112:657, 2011.

Index

Page numbers followed by "*f*" indicate figures, "*t*" indicate tables, and "*b*" indicate boxes.

A

A fibers, 543-544, 543*f*, 543*t*, 548-549, 551
AAE. *See* American Association of Endodontists
AAOS. *See* American Academy of Orthopaedic Surgeons
A-beta fibers, 685, *e*1
Abscess
    acute apical, 30
        description of, 30, 614, 617*f*
        pulpal necrosis with, 708-711
    in apical periodontitis, 641-642, 642*f*
    definition of, 641
    management of, 715-716
    periapical, 642*f*
    swelling with, 710-711, 711*f*
Abutment teeth
    endodontic disease of, 332, 332*f*
    root-treated teeth used as, 506
    survival rates for, 515
Access cavity preparation
    access cavity
        incisal wall of, 152
        visual inspection of, 152-153
    angulations that affect, 164
    anterior teeth, 151-153, 236*f*
        coronal flaring of orifice, 152, 152*f*
        external outline form, 151, 151*f*
        inadequate, 153*f*
        lingual shoulder removal, 152, 152*f*
        pulp chamber roof penetration and removal, 151-152, 151*f*
        restorative margin refinement and smoothing, 153
        straight-line access determination, 152, 153*f*
        visual inspection of access cavity in, 152-153
    in calcified canal teeth, 162-163, 163*f*-164*f*
    cervical dentin bulge removal, 156-157, 158*f*
    challenging cases for, 157-165
    coronal, 335-336, 335*f*, 337*f*-338*f*
    coronal seal for, space adequacy evaluation for, 147
    in crowded teeth, 163-165
    errors in, 160*f*, 165, 166*f*-167*f*, 733*f*
    in heavily restored teeth, 159-162, 161*f*-162*f*
    illumination for, 147
    inadequate
        in anterior teeth, 153*f*
        complications of, 362-363
    instrumentation for
        access cavity wall preparations for, 147
        burs, 148-150, 148*f*-149*f*, 235*f*
        description of, 240
        endodontic explorer, 150, 150*f*, 164*f*
        endodontic spoon, 150, 150*f*
        handpieces, 147-148
        illumination, 147
        magnification, 147

Access cavity preparation *(Continued)*
        Micro-Openers, 146, 146*f*
        ultrasonic unit and tips, 150, 150*f*
    lingual surface for, 146, 146*f*
    magnification for, 147
    mandibular incisors
        central, 183-185, 188*f*
        lateral, 183-185, 188*f*
    mandibular molars, 236*f*
        first, 193-199, 197*f*
        second, 199, 200*f*
    mandibular premolars
        first, 155*f*, 185-192, 191*f*
        second, 192-193, 194*f*
    maxillary canines, 169, 172*f*-173*f*
    maxillary incisors
        central, 165, 167*f*-168*f*
        lateral, 165-166, 170*f*
    maxillary molars
        first, 171*f*-172*f*, 175-177, 179*f*
        second, 177-183, 182*f*-183*f*
        third, 183, 183*f*, 185*f*
    maxillary premolars
        first, 169-173, 175*f*
        second, 173-175, 175*f*-176*f*, 179*f*
    in metalloceramic crown, 159, 162, 162*f*
    with minimal or no clinical crown, 157-159
    "mouse hole" effect, 156, 157*f*
    objectives of, 145
    occlusal surface for, 146, 146*f*
    posterior teeth, 237*f*
        cervical dentin bulge removal, 156-157, 158*f*
        coronal flaring of orifice, 156-157
        external outline form, 154, 154*f*-155*f*
        mandibular first premolars, 155*f*
        pulp chamber roof penetration and removal, 154, 156, 156*f*
        restorative margin refinement and smoothing, 157
        straight-line access determination, 157, 158*f*
        visual inspection of pulp chamber floor, 157, 159*f*
    pulp chamber roof penetration and removal
        in anterior teeth, 151-152, 151*f*
        in posterior teeth, 154, 156, 156*f*
    pulpal irritation caused by, 585
    restorative margin refinement and smoothing
        in anterior teeth, 153
        in posterior teeth, 157
    in rotated teeth, 163-165
    steps involved in, 145-147
        access cavity wall preparation, 147
        cementoenamel junction evaluation, 145-146, 145*f*
        lingual surface, 146, 146*f*
        occlusal tooth evaluation, 145-146

Access cavity preparation *(Continued)*
        pulp chamber wall and flow inspection, 147
        removal of defective restorations and caries before pulp chamber entry, 146-147, 147*f*
        removal of unsupported tooth structure, 147
        space adequacy evaluation for coronal seal, 147
        tapering of cavity walls, 147
        visualization of anatomy, 145
    straight-line
        in anterior teeth, 152, 153*f*
        description of, 145, 145*f*
        in posterior teeth, 157, 158*f*
Accessory canals
    apical, 414*f*
    description of, 132-133, 286
    illustration of, 414*f*
    in mandibular first molars, 133, 133*f*
Acellular afibrillar cementum, 630
Acetaminophen
    analgesic uses of, 117
    nonsteroidal anti-inflammatory drugs and, 121
    in pregnancy, 74
Acetylcholine, 557-558
Actinomyces, in periapical granuloma, 483*f*
Activ GP, 292, 292*f*, 299
Acute apical abscess, 30
    description of, 30, 614, 617*f*
    pulpal necrosis with, 708-711
Acute apical periodontitis, 638, *e*5
    apical bone destruction in, 641
    clinical features of, 641
    description of, 638
    macrophages in, 639
    natural killer cells in, 639
    outcomes of, 641-642
    polymorphonuclear neutrophilic leukocytes in, 638
Acute endodontic pathosis, 83*f*
Acute inflammation, 475
Adaptive immune response, 634-635, 636*f*, 642-643
Adaptive immunity, 633*t*, 634
Adaptive prior image constrained compressed sensing algorithms, 52
A-delta fibers, 685-686, *e*1
Adhesive systems, 844, *e*2
Afferent neurons, 542
Aging, pulp changes caused by, 566
Air emphysema, 749-750, 749*f*-750*f*
Allergic reactions
    to latex, 93-94
    to local anesthetics, 93-94
    sulfite-induced, 94
Allodynia, 550-551, 550*t*, 554, 693-694